Esophageal Surgery

SECOND EDITION

Esophageal Surgery

Edited by

■ F. GRIFFITH PEARSON, MD
Professor, Division of Thoracic Surgery
Department of Surgery
University of Toronto Faculty of Medicine
Senior Surgeon, Division of Thoracic Surgery
The Toronto General Hospital
Toronto, Ontario, Canada

■ JOEL D. COOPER, MD
Chief, Division of Cardiothoracic Surgery
Evarts A. Graham Professor of Surgery
Washington University School of Medicine
St. Louis, Missouri

■ JEAN DESLAURIERS, MD
Professor, Department of Surgery
Laval University Faculty of Medicine
Head, Thoracic Surgery Division
Centre de Pneumologie de l'Hôpital Laval
Ste-Foy, Quebec, Canada

■ ROBERT J. GINSBERG, MD
Chairman and Professor, Division of Thoracic Surgery
Department of Surgery
University of Toronto Faculty of Medicine
Chief, Division of Thoracic Surgery
The Toronto General Hospital
Toronto, Ontario, Canada

■ CLEMENT A. HIEBERT, MD
Chairman Emeritus, Department of Surgery
Maine Medical Center
Portland, Maine

■ G. ALEXANDER PATTERSON, MD
Chief, General Thoracic Surgery
Joseph C. Bancroft Professor of Surgery
Washington University School of Medicine
St. Louis, Missouri

■ HAROLD C. URSCHEL, JR., MD
Professor, Thoracic and Cardiovascular Surgery
University of Texas Southwestern Medical School
Dallas, Texas

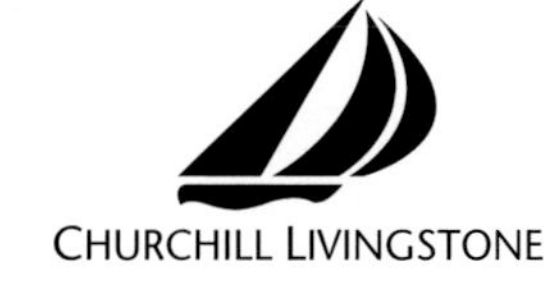

CHURCHILL LIVINGSTONE

An Imprint of Elsevier Science
New York Edinburgh London Philadelphia

CHURCHILL LIVINGSTONE
An Imprint of Elsevier Science

The Curtis Center
Independence Square West
Philadelphia, Pennsylvania 19106

Library of Congress Cataloging-in-Publication Data

Esophageal surgery / F. Griffith Pearson . . . [et al.].—2nd ed.

p. cm.

Includes bibliographical references and index.

ISBN 0–443–07605–7

1. Esophagus—Surgery. I. Pearson, F. Griffith.
[DNLM: 1. Esophagus—surgery. 2. Esophageal Diseases—surgery.
WI 250 E7658 2001]

RD 539.5.E87 2002 617.5′48—dc21

DNLM/DLC 00-058966

Acquisitions Editor: Richard Lampert
Developmental Editor: Melissa Dudlick
Production Manager: Natalie Ware
Manuscript Editor: Carol J. Robins
Illustration Specialists: Rita Martello, Walter Verbitski

ESOPHAGEAL SURGERY ISBN 0–443–07605–7

Printed in the United States of America.

Last digit is the print number: 9 8 7 6 5 4 3 2 1

I thank my wife Hilppa for her patience and ever-present cheerful support. My secretary, Leah Gabriel, was an invaluable resource. Melissa Dudlick, Senior Developmental Editor at WB Saunders, provided a steady stimulus and timely encouragement to our editorial staff during several years of preparation.

F. GRIFFITH PEARSON

To my wife and career-long partner, Janet, whose consistent and unflagging support has made possible all of my professional accomplishments. To my teachers and mentors, especially Griff Pearson, Hermes Grillo, and Ronald Belsey, who have transmitted to me their knowledge, experience, and commitment to the highest standards of clinical care. To my partners and residents over the years for their stimulation and forbearance.

JOEL D. COOPER

This book is dedicated to my wife Debbie and to all the students of Thoracic Surgery.

JEAN DESLAURIERS

My deepest gratitude to Dorrel Granderson for carrying the burden for the second time. To my dear wife, Charlotte, and my children, Karyn, Jordy, and David—thanks for being so patient and understanding during trying times.

ROBERT J. GINSBERG

I wish to thank my secretary, Vicky Bell, for impressive secretarial skills and cheerful assistance. Appreciation also goes to my wife, May Cameron, who, as former head nurse of the thoracic surgical unit at the Toronto General Hospital, had useful insights and suggestions.

CLEMENT A. HIEBERT

I would like to thank my wife Susan—mother, surgeon, scientist, and love of my life. I would also like to acknowledge and thank my four wonderful children—Lachlan, Megan, Brendan, and Caitlan.

G. ALEXANDER PATTERSON

I would like to dedicate my portion of this *Arbeit* to my loving wife Betsey for her understanding of the "time spent away" in thoracic surgery and to my wonderful children—Hal III, Brad, Locke, Amanda, and Susanna—of whom I am extremely proud.

HAROLD C. URSCHEL, JR.

CONTRIBUTORS

Hiroshi Akiyama, MD, PhD
Professor, Department of Surgery, Tokyo Medical University; President, Toranomon Hospital, Tokyo, Japan
Total Gastrectomy and Roux-en-Y Reconstruction

Nasser K. Altorki, MD
Professor of Cardiothoracic Surgery, Weill Medical College of Cornell University; Director, Division of Thoracic Surgery, Department of Cardiothoracic Surgery, Cornell University Medical Center, New York Presbyterian Hospital, New York, New York
En Bloc Resection for Esophageal Carcinoma; Three-Field Lymph Node Dissection for Cancer of the Esophagus

Kathryn D. Anderson, MD, FRCS(Eng)
Professor of Surgery, University of Southern California Keck School of Medicine; Surgeon-in-Chief and Vice President, Surgery, Children's Hospital of Los Angeles, Los Angeles, California
Corrosive Injury

Stephen B. Archer, MD
Assistant Professor of Surgery, Emory University, Atlanta, Georgia
Analysis of Complications in Laparoscopic Antireflux Surgery

Ralph W. Aye, MD
Clinical Assistant Professor, University of Washington School of Medicine; Teaching Attending Physician, Swedish Health Services, University of Washington Medical Center, Seattle, Washington
The Hill Repair

Manjit S. Bains
Attending Surgeon, Thoracic Surgery, Memorial Sloan-Kettering Cancer Center; Professor of Thoracic Surgery, Cornell University Weill Medical College and Graduate School of Medical Sciences, New York, New York
Transabdominal Esophagogastrectomy

Gilles Beauchamp, MD
Professor of Surgery, University of Montreal Faculty of Medicine; Thoracic Surgeon, Maisonneuve-Rosemont Hospital, Montreal, Quebec, Canada
Laser Therapy for Carcinoma of the Esophagus

Italo Braghetto, MD
Professor of Surgery, University of Chile; Chairman, Clinical Hospital, Santiago, Chile
Combined Operations

Carl E. Bredenberg, MD
Professor, University of Vermont College of Medicine, Burlington, Vermont; Surgeon-in-Chief, Maine Medical Center, Portland, Maine
Selection and Placement of Conduits

Patricio Burdiles, MD
Assistant Professor of Surgery, University of Chile; Staff Surgeon, Department of Surgery, Clinical Hospital, Santiago, Chile
Combined Operations

David P. Campbell, MD, BS
Attending Pediatric Surgeon, St. Peter's Hospital and Albany Medical Center Hospital, Albany, New York
Gastroesophageal Reflux in Infants and Children

Alan G. Casson, MB, ChB, MSc, FRCSC, FACS
Professor of Surgery, Dalhousie University Faculty of Medicine; Head, Division of Thoracic Surgery, Queen Elizabeth II Health Science Centre, Halifax, Nova Scotia, Canada
Biology of Esophageal Cancer; Epidemiology of Malignant Neoplasms

Neil Christie, MD
Assistant Professor of Surgery, University of Pittsburgh School of Medicine, Pittsburgh, Pennsylvania
Video-Assisted Approaches for Resection of Carcinoma of the Esophagus

Joel D. Cooper, MD
Chief, Division of Cardiovascular Surgery; Evarts A. Graham Professor of Surgery, Washington University School of Medicine, St. Louis, Missouri
Overview of Operative Techniques

Juan A. Cordero, Jr., MD
Cardiothoracic Surgery Fellow, University of Rochester School of Medicine and Dentistry and The Strong Memorial Hospital, Rochester, New York
Esophageal Intubation

Mario Costantini, MD
Assistant Professor of Surgery, University of Padua, Department of Medical and Surgical Sciences, Padua, Italy
Function Tests

Attila Csendes, MD
Professor of Surgery, University of Chile; Chairman and Staff Surgeon, Department of Surgery, Clinical Hospital, Santiago, Chile
Combined Operations

James B. Cullen, MD, FRCPC
Clinical Professor, University of British Columbia Faculty of Medicine; Medical Director and Head, Department of Pathology and Laboratory Medicine, Vancouver Hospital and Health Sciences Centre, Vancouver, British Columbia, Canada
Pathology of Malignant Neoplasms

Farrokh Dehdashti, MD
Associate Professor of Radiology, Division of Nuclear Medicine, Mallinckrodt Institute of Radiology, Washington University School of Medicine; Associate Radiologist, Barnes-Jewish Hospital, St. Louis, Missouri
Positron Emission Tomography

Steven R. DeMeester, MD
Assistant Professor of Cardiothoracic Surgery, University of Southern California Keck School of Medicine, Los Angeles, California
Physiology of the Lower Esophageal Sphincter; Surgical Palliation of Esophageal Cancer

Tom R. DeMeester, MD
Professor and Chairman, Department of Surgery, University of Southern California Keck School of Medicine; Chief of Surgery, USC University Hospital, Los Angeles, California
Physiology of the Lower Esophageal Sphincter; Function Tests; Laparoscopic Nissen Fundoplication Repair

Nicholas E. Diamant, MD, CM
Professor of Medicine and Physiology, University of Toronto Faculty of Medicine, Toronto, Ontario, Canada
Physiology of Deglutition

Patricia K. Donahoe, MD
Professor of Surgery, Harvard Medical School; Chief of Pediatric Surgical Services, Director of Pediatric Surgical Research Laboratories, and Visiting Surgeon, Department of Pediatric Surgery, Massachusetts General Hospital, Boston, Massachusetts
Esophageal Atresia and Tracheoesophageal Fistula; Other Congenital Disorders in Children

Daniel P. Doody, MD
Associate Professor of Surgery, Harvard Medical School; Visiting Surgeon, Department of Pediatric Surgery, Massachusetts General Hospital, Boston, Massachusetts
Esophageal Atresia and Tracheoesophageal Fistula; Other Congenital Disorders in Children

André Duranceau, MD
Professor of Surgery, University of Montreal Faculty of Medicine; Chief, Thoracic Surgery Service, and Chair, Thoracic Surgery Division, Centre Hospitalier de l'Université de Montreal, Montreal, Quebec, Canada
Esophagectomy for Benign Disease; Pharyngeal and Cricopharyngeal Disorders; Secondary Esophageal Motor Disorders

F. Henry Ellis, Jr., MD, PhD
Professor Emeritus, Department of Surgery, Harvard Medical School; Chief Emeritus, Division of Cardiothoracic Surgery, New England Deaconess Hospital, Boston, Massachusetts
Open Nissen Fundoplication Repair; Vagotomy, Antrectomy, and Roux-en-Y Diversion

Stanley C. Fell, MD
Professor of Cardiothoracic Surgery, Albert Einstein College of Medicine of Yeshiva University; Formerly, Director of Thoracic Surgery, Montefiore Medical Center, Bronx, New York
Esophageal Perforation; Gastric Tubes: Reversed and Nonreversed

Pasquale Ferraro, MD
Assistant Professor, University of Montreal Faculty of Medicine; Thoracic Surgeon and Surgical Director, Lung Transplant Program, Centre Hospitalier de l'Université de Montreal, Montreal, Quebec, Canada
Esophagectomy for Benign Disease; Pharyngeal and Cricopharyngeal Disorders; Secondary Esophageal Motor Disorders

Richard J. Finley, MD, FRCSC, FACCP, FACS
Professor and Head, Department of Surgery, University of British Columbia Faculty of Medicine; Head, Division of Thoracic Surgery, Department of Surgery, and Surgeon in Chief, Vancouver Hospital and Health Sciences Centre, Vancouver, British Columbia, Canada
Achalasia: Thoracoscopic and Laparoscopic Myotomy; Adenocarcinoma of the Esophagus and Esophagogastric Function

Ziv Gamliel, MD
Assistant Professor, University of Maryland School of Medicine; Director, Cardiothoracic ICU, University of Maryland Medical System, Baltimore, Maryland
Video-Assisted Approaches to Staging of Esophageal Carcinoma

Robert J. Ginsberg, MD
Chairman and Professor, Division of Thoracic Surgery, Department of Surgery, University of Toronto Faculty of Medicine; Chief, Division of Thoracic Surgery, The Toronto General Hospital, Toronto, Ontario, Canada
Indications for Surgery for Hiatal Hernia and Gastroesophageal Reflux: The Surgeon's Perspective; Left Thoracoabdominal Cervical Approach; Left Transthoracic Esophagectomy

Allan M. Goldstein
Chief Resident, Pediatric Surgery, Children's Hospital of New York, New York, New York
Esophageal Atresia and Tracheoesophageal Fistula

Sean Grondin, MD
Assistant Professor of Surgery, Section of Thoracic Surgery, Evanston Northwestern University, Chicago, Illinois
Physiology of Esophageal Peristalsis; Laparoscopic Techniques in Reoperation for Failed Repairs

Jeffrey A. Hagen, MD
Associate Professor of Clinical Surgery, University of Southern California Keck School of Medicine; Chief, Section of Thoracic/Foregut Surgery, Los Angeles County–University of Southern California Medical Center, Los Angeles, California
Primary Esophageal Motor Disorders

Bruce H. Haughey, MB, ChB, MS, FRACS, FACS
Director, Division of Head and Neck Surgical Oncology, Department of Otolaryngology–Head and Neck Surgery, Washington University School of Medicine, St. Louis, Missouri
Free Vascularized Grafts in Esophageal Reconstruction

Harry Henteleff, MD, MSC, FRCSC, FACS
Assistant Professor, Dalhousie University Faculty of Medicine; Active Staff, Division of Thoracic Surgery, Queen Elizabeth II Health Sciences Centre, Halifax, Nova Scotia, Canada
Epidemiology of Malignant Neoplasms

Clement A. Hiebert, MD
Clinical Professor, Chairman Emeritus, Department of Surgery, Maine Medical Center, Portland, Maine
Clinical Features; Massive (Paraesophageal) Hiatal Hernia; Belsey Mark IV Repair; Esophageal Diverticula; Selection and Placement of Conduits

Lucius D. Hill, MD*
Clinical Professor of Surgery, University of Washington School of Medicine; Surgeon, Swedish Health Services, University of Washington Medical Center, and Virginia Mason Medical Center, Seattle, Washington
The Hill Repair

Chia Sing Ho, MB, BS, FRCPC
Professor of Radiology, Department of Medical Imaging, University of Toronto Faculty of Medicine; Division Head, Angiography and Intervention Radiology, and Section Head, Gastrointestinal Radiology, Mount Sinai Hospital and University Health Network (Toronto General, Toronto Western, and Princess Margaret Hospitals), Toronto, Ontario, Canada
Radiology, Computed Tomography, and Magnetic Resonance Imaging

John G. Hunter, MD
Professor and Chairman, Department of Surgery, Oregon Health Sciences University School of Medicine, Portland, Oregon
Analysis of Complications in Laparoscopic Antireflux Surgery

David H. Ilson, MD, PhD
Assistant Professor, Cornell University Weill Medical College and Graduate School of Medical Sciences; Assistant Attending Physician, Memorial Sloan-Kettering Cancer Center, New York, New York
Chemotherapy and Radiotherapy as Primary Treatment of Esophageal Cancer

Nasir M. Jaffer, MD, FRCPC
Associate Professor, Department of Medical Imaging, University of Toronto Faculty of Medicine; Mount Sinai Hospital and University Health Network (Toronto General, Toronto Western, and Princess Margaret Hospitals), Toronto, Ontario, Canada
Radiology, Computed Tomography, and Magnetic Resonance Imaging

Glyn G. Jamieson, MB, BS, MS, FRACS, FRCS, FACS
Dorothy Mortlock Professor of Surgery, Department of Surgery, University of Adelaide; Senior Consultant Surgeon and Head, Oesophago-gastric Surgical Unit, Royal Adelaide Hospital, Adelaide, South Australia, Australia
Randomized Controlled Trials for Antireflux Surgery; Adjuvant and Neoadjuvant Therapy for Cancer of the Esophagus

K. Jeyasingham, MB, ChM, FRCS, FRCSE
Honorary Consultant Thoracic Surgeon, Frenchay Hospital, Bristol, United Kingdom
Long-Term Results of Colon Replacement

Owen Korn, MD
Assistant Professor of Surgery, University of Chile; Staff Surgeon, Department of Surgery, Clinical Hospital, Santiago, Chile
Combined Operations

*Deceased.

Robert J. Korst, MD
Assistant Professor of Surgery, Department of Surgery, Cornell University Weill Medical College and Graduate School of Medical Sciences; Assistant Attending Surgeon, Thoracic Service, Memorial Sloan-Kettering Cancer Center, New York, New York
Surgical Palliation of Esophageal Cancer; Unusual Malignancies

Mark J. Krasna, MD
Professor of Surgery, University of Maryland School of Medicine; Chief, Division of Thoracic Surgery, University of Maryland Medical System, Baltimore, Maryland
Video-Assisted Approaches to Staging of Esophageal Carcinoma

Florian Lang, Dr Med
Fellow, Department of Otorhinolaryngology, University of Lausanne Faculty of Medicine; Head and Neck Surgery, Centre Hospitalier Universitaire Vaudois, Lausanne, Switzerland
Esophageal Foreign Bodies in Adults

Simon Y. K. Law, MB, BChir, FRCSEd, FACS
Honorary Clinical Associate Professor, University of Hong Kong; Staff Surgeon, University of Hong Kong Medical Centre, Queen Mary Hospital, Hong Kong, China
Management of Squamous Cell Carcinoma of the Esophagus

Toni Lerut, MD, PhD
Professor of Surgery and Chairman, Department of Thoracic Surgery, Universitaire Ziekenhuizen Leuven, Leuven, Belgium
Belsey Mark IV Repair; Esophageal Diverticula; Three-Field Lymph Node Dissection for Cancer of the Esophagus

Sheryl Lewin, MD
Resident, Department of Surgery, University of Southern California Medical Center, Los Angeles, California
Laparoscopic Nissen Fundoplication Repair

Timothy S. Lian, MD
Department of Otolaryngology–Head and Neck Surgery, Louisiana State University Medical School, New Orleans, Louisiana
Free Vascularized Grafts in Reconstruction

Dorothea Liebermann-Meffert, Dr Med, FACS
Professor, Technische Universität; Surgeon, Department of Surgery, Chirurgische Klinik und Püoliklinik, Klinikum rechts der Isar, Munich, Germany
Anatomy, Embryology, and Histology

Alex G. Little, MD
Professor and Chairman, Department of Surgery, University of Nevada School of Medicine; Chief of Surgery, University Medical Center, Las Vegas, Nevada
Esophageal Bypass

James D. Luketich, MD
Associate Professor of Surgery, University of Pittsburgh School of Medicine; Chief, Division of Thoracic and Foregut Surgery, Presbyterian University Hospital, Pittsburgh, Pennsylvania
Laparoscopic Techniques in Reoperation for Failed Repairs; Video-Assisted Approaches for Resection of Carcinoma of the Esophagus

Victoria A. Marcus, MD, CM, FRCPC
Assistant Professor, McGill University Faculty of Medicine; Pathologist, McGill University Health Centre, Montreal, Quebec, Canada
Pathology of Malignant Esophageal Neoplasms

Jocelyne Martin, MD
Assistant Professor of Surgery, University of Montreal Faculty of Medicine; Chair, Thoracic Oncology Section, Centre Hospitalier de l'Université de Montreal, Montreal, Quebec, Canada
Secondary Esophageal Motor Disorders

Douglas Mathisen, MD
Professor of Surgery, Harvard Medical School; Chief of Thoracic Surgery, Massachusetts General Hospital, Boston, Massachusetts
Ivor Lewis–McKeown Procedures

Sandro Mattioli, MD
Associate Professor, Department of Surgery, Intensive Care and Organ Transplantation, Alma Mater Studiorum–Università di Bologna; Senior Staff Surgeon, Policlinico Sant'Orsola–Malpighi, Bologna, Italy
Open Technique for Dor and Toupet Repairs

Bruce D. Minsky, MD
Professor of Radiation Oncology, Cornell University Weill Medical College and Graduate School of Medical Sciences; Vice Chairman, Department of Radiation Oncology, Memorial Sloan-Kettering Cancer Center, New York, New York
Chemotherapy and Radiotherapy as Primary Treatment of Esophageal Cancer

Philippe Monnier, MD
Professor and Chairman, Department of Otorhinolaryngology, Head and Neck Surgery, University of Lausanne Faculty of Medicine; Centre Hospitalier Universitaire Vaudois, Lausanne, Switzerland
Rigid Esophagoscopy; Esophageal Foreign Bodies in Adults

Darroch W. O. Moores, MD
Clinical Associate Professor, Department of Surgery, Albany Medical College; Attending Thoracic Surgeon, Albany Medical Center; Attending Physician, Department of Thoracic Surgery, St. Peter's Hospital, Albany, New York; and Ellis Hospital, Schenectady, New York
Gastroesophageal Reflux in Infants and Children; Esophageal Intubation

John C. Mullen, MD, MSc
Assistant Clinical Professor, Department of Surgery and Paediatrics, University of Alberta Faculty of Medicine; Staff Surgeon, Division of Cardiothoracic Surgery, W.C. MacKenzie Health Sciences Centre, Edmonton, Alberta, Canada
Vascular Rings

Ninh T. Nguyen, MD
Assistant Professor of Surgery, University of California, Davis, School of Medicine; Director, Minimally Invasive Surgery Program, University of California, Davis, Medical Center, Sacramento, California
Video-Assisted Approaches for Resection of Carcinoma of the Esophagus

Claes Nilsson, MD
Ryan Hill Research Fellow, The Hill Foundation, Seattle, Washington
The Hill Repair

Jean-Baptiste Ollyo, Dr Med
Gastroenterologist, Lausanne, Switzerland
Esophageal Foreign Bodies in Adults

Mark B. Orringer, MD
Professor and Head, Section of Thoracic Surgery, University of Michigan Medical School, Ann Arbor, Michigan
Transhiatal Esophagectomy Without Thoracotomy; Resection of Carcinoma Involving the Cervicothoracic Esophagus: Cervical Exenteration

Denise Ouellette, MD
Associate Professor, University of Montreal Faculty of Medicine, Montreal, Quebec, Canada
Laser Therapy for Carcinoma of the Esophagus

Blake C. Papsin, MD, MSc, FRCS(C), FRCS
Assistant Professor, University of Toronto Faculty of Medicine; Staff Pediatric Otolaryngologist, Department of Otolaryngology, Hospital for Sick Children, Toronto, Ontario, Canada
Esophageal Foreign Bodies in Infants and Children

Bernard J. Park, MD
Senior Clinical Associate in Cardiothoracic Surgery, Weill Medical College of Cornell University; Fellow, Division of Cardiothoracic Surgery, Cornell University Medical Center, New York Presbyterian Hospital, and Memorial Sloan-Kettering Cancer Center, New York, New York
Left Transthoracic Esophagectomy

Philippe Pasche, Dr Med
Associate Professor, University of Lausanne Faculty of Medicine; Department of Otorhinolaryngology, Head and Neck Surgery, Centre Hospitalier Universitaire Vaudois, Lausanne, Switzerland
Esophageal Foreign Bodies in Adults

F. Griffith Pearson, MD
Professor, Division of Thoracic Surgery, Department of Surgery, University of Toronto Faculty of Medicine; Senior Surgeon, Division of Thoracic Surgery, The Toronto General Hospital, Toronto, Ontario, Canada
Pathophysiology of Hiatal Hernia and Gastroesophageal Reflux; Indications for Surgery for Hiatal Hernia and Gastroesophageal Reflux: The Surgeon's Perspective; Peptic Esophagitis, Stricture, and Short Esophagus; Open Gastroplasty; Open Techniques in Reoperation for Failed Repairs; Synchronous Combined Abdominothoracocervical Esophagectomy

Manuel Pera, MD, PhD
Staff Surgeon, Service of Gastrointestinal Surgery; Coordinator, Esophagogastric Cancer Unit, Institute of Digestive Diseases, Hospital Clinic, University of Barcelona Medical School, Barcelona, Spain
Management of Dysplasia and Superficial Carcinoma

Harold G. Preiksaitis, MD, PhD
Associate Professor of Medicine and Physiology, The University of Western Ontario Faculty of Medicine and Dentistry, London, Ontario, Canada
Physiology of Deglutition

Alexandre Radu
Research Fellow, University of Lausanne Faculty of Medicine; Centre Hospitalier Universitaire Vaudois, Lausanne, Switzerland
Rigid Esophagoscopy

Mark Redston, MD, FRCPC
Assistant Professor, University of Toronto Faculty of Medicine; Pathologist, Department of Pathology and Laboratory Medicine, Mount Sinai Hospital, Toronto, Ontario, Canada
Pathology of Malignant Neoplasms

Thomas W. Rice, MD
Head, Section of General Thoracic Surgery, Department of Thoracic and Cardiovascular Surgery, Cleveland Clinic Foundation, Cleveland, Ohio
Endoscopic Esophageal Ultrasound; Flexible Esophagoscopy; Indications for Surgery of the Columnar-Lined Esophagus; Dilation of Peptic Strictures; Overview and Current Status of Laparoscopic Antireflux Surgery; Diagnosis and Staging of Esophageal Carcinoma; Colon Replacement

William G. Richards, PhD
Instructor in Surgery, Harvard Medical School; Research Associate, Brigham and Women's Hospital, Boston, Massachusetts
Physiology of Esophageal Peristalsis

Joel E. Richter, MD
Professor of Medicine, Ohio State University College of Medicine and Public Health; Chairman, Department of Gastroenterology, Cleveland Clinic Foundation, Cleveland, Ohio
Indications for Surgical Referral for Hiatal Hernia and Gastroesophageal Reflux: A Gastroenterologist's Viewpoint

Jorge Rojas, MD
Assistant Professor of Surgery, University of Chile; Staff, Department of Surgery, Clinical Hospital, Santiago, Chile
Combined Operations

Marcel Savary, MD
Honorary Professor, Department of Otolaryngology, Head and Neck Surgery, University of Lausanne Faculty of Medicine; Centre Hospitalier Universitaire Vaudois, Lausanne, Switzerland
Rigid Esophagoscopy; Esophageal Foreign Bodies in Adults

David S. Schrump, MD
Head, Thoracic Oncology Section, Surgery Branch, National Cancer Institute, Bethesda, Maryland
Biology of Esophageal Cancer

Dorry L. Segev, MD
Surgical Research Fellow, Massachusetts General Hospital, Boston, Massachusetts
Other Congenital Disorders in Children

Farid Shamji, MD
Associate Professor, University of Ottawa Faculty of Medicine; Head, Division of Thoracic Surgery, Civic Campus–The Ottawa Hospital, Ottawa, Ontario, Canada
Benign Tumors

Barry A. Siegel, MD
Professor of Radiology and Medicine and Director, Division of Nuclear Medicine, Mallinckrodt Institute of Radiology, Washington University School of Medicine; Nuclear Radiologist-in-Chief, Barnes-Jewish Hospital, St. Louis, Missouri
Positron Emission Tomography

David B. Skinner, MD
Professor of Surgery and Cardiothoracic Surgery, Weill Medical College of Cornell University; President Emeritus, New York Presbyterian Hospital, New York, New York
En Bloc Resection for Esophageal Carcinoma

Alma Smitheringale, MB, BS, FRCS(C)Med
Associate Professor of Otolaryngology, University of Toronto Faculty of Medicine; Staff Pediatric Otolaryngologist, North York General Hospital, and Associate Staff, Toronto General Hospital, Toronto, Ontario, Canada
Esophageal Foreign Bodies in Infants and Children

Joshua R. Sonett, MD
Assistant Professor, University of Maryland School of Medicine; Director, Lung Transplantation, University of Maryland Medical System, Baltimore, Maryland
Video-Assisted Approaches to Staging of Esophageal Carcinoma

Stuart Jon Spechler, MD
Professor of Medicine, Berta M. and Cecil O. Patterson Chair in Gastroenterology, University of Texas Southwestern Medical Center at Dallas Southwestern Medical School; Chief, Division of Gastroenterology, Dallas Veterans Administration Medical Center, Dallas, Texas
Medical Treatment of Gastroesophageal Reflux Disease; Pathophysiology of the Columnar-Lined Esophagus

David J. Sugarbaker, MD
Professor of Surgery, Harvard Medical School; Executive Vice Chairman, Department of Surgery, and Chief, Division of Thoracic Surgery, Brigham and Women's Hospital; Philip L. Lowe Senior Surgeon and Chief, Department of Surgical Services, Dana Farber Cancer Institute, Boston, Massachusetts
Physiology of Esophageal Peristalsis

Lee L. Swanström, MD
Clinical Professor of Surgery, Oregon Health Sciences University; Director, Department of Minimally Invasive Surgery, Legacy Health System, Portland, Oregon
Laparoscopic Toupet Fundoplication; Laparoscopic Gastroplasty

Thomas R. J. Todd, MD
Chairman, Surgery, Shaikh Khalifa Medical Center, Abu Dhabi, United Arab Emirates
Benign Tumors

Victor F. Trastek, MD
Professor of Surgery, Mayo Medical School, Rochester, Minnesota; Chair, Department of Surgery, Mayo Clinic Scottsdale, Scottsdale, Arizona
Management of Dysplasia and Superficial Carcinoma

Harushi Udagawa, MD
Chief, Department of Surgery, Toranomon Hospital, Tokyo, Japan
Total Gastrectomy and Roux-en-Y Reconstruction

David I. Watson, MB, BS, MD, FRACS
Associate Professor of Surgery, Department of Surgery, University of Adelaide Faculty of Medicine; Senior Consultant Surgeon and Director, The Royal Adelaide Centre for Endoscopic Surgery, Royal Adelaide Hospital, Adelaide, South Australia, Australia
Randomized Controlled Trials for Antireflux Surgery

Earle W. Wilkins, Jr., MD
Clinical Professor of Surgery, Emeritus, Harvard Medical School; Senior Surgeon, Massachusetts General Hospital, Boston, Massachusetts
The Historical Evolution of Esophageal Surgery; Rings and Webs; Classic Left Thoracoabdominal Approaches

William G. Williams, MD
Acting Chairman, Division of Cardiovascular Surgery, and Professor, Department of Surgery, University of Toronto Faculty of Medicine; Chief, Pediatric Cardiac Surgery, Hospital for Sick Children, Toronto, Ontario, Canada
Vascular Rings

John Wong, MB, BS, PhD, FRACS, FACS(Hon)
Professor, University of Hong Kong; Head of Surgery, University of Hong Kong Medical Centre, Queen Mary Hospital, Hong Kong, China
Management of Squamous Cell Carcinoma of the Esophagus

Michael G. Wood, MD
Resident, Department of Surgery, University of Southern California Keck School of Medicine, Los Angeles, California
Primary Esophageal Motor Disorders

Manoel Ximenes-Netto, MD, PhD
Professor of Surgery, University of Brasilia School of Medicine; Head, Thoracic Surgery, Hospital de Base do Distrito Federal, and Consultant, Armed Forces Hospital, Brasilia, Brazil
Chagas' Disease; Gastric Tubes: Reversed and Nonreversed

Patrick Yau, MD, FRCS(C)
Consultant, Scarborough Salvation Army Grace Hospital, Scarborough, Ontario, Canada
Adjuvant and Neoadjuvant Therapy for Cancer of the Esophagus

Gregory Zuccaro, Jr., MD
Staff Physician, Department of Gastroenterology and Center for Swallowing and Esophageal Disorders, Cleveland Clinic Foundation, Cleveland, Ohio
Endoscopic Esophageal Ultrasound; Flexible Esophagoscopy

PREFACE

Six years have elapsed since publication of the first editions of *Thoracic Surgery* and *Esophageal Surgery*. In these second editions, all original chapters have been updated and a significant number of new chapters added. Important additions include major advances in the application and acceptance of minimally invasive video-assisted techniques; advances in the technology of imaging with positron emission tomography scanning and ultrasound; the current emphasis on multimodality therapy in the management of many thoracic malignancies (including locally advanced lung and esophageal carcinomas); the expanding field of lung volume reduction surgery and three-field lymphadenectomy for esophageal cancer; and new operative techniques for the management of difficult technical problems, such as resection and reconstruction of the pulmonary artery and superior vena cava.

Otherwise, format and objectives remain the same. Each of the seven medical editors has assumed responsibility for one or more sections in which that particular editor has internationally recognized expertise. Chapter authors were chosen because of their acknowledged expertise in the assigned topic. Content and presentation were designed to create a comprehensive textbook for general reference, with an emphasis on practical guidance for the resident in training and for the established practitioner.

Again, the text has been separated into two volumes in an effort to accommodate the potentially disparate interests of the reader. *Thoracic Surgery* encompasses operative techniques of the airways, lungs, chest wall, and mediastinum. *Esophageal Surgery* will be of interest to general surgeons and gastroenterologists, as well as to thoracic surgeons.

The Department of Surgery at the University of Toronto continues to dominate the background of the editors: Six of the seven current editors hold or have held academic positions in the Division of Thoracic Surgery in Toronto. Many of the individual chapters have been written by graduates of the Toronto training program in general thoracic surgery.

F. GRIFFITH PEARSON

CONTENTS

SECTION VI

Trauma 577

SECTION VII

Neoplasms 637

SECTION VIII

Operative Techniques 793

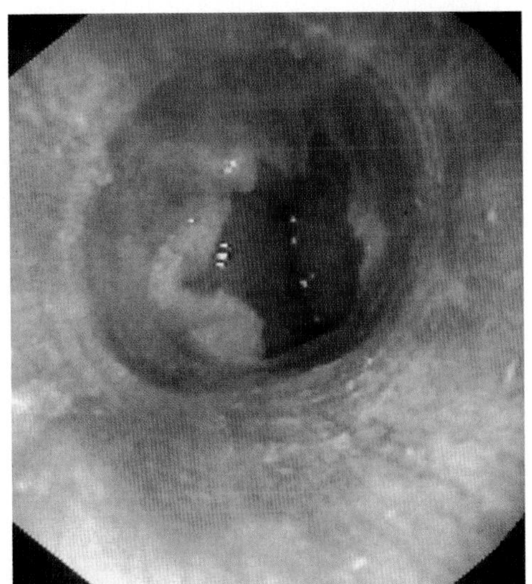

FIGURE 6–10 ■ Normal distal esophagus.

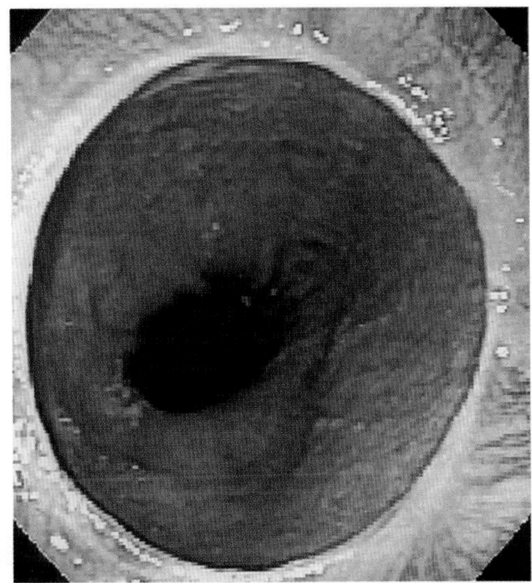

FIGURE 6–11 ■ Distal esophagus, Schatzki's ring, and small hiatal hernia.

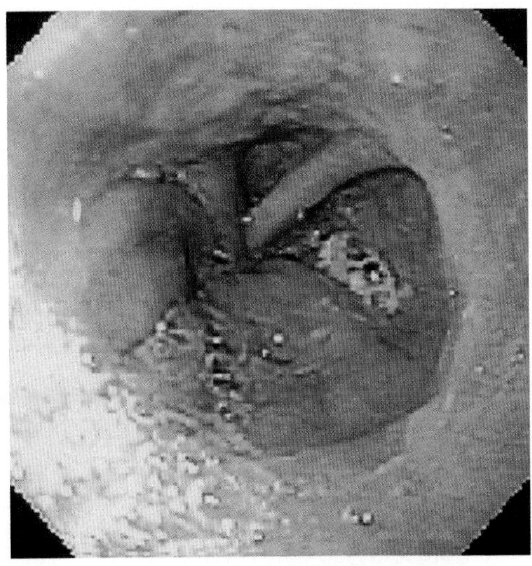

FIGURE 6–12 ■ Small hiatal hernia.

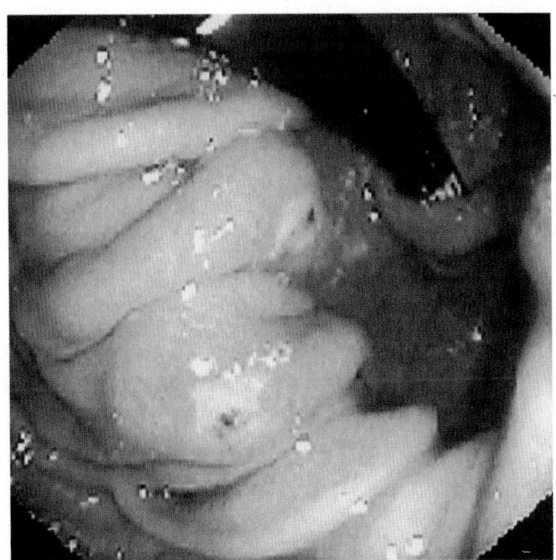

FIGURE 6–13 ■ Retroflexed view, from the stomach, of a large hiatal hernia.

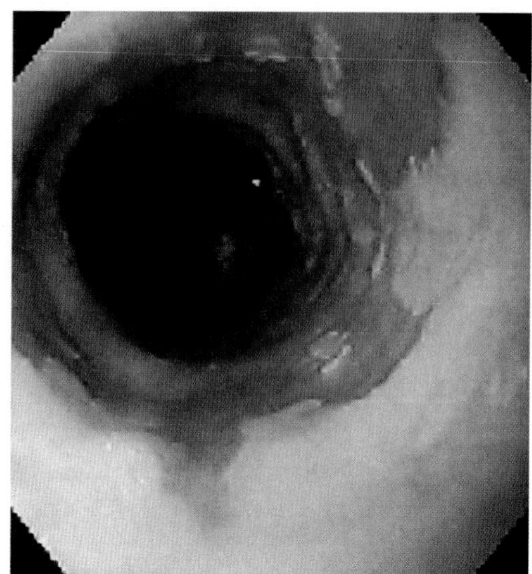

FIGURE 6–14 ■ Long-segment Barrett's esophagus.

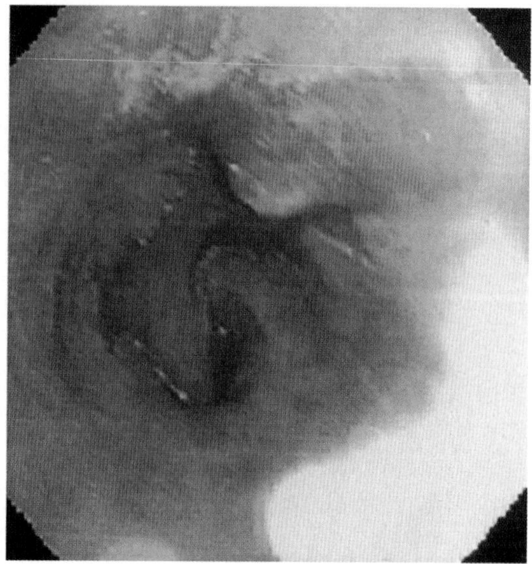

FIGURE 6–15 ■ A nodule in Barrett's esophagus. Biopsy is mandatory to prove this nodule a superficial adenocarcinoma.

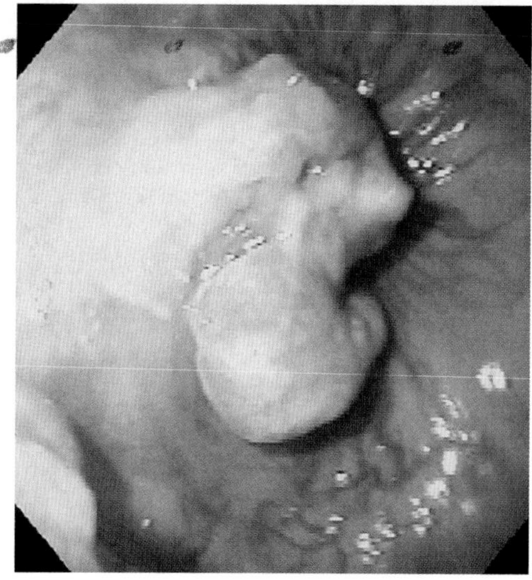

FIGURE 6–16 ■ Squamous cell carcinoma of the esophagus.

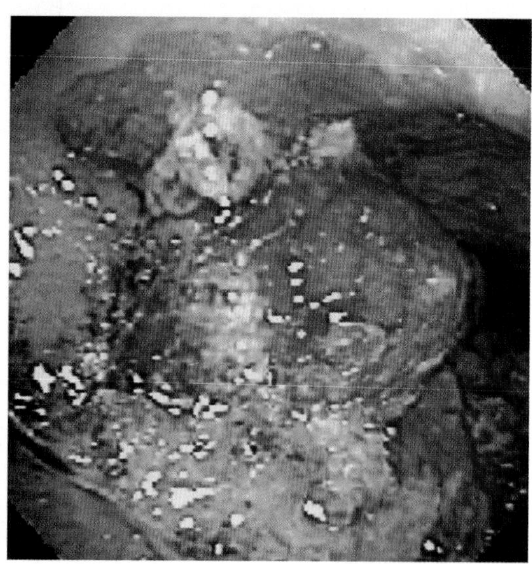

FIGURE 6–17 ■ Barrett's adenocarcinoma.

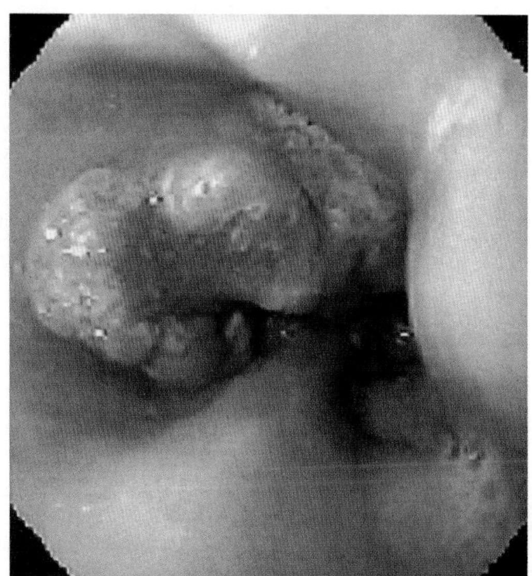

FIGURE 6–18 ■ Adenocarcinoma of the esophagogastric junction.

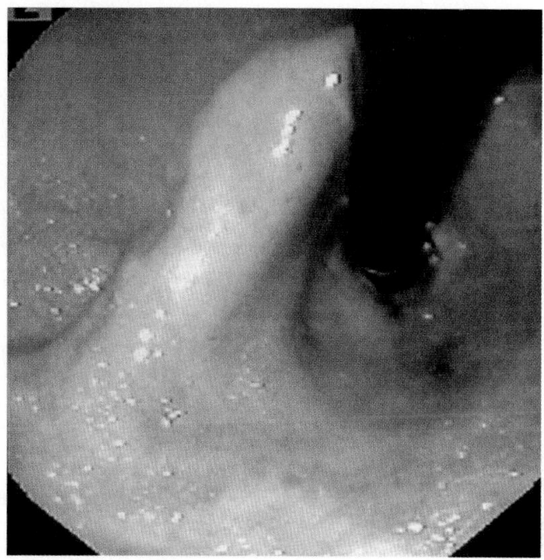

FIGURE 6–19 ■ Retroflexed view within a dilated sigmoid esophagus of achalasia.

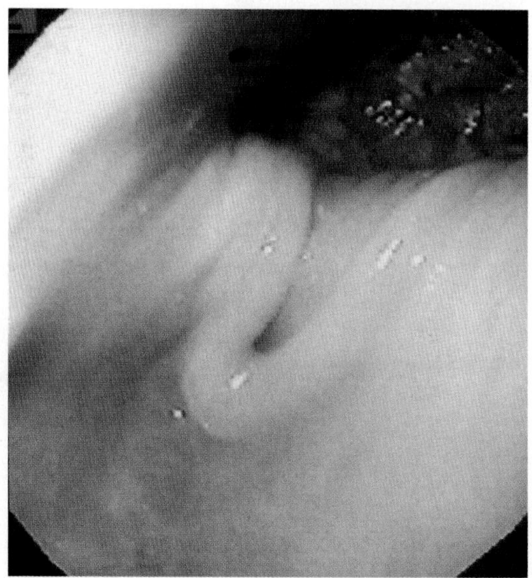

FIGURE 6–20 ■ A large, food-filled epiphrenic diverticulum (at 2 o'clock). The distal esophagus is the small dimple in the center of the figure.

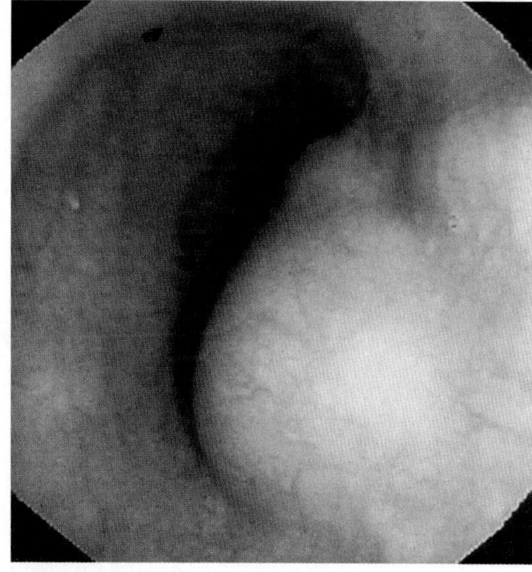

FIGURE 6–21 ■ Leiomyoma of the distal esophagus.

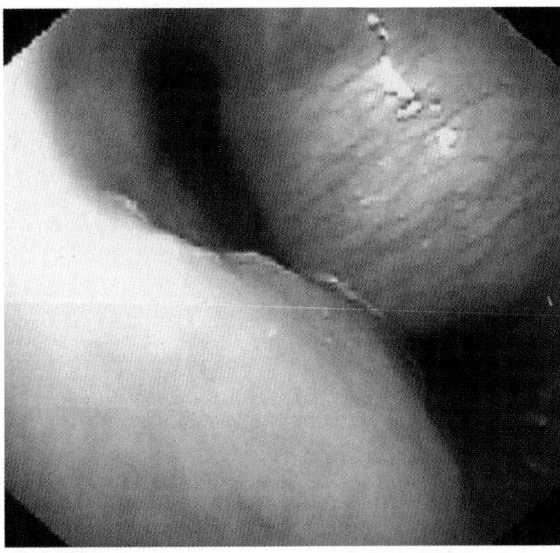

FIGURE 6–22 ■ Vascular ring, the result of an aberrant right subclavian artery.

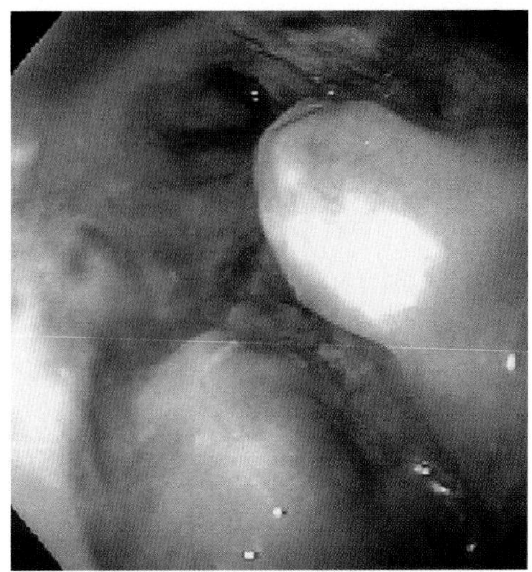

FIGURE 6–23 ■ Esophageal varices.

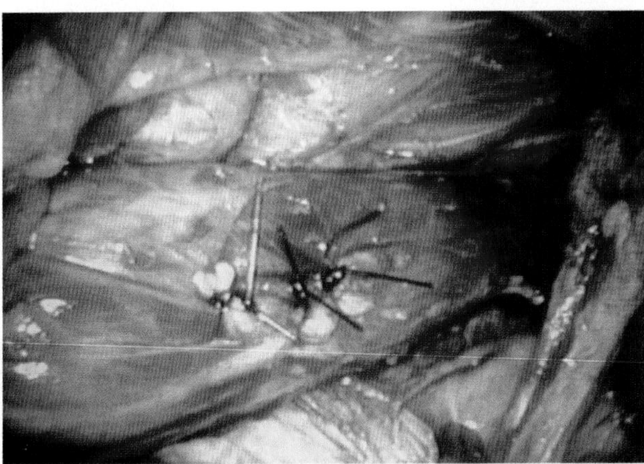

FIGURE 25–7 ■ Repair of an esophageal perforation at the level of the gastroesophageal junction accomplished laparoscopically.

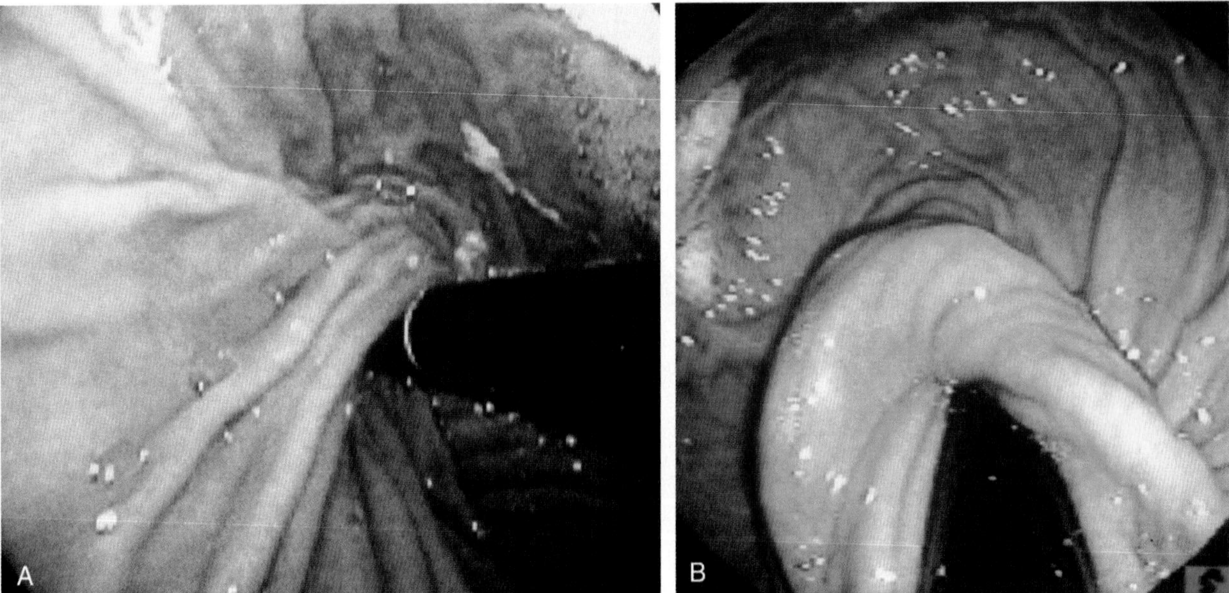

FIGURE 25–10 ■ *A,* Retroflexed endoscopic view of a twisted fundoplication. *B,* Retroflexed endoscopic view of a well-placed fundoplication.

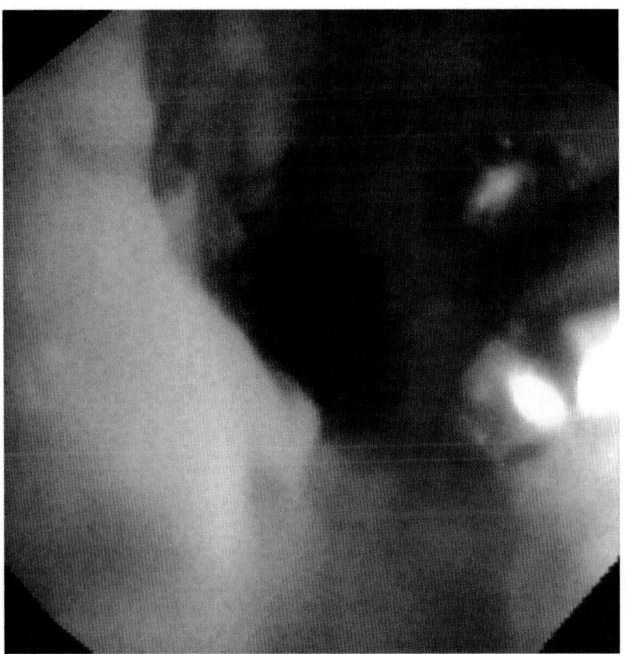

FIGURE 43–2 ■ Esophagoscopy and biopsy, following brush cytology, of a malignant esophageal stricture.

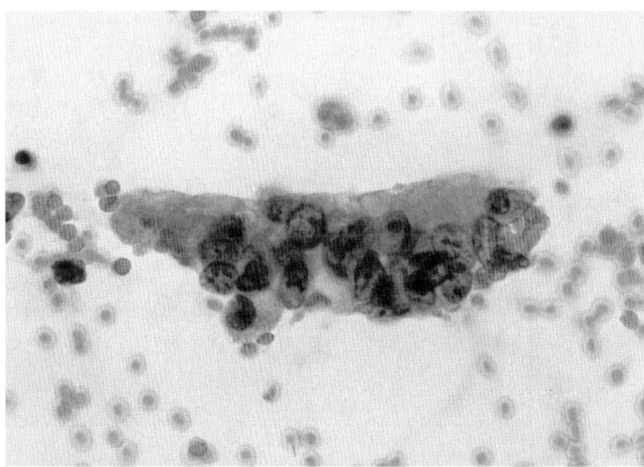

FIGURE 43–3 ■ Adenocarcinoma cells obtained from brushing of Barrett's esophagus. Shown are clusters of neoplastic cells with hyperchromatic, pleomorphic nuclei and loss of polarity but retained columnar configuration and cytoplasmic mucin.

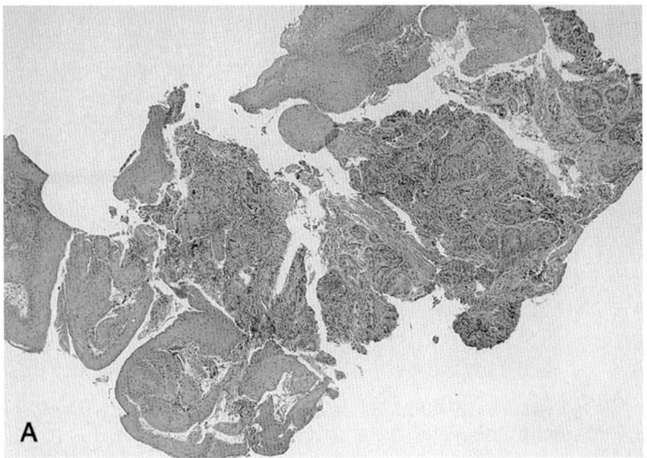

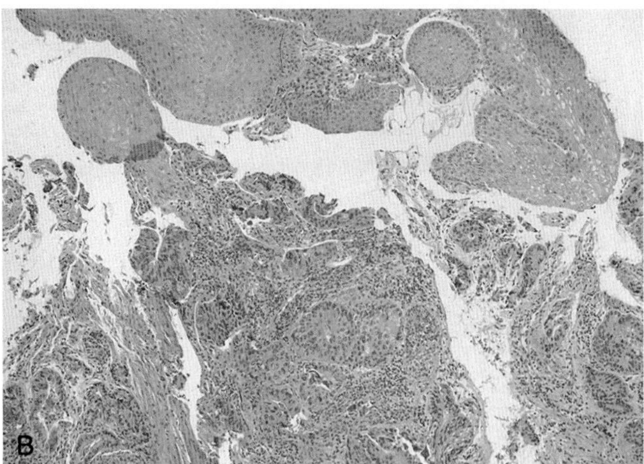

FIGURE 43–4 ■ *A,* Superficial mucosal biopsy demonstrates malignant glands undermining intact squamous mucosa. This is at least intramucosal cancer. No goblet cells are seen. *B,* Higher magnification demonstrates malignant glands infiltrating the lamina propria below the squamous epithelium.

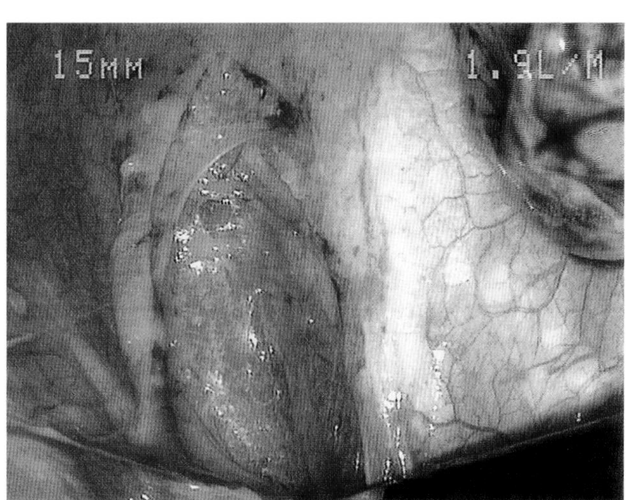

FIGURE 43–15 ■ Upper paraesophageal lymph node dissection.

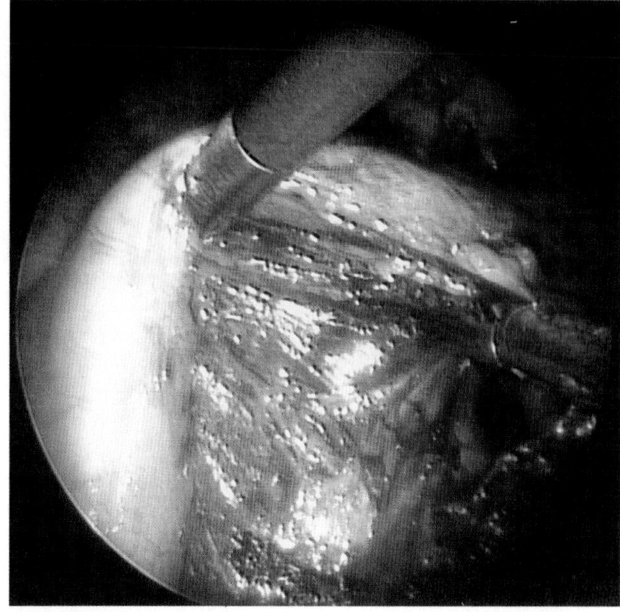

FIGURE 43–16 ■ Subazygous region during lymph node dissection.

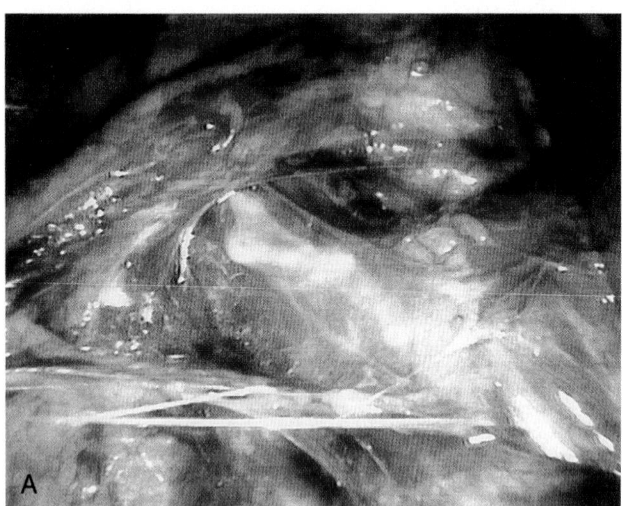

FIGURE 43–17 ■ *A,* Subcarinal lymph node dissection. (From Krasna MJ, Mach M: Atlas of Thoracoscopic Surgery. St. Louis, Quality Medical Publishing, 1993.)

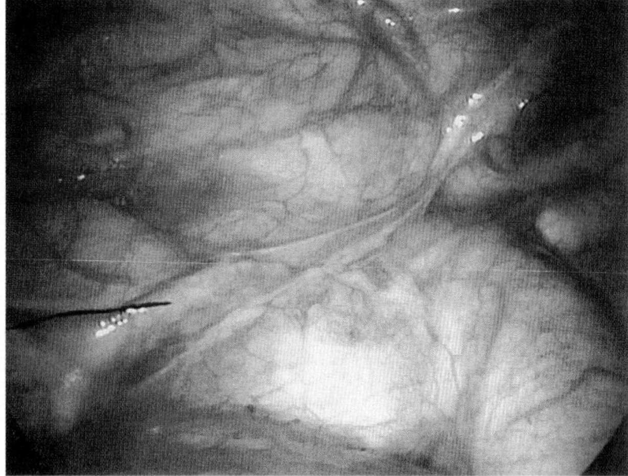

FIGURE 43–19 ■ Exposure of anteroposterior window and lymph nodes at the thoracoscopic lymph node.

I Introduction

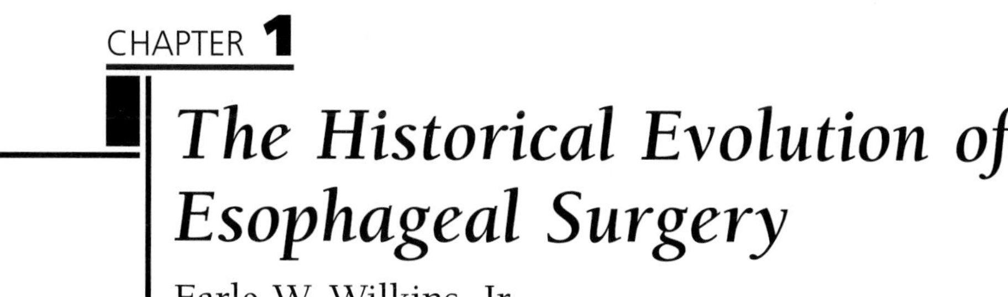

CHAPTER 1

The Historical Evolution of Esophageal Surgery

Earle W. Wilkins, Jr.

Secluded in the posterior mediastinum against the dorsal vertebrae and abutted anteriorly by the heart, the great vessels, and the tracheobronchial airway, the esophagus has always, by its remote inaccessibility, been a major challenge to surgeons. Emslie (1988) has provided perhaps the best perspective of the surgeon's struggle with the esophagus:

> The history of oesophageal surgery is the tale of men repeatedly losing to a stronger adversary yet persisting in this unequal struggle until the nature of the problems became apparent and the war was won.

As we shall see, continuation of the struggle has resulted directly in (1) the founding of the American Association for Thoracic Surgery and (2) the recognition of general thoracic surgery as a necessary subdivision for the appropriate and complete training of the cardiothoracic surgeon.

ORIGINS

"There is no exact date or specific event that marks the birth of chest surgery" (*General Thoracic Surgery: Its History and Development*). That statement is likewise true in the evolution and development of esophageal surgery. It also did not arise de novo in a particular country, nor in a single school of surgery.

Sporadic accounts of surgical procedures on the cervical esophagus are scattered through the millennia dating back to Egyptian times. Brewer (1980) provides a wonderfully detailed reference to the Smith Surgical Papyrus (3000–2500 BC), discovered in 1862 by Edwin Smith and translated and edited in 1930 by Henry Breasted. Case No. 28 describes the treatment, apparently successful, of "a gaping wound of the throat penetrating the gullet." Collis (1982) cites a comment made by Ambroise Paré (1510–1590): "when the oesophagus is being sutured great care should be taken." A marvelous cautionary guideline for the ages!

Vincenz Czerny of Heidelberg, a former assistant of the pioneer Viennese surgeon Theodor Billroth, performed one of the early resections for carcinoma of the cervical esophagus in 1877. Billroth (1871) had demonstrated in dogs that resection with anastomosis of the cervical esophagus was indeed feasible.

Johann von Mikulicz-Radecki, likewise a pupil of Billroth, is described by Olch (1960) as "the father of such endoscopy as we know it today" for his 1881 development with Leiter of an esophagoscope with distal illumination. Such events as these were but preludes to developing attempts at resection of the thoracic esophagus.

ESOPHAGECTOMY

Decades of pioneering surgeons' struggles with resection of the intrathoracic esophagus form a thread that actually traces the historical development of surgery of the esophagus. The anatomic remoteness of the thoracic esophagus along with the physiologic challenge of intraoperative control of respiration presented a double obstacle to successful esophagectomy. It would take some six decades from the time of Billroth's laboratory successes with cervical esophageal resection to a successful resection and intrathoracic anastomosis.

Respiratory Control

Ultimately it was the solution of the problem of control of respiration in the open thorax that permitted substantive advances in the technical challenges of esophageal resection.

In 1904, Mikulicz in Breslau (now Wroclaw, Poland) initiated research into the development of a differential pressure methodology for control of respiration during surgery. His pupil, Ferdinand Sauerbruch (1904), was directly responsible for the negative differential pressure chamber, the complicated system in which the patient and the operating team were closeted in a hermetically sealed space with only the patient's head outside for control of respiration and administration of anesthetic agents. At the same time, Ludolph Brauer (1904) in Marburg, Germany was developing the reverse device: a positive-pressure method that enclosed only the patient's head in a diver's-like helmet. This permitted administering anesthesia with external positive pressure.

A radically different approach came from Samuel Meltzer and John Auer in New York (1909). They devised "continuous respiration without respiratory movements" by means of intratracheal insufflation of a continuous stream of air and anesthetic vapor. Theodore Tuffier (1896) in Paris had earlier reported his development of an intratracheal tube with an inflatable cuff. Development of the methodology of intermittent positive-pressure inflation of the lungs was considered by Leo Eloesser (1970) "the first milestone in chest surgery."

Surgical Techniques

Meade, the thoracic surgical historian, describes "the first successful intrathoracic resection and anastomosis of the esophagus" by Dobromysslow (1901). A 3- to 4-cm segment was resected, the ends were united with two rows of silk sutures, and the anastomosis was wrapped with a large posteriorly based skin flap. Although "complete union of the suture line" was demonstrated at 3 weeks, Meade reported that no further follow-up could be discovered.

The contemporary development of positive-pressure anesthesia permitted the direct transthoracic approach to esophageal resection. The pioneering operation was that of Franz Torek (1913) in New York. He carried out a subtotal, left thoracic resection of the esophagus for a squamous carcinoma of the middle third in a 67-year-old woman. (Dr. Carl Eggers, later a prominent thoracic surgeon, administered the anesthesia.) The patient survived 13 years and was fed orally via a rubber tube that connected her cervical esophagostomy to her gastrostomy. She refused any attempt at plastic antethoracic skin tube reconstruction.

Restoration of alimentary tract continuity following esophageal resection became the principal surgical challenge. Claude Beck (1905) in Cleveland demonstrated in animal experiments that a tube of greater curvature of the stomach could be used to replace the lower esophagus. Cesar Roux (1907) in Lausanne developed the technique of esophagojejunoplasty for distal esophageal stricture. Kelling (1911) in Dresden devised use of the colon for esophageal replacement. In his initial case, an isoperistaltic segment of transverse colon was brought up subcutaneously (its distal end anastomosed to stomach) to the midsternal level in preparation for ultimate skin tube connection to the cervical esophagostomy.

Martin Kirschner (1920) in Leipzig originated the now standard use of a mobilized stomach to replace the esophagus by dividing the left gastric, left gastroepiploic, and short gastric arteries. He planned an antethoracic, subcutaneous placement of the stomach but never succeeded in using it in a patient with carcinoma.

In light of this burst of attempts to treat carcinoma of the esophagus, it is surprising that the final accomplishment of a successful esophagectomy with an intrathoracic esophagogastric anastomosis did not come until 1933. Ohsava in Japan has rather belatedly been given credit for this pioneering success. In 1937, Samuel Marshall in Boston carried out an esophagogastrectomy with reestablishment of continuity by an end-to-side anastomosis. William Adams and Dallas Phemister (1938) in Chicago followed with a similar successful case featuring, for the first time, a two-layer anastomosis using interrupted nonabsorbable sutures, in this case linen.

Edward Churchill and Richard Sweet (1942) in Boston presented a classic report of 11 resections emphasizing preservation of gastric blood supply and the meticulous suturing, with two-layer interrupted fine silk, of the anastomosis as the basis for avoiding leakage or stricture formation at the anastomosis.

Finally, Sweet (1945) and the British surgeon Ivor Lewis (1946) extended esophageal resection for any level of carcinoma within the esophagus, Sweet by the strictly left transthoracic double-rib resection approach and Lewis by separate laparotomy and right thoracic incisions. These surgeons created the anastomosis intrathoracically at the apex of the chest.

With concerns about the consequences of anastomotic leaks within the thorax, other surgeons preferred carrying out the anastomosis in the neck via a separate cervical incision. K. C. McKeown (1972) in England advocated this approach, particularly in high carcinoma where total esophagectomy was in order. Eric Nanson (1975) in Auckland, New Zealand, has been a particular advocate of this operation, combining it with a synchronous two-team approach to abdominothoracocervical esophagectomy, a procedure developed while he was in Bristol, England, with Milnes Walker. He has acknowledged the latter's role (1988): "Professor Milnes Walker encouraged and helped in the development of this operation."

A totally different tack concerning the route of approach to resection of carcinoma of the thoracic esophagus was initiated by Wolfgang Denk (1913) in Vienna. He demonstrated in cadavers that the esophagus could be removed by blunt dissection through a subcostal transhiatal approach combined with a transcervical dissection.

Grey Turner (1933) reported a successful blunt esophagectomy followed by a second-stage completion of an antethoracic skin tube to connect the esophageal and gastric stomas. In his expansive Bradshaw Lecture to the Royal College of Surgeons (1935) he had traced the evolution of his "pull-through" or collo-abdominal technique beginning in 1927. He included a quotation from the English essayist John Ruskin which he found pertinent to his struggles with surgery of the esophagus:

> There is a time and a way in which all things can be done, none shorter—none smoother. For all noble things, the time is long and the way rude.

Ong and Lee (1960) in an innovative approach to esophagopharyngectomy for carcinoma of the hypopharynx or cervical esophagus utilized blunt dissection for removal of the intrathoracic esophagus prior to bringing the stomach through the mediastinum to the neck. LeQuesne and Ranger (1966), in their experience with 10 pharyngolaryngectomy operations—three by triple exposure and seven by blunt dissection of the intrathoracic esophagus—found the latter technique preferable. It was Orringer and Sloan (1978) in Ann Arbor, however, who deserve credit for the resurrection and continuing perfection of the technique of transhiatal-transcervical esophagectomy without thoracotomy. Recent progress in the development of thoracoscopic techniques has added one more facility for this approach.

Alternative Reconstruction Techniques

Gastric Tube

Boerema (1952) in The Netherlands introduced restoration of continuity after esophageal resection utilizing a gastric tube taken from the greater curvature. Gavriliu (1988) in Rumania has recorded extensive experience with 718 of these procedures, first performed by him in 1951. Heimlich (1961) encouraged this technique in North America with his work in replacing the entire esophagus for both malignant and benign stenosis.

Colon

Utilization of the right colon to replace or bypass the entire thoracic esophagus was reintroduced by Mahoney and Sherman (1954). Kelling (1911) and Vulliet (1911) independently had reported early experiences with esophagoplasty using segements of colon. Kergin (1954) reported the successful use of the transverse colon to bypass the esophagus in an unusual situation of esophageal obstruction due to a paraffinoma of the mediastinum, the late result of extrapleural collapse therapy for tuberculosis. Kergin was the first surgeon to use the intrathoracic route for esophageal bypass using the colon.

Goligher and Robin (1954) preferred using the left colon placing the interposed segment in an antiperistaltic fashion. Wilkins (1980), also preferring the left colon but in an isoperistaltic position, suggested that preoperative inferior mesenteric angiography was an enormous help in making the decision regarding the better portion of colon to use.

Jejunum

The greatest experience with use of a long segment of jejunum for replacement of the thoracic esophagus came from Yudin (1944). His reconstructions were largely antethoracic in position. Robertson and Sarjeant (1950) were the first to reconstruct the esophagus with an isoperistaltic segment of jejunum placed in a substernal position through the anterior mediastinum. In general, however, except for short segment interposition procedures for the distal esophagus, the jejunum has not enjoyed popularity as a replacement of the entire thoracic esophagus.

Cervical Skin and Other Grafts

Early management of localized carcinoma of the cervical esophagus and the hypopharynx was provided by Wookey (1942), who used a pioneering two-stage procedure. He resected the carcinoma and replaced the operative defect with a quadrilateral full-thickness flap of cervical skin. This technique has given way to free graft replacement of the cervical esophagus, a natural evolution of the development of microvascular anastomotic techniques. The use of a jejunal autograft was pioneered by Seidenberg and colleagues (1959). An unusual use of a revascularized gastric antrum graft was reported by Hiebert and Cummings (1961).

MANAGEMENT OF ESOPHAGEAL ATRESIA

A detailed account of the history of the evolution of the management of esophageal atresia and tracheoesophageal fistula is presented by Goldstein and colleagues in Chapter 8. Particularly well presented is the description of the evolution and understanding of the principles essential in securing a successful surgical outcome: closure of the fistula and reconstitution of continuity of the alimentary tract.

Early mention of this congenital malformation dates back to Thomas Gibson's *The Anatomy of Human Bodies Epitomized* (1697), which presents remarkably clear accounts of the particulars of the various forms of the anomaly. Credit for the first realistic surgical approach to both the understanding and the management of the complex problem perhaps should be given to Richter (1913). Recognizing the need for gastrostomy for feeding, but also its failure if employed alone, he added intrathoracic ligation of the fistula using positive-pressure anesthesia. The literature is replete for another three decades with descriptions of attempts to handle the challenges of fistula ligation, proximal pouch drainage, and gastrostomy feedings.

Substantive progress finally emerged in the early 1940s, with the not always friendly rivalry of Cameron Haight (1943) in Ann Arbor and William Ladd (1944) at the Boston Children's Hospital. Haight is credited with the first successful primary repair, whereas Ladd accomplished his first success with the construction of an antethoracic skin tube. Leven (1940) at the University of Minnesota had described successful extrapleural ligation of the fistula and cervical esophagostomy and later (1953) described reestablishment of continuity with jejunal interposition. Swenson (1947), who had trained with Ladd, reported a remarkable early 80% success rate with end-to-end anastomosis. The most reliable method of suture of the anastomosis remains a subject of continuing dialogue even today.

With improving additions in preoperative preparation, the use of antibiotics, methods of anesthesia, intraoperative techniques, and postoperative care, primary repair has become more reliable. These same advances have also allowed staged repair in unusually premature or sick infants (Koop and Hamilton, 1965). Foker and Boyle have suggested that it was Richter's approach more than four decades earlier that became the inspiring cornerstone for such staged repairs.

Myers (1986) has supplied a thorough history of the management of esophageal atresia with and without tracheoesophageal fistula from 1670 to 1984.

SURGERY FOR ACHALASIA OF THE ESOPHAGUS

Historically known by various names such as cardiospasm, idiopathic dilatation of the esophagus, or "megaesophagus," achalasia of the esophagus was first described by Willis (1674), who introduced use of a bit of sponge attached to a long strip of whale bone to force impacted food through the narrow distal esophagus. It was Hurst (1927) who gave the condition its present name. He based use of the term "achalasia" on the failure of the distal esophagus to relax. He also devised the rubber tubes filled with mercury used for esophageal dilatation, now recognized as the Hurst dilators, subsequently modified by Maloney with tapering tips.

The surgical approach to relief of the nonrelaxing lower esophageal segment originated in the German and Austrian schools of surgery. A variety of procedures were described, all utilizing the transabdominal approach. There were the Marwedel (1903) and Wendel (1910) operations, full-thickness cardioplasties of the Heineke-Mikulicz type. Heyrofsky (1913) used an esophagogastrostomy side-to-side between the dilated esophagus and the gastric fundus leaving the cardia intact. Gröndahl (1916) modified this concept with a U-shaped incision from dilated esophagus across the cardia to gastric fundus with closure in the fashion of a Finney pyloroplasty.

All of these procedures failed because of a common defect; each procedure resulted in destruction of the lower esophageal sphincter and permitted free gastroesophageal reflux, often with ensuing esophagitis and stricture formation. Many years later, Barrett and Franklin (1949) described this complication and, quite belatedly, all of these procedures began to meet with disfavor.

One operation from this early German era, however, has survived the tests of time—the Heller (1914) esophagomyotomy. This was a procedure not unlike the extramucosal pyloromyotomy of Ramstedt. Heller also approached the distal esophagus abdominally and performed two myotomies, one anterior and one posterior. Zaaijer (1923) recognized that a single myotomy produced equally good results. It is surprising that this very satisfactory procedure was not widely practiced and universally accepted until well after the conclusion of World War II. Today, the modified Heller operation is the standard for the surgical management of achalasia. Video-assisted thoracoscopic and laparoscopic techniques for Heller myotomy have been reported during the last decade.

A common sequel of the Heller myotomy for achalasia has been the development of gastroesophageal reflux. In Europe, Dor and coworkers (1962) and Toupet (1963) developed antireflux repairs with particular application to their use in combination with abdominal Heller esophagomyotomies. The Dor hemifundoplication, in turn, has become an integral part of the popular laparoscopic approach to achalasia.

SURGERY FOR ESOPHAGEAL DIVERTICULUM

The pharyngoesophageal diverticulum was first described by Abraham Ludlow (1767) of Bristol, England, with the unusually titled paper "A case of obstructed Deglutition, from a preternatural Dilatation of, and Bag formed in, the Pharynx." Zenker, for whom the diverticulum came to be named, and von Ziemssen (1877) first described the etiology, pathology, and symptoms. They were less sanguine about therapy: "The radical cure of diverticulum of the esophagus by operative procedure from without is . . . one of our vain wishes." Wheeler (1886) is credited with the first successful resection of the pharyngoesophageal diverticulum.

With early concern for postoperative complications, Goldmann (1909) devised a two-stage method of repair. A modification of the two-stage repair was utilized in the extensive experience of Lahey and Warren (1954): diverticulopexy and mediastinal packing in the first stage and resection of the diverticulum in the second. Harrington (1945) and Sweet (1947) advocated a one-stage operation as the preferred method for the management of diverticula.

The matter of obstruction at the cricopharyngeus had long been a concern in the management of diverticula. Aubin (1936) was the first to propose cricopharyngeal myotomy combined with diverticulectomy. Payne and Clagett (1965) suggested one of the presently favored techniques: one-stage pharyngo-esophageal diverticulectomy with myotomy. The other is diverticulopexy with cricopharyngeal myotomy, pioneered very successfully by Ronald Belsey (1966).

SURGICAL MANAGEMENT OF ESOPHAGEAL PERFORATION

Long before the era of interventional surgery, the entity of postemetic perforation of the esophagus gained renown with the famous case of Baron Jan van Wassenaer, the Grand Admiral of the Dutch fleet. With his stomach overdistended from a hearty meal, he had induced relief-seeking vomiting and immediately experienced excruciating epigastric pain. It is said that he remarked to his servants that his stomach was torn; if true, this was a remarkable bit of self-diagnosis. The eponym for the condition derives from his physician Hermann Boerhaave, who on that evening (October 29, 1723) was called to see the admiral, who succumbed about 18 hours later. The autopsy report, "History of a grievous disease not previously described," highlighted all of the essentials in the pathology of barogenic trauma.

It was more than two centuries later that the preoperative diagnosis of postemetic rupture of the esophagus was made for the first time by Leigh Collis (1944). His patient did not survive the surgical repair. His British colleague Norman Barrett (1947), whose name often appears in this historical account, achieved the first successful repair of a so-called spontaneous perforation of the esophagus. In the United States, Olsen and Clagett (1947) also reported a successful repair.

Mackler (1952), in an experimental and clinical study, concluded that an intraluminal pressure of 5 pounds per square inch was required to cause rupture. He utilized autopsy specimens of the complete esophagus, tied off at either end and subjected to varying pressures, demonstrating that it was the lower extremity of the esophagus that was most likely to rupture.

It has become clear that early diagnosis and prompt surgical intervention are the keys to success. As recorded in the Wassenaer case, abdominal physical findings are often not present.

SURGERY FOR GASTROESOPHAGEAL REFLUX DISEASE

While early efforts to design esophagectomy for carcinoma were pioneered in the German and Austrian schools, advancements in the understanding and surgical management of gastroesophageal reflux disease (GERD) were led by British surgeons. The techniques of esophageal resection and intrathoracic anastomosis had been largely established by the time of World War II, but GERD was not fully understood until early in the decade of the 1950s.

Allison (1951) defined clearly that it was not the sliding hiatal hernia itself that was the crucial pathologic process in GERD but, rather, the reflux of acid peptic gastric secretions that resulted in distal esophageal inflammation and ulceration. He described the first logical anatomic repair, although years later, in a remarkable display of critical self-evaluation (1973), he reported a 49% rate of recurrence—certainly and disappointingly unacceptable.

Meanwhile, Barrett, long considered the dean of British surgeons, was reporting (1950) his experience with columnar lined esophagus with accompanying esophagitis and ulceration. His interpretation that this condition was due to congenital shortening of the esophagus was ultimately proved erroneous, largely as the result of pathologic examination of a case by Allison and Johnstone (1953) of resected nondilatable strictures. In these specimens, normal esophageal musculature was found ensheathing the columnar epithelial lining. Nevertheless, Barrett's name has forever been assigned to this condition.

Years later, Naef and Ozzello (1975) cautioned that the columnar lined esophagus, an acquired lesion, was fraught with a predisposition to malignant change. To this day, controversy regarding the proper management of Barrett's esophagus persists.

With this background, it was clear, certainly to British surgeons, that control of gastroesophageal reflux was the essential requirement in the prevention of GERD. Having spent time working with Barrett, Belsey spent years studying the nature of reflux, with particular emphasis on his direct esophagoscopic observations. This mandatory procedure was always carried out with the patient under topical anesthesia and in the semirecumbent position. By 1952, he had developed a transthoracic technique that restored a 4- to 5-cm segment of intra-abdominal esophagus, and created a 270-degree fundoplication of proximal stomach about the distal esophagus. This constituted the Mark IV operation to prevent gastroesophageal reflux. He did not report this until nine years later with Hiebert (1961). The Mark IV operation remains one of the three basic antireflux surgical repairs.

The second of these successful operations was the transabdominal fundoplication procedure of Rudolf Nissen (1961) of Basel. This technique involved suture approximation of anterior and posterior folds of the gastric fundus anterior to the abdominal segment of esophagus. The technique has often been modified by a number of surgeons, and it remains a mainstay in the prevention of reflux. In addition, it has now become the basis for most laparoscopic operations to prevent GERD.

The third standard operation is the transabdominal posterior gastropexy of Hill (1967). In this operation, the posterior aspect of the gastroesophageal junction is anchored to the median arcuate ligament. In 1978, Hill incorporated intraoperative measurement of lower esophageal sphincteric pressures as his guide to producing the exactly correct sphincteric resistance to reflux. The Hill repair, too, has been adapted to laparoscopic techniques.

A final historical contribution to the management of GERD, when reflux-induced inflammatory intramural scarring has produced esophageal shortening, has been the work of Collis (1957). The Collis cardioplasty technique provides esophageal lengthening by creation of a proximal gastroplasty tube, sometimes termed "neoesophagus," around which is applied a fundoplicating wrap. A popular modern technique has been the combination of a Collis gastroplasty with a Mark IV antireflux repair, first described by Pearson (1971).

THE ESOPHAGUS AND HISTORY

At the outset, it was mentioned that struggles with surgery of the esophagus were to have a poignant place in the history of thoracic surgery. Now let us look at the two critical points in modern surgical times when problems of the esophagus were to result in monumental alterations in our thoracic surgical world.

First, *the aftermath of the 1913 Torek esophagectomy.* Murray (1988) reports that "it is not widely appreciated that Dr. Willy Meyer's description of successful esophageal resection at the annual meeting of the American Medical Association in 1913 was met with indifference" (1914). There was no discussion of this paper. The obvious lack of interest among general physicians for problems concerning the esophagus was the direct impetus for Meyer to take the lead, with a small group of "interested" surgeons, in the formation of the American Association for Thoracic Surgery, the founding organization in the clinical specialty of thoracic surgery. "Thus it was lack of enthusiasm that served to ignite the spark which developed, in time, into the first Society for Thoracic Surgery formed in the world" (Founding of the American Association for Thoracic Surgery, 50th anniversary, 1967).

Second, *response to Donald Paulson's presidential address to the 61st annual meeting of the American Association for Thoracic Surgery in 1981*, "*A Time for Reassessment*" (Paulson, 1981). In this treatise on the imbalances in training of cardiothoracic surgeons, Paulson deplored the decreasing general thoracic experience of residents applying for certification by the American Board of Thoracic Surgery. It was, in particular, the dismally small experience in *esophageal* surgery that dominated his statistics (only six to nine cases annually for the decade 1971–1980). The creation of a Liaison Committee for Thoracic Surgery has led to a more proper balancing of cardiothoracic training and to the development of general thoracic surgical units in many of the leading teaching and research hospitals.

In Canada, it should be noted, the Cardiovascular

and Thoracic Committee of the Royal College offers a Certificate of Special Competence in Thoracic Surgery.

Surgery of the esophagus will always present challenge. With the lessons of history, perhaps we will be better prepared to face and conquer the challenge.

Acknowledgment

The author wishes to acknowledge the careful review of the manuscript by F. G. Pearson, with his historically essential additions to the thread that constitutes one man's memory and understanding of the story.

■ *REFERENCES*

Adams W, Phemister DB: Carcinoma of the lower thoracic esophagus: Report of a successful resection and esophagogastrostomy. J Thorac Surg 7:621, 1938.

Allison PR: Reflux esophagitis, sliding hiatal hernia, and the anatomy of repair. Surg Gynecol Obstet 92:149, 1951.

Allison PR: Hiatus hernia: A 20-year retrospective survey. Ann Surg 178:273, 1973.

Allison PR, Johnstone AS: The oesophagus lined with gastric membrane. Thorax 8:87, 1953.

Aubin A: Un cas de diverticule de pulsion de l'oesophage traité par la résection de la poche associée à l'oesophagotomie extramuqueuse. Ann Otolaryngol 2:167, 1936.

Barrett NR: Report of a case of spontaneous perforation of the oesophagus successfully treated by operation. Br J Surg 35:216, 1947.

Barrett NR, Franklin LH: Concerning the unfavourable late results of certain operations performed in the treatment of cardiospasm. Br J Surg 37:194, 1949.

Barrett NR: Chronic peptic ulcer of the oesophagus and "oesophagitis." Br J Surg 38:175, 1950.

Beck C: Demonstrations of specimens illustrating a method of formation of a prethoracic esophagus. Illinois Med J 7:463, 1905.

Belsey R: Functional disease of the esophagus. J Thorac Cardiovasc Surg 52:164, 1966.

Billroth T: Über die Resektion des Ösophagus. Arch Klin Chir 13:65, 1871.

Boerema I: Oesophagus resection with restoration of continuity by a gastric tube. Arch Chir Nederland 44:120, 1952.

Boerhaave H: Atrocis, nec descripti prius, morbi historia. (Verbatim English translation; Derbes V, Mitchell R.) Bull Am Library A 43:217, 1955.

Brauer L: Über eine wesentliche Vereinfachung der künstlichen Atmug nach Sauerbruch. Z Physiol Chem 41:299, 1904.

Brewer LA III: History of surgery of the esophagus. Am J Surg 139:730, 1980.

Churchill ED, Sweet RH: Transthoracic resection of tumors of the stomach and esophagus. Ann Surg 115:897, 1942.

Collis JL, Humphries DR, Bond WH: Spontaneous rupture of the oesophagus. Lancet 2:179, 1944.

Collis JL: An operation for hiatus hernia with short esophagus. J Thorac Cardiovasc Surg 34:768, 1957.

Collis JL: The history of British oesophageal surgery. Thorax 37:795, 1982.

Czerny V: Neue Operationen. Zentralbl Chir 4:433, 1877.

Denk W: Zur Radikaloperation des Ösophaguskarzinomen. Zentralbl Chir 40: 1065, 1913.

Dobromysslow VD: Ein Fall von transpleuraler Ösophagektomie ein Brustabschnitte. Zentralbl Chir 28:1, 1901.

Dor J, Humbert P, Dor V, et al: L'intétét de la technique de Nissen modifée dans la prevention de reflux après cardiomyotomie extramuqueuse de Heller. Mem Acad Chir (Paris) 88:877, 1962.

Eloesser L: Milestones in chest surgery. J Thorac Cardiovasc Surg 60:157, 1970.

Emslie RG: Perspectives in the development of oesophageal surgery. In Jamieson GG (ed): Surgery of the Oesophagus. Melbourne, Churchill Livingstone, 1988, pp 3–8.

Gavriliu D: The replacement of the oesophagus by a gastric tube. In Jamieson GG (ed): Surgery of the Oesophagus. Melbourne, Churchill Livingstone, 1988, pp 765–775.

Gibson T: The Anatomy of Human Bodies Epitomized, 5th ed. London, Awasham & Churchill, 1697.

Goldmann EE: Die zweideutige Operation von Pulsion Divertikeln der Speiseröhre. Beitr Klin Chir 61:741, 1909.

Goligher JC, Robin IG: Use of left colon for reconstruction of pharynx and oesophagus after pharyngectomy. Br J Surg 42:283, 1954.

Gröndahl NB: Cardiaplastik ved Cardiospasmus. Nor Kirurgisk Forenings 11:236, 1916.

Haight C, Towsley H: Congenital atresia of the esophagus with tracheoesophageal fistula: Extrapleural ligation of fistula and end-to-end anastomosis of esophageal segments. Surg Gynecol Obstet 73:672, 1943.

Harrington SW: Pulsion diverticulum of the hypopharynx at the pharyngoesophageal junction. Surgery 18:66, 1945.

Heimlich HJ: Replacement of the entire esophagus for malignant or benign stenosis. Am J Gastroenterol 35:311, 1961.

Heller E: Extramuköse Cardiaplastik beim chronischen Cardiospasmus mit Dilatation des Ösophagus. Mitt Grenzgeb Med Chir 27:141, 1914.

Heyrofsky H: Casuistik und Therapie der idiopathischen Dilatation der Speiseröhre. Ösophagogastroanastomose. Arch Klin Chir 100:703, 1913.

Hiebert CA, Belsey R: Incompetency of the gastric cardia without radiologic evidence of hiatal hernia. J Thorac Cardiovasc Surg 42:352, 1961.

Hiebert CA, Cummings GO Jr: Successful replacement of the cervical esophagus by transplantation and revascularization of a free graft of gastric antrum. Ann Surg 154: 103, 1961.

Hill LD: An effective operation for hiatal hernia: An eight year appraisal. Ann Surg 166:681, 1967.

Hill LD: Intraoperative measurement of lower esophageal sphincter pressure. J Thorac Cardiovasc Surg 75:368, 1978.

Hurst AF: Treatment of achalasia of the cardia (so-called cardiospasm). Lancet 1:618, 1927.

Kelling G: Ösophagoplastik mit Hilfe des Querkolon. Zentralbl Chir 38:1209, 1911.

Kergin FG: Esophageal obstruction due to paraffinoma of mediastinum. Ann Surg 137:91, 1953.

Kirschner MB: Eines neues Verfahren der Ösophagoplastik. Arch Klin Chir 114: 606, 1920.

Koop CE, Hamilton JP: Atresia of the esophagus: Increased survival with staged procedure in the poor-risk infant. Ann Surg 162:369, 1965.

Ladd W: The surgical treatment of esophageal atresia and tracheoesophageal fistula. N Engl J Med 230:625, 1944.

Lahey FH, Warren K: Esophageal diverticula. Surg Gynecol Obstet 98:1, 1954.

LeQuesne LP, Ranger D: Pharyngolaryngectomy with immediate pharyngogastric anastomosis. Br J Surg 53: 105, 1966.

Leven NL: Congenital atresia of the esophagus with tracheoesophageal fistula: A report of successful extrapleural ligation of fistulous communication and cervical esophagostomy. J Thorac Surg 10:648, 1940.

Leven NL, Varco RL: Experiences with the operative management of delayed restoration of alimentary continuity in children originally treated by the multiple stage procedure for corrections of congenital tracheoesophageal defects. J Thorac Surg 25:16, 1953.

Lewis I: The surgical treatment of carcinoma of the oesophagus: With special reference to a new operation for growths of the middle third. Br J Surg 34:18, 1946.

Ludlow A: A case of obstructed Deglutition, from a preternatural Dilatation of, and Bag formed in, the Pharynx. Med Observ Inquiry 3:85, 1767.

Mackler SA: Spontaneous rupture of the esophagus: Experimental and clinical study. Surg Gynecol Obstet 95:345, 1952.

Mahoney EB, Sherman CD Jr: Total esophagoplasty using intrathoracic right colon. Surgery 35:937, 1954.

Marshall SF: Carcinoma of the esophagus: Successful resection of lower end of esophagus with reestablishment of esophageal gastric continuity. Surg Clin North Am 18:643, 1938.

Marwedel G: Die Aufklappung des Rippenbogens zur Erleichterung operativer Eingriffe in Hypochondrium und im Zwerchfellkuppelraum. Zentralbl Chir 30:938, 1903.

McKeown KC: Trends in oesophageal resection for carcinoma, with special reference to total oesophagectomy. Ann R Coll Surg Engl 51:213, 1972.

Meade RH: A History of Thoracic Surgery. Springfield Ill, Charles C Thomas, 1961.

Meltzer SJ, Auer J: Continuous respiration without respiratory movements. J Exp Med 11:622, 1909.

Meyer W: Extrathoracic and intrathoracic esophagoplasty in connection with resection of the thoracic portion of the esophagus for carcinoma. JAMA 62:100, 1914.

Murray GF: Discussion. In Delarue NC, Wilkins EW Jr, Wong J (eds): International Trends in General Thoracic Surgery: Esophageal Cancer. St. Louis, CV Mosby, 1988, pp 144–146.

Myers NA: The history of esophageal atresia and tracheoesophageal fistula, 1670–1984. Prog Pediatr Surg 20:106, 1986.

Naef AP, Ozzello L: Columnar-lined lower esophagus: An acquired lesion with malignant predisposition: Report on 140 cases of Barrett's esophagus with 12 adenocarcinomas. J Thorac Cardiovasc Surg 70:826, 1975.

Nanson EM: Synchronous combined abdomino-thoraco-cervical oesophagectomy. Aust N Z Surg 45:340, 1975.

Nanson EM: Synchronous combined abdominothoracocervical esophagectomy. In Delarue NC, Wilkins EW Jr, Wong J (eds): International Trends in General Thoracic Surgery: Esophageal Cancer. St. Louis, CV Mosby, 1988, p 219.

Nissen R: Gastropexy and "fundoplication" in surgical treatment of hiatal hernia. Am J Dig Dis 6:954, 1961.

Ohsava T: The surgery of the esophagus (in Japanese). J Jpn Surg Soc 34:1518, 1933.

Olch PD: Johann von Mikulicz-Radecki. Ann Surg 152:923, 1960.

Olsen AM Clagett OT: Spontaneous rupture of the esophagus: Report of a case with immediate diagnosis and successful surgical repair. Postgrad Med 2:417, 1947.

Ong GB, Lee TC: Pharyngogastric anastomosis for oesophago-pharyngectomy for carcinoma of the hypopharynx and cervical esophagus. Br J Surg 48:193, 1960.

Orringer MB, Sloan H: Esophagectomy without thoracotomy. J Thorac Cardiovasc Surg 76:643, 1978.

Paulson DL: A time for reassessment. J Thorac Cardiovasc Surg 82:163, 1981.

Payne WS, Clagett OT: Pharyngeal and esophageal diverticula. Curr Probl Surg 1:31, 1965.

Pearson FG, Langer R, Henderson RD: Gastroplasty and Belsey hiatus hernia repair. J Thorac Cardiovasc Surg 61:50, 1971.

Richter HM: Congenital atresia of the oesophagus: An operation designed for its cure. Surg Gynecol Obstet 27:397, 1913.

Robertson R, Sarjeant TR: Reconstruction of esophagus. J Thorac Surg 20:689, 1950.

Roux C: L'Esophago-jejuno-gastromie, nouvelle operation pour rétrécissement infranchisable de l'esophage. Semaine Med 27:37, 1907.

Sauerbruch JF: Über die physiologischen and physikalischen Grunlagen bei intrathorakalen Eingriffen in meiner pneumatischen Operationkammer. Arch Klin Chir 77:977, 1904.

Seidenberg B, Rosenak SS, Hurwitt ES, et al: Immediate reconstruction of the cervical esophagus by a revascularized isolated jejunal segment. Ann Surg 149:162, 1959.

Sweet RH: Surgical management of carcinoma of the mid-thoracic esophagus. N Engl J Med 233:1, 1945.

Sweet RH: Pulsion diverticulum of the pharyngoesophageal junction: Technic of the one stage operation. A preliminary report. Ann Surg 125:41, 1947.

Swenson O: End-to-end anastomosis of the esophagus for esophageal atresia. Surgery 22:324, 1947.

Torek F: The first successful case of resection of the thoracic portion of the esophagus for carcinoma. Surg Gynecol Obstet 16:614, 1913.

Toupet A: Technique l'oesophago-gastroplastic avec phrenogastropexie appliquée dans la cure radicale des hernias hiatales et comme complement de l'operation d'Heller dans les cardiospasmes. Mem Acad Chir 89:394, 1963.

Tuffier T: Regulation de la pression intrabronchique et de la narcose. Compte-Rendu Soc Biol 3:1086, 1896.

Turner GG: Excision of thoracic oesophagus for carcinoma with construction of extra-thoracic gullet. Lancet 2:1315, 1933.

Turner GG: Carcinoma of the oesophagus: The question of its treatment by surgery. Bradshaw Lecture to Royal College of Surgeons, November 5, 1935. Lancet 1:67, 130, 1936.

von Mikulicz J: Über Operationen in der Brusthöhle mit Hilfe der Sauerbruchschen Kammer. Cited by Eloesser L: Milestones in chest surgery. J Thorac Cardiovasc Surg 60:157, 1970.

Vulliet H: De l'oesophagoplastie et des diverses modifications. Semaine Med 31:529, 1911.

Wendel W: Zur Chirurgie des Ösophagus. Arch Klin Chir 93:311, 1910.

Wheeler WI: Pharyngocele and dilatation of the pharynx, with existing diverticulum at lower part of pharynx lying posterior to the oesophagus. Dublin J Med Sci 82:349, 1886.

Wilkins EW Jr: Long-segment colon substitution for the esophagus. Ann Surg 192:722, 1980.

Willis T: Pharmaceutice Rationalis: Siva Diatriba de Medicamentorum Operationibus in Humano Corpore. Hagae-Comitis. London, 1674.

Wookey H: The surgical treatment of carcinoma of the pharynx and cervical esophagus. Surg Gynecol Obstet 75:499, 1942.

Yudin SS: The surgical construction of 80 cases of artificial esophagus. Surg Gynecol Obstet 78:561, 1944.

Zaaijer HJ: Cardiospasm in the aged. Ann Surg 77:615, 1923.

Zenker FA, von Ziemssen H: Krankheiten des Ösophagus. Handbuch Spezillen Pathol Ther 7:50, 1877.

CHAPTER **2**

Anatomy, Embryology, and Histology

Dorothea Liebermann-Meffert

DEFINITION

The esophagus is the muscular tube that serves as the food passage by connecting the pharynx with the stomach.

SURGICAL ANATOMY

General Features

The esophagus is the narrowest tube of the gastrointestinal tract, spanning the interval between the cricopharyngeal constriction and the most voluminous part of the gut, the stomach (Fig. 2–1). At rest, the tube is collapsed. The configuration is flat in the upper and middle and rounded in the lower portion (Figs. 2–2 and 2–3), presenting mean diameters in transverse sections of 2.5 to 1.6 cm and 2.5 to 2.4 cm, respectively.

Esophageal Bed, Compartments, and Anchors

Unlike the digestive tube, the esophagus has no mesentery and no serosal coating. Its position within the loose, areolar connective tissue of the mediastinum allows the esophagus transverse and longitudinal mobility. Respiration may induce movement over a few millimeters and swallowing as much as the height of one vertebral body (Dodds et al, 1983).

The connective tissue in which the esophagus and trachea are embedded is surrounded by long, continuous sheaths of fibroareolar laminae that cover and bind together the muscles, vessels, and bony constituents of the neck and chest (see Warwick and Williams, 1978). A portion of the deep cervical fascia, the carotid sheath, separates to form the pretracheal (previsceral) fascia anteriorly and the prevertebral (retrovisceral) fascia posteriorly (see Fig. 2–3C). The anterior and posterior space (i.e., the slit-like interval between the various layers of these fasciae) forms a communicating compartment between neck and chest (Pernkopf, 1937; Warwick and Williams, 1978).

The pretracheal space surrounds the vascular structures of the anterior mediastinum and is limited distally by the fibrous tissue of the pericardium. The prevertebral space may extend from the base of the skull down to the diaphragm. This space is lined anteriorly by the continuation of the buccopharyngeal fascia, which spreads downward as a delicate sheath separating the esophagus from the prevertebral fascia. Below the level of the tracheal bifurcation, this space is frequently obliterated.

The stabilizing structures of the esophagus are shown in Figure 2–4. Tiny membranes of different extension connect the trachea, pleura, retrovisceral fascia, and the cranial half of the esophagus. These insert at both lateral and posterior aspects of the esophagus and the tracheal membrane laterally (Liebermann-Meffert, 1997b). They consist of elastic and/or collagen fibers that may contain small smooth muscle bundles or striated muscle fibers. The posterior bundles end in the retrovisceral fascia or blindly within the areolar connective tissue network of the mediastinum. The membranes are all delicate, ranging from 30 to 1000 μm in thickness and 0.5 to 3 cm in craniocaudal extension (Liebermann-Meffert and Duranceau, 1996). They appear much smaller than the coarse "bronchoesophageal" or "pleuroesophageal" muscle cords depicted by Netter (1971) but may be viewed during medianoscopic dissection when the esophagus is exposed from the neck.

Elastically attached by the phrenoesophageal membrane, the distal esophagus traverses the diaphragm through the esophageal hiatus (see Fig. 2–4). At the central margin of the diaphragm, the subdiaphragmatic and the endothoracic aponeuroses blend into "Laimer's ligament" or "Allison's membrane." This structure can be recognized by its well-defined lower edge and its slightly yellow color.

The membrane splits into two sheaths. One sheath extends for 2 to 4 cm upward through the hiatus, where its fibers traverse the esophageal musculature to insert on the submucosa (Eliska, 1973). The second sheath passes down across the cardia, clearly separated from the muscular wall of the gastroesophageal junction by loose areolar connective or fat tissue (Duranceau and Liebermann-Meffert, 1991). At the level of the gastric fundus, the fibers of the membrane blend into the serosa and the gastric musculature, the gastrohepatic ligament, and the dorsal gastric mesentery (Figs. 2–5 and 2–6; see Fig. 2–4). The membrane wraps the gastroesophageal junction completely like a collar that allows the terminal esophagus and the lower esophageal sphincter (LES) to move in relation to the diaphragm and to "slip through the hiatus like in a tendon sheath" (Hayek, 1933).

The phrenoesophageal membrane is composed in equal proportions of elastic and collagenous fiber elements, which guarantee sufficient plasticity to the junction to move up and down with swallows. Stability is provided by the inelastic gastric ligaments that attach the cardia and the posterior fundus wall to the upper

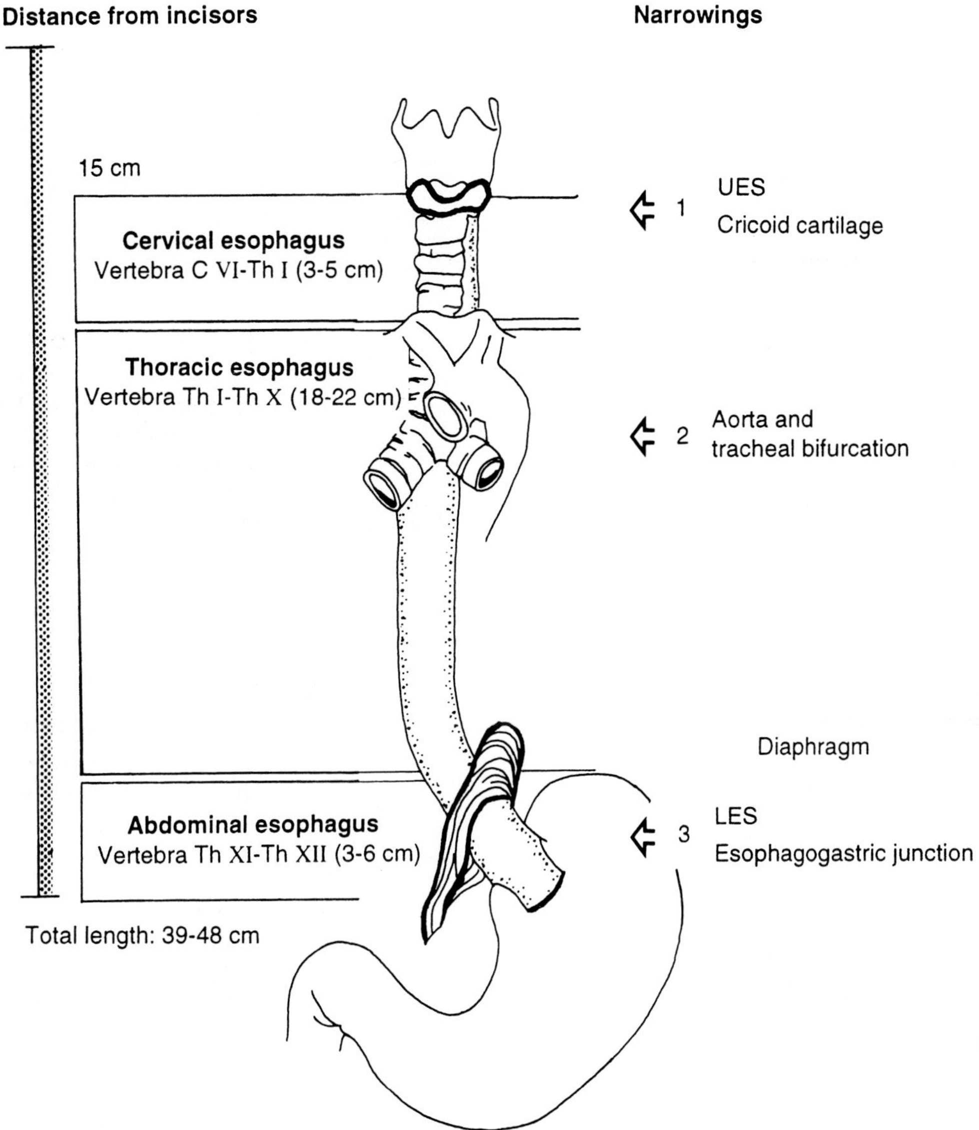

FIGURE 2–1 ■ Classical division of the esophagus and projection to the cervical (C) and thoracic vertebrae (Th) as radiologic landmarks. The lengths and narrowings *(arrows)* of the esophagus are shown. UES, upper esophageal sphincter; LES, lower esophageal sphincter.

retroperitoneal fasciae, as illustrated in Figures 2–4 and 2–6.

Points of Surgical Interest

A number of anatomic features merit the special attention of clinicians and surgeons.

The first of these is the mobile location of the esophagus within the mediastinum. There are no large neurovascular or fibrous structures that tether the esophagus within the chest. Therefore, the esophagus may be subjected to a blunt stripping from the mediastinum if there are no contraindications such as periesophageal tumor invasion (Liebermann-Meffert et al, 1987; Orringer and Orringer, 1983).

A second anatomic peculiarity of clinical interest is the location of the esophagus within defined fascial compartments. Infections spreading from anterior lesions of the esophagus may follow the route of the pretracheal space down to the pericardium. The retrovisceral space, however, is clinically more important. For example, oropharyngeal infections can easily descend through spaces within the various layers of the deep cervical fascia. Necrotizing mediastinitis resulting from peritonsillar or dental abscesses or even wisdom tooth extraction has been reported and may involve a mortality rate of nearly 40% (Marty-Ane et al, 1994; van Straalen et al, 1994). Most instrumental perforations occur in the posterior hypopharynx above the narrowing of the cricopharyngeal sphincter, below which there is no barrier to the spread of infection into the mediastinum. Noninstrumental or spontaneous perforation (Boerhaave's syndrome) and leakage from an esophageal anastomosis behave in a similar way with rapid and disastrous dissemination of sepsis.

A third peculiarity is that, with advancing age, the

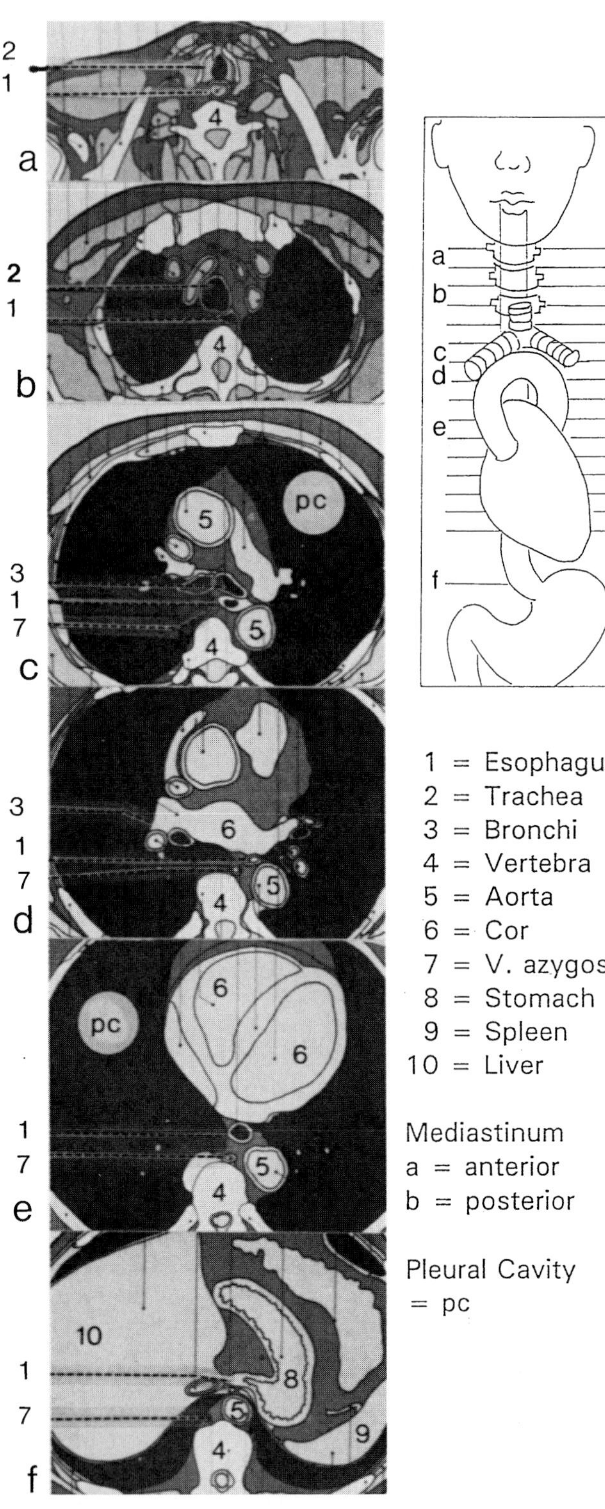

FIGURE 2–2 ■ Positional anatomy of the esophagus shown in computed tomographic representations from the cervical level *(a)* down to the esophagogastric junction *(f)*. The esophagus (1) is shown at various levels of descent *(a–f)*. (From Wegener OH: Whole Body Computerized Tomography. Basel, Karger, 1983.)

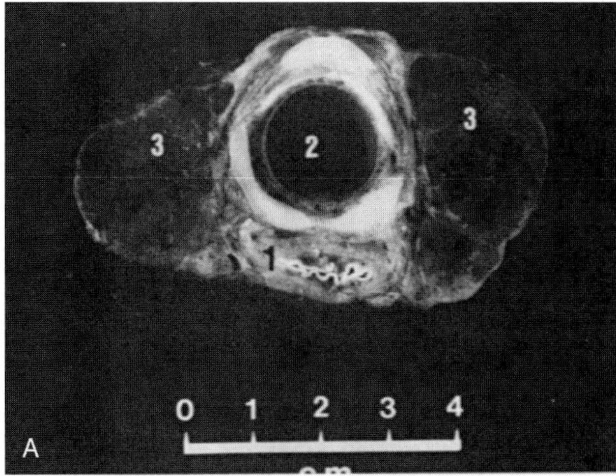

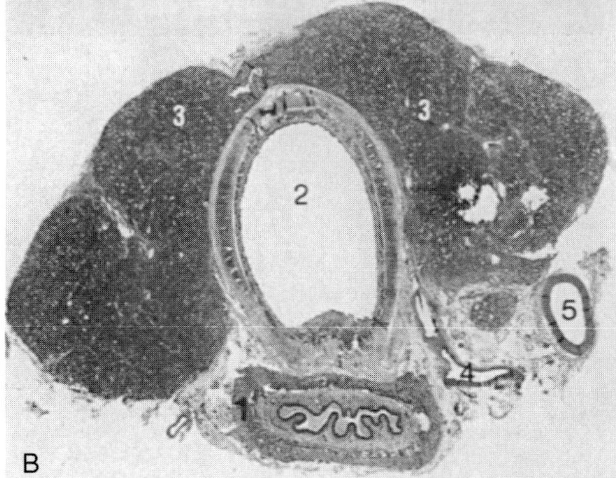

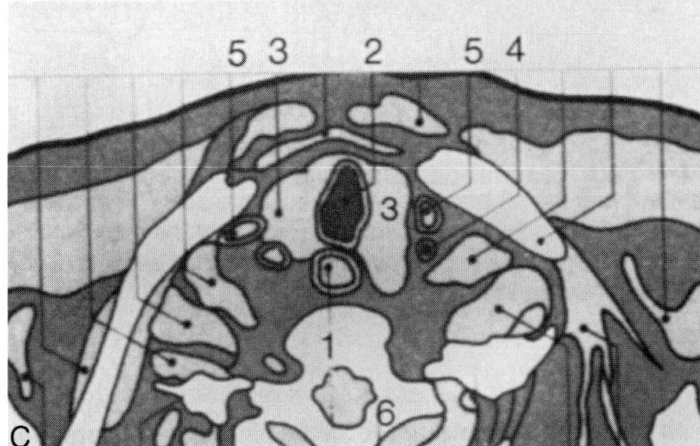

FIGURE 2–3 ■ Transverse section through the mediastinum at a cervical level showing the (1) esophagus, (2) trachea, and (3) thyroid gland in the *(A)* macroscopic, *(B)* histologic, and *(C)* CT aspects. The close positional relationship between the esophagus and trachea and the lack of a distinct dividing tissue is seen as well as the (4) carotid artery, (5) jugular vein, and (6) vertebra. (*A* and *B*, From Liebermann-Meffert D, Siewert JR: Arterial anatomy of the esophagus: A review of literature with brief comments on clinical aspects. Gullet 2:3, 1992. *C*, From Wegener OH: Whole Body Computerized Tomography. Basel, Karger, 1983.)

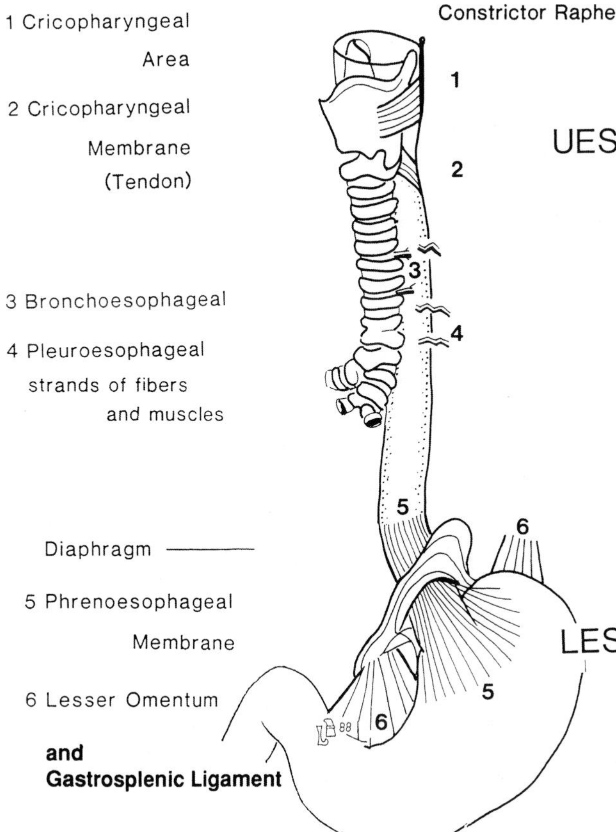

FIGURE 2–4 ■ Anchoring structures of the esophagus. At the upper end, the longitudinal muscle of the esophagus inserts firmly into the cricoid cartilage through the cricopharyngeal tendon (2) and the circular muscle is stabilized by its continuity with the inferior laryngeal constrictor muscles (1), which insert via the raphe to the sphenoid bone. Bundles of solitary elastic, collagen, and muscle fibers connect the esophageal wall transversely to the trachea (3), pleura, and retrovisceral fascia (4). The attachment by the phrenoesophageal membrane (5) is rather mobile, while the posterior gastric ligaments (6) and the lesser omentum (6) yield a tight adherence. LES, lower esophageal sphincter; UES, upper esophageal sphincter.

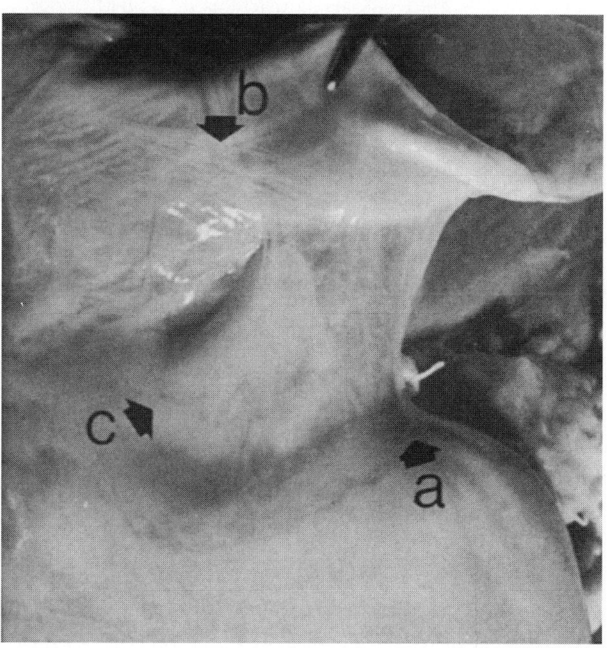

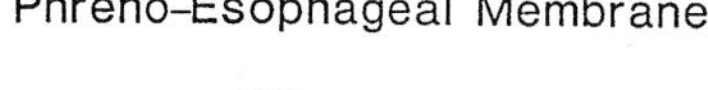

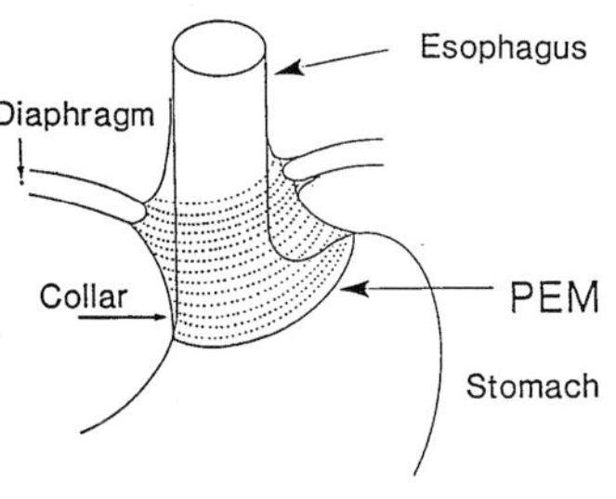

FIGURE 2–5 ■ The phrenoesophageal membrane (PEM) in a human autopsy specimen viewed in situ from the anteriolateral aspect. This structure also became known as Laimer's or Allison's membrane. As shown on the photograph on the left, the lower sheath of the membrane is inserted onto the gastric fundus *(arrow a)*. At the top the diaphragm is held up with a forceps. Diaphragmatic decussating fibers *(arrow b)* and a submembranous inlay of adipose tissue *(arrow c)* are seen. The scheme on the right shows how the PEM wraps the esophagogastric junction with a wide membranous collar. This wrap (dotted lines) is illustrated schematically at the right. (From Duranceau A, Liebermann-Meffert D: Embryology, anatomy, and physiology of the esophagus. In Orringer MB, Zuidema GD [eds]: Shackelford's Surgery of the Alimentary Tract, Vol 1. The Esophagus, 3rd ed. Philadelphia, WB Saunders, 1991, p 3.)

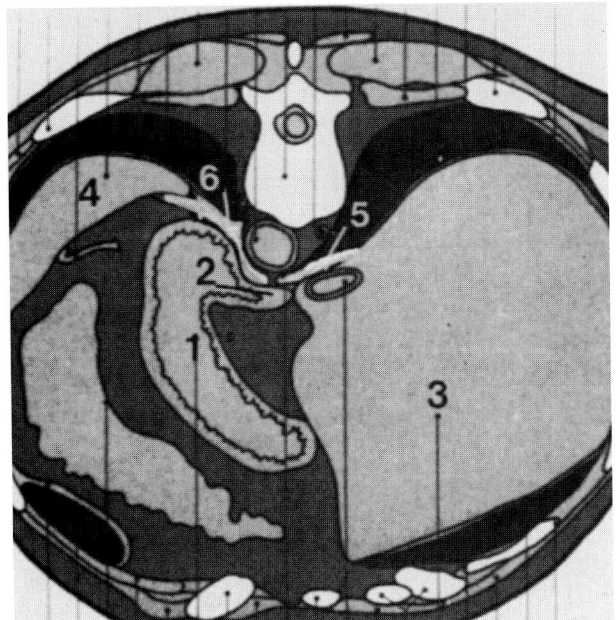

FIGURE 2–6 ■ Tomographic representation of the attachments of the stomach (1) and the relationship of the gastric cardia (2) to the liver (3) and spleen (4), transverse section. Firm ligaments such as the gastrohepatic (5) which continues the lower limb of the phrenicolienal, and the gastrosplenic (6) ligament anchor the cardia and posterior fundus wall to the retroperitoneal tissues and of course, also the LES within the abdominal cavity (From Wegener OH: Whole Body Computerized Tomography. Basel, Karger, 1983.)

elastic fibers of the phrenoesophageal membrane are replaced by inelastic collagenous fiber elements (Eliska, 1973). The loss of elasticity of the membrane in conjunction with a wide hiatus may then result in herniation of the gastroesophageal junction and cardia into the thoracic cavity. Eliska believed that abnormal anchorage of the phrenoesophageal membrane in youth and pathologic accumulation of adipose tissue in the connective tissue space between the phrenoesophageal membrane and the cardia musculature may also contribute to the development of a hiatus hernia (Eliska, 1973).

A sphincter-supporting role has been attributed to the phrenoesophageal ligament and its insertions (Bombeck et al, 1966; Mittal, 1998). This claim could not be confirmed experimentally; complete dissection of the membranes and ligaments and positioning of the LES within the chest by suturing the diaphragm to the midstomach had no effect on either the pressure values or characteristics of the LES (Liebermann-Meffert and Keller, 1985).

Course and Relationship to Other Structures

Three minor esophageal deviations are present. The first one is from the median position (see Fig. 2–3) toward the left at the base of the neck (Fig. 2–7; see Fig. 2–2*a–d*). The second one is at the level of the seventh thoracic vertebra, where the esophagus shifts slightly to the right of the spine (see Fig. 2–2*c*). The third and most prominent angulation is seen just above the esophagogastric junction, where the terminal esophagus shifts to the left (see Fig. 2–1). Because of this deviation, the esophagogastric junction is positioned lateral to the xiphoid process of the sternum and to the left of the spine (see Fig. 2–6). At this point, the fundus and the proximal gastric body extend anterolateral to the body of the vertebra, the greater curvature clearly faces the posterior subdiaphragmatic space, and the anterior gastric wall faces laterally.

This geographic dimension is not adequately displayed in standard anatomy or surgical textbooks, and the local relationships of the area are far better defined by computed tomography (CT). Figure 2–2*a–f* is a CT series by Wegener (1983) that shows the structures surrounding the esophagus as it progresses downward from the neck to the cardia. Macroscopic and histologic aspects of cross-sections of the neck area are also shown in Figures 2–3*A*, *B* and 2–7*A*, *B*. Some other important local relationships, such as the direct contact with the membranous part of

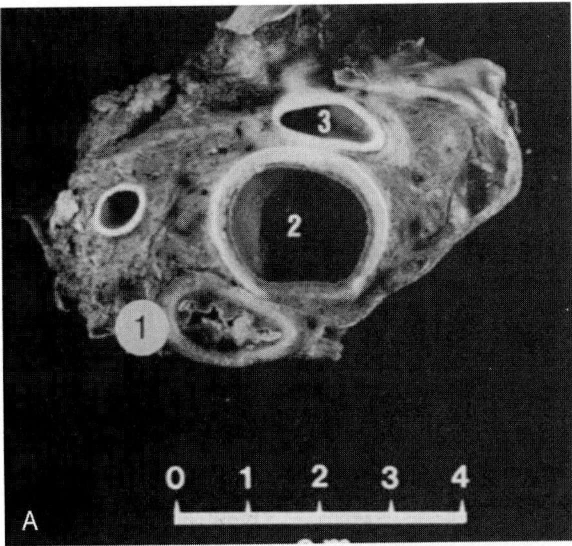

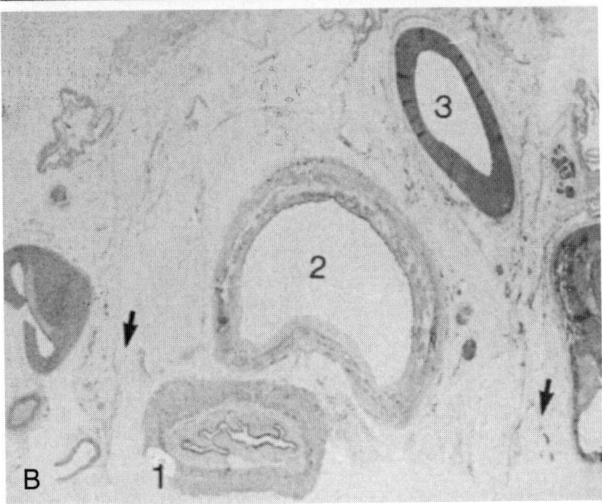

FIGURE 2–7 ■ Transverse section through the mediastinum at a cranial thoracic level showing the (1) esophagus shifted slightly to the left of the (2) trachea in the macroscopic *(A)* and histologic *(B)* aspects. The various branches of the recurrent laryngeal nerve *(arrows)* and the (3) brachiocephalic trunk are seen. (From Liebermann-Meffert D, Siewert JR: Arterial anatomy of the esophagus: A review of literature with brief comments on clinical aspects. Gullet 2:3, 1992.)

the trachea without any boundary tissue and the proximity of the crossing azygos vein to the other vessels and nerves, are presented in the respective sections of this chapter.

Points of Clinical and Surgical Interest

The surgical access to safe removal of the intrathoracic esophagus under direct vision is through the right chest; the azygos vein must usually be divided before the esophagus is dissected free. The cervical esophagus is also vulnerable because of its proximity to the membranous trachea. Because there is no protecting sheath between the two structures (see Figs. 2–3 and 2–7), special care must be taken not to injure the trachea when developing the plane of dissection between esophagus and trachea. Not only periesophageal inflammation or tumor invasion but also the anatomic fibromuscular "fixators" described earlier may occasionally predispose the membranous trachea to surgical injury. The thoracic duct is also vulnerable at this level (Orringer, 1991a, 1991b).

Arteries

Anatomy

Cervical Esophagus. Vascular branches from both the right and left superior and inferior thyroid arteries supply the wall of pharynx, esophagus, and trachea (Fig. 2–8). Compared with the thyroid arteries from which they originate, the vessels supplying the esophagus are small (Shapiro and Robillard, 1950; Vallée et al, 1982). More caudal, paired tracheal arteries give off 2- to 4-cm-long tributaries for the esophagus (Liebermann-Meffert and Siewert, 1992; Liebermann-Meffert et al, 1987), which travel laterally along the esophagus and trachea before they "are joined by anastomotic twigs" (Miura and Grillo, 1966) in the anterior and posterior esophageal wall. Their equal distribution contrasts with Shapiro and Robillard's (1950) claim that a greater number of vessels supplies predominantly the right side of the esophagus. Esophageal branches originating from the superior thyroid artery, the thyroidea ima, the common carotid artery, and the subclavian artery may be present but are far less frequent (Calvet and Poulhes, 1948; Liebermann-Meffert and Siewert, 1992; Liebermann-Meffert et al, 1987; Miura and Grillo, 1966; Vallée et al, 1982).

Thoracic Esophagus. Down to the level of the tracheal bifurcation, the thoracic esophagus is supplied primarily by branches from the right and left inferior thyroid arteries. Further on, the majority of the supplying vessels are derived from an arterial bunch arising at the inflection of the aorta (Liebermann-Meffert et al, 1987; Shapiro and Robillard, 1950). More caudally, most often one singular artery arises from the anterior aspect of the aorta. Although this vessel clearly supplies the most distal part of the trachea and the stem bronchi, small branches also form the esophageal vascularization (Fig. 2–9; see Fig. 2–8). In this region, the vessels are straight and short, connecting tightly the aorta, the trachea, and the esophagus (Liebermann-Meffert et al, 1987). At a variable location, one other unpaired artery may arise from the anterior aortic aspect. This vessel, however, courses obliquely down from its origin (see Fig. 2–9) to divide, still within the mediastinum, into an ascending and a descending branch (Demel, 1924; Liebermann-Meffert and Siewert, 1992; Liebermann-Meffert et al, 1987).

Abdominal Esophagus. The distal esophagus and gastric cardia are nourished by up to 11 small arteries that

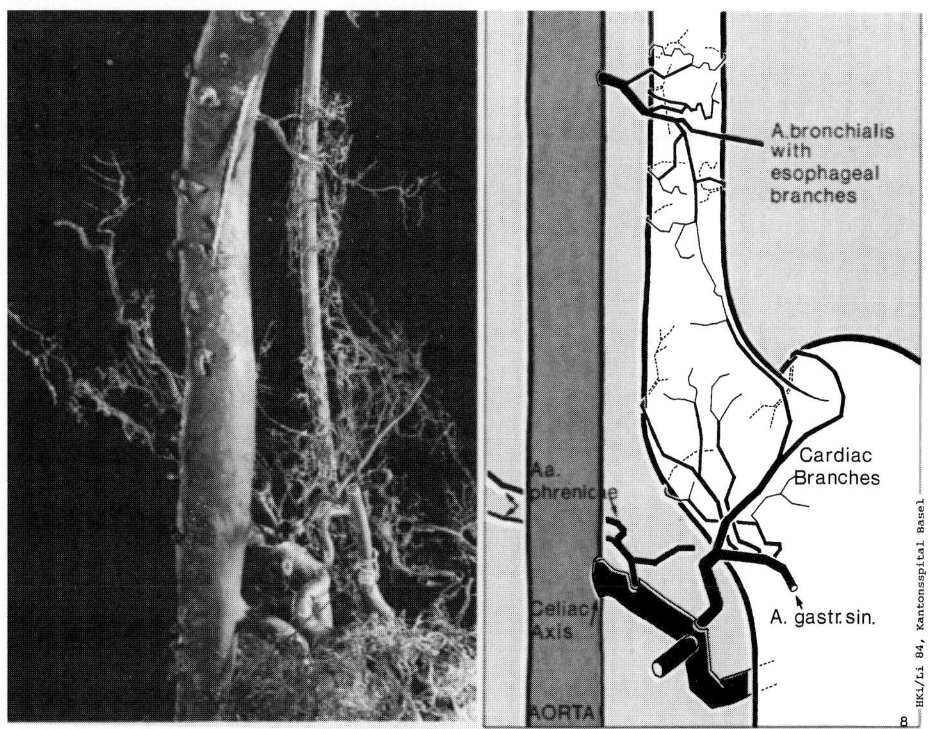

FIGURE 2–8 ■ Arterial cast of thoracic area viewed from the anterior aspect with the bronchial artery deriving from the aorta and giving off smaller branches to form the esophageal network. (Human, Beracryl injection.)

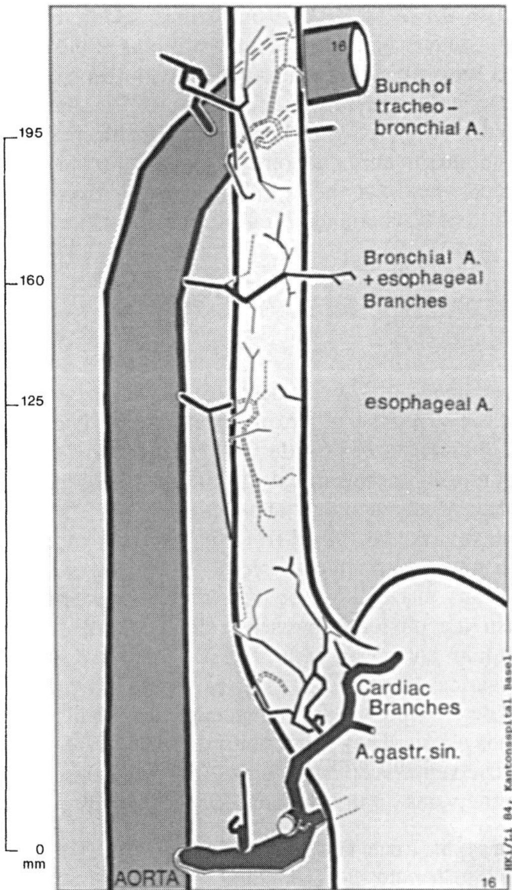

FIGURE 2–9 ■ Most common vascular pattern of blood supply to the esophagus.

originate at intervals from the left gastric artery (Demel, 1924; Liebermann-Meffert and Siewert, 1992; Liebermann-Meffert et al, 1987). These vessels travel straight upward alongside the anterior aspect of the cardia (see Fig. 2–9), following the wall in the longitudinal esophageal axis through the diaphragm to subdivide into periesophageal tributaries before they dip into the muscular layers. The posterior wall of the terminal esophagus receives several large vessels derived from the splenic artery and/or from vessels of the dorsal fundus, but previous claims that nutritional vessels arise from phrenic arteries have not been substantiated (Liebermann-Meffert et al, 1987).

With respect to esophageal vascularization as a whole, the esophagus is an organ of shared vasculature with poor "proper" extrinsic support. In fact, apart from the few "vasa propria" that derive from the aorta directly, the esophagus receives its blood via vessels feeding mainly other organs, such as the thyroid gland, trachea, and stomach. Even though the vessels become minute in the periesophageal tissue, claims of a poor or missing vascularization in the wall of the midesophagus (see in Liebermann-Meffert and Siewert, 1992; Liebermann-Meffert et al, 1987) could not be substantiated because connections within and throughout the submucosa and mucosa form a complete and dense network of fine vessels (Fig. 2–10). At no place is the wall of the esophagus avascular.

Points of Surgical Interest

The mobilized esophagus retains an excellent blood supply over a long distance. It is seldom responsible for a failed anastomosis (Williams and Payne, 1982). This supply is evidently derived from the complete network of vessels within the wall.

Blunt pull-through esophagectomy without thoracotomy for esophageal cancer is relatively safe and involves

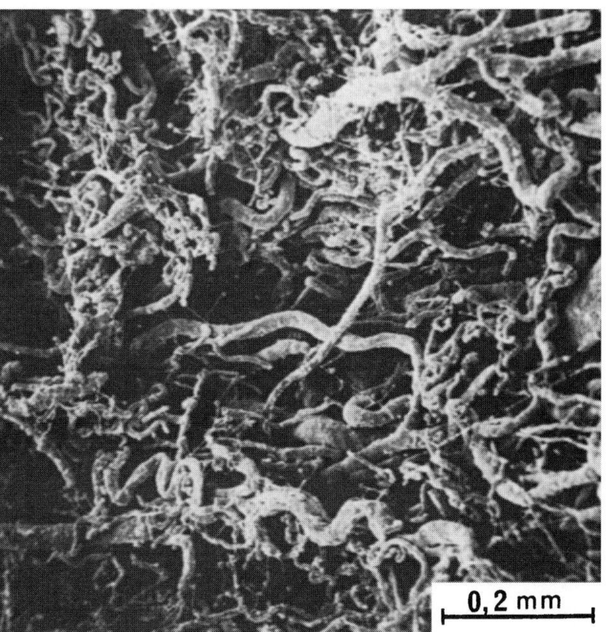

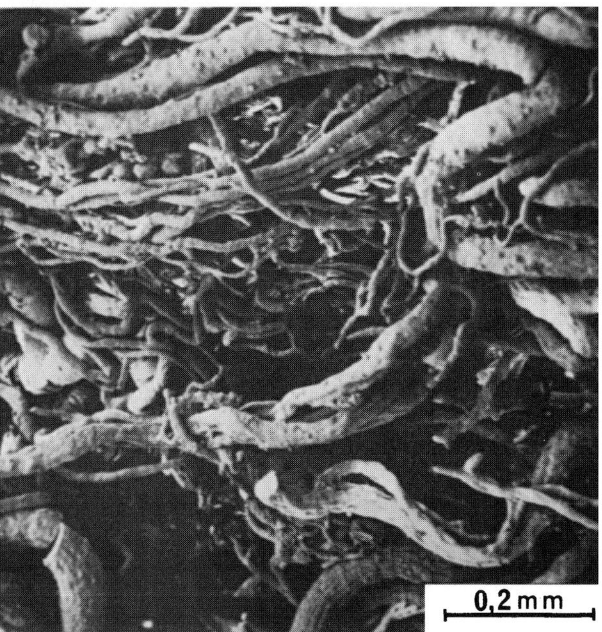

FIGURE 2–10 ■ Intrinsic microvascular esophagus supply seen in a scanning electron micrograph. The arteries and veins are small and form a polygonal network. (Courtesy of Düggelin, M.D., Basel.)

moderate blood loss (Akiyama, 1980; Orringer and Orringer, 1983). When hemorrhage has occurred after stripping of the esophagus, it was from the site of tumor adhesions rather than from the periesophageal vessels (Lam et al, 1982). The ordinarily limited bleeding may occur because the major arteries divide into minute branches at some distance from the esophageal wall, and, when torn, the vessels may benefit from contractile hemostasis (Liebermann-Meffert et al, 1987).

Veins

Anatomy

Intraesophageal. The intraesophageal (intrinsic) veins include the subepithelial plexus, located in the lamina propria of the tunica mucosa (Butler, 1951). The vessels are mainly longitudinally arranged and extend the whole length of the esophageal submucosa (Vianna et al, 1987). The subepithelial plexus receives blood from the adjacent capillaries and drains into the submucous plexus. At the lower end of the esophagus, anastomoses between the systemic and the portal system are obviously present; the thin-walled superficial veins may enlarge in case of portal venous obstruction to form varices.

Vianna and colleagues (1987) described a particular venous arrangement in the lower third of the esophagus and cardia that consists of perforating veins that derive from the small communicating veins of the submucous plexus. They pierce the muscular wall of the esophagus. The veins receive tributaries from the muscle coats and form the veins on the surface of the esophagus.

Extraesophageal. The extraesophageal (extrinsic) veins drain into locally corresponding large vessels, such as the inferior thyroid, which empties into the brachiocephalic veins, the azygos and hemiazygos, the left gastric vein, and the splenic vein.

Points of Surgical Interest

Because of its vicinity to the root of the lung and its lymph nodes, the azygos vein (see Fig. 2–2*c–f*) is one of the initial structures to become involved by the extramural spread of tumors of the midesophagus. In this situation, the azygos vein can be easily damaged during esophageal resection. In blunt pull-through dissection, this vein therefore represents a high risk factor by causing fatal bleeding if the tumor is adherent.

Collateral circulation may exist between the azygos vein and the hemiazygos vein (Wookey, 1940). The hemiazygos vein, if not ligated, can be a source of severe hemorrhage with resection of the esophagus through a right thoracotomy (DeMeester and Levin, 1986).

Lymphatic Pathways

Anatomy

Lymphatic drainage comprises two systems: lymph channels and lymph nodes. The details of these systems, in particular the initial pathways, have received great attention because of the lymphatic spread of malignant tumors.

Lymph capillaries commence in tissue spaces (Fig. 2–11) as a network of endothelial channels or as blind endothelial sacculations (see Bollinger et al, 1985; Partsch, 1988; Zweifach and Prather, 1975). These structures take up fluid, colloid material from the tissue, cell debris, microorganisms, and eventually tumor cells (Casley-Smith in Partsch, 1988; Endrich et al in Liebermann-Meffert and White, 1983). The contents are emptied into collecting lymph channels. Paired semilunar valves within the channels determine the direction of flow. They join to form small trunks that convey the fluid and the other absorbed material through the interpositioned lymph nodes. In its passage through the node, noxious material may be filtered off. Obviously, this system of channels easily provides pathways for tumor spread.

Lymph Vessels of the Esophagus. Because of the considerable technical difficulties of identifying the slender, normally collapsed structures (Lehnert et al, 1985; Mayr and Liebermann-Meffert, 1996), the anatomic knowledge of the esophageal lymphatic system in healthy individuals is still poor and, of course, refers only to sparse studies. Some investigators (Idanov, 1959; Rouvière, 1932; Sakata, 1903) have emphasized the existence of a rich lymphatic

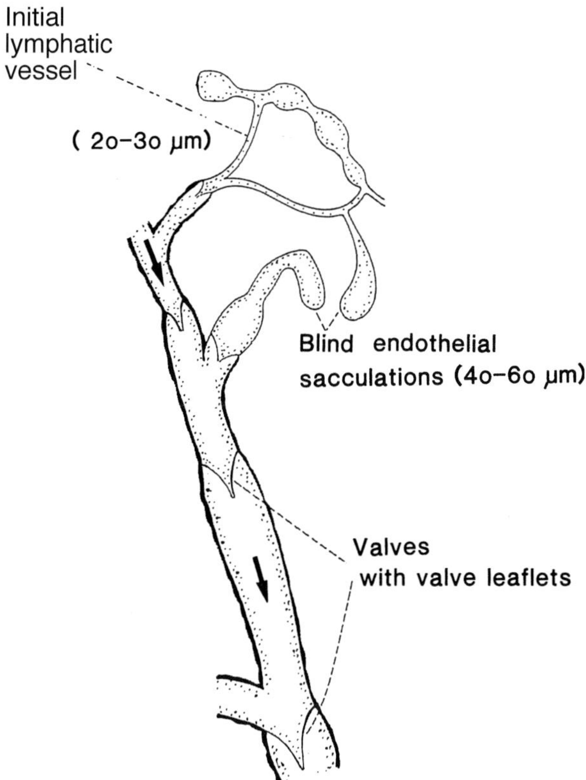

FIGURE 2–11 ■ Initial lymphatic network, which is reconstructed from mesentery preparations. Most probably, this pattern equals that of the esophagus. (Modified from Zweifach BW, Prather JW: Manipulation of pressure in terminal lymphatics in the mesentery. Am J Physiol 228:1326, 1975.)

network in the lamina mucosa and tela submucosa of the esophagus. However, their claims have never been substantiated by convincing or reproducible documentation.

Tiny precapillary spaces may exist in all the levels of the esophageal lamina mucosa, similar to descriptions of interstitial tissues (Casley-Smith in Partsch, 1988), but other authors have stressed the almost complete absence of true lymph capillaries in the upper and middle levels of the lamina mucosa of the human stomach (Lehnert et al, 1985) and esophagus (Mayr and Liebermann-Meffert, 1996). Their transmission electron microscopic studies, however, have confirmed anastomotic lymph capillaries in the lower mucosal levels as well as small vessels in the tela submucosa. Similar to the arrangement suggested by Sakata early in 1903, the submucosal lymphatics of the esophagus appeared to form long channels that parallel the organ axis, giving off occasional branches to the collecting subadventitial and surface trunks.

The principal lymphatic vessel of the body is the thoracic duct, which crosses the chest in front of the spine. The flimsy duct is normally collapsed and then appears, because of numerous strong valves, like a string of beads at preparation. The duct displays width values of 0.5 to 2.0 mm (mean, 1.3) at the distal third, 1.0 to 3.0 mm (mean, 1.7) at the middle, and 1.0 to 4.0 mm (mean, 2.3) at the proximal third (threshold, 4.0 mm) as shown in 500 lymphograms of healthy individuals (Wirth and Frommhold, 1970).

According to the classic anatomic concept, the thoracic duct begins with the cisterna chyli at level L1-2, emerges through the aortic hiatus of the diaphragm, and travels in more than half of cases as a single trunk cranially with the aorta on its left and the azygos vein on its right (Idanov, 1959; Wirth and Frommhold, 1970). The duct turns at the level of T5-6 behind the left mainstem bronchus toward the left. Then it ascends lateroposteriorly to the trachea and esophagus to end at the angle between the left subclavian and jugular veins by draining the lymph into the bloodstream. Anatomic variations are manifold (Wirth and Frommhold, 1970). The close local relationship of the flimsy duct to the esophagus explains its occasional damage during esophageal resection and chylothorax.

Lymph Nodes of the Esophagus. In noncancer autopsy specimens, we found most of the lymph nodes of the thoracic mediastinum piled up around the tracheal bifurcation (Fig. 2–12). These were rather large, dark nodes. Anatomically, it was impossible to determine whether they drain the esophagus or the lungs or whether they transport proximally or distally. There is an accumulation of small nodes in the neck and cardia region, but few lymph nodes are normally present in the lateral and ventral mediastinum of the upper third and in the dorsal mediastinum in the lower third of the thorax. We could not identify the classic chain of lymph nodes along and around the esophagus, as described in textbooks and seen in Netter's (1971) illustration at routine autopsy. This statement is in accordance with that of Wirth and Frommhold (1970), who identified mediastinal lymph nodes in only 5% of 500 normal lymphograms. We found, however, a greater number of lymph nodes of microscopic dimensions cranial to the tracheal bifurcation within the tracheoesophageal groove. With tumor involvement, the classic lymph node arrangement can be seen (Matsubara, 1988).

Points of Surgical Interest

Sakata's (1903) concept that the lymphatics form long channels in the submucosa in which the lymph flows more easily cranially or caudally, respectively, than through the few channels that pierce the muscular coat and that only lymph flows through the subadventitial lymphatics and small trunks into the mediastinal lymph nodes supports the clinical observation that the initial submucosal spread follows the longitudinal axis of the organ (Lehnert et al, 1985). Consequently, primary esophageal tumors may extend over a long distance within the esophageal wall before obstructing the lumen.

The absence of lymphatics from the superficial mucosa and the widely anastomosing plexus within the submucosa may explain why the intramural spread of cancer occurs predominantly in the submucosa; small mucosal malignant lesions may thus be accompanied by extensive tumor spread underneath an intact esophageal mucosa. Free tumor cells may follow the lymphatic channels over a considerably long distance before passing through the muscular coat into regional lymph nodes. This fact may be consistent with the high postoperative recurrence rate at the resection line, including satellite tumors and metastasis in the submucosa far distant from the primary tumor. This means that a tumor-free margin at the resection line in esophagus surgery does not necessarily guarantee radical tumor removal.

Clinical Implications

From the anatomic studies and the clinical observations, it may be deduced (Akiyama, 1980; Lam et al, 1982; Lehnert et al, 1985; Liebermann-Meffert and Duranceau, 1996; Matsubara, 1988) that lymph from areas above the tracheal bifurcation drains mostly cranially toward the thoracic duct, whereas lymph from below the carina flows mainly toward the lower mediastinal, left gastric, and celiac lymph nodes. Flow in the area of the tracheal bifurcation normally seems to be bidirectional (see Fig. 2–12) owing to the embryologic development of the two mesenchymal sources (Hinrichsen, 1990a–1990c; Liebermann-Meffert and Duranceau, 1996). Flow may change under pathologic conditions (tumor invasion). When the lymph vessels become blocked and markedly dilated, either the valves may become incompetent and the flow reversed (Zschiesche, 1963) or a collateral lymphatic circulation may develop (Bruna, 1974); retrograde spread in some malignant tumors may thus be explained. Unfortunately, this possibility also limits the value of establishing normal flow pathways.

Innervation

Anatomy

Vegetative Nervous System. The vegetative nervous system regulates the function of the esophagus, where it

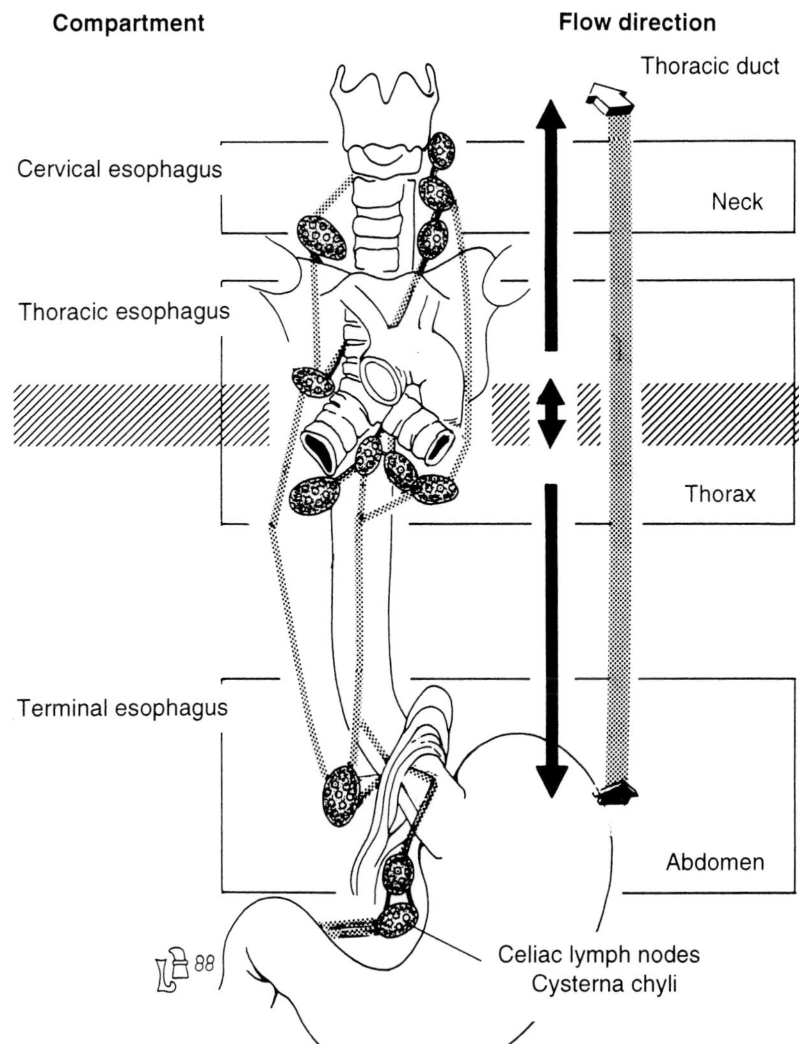

FIGURE 2–12 ■ Concept of lymphatic pathways. Owing to the embryonic development of the lymphatic pathways from two sources, the branchiogenic and the body mesenchyme lymph drains toward two different directions. It presents a bidirectional flow at the tracheal bifurcation, which is the area of embryologic tissue transition. This feature is consistent with clinical observations. The knowledge of lymph flow and the corresponding lymph node distribution is essential in understanding potential spread of malignancy.

controls striated and smooth muscle, glands, and blood vessels. It comprises the peripheral cerebrospinal and the autonomic nerves. These nerves have their roots in central tracts. The innervation has parasympathetic and sympathetic components, which exert antagonistic influences on the esophagus (Cunningham and Sawchenko, 1990; Diamant, 1989).

Parasympathetic Nervous System. The parasympathetic nerve supply comes from the vagus nerves (Fig. 2–13). The esophageal branches of the vagus are motor to the muscular coats and secretomotor to the glands.

The vagus is the paired 10th cranial nerve. Its motor fibers arise in the dorsal vagal nucleus, and sensory fibers derive from the superior and inferior ganglion (ganglion nodosum). The striped fibers that supply the upper part of the esophagus and pharyngoesophageal musculature arise in the nucleus ambiguus (Cunningham and Sawchenko, 1990). Unlike those of smooth muscle, which receive motor input via preganglionic autonomic fibers and synapse on neurons of the myenteric ganglia, the nerve endings of the striped muscle make direct synaptic contacts through motor endplates (Goyal and Cobb, 1981).

Routes of the Vagus Nerves. From their origin in the medulla, the vagus nerves descend and pass through the corresponding jugular foramen. By giving off branches to the pharynx, larynx, and trachea (Fig. 2–14; see Fig. 2–13), these fibers form the cervical plexus that also supplies the proximal esophagus (Goyal and Cobb, 1981).

The bilateral superior laryngeal nerve (SLN) originates from the vagal trunks of the respective side, that is, the ganglion nodosum (see Fig. 2–13). Both nerves descend alongside the carotid arteries before dividing into branches that enter the pharynx in order to supply the intrinsic muscles of the pharynx, hypopharynx, and larynx (Liebermann-Meffert et al, 1999).

Of the inferior (recurrent) laryngeal nerves (RLNs), the right one arises from the vagus nerve in front of the subclavian artery and turns toward posterior around the artery (see Fig. 2–14) to ascend obliquely to the right lateral aspect of the trachea behind the common carotid artery. The right RLN originates from the vagus nerve in front of the aortic arch and surrounds the aorta toward posterior. Both RLNs approach the esophagus during their lateral ascent and give off the same number of nerve branches to both esophagus and trachea (see Figs. 2–13

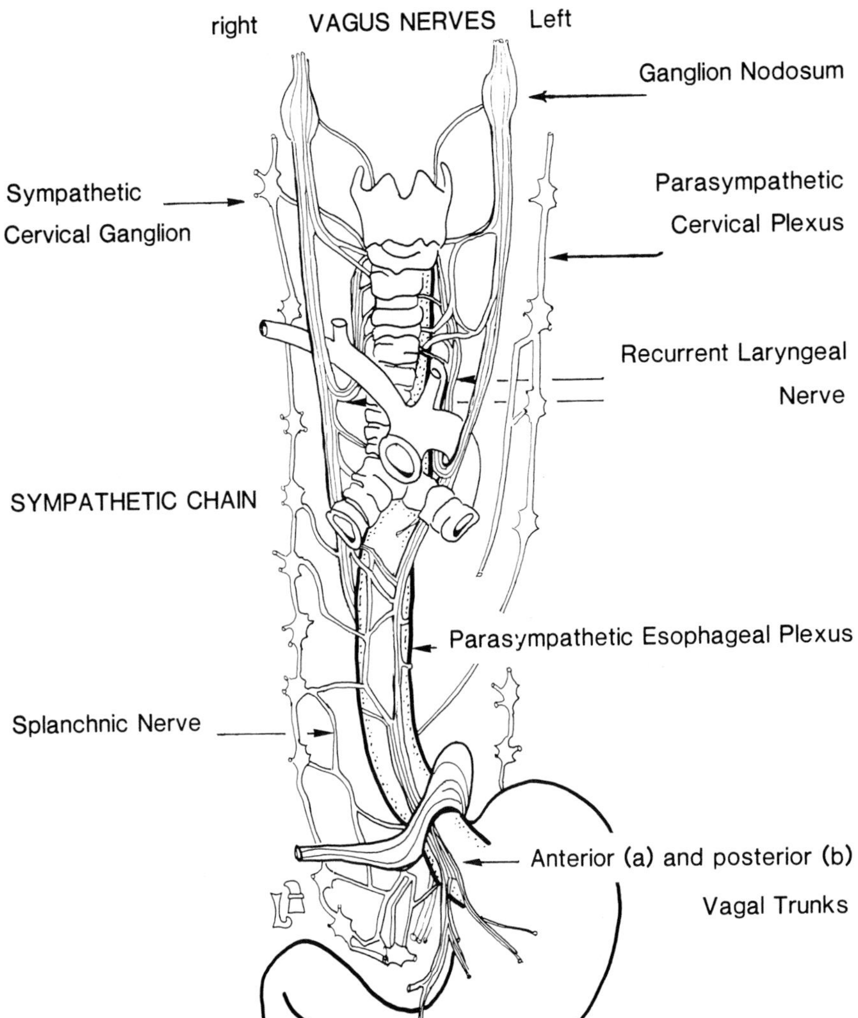

FIGURE 2–13 ■ Topographic relationships between the esophagus and its innervation (schematic drawing shows the situation from the anterior aspect. The dimensions are out of scale.)

and 2–14). Reaching the pharyngoesophageal junction (see Figs. 2–13 and 2–14), both RLNs have obtained an intimate proximity to the wall of the esophagus and trachea. This proximity is particularly pronounced on the left side when the proximal RLNs become positioned below the medial plane of the thyroid gland, which occurs before entering the larynx lateral and just below the cricopharyngeal muscle band. This terminal branch of the RLNs is most often 1.0 to 1.5 mm thick and divides into several branches in order to innervate all the laryngeal muscles, including the vocal and epiglottic muscles (Liebermann-Meffert et al, 1999).

At the level of the tracheal bifurcation, the vagal trunks pass posterior to the roots of the lung and divide into multiple small branches to form pulmonary and esophageal plexuses. Caudal to the tracheal bifurcation, the esophageal vagal trunks break up into a network of fascicles (see Fig. 2–13). The left vagus builds up mainly the anterior and the right vagus the posterior esophageal plexus. At a variable distance from the cardia, the fibers of these plexus reorganize into two thick trunks, which travel down on the anterior and posterior esophageal wall (see Fig. 2–13). Both vagal trunks may now contain fibers from the upper contralateral side. Together with the esophagus, the vagi pass through the diaphragmatic hiatus, where they are barely distinguishable under the phrenoesophageal membrane.

The posterior vagus nerve is often divided into smaller branches that lie 2 to 4 cm distant from the tube and to its right. The anterior vagus nerve runs left side close to the wall toward the anterior gastric wall (Jackson, 1949; Liebermann-Meffert et al, 1997a).

Sympathetic Nervous System. The sympathetic nerve supply comes from the cervical and the thoracic sympathetic chain (see Fig. 2–13). The sympathetic pathways are concerned with the movement of the esophageal tract, contraction of the sphincters, relaxation of the muscular wall, increase in glandular and peristaltic activity, and vasoconstriction (Christensen, 1978).

Routes of the Sympathetic Nerves. The sympathetic trunks are two ganglionated nerve cords that extend from the base of the skull down to the sacrum. They are located lateral to the spine (see Fig. 2–13) and possess 11 to 12 thoracic paravertebral ganglia on each side. The sympathetic innervation of the proximal esophagus is derived from the cervical and upper thoracic ganglia

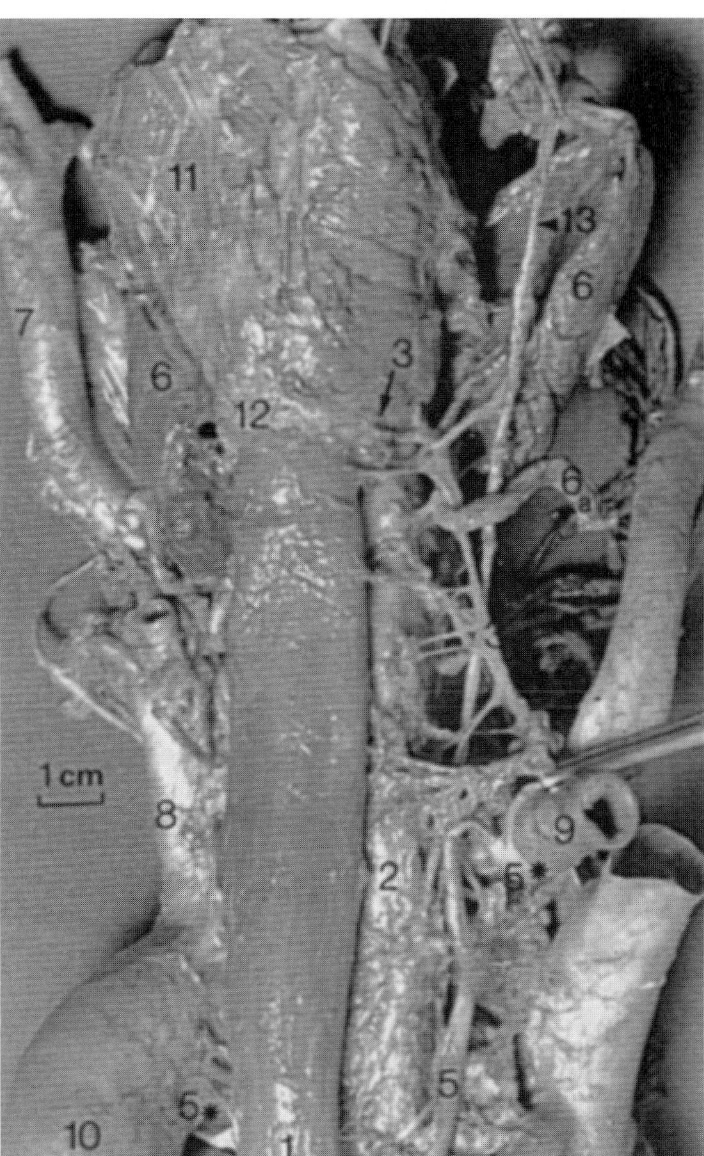

FIGURE 2–14 ■ Posterior aspect of the muscular wall of the esophagus (1) and pharynx (11). The right laryngeal nerve (3), largely removed from its peritracheal tissue bed, is pulled down laterally by tweezers behind its turning point (5*) around the subclavian artery (9). This shows that the ramifications of the recurrent laryngeal nerve enter the lateral wall of the esophagus (1) and trachea (2) by alternating, which was typical. The left thyroid gland (6) is in natural position; the right one (6) is displaced toward posterior. Underneath the lower lobe, the thyroid artery and its vessels (6a) encircle the recurrent laryngeal nerves. The turning point of the left recurrent laryngeal nerve (5*) is seen under the aortic arch (10). Esophagus (1), common carotid artery (7), brachiocephalic trunk (8). Note the venous network on top of the pharyngeal muscle (11), the lower esophageal sphincter (12), and the phrenic nerve (13). (From Liebermann-Meffert D, et al: Recurrent and superior laryngeal nerves: A new look with implications for the esophageal surgeon. Ann Thorac Surg 67: 212, 1999.)

(Cunningham and Sawchenko, 1990). Besides the direct approach to the organ, the fibers form a profuse, delicate network between and around the esophagus (Cunningham and Sawchenko, 1990).

Intramural Innervation. Branches from the periesophageal, parasympathetic, and sympathetic plexus enter the wall of the esophagus together with the blood vessels. They form the intrinsic innervation, which is composed of fine nerve fibers and numerous groups of ganglia. The ganglia lie either between the longitudinal and the circular layers of the tunica muscularis, in which case they are called myenteric or Auerbach's plexus, or in the tela submucosa, in which case they are called submucous or Meissner plexus. The one regulates the contraction of the muscle coats; the other, the peristalsis of the muscularis mucosae and the secretion. All plexus are interconnected by a meshwork of fibers (Kumar and Phillips, 1989).

The number of ganglia is fairly uniform within the esophageal wall (DeSouza et al, 1988; Eckardt and LeCompte, 1978). Near the junctional zone, however, the nerve fascicles become thicker and ganglia accumulate (DeSouza et al, 1988; Kumar and Phillips, 1989).

Points of Clinical Interest

As far as motility disorders are concerned, the frequency of abnormal esophageal contractions in older people may result from age-dependent reduction of ganglion cells within the esophageal wall (Eckardt and LeCompte, 1978), and the partial denervation found may cause increased sensibility of the smooth muscle. Neuropathy in some of the systemic diseases is also associated with loss of myenteric ganglia and uncoordinated esophageal motility (Adams et al, 1976; Heatley et al, 1980; Henderson et al, 1974). Cunningham and Sawchenko (1990) have shown the relationship between vagal lesions and both delayed esophageal emptying and abnormal peristalsis in reflux disease and concluded that vagal nerve dysfunction plays an important role in initiating gastroesophageal reflux.

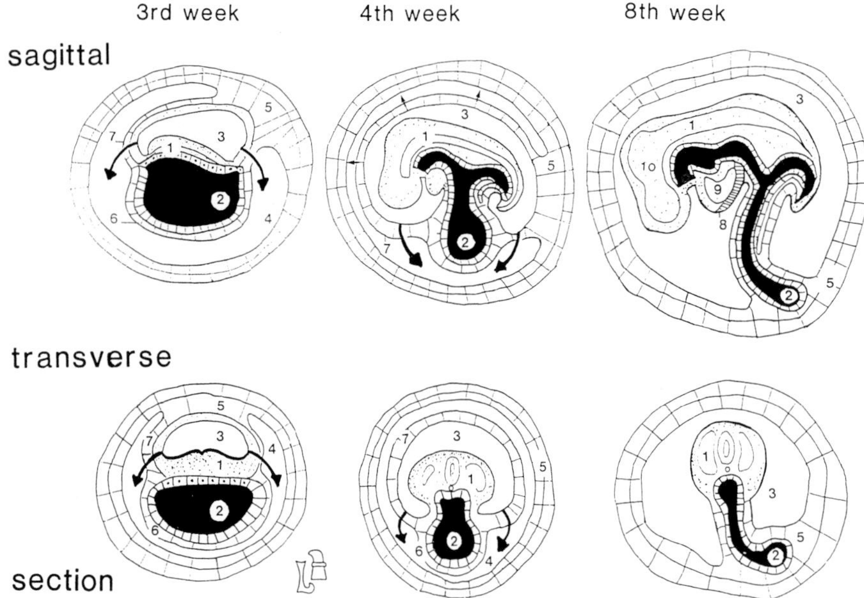

FIGURE 2–15 ■ Formation of the primitive intestinal tube from the regressing yolk sac cavity (2) due to folding of the embryo (1) at the third, fourth, and eighth weeks of gestation. The portion of the yolk sac that has been included in the embryo forms the foregut, midgut, and hindgut. The amniotic cavity (3), extraembryonic coelom (4), extraembryonic mesenchyme and cytotrophoblast (5), somatopleure (6), splanchnopleure (7), septum transversum (8), heart (9), and head and neck area (branchial organs) (10) are shown.

During esophageal resection and goiter operations, the RLNs are at high risk. Injuries involving the SLN and RLNs cause clinical pictures of a variety of transient or even lasting motor and sensory disorders of the pharyngolaryngoesophageal junction area (e.g., hoarseness related to vocal cord palsy and respiration and swallowing failure connected with problems of aspiration and dysphagia).

HUMAN EMBRYOLOGY

The embryo is a bilaminar disk of *ectoderm* and endoderm until the 14th day. The *endoderm*, recognizable at the eighth day of embryonic life, forms the lining of the yolk sac (Fig. 2–15). The third embryonic layer, the *mesoderm*, appears at the 15th day between the two initial layers. It provides the material for the mesenchyme, which differentiates into connective tissues, angioblasts, smooth muscle coats of the gut, and serous coverings. The mesoderm thickens, and by the 21st day of gestation it forms longitudinal masses, the paraxial mesoderm. Until the 31st embryonic day, this material segments progressively from cranial to caudal into cubes of tissue, the somites (Figs. 2–16 and 2–17).

Because of the separation of the endoderm and the ectoderm by the interposition of the intraembryonic mesoderm, the endoderm undergoes extensive changes in order to form the embryonic gut (see Fig. 2–17). Head, tail, and lateral body folds of the embryo compress the dorsal part of the yolk sac, which becomes incorporated as a rim during the fourth week (see Fig. 2–16). Successive growth processes and formation of a "body cylinder" until about the 28th day divide the yolk sac into the intraembryonic part, which represents the origin of the digestive tube (see Fig. 2–17) and its accessory glands, and the extraembryonic part, which regresses and disappears around the 12th week. At this point, the early digestive system divides into foregut, midgut, and hindgut (see Fig. 2–16*B*). The upper endodermal tube is separated from the stomodeal cavity by the buccopharyngeal membrane up to a stage of 4-mm crown-rump (CR) length (26th day).

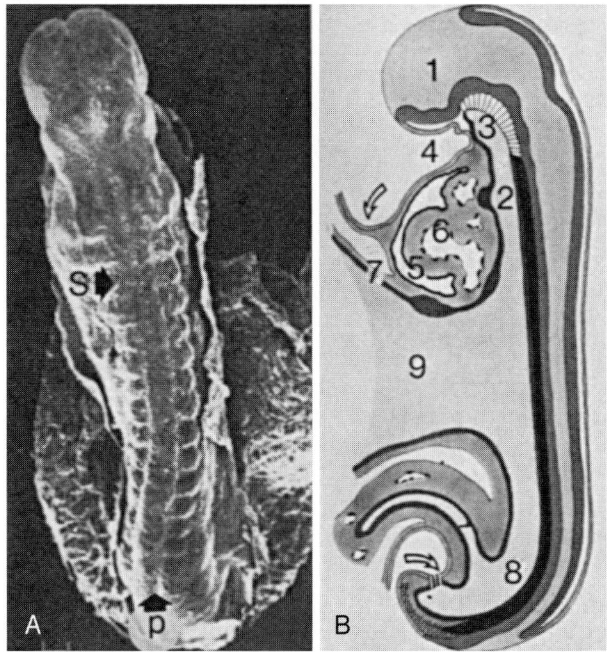

FIGURE 2–16 ■ Formation of the intestinal tube: human embryo, 3 mm long, about 26 days old. *A,* Thirteen paired somites (S) are seen in this scanning electron micrograph. *B,* Schematic counterpart in the sagittal section. Somites are developing from the mesenchymal plate (p). Brain (1), foregut (2), buccopharyngeal membrane (3), stomodeum (4), pericardial coelom (5), heart (6), septum transversum (7), hindgut (8), yolk sac cavity (9) are depicted. Bar is 100 μm. (*A,* From Jirásek JE: Atlas of Human Prenatal Morphogenesis. Nijhoff, Boston, 1982. *B,* From Hinrichsen KV: Human Embryologie. Heidelberg, Springer-Verlag, 1990.)

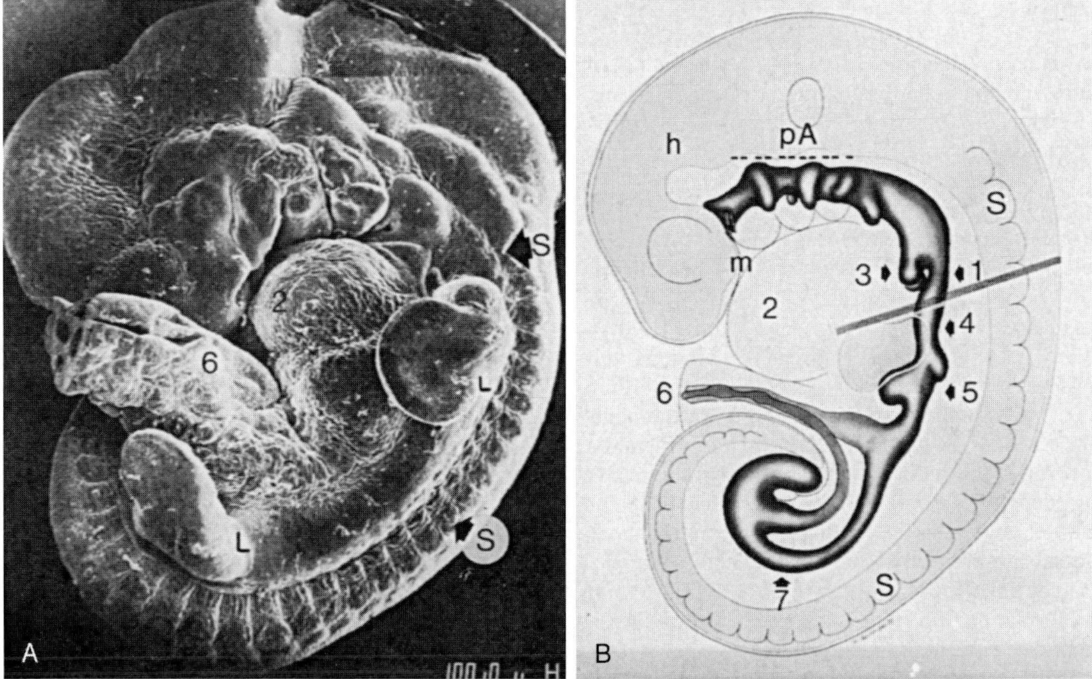

FIGURE 2–17 ■ Progress of intestinal development. *A*, Scanning electron micrograph of human embryo, 10 mm long. 40 days old; completed somite stage (S), primordium of limbs (L), and completed pharyngeal arches (PA). *B*, Schematic illustration (embryo of same age) of the foregut (1), primordium of the heart (2), lung buds (3), area of the future stomach (4), pancreatic buds (5), umbilical cord (6), hindgut (7). Stage of greatest embryologic flexion. The line divides roughly the tissues deriving from the branchiogenic and body mesenchyme. (*A*, From Jirásek JE: Atlas of Human Prenatal Morphogenesis. Boston, Nijhoff, 1983. *B*, Modified from Hinrichsen KV: Human Embryologie. Heidelberg, Springer-Verlag, 1990.)

Foregut

Initially, the foregut is a uniform tube (see Figs. 2–15 and 2–16*B*) that gives rise to the pharynx and its derivatives, trachea and lungs; to the esophagus; and to the stomach and duodenum down to the choledochal duct, liver, biliary system, and pancreas (Hinrichsen, 1990a–1990c; Liebermann-Meffert and Durauceau, 1996; Smith, 1957).

The esophagus, the middle segment of the foregut, is initially very short; it extends from the tracheal groove to the site where the foregut widens to become the stomach (Fig. 2–18). Increasing growth of the tissues of the esophagus, chiefly of its caudal portion, establishes the definite geographic relationships with the surrounding structures by the end of the seventh week (18 to 22 mm in CR length).

The future stomach, which is the distal segment of the foregut, appears as a fusiform dilatation dorsal and caudal to the septum transversum shortly before the tracheal diverticulum develops (Liebermann-Meffert and Duranceau, 1996). The stomach is held in place from this early stage on by the celiac and pancreatic vessel stalks attaching cardia and pylorus to the posterior body wall (Liebermann-Meffert, 1969). Positional changes (see Fig. 2–18) are caused by the asymmetric growth (i.e., mitotic activity) of the stomach, and no evidence has been presented of either esophageal or gastric mechanical rotation (Dankmeijer and Miete, 1961; Hamilton et al, 1978; Kanagasuntheram, 1957; Liebermann-Meffert, 1969; Liebermann-Meffert and White, 1983).

With the extensive growth of the gastric fundus, the esophagogastric junction, which is initially ill defined (see Fig. 2–18), becomes clearly delineated (Duranceau and Liebermann-Meffert, 1991; Liebermann-Meffert, 1966, 1969; Mueller-Botha, 1959). Individual variations in the height of the fundus and the acuteness of the cardiac angle persist during the fetal period.

Formation of the Esophagus

Tunica Muscularis. Morphologically, the mesenchymal cells that give rise to the striated and smooth musculature are identical before the myoblasts differentiate into one of the types. They appear simultaneously in the still undifferentiated mesenchyme on the outer aspect of the esophageal tube in the form of a ring-shaped condensation of elongated nuclei in an embryo 8 to 10 mm in CR length (Fig. 2–19A). They constitute the circular muscle layer of the lamina muscularis of the esophagus long before the musculature appears in the gastric wall.

Tunica Mucosa and Esophageal Lumen. The formation of the primitive gut is indicated by the appearance of the endodermal layer in the blastocyst. Differentiation of the mucosa from the endoderm has been identified in the 2.5-mm CR embryo at about the third week of gestation (Johns, 1952). Subsequently, two or three layers of pseudostratified columnar epithelium line the foregut (see Fig. 2–19*A*, *B*).

During this period, the stratified columnar epithelium

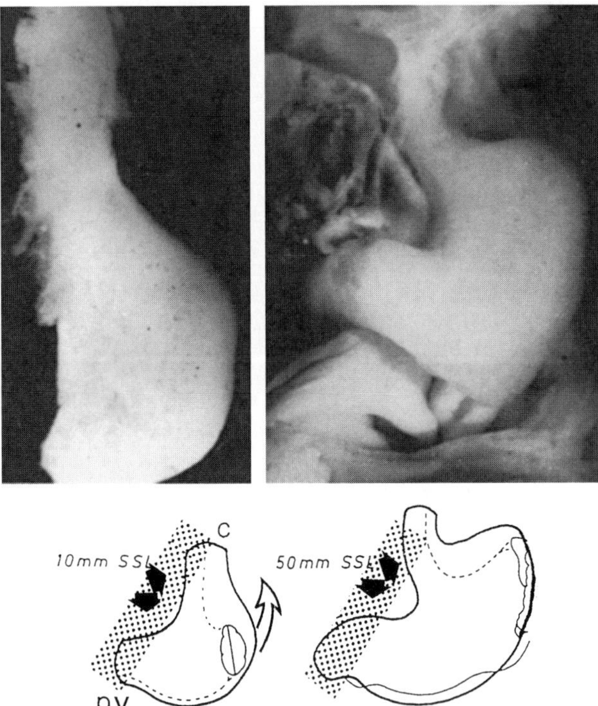

FIGURE 2–18 ■ Macroscopic aspect of the human stomach at 14-mm and 22-mm crown-rump length. The greater curvature undergoes an extensive growth, which will also form the gastric fundus, the cardiac angulation, and the esophagogastric junction. Both cardia (c) and pylorus (py) are tied *(arrows)* by the stalk of the celiac and superior mesenteric vessels. Therefore, growth processes occur mostly at the free margin of the stomach, which is the greater curvature. (From Liebermann-Meffert D: Form und Lageentwicklung des menschlichen Magens und seiner Mesenterien. Acta Anat 72:376, 1969.)

is about four cell layers deep. In the 28-mm CR embryo, large dark cells appear in the basal epithelial cell layer of the middle third of the esophagus. They project toward the lumen to become ciliated columnar cells (Fig. 2–20*A*) while progressing in a cranial and caudal direction. Such ciliated cells develop within the stratified epithelium even in the explanted esophagus from early human fetuses when maintained in organ culture (Menard and Arsenault, 1987).

Finally, in the 60-mm CR embryo, ciliated cells line the entire mucosa of the esophagus except for the upper and lower ends, where the epithelium is made up of a single layer of large columnar cells (Enterline and Thompson, 1984; Johnson, 1910; Mueller-Botha, 1959; Schaller, 1978; Schridde, 1908). The area of the mucin-bearing columnar cells that are in continuity with the gastric mucosa is reduced in the 130-mm CR fetus, and the continuity with the gastric mucosa is lost at about the 140-mm CR stage. However, small discrete patches of columnar epithelium occasionally remain proximal to the esophagogastric junction and in the cervical esophagus until birth (Boerner-Patzelt, 1922; Enterline and Thompson, 1984) (see Fig. 2–20*A–D*).

The stratified squamous epithelium appears in the 90- to 130-mm CR fetus (see Fig. 2–20*B*). This epithelium also migrates from the middle third of the esophagus, spreading cranially and caudally until it has progressively and almost completely replaced the ciliated columnar epithelium in the 250-mm CR fetus (see Fig. 2–20*C*) (Boerner-Patzelt, 1922; Enterline and Thompson, 1984).

The first superficial acini-containing glands have been described in the 60-mm CR fetus. They are numerous in the 210-mm CR fetus and are located chiefly at levels of the cricoid cartilage and terminal esophagus (Enterline and Thompson, 1984; Johns, 1952; Mueller-Botha, 1959). During the last 3 months of gestation, downgrowth of surface epithelium generates submucosal glands (see Fig. 2–20*D*). The formation of the esophageal lumen is largely influenced by the developmental processes of the mucosa (Figs. 2–21 and 2–22; see Fig. 2–19*A–D*). Extensive cell proliferation and vacuolization at the 10- to 21-mm CR stages alter the initially round or elliptical lumen to a narrow and asymmetric bizarre one (Fig. 2–19*A–C*). The changes are most distinct in the upper half of the esophagus. Many, occasionally very large, vacuoles occur in such a manner as to imply solid lumen occlusion. Longitudinal and cross-serial histologic sections, however, show that the lumen remains open (see Figs. 2–19, 2–21, and 2–22) (Liebermann-Meffert and Duranceau, 1996).

Kreuter (1905) believed that esophageal atresia is the consequence if "recanalization" of the lumen does not occur by the formation of vacuoles. Even though none of the subsequent investigators reconfirmed Kreuter's claim, his ideas still appear in surgical and anatomic textbooks.

Since vacuolization of the esophageal mucosa takes place after the trachea and lungs are already fully developed (see in Liebermann-Meffert and Duranceau, 1996), it has also been suggested that atresia of the esophagus may be due to growth defects of the esophagus and the trachea in conjunction with overgrowth of epithelium bulging into the foregut (Smith, 1957). With the disappearance of the vacuoles, the esophageal lumen widens (see Fig. 2–19*D*) but retains the definite large longitudinal folds.

TISSUE ARCHITECTURE AND HISTOLOGY

Apart from the lack of a serosal coating, the construction of the esophagus parallels the basic plan of the tissue organization of the digestive tube. It consists of four layers:

- External fibrous layer
- Intermediate muscular layer
- Intermediate submucous layer
- Internal mucous layer

Tunica Adventitia. Composed of loose connective tissue, the adventitia covers the esophagus and connects it with neighboring structures. The periesophageal tissue contains small vessels, lymphatic channels, and nerve fibers.

Tunica Muscularis. The segment cranial to the esophagus, the laryngopharynx, is marginated posteriorly by the constrictor wall. It is a wide muscular sleeve suspended from the bony structures of the base of the skull, the hyoid bone, and thyroid and cricoid cartilages. The mus-

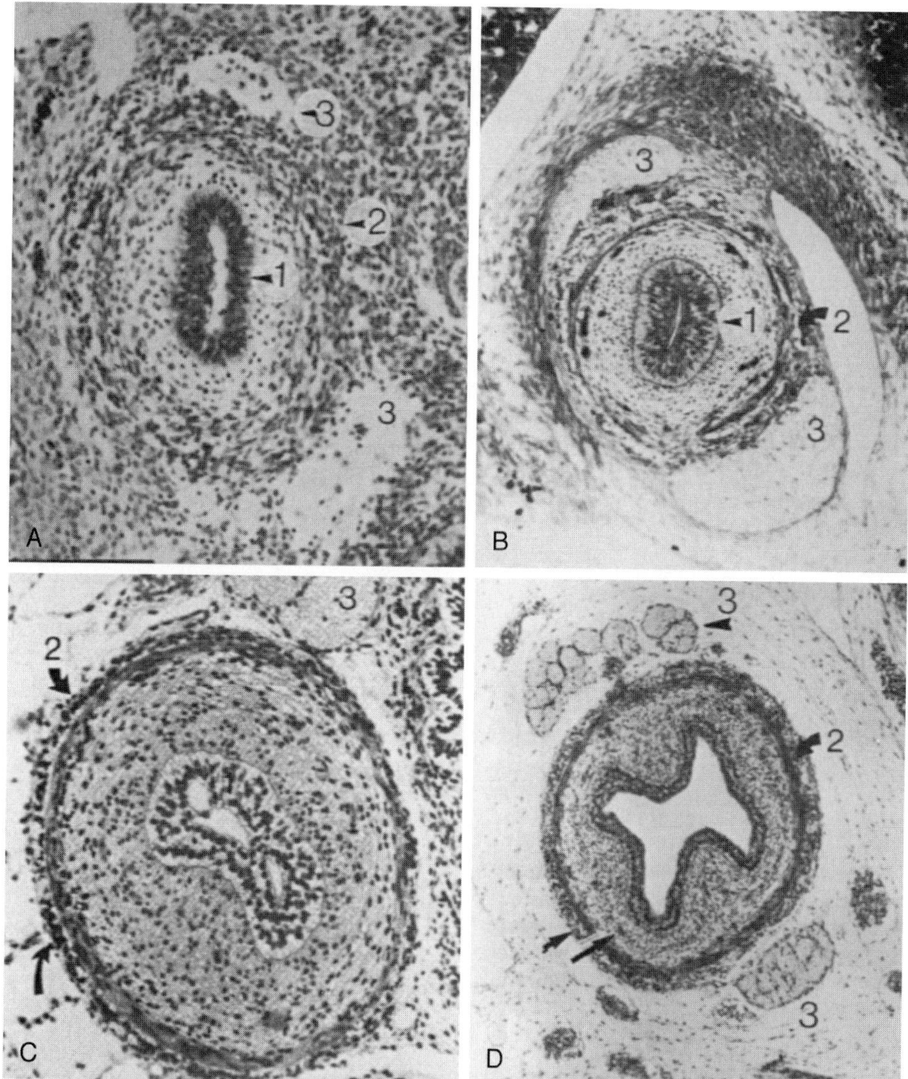

FIGURE 2–19 ■ Transverse section through the esophagus in embryos 8.5 *(A)*, 12.5 *(B)*, 20 *(C)*, and 40-mm *(D)* crown-rump (CR) length. The mucosal epithelium (1) is stratified columnar in the 8.5-mm CR embryo to become multilayered and vacuolized between 12.5-mm and 20-mm CR and columnar in the 40-mm CR stage. The tissue that surrounds the mucosal epithelium is predominantly undifferentiated mesenchyme in the 8.5-mm CR embryo with beginning differentiation of the inner muscle coat identified by the cell condensation (2) and contains pale areas of neural cells exterior to the tube (3). In the 12-mm and 20-mm CR stages, the inner muscular layer is further advanced; the outer longitudinal layer and muscularis mucosae *(arrows)*, however, can be identified only at 40-mm CR length. During this development the extrinsic innervation, in particular the vagus, has become of conspicuous size (3). The developmental changes of the luminal diameter and shape of the esophagus are seen. (*A*, *B*, and *D*, From the collection of Liebermann-Meffert; reprinted from Liebermann-Meffert D, Duranceau A: Anatomy and embryology. In Orringer MB, Zuidema GD [eds]: Shackelford's Surgery of the Alimentary Tract. The Esophagus, Vol I, 4th ed. Philadelphia, WB Saunders, 1996, p 33. *C*, From Enterline H, Thompson J: Pathology of the Esophagus: New York, Springer-Verlag, 1984.)

culature comprises the three constrictors; their muscle bundles spread obliquely upward posteriorly (Figs. 2–23 and 2–24), where they insert into the tela submucosa after crossing the muscle bundles of the opposite side (Liebermann-Meffert, 1995, 1997a, 1997b).

The most caudal of these muscles, the inferior constrictor muscle, consists of two parts: (1) the oblique thyropharyngeal muscle, which overlaps the upper pharyngeal constrictors, and (2) the transverse cricopharyngeal muscle. This arrangement leaves a triangular area (see Fig. 2–24) of sparse musculature (Killian's triangle) (Killian, 1908; Perrott, 1962). The cricopharyngeal muscle is suspended between the cricoid processes (see Fig. 2–24); it is 3 to 4 mm thick, surrounds the narrowest part of the pharynx, and extends for 1 to 2 cm caudally before blending with the circular muscle of the esophagus (see Figs. 2–23 and 2–24).

Two muscular layers support the lumen of the esophagus and provide for its propulsive function. The fibers of the external layer parallel the longitudinal axis of the esophagus; those of the inner layer follow a horizontal plane. The longitudinal layer originates bilaterally from the dorsal plane of the cricoid cartilage. Again, this creates an area of sparse musculature (Laimer's triangle) (Laimer, 1883) (see Fig. 2–24). Subsequently, the muscle bundles join and course straight down the entire esophagus before converging in a more oblique plane along the anterior and posterior gastric wall (Fig. 2–25*A*).

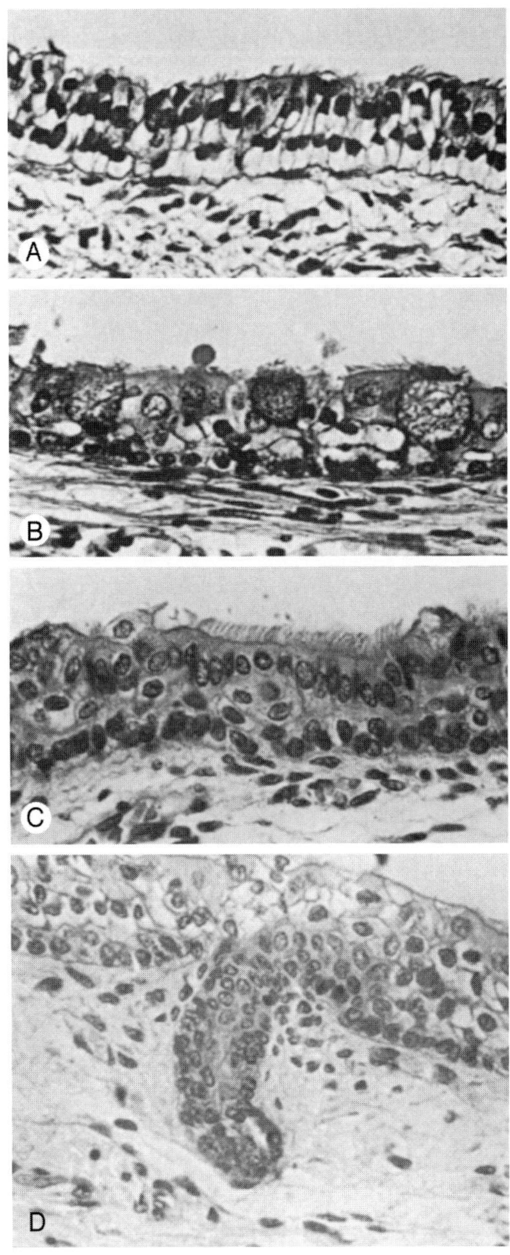

FIGURE 2–20 ■ Sections through the esophagus at different stages of the developing mucosa. *A,* Ciliated pseudostratified mucosa in the 28-mm crown-rump (CR) stage. *B,* Ciliated columnar cells, goblet, and polygonal cells, which represent early squamous replacement, in the 190- to 230-mm CR stage. *C,* Patchy remnants of ciliated epithelium when most of the epithelium is squamous at birth. *D,* Downgrowth of surface epithelium to generate future submucosal glands. (From Enterline H, Thompson J: Diseases of the Esophagus. New York, Springer-Verlag, 1984.)

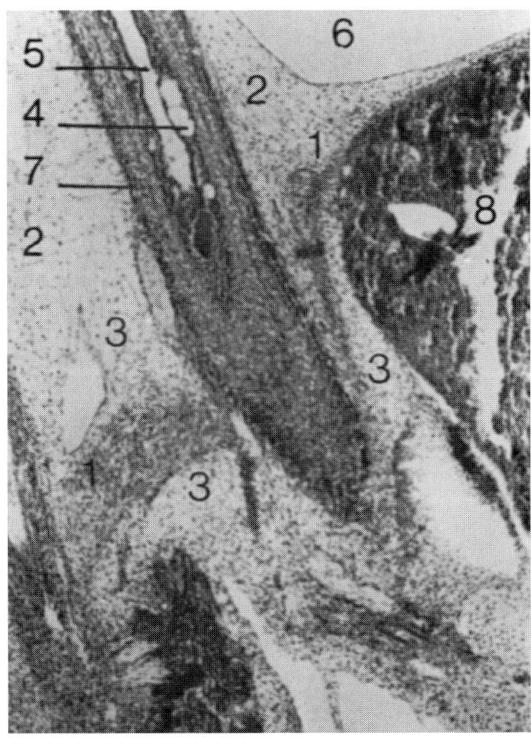

FIGURE 2–21 ■ Sagittal section through a 15-mm crown-rump (CR) long embryo showing the anchoring structures of the esophagogastric junction with developing diaphragmatic musculature (1), undifferentiated mesenchymal tissue (2), and primitive phrenoesophageal membrane (3). The section does display also the vacuoles (4) within the esophageal lumen (5) but not the cardia. The pleural cavity (6), the developing musculature of the esophagus (7), and the liver (8) are seen. (Courtesy of Fernandez de Santos, M.D., Madrid.)

The circular muscle, the inner muscle layer, begins at the level of the cricoid cartilage (see Figs. 2–23 and 2–24) and in descending forms incomplete circles (Liebermann-Meffert et al, 1979).

Both the longitudinal and circular muscle layers have the same muscle thickness of only 1 to 1.5 mm throughout the esophagus; no change occurs with age (Eckardt and LeCompte, 1978; Leese and Hopwood, 1986). Approximately 3 cm cranial to the junction with the stomach, however, the increasing number of muscle fibers of the inner layer produces a progressive muscular thickening (Fig. 2–26; see Fig. 2–25). The fibers at the side of the lesser curvature retain their previous orientation to become the short muscle clasps seen in Figure 2–25*B* (Liebermann-Meffert, 1966; Liebermann-Meffert et al, 1979); those at the greater gastric curvature side become oblique gastric sling fibers (see Fig. 2–25).

The cricopharyngeal muscle and the one to two uppermost centimeters of the cervical esophagus contain predominantly muscle cells of striated type (Liebermann-Meffert and Duranceau, 1996; Liebermann-Meffert and Geissdörfer, 1991; Meyer et al, 1986). Occasionally, isolated small smooth muscle bundles are found in the midst of these muscles. Below this level, the smooth muscle content in the lamina muscularis increases in the

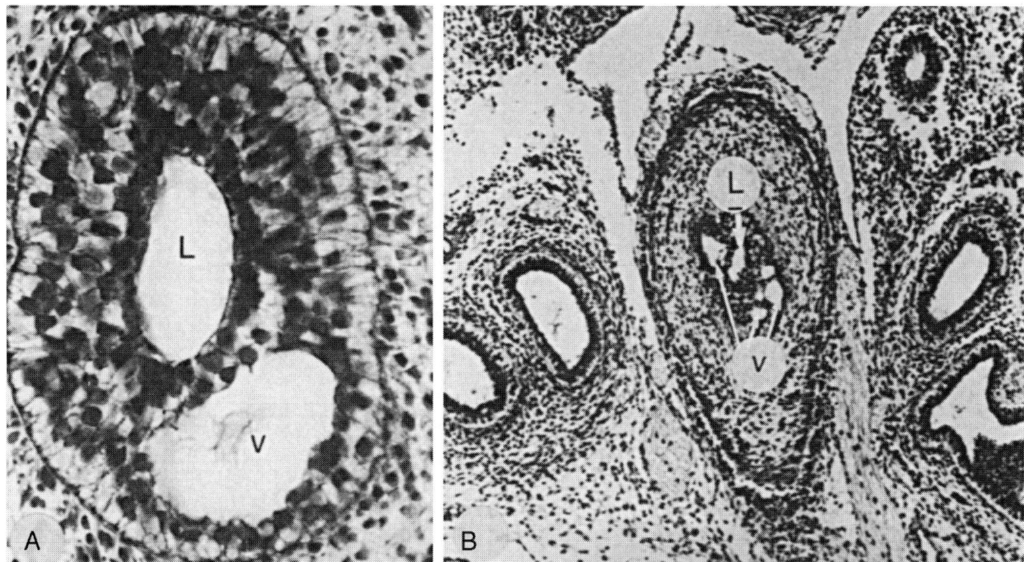

FIGURE 2–22 ■ *A*, Transverse section through the mid-esophagus of a human embryo of 20-mm Crown-rump length. Appearance of vacuoles (v) within the multilayered mucosa. *B*, In the 40-mm stage the vacuoles have increased in size and number to almost occlude the lumen (L). (*B*, Courtesy of Fernandez de Santos, M.D., and Tello Lopes, M.D., Madrid.)

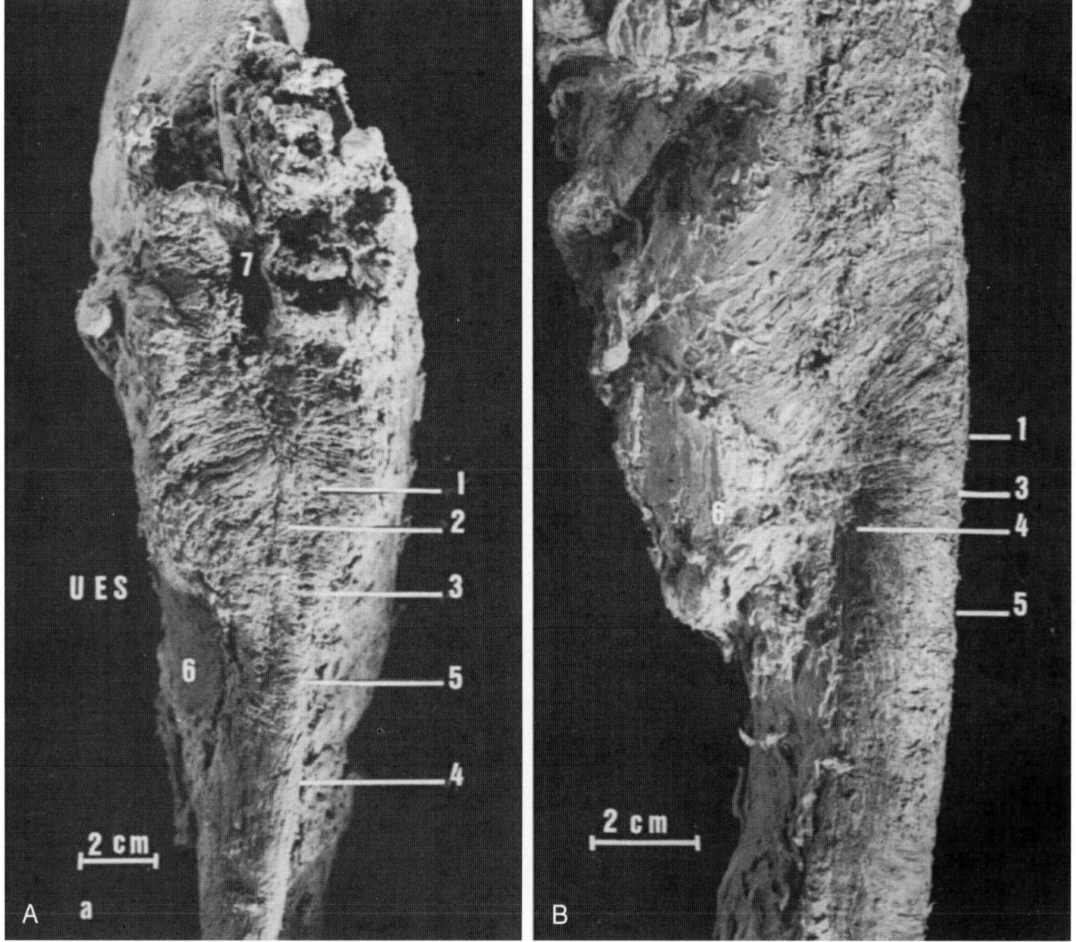

FIGURE 2–23 ■ Arrangement of the muscle fibers at the pharyngoesophageal junction from the *(A)* posterior and *(B)* left lateral aspects. Structures seen are the inferior pharyngeal constrictor muscles (1), pharyngeal line of crossing muscles (raphe) (2), cricopharyngeal muscles (3) that represent the sphincter (UES), longitudinal esophageal muscle (4) with its insertion, circular esophageal muscle (5), medial plane of removed thyroid gland (6), root of tongue (7). (Dry fiber specimen, human.)

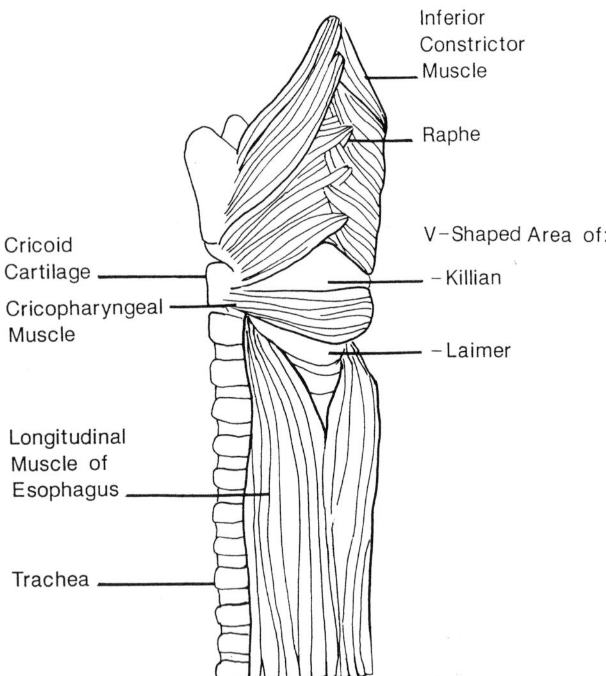

FIGURE 2–24 ■ Muscular architecture of the pharyngoesophageal junction, which is the region of the upper esophageal sphincter. The triangular areas of sparse muscle cover are shown in the scheme. Zenker's diverticulum arises from Killian's triangle. (Modified from Netter FH: Part I. Upper digestive tract. In The Ciba Collection of Medical Illustrations, Vol 3. Digestive System. Ciba Pharmaceutical Embassy, New York, 1971, p 44.)

same proportion as the striated muscle decreases (Figs. 2–27 and 2–28). Smooth muscle appears earlier in the circular muscle layer and in the anterior wall. The transition between both types is neither abrupt nor restricted to individual muscle bundles. Both types of muscle converge without any distinct anatomic septum. Finally, only isolated striated fibers are present in the midst of smooth muscle units (see Fig. 2–27). The transition occurs at the same level in the upper half of the esophagus.

When the esophageal length is defined as 100%, with the cricoid cartilage as a landmark, the transition between the two muscle types is completed in 40% of the total length (see Fig. 2–28) (Liebermann-Meffert and Geissdörfer, 1991). In the neonate and fetus, we found the transition to be more caudal. Below the tracheal bifurcation, no striated muscle cell was ever found in the esophageal wall of our specimens of human adults. The muscularis mucosae of the esophagus is composed entirely of smooth muscle fibers.

Points of Clinical Interest

Anatomically, a sphincter is understood as "a circular or annular muscle surrounding an opening" (Didio and Anderson, 1968) or "a ringlike band of muscle fibers that constricts a passage" (Dorland's, 1974). Sphincters divide the gut into functional segments and are characterized by a resting tone that is higher than that in the adjacent segments.

Upper Esophageal Sphincter. The upper esophageal sphincter (UES) refers to a 2- to 3-mm zone of elevated intraluminal pressure existing between the pharynx and the cervical esophagus. Winans (1972b) showed that the resting pressure is asymmetric both axially and radially. The higher pressure values are recorded anteriorly and posteriorly. This finding is attributed to a flattening of the cricopharyngeal muscle against the ventral plane of the cricoid cartilage. The asymmetric distribution is also explained by the fact that the sphincter, as every endoscopist knows, is not circular (Savary and Miller, 1978).

The cricopharyngeal muscle may be seen as an indenting band with palpable boundaries during surgery (Hiebert, 1975, 1991). This finding coincides with the radiologic view that the UES is "synonymous with the transverse portion of the cricopharyngeal muscle" (Donner et al, 1985; Ekberg, 1991).

Lower Esophageal Sphincter. The existence of the LES, an anatomic sphincter between the esophagus and stomach, has been both accepted and denied for long (Didio and Anderson, 1968; Friedland, 1978; Laimer, 1883; Lerche, 1950; Stelzner and Lierse, 1968). The dilemma is that no circular structure similar to that at the pylorus exists. All the same, with the discovery of a high-pressure zone at the esophagogastric junction in 1956 by Fyke and colleagues and its establishment almost simultaneously in 1967 by Pope and by Winans, the presence of a physiologic sphincter at the lower end of the esophagus became undebatable. In fact, such higher pressures are present in the preterm baby from the 27th week of gestation (Newell et al, 1988).

Approaching the lower end of the esophagus, the inner muscular layer slowly increases in thickness across the junction with the stomach (see Fig. 2–26*A*). It is not a marked thickening and is difficult to palpate. Still, it is twice the 2-mm thickness of the esophageal and gastric musculature (see Fig. 2–26*B*). In this context, one may remember that the LES pressures range from 14.5 to 34 mm Hg or less (Winans, 1972a), whereas for the thicker UES the range is between 30 and 142 mm Hg (Winans, 1972b). A reorganization of the muscle bundles at the terminal esophagus, in particular of those of the inner muscle layer that form the "chassis" of the LES (see Fig. 2–25*B*), is consistent with the change of muscle thickness. The semicircular muscle fibers toward the greater curvature augment and are joined by the gastric sling fibers, which extend upward into the esophagus (Fig. 2–29; see Fig. 2–25) (Liebermann-Meffert et al, 1979). It has been suggested that these fibers exert an antireflux effect at the angle of His (Bombeck et al, 1991).

On the lesser curvature side, the semicircular bundles of the esophagus continue to become the short muscle clasps (Liebermann-Meffert et al, 1979), which, by their anchorage in the tissue along the medial margin of the oblique gastric sling fibers (see Figs. 2–25*B* and 2–29), may contract in a ring-shaped fashion. The muscular arrangement and the corresponding thickening extend upward for 3 to 4 cm and pass beyond the distal end of the esophagus into the stomach wall for another 1 to 2 cm. This extension of the specialized muscle structure is identical to the length given for the functional sphincter

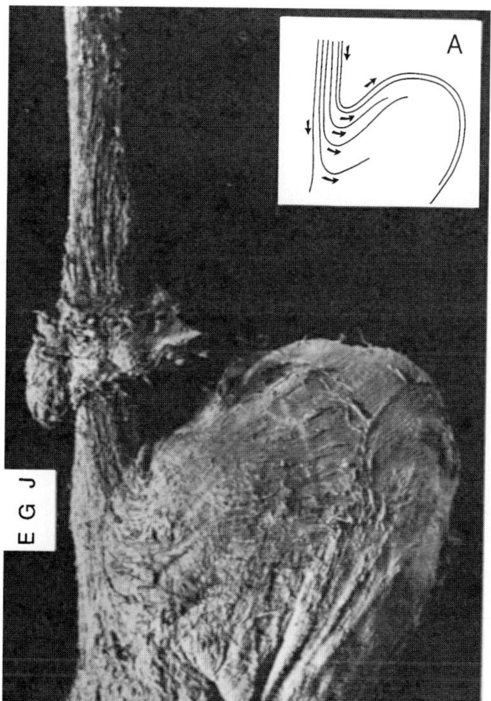

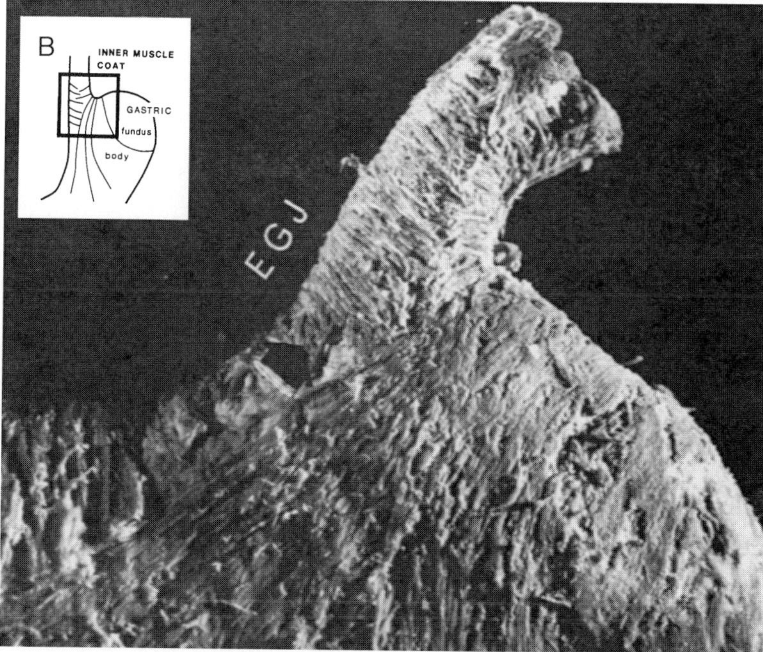

FIGURE 2–25 ■ Arrangement of the muscle fibers at the esophagogastric junction (EGJ) with *(A)* outer longitudinal and *(B)* inner circular layer. The outer layer is composed of multiple muscle bundles following a straight downward orientation. The fibers rarely converge but occasionally split as a result of entering vessels or nerves. Beyond the EGJ the esophageal muscle becomes continuous with the superficial longitudinal bundles of the stomach. Bundles from the right side of the esophagus pass along the lesser curvature; those from the left follow the summit of the fundus along the greater curvature. Bundles from the anterior and posterior esophageal surface, however, fan out and pass to the corresponding gastric surface to blend with the fibers of the underlaying luminal muscular layer of the fundus. The circular fibers of the esophagus *(B)* reorganize to form two components: short muscle clasps on the lesser curve side *(arrow)* and condensed oblique gastric sling fibers that hook around the angle of His and the anterior and posterior gastric surfaces to turn toward the greater gastric curvature. (Dried fiber specimens.) (Fig. *B* from Duranceau A, Liebermann-Meffert D: Embryology, anatomy, and physiology of the esophagus. In Orringer MB, Zuidema GD [eds]: Shackelford's Surgery of the Alimentary Tract, Vol 1. The Esophagus, 3rd ed. Philadelphia, WB Saunders, 1991, p 3.)

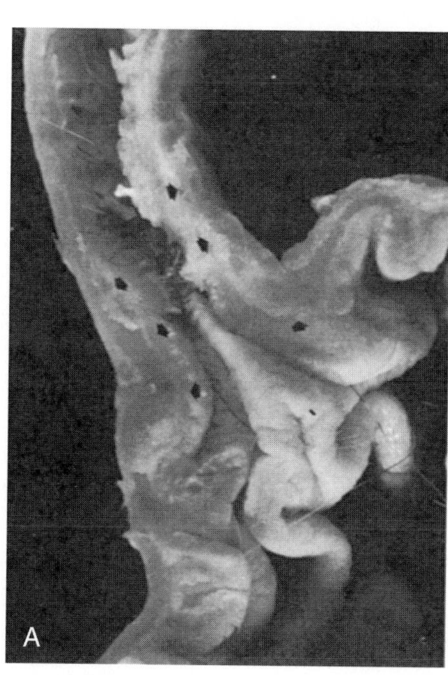

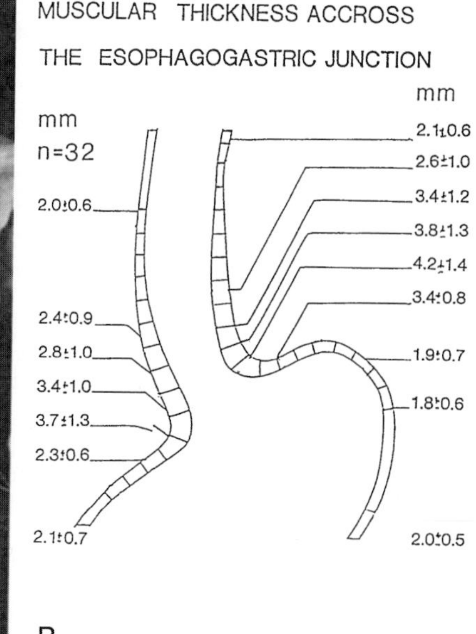

FIGURE 2–26 ■ *A,* Sagittal section through the esophagogastric junction (EGJ) of a formaldehyde-fixed specimen. The progressive, slow change of muscular thicknesses across the EGJ is shown *(arrows)*. *B,* Measurement values are given on the scheme. Thickening shows an axial and radial asymmetry with maximum at the greater curvature. The values are averaged from 32 human kidney donor specimens. (From Duranceau A, Liebermann-Meffert D: Embryology, anatomy and physiology of the esophagus. In Orringer MB, Zuidema GD [eds]: Shackelford's Surgery of the Alimentary Tract, Vol 1. The Esophagus, 3rd ed. Philadelphia, WB Saunders, 1991.)

(Winans, 1972a; Winans and Harris, 1967). Axial and radial asymmetry of the sphincter, as shown when using conventional perfusion manometry techniques (Winans, 1972a; Winans and Harris, 1967) or three-dimensional imaging (Stein et al, 1991, 1995b), coincides with the circumferential difference in muscle architecture (Fig. 2–30).

The LES has been assumed to be positioned at the level of the diaphragm (Mittal, 1998). The muscular structures are, however, precisely at the junction to the stomach and place of the transition line of esophageal into gastric folds (Korn et al, 1997; Liebermann-Meffert et al, 1979; Stein et al, 1995a).

Several points favor the functional muscular structure as constituting the LES. Combined radiomorphologic motility studies using wall markers localized the high-pressure zone to the site of muscular thickening (Liebermann-Meffert et al, 1985). Disruption of the junctional musculature by partial or total myotomy or myectomy (Bombeck et al, 1991; Gahagan, 1962; Siewert et al, 1973; Vandertoll et al, 1966) significantly reduced or abolished LES pressure values. When muscle of the junction is put into a bath, it maintains tonic contraction, whereas the muscle from levels just above or below does not (Christensen, 1991; Siewert et al, 1973).

As a practical matter, the aim of surgery for achalasia is division of the LES musculature. A modified Heller operation uses a myotomy of the anterior wall of the esophagogastric junction. Debate exists about the proper length of the myotomy (Bombeck et al, 1991; Gozzetti et al, 1991). The incision has been commonly recommended to begin at least 10 cm upward on the esophagus and extend at least 3 cm onto the body of the stomach.

To preserve the function of the sphincter and to avoid reflux caused by its disruption, Bombeck and associates (1991) limited the extension of the gastric myotomy to 0.5 cm to avoid damage to the muscular sling of the oblique gastric fibers. Gozzetti and associates (1991)

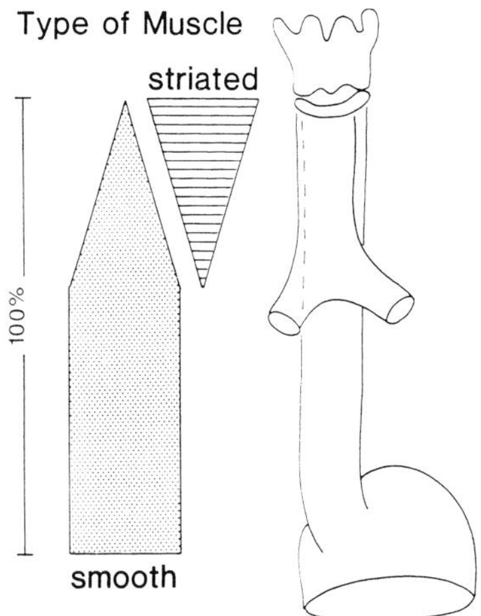

FIGURE 2–28 ■ Location and proportional content of striated and smooth muscle in the esophagus.

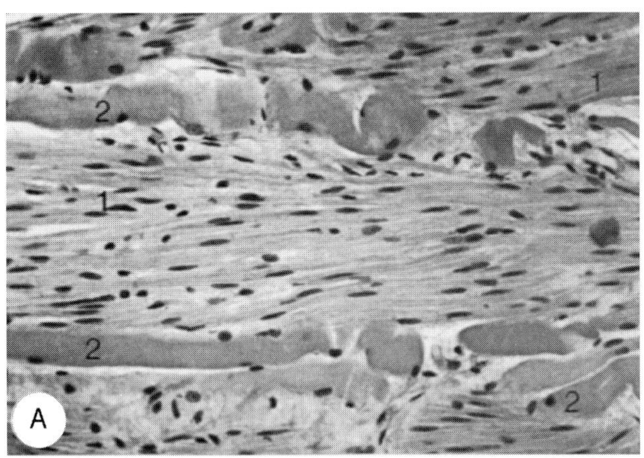

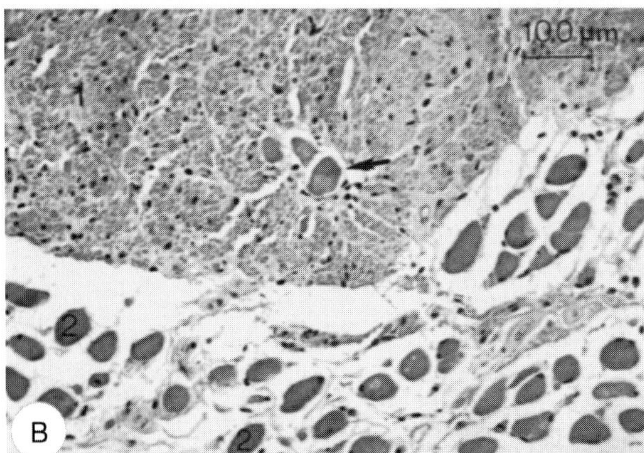

FIGURE 2–27 ■ Longitudinal *(A)* and transverse *(B)* histologic section through the lower area of the cranial third of the human esophagus. In this position the musculature consists mainly of smooth muscle (1) with interwoven striated muscle fibers and bundles (2). One single striated cell within the smooth muscle tissue is shown *(arrow)* (H&E). (From Liebermann-Meffert D, Geissdörfer K: Is the transition of striated into smooth muscle precisely known? In Giuli R, McCallum RW, Skinner DB [eds]: Primary Motility Disorders of the Esophagus: 450 Questions—450 Answers. Paris, Libbey Eurotext, 1991, p 108.)

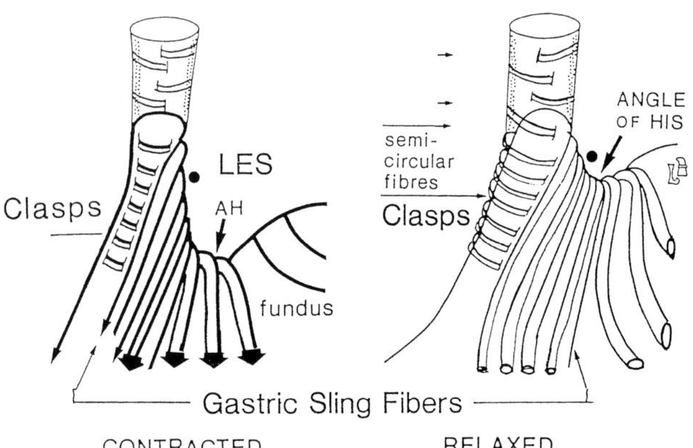

FIGURE 2–29 ■ Schematic illustration of common muscular arrangement at the esophagogastric junction with oblique gastric fiber sling forming the angle of His or the cardiac notch, and the short muscle clasps. Although it may form a ring-like contraction, this arrangement does not at all fit into the traditional concept of a true anatomic sphincter, which is a circular band of muscle. To get rid of old prejudices, to come to terms, and to simplify the fact of the coinciding physiologic sphincter, one may call this structure a false anatomic sphincter. LES, lower esophageal sphincter.

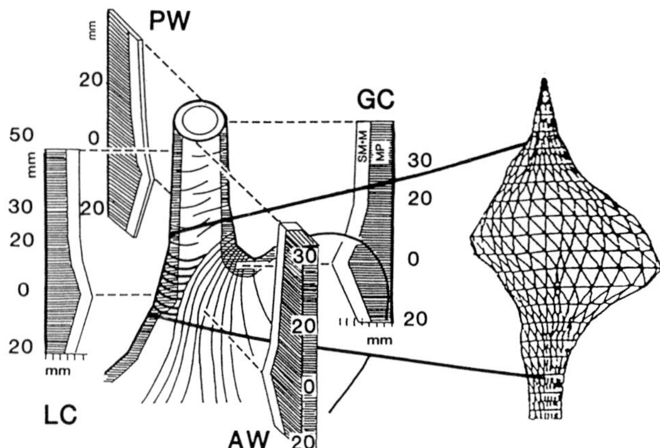

FIGURE 2–30 ■ Schematic showing the correlation between radial thickness of the musculature *(left)* and three-dimensional manometric pressure image *(right)* at the human esophagogastric junction. The thickness across the junction is given in millimeters at the lesser curvature (LC), anterior wall (AW), greater gastric curvature (GC), and posterior wall (PW). Radial pressures at the junction (in millimeters of mercury) are plotted around an axis representing atmospheric pressure. The left side of the positive pressure image corresponds with the lesser curvature, the right one with the greater curvature. Asymmetry of the sphincter is apparent. (From Stein HJ, Liebermann-Meffert D, DeMeester TR, Siewert JR: Three-dimensional pressure image and muscular structure of the human lower esophageal sphincter. Surgery 117:692, 1995.)

questioned the results of this function-preserving procedure and still extended the myotomy to the stomach but divided only the muscular clasps at the lesser curvature, taking great care not to damage the oblique gastric fiber sling.

Tela Submucosa. The submucosa consists of loose connective tissue and contains elastic and collagen fibers, fine blood vessels, networks of lymph channels, nerves, and the deep mucous glands. Esophageal glands are small branching glands of mixed type; their ducts penetrate the muscularis mucosae.

Tunica Mucosa. The mucous layer facing the esophageal lumen consists of the muscularis mucosae, the tunica propria, and the stratified squamous epithelium. The muscularis mucosae is a continuous muscular layer. At rest, it folds the lumen into three or four large longitudinal folds. At the lower end, at the last 2 to 3 cm of the terminal esophagus, it has a greater number of small transversely rippled folds (Eckardt et al, 1980; Liebermann-Meffert et al, 1979). On distention of the lumen, all these folds disappear.

The tunica propria mucosa consists of elastic and collagenous fiber networks and projects into the epithelium to form the papillae. It also contains lymph channels, follicles, and esophageal glands of mucous type or, in the terminal esophagus, glands that resemble cardiac glands. The inner surface is covered by stratified, nonkeratinizing squamous epithelium.

The surface of the esophageal mucosa is reddish in color in its cranial portion and becomes paler toward the lower third of the esophagus. The smooth esophageal mucosa can be easily distinguished from the dark mammillated gastric mucosa.

Points of Clinical Interest

The mucosal transition at the squamocolumnar junction is an objectively recognizable reference point for endoscopists (Savary and Miller, 1978). On fresh anatomic specimens, it is seen as an abrupt demarcation line that shows several small, long or short tongues of squamous epithelium toward the esophagus. The transition, known as the Z line, is normally located near the gastric orifice or just above it (Kramer, 1977). Endoscopic determination is based on differences in color, transparency of the epithelium, mucosal structures, and the epithelial thickness. Proximal extension of a stomach-like or intestine-type columnar epithelium (Barrett's esophagus) is pathologic and is discussed in Chapter 17.

COMMENTS AND CONTROVERSIES

This chapter on esophageal embryology, anatomy, and histology has its roots in observations by the author on human studies, *which are published elsewhere (see Liebermann-Meffert and Duranceau, 1996 and References), rather than information taken from standard anatomic textbooks. Text and references are updated from the first edition. Clinically relevant points are emphasized.*

C.A.H.

REFERENCES

Adams CWM, Brain RHF, Trounce JR: Ganglion cells in achalasia of the cardia. Virchows Arch [A] 372:75, 1976.

Akiyama H: Surgery for carcinoma of the esophagus. Curr Probl Surg 17:53, 1980.

Boerner-Patzelt D: Die Entwicklung der Magenschleimhautinseln im oberen Anteil des Oesophagus von ihrem ersten Auftreten bis zur Geburt. Anat Anz 55:162, 1922.

Bollinger A, Partsch H, Wolfe IHN (eds): The Initial Lymphatics. New York, Thieme, 1985.

Bombeck CT, Dillard DH, Nyhus LM: Muscular anatomy of the gastroesophageal junction and role of the phrenoesophageal ligament. Ann Surg 164:643, 1966.

Bombeck CT, Nyhus LM, Donahue PE: How far should the myotomie extend on the stomach? In Giuli R, McCallum RW, Skinner DB (eds): Primary Motility Disorders of the Esophagus. Paris, Libbey Eurotext, 1991, p 455.

Bruna J: Types of collateral lymphatic circulation. Lymphology 7:61, 1974.

Butler H: The veins of the esophagus. Thorax 6:276, 1951.

Calvet J, Poulhes J: Les artères de l'oesophage. Ann Otolaryngol 65:416, 1948.

Christensen J: The innervation of motility of the esophagus. Front Gastrointest Res 3:18, 1978.

Christensen J: What are the differences between peristalsis in the striated muscle part of the esophagus and that in the smooth muscle part? In Giuli R, McCallum RW, Skinner DB (eds): Primary Motility Disorders of the Esophagus. Paris, Libbey Eurotext, Paris, 1991, p 164.

Cunningham ET, Sawchenko PE: Central neural control of esophageal motility: A review. Dysphagia 5:35, 1990.

Dankmeijer J, Miete M: Sur le développement de l'estomac. Acta Anat 47:384, 1961.

DeMeester TR, Levin B: Cancer of the Esophagus. Orlando, FL, Grune & Stratton, 1986.

Demel R: Die Gefässversorgung der Speiseröhre. Ein Beitrag zur Oesophaguschirurgie. Langenbecks Arch Klin Chir 128:453, 1924.

DeSouza RR, DeCarvalho CAF, Liberti EA, Fujimura I: A quantitative study on the myenteric plexus of the distal end of the human esophagus. Gegenbauers Morphol Jahrb 134:565, 1988.

Diamant NE: Physiology of esophageal motor function. Gastroenterol Clin North Am 18:179, 1989.

Didio LJA, Anderson MC: The Sphincters of the Digestive System: Anatomical, Functional, and Surgical Considerations. Baltimore, Williams & Wilkins, 1968.

Dodds WJ, Stewart ET, Hodges D et al: Movement of the feline esophagus associated with respiration and peristalsis. J Clin Invest 52:1, 1983.

Donner MW, Bosma JF, Robertson DL: Anatomy and physiology of the pharynx. Gastrointest Radiol 10:186, 1985.

Dorland's Illustrated Medical Dictionary, 25th ed. Philadelphia, WB Saunders, 1974.

Duranceau A, Liebermann-Meffert D: Embryology, anatomy, and physiology of the esophagus. In Orringer MB, Zuidema GD (eds): Shackelford's Surgery of the Alimentary Tract, Vol 1. The Esophagus, 3rd ed. Philadelphia, WB Saunders, 1991, p 3.

Eckardt VF, LeCompte P-M: Esophageal ganglia and smooth muscle in the elderly. Dig Dis Sci 23:443, 1978.

Eckardt VF, Adami B, Hücker H, Leeder H: The esophagogastric junction in patients with asymptomatic lower esophageal rings. Gastroenterology 79:426, 1980.

Ekberg O: Is the location of the UES still controversial? In Giuli R, McCallum RW, Skinner DB (eds): Primary Motility Disorders of the Esophagus. Paris, Libbey Eurotext, 1991, p 122.

Eliska O: Phreno-oesophageal membrane and its role in the development of hiatal hernia. Acta Anat 86:137, 1973.

Enterline H, Thompson J: Pathology of the Esophagus. New York, Springer, 1984.

Friedland GW: Historical review of the changing concepts of lower esophageal anatomy: 430 BC–1977. Am J Roentgenol 131:373, 1978.

Fyke FE, Code CF, Schlegel JF: The gastroesophageal sphincter in healthy human beings. Gastroenterologia 86:135, 1956.

Gahagan TH: The function of the musculature of the esophagus and stomach in esophagogastric sphincter mechanism. Surg Gynecol Obstet 114:293, 1962.

Goyal RK, Cobb BW: Motility of the pharynx, esophagus, and esophageal sphincters. In Johnson LR (ed): Physiology of the Gastrointestinal Tract. New York, Raven Press, 1981, p 359.

Gozzetti G, Mattioli S, Pilotti V et al: How far should the myotomy extend on the stomach? In Giuli R, McCallum RW, Skinner DB (eds): Primary Motility Disorders of the Esophagus. Paris, Libbey Eurotext, 1991, p 457.

Hamilton WJ, Mossman HW: Hamilton, Boyd, and Mossman's Human Embryology: Prenatal Development of Form and Function, 4th ed. London, Macmillan, 1978.

Hayek H v: Die Kardia und der Hiatus oesophagus des Zwerchfells. Z Anat Entwicklungsgesch 100:218, 1933.

Heatley RV, Collins J, James PD, Atkinson M: Vagal function in relation to gastrooesophageal reflux and associated motility changes. Br Med J 280:755, 1980.

Henderson RD, Boszko A, van Nostrand SWP: Pharyngoesophageal dysphagia and recurrent nerve palsy. J Thorac Cardiovasc Surg 68:507, 1974.

Hiebert CA: Surgery for cricopharyngeal dysfunction under local anesthesia. Am J Surg 131:423, 1975.

Hiebert CA: Over what length should cricopharyngeal myotomy be performed? In Giuli R, McCallum RW, Skinner DB (eds): Primary Motility Disorders of the Esophagus. Paris, Libbey Eurotext, 1991, p 614.

Hinrichsen KV: Intestinaltrakt. In Hinrichsen KV (ed): Human Embryologie. Lehrbuch und Atlas der vorgeburtlichen Entwicklung des Menschen. Berlin, Springer-Verlag, 1990a, p 305.

Hinrichsen KV: Peripheres Nervensystem. In Hinrichsen KV (ed): Human Embryologie. Lehrbuch und Atlas der vorgeburtlichen Entwicklung des Menschen. Berlin, Springer-Verlag, 1990b, p 449.

Hinrichsen KV: Venen. In Hinrichsen KV (ed): Human Embryologie. Lehrbuch und Atlas der vorgeburtlichen Entwicklung des Menschen. Berlin, Springer-Verlag, 1990c, p 516.

Idanov DA: Anatomie du canal thoracique et des principeaux collecteurs lymphatiques du tronc chez l'homme. Acta Anat 37:20, 1959.

Jackson RG: Anatomy of the vagus nerves in the region of the lower esophagus and the stomach. Anat Rec 103:11, 1949.

Jirásek JE: Altas of Human Prenatal Morphogenesis. Boston, Nijhoff, 1983.

Johns BAE: Developmental changes in the esophageal epithelium in man. J Anat 86:431, 1952.

Johnson FD: The development of the mucous membrane of the esophagus, stomach, and small intestine in the human embryo. Am J Anat 10:521, 1910.

Kanagasuntheram R: Development of the human lesser sac. J Anat 91:118, 1957.

Killian G: Über den Mund der Speiseröhre. Z Ohrenheilkd 55:1, 1908.

Korn O, Stein HJ, Richter TH, Liebermann-Meffert D: Gastroesophageal sphincter: A model. Dis Esoph 10:105, 1997.

Kramer P: Location of the squamocolumnar mucosal junction. Gastroenterology 73:194, 1977.

Kreuter E: Die angeborenen Verschliessungen und Verengerungen des Darmkanals im Lichte der Entwicklungsgeschichte. Dtsch Z Chir 79:1, 1905.

Kumar D, Phillips SF: Human myenteric plexus: Confirmation of unfamiliar structures in adults and neonates. Gastroenterology 96:1021, 1989.

Laimer E: Beitrag zur Anatomie des Oesophagus. Med Jahrb (Wien) 333, 1883.

Lam KH, Cheung C, Wong J, Ong GB: The present state of surgical treatment of carcinoma of the esophagus. J R Coll Surg Edinb 27:315, 1982.

Leese G, Hopwood D: Muscle fiber typing in the human pharyngeal constrictors and oesophagus: The effect of aging. Acta Anat 127:77, 1986.

Lehnert T, Erlandson RA, Decosse JJ: Lymph and blood capillaries of the human gastric mucosa: A morphologic basis for metastasis in early gastric carcinoma. Gastroenterology 89:939, 1985.

Lerche W: The Esophagus and Pharynx in Action: A Study of Structure in Relation to Function. Springfield, IL, Charles C Thomas, 1950.

Liebermann-Meffert D: Die Muskelarchitektur der Magenwand des menschlichen Foeten im Vergleich zum Aufbau der Magenwand des Erwachsenen. Morphol Jahrb 108:391, 1966.

Liebermann-Meffert D: Form und Lageentwicklung des menschlichen Magens und seiner Mesenterien. Acta Anat 72:376, 1969.

Liebermann-Meffert D: The pharyngoesophageal segment: Anatomy and innervation. Dis Esoph 8:242, 1995.

Liebermann-Meffert D: Funktionsstörungen des pharyngo-ösophagealen Übergangs: Funktionelle und chirurgisch orientierte Anatomie. In Fuchs KH, Stein HJ, Thiede A (eds): Gastrointestinale Funktionsstörungen. Diagnose, Operationsindikation, Therapie. Berlin, Springer, 1997a, p 307.

Liebermann-Meffert D: Mobilitätsstörungen des tubulären Ösophagus. In Fuchs KH, Stein HJ, Thiede A (eds): Gastrointestinale Funktionsstörungen. Diagnose, Operationsindikation, Therapie. Berlin, Springer, 1997b, p 349.

Liebermann-Meffert D, Duranceau A: Anatomy and embryology. In Orringer MB, Zuidema GD (eds): Shackelford's Surgery of the Alimentary Tract. The Esophagus, Vol I, 4th ed. Philadelphia, WB Saunders, 1996, p 3.

Liebermann-Meffert D, Geissdörfer K: Is the transition of striated into smooth muscle precisely known? In Giuli R, McCallum RW, Skinner DB (eds): Primary Motility Disorders of the Esophagus: 450 Questions–450 Answers. Paris, Libbey Eurotext, 1991, p 108.

Liebermann-Meffert D, Keller R: Effect of experimental hiatal hernia on peristalsis and lower esophageal sphincter (LES). Gastroenterology 88:1477, 1985.

Liebermann-Meffert D, Siewert JR: Arterial anatomy of the esophagus: A review of literature with brief comments on clinical aspects. Gullet 2:3, 1992.

Liebermann-Meffert D, White H (eds): The Greater Omentum. Anatomy, Physiology, Pathology, Surgery, with a Historical Survey. Embryological Development New York, Springer, 1983, p 13.

Liebermann-Meffert D, Allgöwer M, Schmid P, Blum AL: Muscular equivalent of the lower esophageal sphincter. Gastroenterology 76:31, 1979.

Liebermann-Meffert D, Heberer M, Allgöwer M: The muscular counterpart of the lower esophageal sphincter. In DeMeester TR, Skinner DB (eds): Esophageal Disorders: Pathology and Therapy. New York, Raven Press, 1985, p 1.

Liebermann-Meffert D, Lüscher U, Neff U et al: Esophagectomy without thoracotomy: Is there a risk of intramediastinal bleeding? A study on blood supply of the esophagus. Ann Surg 206:184, 1987.

Liebermann-Meffert D, Walbrun B, Hiebert CA, Siewert JR: Recurrent and superior laryngeal nerves: A new look with implications for the esophageal surgeon. Ann Thorac Surg 67:212, 1999.

Marty-Ane CH, Alauzen M, Alrie P et al: Descending necrotizing mediastinitis. J Thorac Cardiovasc Surg 107:55,1994.

Matsubara T: Computed tomographic evaluation of lymph nodes in cancer of the thoracic esophagus. Dis Esoph 1:109, 1988.

Mayr D, Liebermann-Meffert D: Anatomische Voraussetzungen der lymphogenen Metastasierung des Ösophaguskarzinoms. Inauguraldissertation, TU München, 1996.

Menard D, Arsenault P: Maturation of human fetal esophagus maintained in organ culture. Anat Rec 217:348, 1987.

Meyer GW, Austin RM, Brady CE, Castell DO: Muscle anatomy of the human esophagus. J Clin Gastroenterol 8:131, 1986.

Mittal RK: How can the sphincteric action of the diaphragm in humans be described? What is the relationship between contraction at the esophagogastric junction and increase in intra-abdominal pressure? In Giuli R et al (eds): The Esophagogastric Junction. Paris, Libbey Eurotext, 1998, p 15.

Miura T, Grillo HC: The contribution of the inferior thyroid artery to the blood supply of the human trachea. Surg Gynecol Obstet 123:99, 1966.

Mueller-Botha GS: Organogenesis and growth of the gastroesophageal region in man. Anat Rec 133:219, 1959.

Netter FH: Part I: Upper digestive tract. In: The Ciba Collection of Medical Illustrations, Vol 3. Digestive System. New York, Ciba Pharmaceutical Embassy, 1971, p 44.

Newell SJ, Sarkar PK, Durbin GM et al: Maturation of the lower oesophageal sphincter in the preterm baby. Gut 29:167, 1988.

Orringer MB: Complications of esophageal surgery. In Orringer MB, Zuidema GD (eds): The Esophagus: Shackelford's Surgery of the Alimentary Tract. Philadelphia, WB Saunders, 1991a, p 408.

Orringer MB: Transhiatal esophagectomy without thoracotomy. In Orringer MB, Zuidema GD (eds): The Esophagus: Shackelford's Surgery of the Alimentary Tract. Philadelphia, WB Saunders, 1991b, p 434.

Orringer MB, Orringer JS: Esophagectomy without thoracotomy: A dangerous operation? J Thorac Cardiovasc Surg 85:72, 1983.

Partsch H (ed): Progress in Lymphology XI. New York, Excerpta Medica, 1988.

Pernkopf E: Topographische Anatomie des Menschen. Lehrbuch und Atlas der regionär-stratigraphischen Präparation: I. Band: Allgemeines, Brust, und Brustgliedmasse. Berlin, Urban und Schwarzenberg, 1937.

Perrott JW: Anatomical aspects of hypopharyngeal diverticula. Aust N Z J Surg 31:307, 1962.

Pope CE Jr: A dynamic test of sphincter strength: Its application to the lower esophageal sphincter. Gastroenterology 52:779, 1967.

Rouvière HC: Anatomie des Lymphatiques de L'homme. Paris, Masson, 1932.

Sakata K: Über die Lymphgefässe des Oesophagus und über seine regionalen Lymphdrüsen mit Berücksichtigung der Verbreitung des Carzinoms. Mitt Grenzgeb Med Chit 11:634, 1903.

Savary M, Miller G: The Esophagus: Handbook and Atlas of Endoscopy. Solothurn, Switzerland, Gassmann, 1978.

Schaller G: Die Lumenseite des menschlichen Oesophagus während der Ontogenese. Z Mikrosk Anat Forsch 92:675, 1978.

Schridde H: Ueber die Epithelproliferationen in der embryonalen menschlichen Speiseröhre. Virchows Arch [A] 191:178, 1908.

Shapiro AL, Robillard GL: The esophageal arteries: Their configurational anatomy and variations in relation to surgery. Ann Surg 131:171, 1950.

Siewert JR, Jennewein HM, Waldeck F: Experimentelle Untersuchungen zur Funktion des unteren Oesophagussphinkters nach Intrathorakalverlagerung, Myotomie und zirkulèrer Myektomie. Bruns Beitr Klin Chir 22:818, 1973.

Smith EI: The early development of the trachea and esophagus in relation to atresia of the esophagus and tracheoesophageal fistula. Contrib Embryol Carnegie Inst 36:41, 1957.

Stein HJ, DeMeester TR, Naspetti R et al: Three dimensional imaging of the lower esophageal sphincter in gastroesophageal reflux disease. Ann Surg 214:374, 1991.

Stein HJ, Korn O, Liebermann-Meffert D: Manometric vector volume analysis to assess lower esophageal sphincter function. Ann Chir Gynaecol 84:151, 1995a.

Stein HJ, Liebermann-Meffert D, DeMeester TR, Siewert JR: Three dimensional pressure image and muscular structure of the human lower esophageal sphincter. Surgery 117:692, 1995b.

Stelzner F, Lierse W: Der angiomuskuläre Dehnverschluss der terminalen Speiseröhre. Langenbecks Arch Chir 321:35, 1968.

Vallée B, Hong R, Renelier B et al: Les artères oesophagiennes d'origine cervicale: étude anatomique de 23 dissections. Ann Otolaryngol 99:29, 1982.

Vandertoll J, Ellis FH, Schlegel JF, Code CF: An experimental study of the role of gastric and esophageal muscle in gastroesophageal competence. Surg Gynecol Obstet 122:579, 1966.

van Straalen HCM, Jansveld KA, Michels LFE, Tham TA: Mediastinitis with fistula formation to the left main bronchus. A complication of wisdom tooth extraction. Chest 106:623, 1994.

Vianna A, Hayes PC, Moscoso G et al: Normal venous circulation of the gastroesophageal junction. A route of understanding varices. Gastroenterology 93:876, 1987.

Warwick R, Williams PL (eds): Gray's Anatomy, 35th ed. Edinburgh, Longman, 1978.

Wegener OH: Whole Body Computerized Tomography. Basel, Karger, 1983.

Williams DB, Payne WS: Observations on esophageal blood supply. Mayo Clin Proc 57:448, 1982.

Winans CS: Manometric asymmetry of the lower esophageal high pressure zone. Gastroenterology 62:830, 1972a.

Winans CS: The pharyngoesophageal closure mechanism: A manometric study. Gastroenterology 63:768, 1972b.

Winans CS, Harris LD: Quantitation of lower esophageal sphincter competence. Gastroenterology 52:773, 1967.

Wirth W, Frommhold H: Der Ductus thoracicus und seine Variationen. Lymphographische Studie. Fortschr Roentgenstr 112:450, 1970.

Wookey H: The surgical treatment of midesophageal carcinoma. Br J Surg 27:696, 1940.

Zschiesche W: Kompensationsmechanismen des menschlichen Ductus thoracicus bei Lymphabflussstörungen. Fortschr Med 81:869, 1963.

Zweifach BW, Prather JW: Manipulation of pressure in terminal lymphatics in the mesentery. Am J Physiol 228:1326, 1975.

CHAPTER **3**

Physiology

PHYSIOLOGY OF DEGLUTITION

Harold G. Preiksaitis
Nicholas E. Diamant

In the last two decades, renewed interest in the swallowing mechanism has provided many new insights into the normal physiology and pathophysiology of swallowing. Much attention has focused on the oropharyngeal stage of swallowing. Detailed accounts of these studies can be found in numerous review articles and monographs (Dodds et al, 1989; Goyal and Sivarao, 1999; Jones and Donner, 1991; Kahrilas, 1992; Logemann, 1986; Miller, 1998; Nelson and Richter, 1989; Perlman and Schulze-Delrieu, 1997). It is our intent not to reiterate this material here but to provide an overview of the swallowing mechanism and to cover pharyngeal function specifically as it pertains to normal swallowing. The esophageal swallow mechanism is described in the third part of this chapter, The Lower Esophageal Sphincter.

PHASES OF SWALLOWING

The act of swallowing begins in the mouth and ends when the bolus enters the stomach. Swallowing can be conveniently divided into three or four phases for purposes of study and discussion (Table 3–1).

The *preparatory phase* and the *oral phase* are frequently grouped together as the *oral-preparatory phase*. During this phase, mastication, lubrication with saliva, and the general shaping, preparation, and positioning of the bolus on the tongue occur (preparatory phase). This phase is under voluntary control, and its duration is highly variable. The *oral phase* is dependent on the action of the tongue moving upward and posteriorly, rolling or squeezing the bolus against the palate, propelling it backward past the faucial pillars and thus into the pharynx.

At this point, the *pharyngeal phase* is triggered, and the remainder of the swallow occurs under involuntary control. The bolus is moved rapidly through the pharynx, without aspiration, in approximately 1 second. This phase ends when the bolus crosses the upper esophageal sphincter (UES) and enters the esophagus.

The *esophageal phase* consists of bolus transport to the stomach by esophageal peristaltic contraction, ending when the bolus passes the opened lower esophageal sphincter (LES). This final phase typically lasts 8 to 10 seconds (Goyal and Sivarao, 1999).

ANATOMY

The anatomical structures involved in swallowing consist of bones, cartilage, and neuromuscular elements. The most important structures and their relationships are shown in Figure 3–1. During the oral-preparatory phase, the relevant structural elements would include the mandible; floor of the mouth; teeth; hard and soft palate; many of the muscles of facial expression, especially the perioral muscles; muscles of mastication; and the intrinsic and extrinsic muscles of the tongue. Motor innervation of these muscle groups occurs via the mandibular branch (V3) of the trigeminal nerve (muscles of mastication), the facial nerve (VII, muscles of facial expression), and the hypoglossal nerve (XII, tongue). A total of 20 paired striated muscles contribute to this phase (Jones and Donner, 1991).

Pharyngeal anatomy is more complex. The oropharynx and hypopharynx are formed by three groups of pharyngeal constrictors (superior, middle, and inferior), which form the lateral and posterior walls of a contractile funnel.

Anteriorly, a number of muscular, bony, and cartilaginous elements delimit the pharynx. These include the base of the tongue, uvula, salpingoepiglottic folds, epiglottis, and larynx. The larynx includes the thyroid cartilage, hyoid bone, thyrohyoid membrane, cricoid cartilage and cricothyroid membrane. The *valleculae* are bilateral cavities formed by the space between the base of the tongue and the walls of the pharynx anterior to the epiglottis. Inferiorly, the *piriform sinuses* are formed as bilateral spaces on either side of the larynx, bordered by the lateral insertion of the inferior constrictor and the thyroid cartilage. The nasopharynx is located above the soft palate. The entire pharynx measures 12 to 14 cm in length (Jones and Donner, 1991).

Inferiorly, the UES is formed by the cricopharyngeus arising from the cricoid cartilage and looping around the pharyngoesophageal junction at the cervical level C5 to C6. This muscle has a superior component made up by a small portion of the inferior pharyngeal constrictor above. Between the inferior constrictor and superior components of the cricopharyngeus, the muscle thins somewhat. It is in this thinned area, called the "triangle of Killian," that Zenker's diverticulum can develop. The cricopharyngeus produces the posterior indentation referred to as the "cricopharyngeal bar," commonly seen on barium radiographs (Dodds et al, 1989; Jones and Donner, 1991).

The laryngeal inlet opens to the anterior wall of the

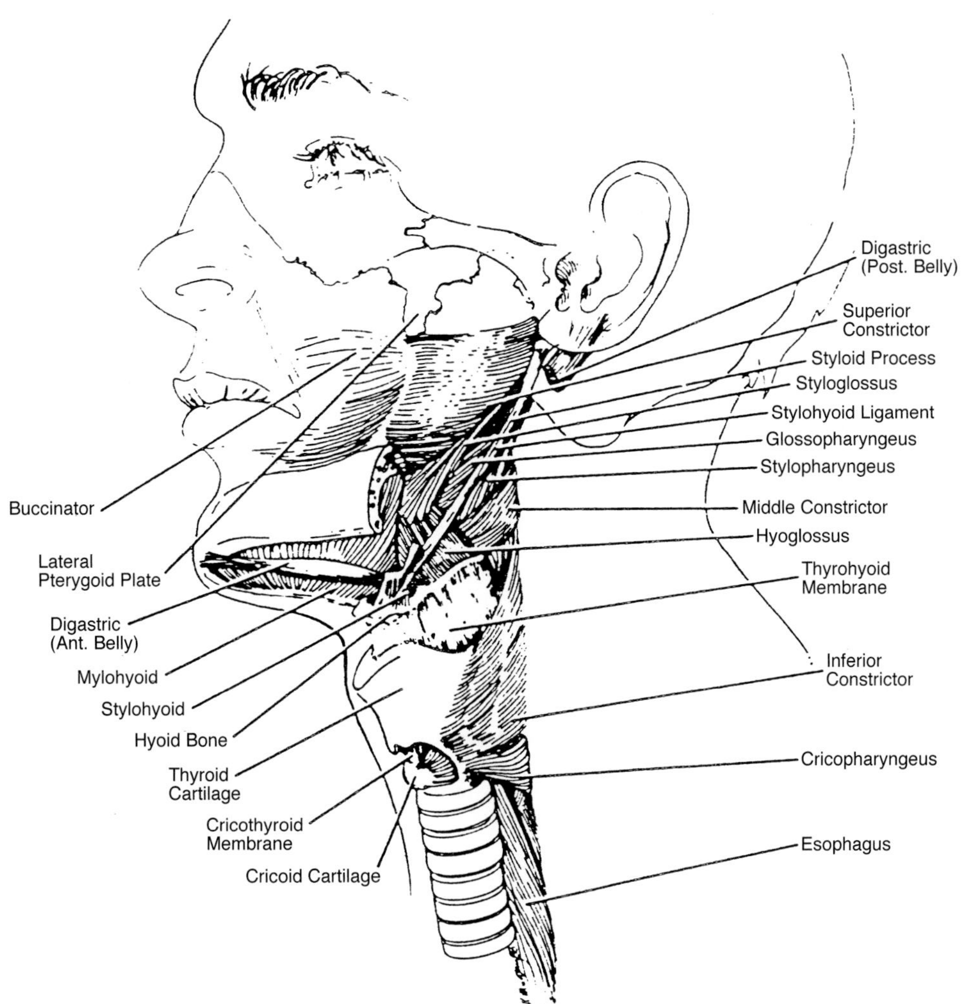

FIGURE 3–1 ■ The main anatomic structures involved in the oropharyngeal phase of swallowing. (From Gelfand, DW, Richter JE: Dysphagia: Diagnosis and Treatment. New York, Igaku-Shoin, 1989, p 13.)

pharynx. The larynx and trachea are suspended by muscles and ligaments from the hyoid bone above and the sternum below. This arrangement affords the mobility needed by these structures to move the laryngeal inlet anteriorly and superiorly out of the path of the bolus during the swallow, which—in addition to closing of the inlet—prevents aspiration (Logemann, 1983).

Twenty-nine pairs of striated muscles are involved in the pharyngeal phase of swallowing (Table 3–2). Motor innervation is dense, with a nerve/muscle fiber ratio comparable to that of the extraocular muscles, to facilitate fine motor control (Dutta and Basmajian, 1960). The major muscles of the pharynx receive their motor innervation from the vagus (X) nerve, except for the stylopharyngeus, which is innervated by the glossopharyngeal nerve (IX). The vagus nerve also controls the intrinsic muscles of the larynx, whereas several nerves control the muscle groups that regulate the essential movement of the hyoid and larynx (V3, VII, C1–C3) during the swallow.

TABLE 3–1 ■ **Four Phases of Swallowing**

Preparatory phase*
Oral phase*
Pharyngeal phase
Esophageal phase

*Often grouped as the oral-preparatory phase.

THE PHARYNGEAL SWALLOW: THE SWALLOW RESPONSE

The pharyngeal swallow is a highly coordinated, complex sequence of motor events normally completed within 1 second (Doty, 1968). Unlike the oral phase, the pharyngeal phase is not under voluntary control; once initiated, it proceeds to completion and cannot be voluntarily interrupted (Doty, 1968; Miller, 1986). It is often referred to as the *swallow reflex*. However, it is not a reflex in the usual sense; it is more correctly viewed as a "patterned response" (Doty, 1968; Miller, 1986). Hence, this reflex is sometimes referred to as the *swallow response*.

The precise stimulus that initiates the swallow response is not known. Direct tactile stimulation of oropharyngeal structures can elicit the swallow response, the tonsillar pillars and posterior wall of the pharynx being most sensitive in humans (Pommerenke, 1928). Factors such as subject age, bolus volume, and temperature can modulate sensitivity of the pharyngeal response (Shaker

TABLE 3–2 ■ **Muscles Involved in the Pharyngeal Phase of Swallowing**

Muscle	*Innervation*
Anterior digastric	Mylohyoid n. V_m
Aryepiglottic	Inferior laryngeal n.
Constrictors	
Superior constrictor	Pharyngeal plexus
Hypopharyngeus (middle)	Pharyngeal plexus
Thyropharyngeus (inferior)	Pharyngeal plexus
Cricopharyngeus (inferior)	Pharyngeal plexus
Cricothyroid	Superior laryngeal n.
Geniohyoid	Hypoglossal n., XII
Hyoglossus	Hypoglossal n., XII
Lateral cricoarytenoid	Inferior laryngeal n.
Levator veli palatini	Pharyngeal plexus
Musculus uvulae	Pharyngeal plexus
Mylohyoid	Mylohyoid n., V_m
Oblique arytenoid	Inferior laryngeal n.
Omohyoid	Ansa cervicalis, C1–3
Palatoglossus	Pharyngeal plexus
Palatopharyngeus	Pharyngeal plexus
Posterior digastric	Facial n., VII
Pterygopharyngeus	Pharyngeal plexus
Salpingopharyngeus	Pharyngeal plexus
Sternohyoid	Ansa cervicalis, C1-3
Sternothyroid	Ansa cervicalis, C1-3
Styloglossus	Hypoglossal n., XII
Stylohyoid	Facial n., VII
Tensor veli palatini	Pharyngeal plexus
Thyroarytenoid	Inferior laryngeal n.
Thyrohyoid	Hypoglossal n., C1
Transverse arytenoid	Inferior laryngeal n.

et al, 1994). The tongue generates large pressures as its base impinges on the posterior pharynx, and this may initiate the swallow (Logemann, 1992). In the case of a volitional swallow, the presence of a bolus facilitates the swallow response. This effect is easily demonstrated by the fact that voluntary repetitive swallowing is difficult to maintain in the absence of a bolus but becomes effortless when liquid or food is present (Doty, 1968). The response must begin precisely as the bolus arrives at the pharynx if aspiration is to be prevented.

Several closely coordinated events ensue (Table 3–3):

1. The nasopharynx is closed from the pharynx by retraction and elevation of the soft palate. Failure of this event can result in nasopharyngeal regurgitation of the bolus.
2. The larynx is elevated and pulled forward under the tongue and out of the path of the bolus while the epiglottis and aryepiglottic folds are repositioned to further shield the larynx from the oncoming bolus.

TABLE 3–3 ■ **The Pharyngeal Swallow Response**

1. The nasopharynx is closed off from the pharynx.
2. The larynx is elevated and pulled forward.
3. Respiration is halted, and the larynx is closed.
4. Tonic vagal excitation to the upper esophageal sphincter is turned off.
5. The upper esophageal sphincter opens.
6. The pharyngeal contraction propels the bolus past the upper esophageal sphincter.

3. The larynx is closed.
4. Tonic vagal excitation to the UES is turned off.
5. The relaxed UES is opened in part by the forward and upward movement of the larynx, which exerts external stretch on the sphincter.
6. The pharyngeal contraction, which assists in propelling the bolus past the UES, is initiated.

NERVOUS CONTROL OF THE SWALLOW MECHANISM

The Central Nervous System

Motor control of the swallowing mechanism resides in the brain stem *swallowing center* (Doty et al, 1967). The center, a bilateral structure located in the medulla and pons, contains a dorsal area of the reticular formation, including the nucleus of the solitary tract and a ventral portion of the reticular substance adjacent to the nucleus ambiguus (Doty, 1968; Jean, 1984, Miller, 1986).

Functionally, the swallowing center can be divided into an afferent reception system, an efferent motor neuron system, and a complex organizing or internuncial system of neurons (Jean, 1984). Its dorsal portion participates in the initiation of swallowing and integration of the swallow sequence. The ventral portion is involved in connecting various motor neuron pools and in coordinating the swallow with other activities, such as respiration.

The swallowing center receives afferent input from the oropharynx and from other structures involved in swallowing and the cerebral cortex to account for the ability to voluntarily initiate a swallow. Cortical input is not essential to the swallow mechanism because swallowing can be evoked after the entire cortex is removed (Miller, 1986). Swallowing is observed in anencephalic infants, who lack neural tissue rostral to the midbrain (Utter, 1928).

Although the cerebral cortex is not essential, the importance of cortical input is highlighted by the fact that direct stimulation of the frontal cortex can elicit a swallow. Magnetic resonance imaging (MRI) and magnetic stimulation studies in humans have demonstrated that recovery of swallowing function following hemispheric stroke is accompanied by increased excitability in the undamaged hemisphere (Hamdy and colleagues, 1998), demonstrating that recovery involves functional plasticity of the cerebral cortex.

The oropharynx, esophagus, and LES are topographically represented within the swallowing center (Jean, 1984). Thus, one group of neurons is active during the pharyngeal swallow, and a second becomes active during the esophageal stage. The swallowing center acts as a "pattern generator," which under the appropriate stimulus executes a well-orchestrated sequence of activation and inhibition of the motor neurons of the many muscle groups participating in the swallow sequence. In addition, the center exerts an overriding function to suspend other activities that utilize the same motor neurons (e.g., respiration, coughing, gagging, chewing, speech) (Doty, 1968).

Efferent Output

The motor neuron pools participating in the swallowing sequence are located mainly in the trigeminal, facial, glossopharyngeal, and hypoglossal nuclei as well as in the nucleus ambiguus (Doty, 1968; Jean, 1984; Miller, 1999). In humans, motor impulses to the pharyngeal region are carried by the recurrent laryngeal nerve, the pharyngeal branches of the vagus nerve, the superior laryngeal nerves, and the cervical nerves via the ansa cervicalis (Doty, 1968). This crossover and density of innervation ensure high-fidelity motor control, accurate sensory information, and perhaps a fail-safe function to help prevent aspiration.

Electromyographic studies of the activation of many of the muscles involved in the pharyngeal swallow indicate that the mylohyoid is the first to become active, followed by the "leading complex" (i.e., activation of the muscles that raise and pull the hyoid bone and larynx anteriorly and superiorly, the muscular base of the tongue, and the superior constrictor) (Doty, 1968; Miller, 1986). The remaining constrictors are activated in sequence to complete the pharyngeal contraction wave. The order of activation of these muscles is in a time-locked sequence; duration can be altered by afferent input, but the sequence remains unchanged (Miller, 1986).

During the first half of the oropharyngeal swallow, the hyoid bone is pulled upward and forward by 10 to 12 mm in each dimension by the coordinated contraction of the mylohyoid, anterior belly of the digastric, the stylopharyngeus muscle, and the geniohyoid (see Table 3–1). This movement of the hyoid bone, by virtue of its attachment to several posterior structures, accomplishes several events critical for the successful completion of the swallow response:

- Elevation of the floor of the mouth
- Horizontal tilting of the epiglottis
- Shortening of the pharyngeal passage
- Opening of the UES (see later)

During the second half of the swallow, the hyoid returns to its resting position by a different path. The infrahyoid muscles move the hyoid posteriorly and downward so that the total trajectory of the hyoid can be described as an ellipse when viewed in the lateral orientation (Fig. 3–2).

Role of Afferent Reception

Sensory information from the oropharynx is carried via extravagal nerves (trigeminal, facial, hyoglossal, and glossopharyngeal) and vagal nerve pathways to the nucleus of the solitary tract (Doty, 1968). Information from various "receptive fields" in the oropharynx may (1) initiate a swallow, (2) alter the threshold for activation of the swallow mechanism, or (3) modify the duration of the swallow sequence.

As mentioned earlier, the presence of a bolus facilitates voluntary swallowing, whereas anesthesia to the entire oral cavity makes it subjectively difficult to initiate a swallow (Miller, 1986). However, Ali and colleagues (1994) demonstrated that anesthesia of the oropharynx in volunteer subjects had little impact on objective measures of the pharyngeal swallow. This apparent paradox remains unexplained.

Others have shown that the characteristics of the swallow bolus, such as volume and viscosity, can independently modify certain characteristics of the pharyngeal swallow sequence (Dantos et al, 1990). For example, increasing bolus volume causes earlier opening of the pharynx and the UES, brought about by the earlier upward and forward laryngeal displacement, whereas increasing bolus viscosity slows pharyngeal transit time and delays UES relaxation and opening. The mechanism responsible for these changes is not completely under-

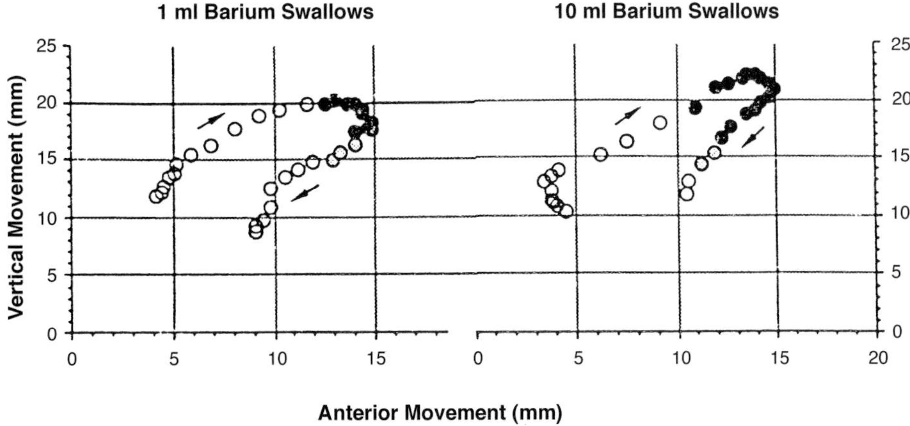

FIGURE 3–2 ■ Elliptical excursion of the hyoid bone during 1-ml and 10-ml liquid swallows viewed in the lateral projection. Each circle is recorded at intervals of one-thirtieth second. *Arrows* indicate the direction of movement. *Open circles* are recorded while the upper esophageal sphincter (UES) is closed. UES opening and closing occur at nearly identical positions for both volumes. The larger volume is associated with persistence of the hyoid position above and anterior to the UES opening coordinates. (From Jacob P, Kahrilas PJ, Logemann JA, et al: Upper esophageal sphincter opening and modulation during swallowing. Gastroenterology 97:1469–1478, 1989.)

stood, but presumably information about the bolus characteristics is carried via afferent innervation to the swallow center, where the appropriate modification of the swallow sequence can occur.

UPPER ESOPHAGEAL SPHINCTER

Because of its crucial role in the normal swallow mechanism, the UES requires special consideration. Between swallows and during the waking state, the UES is tonically closed. UES pressure is maintained by a continuous neural discharge of its motor fibers (Asoh and Goyal, 1978; Doty and Bosma, 1956). This discharge essentially ceases during sleep or with general anesthesia, and UES pressure falls to approximately 10 mm Hg (Kahrilas et al, 1987b). The residual pressure is a result of the elastic component of the muscle.

Because of the position and action of the cricopharyngeus muscle "sling," the UES opening is a slit-like structure with marked radial asymmetry of its intraluminal pressure profile (Welch et al, 1979). The pressures measured in the anterior and posterior directions are significantly greater than the lateral directions. UES pressure increases with inspiration, slow esophageal distention, gagging, and the Valsalva maneuver (Goyal and Siarao, 1989). These mechanisms protect the airway and prevent entry of air into the esophagus. Other factors such as stress, or acidification of the esophageal lumen, also cause increased UES pressure, although not all investigators agree about the effects of esophageal acid perfusion on UES pressure (Cook et al, 1987; Kahrilas, 1992). The presence of the recording catheter itself in the lumen of the UES can significantly increase the pressures, especially during movement of the catheter (Kahrilas et al, 1987a). This makes pressure recording of the UES a technically challenging undertaking.

The sensitivity of the UES to a variety of stimuli may in part explain the "globus" sensation experienced by some individuals. UES pressure falls abruptly in response to rapid esophageal distention, during belching and vomiting (Kahrilas et al, 1986). These "reflexes" permit the decompression of the esophagus and may thus represent protective responses as well.

During swallowing, and under the control of the swallow center, the tonic discharge of motor fibers to the UES ceases and UES pressure falls (Doty and Bosma, 1956; Jacob et al, 1989). Approximately 100 milliseconds later, under the traction force applied by swallow-related laryngeal elevation, the sphincter is "pulled" open to receive the oncoming bolus (Jacob et al, 1989). By altering the extent and pattern of laryngeal elevation, a bolus of larger volume increases the duration of UES opening as well as its diameter (Jacob et al, 1989). The UES returns to its resting tonically contracted state when the pharyngeal contraction arrives at the UES.

In some individuals, the cricopharyngeus muscle appears as a prominent posterior indentation of the pharyngoesophageal junction when viewed laterally during a barium swallow. Whether this finding, sometimes referred as a *cricopharyngeal bar*, represents a true abnormality or a normal variant is still unsettled. Videofluoroscopic analysis of the pharyngeal swallow mechanism has shown that subjects with a "bar" exhibit a decreased open UES diameter. The flow rate across the UES, however, is maintained by an increase in intrabolus pressure (Dantos et al, 1990).

ASPIRATION

Aspiration is defined as the penetration of material into the airway beyond the true vocal cords (Logemann, 1983). Aspiration can occur under the following circumstances:

- *Before* the pharyngeal swallow response is triggered if, for example, material escapes from the mouth into the pharynx during the oral-preparatory phase because of inadequate seal between the soft palate and the tongue
- *During* the pharyngeal swallow if the normal airway protective mechanisms are not functioning adequately
- *After* the swallow if residual material is present in the laryngeal vestibule when respiration resumes

The airway is protected from aspiration during a normal swallow by several mechanisms:

1. The larynx moves anteriorly and superiorly out of the direct path of the bolus.
2. Repositioning of the epiglottis and aryepiglottic folds shields the larynx from intrusion by the bolus.
3. The laryngeal vestibule is closed off by apposition of the true vocal cords, followed by the false vocal cords, the arytenoids, the base of the epiglottis, and, finally, the superior aspect of the epiglottis. The entire sequence occurs in an inferior to superior order.
4. Respiration is momentarily halted during the swallow, resulting in an apneic period of 0.5 to 4 seconds (Preiksaitis et al, 1992).

These various mechanisms must be appropriately coordinated with each other and with the pharyngeal swallow sequence. Hence, several (if not all) of these functions are probably also controlled by the swallow center. Just as for the pharyngeal swallow response, some, but not all of these functions are sensitive to bolus characteristics. For example, closure of the laryngeal vestibule to the level of the arytenoids and base of the epiglottis occurs earlier and lasts longer in the presence of a larger volume bolus, whereas the timing of the descent of the epiglottis is not affected by bolus volume (Logemann et al, 1992).

Despite the modulating effect of bolus volume, videofluoroscopic studies have shown that a large bolus can pass the airway opening before laryngeal closure is complete, emphasizing the importance of other mechanisms that direct the bolus away from the open airway (Logemann et al, 1992). Similarly, in normal adults, the timing of swallows is coordinated with respiration such that almost all swallows occur during the expiratory phase of the respiratory cycle; furthermore, more than 90% of swallows are followed by brief expiratory airflow (Preiksaitis et al, 1992). This timing becomes even more precise if a bolus is present, and it has been hypothesized that the specific reorganization of respiration associated with the swallow may be an additional mechanism to guard against intrusion of swallowed material into the airway (Preiksaitis et al, 1992).

STUDIES OF THE NORMAL SWALLOW AND EVALUATION OF SWALLOWING DISORDERS

Videofluoroscopy and the Modified Barium Swallow

Videofluoroscopic examination of the oral-pharyngeal stage of swallowing has become the "gold standard" for evaluating swallowing pathophysiology. In addition, the use of this technique in studying the swallow mechanism in volunteer subjects has greatly enhanced the present understanding of the normal swallow mechanism.

The videofluoroscopic examination of the oral-pharyngeal swallow, often referred to as a "modified barium swallow," differs from conventional radiologic examination of the upper gastrointestinal tract in several important respects (Logemann, 1983, 1986). Patients are usually seated comfortably to mimic as much as possible their usual eating posture. The videofluoroscopic camera remains fixed instead of following the bolus as it traverses the oropharynx. Specific modifications to the exposure technique are made so that the various structures of the mouth and oropharynx involved in the swallow as well as the larynx and proximal airway structures can be visualized before, during, and after the swallow. Both lateral and anterior views are examined.

The patient is challenged initially with small, calibrated volumes of liquid barium (0.5 to 1.0 ml) with progression to larger boluses (5 to 10 ml) as tolerated. The effect of changing the consistency of the bolus is commonly examined by providing barium paste, cookies, or by mixing contrast material with foodstuffs such as bread or mashed potatoes. With this regimen, abnormalities in the handling and manipulation of the bolus, structural abnormalities, the presence of retained material, and the occurrence and magnitude of aspiration can be assessed.

The modified barium swallow is commonly performed by a radiologist with a speech-swallowing pathologist in attendance. As a result, the examination can be tailored to the specific features of the patient's disorder, and compensatory or rehabilitation strategies can be explored at the same time.

The ability to analyze frame-by-frame computer images of the swallow study has permitted detailed kinematic studies of the oral-pharyngeal structures during the swallow (Jacob et al, 1989). This technique has been extensively used as a research tool to quantify the normal swallow response. It is likely that similar techniques will eventually be used to identify specific swallow abnormalities as well.

Manometry

Although videofluoroscopy provides information about the timing and distance of movement of the bolus and the structures involved in the swallow response, quantitative information about the forces that propel the bolus or relaxation of the UES cannot readily be obtained by this technique. Hence, manometric analysis of the pharyngeal swallow has been of great interest but is a technically difficult undertaking for several reasons.

Manometry employing a conventional perfused system, such as that used to study esophageal pressure changes, does not provide an adequate frequency response for accurate recording of the rapid and large changes in pressure generated in the pharynx (Castell and Dalton, 1992; McConnel et al, 1988). These changes can be as great as 400 mm Hg with rates of rise as great as 4000 mm Hg/second, compared with the esophagus where pressures of up to 200 mm Hg and rates of rise of approximately one tenth of those in the pharynx are usual.

Additional difficulties emerge as a result of the marked radial asymmetry of the UES pressure profile, mentioned previously, and the upward excursion of the UES and other pharyngeal structures during the swallow (Jacob et al, 1989; Welch et al, 1979). By using a perfused catheter modified with a Dent's sleeve device that can transduce pressures over several cm along the catheter and by paying meticulous attention to orienting the sleeve in the anterior-posterior plane, one may be able to avoid some of these difficulties (Nelson and Richter, 1989). This technique provides information of the timing of the pressure waves of the pharynx but is still limited by the frequency response of a perfused catheter system.

The introduction of manometry catheters equipped with solid-state pressure transducers capable of the required frequency response appears to provide the best alternative (Castell and Dalton, 1992; McConnel et al, 1988). Optimal positioning of such catheters remains an issue in obtaining reproducible and accurate results. The combination of manometry with solid-state transducers and concurrent videofluoroscopic visualization of the position and movement of the catheter is ideal and is in use in several centers (McConnel et al, 1988).

In the pharynx, the pressure wave is generated by a combination of the tongue driving force, recorded directly, or transmitted through the bolus and the pharyngeal contraction traveling distally at 9 to 25 cm/second. More distally, in the pharyngoesophageal segment, the pressure recording is more complex because it includes relaxation of the UES and movement of the entire segment relative to the recording device.

Baseline pressure is elevated relative to the pharynx above and the esophagus below, representing the resting pressure of the UES. Typically, a further increase in pressure is seen as an initial positive pressure wave associated with laryngeal elevation. Pressure then falls rapidly as the UES relaxes and frequently dips briefly below atmospheric pressure. This brief negative pressure has been referred to as the *hypopharyngeal suction pump,* or the *Schlukatmung* (German for "swallow-breath"). It is generated by the upward and forward pull of the hyoid bone and laryngeal structures, which applies traction to the UES segment (Jacob et al, 1989). This brief negative pressure may assist in propelling the bolus through the pharyngeal segment. As the UES opens, pressure returns to atmospheric throughout the remainder of UES relaxation. The sequence terminates with a contraction wave occurring in sequence with the pharyngeal contraction before a return to baseline pressure.

Fiberoptic Endoscopy

Fiberoptic endoscopy is a well-established technique for evaluating the esophagus, and is now used to evaluate the pharyngeal swallowing mechanism (Langmore et al, 1988, 1991). Small-caliber fiberoptic scopes of the type used by otolaryngologists for laryngoscopic examination are highly suited to this use. Examinations can be done at the bedside without sedation, and the endoscope is passed transnasally to provide a clear view of the hypopharynx and larynx.

In addition to identifying structural abnormalities by direct inspection, swallowing can be assessed by presenting calibrated boluses of varying consistency in a similar manner to that used in the modified barium swallow. The technique can also be used to assess pharyngeal sensation by puffing air on specific pharyngeal sites (Aviv et al, 1993). Because of the extensive rapid movement of pharyngeal structures during the active swallow, the dynamics are not easily assessed. However, by mixing the bolus with food coloring to provide contrast, one is able to evaluate aspiration or penetration of the bolus before, during, or after the swallow and to demonstrate pooling or abnormal residual material.

Preliminary studies indicate that the technique compares favorably with the modified barium swallow for detecting aspiration but does not provide as thorough an assessment of the entire swallow mechanism (Langmore et al, 1991). Yet, fiberoptic endoscopy can provide detailed information about laryngeal dynamics and vocal cord movement accompanying swallowing not readily available from videofluoroscopy. By utilizing frame-by-frame computer-assisted analysis similar to videofluoroscopy, detailed kinematic studies of laryngeal and vocal cord movement have been made in normal subjects (Shaker et al, 1990).

Ultrasonography

Ultrasonography provides a safe, noninvasive, dynamic modality for studying the swallow mechanism (Sonies and Baum, 1988). Unfortunately, because of the need to "view" structures through a tissue or liquid interface, the only useful position for the transducer is under the chin and study is limited to the oral-preparatory phase of swallowing. Nevertheless, the method has been effective in defining specific swallowing abnormalities of certain disorders, such as cerebral palsy in children and the postpolio syndrome in adults (Kenny et al, 1989; Sonies and Dalakas, 1991).

Other Techniques

Several additional modalities for assessment and study of the swallow mechanism can be utilized, including computed tomography (CT), magnetic resonance imaging (MRI), scintigraphy, sound recording, and analysis of the swallow. These remain largely experimental techniques, and their specific role in the routine evaluation of swallowing disorders or normal physiology remains to be defined.

Last, the value of the bedside clinical examination of swallowing should not be minimized (Logemann, 1983). The fact that most of the swallow events occur too rapidly or cannot be seen by conventional examination of a subject limits the usefulness of simple observation of subjects in defining normal swallowing physiology. However, careful bedside examination of patients with disordered swallowing permits the formulation of reasonable working diagnoses that might be evaluated more efficiently by judicious use of the techniques mentioned earlier.

The use of various diagnostic methods in the evaluation of oropharyngeal dysphagia is the subject of a recent comprehensive review (Cook and Kahrilas, 1999).

CONCLUSION

Swallowing is an extraordinarily complex and yet remarkably coordinated act. It can be divided into four phases: *preparatory, oral, pharyngeal,* and *esophageal.* The pharyngeal phase occurs under the involuntary control of a central nervous system pattern generator and is a highly coordinated, complex sequence of motor events that is normally completed within 1 second. An integral part of this sequence is the timely opening of the UES. While these events occur in a fixed sequence, the duration of swallow events is modulated by afferent nervous signals carrying information about the bolus characteristics. The complexity and speed of swallow-associated events serve to protect the airway from aspiration and limit respiratory compromise.

COMMENTS AND CONTROVERSIES

Drs. Preiksaitis and Diamant are experienced clinicians with major research background in the neurophysiology of the upper gastrointestinal tract. Dr. Diamant continues to direct a multidisciplinary swallowing disorder unit at the Toronto Western Hospital. Dr. Preiksaitis is the director of a similar unit at the University of Western Ontario. These "swallowing centers" are multidisciplinary programs with representation from the specialties of gastroenterology, otolaryngology, thoracic surgery, radiology, speech pathology, and neurophysiology.

Since the first edition, published in 1995, the authors have completely updated their experience in the field, once again providing a clear summary of the current state of knowledge in this complex area. The physiology remains easy for the "non-expert" to follow.

This integrated, sophisticated physiology pertains to important clinical problems—the dysphagia and aspiration that occur due to derangements of function following surgery and/or irradiation in the laryngotracheopharyngeal area. Such disorders commonly occur after head and neck surgery and laryngeal cancer surgery. Aberrations of function also follow resection of the cervical esophagus for esophageal cancer. Dysphagia and aspiration are important complications of recurrent nerve palsy from any cause.

F. G. P.

■ REFERENCES

Ali, G.N., Laundl TM, Wallace KL, et al: Influence of mucosal receptors on deglutitive regulation of pharyngeal and upper esophageal sphincter function. Am J Physiol 267:G644–G649, 1994.

Asoh R, Goyal RK: Manometry and electromyography of the upper esophageal sphincter in the opossum. Gastroenterology 74:514–520, 1978.

Aviv JA, Martin JH, Keen MS, et al: A pulse quantification of supraglottic and pharyngeal sensation: A new technique. Ann Otol Rhinol Laryngol 102:777–780, 1993.

Castell JA, Gideon RM: Esophageal manometry. In Castell DO, Richter JE (eds): The Esophagus, 3rd ed. Philadelphia, Lippincott Williams and Wilkins, 1999, pp 1–32.

Cook IJ, Dent J, Shannon S, Collins SM: Measurement of upper esophageal sphincter pressure: Effect of acute emotional stress. Gastroenterology 93:526–532, 1987.

Cook IJ, Kahrilas PJ: AGA technical review on management of oropharyngeal dysphagia. Gastroenterology 116:455–478.

Dantos RO, Cook IJ, Dodds WJ, et al: Biomechanics of cricopharyngeal bars. Gastroenterology 99:1269–1274, 1990.

Dantos RO, Kern, MK, Massey BT, et al: Effect of swallowed bolus variables on oral and pharyngeal phases of swallowing. Am J Physiol 258:G675–G681, 1990.

Dodds WJ, Stewart ET, Logemann JA: Physiology and radiology of the normal oral and pharyngeal phases of swallowing. Am J Roentgenol 154:953–963, 1989.

Doty RW: Neural organization of deglutition. In Code CF (ed): Handbook of Physiology. Section 6. Alimentary Canal, Vol 4. Washington, D.C., American Physiological Society, 1968, pp 1861–1902.

Doty RW, Bosma JF: An electromyographic analysis of reflex deglutition. J Neurophysiol 19:44–60, 1956.

Doty RW, Richmond WH, Storey AT: Effect of medullary lesions on coordination of deglutition. Exp Neurol 17:91–106, 1967.

Dutta CK, Basmajian JV: Gross and histological structure of the pharyngeal constrictors in the rabbit. Anat Rec 137:127–134, 1960.

Gelfand DW, Richter JE: Dysphagia: Diagnosis and Treatment. New York, Igaku-Shoin, 1989.

Goyal RK, Sivarao DV: Functional anatomy and physiology of swallowing and esophageal motility. In Castell DO, Richter JE (eds): The Esophagus, 3rd ed. Philadelphia, Lippincott Williams and Wilkins, 1999, pp 1–32

Hamdy S, Aziz Q, Rothwell JC, et al: Recovery of swallowing after dysphagic stroke relates to functional reorganization in the intact motor cortex. Gastroenterology 115:1104–1112.

Jacob P, Kahrilas, PJ, Logemann, JA, et al: Upper esophageal sphincter opening and modulation during swallowing. Gastroenterology 97:1469–1478, 1989.

Jean A: Brainstem organization of the swallowing network. Brain Behav Evol 25:109, 1984.

Jones B, Donner MW: Normal and abnormal swallowing: Imaging in diagnosis and therapy. New York, Springer-Verlag, 1991.

Kahrilas PJ, Dent J, Dodds WJ, et al: A method for continuous monitoring of upper esophageal sphincter pressure. Dig Dis Sci 32:121–128, 1987a.

Kahrilas, PJ, Dodds, WJ, Dent J, et al: Effect of sleep, spontaneous gastroesophageal reflux, and a meal on upper esophageal sphincter pressure in normal human volunteers. Gastroenterology 92:466–471, 1987b.

Kahrilas, PJ, Dodds WJ, Dent J, et al: Upper esophageal sphincter function during belching. Gastroenterology 91:133–140, 1986.

Kenny DJ, Casas MJ, McPherson KA: Correlation of ultrasound imaging of oral swallow with ventilatory alterations in cerebral palsied and normal children: Preliminary observations. Dysphagia 4:112–117, 1989.

Langmore SE, Schatz K, Olsen N: Fiberoptic endoscopic examination of swallowing safety: A new procedure. Dysphagia 2:216–219, 1988.

Langmore, SE, Schatz K, Olsen N: Endoscopic and videofluoroscopic evaluations of swallowing and aspiration. Ann Otol Rhinol Laryngol 100:678–681, 1991.

Logemann JA: Evaluation and treatment of swallowing disorders. San Diego, College Hill Press, 1983.

Logemann JA: Manual for the videofluorographic study of swallowing. Boston, College Hill Press, 1986.

Logemann JA: Swallowing physiology and pathophysiology. Otolaryngol Clin North Am 21:613–623, 1992.

Logemann JA, Kahrilas PJ, Cheng J, et al: Closure mechanisms of laryngeal vestibule during swallow. Am J Physiol 262:G338–G344, 1992.

McConnel, FMS, Cerenko D, Mendelsohn MS: Manofluorographic analysis of swallowing. Otolaryngol Clin North Am 21:625–635, 1988.

Miller AJ: Neurophysiologic basis of swallowing. Dysphagia 1:91–100, 1986.

Miller AJ: Neuroscientific Principles of Swallowing and Dysphagia. San Diego, Singular Publishing Group, Inc, 1998.

Nelson, JB, Richter JE: Upper esophageal motility disorders. Gastroenterol Clin North Am 18:195–222, 1989.

Perlman AL, Schulze-Delrieu, KS (eds): Deglutition and Its Disorders: Anatomy, Physiology, Clinical Diagnosis and Management. San Diego, Singular Publishing Group, Inc, 1997.

Pommerenke W: A study of the sensory areas eliciting the swallowing reflex. Am J Physiol 84:36–41, 1928.

Preiksaitis HG, Mayrand S, Robins K, Diamant NE: Coordination of respiration and swallowing: The effect of bolus volume in normal adults. Am J Physiol 263:R624–R630, 1992.

Shaker R, Dodds WJ, Dantos RO, et al: Coordination of deglutitive glottic closure with oropharyngeal swallowing. Gastroenterology 98:1478–1484, 1990.

Sonies BC, Baum BJ: Evaluation of swallowing pathophysiology. Otolaryngol Clin North Am 21:637–648, 1988.

Sonies BC, Dalakas MC: Dysphagia in patients with the post-polio syndrome. N Engl J Med 324:1162–1167, 1991.

Utter O: Ein Fall von Anensephalie. Acta Psychiatr Neurol 3:281–318, 1928.

Welch RW, Luckmann K, Ricks PM, et al: Manometry of the normal upper esophageal sphincter and its alterations in laryngectomy. J Clin Invest 63:1036–1041, 1979.

PHYSIOLOGY OF ESOPHAGEAL PERISTALSIS

William G. Richards
Sean Grondin
David J. Sugarbaker

HISTORICAL NOTE

Systematic study of the physiology of peristalsis has a history of at least 150 years. Cannon (1907) noted that as early as 1839, Reid (1839) had observed a loss of esophageal peristalsis following bilateral vagal section in the rabbit. The first recordings of human esophageal motility during swallowing were obtained by Kronecker and Meltzer in 1883; they measured intraluminal pressure fluctuations using themselves as subjects. These early recordings compare favorably with those obtained using modern manometric equipment (see Fig. 1 in Sanchez et al, 1953). During the last half of the 20th century, the application of newly developed techniques in neurophysiology, neuroanatomy, and pharmacology to the study of esophageal peristalsis has provided many insights into the complex underlying physiologic control mechanisms.

■ HISTORICAL READINGS

Cannon WB: Oesophageal peristalsis after bilateral vagotomy. Am J Physiol 19:436, 1907.

Kronecker H, Meltzer S: Der Schluckmechanismus, seine Erregung und seine Hemmung. Arch Anat Physiol 328, 1883.

Reid J: An experimental investigation into the functions of the eighth pair of nerves, or the glosso-pharyngeal, pneumogastric, and spinal accessory. Edinb Med Surg J 51:269, 1839.

Sanchez GC, Kramer P, Ingelfinger FJ: Motor mechanisms of the esophagus, particularly of its distal portion. Gastroenterology 25:321, 1953.

CHARACTERISTICS OF PERISTALSIS

Definition and Esophageal Anatomy

Esophageal peristalsis is a neuromuscular process responsible for bolus transport between the pharynx and the stomach. It consists of an aboral progressive muscular contraction that is preceded by receptive inhibition in distal esophageal segments and the lower esophageal sphincter (LES). This process involves the coordinated action of the outer longitudinal muscle (LM) and the inner circular muscle (CM) layers, which comprise the muscularis externa. It is controlled by both central and peripheral neuronal mechanisms.

In humans, the source and nature of neuronal control vary along the length of the organ due to regional differences in muscular anatomy. Over the proximal 4% to 5% of the human esophagus, the muscularis externa is composed of striated muscle, which is anatomically continuous with the striated musculature of the upper esophageal sphincter (UES) and the pharynx. In the remainder of the proximal half of the organ, striated and smooth muscle fibers are mixed, the proportion of smooth muscle fibers progressively increasing distally. The distal half of the human esophagus is composed entirely of smooth muscle (Meyer et al, 1986).

Despite this regional variation in muscular anatomy and neural control, the peristaltic wave traverses these segments in a relatively smooth, uninterrupted manner. In fact, esophageal peristalsis is mechanically similar among most vertebrate species, even though muscle composition ranges from entirely smooth in reptiles, birds, and amphibia to entirely striated in many mammals (dogs, sheep, rodents). However, close examination of esophageal peristalsis in humans reveals subtle changes in the force and velocity of the contraction wave as it progresses through these anatomic regions (Clouse and Staiano, 1991; Humphries and Castell, 1977). Aside from humans and other primates, the cat and the American opossum possess mixed striated and smooth esophageal musculature, and these species have been used extensively as model systems to study the physiology of esophageal peristalsis.

Measurement of Esophageal Peristalsis

Analysis of human esophageal peristalsis in both clinical and laboratory settings has generally involved radiographic tracking of a swallowed bolus and intraesophageal manometry. Although specialized strain gauge devices have been developed to measure propulsive force directly (Pope and Horton, 1972), esophageal contractions have been studied primarily by indirect methods using measurements of intraluminal pressure fluctuations. Early manometric methods employed intraesophageal balloon devices (Kramer and Ingelfinger, 1949; Meltzer, 1894; Roman, 1966). Later, intraluminal catheter (Arndorfer et al, 1977; Hollis and Castell, 1972; Pope, 1970; Sanchez et al, 1953; Stef et al, 1974) and microtransducer (Butin et al, 1953; Humphries and Castell, 1977) recording devices were developed.

When a stationary manometric recording device is used, the peristaltic contraction appears as it passes a given esophageal level as the bell-shaped third (Ingelfinger, 1958) or fourth (Butin et al, 1953) wave of the pressure complex observed during liquid swallows. If radiologic imaging is simultaneously used to visualize the progressive occlusion of the lumen during peristalsis, occurrence of the wave correlates with the passage of the tail of the bolus through the region being recorded (Mittal et al, 1990; Ren et al, 1991). The early rising phase of the wave represents an elevation of pressure within the bolus tail, whereas the late rising phase and peak of the wave correspond to the direct pressure exerted by the esophageal musculature on the recording device after the recorded region has been cleared of bolus (Brasseur and Dodds, 1991).

The inhibitory phase of esophageal peristalsis is not always apparent in manometric recordings because of the low or absent resting tone of esophageal musculature. However, potent receptive inhibition associated with esophageal peristalsis becomes apparent if the esophagus is induced to contract (Sifrim et al, 1992) or when a series of swallows is analyzed. Meltzer (1899) noted that in dogs only the last of a series of rapid swallows is followed by esophageal peristalsis. In humans, the frequency and amplitude of peristaltic pressure waves are diminished as the interval between swallows decreases, particularly in distal esophagus (Ask and Tibbling, 1980; Meyer et al, 1981; Vanek and Diamant, 1987).* If the interval between multiple consecutive swallows is short enough, peristalsis is completely inhibited until after the last swallow, when a large amplitude wave is recorded (Ask and Tibbling, 1980).

Long-term manometric recording reveals that in healthy humans approximately half of esophageal contractions are peristaltic and both segmental and simultaneous nonperistaltic contractions are common (Armstrong et al, 1990). Peak pressures average approximately 50 mm Hg in the striated muscle region, are slightly less in the region of transition between striated and smooth muscle fibers, and are slightly higher in the smooth muscle segment. In some records, a region of reduced pressure divides the smooth muscle segment (Clouse and Staiano, 1991; Humphries and Castell, 1977). Propagation velocity is approximately 3 cm/sec in the proximal, 5 cm/sec in middle and 2 cm/sec in distal esophagus (Humphries and Castell, 1977).

Primary and Secondary Peristalsis

Two forms of the esophageal peristaltic contraction have been distinguished on the basis of their mode of initiation (Meltzer, 1906). Primary peristalsis refers to progressive contractions initiated by swallowing; secondary peristalsis is initiated by esophageal distention.

During the pharyngeal phase of swallowing, the UES and LES relax. Primary peristaltic contraction in the esophagus is initiated with the closure of the UES after the swallowed bolus is forced into the esophagus by a pharyngeal contraction. The contraction proceeds along the length of the organ in a progressive, lumen-occluding fashion and terminates with the closure of the LES as the bolus is forced into the stomach.

Secondary peristalsis occurs independently of swallowing in response to local distention (Meltzer and Auer, 1906)† and is associated with UES contraction and LES relaxation (Creamer and Schlegel, 1957; Fleshler et al, 1958). *Transient* distention elicits a propagated contraction (Fleshler et al, 1958), which propels a mobile stimulus (e.g., an injected water bolus) toward the stomach (Creamer and Schlegel, 1957). *Sustained* compliant (isobaric) distention evokes cyclic peristaltic contractions distal to, and irregular simultaneous contractions proximal to, the point of stimulation (Fleshler et al, 1958). The esophageal response to sustained distention by an immobile, obstructing stimulus (e.g., an anchored balloon) consists of contractile responses at the level of (Fleshler et al, 1958; Paterson, 1991) and proximal to the region of the stimulus and a sustained relaxation and cessation of ongoing contractile activity in distal regions including the LES sphincter (Creamer and Schlegel, 1957; Gidda and Goyal, 1985; Kendall et al, 1987). A distally propagated contraction sometimes follows termination of the distending stimulation (Creamer and Schlegel, 1957; Fleshler et al, 1958; but see Paterson et al, 1991).

It has been historically debated whether primary and secondary propagated contractions differ only in terms of the definitional distinction between their modes of initiation or whether they are subserved by distinct motor mechanisms as well. The distinction originally drawn by Meltzer (1906) was based on the observation that in anesthetized dogs a primary peristaltic wave would skip over a ligated or transected esophageal segment and continue in distal segments, whereas a secondary wave would stop at the ligature or transection (Meltzer, 1906; Meltzer and Auer, 1906). Meltzer's interpretation of these findings was that primary peristalsis is directly controlled by a central mechanism, whereas secondary peristalsis is mediated by a chain of peripheral reflexes and is dependent on sequential mucosal stimulation by the bolus. This interpretation, and the derived conclusion that primary and secondary peristalsis must be subserved by different motor mechanisms, have been challenged based on the results of more recent investigations suggesting that both central control and peripheral stimulation contribute to each form of peristalsis.

In contrast to Meltzer's results, Longhi and Jordan (1971) reported that in awake dogs no manometric evidence of peristalsis was detectable in distal esophageal regions in response to swallowing after cervical transection and bolus deviation. This observation was repeated by Janssens and colleagues (1973), who also noted, however, that thoracic transection and bolus deviation did not prevent appearance of primary peristaltic waves in the distal segment in 27% of cases studied. Secondary peristalsis elicited by intraesophageal bolus injection was found to behave in a similar manner. If the bolus was deviated in the cervical esophagus, the peristaltic contraction did not progress beyond the level of transection, whereas peristaltic contractions occurred below thoracic

*Studies in humans (Meyer et al, 1981) and opossums (Gidda and Goyal, 1983) suggest that the effects of rapid swallowing may reflect smooth muscle refractory properties as well as neuronal inhibition.

†Under some circumstances, repetitive secondary contractions may occur spontaneously in association with vague chest pain (Nixon and Koch, 1989a).

levels of transection and bolus deviation in 36% of tests (Janssens et al, 1974).

Hwang (1954) studied lightly anesthetized or awake dogs and found that "no bolus" secondary peristalsis could be elicited in the cervical esophagus, but the threshold pressure or volume of balloon inflation was significantly greater than in the thoracic esophagus. He further noted that proximally initiated secondary peristalsis traversed a region of the esophagus in which the mucosa had been anesthetized with cocaine, although balloon distention in the same region did not elicit peristalsis. Thus, primary and secondary peristalsis are similar in the dog, both involving the combination of a central neuronal control mechanism and peripheral feedback from the bolus. The peripheral component is more crucial to both forms of peristalsis in the cervical portion of the canine esophagus.

Although Meltzer's conclusions concerning dogs are not valid, differences between the motor mechanisms subserving primary and secondary peristalsis are apparent in humans and other species with mixed esophageal musculature. Peristalsis in such species is less bolus-dependent. Cervical bolus deviation in monkeys does not prevent the progression of primary peristalsis, although it reduces the velocity of propagation in distal esophageal segments (Janssens et al, 1976).

In humans, both primary (Dodds et al, 1973; Meltzer, 1899; Richter et al, 1987) and secondary (Fleshler et al, 1958) forms of peristalsis occur in the absence of a bolus. The pressure waves recorded in each case are similar, and both are associated with receptive inhibition (Sifrim et al, 1992; Sifrim and Janssens, 1996), including LES relaxation (Fleshler et al, 1958; Siegel and Hendrix, 1961). Conversely, progression of both primary and secondary peristaltic waves can be inhibited or halted by mechanical stimulation of the pharynx (Lang et al, 1998; Trifan et al, 1996) despite the presence of a bolus (Bardan et al, 1997). However, Patterson (1991) noted that secondary peristalsis in humans exhibits lower contraction amplitude and less sensitivity to atropine compared with primary peristalsis and that the velocity of secondary peristalsis in midthoracic segments is faster than that of primary peristalsis in both humans (Paterson et al, 1991) and opossums (Paterson, 1989; Paterson et al, 1988).

Hellemans and coauthors (1968) noted characteristic patterns of myoelectric discharge associated with striated and smooth muscle segments of monkey esophagus. In recordings from regions where both types of muscle are mixed, both patterns were observed during primary peristalsis; however, only the smooth muscle pattern was observed during secondary peristalsis (Hellemans et al, 1968; Janssens et al, 1976).

Another difference relates to the role of the central nervous system (CNS) in the smooth muscle esophagus. The dependence of primary peristalsis on extramural innervation is indicated by its abolition following bilateral vagotomy and by the findings that cervical esophageal transection in the monkey (Janssens et al, 1976) and curare-induced paralysis of the cervical striated muscle segment in the baboon (Tieffenbach and Roman, 1972) both fail to prevent primary peristaltic contraction of the smooth muscle esophagus. In contrast, secondary peristalsis in the smooth muscle esophagus can be controlled entirely by a local mechanism, surviving bilateral vagal section (Hwang, 1948; Jurica, 1926; Mukhopadhyay and Weisbrodt, 1975), and occurring in vitro in the isolated smooth muscle segment (Christensen, 1970; Christensen and Lund, 1969; Ren and Schulze-Delrieu, 1989).

Modulation of Peristalsis

A number of factors influence the physical characteristics of the peristaltic wave. In general, the mechanism of peristalsis is dynamically modulated to optimize esophageal transport during swallowing under various conditions.

Bolus Effects

Although esophageal peristalsis does occur in the absence of swallowing, the presence and nature of a swallowed bolus can profoundly affect the recorded contraction. Compared with "dry" (no bolus) swallows, "wet" (liquid bolus) swallows are more likely to elicit a peristaltic contraction (Dodds et al, 1973; Meltzer, 1899; Richter et al, 1987) and to result in peristaltic pressure waves in the distal esophagus of greater amplitude and duration and slower propagation velocity (Dodds et al, 1973; Kaye and Wexler, 1981). Increasing bolus viscosity or consistency (solid bolus) is associated with further increases in the frequency of swallow-associated peristaltic contractions, increases in the amplitude and duration of the recorded pressure wave, and in further decreases in peristaltic velocity, compared with water swallows (Dooley et al, 1988, 1990; Keren et al, 1992). These findings suggest that esophageal stimulation by the bolus provides for adaptive modulation of the velocity and force of peristalsis, resulting in a propulsive contraction dynamically optimized for transport of the swallowed material.

It is likely that the mechanisms underlying the effects of bolus presence and viscosity involve pressure applied to the esophagus by the bolus. On the basis of a fluid mechanical analysis of esophageal bolus transport by peristalsis, Brasseur noted that the resistance encountered by the esophageal peristaltic contraction is primarily due to viscous forces and that the pressure gradient generated within a moving bolus is proportional to bolus viscosity (Brasseur, 1987; Brasseur and Dodds, 1991). In addition, a similar modulation of peristalsis (decreased velocity, increased amplitude and duration of pressure wave) has been observed during wet swallows when intrabolus pressure is elevated by partial esophageal obstruction (Mittal et al, 1990),* increased bolus volume (Hollis and Castell, 1975; Mittal et al, 1990), or abdominal compression (Dodds et al, 1974; Ren et al, 1991), and in obese patients with elevated abdominothoracic pressure gradients (Mercer et al, 1985). Because increased intra-abdominal pressure has no effect on peristalsis initiated by "dry" swal-

*Severe or chronic esophageal obstruction results in decreased pressure amplitude and increased frequency of non-peristaltic contractions (Little et al, 1986) and failed propagation (Mittal et al, 1990), indicating that adaptive modulation of peristalsis is disrupted under conditions of pathologic intraesophageal pressure elevation.

lows (Dodds et al, 1974), it is likely that modulation of peristalsis by abdominal compression is mediated by bolus pressure elevation.

This interpretation of bolus effects receives further support from the results of an in vitro experiment. Recording "peristaltic" contractions of isolated opossum esophagus using serosal strain gauges, Ren and Schulze-Delrieu (1989) found that esophageal distention by an intraluminal balloon increased the amplitude and duration of CM contraction elicited by transmural nerve stimulation and decreased the velocity of the propagation.

Effect of a Meal

Twenty-four-hour manometry indicates that the velocity of peristaltic contractions is decreased, and the area under the pressure waveform increased during meal times (Armstrong et al, 1990). Funch-Jensen and Jacobsen (1981) reported a modulation of distal peristaltic waves associated with wet swallows measured during a solid meal compared with the pre-meal fasting state. The effects of a meal on the amplitude, duration, and velocity of the pressure wave were similar to those of increased bolus viscosity or intrabolus pressure and were maximal 10 minutes after the beginning of the meal. A reasonable interpretation of these results in terms of bolus effects is that elevated intragastric pressure caused by distention by accumulation of food contributes to increased intrabolus pressure during subsequent test swallows and thereby mediates modulation of esophageal peristalsis. Further, there may be a hysteresis of modulation effects after repeated solid bolus swallows.

An alternative interpretation attributing the modulation of peristalsis by a meal to the secondary effects of food intake, such as a gastrin response (as proposed by the authors) or elevated blood glucose, is not well supported by available data. The results of in vitro studies suggest that gastrin may enhance the contractility of opossum circular smooth muscle of the LES, but its effect on esophageal body CM is minimal (Cohen and Green, 1973). Furthermore, administration of exogenous pentagastrin has been reported not to affect human esophageal peristalsis (Hollis et al, 1972; Orlando and Bozymksi, 1979). There is evidence that elevated blood glucose may mediate a modulation of esophageal peristalsis similar to the effect of a meal.

During sustained hyperglycemia produced in normal volunteers using a glucose clamp technique, De Boer and associates (1992) recorded peristaltic pressure waves of increased duration and decreased velocity in the distal esophagus (a small increase in pressure wave amplitude was not statistically significant). However, intravenous administration of glucagon, expected to elevate blood glucose, has been reported to significantly *decrease* peristaltic amplitude in the mid and distal human esophagus (Anvari et al, 1989).

Effect of Temperature

Several studies have found that alteration of bolus temperature can modify peristalsis in the distal esophagus. Swallowing of a hot bolus is associated with increased velocity and decreased duration of peristaltic pressure waves compared with those produced by room temperature liquid swallows (Winship et al, 1970), whereas swallowing a cold liquid bolus results in pressure waves of reduced velocity (Kaye et al, 1987; Winship et al, 1970) and amplitude (Kaye et al, 1987; Meyer and Castell, 1981) and increased duration (Kaye et al, 1987; Meyer and Castell, 1981; Winship et al, 1970). Rapid swallowing of very cold liquids can cause transient distal aperistalsis (Winship et al, 1970) and chest pain (Meyer and Castell, 1981). Dooley and co-workers (1990), however, reported no difference in peristalsis among swallows of 5 ml of water at various temperatures.

Effect of Body Position

Body position during manometric recording appears to influence both the amplitude and velocity of the peristaltic wave in a bolus-dependent manner. Compared with a supine position, water swallows in an upright position are associated with smaller peristaltic amplitude, increased velocity in the upper esophagus, and either decreased (Kaye and Wexler, 1981) or unaltered (Dooley et al, 1989) velocity distally. No such differences are observed with a viscous bolus, suggesting that the influence of gravity on the efficiency of the "pharyngeal pump" (Buthpitiya et al, 1987)—and, therefore, on liquid bolus geometry and esophageal stimulation by the bolus—may be responsible for position effects. However, because peristaltic amplitude associated with dry swallows is also significantly decreased in the upright versus the supine position (Kaye and Wexler, 1981), bolus-independent factors probably also play a role.

Effect of pH

It is tempting to speculate that altered esophageal motility in patients with reflux esophagitis may result from a modulation of peristalsis by low intraesophageal pH. However, although failed peristalsis (Kahrilas et al, 1986), reduced peristaltic amplitude (Burns and Venturatos, 1985; Jacob et al, 1990), and increased threshold balloon pressure for elicitation of distal esophageal contractions (Williams et al, 1992) have been observed in reflux patients in the absence of mechanical obstruction, there is little evidence that such effects can be attributed to the presence of refluxed acid. In fact, Corazziari and colleagues (1978) reported that with low pH boluses, *smaller* volumes are required for eliciting secondary peristalsis in the distal esophagus of normal volunteers. Furthermore, amplitude, duration, and velocity of peristalsis are unaffected by acid infusion in either reflux patients or in normal subjects (Burns and Venturatos, 1985; Orr et al, 1984). The results of studies utilizing prolonged acid infusion to produce experimental esophagitis in the opossum (Shirazi et al, 1989), baboon (Sinar et al, 1981), and cat (Spellun et al, 1987) suggest that alteration of peristalsis is secondary to an inflammatory response.

Voluntary Control

Valori and co-authors (1991) reported that peristaltic amplitudes are greater in subjects and patients who are instructed to perform "big gulps" in contrast to "little swallows." Although a "suggestion" effect on wet swallow peristaltic amplitude can be attributed to bolus volume (Hollis and Castell, 1975; Mittal et al, 1990), differences in dry swallow amplitude suggest a degree of voluntary control over peristalsis. The authors propose that biofeedback training may be of therapeutic benefit in some cases of abnormal peristaltic amplitude.

NEUROMUSCULAR CONTROL OF PERISTALSIS

Peristalsis during swallowing involves the coordinated contraction of CM and LM coats. Both coats contract with an aborally increasing latency following the onset of swallowing, but the LM contraction begins sooner and is propagated more rapidly (Sugarbaker et al, 1984b). Mechanically, the CM contraction produces the compressive, lumen-occluding force responsible for the pumping function of the esophagus (Brasseur, 1987). The LM contraction produces esophageal shortening (Edmundowicz and Clouse, 1991), presumably broadening the lumen and increasing the fiber density of the CM in advance of its contraction at each level (Miller et al, 1995), thus improving the efficiency of propulsion. In fact, the traction force applied to the bolus is better correlated to the degree of esophageal shortening distal to the recorded segment than to the amplitude of CM contraction within the segment (Pouderoux et al, 1997).

The muscular events that constitute esophageal peristalsis are coordinated by the autonomic nervous system. The esophagus receives both sympathetic and parasympathetic extrinsic innervation as well as enteric intrinsic innervation. However, striated and smooth esophageal muscle differ in terms of the neuromuscular mechanisms that control peristaltic contraction. The progressive contraction in striated muscle is coordinated by the CNS and is apparently the result of sequential activation of motoneurons innervating progressively more distal esophageal segments. In contrast, smooth esophageal muscle is innervated by postganglionic myenteric neurons. Although the CNS influences motility of the smooth muscle segment via preganglionic efferents, the importance of intramural and/or myogenic control is indicated by the observation that the general patterns of electrical and mechanical activity are preserved in various decentralized and reduced preparations.

Parasympathetic Control

Parasympathetic innervation of the esophagus is provided by the vagus nerves, which represent the major source of extrinsic functional control of the organ. There is considerable evidence that peristaltic contraction in the striated muscle esophagus is programmed centrally and that motor control is mediated by the vagus nerves. Bilateral vagotomy produces a permanent loss of all peristalsis in the esophagus of rabbits (Cannon, 1907) and dogs (Carveth et al, 1962; Hwang et al, 1947).

Roman (1966) sutured the central end of the vagus to the peripheral end of the spinal accessory nerve in sheep, which have striated esophageal musculature. Electromyographic (EMG) recordings were subsequently obtained in awake animals from nonesophageal skeletal muscles that had been innervated by vagal efferent axons. Single unit discharges related to contraction at different esophageal levels were sequentially recorded during peristalsis.

In species possessing smooth esophageal musculature, including the cat (Burgess et al, 1972; Cannon, 1907; Hwang, 1948; Jurica, 1926; Roman and Tieffenbach, 1971; Tieffenbach and Roman, 1972, but see Reynolds et al, 1985), opossum (Ryan et al, 1977), baboon (Tieffenbach and Roman, 1972), and monkey (Cannon, 1907), bilateral vagotomy results in permanent loss of primary peristalsis and paralysis of the striated muscle portion of the esophagus but secondary peristalsis is preserved or recovers in the smooth muscle portion. Electric stimulation of the peripheral end of the cut vagus in anesthetized cats causes increased tone and motility in smooth muscle esophagus (Dodds et al, 1978b; Knight, 1934). As the parameters of stimulation are varied, independent activation of longitudinal and circular smooth muscle may be observed electromyographically (Tieffenbach and Roman, 1972).

Vagal stimulation in anesthetized opossums results in poststimulation propagated contractions (B contractions) in the smooth muscle esophagus (Dodds et al, 1978a; Mukhopadhyay and Weisbrodt, 1975; Sarna et al, 1977; Sugarbaker et al, 1984b). With long-duration stimulus trains, intrastimulus propagated contractions (A contractions) occur in the opossum (Dodds et al, 1978a, 1978b) and cat (Dodds et al, 1978). The propagation velocity of vagal stimulation-produced peristalsis depends on the parameters of stimulation (Gidda et al, 1981) but under some conditions is similar to that of primary peristalsis in intact animals (Dodds et al, 1978a, 1978b; Mukhopadhyay and Weisbrodt, 1975).

When vagal innervation of the smooth muscle is intact, it may participate in the initiation of secondary peristalsis. For example, in monkeys with thoracic esophageal transection, secondary peristaltic contractions initiated by bolus injection into the distal segment often begin in the segment above the transection (Janssens et al, 1976). However, secondary peristalsis initiated by distention in the distal smooth muscle segment in baboons is not accompanied by vagal motor unit activity (Roman and Tieffenbach, 1972).

The inhibitory phase of peristalsis may also be controlled by central commands conveyed in the vagus nerves. Vagally mediated active inhibition of esophageal contractions can be demonstrated using low-level nerve stimulation (Tieffenbach and Roman, 1972) or successive stimulation at varying intervals (Gidda and Goyal, 1983). Gidda and Goyal (1984) recorded electrical activity during swallowing from fibers teased from the central stump of one cut vagus nerve in opossum. Fibers responded with bursts of activity that were bimodally distributed with respect to latency from the initiation of swallowing. Short-latency responses corresponded to smooth muscle inhibition, and long-latency responses to occurrence of the peristaltic contraction at various esophageal levels. The results of these studies suggest that both excitatory and inhibitory components of primary peristalsis in the smooth muscle segment involve vagally mediated CNS control, although CNS influence on secondary peristalsis is relatively weak.

Available anatomic evidence suggests that striated esophageal musculature is controlled by special visceral efferents arising in the nucleus ambiguus. Retrograde labeling with horseradish peroxidase (HRP) indicates that vagal efferent neurons, which innervate the striated muscle esophagus in the dog (Hudson and Cummings, 1985) and the rat (Bieger and Hopkins, 1987; Fryscak et al, 1984), are located in the compact cell column of the rostral nucleus ambiguus (NAc). Motor neurons labeled by injections at cervical, thoracic, and abdominal esophageal levels overlap extensively with no apparent viscerotopic organization, although retrograde transport of two fluorescent dyes from cervical and abdominal esophageal injection sites in rat produces no double-labeled cells and reveals a crude rostrocaudal topography within the compact cell division (Bieger and Hopkins, 1987; Galway et al, 1983). The existence of "bundled" dendrites in this region (Bieger and Hopkins, 1987) provides a potential mechanism for synchronous synaptic activation of groups of motor units.

In the dog, esophageal injection of HRP also labels two distinct groups of cells in the rostral and caudal poles of the dorsal motor nucleus of the vagus (Hudson and Cummings, 1985). However, medullary sites at which low intensity focal electric stimulation elicits esophageal EMG responses in rabbit, although common in the nucleus ambiguus, rarely occur in the dorsal motor nucleus (Lawn, 1964).

Neil and coworkers (1980) reported a similar distribution of label in the rostral and caudal dorsal motor nucleus following injections in the LES of cats, with labeling of ambiguual neurons being less prominent. In the rat, HRP injected at abdominal esophageal levels labels cell bodies in both the nucleus ambiguus and the dorsal motor nucleus. Cervical esophageal injections label only ambiguual neurons, and injections in the proximal stomach label only dorsal motor nucleus neurons (Fryscak et al, 1984). These results suggest that fibers arising in nucleus ambiguus innervate esophageal striated muscle, whereas those arising in the dorsal motor nucleus provide for preganglionic innervation of smooth muscle.

The vagus nerves also provide afferent innervation to the esophagus. Most vagal afferents to the esophagus arise from cell bodies located in the nodose ganglion via fibers in the esophageal branches of the vagus (thoracic) and the superior and recurrent laryngeal nerves (cervical) (Collman et al, 1992; Rodrigo et al, 1982), and they are characterized by highly arborized and laminar nerve endings within the myenteric ganglia (Rodrigo et al, 1975). Central termination of esophageal vagal afferents occurs primarily in the subnucleus centralis (NTSc) (Altschuler et al, 1989) within the nucleus of the tractus solitarius (NTS).

Several classes of esophageal receptors related to vagal afferents have been described. Afferent fibers related to slowly adapting mechanoreceptors located in the muscularis externa of the dog (Satchell, 1984), sheep (Falempin et al, 1978), rat (Andrew, 1956), opossum (Sengupta et al, 1989), and cat (Mei, 1970) esophagus respond during both distention and contraction. Richly innervated muscle spindles, which presumably function as stretch receptors, occur in the striated LM and CM layers of the canine (Asaad et al, 1983) but not the murine (Samarasinghe, 1972) esophagus. Vagal afferents related to warm-sensitive and cold-sensitive thermoreceptors in the abdominal esophagus have also been described (El Ouazzani and Mei, 1982).

In summary, experiments with animals have indicated the crucial nature of the vagal innervation to peristalsis in the esophagus. In striated muscle segments, vagal efferents directly program and control the progressive contraction. It is likely that activation of vagal afferents mediates the initiation of secondary peristalsis (Hwang, 1954) and bolus modulation of the peristaltic contraction by pressure (Roman, 1966) and temperature. Although peristalsis can occur in the smooth muscle segment after denervation or with simultaneous stimulation of decentralized vagus nerves, sequential central motor commands may normally modulate or entrain the peristaltic contraction in this region, as is apparently the case in the smooth muscle esophagus of some birds (Mule, 1991; Postorino et al, 1985).

It is more difficult to discern the role of vagal innervation in the control of peristalsis in humans. However, disordered peristalsis is associated with autonomic neuropathy in diseases such as diabetes (Channer et al, 1985; Loo et al, 1985; Russell et al, 1983) and dysautonomia (Linde and Westover, 1962). Cunningham and associates (1991) reported that 44% of patients with reflux who underwent testing exhibited abnormal vagal function and also experienced prolonged esophageal transit.

Sympathetic Control

Sympathetic efferent fibers innervating the esophagus arise in the cervical, thoracic chain and celiac ganglia (Hudson and Cummings, 1985). The esophageal musculature apparently does not receive direct efferent sympathetic innervation, however, as noradrenergic terminals demonstrated in the dog (Jacobowitz and Nemir Jr, 1969), cat, and monkey (Baumgarten and Lange, 1969) esophagus by histofluorescence techniques are largely confined to the myenteric ganglia. Correspondingly, Knight (1934) reported that electrical stimulation of sympathetic ganglia in cats produces no direct mechanical response but results in proximal augmentation and distal inhibition of esophageal contractions produced by vagal nerve stimulation.

The finding that sympathetic stimulation produces opposite modulatory effects in different esophageal regions suggests that more than one adrenergic receptor type may be present in esophageal muscle. In isolated strips of smooth muscle from the cat distal esophagus in vitro, α-adrenergic receptor stimulation produces contraction of LM (Christensen and Daniel, 1966) or CM, while β-adrenergic receptor stimulation inhibits CM contractions elicited with cholinergic agonists (Christensen and Daniel, 1968). Similarly, specific β-adrenergic agonists decrease the amplitude of peristaltic pressure waves in humans (Lyrenas and Abrahamsson, 1986), and noradrenaline is capable of producing both contraction and relaxation of human esophageal smooth muscle strips in vitro (Ellis et al, 1960).

Sympathetic nerves have also been found to provide spinal afferent innervation to the esophagus. Injections of fast blue into striated, smooth, and LES muscle segments of cats label cell bodies in C1-T8, C5-L2, and T1-L3 dorsal root ganglia, respectively (Collman et al, 1992). Clerc and Mei (1983) recorded excitatory unit responses to esophageal stretch and manipulation in feline thoracic spinal ganglia related to low threshold, slowly adapting mechanoreceptors located in the esophageal muscularis externa. These results suggest that sympathetic innervation may provide for modulation of esophageal peristalsis via a spinal reflex mechanism. However, no anatomic or physiologic evidence for such a reflex has been reported.

Jurica (1926) found that bilateral splanchnicectomy had no effect on esophageal motility in cats. Similarly, bilateral upper thoracic sympathectomy in humans does not appear to affect esophageal peristalsis (Soffer et al, 1988). On the other hand, Sengupta and associates (1990) recorded high threshold esophageal mechanoreceptive units from opossum sympathetic nerve fibers and suggested that they may serve a nociceptive function. Spinal reflexes linked to activation of such units by extreme intraesophageal pressure elevation may account for disrupted peristalsis observed during severe or chronic esophageal obstruction (Little et al, 1986; Mittal et al, 1990).

Central Nervous System Control

Although the stereotyped nature of the deglutition reflex implies the existence of a central pattern generator, the nature and location of involved brain circuitry have not been clearly established. Jean and colleagues have described a medullary swallowing center mediating CNS control of swallowing in sheep and have suggested that a group of units located in the NTS and the surrounding reticular formation, the dorsal region, control the patterning of both oropharyngeal and esophageal stages of swallowing (Jean, 1972a). These units fire in relation to swallowing-related muscular contractions and project to relevant motor nuclei.

"Early" units are located rostrally in the dorsal region and fire in relation to oropharyngeal muscle contraction. They project directly to motor neurons in the nucleus ambiguus and via a relay in the ventral region of the swallowing center to the motor trigeminal, facial, and hypoglossal nuclei (Amri et al, 1984; Jean et al, 1983). "Late" and "very late" firing units are located more caudally in the dorsal region and exhibit activity related to the esophageal stage of swallowing. Delayed excitation by these pre-motor neurons and direct inhibition in response to swallowing (Zoungrana et al, 1997) apparently both contribute to the timing of esophageal ambiguual motor neuron activation.

Caudally placed lesions in the dorsal region selectively abolish the esophageal stage of the deglutition reflex (Jean, 1972b). Units in this region receive afferent input from esophageal levels to which they apparently provide motor control. Thus, vagal sensory and motor nuclei related to striated muscle esophagus may be monosynaptically (Loewy and Spyer, 1990) and/or disynaptically (Cunningham and Sawchenko, 1989) connected and may represent a vagovagal reflex pathway. However, although the activity of esophageal afferents may trigger or modify peristalsis (Jean, 1984), it is not essential to central circuitry responsible for programming the sequential contraction.

Peripheral motor paralysis with curare does not alter the timing of unit firing, indicating that central patterning rather than peripheral feedback is responsible for sequential motor commands (Jean, 1972a). It is not clear, however, whether such patterning arises from the synaptic arrangement of dorsal region neurons or is projected from elsewhere in the brain.

A discrete pathway from the NTSc to rostral nucleus ambiguus has been identified in the rat and may represent esophageal command neurons homologous to the dorsal region in sheep (Barrett et al, 1994; Cunningham and Sawchenko, 1989). NTSc neurons receive esophageal vagal afferents (Altschuler et al, 1989), creating the anatomic substrate for a bilateral disynaptic circuit that likely mediates initiation of secondary peristalsis and bolus modulation in striated muscle esophagus (Lu and Bieger, 1998a). However, several lines of evidence converge to suggest that NTSc neurons, in addition to providing an excitatory relay in a reflex arc, also integrate peripheral and central inputs and comprise a pattern generator for propagated contraction through the striated muscle esophagus. These neurons respond to a biochemically diverse set of inputs and contain an array of putative transmitters and neuromodulators. Diffuse excitatory stimulation or disinhibition of the region produces rhythmic activity phase-locked to propulsive esophageal contractions. These neurons may constitute a motor pattern generator for esophageal peristalsis by virtue of intrinsic membrane properties, chemical coding, and synaptic connectivity to each other and to motor neurons.

Esophageal vagal afferents probably use glutamate as a transmitter (Schaffar et al, 1997) to excite NTSc neurons via *N*-methyl-D-aspartate (NMDA) (Broussard et al, 1995) and non-NMDA excitatory amino acid receptors (Lu and Bieger, 1998b). Bath application of NMDA to brainstem slice preparations induces rhythmic bursting of NTS neurons (Tell and Jean, 1990, 1993), whereas microinjections of S-glutamate in the NTSc in vivo can elicit single, propulsive esophageal contractions (Bieger, 1984).

Muscarinic cholinergic agonists microinjected into NTSc produce repetitive propulsive or simultaneous esophageal contractions (Lu et al, 1997). Muscarinic receptor antagonism in NTSc reduces neuronal and esophageal responses to distention (Lu and Bieger, 1998b) and eliminates the esophageal phase of evoked swallowing (Bieger, 1984; Wang and Bieger, 1991a). Although abundant choline acetyltransferase immunoreactive nerve fibers innervate the NTSc (Ruggiero et al, 1990), the source of cholinergic input to these neurons is not yet clear.

NTSc neurons also receive a tonic GABAergic inhibition, which apparently maintains the motor circuit in a quiescent state (Broussard et al, 1996; Wang and Bieger, 1991a). Rhythmic esophageal contractions are elicited by local application of the GABAA receptor antagonist bicuculline in the NTSc (Wang and Bieger, 1991a). Subthreshold bicuculline doses enhance coupling of propulsive esophageal responses to evoked pharyngeal contractions (Wang and Bieger, 1991a), implying that coordination of buccopharyngeal and esophageal phases of swallowing involves NTSc disinhibition. Possible mediators of such coordination would include populations of neurons identified in the intermediate and interstitial NTS subnuclei that project to both esophageal and pharyngeal premotor neurons (Broussard et al, 1998).

NTSc neurons projecting to esophageal motor neurons appear to utilize a variety of neurotransmitter and neuromodulator substances, including glutamate and/or aspartate (Wang et al, 1991b, 1993), somatostatin (Broussard et al, 1998; Cunningham et al, 1991; Wang et al, 1993;), enkephalin (Cunningham et al, 1991), and nitric oxide (NO) (Broussard et al, 1995; Wiedner et al, 1995). Esophageal motor neurons in the NAc are excited by glutamate and acetylcholine (via nicotinic receptors); earlier cholinergic excitation potentiates the glutamate response (Wang et al, 1991a). NMDA receptor activation, presumably by glutamate, is crucial to motor neuron excitation (Wang et al, 1991b). One potential source of cholinergic input has been located in the medullary reticular formation, where some neurons that are retrogradely labeled by NAc tracer injections are also immunoreactive for choline acetyltransferase (Zhang et al, 1993).

Colocalization of somatostatin with enkephalin has been demonstrated in some neurons (Cunningham et al, 1991), and most of the cells in this projection contain the synthetic enzyme for NO. Somatostatin gates motor neuronal NMDA receptor activation (Wang et al, 1993) and inhibits nicotinic cholinoceptor activation (Wang et al, 1991b), whereas NO may potentiate nicotinic neurotransmission (Briggs, 1992). No role has yet been postulated for enkephalin in this pathway, however, and it is unknown how these various neurochemical interactions might relate to modulation or patterning of motor neuron output or affect rhythmicity of the circuit.

The orderly and oriented structure, synaptic connectivity (Hopkins, 1995), and rostral-to-caudal topographic arrangement (Bieger and Hopkins, 1987) of motor neurons imply that cellular architecture within the NAc may contribute to propagation of peristalsis in striated muscle esophagus. In addition, though, the presence of calcitonin gene-related peptide (CGRP) (Lee et al, 1992) and galanin (Kuramoto et al, 1996) in these cholinergic motor neurons and coinnervation of esophageal motor endplates by enteric interneurons (see later) suggest that neurochemical coding at the level of the neuromuscular junction may also play a role.

Central control of peristalsis in animals with smooth muscle esophagus is less well characterized. Systemic administration of nicotine elicits striated and smooth muscle esophageal peristalsis in cats without oropharyngeal activation via a central, vagus nerve-dependent mechanism (Greenwood et al, 1992). Although this observation suggests that the esophageal stage of swallowing is controlled by a discrete central circuit, the details of such a circuit have not been elucidated.

Enteric Nervous System Control

Enteric Neuroanatomy

The esophagus is innervated by two interconnected plexuses: a submucosal plexus within the submucosa and a myenteric plexus between the LM and CM layers of the muscularis externa. Several anatomic features distinguish the enteric innervation of the esophagus from that of the rest of the gut.

The esophageal submucosal plexus consists of a network of fibers and contains few (Christensen et al, 1983) or no (Jacobowitz and Nemir Jr, 1969; Asaad et al, 1983) ganglion cells. The myenteric plexus contains numerous ganglia, but unlike most other regions of the gut (Christensen et al, 1983), these are irregularly arranged in relation to fiber bundle crossings.

The function of ganglion cells observed in striated muscle regions (Asaad et al, 1983; Bremner et al, 1970; Floyd, 1973; Jacobowitz and Nemir Jr, 1969; Marklin et al, 1979; Samarasinghe, 1972;) is not known, although it has been suggested that they may be second-order secretomotor neurons innervating the submucosa (Asaad et al, 1983). In smooth muscle regions, many ganglion cells are undoubtedly postganglionic motor neurons innervating the muscle layers. These are probably Dogiel type I neurons, which are innervated by club-like or bud-like endings of nonmyelinated fibers (Rodrigo et al, 1975). In the opossum, the density of nerve cells and ganglia decreases aborally along the smooth muscle esophagus, becoming minimal at the lower sphincter (Christensen and Robison, 1982; Marklin et al, 1979), but the relationship of this gradient to apparent regional gradients of transmitter release in vitro (e.g., Crist et al, 1984a) is unclear.

In Vitro Studies of Enteric Activation

Many details of the pharmacology of enteric innervation of esophageal smooth muscle have been elucidated using in vitro preparations, which offer the advantages that LM and CM may be studied separately and that bath concentrations of agents can be precisely controlled. To a large extent, the principal features of smooth muscle motility are preserved.

The excised esophagus may be stimulated electrically or by intraluminal balloon inflation, producing responses similar to those induced by vagal stimulation or distention, respectively, in vivo (Christensen and Lund, 1969):

- An intrastimulus "on" (A) contraction at and proximal to the point of stimulation
- An intrastimulus longitudinal shortening (duration response)
- A post-stimulus, distally propagated "off" (B) contraction

In isolated strips of smooth muscle from animal (Chan and Diamant, 1976; Christensen and Lund, 1969; Crist et al, 1984b) or human (Bennett and Stockley, 1975; McKirdy and Marshall, 1985; Tottrup et al, 1990a) esophagus, enteric nerve activation may be achieved by electric field stimulation (EFS). When stimulation parameters are appropriately adjusted, all responses to EFS are abolished by tetrodotoxin, suggesting that they are mediated by activation of intramural nerves. EFS produces intrastimulus "on" and post-stimulus "off" contractions of CM rings or strips. Intrastimulus inhibition is apparent as a relaxation response when a tone exists (Bennett and Stockley, 1975) or is induced in CM strips (Behar et al, 1989; Tottrup et al, 1990a) and often masks "on" contractions at low stimulation frequencies. CM "off" contractions are generally considered to be analogous to the peristaltic CM contraction in the intact organ, as both contractions follow a period of neurogenic inhibition.

Exposure of LM strips to EFS results in duration contractions (Christensen and Lund, 1969; Lund and Christensen, 1969; Tottrup et al, 1990a) and, at high frequencies, *extended-duration* contractions, which outlast stimulation and which are more prolonged distally (Crist et al, 1986). Extended-duration LM contractions have also been observed in the distal opossum esophagus in vivo in association with peristalsis produced by both swallowing and vagal stimulation (Sugarbaker et al, 1984b).

Acetylcholine

There is considerable evidence that acetylcholine appears to be an excitatory neurotransmitter used by esophageal postganglionic enteric neurons, and it acts at muscarinic receptors on smooth muscle cells. Pharmacologic stimulation of cholinergic mechanisms generally enhances peristalsis, whereas muscarinic antagonism diminishes it. In humans, cholinergic stimulation with bethanechol increases primary peristaltic amplitude and decreases its velocity (Hollis and Castell, 1976; Humphries and Castell, 1981). Intravenous (Ceccatelli et al, 1988; Corazziari et al, 1989; Gilbert et al, 1987) but not oral (Gilbert et al, 1987; Wallin et al, 1987) cisapride enhances peristaltic amplitude and duration in an atropine-sensitive manner.

Cholinergic agonists also cause atropine-sensitive contractions of isolated strips of LM (Christensen and Daniel, 1966) and CM (Behar et al, 1989; Christensen and Daniel, 1968; Nelson and Mangel, 1979) from animal and human (Bennett and Stockley, 1975; Ellis et al, 1960; Tottrup et al, 1990c) esophagus. Physostigmine and metoclopramide affect distal primary peristalsis by increasing the amplitude, duration, and propagation velocity of contraction (DiPalma et al, 1987; Gidda and Buyniski, 1986; Tolu et al, 1988),* and enhance the amplitude of "off" contractions in humans (McKirdy and Marshall, 1985) and cats (Behar et al, 1989) CM strips.

Muscarinic antagonism with intravenous (Dodds et al, 1981; Jaup et al, 1982; Marzio et al, 1989) or intramuscular (Kantrowitz et al, 1966) atropine decreases the incidence and amplitude (by about 60%) of primary peristalsis in humans. In the opossum, intravenous atropine abolishes esophageal shortening associated with swallowing, although nonmuscarinic and/or myogenic LM contractions are associated with balloon distention in some animals (Paterson, 1997a).

In in vitro experiments, LM duration contractions are antagonized by atropine (Crist et al, 1986; Lund and Christensen, 1969; Murray et al, 1991; Tottrup et al, 1990a). In CM strips, "on" contractions are 90% abolished by atropine (Crist et al, 1984b; Richards et al, 1995), but the role of cholinergic mechanisms in "off" responses differs among various species studied.

In the opossum, although cholinergic agonists enhance the CM "off" contraction (Christensen et al, 1991; Cohen and Green, 1974), atropine has little effect on the response of untreated strips (Crist et al, 1984b; Lund and Christensen, 1969). In contrast, "off" responses are totally abolished in cat CM (Behar et al, 1989; Leander et al, 1982) and up to 90% inhibited in human CM strips (Tottrup et al, 1990a) by atropine.

The M_1 muscarinic receptor antagonist pirenzepine disrupts primary peristalsis in the human distal esophagus (Jaup et al, 1982), whereas selective M_2 (but not M_1) receptor blockade disrupts smooth muscle primary peristalsis in opossum (Gilbert and Dodds, 1986) and cat (Blank et al, 1989).

Catecholamines

As previously mentioned, adrenergic innervation has not been found to contribute substantially to the normal control of peristalsis; dopaminergic innervation is probably not involved in the control of peristalsis either. Exogenous dopamine produces tetrodotoxin-resistant contractile responses and reduces EFS-produced "off" response amplitude in opossum CM strips. However, haloperidol and bulbocapnine do not affect EFS-produced "off" responses, although they antagonize the effects of exogenous dopamine (de Carle and Christensen, 1976). In feline esophageal smooth muscle, dopamine histofluorescence is lacking (Baumgarten and Lange, 1969), and exogenous dopamine does not affect EFS-produced responses (Behar et al, 1989).

However, there is good evidence for both noncholinergic excitatory and nonadrenergic inhibitory innervation of esophageal smooth muscle. In particular, the data suggest that neuropeptides and nitric oxide may function as nonadrenergic, noncholinergic (NANC) neurotransmitters in the esophagus.

Nitric Oxide

Nitric oxide relaxes smooth muscle and is a candidate mediator of NANC inhibition in the esophagus and the LES. It is synthesized from L-arginine by nitric oxide synthase (NOS). This enzyme can be detected in myenteric nerves throughout the esophagus, being relatively more abundant in smooth muscle regions (Fang and Christensen, 1994; Ny et al, 1994).

In cats and monkeys, 35% to 40% of esophageal myenteric ganglion cells are immunoreactive for NOS. Immunoreactive fibers course through striated regions parallel to muscle fibers and form dense plexuses in smooth muscle regions, with equal density in CM and LM coats (Rodrigo et al, 1998). In the human esophagus, more than half of ganglion cells contain NOS (Singaram et al, 1994), as do abundant varicose fibers throughout circular (Richards et al, 1995) and, to a lesser extent, longitudinal smooth muscle (Singaram et al, 1994).

*Interestingly, metoclopramide does not affect esophageal motility in patients with erosive reflux esophagitis (Grande et al, 1992).

Competitive inhibition of NO synthesis by intravenous administration of L-arginine analogs increases primary peristaltic velocity and decreases contraction amplitude in the opossum and cat in vivo (Anand and Paterson, 1994; Yamato et al, 1992; Xue et al, 1996, but see Tottrup et al, 1991). Primary peristalsis is abolished in the opossum when NOS inhibition is combined with atropine (Anand and Paterson, 1994). NOS inhibition also abolishes vagal stimulation–produced B contractions and post-balloon distention-propagated contractions along with the characteristic hyperpolarization-depolarization sequence normally recorded in CM (Anand and Paterson, 1994; Yamato et al, 1992).

In healthy humans, NOS inhibitors increase the amplitude of peristaltic waves distally and increase velocity proximally (Hirsch et al, 1998), whereas recombinant hemoglobin, which binds NO, increases peristaltic velocity and contraction amplitude and duration (Murray et al, 1995). Inhibitory L-arginine analogs also abolish (and L-arginine restores) EFS-produced "off" contractions of CM preparations from the opossum (Knudsen et al, 1991; Murray et al, 1991; Yamato et al, 1992) and human (Richards et al, 1995) esophagus in vitro. These results suggest that NO synthesis mediates neurogenic inhibition of esophageal CM, which normally controls the velocity of peristalsis in the smooth muscle segment, and accounts for delayed, post-stimulus contractions in vitro.

Available biophysical evidence obtained by whole-cell patch-clamp of dispersed circular smooth muscle cells indicates that NO hyperpolarizes muscle cells by activating a calcium-dependent potassium current (Jury et al, 1996; Murray et al, 1995) and/or by suppressing a calcium-activated chloride current (Zhang et al, 1998) via a cyclic guanosine monophosphate (cGMP)–dependent mechanism.

Peptides

A variety of neuropeptides have been localized in enteric neurons and nerve fibers innervating esophageal muscle, including (1) vasoactive intestinal polypeptide (VIP), (2) CGRP, (3) galanin, (4) substance P (SP), (5) neuropeptide Y, and (6) met-enkephalin (Singaram et al, 1991). The pattern of peptidergic innervation of the human esophagus is distinct relative to other regions of the gut (Wattchow et al, 1987). Evidence to date is consistent with a role for several of these peptides in mediating modulation of peristalsis in the esophagus.

Substance P

Immunoreactive SP has been localized in neuronal processes within cat (Leander et al, 1982; Rodrigo et al, 1985), monkey (Rodrigo et al, 1985), opossum (Christensen et al, 1989; Domoto et al, 1983), and human (Singaram et al, 1991; Wattchow et al, 1987, 1988) smooth muscle esophagus. Exogenous SP causes contraction and enhances EFS-produced responses in CM strips (Leander et al, 1982; Richards et al, 1992; Sugarbaker et al, 1993). In human CM strips, the SP antagonist spantide II or SP tachyphylaxis inhibits the atropine-resistant component of "off" contractions (Sugarbaker et al, 1993). In opossum LM strips, exogenous SP produces contraction and SP tachyphylaxis abolishes the extended-duration response to high-frequency EFS (Crist et al, 1986). These results suggest that SP innervation of the smooth muscle esophagus may contribute to and/or may modulate the peristaltic contraction.

Calcitonin Gene-Related Peptide

CGRP-immunoreactive nerves have been localized in the rat, cat, monkey (Rodrigo et al, 1985), opossum (Christensen et al, 1995; Rattan et al, 1988), and human (Singaram et al, 1991) esophagus. Although CGRP nerves have been associated with a sensory function (Green and Dockray, 1987; Parkman et al, 1989; Rodrigo et al, 1985), inhibitory motor properties have also been noted in the cat (Parkman et al, 1989) and opossum (Rattan et al, 1988), apparently acting both directly at the level of smooth muscle and by stimulating other NANC inhibitory nerves. In opossum CM strips in vitro, exogenous CGRP diminishes amplitude and prolongs latency of "off" contractions. The inhibitor peptide CGRP8-37 increases amplitude and diminishes latency, implying a release from endogenous CGRP-mediated inhibition (Aliye et al, 1997). CGRP colocalizes with NOS in human (Singaram et al, 1994) esophageal enteric nerves. CGRP- and NOS-containing fibers demonstrate similar graded distribution in the opossum, being more abundant proximally in the CM and distally in the LM of the smooth muscle segment (Christensen et al, 1995). These results suggest that CGRP may mediate inhibitory modulation of smooth muscle peristalsis.

CGRP and SP appear to be colocalized in some LES enteric neurons (Parkman et al, 1989) and in other viscera (Maggi and Meli, 1988), but this is apparently not the case in the esophageal body (Rodrigo et al, 1985).

Vasoactive Intestinal Polypeptide

VIP has been postulated to be an inhibitory NANC neurotransmitter in humans (Ny et al, 1995), cat (Biancani et al, 1984) and opossums (Goyal and Rattan, 1980) LES, but its role in esophageal peristalsis is less clear. Intraaortic VIP in the opossum stimulates esophageal body smooth muscle contractions, which are often (65%) peristaltic (Rattan et al, 1982). However, its in vitro effects on cat esophageal body CM are inhibitory (Behar et al, 1989).

In the human esophagus, 27% of myenteric ganglion cells exhibit VIP immunoreactivity and 92% of ganglion cells are associated with VIP immunoreactive nerve terminals (Singaram et al, 1994). Achalasia is associated with a loss of nerves containing VIP from esophageal tissue (Aggestrup et al, 1983) and in some patients with achalasia and scleroderma, symptomatic relief (including augmented peristalsis) has been achieved with transcutaneous nerve stimulation, a procedure that significantly elevates plasma VIP levels (Kaada, 1987).

VIP colocalizes with NOS in some myenteric nerves, and there is evidence that VIP may act synergistically with NO in producing relaxation of gastrointestinal smooth muscle (Murthy et al, 1996). Synergism of this nature in the esophagus has not been reported, although 14% of NOS-containing neurons in human esophageal myenteric ganglia are VIP immunoreactive (Singaram et al, 1994).

Galanin

In the opossum, 54% of NOS-positive myenteric ganglion cells are immunoreactive for galanin (Christensen and Fang, 1994). Although only 10% of NOS-containing cells are coreactive for galanin in human esophageal myenteric ganglia, 64% are associated with galanin immunoreactive nerve terminals (Singaram et al, 1994). However, the significance of this peptide's colocalization with NOS and its role in the control of esophageal motility remain unclear.

In striated muscle esophagus of the rat, NOS-containing terminals coinnervate motor endplates (Worl et al, 1994), and 91% of these terminals are also galanin-immunoreactive (Kuramoto et al, 1999). These neurons are of enteric origin, and many are also immunoreactive for VIP (Worl et al, 1998). In addition to direct synaptic contacts on striated muscle, they exhibit presynaptic contacts on CGRP immunoreactive nerve fibers at motor endplates (Worl et al, 1997), which have been demonstrated to be ambiguual motor neurons (Lee et al, 1992). These results are suggestive of a complex enteric influence on motility in striated muscle esophagus. For example, the aborally increasing density of coinnervated endplates along the length of the esophagus (Worl et al, 1994) suggests that these enteric neurons may mediate descending inhibition. However, no details concerning functional enteric influence on peristalsis have been reported in the rat, nor has the generality of this pattern of striated muscle innervation been demonstrated in humans or other species.

Enkephalins

Met-enkephalin analogs administered intravenously (Jian et al, 1987) or intramuscularly (Stacher et al, 1982) increase the amplitude, duration, and velocity of distal primary peristalsis in human subjects, suggesting that opioid stimulation interrupts esophageal inhibitory mechanisms. However, the role of endogenous met-enkephalin in the esophagus (Singaram et al, 1991) is unclear because neither naloxone (Mittal et al, 1986) nor enkephalinase inhibitors (Chaussade et al, 1988) affect peristaltic contractions.

One possibility is that enkephalin may be a mediator or modulator of sympathetic control of esophageal motility, in which case such pharmacologic manipulation might require simultaneous sympathetic activation to produce a detectable effect on motility. Consistent with this interpretation are the restriction of both met-enkephalinergic (Singaram et al, 1991) and noradrenergic (Baumgarten and Lange, 1969; Jacobowitz and Nemir Jr, 1969) esophageal innervation to myenteric ganglia, a modulatory effect of sympathetic ganglion stimulation on esophageal motility (Knight, 1934) and a suspected sympathetic function of enkephalins in the proximal gut (Bachoo et al, 1987).

Myogenic Control

Control of peristalsis in the smooth muscle segment may also involve a myogenic component. Sarna and coworkers (1977) demonstrated that esophageal smooth muscle is capable of propagated contraction independent of neural influence. Direct stimulation of esophageal smooth muscle in vivo in opossums causes a bidirectionally propagated contraction. This response is not blocked by intra-arterial tetrodotoxin, indicating a myogenic mechanism, and is facilitated by factors that would be expected to depolarize esophageal smooth muscle (e.g., intra-arterial infusion of potassium chloride or tetraethylammonium, death) (Sarna et al, 1977). Ultrastructural examination reveals that circular smooth muscle cells from the opossum esophageal body are connected to adjacent muscle cells by numerous gap junctions (Daniel and Posey-Daniel, 1984). Thus, it is likely that propagated contraction in circular smooth muscle is at least partly mediated by electrotonic spread of activation. Circular smooth muscle cells are also connected by gap junctions to interstitial cells of Cajal. Because neuronal varicosities innervate both muscle cells and interstitial cells, it has been suggested that the latter may mediate some neurogenic responses in this tissue (Daniel and Posey-Daniel, 1984).

The findings that longitudinal smooth muscle is not commonly associated with gap junctions (Daniel et al, 1976) and that vagal stimulation produces simultaneous LM contraction indicate that sequential LM contraction during swallowing is probably neurally controlled and depends on central patterning (Sugarbaker et al, 1984b). However, apparently myogenic esophageal shortening and propagated LM contraction have been observed in an opossum in vitro preparation in response to balloon distention and long-duration electrical pulses, respectively (Paterson, 1997a).

Myogenic mechanisms may also contribute to bolus modulation of peristalsis. For example, the force and power developed by esophageal CM during "off" contractions depend on its degree of stretch (determined in vivo by bolus volume and viscosity) prior to contraction and on the force against which it contracts (determined by intrabolus pressure), other factors being equal (Cohen and Green, 1973; Tottrup et al, 1990c).

Electrophysiology of Esophageal Muscle

Electromyography reveals that peristaltic contraction in both striated and smooth muscle is associated with action potential discharge. Electrical activity in striated (canine) esophageal muscle precedes the arrival of the peristaltic pressure wave at the site of recording, attains a peak frequency coincident with peak pressure, and dies out as resting pressure is restored (Arimori et al, 1970; Hellemans and Vantrappen, 1967). Esophageal striated muscle fibers are characterized as "twitch" type by morphologic (Samarasinghe, 1972) and physiologic (Dodds et al, 1978) criteria, but they are innervated by nonmyelinated axon terminals of central motor neurons at unusual motor endplate synapses, where more than one terminal often innervates the same endplate (Samarasinghe, 1972).

In smooth (opossum) esophageal muscle, spike bursts are associated primarily with the initial rising phase of the primary (Rattan et al, 1983) and secondary (Paterson, 1989) peristaltic pressure complex. Direct-current recording with serosal suction electrodes reveals that peristalsis is associated with initial hyperpolarization followed by depolarization, spike burst, and contraction (Paterson, 1989; Rattan et al, 1983). In this situation, both LM and CM activity are recorded; recording separately from each muscle layer reveals that LM exhibits only depolarization, whereas the hyperpolarization-depolarization sequence is associated with CM (Sugarbaker et al, 1984a). Serosal recordings from the isolated smooth muscle esophagus in vitro during balloon inflation reveal proximal "on" and distal propagated "off" bursts of action potentials (Christensen, 1970).

In vitro recordings of CM membrane potential using intracellular microelectrode (Chan and Diamant, 1976; Crist et al, 1987; Daniel et al, 1977; Decktor and Ryan, 1982; Du et al, 1991) or sucrose gap (Serio and Daniel, 1988) techniques have shown that CM cells (or syncytia) respond to EFS with *inhibitory (hyperpolarizing) junction potentials* (IJPs), often followed by *excitatory (depolarizing) junction potentials* (EJPs). IJPs are inhibited by tetrodotoxin (Daniel et al, 1977) and nitric oxide synthesis inhibitors (Du et al, 1991). Measurements of input resistance during the IJP and of its reversal potential (Jury et al, 1985; Kannan et al, 1985) suggest mediation by an increased K^+ conductance. However, decreased chloride conductance has also been proposed as a mechanism (Crist et al, 1991).

It has been suggested that anode-break "rebound" from membrane hyperpolarization contributes to post-stimulus excitation and "off" contractions (Wood and Marsh, 1973); however, the voltage dependence of inactivation of relevant membrane channels has not been described in esophageal smooth muscle. Whatever the contribution of membrane potential rebound may be, it is likely that EFS-produced release of excitatory transmitters (e.g., acetylcholine and/or substance P) also contributes to post-stimulation depolarization (see earlier). Although delayed CM depolarization requires NO-mediated inhibition, depolarization per se does not (Conklin et al, 1991; Du et al, 1991).

A number of studies have established the dependence of esophageal smooth muscle contraction on the extracellular Ca^{2+} concentration. The force generated by opossum CM strips in response to EFS is maximal at 2.5 mM bath concentrations of Ca^{2+} and is reduced at lower concentrations (Cohen and Green, 1973). Opossum esophageal LM and CM contractions are abolished in Ca^{2+}-free medium and in medium containing excess Mg^{2+}, although restoration of contractile responses in CM, but not in LM, by addition of strontium suggests that different Ca^{2+}-dependent mechanisms may mediate contraction in the two layers (de Carle et al, 1977). In vitro EFS-produced contractions of feline CM are also abolished by removal of Ca^{2+} from the medium (Biancani et al, 1987).

Ca^{2+} channel blockers (primarily nifedipine, diltiazem, and verapamil) have been used experimentally and clinically (Castell, 1985) and have been found to reduce peristaltic amplitude in normal human subjects (Konrad-Dalhoff et al, 1991; Smout et al, 1992) and in patients with achalasia (Blackwell et al, 1981; Triadafilopoulos et al, 1991), nutcracker esophagus (Richter et al, 1984), and diffuse spasm (Blackwell et al, 1981).

Mechanism of Propagation

It is clear that the CNS controls peristaltic contraction of LM and striated CM, although most of the details of the responsible central circuitry remain to be elucidated. The mechanisms controlling propagated contraction of circular smooth muscle are less clear. It has been suggested that peristaltic progression through the smooth muscle segment may be due to regional gradients in the physiologic properties of the smooth muscle and its innervation. Of particular interest is the finding that the latency of "off" contractions is longer in strips of CM taken from distal segments than in those from proximal segments (Weisbrodt and Christensen, 1972).

Although the magnitude of this latency gradient depends on the parameters of EFS employed (Christensen et al, 1991; Crist et al, 1984a), its existence in isolated strips corresponds to graded duration of the inhibitory effects of vagal stimulation in vivo (Gidda and Goyal, 1985). Spatial gradients of CM and LM response duration (Crist et al, 1986), membrane potential (Decktor and Ryan, 1982, but see Crist et al, 1987), potassium content (Schulze et al, 1977; Schulze et al, 1978), refractory properties (Weisbrodt and Christensen, 1972), acetylcholine release (Crist et al, 1984a; Gilbert and Dodds, 1986), and SP sensitivity (Richards et al, 1992) and release (Crist et al, 1986) have also been reported, based on examination of strips of CM or LM from different levels of the esophagus. However, the role of these gradients in vivo has not been clearly established.

The data suggest that control of smooth muscle peristalsis involves a combination of myogenic and neurogenic mechanisms. Excitation and contraction of circular smooth muscle would be expected to spread electronically from an area of local excitation. The contraction would be unidirectional by virtue of distally oriented *neurogenic inhibition* (mediated by NO), which would also mediate control of propagation velocity. Neurogenic depolarization would sustain propagation (acetylcholine). The relatively short time scale of the action of NO and acetylcholine would implicate these substances in the short-term (intraswallow) modulation of contraction amplitude and velocity, whereas longer-term modulation (e.g., over the course of a meal) probably involves enteric neuropeptides.

The balance between neurogenic excitatory and inhibitory processes apparent in the control of normal peristalsis at both central and peripheral levels provides a framework for interpretation of esophageal dysfunction in disease. In particular, esophageal primary motor disorders (Konturek et al, 1995; Mearin et al, 1993; Paterson, 1997b; Tottrup et al, 1990b; Wattchow and Costa, 1996;) and gastroesophageal reflux disease (Ceccatelli et al, 1988; Janssens and Sifrim, 1997; Rossiter et al, 1991; Wienbeck and Li, 1989) may be associated with disruptions of this balance. Further work elucidating the normal physiology of esophageal function will continue to direct development and evaluation of new therapies for such disorders.

Acknowledgment

The authors wish to thank Mary Sullivan Visciano for editorial assistance.

■ REFERENCES

Aggestrup S, Uddman R, Sundler F, et al: Lack of vasoactive intestinal polypeptide nerves in esophageal achalasia. Gastroenterology 84:924, 1983.

Aliye UC, Murray JA and Conklin JL: Effects of calcitonin gene-related peptide on opossum esophageal smooth muscle. Gastroenterology 113:514, 1997.

Altschuler SM, Bao X, Bieger D, et al: Viscerotopic representation of the upper alimentary tract in the rat: Sensory ganglia and nuclei of the solitary and spinal trigeminal tracts. J Comp Neurol 283:248, 1989.

Amri M, Car A, Jean A: Medullary control of the pontine swallowing neurones in sheep. Exp Brain Res 55:105, 1984.

Anand N, Paterson WG: Role of nitric oxide in esophageal peristalsis. Am J Physiol 266:G123, 1994.

Andrew BL: The nervous control of the cervical oesophagus of the rat during swallowing. J Physiol (Lond) 134:729, 1956.

Anvari M, Richards D, Dent J, et al: The effect of glucagon on esophageal peristalsis and clearance. Gastrointest Radiol 14:100, 1989.

Arimori M, Code CF, Schlegel JF, et al: Electrical activity of the canine esophagus and gastroesophageal sphincter. Am J Dig Dis 15:191, 1970.

Armstrong D, Emde C, Bumm R, et al: Twenty-four-hour pattern of esophageal motility in asymptomatic volunteers. Dig Dis Sci 35:1190, 1990.

Arndorfer RC, Stef JJ, Dodds WJ, et al: Improved infusion system for intraluminal esophageal manometry. Gastroenterology 73:23, 1977.

Asaad K, Abd-El Rahman S, Nawar NNY, et al: Intrinsic innervation of the oesophagus in dogs with special reference to the presence of muscle spindles. Acta Anat 115:91, 1983.

Ask P, Tibbling L: Effect of time interval between swallows on esophageal peristalsis. Am J Physiol 238:G485, 1980.

Bachoo M, Ciriello J, Polosa C: Effect of preganglionic stimulation on neuropeptide-like immunoreactivity in the stellate ganglion of the cat. Brain Res 400:377, 1987.

Bardan E, Xie P, Ren J, et al: Effect of pharyngeal water stimulation on esophageal peristalsis and bolus transport. Am J Physiol 272:G265, 1997.

Barrett RT, Bao X, Miselis RR, et al: Brain stem localization of rodent esophageal premotor neurons revealed by transneuronal passage of pseudorabies virus. Gastroenterology 107:728, 1994.

Baumgarten HG, Lange W: Adrenergic innervation of the oesophagus in the cat *(Felis domestica)* and rhesus monkey *(Macacus rhesus)*. Z Zellforsch 95:529, 1969.

Behar J, Guenard V, Walsh JH, et al: VIP and acetylcholine: Neurotransmitters in esophageal circular smooth muscle. Am J Physiol 257:G380, 1989.

Bennett A, Stockley HL: The intrinsic innervation of the human alimentary tract and its relation to function. Gut 16:443, 1975.

Biancani P, Hillemeier C, Bitar KN, et al: Contraction mediated by Ca^{2+} influx in esophageal muscle and by Ca^{2+} release in the LES. Am J Physiol 253:G760, 1987.

Biancani P, Walsh JH, Behar J: Vasoactive intestinal polypeptide a neurotransmitter for lower esophageal sphincter relaxation. J Clin Invest 73:963, 1984.

Bieger D: Muscarinic activation of rhombencephalic neurones controlling oesophageal peristalsis in the rat. Neuropharmacology 23:1451, 1984.

Bieger D, Hopkins DA: Viscerotopic representation of the upper alimentary tract in the medullar oblongata in the rat: The nucleus ambiguus. J Comp Neurol 262:546, 1987.

Blackwell JN, Holt S, Heading RC: Effect of nifedipine on oesophageal motility and gastric emptying. Digestion 21:50, 1981.

Blank EL, Greenwood B, Dodds WJ: Cholinergic control of smooth muscle peristalsis in the cat esophagus. Am J Physiol 257:G517, 1989.

Brasseur JG: A fluid mechanical perspective on esophageal bolus transport. Dysphagia 2:32, 1987.

Brasseur JG, Dodds WJ: Interpretation of intraluminal manometric measurements in terms of swallowing mechanics. Dysphagia 6:100, 1991.

Bremner CG, Shorter RG, Ellis Jr FH: Anatomy of feline esophagus with special reference to its muscular wall and phrenoesophageal membrane. J Surg Res 10:327, 1970.

Briggs CA: Potentiation of nicotinic transmission in the rat superior cervical sympathetic ganglion: Effects of cyclic GMP and nitric oxide generators. Brain Res 573:139, 1992.

Broussard DL, Bao X, Altschuler SM: Somatostatin immunoreactivity in esophageal premotor neurons of the rat. Neurosci Lett 250:201, 1998.

Broussard DL, Bao X, Li X, et al: Co-localization of NOS and NMDA receptor in esophageal premotor neurons of the rat. Neuroreport 6:2073, 1995.

Broussard DL, Li X, Altschuler SM: Localization of GABAA alpha 1 mRNA subunit in the brainstem nuclei controlling esophageal peristalsis. Brain Res Mol Brain Res 40:143, 1996.

Broussard DL, Lynn RB, Wiedner EB, et al: Solitarial premotor neuron projections to the rat esophagus and pharynx: Implications for control of swallowing. Gastroenterology 114:1268, 1998.

Burgess JN, Schlegel JF, Ellis Jr FH: The effect of denervation on feline esophageal function and morphology. J Surg Res 12:24, 1972.

Burns TW, Venturatos SG: Esophageal motor function and response to acid perfusion in patients with symptomatic reflux esophagitis. Dig Dis Sci 30:529, 1985.

Buthpitiya AG, Stroud D, Russell CO: Pharyngeal pump and esophageal transit. Dig Dis Sci 32:1244, 1987.

Butin JW, Olsen AM, Moersch HJ, et al: A study of esophageal pressures in normal persons and patients with cardiospasm. Gastroenterology 23:278, 1953.

Cannon WB: Oesophageal peristalsis after bilateral vagotomy. Am J Physiol 19:436, 1907.

Carveth SW, Schlegel JF, Code CF, et al: Esophageal motility after vagotomy, phrenicotomy, myotomy, and myomectomy in dogs. Surg Gynecol Obstet 114:31, 1962.

Castell DO: Calcium-channel blocking agents for gastrointestinal disorders. Am J Cardiol 55:210B, 1985.

Ceccatelli P, Janssens J, Vantrappen G, et al: Cisapride restores the decreased lower oesophageal sphincter pressure in reflux patients. Gut 29:631, 1988.

Chan WW-L, Diamant NE: Electrical off response of cat esophageal smooth muscle: An analog simulation. Am J Physiol 246:233, 1976.

Channer KS, Jackson PC, O'Brien I, et al: Oesophageal function in diabetes mellitus and its association with autonomic neuropathy. Diabet Med 2:378, 1985.

Chaussade S, Hamm R, Lecomte JM, et al: Effects of an enkephalinase inhibitor on esophageal motility in man. Gastroenterol Clin Biol 12:793, 1988.

Christensen J: Patterns and origin of some esophageal responses to stretch and electrical stimulation. Gastroenterology 59:909, 1970.

Christensen J, Arthur C, Conklin JL: Some determinants of latency of off-response to electrical field stimulation in circular layer of smooth muscle of opossum esophagus. Gastroenterology 77:677, 1991.

Christensen J, Daniel EE: Electric and motor effects of autonomic drugs on longitudinal esophageal smooth muscle. Am J Physiol 211:387, 1966.

Christensen J, Daniel EE: Effects of some autonomic drugs on circular esophageal smooth muscle. J Pharmacol Exp Ther 159:243, 1968.

Christensen J, Fang S: Colocalization of NADPH-diaphorase activity and certain neuropeptides in the esophagus of opossum *(Didelphis virginiana)*. Cell Tissue Res 278:557, 1994.

Christensen J, Fang S, Rick GA: NADPH-diaphorase–positive nerve fibers in smooth muscle layers of opossum esophagus: Gradients in density. J Auton Nerv Syst 52:99, 1995.

Christensen J, Lund GF: Esophageal responses to distention and electrical stimulation. J Clin Invest 48:408, 1969.

Christensen J, Rick GA, Robison BA, et al: Arrangement of the myenteric plexus throughout the gastrointestinal tract of the opossum. Gastroenterology 85:890, 1983.

Christensen J, Robison BA: Anatomy of the myenteric plexus of the opossum esophagus. Gastroenterology 83:1033, 1982.

Christensen J, Williams TH, Jew J, et al: Distribution of immunoreactive substance P in opossum esophagus. Dig Dis Sci 34:513, 1989.

Clerc N, Mei N: Thoracic esophageal mechanoreceptors connected with fibers following sympathetic pathways. Brain Res Bull 10:1, 1983.

Clouse RE, Staiano A: Topography of the esophageal peristaltic pressure wave. Am J Physiol 261:G677, 1991.

Cohen S, Green F: The mechanics of esophageal muscle contraction:

Evidence of an inotropic effect of gastrin. J Clin Invest 52:2029, 1973.

Cohen S, Green F: Force-velocity characteristics of esophageal muscle: Effect of acetylcholine and norepinephrine. Am J Physiol 226:1250, 1974.

Collman PI, Tremblay L, Diamant NE: The distribution of spinal and vagal sensory neurons that innervate the esophagus of the cat. Gastroenterology 103:817, 1992.

Conklin JL, Du CA, Schulze-Delrieu K, et al: Hypertrophic smooth muscle in the partially obstructed opossum esophagus: Excitability and electrophysiological properties. Gastroenterology 101:657, 1991.

Corazziari E, Bontempo I, Anzini F: Effects of cisapride on distal esophageal motility in humans. Dig Dis Sci 34:1600, 1989.

Corazziari E, Pozzessere C, Dani S, et al: Intraluminal pH and esophageal motility. Gastroenterology 75:275, 1978.

Creamer B, Schlegel J: Motor responses of the esophagus to distention. J Appl Physiol 10:498, 1957.

Crist J, Gidda JS, Goyal RK: Intramural mechanism of esophageal peristalsis: Roles of cholinergic and noncholinergic nerves. Proc Natl Acad Sci U S A 81:3595, 1984a.

Crist J, Gidda JS, Goyal RK: Characteristics of "on" and "off" contractions in esophageal circular muscle in vitro. Am J Physiol 246:G137, 1984b.

Crist J, Gidda JS, Goyal RK: Role of substance P nerves in longitudinal smooth muscle contractions of the esophagus. Am J Physiol 250:G336, 1986.

Crist J, Surprenant A, Goyal RK: Intracellular studies of electrical membrane properties of opossum esophageal circular smooth muscle. Gastroenterology 92:987, 1987.

Crist JR, He XD, Goyal RK: Chloride-mediated inhibitory junction potentials in opossum esophageal circular smooth muscle. Am J Physiol 261:G752, 1991.

Cunningham ET Jr, Sawchenko PE: A circumscribed projection from the nucleus of the solitary tract to the nucleus ambiguus in the rat: Anatomical evidence for somatostatin-28-immunoreactive interneurons subserving reflex control of esophageal motility. J Neurosci 9:1668, 1989.

Cunningham ET Jr, Simmons DM, Swanson LW, et al: Enkephalin immunoreactivity and messenger RNA in a discrete projection from the nucleus of the solitary tract to the nucleus ambiguous in the rat. J Comp Neurol 307:1, 1991.

Cunningham KM, Horowitz M, Riddell PS, et al: Relations among autonomic nerve dysfunction, oesophageal motility, and gastric emptying in gastro-oesophageal reflux disease. Gut 32:1436, 1991.

Daniel EE, Daniel VP, Duchon G, et al: Is the nexus necessary for cell-to-cell coupling of smooth muscle? J Membr Biol 28:207, 1976.

Daniel EE, Posey-Daniel V: Neuromuscular structures in opossum esophagus: Role of interstitial cells of Cajal. Am J Physiol 246:G305, 1984.

Daniel EE, Taylor GS, Daniel VP, et al: Can nonadrenergic inhibitory varicosities be identified structurally? Can J Physiol Pharmacol 55:243, 1977.

De Boer SY, Masclee AM, Lam WF, et al: Effect of acute hyperglycemia on esophageal motility and lower esophageal sphincter pressure in humans. Gastroenterology 103:775, 1992.

de Carle DJ, Christensen J: A dopamine receptor in esophageal smooth muscle of the opossum. Gastroenterology 70:216, 1976.

de Carle DJ, Christensen J, Szabo AC, et al: Calcium dependence of neuromuscular events in esophageal smooth muscle of the opossum. Am J Physiol 232:E547, 1977.

Decktor DL, Ryan JP: Transmembrane voltage of opossum esophageal smooth muscle and its response to electrical stimulation of intrinsic nerves. Gastroenterology 82:301, 1982.

DiPalma JA, Perucca PJ, Martin DF, et al: Metoclopramide effect on esophageal peristalsis in normal human volunteers. Am J Gastroenterol 82:307, 1987.

Dodds WJ, Christensen J, Dent J, et al: Esophageal contractions induced by vagal stimulation in the opossum. Am J Physiol 235:E392, 1978a.

Dodds WJ, Dent J, Hogan WJ, et al: Effect of atropine on esophageal motor function in humans. Am J Physiol 240:G290, 1981.

Dodds WJ, Hogan WJ, Reid DP, et al: A comparison between primary esophageal peristalsis following wet and dry swallows. J Appl Physiol 35:851, 1973.

Dodds WJ, Hogan WJ, Stewart ET, et al: Effects of increased intra-abdominal pressure on esophageal peristalsis. J Appl Physiol 37:378, 1974.

Dodds WJ, Stef JJ, Stewart ET, et al: Responses of feline esophagus to cervical vagal stimulation. Am J Physiol 235:E63, 1978b.

Domoto T, Jury J, Berezin I, et al: Does substance P comediate with acetylcholine in nerves of opossum esophageal muscularis mucosa? Am J Physiol 245:G19, 1983.

Dooley CP, Di Lorenzo C, Valenzuela JE: Esophageal function in humans: Effects of bolus consistency and temperature. Dig Dis Sci 35:167, 1990.

Dooley CP, Schlossmacher B, Valenzuela JE: Effects of alterations in bolus viscosity on esophageal peristalsis in humans. Am J Physiol 254:G8, 1988.

Dooley CP, Schlossmacher B, Valenzuela JE: Modulation of esophageal peristalsis by alterations of body position: Effect of bolus viscosity. Dig Dis Sci 34:1662, 1989.

Du C, Murray J, Bates JN, et al: Nitric oxide: mediator of NANC hyperpolarization of opossum esophageal smooth muscle. Am J Physiol 261:G1012, 1991.

Edmundowicz SA, Clouse RE: Shortening of the esophagus in response to swallowing. Am J Physiol 260:G512, 1991.

El Ouazzani T, Mei N: Electrophysiologic properties and role of the vagal thermoreceptors of lower esophagus and stomach of cat. Gastroenterology 83:995, 1982.

Ellis FG, Kauntze R, Trounce JR: The innervation of the cardia and lower oesophagus in man. Br J Surg 47:466, 1960.

Falempin M, Mei N, Rousseau JP: Vagal mechanoreceptors of the inferior thoracic oesophagus, the lower oesophageal sphincter and the stomach in the sheep. Pflugers Arch 373:25, 1978.

Fang S, Christensen J: Distribution of NADPH diaphorase in intramural plexuses of cat and opossum esophagus. J Auton Nerv Syst 46:123, 1994.

Fleshler B, Hendrix TR, Kramer P, et al: The characteristics and similarity of primary and secondary peristalsis in the esophagus. J Clin Invest 38:110, 1958.

Floyd K: Cholinesterase activity in sheep oesophageal muscle. J Anat 116:357, 1973.

Fryscak T, Zenker W, Kantner D: Afferent and efferent innervation of the rat esophagus: A tracing study with horseradish peroxidase and nuclear yellow. Anat Embryol 170:63, 1984.

Funch-Jensen P, Jacobsen E: Esophageal peristalsis before, during, and after food intake in healthy people. Scand J Gastroenterol 16:209, 1981.

Galway G, Bieger D, Scott TM: Identification of nucleus ambiguus motor neurons innervating the rat oesophagus by means of retrograde double labelling with fluorescent dyes (Abstract). J Anat 137:436, 1983.

Gidda JS, Buyniski JP: Swallow-evoked peristalsis in opossum esophagus: Role of cholinergic mechanisms. Am J Physiol 251:G779, 1986.

Gidda JS, Cobb BW, Goyal RK: Modulation of esophageal peristalsis by vagal efferent stimulation in opossum. J Clin Invest 68:1411, 1981.

Gidda JS, Goyal RK: Influence of successive vagal stimulations on contractions in esophageal smooth muscle of opossum. J Clin Invest 71:1095, 1983.

Gidda JS, Goyal RK: Swallow-evoked action potentials in vagal preganglionic efferents. J Neurophysiol 52:1169, 1984.

Gidda JS, Goyal RK: Regional gradient of initial inhibition and refractoriness in esophageal smooth muscle. Gastroenterology 89:843, 1985.

Gilbert RJ, Dodds WJ: Effect of selective muscarinic antagonists on peristaltic contractions in opossum smooth muscle. Am J Physiol 250:G50, 1986.

Gilbert RJ, Dodds WJ, Kahrilas PJ, et al: Effect of cisapride, a new prokinetic agent, on esophageal motor function. Dig Dis Sci 32:1331, 1987.

Goyal RK, Rattan S: VIP as a possible neurotransmitter on non-cholinergic non-adrenergic inhibitory neurones. Nature 288:378, 1980.

Grande L, Lacima G, Ros E, et al: Lack of effect of metoclopramide and domperidone on esophageal peristalsis and esophageal acid clearance in reflux esophagitis: A randomized, double-blind study. Dig Dis Sci 37:583, 1992.

Green T, Dockray GJ: Calcitonin gene-related peptide and substance P in afferents to the upper gastrointestinal tract in the rat. Neurosci Lett 76:151, 1987.

Greenwood B, Blank E, Dodds WJ: Nicotine stimulates esophageal peristaltic contractions in cats by a central mechanism. Am J Physiol 262:G567, 1992.

Hellemans J, Vantrappen G: Electromyographic studies on canine esophageal motility. Am J Dig Dis 12:1240, 1967.

Hellemans J, Vantrappen G, Valembois P, et al: Electrical activity of striated and smooth muscle of the esophagus. Am J Dig Dis 13:320, 1968.

Hirsch DP, Holloway RH, Tytgat GN, et al: Involvement of nitric oxide in human transient lower esophageal sphincter relaxations and esophageal primary peristalsis. Gastroenterology 115:1374, 1998.

Hollis JB, Castell DO: Amplitude of esophageal peristalsis as determined by rapid infusion. Gastroenterology 63:417, 1972.

Hollis JB, Castell DO: Effect of dry swallows and wet swallows of different volumes on esophageal peristalsis. J Appl Physiol 38:1161, 1975.

Hollis JB, Castell DO: Effects of cholinergic stimulation on human esophageal peristalsis. J Appl Physiol 40:40, 1976.

Hollis JB, Levine SM, Castell DO: Differential sensitivity of the human esophagus to pentagastrin. Am J Physiol 222:870, 1972.

Hopkins DA: Ultrastructure and synaptology of the nucleus ambiguus in the rat: The compact formation. J Comp Neurol 360:705, 1995.

Hudson LC, Cummings JF: The origins of innervation of the esophagus of the dog. Brain Res 326:125, 1985.

Humphries TJ, Castell DO: Pressure profile of esophageal peristalsis in normal humans as measured by direct intraesophageal transducers. Dig Dis Sci 22:641, 1977.

Humphries TJ, Castell DO: Effect of oral bethanechol on parameters of esophageal peristalsis. Dig Dis Sci 26:129, 1981.

Hwang K: On tertiary peristalsis of esophagus of the cat (Abstract). Am J Physiol 159:574, 1948.

Hwang K: Mechanisms of transportation of the content of the esophagus. J Appl Physiol 6:781, 1954.

Hwang K, Essex HE, Mann FC: A study of certain problems resulting from vagotomy in dogs with special reference to emesis. Am J Physiol 149:429, 1947.

Ingelfinger FJ: Esophageal motility. Physiol Rev 38:533, 1958.

Jacob P, Kahrilas PJ, Vanagunas A: Peristaltic dysfunction associated with nonobstructive dysphagia in reflux disease. Dig Dis Sci 35:939, 1990.

Jacobowitz D, Nemir Jr P: The autonomic innervation of the esophagus of the dog. J Thorac Cardiovasc Surg 58:678, 1969.

Janssens J, De Wever I, Vantrappen G, et al: Peristalsis in smooth muscle esophagus after transection and bolus deviation. Gastroenterology 71:1004, 1976.

Janssens J, Sifrim D: New insights in the pathophysiology of primary motility disorders of the esophagus. Verh K Acad Geneeskd Belg 59:209, 1997.

Janssens J, Valembois P, Hellemans J, et al: Studies on the necessity of a bolus for the progression of secondary peristalsis in the canine esophagus. Gastroenterology 67:245, 1974.

Janssens J, Valembois P, Vantrappen G, et al: Is the primary peristaltic contraction of the canine esophagus bolus-dependent? Gastroenterology 65:750, 1973.

Jaup BH, Abrahamsson H, Virtanen R, et al: Effect of pirenzepine compared with atropine and L-hyoscyamine on esophageal peristaltic activity in humans. Scand J Gastroenterol 17:233, 1982.

Jean A: Localisation et activite des neurones deglutiteurs bulbaires. J Physiol Paris 64:227, 1972a.

Jean A: Effet de lesions localisees du bulbe rachidien sur le stade oesophagien de la deglutition. J Physiol Paris 64:507, 1972b.

Jean A: Control of the central swallowing program by inputs from the peripheral receptors: A review. J Auton Nerv Syst 10:225, 1984.

Jean A, Amri M, Calas A: Connections between the ventral medullary swallowing area and the trigeminal motor nucleus of the sheep studied by tracing techniques. J Auton Nerv Syst 7:87, 1983.

Jian R, Janssens J, Vantrappen G, et al: Influence of metenkephalin analogue on motor activity of the gastrointestinal tract. Gastroenterology 93:114, 1987.

Jurica EJ: Studies on the motility of the denervated mammalian esophagus. Am J Physiol 77:371, 1926.

Jury J, Boev KR, Daniel EE: Nitric oxide mediates outward potassium currents in opossum esophageal circular smooth muscle. Am J Physiol 270:G932, 1996.

Jury J, Jager LP, Daniel EE: Unusual potassium channels mediate nonadrenergic noncholinergic nerve-mediated inhibition in opossum esophagus. Can J Physiol Pharmacol 63:107, 1985.

Kaada B: Successful treatment of esophageal dysmotility and Raynaud's phenomenon in systemic sclerosis and achalasia by transcutaneous nerve stimulation: Increase in plasma VIP concentration. Scand J Gastroenterol 22:1137, 1987.

Kahrilas PJ, Dodds WJ, Hogan WJ, et al: Esophageal peristaltic dysfunction in peptic esophagitis. Gastroenterology 91:897, 1986.

Kannan MS, Jager LP, Daniel EE: Electrical properties of smooth muscle cell membrane of opossum esophagus. Am J Physiol 248:G342, 1985.

Kantrowitz PA, Siegel CI, Hendrix TR: Differences in motility of the upper and lower esophagus in man and its alteration by atropine. Bull Johns Hopkins Hosp 118:479, 1966.

Kaye MD, Kilby AE, Harper PC: Changes in distal esophageal function in response to cooling. Dig Dis Sci 32:22, 1987.

Kaye MD, Wexler RM: Alteration of esophageal peristalsis by body position. Dig Dis Sci 26:897, 1981.

Kendall GP, Thompson DG, Day SJ, et al: Motor responses of the oesophagus to intraluminal distension in normal subjects and patients with oesophageal clearance disorders. Gut 28:272, 1987.

Keren S, Argaman E, Golan M: Solid swallowing versus water swallowing: Manometric study of dysphagia. Dig Dis Sci 37:603, 1992.

Knight GC: The relation of the extrinsic nerves to the functional activity of the oesophagus. Br J Surg 22:155, 1934.

Knudsen MA, Svane D, Tottrup A: Importance of the L-arginine–nitric oxide pathway in NANC nerve function of the opossum esophageal body. Dig Dis Sci 9:365, 1991.

Konrad-Dalhoff I, Baunack AR, Ramsch KD, et al: Effect of the calcium antagonists nifedipine, nitrendipine, nimodipine and nisoldipine on oesophageal motility in man. Eur J Clin Pharmacol 41:313, 1991.

Konturek JW, Gillessen A, Domschke W: Diffuse esophageal spasm: A malfunction that involves nitric oxide? Scand J Gastroenterol 30:1041, 1995.

Kramer P, Ingelfinger FJ: I. Motility of the human esophagus in control subjects and in patients with esophageal disorders. Am J Med 7:168, 1949.

Kronecker H, Meltzer S: Der Schluckmechanismus, seine Erregung und seine Hemmung. Arch Anat Physiol 328, 1883.

Kuramoto H, Kato Y, Sakamoto H, et al: Galanin-containing nerve terminals that are involved in a dual innervation of the striated muscles of the rat esophagus. Brain Res 734:186, 1996.

Kuramoto H, Kawano H, Sakamoto H, et al: Motor innervation by enteric nerve fibers containing both nitric oxide synthase and galanin immunoreactivities in the striated muscle of the rat esophagus. Cell Tissue Res 295:241, 1999.

Lang IM, Medda BK, Ren J, et al: Characterization and mechanisms of the pharyngoesophageal inhibitory reflex. Am J Physiol 275:G1127, 1998.

Lawn AM: The localization, by means of electrical stimulation, of the origin and path in the medulla oblongata of the motor nerve fibres of the rabbit oesophagus. J Physiol (Lond) 174:232, 1964.

Leander S, Brodin E, Hakanson R, et al: Neuronal substance P in the esophagus: Distribution and effects on motor activity. Acta Physiol Scand 115:427, 1982.

Lee BH, Lynn RB, Lee HS, et al: Calcitonin gene-related peptide in nucleus ambiguus motoneurons in rat: Viscerotopic organization. J Comp Neurol 320:531, 1992.

Linde LM, Westover JL: Esophageal and gastric abnormalities in dysautonomia. Pediatrics 29:303, 1962.

Little AG, Correnti FS, Calleja IJ, et al: Effect of incomplete obstruction on feline esophageal function with a clinical correlation. Surgery 100:430, 1986.

Loewy AD, Spyer KM: Vagal preganglionic neurons. In Loewy AD, Spyer KM (eds): Central Regulation of Autonomic Functions. New York, Oxford University Press, 1990, pp 68–87.

Longhi EH, Jordan Jr PH: Necessity of a bolus for propagation of primary peristalsis in the canine esophagus. Am J Physiol 220:609, 1971.

Loo FD, Dodds WJ, Soergel KH, et al: Multipeaked esophageal peristaltic pressure waves in patients with diabetic neuropathy. Gastroenterology 88:485, 1985.

Lu W, Zhang M, Neuman RS, et al: Fictive oesophageal peristalsis evoked by activation of muscarinic acetylcholine receptors in rat nucleus tractus solitarii. Neurogastroenterol Motil 9:247, 1997.

Lu WY, Bieger D: Vagovagal reflex motility patterns of the rat esophagus. Am J Physiol 274:R1425, 1998a.

Lu WY, Bieger D: Vagal afferent transmission in the NTS mediating reflex responses of the rat esophagus. Am J Physiol 274:R1436, 1998b.

Lund GF, Christensen J: Electrical stimulation of esophageal smooth muscle and effects of antagonists. Am J Physiol 217:1369, 1969.

Lyrenas E, Abrahamsson H: Beta adrenergic influence on oesophageal peristalsis in man. Gut 27:260, 1986.

Maggi CA, Meli A: The sensory-efferent function of capsaicin-sensitive nerves. Gen Pharmacol 19:1, 1988.

Marklin GF, Krause WJ, Cutts JH: Structure of the esophagus in the adult opossum, *Didelphis virginiana*. Anat Anz 145:249, 1979.

Marzio L, Pieramico O, Neri M, et al: Comparative study of the effects of cimetropium bromide and atropine on human esophageal motor functions. Digestion 44:117, 1989.

McKirdy HC, Marshall RW: Effect of drugs and electrical field stimulation on circular muscle strips from human lower oesophagus. Q J Exp Physiol 70:591, 1985.

Mearin F, Mourelle M, Guarner F, et al: Patients with achalasia lack nitric oxide synthase in the gastro-oesophageal junction. Eur J Clin Invest 23:724, 1993.

Mei N: Mecanorecepteurs vagaux digestifs chez le chat. Exp Brain Res 11:502, 1970.

Meltzer SJ: Recent experimental contributions to the physiology of deglutition. N Y Med J 59:389, 1894.

Meltzer SJ: On the causes of the orderly progress of the peristaltic movements in the oesophagus. Am J Physiol 2:266, 1899.

Meltzer SJ: Secondary peristalsis of the esophagus: A demonstration on a dog with a permanent esophageal fistula. Proc Soc Exp Biol Med 4:35, 1906.

Meltzer SJ, Auer J: Vagus reflexes upon oesophagus and cardia. Br Med J 2:1806, 1906.

Mercer CD, Rue C, Hanelin L, et al: Effect of obesity on esophageal transit. Am J Surg 149:177, 1985.

Meyer GW, Austin RM, Brady CE III, et al: Muscle anatomy of the human esophagus. J Clin Gastroenterol 8:131, 1986.

Meyer GW, Castell DO: Human esophageal response during chest pain induced by swallowing cold liquids. JAMA 246:2057, 1981.

Meyer GW, Gerhardt DC, Castell DO: Human esophageal response to rapid swallowing: Muscle refractory period or neural inhibition? Am J Physiol 241:G129, 1981.

Miller LS, Liu J, Colizzo FP, et al: Correlation of high-frequency esophageal ultrasonography and manometry in the study of esophageal motility. Gastroenterology 109:832, 1995.

Mittal RK, Frank EB, Lange RC, et al: Effects of morphine and naloxone on esophageal motility and gastric emptying in man. Dig Dis Sci 31:936, 1986.

Mittal RK, Ren J, McCallum RW, et al: Modulation of feline esophageal contractions by bolus volume and outflow obstruction. Am J Physiol 258:G208, 1990.

Mukhopadhyay AK, Weisbrodt NW: Neural organization of esophageal peristalsis: Role of vagus nerve. Gastroenterology 68:444, 1975.

Mule F: The avian oesophageal motor function and its nervous control: Some physiological, pharmacological and comparative aspects. Comp Biochem Physiol A 99:491, 1991.

Murray J, Du C, Ledlow A, et al: Nitric oxide: Mediator of nonadrenergic noncholinergic responses of opossum esophageal muscle. Am J Physiol 261:G401, 1991.

Murray JA, Ledlow A, Launspach J, et al: The effects of recombinant human hemoglobin on esophageal motor functions in humans. Gastroenterology 109:1241, 1995.

Murray JA, Shibata EF, Buresh TL, et al: Nitric oxide modulates a calcium-activated potassium current in muscle cells from opossum esophagus. Am J Physiol 269:G606, 1995.

Murthy KS, Grider JR, Jin JG, et al: Interplay of VIP and nitric oxide in the regulation of neuromuscular function in the gut. Ann N Y Acad Sci 805:355, 1996.

Nelson DO, Mangel AW: Acetylcholine induced slow-waves in cat esophageal smooth muscle. Gen Pharmacol 10:19, 1979.

Niel JP, Gonella J, Roman C: Localisation par la technique de marquage a la peroxydase des corps cellularies des neurones ortho et parasympathiques innervant le sphincter oesophagien inferieur du chat. J Physiol Paris 76:591, 1980.

Nixon TE, Koch KL: Recurrent autonomous esophageal peristalsis in patients with chest discomfort. Dig Dis Sci 34:497, 1989.

Ny L, Alm P, Ekstrom P, et al: Nitric oxide synthase–containing, peptide-containing, and acetylcholinesterase-positive nerves in the cat lower oesophagus. Histochem J 26:721, 1994.

Ny L, Larsson B, Alm P, et al: Distribution and effects of pituitary adenylate cyclase activating peptide in cat and human lower oesophageal sphincter. Br J Pharmacol 116:2873, 1995.

Orlando RC, Bozymksi EM: The effects of pentagastrin in achalasia and diffuse esophageal spasm. Gastroenterology 77:472, 1979.

Orr WC, Johnson LF, Robinson MG: Effect of sleep on swallowing, esophageal peristalsis, and acid clearance. Gastroenterology 86:814, 1984.

Parkman HP, Reynolds JC, Elfman KS, et al: Calcitonin gene-related peptide: A sensory and motor neurotransmitter in the feline lower esophageal sphincter. Regul Pept 25:131, 1989.

Paterson WG: Electrical correlates of peristaltic and nonperistaltic contractions in the opossum smooth muscle esophagus. Gastroenterology 97:665, 1989.

Paterson WG: Neuromuscular mechanisms of esophageal responses at and proximal to a distending balloon. Am J Physiol 260:G148, 1991.

Paterson WG: Studies on opossum esophageal longitudinal muscle function. Can J Physiol Pharmacol 75:65, 1997a.

Paterson WG: Esophageal and lower esophageal sphincter response to balloon distention in patients with achalasia. Dig Dis Sci 42:106, 1997b.

Paterson WG, Hynna-Liepert TT, Selucky M: Comparison of primary and secondary esophageal peristalsis in humans: Effect of atropine. Am J Physiol 260:G52, 1991.

Paterson WG, Rattan S, Goyal RK: Esophageal responses to transient and sustained esophageal distension. Am J Physiol 255:G587, 1988.

Pope CE II: Effect of infusion on force of closure measurements in the human esophagus. Gastroenterology 58:616, 1970.

Pope CE II, Horton PF: Intraluminal force transducer measurements of human oesophageal peristalsis. Gut 13:464, 1972.

Postorino A, Fileccia R, Serio R, et al: Contribution of peripheral and central mechanisms to the oesophageal primary peristalsis. Boll Soc Ital Biol Sper 61:727, 1985.

Pouderoux P, Lin S, Kahrilas PJ: Timing, propagation, coordination, and effect of esophageal shortening during peristalsis. Gastroenterology 112:1147, 1997.

Rattan S, Gidda JS, Goyal RK: Membrane potential and mechanical responses of the opossum esophagus to vagal stimulation and swallowing. Gastroenterology 85:922, 1983.

Rattan S, Gonnella P, Goyal RK: Inhibitory effect of calcitonin gene-related peptide and calcitonin on opossum esophageal smooth muscle. Gastroenterology 94:284, 1988.

Rattan S, Grady M, Goyal RK: Vasoactive intestinal peptide causes peristaltic contractions in the esophageal body. Life Sci 30:1557, 1982.

Reid J: An experimental investigation into the functions of the eighth pair of nerves, or the glosso-pharyngeal, pneumogastric, and spinal accessory. Edinb Med Surg J 51:269, 1839.

Ren J, Schulze-Delrieu K: Modulation of esophageal contractions by distension in vitro. Dig Dis Sci 34:503, 1989.

Ren JL, Dodds WJ, Martin CJ, et al: Effect of increased intra-abdominal pressure on peristalsis in feline esophagus. Am J Physiol 261:G417, 1991.

Reynolds RP, El-Sharkawy TY, Diamant NE: Oesophageal peristalsis in the cat: The role of central innervation assessed by transient vagal blockade. Can J Physiol Pharmacol 63:122, 1985.

Richards WG, Kee KA, Sugarbaker DJ: Role of substance P in in vitro responses of opossum esophageal circular muscle (Abstract). Gastroenterology 103:1406, 1992.

Richards WG, Stamler JS, Kobzik L, et al: Role of nitric oxide in human esophageal circular smooth muscle in vitro. J Thorac Cardiovasc Surg 110:157, 1995.

Richter JE, Spurling TJ, Cordova CM, et al: Effects of oral calcium blocker, diltiazem, on esophageal contractions: Studies in volunteers and patients with nutcracker esophagus. Dig Dis Sci 29:649, 1984.

Richter JE, Wu WC, Johns DN, et al: Esophageal manometry in 95 healthy adult volunteers: Variability of pressures with age and frequency of "abnormal" contractions. Dig Dis Sci 32:583, 1987.

Rodrigo J, de Felipe J, Robles-Chillida EM, et al: Sensory vagal nature and anatomical access paths to esophagus laminar nerve endings in myenteric ganglia: Determination by surgical degeneration methods. Acta Anat 112:47, 1982.

Rodrigo J, Hernandez CJ, Vidal MA, et al: Vegetative innervation of the esophagus: II. Intraganglionic laminar endings. Acta Anat 92:79, 1975.

Rodrigo J, Polak JM, Fernandez L, et al: Calcitonin gene-related peptide immunoreactive sensory and motor nerves of the rat, cat, and monkey esophagus. Gastroenterology 88:444, 1985.

Rodrigo J, Uttenthal LO, Peinado MA, et al: Distribution of nitric oxide synthase in the esophagus of the cat and monkey. J Auton Nerv Syst 70:164, 1998.

Roman C: Controle nerveux du peristaltisme oesophagien. J Physiol Paris 58:79, 1966.

Roman C and Tieffenbach L: Motricite de l'oesophage a musculeuse lisse apres bivagotomie: Etude electromyographique (E.M.G.). J Physiol Paris 63:733, 1971.

Roman C, Tieffenbach L: Enregistrement de l'activite unitaire des fibres motrices vagales destinees a l'oesophage du babouin. J Physiol Paris 64:479, 1972.

Rossiter A, Guelrud M, Souney PF, et al: High vasoactive intestinal polypeptide plasma levels in patients with Barrett's esophagus. Scand J Gastroenterol 26:572, 1991.

Ruggiero DA, Giuliano R, Anwar M, et al: Anatomical substrates of cholinergic-autonomic regulation in the rat. J Comp Neurol 292:1, 1990.

Russell COH, Gannan R, Coatsworth J, et al: Relationship among esophageal dysfunction, diabetic gastroenteropathy, and peripheral neuropathy. Dig Dis Sci 28:289, 1983.

Ryan JP, Snape Jr WJ, Cohen S: Influence of vagal cooling on esophageal function. Am J Physiol 232:E159, 1977.

Samarasinghe DD: Some observations on the innervation of the striated muscle in the mouse oesophagus-an electron microscope study. J Anat 112:173, 1972.

Sanchez GC, Kramer P, Ingelfinger FJ: Motor mechanisms of the esophagus, particularly of its distal portion. Gastroenterology 25:321, 1953.

Sarna SK, Daniel EE, Waterfall WE: Myogenic and neural control systems for esophageal motility. Gastroenterology 73:1345, 1977.

Satchell PM: Canine oesophageal mechanoreceptors. J Physiol (Lond) 346:287, 1984.

Schaffar N, Rao H, Kessler JP, et al: Immunohistochemical detection of glutamate in rat vagal sensory neurons. Brain Res 778:302, 1997.

Schulze K, Conklin JL, Christensen J: A potassium gradient in smooth muscle segment of the opossum esophagus. Am J Physiol 232:270, 1977.

Schulze K, Hajjar J-J, Christensen J: Regional differences in potassium content of smooth muscle from opossum esophagus. Am J Physiol 235:709, 1978.

Sengupta JN, Kauvar D, Goyal RK: Characteristics of vagal esophageal tension-sensitive afferent fibers in the opossum. J Neurophysiol 61:1001, 1989.

Sengupta JN, Saha JK, Goyal RK: Stimulus-response function studies of esophageal mechanosensitive nociceptors in sympathetic afferents of opossum. J Neurophysiol 64:796, 1990.

Serio R, Daniel EE: Electrophysiological analysis of responses to intrinsic nerves in circular muscle of opossum esophageal muscle. Am J Physiol 254:G107, 1988.

Shirazi S, Schulze-Delrieu K, Custer-Hagen T, et al: Motility changes in opossum esophagus from experimental esophagitis. Dig Dis Sci 34:1668, 1989.

Siegel CI, Hendrix TR: Evidence for the central mediation of secondary peristalsis in the esophagus. Bull Johns Hopkins Hosp 108:297, 1961.

Sifrim D, Janssens J: Secondary peristaltic contractions, like primary peristalsis, are preceded by inhibition in the human esophageal body. Digestion 57:73, 1996.

Sifrim D, Janssens J, Vantrappen G: A wave of inhibition precedes primary peristaltic contractions in the human esophagus. Gastroenterology 103:876, 1992.

Sinar DR, Fletcher JR, Cordova CC, et al: Acute acid-induced esophagitis impairs esophageal peristalsis in baboons (Abstract). Gastroenterology 80:1286, 1981.

Singaram C, Sengupta A, Sugarbaker DJ, et al: Peptidergic innervation of the human esophageal smooth muscle. Gastroenterology 101:1256, 1991.

Singaram C, Sengupta A, Sweet MA, et al: Nitrinergic and peptidergic innervation of the human oesophagus. Gut 35:1690, 1994.

Smout AJ, Devore MS, Dalton CB, et al: Effects of nifedipine on esophageal tone and perception of esophageal distension. Dig Dis Sci 37:598, 1992.

Soffer EE, Schneiderman J, Schwartz I, et al: Effects of upper dorsal sympathectomy on esophageal motility in humans. Dig Dis Sci 33:157, 1988.

Spellun JS, Neslin NR, Behar J, et al: Changes in esophageal contraction secondary to experimental esophagitis in the cat (Abstract). Gastroenterology 92:1650, 1987.

Stacher G, Bauer P, Steinringer H, et al: Dose-related effects of the synthetic met-enkephalin analogue FK 323-824 on esophageal motor activity in healthy humans. Gastroenterology 83:1057, 1982.

Stef JJ, Dodds WJ, Hogan WJ, et al: Intraluminal esophageal manometry: An analysis of variables affecting recording fidelity of peristaltic pressures. Gastroenterology 67:221, 1974.

Sugarbaker DJ, Kee KA, Richards WG: Role of substance P in in vitro contraction of human esophageal circular smooth muscle (ECSM) (Abstract). Gastroenterology 104:A587, 1993.

Sugarbaker DJ, Rattan S, Goyal RK: Mechanical and electrical activity of esophageal smooth muscle during peristalsis. Am J Physiol 246:G145, 1984a.

Sugarbaker DJ, Rattan S, Goyal RK: Swallowing induces sequential activation of esophageal longitudinal smooth muscle. Am J Physiol 247:G515, 1984b.

Tell F, Jean A: Rhythmic bursting patterns induced in neurons of the rat nucleus tractus solitarii, in vitro, in response to *N*-methyl-D-aspartate. Brain Res 533:152, 1990.

Tell F, Jean A: Ionic basis for endogenous rhythmic patterns induced by activation of *N*-methyl-D-aspartate receptors in neurons of the rat nucleus tractus solitarii. J Neurophysiol 70:2379, 1993.

Tieffenbach L, Roman C: Role de l'innervation extrinseque vagale dans la motricite de l'oesophage a musculeuse lisse: Etude electromyographique chez le chat et le babouin. J Physiol Paris 64:193, 1972.

Tolu E, Mameli O, Soro P, et al: Physostigmine and metoclopramide in oesophageal peristaltic spread in man. Pharmacol Res Commun 20:869, 1988.

Tottrup A, Forman A, Funch-Jensen P, et al: Effects of transmural field stimulation in isolated muscle strips from human esophagus. Am J Physiol 258:G344, 1990a.

Tottrup A, Forman A, Funch-Jensen P, et al: Effects of postganglionic nerve stimulation in oesophageal achalasia: An in vitro study. Gut 31:17, 1990b.

Tottrup A, Forman A, Uldbjerg N, et al: Mechanical properties of isolated human esophageal smooth muscle. Am J Physiol 258:G338, 1990c.

Tottrup A, Knudsen MA, Gregersen H: The role of the L-arginine-nitric oxide pathway in relaxation of the opossum lower oesophageal sphincter. Br J Pharmacol 104:113, 1991.

Triadafilopoulos G, Aaronson M, Sackel S, et al: Medical treatment of esophageal achalasia: Double-blind crossover study with oral nifedipine, verapamil, and placebo. Dig Dis Sci 36:260, 1991.

Trifan A, Ren J, Arndorfer R, et al: Inhibition of progressing primary esophageal peristalsis by pharyngeal water stimulation in humans. Gastroenterology 110:419, 1996.

Valori RM, Hallisey MT, Dunn J: Power of oesophageal peristalsis can be controlled voluntarily. Gut 32:236, 1991.

Vanek AW, Diamant NE: Responses of the human esophagus to paired swallows. Gastroenterology 92:643, 1987.

Wallin L, Kruse-Andersen S, Madsen T, et al: Effect of cisapride on the gastro-oesophageal function in normal human subjects. Digestion 37:160, 1987.

Wang YT, Bieger D: Role of solitarial GABAergic mechanisms in control of swallowing. Am J Physiol 261:R639, 1991a.

Wang YT, Bieger D, Neuman RS: Activation of NMDA receptors is necessary for fast information transfer at brainstem vagal motoneurons. Brain Res 567:260, 1991b.

Wang YT, Neuman RS, Bieger D: Nicotinic cholinoceptor-mediated excitation in ambigual motoneurons of the rat. Neuroscience 40:759, 1991a.

Wang YT, Neuman RS, Bieger D: Somatostatin inhibits nicotinic cholinoceptor-mediated excitation in rat ambigual motoneurons in vitro. Neurosci Lett 123:236, 1991b.

Wang YT, Zhang M, Neuman RS, et al: Somatostatin regulates excitatory amino acid receptor-mediated fast excitatory postsynaptic potential components in vagal motoneurons. Neuroscience 53:7, 1993.

Wattchow DA and Costa M: Distribution of peptide-containing nerve fibres in achalasia of the oesophagus. J Gastroenterol Hepatol 11:478, 1996.

Wattchow DA, Furness JB, Costa M: Distribution and coexistence of peptides in nerve fibers of the external muscle of the human gastrointestinal tract. Gastroenterology 95:32, 1988.

Wattchow DA, Furness JB, Costa M, et al: Distributions of neuropeptides in the human esophagus. Gastroenterology 93:1363, 1987.

Weisbrodt NW, Christensen J: Gradients of contractions in the opossum esophagus. Gastroenterology 62:1159, 1972.

Wiedner EB, Bao X, Altschuler SM: Localization of nitric oxide synthase in the brain stem neural circuit controlling esophageal peristalsis in rats. Gastroenterology 108:367, 1995.

Wienbeck M, Li Q: Cisapride in gastro-oesophageal reflux disease: Effects on oesophageal motility and intra-oesophageal pH. Scand J Gastroenterol Suppl 165:13, 1989.

Williams D, Thompson DG, Marples M, et al: Identification of an abnormal esophageal clearance response to intraluminal distention in patients with esophagitis. Gastroenterology 103:943, 1992.

Winship DH, Viegas de Andrade SR, Zboralske FF: Influence of bolus temperature on human esophageal motor function. J Clin Invest 49:243, 1970.

Wood JD, Marsh DR: Effect of atropine, tetrodotoxin and lidocaine on rebound excitation of guinea-pig small intestine. J Pharmacol Exp Ther 184:590, 1973.

Worl J, Fischer J, Neuhuber WL: Nonvagal origin of galanin-containing nerve terminals innervating striated muscle fibers of the rat esophagus. Cell Tissue Res 292:453, 1998.

Worl J, Mayer B, Neuhuber WL: Nitrergic innervation of the rat esophagus: Focus on motor endplates. J Auton Nerv Syst 49:227, 1994.

Worl J, Mayer B, Neuhuber WL: Spatial relationships of enteric nerve fibers to vagal motor terminals and the sarcolemma in motor endplates of the rat esophagus: A confocal laser scanning and electron-microscopic study. Cell Tissue Res 287:113, 1997.

Xue S, Valdez D, Collman PI, et al: Effects of nitric oxide synthase blockade on esophageal peristalsis and the lower esophageal sphincter in the cat. Can J Physiol Pharmacol 74:1249, 1996.

Yamato S, Spechler SJ, Goyal RK: Role of nitric oxide in esophageal peristalsis in the opossum. Gastroenterology 103:197, 1992.

Zhang M, Wang YT, Vyas DM, et al: Nicotinic cholinoceptor-mediated excitatory postsynaptic potentials in rat nucleus ambiguus. Exp Brain Res 96:83, 1993.

Zhang Y, Vogalis F, Goyal RK: Nitric oxide suppresses a $Ca^{(2+)}$-stimulated Cl^- current in smooth muscle cells of opossum esophagus. Am J Physiol 274:G886, 1998.

Zoungrana OR, Amri M, Car A, et al: Intracellular activity of motoneurons of the rostral nucleus ambiguus during swallowing in sheep. J Neurophysiol 77:909, 1997.

PHYSIOLOGY OF THE LOWER ESOPHAGEAL SPHINCTER

Steven R. DeMeester

Tom R. DeMeester

Today we know that a person is able to be suspended in the weightless environment of outer space, eat a meal, and not regurgitate food back into the esophagus or mouth. Similarly, we have all witnessed an acrobat who can hang upside down while swinging on a trapeze and also not regurgitate. From these and other circumstances, it is intuitively clear that a one-way valve mechanism must exist between the esophagus and stomach so that, despite a variety of maneuvers and circumstances, gastric contents are prevented from refluxing into the esophagus. The nature of this valve mechanism has been extensively studied, yet it represents an area of controversy that continues to some extent today.

HISTORICAL BACKGROUND

In 1719, Helvetius described a morphologic sphincter at the cardioesophageal junction; subsequently, other anatomists both confirmed and disputed his findings (Marchand, 1955). In the early 1900s, Chevalier Jackson, unconvinced of the presence of an anatomic sphincter within the lower esophagus, suggested that the diaphragm exerts a pinchcock effect on the esophagus and in this way acts as a sphincter. Others proposed that the manner in which the esophagus joins the stomach forms a flap-valve mechanism, which functions as the sphincter.

Subsequently, Fyke and colleagues (1956) clarified this paradox by demonstrating that the sphincter is a physiologic rather than an anatomic structure. In their landmark human study, these investigators measured the pressure within a series of balloons that were sequentially withdrawn from the stomach into the esophagus and noted that the sphincter represented a high-pressure zone located in the distal esophagus. This high-pressure zone was found to be subject to changes in intra-abdominal pressure in its distal portion and to intrathoracic pressure in its proximal portion. Furthermore, these investigators demonstrated that the high-pressure zone relaxed with swallowing.

These initial observations and conclusions remain valid today, although current technology permits a much more detailed evaluation of the function and dysfunction of what now is referred to as the lower esophageal sphincter (LES). Interestingly, in our modern understanding of the antireflux barrier we have integrated the various proposed mechanisms, including the LES, the pinchcock action of the diaphragm, and the flap-valve effect of the angle of His.

SIGNIFICANCE OF THE LOWER ESOPHAGEAL SPHINCTER

The gastrointestinal tract, considered in its simplest form, is actually a long, continuous hollow tube designed to allow the ingestion, digestion, and absorption of protein, carbohydrates, and fats and the elimination of residue. Different areas of the gastrointestinal tract function in concert to allow this process to take place, yet each of these areas, or compartments, has its own unique task. To perform its task and contribute to the overall mission of the gastrointestinal tract, each compartment has a pumping mechanism to propel luminal contents into a receptacle or reservoir portion of that compartment, a sphincter to separate the pump from the reservoir, and the ability to maintain within the reservoir a distinct chemical, enzymatic, and pH environment appropriate to its function (DeMeester et al, 1999).

In the human gastrointestinal tract are four valves or sphincters:

- UES
- LES
- Pylorus
- Ileocecal valve

The LES represents the barrier that confines the gastric environment to the stomach and protects the acid-sensitive squamous esophageal mucosa from injury due to reflux of gastric contents back into the esophagus. Like any valve, failure of the LES can occur in two completely opposite ways, leading to two distinct clinical disease entities. Regardless of the type of LES failure, the secondary effects are produced proximally in the esophagus. Failure of the LES to relax, or open appropriately, leads to the inability of the esophagus to propel food into the stomach, esophageal distention, and the condition known as *achalasia*. On the other hand, incompetence of the LES leads to an increased reflux of gastric contents into the esophagus, esophageal mucosal injury, and the condition known as *gastroesophageal reflux disease*.

ANATOMY

The Lower Esophageal Sphincter

The LES exists primarily as a manometrically identifiable high-pressure zone located in the distal esophagus. From a practical standpoint, there are no anatomic landmarks that allow visible identification of the LES. The smooth muscle in the lower esophagus and in the region of the LES outwardly look the same and are composed of the same inner circular and outer longitudinal layers. However, detailed studies of the human gastroesophageal junction by Liebermann-Meffert and colleagues (1979) suggest that there is an asymmetric thickening of the muscularis propria in the distal esophagus below the diaphragm but above the angle of His.

In a series of autopsies, these authors recorded a gradual increase in muscle thickness from 2.1 ± 0.6 mm in the esophagus to 4.2 ± 1.4 mm at an area they called the "gastroesophageal ring." This ring, or site of maximal muscle thickness, was asymmetric and angled obliquely upward from the lesser to the greater curvature side of the stomach. Maximal muscle thickness occurred over a distance of 31.4 mm along the greater curvature but was shorter and thinner along the lesser curvature. The authors speculated that perhaps this area of increased muscular thickness in the distal esophagus corresponds to the manometrically defined high-pressure zone, or LES, known to be located in this same region.

Neural Regulation

Innervation of the esophagus and LES is by both sympathetic and parasympathetic branches. The major neural network, the myenteric plexus, lies between the longitudinal and circular muscle layers. Efferent stimuli reach the LES via the vagus nerves and the myenteric plexus. Swallow-induced sphincter relaxation is mediated centrally from the dorsal motor nucleus of the vagus nerve. The vagal fibers involved in LES relaxation enter the esophagus proximal to the sphincter and are unaffected by high abdominal truncal vagotomy.

Within the LES, acetylcholine functions as the presynaptic neurotransmitter, whereas nitric oxide and perhaps vasoactive intestinal peptide (VIP) act as postsynaptic neurotransmitters (Yamato et al, 1992). Atropine has been shown to reduce but not eliminate the resting tone of the LES, suggesting that the vagus nerves are only partially involved in LES tone production (Dodds et al, 1981; Mittal, et al, 1995).

Recent studies in patients with achalasia have implicated a subclass of nitric oxide synthesizing enteric neurons in the LES and gastric fundus as playing a pivotal role in LES relaxation (De Giorgio et al, 1999). De Giorgio's group noted that in smooth muscle from normal human LES and gastric fundus, stains for nitric oxide–releasing neurons were positive in nerve processes distributed to the muscle layer and myenteric ganglia; here they formed a dense plexus surrounding the myenteric neurons. Interestingly, the investigators found that in patients with achalasia the density of nitric oxide staining nerve fibers and ganglion cells was dramatically reduced. Consequently, it is thought that nitric oxide–releasing neurons are crucial to appropriate LES relaxation.

Gastric Sling Fibers and the Phrenoesophageal Ligament

The sling, or oblique, fibers of the stomach are located below the LES and are arranged in a "C-shaped" fashion. The open end of the "C" is oriented toward the lesser curve of the stomach. This configuration contributes to the formation of a "flap-valve" mechanism that potentially augments LES function and participates in the barrier against gastroesophageal reflux. The phrenoesophageal ligament attaches to the distal esophagus and anchors the esophagus to the crural diaphragm (Liebermann-Meffert et al, 1979; Mittal and Balaban, 1997).

The Diaphragm

The diaphragm is composed of both a costal and a crural portion. Evidence, primarily from studies in dogs, suggests that the two parts of the diaphragm are embryologically and functionally distinct. The costal portion is attached to the ribs and originates embryologically from the lateral body wall. It functions primarily as a respiratory muscle, and contraction causes flattening of this portion of the diaphragm along with expansion of the

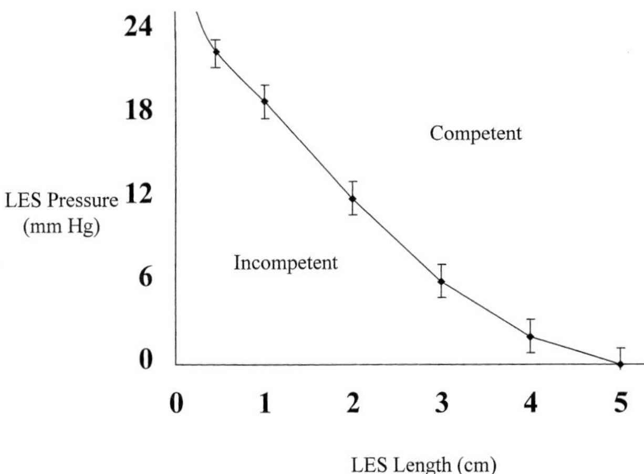

FIGURE 3–3 ■ Competency of the lower esophageal sphincter (LES) is dependent on adequate resistance to flow across the normal pressure gradient that exists from the intra-abdominal stomach to the intrathoracic esophagus. The resistance to flow imposed by the LES, and thereby the likelihood of competency of the LES, is dependent on the integral relationship between LES length and pressure. A longer LES requires a lower resting pressure to maintain competency; however, even a very high pressure may be inadequate to maintain competency in a valve less than 1 cm in length.

lower rib cage (Mittal and Balaban, 1997). In contrast, the crural portion of the diaphragm is attached to the vertebral column and develops from the dorsal mesentery of the esophagus. It forms a canal through which the esophagus passes into the abdomen. This canal is approximately 2 cm long and encircles the proximal portion of the LES (Mittal and Balaban, 1997). Because the LES is normally about 4 cm long, part of the LES lies in the esophageal hiatus and part is intra-abdominal. Crural contraction produces hiatal closure and results in a pinchcock-like constriction around the esophagus.

In dogs, Monges and colleagues (1978) demonstrated dissociation between the electrical activity of the costal and crural portions of the diaphragm. During episodes of vomiting, the researchers noted electrical inactivity (relaxation) of the crura, yet vigorous, simultaneous contraction of both the costal diaphragm and the rectus abdominis muscle. De Troyer and colleagues (1982) carried this concept further again in dogs and found that the costal and crural portions of the diaphragm were innervated differently. The phrenic nerve supplied the costal diaphragm, whereas the lower segmental nerves supplied the crural diaphragm. Whether this applies to the human diaphragm is unclear.

PHYSIOLOGY

The Lower Esophageal Sphincter

Physiologically, the LES functions as the major barrier against reflux of gastric contents from the positive-pressure environment of the abdomen to the negative-pressure environment of the thorax. This barrier is normally present except after a swallow, when the LES relaxes to allow passage of material into the stomach. The LES also relaxes during episodes of gaseous fundic distention to allow venting of the gas. The ability of the LES to maintain this barrier against reflux is dependent on the resistance to flow created by the LES.

Essentially, the competency of the LES is a function of the pressure within the LES and the length over which that pressure is applied (Bonavina et al, 1986). The shorter the overall length of the sphincter, the higher the pressure must be to maintain sufficient resistance to prevent reflux. Consequently, even a normal sphincter pressure may be inadequate to maintain competency in the setting of a short abdominal sphincter length, or overall sphincter length. The integral relationship between length and pressure for function of the LES is demonstrated in Figure 3–3.

Manometry

The important sphincter characteristics of length and pressure are determined by a catheter that has multiple pressure-sensing sites. Both water-perfused and solid-state catheters are available, and each has certain advantages. The pressure and length of the LES can be determined by a *stationary* or by a slow, *motorized* pull-through technique (Fig. 3–4). Normal values for LES pressure and length have been determined in asymptomatic volunteers (Table 3–4) (Zaninotto et al, 1988).

Pressure

The LES is primarily a physiologic rather than an anatomic structure, and it is the intrinsic tone or pressure of the LES that allows one to identify its presence manometrically. The normal resting pressure of the LES varies from 10 to 30 mm Hg above gastric pressure. In our laboratory, we have chosen to measure the resting LES pressure at the respiratory inversion point and record it as the mean of the maximal and minimal pressures at that point.

Various substances, including certain foods, hormones, peptides, and drugs, affect LES pressure. Some of the common agents known to lower LES pressure include caffeine, nicotine, alcohol, fat, chocolate, and pepper-

TABLE 3–4 ■ **Normal Parameters of the Lower Esophageal Sphincter in 50 Healthy Volunteers[13]**

	Mean	*Median*	*Standard Deviation*	*Fifth Percentile*
Pressure (mm Hg)	14.87	13.8	5.14	8
Abdominal length (cm)	2.18	2.2	0.72	1.1
Overall length (cm)	3.65	3.6	0.68	2.6

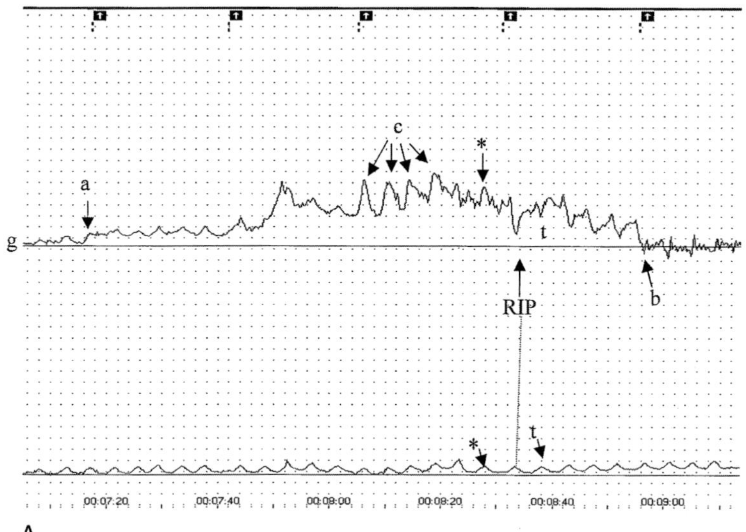

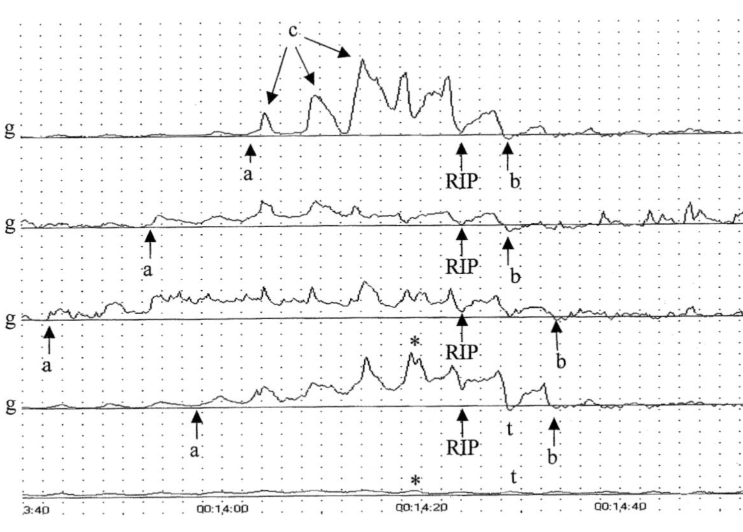

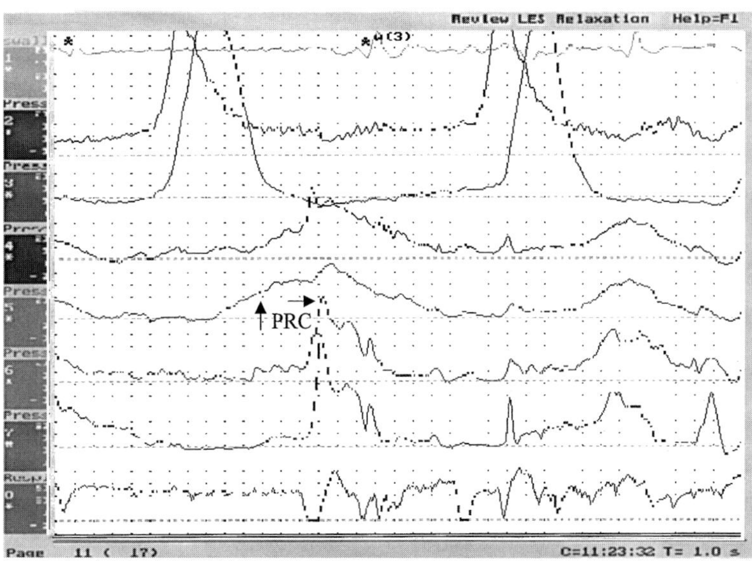

FIGURE 3–4 ■ Pull-through techniques. (a, start of sphincter; b, end of sphincter; c, crural impressions; g, gastric baseline pressure; RIP, respiratory inversion point; positive deflection associated with inspiration (intra-abdominal location); t, negative deflection associated with inspiration [intrathoracic location]).

The three important characteristics of LES (pressure, total length, abdominal length) are determined by a pressure-sensitive motility catheter. All pressures are referenced to gastric baseline pressure. A rise above gastric baseline pressure signals the start of the sphincter; a drop below gastric baseline pressure signifies that the catheter has left the sphincter and has entered the intrathoracic esophagus. In our laboratory, we determine the resting pressure of the sphincter at the point where the pressure change associated with inspiration changes from positive (intra-abdominal location) to negative (intrathoracic location)—the respiratory inversion point (RIP). We measure the LES resting pressure as the mean of the maximum and minimum pressures at the RIP in each channel. We measure intra-abdominal sphincter length from the start of the sphincter to the RIP (a→RIP). Total sphincter length includes both intra-abdominal and intrathoracic portions of the sphincter (a→b).

A, Stationary pull-through technique. A catheter with pressure sensors positioned 1 cm apart is placed so that all the sensors are in the stomach. It is then withdrawn at 1 cm increments; as each sensor passes through the LES, a pressure tracing is generated. (*Arrows* mark locations where the catheter was withdrawn manually 1 cm.) The length and pressure values from each channel are then averaged to give the overall values for the LES. For clarity, only one channel is shown. Total sphincter length is 4 cm (a→b); intra-abdominal length is 3 cm (a→RIP).

B, Slow motorized pull-through technique. The catheter has four sensors radially located at the same level on the catheter. All four are initially positioned in the stomach and then withdrawn through the LES. Instead of manually withdrawing the catheter in 1-cm increments; however, a machine withdraws the catheter at a constant, slow rate. The advantages are that this slow, steady withdrawal usually does not stimulate a swallow by the patient and the sphincter is seen simultaneously in four channels. Length of the sphincter with this technique is determined by time, since the speed of withdrawal is constant at 1 mm/second. Each *dotted line* represents 2 seconds (2 mm). With this technique, some degree of asymmetry is often noted in the LES.

C, Relaxation study. The normal LES should relax to gastric baseline pressure with a swallow. In this normal tracing, the motility catheter has four radially positioned sensors recorded on channels 4 to 7. Channel 1 is the swallowing microphone, and channels 2 and 3 are in the distal body of the esophagus. A swallow recorded by the microphone at the *asterisk* (*) is followed by a peristaltic wave in the body of the esophagus. Relaxation in the LES occurs with initiation of the swallow. Consequently, the LES is open when the peristaltic wave reaches the distal esophagus. A postrelaxation contraction (PRC) occurs at the conclusion of the swallow.

mint. The resting tone of the LES is also influenced by circadian rhythm and is reported to be highest at night (Dent et al, 1980). It is interesting that the resting tone of the LES is produced by the muscles of the sphincter existing in a state of partial depolarization (Daniel et al, 1976). This tone is at least in part an intrinsic property of the muscle itself, since it is not ablated by the nerve-blocking agent tetrodotoxin and is only partially reduced by atropine (Dodds et al, 1981; Goyal and Rattan, 1976). Animal work suggests that intrinsic tone in the LES is mediated by shifts of intracellular stores of calcium within the sphincter muscle (Biancani et al, 1987). Deficits in sphincter pressure compromise the competency of the sphincter, and clinical studies suggest that this is the leading cause of a defective sphincter.

Length

In normal subjects, the manometrically determined overall length of the LES varies from 4 to 6 cm, with one half to two thirds exposed to intra-abdominal pressure and the remainder exposed to intrathoracic pressure. The point of transition from the positive-pressure abdominal environment to the negative-pressure intrathoracic environment is recognized manometrically by the point at which the respiratory pressure waveforms invert. The portion of the sphincter distal to the respiratory inversion point represents the intra-abdominal length of the sphincter.

An adequate length of LES exposed to the abdominal environment is important for the LES to remain competent under conditions of varying intra-abdominal pressures. This has been demonstrated both clinically and experimentally (DeMeester et al, 1979; Pellegrini et al, 1976). In an experimental model, when the intra-abdominal sphincter length was reduced to less than 1 cm, the sphincter became incompetent regardless of the sphincter pressure (DeMeester et al, 1979). Further clinical and experimental studies have also demonstrated the importance of overall sphincter length. Bonavina and coauthors found that sphincter competency was markedly impaired when the overall length became less than 2 cm (Bonavina et al, 1986). Consequently, sphincter resting pressure, overall length, and abdominal length are important, independent factors in sphincter competency and should be assessed as part of esophageal manometry.

Vector Volume

One problem with measuring LES length and pressure is that most sphincters are asymmetric. For more detailed information about the length and pressure characteristics of the LES, a computer image can be generated from a series of pressure measurements taken simultaneously from four quadrants at 1-cm intervals throughout the sphincter (Fig. 3–5). The calculated volume of the computer-generated image correlates with the overall resistance of the LES to reflux, now referred to as the "sphincter pressure vector volume" (Stein et al, 1991).

Without the aid of computer software programs, vector volume is difficult and time-consuming to calculate. However, using computer-calculated vector volumes for both the intra-abdominal portion and the total sphincter, Wetscher and associates found that it was simple, reliable, and superior to the usual stepwise pull-back procedure for evaluating LES competency (Wetscher et al, 1996).

The Diaphragm

The esophagus passes into the abdomen through a canal formed primarily by the right crus of the diaphragm. In the late 1950s, Marchand (1957) studied the forces responsible for the production of reflux and, in particular, the role of the pressure gradient generated between the abdomen and chest by diaphragmatic function.

Boyle and coauthors (1985) used a cat model to demonstrate that although the costal portion of the diaphragm creates a pressure gradient between the chest and

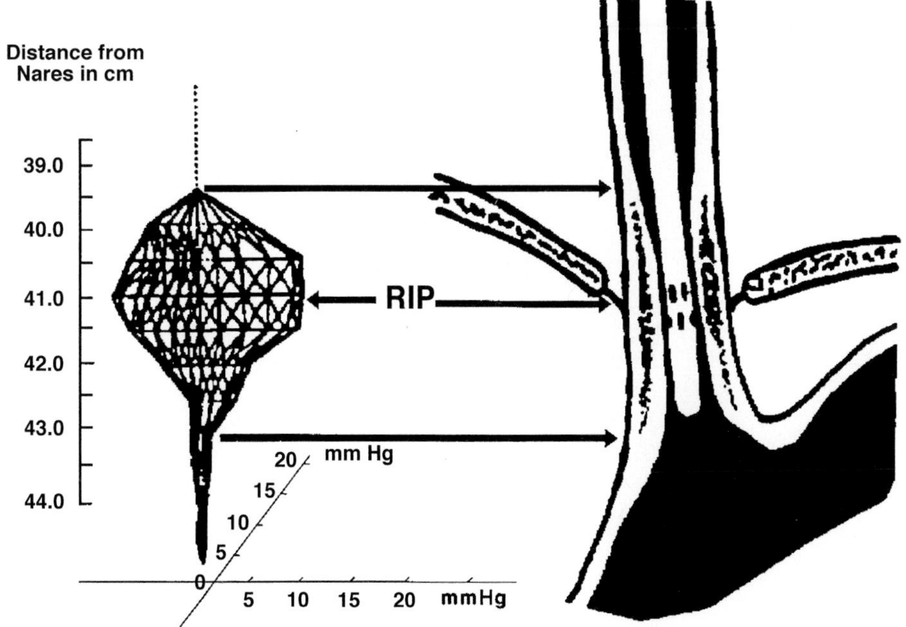

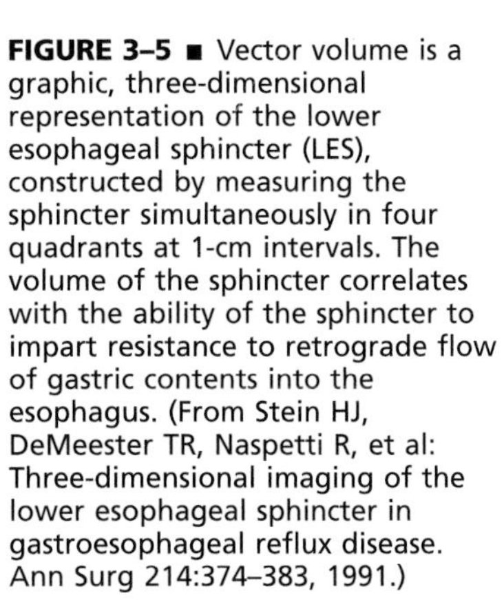
FIGURE 3–5 ■ Vector volume is a graphic, three-dimensional representation of the lower esophageal sphincter (LES), constructed by measuring the sphincter simultaneously in four quadrants at 1-cm intervals. The volume of the sphincter correlates with the ability of the sphincter to impart resistance to retrograde flow of gastric contents into the esophagus. (From Stein HJ, DeMeester TR, Naspetti R, et al: Three-dimensional imaging of the lower esophageal sphincter in gastroesophageal reflux disease. Ann Surg 214:374–383, 1991.)

the abdomen favoring reflux, the pinchcock action of the crural diaphragm contributes to the production of a pressure gradient across the distal esophagus, preventing reflux.

Subsequently, Mittal and colleagues (1990) reported a series of studies that further clarified the synergistic relationship between the crural portion of the diaphragm and the LES. By monitoring crural electromyographic (EMG) activity simultaneously with gastric and LES pressure, they noted that during periods of increased abdominal pressure produced by straight-leg raising, straining, or abdominal compression, LES pressure increased more than gastric pressure, and this increase coincided with tonic contraction of the crural diaphragm. Atropine inhibited LES resting pressure substantially but had no effect on peak LES pressure during episodes of increased abdominal pressure or on tonic crural contraction, as demonstrated by EMG. Mittal's group concluded that the crural diaphragm is responsible for increased resistance to gastroesophageal reflux during various physiologic events that increase intra-abdominal pressure, such as coughing, straining, and deep breathing.

In another report, Klein and colleagues (1993) found a sphincter-like thoracoabdominal high-pressure zone after esophagogastrectomy, which they attributed to crural function. This action of the crural diaphragm can best be observed during a videoesophagram. In normal, upright subjects the flow of barium through the hiatus is halted during deep inspiration and resumes during expiration.

PATHOPHYSIOLOGY

Gastroesophageal Reflux Disease

The Defective Lower Esophageal Sphincter

The common denominator for virtually all episodes of gastroesophageal reflux is a loss of LES resistance, with subsequent retrograde flow of gastric contents into the esophagus along a pressure gradient from the abdomen to the chest. Patients with severe gastroesophageal reflux disease (GERD) usually have permanent defects in LES barrier function, whereas normal subjects and patients with early GERD have reflux because of a transient loss of LES resistance.

The most common cause of a permanently defective sphincter is an inadequate pressure (Zaninotto et al, 1988) (Fig. 3–6). However, an inadequate abdominal or overall sphincter length can compromise the competence of a sphincter even if the resting pressure is normal. If only one component of the LES is defective, the prevalence of increased esophageal exposure to refluxed gastric juice is 69% to 76%. However, when all three components are defective, GERD is almost inevitable (Zaninotto et al, 1988).

The finding of a permanently defective LES has several important implications for the clinician. Most important, it predicts that the patient is more likely to have complications from GERD, including the development of esophagitis, peptic stricture, and Barrett's esophagus (Fig. 3–7). Furthermore, injury and impairment of esophageal body function is most likely to occur in patients with a permanently defective LES. Esophageal body dysfunction results in ineffective clearance of refluxed gastric juice and more severe mucosal injury. In addition, esophageal body dysfunction can lead to episodes of aspiration that can ultimately result in progressive pulmonary failure.

Hiatal Hernia

Most patients with moderate to severe GERD have a hiatal hernia, and the presence of a hiatal hernia has been shown to be an independent predictor of esophagitis (Sontag et al, 1991). Normally, diaphragmatic crural pressure is superimposed on the LES to augment the antireflux function of the LES, particularly during episodes of coughing, straining, and deep breathing. In patients with a hiatal hernia, the fundus of the stomach rather than the LES is positioned within the crural tunnel. In this

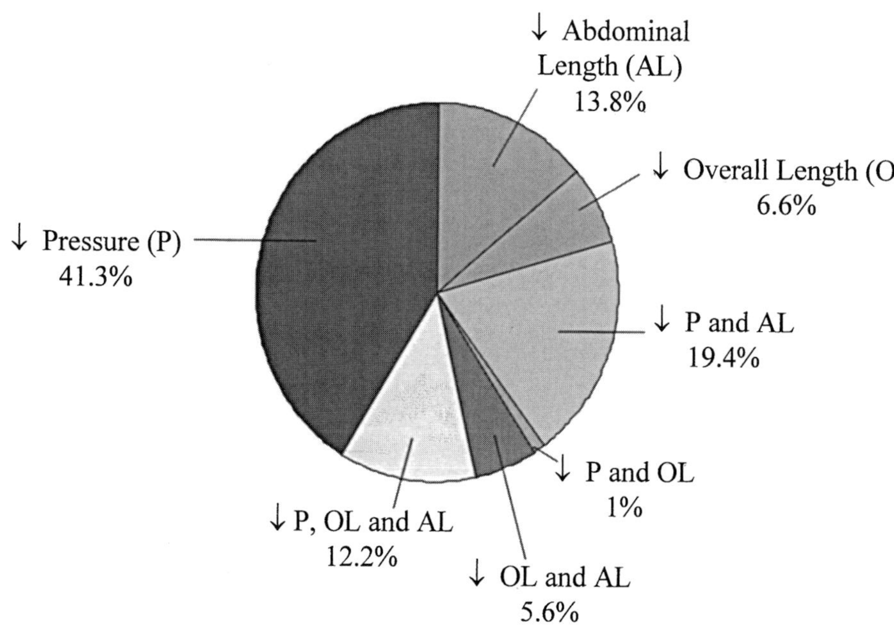

FIGURE 3–6 ■ Specific abnormalities of the lower esophageal sphincter (LES) detected in 196 patients with abnormal esophageal acid exposure by 24-hour pH testing. An inadequate resting pressure is the most common deficit noted in patients with reflux disease. (AL, abdominal length; OL, overall length; P, resting pressure.)

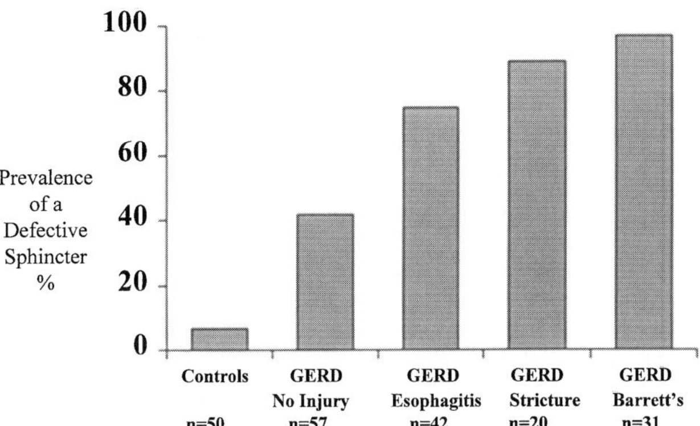

FIGURE 3–7 ■ Prevalence of a defective lower esophageal sphincter (LES) in patients with increasing degrees of mucosal injury related to gastroesophageal reflux disease (GERD). Patients with a defective LES are at risk for complications from reflux disease.

situation, the stomach may become compartmentalized by the crura. Pressurization within the herniated fundus can occur as a consequence of air trapped above the crura and may overpower the LES, allowing reflux of gastric juice into the esophagus.

In addition, loss of the normal angle of His that accompanies the development of a sliding hiatal hernia distorts the geometry of the gastroesophageal junction and impairs LES function. This fact was elegantly demonstrated in a study by Marchand in the 1950s (Marchand, 1955). In this study, the pylorus in a series of young male cadavers was cannulated and the stomach distended with water until the water was seen to escape from the esophagus. Normally, 28 cm of water pressure was necessary to produce gastroesophageal reflux, as evidenced by visualization of fluid escape from the esophagus in these cadavers. However, altering the geometry of the angle of His significantly changed the pressure necessary to induce reflux. When the angle of His was abolished, reflux occurred at only 3 cm of water pressure. In contrast, augmenting the angle of His by resecting the left hemidiaphragm resulted in a requirement for 42 cm of water pressure in order for reflux to occur. Marchand also noted that interference with normal receptive relaxation of the stomach allowed reflux to occur at 9 cm of water pressure.

Along similar lines, Ismail and colleagues (1995) compared the yield pressure at which the cardia opened in response to gastric distention in subjects with and without reflux and with varying sizes of a hiatal hernia. They noted that yield pressure dropped progressively with increasing size of the hiatal hernia (Fig. 3–8).

Independent of problems with reflux, a hiatal hernia can also produce symptoms of dysphagia and regurgitation (Kaul et al, 1990). As seen in manometric studies, the presence of a hiatal hernia is often noted by the detection of a "double hump" in the pressure tracing of the LES (Fig. 3–9).

The Phrenoesophageal Ligament

Although most patients with GERD have a hiatal hernia, many individuals with a hiatal hernia have no reflux. Clearly, the mere presence of a hernia does not always lead to increased esophageal acid exposure.

One potential explanation is that the point of attachment of the phrenoesophageal ligament may influence the likelihood of development of abnormal gastroesophageal reflux (Fig. 3–10). Fluctuations in intra-abdominal pressure can be transmitted by the hernia sac to the abdominal portion of the LES, even though anatomically it may be positioned within the posterior mediastinum. If the attachment of the phrenoesophageal ligament remains high on the LES, the intra-abdominal length of the LES is preserved. In this setting, esophageal acid exposure, as determined by 24-hour pH monitoring, is likely to be normal (Kaul et al, 1990). In many patients, however, the phrenoesophageal ligament becomes attenuated during development of a hiatal hernia, and its remaining point of attachment to the LES is low. In this setting the abdominal portion of the LES is short, and with increased intra-abdominal pressure the ligament may act as a distracting force and further compromise the function of the LES.

The Stomach

In normal subjects without increased esophageal acid exposure on 24-hour pH monitoring, episodes of reflux occur most frequently during the postprandial period, when the stomach is distended (Mason et al, 1998). Ingestion of excessive food or air results in gastric dilatation. As the stomach distends, the LES is "taken up" into the stretched fundus much in the way that the neck of a balloon shortens as the balloon is inflated (Fig. 3–11). With shortening of the LES, the likelihood of competency progressively decreases (Fig. 3–12). In addition, the force vectors produced by gastric distention vary according

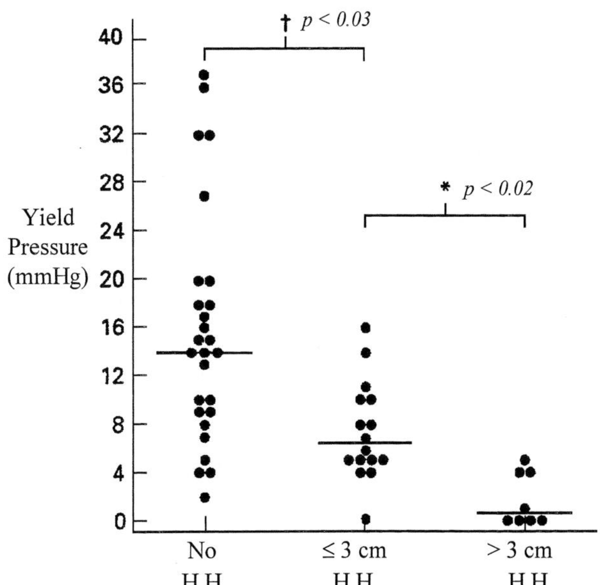

FIGURE 3–8 ■ Relationship between hiatal hernia (H.H.) and yield pressure of the lower esophageal sphincter during endoscopy. *Bars* represent medians; $*P < .002$; $\dagger\ P < .003$ (Mann-Whitney U test). (From Ismail T, Bancewicz J, Barlow J: Yield pressure, antomy of the cardia and gastro-oesophageal reflux. Br J Surg 82:943–947, 1995.)

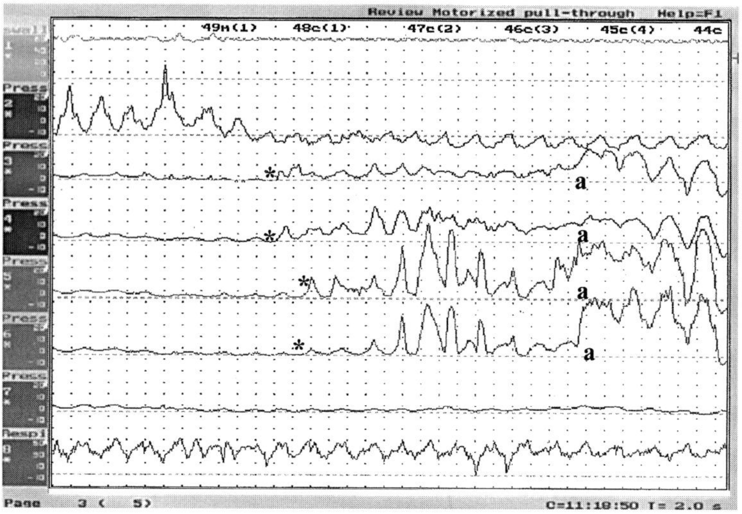

FIGURE 3–9 ■ Slow motorized pull-through tracing of the lower esophageal sphincter in a patient with a hiatal hernia demonstrating a characteristic "double hump." The catheter has four sensors (channels 3 to 6), positioned at the same level and oriented in separate directions. Typically, there is a rise above gastric baseline pressure with the onset of crural impressions or impingement on the herniated portion of the stomach (*asterisk*) (see Fig. 3–10). This is followed by a plateau period while the catheter is in the portion of herniated stomach above the diaphragm (best seen in channels 3 and 4). At the true start of the sphincter (a), the pressure rises further.

to the geometry of the cardia. Consequently, the forces associated with gastric distention are applied more directly to the LES when a hiatal hernia is present than when a proper angle of His exists (Ismail et al, 1995). With continued shortening of the LES by gastric distention, a point is reached, usually at about 1 cm, when the LES pressure drops precipitously and reflux occurs (Pettersson et al, 1980).

After gastric venting, LES length is restored and the barrier function is reestablished until gastric distention again compromises the LES, and further venting and reflux occurs. This sequence is responsible for the common complaints of bloating and repetitive belching in patients with GERD. In normal subjects, belching precipitates almost all reflux episodes; in patients with GERD, however, belching is an important but decreasing cause of reflux as the severity of the disease, reflected by the grade of esophagitis, worsens (DeMeester et al, 1999). This suggests that GERD may be initiated by the stomach secondary to gastric distention from overeating and from delayed gastric emptying due to the ingestion of fried or fatty foods. Repetitive reflux episodes cause mucosal damage and, ultimately, an inflammatory injury of the underlying LES muscle. Consequently, there can be a progressive injury to the LES that eventually leads to permanent incompetence (Zaninotto et al, 1989).

Transient Relaxation of the Lower Esophageal Sphincter

Dent and colleagues (1980) studied 10 healthy volunteers and noted that in these asymptomatic subjects, reflux

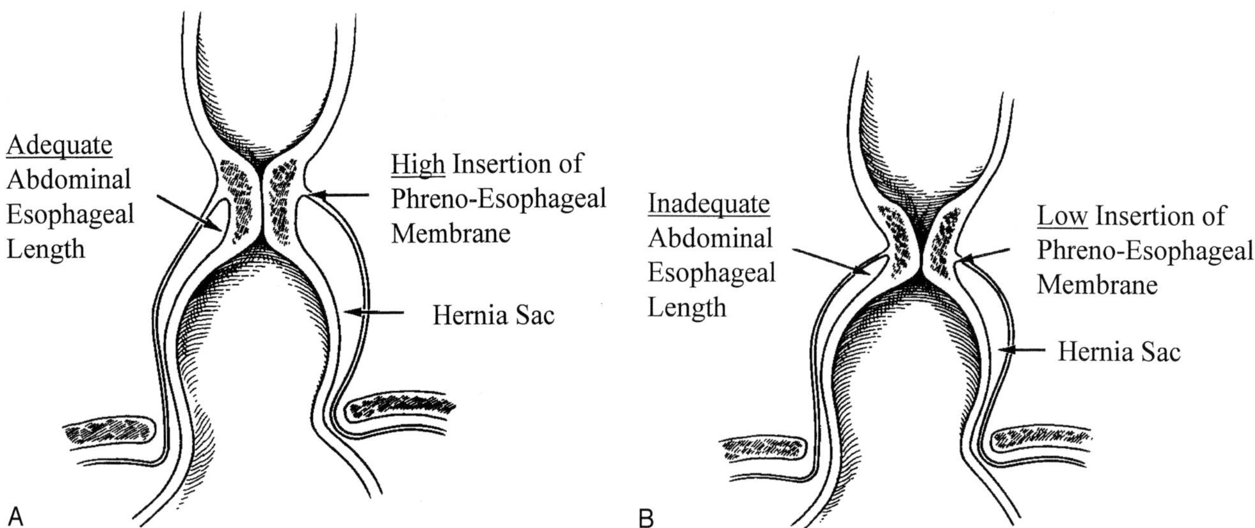

FIGURE 3–10 ■ *A*, High insertion of the phrenoesophageal membrane onto the esophagus allows an adequate length of the lower esophageal sphincter (LES) to be exposed to intra-abdominal pressure transmitted through the hernia sac. *B*, Low insertion of the phrenoesophageal membrane onto the esophagus with an inadequate length of the LES exposed to intra-abdominal pressure. In addition, this anatomic arrangement leads to distraction and further mechanical disadvantage of the sphincter with distention of the herniated portion of stomach. (From DeMeester TR, Lafontaine E, Joelsson BE, et al: Relationship of a hiatal hernia to the function of the body of the esophagus and the gastroesophageal junction. J Thorac Cardiovasc Surg 82:547–558, 1981.)

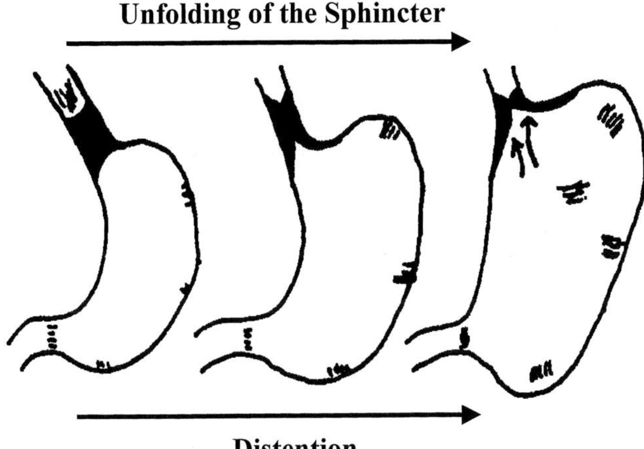

FIGURE 3–11 ■ Schematic illustration of the pathogenesis of early gastroesophageal reflux disease. Distention of the stomach from overeating, aerophagia, or delayed gastric emptying, with or without a rise in intragastric pressure, results in shortening of sphincter length as it is taken up by the distended stomach. A point is reached when sphincter length is no longer adequate for competency, causing a precipitous drop in sphincter pressure, loss of sphincter resistance, and reflux. The process of taking up the sphincter by the distended fundus exposes the squamous epithelium within the sphincter to gastric juice and may result in mucosal injury and to the development of carditis.

episodes occurred in the recumbent position during episodes of transient LES relaxation. These episodes have subsequently been termed "transient LES relaxations" (TLESRs). Identifying TLESRs requires differentiating them from normal swallow-induced LES relaxation. Complicating understanding even further was the finding by Trifan and colleagues (1995) that a pharyngeal stimulus can cause LES relaxation in the absence of esophageal peristalsis, an event that mimics a TLESR.

A current controversial issue pertains to the frequency and importance of TLESRs in normal people and in patients with GERD and to how to define and determine a TLESR. Nonetheless, TLESRs have been implicated as the major mechanism of reflux in patients with a normal LES and as an important cause of reflux in patients with GERD. The proportion of reflux episodes ascribed to TLESRs may vary inversely with the severity of GERD, presumably because of the increasing prevalence of LES deficits in patients with advanced disease (Mittal et al, 1995).

Gastric distention is known to be a potent stimulus for TLESRs. Some investigators think that TLESRs are a reflex event primarily mediated by the vagus nerve and are stimulated by receptors in the gastric fundus and the pharynx (Mittal et al, 1997). However, given that gastric distention contributes to shortening of the length of the LES, perhaps TLESRs are a mechanical event that occurs as a result of the sudden loss of LES competency when a crucial length of LES is reached during progressive gastric distention. The increased frequency of swallowing seen in patients with GERD, in an effort to clear refluxed gastric juice from the esophagus, results in recurrent episodes of gastric distention from the swallowed air. This may explain why TLESRs seem to occur more commonly in patients with GERD. If TLESRs are actually a mechanical event secondary to gastric distention, a better term for these events might be "transient sphincter shortenings."

Interestingly, fundoplication has been demonstrated to substantially reduce the frequency of TLESRs as well as the likelihood that reflux will occur in conjunction with the event (Ireland et al, 1993). This lends further support to a mechanical rather than a neural cause of these events. Further studies should help clarify the etiology and significance of these events in both normal subjects and patients with GERD.

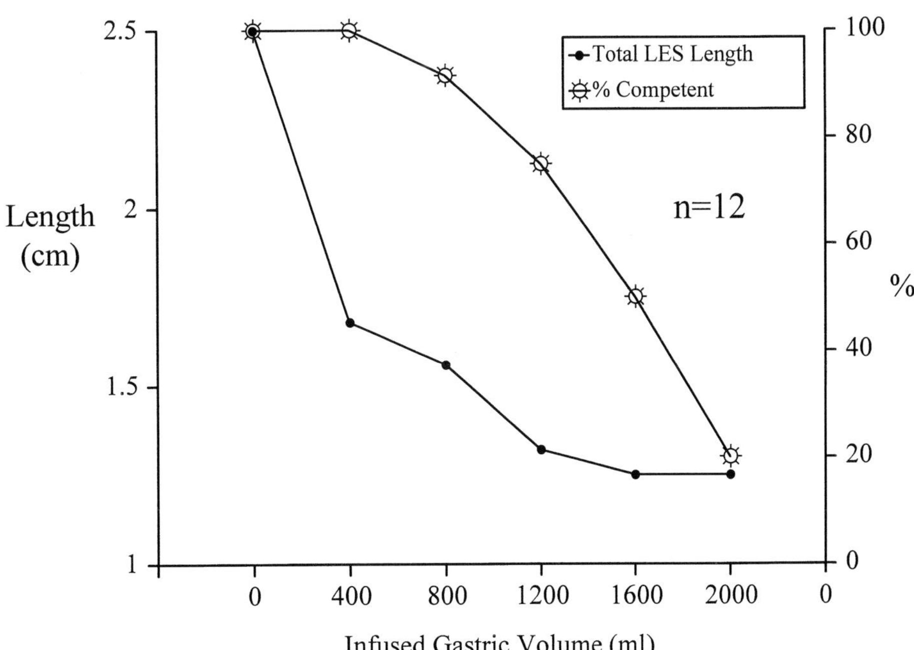

FIGURE 3–12 ■ Representation of changes in length of the lower esophageal sphincter (LES) and competency with saline infusion into the stomachs of anesthetized baboons. The pylorus has been clamped shut. As saline is infused, progressive shortening of sphincter length and a corresponding loss of sphincter competency result.

Antireflux Surgery

Symptoms in patients with permanent LES incompetence are difficult to control with medical therapy. However, fundoplication reestablishes the LES barrier to reflux, prevents shortening of the sphincter during gastric distention, and improves gastric emptying (Mason et al, 1997; Vu et al, 1999). In addition to the safety and longevity of an antireflux operation, new, minimally invasive approaches have shortened the hospital stay, decreased the discomfort associated with the procedure, and allowed earlier return to work and full activity.

Achalasia

Achalasia of the esophagus is a motor disorder characterized by incomplete swallow-induced relaxation of the LES with or without increased resting LES pressure and the absence of esophageal body contractility. The cause is unknown but may represent the consequences of a viral infection or autoimmune process. Ultimately, there is degeneration of the myenteric plexus and a marked reduction in nitric oxide–secreting myenteric ganglion cells in both the LES and the gastric fundus (De Giorgio et al, 1999). The process probably begins in the LES, perhaps as a consequence of inflammatory changes in the intrinsic esophageal neural network (Goldblum et al, 1996). Loss of esophageal body function may be a secondary event, since in some patients disruption of the LES by balloon dilatation or surgical myotomy has resulted in return of peristalsis.

Hypertensive Lower Esophageal Sphincter

Similar to achalasia, the condition called hypertensive LES features an elevated resting LES pressure but complete LES relaxation with a swallow. Peristalsis in the esophageal body is usually normal.

Most patients present with complaints of solid food dysphagia although usually videoesophagraphic and endoscopic findings are relatively normal. The diagnosis is made only by esophageal manometry. The natural history of this condition is not known with certainty. Perhaps, in some patients, this condition represents the earliest manifestations of achalasia or another named motility disorder. In some patients, LES injection with botulinum toxin or surgical myotomy relieves dysphagia.

■ REFERENCES

Biancani P, Hillemeier C, Bitar KN, Makhlouf GM: Contraction mediated by Ca^{2+} influx in esophageal muscle and by Ca^{2+} release in the LES (Abstract). Am J Physiol 253:G760–G766, 1987.

Bonavina L, Evander A, DeMeester TR, et al: Length of the distal esophageal sphincter and competency of the cardia. Am J Surg 151:25–34, 1986.

Boyle JT, Altschuler SM, Nixon TE, et al: Role of the diaphragm in the genesis of lower esophageal sphincter pressure in the cat. Gastroenterology 88:723–730, 1985.

Daniel EE, Taylor GS, Holman ME: The myogenic basis of active tension in the lower esophageal sphincter (Abstract). Gastroenterology 70:874, 1976.

De Giorgio R, Simone MP, Stranghellini V, et al: Esophageal and gastric nitric oxide synthesizing innervation in primary achalasia. Am J Gastroenterol 94:2357–2362, 1999.

DeMeester TR, Wernly JA, Bryant GH, et al: Clinical and in vitro analysis of determinants of gastroesophageal competence: A study of the principles of antireflux surgery. Am J Surg 137:39–46, 1979.

DeMeester TR, Lafontaine E, Joelsson BE, et al: Relationship of a hiatal hernia to the function of the body of the esophagus and the gastroesophageal junction. J Thorac Cardiovasc Surg 82:547–558, 1981.

DeMeester TR, Peters JH, Bremner CG, Chandrasoma P: Biology of gastroesophageal reflux disease: Pathophysiology relating to medical and surgical treatment (Abstract). Annu Rev Med 50:469–506, 1999.

Dent J, Dodds WJ, Friedman RH, et al: Mechanism of gastroesophageal reflux in recumbent asymptomatic human subjects. J Clin Invest 65:256–267, 1980.

De Troyer A, Sampson M, Sigrist S, Macklem PT: Action of costal and crural parts of the diaphragm on the rib cage in dog. J Appl Physiol 53:30–39, 1982.

Dodds WJ, Dent J, Hogan WJ, Arndorfer RC: Effect of atropine on esophageal motor function in humans. Am J Physiol 240:G290–G296, 1981.

Fyke FE Jr, Code CF, Schlegel JF: The gastroesophageal sphincter in healthy human beings. Gastroenterologia 86:135–150, 1956.

Goldblum JR, Rice TW, Richter JE: Histopathologic features in esophagomyotomy specimens from patients with achalasia. Gastroenterology 111:648–654, 1996.

Goyal RK, Rattan S: Genesis of basal sphincter pressure: Effect of tetrodotoxin on lower esophageal sphincter pressure in opossum in vivo. Gastroenterology 71:62–67, 1976.

Ireland AC, Holloway RH, Toouli J, Dent J: Mechanisms underlying the antireflux action of fundoplication. Gut 34:303–308, 1993.

Ismail T, Bancewicz J, Barlow J: Yield pressure, anatomy of the cardia and gastro-esophageal reflux (Abstract). Br J Surg 82:943–947, 1995.

Kaul BK, DeMeester TR, Oka M, et al: The cause of dysphagia in uncomplicated sliding hiatal hernia and its relief by hiatal herniorrhaphy: A roentgenographic, manometric, and clinical study. Ann Surg 211:406–410, 1990.

Klein W, Parkman H, Dempsey D, Fisher R: Sphincter-like thoracoabdominal high pressure zone after esophagogastrectomy (Abstract). Gastroenterology 105:1362–1369, 1993.

Liebermann-Meffert D, Allgower M, Schmid P, Blum AL: Muscular equivalent of the lower esophageal sphincter. Gastroenterology 76:31–38, 1979.

Marchand P: The gastro-esophageal 'sphincter' and the mechanism of regurgitation. Br J Surg 42:504–513, 1955.

Marchand P: A study of the forces productive of gastroesphageal regurgitation and herniation through the diaphragmatic hiatus (Abstract). Thorax 12:189–202, 1957.

Mason RJ, Oberg S, Bremner CG, et al: Postprandial gastroesophageal reflux in normal volunteers and symptomatic patients. J Gastrointest Surg 2:342–349, 1998.

Mason RJ, DeMeester TR, Lund RJ, et al: Nissen fundoplication prevents shortening of the sphincter during gastric distention. Arch Surg 132:719–724, 1997 [discussion, 724–726].

Mittal RK, Fisher M, McCallum RW, et al: Human lower esophageal sphincter pressure response to increased intra-abdominal pressure. Am J Physiol 258:G624–G630, 1990.

Mittal RK, Holloway R, Dent J: Effect of atropine on the frequency of reflux and transient lower esophageal sphincter relaxation in normal subjects. Gastroenterology 109:1547–1554, 1995.

Mittal RK, Balaban DH: The esophagogastric junction (Review). N Engl J Med 336:924–932, 1997.

Mittal RK, Holloway RH, Penagini R, et al: Transient lower esophageal sphincter relaxation (Review). Gastroenterology 109:601–610. 1995.

Mittal RK, Chiareli C, Liu J, et al: Atropine inhibits gastric distension and pharyngeal receptor mediated lower oesophageal sphincter relaxation. Gut 41:285–290, 1997.

Monges H, Salducci J, Naudy B: Dissociation between the electrical activity of the diaphragmatic dome and crura muscular fibers during esophageal distension, vomiting and eructation: An electromyographic study in the dog. J Physiol (Paris) 74:541–554, 1978.

Pellegrini CA, DeMeester TR, Skinner DB: Response of the distal esophageal sphincter to respiratory and positional maneuvers in humans. Surg Forum 27:380–382, 1976.

Pettersson GB, Bombeck CT, Nyhus LM: The lower esophageal sphincter: Mechanisms of opening and closure. Surgery 88:307–314, 1980.

Sontag SJ, Schnell TG, Miller TQ, et al: The importance of hiatal hernia in reflux esophagitis compared with lower esophageal sphincter pressure or smoking. J Clin Gastroenterol 13:628–643, 1991; comment, 13:617–619.

Stein HJ, DeMeester TR, Naspetti R, et al: Three-dimensional imaging of the lower esophageal sphincter in gastroesophageal reflux disease. Ann Surg 214:374–83, 1991 [discussion, 383–384].

Trifan A, Shaker R, Ren J, et al: Inhibition of resting lower esophageal sphincter pressure by pharyngeal water stimulation in humans. Gastroenterology 108:441–446, 1995.

Vu MK, Straathof JW, v d Schaar PJ, et al: Motor and sensory function of the proximal stomach in reflux disease and after laparoscopic Nissen fundoplication. Am J Gastroenterol 94:1481–1489, 1999.

Wetscher GJ, Hinder RA, Perdikis G, et al: Three-dimensional imaging of the lower esophageal sphincter in healthy subjects and gastroesophageal reflux. Dig Dis Sci 41:2377–2382, 1996.

Yamato S, Spechler SJ, Goyal RK: Role of nitric oxide in esophageal peristalsis in the opossum. Gastroenterology 103:197–204, 1992.

Zaninotto G, DeMeester TR, Schwizer W, et al: The lower esophageal sphincter in health and disease. Am J Surg 155:104–111, 1988.

Zaninotto G, DeMeester TR, Bremner CG, Smyrk TC, Cheng SC: Esophageal function in patients with reflux-induced strictures and its relevance to surgical treatment. Ann Thorac Surg 1989;47:362–70.

Investigation of Esophageal Disease

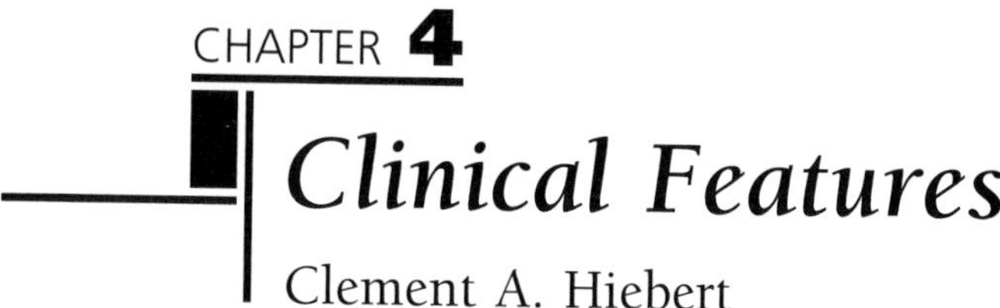

CHAPTER 4

Clinical Features

Clement A. Hiebert

NORMAL ESOPHAGEAL FUNCTION

As organs go, the esophagus is a shy performer, a sensory void between the pleasures of an appraising palate and the lingering contentment of an agreeably full stomach. For years the esophagus was dismissed as a drainpipe to the stomach, a place where the digestive tract got down to serious business, a respectable place on which the subspecialty of gastroenterology could stake its identity. The gullet became a Cinderella when cineradiography, flexible endoscopy, and motility and pH studies provided rewarding tools for investigating esophageal disease, tools that refined the concepts that surgeons such as Allison (1951), Belsey (1952), and Barrett (1954) had correctly understood by relating the patient's symptoms to the findings at rigid esophagoscopy half a century ago.

This chapter is concerned with features of esophageal disease that can be defined at the bedside. To search for what is abnormal, one must have a sure sense of what is normal. The functions of the esophagus are as follows:

1. Smoothly transporting liquids and food from the pharynx to the stomach.
2. Protecting the esophageal mucosa from gastric contents.
3. Defending the airway from exposure to esophageal contents.
4. Venting of gastric and esophageal gas.
5. Vomiting, under suitably wretched circumstances.

ESOPHAGEAL DYSFUNCTION

Each esophageal symptom represents a maloccurrence in one or more of these assignments. Deviation from the normal is often subtle, and the quality of the recorded history depends on the patient's sensitivity to the dysfunction, an ability to articulate the matter, and the physician's willingness to listen, elicit, and arrange the symptoms into a plausible portrait of an illness. Consider the compelling history with which Phillip Allison (1951) launched the modern era of antireflux surgery:

> A 59-year-old woman complains that for 6 years she has suffered from intense burning pain behind the lower part of the sternum, which rises up toward, or even into, the neck. The pain may spread into the jaw, the ear, or the hard palate, or radiate through to the back between the shoulder blades or down the arm. It comes on especially when she exerts herself stooping forward, as in washing the floor, bending over the washtub, poking the fire, or fastening her shoes. It wakes her in the middle of the night, especially if she is sleeping on her back or her right side, and she seeks relief from what she describes as an agonizing pain by sitting upright and taking a few sips of water, milk, or alkaline mixture. She says that her throat usually feels dry and burning. When she swallows, she may be conscious of the passage of food down the gullet; it may cause a feeling of soreness, a pain that is immediately relieved as the bolus passes into the stomach. If she bends forward after a meal, food or sour liquid rises into her throat and has to be swallowed again. Her husband says that for belching she takes first prize. She has tried all the advertised stomach medicines with only temporary relief and has finally been told that "the nerve of her stomach has been upset by the change of life."

For polished medical prose, Allison's history of a present illness is unsurpassed. The surgeon has gotten inside his patient, exposed the gastroesophageal junction, and bared its abnormality.

The history should contain clues so that the reading of it provides tentative answers to three questions:

1. *Which organ is sick*? Which component has failed? Is the likely culprit muscle, mucosa, or a sphincter?
2. *What is wrong*? What is the pathologic process: cancer? spasm? reflux? a congenital abnormality?
3. *How severe is the process*? How far has it gone? Has a cancer spread beyond the logical perimeter of the surgeon's scalpel? Does the reflux qualify for surgical relief?

Dysphagia

Dysphagia is the signature symptom of the gullet. Unlike substernal pain, regurgitation, bleeding, aspiration, and other symptoms that mimic those of the heart, gallbladder, stomach, or duodenum, swallowing complaints are always foregut complaints. When one is inquiring about the possibility of a swallowing disorder, it is well to frame

the question so that the patient understands that at issue is the sticking of food at any level between the Adam's apple and the xiphoid—an important issue because an occasional patient regards the throat as the "end-all" of swallowing.

Like the malady itself, the word *dysphagia* strikes two notes: perception (difficult) and process (eating). A useful way of looking at dysphagia is to regard the intensity of the complaint as a function of both the sensitivity of the patient and the severity of the affliction. Dysphagia is a continuum, bracketed by the half-noticed hesitation of food on its journey to the stomach on the one hand and by the wretchedness of total blockage on the other. One individual with heightened awareness of swallowing events may fret about a sensation that defies definition by barium and motility studies, whereas another is oblivious of symptoms leading to a stricture that may have taken years to mature. Skinner and Belsey (1988) noted that 20% of patients with benign stricture are unaware of antecedent reflux.

Perceptive patients can accurately identify the level of a mechanical obstruction, except for problems in the lower third that may be felt to be in the neck. The opposite does not happen; impedance in the cervical esophagus is never sensed lower down.

Another characteristic of dysphagia is the variable character of the triggering bolus: the person with esophageal cancer is intolerant of solid food. In patients with achalasia, both liquids and solids are delayed at the cardia. Liquids alone, especially at the extremes of temperature, may profoundly alter esophageal motor function (Meyer and Castell, 1981; Winship et al, 1970).

Dysphagia lusoria, compression of the esophagus by a congenital vascular anomaly, was first described by Bayford in 1787; see Asherson (1979). The most common of several types of vascular rings is an aberrant right subclavian artery that passes posterior to the esophagus. According to Gross (1955), the dysphagia associated with this anomaly begins usually after the age of 1 year and is manifested by feeding problems, stridor, and respiratory infections. The symptoms are worsened by neck flexion (Edwards, 1959).

At the outset, dysphagia may be abrupt and total, as when a previously silent lower esophageal ring or stricture becomes plugged with imperfectly chewed steak and the anxious patient comes to the emergency department, coughing, retching, and pressing a handkerchief soaked with mucus to the mouth. More often, the onset is insidious, only later recalled as a "catch" at the manubrium that was eased by a sip or two of water. If the symptom was reported at all, the chances were good that the physician dismissed it as just another "lump in the throat." Skinner and Belsey (1988) observed that by the time the symptom of dysphagia is recognized for what it is, fully half of the patients with cancer have metastases.

The association of weight loss and progressive dysphagia is ominous and pathognomonic of cancer when the duration of symptoms is less than 3 months and the patient is older than 50 years of age. By contrast, the development of a benign stricture in an adult may take years to develop, and alterations in appetite or weight are less likely. A lengthy history of esophageal symptoms does not automatically exclude malignancy, as when, for example, cancer complicates achalasia or when it develops in a columnar lined esophagus consequent to long-standing reflux.

Odynophagia

Odynophagia is a painful term for painful swallowing: it smacks of pretension, as do the terms *masticating, deglutition*, and *eructation*. We certainly don't hear of odyno-anything else. Either "esoph-algia" or "esopha-phag-algia" would get the idea across, but neither is likely to catch hold with physicians who cannot agree whether to spell *oesophagus* with an *e* or an *o*.

Swallowing may cause pain in a healthy person when the bolus is the wrong size or of the wrong consistency. The esophagus may flinch if the bolus is too hot, less commonly when it is too cold. For practical purposes, however, painful swallowing means either cramped muscle or sore mucosa. Cramped muscle may figure in the painful passage or impaction of a bolus (see Chapter 32); the present discussion is limited to mucosal injury.

Although the esophagus may be brutalized by swallowing caustic or highly acid material, a more common burn in the Western world is that caused by a medicinal tablet that fails to make it to the stomach. One patient described the sensation as a "burr that got stuck." The fault may be inadequate salivary lubrication or an insufficient flush of water. The pill may be too large or too harsh. Common offenders are tetracycline, potassium iodide, quinidine along with ascorbic acid tablets. Transit times of various medicines have been discussed by Hey, and colleagues (1982). The elderly are especially susceptible, perhaps because they use more medicine and because esophageal clearance is less reliable. Taking medicine in the supine position is to be avoided.

Swallowing pain is very common in patients undergoing chemotherapy or radiation treatment. Brereton and coworkers (1979) state that moderate to severe esophagitis afflicts more than half of patients who receive combined treatment. Patients with acquired immunodeficiency syndrome (AIDS) and individuals with a compromised immune system are vulnerable to infections, commonly, *Candida*, herpes simplex, cytomegalovirus and, less commonly, mucosal tuberculosis.

Painful swallowing is usually seen after withdrawal of a foreign body, particularly one that may have scratched or impaled itself on the esophageal wall. In such a circumstance, the patient may be convinced that the foreign body has yet to be removed. The patient who has undergone multiple biopsy procedures or who has had an esophagoscopy that was difficult or prolonged may experience a similarly unpleasant and gritty sensation on attempting to swallow. This problem is invariably present when the esophageal wall has been breached, either "spontaneously" or from instrumentation.

Globus Hystericus

Globus hystericus is the perception of a lump in a throat that is actually clean as a whistle. Over the years, the fortunes of globus hystericus have waxed and waned as

motility laboratories and psychiatric centers have offered a succession of promising studies that just as often were abandoned. Is it a phantom lump that is felt with swallowing or the sense of a mass when the throat is at rest? The suggestion has been made that a name change is in order. Because hysteria is ostensibly not present, the proper name is *globus*—period (Castell, 1992). That notion has its own problems, for when was the last time a patient, in Latin or in English, likened the sensation to a ball?

The important concept is to maintain a keen ear and open mind and to use common sense. A 20-year-old male college student, shattered by the loss of a girlfriend, does not require the same workup for a month-long sensation of a lump in the throat and 7-pound weight loss that would be mandated by those symptoms in a 65-year-old alcoholic who smokes three packs of cigarettes a day.

Heartburn

Approximately 50% of American adults have consumed antacids, and 75% of those users do so two to six times a day (Graham et al., 1983). Of heavy antacid users, 80% seek relief from heartburn, and the task of the physician is to determine when the symptom is trivial and when it is less likely so. Unfortunately, it is the gullet's lot that the severity of its symptoms does not necessarily reflect the severity of the disease or the pathologic process.

To capture the essence of heartburn, the patient's own words are preferable to trite and presumptive descriptors, such as "symptoms of esophagitis" or "complaints of reflux." Aside from the fact that heartburn is not to be equated with esophagitis (Hiebert and Belsey, 1961; Mattioli et al, 1989), such phrases tell us more about the harried state of the interviewer than about the character of the patient's symptom. Using the patient's own words is better and affirms that the physician took time to connect with an ailing fellow human and to experience a measure of the distress (and sometimes the humor) inherent in the response to "What bothers you the most?" A sample of complaints taken from office records:

- "Exploding—burning pressure in the chest."
- "Sour stomach and acid coming through mouth–nose."
- "When I eat I have to wash my solid food down with liquids, and when I do, it pains where my esophagus narrows as the liquid pushes my food down."
- "Pain in the pity [sic] of my stomach."
- "Heartburn and gas and pain in the stomach. The pain in my stomach hurts when I cough and sometimes when I breathe and when I bend down. I feel like throwing up mostly all the time at work."
- "Heartburn follows 20 minutes to 1 hour after meals, sometimes accompanied by a sharp pain in my back and chest."
- "Heartburn and pukus."
- ". . . when the acid gets bad, it backs up to my mouth and gets me sick. When I bend over, it really bothers me. Sometimes the pain is so bad it wakes me out of a dead sleep."
- "Pain in left upper chest for one-half hour to one hour after eating . . . pain in armpits when arms used."
- "Gas and heartburn wake me up from 4 to 6 AM."
- "Heartburn when I bend over to brush my teeth."
- "I can almost taste the acid at the bottom of my esophagus."

Several patients noted burning chest pain during sexual intercourse, and one mother experienced the problem when lifting a child from his cot. A 17-year-old baseball pitcher reported heartburn when leaning over to finger the rosin bag but made the most of his affliction after discovering the advantage of regurgitated mucus on his curve ball.

Although the patient with disordered motor activity may experience overlapping pain, heartburn is most often the expression of a mucosal burn from refluxed acid-pepsin. *The pathognomonic hallmark of heartburn caused by gastroesophageal reflux is the initiation or exacerbation of pain on stooping, bending, or lying down.*

Patients usually discover that sitting up or rinsing the gullet with alkali is helpful. Many individuals express a preference for one side when lying in bed. The physician should search for the clue of posturally aggravated symptoms on recumbency and relief on assumption of an upright position, with the same directed interest as exercised, say, in ferreting out a history of fatty meals precipitating right subcostal pain radiating to the right subscapular region when gallstones are suspected.

The flare of heartburn characteristically begins 20 minutes to 2 hours following a large, fatty, or spicy meal. Chocolate, fruit juices, and alcoholic drinks are notorious provokers as, to a lesser degree, are beverages containing caffeine. Tobacco stokes the reflux furnace. "Another reason for not smoking while lying down in bed," notes Spiro (1983).

A useful method (tested over 25 years) for defining the boundaries of a symptom such as heartburn is to ask the patient to shade in where it hurts on a line sketch of the human figure (Fig. 4–1). Advantages of this method are (1) a swift and accurate portrayal of the area of pain and (2) an opportunity for the physician to subtract the post-treatment picture from the original sketch and thereby forge maps of the true reference area of esophageal complaints.

Heartburn is most commonly sensed in the lower substernal and subxiphoid regions. Belsey (Skinner and Belsey, 1988) finds that patients often point with the index finger to a spot high in the epigastrium, the same signal seen during endoscopy with topical anesthesia as the instrument slides by the irritated lower esophageal segments. Spiro (1983) notes a hand over the heart to be the giveaway. Judging from several hundred pain portraits prepared by our patients, the unabridged gesture would require both hands (see Fig. 4–1).

Vanishing Heartburn

Vanishing heartburn is not always something to cheer about. To be sure, there are seasonal fluctuations of the symptom in some individuals and variability of closeness

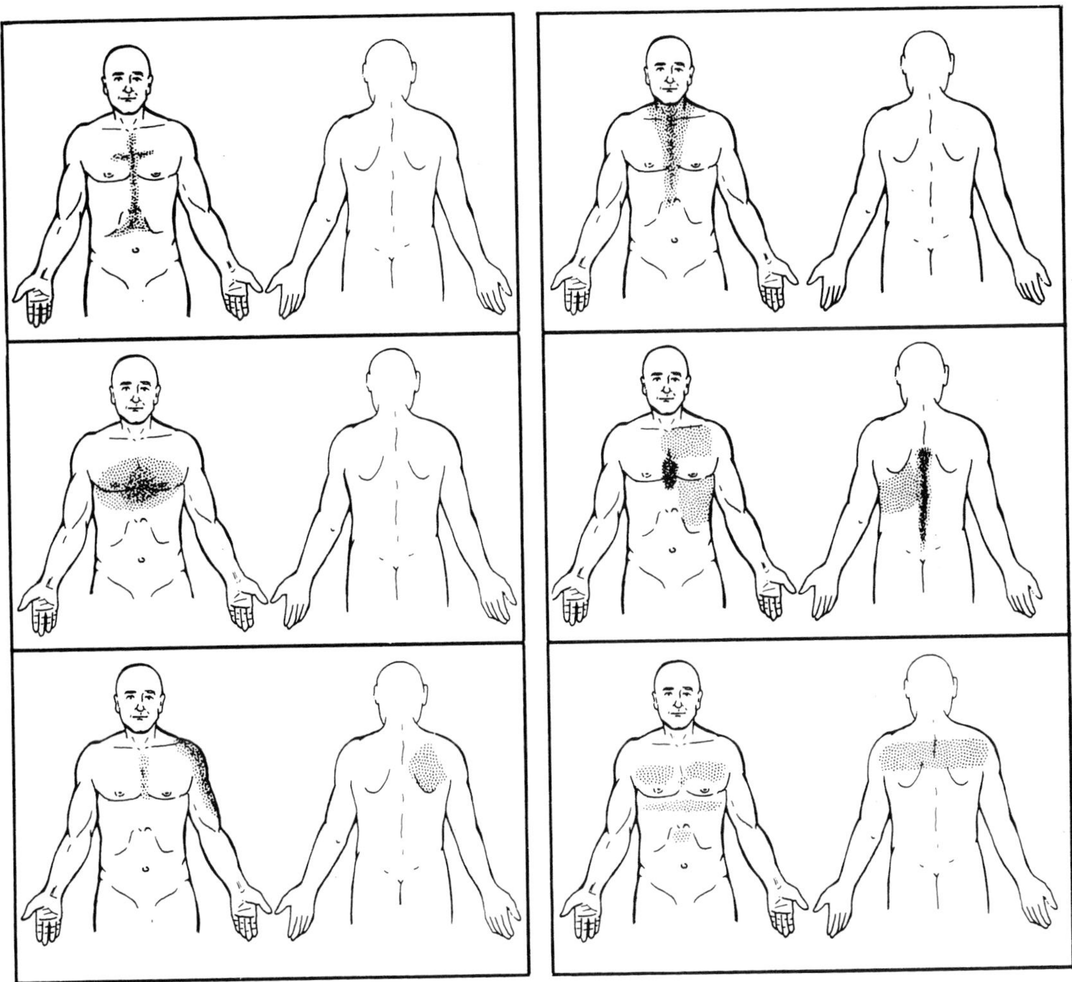

FIGURE 4–1 ■ Various pain patterns of gastroesophageal reflux. Patients shaded in the original sketches to indicate the location of the discomfort. (From Hiebert CA: Evaluation and treatment of hiatal hernia and gastroesophageal reflux. In Zuidema GD [ed]: Shackelford's Surgery of the Alimentary Tract, 3rd ed. Philadelphia, WB Saunders, 1991, p. 168.)

in following doctors' instructions to account for changes in other patients. Most patients discover the influence of certain foods and assume anatomically helpful positions both by day and at night.

A more ominous regression of heartburn is occasionally seen in Barrett's esophagus, when an adenocarcinoma at the cardia that is too small to cause dysphagia is, nevertheless, able to block reflux. "Spontaneous" regression of heartburn may also occur when severe gastroesophageal reflux is reduced by development of a fibrotic stricture. In my experience, the clinical clue of vanishing heartburn is a retrospective sign.

Regurgitation

Regurgitation is the passive return of swallowed material to the pharynx or mouth when the stomach or esophagus is overfilled, obstructed, hypotonic, or valveless. The level of the problem is usually clear from the patient's description of the color, taste, and character of the material and the timing of its appearance. For example, was it green and bitter, clear and frothy, or essentially unchanged from when it was swallowed? Was the interval between ingestion and regurgitation a day, several hours, a few seconds, or instantaneous?

Regurgitation from the stomach is most often the consequence of a patulous esophagogastric junction, either with or without a hiatal hernia. One telltale history is the victim's awakening from sound sleep with a paroxysm of coughing and choking that is relieved by sitting up and swallowing a glass of water or taking an antacid mixture. If the expectorated material is viewed, it would likely be reported to be green and stringy. Streaks of blood suggest the possibility of ulcerative esophagitis; the smell of yeast, achalasia. Occasional patients with gastroesophageal reflux describe the experience of "waterbrash," a sudden filling of the mouth with clear salty fluid consistent with massive salivation triggered by reflux.

Regurgitation occurs also in the daytime. It is posturally aggravated, and the patient soon learns to avoid bending over after eating. This situation may be difficult if the patient's work requires bending and lifting, as it did for an employee of a paper company who was required to empty heavy containers of dye; in straining to do his assignment, he sometimes regurgitated and added un-

specified coloring to the concoction in the vats beneath him. Another man with reflux symptoms recalled how, when he was a youth, his ability to regurgitate at will earned him a reputation as a trackside entertainer. He and his classmates would pause on their way to school on a bridge above the train tracks while he emptied the contents of his stomach into the smokestack on any designated passing train.

In a less dramatic but potentially disabling circumstance, gross incompetency of the gastroesophageal junction may present during the postoperative period of a patient who has undergone an abdominal operation and passively regurgitates because of imposed recumbency. The unwitting house officer who assumes obstruction to be the basis of the reported "vomiting" may pass a nasogastric tube, and subsequent esophagitis may then be attributed to tube trauma rather than to occult reflux exacerbated or provoked by the patient's supine position.

Rumination

To the ordinarily constituted person, the thought of reswallowing regurgitated food and ferments disgusts and, at the very least, smacks of behavior befitting a grass-chewing animal (Long, 1929). Until recently, rumination was thought to be the symptom of a mental disorder and that infants who ruminated were starved for love (Menking et al., 1969). The mortality of the inevitable delay was as high as 20%.

Luschka (1857) found through anatomic dissection that ruminators have a 3- to 4-cm pouch of forestomach situated above the diaphragm, but the diagrams today are said by Herbst et al (1971) to look less like the anatomy of a cow than like the thoracic component of a sliding hiatal hernia. Regurgitation and rumination in infants and children should suggest chalasia or hiatal hernia (Hiebert and Belsey, 1961; Skinner and Belsey, 1967).

Together with failure to thrive and aspiration, this triad of symptoms is pathognomonic of worrisome gastroesophageal reflux. The trick is to distinguish between the infant "mewling and puking in [his mother's] arms" (Shakespeare, *As You Like It*, 1599) and the infant destined for esophagitis, malnourishment, and aspiration pneumonia.

Vomiting

In contrast to the passive character of regurgitation and rumination, vomiting is one of life's most wretched moments. The prostrating nausea, the groaning, the reeking ferments cascading through mouth and nose is misery out of proportion to the usual physiologic innocence of the event. Vomiting is the proclaiming act of the unwell. It is of interest to the esophageal specialist, however, in four urgent circumstances.

The first occurs in the person with *Boerhaave syndrome* when, following a prodigious meal, vomitus pours into the mediastinum and pleural space through a rent in the lower esophageal wall. Another form of injury is the *Mallory-Weiss syndrome*, in which retching and stretching of the gastroesophageal junctional mucosa may result in brisk bleeding (Mallory and Weiss, 1929; Bubrick et al, 1980). A third circumstance is the retching and vomiting that is noted in 57% (Treacy and Jamieson, 1988) of patients with obstruction of a massive *hiatal hernia*. Finally, vomiting can mean *bowel obstruction* following any thoracoabdominal operation.

Aspiration and Respiratory Symptoms

Inhalation of esophageal contents may result in mere hoarseness if the contact with the larynx is fleeting in duration, minor in quantity, and nearly neutral in terms of pH. In contrast, repetitive nocturnal inhalation of even a few milliliters of stomach contents, of the fetid contents of Zenker's diverticulum, or of contents of a chronically obstructed esophagus may inoculate the lungs with an intolerable burden of pathogenic organisms or corrosive chyme. Consequences include cough, stridor, bouts of pneumonia, progressive pulmonary fibrosis, and respiratory insufficiency. The patient may present with respiratory symptoms and may be altogether oblivious of esophageal ones. In time, the larynx and proximal airway become inured to the presence of foreign material so that the patient who is aspirating may tolerate bronchoscopy without topical anesthesia.

Chronic aspiration is a feature of the infant hiatal hernia syndrome and may be manifested by stridor, choking spells, and bouts of pneumonia (Lilly and Randolph, 1968). Asthma in the adult is less likely to be a consequence of insidious aspiration. Skinner and Belsey (1988) note that the reversal of pulmonary symptoms concomitant with correction of the esophageal pathology is a dramatic argument for the correctness of the ascription. Castell (1992) has presented an excellent review of the subject.

Bleeding and Anemia

Bleeding from the esophagus is more often a trickle than a torrent. Exceptions include the painless catastrophic cascade of bright clots and blood from eroded esophageal varices, penetration of a Barret's ulcer into an esophageal branch of the aorta, encroachment on the aorta by an esophageal malignancy or foreign body, and fistulous communication with an aortic aneurysm.

Gastric sources of major hemorrhage include the Mallory-Weiss syndrome (already mentioned) and the discrete ulcer at the hiatal rim or diffuse erosions within the throttled pouch of a massive incarcerated hiatal hernia (Cameron, 1976; Trastek et al, 1996). As a rule, bleeding that is bright red has had less of a chance to react with gastric acid, either because the source is intraesophageal or because the loss is massive. A "coffee-grounds" appearance, however, indicates a lesser bleeding episode or bleeding that is within the stomach.

The most common source of esophageal bleeding is from ulcerative esophagitis secondary to gastroesophageal reflux. It is almost always insidious and reveals itself through occult blood in the stool or in the presence of a chronic microcytic anemia. Other sources of gastrointestinal tract bleeding must be sought before one attributes the problem to reflux. The same recommendation holds for erosions and ulcerations associated with a massive incarcerated hiatal hernia (Maziak et al, 1998). Blood loss anemia is one of the common stigmata of hiatal hernia in the very young. In a series of childhood hernias, Belsey found that 50% of the patients were anemic (Skinner and Belsey, 1988). Bleeding from esophageal cancer is also likely to be insidious and noticed by the patient only when regurgitated mucus and food is blood-streaked. Gastric contents may resemble coffee grounds, but hematemesis is rare.

Bleeding from benign growths is most unusual, the important exception being hemangiomas, for which Govoni (1982) reports a 20% incidence of bleeding. A leiomyoma remains submucosal, unlike its gastric cousin, which is notorious for erosion and serious hemorrhage.

Finally, the syndrome of Plummer-Vinson (Vinson, 1922) must be mentioned. We do not hear much about this syndrome anymore, but at one time the combination of a hypochromic anemia, upper esophageal web, and brittle fingernails in a middle-aged woman was a recognized entity.

Belching

The act of belching requires air to have been swallowed, an esophageal wall under tension, and leaky sphincters. The cardia shares the subtle and important capacity to tell the difference between liquid and gas with the mucosquamous junction at the opposite end of the gastrointestinal tract. Belching is partially under cerebral control (Dent et al, 1980) and partly susceptible to the whims of a puckish tube that waits for a pause in dinner party conversation to loosen the cricopharyngeal collar and relieve the tension (Holloway and Dodds, 1988). This violation of an understanding between owner and organ may be embarrassing, but the consequences are ordinarily social, not physiologic.

Excessive belching is another matter and may be viewed as an indicator of increased voluntary or involuntary dry swallows taken to clear the esophagus. By way of illustration, an 84-year-old man consulted his physician when his wife of many years became concerned about his newly acquired habit of belching. On the strength of this sign alone, he was sent to an ear, nose, and throat surgeon; a barium swallow eventually resulted in the removal of a lower-third esophageal cancer (my case).

Some patients with achalasia state that they are unable to belch. This problem results from an esophagus that is overstretched already and incapable of moving a pocket of gas through either sphincter (de Carle, 1988).

Hiccups

Hiccups are involuntary diaphragmatic contractions with the vocal cords adducted. They are a common human experience with no obvious purpose, and what causes them remains a mystery. The sporadic form is at worst an annoyance and an embarrassment. When hiccups persist for days they cripple and exhaust.

Ideas for obtaining relief abound, and because anecdotal reports have suggested the culprit to be esophageal distention or reflux, surgeons have occasionally attempted operative relief. Skinner and Belsey (1988) report relief of intractable hiccups in a middle-aged man with esophagitis following colon substitution for the stenotic and inflamed gullet. In a Mayo Clinic study of 220 cases of chronic hiccups, Souadjian and Cain (1968) found that 26% had a diaphragmatic hernia. However, I have seen hiccups persist after esophagectomy (my case).

Nutritional Depletion and Avitaminosis

The esophagus can be narrowed to a diameter of 3 or 4 mm; if the process is benign, the patient may remain the picture of health. On the other hand, a cancer that barely encroaches on the lumen may be associated with wasting and shriveling of the flesh. Almost from the onset of dysphagia, esophageal cancer proclaims its presence by a haunting visceral aversion to food, not explained by swallowing limitations.

Weight loss may also be seen in patients with achalasia of either the upper or the lower esophageal sphincter, but anorexia is less prominent. Weight gain following correction of the problem is the rule. Wasting with listlessness in infants with hiatal hernia may be striking and is termed "failure to thrive" by pediatric surgeons (Lilly and Randolph, 1968). Hiebert (1977) reported an instance of clinical scurvy in a patient with hiatal hernia and esophagitis who became obsessed with the idea that an "acid condition" should be treated by total avoidance of acid-containing food and liquid.

Malnutrition, iron deficiency anemia, glossitis, fissures at the angles of the mouth, atrophic oral mucosa, brittle spoon-shaped nails, and thin membranous webbing of the cervical esophagus were the principal stigmata of the Plummer-Vinson or Patterson-Kelly syndrome (Vinson, 1922).

Esophageal Angina

An estimated 10% to 20% of patients with gastroesophageal reflux present with distress that is clinically indistinguishable from that of angina pectoris (Castell, 1984; Vantrappen et al, 1987). The pain, described as "squeezing," a "heavy pressure," or "tightness," can be severe and radiate from the precordium to the interscapular area, neck, jaws, ear, and one or both arms. If the sometimes ashen and perspiring patient reports the pain to have been triggered by exertion or emotional events, the cardiologist will be early on the scene. Confusion follows the discovery of normal electrocardiogram (ECG) and myocardial enzymes, and the problem may be shared with a gastrointestinal consultant or psychiatrist.

Fabricius (1737) cited the 2nd century surgeon, Galen, as naming the uppermost portion of the stomach the "cardia" because he thought that neighboring organs were likely to have overlapping symptoms. Seventeen hundred years later, Nazum (1947) found hiatal hernia to be present in 25% of 100 patients with a diagnosis of angina pectoris. Belsey (1952) warned about confusion of the symptoms of aortic valvular stenosis with hiatal hernia. Hiebert and Belsey (1961) noted that reflux occurs without hiatal hernia and in that circumstance pain in the precordium, neck, jaw, and arm is likely to be mistaken for angina.

The more recent literature is replete with reports of efforts to sort out pain in the heart and esophagus with objective studies (Benjamin and Castell, 1983; Castell, 1984; Chobanian et al, 1986; Davies et al, 1982; Kline et al, 1981; Rasmussen et al, Richter et al, 1986a, 1986b, 1989). Despite extensive screening of patients with apparent angina and normal coronaries using motility, pH, isotope, radiologic, and provocative studies, a sensitive and specific discriminator has yet to be found. Castell (1984) reminds us that the mere presence of an esophageal motility of pH aberration is insufficient proof unless the pain that mimics angina presents simultaneously with the abnormality on the tracing. Equipment for ultralong-term monitoring is what is needed. Until such equipment is available, a chronicle of the patient's perception is available for the asking.

The following clinical features incrementally suggest that the esophagus—rather than the heart, or for that matter, larynx, thyroid, stomach, duodenum, pancreas, gallbladder, thoracic outlet, pleura, ribs, or spine—is the source of atypical pain:

1. Posturally aggravated symptoms.
2. A history of dysphagia.
3. Substernal pain limited to the midline and radiating to the interscapular area.
4. Pain lasting for days.
5. A history of antacid use.
6. Relief of pain with belching.
7. Slow relief of pain with nitroglycerine. Pope (1983) notes that it usually takes longer (8 to 10 minutes) for nitroglycerine to relieve esophageal "colic" than to relieve angina pectoris (2 to 3 minutes).
8. Youthfulness.
9. Pain that awakens the patient from a sound sleep.
10. Relief with a swallow of 10 ml of 2% viscous xylocaine (Hiebert, unpublished observation).

Hypochondriasis

Persistent, emotionally distraught patients with elusive esophageal symptoms have frustrated physicians for more than a hundred years. Sir William Osler wrote of the problem in his textbook of medicine in 1892: "Esophagismus is met with hysterical patients and hypochondriacs . . . The idiopathic form is found in females of a marked neurotic habit, but may also occur in elderly men." Eighty-one years later, in his 1973 address to the American Surgical Association on the subject of a 20-year experience with 898 patients with hiatal hernia, Allison (1973) noted that approximately 25% of his patients suffered from anxiety or emotional disturbances. He offered as an afterthought, "Impressions over the years would have put the figures more in the region of 75 percent."

More recently, with the advent of motility studies and technicians to take the pulse of the gullet and report on its pH, many patients with atypical chest pain were spared a psychiatric label by the discovery of a spastic esophagus or occult reflux. In fact, the word *hypochondriac* refers to the area beneath the cartilaginous arch where the lower esophagus finds expression. Even so, the hope that curbing spasm or reflux would purge the gullet of one of its last remaining "gremlins" has not occurred (Richter et al, 1986a, 1986b).

CONCLUSIONS

Each of the foregoing features of esophageal disease must be evaluated by the physician. The interview with the patient is a solo project. It requires time. Properly done, it allows the surgeon to get "inside" the patient without making an incision. The intention is to make the depiction so accurate that, were the record shown to the patient, the response would be "Yes, that's just the way it happened," or "It's just how I feel." Relegating the definitive history to others or hastily asking questions solely to satisfy the hospital record committee may be excusable in times of emergency, but a physician's habitual detachment diminishes both the process and the conclusions.

■ REFERENCES

Allison PR: Reflux esophagitis, sliding hiatal hernia, and the anatomy of repair. Surg Gynecol Obstet 92:419, 1951.

Allison PR: Hiatus hernia: A 20-year retrospective survey. Ann Surg 178:273, 1973.

Asherson DB: His syndrome and sign of dysphagia lusoria. Ann R Coll Surg Eng 61:63, 1979.

Barrett NR: Hiatus hernia: A review of some controversial points. Br J Surg 42:231, 1954.

Belsey R (ed): Hiatus hernia. In Modern Trends in Gastroenterology. London, Butterworth, 1952, p 163.

Benjamin SB, Castell DO: Chest pain of esophageal origin: Where are we and where should we go? Arch Intern Med 143:772, 1983.

Brereton HD, Kent CJ, Johnson RE: Chemotherapy and radiation therapy for small cell carcinoma of the lung: A remedy for past therapeutic failure. In Muggia F, et al (eds): Lung Cancer: Progress in Therapeutic Research. New York, Raven Press, 1979.

Bubrick MP, Lundeen JW, Onstad GR et al: Mallory-Weiss syndrome: Analysis of fifty-nine cases. Surgery 88:400, 1980.

Cameron AJ: Incidence of iron deficiency anemia in patients with large diaphragmatic hernia. Mayo Clin Proc 51:767, 1976.

Castell DO: Esophageal chest pain (Editorial). Am J Gastroenterol 79:969, 1984.

Castell DO: The Esophagus. Boston, Little, Brown, 1992.

Chobanian SJ, Benjamin SB, Curtis DJ et al: Systematic esophageal evaluation of patients with noncardiac chest pain. Arch Intern Med 146:1505, 1986.

Davies HA, Jones DB, Rhodes J: "Esophageal angina" as the cause of chest pain. JAMA 248:2274, 1982.

de Carle DJ: Achalasia. In Gamieson GG (ed): Surgery of the Oesophagus. New York, Churchill Livingstone, 1988, p 465.

Dent J, Dodds WJ, Friedman RH et al: Mechanism of gastroesophageal reflux in recumbent asymptomatic human subjects. J Clin Invest 65:256, 1980.

Edwards FR: Vascular compression of the trachea and oesophagus. Thorax 14:187, 1959.

Fabricius ab Aquapendente N: De Gula, Ventriculo, Intestinis Tractus. Patavu, Opera Omnia Luduni Batavorum, 1737.

Govoni AF: Hemangiomas of the esophagus. Gastrointest Radiol 7:113, 1982.

Graham DY, Smith JL, Patterson DJ: Why do apparently healthy people use antacid tablets? Am J Gastroenterol 78:257, 1983.

Gross RE: Arterial malformations which cause compression of the trachea and esophagus. Circulation 11:124, 1955.

Herbst J, Friedland GW, Zboralske FF: Hiatal hernia and "rumination" in infants and children. J Pediatr 78:261, 1971.

Hey H, Jorgensen F, Sorensen K, et al. Oesophageal transit of six commonly used tablets and capsules. Br Med J 285:1717, 1982.

Hiebert CA: Gastroesophageal reflux and ascorbic acid insufficiency. Ann Thorac Surg 24:108, 1977.

Hiebert CA, Belsey R: Incompetency of the gastric cardia without radiologic evidence of hiatal hernia. J Thorac Cardiovasc Surg 42:352, 1961.

Holloway RH, Dodds WJ: Pathogenesis, In Jamieson GG (ed): Surgery of the Oesophagus. New York, Churchill Livingstone, 1988.

Janssens J, Vantrappen G, Ghillebert G: 24-Hour recording of esophageal pressure and pH in patients with noncardiac chest pain. Gastroenterology 90:1978, 1986.

Kline M, Chesue R, Sturdevant RAL, McCallum RW: Esophageal disease in patients with angina-like chest pain. Am J Gastroenterol 75:116, 1981.

Lilly JR, Randolph JG: Hiatal hernia and gastroesophageal reflux in infants and children. J Thorac Cardiovasc Surg 55:42, 1968.

Long CF: Rumination in man. Am J Med Sci 178:814, 1929.

Luschka H von: Das antrum, cardiacum des menschlichen magens. Arch Path Anat 9:427, 1857.

Mallory GK, Weiss S: Hemorrhages from lacerations of the cardiac orifice of the stomach due to vomiting. Am J Med Sci 178:506, 1929.

Mattioli S, Pilotti V, Spangaro M, et al: Reliability of 14-hour home esophageal pH monitoring in diagnosis of gastroesophageal reflux. Dig Dis Sci 34:71, 1989.

Maziak DE, Todd RJ, Pearson FG: Massive hiatus hernia: Evaluation and surgical management. J Thorac Cardiovasc Surg 115:53, 1998.

Menking M, Wagnitz JG, Burton JJ, et al: Rumination: A near fatal psychiatric disease of infancy. N Engl J Med 280:802, 1969.

Meyer GW, Castell DO: Human esophageal response during chest pain induced by swallowing cold liquids. JAMA 246:2057, 1981.

Nazum R: Hernia of the esophageal hiatus: Its relation to angina pectoris. Am Heart J 33:724, 1947.

Osler W: Principles and Practice of Medicine. New York, Appleton, 1892.

Pope CE: Symptoms of esophageal disease. In Sleisinger MH, Fordtran JS (eds): Gastrointestinal Disease, 3rd ed. Philadelphia, WB Saunders, 1983.

Rasmussen K, Ravnsbaek J, Funch-Jensen P, et al: Oesophageal spasm in patients with coronary artery spasm. Lancet 1:174 1986.

Richter JE, Barish CF, Castell DO: Abnormal sensory perception in patients with esophageal chest pain. Gastroenterology 91:845, 1986a.

Richter JE, Obrecht WF, Bradley LA, et al: Psychological comparison of patients with nutcracker esophagus and irritable bowel syndrome. Dig Dis Sci 31:131, 1986b.

Richter JF, Bradley LA, Castrell DO: Esophageal chest pain: Current controversies in pathogenesis, diagnosis, and therapy. Ann Intern Med 110:66, 1989.

Skinner DB, Belsey RH: Surgical management of esophageal reflux and hiatus hernia: Long-term results with 1,030 patients. J Thorac Cardiovasc Surg 53:33, 1967.

Skinner DB, Belsey RHR: Management of Esophageal Disease. Philadelphia, WB Saunders, 1988, p 522.

Souadjian JV, Cain JC: Intractable hiccup. Postgrad Med 43:72, 1968.

Spiro HM: Clinical Gastroenterology, 3rd ed. New York, Macmillan, 1983.

Trastek VF, Allen MS, Deschamps C, et al: Diaphragmatic hernia and associated anemia: Response to surgical treatment. J Thorac Cardiovasc Surg 112:1340, 1996.

Treacy J, Jamieson GG: Para-oesophageal hernia. In Jamieson GG (ed): Surgery of the Oesophagus. New York, Churchill Livingstone, 1988, p 1.

Vantrappen G, Janssens J, Ghillebert G: The irritable oesophagus: A frequent cause of angina-like pain. Lancet 2:1232, 1987.

Vinson PP: Hysterical dysphagia. Minn Med 5:107, 1922.

Winship DH, Andrade SR, Zboralske FF: Influence of bolus temperature on human esophageal motor function. J Clin Invest 49:243, 1970.

CHAPTER **5**

Imaging

RADIOLOGY, COMPUTED TOMOGRAPHY, AND MAGNETIC RESONANCE IMAGING

Nasir M. Jaffer
Chia Sing Ho

Major technologic advances in diagnostic imaging in the past 2 decades have significantly enhanced our ability to evaluate diseases of the esophagus. Although fluoroscopy and barium studies remain useful, the newer diagnostic techniques provide significant additional diagnostic capabilities unavailable from conventional imaging. For example, nuclear medicine assesses and quantifies the functional abnormalities of the esophagus and positron emission tomography (PET) can detect neoplastic mediastinal nodes even when the nodal enlargement is minimal or negligible. Computed tomography (CT) and magnetic resonance imaging (MRI) display esophageal neoplasms and their extent in three dimensions. Endoscopic ultrasound (EUS) has been used for its unique ability to depict the finer details of the esophageal wall and to trace tumor origin and local extension (Tio and Tytgat, 1986).

Since the 1990s, rapid advances in digital technology in imaging and telecommunication have significantly changed the way medical imaging is managed. Diagnostic images can be captured, archived, and distributed to desired locations for viewing in a system called Picture Archive and Communication System (PACS). The images can also be viewed on demand at desktop computers or workstations connected to the PACS network. This depends on acquisition or conversion of images in the digital format. Images from the new imaging modalities (CT, MRI, and the newer generation of ultrasound scanners) are produced in digital format and, recently, even the conventional chest and abdominal radiographs as well. Analogue images (films) can also be converted to the digital format to be managed by PACS. To practicing clinicians, the ability to receive images from elsewhere at their own offices and convenience makes their daily activities much more efficient.

Digital images can also be sent through fast modem (cable modem or DSL phone lines) or the Internet (when formatted in web-based language). This capability greatly facilitates consultation for out-of-town or overseas patients. The digital or information revolution has reached a clinical level that has benefited and will continue to benefit both patients and physicians.

Conventional radiology, including contrast study by fluoroscopy, CT, and MRI, is described in this subchapter; PET and EUS are described in subsequent subchapters. Also highlighted are their roles and findings in esophageal disorders often encountered in the practice of thoracic surgery.

TECHNIQUES OF EXAMINATION

Chest Radiograph

Routine posteroanterior (PA) and lateral chest films are often obtained to assess pleural or pulmonary involvement of acute esophageal diseases or postoperative changes. When mediastinal involvement due to esophageal diseases is sought, an overpenetrated PA chest film with barium in the esophagus may be useful. This technique to assess the mediastinum is now less frequently employed because of the availability of computed radiography and CT.

Contrast Studies

Barium is the most commonly used contrast agent for fluoroscopic examination of the esophagus and the rest of the gastrointestinal tract. It permits a safe, expedient study of the esophageal mucosa, luminal distensibility, motility, and any anatomic pathology. However, when examining a patient for esophageal perforation, the examiner should first use a water-soluble contrast agent such as diatrizoate meglumine/diatrizoate sodium (Gastrografin) (Dodds et al, 1982) or ioxaglate meglumine/ioxaglate sodium (Hexabrix). If no esophageal leakage is shown, the study should be complemented by barium swallow. A large esophageal perforation or leak may be missed by using Gastrografin alone; the extravasated Gastrografin, a less radiopaque contrast medium than barium, is immediately diluted by fluid contained in a large cavity and rendered fluoroscopically invisible.

Water-soluble contrast medium is unable to detect 15% to 25% of thoracic and 50% of cervical perforations (Foley et al, 1982; James et al, 1975; Love and Berkow, 1978; Meyers and Ghahremani, 1975; Phillips and Cunningham, 1984; Vessal et al, 1975). On the other hand, extraluminal barium in the mediastinum incites a granulomatous and fibrotic reaction and interferes with subsequent imaging with CT or fluoroscopy and should be avoided as much as possible.

Routine Barium Study

With the patient in both upright and recumbent positions, the esophagus is examined to evaluate its anatomic details and its motility pattern. Air-contrast views showing mucosal details are obtained with the patient in the upright left posterior oblique (LPO) position. The patient is asked to swallow a cup (4 ounces) of high-density barium E-Z-HD (E-Z-M Co., Westbury, N.Y). With rapid swallowing, air is trapped within the esophagus and produces a double-contrast mucosal relief of the esophagus (Fig. 5–1).

In the recumbent position, the patient lies in a prone right anterior oblique (RAO) position and drinks a low-density barium suspension. In this position, esophageal motility is studied without the influence of gravity. In addition, the esophagus can be fully distended by barium for diagnosis of early strictures. This technique is modified to enhance its sensitivity in the following conditions.

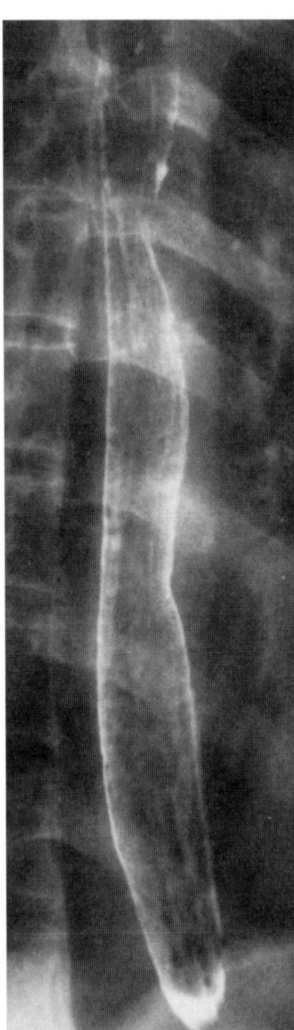

FIGURE 5–1 ■ Normal air-contrast esophagogram. Note the fine mucosal relief.

Varices. Varices are best seen on mucosal relief view of the partially collapsed esophagus with the patient in a recumbent position. This condition can be induced by intravenous (IV) injection of an anticholinergic drug such as hyoscine butylbromide (Buscopan) to paralyze the esophagus (Cockerill et al, 1976; Dalinka et al, 1972).

Tube Esophagogram. The mucosal detail is better delineated with this technique, which is also useful for confirming the diagnosis of tracheoesophageal (TE) fistulas or esophageal leak. For better double-contrast study of mucosal details, a small red rubber catheter is passed orally into the proximal thoracic esophagus. The patient swallows a high-density barium suspension as air is gently insufflated through the catheter. Controlled double-contrast views of the esophagus in various projections can be obtained.

When a TE fistula or esophageal leak is suspected in an uncooperative patient or one who aspirates, placing a nasogastric tube in the esophagus facilitates the examination. With the patient lying on the right side, barium is injected via the nasogastric tube to outline the upper esophagus (Levine et al, 1974). In the newborn a small radiopaque tube is inserted to confirm esophageal atresia or TE fistula. The upper esophageal pouch is indicated by the end of the tube. If necessary, 1 to 2 ml of barium is instilled into the pouch through the tube to confirm the diagnosis.

Marshmallow Swallow. Patients with dysphagia may show no abnormality on barium esophageal examinations. However, a barium-coated marshmallow ingested during fluoroscopy may help to uncover the presence of a mild esophageal stricture (Fig. 5–2), which impedes its passage (Danielson and Hunter, 1985; Somers et al, 1986).

Video Fluoroscopy. To study the motility of the esophagus, video fluoroscopy has supplanted the use of cineradiography because of its convenience, lower cost, and, more important, reduced radiation dose to the patients. Assessment of esophageal motility is centered at three regions: the hypopharynx, the body of the esophagus, and the gastroesophageal (GE) junction.

In the hypopharynx, a video recording is made in the frontal and lateral positions, with the patient upright or sitting. Peristalsis of the body of the esophagus is evaluated with the patient lying in the RAO position and swallowing the barium one mouthful at a time at, minimally, 15-second intervals. The emptying of the GE junction is evaluated in both the upright and recumbent positions.

Air-Contrast Upper Gastrointestinal Series

In patients with lower esophageal strictures, an air-contrast upper gastrointestinal series should be obtained during the esophageal study to evaluate the fundus of the stomach. The patient swallows a high-density barium suspension (E-Z-HD), followed by gas-producing granules; these liberate carbon dioxide on contact with gastric acid. The patient is rotated 360 degrees on the fluoro-

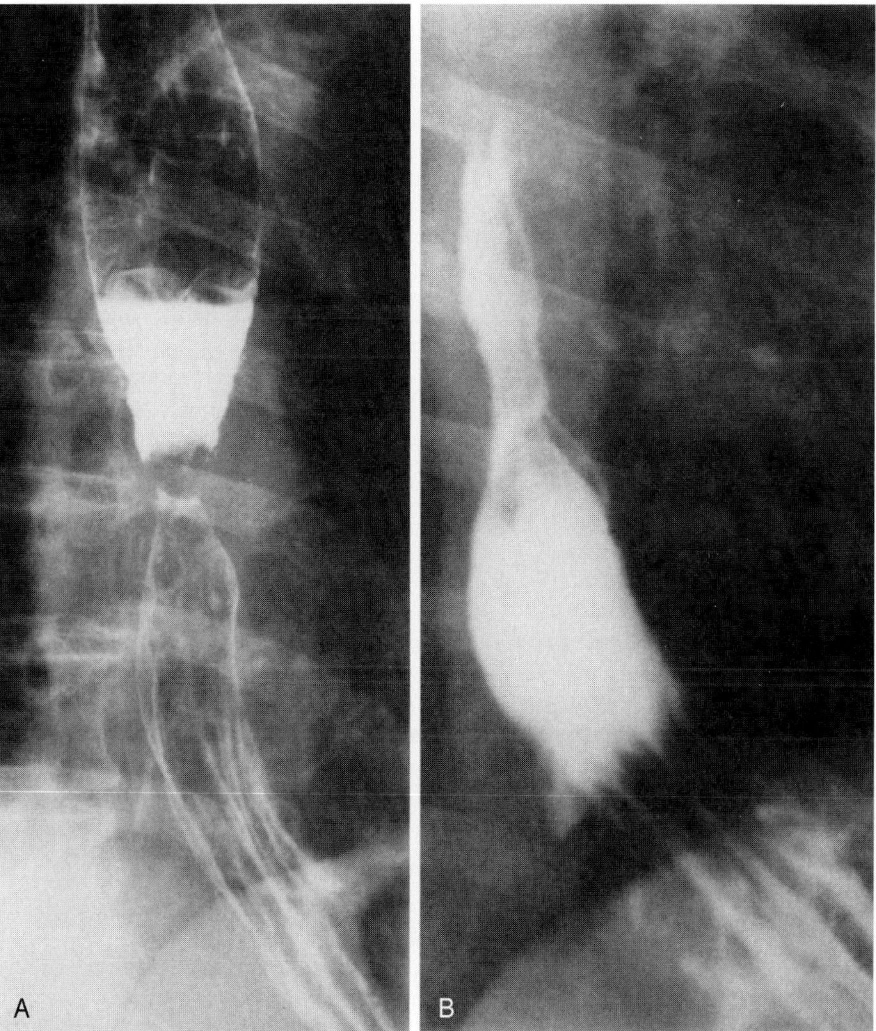

FIGURE 5–2 ■ Marshmallow swallow for detection of peptic stricture. *A*, Marshmallows are held up by the stricture. A hiatal hernia is present, as evidenced by the enlarged mucosal folds (rugal folds). *B*, The stricture is less evident without the marshmallow.

scopic table to coat the gastric mucosa with barium while the carbon dioxide maintains gastric distention. At least four basic views of the stomach are obtained:

1. Supine LPO view, to show air contrast of the antrum and distal body.
2. Right posterior oblique (RPO) view, with the patient semiupright (Shatzki's view) for demonstration of upper body and cardia in double contrast.
3. Prone RAO view, for double-contrast study of the upper body and single-contrast study of the distal body, antrum, and duodenum.
4. Upright LPO view, for further evaluation of upper body and compression of the stomach and cap. If the duodenal cap and loop are not satisfactorily demonstrated, special efforts are made to show them in both double-contrast and single-contrast views.

Sinogram or Fistulogram

Water-soluble contrast 60% diatrizoate (Hypaque) is injected into a sinus or fistulous tract to identify an esophageal fistula or leakage or the size of an empyema. Anteroposterior (AP) and lateral projections of the contrast collection are obtained for evaluation of its size and location. Evidence of fistulous communication of the sinus tract with the bronchial tree (Fig. 5–3) is noted during fluoroscopy and is often signaled by coughing. Should this occur, injection of diatrizoate must be replaced with a low-osmolar-contrast agent such as ioxaglate meglumine or iohexol (Omnipaque). A high-osmolar-contrast agent, such as diatrizoate, can induce acute pulmonary edema (Dodds et al, 1982).

Computed Tomography

CT scanning allows three-dimensional evaluation of the esophagus in relation to its adjacent structures. CT is often used for assessing extraluminal involvement of esophageal malignancy both for preoperative staging and postoperative surgical complications. The oncologist also finds it useful for assessing a patient's response to chemotherapy. Rarely, it has been used to assess benign lesions of the esophagus (such as leiomyoma), duplication cysts, or foreign body ingestion.

CT has undergone many technical changes since its introduction in 1972. The current "helical scanners" were introduced to clinical use in 1991 and represented a new technologic advancement. The table moves along the longitudinal axis of the body while the x-ray tube rotates around its transverse axis. Scanner tables do not move

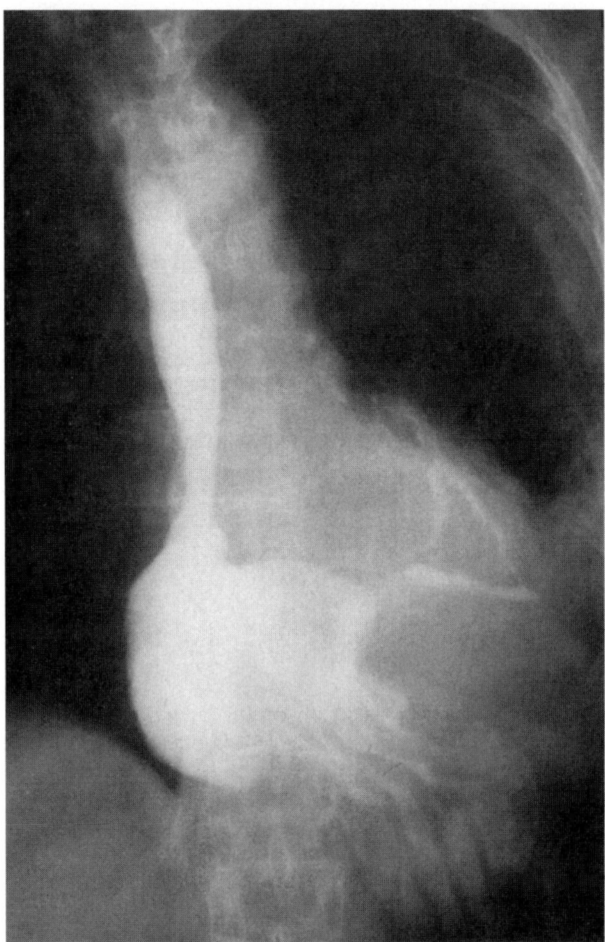

FIGURE 5–3 ■ Gastrobronchial fistula. After hiatal hernia repair, breakdown of the fundus of the stomach leads to fistula of the bronchial tree.

while the x-ray tube rotates around the body; they move incrementally after each rotation. With helical or spiral scanning, a series of thinner image slices are made from the volumetric CT data collected from a single row of detectors. These are used for reconstruction into thicker image slices to increase the resolution of the structures under examination.

During the late 1990s, even faster scanners (i.e., multislice scanners) were produced for clinical use (e.g., GE Light Speed, Toshiba Acquilon, Siemens Somatom plus IV volume zoom). This latest technology uses multiple rows instead of a single row of detectors, and x-ray tube cooling is not required. Thus, four images are acquired with each 360-degree rotation of the x-ray tube. This increase in the scanning speed by 3-fold to 6-fold is achieved without sacrifice of image quality. The end result is significant reduction of the time required for scanning the body; larger areas of the body can now be scanned with a single breath-hold.

For example, the chest can be imaged using 1.25-mm scan slices with a 19-second single breath-hold (useful for pulmonary embolism); the entire chest, abdomen, and pelvis can be scanned using 5-mm scan slices with a 17-second single breath-hold (useful for follow-up in patients with cancer). The combination of speed and high resolution allows for improved diagnosis and increase in patient throughput. Small structures such as lymph nodes and even bronchial arteries are seen with increased frequency (Fig. 5–4).

The fast rate of scanning has also allowed for the development of a new technique: CT fluoroscopy. CT fluoroscopy permits real-time imaging of the biopsy needle and enhances the radiologist's ability to sample small lesions in the body (Katada et al, 1996; Meyers, 1998).

Another improvement in CT is the method of viewing of the many slices of images. By viewing them with a computer workstation, the imaging specialist can now accurately differentiate small structures such as vessels, pulmonary or liver metastases, or mediastinal lymph nodes that were previously difficult to distinguish. In certain cases, three-dimensional reconstruction of the volumetric data can produce images similar to anatomic models for better understanding of the pathologic process (Fig. 5–5).

Despite these advances, CT has played little role in tissue characterization of esophageal lesions, except for water-density lesions (Fig. 5–6) (e.g., duplication cysts). It has no role in the diagnosis of mucosal lesions and only a limited role in early stage T1, T2, or even T3 esophageal cancers. CT has been most useful in assessment of submucosal esophageal lesions seen on barium studies or at endoscopy and staging of advanced esophageal carcinoma (T4) for local invasion and distant metastasis.

CT Scanning Technique. CT of the esophagus should always include the supraclavicular region, chest, and upper abdomen. IV contrast (100 ml of Omnipaque or Isovue) is administered with an automated injector to enhance the vascular structures. When possible, Esopho-CAT (E-Z-EM; Westbury, N.Y.), a 1% barium oral contrast

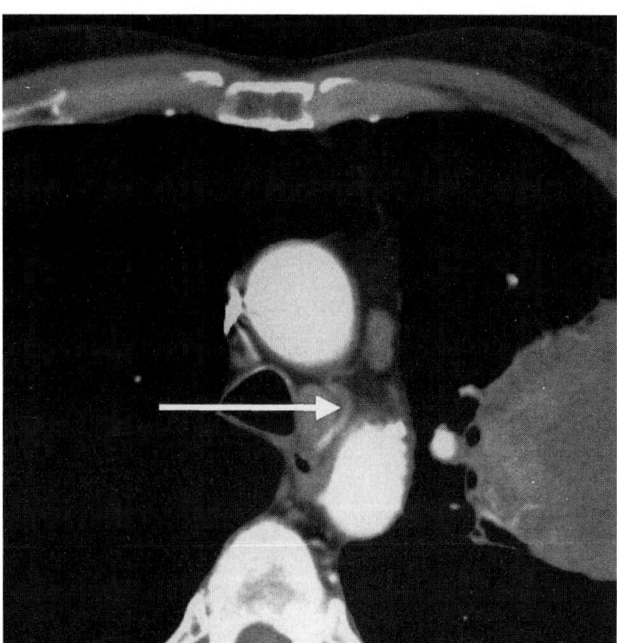

FIGURE 5–4 ■ Bronchial artery (*arrow*) at the level of the aortopulmonary window.

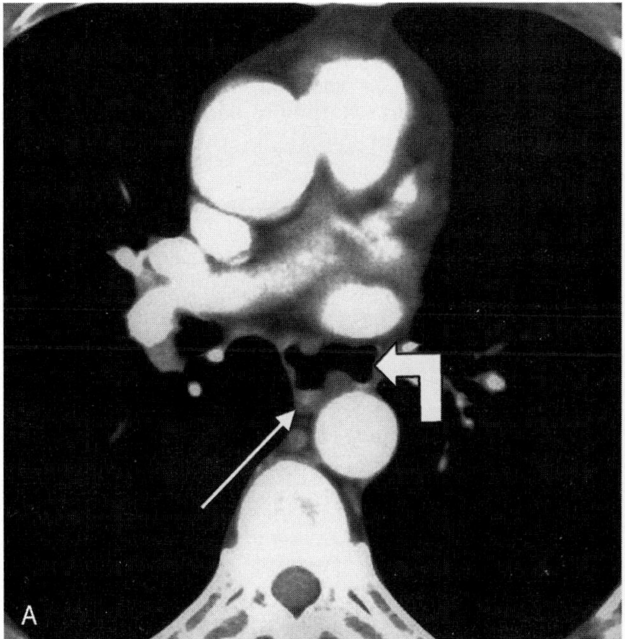

FIGURE 5–5 ■ Diverticulum. *A*, a distal esophageal diverticulum (*angled arrow*) is communicating with the barium-filled esophagus (*straight arrow*). *B*, Posterior view of a three-dimensional, surface-rendered image of the distal esophageal diverticulum (D) (*arrowhead*). Indentations made by the aorta (Ao) (*straight arrow*) and left main stem bronchus (LMB) (*curved arrow*) are shown.

medium, is given to opacify the esophagus. The gastric fundus should be distended with either barium or air using effervescent granules or a large amount of water (~500 ml) given to the patient just before scanning. For patients with TE fistula or perforation, a low osmolar water-soluble contrast medium (Hexabrix, Omnipaque, or Isovue) should be used to prevent mediastinitis and aspiration pneumonia.

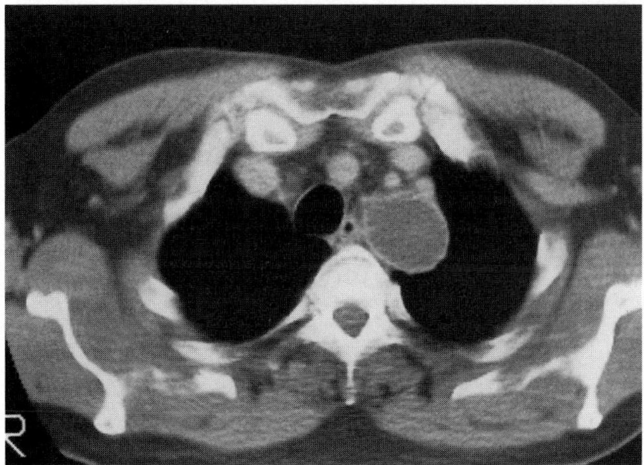

FIGURE 5–6 ■ Upper esophagus. CT scan of the upper esophagus showing a well-defined fluid-containing cavity to the left of the esophagus, which at surgery was found to be esophageal duplication.

The scanning parameters depend on the available equipment. With the GE QX/I Light Speed Scanner, we scan at 5-mm thickness with a 2.5-mm scan interval from the cricoid cartilage to the upper abdomen to include the middle portion of the kidneys. The area scanned includes most of the lymphatic drainage area of the esophagus and possible sites of metastasis for esophageal carcinoma.

Anatomic Levels. The absence of a serosal covering around the esophagus allows for a rapid spread of tumor to the adjacent mediastinal structures. Therefore, the anatomic relationship of the esophagus to the various mediastinal structures is important in CT assessment of an esophageal tumor. The key anatomic levels are outlined:

1. *Upper mediastinum.* This level extends from the thoracic inlet to the carina. The trachea is anteriorly located and normally not indented by the esophagus.
2. *Aortic arch.* The arch displaces the esophagus and trachea from the left to the midline.
3. *Carina.* The esophagus lies in the midline immediately behind the carina and left mainstem bronchus. Like the trachea in the thorax, the left mainstem bronchus is never indented posteriorly by the esophagus.
4. *Left atrium.* This level lies immediately anterior to the esophagus, and a fat plane may or may not exist between them.
5. *Lower mediastinum.* The esophagus has moved anteriorly and to the left and now lies anterior to the descending aorta.

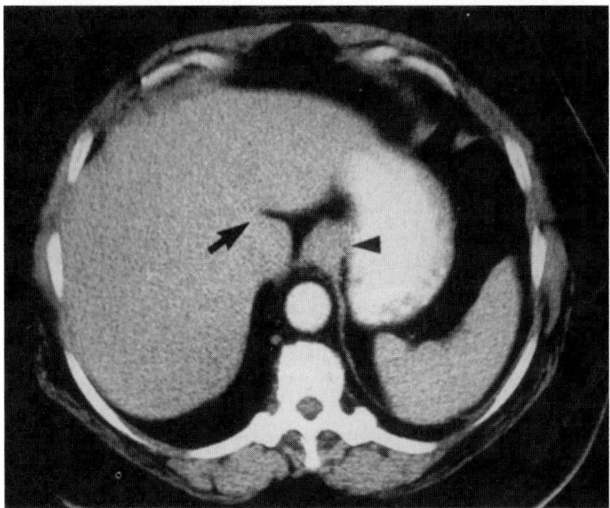

FIGURE 5–7 ■ Gastroesophageal (GE) junction. CT scan of the liver showing a cleft on its medial surface. *Arrow* marks the insertion of the gastrohepatic ligament. The GE junction (*arrowhead*) appears as a soft tissue density at the medial border of the stomach.

6. *Diaphragmatic hiatus.* The diaphragmatic crus is seen encircling the esophagus as it enters from the thorax into the abdomen. There is no normal fat surrounding the esophagus at this level.

7. *GE junction.* The upper portion of the lesser omentum or gastrohepatic ligament encircles the intra-abdominal esophagus. The ligament extends to the liver, inserting into the fissure for the ligamentum venosum, and can be recognized on the CT as an indentation or cleft on the posteromedial surface of the liver (Fig. 5–7). This cleft defines the GE junction on the CT scan.

Lymphatic Drainage. The primary lymphatic drainage of the esophagus is oriented along its long axis. A dense network of lymphatic vessels within the mucosa and submucosa communicates freely with lymphatic channels in the muscular layers of the esophagus. The lymphatic drainage extends through the esophagus into the cervical, mediastinal, and upper abdominal lymph nodes (Meyers, 1998). The most relevant regions of lymph nodes include the following:

- Cervical esophagus: the cervical nodes, including the supraclavicular nodes
- *Upper and middle intrathoracic esophagus:* the periesophageal, paratracheal, and subcarinal lymph nodes
- *Lower intrathoracic esophagus:* the lower mediastinal nodes and perigastric lymph nodes, excluding the celiac artery
- *GE junction:* the gastric lymph nodes, along left gastric, splenic or celiac arteries

Normal CT Features and Diagnostic Pitfalls. The normal esophageal wall should not exceed 3 to 5 mm and is best assessed when distended with air or barium. The oblique course of the GE junction, which is sometimes collapsed, is more difficult to assess on CT. This is further compounded when a hiatal hernia exists. Tumors at the level of the GE junction are best assessed with air or water distention of both the gastric fundus and the esophagogastric junction and scanning in decubitus or prone position (Doyle and Simpson, 1994) (Fig. 5–8).

Magnetic Resonance Imaging

Since its introduction into clinical practice in 1982, MRI has become an indispensable modality for detection and diagnosis of diseases of the brain, the spinal cord, and the musculoskeletal system. Its contribution in the hollow viscera, including the esophagus, however, has so far been limited.

There are several disadvantages to MRI of the esophagus:

1. The presence of motion artifacts. Even though peristalsis is less a problem in imaging the esophagus than in imaging the remaining gastrointestinal tract, spontaneous swallowing motion is still a significant degrading factor during the 5 to 10 minutes of imaging time. In addition, respiratory and cardiac motion artifacts also contribute to the degradation of image quality. Faster scanning will undoubtedly bring about significant improvement.
2. The inferiority of MRI's spatial resolution compared with that of CT.
3. The incremental cost of MRI over CT or other imaging modalities under the current economically constrained environment.

MRI does have a few advantages:

1. MRI can image the entire length of the esophagus and show the topographic relationship in the coronal and sagittal planes (Fig. 5–9). This view can provide additional valuable information for radiation therapy planning for esophageal carcinoma. With the introduction of multislice CT scanners, similar coronal and sagittal reconstruction can be achieved if needed.
2. Another advantage over CT is the ability of MRI to distinguish tumor recurrence from postoperative fibrosis in postsurgical patients with cancer. Fibrosis has a low signal intensity on T2-weighted images and a delayed signal or no signal on T1-weighted images enhanced with gadolinium–diethylene-tetramine-pentaacetic acid (Gd-DTPA). For one to take full advantage of these changes, comparison with a baseline post-treatment MR image would be useful.

Relatively few articles have been published on MRI of the esophagus, reflecting its limited clinical role. Lehr and associates (1988) described a prospective study that assessed resectability of esophageal cancer by CT and MRI and reported a sensitivity and specificity for both methods in the range of 60%. They questioned the value of these two modalities for planning surgery or for stratification to different therapeutic arms in comparative studies.

Since their report, major technologic innovations have occurred in MRI, and clinical application with the new generation of technology is still being evaluated. For example, by using an endoluminal coil in a patient placed in a 1.5-tesla (T) superconductive magnet, one can distin-

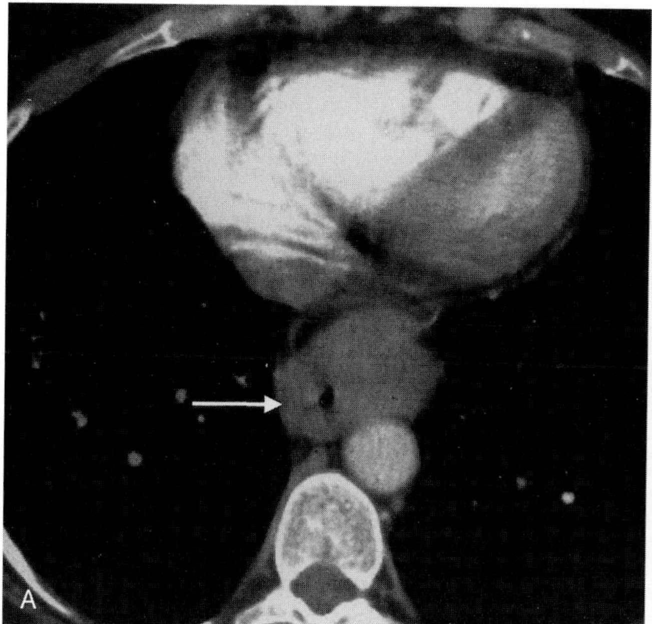

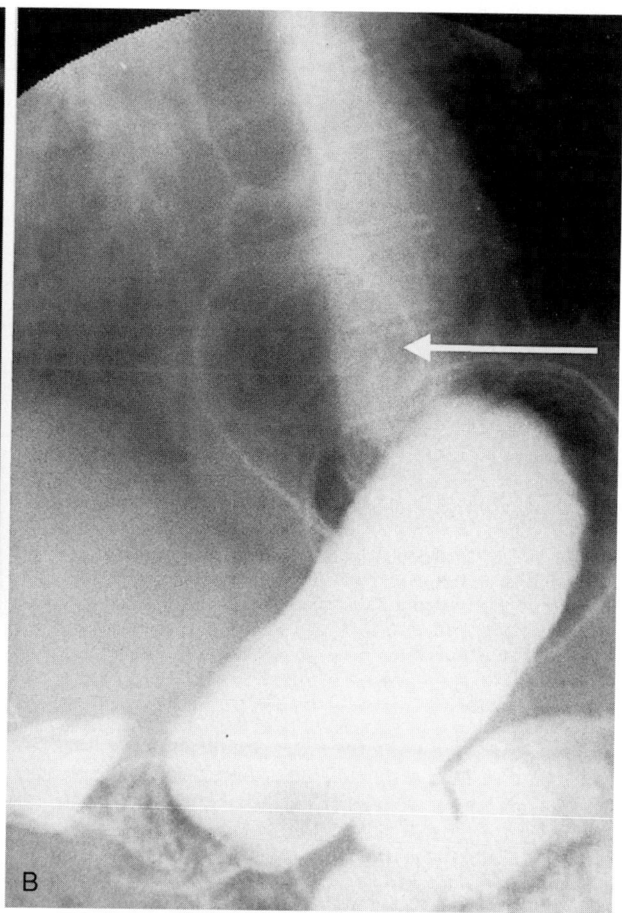

FIGURE 5–8 ■ *A*, Large mass seen in the distal esophagus (*arrow*) on a CT scan. *B*, A double-contrast upper gastrointestinal barium study shows a large hiatal hernia (*arrow*) but no esophageal lesion.

guish different layers of the esophagus in both T1-weighted and T2-weighted images and can determine cancer invasion of the esophageal wall (Ozawa et al, 2000).

Another area of new research and development is *endoscopic MRI*, a technique that combines the use of endoscopy and MRI. With this method, a prototype MRI endoscope connected to a 1.5-T MRI scanner was used. A preliminary report (Inui et al, 1995) shows that the normal gastrointestinal wall consists of three layers, and tumors are visualized as having a low signal intensity on both T1-weighted and T2-weighted sequences. Destruction of the wall layers was found to be characteristic of malignancy. In another study (Kulling et al, 1998), the results of endoscopic MRI and EUS in patients with esophageal cancer were found to be comparable in their ability to detect mural invasion.

A third area of MRI research is *functional MRI*, which attempts to identify cortical activities with esophageal function. Although this is of significant theoretical interest, application to thoracic surgery is limited.

It is reasonable to limit MRI of the esophagus to problem solving, such as postoperative changes versus tumor recurrence. More imaging research is needed before indications for routine clinical use can be defined. To this end, research in prospective comparative studies between the newer imaging modalities and the use of IV and oral contrast agents will be helpful.

RADIOLOGIC FINDINGS

Hiatal Hernia

A hiatal hernia is formed when a part of the stomach migrates above the diaphragm through the esophageal hiatus. Three types of hiatal hernias are recognized:

- Type I, or sliding
- Type II, or paraesophageal
- Type III, or mixed

The GE junction is above the diaphragm in sliding hiatal hernia but remains in normal position in a type II paraesophageal hernia. The type III (mixed) hernia begins as a sliding hernia and becomes a paraesophageal hernia when it is large enough to develop a rolling, paraesophageal component, which may undergo organoaxial volvulus. Ninety-nine percent of hiatal hernias are type I, and only 1% belong to the paraesophageal or mixed categories (Dodds, 1983).

Type I: Sliding Hiatal Hernia

Moderate and large type I hiatal hernias are obvious on barium studies and can be recognized as large soft tissue shadows behind the cardiac silhouettes on both the PA and lateral chest radiographs. A small type I hiatal hernia is easily recognized on barium studies when gastric mucosa, or a Schatzki ring, is seen above the diaphragm (Fig. 5–10). Because the hernia has no peristalsis, its

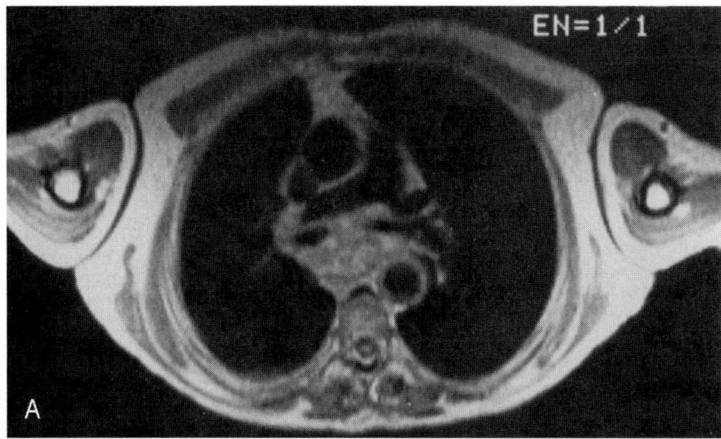

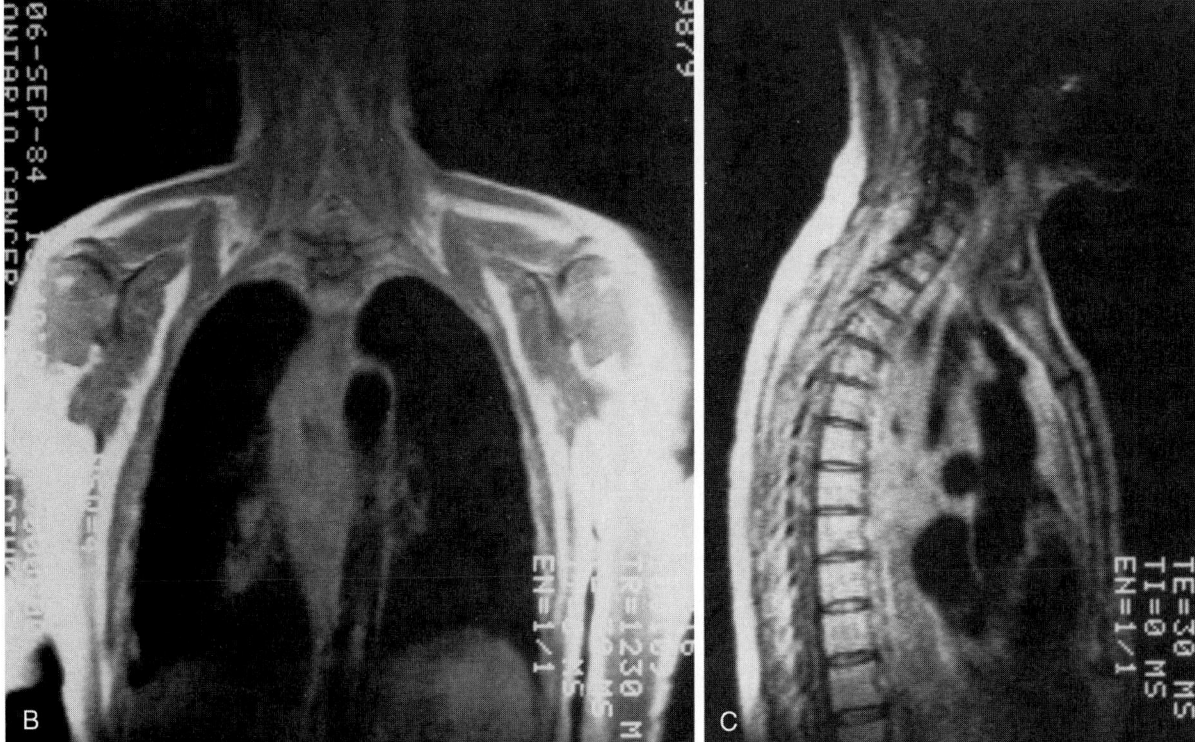

FIGURE 5–9 ■ Magnetic resonance image of the thorax showing a midesophageal carcinoma in the axial (*A*), coronal (*B*), and parasagittal (*C*) planes. Proton-weighted spin-echo pulse sequences are used. The relation between the tumor and the spinal cord is clearly defined. This anatomic information is very valuable to the radiation oncologist in directing the radiation beams.

presence can be confirmed on fluoroscopy by an inability to observe peristalsis in that segment.

It is important to distinguish a *fixed* from a *reducible* sliding hiatal hernia if surgical treatment is considered. A fixed hiatal hernia is seen in both upright and recumbent positions and is caused by either esophageal shortening from esophagitis and scar or from incarceration of a large hernia above the diaphragmatic hiatus. A sliding hernia "reduces" and is not apparent in the upright position.

Type II: Paraesophageal Hiatal Hernia

Paraesophageal hiatal hernia (Fig. 5–11) occurs as a result of weakness or defect in the phrenoesophageal membrane that allows part of the stomach to migrate to the thorax. Despite its rare occurrence, paraesophageal hernia is more prone to complications such as incarceration, strangulation, or infarction. In view of these complications, many surgeons recommend elective surgery even for asymptomatic type II hernias. Radiologically, both AP and lateral projections of the GE junction are required in order to accurately determine the location of the GE junction.

Type III: Mixed Sliding and Paraesophageal Hiatal Hernia

Progressive increase in size of a paraesophageal hiatal hernia enlarges the esophageal hiatus, resulting in formation of a sliding hernia in addition (Skinner, 1985). A long air-fluid level sometimes may be present behind the cardiac silhouette on a plain chest film to suggest its presence. This finding is particularly prevalent when most of the stomach has herniated and has undergone

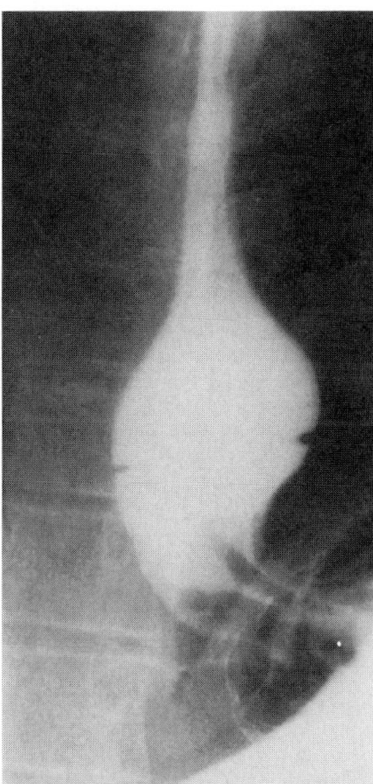

FIGURE 5–10 ■ Schatzki's ring. This mucosal ring marks the squamosal columnar junction and usually indicates the presence of a hiatal hernia.

volvulus ("upside-down" stomach). This condition may cause obstruction when part of the stomach begins to descend through the hiatus, causing torsion, volvulus, or infarction (Gerson and Lewicki, 1976).

Reflux Esophagitis and Peptic Stricture

Fluoroscopic demonstration of reflux on barium study is unreliable. Reflux is seen on barium studies in 40% of asymptomatic volunteers (Skinner and Camp, 1967) and in only 20% to 40% of patients with proven reflux esophagitis (Dodds et al, 1981; Ott et al, 1981, 1982). This poor correlation is explained by the intermittent nature of reflux and the brief duration of fluoroscopy. A more reliable test for reflux is esophageal scintigraphy using ^{99m}Tc-sulfur colloid or intraesophageal pH monitoring (Dodds et al, 1976). It is relevant to determine how long the esophagus takes to clear the refluxed barium. This information is easily obtainable during fluoroscopy. It is believed that prolonged stasis of gastric contents in the esophagus is more harmful than transient stasis.

Early radiologic changes in reflux esophagitis are best shown by double-contrast radiograph (Fig. 5–12). These include thickening of mucosal folds, mucosal granularity, and superficial ulcerations. In some instances, these mucosal abnormalities may be accompanied by motor dysfunction seen on fluoroscopy: loss of primary peristalsis with or without frequent, nonperistaltic contractions (Olsen and Schlegel, 1965).

Severe or long-standing esophagitis may result in esophageal stricture and is invariably associated with a hiatal hernia (Fig. 5–13). At an early stage of reflux esophagitis, a hiatal hernia may not be demonstrated. However, fibrosis in a peptic stricture is associated with both luminal narrowing and longitudinal shortening. Consequently, a part of the stomach (hernia) is pulled up (Fig. 5–14). This association is so constant that malig-

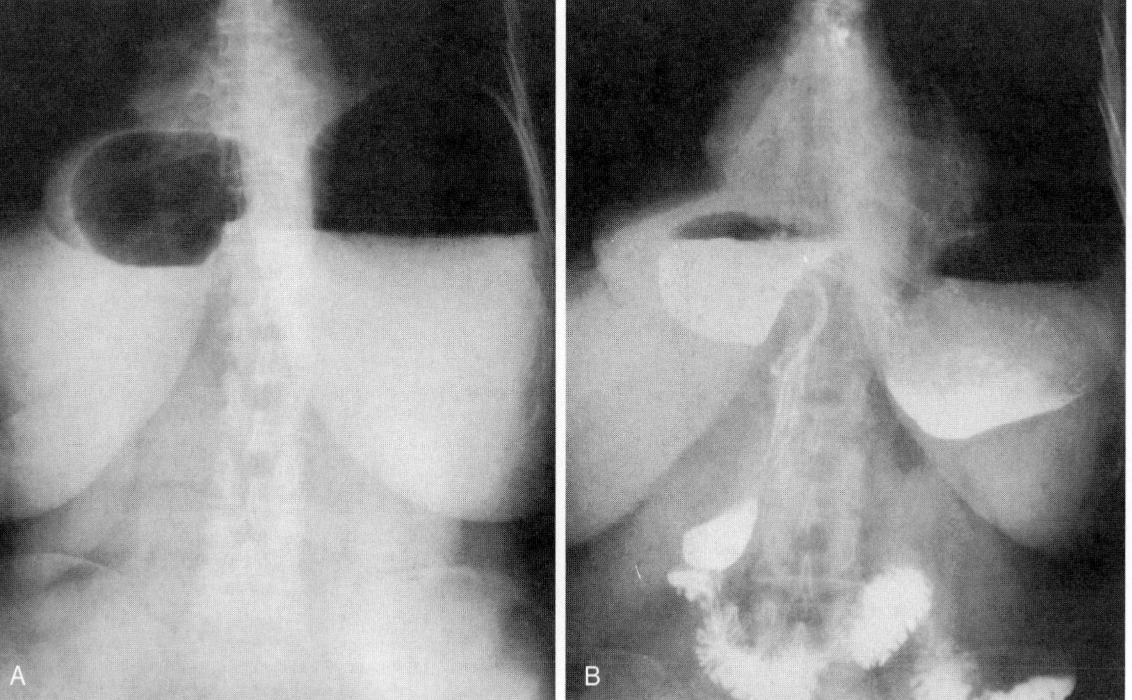

FIGURE 5–11 ■ Paraesophageal hernia with obstruction. *A*, Note the two large air-fluid levels on plain film of the abdomen. *B*, Barium swallow shows that the air-fluid level on the left is caused by a distended fundus of the stomach. The gastroesophageal junction is below the hiatus. The body of the esophagus has herniated through the hiatus into the thorax and forms the second air-fluid level.

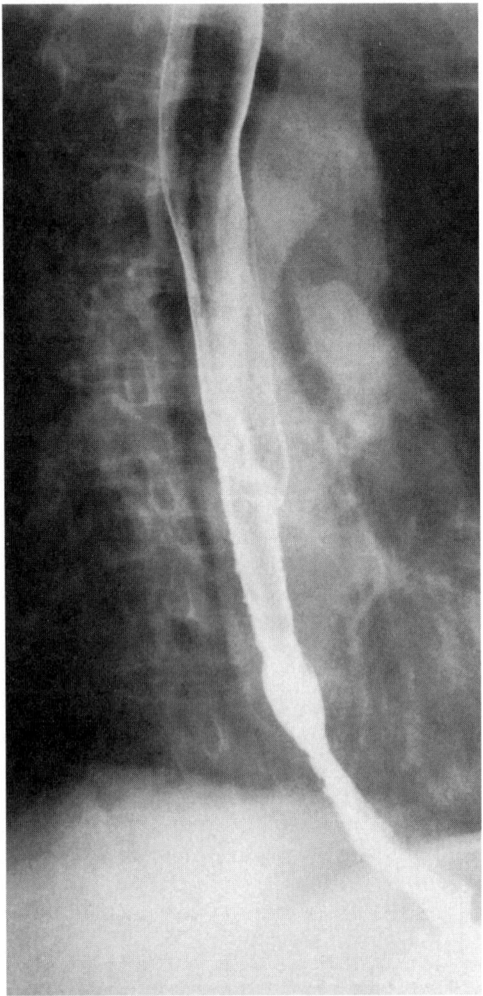

FIGURE 5–12 ■ Peptic esophagitis. The air-contrast esophagogram shows as a long segment of narrowing at the distal esophagus together with mucosal ulcerations in the stricture area.

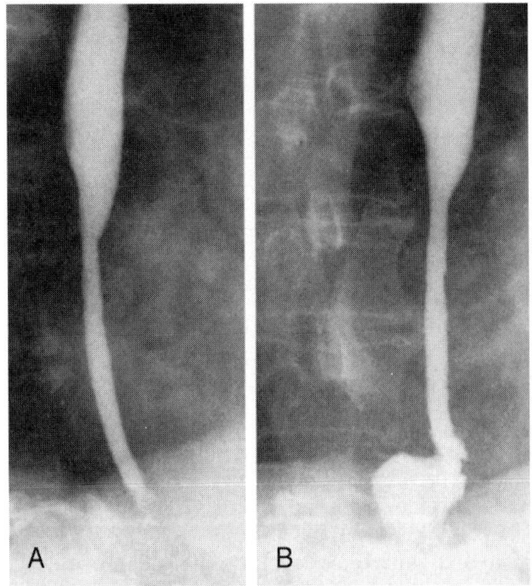

FIGURE 5–13 ■ A hiatal hernia is present distally in the recumbent *(B)* but not in the upright *(A)* position.

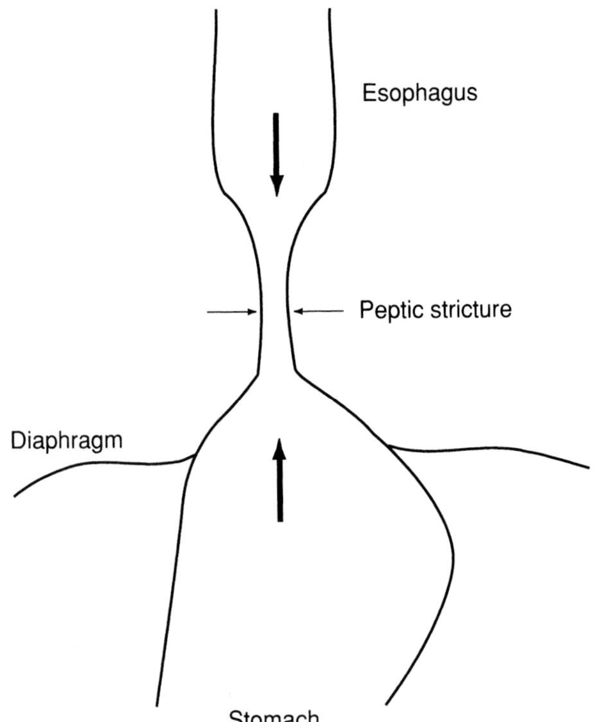

FIGURE 5–14 ■ Diagram showing the effect of a peptic stricture on the stomach. The fibrosis of the stricture results in narrowing and shortening of the esophagus. Consequently, part of the stomach is pulled up to the thorax, forming a hiatal hernia, even though this condition may not have been present at the inception of peptic esophagitis.

nancy must be suspected in any esophageal stricture if conscientious efforts fail to demonstrate a hiatal hernia (Ho and Rodrigues, 1980). Esophageal strictures are best shown with a single-contrast esophagogram obtained with the patient drinking barium in the recumbent, prone oblique position. The barium study, especially when incorporated with a marshmallow swallow, may occasionally uncover mild or early strictures that may elude endoscopic detection (Ott et al, 1985).

Another consequence of long-standing reflux esophagitis is Barrett's esophagus, or metaplasia of squamous to columnar epithelium in the distal esophagus (Adler, 1963). Radiologically, deep ulcers or strictures are seen at the columnar squamosal junction, often located in the distal or midesophagus, depending on the extent of columnar replacement. The stricture may be ring-like or long and tapered. Invariably, a hiatal hernia is shown on barium study. A reticular mucosal pattern has also been described in Barrett's esophagus (Levine et al, 1983) but is not consistently present. This condition is associated with an increased risk of esophageal cancer and requires periodic endoscopic surveillance with biopsy and cytology (Harle et al, 1985).

Differential Diagnosis

Radiation Stricture

Radiation treatment of mediastinal malignancies with doses of 3000 to 5000 cGy may cause radiation esophagitis. If the radiation is combined with doxorubicin (Adriamycin) chemotherapy, radiation dosage as low as 500 cGy is sufficient to cause radiation injury (Boal et al, 1979). This problem is probably the result of the inhibiting action of doxorubicin on DNA repair, which decreases the chances of cellular recovery from sublethal radiation damage (Greco et al, 1976).

Radiation changes are confined to the portal of radiation. Early radiation esophagitis occurs 2 to 3 weeks after radiation and includes thickening of the mucosal folds and an irregular, serrated esophageal contour caused by mucosal ulcerations or sloughing. Late changes may be evident 3 to 4 months later, although radiation stricture occurring 18 months later has also been reported (Goldstein et al, 1975). Radiation strictures are smooth and concentric with tapering margins. Esophageal airway fistulas may complicate radiation treatment as long as 4 years after completion of therapy (Lepke and Libshitz, 1983).

Caustic Stricture

Ingestion of either strong acid or alkali causes severe esophageal injury, resulting in esophageal stricture. Alkaline liquid, such as lye (sodium hydroxide), causes esophageal damage by liquefaction necrosis (Goldman and Weigert, 1973; Kirsh and Ritter, 1976). In contrast, acid ingestion causes esophageal injury by coagulative necrosis, forming a protective eschar that may limit further tissue penetration.

Radiologically, caustic strictures tend to be long and smooth with tapering margins (Fig. 5–15); they may also be focal, affecting the cervical or thoracic esophagus. At times, the stricture may appear irregular and may acquire an eccentric sacculation caused by asymmetric scarring. In 20% of patients with corrosive esophagitis from lye ingestion, the stomach may be severely injured, resulting in a linitis plastica appearance (Francine, 1973).

Early and moderate changes caused by corrosive ingestion such as hyperemia, edema, and superficial sloughing of the mucosa may not be detected on barium studies in 20% to 30% of patients (Stannard, 1978). However, endoscopic examination of a tight stricture may be limited and a barium study is more informative (Neimark and Rogers, 1985).

Neoplastic Stricture

Primary carcinoma of the esophagus is the most important condition to be differentiated from reflux peptic stricture. Infiltrative carcinoma usually causes irregular narrowing, with ulcerated mucosa and abrupt, well-defined proximal and distal margins or "shouldering" (Fig. 5–16). However, infiltrative cancer of the esophagus may mimic a benign stricture (Fig. 5–17*A*) with more smooth-looking mucosa and gradually tapering borders (Goldstein et al, 1981). Strictures of this type at the distal esophagus require evaluation for the presence of a hiatal hernia. Although the presence of a hernia does not exclude malignancy, its absence strongly suggests it (Ho and Rodrigues, 1980). The fundus of the stomach should be carefully examined for tumor because many distal

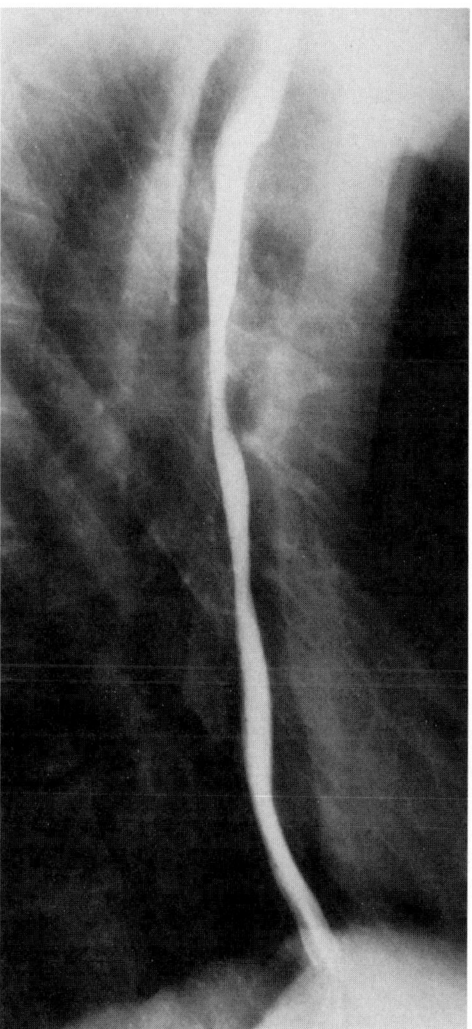

FIGURE 5–15 ■ Long esophageal stricture caused by caustic ingestion.

esophageal cancers arise from the stomach (see Fig. 5–17*B*).

Secondary lesions may cause mediastinal nodal enlargement and may compress the esophagus, resulting in a smooth, gradually tapering stricture, mimicking peptic stricture. Sometimes the esophagus is both narrowed and displaced by a mediastinal mass. The history of known primary malignancy and CT demonstration of mediastinal lymphadenopathy often differentiate malignant from benign peptic stricture.

Postoperative Strictures

Previous antireflux surgery, a Sugiura operation, or post-endoscopic sclerotherapy may all result in narrowing of the esophagus (Agha, 1984).

After an antireflux operation, the esophagus is narrowed at the GE junction, where the gastric wraparound is evident as an adjacent soft tissue density (Fig. 5–18).

In a Sugiura operation, the esophagus is transected for the treatment of esophageal varices. The postoperative anastomotic narrowing is short, circumferential, and well demarcated (Fig. 5–19).

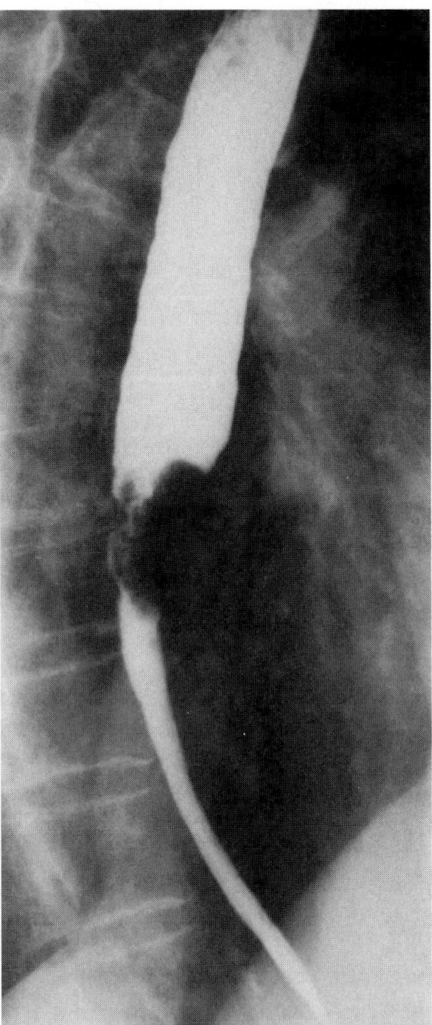

FIGURE 5–16 ■ Carcinoma of the esophagus. The carcinoma has caused an abrupt filling defect in the esophagogram. The central lumen is narrowed and is irregular, reflecting ulceration of the mass.

Esophageal strictures caused by endoscopic injection of sclerosants for the treatment of varices are usually short but may be extensive in severe cases. CT in these patients may reveal esophageal wall thickening and para-esophageal mediastinal inflammation. The wall thickening on an enhanced CT scan has a characteristic laminated appearance (outer high-attenuation and inner low-attenuation regions) (Halden et al, 1983; Mauro et al, 1986).

Drug-Induced Stricture

When lodged in the esophagus for a prolonged period of time, certain drugs may cause esophagitis, leading to stricture. The commonly encountered drugs include potassium chloride (Slow-K) (Lubbe et al, 1979; Teplick et al, 1980), quinidine, Clinitest reagent tablets, and tetracycline. Of these, potassium chloride and quinidine are more likely to cause strictures. Radiologically, these strictures are short in patients with cardiomegaly, which may compress the esophagus and delay the normal passage of the food bolus.

Strictures Associated with Dermatologic Diseases

Epidermolysis bullosa dystrophica and benign mucous membrane pemphigoid are two skin conditions that form recurrent bullous eruptions on the mucous membranes. Both conditions affect the oropharynx and the upper esophagus and may cause strictures. In epidermolysis bullosa, the bullous formation is caused by the separation of epidermis from the dermis after minimal trauma, which heals with severe scarring. In view of this, barium is a much safer examination than endoscopy, the use of which should be minimized (Hadley and MacDonald, 1960; Tishler et al, 1983). In mucous membrane pemphigoid, the use of endoscopy does not pose a similar threat and is helpful in identifying the early discrete bullae and mucosal changes. The pemphigoid strictures are located in the cervical and upper esophagus and may appear web-like in barium studies.

Crohn's Disease

Esophageal involvement by Crohn's disease is rare and often symptomatic. It is almost always accompanied by small bowel or colonic involvement. Characteristic radiologic changes of Crohn's disease seen in the intestine are also noted in the esophagus: aphthous ulcerations, mucosal edema, deep ulceration, and cobblestone appearance. Long segmental strictures may complicate the disease and usually affect the distal third of the esophagus. Rarely, intramural fistulas may be seen, as may esophagobronchial fistulas (Cynn et al, 1975; Ghahremani et al, 1983).

Trauma

Esophageal trauma may result from blunt or penetrating injury to the chest, esophageal surgery, instrumentation, or ingested foreign bodies. A sudden increase in intraesophageal pressure (e.g., severe retching or vomiting) may also cause esophageal trauma. The role of radiology depends on the cause and extent of esophageal injury.

Mucosal Tear (Mallory-Weiss)

Sudden increase in the intraluminal pressure of the esophagus, as a result of severe vomiting, may cause a linear mucosal tear at or near the cardia or distal esophagus. The main presenting symptom is hematemesis, which is usually self-limiting within 48 to 72 hours (Ansari, 1975; Knaver, 1976). Although double-contrast radiography can occasionally outline the tear as a shallow, linear collection of barium, endoscopy is the method of choice for diagnosis, as it is for other causes of upper gastrointestinal bleeding. In most instances, barium examination is not performed.

Esophageal Hematoma

Most esophageal hematomas originate from mucosal trauma. Mucosal lacerations may become partially or completely occluded by edema or blood clot, but continued submucosal or intramural bleeding results in esophageal hematomas. Spontaneous esophageal hematomas may also occur in coagulation disorders or as a result of overzealous anticoagulation therapy. Spontaneous hematomas tend to spare the distal esophagus and occur at multiple sites (Shay et al, 1981).

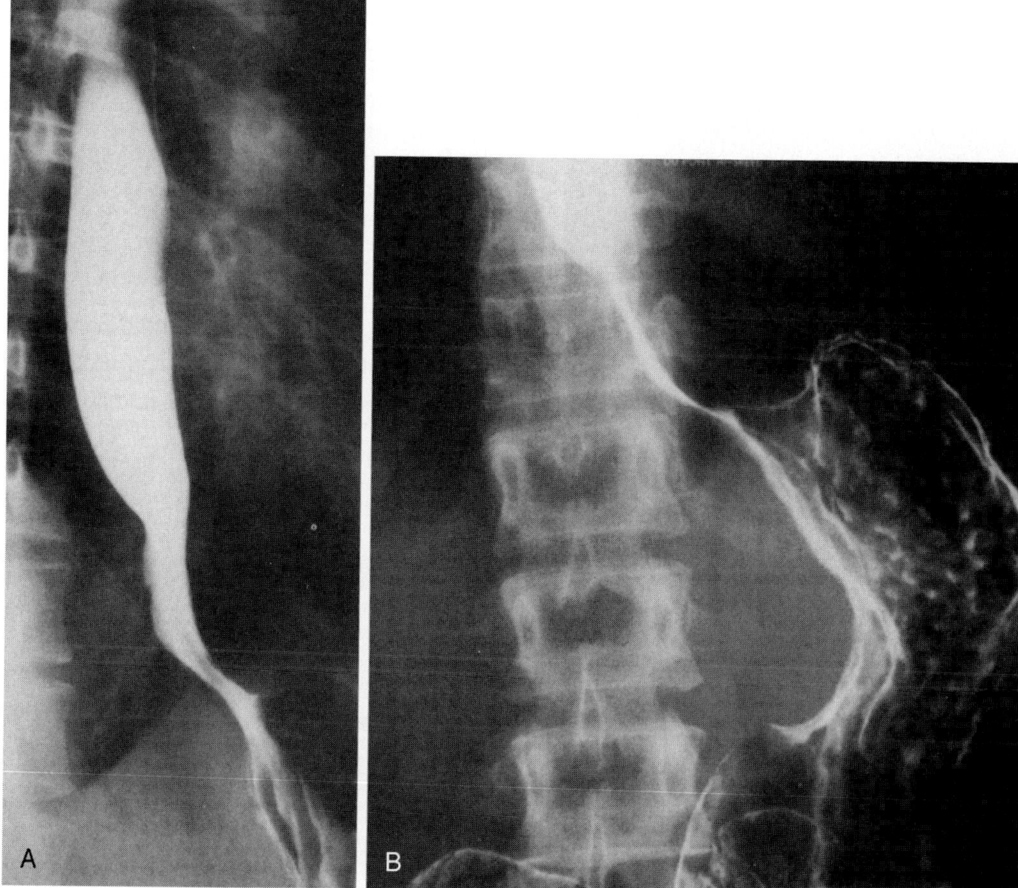

FIGURE 5–17 ■ Malignant stricture of the distal esophagus caused by submucosal spread of primary carcinoma of the stomach. *A*, Smooth esophageal stricture with gentle tapering and the absence of a hiatal hernia. Malignancy was suggested on radiographic ground, but both repeated endoscopy and biopsy findings were negative for malignancy. Manometry shows a hypertensive lower esophageal sphincter. *B*, Air-contrast view of fundus of the stomach shows extensive infiltrative carcinoma.

The patient presents with sudden onset chest pain or dysphagia or both; the pain can be severe, like that of myocardial infarction or dissecting aneurysm. Esophageal hematoma may also result from sclerotherapy for esophageal varices.

Barium study shows a smooth, elongated submucosal filling defect (Fig. 5–20). Sometimes contrast medium escapes through the mucosal tear into the hematoma (Fig. 5–21) and produces "a double-barrel" appearance (Lowman et al, 1969).

The diagnosis is made from the history and is confirmed, if necessary, by CT. CT is useful in assessing the intramural nature and the extent of the hematoma. It is performed with oral contrast medium enhancement to assess the luminal narrowing. Usually, IV contrast medium is not given (Fig. 5–22). The hematoma has high attenuation CT values on nonenhanced CT (Fig. 5–23), with smooth margins and minimal mediastinal changes.

Because management is conservative, a subsequent CT or barium study in 1 to 2 weeks is suggested to assess resolution of the hematoma.

Esophageal Perforation

Esophageal rupture is the most serious consequence of trauma to the esophagus; it may rapidly become fatal if left untreated. Even with proper treatment, the condition may be associated with a high morbidity and mortality. Esophageal endoscopy accounts for 80% of all esophageal perforations, and the estimated incidence of perforation from the procedure is 1 in 1000 (Meyers and Ghahremani, 1975). Other traumatic causes include pneumatic dilatations (Stewart et al, 1979), nasogastric or endotracheal intubations, and insertions of Celestin tubes (Ghahremani et al, 1980) or Sengstaken-Blakemore tubes (Rubin et al, 1982).

Esophageal perforation occurs commonly at the distal esophagus and in the posterior wall of the cervical esophagus at or near the level of the cricopharyngeus. The presence of Zenker's diverticulum, cervical lordosis, or an osteophyte increases the risk of perforation (Leigh and Achord, 1964). Pre-existing disease at the distal esophagus often accounts for perforations at this site.

Spontaneous rupture of the esophagus (Boerhaave syndrome) is a full-thickness perforation of the normal esophagus and is caused by sudden increase of intraluminal pressure in the esophagus. Most cases occur from severe retching or vomiting after a drinking binge; however, other causes such as weight lifting, coughing, seizure, and status asthmaticus have also been reported (Panaro and Leslie, 1960). Most perforations occur at the

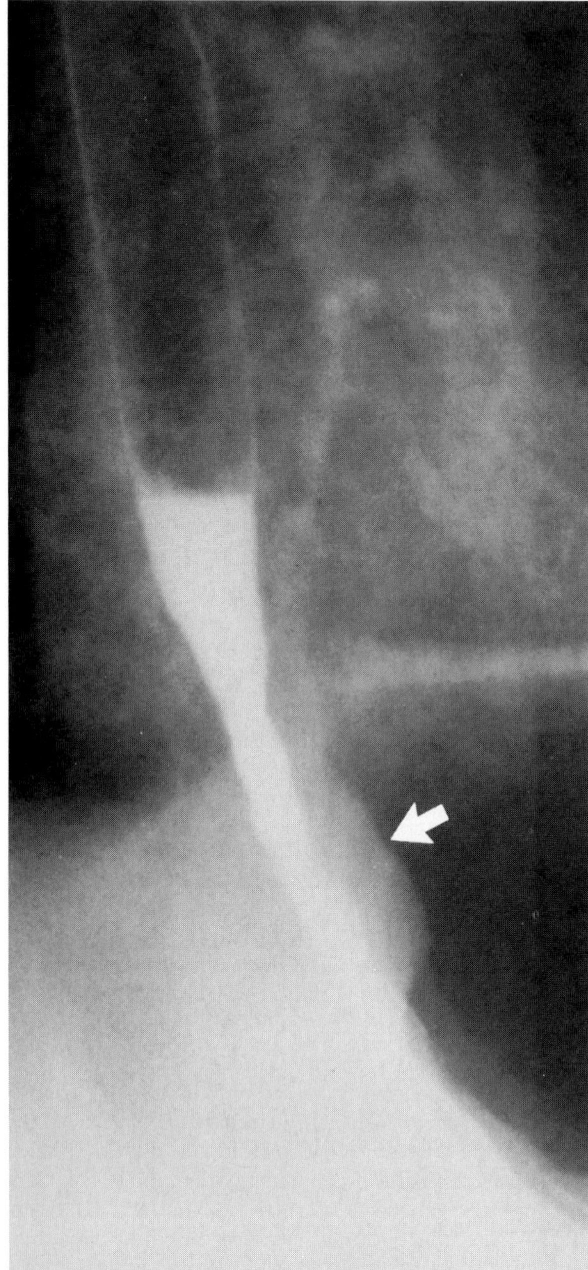

FIGURE 5–18 ■ Radiographic appearance after hiatal hernia repair and Nissen fundoplication. Note the soft tissue density anterior to the narrow segment of the esophagus, which is wrapped around by the fundoplication (*arrow*).

GE junction, with 65% on the left, 25% on the right, and 10% occurring bilaterally.

The diagnosis may be made on chest radiography, CT of the thorax, or contrast studies. Subcutaneous emphysema can be seen on an AP or lateral chest film within 1 hour after perforation of the cervical esophagus. Air may track down along the fascial planes from the neck to the chest, and pneumomediastinum can be seen (Love and Berkow, 1978). Prevertebral air, or widening of the prevertebral space, may be observed on a lateral radiograph of the neck (Figs. 5–24 and 5–25). Air-fluid level or mottled gas shadow may be seen in the prevertebral space if infection occurs or abscess forms. A water-soluble contrast study of the esophagus confirms the perforation.

In perforation of the thoracic esophagus, abnormal findings on a chest radiograph, predominantly pneumomediastinum, are noted in 90% of patients. Surgical emphysema of the neck may also be evident as air tracks upward, within hours. In 75% to 90% of patients with esophageal perforation, pleural effusion or hydropneumothorax is found. Free air in the abdomen may be seen if the perforation involves the intra-abdominal segment of the esophagus.

On CT scans, pneumomediastinum (Fig. 5–26) and secondary signs (e.g., mediastinal fluid and pleural effusions) are more often seen and may help to localize the site of perforation. When the diagnosis is in question, a contrast study should be performed using water-soluble contrast (Gastrografin) for the initial swallow. However,

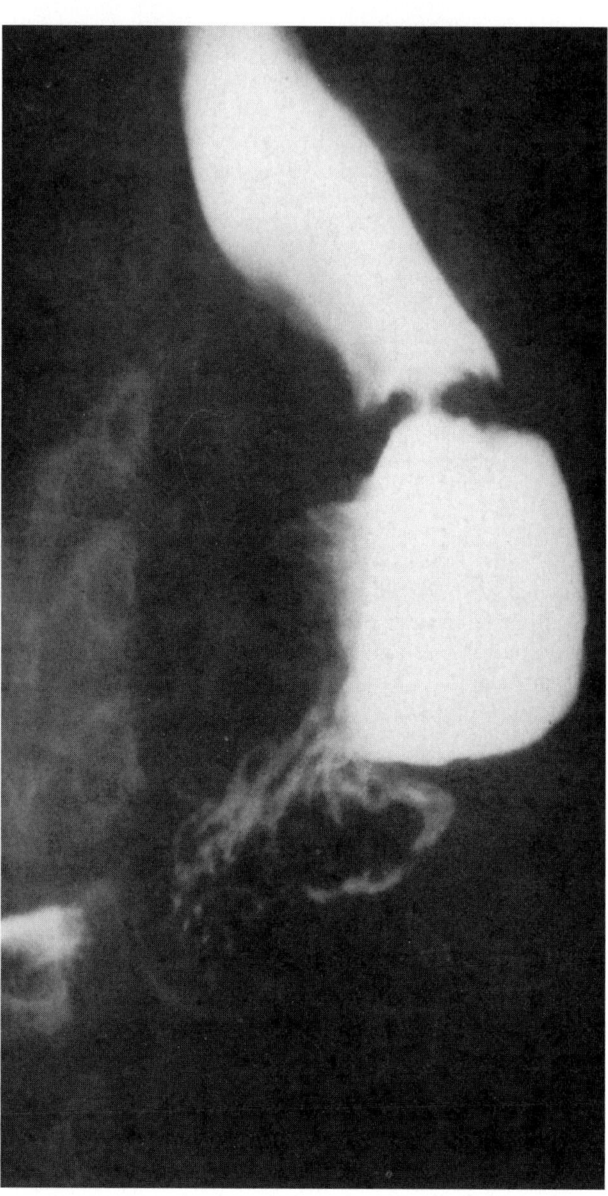

FIGURE 5–19 ■ Postoperative anastomotic stricture. Typical postsurgical stricture following esophagogastrectomy, short and circumferential.

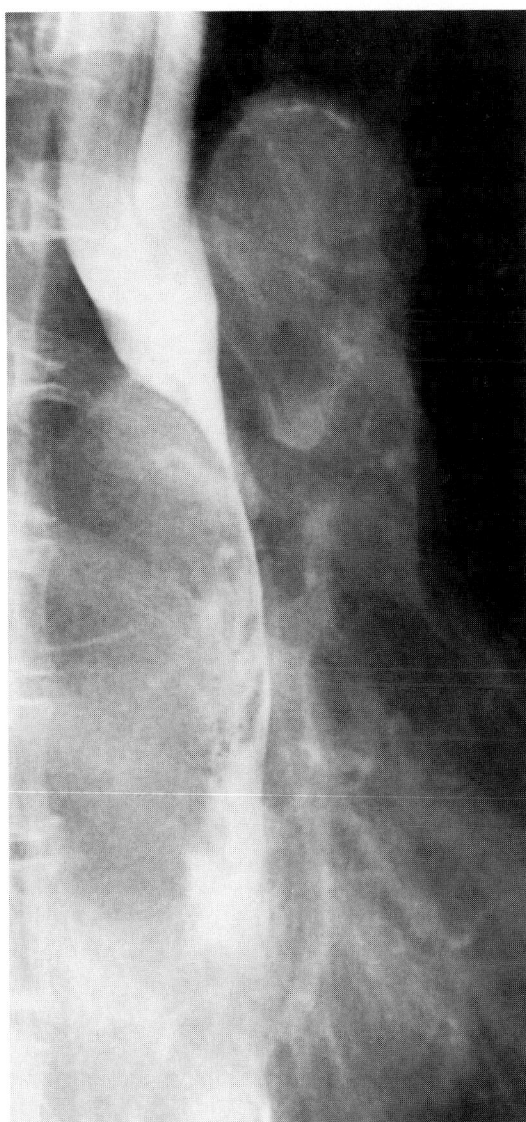

FIGURE 5–20 ■ Barium examination of the esophagus shows a long, smooth submucosal hematoma in a patient who had undergone sclerotherapy for varices 1 week earlier.

this should be followed with barium if the Gastrografin study shows no perforation (see Contrast Studies, earlier, for rationale). Even if barium escapes into the mediastinum, its deleterious effect is more than offset by the benefit of earlier diagnosis and treatment of a potentially life-threatening situation. An important technique of examination is to obtain, if possible, two perpendicular views of the esophagus (AP, lateral) to prevent small perforations from being obscured by barium within the esophagus.

Foreign Body Impaction

By far, the majority (80% or more) of foreign body impaction occurs in children as a result of accidental ingestion. The objects include fish or chicken bones, dentures, and metallic objects (e.g., needles and coins) or unchewed food boluses (Nandi and Ong, 1978). Fish or animal bones may sometimes be visible on a lateral radiograph of the neck. Endoscopy, however, is preferred for confirmation and removal of the foreign bodies.

Occasionally, the foreign body may lead to delayed perforation of the esophagus, with inflammatory changes or abscess formation in the mediastinum. In such cases, patients may present with dysphagia, prompting a barium examination. Contrast studies may show the site of perforation or changes on the esophagogram suggesting an extraluminal mass in cases of late, missed perforation (Fig. 5–27). CT shows not only the foreign body but also mediastinal changes (Fig. 5–28). CT is usually performed without oral contrast medium enhancement, but some-

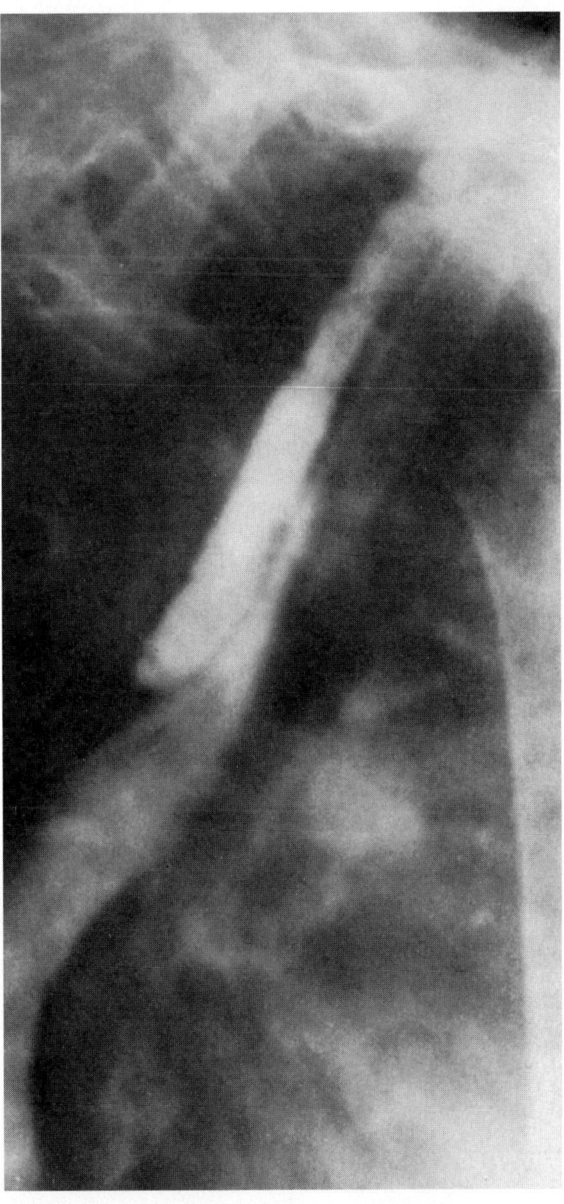

FIGURE 5–21 ■ Intramural dissection of the esophagus resulting from esophagoscopy. The appearance of a "double-barreled" esophagus is the result of perforation and dissection of the mucosa from trauma. Note the long linear radiolucency between the two lumina. The false lumin ends abruptly and is separated from the true lumen by a long esophageal mucosal stripe. Barium in the false lumen may remain after swallowing of water.

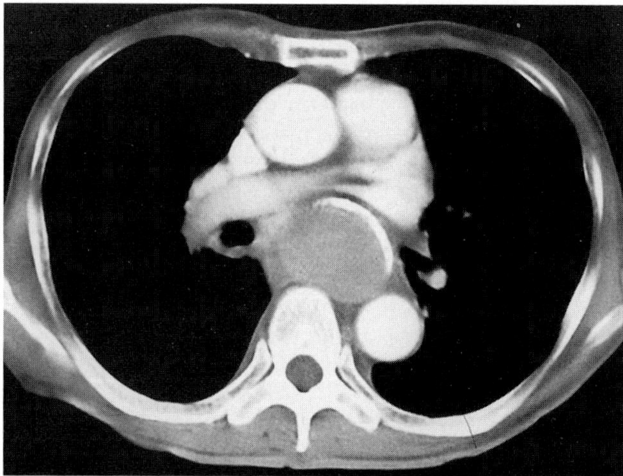

FIGURE 5–22 ■ CT scan of the intramural hermatoma in the esophagus of same patient. Note the curvilinear barium in a compressed esophagus.

times oral and IV contrast media may be given to show the relationship of the high-density foreign body to the esophagus and mediastinal structures.

If a mediastinal abscess is present, it may be amenable to percutaneous aspiration under CT guidance. The actual removal of the foreign body can be accomplished in a separate operation.

After removal of an impacted foreign body from the esophagus, another barium examination of the esophagus is indicated to exclude pre-existing lesions (e.g., esophageal stricture and Schatzki's ring).

In recent years, radiologists have successfully removed blunt foreign bodies by means of a wire basket or Foley catheter balloon under fluoroscopic guidance (Campbell and Davis, 1979; Shaffer et al, 1986). IV Glucagon (Eli Lilly, Indianapolis) has also been given to lower the pressure of the lower esophageal sphincter (LES) for dislodging impacted foreign bodies. This measure has

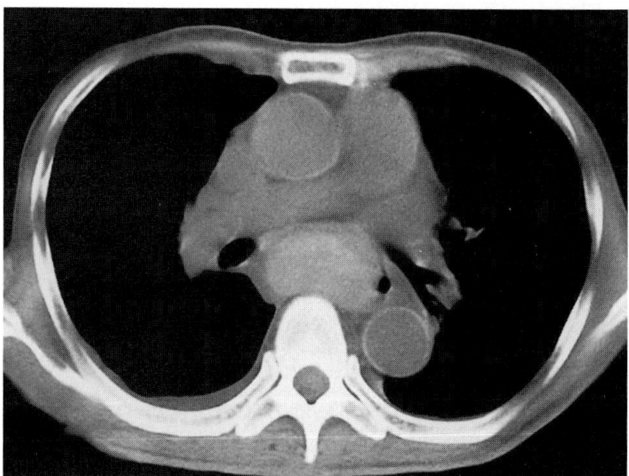

FIGURE 5–23 ■ A nonenhanced CT scan shows a high attenuation of the submucosal hematoma within the esophagus. The patient had undergone sclerotherapy for varices 1 week earlier.

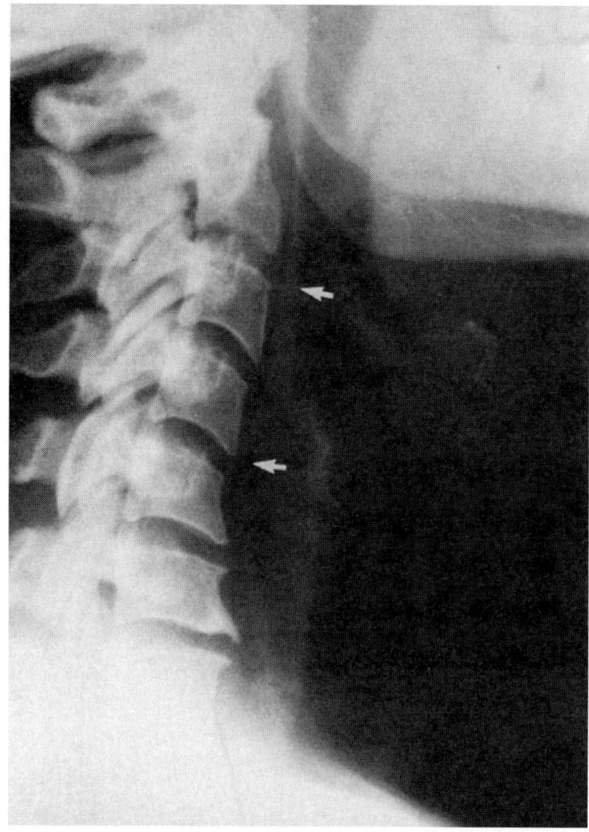

FIGURE 5–24 ■ Esophageal perforation from foreign body ingestion. Note the presence of prevertebral free air (*arrows*) caused by perforation from ingestion of a chicken bone.

been reported to be successful in 35% to 50% of the cases (Ferrucci and Long, 1977; Trenkner et al, 1983). Other radiologists have advocated the use of a gas-forming agent to distend the esophagus above the impacted foreign body to facilitate disimpaction (Rice et al, 1983). This sudden increase in intraluminal pressure in the esophagus may cause esophageal perforation and should not be used for foreign bodies impacted for more than 24 hours.

Because the noninvasive methods have not been consistently successful, endoscopic management remains the principal method of treatment of foreign bodies impacted in the esophagus.

Motor Disorders

Motility disorders of the esophagus occur frequently and are easily recognized on fluoroscopy or manometry. The common complaints of patients with motility disorders are dysphagia or chest pain, frequently aggravated by swallowing cold liquids. Correlating motor dysfunction with symptoms remains a challenge, in that many patients with motor abnormalities are asymptomatic. The following functional abnormalities of the esophagus are recognized on fluoroscopy.

Pharyngeal Dysfunction

Motor abnormality in the region of the pharynx usually results in aspiration, misdirection of barium to the nasal pharynx, or inability to relax the cricopharyngeus. Crico-

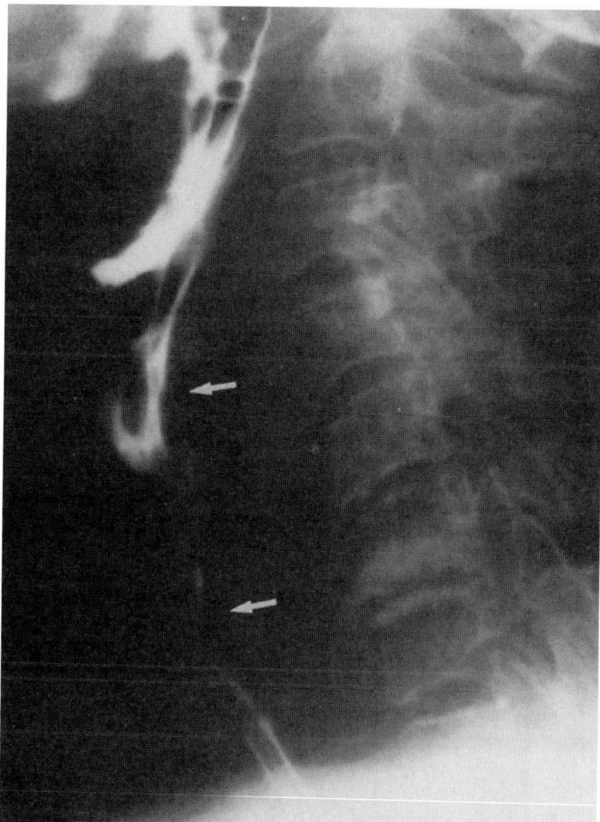

FIGURE 5–25 ■ Retropharyngeal abscess. Note the increase in the retropharyngeal space between the spine and the barium-filled pharynx (*arrow*).

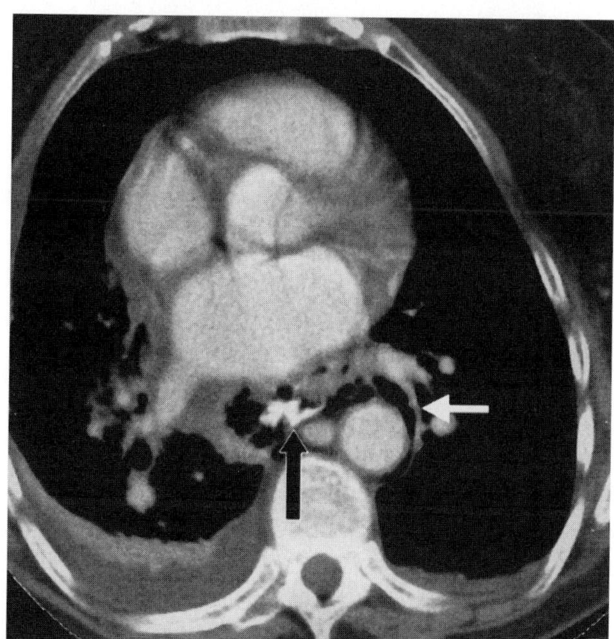

FIGURE 5–26 ■ The patient had undergone Boorhave's transection of the esophagus. CT scan shows the pneumomediastinum around the distal thoracic aorta (*white arrow*). The contrast medium–filled esophagus is seen in between the aorta and extravasated water-soluble contrast medium in the mediastinum (*black arrow*).

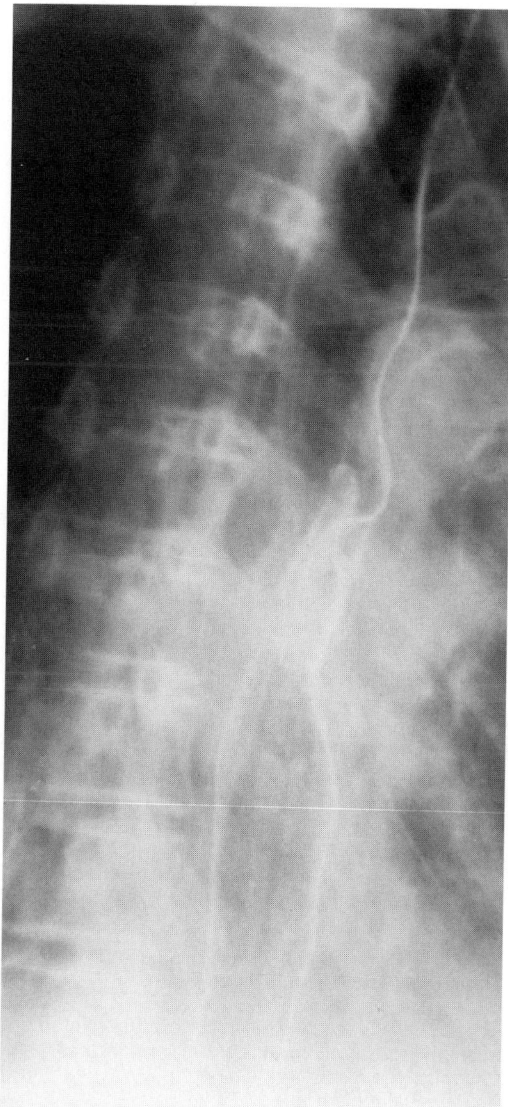

FIGURE 5–27 ■ Barium swallow study shows extramucosal indentation along the left aspect of esophagus at the level of the carina (*arrow*).

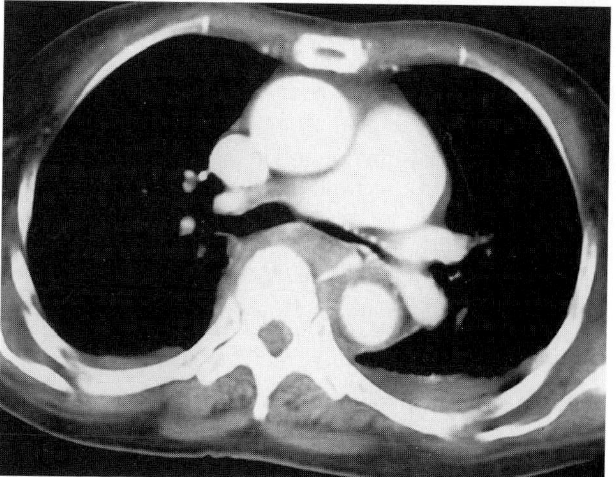

FIGURE 5–28 ■ CT scan at the level of the carina shows a triangle-shaped, high-attenuation chicken bone outside the esophagus (*arrow*). At surgery, a large mediastinal abscess around the bone was also drained.

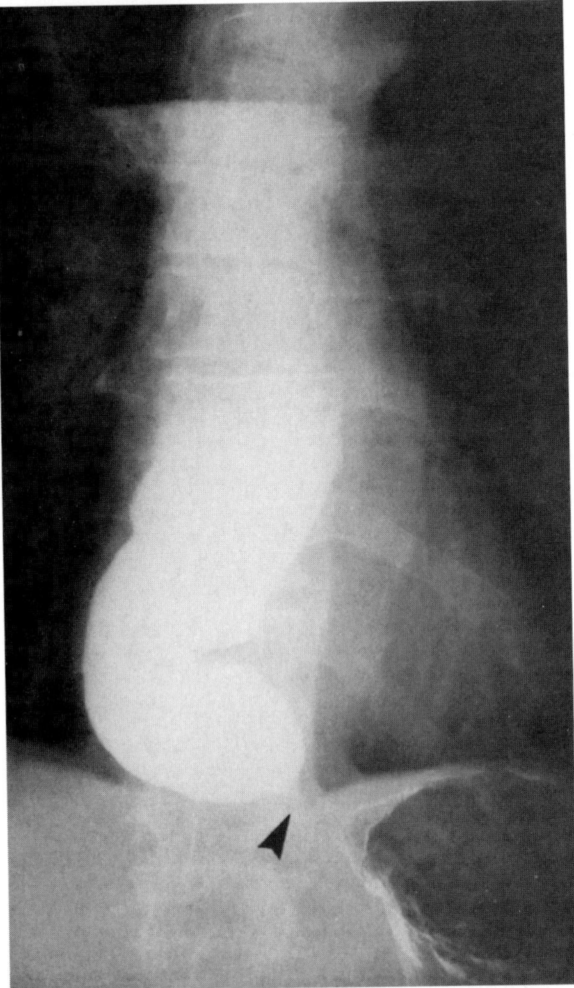

FIGURE 5–29 ■ Advanced achalasia. Note the dilated and tortuous esophagus with an air-barium level in the midesophagus. The distal end is tapered (*arrowhead*) at the gastroesophageal junction.

pharyngeal dysfunction may cause posterior indentation of the barium column at the corresponding level in the early stage and a diverticulum in the later stages of evolution of Zenker's diverticulum.

Interruption of Primary Peristalsis

Normal peristalsis is manifested as a stripping wave beginning at the cricopharyngeal level and progressing to the GE junction. Interruption of the normal wave may occur at the level of the aortic arch, with the barium bolus subsequently cleared by secondary waves. Although abnormal, such interruption is nonspecific and occurs often in older adults.

Nonperistaltic Contractions

Nonperistaltic contractions are nonpropulsive, and the barium bolus remains in the esophagus after ingestion in the recumbent position. The contractions may be either feeble or vigorous or single or repetitive.

Aperistalsis

With the patient in the upright position, barium passage is influenced mainly by gravity rather than by peristalsis. When the patient is recumbent, however, aperistalsis is easily noted as the esophagus appears motionless and the barium bolus remains stationary. Aperistalsis can be transient as in acute esophagitis (Simeone et al, 1977) or permanent as in scleroderma and achalasia.

Lower Esophageal Sphincteric Abnormalities

Abnormal LES pressures may be high or low. Low LES pressure is often associated with reflux, but high LES pressure is not evident on fluoroscopy unless it is associ-

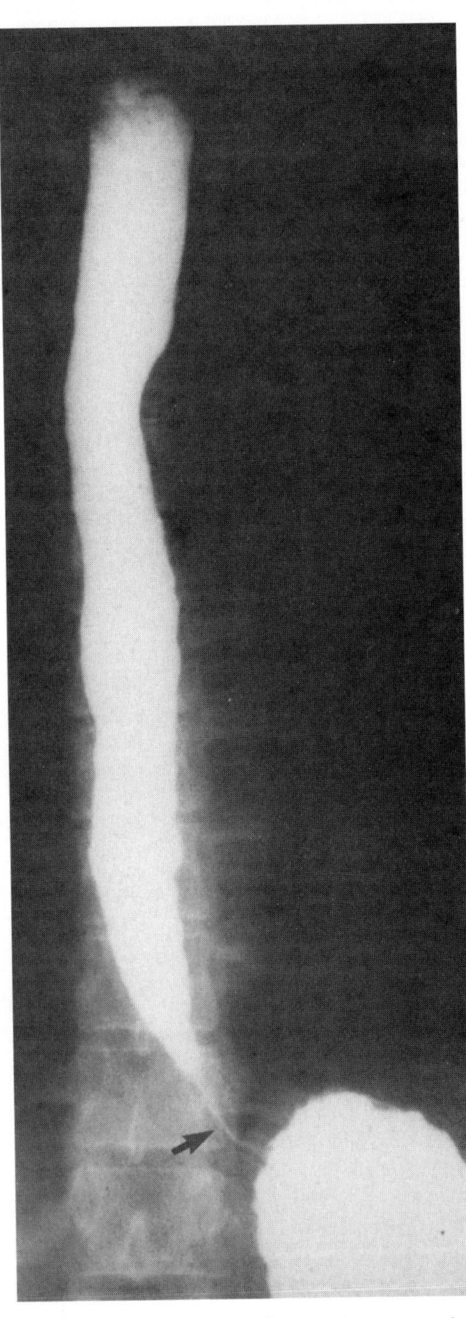

FIGURE 5–30 ■ Early achalasia. The esophagogram is taken with the patient in the recumbent position. Note the filling of the entire esophagus and the gentle tapering of the distal end (*arrow*). No peristalsis was noted on fluoroscopy, and barium remained in the esophagus for a prolonged period. With the patient in the upright position, barium emptied into the stomach intermittently because of gravity.

ated with abnormal relaxation. In the latter case, delay in barium emptying at the GE junction is noted in both the upright and recumbent positions. Similar delay may also be seen in normal LES resting pressure with failure of relaxation.

The radiologic findings of common esophageal motor disorders are described next.

Achalasia. This disease affects the entire esophagus and is characterized by aperistalsis and absence of relaxation of the LES. Patients with long-standing (20 years or more) achalasia have an increased incidence of squamous cell carcinoma, which usually assumes the polypoid type.

Radiologically, the changes are more marked in the advanced stage. The esophagus is dilated and elongated and assumes a "sigmoid" shape (Fig. 5–29). It appears on a chest radiograph as an enlarged right mediastinal shadow, sometimes with an air-fluid level seen in the posterior mediastinum. In the early stage, the esophagus is of normal size. In both early and late stages, the esophagus just above the GE junction tapers to produce a beak-like appearance (Fig. 5–30). With the patient in the upright position, barium empties by gravity and the GE sphincter relaxes intermittently when the height of barium in the esophagus reaches a certain level (Fig. 5–31).

Fluoroscopically, aperistalsis and delayed emptying of barium at the GE junction are noted. In some patients, the esophagus may show repetitive, simultaneous nonperistaltic contractions, so-called vigorous achalasia (Bondi et al, 1972). The radiologic and manometric changes of achalasia may be mimicked by Chagas' disease and by carcinoma of the stomach. In both conditions, the myenteric plexus is destroyed (by tumor or parasite—*Trypanosoma cruzi* in Chagas' disease). Chagas' disease is endemic in South America, and affected patients also have cardiomegaly and megacolon.

Diffuse Spasm. Patients with diffuse esophageal spasms complain of chest pain or dysphagia and have high-amplitude repetitive, nonperistaltic esophageal contractions following 30% of swallows (Cohen, 1979). In contrast to achalasia, peristalsis is present and is interspersed with the nonperistaltic contractions. In most cases, the LES relaxes normally, although occasionally manometric pressure may be high; sometimes the LES may fail to relax on swallowing. In some instances, diffuse spasm is associated with a thickened esophageal wall (Fig. 5–32), which can be identified as a thick soft tissue stripe alongside a barium-filled esophagus (Gonzalez, 1973).

Nutcracker Esophagus. Patients have chest pain associated with very high manometric amplitude peristaltic waves (>180 mm Hg; normal < 125 mm Hg) (Benjamin et al, 1979). Fluoroscopic findings in this condition are

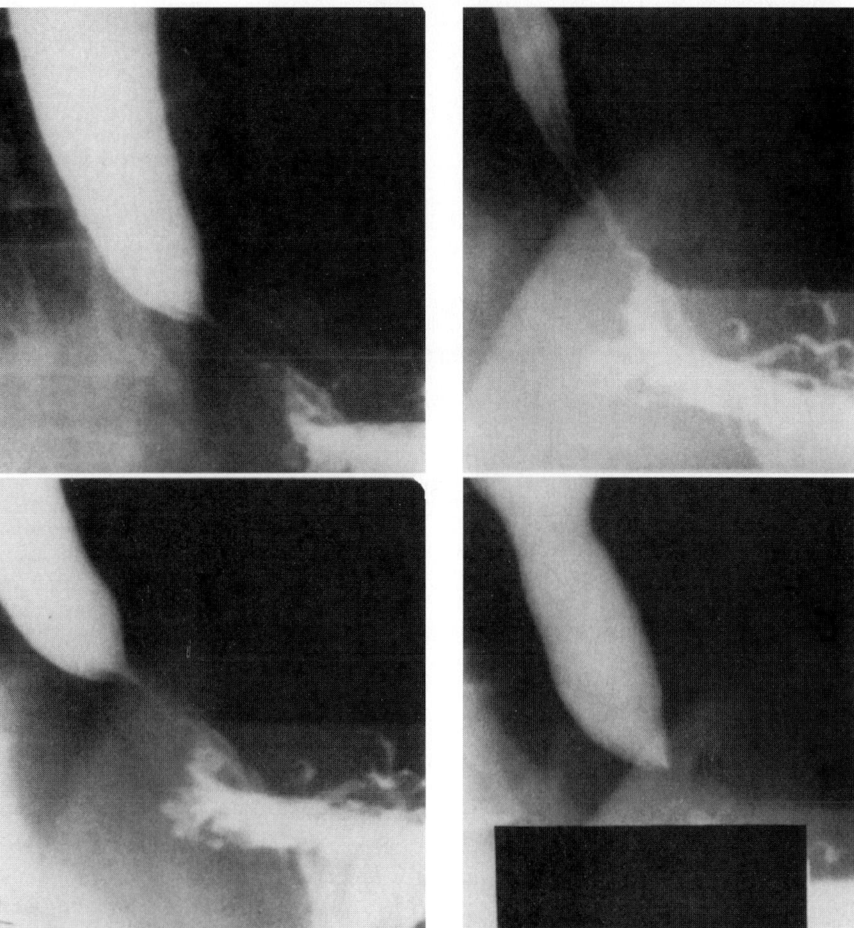

FIGURE 5–31 ■ Spot films of the gastroesophageal junction in a patient with achalasia showing different stages of emptying, with the patient in the upright position.

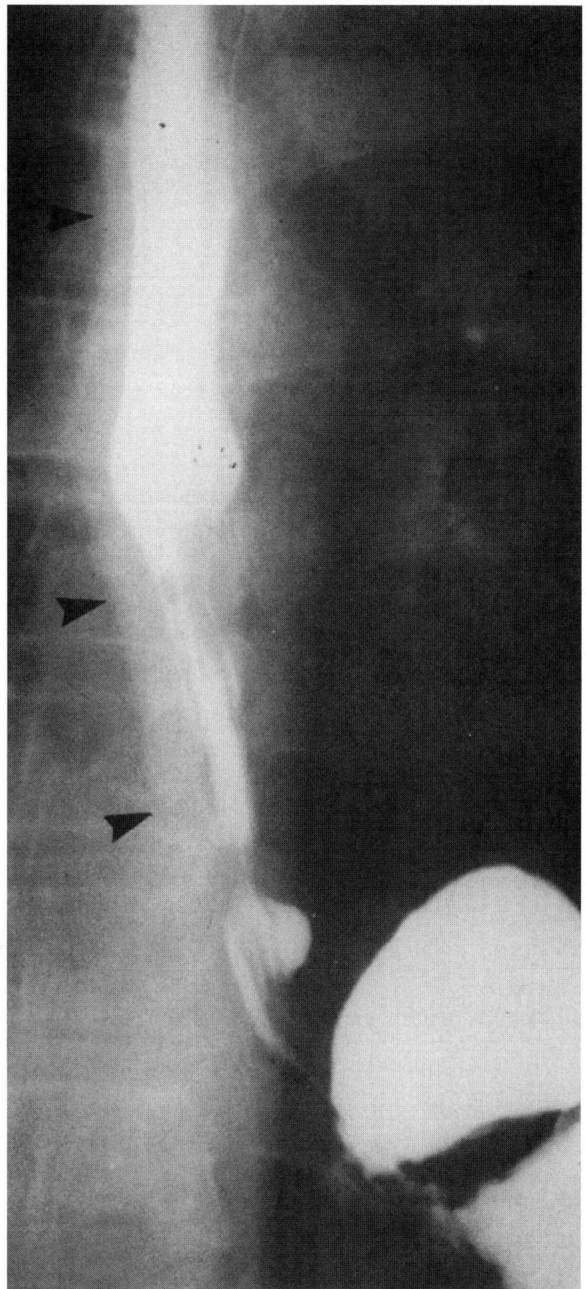

FIGURE 5–32 ■ Diffuse esophageal spasm. There is marked disordered contraction in the distal esophagus. The esophageal wall is thickened, and its outer wall is outlined by the pleural esophageal stripe (*arrowheads*).

normal. The diagnosis is made by manometry (Ott et al, 1986).

Nonspecific Esophageal Motor Disorders. Intermittent motor disorders such as aperistalsis, repetitive nonperistaltic contractions, and occasional failure of relaxation of the LES are sometimes encountered during fluoroscopy. Some patients have chest pain or dysphagia, and others do not. Because the correlation of these disorders with symptoms is poor, the disorders are usually considered nonspecific in asymptomatic patients.

Scleroderma. Esophageal involvement by scleroderma is characterized by atrophy and fibrosis of the smooth muscle of the distal two thirds of the esophagus. The esophagus is involved in 75% of patients with the disease. The GE junction is patulous, and the LES pressure is low. Peristalsis is absent in the distal two thirds of the esophagus, and fluoroscopy frequently shows gastroesophageal reflux. In advanced cases, distal esophageal stricture with a hiatal hernia may be the result of reflux esophagitis (Fig. 5–33).

Esophageal Diverticulum. Two types of esophageal diverticula are described:

1. A *pulsion* diverticulum is a mucosal outpouching through a weakness in the esophageal muscular wall and represents a false diverticulum.
2. A *traction* diverticulum is a true diverticulum containing both a mucosal and a muscular layer and is caused by focal fibrosis in the periesophageal tissue.

Midesophageal diverticula are usually traction in origin; Zenker's and epiphrenic diverticula are usually pulsion in nature.

Radiologically, traction diverticula may have a pointed base and tend to empty well. Pulsion diverticula tend to retain barium and are often associated with motor dysfunction. Pulsion diverticula have a wide neck and rounded contour and may retain barium after the esophagus has contracted. Diverticula may attain a large size and simulate a large soft tissue density in the mediastinum seen on plain chest radiographs (Fig. 5–34).

Esophageal Neoplasms

Benign Neoplasms

Leiomyoma is the most common benign esophageal neoplasm, accounting for more than 50% of benign esophageal lesions (Attah and Hajdu, 1968; Plachta, 1962). Other benign esophageal neoplasms are much less common and include papilloma, adenoma, lipoma, and fibrovascular polyps.

Leiomyoma. More than 60% of leiomyomas occur in the distal third of the esophagus, 30% in the middle third, and only 10% in the upper third (Green et al, 1959). Most lesions are solitary, but multiple tumors occur in 3% to 4% of patients (Seremetis et al, 1976). Lesions are usually small and discrete, but rare giant leiomyomas weighing more than 1000 g have been reported (Tsuzuki et al, 1971).

Most leiomyomas are asymptomatic, especially when small. Even with a large tumor, the patient may have only occasional symptoms, such as dysphagia and chest pain. Bleeding from esophageal leiomyoma is uncommon because the mucosa rarely ulcerates. Equally rare is the malignant transformation of leiomyomas (Glanz and Grunebaum, 1977). Large leiomyomas may be recognized on a chest radiograph as a posterior mediastinal mass (Fig. 5–35*A*), which may rarely contain amorphous calcifications. In contrast studies, the tumor has the following features:

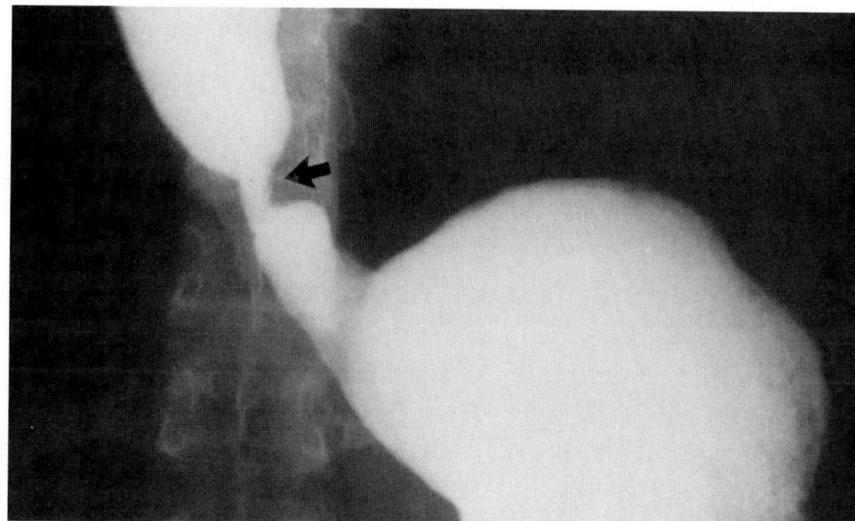

FIGURE 5–33 ■ Involvement of the esophagus in a patient with scleroderma. Note the patulous gastroesophageal junction and the presence of a small hiatal hernia. A short distal esophageal stricture (*arrow*) is present as a result of reflux esophagitis.

1. An eccentric filling defect may be seen to be indenting one side of the esophageal lumen with smooth mucosa (see Fig. 5–35*B*), typical of an extramucosal, intramural lesion in the gastrointestinal tract (Schatzki and Hawes, 1942). Viewed en face, the lesion may appear ovoid, round, or crescent shaped. Viewed in profile, the upper and lower borders of the lesion form either a right angle or an obtuse angle with the adjacent esophageal wall (Stein and Margulls, 1975).

2. Although a leiomyoma indents the esophagus, a large portion is exophytic and extends away from the lumen and into the mediastinum (Griff and Cooper, 1967).

3. Ten percent of leiomyomas may grow concentrically and produce an annular lesion indistinguishable from a carcinoma (Seremetis et al, 1976). Occasionally, a leiomyoma at the GE junction may extend into the cardia, again simulating esophageal malignancy (Schung, 1952).

FIGURE 5–34 ■ *A*, Chest film of large mediastinal mass caused by a large esophageal diverticulum (*arrows*). *B*, Barium swallow shows the large esophageal diverticulum that contracts during fluoroscopy.

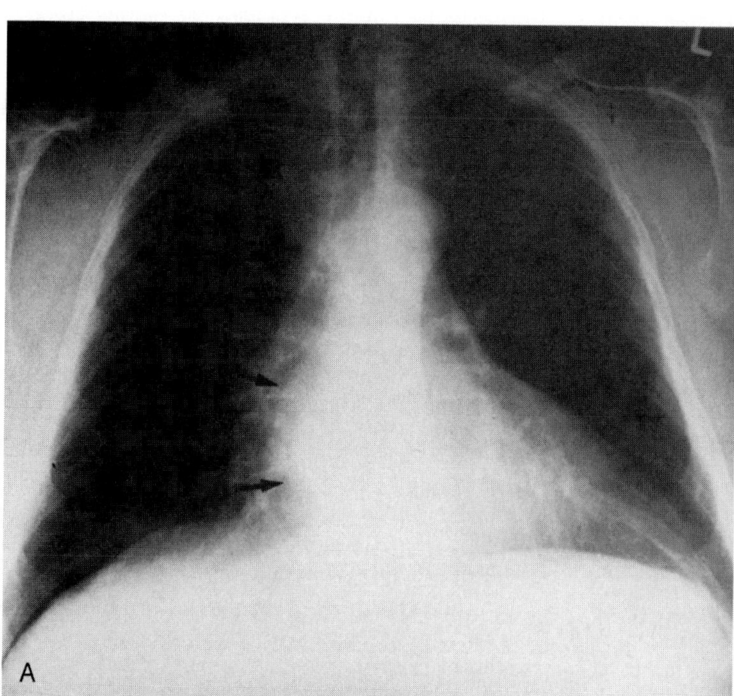

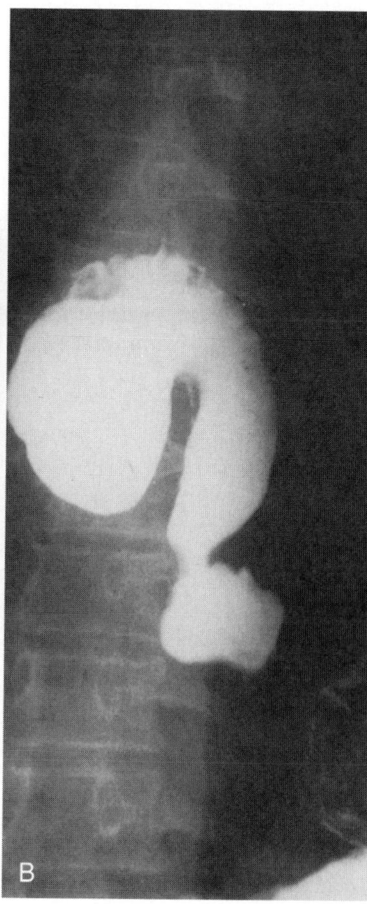

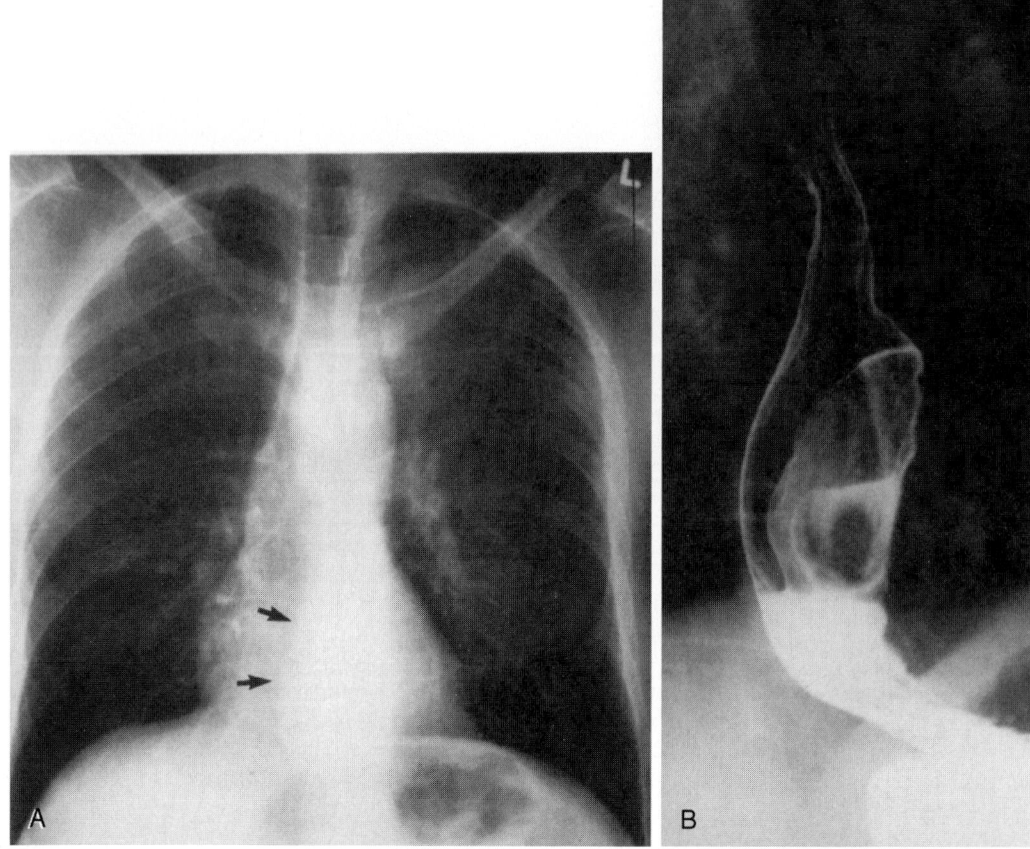

FIGURE 5–35 ■ Leiomyoma of the esophagus. *A*, Note the posterior mediastinal mass (*arrows*) on the posteroanterior chest x-ray film. *B*, Large intramural extramucosal filling defect caused by the large leiomyoma. Note the smooth surface of the leiomyoma.

4. A rare form of diffuse esophageal leiomyoma may involve the entire esophagus, with hypertrophy and thickening of its smooth muscle but with discrete lesions (Fernandes et al, 1975). This form of leiomyoma is associated with motility disorders, as seen in achalasia or diffuse spasm.

Both CT and MRI are useful in displaying a large leiomyoma and its relationship to the neighboring mediastinal structures. However, when the radiologic features of the lesion mimic carcinoma, endoscopy or EUS may be helpful. Endoscopy confirms normal mucosa overlying the submucosal lesion; endoscopic ultrasound demonstrates both the submucosal origin and the extramural extension. CT, MRI, and EUS are useful in differentiating a duplication cyst from a leiomyoma because they all identify the fluid content in a duplication cyst.

Fibrovascular Polyp. This uncommon benign lesion is characterized by a pedunculated, large intraluminal mass arising from the cervical esophagus. The tumor is composed of varying amounts of fibrovascular and adipose tissue covered by a normal mucosa. It may cause obstruction, bleeding, or anemia. Sometimes, the patient complains of a dragging discomfort behind the tongue. Occasionally, the patient may vomit a sausage-shaped mass into the mouth (Burrell and Toffler, 1973; Lolley et al, 1976).

The key radiologic feature is a large, elongated, sometimes mobile intraluminal filling defect. The pedicle is often obscured by the size of the mass. A very large fibrovascular polyp may widen the esophagus, and ripples of incoordinated contractions are seen, reflecting the futile attempts the esophagus makes to rid itself of the tumor bolus (Fig. 5–36). Despite their size, giant fibrovascular polyps have been missed on esophagoscopy, and a barium study may be more diagnostic.

Malignant Neoplasms

By far, the most common primary esophageal malignancy is carcinoma; lymphoma and sarcoma are rare. Most metastatic tumors involve the esophagus by direct extension (stomach and lung cancers). Hematogenous spread can also occur, usually in the late stages of the primary malignancy (melanoma, breast cancer).

Esophageal Carcinoma. This neoplasm comprises 1% of all cancers and 7% of gastrointestinal malignancies (Livingstone and Skinner, 1985). Both squamous carcinoma and adenocarcinoma may have similar gross morphology: infiltrative, ulcerative, polypoid, or superficial spreading. The infiltrative growth involves the muscular wall and narrows the lumen. The polyploid, or fungating, type produces an intraluminal esophageal mass. The ulcerative lesion is flat with central ulcerations. The superficial

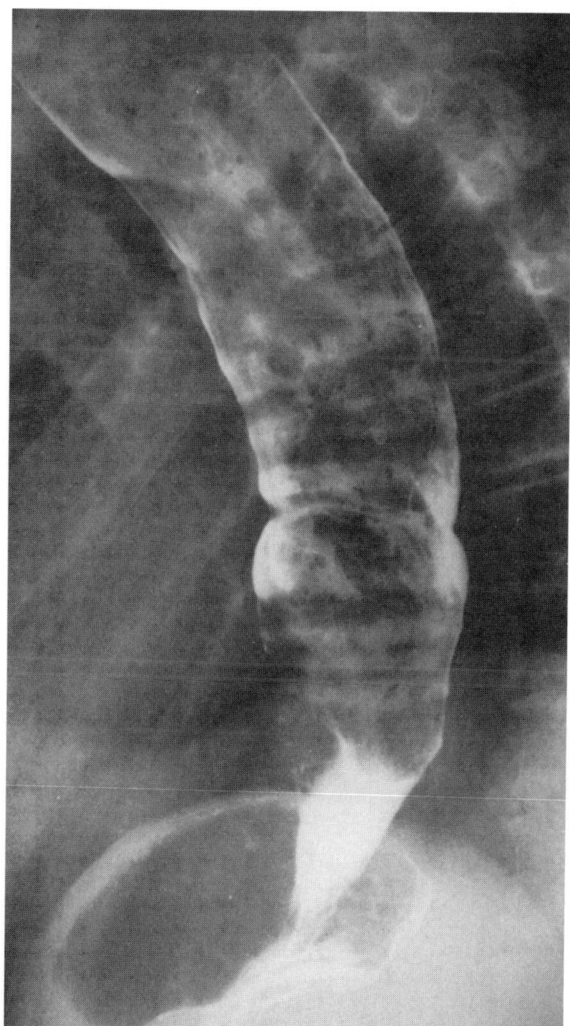

FIGURE 5–36 ■ Giant fibrovascular polyp of the esophagus. Note the large, elongated filling defect, which also enlarges the esophagus. Ripples of barium across the esophagus represent tertiary contractions by which the esophagus attempts, in vain, to rid itself of the mass.

spreading type involves the mucosa but spares the deeper structures.

The term *early carcinoma* is a histologic diagnosis and refers to a cancerous lesion involving the mucosa or mucosa and submucosa only; such early cancers can assume any of the preceding morphologic features. Squamous carcinomas are located predominantly in the upper third (20%) and middle third (50%) of the esophagus. In contrast, adenocarcinoma is usually found in the distal esophagus, at the GE junction. Adenocarcinoma may originate from the stomach and spread proximally to involve the distal esophagus. Adenocarcinoma may also arise from the abnormal columnar epithelium in patients with Barrett's esophagus. In such cases, the tumor may be more proximally located in the thoracic esophagus.

Early cancer appears as small intraluminal plaque-like or polypoid protrusions (Fig. 5–37) or as an area of discrete ulceration. It is best shown on a double-contrast esophagogram. Occasionally, a large polypoid carcinoma may fall into this early stage if it has not invaded the underlying mucosa and submucosa.

Patients with advanced esophageal cancer may have abnormal chest radiographs showing a widened retrotracheal stripe, a hilar or retrocardiac mass, or an air-fluid level in the esophagus (Lindell et al, 1979). Although nonspecific for malignancy, these signs should alert the clinician to a significant esophageal pathologic process and the need for further diagnostic imaging. Barium studies usually reflect the gross pathology of esophageal cancers.

Infiltrative Type. The infiltrative type of radiologic pattern is most commonly seen. Depending on the extent

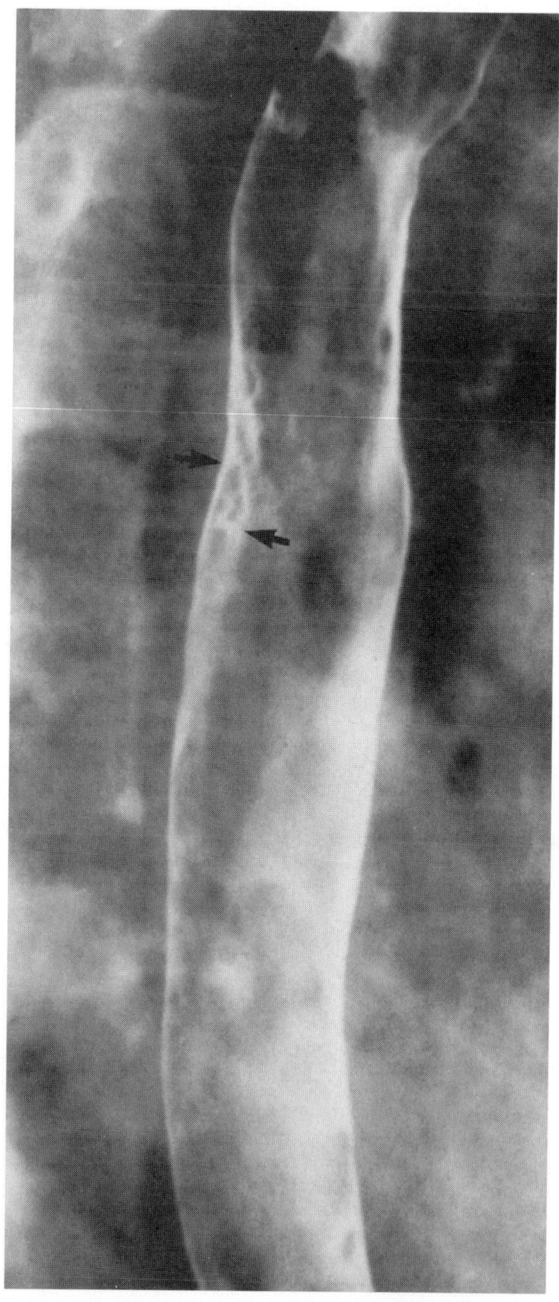

FIGURE 5–37 ■ Early carcinoma. An air esophagogram (*arrows*), with a nasogastric tube inserted in the upper esophagus, demonstrates an area of mucosal defect, suggesting the presence of plaques. Biopsy of area showed early carcinoma.

of circumferential infiltration, the esophageal lumen is eccentrically or concentrically narrowed (Fig. 5–38). The contour of the narrowed segment is irregular because of ulceration on the tumor surface. At either end of the narrowed segment, an indentation caused by the margin of the tumor may be observed. Occasionally, these indentations form shelf-like borders on both sides and produce an "apple core" appearance. Rarely, a gentle tapering edge is seen, together with a normal-looking mucosal pattern mimicking a benign stricture (Goldstein et al, 1981).

On occasion, neither endoscopy nor biopsy may secure the diagnosis. In this rare situation, operative diagnosis is required (see Fig. 5–15*A*). In advanced cases the esophageal lumen is severely or completely occluded, resulting in dilatation of the proximal esophagus.

Polypoid Type. The polypoid type appears as a large filling defect (>3.5 cm) within the lumen of the esophagus (Fig. 5–39). The tumor mass often contains areas of ulceration from tumor necrosis, resulting in an uneven contour; in contrast, a benign polypoid lesion such as fibrovascular polyp has a smooth surface and contour.

Ulcerative Type. The ulcer is often large and replaces most of the tumor mass (Fig. 5–40). When shown in profile, this type appears as a well-defined meniscoid ulcer with a radiolucent rim surrounding it (Gloyna et al, 1977). The rim may not be obvious when the lesion is seen en face, and the optimal profile view should be obtained by turning the patient during fluoroscopy.

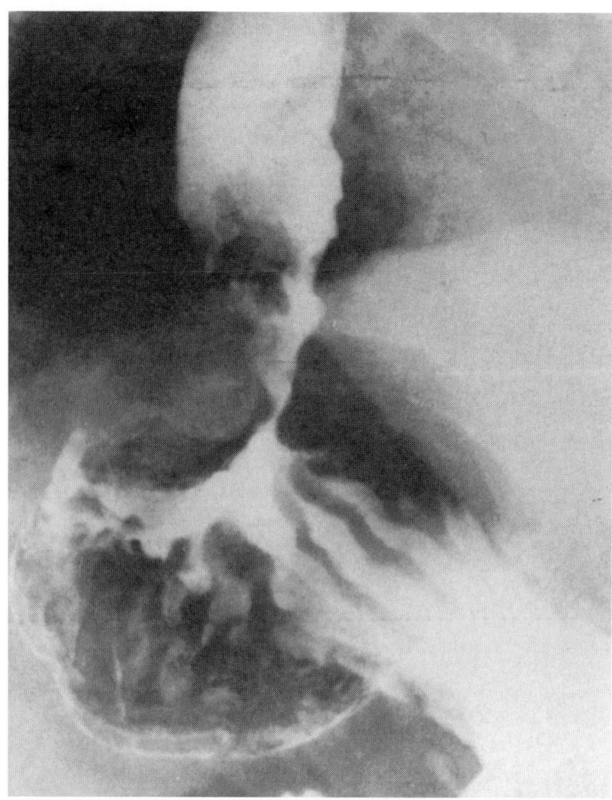

FIGURE 5–39 ■ Fungating carcinoma of the esophagus. A large filling defect in the distal esophagus extends to involve the fundus.

Varicoid Type. The varicoid type is produced by diffuse submucosal spread of the tumor, resulting in marked thickening and tortuosity of the mucosal folds, simulating esophageal varices (Fig. 5–41) (Lawson et al, 1969). Despite such diffuse disease, the patient may not have dysphagia. Differentiation from true varices can be made by the tumor location (middle or upper third) and its failure to change size with peristalsis or respiration. The demarcation between varicoid tumor and the adjacent normal mucosa is more distinct and abrupt than for varices.

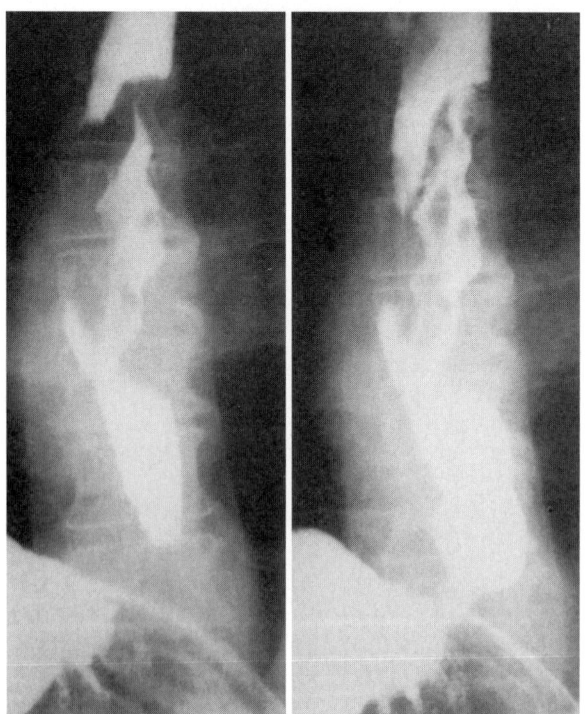

FIGURE 5–38 ■ Infiltrative carcinoma of the esophagus, with narrowing of the lumen and shelf-like indentation on the proximal end of the stricture.

Other Changes. Contrast studies also reflect other changes caused by tumor invasion in advanced malignancy. For example, large mediastinal lymphadenopathy may cause extrinsic encroachment and deviation of the esophagus. In 5% to 10% of the cases, an esophageal-airway fistula (involving mainly the trachea or the left main bronchus) may develop, often after radiation treatment (Fitzgerald et al, 1981). Even more rarely, the pericardium may be invaded, resulting in esophagopericardial fistula (Fig. 5–42).

In rare instances, the cancer may spread through submucosal lymphatics to other locations in the esophagus (Steiner et al, 1984) or to the fundus of the stomach (Glick et al, 1986). Esophageal carcinoma can metastasize to other parts of the esophagus or stomach and be evident as small, polypoid masses or plaque-like or ulcerated lesions distant from the main tumor. Gastric metastases manifest as large submucosal fundic lesions, with or without ulceration, and may mimic leiomyomas. A dou-

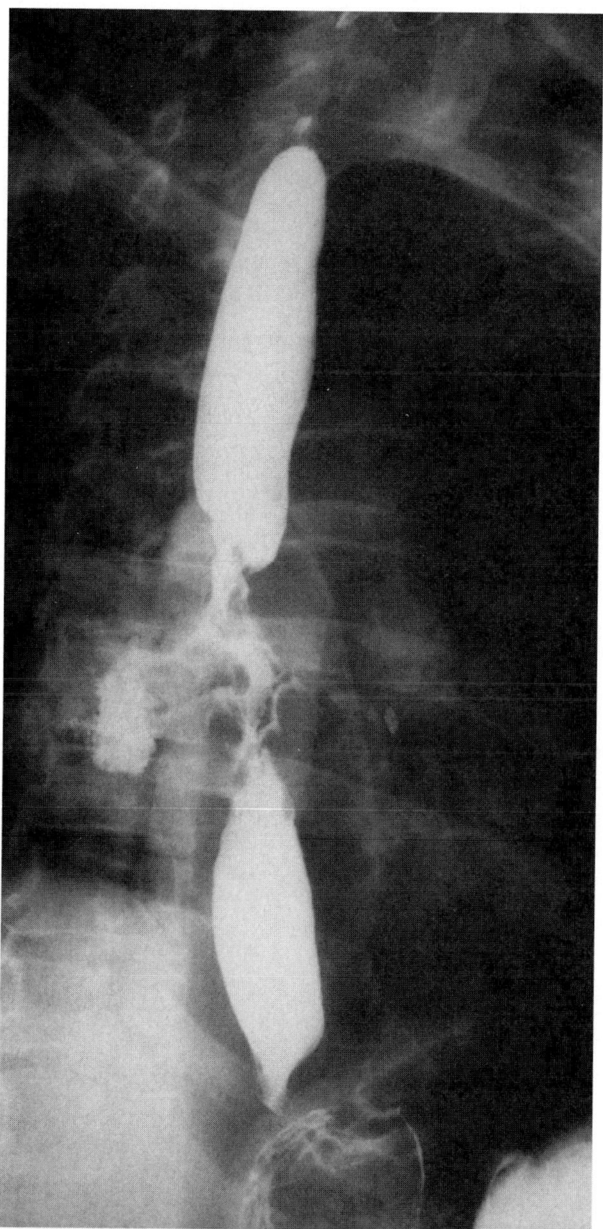

FIGURE 5–40 ■ Carcinoma of the esophagus with perforation. The large carcinoma in the midesophagus has ulcerated, and a large ulcer extends beyond the lumen of the esophagus.

ble-contrast study of the esophagus and stomach is therefore an important part of staging.

Lymphoma. Primary lymphoma of the esophagus is very uncommon. More often, the esophagus is invaded by lymphomatous mediastinal nodes or spread from the stomach in patients with widespread disease. Barium studies reveal extrinsic compression from the mediastinal nodal enlargement or segmental narrowing of the distal esophagus from tumor extension, as in gastric carcinoma. Intrinsic lymphoma of the esophagus may present features of a submucosal carcinoma, that is, as enlargement of esophageal folds or as multiple discrete submucosal nodules or strictures.

Leiomyosarcoma. Leiomyosarcoma is a rare malignant tumor accounting for less than 1% of all malignant growths in the esophagus (Goodner, 1963). Like leiomyoma, leiomyosarcoma has a tendency for exophytic growth and may be asymptomatic despite its large size (Lyons and Garlock, 1951). In barium studies, the tumor appears as a large intraluminal mass enlarging the esophageal lumen because of its expansile growth. The exophytic component may be noted in a chest radiograph as a mediastinal mass. These two features are rarely seen in esophageal carcinoma. Leiomyosarcoma may rarely assume an infiltrative growth pattern causing narrowing

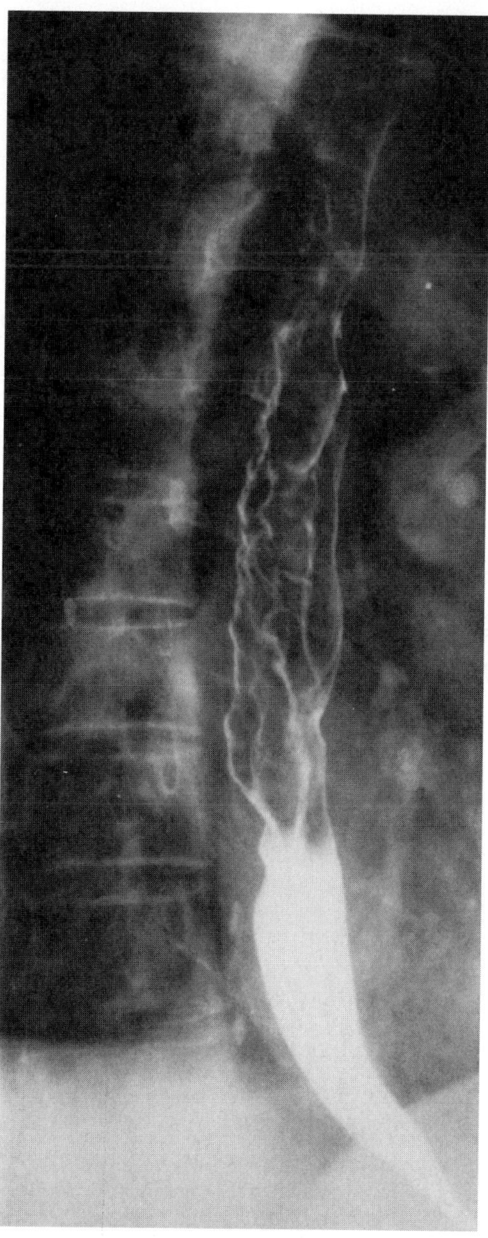

FIGURE 5–41 ■ Varicoid carcinoma of the esophagus. Note the thickened, nodular, longitudinal folds of the esophagus with features of varices. The absence of involvement in the proximal and distal esophagus, however, should exclude the diagnosis of varices. The absence of any changes on fluoroscopy favors carcinoma.

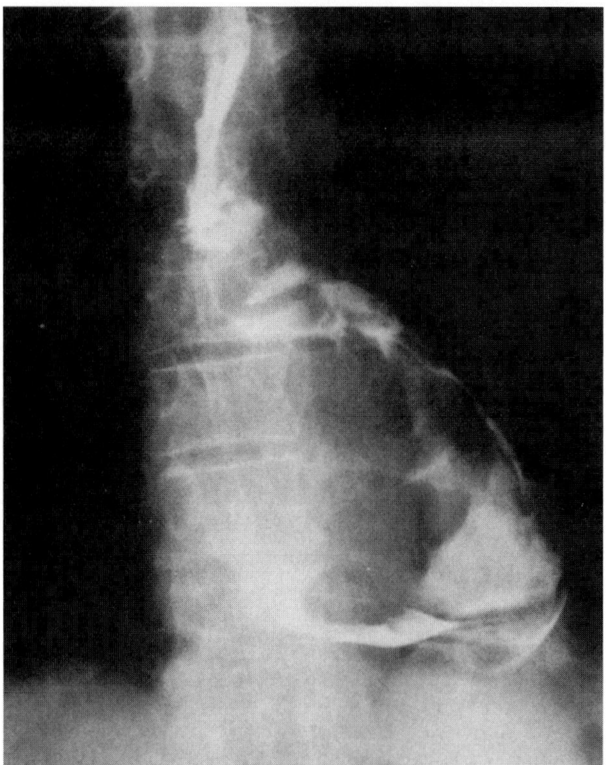

FIGURE 5–42 ■ Esophageal pericardial fistula. A carcinoma of the esophagus has eroded into the pericardium. Barium swallow outlines the pericardial cavity. No arrhythmia was associated with the study.

of the esophagus and obstructive symptoms, mimicking carcinoma of the esophagus.

Malignant Melanoma. The prognosis is poor because of early metastases, and the radiologic features are those of polyploid growth (single or multiple). Rarely, the center of the tumor may ulcerate and a bull's-eye appearance can be identified, as with melanomas in other parts of the gastrointestinal tract (Fig. 5–43).

Kaposi's Sarcoma and Leukemia. In both diseases, esophageal involvement occurs in the late stage and the lesions usually appear in the esophagogram as discrete, multiple, submucosal nodules. Occasionally, leukemic nodules may be bulky or submucosal masses may coalesce to form irregular strictures.

Metastases. Esophageal metastases are the result of direct spread from malignancies arising from the adjacent organs, such as lung, stomach, and mediastinal lymph nodes. Lymphatic spread to mediastinal nodes also results from primary cancers of the head and neck, breast, and pancreas. Hematogenous spread of tumor to the esophagus is extremely rare.

Esophagograms show the extrinsic lesion displacing or compressing the esophagus. When the esophagus becomes infiltrated by tumor extension, the surface of the affected area may show a serrated or tethered appearance. When tumor infiltration is extensive and the esophagus becomes completely encased, distinction from a primary esophageal cancer may be impossible. Stomach cancer extending from the fundus of the stomach to involve the lower esophagus may mimic achalasia or benign peptic stricture as it presents as a narrowed segment of varying lengths. Esophageal motility may be affected and simulate achalasia as well. The presence of a mass lesion in the gastric fundus is the main distinguishing feature and should always be sought in patients with lower esophageal strictures.

CANCER STAGING

CT, MRI, and, more recently, EUS have all been used to determine the clinical stage of carcinoma. Staging is use-

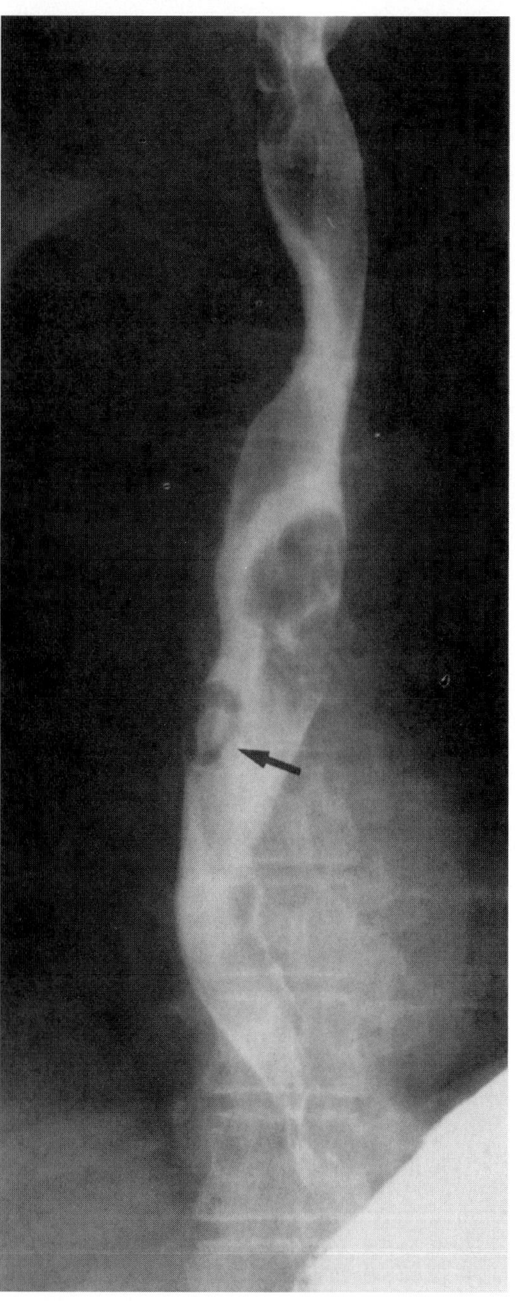

FIGURE 5–43 ■ Metastatic melanoma to the esophagus. Notice the bull's-eye lesion (*arrow*) in the distal esophagus. The central barium collection, surrounded by a rim of radiolucency, is caused by a large ulceration in the melanoma.

ful for assessing the outcome of the different treatment methods. Preliminary results comparing the accuracy in predicting resectability by MRI and CT show no difference between the two modalities (Takashima et al, 1991). A 1991 study comparing endoscopic ultrasound and CT in their ability to assess operability showed endoscopic ultrasound to be more accurate (Ziegler et al, 1991). For esophageal cancer, the more recent recommendations of the International Union Against Cancer and the American Joint Committee on Cancer are based on the tumor, node, metastasis (TNM) classification (Rice et al, 1991). They no longer place any significance on the length, size, or site of the tumor; only depth of esophageal wall invasion is considered for evaluation of the tumor (T). EUS evaluation is limited to the tumor and its local extension, including the adjacent nodes (N). Distant metastases (M) are assessed by both CT and MRI but not by EUS.

Because CT is more widely used, findings used for CT staging are given in the following text.

Esophageal Wall Thickness

The normal thickness is 3 to 5 mm. Asymmetric thickening is usually seen in esophageal carcinoma (Fig. 5–44) (Halber et al, 1979; Moss et al, 1981). Benign processes, on the other hand, tend to produce smooth symmetric and circumferential wall thickening.

Tumor Size

Tumors larger than 5 cm are automatically classified beyond T1 stage. It is generally accepted that CT is more reliable than barium or endoscopy in assessing the length of the lesion (Thompson et al, 1983). The actual difference in length as measured by CT versus that derived by radiographic or endoscopic measurement can be as much as 6 cm.

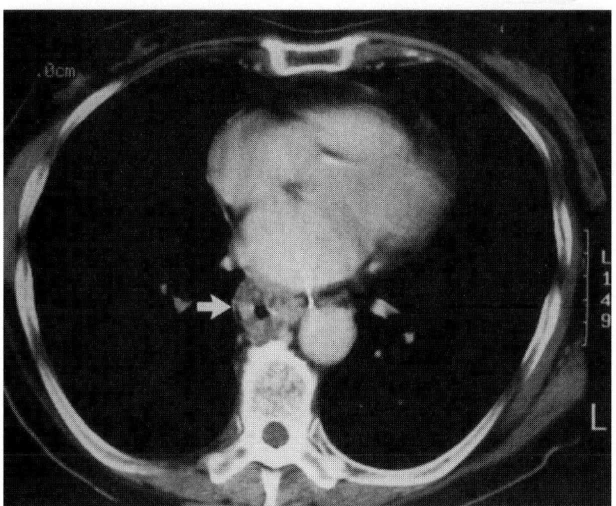

FIGURE 5–44 ■ Carcinoma of the esophagus. CT scan shows marked thickening of the esophageal wall (*arrow*) caused by tumor infiltration.

Periesophageal Invasion

Tumor invasion to adjacent structures is best evaluated by the presence of a fat plane separating the esophagus from the adjacent tissue. Tumor extension into the periesophageal fat may manifest as strand-like areas of soft tissue density producing a feathery appearance within the fat (Coulamb et al, 1981). The presence of a normal-looking fat plane generally indicates absence of tumor invasion. However, the normal fat plane may be absent in the thin and emaciated patient, even without periesophageal tumor extension. Invasion of periesophageal structures such as the trachea and bronchus is determined by tumor indentation of these tubular structures.

Vascular Invasion. The esophagus is intimately related to the aortic arch, most of the descending thoracic aorta, the pulmonary artery, and the left atrium. Neoplastic invasion of these structures makes the tumor unresectable (Fig. 5–45).

The obliteration of mediastinal fat surrounding these vascular structures on CT has been used to suggest tumor invasion. Picus and associates (1983) showed that invasion was unlikely if tumor involved less than 25% of the aortic circumference and highly likely if tumor involved over 90%. However, several studies have shown that the sensitivity of these criteria ranged between 50% and 100% (Becker et al, 1986; Halvorsen and Thompson, 1989; Quint et al, 1985). Therefore, obliteration of these planes cannot be used for reliable prediction of neoplastic invasion of the aorta.

Pericardial invasion by esophageal carcinoma is seen in about 1% of autopsy cases (Postlethwait, 1986). The CT signs include obliteration of fat planes between the pericardium and the tumor, provided the normal fat planes are present above and below the tumor mass. In cachectic patients, in whom no fat planes are seen, this CT sign is not useful.

Tracheobronchial Invasion. Tracheobronchial invasion by esophageal carcinoma may not only render the tumor unresectable but may also lead to severe complications such as TE fistula. In the past, contrast medium–enhanced studies were necessary to demonstrate the fistula (Fig. 5–46); however, with the new multislice CT helical scanners, such fistulas can be visualized (Fig. 5–47) and may be treated with a covered endoprosthesis.

Diaphragmatic Invasion. It is generally agreed that CT is inaccurate in assessing invasion of the diaphragm by esophageal tumor (Quint et al, 1994). Clinically, diaphragmatic invasion does not preclude tumor resection.

Lymphadenopathy

Esophageal carcinoma metastasizes to regional lymph node groups within the thorax and to distant nodes outside, for example, the supraclavicular nodes and abdominal lymph nodes including the aortocaval lymph nodes (Fig. 5–48). The size, number, and CT appearance of lymph nodes have been used to determine if metastasis is present. Metastatic nodes are generally not calcified

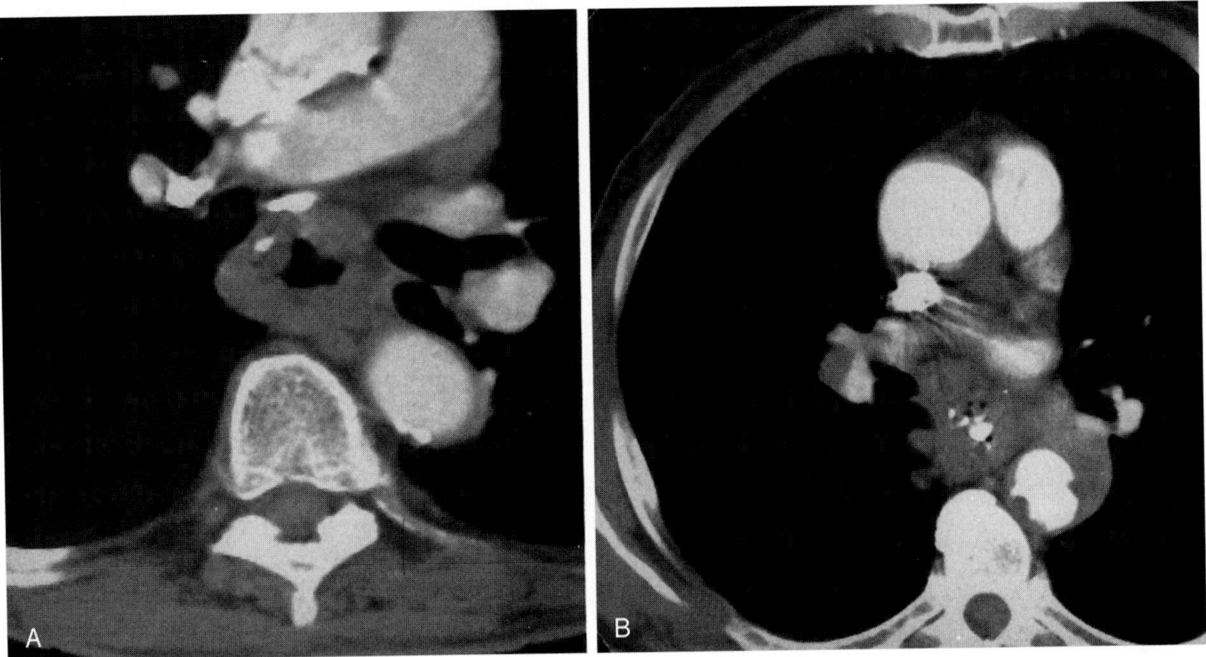

FIGURE 5–45 ■ *A*, Large esophageal carcinoma invading the main right pulmonary artery. *B*, Unresectable esophageal carcinoma has encircled more than 270 degrees in circumference of the distal thoracic aorta. (Compare with *A*.)

and may have homogeneous or inhomogeneous CT density (with necrosis).

Supraclavicular nodes should be considered enlarged when their transverse diameter equals or is greater than 5 mm (Coulomb et al, 1981). Supraclavicular metastasis may be found in 22% of patients with squamous cell carcinoma and only 10% of patients with adenocarcinomas undergoing CT staging of esophageal carcinoma.

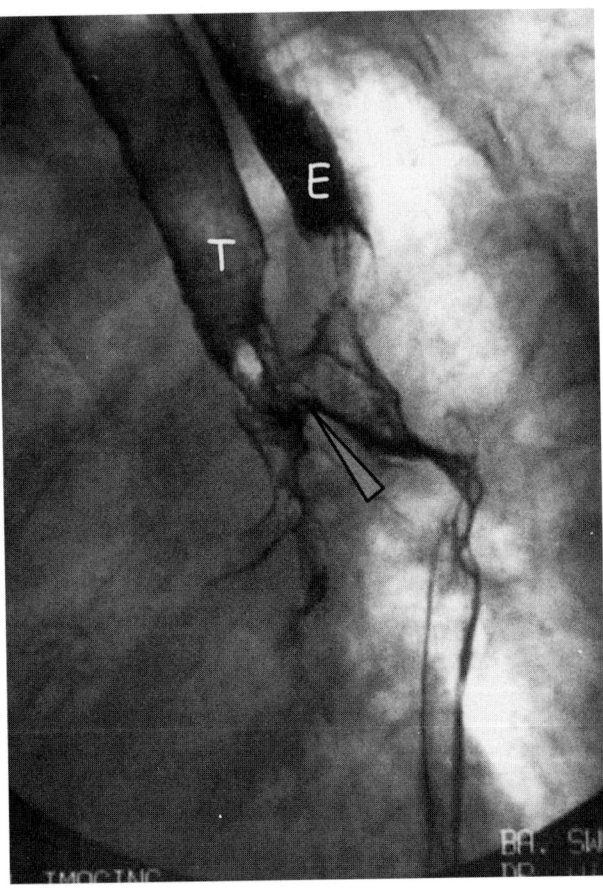

FIGURE 5–46 ■ A barium study of the same patient, showing the fistula *(arrowhead)*. (E, esophagus; T, trachea.)

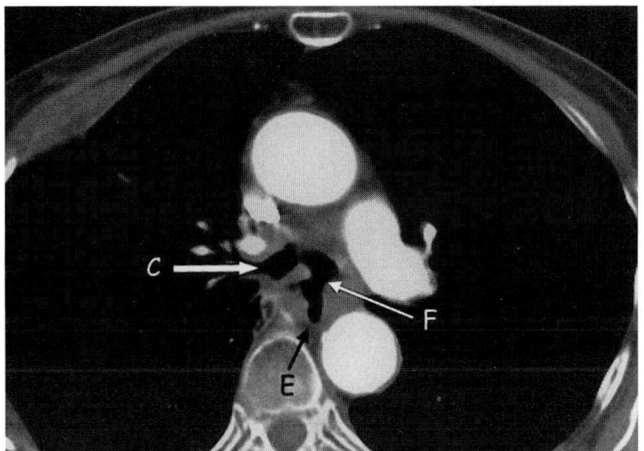

FIGURE 5–47 ■ Spiral thin-slice CT scan at the level of the carina (C) shows a fistula (F) between the esophagus (E) and the left main stem bronchus.

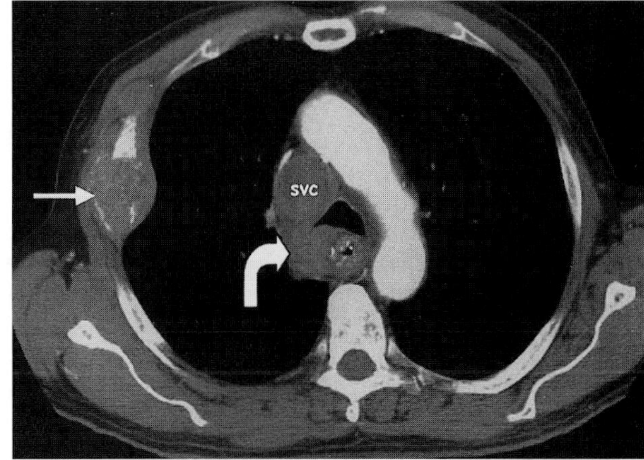

FIGURE 5–49 ■ CT scan at the level of the carina shows a large esophageal mass (*curved arrow*) invading the superior vena cava (SVC) and bronchi. Osteolytic metastasis (*straight arrow*) expanding the rib is visible.

Mediastinal or abdominal lymph nodes larger than 10 to 15 mm are considered abnormal, except for retrocrural nodes, which should not be greater than 6 mm (Quint et al, 1994). Most authors using these criteria report a specificity of about 90% but a sensitivity of only 40% to 60% (Thompson et al, 1994). The relatively low sensitivity is mainly caused by normal nodes harboring metastasis and some abnormally large lymph nodes occurring as a result of some benign inflammatory mediastinal process. CT-fluoroscopy, where available, can be used to guide needle biopsy of lymph nodes and increase the sensitivity.

Distant Metastasis

Esophageal carcinoma also metastasizes to liver, lung, adrenals, peritoneum, and, rarely, bones.

Liver metastases, which are of low attenuation and usually focal, are found in about 10% of patients undergoing CT for preoperative evaluation. These lesions have to be differentiated from other benign lesions such as hemangiomas. The presence of uniformly enhancing margins surrounding a liver lesion is in favor of malignancy. Triphasic contrast scanning (noncontrast, arterial and venous phases) of the liver used with high-resolution CT increases the sensitivity and specificity of detection of liver metastasis.

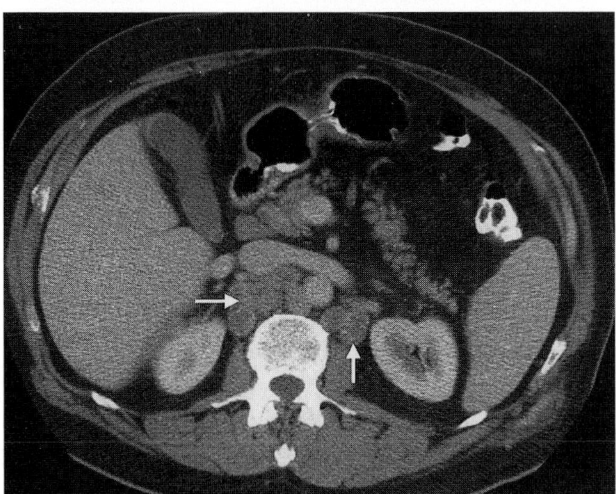

FIGURE 5–48 ■ Low attenuation aortocaval lymphadenopathy *(arrows)* in the retroperitoneum in a patient with esophageal carcinoma.

Pulmonary metastases, seen as noncalcified nodules, are best detected by CT. Peritoneal metastases are suspected when ascites or nodular peritoneal lesions are seen. Esophageal carcinoma rarely metastasizes to bone (Fig. 5–49).

Predicting Prognosis

CT has also been used for predicting prognosis for survival. Halvorsen and colleagues (1986) found poorer survival for patients with subdiaphragmatic spread compared with those with mediastinal spread only (90 days versus 7 months). The mean survival was 1.7 years if no metastases were found.

POSTOPERATIVE APPEARANCE

The esophagus is often examined after surgical or interventional procedures for its anatomic integrity and functional alteration. Interpretation of any radiologic examination requires an understanding of the nature and complications of these procedures. The postoperative radiologic appearance of the commonly encountered procedures is described next.

Antireflux Surgery

Surgical treatment for reflux is performed in patients with severe esophagitis refractory to medical management or with complications such as peptic stricture, bleeding, or Barrett's esophagus. Antireflux surgery aims at creating a valvular action at the GE junction to prevent reflux. This aim is achieved through a fundoplication that wraps around the GE junction (Butterfield, 1961).

Three surgical methods have been developed for fundoplication: (1) an approach from the abdomen (Hill posterior gastropexy), (2) an approach from the thorax (Belsey Mark IV repair), and (3) an approach from either the abdomen or the thorax (Nissen fundoplication). (Details of these procedures are described in Chapters 20 to 22.)

It suffices to suggest that in Nissen fundoplication the distal esophagus is "wrapped around" 360 degrees; in the Belsey repair, 270 degrees; and in the Hill procedure, 180 degrees or less. The Hill procedure also includes suturing of the proximal lesser curvature to the median arcuate ligament (posterior gastropexy).

In patients with irreducible hiatal hernia caused by shortening of the esophagus, a Collis gastroplasty is performed (Collis, 1954; Pearson et al, 1971). This procedure consists of two components: lengthening of the esophagus through dividing the fundus by a row of staples and creating an antireflux wrap around the newly formed gastroplasty tube.

Radiologic features of both the Nissen and Hill operations are similar, with the distal esophagus showing a short segment of smooth narrowing resulting from the fundoplication (Fig. 5–50). The fundoplication appears as a smooth mass lesion at the site of narrowing and is smaller in the Hill gastropexy. In the Belsey Mark IV operation, the narrowed intra-abdominal portion of the esophagus has two distinct angles, one when the wraparound is sutured to the esophagus and the diaphragm and a lower one when the fundus is pulled toward the esophagus (Feigin et al, 1974). These angles are best seen in an RAO view of the fundus of the stomach. In a Collis gastroplasty, the newly created gastric tube may show a row of staples.

Complications in the early postoperative period include leakage and obstruction at the fundoplication. Both complications can be demonstrated by contrast study. If leakage is present and the extent of leakage into the mediastinum and pleura is to be evaluated, CT of the thorax is performed. Late complications include suture breakdown with disruption of the wrap-around and recurrence of the hiatal hernia and GE reflux (Fig. 5–51). The fundoplication may also be too tight, and the patient complains of dysphagia or bloating because of an inability to belch (DeMeester et al, 1974). The degree of narrowing at the "wraparound" should be evaluated with a marshmallow swallow. A very narrowed segment at the fundoplication, shown in a contrast radiograph, does not necessarily imply dysphagia; however, if a marshmallow fails to pass through the narrowed segment, the cause of clinical symptoms may be ascertained.

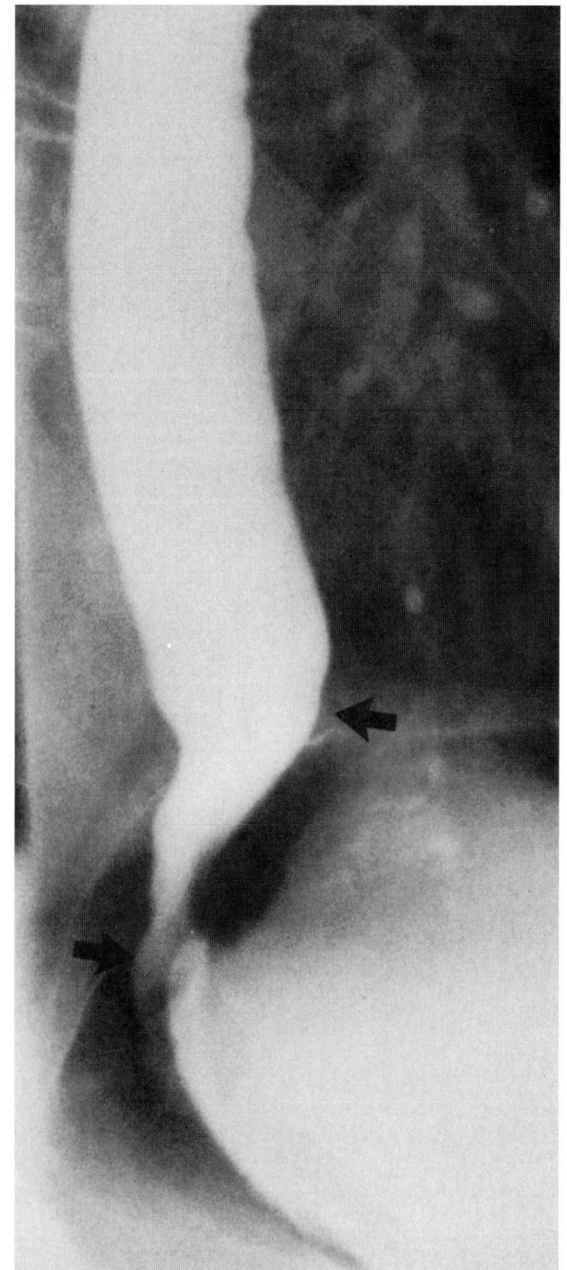

FIGURE 5–50 ■ Radiographic appearance of the esophagus after Belsey Mark IV repair. Note the angulation and narrowing (*arrow*) of the distal esophagus, which is wrapped around by the fundoplication.

Cancer Surgery

Because patients with carcinoma of the esophagus usually present late, surgical treatment is performed more often for palliation than for cure. Esophagogastrectomy is performed for palliation as well as for cure; esophageal bypass surgery (gastric tubes and colonic interposition) is a palliative procedure for cancer, severe esophageal dysfunction, or strictures.

Esophagogastrectomy

Distant metastases and aortic or tracheobronchial invasion by tumor are contraindications to surgery, but mediastinal adenopathy is not. At surgery, the diseased esophagus is removed and the stomach mobilized and pulled into the thorax for anastomosis with the upper esophagus. Depending on the approach, the stomach may lie in the right hemithorax (Ivor Lewis procedure) or in the posterior mediastinum (transhiatal or transabdominal approach). To prevent reflux, a small fundoplication or invagination of a short segment of the esophagus at the level of anastomosis is sometimes performed. A pyloroplasty is also added to improve gastric emptying.

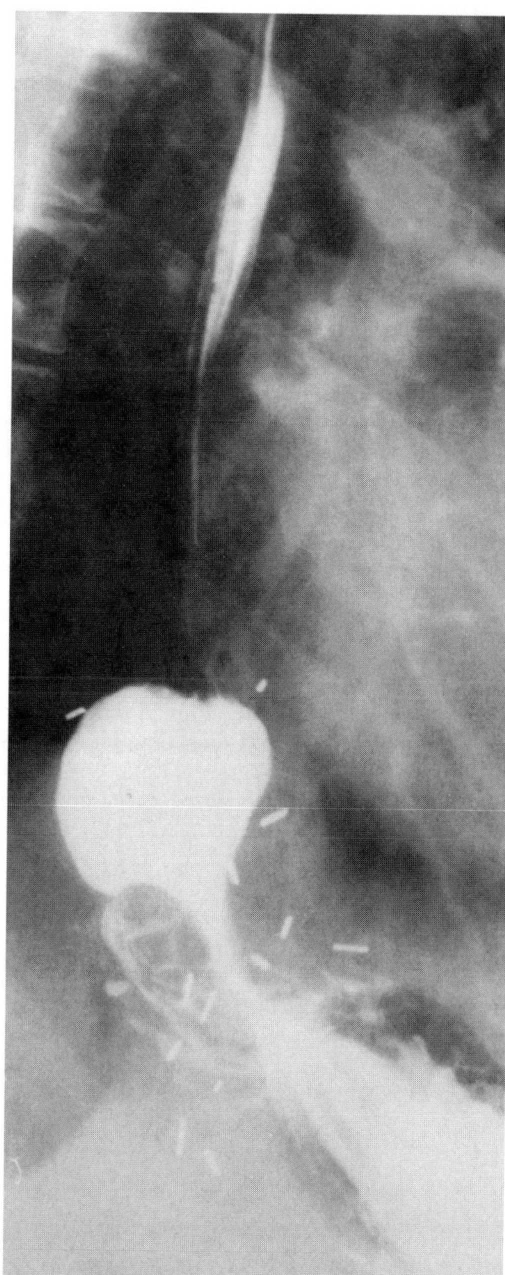

FIGURE 5–51 ■ Complication after hiatal hernia repair. The gastric portion of the wraparound has partially slipped, forming a recurrence of hiatal hernia.

Contrast examination is performed before oral feeding in the postoperative period. The study is focused on detection of leakage at the anastomotic site and gastric emptying. To demonstrate a small anastomotic leak, contrast medium must adequately fill the anastomotic site. This procedure may require placing the patient in the Trendelenburg position to pool the medium at the site of anastomosis. If the contrast agent does not empty into the small bowel, a delayed film of the thorax and upper abdomen is useful to assess the residual amount of contrast agent remaining in the stomach.

Although a water-soluble contrast esophagogram better defines the site of anastomotic leakage, CT is routinely used in assessing other complications, such as pleural extension and mediastinal abscess formation (Fig. 5–52). It also aids in planning management of these complications (Reichle et al, 1993). As with preoperative CT, the esophagus and stomach must be adequately distended with oral contrast medium, water, or air to avoid misinterpretation of a collapsed anastomosis or stomach as tumor recurrence. Postoperative changes include wall thickening; increased density of mediastinal fat caused by edema from surgery or radiation; fluid collections resulting from anastomotic leak or, rarely, thoracic duct injury; and effusions in pericardial and pleural spaces.

Follow-up barium examination is performed for tumor recurrence at the anastomotic site, usually prompted by obstructive symptoms. Recurrent tumor at the anastomosis takes the form of nodular narrowing (Fig. 5–53), whereas postoperative stricture is characteristically short and concentric (see Fig. 5–19). Comparison with the immediate postoperative barium study is useful when the radiologic features are not conclusive for distinction.

Tumor recurrence and distant metastasis are best evaluated with CT. Tumor recurrence presents as soft tissue masses in the mediastinum (Fig. 5–54) or as intramural nodular wall thickening of the stomach or esophagus at, or even distant from, the anastomosis. Distant metastasis occurs at sites similar to those described with the primary tumor.

Esophageal Bypass Surgery

Bypass provides an alternative food passage when the esophagus is completely obstructed by cancer or made dysfunctional by severe stricture or motor disorders. The stomach, small bowel, and colon have been used for this purpose.

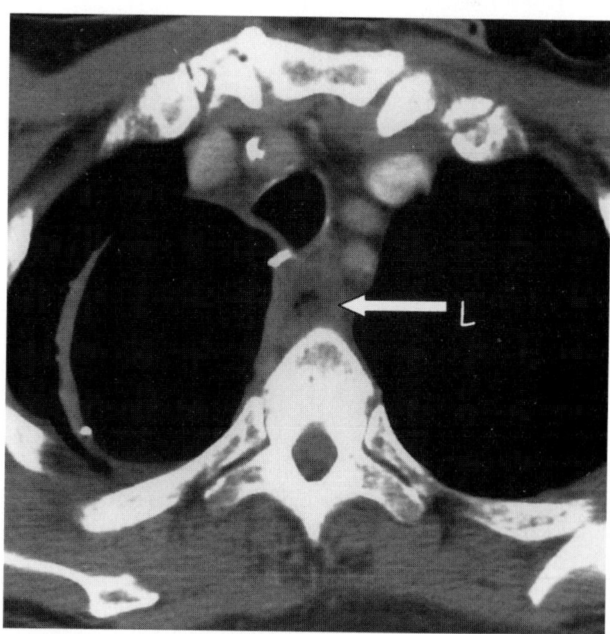

FIGURE 5–52 ■ CT scan of the upper mediastinum showing mediastinal abscess (*arrow*) in a patient who had undergone an Ivor Lewis procedure.

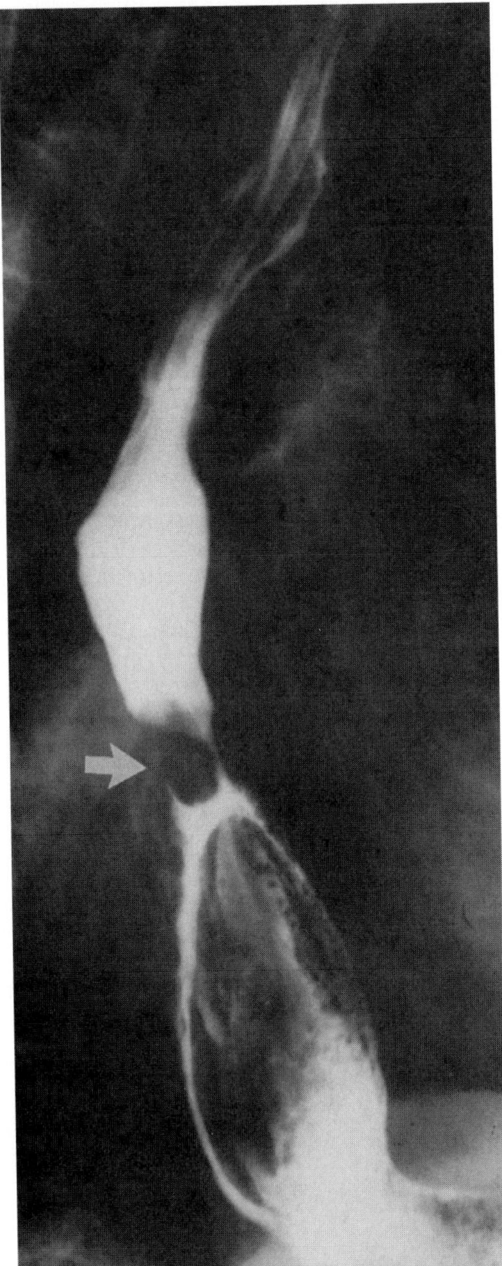

FIGURE 5–53 ■ Tumor recurrence at esophagogastrectomy. Note the length of the narrowing at the esophagogastrectomy (*arrow*) and the presence of mass effect on the proximal esophagus.

Gastric Tube

A conduit or gastric tube is constructed from the greater curvature of the stomach by separating a part of it from the remaining stomach. This tube is mobilized and brought superiorly into the thorax for anastomosis with the cervical esophagus. Two methods have been described for connecting the gastric tube to the cervical esophagus. In the *Heimlich reversed gastric tube*, the base is attached to the fundus and the antral end is brought up superiorly for anastomosis. In contrast, the *Beck bypass* has its base in the gastric antrum and its fundal end is elevated to the nose.

A gastric tube procedure is a simpler operation than colonic or jejunal interposition, and the blood supply of the gastric tube is better preserved. Postoperative study with contrast medium is performed to identify leakage at the anastomotic sites, most often in the neck. The staple line of the gastric tube may sometimes be seen.

Colonic Interposition

For severe peptic strictures, inoperable esophageal carcinomas, or severe neuromuscular disorders refractory to conventional treatment, colonic interposition represents a last resort to restore esophageal function. The diseased esophagus is replaced by a segment of the colon that acts as a conduit for food passage. The right, transverse, or left colon can be mobilized for interposition either in the posterior or, more often, anterior mediastinum (Fig. 5–55). A pyloroplasty is often performed to facilitate gastric emptying (Agha and Orringer, 1984).

A postoperative contrast study is performed to assess the integrity of the upper and lower anastomoses. Because the transit of contrast medium through the colonic segment is slow, the fluoroscopic table is tilted to expedite the study for the lower anastomosis. Postoperative leak occurs more frequently at the upper anastomosis and may lead to stricture at a later date (Larson et al, 1985). Such stricture is often resistant to treatment by dilatation. Ischemic changes in the interposed colon may lead to ulcerations, edema, and loss of haustral pattern.

Other complications include mediastinal or abdominal abscesses, which are best studied by CT. When appropriate, percutaneous drainage of the abscess may be performed, obviating a surgical intervention under general anesthesia. When the colonic segment is too long, delayed transit to the stomach may occur. More remote but less frequent complications are diverticulitis and small bowel obstruction.

Heller Myotomy

The Heller myotomy, the classic treatment of achalasia, consists of a longitudinal incision through the LES to 6 cm proximal above the cardia. Some surgeons incorporate an antireflux operation after a Heller myotomy to prevent reflux. Postoperative barium study shows no further hold-up at the GE junction, which may be transformed into an eccentric outpouching from bulging of the mucosa through the myotomy, above the diaphragm.

Sugiura Procedure

Originated in Japan, this is a two-part operation for devascularization of esophageal varices (Sugiura and Futagawa, 1973). The paraesophageal varices from the esophageal hiatus to the level of the left inferior pulmonary veins are ligated. Ligation is followed by transection of the esophagus at the level of the diaphragm. An abdominal devascularization is also performed with splenectomy, selective vagotomy, and pyloroplasty. The operation carries a lower incidence of encephalopathy and recurrent variceal bleeding compared with a portocaval shunt (Sugiura and Futagawa, 1973). Postoperative com-

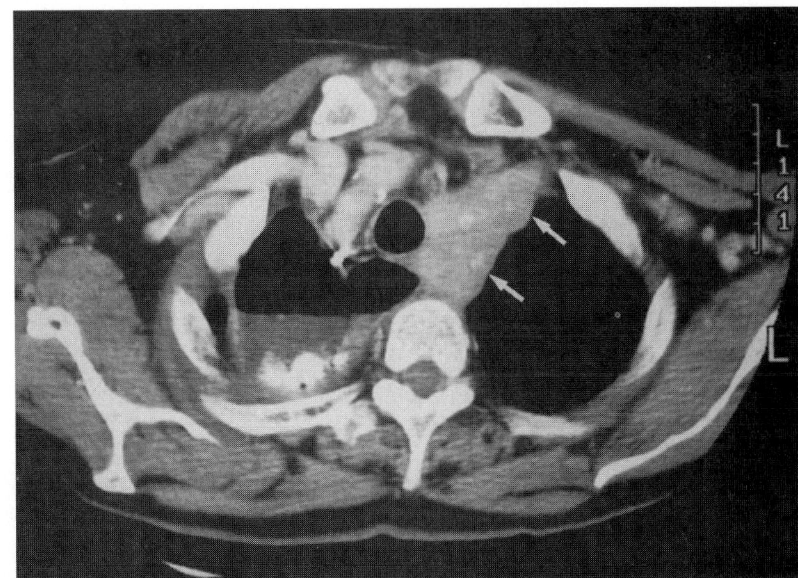

FIGURE 5–54 ■ Superior mediastinal lymphadenopathy resulting from tumor extension. CT scan shows marked nodal enlargement (*arrow*) encasing the major branches of the aorta. The patient had undergone esophagogastrectomy. Note the stomach pull-up in the right.

plications may result from suture breakdown leading to esophageal leakage and mediastinitis. The transection site may become narrowed after the operation (Koyama et al, 1980).

Nonsurgical Procedures

Dilatation

Pneumatic dilatation of the LES is effective in relieving dysphagia in patients with achalasia. The procedure is performed under fluoroscopy to ensure proper positioning of the balloon at the GE junction, which is identifiable by a notch in the distended balloon. A 1% to 4% incidence of esophageal perforation has been reported (Okike et al, 1979). Perforation is usually associated with chest pain or fever. However, because of heavy sedation, some patients may complain later, and Gastrografin or barium study may not reveal the perforation (Zegel et al, 1979). Should symptoms persist, another examination later is justified because leakage may become more apparent after subsidence of edema.

For peptic esophageal strictures, bougienage with different dilators or with a Grunzig-type balloon may be introduced perorally and under fluoroscopic control. Postdilatation contrast studies are routinely performed to exclude leakage, as in pneumatic dilatation.

Intubations

Plastic Tubes. Celestin tube placement across an obstructing esophageal cancer may bring about relief of dysphagia for patients with advanced cancer and limited life expectancy. A contrast study after insertion should show satisfactory tube position (bridging across the obstruction) with contrast medium flowing through the Celestin tube. The tube can be blocked by a food bolus (Fig. 5–56) and may migrate after insertion. An esophageal leak may occur early after insertion as a result of forceful insertion or late from erosion.

Metallic Stents. Since the early 1990s, self-expandable metallic stents have been gradually gaining acceptance by gastroenterologists and thoracic surgeons. Covered metallic stents are used for palliative treatment of bronchoesophageal (Fig. 5–57) or TE fistula due to malignancy (Raijman and Lynch, 1997) and for relieving malignant esophageal obstruction (Song et al, 1998).

In a small series of prospective randomized study of patients with unresectable esophageal cancers, the efficacy, ease of implantation, cost-effectiveness, patency, and complications between plastic and metallic stents were studied. The metallic Wallstent was found to be superior in terms of ease of implantation, long-term patency, and fewer complications (Sanyika et al, 1999). The study also found it more expensive to implant metallic rather than plastic stents.

Expandable metallic stents can be placed using either endoscopic or fluoroscopic control. Endoscopic insertion requires heavy sedation or even general anesthesia; fluoroscopic insertion requires heavy conscious sedation only, and patients can be discharged on the same day of insertion. The success rate of metallic stent insertion is high, and complications are few. Serious complications include stent occlusion, migration, and delayed massive bleeding (Song et al, 1994).

The advantages of metallic over plastic stents are convincing, and the only drawback appears to be the greater cost compared with the plastic tubes. Considering the improved morbidity and quality of life, the incremental cost appears to be generally accepted worthwhile.

COMMENTS AND CONTROVERSIES

This concise, comprehensive subchapter by Drs. Jaffer and Ho presents information in a unique fashion. The authors have outlined the modalities used for investigation of esophageal disease and then provide detailed and practical information for each surgical condition that may afflict the esophagus. These include common problems such as gastroesophageal reflux disease and its complications,

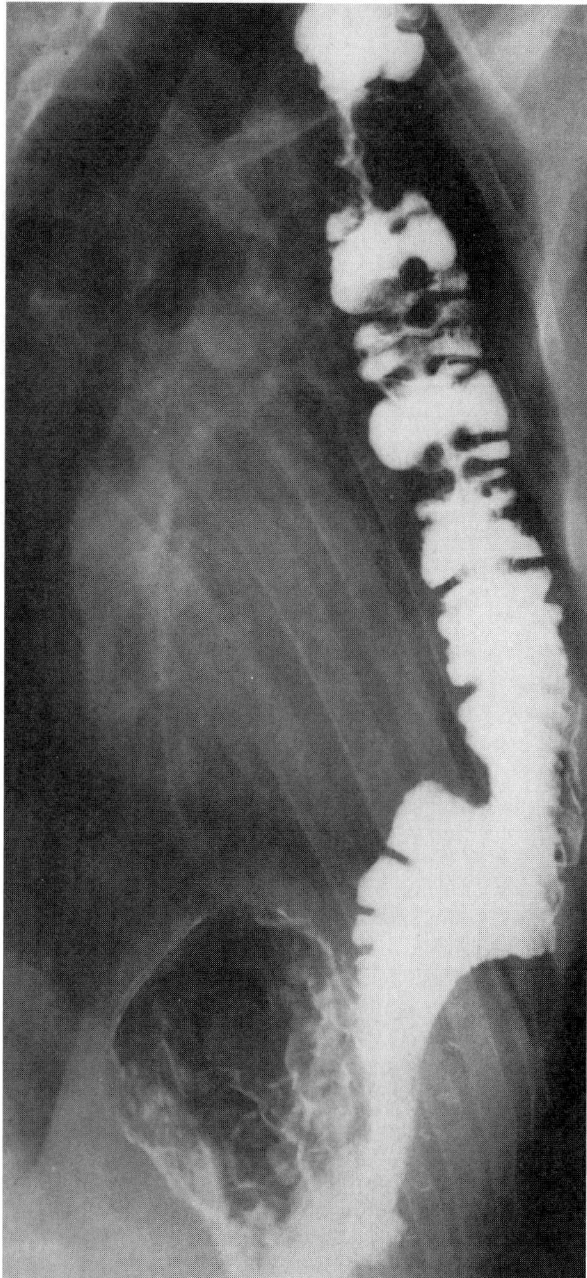

FIGURE 5–55 ■ Colonic interposition. A colonic segment is placed in the anterior mediastinum to replace the severe caustic stricture seen in Figure 5–13.

esophageal trauma, motor disorders of the esophagus, and neoplasia. On reviewing this subchapter, it becomes apparent that consultation between radiologist and surgeon is often critical to obtaining the best radiologic examination and interpretation. I have had the benefit of working closely with Dr. Ho at Toronto General Hospital for the past 20 years, and he has educated all our staff regarding the value of advance consultation with the radiologist when requesting imaging procedures, particularly with complex or unusual cases. It is equally instructive for the resident or staff to accompany the patient to the examination in many instances.

The authors have drawn attention to several important advances in the field that have developed since publication of the first edition of this book. Advances in digital technology have revolutionized film storage systems and image transmission. The Picture Archive Communication System (PACS), using cable modem or DSL phone lines, allows rapid transmission of images to monitor screens on nursing units, physician's offices, and so on. Images can be transmitted over the Internet, using Web-based language for consultation, anywhere in the world.

Major advances have occurred in the speed and resolution of CT scans such that a much larger field can be scanned during a single breath-hold: 1.25-mm cuts of the entire chest in 19 seconds and 5-mm cuts of the entire

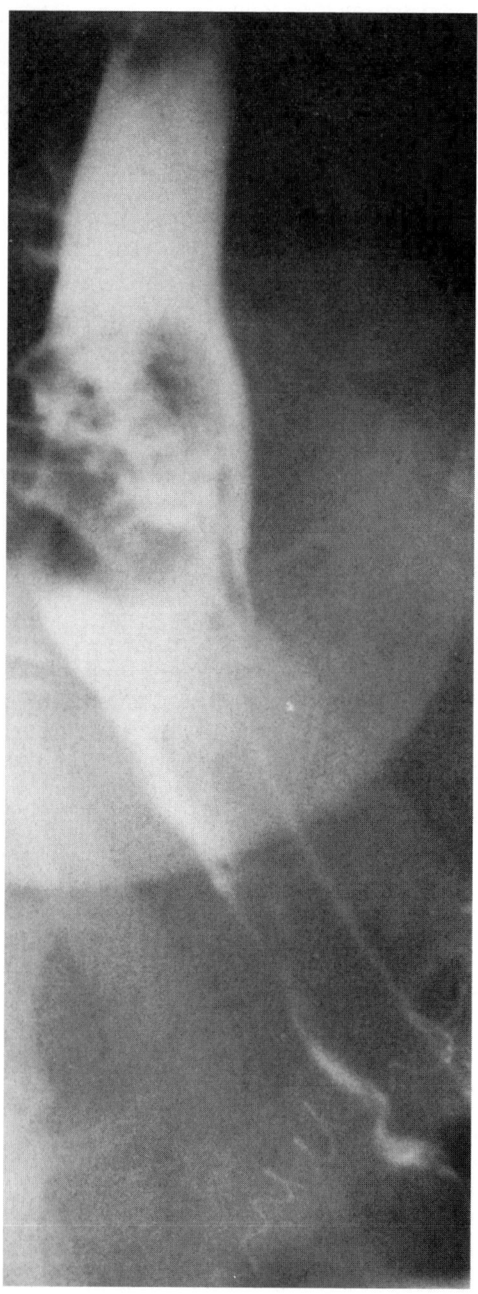

FIGURE 5–56 ■ Celestin tube insertion. Large filling defect proximal to the Celestin tube indicates obstruction by a large food bolus.

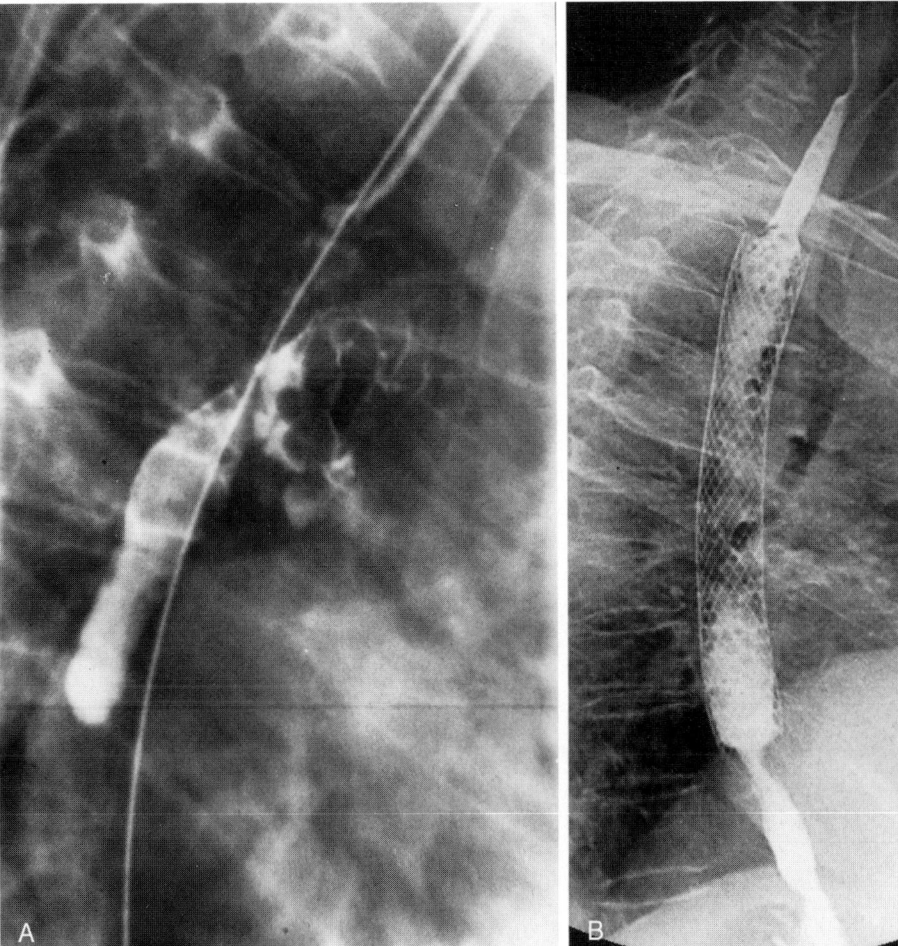

FIGURE 5–57 ■ *A*, Bronchoesophageal fistula caused by carcinoma of the esophagus. Contrast medium injected into esophagus just before stent insertion shows communication with the bronchial tree. *B*, Bronchoesophageal fistula after insertion of a covered Wallstent. Note complete obliteration of the fistula and passage of barium to the stomach without obstruction.

chest, abdomen, and pelvis in 15 seconds. For example, the improved resolution in chest scans now makes CT valuable in the diagnosis of pulmonary embolism.

During the past 5 years, the development of "CT fluoroscopy" has greatly facilitated CT-guided biopsy by radiologists, who now seem capable of obtaining a needle sample from tiny lesions in the most obscure and difficult locations.

F. G. P.

■ KEY REFERENCES

Levine S (ed): Radiology of the Esophagus. Philadelphia, WB Saunders, 1989.

This monograph on radiology of the esophagus gives a detailed account of examination technique and normal anatomy. It is an excellent text on double-contrast examination of the esophagus and includes subjects related to thoracic surgery (e.g., trauma and postoperative esophagus). Also included is a discussion of clinical management for most esophageal diseases. The book provides a broader perspective of esophageal disorders.

Meyers MA (ed): Neoplasms of the Digestive Tract: Imaging, Staging and Management. New York, Lippincott-Raven, 1998.

This publication on imaging, management, and treatment of tumors of the gastrointestinal tract is written by several experts in the different fields of imaging modalities. It is a complete book on all imaging modalities (contrast studies, EUS, CT, and MRI) for diagnosis and staging of tumors. Also included are current surgical and oncologic treatment options for gastrointestinal tumors that include the esophagus.

Stewart ET, Dodds WJ: Radiology of the esophagus. In Freeny PC, Stevenson GW (eds): Margulis and Berhennes' Alimentary Tract Radiology, 5th ed. St. Louis, Mosby–Year Book, 1994, p 192.

This comprehensive chapter on radiology of the esophagus includes examination techniques and has an excellent section on motor disorders of the esophagus. The different esophageal diseases are described, and excellent illustrations are provided.

■ REFERENCES

Adler RH: The lower esophagus lined by columnar epithelium: Its association with hiatal hernia, ulcer, stricture, and tumor. J Thorac Cardiovasc Surg 45:13, 1963.

Agha FP: The esophagus after endoscopic injection sclerotherapy: Acute and chronic changes. Radiology 49:639, 1984.

Agha FP, Orringer MB: Colonic interposition: Radiographic evaluation. Am J Roentgenol 142:703, 1984.

Allen RE, Thoshinsky MJ, Stallone RJ, Hunt TK: Corrosive injuries of the stomach. Arch Surg 100:409, 1970.

Ansari A: Mallory-Weiss syndrome revisited. Am J Gastroenterol 64:460, 1975.

Attah EB, Hajdu SI: Benign and malignant tumors of the esophagus at autopsy. J Thorac Cardiovasc Surg 5:396, 1968.

Becker CD, Barbier P, et al: CT evaluation of patients undergoing transhiatal esophagectomy for cancer. J Comput Assist Tomogr 4:114, 1986.

Benjamin SB, Gerhardt DC, Castell DO: High amplitude persistent esophageal contractions associated with chest pain and/or dysphagia. Gastroenterology 77:478, 1979.

Boal DKB, Newburger PE, Teele RL: Esophagitis induced by combined Adriamycin and radiation. Am J Roentgenol 132:567, 1979.

Bondi JL, Godwin DH, Garrett JM: Vigorous achalasia. Am J Gastroenterol 58:145, 1972.

Burrell M, Toffler R: Fibrovascular polyp of the esophagus. Am J Dig Dis 18:714, 1973.

Butterfield WC: Current hiatal hernia repairs: Similarities, mechanisms, and extended indications—an autopsy study. Surgery 69:910, 1961.

Campbell JB, Davis WS: Catheter technique for extrication of blunt esophageal foreign bodies. Radiology 108:438, 1979.

Cockerill EM, Miller RE, Chernish SM et al: Optimal visualization of esophageal varices. Am J Roentgenol 126:512, 1976.

Cohen S: Motor disorders of the esophagus. N Engl J Med 301:184, 1979.

Collis JL: An operation for hiatus hernia with short esophagus. J Thorac Cardiovasc Surg 34:768, 1954.

Coulamb M, Lebas JD, Sarrazin R, Geindre M: Computed tomography and esophageal carcinoma [French]. J Radiol 62:475, 1981.

Cynn WS, Chon H, Gureghian PA, Levin BL: Crohn's disease of the esophagus. Am J Roentgenol 125:359, 1975.

Dalinka MK, Smith EH, Wolfe RD, et al: Pharmacologically enhanced visualization of oesophageal varices by Pro-Banthine: A preliminary report. Radiology 102:281, 1972.

Danielson KS, Hunter TB: Barium capsules. Am J Roentgenol 144:414, 1985.

DeMeester TR, Johnson LF, Kent AH: Evaluation of current operations for the prevention of gastroesophageal reflux. Ann Surg 180:511, 1974.

Dodds WJ: Esophagus and oesophago-gastric region. In Margulis AR, Burhenne HJ (eds): Alimentary Tract Radiology, 3rd ed. St. Louis, CV Mosby, 1983, p 529.

Dodds WJ, Hogan WJ, Helm JF, Dent J: Pathogenesis of reflux esophagitis. Gastroenterology 81:376, 1981.

Dodds WJ, Hogan WJ, Miller WN: Reflux esophagitis. Dig Dis 21:49, 1976.

Dodds WJ, Stewart ET, Vlyman WJ: Appropriate contrast media for evaluation of esophageal disruption. Radiology 144:439, 1982.

Doyle GJ, Simpson W: Technical report: Prone scanning in the CT assessment of esophageal carcinoma. Clin Radiol 49:209–210, 1994.

Feigin DS, James AE, Stitik FP, et al: The radiological appearance of hiatal hernia repairs. Radiology 110:71, 1974.

Fernandes JP, Mascarenhas KJ, daCosta JC, Correia JP: Diffuse leiomyomatosis of the esophagus: A case report and review of the literature. Am J Dig Dis 20:684, 1975.

Ferrucci JF, Long JA: Radiologic treatment of esophageal food impaction using intravenous glucagon. Radiology 125:25, 1977.

Fitzgerald RH, Bartles DM, Parker EF: Tracheoesophageal fistulas secondary to carcinoma of the esophagus. J Thorac Cardiovasc Surg 82:194, 1981.

Foley MJ, Ghahremani GG, Rogers LF: Reappraisal of contrast media used to detect upper gastrointestinal perforations. Radiology 144:231, 1982.

Francine EA: Caustic damage of the gastrointestinal tract: Roentgen features. Am J Roentgenol 118:77, 1973.

Gerson DE, Lewicki AM: Intrathoracic stomach: When does it obstruct? Radiology 119:257, 1976.

Ghahremani GG, Turner MA, Port RB: Iatrogenic intubation injuries of the upper gastrointestinal tract in adults. Gastrointest Radiol 5:1, 1980.

Ghahremani GG, Gore RM, Breuer RI, Larson RH: Esophageal manifestations of Crohn's disease. Gastrointest Radiol 7:199, 1983.

Glanz I, Grunebaum M: The radiological approach to leiomyoma of the esophagus with a long-term follow-up. Clin Radiol 28:197, 1977.

Glick SN, Teplick SK, Levine MS, Caroline DF: Gastric cardia metastasis in esophageal carcinoma. Radiology 160:627, 1986.

Gloyna RE, Zornoza J, Goldstein HM: Primary ulcerative carcinoma of the esophagus. Am J Roentgenol 129:599, 1977.

Goldman LP, Weigert JM: Corrosive substance ingestion: A review. Am J Gastroenterol 79:85, 1973.

Goldstein HM, Rogers LF, Fletcher GH, Dodd GD: Radiological manifestations of radiation-induced injury to the normal upper gastrointestinal tract. Radiology 117:135, 1975.

Goldstein HM, Zornoza J, Hopens T: Intrinsic diseases of the adult esophagus: Benign and malignant tumors. Semin Roentgenol 16:183, 1981.

Gonzalez G: Diffuse esophageal spasm. Am J Roentgenol 117:251, 1973.

Goodner JT, Miller TR, Watson WL: Sarcoma of the esophagus. Am J Roentgenol 89:132, 1963.

Greco FA, Brereton HD, Kent H, et al: Adriamycin and enhanced radiation reaction in normal esophagus and skin. Ann Intern Med 85:294, 1976.

Green AE, Brogdon BG, Crow NE, Swearingen AG: Leiomyoma of the esophagus. Am J Roentgenol 82:1058, 1959.

Griff LC, Cooper J: Leiomyoma of the esophagus presenting as a mediastinal mass. Am J Roentgenol 101:472, 1967.

Hadley M, MacDonald AF: Epidermolysis bullosa. Br J Radiol 33:646, 1960.

Halber MD, Daffner RH, Thompson WM: CT of the oesophagus: I. Normal appearance. Am J Roentgenol 133:1047, 1979.

Halden WJ, Harnsberger JR, Mancuso AA: Computed tomography of esophageal varices after sclerotherapy. Am J Roentgenol 140:1195, 1983.

Halvorsen RA, Magruder-Habib K, Foster WL, et al: Esophageal cancer staging by CT: Long-term follow-up study. Radiology 161:147, 1986.

Halvorsen RA, Thompson WM: CT of esophageal neoplasms. Radiol Clin North Am 27:657, 1989.

Harle IA, Finley RJ, Belsheim M: Management of adenocarcinoma in a columnar-lined esophagus. Ann Thorac Surg 40:330, 1985.

Ho CS, Rodrigues PR: Lower esophageal strictures: Benign or malignant? J Can Assoc Radiol 31:110, 1980.

Inui K, Nakazawa S, Yoshino J, et al: Endoscopic MRI: Preliminary results of a new technique for visualization and staging of gastrointestinal tumors. Endoscopy 27:480, 1995.

James AE, Montali RJ, Chaffee V, et al: Barium or Gastrografin: Which contrast media for diagnosis of esophageal tear? Gastroenterology 68:1103, 1975.

Katada K, Kato K, et al: Guidance with real time CT fluoroscopy. Radiology 200:851, 1996.

Kirsh MM, Ritter F: Caustic ingestion and subsequent damage to the oropharyngeal and digestive passages. Ann Thorac Surg 21:74, 1976.

Knaver CM: Mallory-Weiss syndrome: Characterization of 75 Mallory-Weiss lacerations in 528 patients with upper gastrointestinal hemorrhage. Gastroenterology 71:5, 1976.

Koyama K, Tajagu Y, Ouchi K, Sato T: Results of esophageal transection for esophageal varices: Experience in 100 cases. Am J Surg 139:204, 1980.

Kulling D, Feldman DR, Kay CL, et al: Local staging of esophageal cancer using endoscopic magnetic resonance imaging: Prospective comparison with endoscopic ultrasound. Endoscopy 30:745, 1998.

Larson TC, Shuman LS, Libshitz HI, McMurtrey MJ: Complications of colonic interposition. Cancer 56:681, 1985.

Lawson TL, Dodds WJ, Shelf DJ: Carcinoma of the esophagus simulating varices. Am J Roentgenol 107:83, 1969.

Lehr L, Rupp N, Siewert JR: Assessment of resectability of esophageal cancer by computed tomography and magnetic resonance imaging. Surgery 103:344, 1988.

Leigh TF, Achord JL: Pharyngeal and esophageal perforations during instrumentation. Am J Roentgenol 91:757, 1964.

Lepke RA, Libshitz HI: Radiation-induced injury of the esophagus. Radiology 148:375, 1983.

Levine MS, Kressel HY, Caroline DF, et al: Barrett's esophagus: Reticular pattern of the mucosa. Radiology 147:663, 1983.

Levine MS, Kressel HI, Laufer I, et al: The tube esophagogram: A technique for obtaining a detailed double-contrast examination of the esophagus. Am J Roentgenol 142:711, 1974.

Levine S (ed): Radiology of the Esophagus. Philadelphia, WB Saunders, 1989.

Lindell MM, Hill CA, Libshitz HI: Esophageal cancer: Radiographic chest findings and their prognostic significance. Am J Roentgenol 133:461, 1979.

Livingstone EM, Skinner DB: Tumors of the esophagus. In Berk JE (ed): Gastroenterology. Philadelphia, WB Saunders, 1985, p 818.

Lolley D, Razzuk MA, Urschel HC: Giant fibrovascular polyp of the esophagus. Ann Thorac Surg 22:383, 1976.

Love L, Berkow AE: Trauma to the oesophagus. Gastrointest Radiol 2:305, 1978.

Lowman RM, Goldman R, Stern H: The roentgen aspects of intramural dissection of the esophagus. Radiology 95:379, 1969.

Lubbe WF, Cadogan ES, Kannemeyr AHR: Esophageal ulceration due to slow-release potassium in the presence of left atrial enlargement. N Z Med J 90:377, 1979.

Lyons AS, Garlock JH: Leiomyosarcoma of the esophagus: Report of the first successful resection. Surgery 29:281, 1951.

Mauro MA, Jaques PF, Swantkowski TM, et al: CT after uncomplicated esophageal sclerotherapy. Am J Roentgenol 147:57, 1986.

Meyers MA (ed): Neoplasms of the Digestive Tract: Imaging, Staging and Management. New York, Lippincott-Raven, 1998.

Meyers MA, Ghahremani GG: Complications of fiberoptic endoscopy: I. Esophagoscopy and gastroscopy. Radiology 115:293, 1975.

Moss AA, Schnyder P, Thoeni R, Margulls AR: Esophageal carcinoma: Therapy staging in computed tomography. Am J Roentgenol 136:1051, 1981.

Nandi P, Ong GB: Foreign bodies in the esophagus: Review of 2,394 cases. Br J Surg 65:5, 1978.

Neimark S, Rogers A: Chemical injury of the esophagus. In Berk JA (ed): Bockus Gastroenterology, 4th ed. Philadelphia, WB Saunders, 1985, p 769.

Okike N, Payne WS, Neufeld DM, et al: Esophagomyotomy versus forceful dilatation for achalasia of the esophagus: Results in 899 patients. Ann Thorac Surg 28:119, 1979.

Olsen AM, Schlegel JF: Motility disturbances caused by esophagitis. J Thorac Cardiovasc Surg 50:607, 1965.

Ott DJ, Chen YM, Wu WC, Gelfand DW: Endoscopic sensitivity in the detection of esophageal strictures. J Clin Gastroenterol 7:121, 1985.

Ott DJ, Dodds WJ, Wu WC, et al: Current status of radiology in evaluating for gastroesophageal reflux disease. J Clin Gastroenterol 4:365, 1982.

Ott DJ, Richter JE, Wu WC, et al: Radiologic and manometric correlation in "nutcracker esophagus." Am J Roentgenol 147:692, 1986.

Ott DJ, Wu WC, Gelfand DW: Reflux esophagitis revisited: Prospective analysis of radiologic accuracy. Gastrointest Radiol 6:1, 1981.

Ozawa S, Imai Y, Suwa T, Kitajima M: What's new in imaging? New magnetic resonance imaging of esophageal cancer using an endoluminal surface coil and antibody-coated magnetite particles. Recent Results Cancer Res 155:73, 2000.

Panaro VA, Leslie ES: Spontaneous rupture of the esophagus. Radiology 84:252, 1960.

Pearson FG, Langer B, Henderson RD: Gastroplasty and Belsey hiatus hernia repair: An operation for the management of peptic stricture with acquired short esophagus. J Thorac Cardiovasc Surg 61:50, 1971.

Phillips LG, Cunningham J: Oesophageal preparation. Radiol Clin North Am 22:607, 1984.

Picus D, Balfe DM, Koehler IE, et al: Computed tomography in the staging of oesophageal carcinoma. Radiology 146:433, 1983.

Plachta A: Benign tumors of the esophagus: Review of literature and report of 99 cases. Am J Gastroenterol 38:639, 1962.

Postlethwait RW: Surgery of the Esophagus, 2nd ed. Norwalk, CT, Appleton-Century-Crofts, 1986, pp 369–442.

Quint LE, Glazer GM, Orringer MB: CT and MR staging of tumors of the esophagus and gastroesophageal junction and detection of postoperative recurrence. In Freeny O, Stevenson G (eds): Margulis and Burhenne's Alimentary Tract Radiology, 5th ed. St. Louis, Mosby–Year Book, 1994.

Quint LE, Glazer GM, Orringer MB, Gross BH: Esophageal carcinoma: CT findings. Radiology 155:171, 1985.

Rafal RB, Markisz JA: Magnetic resonance imaging of an esophageal duplication cyst. Am J Gastroenterol 86:1809, 1991.

Raijman I, Lynch P: Coated expandable esophageal stents in the treatment of digestive-respiratory fistulas. Am J Gastroenterol 92:2188, 1997.

Reichle RL, Fishman EK, Nixon MA, et al: Evaluation of the postsurgical esophagus after partial esophagogastrectomy for esophageal cancer: Normal postoperative appearance and complications. Invest Radiol 8:247, 1993.

Rice BT, Spiegel PK, Dombrowski PJ: Acute esophageal food impaction treated by gas-forming agent. Radiology 146:299, 1983.

Rice TW, Boyce GA, Sivak MV, et al: Esophageal carcinoma: Esophageal ultrasound assessment of preoperative chemotherapy. Ann Thorac Surg 53:972, 1992.

Rice TW, Boyce GA, Sivak MV: Esophageal ultrasound and the preoperative staging of carcinoma of the esophagus. J Thorac Cardiovasc Surg 101:536, 1991.

Rubin SA, Winsett MZ, Diner WC: Intrathoracic gastric balloon: Radiographic recognition of esophageal perforation. Gastrointest Radiol 7:311, 1982.

Sanyika C, Corr P, Haffejee A: Palliative treatment of esophageal carcinoma—efficacy of plastic versus expandable stents. S Afr Med J 89:640, 1999.

Schatzki R, Hawes LE: The roentgenological appearance of extramucosal tumors of the esophagus: Analysis of intramural extramucosal lesions of the gastrointestinal tract in general. Am J Roentgenol 48:1, 1942.

Schung GE: Leiomyoma of the cardioesophageal junction. Arch Surg 65:342, 1952.

Seremetis MG, Lyons WS, DeGuzman VC, Peabody JW: Leiomyomata of the esophagus: An analysis of 838 cases. Cancer 38:2166, 1976.

Shaffer HA, Alford BA, deLange EE et al: Basket extraction of esophageal foreign bodies. Am J Roentgenol 147:1010, 1986.

Shay SS, Berendson RA, Johnson LF: Esophageal hematoma: Four new cases, a review, and proposed etiology. Dig Dis Sci 26:1019, 1981.

Simeone JF, Burrell M, Toffler R, Smith GJW: Aperistalsis and esophagitis. Radiology 123:9, 1977.

Skinner DB: Hernia (hiatal, traumatic, and congenital). In Berk JE (ed): Bockus Gastroenterology, 4th ed. Philadelphia, WB Saunders, 1985, p 705.

Skinner DB, Camp TF: Measurement of gastroesophageal reflux in the evaluation of hiatus hernia and chest pain in the fliers. Aerospace Med 8:846, 1967.

Somers S, Stevenson GW, Thomson G: Comparison of endoscopy and barium swallow with marshmallow in dysphagia. J Can Assoc Radiol 37:73, 1986.

Song HY, Do YS, Han YM, et al: Covered expandable esophageal metallic stent tubes: Experiences in 119 patients. Radiology 193:689, 1994.

Stannard MW: Corrosive esophagitis in children. Am J Dis Child 132:596, 1978.

Stein LA, Margulis AR: The spheroid sign: A new sign for accurate differentiation of intramural from extramural masses. Am J Roentgenol 123:420, 1975.

Steiner H, Lammer J, Hackl A: Lymphatic metastases to the esophagus. Gastrointest Radiol 9:1, 1984.

Stewart ET, Dodds WJ: Radiology of the esophagus. In Freeny PC, Stevenson GW (eds): Margulis and Berhennes' Alimentary Tract Radiology, 5th ed. St. Louis, Mosby–Year Book, 1994, p 192.

Stewart ET, Miller WN, Hogan WJ, Dodds WJ: Desirability of roentgen esophageal examination immediately after pneumatic dilatation for achalasia. Radiology 130:589, 1979.

Sugiura M, Futagawa S: A new technique for treating esophageal varices. J Thorac Cardiovasc Surg 66:677, 1973.

Takashima S, Takeuchi N, Shiozaki H, et al: Carcinoma of the esophagus: CT vs MR imaging in determining resectability. AJR Am J Roentgenol 156:297, 1991.

Teplick JG, Teplick SK, Ominsky RS, Haskin ME: Oesophagitis caused by oral medication. Radiology 134:23, 1980.

Thompson WM, Halvorsen RA, Foster WL, et al: Computed tomography for staging esophageal and gastroesophageal cancer: Reevaluation. Am J Roentgenol 141:951, 1983.

Thompson WM, Halvorsen RA Jr: Staging esophageal carcinoma II: CT and MRI. Semin Oncol 21:447, 1994.

Tio TL, Tytgat NJ: Endoscopic ultrasonography of normal and pathologic upper gastrointestinal wall structure: Comparison of studies in vivo and in vitro with histology. Scand J Gastroenterol 21(Suppl 123):27, 1986.

Tishler JM, Han SY, Helman CA: Esophageal involvement in epidermolysis bullosa dystrophica. Am J Roentgenol 141:1283, 1983.

Trenkner SW, Maglinte DDT, Lehman GA, et al: Esophageal food impaction: Treatment with glucagon. Radiology 149:401, 1983.

Tsuzuki T, Kakegawa T, Atimori M, et al: Giant leiomyoma of the esophagus and cardia weighing more than 1000 grams. Chest 60:396, 1971.
Vessal K, Montali RJ, Larson SM, et al: Evaluation of barium and Gastrografin as contrast media for the diagnosis of oesophageal ruptures or complications. Am J Roentgenol 123:307, 1975.
White CS, Templeton PA, Attar S: Esophageal perforation: CT findings. AJR Am J Roentgenol 160:767, 1993.
Zegel HG, Kressel HY, Levine GM, Rosato EF: Delayed perforation after dilatation for the treatment of achalasia. Gastrointest Radiol 4:219, 1979.
Ziegler K, Sanft C, Zeitz M, et al: Evaluation of endosonography in TN staging of esophageal cancer. Gut 32:16, 1991.

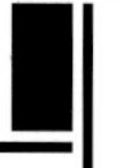

POSITRON EMISSION TOMOGRAPHY

Farrokh Dehdashti
Barry A. Siegel

BASIC PRINCIPLES

Over the past decade, positron emission tomography (PET) has evolved from a research tool into a highly useful clinical tool. PET is a functional imaging modality that uses biologically active compounds labeled with positron-emitting radionuclides and produces images reflecting biochemical and physiologic processes in normal and diseased tissues. Unlike anatomically based imaging techniques, which rely on structural changes for detection of disease, PET has the ability to detect changes in physiologic and biochemical processes associated with many disease processes. Because the biochemical and physiologic changes of disease often precede—and may be more specific than—the associated structural changes, PET offers the potential to detect disease before any structural abnormality is apparent and to exclude the presence of disease in an anatomically altered structure.

PET has several advantages when compared with conventional nuclear medicine imaging methods, such as planar scintigraphy and single-photon emission computed tomography (SPECT); these advantages are largely related to the mode of decay of the radionuclides used for PET. Positrons are the positively charged, antimatter equivalents of electrons. When a positron is emitted from an unstable nucleus, the particle travels a short distance before interacting with an electron through a process known as annihilation. Both the positron and the electron are converted into energy in the form of two 511-keV photons, emitted in nearly opposite directions (to achieve conservation of momentum). PET imaging is based on the nearly simultaneous detection of these two high-energy photons with opposed radiation detectors, operated in coincidence mode. When an event is registered by both detectors, the origin of the positron decay can be localized within the volume seen simultaneously by the two detectors.

In a modern PET scanner, there are typically several rings consisting of multiple radiation detectors, with each detector operating in coincidence with many detectors on the opposite side of the ring. The data obtained from the recording of a large number of coincident events can be reconstructed into a cross-sectional image by the same general method (filtered backprojection) utilized in computed tomography (CT). The intrinsic radiation detection efficiency of a PET scanner is much greater than that of a conventional gamma camera because positional information in PET is obtained without the need for the lead collimators used in conventional radionuclide imaging. In addition, the resolution of PET scanners is superior to that of the conventional gamma cameras. The typical resolution of PET images reconstructed for clinical studies is in the range of 5 to 10 mm (versus 15 to 20 mm for typical SPECT images) (Budinger, 1998).

One of the most important characteristics of PET is the ability to correct for attenuation of emitted photons within the patient and provide precise quantification of the regional distribution of radioactive tracer. This is typically done by the use of a ring source or rotating-rod source of a long-lived positron-emitting radionuclide (germanium 68 in equilibrium with gallium 68) surrounding the patient to obtain a transmission image of the subject. The ability to provide precise quantification has been one of the most important strengths of PET as a research tool for investigating regional physiology and biochemistry.

Although conventional nuclear medicine imaging also evaluates regional physiology and biochemistry, PET offers the ability to assess a wider variety of biologic processes. This is because many biologically relevant molecules can be radiolabeled with the radionuclides commonly used for PET:

- Oxygen 15 (O-15) ($T_{1/2}$ = 123 seconds)
- Nitrogen 13 (N-13) ($T_{1/2}$ = 10 minutes)
- Carbon 11 (C-11) ($T_{1/2}$ = 20 minutes)
- Fluorine 18 (F-18) ($T_{1/2}$ = 110 minutes)

The first three of these radionuclides can be substituted directly for the corresponding stable atoms, and fluorine-18 can be substituted for hydrogen or a hydroxyl group in many organic compounds.

Many different physiologic and biochemical parameters, including blood flow, blood volume, oxidative metabolism, glucose metabolism, protein synthesis, and various aspects of receptor function (Tewson and Krohn, 1998) can be assessed using a wide variety of radiopharmaceuticals prepared with these radionuclides.

F-18 FLUORODEOXYGLUCOSE

The current clinical applications of PET in oncology are chiefly focused on the assessment of glucose metabolism with the radiolabeled glucose analog 2-[F-18]fluoro-2-deoxy-D-glucose (FDG) (Som et al, 1980). Like glucose, FDG is taken up by cellular glucose transport mechanisms and undergoes phosphorylation by hexokinase to FDG-6-phosphate; unlike glucose-6-phosphate, however, FDG-6-phosphate is not further metabolized through glycolytic or glycogen-synthetic pathways, and, because it is charged, cannot diffuse out of the cell. In cells (including most malignant tumor cells) with little or no glucose-6-phosphatase activity to reconvert FDG-6-phosphate to FDG, the tracer thus becomes metabolically "trapped" within the cell. The cellular level of F-18 radioactivity is related to the rate of glucose uptake and utilization by the cell. The use of FDG as a tracer for tumor detection is based on the knowledge that most malignant tumors have a higher rate of glucose utilization compared with normal tissues (Warburg, 1930).

Although the mechanisms of increased tumor uptake of FDG are not fully understood, it has been shown that malignant transformation of several cell lines is associated with a more rapid rate of glucose transfer across cell membranes, increased activities of glycolytic enzymes, or both (Monakhov et al, 1978; Pauwels et al, 1998; Smith, 1998; Weber et al, 1984).

FDG-PET involves no specific patient preparation other than fasting for at least 4 hours, preferably overnight. This is because tumor uptake of FDG is competitively inhibited by hyperglycemia. Additionally, postprandial hyperinsulinemia further reduces tumor uptake of FDG because it results in preferential uptake of the tracer in skeletal muscle and adipose tissue. Satisfactory oncologic FDG imaging may not be possible in some patients with diabetes mellitus.

After intravenous (IV) injection of FDG, imaging is begun approximately 45 minutes later. Excreted activity in the urinary tract can obscure small adjacent tumor foci or can be confused with tumor. For abdominopelvic imaging, some PET facilities thus routinely use one or more of the following: IV hydration, IV administration of furosemide, and insertion of a Foley catheter into the urinary bladder. Muscle uptake of FDG, particularly in the cervical strap muscles and paravertebral muscles, is occasionally quite prominent and can obscure tumor foci. Uptake of FDG in the esophagus, stomach, small intestine, and colon is a highly variable, but normal, finding on PET images. The tracer is localized in the wall of the visualized gut rather than within the lumen. This normal uptake can usually be distinguished from disease by the distribution of activity.

FDG-PET IN ESOPHAGEAL CANCER

Staging

Accurate staging of esophageal cancer is extremely important, both for selecting appropriate therapy and for predicting prognosis. The anatomic imaging methods traditionally used for staging of esophageal cancer, such as CT and endoscopic ultrasonography (EUS), have significant limitations. As noted earlier, PET provides functional information that has been shown to be complementary to that provided by conventional imaging techniques. PET using FDG has been successfully used in evaluating many different malignant tumors (Rigo et al, 1996).

Although only limited data pertaining to the use of FDG-PET in esophageal cancer are available, the published reports suggest an important role of PET in this disease. The earliest report of the use of FDG-PET in esophageal cancer by Fukunaga and associates (1994) demonstrated that quantitative FDG-PET provides valuable prognostic information in patients with primary esophageal carcinoma. These investigators more recently demonstrated that patients with tumor standardized uptake values (SUVs) greater than 7.0 had worse prognosis than those with tumor SUVs less than 7.0 (Fukunaga et al, 1998). More recently, Luketich and colleagues (1999) reported that the extent of disease detected by FDG-PET at initial presentation is useful for stratifying survival. The 30-month survival of patients with PET evidence of local disease was longer (60% versus 20%) than patients with PET evidence of distant disease ($P = .01$).

Fukunaga and associates (1994) also found a good correlation between the hexokinase activity, assessed histochemically in the resected tumor, and the preoperative tumor FDG uptake. These investigators did not evaluate the use of FDG-PET in pretreatment staging of esophageal cancer. This has been the focus of several subsequent clinical studies, however, and FDG-PET is now used routinely in many institutions for staging of esophageal cancer (Block et al, 1997; Flamen et al, 2000b; Flanagan et al, 1997; Kole et al, 1998; Luketich et al, 1997, 1999; Meltzer et al, 2000; Rankin et al, 1998; Yeung et al, 1999).

Primary Tumor (T Stage)

The T stage is dependent on the depth of primary tumor infiltration into or through the esophageal wall. FDG-PET is a functional imaging technique with limited capability for delineation of normal anatomic structures and, therefore, cannot reliably determine the extent of tumor spread through the esophageal wall or tumor invasion of the adjacent structures. However, a heterogeneous pattern of FDG uptake at the primary site has been reported to be suggestive of local extension of the tumor.

Despite this inability of FDG-PET to accurately depict the local extent of the primary tumor, several reports have shown that FDG-PET has a somewhat higher sensitivity (95% to 100%) than CT (81% to 92%) for detection of primary esophageal cancer (Block et al, 1997; Flamen et al, 2000b; Flanagan et al, 1997; Kole et al, 1998; Luketich et al, 1997; McAteer, 1999; Rankin et al, 1998; Yeung et al, 1999). The intensity of FDG uptake in primary lesions, assessed by the semiquantitative SUV, is similar with squamous cell carcinomas and adenocarcinomas (Yeung et al, 1999). Primary tumors not detected by FDG-PET typically are very small T1 lesions. None of the currently used imaging techniques can reliably distinguish tumor from inflammatory disease or detect microscopic disease; therefore, histopathologic examination of the resected specimen remains the "gold standard" for T-stage determination.

Regional Lymph Node Metastases (N Stage)

The rich network of lymphatics along the entire esophagus and the absence of serosa contribute to the high prevalence of lymph node involvement in patients with esophageal cancer at initial presentation. Metastatic spread is commonly seen to regional and distant lymph nodes before widespread dissemination of esophageal cancer. Information about the lymph node status is essential for selection of therapy, and lymph node involvement implies a higher likelihood of systemic disease and a poor prognosis (Roth et al, 1993). The limited ability of conventional imaging methods to detect metastatic disease in normal-sized lymph nodes and to distinguish metastatic disease from reactive or inflammatory changes in enlarged lymph nodes often leads to inaccurate preoperative staging.

Several clinical studies indicate that FDG-PET can improve preoperative nodal staging of patients with esophageal cancer (Table 5–1). The results have been quite variable from institution to institution, however, likely reflecting differences in scanning technique. Overall, the results suggest that the sensitivity of FDG-PET is still too low for it to substitute for nodal sampling in patients otherwise considered to have resectable disease.

In our initial study of 36 patients at Washington University, we found that FDG-PET was more accurate than CT (76% versus 45%) in determining the presence or absence of lymph node involvement in the subset of 29 patients who underwent esophagectomy with curative intent (Flanagan et al, 1997). In a subsequent report of 58 patients, we confirmed that FDG-PET was more sensitive than CT for detection of regional nodal involvement in the subset of 35 patients who underwent complete resection of their esophageal cancer (Block et al, 1997). In 14 patients, there was no metastatic involvement of lymph nodes. PET was falsely positive in three of these patients, and CT was falsely positive in three different patients. Of the 21 patients with metastases to adjacent lymph nodes, PET showed metastases in 11 (52%) and CT was positive in only 6 (28%). Metastatic disease in lymph nodes not adjacent to the primary tumor was documented in 8 of the 21 patients. PET correctly identified the involved lymph nodes in 2 patients; however, CT did not identify disease in any of involved lymph nodes (Block et al, 1997).

Luketich and colleagues (1997) have reported that non–attenuation-corrected FDG-PET correctly detected locoregional disease in 9 of 20 patients (45%) with esophageal cancer. Kole and co-workers (1998) demonstrated that FDG-PET is superior to CT (sensitivity 92% versus 38%) in the detection of nodal involvement. One small study by Rankin and associates (1998) demonstrated that CT may be superior to FDG-PET in the detection of regional nodal disease located very close to the primary tumor. In the detection of metastatic disease involving the periesophageal lymph nodes, CT identified disease in four of eight (50%); however, PET was positive in one of these four patients and in two additional patients (3/8 [37%]). In the detection of left gastric nodes in patients with gastroesophageal cancer, CT identified disease in five of nine (55%) and PET in one of nine patients.

More recently, Yeung and associates (1999) reported relatively poor sensitivity for both FDG-PET (28%) and CT (25%) for detection of perigastric and periesophageal nodal metastases. Similar results have been reported by others (Flamen et al, 2000b) (see Table 5–1). In a study with a partial-ring PET scanner (ECAT ART), non–attenuation-corrected FDG-PET had a lower sensitivity than CT (41% versus 87%) but higher specificity (88% versus 43%) for detection of locoregional nodal involvement (Meltzer et al, 2000).

In all of these reports, the false-negative results with FDG-PET were mainly related to small tumor burden, typically lesions less than 1 cm in diameter. In addition, when involved lymph nodes were in close proximity to the primary tumor, the activity within the nodes often could not be distinguished from the intense activity in the primary tumor (Flanagan et al, 1997; Rankin et al,

TABLE 5–1 ■ **Accuracy of FDG-PET and CT for Detection of Regional Lymph Node Involvement in Esophageal Cancer**

		Sensitivity (%)		*Specificity (%)*	
Study (Year)	*No. of Patients Total/Surgery**	*PET*	*CT*	*PET*	*CT*
Flanagan et al (1997)	36/29	72	28	82	73
Block et al (1997)†	58/35	52	28	78	78
Luketich et al (1997)	35/21	45	NA	100	NA
Kole et al (1998)	26/22	92	38	88	100
Rankin et al (1998)	25/18	37	50	90	80
Yeung et al (1999)	67/NA	28	25	99	98
Flamen et al (2000b)	74/39	33	0	89	100
Meltzer et al (2000)	47/37	41	87	88	43

*Number of patients who underwent surgical resection of esophageal cancer.
†The PET and CT results of some of these patients have also been reported by Flanagan and coworkers (1997).
NA, information not reported.

1998). The false-positive results were typically related to inflammatory disease; it is well documented that FDG uptake can be seen in areas of active inflammation or infection, presumably reflecting the increased glucose utilization of leukocytes (Kubota et al, 1994). Evidence of granulomatous disease, such as the finding of nodal calcification on CT, may help to indicate that abnormal FDG uptake is more likely caused by inflammatory disease than lymph node metastasis.

Distant Metastatic Disease (M Stage)

Esophageal cancer typically metastasizes to distant lymph nodes, liver, and lung before metastasizing to other organs. Although, the reported experience is limited, FDG-PET has been quite useful in identifying unsuspected distant metastatic disease.

Several reports have shown that FDG-PET is more sensitive than conventional imaging techniques for demonstrating the true extent of metastatic disease. In 36 patients with esophageal cancer, we demonstrated that FDG-PET correctly identified distant metastases in five of seven patients (71%) with metastatic disease; CT did not detect metastases in any of these seven patients (Flanagan et al, 1997). All five metastatic foci detected by PET were in supraclavicular lymph nodes and were confirmed by biopsy. Metastatic disease not detected by PET was discovered at laparotomy in the remaining two patients, with demonstration of a small hepatic lesion and a small pancreatic lesion, respectively.

In a later report, we confirmed that FDG-PET was superior to CT (sensitivity of 100% versus 29%) in detection of unsuspected distant metastatic disease (Block et al, 1997). FDG-PET correctly identified all 17 patients with distant metastatic disease, whereas CT detected metastases in only 5 of these patients. In 11 of the 17 patients, metastatic disease was confirmed by minimally invasive procedures, such as percutaneous biopsy or mediastinoscopy.

Similarly, Luketich and colleagues (1997), in a study of 35 patients with esophageal cancer, demonstrated that non–attenuation-corrected FDG-PET correctly identified metastatic disease in seven of eight patients (88%) with distant disease. A 2-mm hepatic lesion was missed by FDG-PET in the remaining patient. FDG-PET facilitated treatment planning in up to 20% of patients by demonstrating unsuspected distant metastatic disease.

Kole and associates (1998) also demonstrated the superiority of FDG-PET over CT in the detection of distant metastatic disease (eight patients versus five patients). Rankin and coworkers (1998) reported that FDG-PET demonstrated distant disease not detected by CT in seven patients. In their study, both CT and FDG-PET detected distant disease in liver (same patients [n = 3] and different patients [n = 1]) and peritoneum.

Yeung and associates (1999) reported that FDG-PET disclosed distant metastases not seen on CT in 20% of their patients. The FDG-PET results led to a change in management in 14% of patients.

In a prospective study of 91 patients (100 PET scans) with esophageal cancer, Luketich and colleagues (1999) demonstrated that non–attenuation-corrected FDG-PET has higher sensitivity (69% versus 46%) and specificity (93% versus 74%) than CT for detection of distant metastatic disease. Similar results have been reported by others (Flamen et al, 2000b; Meltzer et al, 2000).

One of the important uses of FDG-PET in patients with esophageal cancer is identifying sites of local or distant metastatic disease that can be confirmed with a minimally invasive surgical procedure (Fig. 5–58) (Block et al, 1997; Flanagan et al, 1997; Luketich et al, 1997, 1998, 1999). As a result, both the cost and the morbidity of unnecessary extensive surgical interventions can be avoided.

Assessment of Response to Therapy

Although surgery is the mainstay of treatment of esophageal cancer, the long-term outcome with surgery alone is dismal. Regional or systemic recurrences are common

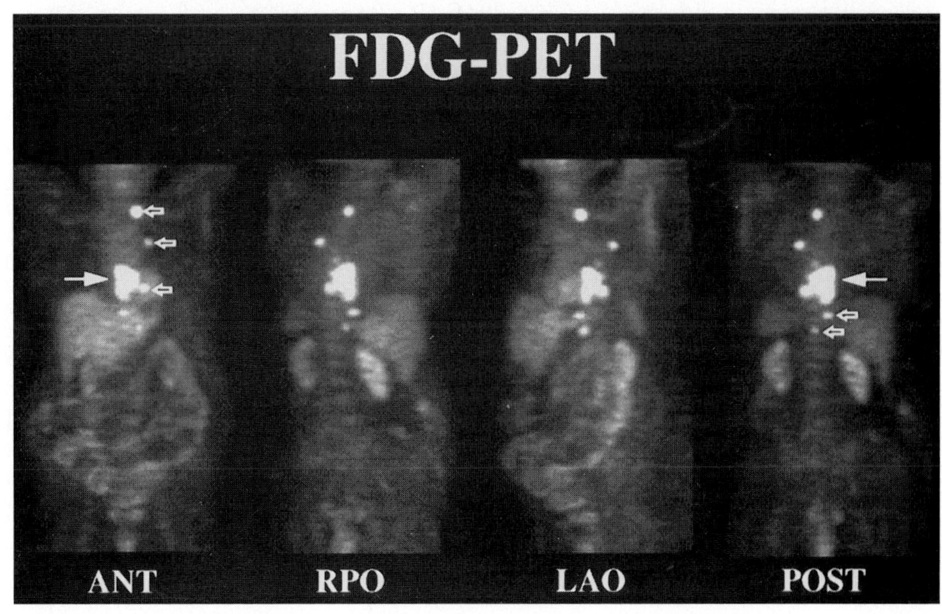

FIGURE 5–58 ■ Use of FDG-PET for staging of esophageal cancer. Anterior (ANT), right posterior oblique (RPO), left anterior oblique (LAO), and posterior (POST) reprojection images of the torso demonstrate markedly increased accumulation of FDG within a large lobulated distal esophageal cancer *(solid arrow)*. Markedly increased accumulation of FDG also is seen in multiple lymph node metastases, including supraclavicular, para-aortic, periesophageal, gastrohepatic, and celiac nodes *(open arrows)*. The diagnosis of metastatic disease was confirmed by biopsy of the left supraclavicular lymph node.

after surgical resection alone. There is thus considerable effort devoted to developing multimodality therapeutic approaches, combining surgery with neoadjuvant or adjuvant chemotherapy, radiation therapy, or both. Patients with unresectable disease are treated with definitive chemotherapy and radiation therapy (or combination therapy).

The degree of response after chemotherapy and radiation therapy is a strong predictor of long-term survival (Thomas, 1997). Patients with complete response to chemotherapy and radiation therapy have longer survival than those with partial or no response. Reliable assessment of the effectiveness of therapy often is not possible with conventional imaging techniques. A delay of several weeks after completion of therapy is typically required to determine its effectiveness. Disease progression is often detected at a time when further therapy cannot effectively eradicate the disease. Therefore, the ability to monitor response to therapy early during treatment would be very important. If nonresponders can be distinguished from responders early after institution of therapy, more aggressive treatment could be substituted in the patients who are not likely to respond to standard therapy. Additionally, the morbidity of treatment destined to fail could be avoided.

FDG-PET can be used to monitor the effects of therapy in several different types of cancer. With effective therapy, FDG uptake in tumors declines rapidly (Fig. 5–59); with

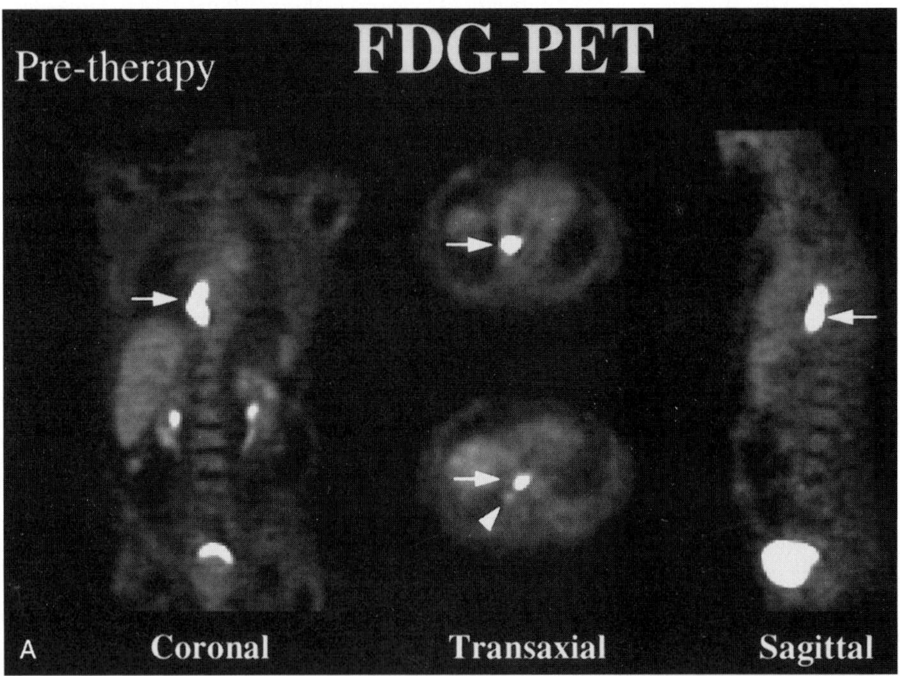

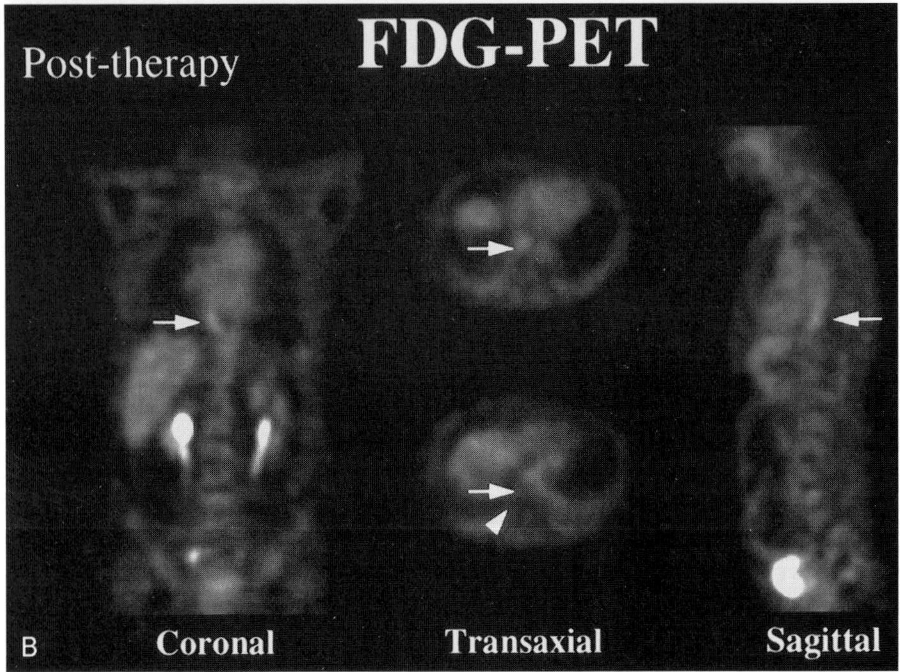

FIGURE 5–59 ■ Use of FDG-PET for evaluation of response to therapy: *A*, Coronal, transaxial, and sagittal FDG-PET images obtained before treatment demonstrate markedly increased FDG accumulation in the distal esophageal cancer *(arrow)*. Moderately increased accumulation of FDG also is seen in a para-aortic lymph node *(arrowhead)*. *B*, After chemoradiation, similar images show almost complete resolution of the increased activity previously noted in the primary esophageal cancer *(arrow)* and in the lymph node metastasis *(arrowhead)*. Esophagectomy revealed no viable tumor cells.

ineffective treatment, FDG uptake does not decline as much or can increase (Wahl et al, 1993). Changes in FDG uptake occur earlier than do corresponding changes on CT.

Couper and coworkers (1998) reported findings in 13 patients with esophageal or gastric cancer who underwent FDG-PET before and after two to three cycles of neoadjuvant chemotherapy. Six of these patients showed a greater than 30% decline in tumor FDG uptake and subsequently experienced improvement in their symptoms. CT changes suggestive of partial response were seen in only four of these six patients. Five patients showed a reduction in tumor FDG uptake of up to 30%; three of these patients experienced improvement in dysphasia, but none had CT evidence of response. The remaining two patients who demonstrated increases in tumor FDG uptake during treatment had no clinical or radiologic evidence of response. Clinical follow-up in the six patients who underwent surgical resection of their tumors after chemotherapy revealed that the patients with increasing tumor FDG uptake had the shortest survival. Two patients with 36% and 54% reductions in FDG uptake within their tumors after therapy were alive and disease free at 24 and 15 months, respectively.

This study demonstrated that FDG-PET has the potential to assess treatment effectiveness shortly after initiation of therapy. Moreover, it appears that the magnitude of the change in tumor FDG uptake after therapy may have prognostic significance in patients with esophageal cancer. Similar preliminary results have been reported by Weber and associates (1999). Further studies are needed to fully define the use of FDG-PET in assessment of response to therapy.

Recurrent Disease

Flamen and colleagues (2000a) studied the use of FDG-PET in restaging of suspected recurrent esophageal cancer after initial curative resection in 41 patients, 33 of whom were shown to have recurrent disease. By comparison with conventional imaging (CT and EUS), FDG-PET provided additional information in 11 of the 41 patients (27%); PET correctly detected recurrent disease in 5 patients with equivocal or negative conventional imaging results and upstaged disease in 5 additional patients (local recurrence to metastatic disease). In an additional patient with equivocal conventional imaging, PET correctly excluded recurrent disease.

OTHER RADIOPHARMACEUTICALS

Several other radiopharmaceuticals have shown promise as agents for detection or biologic characterization of malignant tumors, including:

- Tracers for evaluation of amino acid metabolism and protein synthesis (C-11 methionine) (Reinhardt et al, 1997)
- DNA synthesis (C-11 thymidine) (Shields et al, 1998)
- Tumor hypoxia (F-18 fluoromisonidazole) (Koh et al, 1995)
- Receptor expression (F-18 fluoroestradiol) (Dehdashti et al, 1995)

These agents have not been studied in patients with esophageal cancer. There has been interest in the use of C-11 choline for tumor imaging (Hara et al, 1998); its uptake into cells presumably reflects its incorporation into phosphatidylcholine, a cell membrane constituent, and its increased uptake in tumor cells is thought to be related to their more rapid rate of duplication. Kobori and coworkers (1999) have reported that PET with C-11 choline is more effective than FDG-PET in detecting mediastinal lymph node metastases of esophageal cancer.

■ *REFERENCES*

Block MI, Sundaresan SR, Patterson GA, et al: Improvement in staging of esophageal cancer with the addition of positron emission tomography. Ann Thorac Surg 64:770–777, 1997.

Budinger TF: PET instrumentation: What are the limits? Semin Nucl Med 28:247–267, 1998.

Couper GW, McAteer D, Wallis F, et al: Detection of response to chemotherapy using positron emission tomography in patients with oesophageal and gastric cancer. Br J Surg 85:1403–1406, 1998.

Dehdashti F, Mortimer JE, Siegel BA, et al: Positron tomographic assessment of estrogen receptors in breast cancer: Comparison with FDG-PET and in vitro receptor assays. J Nucl Med 36:1766–1774, 1995.

Flamen P, Lerut A, Van Cutsem E, et al: The utility of positron emission tomography for the diagnosis and staging of recurrent esophageal carcinoma. J Thorac Cardiovasc Surg 120:1085–1092, 2000a.

Flamen P, Lerut A, Van Cutsem E, et al: Utility of positron emission tomography for the staging of patients with potentially operable esophageal carcinoma. J Clin Oncol 18:3202–3210, 2000b.

Flanagan FL, Dehdashti F, Siegel BA, et al: Staging of esophageal cancer with FDG-PET. AJR Am J Roentgenol 168:417–424, 1997.

Fukunaga T, Enomoto K, Okazumi S, et al: Analysis of glucose metabolism in patients with esophageal cancer by PET: Estimation of hexokinase activity in the tumor and usefulness for clinical assessment using FDG. Nippon Geka Gakka Zasshi 95:317–325, 1994.

Fukunaga T, Okazumi S, Koide Y, et al: Evaluation of esophageal cancers using fluorine-18-fluorodeoxyglucose PET. J Nucl Med 39:1002–1007, 1998.

Hara T, Kosaka N, Kishi H: PET imaging of prostate cancer using carbon-11-choline. J Nucl Med 39:990–995, 1998.

Kobori O, Kirihara Y, Kosaka N, Hara T: Positron emission tomography of esophageal carcinoma using ^{11}C-choline and ^{18}F-fluorodeoxyglucose: A novel method of preoperative lymph node staging. Cancer 86:1638–1648, 1999.

Koh WJ, Bergman KS, Rasey JS, et al: Evaluation of oxygenation status during fractionated radiotherapy in human non–small cell lung cancers using [F-18]fluoromisonidazole positron emission tomography. Int J Radiot Oncol Biol Phys 33:391–398, 1995.

Kole AC, Plukker JT, Nieweg OE, et al: Positron emission tomography for staging oesophageal and gastroesophageal malignancy. Br J Cancer 74:521–527, 1998.

Kubota R, Kubota K, Yamada S, et al: Microautoradiographic study for the differentiation of intratumoral macrophages, granulation tissues and cancer cells by the dynamics of fluorine-18–fluorodeoxyglucose uptake. J Nucl Med 35:104–112, 1994.

Luketich JD, Friedman DM, Weigel TL, et al: Evaluation of distant metastases in esophageal cancer: 100 consecutive positron emission tomography scans. Ann Thorac Surg 68:1133–1137, 1999.

Luketich JD, Schauer PR, Meltzer CC, et al: Role of positron emission tomography in staging esophageal cancer. Ann Thorac Surg 64:770–777, 1997.

Luketich JD, Schauer P, Urso K, et al: Future directions in esophageal cancer. Chest 113:120S–122S, 1998.

McAteer D, Wallis F, Cooper G, et al: Evaluation of ^{18}F-FDG positron emission tomography in gastric and oesophageal carcinoma. Br J Radiol 72:525–529, 1999.

Meltzer CC, Luketich JD, Friedman D, et al: Whole-body FDG positron emission tomographic imaging for staging esophageal cancer. Comparison with computed tomography. Clin Nucl Med 25:882–887, 2000.

Monakhov NK, Neisfadt EL, Shavlovskii MM, et al: Physiochemical properties and isoenzyme composition of hexokinase from normal and malignant human tissue. J Natl Cancer Inst 61:27–34, 1978.

Pauwels EKJ, McReady VR, Stoot JHMB, et al: The mechanism of accumulation of tumour-localising radiopharmaceuticals. Eur J Nucl Med 25:277–305, 1998.

Rankin SC, Taylor H, Cook GJR, et al: Computed tomography and positron emission tomography in the preoperative staging of oesophageal carcinoma. Clin Radiol 53:659–665, 1998.

Reinhardt MJ, Kubota K, Yamada S, et al: Assessment of cancer recurrence in residual tumors after fractionated radiotherapy: A comparison of fluorodeoxyglucose, L-methionine and thymidine. J Nucl Med 38:280–287, 1997.

Rigo P, Paulus P, Kaschten BJ, et al: Oncological applications of positron emission tomography with fluorine-18 fluorodeoxyglucose. Eur J Nucl Med 23:1641–1674, 1996.

Roth JA, Putnam JB Jr, Rich TA, Forastiere AA: Cancer of the esophagus. In Devita VT Jr, Hellman S, Rosenberg SA (eds): Cancer: Principles and Practice of Oncology, 5th ed. Philadelphia, JB Lippincott, 1997, pp 980–1021.

Shields AF, Mankoff DA, Link JM, et al: [C-11]thymidine and FDG to measure therapy response. J Nucl Med 39:1757-1762, 1998.

Smith TAD: FDG uptake, tumour characteristics, and response to therapy: A review. Nucl Med Commun 19:97–105, 1998.

Som P, Atkins HL, Bandoypadhyay D, et al: A fluorinated glucose analog, 2-fluoro-2-deoxy-D-glucose (F-18): Nontoxic tracer for rapid tumor detection. J Nucl Med 21:670–675, 1980.

Tewson TJ, Krohn KA: PET radiopharmaceuticals: State-of-the-art and future prospects. Semin Nucl Med 28:221–234, 1998.

Thomas CR Jr: Biology of esophageal cancer and the role of combined modality therapy. Surg Clin North Am 77:1139–1167, 1997.

Wahl RL, Zasadny KR, Helvie MA, et al: Metabolic monitoring of breast cancer chemohormonotherapy using positron emission tomography: Initial evaluation. J Clin Oncol 11:2101–2111, 1993.

Warburg O: The Metabolism of Tumors. London, Arnold Constable, 1930, pp 75–327.

Weber MJ, Nakamura KD, Salter DW: Molecular events leading to enhanced glucose transport in Rous sarcoma virus–transformed cells. Fed Proc 43:2246–2250, 1984.

Weber WA, Ott K, Fink U, et al: FDG-PET for monitoring neo-adjuvant chemotherapy of adenocarcinomas of the distal esophagus. J Nucl Med 40:136p, 1999.

Yeung HWD, Macapinlac HA, Mazumdar M, et al: FDG-PET in esophageal cancer: Incremental value over CT. Clin Positron Imag 4:213–221, 1999.

ENDOSCOPIC ESOPHAGEAL ULTRASOUND

Thomas W. Rice
Gregory Zuccaro, Jr.

Endoscopic esophageal ultrasound (EUS) extends endoscopic examination of the esophagus beyond the epithelium into the esophageal wall and periesophageal tissues. The diagnostic capabilities of surface ultrasound are broadened by the endoscopic placement of ultrasound transducers adjacent to the esophageal mucosa. The marriage of esophagoscopy and ultrasound provides unprecedented imaging of this previously "silent" area. EUS is the most significant advancement in the diagnosis of esophageal disease since the introduction of flexible fiberoptic endoscopy.

FUNDAMENTALS OF ULTRASOUND

Vibration within a medium produces cyclic compression and rarefaction (expansion) of molecules within the medium. This results in a wave of energy transmitted through the medium. The number of cycles (compression and rarefaction) of a wave occurring in 1 second is the frequency and is measured in hertz (Hz). The frequency of sound waves audible to the human ear is between 20 and 20,000 Hz. Waves with higher frequencies (20,000+ Hz) are ultrasound waves. Frequencies used in medical ultrasound imaging range from 1 million to 20 million Hz (1 to 20 MHz).

Ultrasound waves are produced by the electrical excitation of a piezoelectric crystal. Application of a voltage across the crystal deforms it. Alternating electrical energy vibrates the crystal and produces ultrasound waves. If an ultrasound wave deforms the crystal, electrical energy is produced. The ability to convert electrical energy into sound energy and conversely to convert sound energy into electrical energy allows these crystals to function as both transmitters and receivers (i.e., as transducers). Because transducers are responsive to a limited range of frequencies, more than one transducer may be required for an ultrasound examination.

Speed of an ultrasound wave through tissue is defined by the relationship

$$V = (K/p)^{1/2}$$

where V is the velocity of the ultrasound wave, K is the bulk modulus of the tissue (a measure of stiffness), and p is the density of the tissue.

Resistance to passage of a wave through tissue is called the acoustic impedance (Z), which is defined by the relationship

$$\begin{aligned} Z &= p\,V \\ &= (p\,K)^{1/2} \end{aligned}$$

Ultrasound waves travel best through dense or elastic tissues. Energy is absorbed as an ultrasound wave passes through tissue. The amount of absorption is determined by tissue characteristics and the frequency of the ultrasound wave. The higher the frequency, the greater the absorption.

Diagnostic capabilities of ultrasound are determined by interactions that occur as an ultrasound wave encounters different tissues. As an ultrasound wave passes from one tissue to the next, a portion of the wave is transmitted into the new tissue and a portion is reflected. The reflected ultrasound wave is received by the transducer and processed, providing the diagnostic information of ultrasound. The difference in acoustic impedance between the two tissues and the angle at which the ultrasound wave enters the new medium (angle of incidence) determine the portion of the wave that is reflected and the portion that is transmitted.

When acoustic impedances are similar, the majority of the ultrasound wave is transmitted. Soft tissues have excellent transmission qualities; density and velocity vary only by 12% to 14% between different soft tissues. Because the acoustic impedance is the product of velocity and density, the product of these small changes results in a 22% difference in the acoustic impedance between fat and muscle (Kimmey and Martin, 1992). Useless bright echo images are produced when an ultrasound wave encounters air or bone. Air is very compressible and has a low density, whereas bone, although dense, has a low compressibility and a high reflectivity. These properties account for the poor transmission of ultrasound waves from tissue to air or tissue to bone. The amount of reflected ultrasound wave is also related to the angle of incidence; as the angle of incidence increases, less sound is reflected. In addition, ultrasound waves are bent as they travel from one tissue to the next. This process is refraction.

As an ultrasound wave passes through tissue, energy is lost; this process is called *attenuation*. Absorption, reflection, and refraction are major causes of attenuation. Some ultrasound energy is lost by the process of scattering *(diffusion)*. Diffusion occurs when a sound wave encounters heterogenous tissue. Tiny particles within tissue (such as fat in muscle) that are smaller than the ultrasound wavelength scatter the ultrasound wave. Attenuation increases as more tissues are encountered and as the wave travels farther from the source. Therefore, if the returning ultrasound wave is not processed, the same tissue would image differently, depending on its distance from the transducer. The intensity of the returning waves is amplified *(gain)* to ensure that distant waves are correctly represented. Attenuation increases as ultrasound frequency increases.

Resolution is the ability to discriminate different tissues with ultrasound waves. *Depth* or axial resolution is the ability to differentiate between two tissues along the path of the ultrasound wave. *Lateral resolution* is the ability to distinguish between adjacent tissues. Transducer characteristics and focus determine resolution. Higher frequencies allow for better resolution but decrease tissue penetration.

Pulse-echo technique is used in endoscopic ultrasound. Ultrasound waves are emitted for a brief period, followed by a listening period during which the reflected ultrasound waves are received. Returning sound waves are displayed so that brightness is proportional to the amplitude of the returning ultrasound waves. This is *B-mode* ultrasound. Because amplitude is presented in a range from white to gray to black, this ultrasound display is also called *gray-scale* ultrasound. Individual scans are shown at a rate such that the eye cannot detect single images (12 per second). This fast-frame display is real-time ultrasound and allows tissue to be studied temporally as well as spatially.

INSTRUMENTS AND TECHNIQUES

The forward oblique endoscopic view of EUS is inadequate for complete endoscopic inspection of the upper gastrointestinal tract. Therefore, every ultrasound study should be preceded by a standard flexible videoscopic upper gastrointestinal examination. This provides precise location and mucosal definition (including biopsy) of the esophageal lesion and guides the ultrasound examination. IV administration of a narcotic (e.g., meperidine) and a benzodiazepine (e.g., midazolam) usually provides adequate sedation. The ultrasound endoscope is passed under direct vision through the oropharynx and hypopharynx. Care must be exercised because the distal tip containing the transducer is rigid; however, the newest ultrasound endoscopes are less bulky and much easier to pass. For complete examination, the endoscope must be passed beyond the esophagus and into the stomach.

The principal instrument used in EUS is the radial mechanical ultrasound endoscope (Fig. 5–60). The ultrasound transducer is housed in the tip of the endoscope. It rotates at a speed of seven revolutions per minute to produce a 360-degree sector scan perpendicular to the transducer tip. Because the transducer is adjacent to the tissues to be examined, higher frequencies than those used in extracorporeal ultrasound can be employed.

In most models, two frequencies are available. One transducer images at 7.5 MHz, the other at 12 MHz. The 7.5-MHz transducer allows adequate study to a depth of 4 to 5 cm, the 12-MHz transducer to a depth of 1 to 2 cm. An acoustic interface between the transducer and the tissue being examined must be obtained to ensure good-quality images. This is most commonly accomplished by covering the tip of the endoscope with a latex balloon that can be filled with water to provide an excellent acoustic interface (see Fig. 5–60).

A less commonly employed technique, necessary in patients with latex allergies, is the rapid insufflation of the esophageal lumen with water. This provides an excellent (but transient) acoustic interface without the tissue compression that can occur with the latex balloon. Located behind the transducer is the endoscope tip. This endoscope provides a limited field of view in a forward oblique direction. A 2-mm suction channel is oriented at this oblique angle.

The control section contains deflection controls and air/water and suction valves identical to those on a standard endoscope (see Fig. 5–60). A water inflation/deflation system for the balloon is incorporated into the air/

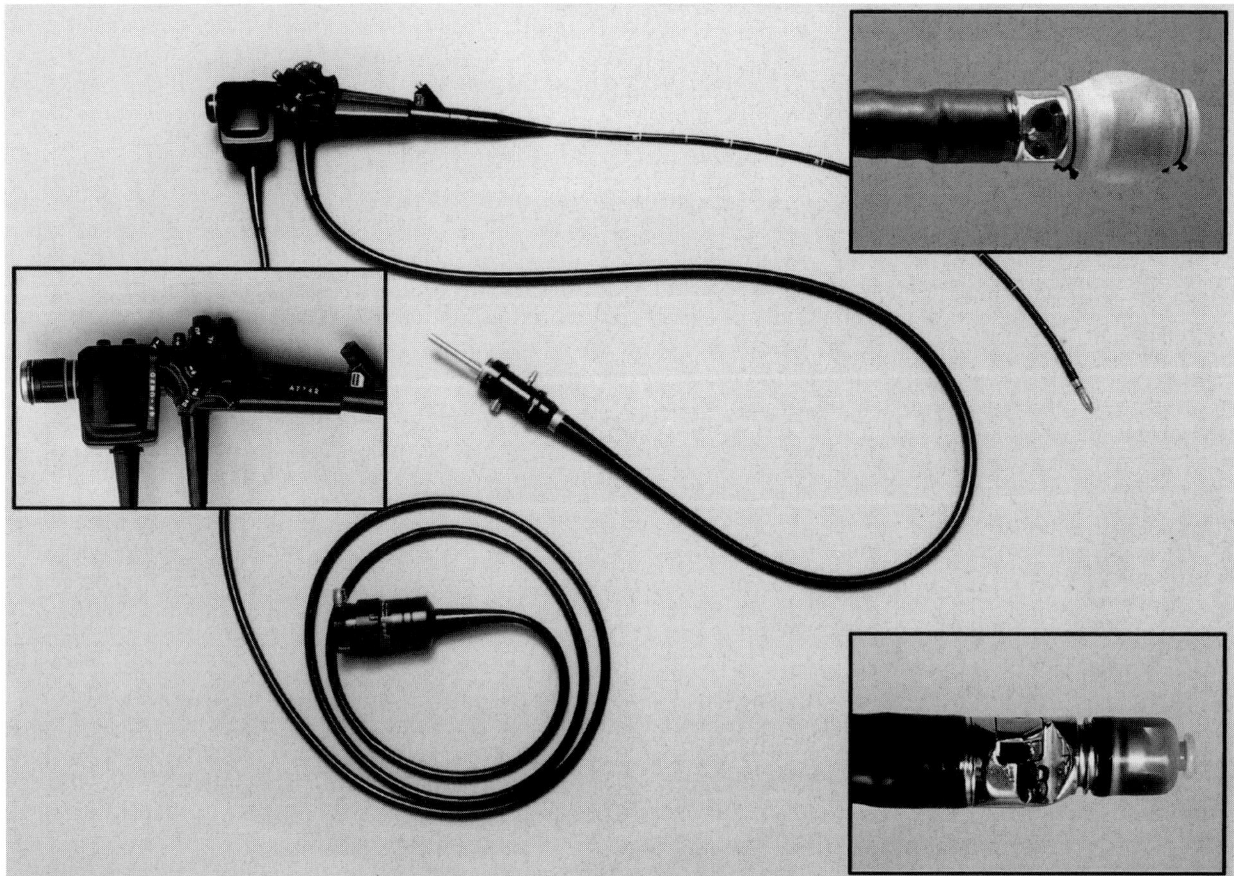

FIGURE 5–60 ■ The Olympus GF-UM20 ultrasound endoscope. *Top right inset,* Distal tip of the ultrasound endoscope with the water-inflated contact balloon. *Bottom right inset,* Uncovered distal tip. *Left inset,* Control section and drive motor.

water and suction valve mechanisms. The motor and drive mechanism, which rotates the ultrasound transducer, are housed in the control section. Current ultrasound endoscopes are totally immersible.

The radial mechanical blind probe (Fig. 5–61) is available for evaluation of esophageal strictures. This echoendoscope provides images similar to larger diameter radial mechanical echoendoscopes but no endoscopic optical capabilities. It is under 8 mm in diameter. Miniature ultrasound catheter probes (see Fig. 5–61) can be passed through the biopsy channel of a therapeutic esophagoscope and advanced through strictures. These 20-MHz probes can accurately image the esophageal wall; however, their poor depth of penetration prohibits accurate assessment of periesophageal tissue and lymph node status (Binmoeller et al, 1995; Hunerbein et al, 1998; McLoughlin et al, 1995; Menzel et al, 1999).

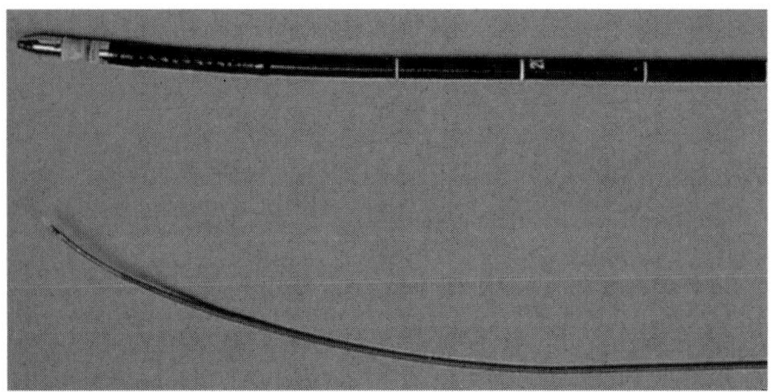

FIGURE 5–61 ■ The 8-mm radial mechanical blind probe and miniature ultrasound probe.

These instruments are used in conjunction with an image processor (Fig. 5–62). The controls of the image processor allow adjustment of gain, contrast, and sensitivity time control that regulates the strength of the returning echo. On-screen calibration and labeling can be done with the image processor. The image may be displayed on a video monitor or stored in a computer, on videotape, or on instant film. The image processor has been refined and miniaturized with successive generations of endoscopic ultrasound equipment. Current models are rack-mounted and weigh about 80 pounds.

In contrast to the radial mechanical scanner, the curvilinear electronic echoendoscope (Fig. 5–63) produces a field slightly over 100 degrees in an oblique forward direction. It uses transducers with 5- or 7.5-MHz scanning frequencies, allowing a 5- to 10-cm depth of penetration. Advantages include a system that provides color Doppler and direct visualization of cytology needles passed into and beyond the esophageal wall.

Radial mechanical and electronic linear systems have increased both accuracy and complexity of EUS. For diagnostic studies, the radial mechanical scanner is preferable because of its 360-degree range. It is the reason this echoendoscope system remains the "workhorse" of

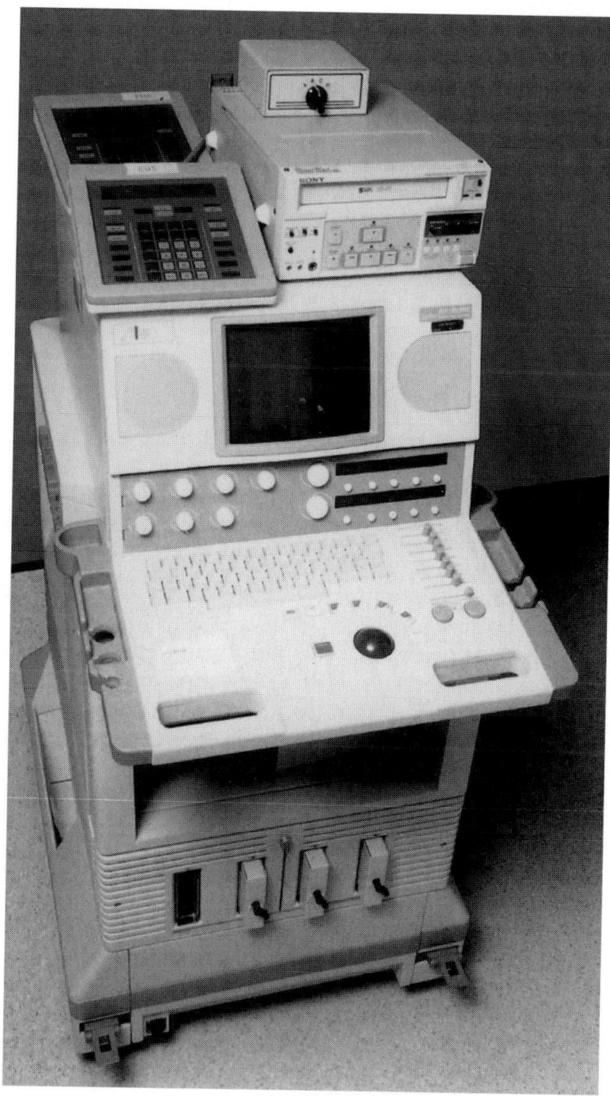

FIGURE 5–62 ■ The Olympus EU-M20 image processor is rack-mounted in a standard cart, which includes the essential endoscopic equipment. The keyboard can be used to mark and measure ultrasound findings.

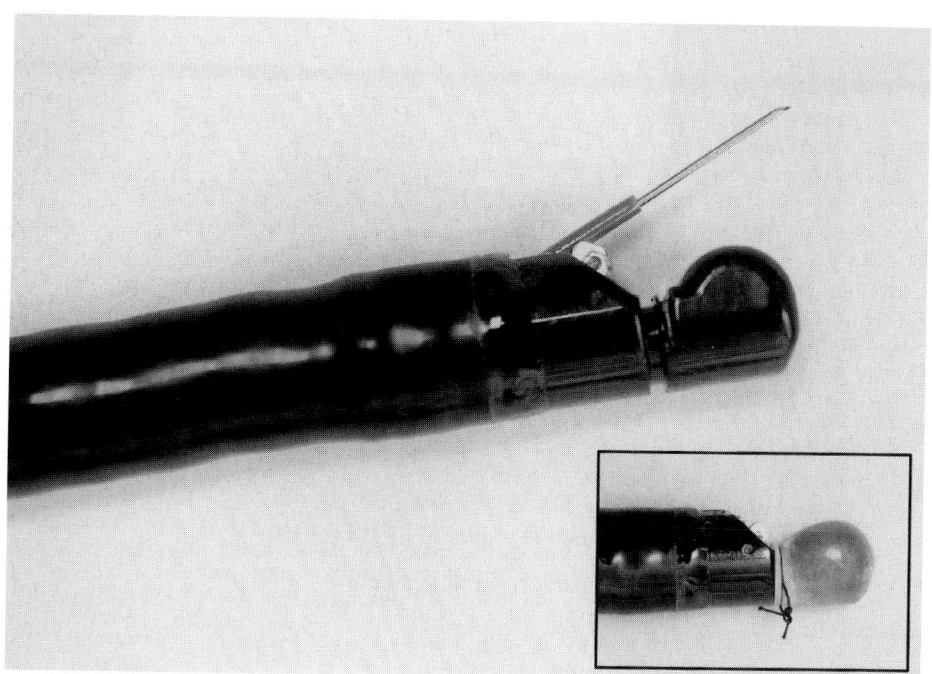

FIGURE 5–63 ■ The curvilinear electronic endoscope. The optics and operating channel, through which a fine needle is passed, are positioned behind the linear ultrasound transducer. *Inset*, The distal tip of the linear ultrasound endoscope is covered with a water-inflated contact balloon.

EUS. When a tissue sample for cytologic evaluation is required, however, the radial mechanical scanner cannot safely direct passage of a needle into the esophageal wall or adjacent tissue. Therefore, a second instrument, the electronic linear echoendoscope, powered by a separate and costly system, is employed. Although it is possible to perform both diagnosis and fine-needle aspiration with the electronic linear echoendoscope alone, the limitation in viewing field requires significant torque on the insertion tube to image the esophageal wall and adjacent tissues to 360 degrees.

ULTRASOUND ANATOMY

A normal esophagus is usually viewed by EUS as five discrete layers (Fig. 5–64). These layers are projected as alternating hyperechoic (white) and hypoechoic (black) rings. Studies have demonstrated that the five layers seen by EUS correspond to (1) the balloon-mucosa interface, (2) the mucosa deep to this interface, (3) the submucosa and the acoustic interface between the submucosa and muscularis propria, (4) the muscularis propria minus the acoustic interface between the submucosa and the muscularis propria, and (5) the periesophageal tissue (Bolondi et al, 1986; Kimmey et al, 1989). For clinical evaluation, these layers represent the superficial mucosa, the deep mucosa, the submucosa, the muscularis propria, and the periesophageal tissue.

Overdistention of the examining balloon or the transducer too close to the esophageal wall may result in the appearance of only a three-layer esophageal wall on the ultrasound image (the superficial mucosa, deep mucosa, and submucosa are compressed into one hyperechoic layer). The thickness of each layer is nearly equal and does not represent the thicknesses of the tissue layer but, rather, the time it takes the ultrasound wave to traverse this layer.

INDICATIONS

Staging of Esophageal Carcinoma

The stage of an esophageal carcinoma, defined by its anatomic extent, is the best predictor of outcome for patients with esophageal carcinoma. Recent refinements in the staging of esophageal carcinoma have resulted in a TNM-based staging system (Table 5–2) (Fleming et al, 1998). The primary tumor (T) is defined only by the depth of invasion; EUS is ideal for this determination.

T1 tumors are confined to the submucosa or more superficial esophageal layers. T2 tumors invade into but do not breach the muscularis propria. T3 tumors invade beyond the esophageal wall and into the paraesophageal tissue but do not invade adjacent structures. T4 tumors directly invade structures in the vicinity of the esophagus.

Regional lymph nodes (N) are characterized only by the presence or absence of metastases in lymph nodes in the area of the primary tumor. Regional lymph nodes are characterized by the presence (N1) or absence (N0) of metastases. Distant sites (M) are also characterized by the presence (M1) or absence (M0) of metastases.

Recent revisions of the staging system for esophageal carcinoma subdivide distant metastatic carcinomas (M1) into M1a (distant, nonregional lymph node metastases) and M1b (other distant metastases). M1a disease is further classified by tumor location; M1a tumors of the upper thoracic esophagus have metastasized to cervical nodes and M1a tumors of the lower thoracic esophagus

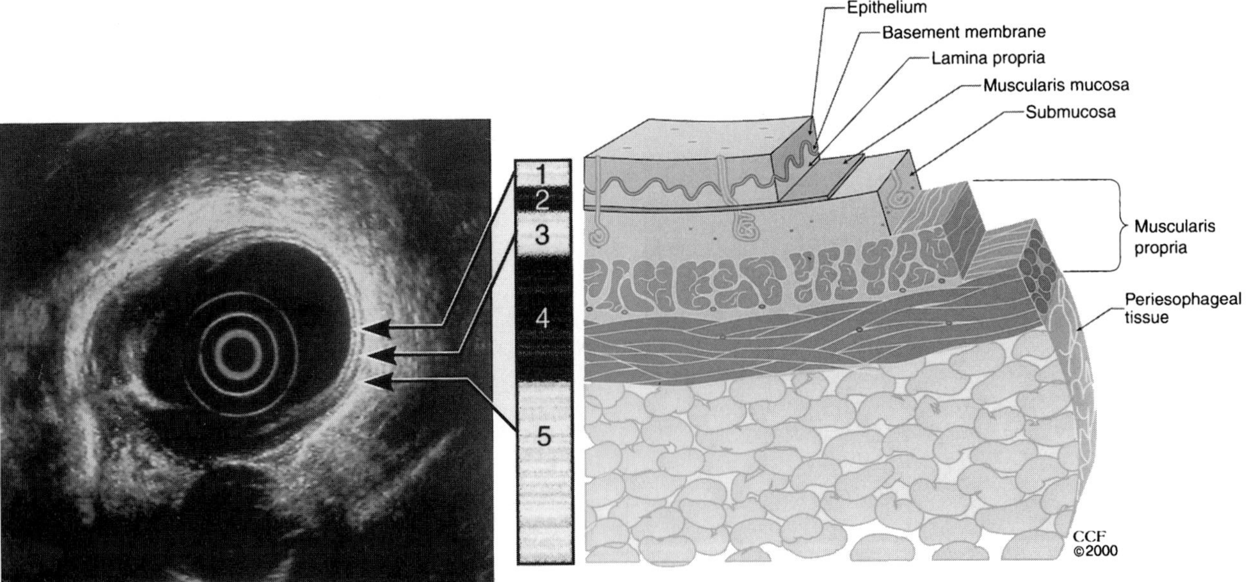

FIGURE 5–64 ■ The esophageal wall is visualized as five alternating layers of differing echogenicity by endoscopic esophageal ultrasonography (EUS). The first (inner) layer is hyperechoic (white) and represents the superficial mucosa (epithelium and lamina propria). The second layer is hypoechoic (black) and represents the deep mucosa (muscularis mucosae). The third layer is hyperechoic and represents the submucosa. The fourth layer is hypoechoic and represents the muscularis propria. The fifth layer is hyperechoic and represents the periesophageal tissue. The thickness of ultrasound layers does not equal the actual thickness of the anatomic layers. (Courtesy of Cleveland Clinic Foundation, © 2001.)

TABLE 5–2 ■ **Tumor-Node-Metastasis (TNM) Staging of Esophageal Carcinoma**

T	**Primary Tumor**	
	TX	Tumor cannot be assessed.
	T0	No evidence of tumor
	Tis	High-grade dysplasia
	T1	Tumor invades the lamina propria, muscularis mucosa, or submucosa. It does not breach the submucosa.
	T2	Tumor invades into and not beyond the muscularis propria.
	T3	Tumor invades the periesophageal tissue but does not invade adjacent structures.
	T4	Tumor invades adjacent structures.
N	**Regional Lymph Nodes**	
	NX	Regional lymph nodes cannot be assessed.
	N0	No regional lymph node metastases
	N1	Regional lymph node metastases
M	**Distant Metastasis**	
	MX	Distant metastases cannot be assessed.
	M0	No distant metastases
	M1a	Upper thoracic esophagus metastatic to cervical lymph nodes
		Lower thoracic esophagus metastatic to celiac lymph nodes
	M1b	Upper thoracic esophagus metastatic to other nonregional lymph nodes or other distant sites
		Midthoracic esophagus metastatic to either nonregional lymph nodes or other distant sites
		Lower thoracic esophagus metastatic to other nonregional lymph nodes or other distant sites

Stage Groupings			
Stage 0	Tis	N0	M0
Stage I	T1	N0	M0
Stage IIA	T2	N0	M0
	T3	N0	M0
Stage IIB	T1	N1	M0
	T2	N1	M0
Stage III	T3	N1	M0
	T4	Any N	M0
Stage IVA	Any T	Any N	M1a
Stage IVB	Any T	Any N	M1b

have metastasized to celiac lymph nodes. There is no M1a subdivision for midthoracic esophageal carcinomas because midthoracic tumors metastatic to nonregional lymph nodes have a prognosis equivalent to tumors metastatic to other distant sites.

TNM descriptors with similar behavior and prognosis are grouped into stages (see Table 5–2).

The examination for staging must be done before treatment to determine clinical stage. Detailed images of the esophageal wall by EUS make it the most accurate modality for determination of depth of tumor invasion (T) before treatment (Figs. 5–65 through 5–68). Experience with both examination techniques and ultrasound interpretations is critical to accurately determine depth of tumor invasion. Seventy-five to 100 examinations are required before competence is obtained (Fockens et al, 1996; Schlick et al, 1999).

A review of 21 series showed the accuracy of EUS for T determination was 84% (Rösch et al, 1995). Accuracy is not constant and varies with T stage. In this meta-analysis, accuracy for T1 carcinomas was 83.5%, with 16.5% of tumors overstaged; accuracy for T2 was 73%, with 10% understaged and 17% overstaged; accuracy for T3 was 89%, with 5% understaged and 6% overstaged; and accuracy for T4 was 89%, with 11% understaged. A review of the literature shows variation in accuracy with T stage: 75% to 82% for T1, 64% to 85% for T2, 89% to 94% for T3, and 88% to 100% for T4 (Saunders et al, 1997).

In the evaluation of regional lymph node status, size, nodal shape, internal echo characteristics, and border are assessed (Fig. 5–69). Large (>1 cm), round, hypoechoic, nonhomogeneous, sharply bordered lymph nodes are more likely malignant; small, oval or angular, hyperechoic, homogeneous lymph nodes with indistinct borders are more likely benign. In a retrospective review of 100 EUS examinations, the EUS determination of N was 89% sensitive, 75% specific, and 84% accurate (Catalano et al, 1994). The positive predictive value of EUS for N1 disease was 86%; the negative predictive value was 79%.

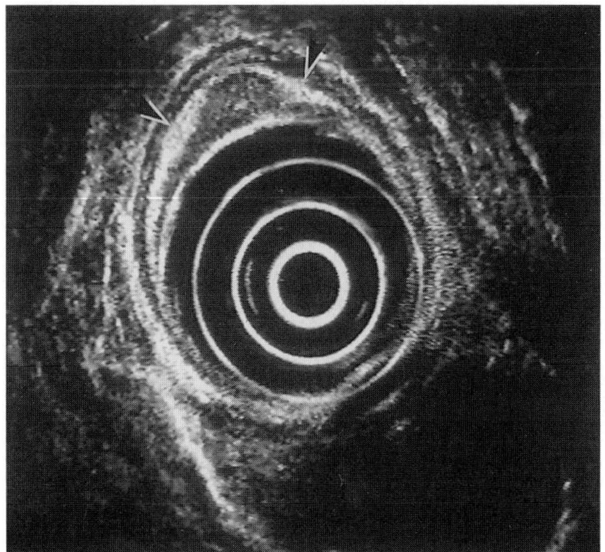

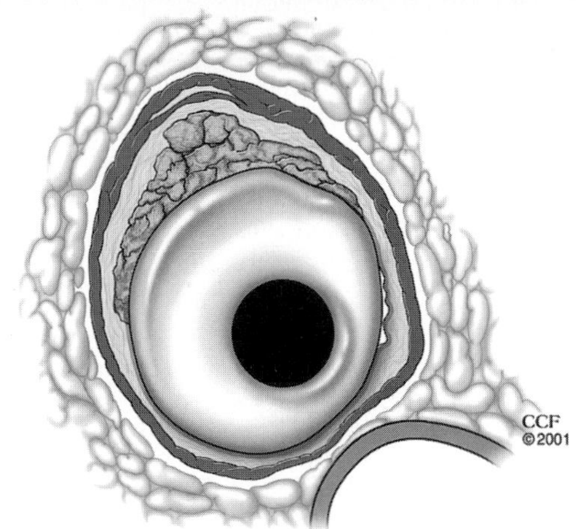

FIGURE 5–65 ■ A T1 esophageal carcinoma. *Top*, A T1 tumor as seen by EUS. The hypoechoic (black) tumor invades the hyperechoic (white) third ultrasound layer (submucosa) but does not breach the boundary between the third and fourth ultrasound layers (*arrows*). *Bottom*, A T1 tumor invades but does not breach the submucosa. (Courtesy of Cleveland Clinic Foundation, © 2001.)

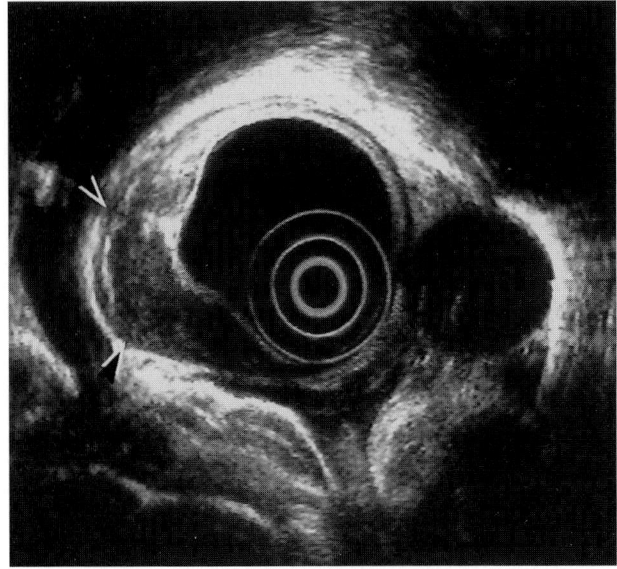

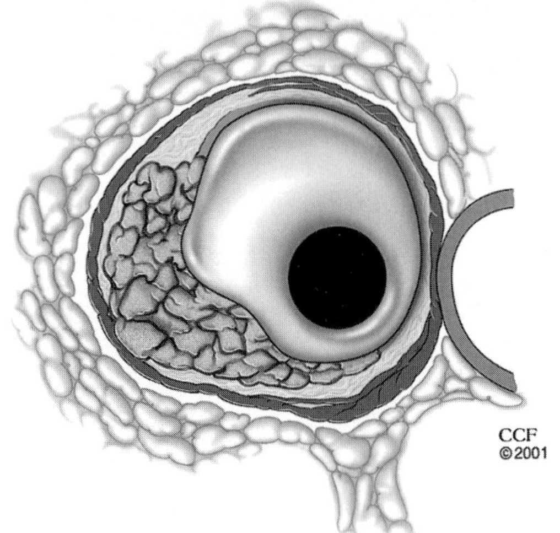

FIGURE 5–66 ■ A T2 esophageal carcinoma. *Top*, A T2 tumor as seen by EUS. The hypoechoic (black) tumor invades the hypoechoic (black) fourth ultrasound layer (muscularis propria) but does not breach the boundary between fourth and fifth ultrasound layers (*arrows*). *Bottom*, A T2 tumor invades but does not breach the muscularis propria. (Courtesy of Cleveland Clinic Foundation, © 2001.)

A patient was 24 times more likely to have N1 disease if EUS detected regional lymph nodes. The single most sensitive predictor in detecting N1 was a hypoechoic internal echo pattern, followed by a sharp border, a round shape, and size greater than 1 cm. When all four factors are present, the accuracy of N1 detection is 80% to 100%. Unfortunately, all four features are present in only 25% of N1 nodes (Bhutani et al, 1997).

In a meta-analysis of 21 series, the accuracy of EUS determination of N was 77%; for N0, 69%; and for N1, 89% (Rösch et al, 1995). The ability to use EUS to diagnose nodal metastases varies with location. It is better in the assessment of celiac nodes (accuracy, 95%; sensitivity, 83%; specificity, 98%; positive predictive value, 91%; and negative predictive value, 97%) than in mediastinal nodes (accuracy, 73%; sensitivity, 79%; specificity, 63%; positive predictive value, 79%; and negative predictive value, 63%) (Catalano et al, 1999).

Comparison of the echo characteristics of the tumor and regional lymph nodes is useful for EUS lymph node evaluation. The relationship of T to N1 must be considered during EUS examinations. Incidence of N1 disease increases with deeper tumor invasion. For a patient with a poorly differentiated adenocarcinoma, the probability of N1 disease is 17% for T1 tumors, 55% for T2, 83% for T3, and 88% for T4 (Rice et al, 1998). In T3 and T4 carcinomas, an EUS assessment of N0 does not ensure absence of N1 disease.

Endosonography-directed fine-needle aspiration (EUS FNA) further defines clinical staging by adding tissue

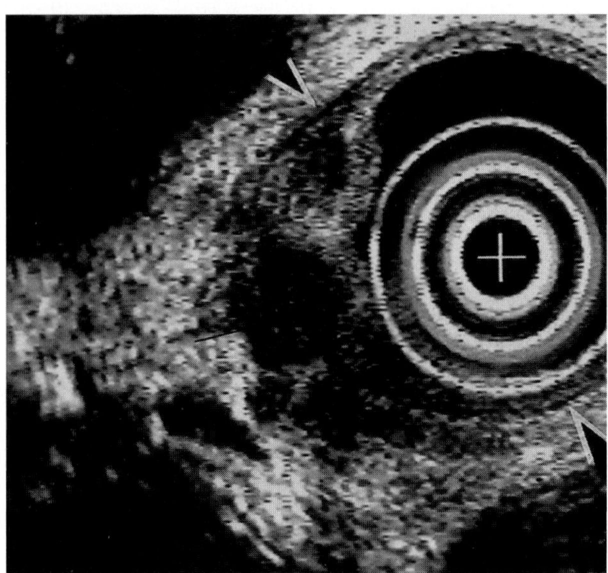

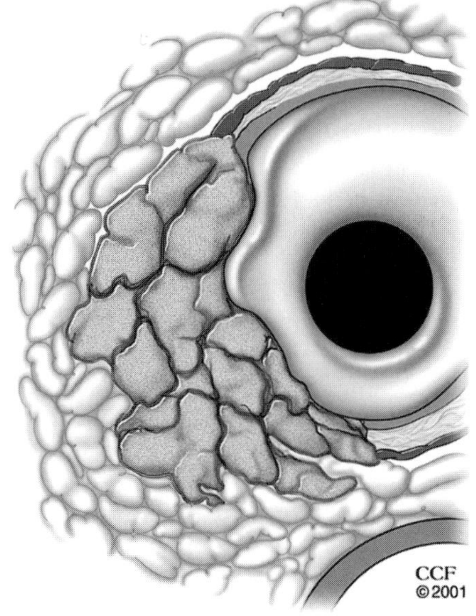

FIGURE 5–67 ■ A T3 esophageal carcinoma. *Top*, A T3 tumor as seen by EUS. The hypoechoic (black) tumor breaches the boundary between the fourth and fifth ultrasound layers *(arrows)* and invades the hyperechoic (white) fifth ultrasound layer (periesophageal tissue). *Bottom*, A T3 tumor invades the periesophageal tissue but not adjacent structures. (Courtesy of Cleveland Clinic Foundation, © 2001.)

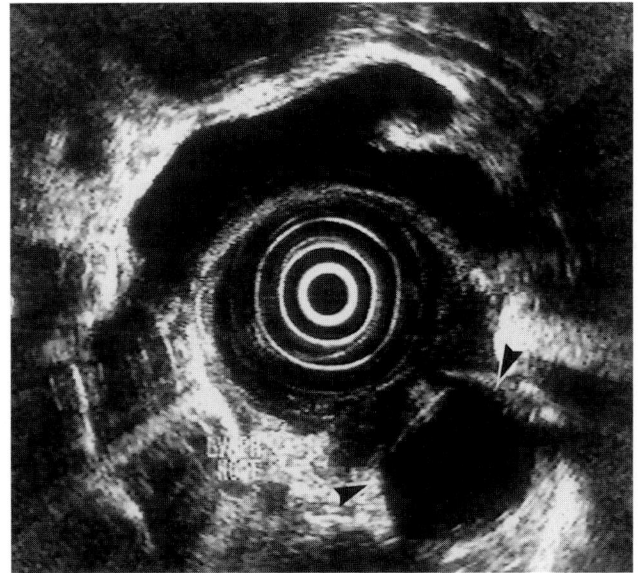

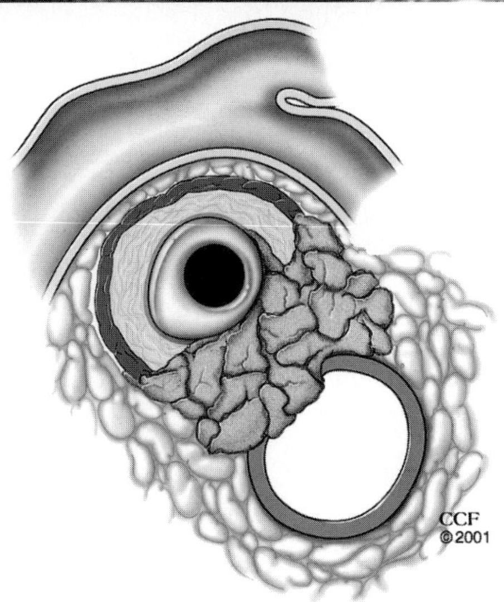

FIGURE 5–68 ■ A T4 esophageal carcinoma. *Top*, A T4 tumor as seen by EUS. The hypoechoic (black) tumor invades the aorta. The tumor breaches the boundary between the periesophageal tissue and the aortas (*arrows*). *Bottom*, A T4 tumor invades the aorta. (Courtesy of Cleveland Clinic Foundation, © 2001.)

sampling to EUS findings (Fig. 5–70). EUS FNA is the gold standard for the assessment of regional (N1) and nonregional (M1a and M1b) lymph nodes. If the primary tumor does not lie in the needle's path, EUS FNA is indicated in all lymph nodes that are abnormal by EUS examination. A 21-gauge needle with a 10-ml syringe and continuous suction provide excellent cytologic results (Bhutani et al, 1999). EUS FNA accuracy in determination of lymph node status was reported with a sensitivity of 92%, specificity of 93%, positive predictive value of 100%, and negative predictive value of 86% (Wiersema et al, 1997). The combination of EUS and EUS FNA of celiac lymph nodes deemed positive by EUS had a sensitivity of 72%, a specificity of 97%, a positive predictive value of 95%, and a negative predictive value of 82% (Reed et al, 1999). EUS FNA confirmed M1a disease in 88% of patients.

EUS has limited value in the screening for distant metastases (M1b). The distant organ must be in direct contact with the upper gastrointestinal tract for EUS to be useful (e.g., the left lateral segment of the liver and retroperitoneum are two sites).

EUS may be used to determine stage after therapy (re-treatment stage). Re-treatment stage is typically determined after induction therapy before surgery. Theoretically, the advantage of re-treatment staging is the avoidance of surgery in patients who have no residual cancer (T0 N0 M0) after induction therapy. EUS has been applied in multiple clinical series for this purpose.

Early series indicated that EUS was very accurate in determining T after chemotherapy; however, in these series, the presurgical therapy was largely ineffective in causing pathologic downstaging. Therefore, EUS was accurate by merely indicating that no significant change

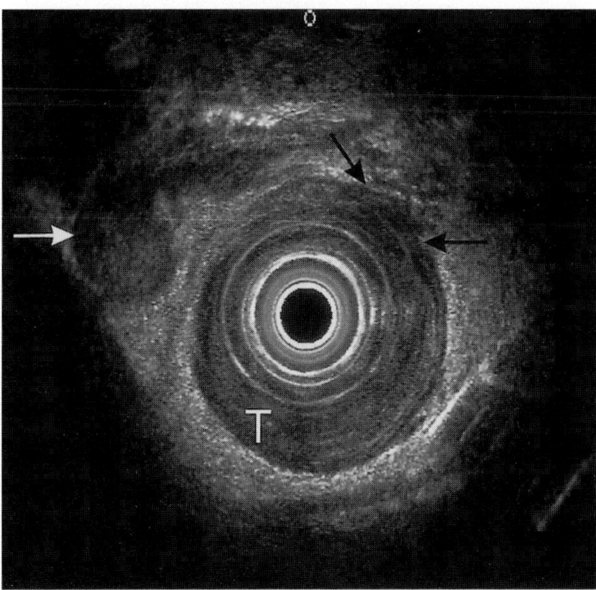

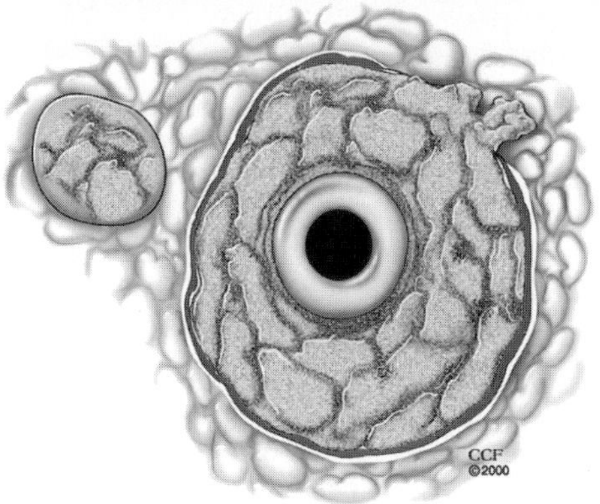

FIGURE 5–69 ■ A T3N1 esophageal carcinoma. *Top*, The T3 tumor (T) obliterates the ultrasound anatomy at this level. At 1 o'clock (*black arrows*), the tumor breaks through the fourth ultrasound layer and invades the fifth ultrasound. An N1 regional lymph node (*white arrow*), close to the primary tumor, is large (2.2 cm in diameter), round, hypoechoic, and sharply demarcated. *Bottom*, A T3N1 tumor breaches the muscularis propria to invade the periesophageal tissue and metastasizes to a regional lymph node. (Courtesy of Cleveland Clinic Foundation, © 2000.)

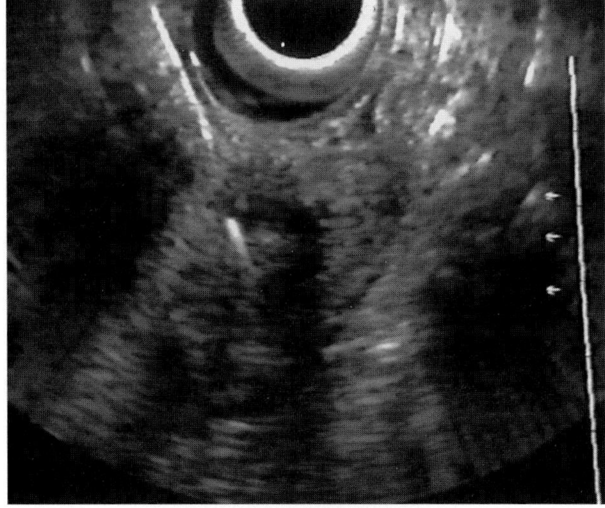

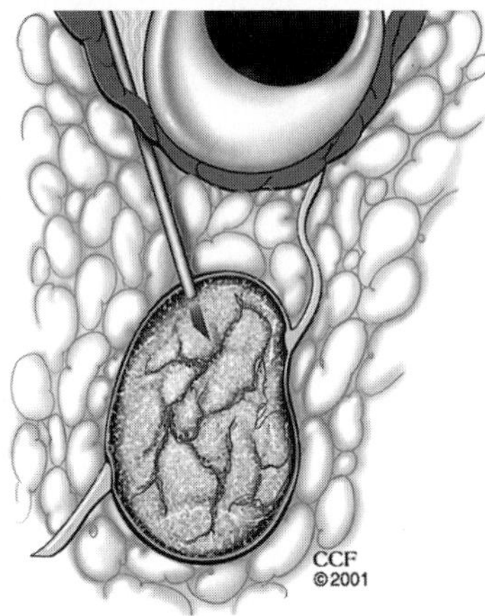

FIGURE 5–70 ■ *Top and bottom,* EUS-directed, fine-needle aspiration of an N1 regional lymph node. (Courtesy of Cleveland Clinic Foundation, © 2001.)

had occurred (Adelstein et al, 1994; Hordijk et al, 1993; Roubein et al, 1993).

In two earlier series in which radiation was accompanied by chemotherapy, accuracy of determination of T was again high (72% to 78%), but the prevalence of pathologic T0 was low or not reported (Dittler et al, 1994; Giovannini et al, 1997). Accuracy of T determination can be attributed primarily to a lack of tumor response to chemoradiotherapy.

Later series have incorporated more aggressive regimens of chemoradiotherapy with higher rates of significant downstaging of tumor and pathologic T0 N0. In these series, up to 31% of patients were classified as having pathologic T0 N0 after chemoradiotherapy (Zuccaro et al, 1999). EUS was reported inaccurate in determining T (27% to 59%) (Beseth et al, 2000; Bowrey et al, 1999; Isenberg et al, 1998; Laterza et al, 1999; Zuccaro et al, 1999).

The most common mistake made in determining T was overstaging. EUS is unable to distinguish tumor from inflammation and fibrosis produced by chemoradiotherapy. Similar difficulties in distinguishing tumor from post-chemoradiotherapy inflammation and fibrosis have also been reported with EUS staging of rectal cancers (Fleshman et al, 1992). However, the reduction of tumor size as measured by EUS as a decrease of maximal tumor cross-sectional area is a predictor of improved survival after induction chemoradiotherapy (Chak et al, 2000; Shinkai et al, 2000).

EUS accuracy for N staging after chemoradiotherapy has been reported at 58% to 71% (Beseth et al, 2000; Bowrey et al, 1999; Laterza et al, 1999; Zuccaro et al, 1999). The accuracy of N determination after chemoradiotherapy is lower than that for the initial determination. This is because of alteration in ultrasound appearance of nodes after chemoradiotherapy to the extent that established EUS criteria do not apply and residual foci of cancer within the nodes are too small for detection by any modality other than pathologic analysis.

EUS has been useful in the diagnosis and restaging of patients with malignant strictures and anastomotic recurrences that are not endoscopically visible (Catalano et al, 1995; Faigel et al, 1998; Lightdale et al, 1989).

DIAGNOSIS

Benign Esophageal Disease

Detailed examination of the esophageal wall by EUS has improved the diagnosis of benign esophageal tumors. EUS identification of intramural masses relies on both the layer from which the tumor arises (Table 5–3) and the ultrasound characteristics of the tumor. Homogeneous lesions that are anechoic, of intermediate echogenicity, or hyperechoic are almost exclusively benign (Kawamoto et al, 1997). A heterogeneous echo pattern may be seen in benign tumors, but this endosonographic finding, particularly in lesions greater than 3 to 4 cm in largest diameter, may be indicative of malignancy.

Cysts are echo-free, rounded, and sometimes septated (Yasuda et al, 1992). Lipomas are homogeneous, intensely hyperechoic lesions. Lipomas can often be recognized by endoscopy alone; they frequently have a yellow tint and are soft and pliable when probed. Granular cell

TABLE 5–3 ■ **Endoscopic Ultrasound Classification of Esophageal Tumors**

EUS Layer	*Esophageal Tumor*
First/second (mucosa/ deep mucosa)	Fibrovascular polyp Retention cyst Squamous papilloma Tis esophageal cancer
Third (submucosa)	Lipoma Fibroma Neurofibroma Granular cell tumor T1 esophageal cancer
Fourth	Leiomyoma* T2 esophageal cancer

*Leiomyomas may also arise from the second ultrasound layer (muscularis mucosa), but these tumors are much more common from the fourth ultrasound layer.

EUS, endoscopic ultrasound.

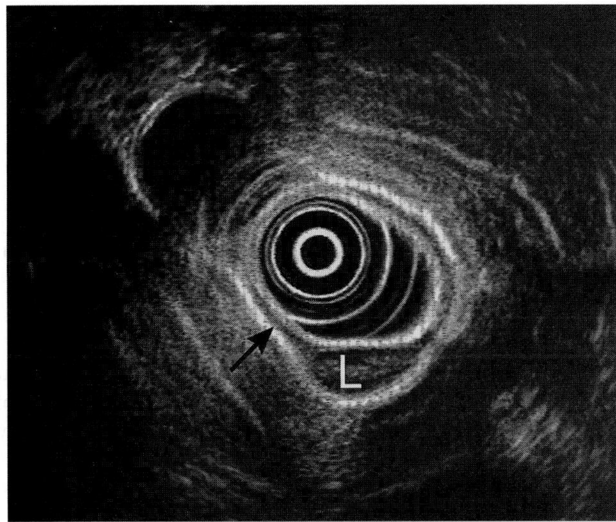

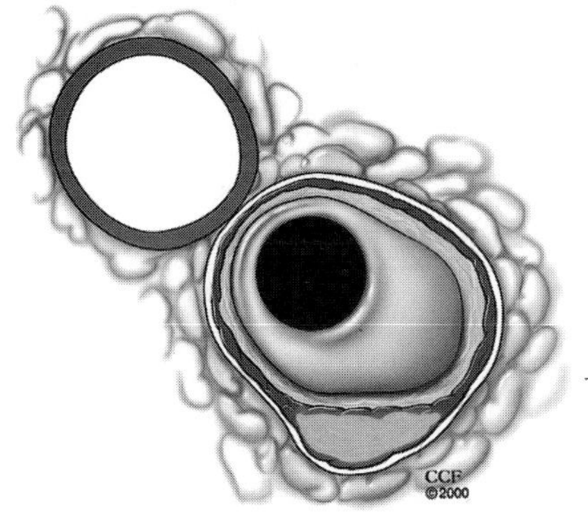

FIGURE 5–71 ■ An esophageal leiomyoma. *Top*, EUS of this most common benign tumor demonstrates a hypoechoic, homogeneous, well-demarcated tumor with no associated lymphadenopathy. EUS balloon overdistention blends the first three ultrasound layers into one hyperechoic layer. The tumor arises from and is confined to the fourth ultrasound layer (*arrow*). *Bottom*, A benign leiomyoma arises from and is confined to the muscularis propria. (Courtesy of Cleveland Clinic Foundation, © 2000.)

tumors are typically found in the third ultrasound layer and may be hypoechoic or intermediate echogenic but generally less hyperechoic than lipomas (Goldblum et al, 1996; Palazzo et al, 1997; Tada et al, 1990). The most common benign esophageal tumors are smooth muscle tumors of the distal esophagus; more than 70% of patients with benign intramural esophageal tumors referred for EUS have leiomyomas. EUS displays hypoechoic tumors arising from the fourth ultrasound layer (muscularis propria) (Fig. 5–71). Because routine endoscopic biopsy specimens reveal only normal overlying squamous mucosa, EUS is the most helpful test in establishing the nature of the lesion. EUS findings that suggest malignant degeneration are larger than 4 cm and have irregular borders, mixed internal echo patterns, or associated lymphadenopathy (Tio et al, 1990).

On EUS studies, esophageal varices have the typical appearance of blood vessels. They appear as tubular, round, or serpiginous echo-free structures. They may be visualized within the submucosal layer of the esophageal wall or in tissues adjacent to the esophagus. These EUS patterns change after sclerosis. Intravariceal sclerosis fills the varix with echogenic material representing thrombus. Paravariceal injection leads to obliteration of the varix with hypoechoic extravariceal thickening.

EUS findings in achalasia are controversial. A thickened esophageal wall is seen in most patients; however, the slight increase in the mean size of the muscularis propria is not helpful in the diagnosis of achalasia (Barthet et al, 1998). This excessive thickening may be artifactual. In a dilated and convoluted esophagus, the ultrasound transducer may orient at an angle oblique to the esophageal wall, giving a false appearance of wall thickening (Falk et al, 1994; Van Dam, 1998). The main role of EUS in achalasia is to exclude other mural abnormalities and pseudoachalasia.

EUS has not been useful in the surveillance of patients with columnar-lined esophagus. Mucosal definition by EUS cannot differentiate dysplasia from intramucosal carcinoma (Falk et al, 1994; Waxman 1997). Improvements in ultrasound and balloon technology may resolve this problem (Gillard, 1999; Inoue et al, 1998).

Paraesophageal Disease

EUS has been used to examine mediastinal lymph nodes in patients with bronchogenic carcinoma (Gress et al, 1997; Kondo et al, 1990; Potepan et al, 1996). For this purpose, EUS has a reported positive predictive value of 77%, a negative predictive value of 93%, and an overall accuracy of 92%, using criteria similar to those for regional lymph node evaluation in esophageal carcinoma. However, anatomic constraints limit its usefulness for evaluation of lymph nodes in proximity to the airway. EUS-directed fine-needle aspiration provides cytologic differentiation between benign and malignant lymphadenopathy (Mishra et al, 1999). EUS-directed fine-needle aspiration has been successful in identifying solid lesions of the mediastinum and lung (Fritscher-Ravens et al, 1999; Hunerbein et al, 1998b, 1998c; Pedersen et al, 1996).

EUS has proved useful in the diagnosis of foregut cysts (Rice, 1992; Van Dam et al, 1992). These cysts are generally hypoechoic and located outside the esophageal wall (Fig. 5–72). They may occasionally be found within the esophageal wall. If foregut cysts contain proteinaceous material, they may have a hyperechoic or an inhomogeneous (hyperechoic and hypoechoic) ultrasound appearance. Extrinsic esophageal compression may also be characterized with EUS (Silva et al, 1988). However, examination of structures distant from the esophagus is best performed with transducers of lower frequencies. Transesophageal cardiac ultrasound provides better definition of these structures using probes with frequencies of 3 to 5 MHz.

COMMENTS AND CONTROVERSIES

Drs. Rice and Zuccaro have provided a comprehensive and informed review of the current and evolving roles of endoscopic esophageal ultrasound (EUS) in evaluation

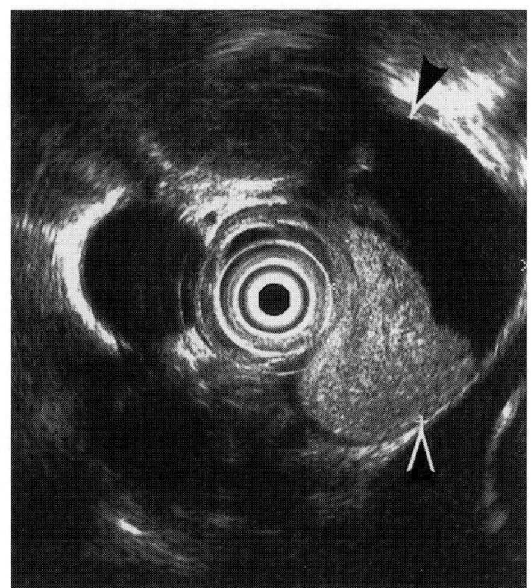

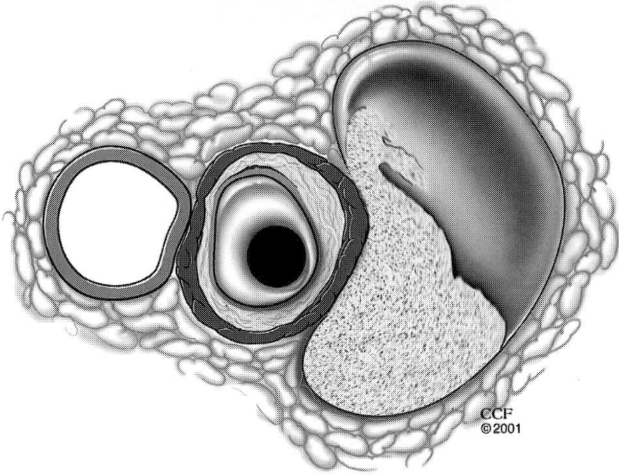

FIGURE 5–72 ■ A foregut cyst. *Top*, EUS demonstrates a mass (*arrows*) adjacent to the trachea and esophagus. The cyst has two components, one hyperechoic (white) representing proteinaceous material and one hypoechoic (black) representing fluid. *Bottom*, A foregut cyst is in close proximity to the esophagus and trachea. (Courtesy of Cleveland Clinic Foundation, © 2001.)

of both benign and malignant esophageal diseases. The perspectives elaborated represent the extensive clinical experience of a thoracic surgeon (Rice) and gastroenterologist (Zuccaro) working closely together in the investigation and management of esophageal cancer in the earliest, asymptomatic states. The importance of a preliminary flexible endoscopy is appropriately emphasized. It is evident that EUS is the most accurate determinant of tumor T status.

EUS has proved valuable in the diagnosis of several benign conditions. The most common among these is leiomyoma of the muscular wall of the esophagus. The EUS appearance is diagnostic—a homogeneous, hypoechoic lesion of regular configuration and smoother margins arising in the muscularis propria. The EUS appearance confirms a provisional diagnosis based on the esophagogram and endoscopy. In the absence of symptoms, such cases may be confidently managed conservatively with interval follow-up, which may include repeated EUS. Foregut cysts also have a characteristic EUS appearance and may be treated conservatively in the absence of symptoms. "Pseudo-achalasia" caused by neoplasm at the esophagogastric junction can be clearly distinguished from true achalasia when uncertainty exists.

In experienced hands, EUS can be completed in approximately 20 minutes. The instrumentation and technology continue to improve in safety and quality.

F. G. P.

■ REFERENCES

Adelstein DJ, Rice TW, Boyce GA, et al: Adenocarcinoma of the esophagus and gastroesophageal junction: Clinical and pathologic assessment of response to induction chemotherapy. Am J Clin Oncol 17:14, 1994.

Barthet M, Mambrini P, Audibert P, et al: Relationships between endosonographic appearance and clinical or manometric features in patients with achalasia. Eur J Gastroenterol Hepatol 10:559, 1998.

Beseth BD, Bedford R, Isacoff WH, et al: Endoscopic ultrasound does not accurately assess pathologic stage of esophageal cancer after neoadjuvant chemoradiotherapy. Am Surgeon 66:827, 2000.

Bhutani MS, Hawes RH, Hoffman BJ: A comparison of the accuracy of echo features during endoscopic ultrasound (EUS) and EUS-guided fine needle aspiration for diagnosis of malignant lymph node invasion. Gastrointest Endosc 45:474, 1997.

Bhutani MS, Suryaprasad S, Moezzi J, et al: Improved technique for performing endoscopic ultrasound fine needle aspiration of lymph nodes. Endoscopy 31:550, 1999.

Binmoeller KF, Seifert H, Seitz U, et al: Ultrasonic esophagoprobe for TNM staging of highly stenosing esophageal carcinoma. Gastrointest Endosc 41:547, 1995.

Bolondi L, Casanova P, Santi V, et al: The sonographic appearance of the normal gastric wall: An in vivo study. Ultrasound Med Biol 12:991, 1986.

Bowrey DJ, Clark GW, Roberts SA, et al: Serial endoscopic ultrasound in the assessment of response to chemoradiotherapy for carcinoma of the esophagus. J Gastrointest Surg 3:462, 1999.

Catalano MF, Sivak MV Jr, Rice TW, et al: Endosonographic features predictive of lymph node metastases. Gastrointest Endosc 40:442, 1994.

Catalano MF, Sivak MV Jr, Rice TW, et al: Postoperative screening for anastomotic recurrence of esophageal carcinoma by endoscopic ultrasonography. Gastrointest Endosc 42:540, 1995.

Catalano MF, Alcocer E, Chak A, et al: Evaluation of metastatic celiac axis lymph nodes in patients with esophageal carcinoma: Accuracy of EUS. Gastrointest Endosc 50:352, 1999.

Chak A, Canto MI, Cooper GS, et al: Endosonographic assessment of multimodality therapy predicts survival of esophageal carcinoma patients. Cancer 88:1788, 2000.

Dittler HJ, Fink U, Siewert GR: Response to chemotherapy in esophageal cancer. Endoscopy 26:769, 1994.

Faigel DO, Deveney C, Phillips D, et al: Biopsy-negative malignant esophageal stricture: Diagnosis by endoscopic ultrasound. Am J Gastroenterol 93:2257, 1998.

Falk GW, Catalano MF, Sivak MV Jr, et al: Endosonography in the evaluation of patients with Barrett's esophagus and high-grade dysplasia. Gastrointest Endosc 40:207, 1994.

Falk GW, Van Dam J, Sivak MV, et al: Endoscopic ultrasonography (EUS) in achalasia. Gastrointest Endosc 37:241, 1991.

Fleming ID, Cooper JS, Henson DE, et al (eds): Digestive system: Esophagus. In AJCC Cancer Staging Manual, 5th ed. Philadelphia, Lippincott-Raven, 1998, p 65.

Fleshman JW, Myerson RJ, Fry RD, et al: Accuracy of transrectal ultrasound in predicting stage of rectal cancer before and after preoperative radiation therapy. Dis Colon Rectum 35:823, 1992.

Fockens P, Van den Brande JHM, van Dullemen HM, et al: Endosonographic T-staging of esophageal carcinoma: A learning curve. Gastrointest Endosc 44:58, 1996.

Fritscher-Ravens A, Petrasch S, Reinacher-Schick A, et al: Diagnostic value of endoscopic ultrasonography-guided fine-needle aspiration cytology of mediastinal masses in patients with intrapulmonary lesions and diagnostic bronchoscopy. Respiration 66:150, 1999.

Gillard V: Evaluation of polyps by endoscopic ultrasonography (EUS): Implications for endotherapy. Acta Gastroenterol Belg 62:196, 1999.

Giovannini M, Seitz FJ, Thomas P, et al: Endoscopic ultrasonography for assessment of response to combined radiation therapy and chemotherapy in patients with esophageal cancer. Endoscopy 29:4, 1997.

Goldblum JR, Rice TW, Zuccaro G Jr, et al: Granular cell tumors of the esophagus: A clinical and pathologic study of 13 cases. Ann Thorac Surg 62:860, 1996.

Gress FG, Savides TJ, Sandler A, et al: Endoscopic ultrasonography, fine-needle aspiration biopsy guided by endoscopic ultrasonography, and computed tomography in the preoperative staging of non–small-cell lung cancer: A comparison study. Ann Intern Med 127:604, 1997.

Hordijk ML, Kok TC, Wilson JHP, et al: Assessment of response of esophageal carcinoma to induction chemotherapy. Endoscopy 25:592, 1993.

Hunerbein M, Ghadimi BM, Haensch W, et al: Transendoscopic ultrasound of esophageal and gastric cancer using miniaturized ultrasound catheter probes. Gastrointest Endosc 48:371, 1998a.

Hunerbein M, Dohmoto M, Haensch W, et al: Endosonography-guided biopsy of mediastinal and pancreatic tumors. Endoscopy 30:32, 1998b.

Hunerbein M, Ghadimi BM, Haensch W, et al: Transesophageal biopsy of mediastinal and pulmonary tumors by means of endoscopic ultrasound guidance. J Thorac Cardiovasc Surg 116:554, 1998c.

Inoue H, Kawano T, Takeshita K, et al: Modified soft-balloon methods during ultrasonic probe examination for superficial esophageal cancer. Endoscopy 30:A41, 1998.

Isenberg G, Chak A, Canto MI, et al: Endoscopic ultrasound in restaging of esophageal cancer after neoadjuvant chemoradiation. Gastrointest Endosc 48:158, 1998.

Kawamoto K, Yamada Y, Utsunomiya T, et al: Gastrointestinal submucosal tumors: Evaluation with endoscopic US. Radiology 205:733, 1997.

Kimmey MB, Martin RW: Fundamentals of endosonography. Gastrointest Endosc Clin North Am 2:557, 1992.

Kimmey MB, Martin RW, Haggitt RC, et al: Histologic correlates of gastrointestinal ultrasound images. Gastroenterology 96:433, 1989.

Kondo D, Imaizumi M, Abe T, et al: Endoscopic ultrasound examination for mediastinal lymph node metastases of lung cancer. Chest 98:586, 1990.

Laterza E, deManzoni G, Guglielmi A, et al: Endoscopic ultrasonography in the staging of esophageal carcinoma after preoperative radiotherapy and chemotherapy. Ann Thorac Surg 67:1466, 1999.

Lightdale CJ, Botet JF, Kelson DP, et al: Diagnosis of recurrent upper gastrointestinal cancer at the surgical anastomosis by endoscopic ultrasound. Gastrointest Endosc 35:407, 1989.

McLoughlin RF, Cooperberg PL, Mathieson JR, et al: High resolution endoluminal ultrasonography in the staging of esophageal carcinoma. J Ultrasound Med 14:725, 1995.

Menzel J, Hoepffner N, Nottberg H, et al: Preoperative staging of esophageal carcinoma: Miniprobe sonography versus conventional endoscopic ultrasound in a prospective histopathologically verified study. Endoscopy 31:291, 1999.

Mishra G, Sahai AV, Penman ID, et al: Endoscopic ultrasonography with fine-needle aspiration: An accurate and simple diagnostic modality for sarcoidosis. Endoscopy 31:377, 1999.

Palazzo L, Landi B, Cellier C, et al: Endosonographic features of esophageal granular cell tumors. Endoscopy 29:850, 1997.

Pedersen BH, Vilmann P, Folke K, et al: Endoscopic ultrasonography and real-time guided fine-needle aspiration biopsy of solid lesions of the mediastinum suspected of malignancy. Chest 110:539, 1996.

Potepan P, Meroni E, Spagnoli I, et al: Non-small cell lung cancer: Detection of mediastinal lymph node metastases by endoscopic ultrasound and CT. Eur Radiol 6:19, 1996.

Reed CE, Misha G, Sarai AV, et al: Esophageal cancer staging: Improved accuracy by endoscopic ultrasound of celiac lymph nodes. Ann Thorac Surg 67:319, 1999.

Rice TW: Benign neoplasm and cysts of the mediastinum. Semin Thorac Cardiovasc Surg 4:25, 1992.

Rice TW, Zuccaro G Jr, Adelstein DJ, et al: Esophageal carcinoma: Depth of tumor invasion is predictive of regional lymph node status. Ann Thorac Surg 65:787, 1998.

Rösch T: Endosonographic staging of esophageal cancer: A review of literature results. Gastrointest Endosc Clin North Am 5:537, 1995.

Roubein LD, DuBrow R, David C, et al: Endoscopic ultrasonography in the quantitative assessment of response to chemotherapy in patients with adenocarcinoma of the esophagus and esophagogastric junction. Endoscopy 25:587, 1993.

Saunders HS, Wolfman NT, Ott DJ: Esophageal cancer: Radiologic staging. Radiol Clin North Am 35:281, 1997.

Schlick T, Heintz A, Junginger T: The examiner's learning effect and its influence on the quality of endoscopic ultrasonography in carcinoma of the esophagus and gastric cardia. Surg Endosc 13:894, 1999.

Shinkai M, Niwa Y, Arisawa T, et al: Evaluation of prognosis of squamous cell carcinoma of the oesophagus by endoscopic ultrasonography. Gut 47:120, 2000.

Silva SA, Kouzu T, Ogino Y, et al: Endoscopic ultrasonography of oesophageal tumors and compressions. J Clin Ultrasound 16:149, 1988.

Tada S, Iida M, Yao T, et al: Granular cell tumor of the esophagus: Endoscopic ultrasonography demonstration and endoscopic removal. Am J Gastroenterol 85:1507, 1990.

Tio TL, Tytgat GN, den Hartog Jager FC: Endoscopic ultrasonography for the evaluation of smooth muscle tumors in the upper gastrointestinal tract: An experience with 42 cases. Gastrointest Endosc 36:342, 1990.

Van Dam J, Rice TW, Sivak MV Jr, et al: Endoscopic ultrasonography and endoscopically guided needle aspiration for the diagnosis of upper gastrointestinal tract foregut cysts. Am J Gastroenterol 87:762, 1992.

Van Dam J: Endosonographic evaluation of the patient with achalasia. Endoscopy 30:A48, 1998.

Waxman I: Endosonography in columnar-lined esophagus. Gastroenterol Clin North Am 26:607, 1997.

Wiersema MJ, Vilmann P, Giovannini M, et al: Endosonography-guided fine-needle aspiration biopsy: Diagnostic accuracy and complication assessment. Gastroenterology 112:1087, 1997.

Yasuda K, Nakajima M, Kawai K: Endoscopic ultrasonographic imaging of submucosal lesions of the upper gastrointestinal tract. Gastrointest Endosc Clin North Am 2:615, 1992.

Zuccaro G Jr, Rice TW, Goldblum JR, et al: Endoscopic ultrasound cannot determine suitability for esophagectomy after aggressive chemoradiotherapy for esophageal cancer. Am J Gastroenterol 94:906, 1999.

CHAPTER **6**

Esophagoscopy

RIGID ESOPHAGOSCOPY

Marcel Savary
Alexandre Radu
Philippe Monnier

HISTORICAL NOTE

The first rigid esophagoscopies were performed more than 100 years ago (Bevan, 1868; Kussmaul, 1870; Mikulicz, 1881; Waldenburg, 1870); even at that time, their purpose was both diagnostic and therapeutic.

As a result of constant improvements in instrumentation (diverse endoscopes with various lengths and diameters, distal lighting, cold light, magnifying wide-angle optics, capacity for aspiration, insufflation of air, photodocumentation, video recording, and laser application), rigid esophagoscopy today permits complete examination of the entire esophagus, regardless of the patient's age and without contraindications except those that apply for anesthesia. It permits comprehensive analysis of mucosal lesions by means of photography, video recording, biopsy, and sampling of cytologic and microbiologic material with high accuracy. It makes possible therapeutic measures such as removal of foreign bodies or impacted food boluses, dilatation of strictures, intubation or palliative laser resection of malignant tumors, sclerosing injections, endoscopic hemostasis, photodynamic therapy, and mucosal ablation.

Nowadays esophagoscopy has become an explorative and therapeutic method whose value must be established by the basic criteria of risk and success. Success and complication rates must be estimated from global series, including diagnostic and therapeutic procedures performed at all age levels, with no preselection of patients, and with account taken of the need to train endoscopists.

■ *HISTORICAL READINGS*

Bevan L: The esophagoscope. Lancet 1:470, 1868.
Kussmaul J: Ueber Magenspiegelung. Verh Med Wochenschr 12:271, 1870.
Mikulicz J: Ueber Gastroskopie und Oesophagoskopie. Zentralbl Chir 43:673, 1881.
Waldenburg L: Oesophagoskopie. Klin Wochenschr 47:578, 1870.

INDICATIONS AND CONTRAINDICATIONS

Every symptom of long duration that may lead to suspicion of an esophageal disease warrants esophagoscopy, even when radiology shows no positive findings.

The contraindications listed in old textbooks (paresis of the recurrent laryngeal nerve, esophageal varices, diverticulum, aortic aneurysm, corrosive esophagitis, hematemesis, kyphoscoliosis) have become obsolete. However, the endoscopist must be aware of the fact that there are circumstances during endoscopy that require cessation of the examination: impassable strictures, serious acute and corrosive lesions, esophageal varices with erosive esophagitis, and severe pulsatile compression. Such incomplete endoscopies occur relatively frequently (0.8% to 2% of cases) and are responsible for most of the failures of esophagoscopy (Savary and Rivier, 1971). Endoscopy that cannot be completed owing to abnormal anatomic conditions is rare if appropriate instrumental and anesthetic techniques are at hand. Unsuccessful endoscopy can also occur when the endoscopist's ability does not meet the required standard. From a diagnostic standpoint, success depends on the following factors:

1. Complete mastery of the endoscopic methods with all instruments (both flexible and rigid) and various types of anesthesia.
2. Systematic and critical examination of the esophagus.
3. Endoscopic knowledge of the normal esophagus, its anatomy, and its behavior with regard to respiratory movements, contact with the endoscope, inflation of air, mobilization, and dilatation.
4. Recognition of minor changes in the esophageal mucosa.
5. Exact knowledge of the endoscopic appearance of the various esophageal diseases.

Failed endoscopy may also occur in diagnostic and therapeutic operations; 94% of esophageal biopsies performed are successful, when a rigid endoscope with angled biopsy forceps is available (Savary and Rivier, 1971). Removal of food particles is virtually always successful when the rigid endoscope is used. In isolated cases in elderly patients, the operation can take so long that it can be carried out only by mechanical ventilation with the use of general anesthesia. Foreign bodies, in children as well as in adults, can be removed in more than 95% of cases with a minimum of risk (Brossard et al, 1991). Foreign bodies that occur in association with severe hematemesis must be treated primarily surgically without prior endoscopy.

Complications

Since the introduction of esophagoscopy, complications have been reported from the diagnostic, therapeutic, and especially the preventive points of view. The major danger is esophageal perforation with the distal end of the instrument. Chevalier Jackson's advice—"seek the lumen and follow it"—is still valid today (Jackson and Jackson, 1934, 1950; Terracol, 1951).

For the rigid esophagoscope, the risk of endoscopic trauma from the distal end of the tube has practically disappeared since the development of instruments with cold-light illumination, wide-angle Hopkins optics, and capacity for inflation with air and the use of general anesthesia with intubation and curarization. Today the rigid instruments carry another risk during endoscopy of the lower esophagus. When the patient's position is incorrect and spondylosis of the spine is present, injury to the rear wall of the upper esophagus can result from cervical osteophyte projections during examination of the cardia (Fig. 6–1). Biopsy or removal of food particles or foreign bodies presents no danger if the correct technique with the suitable instrument is used (Brossard et al, 1991).

Vagal reflexes as well as coronary circulatory disturbances can be observed during the examination (Berci, 1976; Kumagai and Makuuchi, 1987). In patients with cardiovascular disease, the heart should be under continuous monitoring during operations in the area of the cardia, especially during prolonged endoscopic intervention (removal of impacted food bolus).

The type of esophagoscopy (diagnostic versus therapeutic), the expertise of the endoscopist (senior or young resident), and the patient's age (young versus old) play a key role in assessing the risk involved in an esophagoscopic procedure. In endoscopic examinations for purely diagnostic purposes, the complication rate today appears to be nearly the same for the fiberscope and the rigid instruments. As far as perforation is concerned, this risk should be less than 1 per 2000 diagnostic procedures (Dawson and Cockel, 1981; Savary and Rivier, 1971; Schweizer et al, 1991).

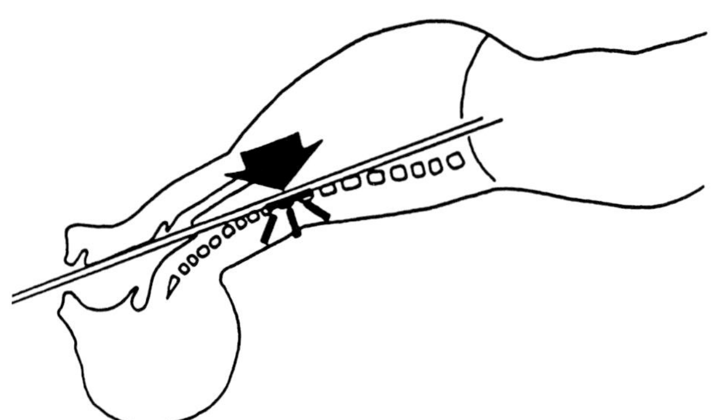

FIGURE 6–1 ■ Lever mechanism of the rigid esophagoscope during examination of the cardia: there is danger that the posterior wall of the esophagus may be split if spondylosis with ventral peaks is present.

For therapeutic esophagoscopies, including removal of foreign bodies or food particles, dilatation of strictures, and palliative therapy for malignant tumors by laser or intubation, the risk of perforation ranges between 2 and 3 per 100 endoscopies (Dawson and Cockel, 1981). As for the palliative treatment of malignant tumors (intubation or laser tumorectomy), the risk for perforation can reach 4.5%, with a related mortality rate of 0.9% (Hugonnet et al, 1988; Schweizer et al, 1991).

The endoscopist's desire to reduce to a minimum the number of contraindications to the use of esophagoscopy and to limit the number of diagnostic and therapeutic failures is offset by an increased risk for the patient. The comparison between rate of success and complication rate, when established under precise conditions, is a valid measure of the expertise of an endoscopy group, the quality of its methods, instruments, and equipment and the excellence of its teaching.

TECHNIQUE: PREPARATION

The indication for rigid esophagoscopy plays a major role in the selection of room, staffing, equipment, instrumentation, and method and type of anesthesia. Before the examination, a discussion with the patient and information from the attending physician are of great importance. If available, the chest x-ray and upper gastrointestinal (GI) series should be obtained. Before an endoscope is introduced, the patient must be checked for the following:

1. The mouth, with attention to condition of the teeth and to function of the mandibular joints.
2. The neck, for asymmetry or lymph node or thyroid enlargement.
3. The spine, for function of the atlanto-occipital joint and range of mobility of the cervical spine.

The patient must have an empty stomach, except in emergency endoscopy, for removal of a foreign body or an impacted food bolus. Dentures, when present, are removed. A bleeding disorder should be ruled out. In case of foreign body or food impaction, radiographic examination with barium is contraindicated, but a chest x-ray and a neck profile should be available to help locate the foreign body and to look for the presence of a cervical or mediastinal emphysema. The patient's temperature should be taken before endoscopy for removal of a foreign body.

EQUIPMENT

To solve various diagnostic and therapeutic problems with safety and efficiency, endoscopists should have three different types of instruments at their disposal:

1. A rigid, open "full-lumen" tube (Haslinger or Chevalier Jackson type).
2. A rigid esophagoscope with Hopkins or Lumina optics ("universal" Storz or Wolf type).
3. A fiberscope.

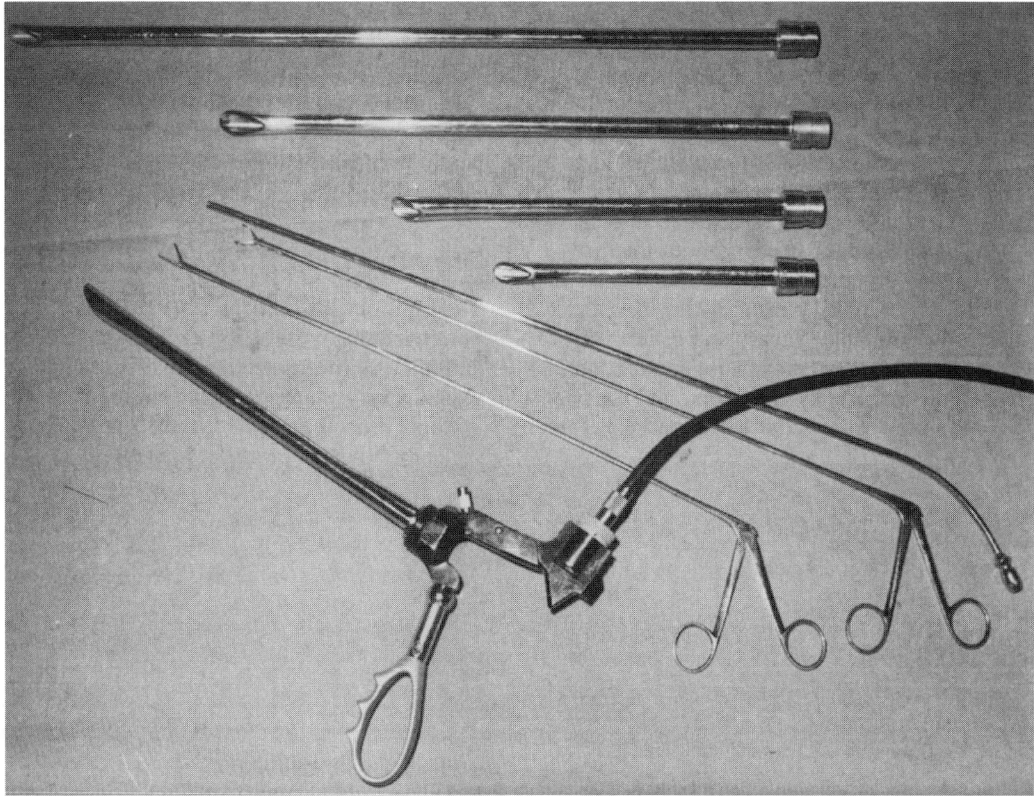

FIGURE 6–2 ■ Rigid, "full-lumen" open esophagoscope (Haslinger type) for extraction of foreign bodies and impacted food boluses.

Rigid, Full-Lumen Open Tube

The removal of impacted food or foreign bodies calls for open esophagoscopes of various lengths and diameters, which allow the operation to proceed freely and under stable conditions. The Haslinger open tube and the Chevalier Jackson esophagoscope with full lumen are good examples of suitable instruments for this purpose (Fig. 6–2). They enable the various endoscopic operations (palpation, axial and lateral mobilization, cutting up, turning, and orientation of the foreign body) to be carried out under good conditions for stability and free maneuverability. The different diameters and lengths of the instruments make operation possible regardless of the location of the obstruction or the age of the patient. The proximal cold-light illumination and magnifying glass of the Haslinger tube allow an excellent view, whereas the handle and rigid tube lend the necessary stability in the extraction of the foreign body.

Rigid Esophagoscope with Hopkins or Lumina Optics ("Universal" Storz or Wolf Model)

In 1958, K. Storz, a manufacturing company in Tüttlingen, Germany, introduced a "universal" esophagoscope (Heidelberg model). This long, rigid, open esophagoscope had the capacity for aspiration, inflation with air, photography, and cinematography through a magnifying optic system (Fig. 6–3). Between the date of its introduction and the general use of forward-viewing fiberscopes (1973 to 1975), this instrument allowed the precise endoscopic description of various esophageal lesions, including reflux esophagitis and Barrett's esophagus (Mounier-Kuhn and Gaillard, 1965; Savary, 1968a–c, 1970; Savary and Naef, 1976).

In addition to stability, the instrument's rigidity makes it possible to shift the axis of the esophagus. Thereby, one can maneuver mucosal lesions into view, which is important in performing precise and selective biopsies, especially in the sphincter regions. The rigid and angled biopsy forceps mounted on a wide-angled Hopkins optical system makes it possible to obtain large biopsy specimens, with an accuracy of 94% in malignant tumors (Savary and Rivier, 1971).

Because these endoscopes may also be used as an open tube, precise and safe endoscopic operations are possible. In view of their excellent instrumental accessories, the Storz and Wolf rigid esophagoscopes remain suitable for therapeutic and surgical endoscopy in adults as well as in children and for difficult diagnostic situations (esophageal diseases associated with food impaction). Because of the rigidity of the instruments, in approximately 2% of cases spondylosis or stiffness of the cervical spine make examination of the esophagogastric junction impossible (Savary and Rivier, 1971). In compensation, they always permit precise exploration of the oropharynx, the hypopharynx, the larynx, and the pharyngoesophageal junction, especially when pathology of these regions is present.

The main inconvenience related to the use of the rigid Storz or Wolf esophagoscope is the necessity for technical

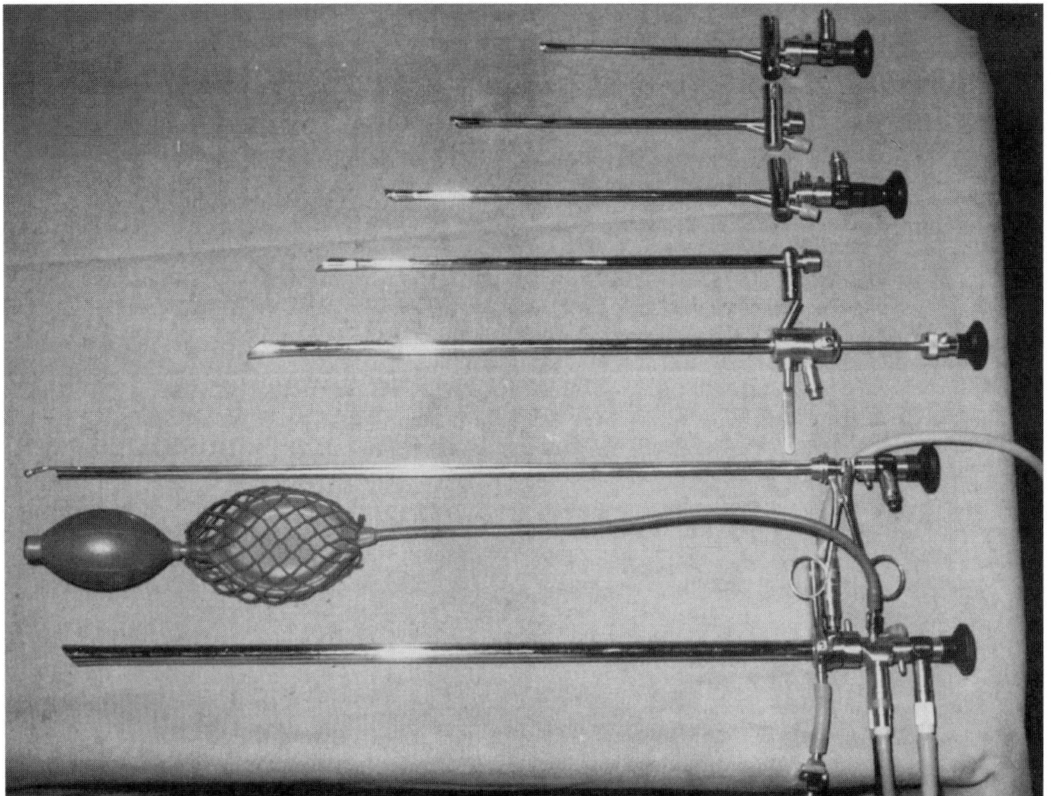

FIGURE 6–3 ■ "Universal" Storz esophagoscope. The tube is available in various diameters with corresponding instrumentational accessories.

training of the endoscopist and the requirement of general anesthesia for the patient. Therefore, in adults these instruments are reserved mainly for therapeutic and surgical endoscopy and for diagnostic exploration, when fiberoptic endoscopy has failed to achieve a precise and complete diagnosis. In addition, their optical qualities, their capacity to carry out large-sample, precise, and selective biopsy, and their ability to provide perfect exploration of the mouth, the pharynx, and the hypopharynx have made these instruments the most suitable for upper aerodigestive panendoscopy in the fields of oncology, traumatology, and congenital malformations (see later).

In infants and preschool children, rigid optical esophagoscopes remain the most convenient instruments for therapeutic purposes and for some diagnostic procedures as well.

PROCEDURES

To solve the various problems in diagnosis and therapy in both ambulatory and hospitalized patients of all ages, endoscopists must be able to utilize different methods. Most important is the selection of the best one for each individual patient and problem. The following points must be considered:

1. Indications for endoscopy.
2. Circumstances of the procedure (emergency endoscopy; perioperative endoscopy).
3. Difficulties that can be foreseen.
4. Age and general condition of the patient.

In accordance with these points, the endoscopist selects the type of examination room, equipment, type of anesthesia or sedation, appropriate positioning of the patient, and necessary instruments.

Rigid Esophagoscopy

Examination Room

Rigid esophagoscopes are surgical instruments devoted mainly to difficult diagnostic investigations and therapeutic procedures. They must be used exclusively in operating rooms set up for surgical endoscopy or in endoscopy units supplied with adequate equipment for general anesthesia, patient monitoring, resuscitation, and recovery.

Staff

The staff must be a surgical one, including an anesthetist, a fully instructed instrument nurse, an endoscopist, and an assistant who is in charge of positioning and stabilizing the patient. A clinical pathologist must be available.

Equipment

In addition to the equipment required for general anesthesia, monitoring of the patient, and resuscitation, the endoscopist must have available rigid endoscopes and fiberscopes of various sizes with the appropriate attachments and accessories for biopsy, cytologic and microbiologic sampling, removal of foreign bodies and food particles, sclerosing injections, esophageal dilatation, and tumor intubation. Optimally, equipment for photography and video recording should be on hand as well as a neodymium:yttrium-aluminum-garnet (Nd:YAG) and potassium titanyl phosphate (KTP) laser and an argon ion-pumped dye or a diode laser for photodynamic therapy. Performance of upper aerodigestive panendoscopy requires the use of laryngoscopes and bronchoscopes with solutions for vital stainings (toluidine blue and Lugol solution).

Patient Positioning and Examination Technique

The Chevalier Jackson method, described for rigid esophagoscopy, has never been improved upon (Jackson, 1915; Jackson and Jackson, 1934, 1950). The patient lies supine on a horizontal table. The head, neck, and upper thoracic area project beyond the table so that the cervical spine and upper thoracic spine are entirely free and can move unhindered during examination of the cardia (Fig. 6–4*A*). The head is held by an assistant, seated to the left of the patient, who is responsible for the progressive changes in the patient's position during the examination. During esophagoscope insertion, the patient's head is held high (neck flexed) with maximal atlanto-occipital extension, eliminating the angle between mouth and pharynx (Fig. 6–4*B*). As the instrument reaches the aortic narrowing, the patient's head and cervical spine are slowly lowered (Fig. 6–4*C*). While the cardia is examined, the head and neck are lowered again below the level of the table and slightly shifted to the right (Fig. 6–4*D* and *E*).

The endoscope is held with the right hand while the left hand keeps the patient's mouth open, the left thumb resting between instrument and upper teeth. The left thumb directs the distal end of the instrument while the right hand only supports its proximal end. The esophagoscope is introduced vertically, passing the right corner of the patient's mouth to the right amygdaloglossal sulcus. In this way, the gingivoglossal groove, the base of the tongue, the lingual valleculae, the epiglottis, the pharyngoepiglottic fold, the larynx, and the two piriform sinuses can be inspected from top to bottom. The left thumb is then used to slowly shift the distal end of the endoscope toward the median line, which brings the cricopharyngeal sphincter into view, transversally presenting its posterior lip. While the endoscopist is inflating the hypopharynx with air and applying a slight forward pressure with the left thumb, the cricopharyngeal sphincter can be passed without difficulty and the endoscope then drops into the esophagus under its own weight.

As soon as the cervical esophagus is reached, the position of the instrument is tilted to an angle of 45 degrees. If the patient's position is correct, one can, while inflating with air, recognize the upper cervicothoracic esophagus for a distance of about 10 cm, which is in the exact line of the esophagoscope. The humps of the posterior wall caused by the cervical vertebrae can be recognized. If there is a pronounced spondylosis, the endoscopy must be carried out with great care because during examination of the cardia the rigid tube becomes a lever resting on these spondylotic ridges (see Fig. 6–1). If abnormal resistance appears during advancement of the endoscope, the examination should be interrupted and continued with a fiberscope.

When the aortic narrowing is reached, the instrument is brought into a horizontal position. By inflating the esophagus with air, one can again recognize a 5- to 6-cm segment whose pulsatile movements on the anterior wall are due to the aortic arch and to the heart. The instrument, which had previously lain horizontally, then assumes an inclined position so that a direct view of the longer third of the esophagus is obtained.

The patient's neck and upper chest must now be below the level of the table ("high-low" of Chevalier Jackson) (see Fig. 6–4*D*). If this movement is not carried out correctly, the lumen can no longer be seen, as the instrument touches the rear wall of the esophagus. If both patient and instrument are in the correct position, the lower thoracic esophagus comes, with inflation, into view down to the cardia. To examine the esophagogastric junction, the endoscopist must guide the instrument around a curve toward the front and the left. Therefore, the patient's head and neck must be shifted to the right (see Fig. 6–4*A*). By inflating the distal esophagus with air, the endoscopist can carefully investigate the entire transitional zone—the lower esophageal sphincter, the Z line, and the esophageal hiatus.

During withdrawal of the endoscope, the same positions of the patient and movements of the endoscope must occur in reverse sequence. While looking for possible injuries, the endoscopist must pay special attention to the rear wall of the esophagus in the cervical segment and to the posterior lip of the cricopharyngeal sphincter.

Upper Aerodigestive Panendoscopy

Patients with head and neck cancer are at high risk for development of synchronous or metachronous carcinomas in the upper aerodigestive tract, such as in the esophagus and bronchi (Andrieu-Guitrancourt et al, 1975; Cachin, 1972; Cahan et al, 1976; Dargent et al, 1972; Derrick et al, 1980; Pradoura, 1981; Strigenz et al, 1987; Thompson et al, 1978; Vrabec, 1979; Warren and Gates, 1932). In western Europe, the 5-year cumulative risk for development of a second tumor in patients with head and neck cancer appears to be 30%, whereas the 5-year cumulative risk for development of a third tumor in patients with two cancers is 50% (Pasche et al, 1984; Savary et al, 1991). Most of the simultaneous second primary cancers are asymptomatic at the time of the first medical consultation. Therefore, upper aerodigestive panendoscopy has been proposed for patients with head and neck cancer as a workup and staging procedure before the first treatment is planned (Savary et al, 1979).

This oncologically oriented upper aerodigestive tract panendoscopy must provide a complete examination of the airway and of the upper digestive tract, which is lined with squamous mucosa. It is carried out in two steps:

1. For the mouth, pharynx, and larynx, a wall-fixed surgical microscope is used with an angled laryngeal mirror or a 90-degree optical (von Stuckrad) laryngoscope.

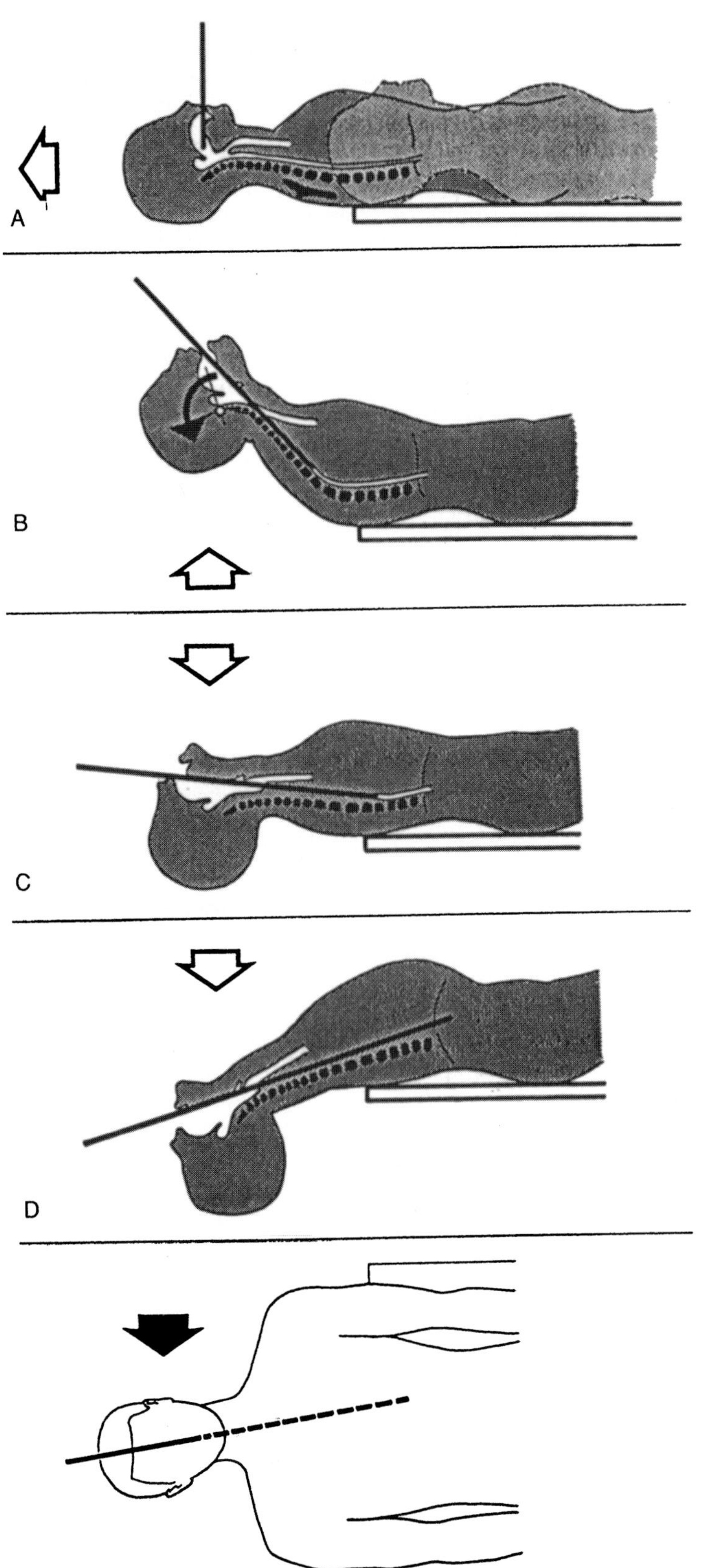

FIGURE 6–4 ■ Esophagoscopy with rigid instruments. *(A)*, Positioning of the patient: the upper part of the body projects beyond the table above the shoulder blades. *(B)*, Atlanto-occipital extension and cephalocervical elevation. *(C)*, Slow descent of head and neck to the horizontal plane. *(D)*, Further descent of head and neck below the horizontal plane. *(E)*, Displacement of head and neck to the right.

2. For the hypopharynx, esophagus, trachea, and bronchi, both rigid and fiberoptic endoscopes are used under general anesthesia (Savary et al, 1983).

For a careful oncologic exploration of the squamous mucosa of the upper digestive system, the rigid "universal" Storz or Wolf esophagoscope appears more suitable than a fiberscope; it permits (1) complete unfolding of the mucosa; (2) high-power exploration of the base of the tongue, the lingual valleculae, both sides of the epiglottis, the larynx, both piriform fossae, and the pharyngoesophageal junction; (3) precise application of vital staining with toluidine blue; and (4) selective and large biopsies. The screening power of upper digestive system rigid endoscopy using wide-angle optics, vital staining, and angled biopsy forceps mounted on Hopkins optics appears particularly suitable for oncologic purposes, provided that the endoscopist is fully aware of the endoscopic aspects of early oral, pharyngeal, and esophageal carcinomas (Endo et al, 1971; Monnier et al, 1981b).

In patients with head and neck cancer, oncologically oriented upper aerodigestive panendoscopy has been proposed as both a diagnostic and a surveillance procedure, at first during the pretherapy evaluation and later during the control evaluation 2 years after the initial treatment (Fig. 6–5). The detection rate of the pretherapy panendoscopy has been reported to be as high as 32% of the number of synchronous second tumors and 24% based on the number of affected patients (Brossard and Monnier, 1991). For 2-year control panendoscopy, the rate has been estimated at 19% based on the number of primary tumors and at 15% based on the number of affected patients (Pasche and Monnier, 1991). When performed in asymptomatic patients with normal otolaryngologic findings and normal chest x-ray and sputum cytology, the yield of 2-year control panendoscopy still reached 15% based on number of second primary tumors and 12% based on number of affected patients in the same clinical study (Pasche and Monnier, 1991).

In addition to oncologic applications, upper aerodigestive panendoscopy has proved useful for investigation of intrathoracic congenital malformations as well as in cases of cervical and thoracic trauma with mediastinal emphysema (Pasche and Monnier, 1990).

Pediatric Esophagoscopy

Despite the development of small-diameter fiberscopes, the rigid instrument remains the most suitable for diagnostic and therapeutic esophagoscopies in neonates, infants, and preschool children. General anesthesia with endotracheal intubation is necessary to prevent discomfort, to ensure immobility of the patient, and to maintain a perfect control of respiratory function. In children, the necessity of general anesthesia as well as the high flexibility of the cervicothoracic spine offsets the main advantages of the fiberscope for esophagoscopy. Thanks to the technical advances that have been made in rigid pediatric esophagoscopy (e.g., wide range of diameters, high optical quality, and capacity for aspiration, insufflation, photography, video recording, biopsy, removal of foreign bodies), exact diagnostic and therapeutic esophagoscopy can be performed even on premature babies. The examination technique is the same as that used for adults.

Perioperative Esophagoscopy

During surgery, esophagoscopy may be used to locate a lesion that cannot be palpated by the surgeon, to check an anastomosis, to introduce a feeding tube into the esophagus and stomach under direct vision, or to remove a foreign body. The method and the instrument are selected according to the surgical situation and the indications for esophagoscopy.

Fiberscope

Perioperative fiberscopy presents no difficulty regardless of the patient's position, and thus the fiberscope appears to be the most suitable instrument. The anesthetist places the endotracheal tube in the left corner of the patient's mouth and in the left amygdaloglossal sulcus and is responsible for maintaining sufficient curarization. With atlanto-occipital extension and raising of the head and neck, the fiberscope is introduced with the right hand while the left hand moves the endotracheal tube toward the front with the help of a curved McIntosh spatula inserted into the hypopharynx. During the examination, one must be careful not to inflate with too much air, which may interfere with the surgeon's work in the abdomen.

Rigid Esophagoscope

Perioperative rigid esophagoscopy is much more difficult than fiberscopy for the anesthetist as well as for the surgeon. It is possible only if the patient is positioned accordingly, as discussed earlier. This technique must be

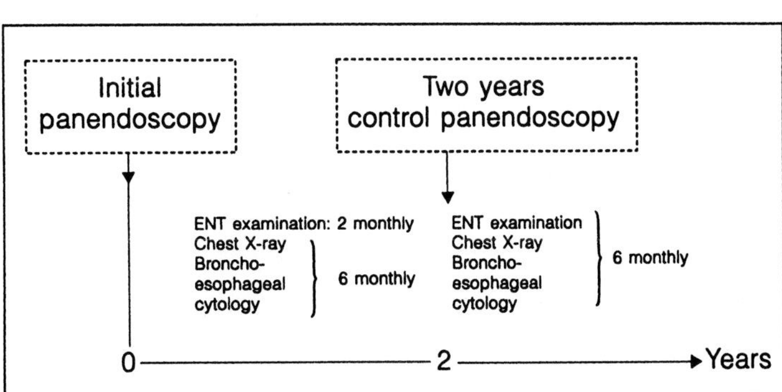

FIGURE 6–5 ■ Standard diagnostic and follow-up procedure for patients with head and neck cancer. ENT, ear-nose-throat.

used only in therapeutic maneuvers (e.g., extraction of a foreign body or difficult transanastomotic intubation under direct vision).

Retrograde Esophagoscopy

With the recent technical progress in esophageal dilatation, indications for retrograde esophagoscopy through a gastric stoma have practically disappeared. When performed with rigid endoscopes, retrograde esophagoscopy in the past presented major difficulties (Terracol, 1951; Tucker, 1924), which were eliminated by the introduction of the fiberscope with capacity for air inflation. After being introduced into the stomach, the fiberscope can easily be guided along the lesser curvature to the cardia and through it into the esophagus.

Mucosal Staining Methods

Lugol's Iodine Solution

When applied in vivo or in vitro to the esophageal squamous mucosa, 1.5% Lugol's solution produces a brown stain as a result of storage of the iodine in the glycogen granules of normal squamous cells (Voegeli, 1966). This staining method has been proposed for detecting areas of gastric or columnar metaplasia, which do not stain and stand out clearly against the surrounding brown-stained esophageal mucosa (Mainguet and Savary, 1982). In contrast, areas of acanthotic hyperplasia (benign epithelial hyperplasia with high glycogen content) give a positive dark brown stain (Clemonçon, 1974).

The main indication for mucosal staining with Lugol is to demonstrate squamous dysplastic and carcinomatous changes in the esophageal mucosa. Unlike normal mucosa, dysplasia and intramucosal carcinoma do not take up the stain because of the lack of glycogen in undifferentiated squamous cells (Mainguet and Savary, 1982; Mandard et al, 1980; Mori et al, 1993; Voegeli, 1966).

Complications related to the use of Lugol's iodine solution during esophagoscopy remain hypothetical, provided that iodine hypersensitivity has been ruled out and that a total amount of 5 ml of a 3% aqueous solution is not exceeded (Mainguet and Savary, 1982).

Aqueous Toluidine Blue Solution

When applied on smooth surfaces of the squamous upper digestive mucosa (mouth, pharynx, esophagus), a 1% aqueous toluidine blue solution reveals zones of increased mitotic activity. This metachromatic stain of the thiazine group has the property of fixing itself on ribonucleic acid (RNA) and deoxyribonucleic acid (DNA) (Fontolliet and Monnier, 1991; Mainguet and Savary, 1982; Mashberg, 1981; Savary and Miller, 1978; Savary et al, 1983; Richart, 1963; Shedd et al, 1965; Strong et al, 1968; Vaughan, 1972). It penetrates a carcinomatous epithelium to a depth of about four to six epithelial layers (Monnier et al, 1981a).

The following steps must be taken to obtain an optimal result:

1. Abundant washing with 1% aqueous solution of acetic acid in order to attain mucolysis and to remove food residues.
2. Application of aqueous 1% toluidine blue solution for 1 minute on the mucosa to be stained.
3. Repeated washing and aspiration with 1% acetic acid solution until the excess stain is removed and the rinse liquid becomes clear.

False-positive responses are due to food particles, mucosal erosions, chronic inflammation, and ciliated respiratory epithelium. False-negative responses are limited to severe dysplasia with parakeratosis and submucosal tumoral extension (Fontolliet and Monnier, 1991; Monnier et al, 1981a). The main advantages of using toluidine blue staining during esophagoscopy performed for oncologic purposes are (1) to detect dysplastic or carcinomatous mucosal changes, (2) to clearly delineate the mucosal extension of a cancer, (3) to detect satellite carcinomatous lesions, and (4) to precisely indicate the sites for biopsy.

Biopsy of the Esophagus

The technique of esophageal biopsy depends on the endoscopic method used—rigid esophagoscopy or fiberscopy.

Rigid Esophagoscope

With the rigid esophagoscope, biopsy is performed by using an angled forceps mounted on a wide-angle Hopkins optical system. The biopsy specimens are large, can include the muscularis mucosae, and can be easily oriented. The basic rules for safety were specified long ago (Jackson and Jackson, 1950; Terracol, 1951):

1. Esophageal biopsies are performed only on previously recognized mucosal lesions. The combination of biopsy forceps with an optical system is indispensable. Blind suction biopsy should be avoided in the esophagus.
2. A submucosal process may be sampled for biopsy only when it is causing a *recognizable* mucosal lesion.
3. Biopsy of macroscopically healthy mucosa must be performed with care (because of the risk of tearing). The same holds true for mucosal scars, corrosive injuries, or areas of radiotherapy.

The technique of esophageal biopsy is based on the fact that the success of a biopsy depends on the site of origin. Thus, the biopsy site must be selective. This implies the following:

1. One must examine the lesion at a distance while avoiding contact with the endoscope, which may produce bleeding. The lesion must be "prepared" (to eliminate retained food and necrotic tissue); the esophagus should be washed out, tamponaded (if it is bleeding), and inflated.
2. After the biopsy site has been precisely determined, endoscopic contact is made with the lesion.
3. Stability between the mucosal lesion and the biopsy forceps is then established. This condition is always fulfilled when rigid instruments are used in patients under general anesthesia and curarization but may be difficult to achieve when fiberscopes are used.

4. The mucous membrane is pushed into the mouth of the esophagoscope by the higher intrathoracic pressure related to general anesthesia, and an exact selective biopsy can be performed.

A single biopsy sample, precisely taken, should be sufficient with use of the rigid instrument. For malignant tumors, the success rate is 90% for the first specimen taken; the second specimen increased the positive result by only 2% in a series of 447 consecutive cases. In this same series, esophageal biopsy with the rigid instrument produced only two complications (bleeding), with no perforations and no deaths (Savary and Miller, 1978).

Fiberscope

With fiberscopes, the flexible biopsy forceps introduced through a flexible instrument in a conscious patient makes the problem of stability more difficult. The biopsy specimens are smaller and rarely include submucosal tissue. Whereas multiple biopsies give no better results with rigid instruments, 4 to 10 samples must be taken from any lesion when fiberscopes are used (Kumagai and Makuuchi, 1987). Even when the basic rules for efficiency are observed, the rate of success for fiberoptic esophageal biopsy usually ranges between 75% and 85% in cases of malignant tumors (Vilardell, 1972). However, the risk of complications is very low when traditional forceps are used with fiberscopes.

Cytology

After the oral cavity, the esophagus is the part of the gastrointestinal tract that is most suitable for cytologic examination (Prolla and Kirsner, 1972). In cases of esophageal carcinoma, the accuracy of the cytologic examination is as high as 90% (Vilardell, 1974). However, because endoscopic biopsy has a success rate of over 90% for malignant tumors, cytology is rarely used in practice.

During esophagoscopy, material for cytologic studies can be productively obtained by using a gauze swab or by direct brushing of the lesion (Berci, 1976; Vilardell, 1974). The brush is then withdrawn just into the tip of the suction channel. The endoscope with brush in place is removed from the patient, and the brush is immediately streaked onto the slide, which is washed out in a 65% alcohol solution. With the rigid esophagoscope, the same technique is used with a swab (Debray et al, 1959).

Cytologic examination has proved to be helpful in Barrett's esophagus when it is associated with stricture. The area at risk for adenocarcinoma is usually located at the distal end and below the stricture (Robey et al, 1988; Savary and Miller, 1978).

When used as a screening method for early detection of esophageal cancer, exfoliative cytologic material is usually sampled without endoscopy with either a nylon brush inside a standard nasogastric tube (Dowlatsahi et al, 1985) or an encapsulated sponge attached to a thread (Greenebaum et al, 1984; Pasche et al, 1991; Shu Yi-Jing, 1983). When used in the course of a screening program for high-risk esophageal cancer (high-risk geographic areas for esophageal cancer, patients primarily treated for ear-nose-throat cancer, patients with Barrett's esophagus), the value of esophageal exfoliative cytology has been well established (Dowlatsahi et al, 1985; Greenebaum et al, 1984; Geisinger et al, 1992; Pasche et al, 1991; Shu Yi-Jing, 1983).

Endoscopic Hemostasis

The necessity for hemostasis may arise (1) when hemorrhage is caused by an endoscopic procedure (biopsy, polypectomy, sclerotherapy) or (2) when spontaneous bleeding occurs (varices, ulcers, malignant tumor).

Before any endoscopic operation, coagulation time must be determined if the patient's history gives a reason to suspect a bleeding disorder. The rules concerning esophageal biopsy and endoscopic tumor resection must be observed because there is no guarantee that hemorrhage can be controlled endoscopically, no matter which instrument is used.

The open-tube rigid esophagoscope allows:

1. Efficient clearance of blood with large suction tubes.
2. Removal of blood clots.
3. Introduction of a vasocontrictive swab with epinephrine solution.
4. When necessary, use of bipolar electrocoagulation, an Nd:YAG laser, or sclerotherapy with 1% ethoxysclerol (3 ml maximum dose) injected as close as possible to the point of bleeding.

In case of failure, local tamponade is applied and the patient is prepared for operation and surgical control.

Endoscopic Treatment of Esophageal Tumors

Small, benign esophageal mucosal and submucosal tumors, such as papillomas, granulomatous polyps, fibromas, lipomas, granular cell tumors, or cysts, can be resected by using large biopsy forceps, electrosurgical snares, or diathermy loops. After biopsy, they can also be destroyed with the Nd:YAG or KTP laser. In all instances, submucosal injection of an isotonic saline solution is advised to expand the distance between the tumor and the muscular layer.

For lesions arising within the muscular layer, such as myomas, the endoscopic resection always involves a risk for esophageal perforation because the esophagus has no serosa (Jackson and Jackson, 1950). However, when they develop in the submucosal layer (small, pedunculated, or largely protruding tumors), endoscopic resection of myomas with an electrical snare after dissection with an electrosurgical cutter has been proposed (Kumagai and Makuuchi, 1987).

In the case of malignant tumors, the conventional therapy is surgical resection with or without radiation therapy or chemotherapy. These radical procedures, however, carry a certain rate of morbidity and mortality and may even be proscribed in patients with limited cardiac and pulmonary functions. This consideration led to the development of several minimally invasive and nonmutilating endoscopic techniques, such as (1) *argon plasma coagulation,* (2) *multipolar electrocoagulation,* (3) *mucosec-*

tomy, and (4) *photodynamic therapy.* Each of these therapies can easily be performed on an outpatient basis.

The main interest in using these new modalities is the cure of early superficial carcinomas, which do not invade the muscularis mucosae, and of the premalignant changes associated with Barrett's esophagus. In contrast, their application in the palliation of bulky obstructing and invasive malignancies has shown no significant benefit, compared with other standard modalities, such as endoprosthesis and thermal Nd:YAG laser vaporization.

Argon Plasma Coagulation

Argon plasma coagulation (APC) is a noncontact thermal modality in which energy is transmitted to the tissue through ionized argon gas. This technique involves (1) an argon gas source, (2) a high-frequency generator needed for ionization of argon and coagulation of the target tissue, and (3) a probe with an applicator to direct the gas flow and the electrical current to the lesion through the operating channel of a flexible endoscope.

Because of an electrically insulating steam layer that causes the argon plasma to move automatically to another point of the tissue surface, this modality has the theoretical advantage of inducing a homogeneous and controllable penetration depth varying from 0.5 to 3.0 mm, according to the parameters of application (Farin and Grund, 1994).

On the basis of clinical experience accumulated so far, it appears that the most relevant indication for the application of argon plasma coagulation is the treatment of intestinal metaplasia and dysplasia associated with Barrett's esophagus. The modality must be applied in a long-term, acid-controlled environment in order to achieve a squamous restoration of the esophageal epithelium. Moreover, the dose of the acid suppression medication seems to play an important role in the rate of a durable mucosal re-epithelialization.

Van Laethem and colleagues (1998) and Byrne and coworkers, (1998) reported on 31 and 30 patients, respectively, with histologically confirmed Barrett's mucosa treated with argon plasma coagulation in combination with continuous antireflux therapy at standard doses (omeprazole, 10 to 40 mg/day). Eradication of Barrett's esophagus was achieved in only 61% and 70%, respectively, of patients because of the presence of residual Barrett's glands underneath the newly formed squamous epithelium. In contrast to these findings, Schultz and coworkers (2000) described 73 patients who underwent ablation of Barrett's esophagus using argon plasma coagulation in combination with intensive, high-dose acid-suppressive medication (omeprazole, 40 mg 3 times a day). Complete squamous regeneration with no relapse was achieved in all but one of the cases after a mean of two sessions and a mean follow-up period of 12 months. Because it is not known whether regenerated squamous epithelium is stable over longer follow-up periods, a regular schedule of endoscopic surveillance should be recommended after ablation of Barrett's esophagus.

Multipolar Electrocoagulation

Multipolar electrocoagulation (MPEC) has been used in combination with antiacid medication for the treatment of Barrett's esophagus. Sharma and coauthors (1999) reported their results in 11 patients who all had an initial complete response with no evidence of Barrett's mucosa endoscopically and histologically after a mean of 9.5 sessions. At the time of their last evaluation (mean follow-up, 36 months), however, three patients showed a relapse of intestinal metaplasia.

The major concern with this contact technique is to achieve a homogeneous ablation, because the depth of injury is difficult to determine as it depends on multiple factors, such as the amount of energy delivered, the force of application, and the duration of contact.

Mucosectomy

Endoscopic mucosal resection (EMR) represents an important advance in both diagnostic and therapeutic measures for superficial malignant and premalignant esophageal lesions. This technique has the specific advantage over other endoscopic methods of providing tissue specimens for histologic analysis, including confirmation of lateral security margins and depth of tumor invasion.

Several techniques have been developed using the principles of first lifting, then sectioning the lesion. Inoue and associates (1993) proposed the *cap-fitted procedure,* consisting of a cap inserted at the tip of an endoscope. Once suctioned into the cap, the lesion is captured and snared tightly by a snare device inserted through the biopsy channel of the endoscope. Resection of the mucosal lesion is then performed with high-frequency electrocautery.

Nijhawan and Wang (2000) described a technique using a barbed snare inserted through one of the channels of an endoscope and placed around the elevated region while a grasping forceps, introduced through the other channel, is used to pull the lesion into the snare loop. The resulting bulk is then removed by standard electrocautery and retrieved.

Both techniques involve injection of physiologic saline solution into the submucosa in order to separate the target lesion from the underlying layer and thus prevent damage to the muscularis propria and minimize thermal trauma. Furthermore, this procedure has a prognostic value, since inability to elevate the mucosa raises suspicion of deeper invasion of the lesion. Despite relatively short follow-up periods and a small number of patients, these methods are associated with encouraging preliminary clinical results, especially for early cancer and high-grade dysplasia in patients with Barrett's esophagus (Ell et al, 2000; Takeshita et al, 1997).

The aforementioned techniques produce the so-called piecemeal resection, which yields only relatively small pieces with a mean size of 1.5 cm in diameter. Therefore, correct identification and orientation of the multiple pieces of a resected specimen by the pathologist are difficult to achieve. Moreover, in the case of extended superficial lesions, there is a potential risk of perforation because the muscularis propria may be damaged by repeated resections performed in the same area. These techniques also have the disadvantage of requiring multiple sessions. It is, however, important to perform a complete ablation of the lesion in one session because scarring

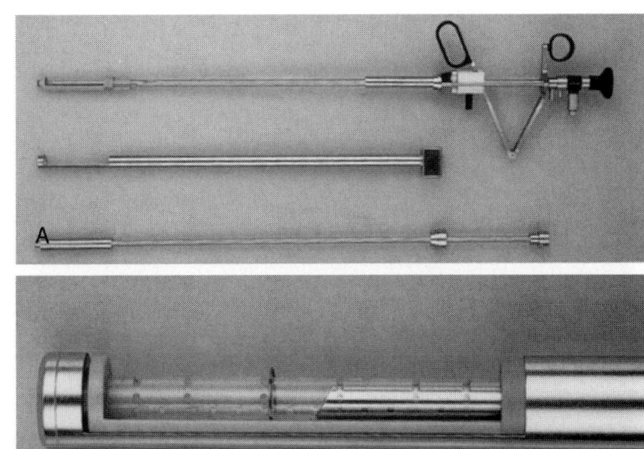

FIGURE 6–6 ■ Prototype of rigid esophagoscope for mucosectomy. *A (top),* The instrument consists of three pieces: (1) the outer tube (middle), (2) the inner tube with obturator (bottom), and (3) the resection device (top). *B,* Close-up view of the resection device (plastic window with holes, resection wire loop) inside the outer tube. The 30-degree angulated telescope is also visible.

may induce adherences to the muscular layer, thus making other resection attempts more difficult.

In an effort to overcome these drawbacks, our group has been evaluating a promising new method of mucosectomy based on the use of a modified rigid esophagoscope, allowing the resection of a single mucosal specimen of several square centimeters in size (Fig. 6–6). The instrument consists of an outer tube 17 mm in diameter at the distal end of which a window of 6 cm in length over 200 degrees has been cut out. The dimension of the window can vary according to the size of the lesion to be resected. Introduction of the outer tube in the esophagus is achieved under visual control with an inner tube and a zero-degree straightforward telescope.

Once at the level of the lesion, the inner tube is removed and replaced by the resectoscope. It consists of a transparent window and a resection wire loop that can be moved from the distal toward the proximal part of the window. An angulated 30-degree telescope attached to the resectoscope allows side viewing through the window and accurate targeting of the lesion. Suction is then turned on, creating a negative pressure within the resection device and thus allowing the mucosa to be aspirated through the holes drilled into the window. The wire loop is connected to a high-frequency surgical device that permits resection of the mucosa. The space between the window and the wire loop is chosen precisely (~1 mm), corresponding to a depth of resection that does not damage the muscular layer.

The wire loop is thin enough (0.3 mm) to minimize the thermal damage. Once mucosal ablation is completed, the resectoscope is removed from the esophagus together with the outer tube under continuous suction to keep the resected mucosal piece attached to the window. Macroscopic and histologic results in a sheep animal model show that mucosectomy using a rigid esophagoscope is feasible and safe and permits the resection of about 10 cm^2 in a single piece of tissue (Grosjean, 1998). An endoscopic view of the sheep esophagus before and after mucosectomy is presented in Figure 6–7. Figure 6–8 shows an esophageal specimen resected with our technique. Up to now, we have performed, overall, more than 100 mucosectomies in the animal model with reproducible results in terms of accurate histologic depth of the resected specimens without occurrence of perforation. Therefore, we feel very confident of an imminent application of this method in a clinical study.

All these new ablative procedures need to be further assessed in precisely controlled and randomized long-term studies, including large numbers of patients before they can be considered as a treatment alternative in early superficial esophageal cancers. Avoidance of complications, such as perforation and stenosis, is another aspect that has to be achieved (Yoshida et al, 1995).

Although the occurrence of perforation depends, in part, on the endoscopist's skills, stenosis is a common result of large circumferential resected areas, as required in Barrett's esophagus. This problem might be solved by using additional therapies that have the potential to bring about a more satisfying result. Ohmura and co-workers (1998) reported on the successful use of a temporary stenting that could be easily removed after a short period of time. At the time of resection, topical application of mitomycin-C, an antimetabolite that inhibits fibroblast proliferation and angiogenesis, has shown promising effects on laryngeal and tracheal stenosis. Thus, it might also be an interesting option in preventing stricture formation in the esophagus (Rahbar et al, 2001).

Photodynamic Therapy

The principle of photodynamic treatment is the sensitization of tumor cells to a light beam with a dye or photosensitizer. The interaction of the light beam and the dye in the tumor cells leads to their destruction. This type of therapy is used essentially for the treatment of early carcinomas of the esophagus (in situ and microinvasive squamous cell carcinomas), in which the malignant infiltration does not extend beyond the lamina muscularis mucosae and the risk of distant metastasis is very low (Endo et al, 1986). There is no interest in the use of phototherapy for palliative therapy of infiltrating and obstructive tumors of the esophagus. In fact, in these cases, relief of obstruction by vaporization with an Nd:YAG laser or tumor intubation by a prosthesis gives the best results.

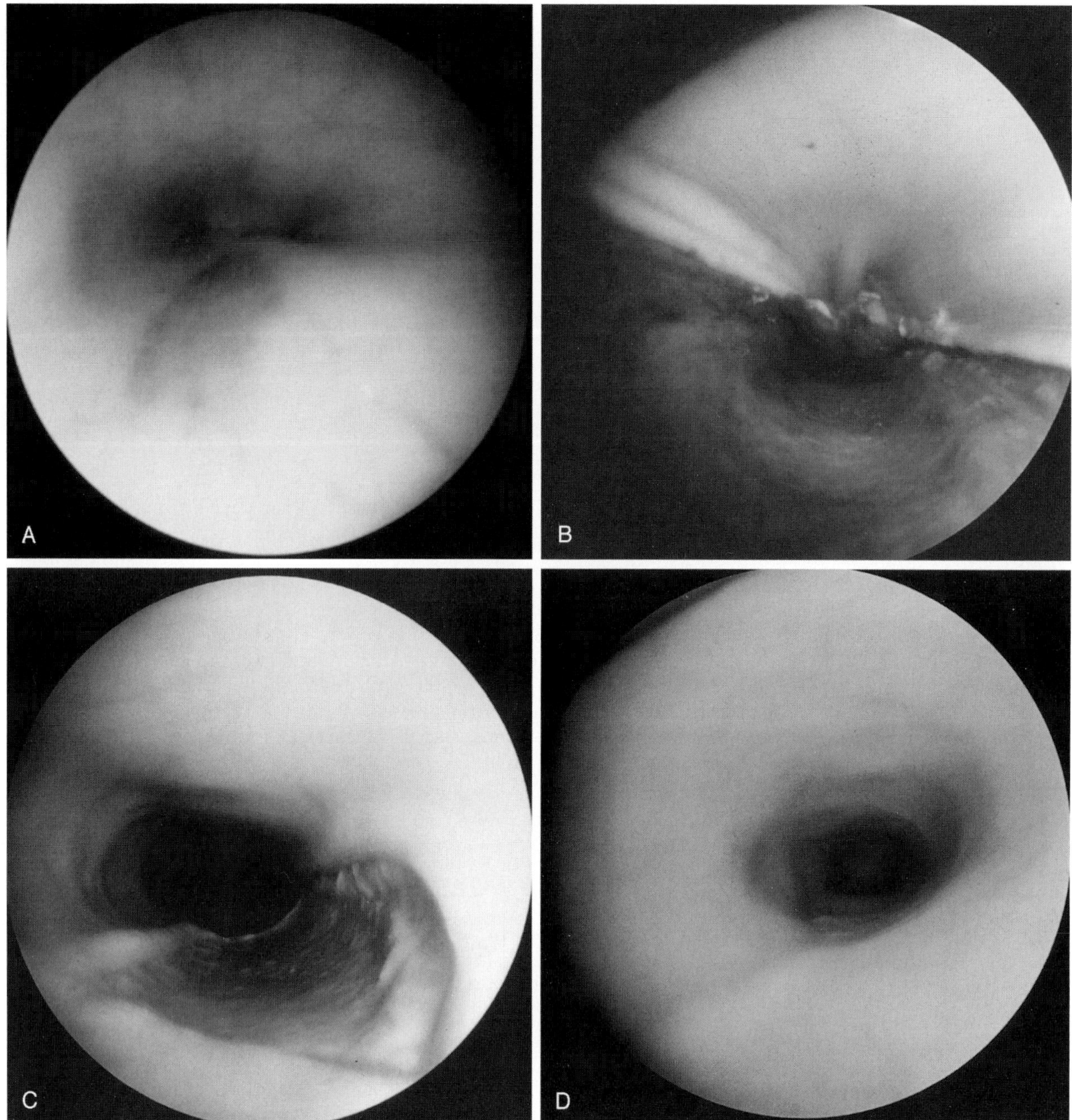

FIGURE 6–7 ■ Endoscopic view of a sheep esophagus before and after mucosal resection with a modified rigid esophagoscope. *A,* Before resection. An artificially stained area is seen on the esophageal wall. *B,* Immediately after resection. The resected area corresponds exactly to the size of the window. *C,* One month after resection. Partial re-epithelialization of the initially ulcerated area is seen. *D,* Two months after resection. Complete re-epithelialization of the resected area and a small scar are visible.

Photodynamic therapy should be prescribed only by agreement of a team that includes surgeons, oncologists, and radiotherapists. At the time of therapy, the photosensitizer, usually a porphyrin derivative, is injected intravenously some hours or days before the irradiation (Savary et al, 1993). The light is produced by an argon laser connected to cylinders with an irradiation window of 180 to 240 degrees (Wagnières et al, 1990). These irradiators are introduced into the esophagus orally and allow therapy of the tumors, which can be hemicircumferential and extend for up to 5 cm. The duration of the irradiation is 10 to 30 minutes.

Side effects and complications are linked to the lack of selectivity of the photosensitizer and are due essentially to the photosensitivity of the skin to sunlight (from 6 weeks to 3 months, depending on the photosensitizer used) and stenoses of the esophagus or esophagobronchial fistula (Monnier et al, 1990).

Between September 1984 and March 2001, we treated 19 in situ carcinomas and 33 microinvasive squamous cell carcinomas, for a total of 52 early carcinomas of the esophagus. The overall success rate was 75% (39 of 52 cases). The results are significantly better for in situ carcinomas with a complete cure in 17 of 19 (90%)

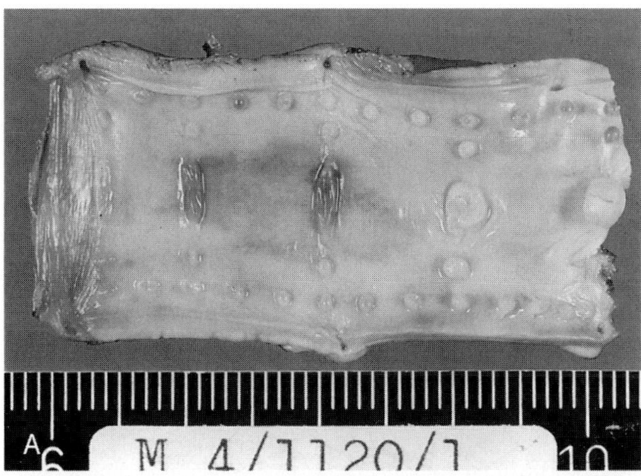

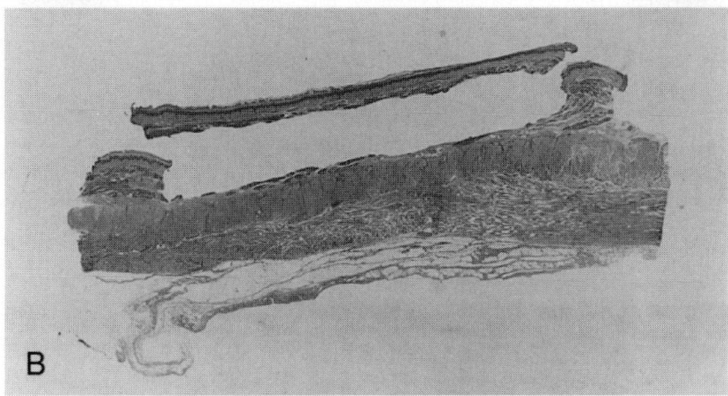

FIGURE 6–8 ■ Esophageal specimen after mucosal resection. *A,* Macroscopic view. The artificially stained area is totally removed in a single piece. The visible blebs are due to the suction of the mucosa through the holes of the window of the resection device. *B,* Histologic view of the mucosal specimen and the corresponding resected area of the esophageal wall. The section is performed precisely at the junction between the submucosa and the inner layer of the muscularis propria.

patients as compared to microinvasive carcinomas with a complete cure rate of 66% (22 of 33 cases). The mean follow-up is 28 months.

In addition to esophageal mucosectomy (Inoue and Endo, 1990), photodynamic therapy may represent an alternative treatment for early carcinomas of the esophagus in patients in poor general condition.

■ REFERENCES

Andrieu-Guitrancourt J, Brossard-Legrand M, Happich J, et al: Endoscopie systématique de l'oesophage au cours des cancers buccaux, pharyngés et laryngés. Ann Otolaryngol Chir Cervicofac 92:659, 1975.

Berci G: Endoscopy. Appleton & Lange, East Norwalk, CT, 1976.

Bevan L: The esophagoscope. Lancet 1:470, 1868.

Brossard E, Monnier P: The contribution of panendoscopy in the pretherapeutic screening of bucco-pharyngo-esophageal cancer. Acta Endosc 21:599, 1991.

Brossard E, Ollyo J-B, Monnier P: Foreign bodies in the esophagus: Diagnosis and treatment. Acta Endosc 21:655, 1991.

Byrne JP, Armstrong GR, Attwood SE: Restoration of the normal squamous lining in Barrett's esophagus by argon beam plasma coagulation. Am J Gastroenterol 93:1810, 1998.

Cachin Y: Cancers multiples concomitants des voies aéro-digestives supérieures. J Fr Otorhinolaryngol 3:667, 1972.

Cahan WG, Castro B, Rosen PP, et al: Separate primary carcinomas of the esophagus and head and neck region in the same patient. Cancer 37:85, 1976.

Clemençon G, Gloor R: Benign epithelial hyperplasia of the esophagus. Endoscopy 6:214, 1974.

Dargent M, Hoel P, Pierluca P: Résultats d'une étude nécropsique de la muqueuse oesophagienne chez des sujets ayant présenté des cancers de la sphère ORL. Bull Acad Natl Med (Paris) 156:408, 1972.

Dawson J, Cockel R: Oesophageal perforation at fiberoptic gastroscopy. Br Med J 283:583, 1981.

Debray C, Hardouin JP, Deporte A, et al: Le procédé de la mèche: Technique de cytodiagnostic des épithéliomas de l'oesophage. Arch Fr Mal App Dig 48:335, 1959.

Derrick JH, Wagenfeld FCS, Harwood AR: Second primary respiratory tract malignancies in glottic carcinoma. Cancer 16:1883, 1980.

Dowlatsahi K, Lester E, Bibbo M, et al: Brush cytology of the early detection of esophageal carcinoma among patients with upper aerodigestive malignancies. Laryngoscope 95:971, 1985.

Ell C, May A, Gossner L, et al: Endoscopic mucosal resection of early cancer and high-grade dysplasia in Barrett's esophagus. Gastroenterology 118:670, 2000.

Endo M, Kobayashi S, Susuki H, et al: Diagnosis of early esophageal cancer. Endoscopy 2:61, 1971.

Endo M, Takeshita K, Yoshibo M: How can we diagnose the early stage of esophageal cancer? Endoscopic diagnosis. Endoscopy 18:11, 1986.

Farin G, Grund KE: Technology of argon plasma coagulation with particular regard to endoscopic applications. Endosc Surg 2:71, 1994.

Fontolliet C, Monnier P: The histological reliability of vital staining with toluidine blue. Acta Endosc 21:617, 1991.

Geisinger KR, Teot LA, Richter JE: A complete cytopathologic and histologic study of atypia, dysplasia and adenocarcinoma in Barrett's esophagus. Cancer 69:8, 1992.

Greenebaum E, Schreiber K, Shu Y, et al: Use of esophageal balloon in the diagnosis of carcinomas of the head, neck, and upper gastrointestinal tract. Acta Endosc 28:9, 1984.

Grosjean P: La mucosectomie endoscopique oesophagienne: Étude préclinique. In Huber H (ed): Problèmes Actuels d'Otorhinolaryngologie. Bern, 1998, pp 293–302.

Hugonnet B, Monnier P, Savary M: Le traitement endoscopique palliatif du cancer de l'oesophage: Indications, modalités, résultats. Med Hyg 46:3074, 1988.

Inoue H, Endo M: Endoscopic esophageal mucosal resection using a transparent tube. Surg Endosc 4:198, 1990.

Inoue H, Takeshita K, Hori H, et al: Endoscopic mucosal resection with a cap-fitted panendoscope for esophagus, stomach, and colon mucosal lesions. Gastrointest Endosc 39:58, 1993.

Jackson C: Peroral endoscopy and Laryngeal Surgery. St. Louis, The Laryngoscope Company, 1915.

Jackson C, Jackson CL: Bronchoesophagology. Philadelphia, WB Saunders, 1950.

Jackson C, Jackson CL: Bronchoscopy, Esophagoscopy, and Gastroscopy. Philadelphia, WB Saunders, 1934.

Kumagai Y, Makuuchi H: Practical Fiberoptic Esophagoscopy. Tokyo, Igaku-Shoin, 1987.

Kussmaul J: Ueber Magenspiegelung. Verh Med Wochenschr 12:271, 1870.

Mainguet P, Savary M: Practical Applications of Mucosal Staining in Digestive Endoscopy. Brussels, SmithKline, 1982.

Mandard AM, Tourneux J, Gignoux M, et al: In situ carcinoma of the esophagus: Macroscopic study with particular reference to the Lugol test. Endoscopy 12:51, 1980.

Mashberg A: Tolonium (toluidine blue) rinse—a screening method for recognition of squamous carcinoma (continuing study of oral cancer IV). JAMA 245:2408, 1981.

Mikulicz J: Ueber Gastroskopie und Oesophagoskopie. Zentralbl Chir 43:673, 1981.

Monnier P, Savary M, Fontolliet C, et al: Photodetection and photodynamic therapy of "early" squamous cell carcinomas of pharynx, oesophagus and tracheobronchial tree. Laser Med Sci 5:149, 1990.

Monnier P, Savary M, Pasche R: Contribution of toluidine blue to bucco-pharyngo-esophageal cancerology. Acta Endosc 11:299, 1981a.

Monnier P, Savary M, Pasche R, et al: Intraepithelial carcinoma of the oesophagus: Endoscopic morphology. Endoscopy 13:185, 1981b.

Mori M, Adachi Y, Matsushima T, et al: Lugol staining pattern and histology of esophageal lesions. Am J Gastroenterol 88:701, 1993.

Mounier-Kuhn P, Gaillard J: La Pathologie de Reflux Gastrooesophagien. Oesophagites et Stenoses Peptiques. Paris, Arnette, 1965.

Nijhawan PK, Wang KK: Endoscopic mucosal resection for lesions with endoscopic features suggestive of malignancy and high-grade dysplasia within Barrett's esophagus. Gastrointest Endosc 52:328, 2000.

Ohmura K, Nagashima R, Takeda H, Takahashi T: Temporary stenting with metallic endoprosthesis for refractory esophageal stricture secondary to cylindrical resection of carcinoma. Gastrointest Endosc 48:214, 1998.

Pasche P, Monnier P: Is 2-years control panendoscopy justified in head and neck cancer patient? Acta Endosc 21:623, 1991.

Pasche P, Monnier P: La place de l'endoscopie ORL dans le bilan des malformations trachéo-bronchiques. In Aktuelle Probleme der Otorhinolaryngologie. Bern, Hans Huber AG, 1990.

Pasche P, Pellissier S, Gloor E, et al: The contribution of bronchial and esophageal cytology in the follow-up of head and neck cancer. Acta Endosc 21:631, 1991.

Pasche R, Savary M, Monnier P: Le risque de seconde localisation tumorale chez le porteur d'un cancer de la bouche, du pharynx et du larynx. In Aktuelle Probleme der Otorhinolaryngologie. Bern, Hans Huber AG, 1984.

Pradoura JP: L'Oesophage du Cancéreux ORL. Marseille, France, Institute Paoli-Calmettes, 1981.

Prolla JC, Kirsner BJ: Handbook and Atlas of Exfoliative Cytology. Chicago, University of Chicago Press, 1972.

Rahbar R, Shapshay SM, Healy GB: Mitomycin: Effects on laryngeal and tracheal stenosis, benefits, and complications. Ann Otol Rhinol Laryngol 110:1, 2001.

Richart RM: A clinical staining test for the in vivo delineation of dysplasia and carcinoma in situ. Am J Obst Gynecol 86:703, 1963.

Robey SS, Hamilton SR, Gupta PK, et al: Diagnostic value of cytopathology in Barrett esophagus and associated carcinoma. Am J Clin Pathol 88:493, 1988.

Savary M: L'endobrachy-oesophage (esophagus lined with columnar epithelium): À propos de 43 observations endoscopiques. Ther Umschau 28:148, 1970.

Savary M: Les hernies hiatales compliquées: endoscopie: Importance du prélèvement histologique dans le bilan préthérapeutique. Med Hyg 26:799, 1968a.

Savary M: Les hernies hiatales non compliquées: endoscopie: Maladie peptique oesophagienne et gastrites herniaires. Med Hyg 26:789, 1968b.

Savary M: L'aspect endoscopique du vestibule gastro-oesophagien. ORL Otorhinolaryngol Relat Spec 1968c.

Savary M, Crausaz PH, Monnier P: La place de l'endoscopie totale aérodigestive supérieure en cancérologie. Schweiz Med Wochenschr 109:838, 1979.

Savary M, Miller G: The Esophagus: Handbook and Atlas of Endoscopy. Solothurn, Switzerland, Gassmann AG, 1978.

Savary M, Monnier P, Pasche R: Les cancers oro-pharyngo-laryngés: Le bilan endoscopique. Helv Chir Acta 50:509, 1983.

Savary M, Monnier P, Pasche R, et al: Multiple primaries malignancies. In Advances in Otorhinolaryngology: Bearing of Basic Research on Clinical Otolaryngology. Bern, Karger AG, 1991.

Savary JF, Monnier P, Wagnières G, Fontolliet C: Preliminary clinical studies of photodynamic therapy with m-THPC as a photosensitizing agent for the treatment of early pharyngeal, esophageal, and bronchial carcinomas. SPIE Meeting Proceedings, Photodynamic Therapy of Cancer, 1993, Bellingham, WA.

Savary M, Naef AP: Le carcinome oesophagien "in situ." J Fr Otorhinolaryngol 25:669, 1976.

Savary M, Rivier A: Possibilités et limites de l'oesophagoscopie. Med Hyg 29:1658, 1971.

Schultz H, Miehlke S, Antos D, et al: Ablation of Barrett's epithelium by endoscopic argon plasma coagulation in combination with high-dose omeprazole. Gastrointest Endosc 51:659, 2000.

Schweizer V, Monnier P, Ollyo JB: The risk of perforation during rigid oesobronchoscopy. Acta Endosc 21:593, 1991.

Segal A, Willemot J: Naissance et développement de l'otorhinolaryngologie dans l'histoire de la médecine. Acta Otorhinolaryngol Belg 35:393, 1981.

Sharma P, Bhattacharyya A, Garewal HS, Sampliner RE: Durability of new squamous epithelium after endoscopic reversal of Barrett's esophagus. Gastrointest Endosc 50:159, 1999.

Shedd DP, Hukill PB, Bahn S: In vivo staining properties of oral cancer. Am J Surg 110:631, 1965.

Shu Yi-Jing H: Cytopathology of the esophagus: An overview of esophageal cytopathology in China. Acta Cytol 27:7, 1983.

Strigenz MA, Toohill RJ, Grossmann TW: Association of laryngeal and pulmonary malignancies: A continuing challenge. Ann Otol Rhinol Laryngol 96:621, 1987.

Strong MS, Vaughan CW, Incze J: Toluidine blue in the management of carcinoma of the oral cavity. Arch Otolaryngol 87:527, 1968.

Takeshita K, Tani M, Inoue H, et al: Endoscopic treatment of early oesophageal or gastric cancer. Gut 40:123, 1997.

Terracol J: Les Maladies de l'Oesophage. Paris, Masson, 1951.

Thompson WM, Oddson TE, Kelvin P, et al: Synchronous and metachronous squamous cell carcinomas of the head, neck, and esophagus. Gastrointest Radiol 3:123, 1978.

Tucker G: The Retrograde Esophagoscopy. Philadelphia, WB Saunders, 1924.

Van Laethem JL, Cremer M, Peny MO, et al: Eradication of Barrett's mucosa with argon plasma coagulation and acid suppression: Immediate and mid term results. Gut 43:747, 1998.

Vaughan CW: Supravital staining in early diagnosis of carcinoma. Otolaryngol Clin North Am 5:301, 1972.

Vilardell F: Exfoliative cytology. In Bockus HL (ed): Gastroenterology: Section II. The Esophagus. Philadelphia, WB Saunders, 1974.

Vilardell F: Cancer de l'oesophage. Arch Fr Mal Appl Dig 61:265, 1972.

Voegeli R: Die Schillersche Iodprobe in Rahmen der Oesophagus Diagnostik. ORL J Otorhinolaryngol Relat Spec 28:230, 1966.

Vrabec DP: Multiple primary malignancies of the upper aerodigestive system. Ann Otol Rhinol Laryngol 88:846, 1979.

Wagnières G, Monnier PH, Savary M, Van den Bergh H: Photodynamic therapy of early cancer in the upper aerodigestive tract and bronchi. Instrumentation and clinical results. SPIE Meeting Proceedings, Future Directions and Applications in Photodynamic Therapy, 1990, Bellingham, WA.

Waldenburg L: Oesophagoskopie. Klin Wochenschr 47:578, 1870.

Warren S, Gates O: Multiple primary malignant tumors: A survey of the literature and statistical study. Am J Cancer 16:1358, 1932.

Yoshida M, Hanashi T, Momma K, et al: Endoscopic mucosal resection for radical treatment of esophageal cancer. Jpn J Cancer Chemother 22:847, 1995.

FLEXIBLE ESOPHAGOSCOPY

Thomas W. Rice
Gregory Zuccaro, Jr.

Although esophagoscopy has been practiced for more than 130 years, it was not until the introduction of the flexible fiberoptic endoscope in the 1970s that esophagoscopy became a routine and practical investigation. Refinements in optics, imaging, and instrumentation have further increased its diagnostic and therapeutic capabilities. Esophagoscopy allows evaluation of symptoms, planned therapy, and treatment assessment. This is accomplished by luminal examination of the esophagus with direct evaluation of the mucosa and indirect appraisal of extramucosal structures. The potential for therapeutic esophagoscopy is limitless, and an ever-increasing number of procedures are being performed with the video esophagoscope. Flexible fiberoptic video esophagoscopy has nearly eliminated the need for rigid esophagoscopy.

INSTRUMENTS

A flexible fiberoptic video esophagoscope has five components: (1) the video camera, (2) the control section, (3) the insertion tube, (4) the bending section, and (5) the distal tip (Fig. 6–9). A miniature video camera attached to the flexible fiberoptic endoscope has revolutionized imaging, allowing further diagnostic and therapeutic advances. The control section, which houses the controls for deflection of the bending section and the suction and air insufflation/water irrigation valves, is approximately 0.3 meter long. The insertion tube, the bending section, and the distal tip, which are inserted into the patient, have an overall working length of approximately 1 meter. These sections house the optic bundles and the instrument-suction and air-water channels.

Optic bundles are two types: the *light guide* (LG) and the *optic guide* (OG). Light guide bundles are designed for maximal light transmission and are incapable of producing an image. Adequate illumination is provided by endoscopes with one light guide bundle. However, a second light guide bundle in specialized endoscopes produces a sharper, brighter image and minimizes instrument shadowing. Optic guide bundles transmit the image;

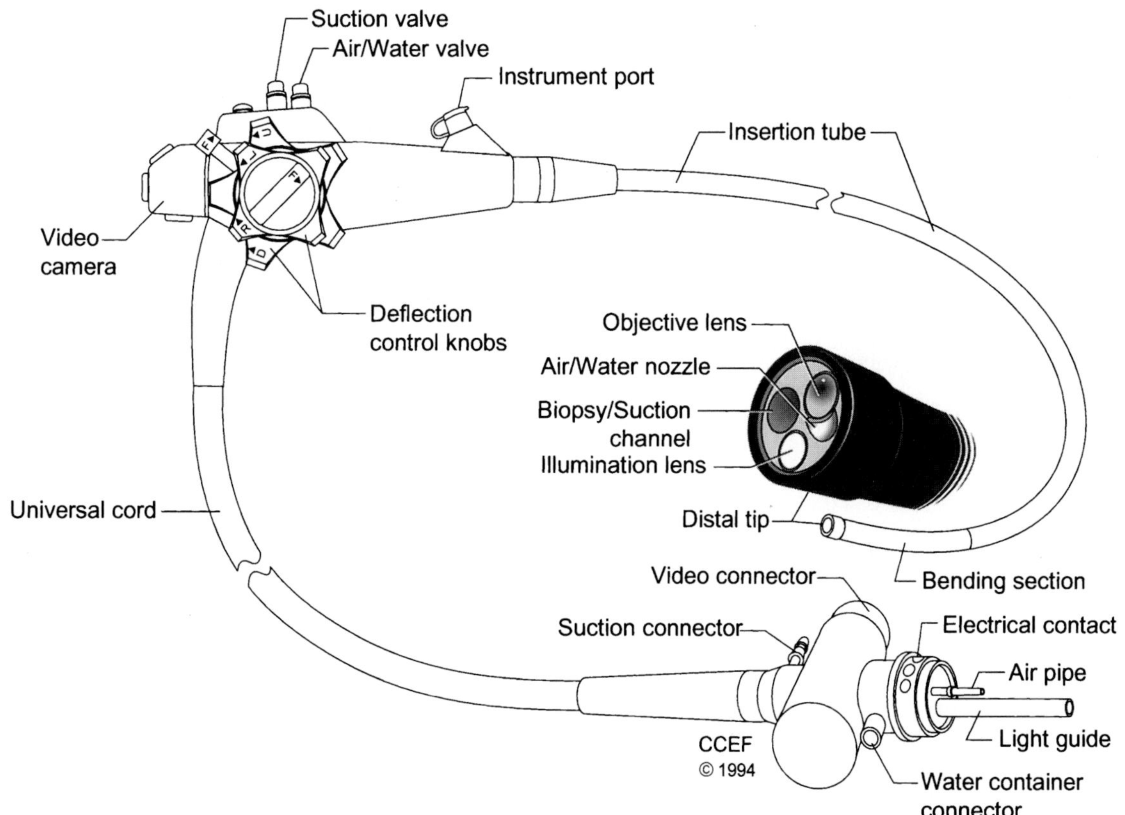

FIGURE 6–9 ■ Flexible fiberoptic videoscope. (Courtesy of Cleveland Clinic Foundation.)

its design characteristics determine the resolution of the endoscope (Chen and Kovacs, 1997).

The diameter of the insertion tube, the bending section, and the distal tip are determined by the size of the optic bundles and the channels. The outside diameter (OD) of the insertion tube of a pediatric endoscope is as little as 5.3 mm. In these units, the inside diameter (ID) of the instrument channel is usually 2 mm. This channel must be used for air, water, suction, and instrumentation. The OD of adult endoscopes ranges from 9 to 11 mm, and the ID of the instrument-suction channel is 2.2 to 2.8 mm. Generally, there is a separate channel for air and water. For therapeutic procedures, endoscopes of 12.8 mm OD with two instrument channels of 2.8 mm and 3.7 mm ID are available.

Forward-viewing endoscopes that provide a 120-degree field of vision are used for esophagoscopy. Depth of field is 3 to 100 mm. Objects closer than 3 mm to the distal tip are not in view; objects farther than 100 mm from the distal tip are not in focus. The bending section is capable of being deflected through 210 degrees in an upward direction, 90 degrees in a downward direction, and 100 degrees to the right or left. The direction of the distal tip deflection is respective to the control section of the endoscope when the insertion tube is straight.

Illumination is provided by a light source. Low-output halogen sources (150 W) are adequate for nonvideo systems. However, high-output xenon systems (300 W) are required for optimum examinations with video endoscopes. The light source also contains an air pump for pressurization of water irrigation and air insufflation systems. The universal cord connects the endoscope to the light source.

An ever-increasing number of endoscopic instruments are designed for use through the instrument channel of these endoscopes. An abbreviated list includes biopsy forceps, cytology brushes, aspiration needles, curets, retrieval forceps and baskets, magnetic extractors, polypectomy snares, coagulation electrodes, injection needles, guidewires, balloon catheters, suture cutters, scissors, and knives. A wide variety of dilators and expandable metal prostheses are available for management of esophageal strictures.

TECHNIQUE OF EXAMINATION

Esophagoscopy should be performed in an endoscopy suite designed for the use as well as the preparation and postprocedural care of the patient. Most endoscopic esophageal examinations may be conducted in the outpatient setting with the patient conscious and sedated. Preparation is crucial to ensure good outcome. The night before the procedure, the patient is instructed to take a light dinner and take nothing by mouth (NPO) after midnight if the examination is scheduled before noon. For an afternoon examination, a fluid breakfast may be taken early in the morning, after which the patient should remain on NPO status. Patients with achalasia should receive clear fluids 24 to 48 hours before the procedure. Those with significant emptying abnormalities may require esophageal lavage prior to a clear fluid restriction. Complex examinations should be performed early in the day. This allows time for adequate observation and management of any complications that may arise.

It is prudent that the endoscopist take an appropriate history, perform a pertinent physical examination, and review relevant investigations. The patient should receive detailed instructions to ensure full cooperation during the procedure and to allow informed consent to be given.

Before the procedure, a peripheral intravenous (IV) catheter is inserted. Before the examination of patients with valvular heart disease or implanted prosthetic material, prophylactic antibiotics are administered via the IV catheter. IV medication consisting of a narcotic analgesic and a minor tranquilizer (meperidine, 25 to 100 mg, and midazolam, 1 to 4 mg IV), provides sufficient sedation so that the patient is comfortable and cooperative but not stuporous or combative (Bianchi Porro et al, 1988; Carrougher et al, 1993). The indwelling IV catheter allows additional medication to be given if the initial dose is inadequate or if a prolonged procedure calls for further medication. If rapid reversal of sedation is required, IV access is crucial for the immediate administration of naloxone (0.4 mg) and flumazenil (0.2–1.0 mg) (Birkenfeld et al, 1989). These examinations are rarely performed without sedation. Topical anesthesia (4% lidocaine [Xylocaine Viscous] gargle or 1% topical spray) is optional.

Continuous monitoring of oxygen saturation (percutaneous), blood pressure (noninvasive), and electrocardiogram (ECG) is mandatory in all patients (Dark et al, 1990; Hayward et al, 1989). Supplemental oxygen should be delivered by nasal prongs.

A right-handed endoscopist holds the endoscope in the left hand. The junction of the universal cord and the control section hangs in the web space between the thumb and index finger. The left thumb is used to manipulate the "up" and "down" control knobs. Right and left deflection is accomplished by flexion and extension of the left wrist, rotation of the elbow, and raising or lowering the left shoulder. The "right-left" control knob is infrequently required for this deflection. The left index finger controls the upper valve (suction). Although the left index finger may also be used to operate the lower valve (air/water), it is practical to use the left middle finger to control this lower valve separately. The ring and little fingers of the left hand support the lower portion of the control section. The right hand is used to introduce and advance the endoscope and to manipulate instruments within the instrument channel.

Upper gastrointestinal (GI) endoscopy is performed with the patient in the left lateral decubitus position. It is best to introduce the endoscope under direct visualization. Using the videoscope enhances direct vision passage of the endoscope. *Blind passage* has distinct disadvantages and is more likely to result in injury to both endoscopist (bite injuries) and patient. Blind passage does not allow examination of the oropharynx, hypopharynx, or upper esophagus. With the patient's head flexed, the endoscope is placed on the posterior portion of the tongue. It is then visually guided into the posterior portion of the oropharynx, where the epiglottis is visualized. The endoscope is then passed over the epiglottis and larynx, where the piriform sinuses come into view. The vocal cords and their mobility should be routinely inspected.

Keeping the endoscope on the posterior pharyngeal wall and as close to the midline as possible, the patient is asked to swallow. This opens the cricopharyngeus, and the endoscope can be advanced through this rosette of tissue into the upper esophagus. If the endoscope cannot be passed into the esophagus, it is usually because the endoscope has been deflected into the left piriform sinus. By withdrawal of the endoscope into the hypopharynx, this maneuver may be attempted again. It is also possible to manipulate the endoscope tip out of the piriform sinus into the esophagus. This is accomplished by rotating the endoscope tip to the midline (to the right), dislodging it from the piriform sinus. If the patient is asked to swallow during this process, the endoscope can usually be advanced into the upper esophagus.

The cricopharyngeus and upper esophagus are the most difficult areas to examine. Careful viewing at the time the endoscope is removed adds to the initial observations seen at its insertion. Examination of the esophagus is carried out with air insufflation sufficient to distend the esophagus. Excessive insufflation causes patient discomfort, retching, or vomiting. Complete examination of the duodenum and stomach, with retroflexed inspection of the gastric cardia, should be included with every esophagoscopy.

It is preferable that the patient recover in a monitored setting. Once the sedation has worn off, the patient should be questioned concerning odynophagia, dysphagia, and chest pain. If these are present or if they occur within the next 24 to 48 hours, the physician who performed the procedure should be contacted immediately. The patient must be accompanied by and driven home by a companion.

ANATOMY

The esophagus begins at the cricopharyngeus and ends at the esophagogastric junction. In the adult, it is approximately 25 to 30 cm long. Because the normal esophagus is a relatively straight mucosal-lined muscular tube, it possesses no intrinsic markings and there are few extrinsic landmarks (Fig. 6–10) (see Color Plate). For recording purposes, endoscopic findings are measured as a distance in centimeters from the incisor teeth. The cricopharyngeus is encountered at 15 to 18 cm from the incisor teeth. The esophagus passes into the mediastinum at 18 to 20 cm.

The next landmark is the indentation of the anterior and left lateral wall of the esophagus produced by the aortic arch. This physiologic narrowing and the transmitted aortic pulsation are usually seen approximately 25 cm from the incisors. The left pulmonary hilum, which lies below the aortic arch, does not generally cause any recognizable extrinsic compression of the esophagus. Approximately 30 to 35 cm from the incisors, the pulsations of the left atrium are transmitted to the anterior esophageal wall. At 40 to 45 cm, the diaphragmatic hiatus is encountered. One can confirm this position by asking the patient to sniff or to perform a Valsalva maneuver that will cause the esophagus to be pinched by the contracting

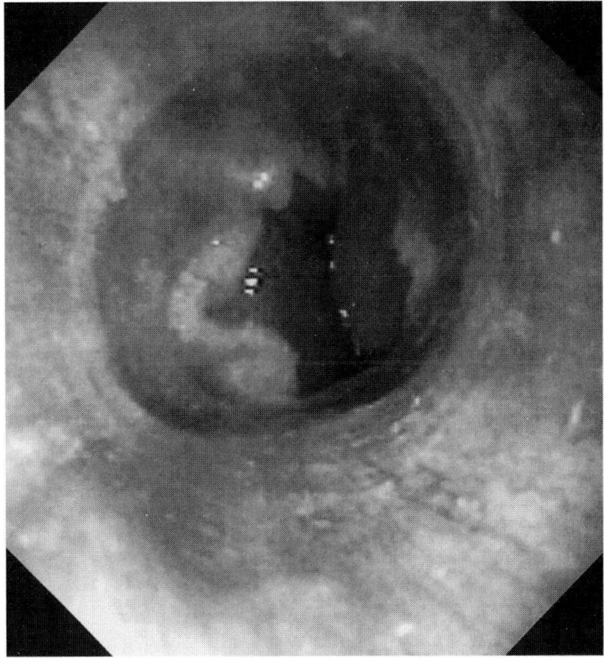

FIGURE 6–10 ■ Normal distal esophagus. (See Color Plate.)

diaphragm. The intra-abdominal portion of the esophagus is 1 to 3 cm long. Typically, it is not appreciated endoscopically. Immediately after the endoscope passes through the diaphragm, the stomach is entered. The lower esophageal sphincter (LES) is not identifiable at esophagoscopy.

The esophageal lumen can be distended to 2 cm in anterior-posterior (AP) diameter and 3 cm in lateral diameter. An undistensible or redundant dilated esophagus is a sign of esophageal pathology. During esophagoscopy, esophageal distention is crucial because it allows assessment of the mucosa. The esophageal mucosa is a pearly gray, homogeneous color with a pale, dull appearance. Submucosal vessels can be seen to course longitudinally in the esophageal wall. These vessels are absent in the distal 2 to 3 cm of the esophagus. In the lower third of the esophagus, longitudinal folds can sometimes be seen. The abrupt transition from the squamous epithelium of the esophagus to the shiny, velvety, salmon pink-orange mucosa of the stomach marks the squamocolumnar junction. Recognition of this transition, along with documenting its location, is essential in the diagnosis of Barrett's esophagus. Islands of gastric mucosa may be seen throughout the esophageal body and must be distinguished from the normal squamocolumnar junction.

Inspection of the esophagus includes evaluation of peristalsis. If the patient is asked to swallow when the endoscope is positioned in the proximal esophagus, primary esophageal waves can be seen to traverse the length of the esophagus. The endoscope, especially with insufflation, stimulates secondary waves, which can be observed to progress from the point of stimulation to the distal esophagus. In patients with certain motility disorders, tertiary nonpropulsive waves can be seen at esophagoscopy.

INDICATIONS AND CONTRAINDICATIONS

Esophagoscopy is indicated in the evaluation of dysphagia, odynophagia, heartburn, regurgitation, atypical chest pain, and upper GI bleeding. It is useful in the definition of abnormalities seen on the barium esophagram and chest roentgenogram (Tabibian, 1991). Strictures, diverticula of the esophageal body, ulcers, tumors, intramural masses, varices, hiatal hernias, and aspiration pneumonia may all require further evaluation at esophagoscopy. Established esophageal diseases (e.g., esophagitis, chemical injuries, infections, achalasia, scleroderma, diffuse esophageal spasm, and esophageal neoplasms) may require esophagoscopy during management. Esophagoscopy is the best means of surveillance of patients at risk for esophageal malignancy. Patients with Barrett's esophagus and known esophageal malignancy should undergo routine endoscopy and biopsy. Esophagoscopy is also indicated in the postoperative evaluation of patients who have undergone resection or repair of esophageal disorders.

Therapeutic esophagoscopy is indicated for (1) dilatation of strictures, (2) coagulation of upper GI bleeding sites, (3) laser ablation of esophageal malignancies, (4) placement of esophageal stents, (5) removal of foreign bodies, and (6) sclerosis of esophageal varices. The role of endoscopic mucosal ablation or resection is still being defined (Ell et al, 2000; Gossner et al, 1998 and 1999; Grade et al, 1999; Overholt and Panjehpour, 1996).

Endoscopy is contraindicated in the following: (1) uncooperative or moribund patients, (2) patients with severe cardiac or pulmonary compromise, and (3) patients with certain vertebral diseases (Welsh et al, 1989). Age is not a contraindication to esophagoscopy (Brussaard and Vandewoude, 1988). All examinations should be performed by an experienced endoscopist with appropriate equipment.

ESOPHAGEAL DISORDERS

Gastroesophageal Reflux Disease

Hiatal hernia, reflux esophagitis, Schatzki's ring, peptic stricture, and Barrett's esophagus are part of the *broad spectrum* of endoscopic findings seen at esophagoscopy in patients with gastroesophageal reflux disease (GERD). Understanding the esophagogastric junction (EGJ) and its anatomic landmarks is critical to the endoscopist in identifying a hiatal hernia and in diagnosing the complications of GERD. The *EGJ* can be defined as the point where the tubular esophagus joins the saccular stomach. It can either be muscular or mucosal. *Muscular EGJ* is defined manometrically as the distalmost portion of the LES. The LES is a 2- to 4-cm zone of increased pressure that is higher than the pressure in the stomach or esophageal body. Although the LES can be defined physiologically, no distinct anatomic structure has been identified.

Endoscopically, the proximal margin of the gastric folds has been shown to closely approximate the muscular EGJ (McClave and Boyce, 1987). The mucosal EGJ, which normally lies within the LES, does not correspond to the muscular EGJ and is usually 1 to 2 cm above the muscular junction. If the muscular EGJ is used to define the limits of the esophagus, the distal 1 to 2 cm of the esophagus is lined by columnar epithelium that is either gastric, cardiac, or fundic. It is for this reason that, in the absence of intestinal metaplasia, many physicians require at least 3 cm of columnar epithelium above the EGJ before the diagnosis of Barrett's esophagus is accepted.

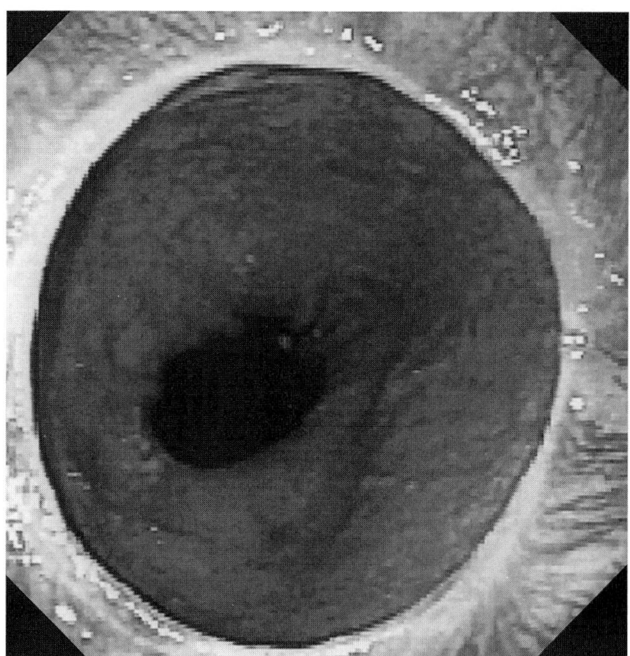

FIGURE 6–11 ■ Distal esophagus, Schatzki's ring and small hiatal hernia. (See Color Plate.)

Diagnosis of a type I hiatal hernia requires that the esophagogastric junction be displaced above the diaphragm (Figs. 6–11 to 6–13) (see Color Plate). Generally,

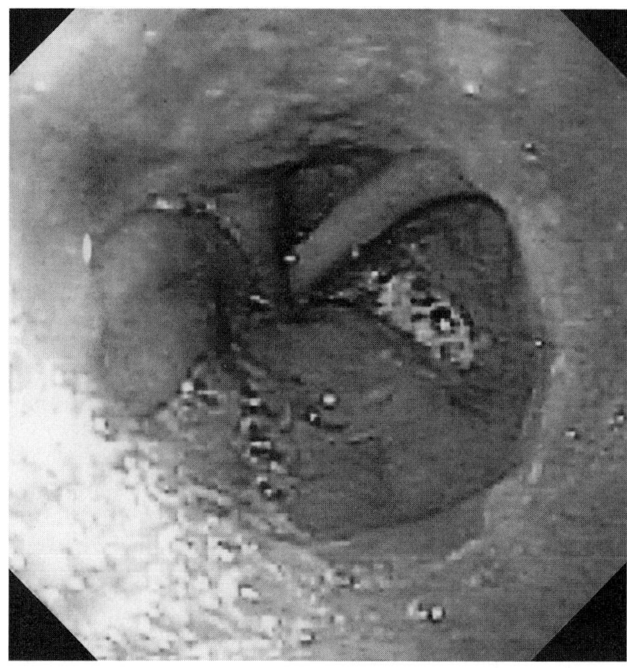

FIGURE 6–12 ■ Small hiatal hernia. (See Color Plate.)

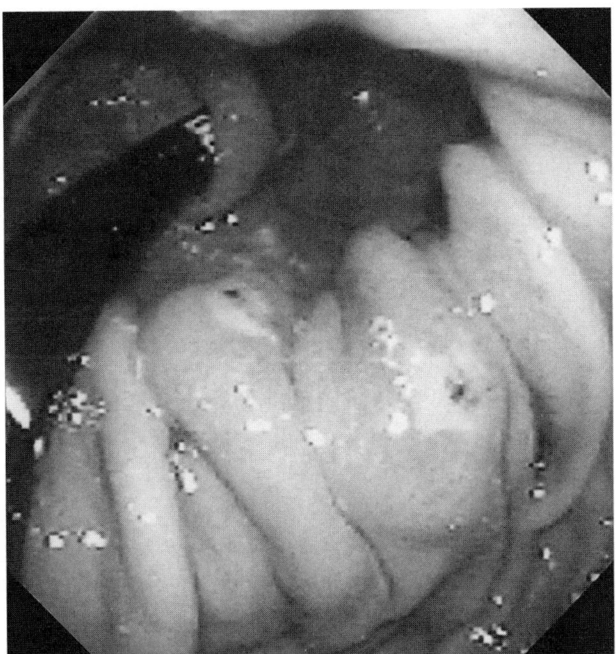

FIGURE 6–13 ■ Retroflexed view, from the stomach, of a large hiatal hernia. (See Color Plate.)

the squamocolumnar junction is used to visually identify the esophagogastric junction. Large hiatal hernias are easily appreciated because the squamocolumnar junction is seen well above the diaphragm and the diaphragmatic impression is located about the intrathoracic portion of the stomach. Smaller hiatal hernias are sometimes easier to verify with the retroflexed esophagoscope in the stomach.

Reflux esophagitis can be visually graded; however, a description that includes "redness" is subjective and is not useful. Common endoscopic grading systems include those of Hetzel and co-workers (1988), Savary-Miller (Ollyo JB et al, 1990), and Sonnenberg and colleagues (1982) (Table 6–1). All cases of suspected reflux esophagitis should be confirmed by biopsy.

Schatzki's ring, located at the squamocolumnar junction, is a benign disorder presenting with dysphagia (see Fig. 6–11). Histologically, the ring is the result of fibrosis in the lamina propria, the muscularis propria or the submucosa. Endoscopically, a Schatzki's ring appears as a circumferential constriction at the squamocolumnar junction with maximal esophageal distension. An associated hiatal hernia is always present, but reflux esophagitis is seen only rarely.

Esophagoscopy is crucial in the diagnosis of peptic esophageal strictures. A diagnosis can be obtained at endoscopy in 90% to 95% of patients (Eastman et al, 1978, Webb et al, 1984). Cytologic brushings of the stricture must be added to random biopsy specimens to reach this level of diagnostic accuracy. Endoscopy, biopsy, and dilatation can be safely performed together (Barkin et al, 1981). After dilatation, careful endoscopic examination of the stricture and the distal GI tract is required.

Barrett's esophagus is easily identified if the squamocolumnar junction has retreated well above the gastroesophageal junction (Fig. 6–14) (see Color Plate).

TABLE 6–1 ■ **Endoscopic Grading Systems of Esophagitis**

Hetzel	
Grade 0	Normal-appearing mucosa on endoscopy
Grade 1	Mucosal edema, hyperemia, and/or friability of the mucosa
Grade 2	Superficial erosions involving less than 10% of the mucosal surface of the last 5 cm of the esophageal squamous mucosa
Grade 3	Superficial erosions and ulcerations involving 10% to 50% of the distal esophagus
Grade 4	Deep peptic ulceration anywhere in the esophagus or confluent erosions involving more than 50% of the distal esophageal squamous mucosa
Sonnenberg	
Grade 1	(Mild) isolated linear or round erosions
Grade 2	(Severe) confluence of erosions involving the total luminal circumference
Grade 3	(Complicated) grade 1 or grade 2 erosions associated with deep ulcers, strictures, or Barrett's esophagus
Savary-Miller	
Grade I	Single, erosive or exudative lesion, oval or linear, taking only one longitudinal fold
Grade II	Noncircular, multiple erosions or exudative lesion, taking more than one longitudinal fold, with or without confluence
Grade III	Circular erosive or exudative lesion
Grade IV	Chronic lesions: ulcers, strictures, or short esophagus, isolated or associated with lesions grades I to III
Grade V	Barrett's epithelium isolated or associated with lesions grades I to III

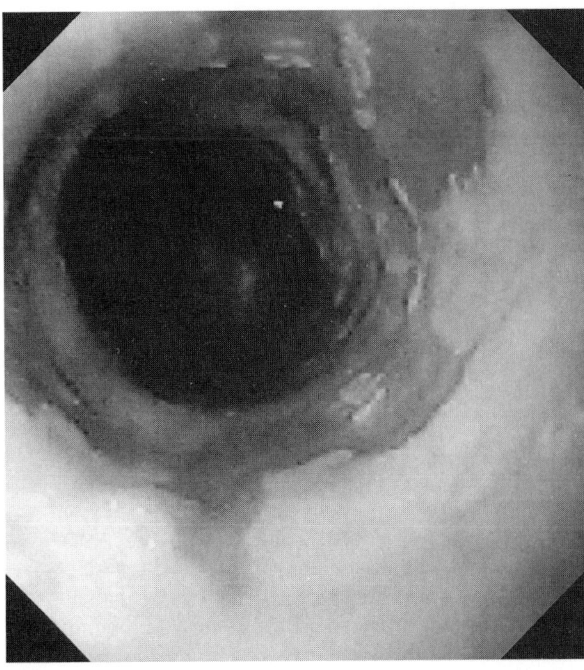

FIGURE 6–14 ■ Long-segment Barrett's esophagus. (See Color Plate.)

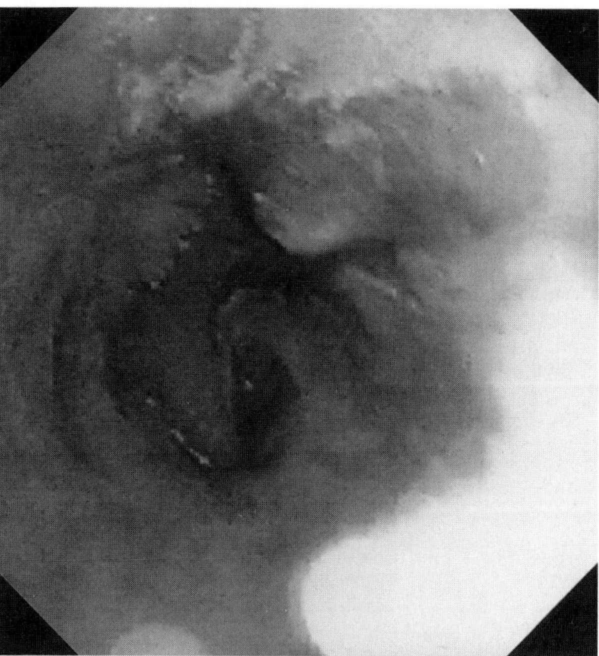

FIGURE 6–15 ■ A nodule in Barrett's esophagus. Biopsy is mandatory to prove this nodule a superficial adenocarcinoma. (See Color Plate.)

Short-segment Barrett's esophagus is a columnar-lined esophagus that is less than 3 cm in length. Biopsy is indicated in all suspected cases of Barrett's esophagus to confirm the diagnosis and to assess dysplasia. If a biopsy specimen from the esophagus shows specialized epithelium with goblet cells or columnar epithelium overlying either the submucosal glands or the squamous-lined duct of these glands, a diagnosis of Barrett's esophagus is established. In the absence of intestinal metaplasia, if either cardiac or fundic epithelium is present overlying submucosal glands or squamous-lined ducts, a diagnosis of Barrett's esophagus is also established.

A metaplasia-dysplasia-carcinoma sequence, similar to that described in the colon, is thought to be present in Barrett's esophagus (Hamilton et al, 1987). Dysplasia is unequivocally neoplastic epithelium confined within the basement membrane of the glands from which it arose. Once a diagnosis of Barrett's esophagus is established, patients should be placed into a cancer surveillance program, with identification of epithelial dysplasia as the surveillance goal. There are considerable variations in the instrumentation, technique, and timing of surveillance endoscopy (Falk et al, 1999, 2000; Katz et al, 1998; van Sandick et al, 2000). A safe, accepted protocol is esophagoscopy and biopsy every 2 years. This is accomplished using jumbo biopsy forceps to obtain four-quadrant biopsies at 2-cm intervals along the entire columnar lining. Any ulcer, nodule, or mass should be biopsied separately (Fig. 6–15) (see Color Plate).

Histologically, a diagnosis of dysplasia is based on both architectural and cytologic changes that suggest a neoplastic transformation. Dysplasia classification is a modification of the classification for dysplasia in inflammatory bowel disease (Riddell et al, 1983) and has been applied to Barrett's esophagus:

1. *Negative for dysplasia*: The mucosal architecture is within normal limits and, on cytologic examination, there is little nuclear hyperchromatism or pleomorphism.
2. *Indefinite for dysplasia*: In areas adjacent to erosions or ulcerations, inflammatory reactive changes may be difficult to differentiate from low-grade dysplasia. In general, true dysplasia is characterized by more prominent nuclear enlargement and hyperchromasia as well as more irregular nuclear contours and nuclear crowding than is seen in inflammatory repair. Because it is often difficult to differentiate between these two, however, the term "indefinite for dysplasia" is acceptable.
3. *Positive for dysplasia*: Biopsy specimens show both cytologic and architectural abnormalities suggesting neoplastic transformation. Both low-grade and high-grade dysplasia are recognized, depending on the severity of the changes.
4. *Intramucosal carcinoma*: The carcinoma has penetrated through the glandular basement membrane and into the lamina propria, but there is no invasion beyond the muscularis mucosae into the submucosa.

Despite these criteria, there are still considerable interobserver variations in the diagnosis of dysplasia. In a consensus conference, intramucosal carcinoma and high-grade dysplasia showed the best interobserver agreement in this histologic classification, with 85% and 87% agreement in successive reviews of selected cases (Reid et al, 1988). In this study, "negative for dysplasia" showed only 71% and 72% agreement among experienced GI pathologists.

Esophageal Carcinoma

Flexible esophagoscopy is the procedure of choice for the diagnosis of esophageal carcinoma (Figs. 6–16 to 6–18)

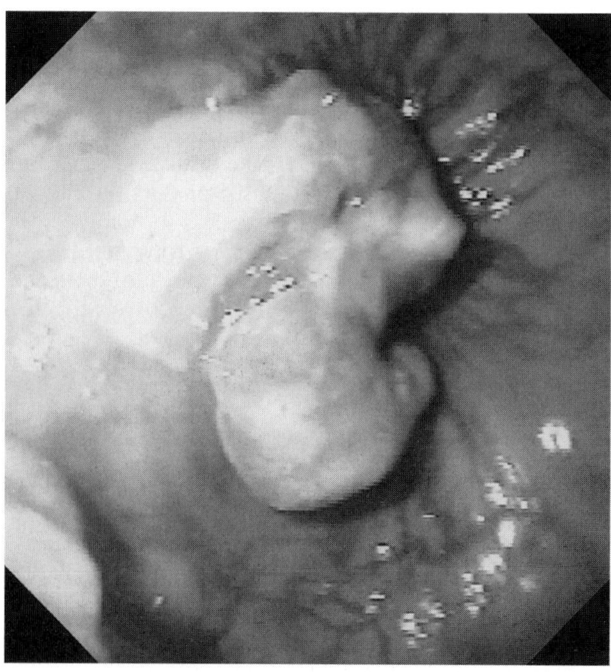

FIGURE 6–16 ■ Squamous cell carcinoma of the esophagus. (See Color Plate.)

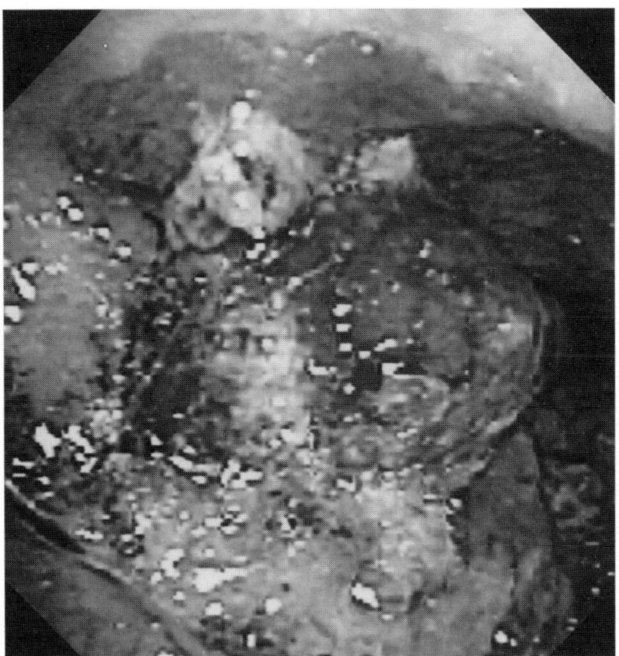

FIGURE 6–17 ■ Barrett's adenocarcinoma. (See Color Plate.)

(see Color Plate). Modern endoscopy equipment provides excellent visualization of all areas of the upper GI tract, including the cervical esophagus, esophagogastric junction, and gastric cardia. In addition, flexible endoscopy permits assessment of the GI tract distal to obstructing esophageal cancer in approximately 80% of patients (Cheung et al, 1988). Inspection of the mucosa distant from the primary tumor site allows detection of intramural metastases, which are associated with advanced tumor stage and decreased survival. Intramural metastases have been reported in 12% of patients with squamous cell carcinoma of the esophagus (Takubo et al, 1990).

A clinical diagnosis of esophageal carcinoma requires tissue confirmation prior to treatment. Improved equipment and techniques have increased the diagnostic capabilities of fiberoptic endoscopic biopsy from 70% to 80% to nearly 100% (Graham et al, 1982; Lal et al, 1992; Prolla et al, 1977; Witzel et al, 1976). The number of biopsy specimens obtained increases the diagnostic yield from 93% for one specimen to 98% to 100% with six or seven specimens. Lusink and colleagues (1983) reported flexible endoscopy unreliable in the diagnosis of adenocarcinoma of the lower esophagus due to inflammation of the mucosa and tumor infiltration of the submucosa. More recent work reports that neither site nor type of malignancy adversely affects diagnostic yield (Lal et al, 1992). The area biopsied within an esophageal lesion has not been reported to influence diagnostic accuracy. If an esophageal ulcer is encountered, however, experience with gastric ulcers shows the combination of biopsies from the rim of the ulcer and the ulcer crater provides a 95% diagnostic accuracy (Hatfield et al, 1975). Larger biopsy forceps produce larger volumes but not deeper tissue samples. Biopsy forceps with a centering needle may obtain deeper biopsy specimens (Bernstein et al, 1995).

Endoscopic cytology brushings of esophageal lesions are easily obtained and should be considered for all lesions. Brush cytology has a reported accuracy of 80% to 97% and a false-positive rate of 0.3% to 2.0% (Chambers et al, 1986; Kasugai et al, 1978, O'Donoghue et al, 1992; Prolla et al, 1977; Witzel et al, 1976). O'Donoghue and colleagues (1992) analyzed both endoscopic brush cytology and biopsy and reported a sensitivity of 81% and 87%, a specificity of 98% and 99%, and a positive predictive value of 92% and 96%, respectively, in the diagnosis of esophageal malignancies. Brush cytology is particularly helpful when adequate biopsy samples are difficult to obtain, such as with small superficial cancers or strictures. It has been reported that when obstructing lesions preclude biopsy, cytologic examination may provide a diagnosis in 75% of patients (Cusso et al, 1989). With the addition of brush cytology to biopsy, the diagnostic yield of endoscopy is increased by as much as 21%. Cytology specimens should be obtained before biopsy. Accuracy of brush cytology is reduced from 94% to 83% if it is done after biopsy (Zargar et al, 1991). The accuracy of endoscopic biopsy is not altered by preceding brush cytology. Brush cytology is complementary to biopsy and may be used to improve diagnostic yield.

Endoscopic fine-needle aspiration may be helpful in the diagnosis of mucosal and submucosal esophageal lesions. This procedure should be reserved for deeper lesions and for those that remain undiagnosed by both biopsy and brush cytology (Graham et al, 1989, Layfield et al, 1992).

Rigid esophagoscopy allows large biopsy specimens to be obtained and may permit assessment of fixation of an esophageal carcinoma. Without insufflation and magnification, the esophageal assessment may be difficult and incomplete. Examination of the entire esophagus with

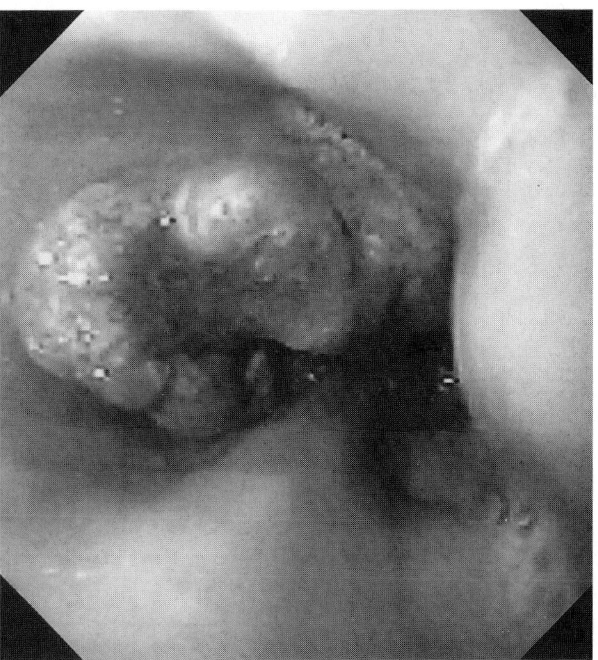

FIGURE 6–18 ■ Adenocarcinoma of the esophagogastric junction. (See Color Plate.)

rigid esophagoscopy was possible in only 79% of patients with esophageal carcinoma (Bacon and Hendrix, 1992). Passage of the rigid scope through a tumor is reported to increase the risk of perforation from negligible levels to 1.13% (Ritchie et al, 1992).

Although rigid esophagoscopy may be as likely as flexible esophagoscopy to allow passage of the instrument through the carcinoma, examination of the esophagogastric junction is inferior. Examination of the stomach and duodenum is not possible with rigid esophagoscopy. General anesthesia is usually required for this examination. Since flexible endoscopy provides more information, is safer, easier to perform, less expensive, and better tolerated than rigid esophagoscopy, rigid esophagoscopy should be reserved for failures of flexible fiberoptic esophagoscopy (Glaws et al, 1996).

Motility Disorders

Endoscopy is indicated in achalasia to exclude the mucosal complications of stasis esophagitis and squamous cell carcinoma (Fig. 6–19) (see Color Plate). Careful inspection of the stomach with a retroflexed examination of the EGJ is necessary to rule out an obstructing carcinoma of the cardia masquerading as achalasia. Endoscopy is indicated in diffuse esophageal spasm (DES) to exclude other disorders that may be misdiagnosed as DES. Endoscopic findings of scleroderma are those of GERD. The lack of peristalsis and monilial esophagitis in advanced cases may be recognized at endoscopy.

Diverticula

Esophagoscopy has limited use in the direct evaluation of thoracic and epiphrenic diverticula which frequently form as a consequence of an esophageal motility disorder

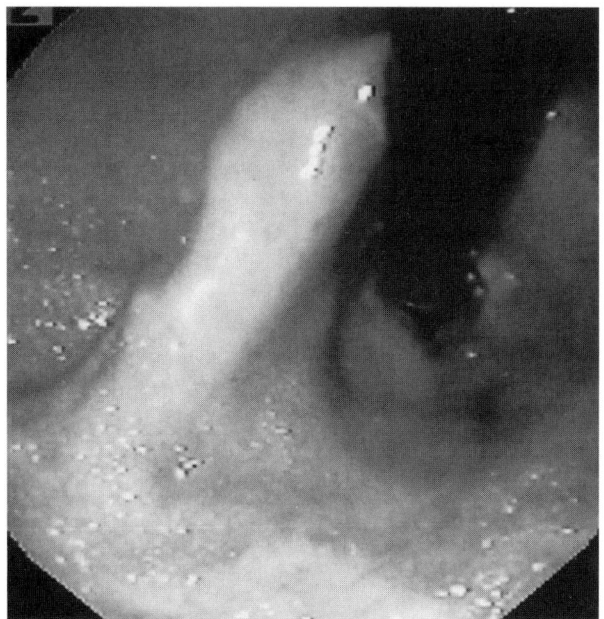

FIGURE 6–19 ■ Retroflexed view within a dilated sigmoid esophagus of achalasia. (See Color Plate.)

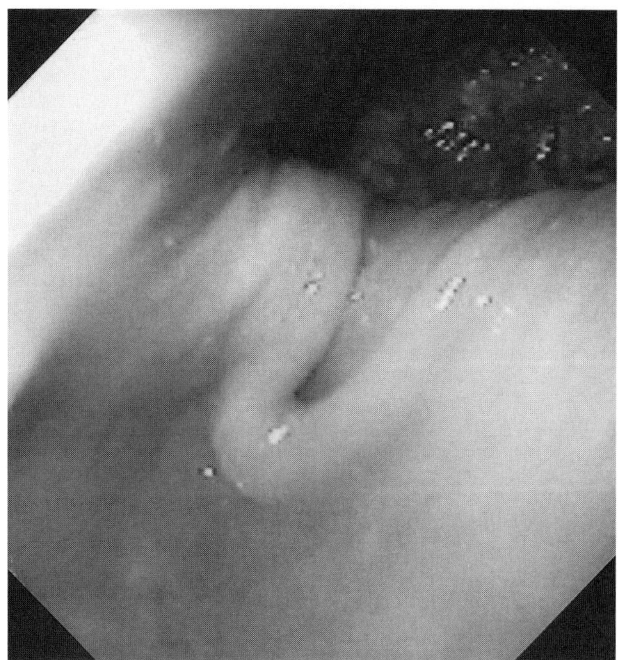

FIGURE 6–20 ■ A large, food-filled epiphrenic diverticulum (at 2 o'clock). The distal esophagus is the small dimple in the center of the figure. (See Color Plate.)

(Baker et al, 1999). Therefore, although endoscopy may not be essential in the evaluation of the diverticulum itself, it is useful and mandated in the assessment of the underlying motility disorder (Fig. 6–20) (see Color Plate).

Intramural and Periesophageal Tumors

At esophagoscopy, an intramural or periesophageal tumor appears as an extramucosal mass bulging into the lumen with no involvement of the esophageal mucosa (Figs. 6–21 and 6–22) (see Color Plate). Intramural tumors are usually mobile, and the esophagoscope can generally pass without obstruction. It is difficult to distinguish these uncommon tumors at esophagoscopy. There are few features or locations that are pathognomonic for any tumor. Detailed examination of the esophageal wall provided by endoscopic esophageal ultrasound has proved invaluable in diagnosis. If the overlying mucosa is normal, biopsy should be avoided, because it may complicate enucleation.

Esophageal Varices

Esophageal varices have variable appearances at esophagoscopy, depending on their complexity and previous treatment (Fig. 6–23) (see Color Plate). They can lie deep in the muscular wall or may be entirely extraluminal; they may not be visible at esophagoscopy. In a patient with known varices, a complete upper GI endoscopy is required during each bleeding episode to exclude other common sources of upper GI bleeding. Sclerotherapy is an effective means of bleeding control. No single sclerosing agent has been demonstrated to be superior (Kochhar

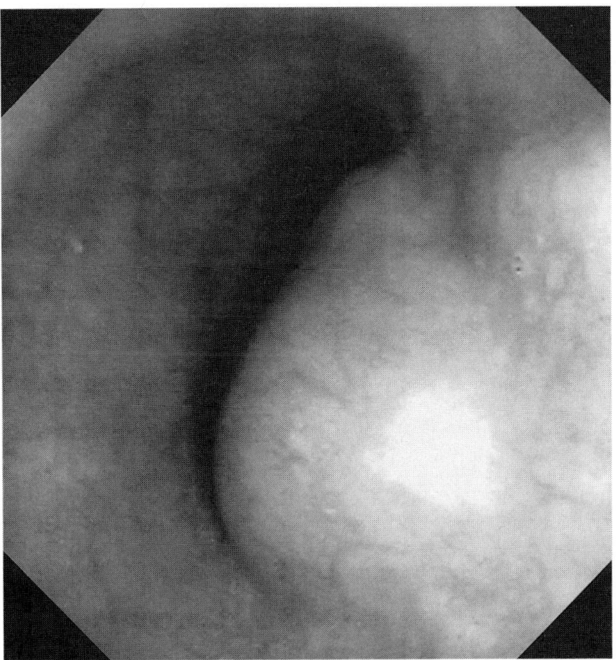

FIGURE 6–21 ■ Leiomyoma of the distal esophagus. (See Color Plate.)

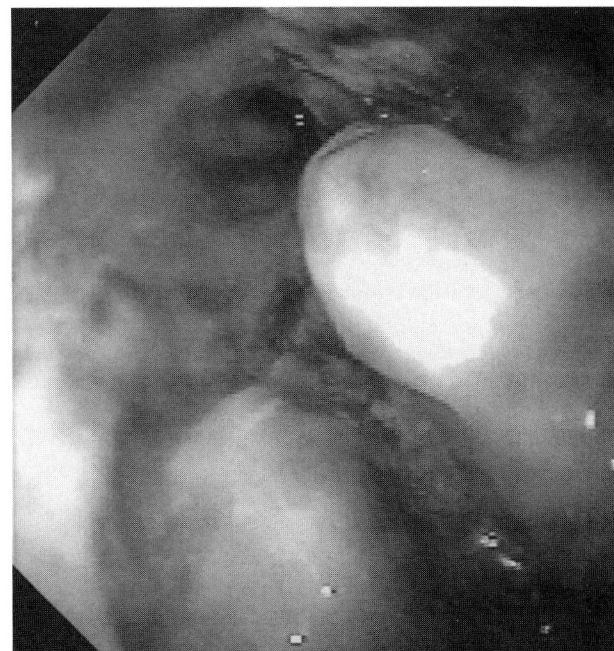

FIGURE 6–23 ■ Esophageal varices. (See Color Plate.)

et al, 1990). Variceal sclerotherapy may be complicated by fever, chest pain, dysphagia, ulcers, and perforation. Complications have been reported to be less frequent with rubber band ligation (Steigmann et al, 1992).

COMPLICATIONS

Flexible fiberoptic esophagoscopy is an extremely safe procedure. The overall complication rate for upper GI endoscopy is in the range of 0.1%. Mortality rate is less than 0.005% (Pasricha et al, 1994). The most frequent complications are cardiopulmonary. Careful monitoring and oxygen supplementation during the procedure may minimize these complications.

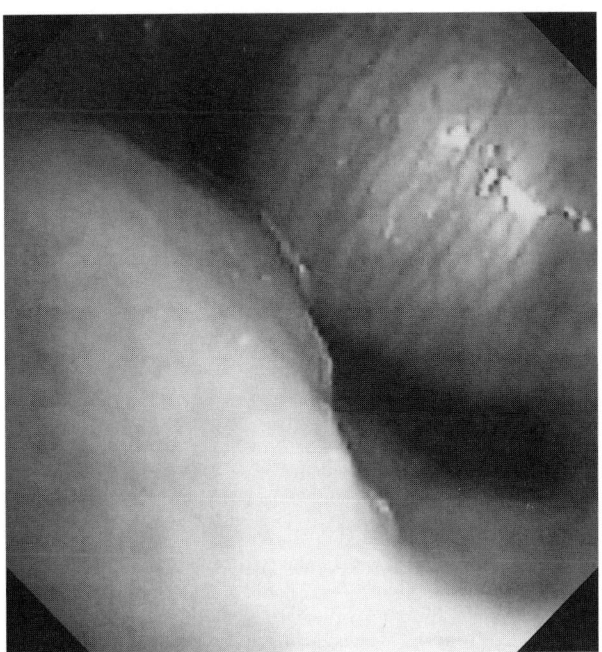

FIGURE 6–22 ■ Vascular ring, the result of an aberrant right subclavian artery. (See Color Plate.)

Esophageal perforation is the most feared complication of esophagoscopy. Replacement of rigid endoscopy with flexible fiberoptic endoscopy has significantly reduced perforations (from 0.11% or more to 0.03%) but has not eliminated them. Perforations are more likely to occur during complex examinations, therapeutic esophagoscopy, or in the presence of significant esophageal pathology. Prompt recognition and treatment minimizes morbidity and mortality. Perforation should be suspected in a patient who complains of excessive and prolonged pain following esophagoscopy. Subcutaneous emphysema and a pneumothorax may be detected on physical examination. An urgent chest roentgenogram will demonstrate a hydropneumothorax and possibly mediastinal and subcutaneous emphysema. Early surgical intervention is required with lavage and debridement of the mediastinum and pleural cavity, repair of the perforation, and surgical management of the underlying pathology. Rarely, there may be a contained leak with free, preferential drainage into the esophagus, which may be managed nonsurgically.

Other less frequent complications of esophagoscopy include bacteremia, cerebral abscess, septic arthritis, bacterial endocarditis, bleeding, and equipment failure (Katz, 1967).

COMMENTS AND CONTROVERSIES

Rice and Zuccaro note that flexible esophagoscopy has almost completely supplanted rigid endoscopy in current practice. Indeed, the experience and skills required for rigid endoscopy today are limited to relatively few thoracic, esophageal, and ear-nose-throat surgeons. Unfortunately, in many surgical units in North America and Europe, the operating esophageal surgeon may do little or no esophagoscopy for his or her own surgical patients. Regardless of the expertise of the referring "endoscopist–gastroenterologist," this practice puts the surgeon at a decided disadvantage; errors in endoscopic interpretation may adversely affect the surgical procedure, and no one will learn better from such errors than the responsible surgeon. Drs. Rice and Zuccaro clearly support and emphasize importance of esophagoscopy being done by the operating surgeon.

A clear and methodical technique is outlined that defines the anatomic features observed at each level of the examination. The authors recommend that the scope be introduced and advanced through the mouth and into the hypopharynx under video display rather than indirectly or blindly. Importantly, this technique permits examination of the pharynx, the hypopharynx and piriform sinuses, and the superior aspect of the larynx. The authors note the difficulty in clear visualization of the mucosal surfaces of the cricopharyngeal channel, since the upper sphincter opens for brief moments during episodes of swallowing. The technique of rigid endoscopy, described by Savary and Monnier in the preceding subchapter, affords excellent visualization of this cricopharyngeal region, and is much more sensitive in identifying abnormalities such as islands of ectopic columnar epithelium, which most commonly occur at this level.

The definitions of dysplasia and malignancy in Barrett's columnar epithelium reflect the current opinion of pathologists with interest and expertise in this important field. The term "carcinoma in situ" is no longer used. Intramucosal malignancy and severe dysplasia are not synonymous descriptors. Invasive cancer is defined by invasion of the basement membrane of the epithelial layer, whereas high-grade dysplasia is cytologic malignant cells confined to the epithelium.

The flexible esophagoscope is ideally suited for perioperative or intraoperative endoscopy. In the present era of laparoscopic antireflux surgery, the flexible scope may be positioned during the procedure in order to identify precise levels of anatomy such as the esophagogastric junction; the light at the end of the scope is visible through the esophageal wall, and the end of the scope itself can be felt with a laparoscopic probe (Awad, 2000).

I believe that many practitioners underestimate the potential role of rigid endoscopy today. Although it is obvious that rigid instrumentation is frequently necessary for the removal of foreign bodies, there are real benefits to rigid instrumentation in a number of other selected circumstances that are clearly presented in the preceding subchapter on rigid esophagoscopy by Savary and Monnier. They clarify the indications for both rigid and flexible esophagoscopy. Monnier is currently working with a modified Storz esophagoscope-resectoscope, which allows an endoscopic resection of mucosa and submucosa (at a precise depth level) in any region of the esophagus. An excellent specimen is obtained for the pathologist, and this is a superior alternative to current ablative *methods of endoscopic removal for severe dysplasia, mucosal carcinoma, or Barrett's mucosa with intestinal metaplasia (cautery coagulation, photodynamic therapy).*

REFERENCE

Awad ZT, Filipi CJ, Mittal SK, et al: Left side thoracoscopically assisted gastroplasty: A new technique for managing the shortened esophagus. Surg Endosc 14:508–512, 2000.

F. G. P.

REFERENCES

Bacon CK, Hendrix RA: Open tube versus flexible esophagoscopy in adult head and neck endoscopy. Ann Otol Rhinol Laryngol 101:147, 1992.

Baker ME, Zuccaro G Jr, Achkar E, et al: Esophageal diverticula: Patient assessment. Semin Thorac Cardiovasc Surg 11:326, 1999.

Barkin JS, Taub S, Rogers AI: The safety of combined endoscopy, biopsy and dilation in esophageal strictures. Am J Gastroenterol 76:23, 1981.

Bernstein DE, Barkin JS, Reiner DK, et al: Standard biopsy forceps versus large-capacity forceps with and without needle. Gastrointest Endosc 41:573, 1995.

Bianchi Porro G, Baroni S, Parente F, et al: Midazolam versus diazepam as premedication for upper gastrointestinal endoscopy: A randomized, double-blinded, crossover study. Gastrointest Endosc 34:252, 1988.

Birkenfeld S, Federico C, Dermansky-Avni Y, et al: Double-blind controlled trial of flumazenil in patients who underwent upper gastrointestinal endoscopy. Gastrointest Endosc 35:519, 1989.

Brussaard CC, Vandewoude MF: A prospective analysis of elective upper gastrointestinal endoscopy in the elderly. Gastrointest Endosc 34:118, 1988.

Carrougher JG, Kadakia S, Shaffer RT, et al: Venous complications of midazolam versus diazepam. Gastrointest Endosc 39:396, 1993.

Chambers LA, Clark WE 2nd: The endoscopic diagnosis of gastroesophageal malignancy: A cytologic review. Acta Cytol 30:110, 1986.

Chen YK, Kovacs BJ: The structure and function of the endoscope. In DiMarino AJ, Benjamin SB (eds): Gastrointestinal Disease: An endoscopic approach. Malden, MA, Blackwell Science, 1997, p 25.

Cheung HC, Siu KF, Wong J: A comparison of flexible and rigid endoscopy in evaluating esophageal cancer patients. World J Surg 12:117, 1988.

Cusso X, Monés-Xiol J, Vilardell F: Endoscopic cytology of cancer of the esophagus and cardia: A long-term evaluation. Gastrointest Endosc 35:321, 1989.

Dark DS, Campbell DR, Wesselium LJ: Arterial desaturation during gastrointestinal endoscopy. Am J Gastroenterol 85:1317, 1990.

Eastman MC, Gear MW, Nicol A: An assessment of the accuracy of modern endoscopic diagnosis of oesophageal stricture. Br J Surg 65:182, 1978.

Ell C, May A, Gossner L, et al: Endoscopic mucosal resection of early cancer and high-grade dysplasia in Barrett's esophagus. Gastroenterology 118:670, 2000.

Falk GW, Rice TW, Goldblum JR, et al: Jumbo biopsy forceps protocol still misses unsuspected cancer in Barrett's esophagus with high-grade dysplasia. Gastrointest Endosc 49:170, 1999.

Falk GW, Ours TM, Richter JE: Practice patterns for surveillance of Barrett's esophagus in the United States. Gastrointest Endosc 52:197, 2000.

Glaws WR, Etzkorn KP, Wening BL, et al: Comparison of rigid and flexible esophagoscopy in the diagnosis of esophageal disease: Diagnostic accuracy, complications and costs. Ann Otol Rhino Laryngol 105:262, 1996.

Gossner L, Stolte M, Sroka R, et al: Photodynamic ablation of high-grade dysplasia and early cancer in Barrett's esophagus by means of 5-aminolevulinic acid. Gastroenterology 114:448, 1998.

Gossner L, May A, Stolte M, et al: KTP laser destruction of dysplasia and early cancer in columnar-lined Barrett's esophagus. Gastrointest Endosc 49:8, 1999.

Grade AJ, Shah IA, Medlin SM, et al: The efficacy and safety of argon plasma coagulation therapy in Barrett's esophagus. Gastrointest Endosc 50:18, 1999.

Graham DY, Schwartz JT, Cain GD, et al: Prospective evaluation of biopsy number in the diagnosis of esophageal and gastric carcinoma. Gastroenterology 82:228, 1982.

Graham DY, Tabibian N, Michaletz PA, et al: Endoscopic needle biopsy: A comparative study of forceps biopsy, two different types of needles, and salvage cytology in gastrointestinal cancer. Gastrointest Endosc 35:207, 1989.

Hamilton SR, Smith RR: The relationship between columnar epithelial dysplasia and invasive carcinoma arising in Barrett's esophagus. Am J Clin Pathol 87:301, 1987.

Hatfield AR, Slavin G, Segal AW, et al: Importance of the site of endoscopic gastric biopsy in ulcerating lesions of the stomach. Gut 16:884, 1975.

Hayward SR, Sugawa C, Wilson RF: Changes in oxygenation and pulse rate during endoscopy. Am Surg 55:198, 1989.

Hetzel DJ, Dent J, Reed WD, et al: Healing and relapse of severe peptic esophagitis after treatment with omeprazole. Gastroenterology 95:903, 1988.

Kasugai T, Kobayashi S, Kuno N: Endoscopic cytology of the esophagus, stomach and pancreas. Acta Cytol 22:327, 1978.

Katz D: Morbidity and mortality in standard and flexible gastrointestinal endoscopy. Gastrointest Endosc 15:134, 1967.

Katz D, Rothstein R, Schned A, et al: The development of dysplasia and adenocarcinoma during endoscopic surveillance of Barrett's esophagus. Am J Gastroenterol 93:536, 1998.

Kochhar R, Goenka MK, Mehta S, et al: A comparative evaluation of sclerosants for esophageal varices: A prospective randomized controlled study. Gastrointest Endosc 36:127, 1990.

Lal N, Bhasin DK, Malik AK, et al: Optimal number of biopsy specimens in the diagnosis of carcinoma of the oesophagus. Gut 33:724, 1992.

Layfield LJ, Reichman A, Weinstein WM: Endoscopically directed fine needle aspiration biopsy of gastric and esophageal lesions. Acta Cytol 36:69, 1992.

Lusink C, Sali A, Chou ST, et al: Diagnostic accuracy of flexible endoscopic biopsy in carcinoma of the oesophagus and cardia. Aust N Z J Surg 53:545, 1983.

McClave SA, Boyce HW Jr, Gottfried MR: Early diagnosis of columnar-lined esophagus: A new endoscopic criterion. Gastrointest Endosc 33:413, 1987.

O'Donoghue J, Waldron R, Gough D, et al: An analysis of the diagnostic accuracy of endoscopic biopsy and cytology in the detection of oesophageal malignancy. Eur J Surg Oncol 18:332, 1992.

Ollyo JB, Lang F, Fontolliet C, et al: Savary-Miller new endoscopic grading of reflux oesophagitis: A simple, reproducible, logical, complete and useful classification. Gastroenterology 89:A100, 1990.

Overholt BF, Panjehpour M: Photodynamic therapy for Barrett's esophagus: Clinical update. Am J Gastroenterol 91:1719, 1996.

Pasricha PJ, Fleischer DE, Kalloo AN, et al: Endoscopic perforations of the upper GI tract: A review of their pathogenesis, prevention and management. Gastroenterology 106:787, 1994.

Prolla JC, Reilly W, Kirsner JB, et al: Direct-vision endoscopic cytology and biopsy in the diagnosis of esophageal and gastric tumors: current experience. Acta Cytol 21:399, 1977.

Reid BJ, Haggitt RC, Rubin CE, et al: Observer variation in the diagnosis of dysplasia in Barrett's esophagus. Hum Pathol 19:166, 1988.

Riddell RH, Goldman H, Ransohoff DF, et al: Dysplasia in inflammatory bowel disease: Standardized classification with provisional clinical applications. Hum Pathol 14:931, 1983.

Ritchie AJ, McManus K, McGuigan J, et al: The role of rigid oesophagoscopy in oesophageal carcinoma. Postgrad Med 68:892, 1992.

Tabibian N: Endoscopy versus x-ray studies of the gastrointestinal tract: Future health care implications. South Med J 84:219, 1991.

Takubo K, Sasajima K, Yamashita K, et al: Prognostic significance of intramural metastasis in patients with esophageal carcinoma. Cancer 65:1816, 1990.

Sonnenberg A, Lepsien G, Muller-Lissner SA, et al: When is esophagitis healed? Esophageal endoscopy, histology and function before and after cimetidine treatment. Dig Dis Sci 27:297, 1982.

Steigmann GV, Goff JS, Michaletz Onody PA, et al: Endoscopic sclerotherapy as compared with endoscopic ligation for bleeding esophageal varices. N Engl J Med 326:1527, 1992.

van Sandick JW, Bartelsman JF, van Lanschott JJ, et al: Surveillance of Barrett's oesophagus: Physicians' practices and review of current guidelines. Eur J Gastroenterol Hepatol 12:111, 2000.

Webb WA, McDaniel L, Jones L: The use of endoscopy in assessment and treatment of peptic strictures of the esophagus. Am Surg 50:476, 1984.

Welsh LW, Welsh JJ, Chinnici JC: Endoscopic problems due to certain vertebral diseases. Ann Otol Rhinol Laryngol 98:597, 1989.

Witzel L, Halter F, Gretillat PA, et al: Evaluation of specific value of endoscopic biopsies and brush cytology for malignancies of the esophagus and stomach. Gut 17:375, 1976.

Zargar SA, Khuroo MS, Jan GM, et al: Prospective comparison of the value of brushing before and after biopsy in the endoscopic diagnosis of gastroesophageal malignancy. Acta Cytol 35:549, 1991.

CHAPTER 7

Function Tests

Tom R. DeMeester

Mario Costantini

Esophageal surgery for benign diseases is one of the most challenging fields in that it alters or reconstructs anatomy in an effort to improve function. The outcome is assessed on the ability of the procedure to provide complete and permanent relief of all symptoms and complications of the esophageal abnormality. Preoperative symptoms are often severe without evidence of anatomic or histologic alterations. Usually, anatomic and histologic changes occur late and represent the end stage of altered function. Further, symptoms of esophageal diseases (i.e., dysphagia, heartburn, regurgitation, belching, epigastric and retrosternal pain) are often nonspecific and occur in a variety of esophageal as well as gastric and duodenal disorders. On the other hand, atypical symptoms of esophageal diseases (wheezing, choking, coughing, and chest pain) can mimic other organ abnormalities (DeMeester et al, 1990). Consequently, a precise diagnosis must be made prior to any surgical therapy, since its purpose is to improve the performance of a malfunctioning organ that will remain in the patient. Achievement of this result depends on an accurate understanding of the pathophysiologic mechanism causing the patient's abnormality. This understanding requires the use of esophageal function tests.

The tests available can be divided into several types: (1) tests to evaluate the motor function and clearing ability of the gullet, (2) tests to evaluate upper and lower sphincter function, (3) tests to evaluate exposure of the esophagus to gastric juice, and (4) tests to document the relationship between symptoms and esophageal function. Since esophageal function is closely related to foregut function, there is, on occasion, a need for tests to evaluate gastroduodenal function.

HISTORICAL NOTE

Esophageal function tests were first performed more than a century ago when Kronecker and Meltzer began performing esophageal manometry in 1883, using a large balloon system, and discovered peristalsis. This was more than a decade before the discovery by Roentgen, in 1895, of x-rays and the first studies on esophageal peristalsis with radiopaque swallowed substances (Cannon and Moser, 1898). These early, balloon-based manometric systems were limited in their accuracy. Despite this, they were used for several decades and allowed for important advancements in the understanding of esophageal physiology, namely the identification of the lower esophageal sphincter (Fyke et al, 1956). The demonstration that the size of the balloon influenced the fidelity of the recordings led to the introduction, in the 1960s, of small, multilumen, nonperfused, fluid-filled catheters with their terminal openings separated from each other, allowing measurement of pressure events at different points along the gullet. Subsequently, it was shown that these nonper-

TESTS TO EVALUATE ESOPHAGEAL MOTOR DISORDERS AND GASTROESOPHAGEAL REFLUX

Evaluation of Esophageal Motor Function and Clearance

1. Esophageal manometry (body evaluation)
2. 24-hour motility monitoring
3. Esophageal scintigraphy
4. Acid clearing test
5. Video radiograph with liquid and solid barium

Evaluation of Lower Esophageal Sphincteric Function

1. Esophageal manometry
2. Standard acid reflux test

Evaluation of Upper Esophageal Sphincteric Function

1. Esophageal manometry
2. Video radiograph with liquid barium

Detection of Abnormal Exposure of Distal Esophagus to Gastric Juice

1. 24-hour pH monitoring

Relationship Between Symptoms and Esophageal Dysfunction

1. Pharmacologic provocative test (bethanechol, edrophonium)
2. Balloon distention test
3. Acid perfusion test (Bernstein test)
4. 24-hour pH monitoring
5. 24-hour motility monitoring

Evaluation of Gastroduodenal Function

1. 24-hour pH monitoring of the stomach
2. Gastric acid analysis
3. Gastroduodenal manometry
4. Gastric emptying study
5. Cholescintigraphy

fused catheters presented high variability and were still inaccurate. Constant perfusion of the catheters was introduced by means of a mechanical type of infusion pump, but the perfusion rate was shown to heavily influence the fidelity of the recordings.

The introduction of the noncompliant pneumohydraulic infusion pump (Arndorfer et al, 1977), in which a constant, small volume of distilled water is delivered through a capillary system by means of a constant pressure, represents the birth of modern esophageal manometry as it is routinely performed today. Most esophageal laboratories use these low-compliance infused systems, with multilumen catheters in which lateral openings ("side holes") are located at different levels and are arranged in different directions, to study the entire length of the esophagus and compensate for radial asymmetry of the sphincters.

After the first description of peptic esophagitis by Winkelstein in 1935, several tests were designed to assess the competency of the gastroesophageal junction (standard acid reflux test; Tuttle and Grossman, 1958), the esophageal sensitivity to acid (acid perfusion test; Bernstein, 1958), or the ability of the esophagus to clear acid (acid clearance test; Booth et al, 1968). In 1964, however, the concept of pH monitoring was introduced for peptic ulcer disease (Miller, 1964). In 1974, Johnson and DeMeester applied the concept of pH testing to esophageal disease and monitored patients for a 24-hour period. This allowed quantitation of esophageal acid exposure and provided direct correlation of a reflux episode with spontaneously occurring symptoms. Today the test has been standardized and forms the basis of the diagnosis of gastroesophageal reflux disease. This test opened the era of 24-hour monitoring of a variety of foregut functions in an ambulatory setting.

In the late 1980s, development of computer systems and the widespread use of miniaturized pressure transducers allowed monitoring of esophageal motility for a complete circadian cycle. This test can be performed together with 24-hour pH monitoring of the distal esophagus and the stomach, allowing complete foregut monitoring (Stein and DeMeester, 1992).

■ *HISTORICAL READINGS*

DeMeester TR, Wang CI, Wernly JA, et al: Technique, indications and clinical use of 24-hour esophageal pH monitoring. J Thorac Cardiovasc Surg 79:656, 1980.

Stein HJ, DeMeester TR: Indications, technique, and clinical use of ambulatory 24-hour esophageal motility monitoring in a surgical practice. Ann Surg 217:128, 1993.

Stein HJ, DeMeester TR, Hinder RA: Outpatient physiologic testing and surgical management of foregut motility disorders. Curr Probl Surg 24:418, 1992b.

STATIONARY ESOPHAGEAL MANOMETRY

Technique

In the last 25 years, several technical improvements have allowed esophageal manometry to be more widely used in clinical practice. At present, esophageal manometry is the gold standard for assessment of function of the lower esophageal sphincter (LES) and body of the esophagus. It has allowed for the identification of primary esophageal motility disorders (achalasia), diffuse esophageal spasm, nutcracker esophagus, and hypertensive LES as well as of systemic disorders affecting the esophagus, such as scleroderma, dermatomyositis, mixed connective tissue disease, diabetes, and alcoholic neuropathy. In gastroesophageal reflux disease (GERD), esophageal manometry is used to identify a defective LES and deterioration of esophageal body function.

Esophageal manometry is performed using electronic pressure-sensitive transducers or water-perfused catheters with lateral side holes, connected to external transducers. Electronic microtransducers have become popular because they are small enough to be carried in a 7 French catheter, are independent of posture, and can be directly connected to a recording device. For these reasons, they are ideally suited for ambulatory manometry. The major drawbacks are their high cost (about \$1500 per transducer, or \$5000 to \$8000 per catheter) and their fragility.

Low-compliance, water-perfused catheters constitute the most widely used system for stationary manometry. These catheters are made by combining three to eight capillary tubes 0.8 mm in inner diameter, with side openings at different levels. Side holes arranged radially at the same level are ideal for measuring circumferential pressures around the LES and upper esophageal sphincters (UES). Side holes spaced 5 cm apart are necessary for studying esophageal peristaltic activity. To obtain maximal information during a single intubation and a minimum number of swallows, most laboratories use an 8-lumen catheter with four side holes at the same level arranged at 90 degrees to each other and the remaining four placed at 5-cm intervals along the length of the catheter. The rate of water infusion must be adjusted to obtain reliable and reproducible pressure tracings. This adjustment is best achieved by a low-compliance pneumohydraulic capillary infusion system, with a constant rate of 0.6 ml/minute (Arndorfer, 1977).

The study is performed after an overnight fast. The catheter is passed through the nose and esophagus into the stomach, and the gastric pressure pattern is confirmed. To identify the high-pressure zone of the LES, the catheter is withdrawn across the cardia (Fig. 7–1*A*).

As the pressure-sensitive station is brought across the gastroesophageal junction, a rise in pressure on the gastric baseline identifies the beginning of the LES. The respiratory inversion point (RIP) is identified when the positive excursions that occur with breathing in the abdominal cavity change to negative deflections in the thorax. The RIP serves as a reference point at which the amplitude of LES pressure and the length of the sphincter exposed to abdominal pressure are measured. As the pressure-sensitive station is withdrawn into the body of the esophagus, the upper border of the LES is identified by the drop in pressure to the esophageal baseline. From these measurements, the pressure, abdominal length, and overall length of the sphincter are determined (Fig. 7–1*B*). To account for the asymmetry of the sphincter (Winans, 1977), the pressure profile is repeated with each transducer, and the average values for sphincter pressure above gastric baseline, overall sphincter length, and ab-

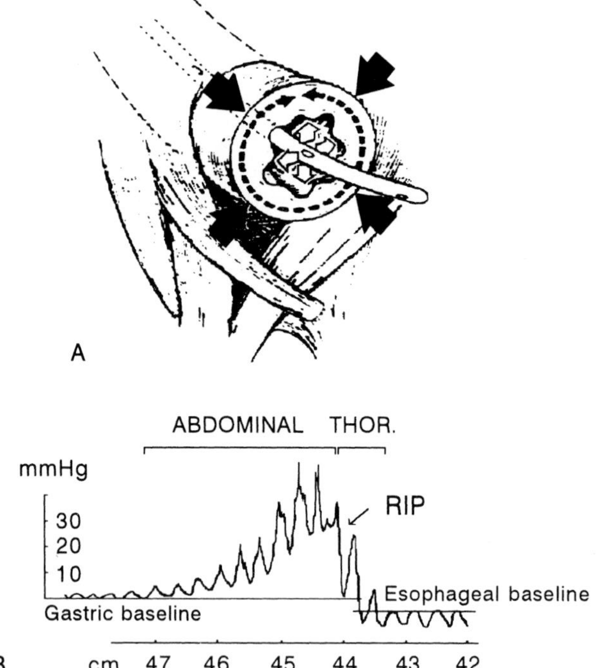

FIGURE 7–1 ■ *A,* Schematic illustration showing how lower esophageal sphincter (LES) pressure is measured with a perfused catheter system. The outflow of the perfusate through the side holes *(white arrows)* is restricted by the circular muscle tone of the cardia (dotted line) and the externally applied intra-abdominal pressure *(gray arrows). B,* The length of the abdominal and thoracic portion of the LES can be measured on the pressure record by identifying the point where respiratory excursion changes from positive to negative. This point, the respiratory inversion point (RIP) is the point at which the resting pressure of the LES is measured.

dominal length of the sphincter are calculated (Zaninotto, et al, 1988a).

To improve the station pull-through technique, a new method (the slow motorized pull-through technique) has been introduced to evaluate the LES. The catheter is pulled back at a slow constant rate (1.0 mm/second) using a motor and recording pressure from the four radial side holes. This technique is quick, taking about 1 minute for a passage through the sphincter, and is well accepted by the patient. It allows high-fidelity tracings without swallowing artifacts, even in the most difficult patients (Fig. 7–2). Because the pull-through is performed in a continuous mode, it provides an accurate determination of sphincter length without the approximation (± 0.5 to 1.0 cm) given by the station pull-through technique. Because the patient is allowed to breathe normally, it is possible to locate the RIP, from which the abdominal length can be calculated. Since the technique is independent of the operator, it lends itself to automated computer analysis. Comparison of the technique with the traditional station pull-through in a group of healthy volunteers and patients with different esophageal disorders reveals a good correlation for pressure overall and abdominal length (Costantini et al, 1992a).

By using the four radially oriented side holes positioned at the same level, one can also construct a three-dimensional pressure image of the sphincter by plotting the pressure values radially around an axis representing the gastric baseline (Stein et al, 1991a). For visual purposes, one can enhance the three-dimensional image by applying a cubic curve smoothing interpolation, which retains the original data points while adding intermediate ones to give a smoother surface to the three-dimensional sphincter image and improve its readability (Fig. 7–3).

The volume circumscribed by the three-dimensional sphincter image, the *vector volume* (Bombeck et al, 1987), integrates pressures exerted over the entire length and circumference of the sphincter into one number, representing sphincter resistance to reflux of gastric contents. This measure can be calculated using standard trigonometric formulas and is expressed in units of mm $Hg^2 \cdot$ mm. With the stationary pull-through or the slow motorized pull-through technique, the RIP can be identified and the intrathoracic and intra-abdominal portions of the volume (i.e., the portion of sphincter pressure vector volume located above and below the RIP) can be

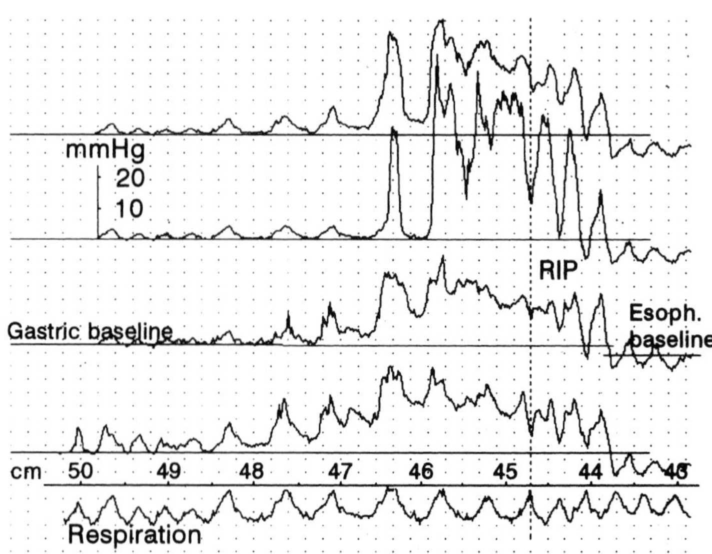

FIGURE 7–2 ■ Manometric tracing of lower esophageal sphincter (LES) pressure obtained with four side holes located at the same level and positioned radially at 90 degrees to each other. The slow motorized pull-through technique was used. The asymmetry of the sphincter is evident, in that the sphincter is longer in the lower tracing and the pressure is higher in the upper tracing. (RIP, respiratory inversion point.)

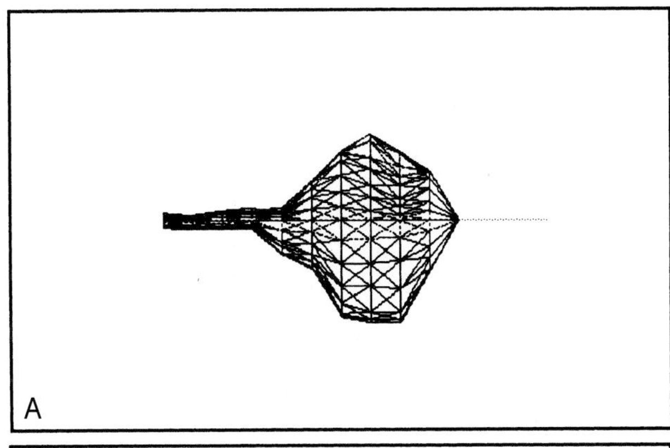

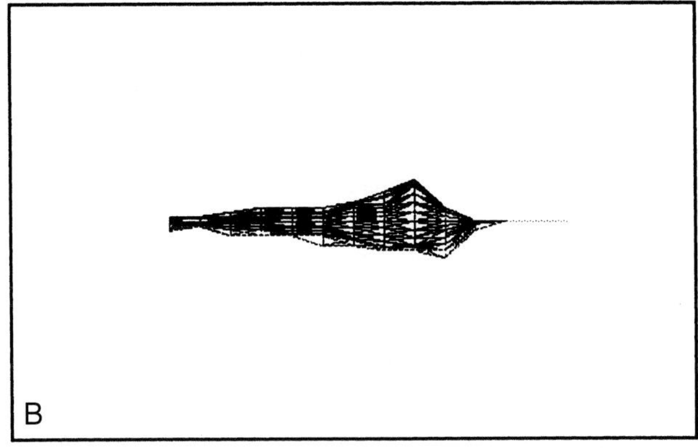

FIGURE 7–3 ■ Computerized three-dimensional image of the lower esophageal sphincter (LES) in a healthy volunteer *(A)* and a patient with Barrett's esophagus *(B)*. A catheter with four to eight radial side holes is withdrawn through the gastroesophageal junction. The radially measured pressures are plotted around an axis representing gastric baseline pressure. The volume inscribed by the three-dimensional image (sphincter vector volume) can be calculated, giving the best estimate of the LES mechanical effectiveness in the prevention of reflux of gastric juice from the stomach into the esophagus. (From Stein HJ, DeMeester TR, Naspetti R, et al: Three-dimensional imaging of the lower esophageal sphincter in gastroesophageal reflux disease. Ann Surg 214:374, 1991.)

calculated separately. Validation studies have shown that calculation of the sphincter pressure volume based on four radial transducers is sufficient to reliably evaluate sphincter resistance. Table 7–1 shows the values of LES pressure, overall length, length of the abdominal segment, and sphincter vector volume in 50 asymptomatic subjects with the range of normality in our laboratory.

TABLE 7–1 ■ **Normal Lower Esophageal Sphincter Parameters in 50 Healthy Volunteers**

			Percentile		
	Mean	*SEM*	*Median*	*5th*	*95th*
Pressure (mm Hg)	13.8	0.7	13.0	8	26.5
Overall length (cm)	3.7	0.2	3.6	2.6	5.4
Abdominal length (cm)	2.2	0.2	2.0	1.1	3.4
Intra-abdominal SVV ($mm\ Hg^2 \cdot mm$)	3,613	531	2,012	684	12,918
Total SVV ($mm\ Hg^2 \cdot mm$)	5,723	843	3,667	1,212	16,780

SEM, standard error of the mean; SVV, sphincter vector volume.

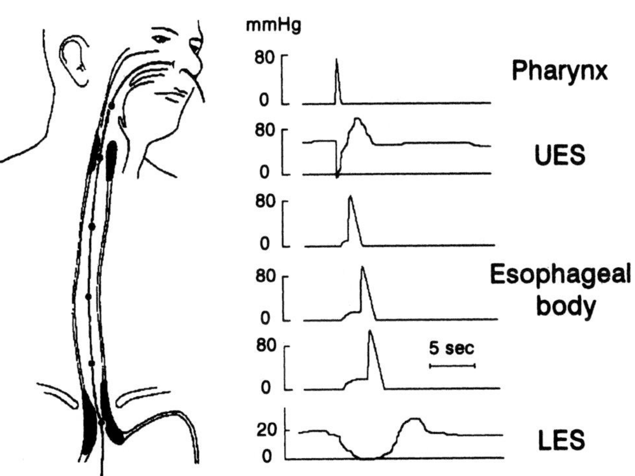

FIGURE 7–4 ■ Schematic representation of normal esophageal peristalsis initiated by a pharyngeal swallow and coordinated with relaxation of the upper esophageal sphincter (UES) and the lower esophageal sphincter (LES).

For the evaluation of sphincter relaxation and postrelaxation characteristics, the side holes located 5 cm apart are used; one side hole is positioned within the high pressure zone, with a distal one located in the stomach and a proximal one within the esophageal body. Five to ten wet swallows (5 ml of water) are performed. In the normal situation, the sphincter pressure should drop to the level of gastric pressure during each wet swallow.

The function of the esophageal body is assessed with the five recording sites located at various levels in the esophagus. To standardize the procedure, the most proximal pressure transducer is located 1 cm below the well-defined cricopharyngeal sphincter, with the distal orifices trailing at 5-cm intervals over the whole length of the esophagus. By this method, a pressure response throughout the whole esophagus can be obtained on swallowing (Fig. 7–4). The response to 10 wet swallows is recorded. Amplitude, duration, and morphology (i.e., number of peaks and repetitive contractions following each swallow) are calculated at all recorded levels of the esophageal body. The delay between the onset or peak of esophageal contractions at the various levels in the esophagus is used to calculate the speed of wave propagation. For computer-read records, the peak of esophageal contraction is used to calculate the speed.

The esophageal contraction waves following a swallow are classified as (1) *peristaltic*, (2) *simultaneous*, (3) *interrupted*, or (4) *dropped* (Fig. 7–5). Modern computer technology allows an objective and quick analysis of these parameters (Zaninotto et al, 1988b). Figure 7–6 shows a report of the esophageal body motility analysis obtained by the computer. Table 7–2 reports manometric values at different esophageal levels obtained in a group of 136 healthy subjects with a wide age range. They form the reference values for our laboratory (Costantini et al, 1992b).

It is important to know that recorded manometric pressures are affected by such variables as age, posture, bolus characteristic, catheter diameter, swallowing frequency, and compliance of the perfusion system (Hollis

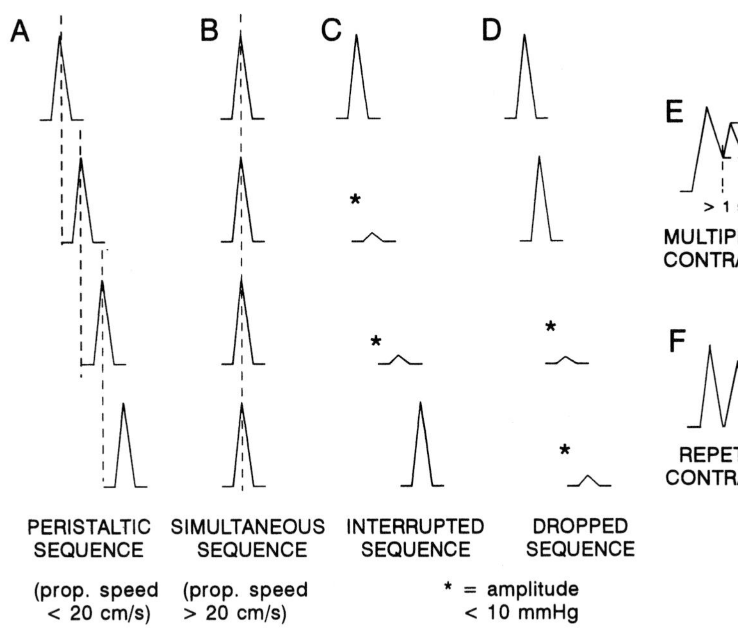

FIGURE 7–5 ■ Graphic representation of the classification of esophageal contraction waves on stationary manometry. *A*, A complete peristaltic sequence is a series of detectable contractions at each esophageal level, with a progression speed slower than 20 cm/sec (i.e., the time between the peak axes of two adjacent contractions). *B*, Simultaneous sequence is a series of detectable contractions at each esophageal level, with a progression speed faster than 20 cm/sec. *C*, An interrupted sequence is a series of detectable contractions in which an initial contraction is followed by no detectable contractions (<10 mm Hg) with a normal contraction subsequently reappearing. *D*, Dropped sequence is a series of detectable contractions in which an initial contraction is followed by *no* detectable contractions (<10 mm Hg). The morphology of the contractions is classified as normal, multipeaked, or repetitive. The difference between multipeaked *(E)* and repetitive *(F)* contractions is that the pressure between two consecutive peaks returns to the baseline in the latter.

and Castell, 1975; Lydon et al, 1975; Richter et al, 1987). Because these parameters are not necessarily standardized among various laboratories, they must be controlled within the individual laboratory. Each laboratory should define its own normal values from volunteers who have no subjective or objective evidence of a foregut disorder; alternatively, one laboratory may adopt the normal values of another laboratory, provided that it employs identical procedures and equipment.

The position, length, and pressure of the UES are evaluated by a stationary pull-through technique, using 0.5 to 1.0 cm increments, from the cervical esophagus to the pharynx. The rapid pull-through technique should be avoided. It gives pressure values consistently higher than the station pull-through technique, probably because of catheter irritation as it is rapidly withdrawn (Hellemans et al, 1981). To account for the anatomic asymmetry of the UES (Welch et al, 1979), the values obtained from the side holes oriented in the different directions must be averaged. One may evaluate the function of the UES on swallowing by placing one side hole of the catheter in the pharynx, one in the sphincter, and one in the upper esophagus. Because of the short duration of the pharyngeal swallowing phase (1.5 seconds), high-speed graphic recordings (50 mm/second) are necessary in order to evaluate the coordination of cricopharyngeal relaxation with hypopharyngeal contraction. Normally, pharyngeal contractions reach 50 to 60 mm Hg and are coordinated with complete UES relaxation (i.e., a fall in the sphincter pressure to the less-than-atmospheric intraesophageal pressure).

Movement of the UES orad during swallowing (2 to 3

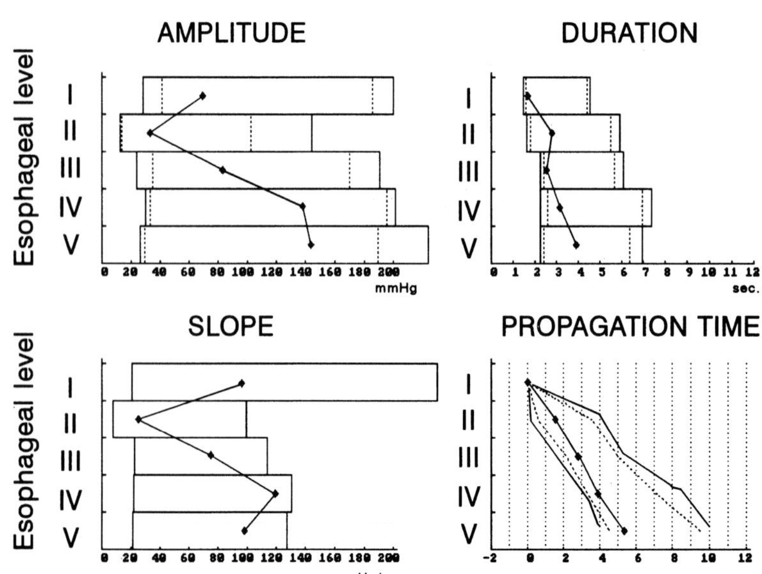

FIGURE 7–6 ■ Computerized printout of an esophageal body motility study. Median patient values are related to the normal range obtained in healthy volunteers. (2.5th and 97.5th percentile, *solid lines*; 5th and 95th percentile, *dotted lines*.)

TABLE 7–2 ■ **Median Values and Range of Normality (5th to 95th Percentiles) for Manometric Parameters of Esophageal Body Obtained by Wet and Dry Swallows in 136 Normal Subjects**

Parameter	*Level*	*Wet Swallows*	*Dry Swallows*
Amplitude (mm Hg)	I	88 (40–177)	74 (26–154)
	II	40 (14–94)	28 (14–74)
	III	76 (30–164)	52 (26–142)
	IV	93 (38–180)	61 (20–148)
	V	93 (36–190)	78 (22–172)
Duration (seconds)	I	2.3 (1.5–4.3)	2.3 (1.5–3.9)
	II	3.1 (1.8–4.8)	2.8 (1.0–4.5)
	III	3.3 (2.4–5.2)	3.1 (1.8–4.6)
	IV	3.6 (2.6–5.7)	3.4 (2.0–5.6)
	V	3.7 (2.4–7.0)	3.6 (2.4–6.4)
Velocity (cm/second)	I–II	2.4 (1.5–4.6)	2.8 (1.6–6.2)
	II–III	2.8 (1.9–6.2)	3.1 (1.9–8.3)
	III–IV	3.8 (1.9–8.3)	4.5 (1.8–8.3)
	IV–V	2.6 (1.3–8.3)	3.5 (1.7–12.5)
	I–V	2.9 (2.1–4.0)	3.5 (2.2–5.0)
% Simultaneous	I–II	0 (0–10)	0 (0–10)
	II–III	0 (0–10)	0 (0–20)
	III–IV	0 (0–10)	0 (0–20)
	IV–V	0 (0–10)	0 (0–40)
% Interrupted	I	0 (0–0)	0 (0–10)
	II	0 (0–20)	0 (0–30)
	III	0 (0–10)	0 (0–30)
	IV	0 (0–10)	0 (0–30)
	V	0 (0–10)	0 (0–30)
% Dropped	II	0 (0–10)	0 (0–20)
	III	0 (0–10)	0 (0–30)
	IV	0 (0–10)	0 (0–30)

cm) may give a misleading impression of its relaxation, since a single side hole, positioned in the center of the UES at rest, may actually lay in the cervical esophagus during a swallow (Kahrilas et al, 1988a). To obviate this problem, we use a dedicated special catheter assembly consisting of eight side holes located at 1.0-cm intervals, oriented radially around the catheter. Experience has shown this procedure to be useful in evaluating the UES relaxation and the pharyngoesophageal coordination (Fig. 7–7). An alternative approach is the use of a particular type of sleeve sensor (Kahrilas et al, 1987) made especially for the evaluation of UES relaxation over long periods of time. This device is a reliable indicator of UES relaxation. Its disadvantages are its slow response rate to pressure rises and its large caliber. Both must be taken into account in evaluating resting pressure values.

Water-perfused catheters, even with low compliance and good pressure rise rate (>200 mm Hg/second), may be inadequate in studying rapid changes in pharyngeal pressure that reach up to 500 mm Hg/second. Therefore, some authors advocate the use of solid-state microtransducers for this purpose (Castell et al, 1990). Because of their intrinsic construction characteristics, these transducers cannot be assembled closely enough to each other without making the probe rigid and unusable for intubation. Currently, the minimum possible distance between transducers is 3 cm. To overcome this problem, two adjacent probes had been used in some studies (Dantas et al, 1990a).

Clinical Application

Stationary esophageal manometry, performed as described, is indicated when

1. A motility disorder of the esophageal body and/or the LES is suspected from complaints of dysphagia, regurgitation, or chest pain.
2. A comprehensive evaluation of the antireflux mechanism in GERD is desired.
3. A disturbance of the pharyngoesophageal phase of swallowing is suspected.

Functional Disorders of the Esophageal Body and Lower Esophageal Sphincter

Abnormalities occurring in the esophageal body or the LES can give rise to a number of disorders in the esophageal phase of swallowing. These disorders result from either a direct deterioration of esophageal muscle func-

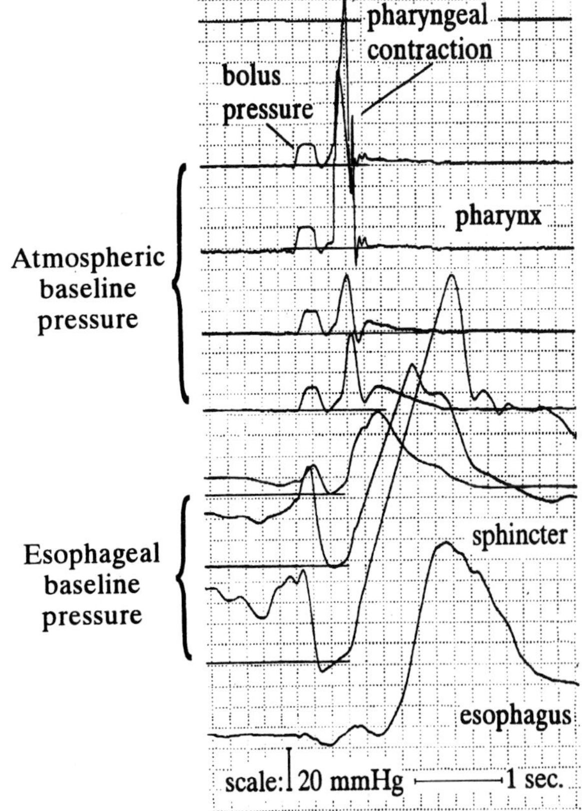

FIGURE 7–7 ■ Normal cricopharyngeal recording made with a catheter having side holes spaced 1 cm apart. This technique shows the relation of pharyngeal contractions to the relaxation of the upper esophageal sphincter and response in the cervical esophagus. The typical intrabolus pressure is evident before the upstroke of pharyngeal contractions. (From DeMeester TR, Crookes PF: Benign and malignant disease of the esophagus. In Levine BA, Copeland EM III, Howard RJ, et al [eds]: Current Practice of Surgery. New York, Churchill Livingstone 1993, p 14.)

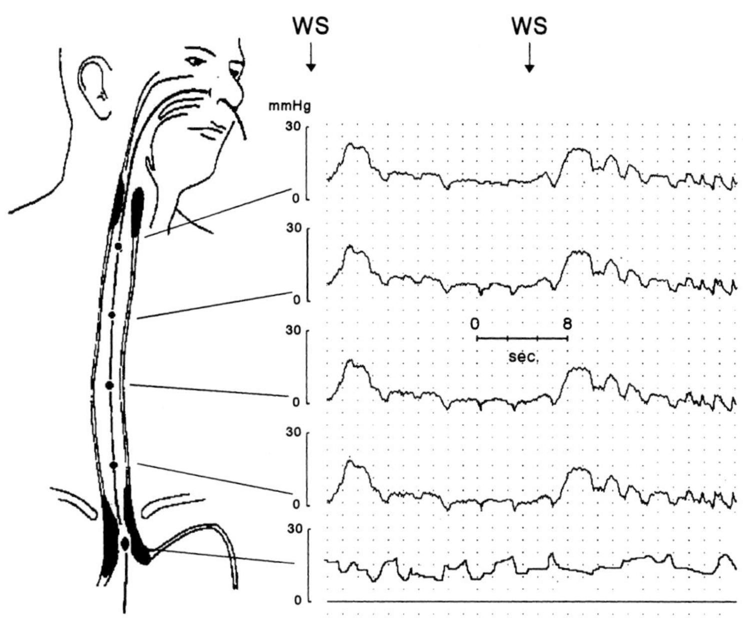

FIGURE 7–8 ■ Esophageal motility in a patient with achalasia, showing the typical features: absence of peristaltic progression in the esophageal body and the inability of the lower esophageal sphincter to completely relax on swallowing. (WS, wet swallow.)

tion or a more generalized neural, muscular, or systemic disease such as progressive systemic sclerosis, dermatomyositis, or myasthenia gravis. With the introduction of esophageal manometry, a number of primary esophageal motility disorders have been classified as separate disease entities. These specific primary disorders are (1) achalasia, (2) diffuse or segmental esophageal spasm, (3) high-amplitude peristaltic esophageal contractions, the so-called nutcracker esophagus, (4) the hypertensive LES, and (5) ineffective esophageal motility. The term *nonspecific esophageal motor disorder* includes patients whose manometric features are clearly abnormal but defy classification into one of the major groups.

The pathogenesis, clinical aspects, and treatment of these conditions are explained in Chapter 34. Here we briefly review their motility patterns and manometric diagnostic criteria.

Achalasia

The classic pattern includes the loss of progressive peristalsis in the body of the esophagus and failure of the LES to relax on deglutition (Fig. 7–8). The contractions recorded at different esophageal levels are simultaneous and usually of low amplitude. Other features include elevation of intraluminal esophageal pressure and hypertension of the LES. The combination of peristaltic failure and nonrelaxation of the sphincter causes a functional holdup of ingested material in the esophagus and results in dilatation of the esophageal body. With time, the functional disorder results in anatomic alterations, which show on radiographic studies as a dilated esophagus with a tapering, beaklike narrowing of the distal end. Usually, the air fluid level in the esophagus reflects the degree of resistance imposed by the nonrelaxing sphincter. As the disease progresses, the esophagus becomes massively dilated and tortuous.

A subgroup of patients with otherwise typical features of classic achalasia show simultaneous contractions of the esophageal body, which may be of high amplitude. This manometric pattern has been termed *vigorous achalasia*, and chest pain episodes are a common complaint in these patients (Bondi et al, 1972). In patients with advanced disease, the radiographic study can show a corkscrew deformity of the esophagus and diverticulum formation.

Diffuse and Segmental Esophageal Spasm

This manometric abnormality occurs relatively infrequently. Its incidence is approximately one-fifth that of achalasia. It may involve the total length of the esophageal body but is usually confined to the smooth muscle in the distal two thirds. In segmental esophageal spasm,

> **ESOPHAGEAL MOTILITY DISORDERS**
>
> **Primary**
>
> 1. Achalasia, vigorous achalasia.
> 2. Diffuse and segmental esophageal spasm.
> 3. Nutcracker esophagus.
> 4. Hypertensive lower esophageal sphincter.
> 5. Ineffective esophageal motility.
> 6. Nonspecific esophageal motility disorders.
>
> **Secondary**
>
> 1. Collagen vascular diseases (e.g., progressive systemic sclerosis, polymyositis and dermatomyositis, mixed connective tissue disease, systemic lupus erythematosus).
> 2. Chronic idiopathic intestinal pseudo-obstruction.
> 3. Neuromuscular diseases.
> 4. Endocrine and metastatic disorders.
> 5. Alcoholic neuropathy.

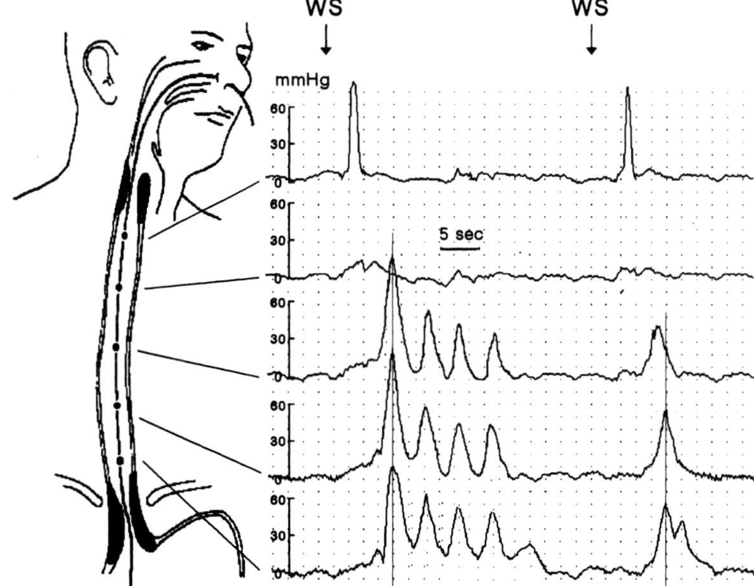

FIGURE 7–9 ■ Esophageal body motility in a patient with diffuse esophageal spasm. The motor disorder is characterized by an increased percentage of simultaneous contractions (>20%). The contraction can be repetitive and multipeaked, with high amplitude and long duration. The second level from the top is at the junction of striated and smooth muscle where contractions are normally of low amplitude. (WS, wet swallow.)

the manometric abnormalities are confined to a short segment of the smooth muscle esophagus.

The classic motility finding in these patients is characterized by the frequent occurrence of simultaneous and repetitive esophageal contractions, which may be of abnormally high amplitude or long duration (Fig. 7–9). Key in the diagnosis of diffuse esophageal spasm is that the esophagus usually retains some degree of peristaltic performance, thus distinguishing it from achalasia. A criterion of 20% or more simultaneous contractions in response to wet swallows has been used to justify the diagnosis of diffuse esophageal spasm. The LES in patients with the disease usually shows normal resting pressure and relaxation on deglutition. A hypertensive sphincter with poor relaxation may also be present (Richter and Castell, 1984) and may make differentiation from vigorous achalasia difficult.

Nutcracker Esophagus

Esophageal manometric studies in patients with chest pain of a noncardiac origin have shown that a large proportion of these patients have peristaltic esophageal contractions of exceedingly high amplitude. In the late 1970s, this disorder was termed *nutcracker* or *super-squeezer esophagus*. Other terms used to describe this entity are *hypertensive peristalsis* or *high-amplitude peristaltic contractions* (Benjamin et al, 1979). It is the most frequent of the primary esophageal motility disorders.

By definition, nutcracker esophagus is a manometric abnormality in patients with chest pain and/or dysphagia and is characterized by peristaltic esophageal contractions of amplitude that exceeds the 95th percentile of a healthy population (Fig. 7–10). Contraction amplitudes in these patients can easily be above 400 mm Hg. Patients with peristaltic waves of excessively long duration are

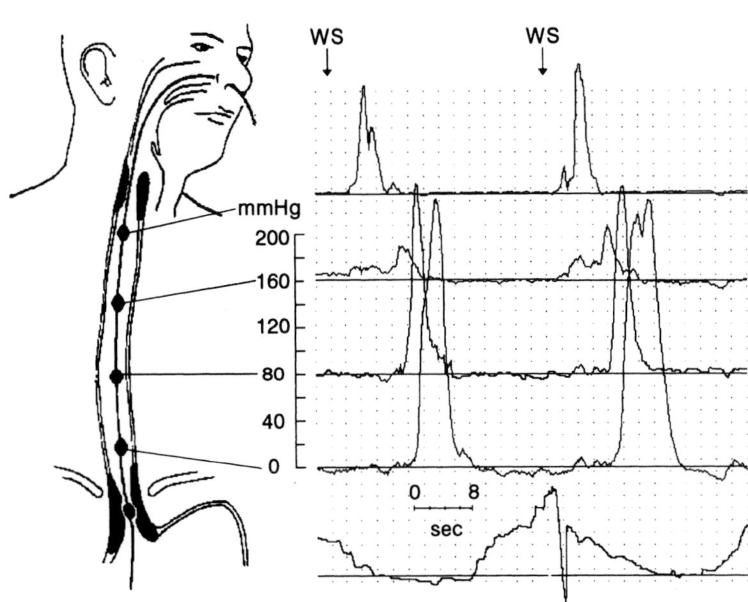

FIGURE 7–10 ■ Esophageal motility in a patient with nutcracker esophagus. Esophageal contractions are always peristaltic, with high amplitude (>180 mm Hg). Relaxation of the lower esophageal sphincter is maintained. (WS, wet swallow.)

also considered to have nutcracker esophagus. So far, the cause of peristaltic contractions with high amplitude or long duration in the pathogenesis of noncardiac chest pain or dysphagia has not been established.

Hypertensive Lower Esophageal Sphincter

An LES of high pressure was first described as a separate entity by Code and colleagues (1960) in patients with chest pain or dysphagia. The disorder is characterized by elevated basal pressure of the LES with normal relaxation and normal wave progression in the body of the esophagus. About 50% of these patients have associated motility disorders of the esophageal body, particularly nutcracker esophagus and diffuse esophageal spasm, which may account for the symptoms. In the remainder, the disorder exists as an isolated abnormality of the distal esophageal sphincter. Symptoms can be caused by a prolonged postrelaxation contraction of the LES in addition to the hypertensive sphincter. Our criteria for the diagnosis of a hypertensive-hypercontracting LES are listed in the following box (Eypasch et al, 1990a).

DIAGNOSTIC CRITERIA FOR A HYPERCONTRACTING LOWER ESOPHAGEAL SPHINCTER

1. Dysphagia and chest pain as the predominant symptoms.
2. Lower esophageal mean resting pressure > 25 mm Hg.
3. Mean duration of postrelaxation contractions > 14 seconds
4. Mean slope of postrelaxation contraction pressure rise under 25 mm Hg/second.
5. No other primary esophageal motor disorders.
6. No endoscopic or radiographic evidence of an organic cause for the symptoms.

From Eypasch EP, Stein HJ, DeMeester TR, et al: The hypercontracting-hypertensive lower esophageal sphincter as a cause of dysphagia and chest pain. In Little AG, Ferguson MK, Skinner DB (eds): Diseases of the Esophagus, Vol II: Benign Diseases. Mount Kisco, NY, Futura Publishing Company, 1990, p 351.

Ineffective Esophageal Motility

Castell (2000) has introduced a new specific esophageal motility disorder called *ineffective esophageal motility.* This is defined as a contraction abnormality of the distal esophagus where the sum total of the number of low-amplitude contractions (<30 mm Hg) and nontransmitted contractions exceeds 30% of wet swallows. This abnormality is the most common manometric finding in patients with GERD and may be secondary to inflammatory injury of the esophageal body due to increased exposure to gastric juice. When present, the abnormality contributes to increased esophageal acid exposure due to a loss of effective esophageal acid clearance. At present, the process causing the altered motility appears to be irreversible once it has occurred.

Nonspecific Esophageal Motility Disorders

Many patients complaining of dysphagia or chest pain of noncardiac origin demonstrate a variety of esophageal contraction patterns on esophageal manometry that are clearly out of the normal range but do not meet the criteria of a classic primary esophageal motility disorder. Esophageal manometry in these patients frequently shows an increased number of multipeaked or repetitive contractions, contractions of prolonged duration, nontransmitted pharyngeal contractions, interrupted contraction waves, or contractions of low amplitude. These motility abnormalities have been termed *nonspecific* esophageal motility disorders. The significance of these abnormal contractions in the etiology of chest pain or dysphagia is still unclear.

There is considerable overlap in the classification of patients with esophageal motor abnormalities. A clear distinction between the classic primary esophageal motility disorders and so-called nonspecific esophageal motility disorders is often impossible. Patients with a diagnosis of nutcracker esophagus often have only nonspecific esophageal motility abnormalities when studied repeatedly, and progression from a nonspecific esophageal motility disorder to classic diffuse esophageal spasm during the natural course of the disease has been demonstrated (Dalton et al, 1988). Therefore, the finding of a nonspecific esophageal motility disorder may represent only a manometric marker of an intermittent more severe esophageal motor abnormality.

The boundaries between classic esophageal motility disorders of achalasia, diffuse esophageal spasm, nutcracker esophagus, and hypertensive LES are also vague. Differentiation of vigorous achalasia and diffuse esophageal spasm can be difficult, and intermediate types exist. Progression of diffuse esophageal spasm to achalasia has been observed (Vantrappen et al, 1979), and peristalsis may return in patients with classic achalasia after a Heller myotomy or balloon dilatation (Mellow, 1976). These observations support the concept that primary esophageal motility disorders may represent different expressions of a common underlying esophageal pathology.

Secondary Esophageal Motor Disorders

Although the most common disease leading to secondary deterioration of esophageal body function is long-standing GERD, the term usually denotes an esophageal motility disorder resulting from a generalized neural, muscular, or systemic metabolic disturbance. The esophagus is particularly affected by almost any of the collagen vascular disorders; the most common are progressive systemic sclerosis, mixed connective tissue disease, and polymyositis or dermatomyositis.

Eighty percent of patients with progressive systemic sclerosis have an esophageal motor abnormality. In most cases, the disease follows a prolonged course and usually affects only the smooth muscle in the distal two thirds of the esophagus. Typical findings on esophageal manometry are normal peristalsis in the proximal striated muscle, with weak or absent peristalsis in the distal smooth muscle portion (Fig. 7–11). LES pressure is progressively

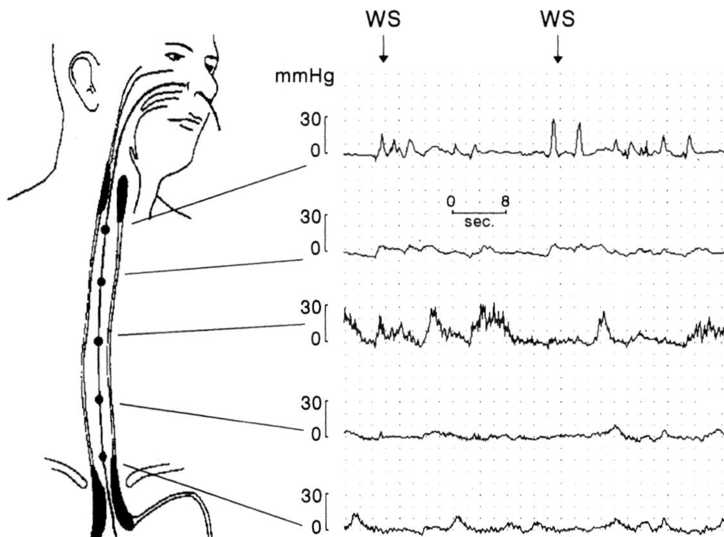

FIGURE 7–11 ■ Esophageal motility in a patient with progressive systemic sclerosis. A weak motor activity is maintained in the upper esophagus; in the distal two thirds (smooth muscle), any detectable activity in response to swallow is virtually absent. (WS, wet swallow.)

weakened as the disease advances, resulting in increased esophageal exposure to gastric juice due to a mechanically defective LES and poor clearance function of the esophageal body (Orringer et al, 1976; Zaninotto et al, 1989).

In patients with polymyositis or dermatomyositis, the upper striated muscle portion is the major site of esophageal involvement causing aspiration, nasopharyngeal regurgitation, and cervical dysphagia. Mixed connective tissue disease shows a mixture of the manometric findings of progressive systemic sclerosis and polymyositis.

GASTROESOPHAGEAL REFLUX DISEASE

GERD is a common foregut disorder, complicated by esophagitis, stricture, or Barrett's esophagus in about 50% of affected patients. The basic pathophysiologic abnormality in this condition is an increased esophageal exposure to gastric juice, for which there are three known causes. The first is a mechanically defective LES, accounting for about 60% of cases of GERD (Zaninotto et al, 1988a). The identification of this cause is important because medical therapy in this situation is plagued by high failure and relapse rates (Lieberman, 1987). The other two causes are inefficient esophageal clearance of refluxed gastric juice and abnormalities of the gastric reservoir that augment physiologic reflux, such as gastric dilatation and persistent gastric reservoir.

Incompetence of the Lower Esophageal Sphincter

Failure of the LES is caused by inadequate pressure, overall length, or abdominal length (that is, of the portion exposed to the positive pressure environment of the abdomen measured on manometry) (Bonavina et al, 1986; Zaninotto et al, 1988a). The probability of increased exposure to gastric juice is 69% to 76% if one component of the sphincter is abnormal, 65% to 88% if two components are abnormal, and 92% if all three are abnormal. This finding indicates that the failure of one or two of the components of the sphincter may be compensated for by the clearance of the esophageal body. Failure of all three sphincter components inevitably leads to increased esophageal exposure to gastric juice.

The most common cause of a mechanically defective LES is inadequate sphincter pressure, probably related to an abnormality of myogenic function. However, the efficiency of a normal sphincter pressure can be nullified by an inadequate abdominal length or an abnormally short overall resting length of the sphincter. An adequate abdominal length of sphincter is important in preventing reflux caused by increases in intra-abdominal pressure, and an adequate overall length is important in increasing the resistance to reflux caused by gastric dilatation. Therefore, patients with a low sphincter pressure or those with a normal pressure but a short abdominal length are unable to protect against reflux caused by fluctuations of intra-abdominal pressure that occur with daily activities or changes in body position. Patients with a low sphincter pressure or those with a normal pressure and abdominal length but short overall length are unable to protect against reflux related to further shortening of the sphincter caused by gastric dilatation as a result of outlet obstruction, aerophagia, or gluttony. Persons with short overall length commonly suffer from reflux caused by further shortening of the sphincter that occurs with eating (i.e., postprandial reflux) (DeMeester et al, 1999).

The overall competency of the LES is well represented by the calculation of the sphincter vector volume that combines pressures exerted over the entire length of the sphincter. When measured in a large number of patients, total and abdominal sphincter vector volumes were found to be markedly lower in patients with increased esophageal acid exposure compared with healthy volunteers, and volume decreased with increased severity of mucosal injury (Stein et al, 1991a). Comparing sphincter vector volume with standard sphincter parameters (i.e., resting pressure, overall and abdominal length), we found that sphincter vector volume had no significant advantage in detection of a defective sphincter in patients with advanced complications of GERD. Sphincter vector volume

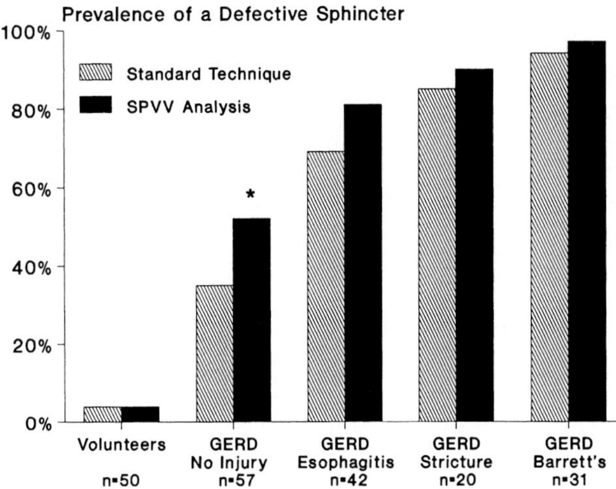

FIGURE 7–12 ■ Comparison of standard manometric techniques and sphincter pressure vector volume (SPVV) analysis in the identification of a mechanically defective lower esophageal sphincter. SPVV identifies a significantly higher number of patients with defective sphincter in the group of patients without complications of gastroesophageal reflux disease. *Asterisk*, $P < .05$ versus standard manometry. (From Stein HJ, DeMeester TR, Naspetti R, et al: Three-dimensional imaging of the lower esophageal sphincter in gastrointestinal reflux disease. Ann Surg 214:374, 1991.)

did have a greater sensitivity than standard manometry in identifying a mechanically defective sphincter in patients with increased esophageal acid exposure but no mucosal damage (Fig. 7–12).

Transient loss of the LES can be a functional problem of the gastric reservoir. Ingestion of excessive air or food can result in gastric dilatation and, if the active relaxation reflex has been lost, in increased intragastric pressure. When the stomach is distended, the vectors produced by gastric wall tension pull on the gastroesophageal junction with a force that varies according to the geometry of the cardia; that is, the forces are applied more directly when a hiatal hernia exists than when a proper angle of His is present. These forces pull on the terminal esophagus, causing it to be "taken up" into the stretched fundus, thereby reducing the length of the high-pressure zone. This process continues until a critical length is reached, usually about 1 to 2 cm, when the pressure drops precipitously and reflux occurs. If only the pressure—and not the length—of the high-pressure zone is measured, as with a Dent sleeve, this event appears as a spontaneous dissipation, or "relaxation," of the high-pressure zone.

The mechanism by which gastric distention contributes to shortening of the high-pressure zone, so that its pressure drops and reflux occurs, provides a mechanical explanation for transient relaxations of the LES without invoking a neuromuscular reflex. Rather than a transient muscular relaxation, there is a mechanical shortening of the high-pressure zone, secondary to progressive gastric distention, to the point where competence is lost. Consequently, non-swallow–induced relaxations of a normal high-pressure zone are inappropriately termed transient lower *relaxations*; instead, they should be called transient LES *shortenings*. These transient sphincter shortenings occur in the initial stages of GERD and are the mechanisms responsible for the early complaint of excessive postprandial reflux.

Esophageal Clearance of Refluxed Material

A second cause of increased esophageal exposure to gastric juice is inefficient esophageal clearance of refluxed material (Joelsson et al, 1982). This problem can result in an abnormal esophageal exposure to gastric juice in individuals who have a mechanically normal LES and normal gastric function by ineffectual clearing of physiologic reflux episodes. This situation is relatively rare, and ineffectual clearance is more apt to be seen in association with a mechanically incompetent cardia, in which case it augments the esophageal exposure to gastric juice by prolonging the duration of each reflux episode. As discussed previously, the motility abnormality that occurs in GERD has been termed by Castell as *ineffective esophageal motility disorder*.

Manometry of the esophageal body can detect failure of esophageal clearance by analysis of the pressure amplitude and speed of progression of the peristaltic wave through the esophagus. The work of Kahrilas and colleagues (1988b) has shown that the amplitude of an esophageal contraction required to clear the esophagus of barium varies according to the level. Lower segments require a greater amplitude (30 to 40 mm Hg) than upper segments. Inadequate amplitude results in ineffective clearance. Increased esophageal clearance as a result of increased swallowing may compensate for a mechanically defective sphincter with an abnormality of one or two of its critical components but is unlikely to compensate for three abnormal components.

PHARYNGOESOPHAGEAL SWALLOWING DISORDERS

Disorders of the pharyngoesophageal phase of swallowing are relatively uncommon. They result from a discoordination of the neuromuscular events during the act of swallowing and the inability to propel the swallowed material from the oropharynx into the cervical esophagus. Zenker's diverticulum or a cricopharyngeal bar is often, but not always, present.

The rapidity of the oropharyngeal phase of swallowing, the movement of the gullet, and the asymmetry of the cricopharyngeus account for the difficulty in assessing abnormalities of esophagopharyngeal swallowing disorders with manometric techniques. However, carefully performed motility studies may demonstrate incoordination and incomplete relaxation of the UES during swallowing. This pattern is the feature of many neurologic diseases, including cerebrovascular accident and trauma (head injury and iatrogenic nerve injury) (Duranceau et al, 1988). It may result in failure of the pharynx to empty or cause nasal regurgitation and aspiration. It may, but not always, cause dysphagia. In other patients, particularly those with a history of poliomyelitis, the pressure generated by the pharynx can be subnormal. This condition is important to identify, because the

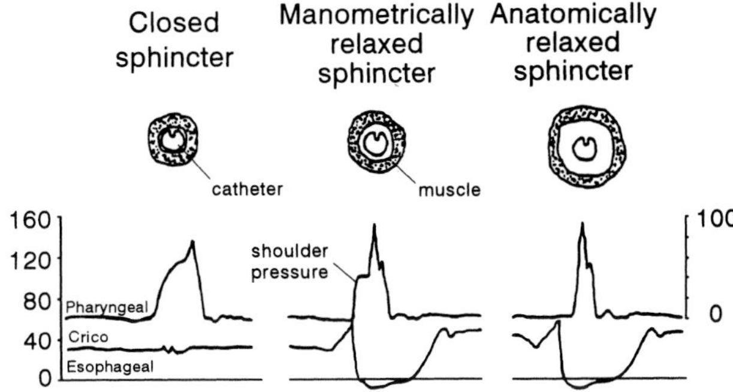

FIGURE 7–13 ■ The intrabolus pressure or shoulder pressure in the hypopharynx, in a manometrically relaxed but incomplete anatomically relaxed upper esophageal sphincter (UES). The shoulder on the pharyngeal pressure wave indicates increased resistance to the passage of a bolus through the pharyngoesophageal segment caused by pathology of the cricopharyngeal and cervical esophageal muscle resulting in poor compliance and incomplete anatomic relaxation. (From Stein HJ, DeMeester TR, Hinder RA: Outpatient physiologic testing and surgical management of foregut motility disorders. Curr Probl Surg 24:441, 1992.)

presence of a profound loss of pharyngeal pressure may be helped by a cricopharyngeal myotomy.

It has been difficult to consistently demonstrate motility abnormalities in patients with cervical dysphagia, cricopharyngeal bar, or Zenker's diverticulum. Some studies (Cook et al, 1989; Dantas et al, 1990) focused attention on the role of reduced compliance of the UES and cervical esophagus in the pathophysiology of these disorders, making a distinction between a "manometrically relaxed" and "anatomically relaxed" sphincter (Fig. 7–13). Combined radiographic and manometric studies have highlighted the importance of the intrabolus pressure, detected as a "shoulder" or "hump" just before the upstroke of hypopharyngeal pressure wave as an indication of a manometrically relaxed but incompletely anatomically relaxed sphincter. In two separate studies of patients with Zenker's diverticulum and cricopharyngeal bar (Cook et al, 1990; Dantas et al, 1990b), the intrabolus pressure was found to be elevated despite complete manometric relaxation of the UES. This phenomenon is attributed to decreased compliance of the striated muscle in the cervical esophagus. It allows manometric relaxation but incomplete opening of the sphincter and a higher driving pressure transmitted to the bolus by the tongue and soft palate to compensate for the loss of compliance of the upper esophagus.

Loss of compliance of the pharyngocervical esophageal segment may be the most common abnormality in patients with pharyngeal dysphagia, with or without Zenker's diverticulum. Increasing the diameter of this noncompliant segment by a surgical myotomy reduces the resistance it imposes to the bolus transport into the esophagus. Manometrically, this procedure results in the disappearance of the "shoulder" in the pharyngeal contraction (Fig. 7–14).

With extensive study, Mason and co-workers (1998) have clarified pharyngeal swallowing disorders and have emphasized that pharyngeal swallowing is a mechanical process. It requires the thyrohyoid muscle groups to elevate the larynx, the glossopharyngeal musculature to propel the bolus, the cricopharyngeus to relax, and the cervical esophageal muscle to be compliant (Asoh and Goyal, 1978; Cook et al, 1989; Ekberg, 1986; Kahrilas et al, 1988; Mason et al, 1998; Palmer et al, 1989; Shipp et al, 1970). This equates mechanically to three primary forces:

1. A traction force ($F_{traction}$), due to the contractions of the thyrohyoid muscles, resulting in the anterior-superior movement of the hyoid bone and, in turn, elevation of the larynx.
2. A muscle force (F_{muscle}), due to the active and passive tone within the inferior constrictor, cricopharyngeal, and cervical esophageal muscles, which resist sphincter opening.
3. A bolus force (F_{bolus}) generated by the glossopharyngeal muscles, which propel the bolus into the pharyngoesophageal segment.

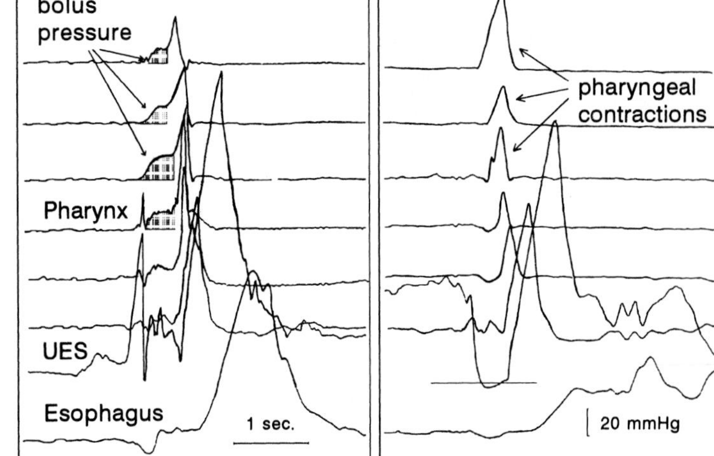

FIGURE 7–14 ■ Pharyngoesophageal manometric tracing in a patient with Zenker's diverticulum before and after diverticulectomy and myotomy. A nonrelaxing upper esophageal sphincter and a prominent bolus or shoulder pressure are evident in the preoperative recording. Myotomy increased the compliance of the pharyngoesophageal segment, with complete disappearance of the shoulder pressure in the pharyngeal contractions.

For opening of the UES to occur, the following must be true:

$$F_{\text{traction}} - F_{\text{muscle}} + F_{\text{bolus}} \geq 0 \text{ (atm pressure)}$$

or

$$F_{\text{traction}} + F_{\text{bolus}} \geq F_{\text{muscle}}$$

where atm is atmospheric.

Manometry can measure the forces involved in the transfer of a bolus from the hypopharynx into the esophagus and the resistance to flow imposed by a noncompliant cricopharyngeal and cervical esophageal muscle. These measurements provide insight into the mechanical deficiencies of the various steps in the swallowing process and a logical basis for therapy. Surgeons have the ability to substantially alter the F_{muscle} and, possibly, the F_{traction} force. Manometry of the pharyngoesophogeal segment can identify manometric markers of pharyngeal swallowing that can serve as a guide to the selection of patients who would benefit from a cricopharyngoesophageal myotomy.

Manometry of the pharyngoesophageal segment (Mason et al, 1998) can be used to measure pressure associated with three different physical conditions of the UES (Fig. 7–15):

- Cavity or opening pressure
- Hydrodynamic or intrabolus pressure
- Contact or closing pressure

The mechanics of pharyngeal swallowing consist of a closed, an opening, an open, and finally a reclosing of the UES. The pressure sequence during a swallow is from a closing, to an opening, to a hydrodynamic, and finally back to a closing pressure. The cavity or opening pressure

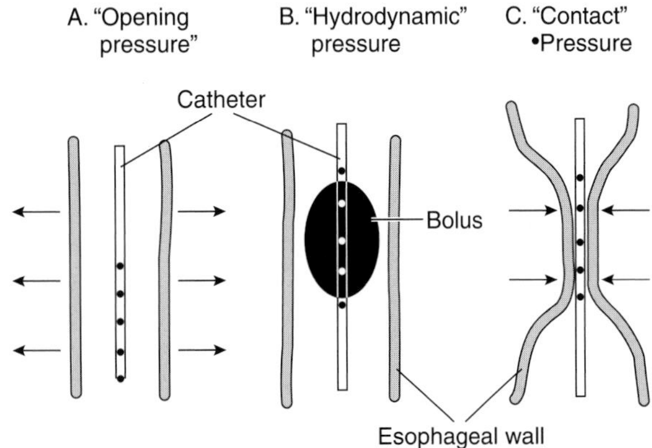

FIGURE 7–15 ■ Diagrammatic representation of the manometry catheter during the three different physical conditions of the upper esophageal sphincter. *Arrows* indicate the direction of movement of the esophageal walls relative to the catheter. *A*, The esophageal walls are distracted away from the catheter. During this phase, a falling pressure is recorded. *B*, A bolus surrounds the pressure transducer on its passage through the pharyngoesophageal segment. During this phase, the pressure reflects the intrabolus pressure. *C*, The esophageal or pharyngeal muscles contract and compress the catheter. During this phase of the swallow, a rising pressure is recorded.

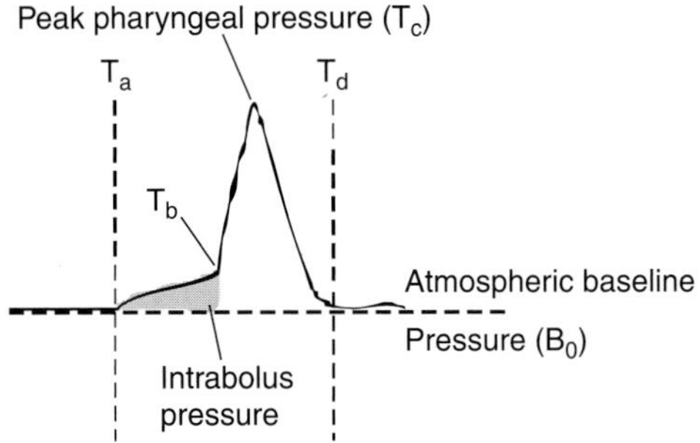

FIGURE 7–16 ■ Schematic diagram of a typical pharyngeal pressure tracing. T_a represents arrival of the bolus head; T_b, the bolus tail; T_c, peak pressure of the pharyngeal-stripping wave; T_d, completion of the pharyngeal pressure wave; and B_0, baseline atmospheric pressure.

reflects the pressure within the UES caused by the walls being pulled open (Fig. 7–15*A*). During this phase, the walls of the pharyngoesophageal segment are no longer in contact with the catheter and air fills the space. After the UES is opened, the bolus flows into the pharyngoesophageal segment, producing a hydrodynamic or intrabolus pressure. This pressure reflects the forces applied on the bolus as it passes through the UES and into the cervical esophagus (Fig. 7–15*B*). The pharyngeal stripping wave closely follows the tail of the bolus, and as the pharyngeal and cricopharyngeal muscles squeeze down on the catheter, a contact or closing pressure occurs (Fig. 7–15*C*).

The characteristic feature of the pressure tracing in the proximal pharyngoesophageal segment is that before the swallow the catheter lies freely in the hypopharynx, exposed to atmospheric pressure. After the swallow is completed, the pressure tracing returns to atmospheric pressure (Fig. 7–16). The onset of a swallow (T_a) is identified by a rise in pressure >2 mm Hg above the atmospheric baseline pressure (B_0). This is caused by the movement of the bolus into the pharyngoesophageal segment. A second steeper slope (T_b) occurs as the tail of the bolus passes the pressure port ahead of the pharyngeal stripping wave. The peak of this slope is the closing pressure of the pharyngeal wall on the pressure port and is the highest amplitude attained during a pharyngeal contraction (T_c). This is followed by a decline back to the resting pressure (T_d). The pharyngeal stripping or clearing wave can be assessed by noting the time interval between successive peak pharyngeal pressures recorded by different channels. One can measure the total duration of the pharyngeal event by noting the time interval between T_a and T_d.

The cricoesophageal muscle or UES is closed at rest. At the onset of a swallow, the port in the proximal UES exhibits at rise in pressure, reflecting the upward motion of the tonically contracted sphincter on the manometry catheter (T_0) (Fig. 7–17). When this occurs, pressure ports in the more distal sphincter may exhibit an immediate pressure fall consistent with the port slipping caudally out of the sphincter into the esophagus as the larynx is elevated. Following this rise in pressure in the more proximal portion of the sphincter, a decline in pressure is observed with the relaxation of the sphincter.

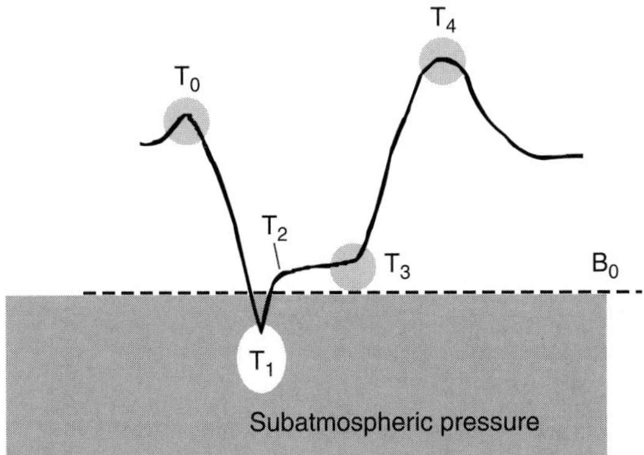

FIGURE 7–17 ■ Schematic diagram of a typical upper esophageal sphincter pressures tracing illustrating the distal pharyngoesophageal segment. T_0 represents the beginning of the swallow; T_1 complete opening of the sphincter (with complete opening, pressure is subatmospheric); T_2, transition from a subatmospheric to a supra-atmospheric pressure as the head of the bolus flows into the sphincter; T_3, the bolus tail ahead of the pharyngeal stripping wave; T_4, peak pressure following luminal closure by the pharyngeal stripping wave; and B_0, baseline atmospheric pressure.

As the traction forces begin to dominate, the rate of the pressure drop increases and a "checkmark" or kink in the pressure tracing may be generated. (Brasseur et al, 1996; McConnel et al, 1988a, 1988b, 1988c; Shaker et al, 1997). This is due to the traction forces overcoming the muscular forces, causing the sphincter walls to separate with the creation of a gap. The pressure becomes subatmospheric as the walls of the sphincter are pulled apart to create this expanding space. This drop to subatmospheric pressure within the pharyngoesophageal segment implies sphincter opening. (Brasseur et al, 1996; Cook et al, 1989; McConnel et al, 1988a, 1988b, 1988c). As the fluid bolus enters the open sphincter, the pressure rises from the subatmospheric drop to a supra-atmospheric pressure (T_2). As the bolus tail leaves the segment, there is again an abrupt rise in pressure (T_3), representing closure of the esophageal lumen against the pressure ports. The maximum pressure reached in this rapid ascent is due to the passage of the pharyngeal stripping wave (T_4) through the cricopharyngeal muscle and into the cervical esophagus. Sphincter opening is defined as "normal" if the pressure at T_1 became subatmospheric and as "impaired" if this does not occur. For a normal subatmospheric intrasphincteric pressure drop to occur, there must be complete sphincter relaxation.

The resistance to pharyngoesophageal flow relates to the compliance of the cricopharyngeal and cervical esophageal muscles and the amplitude of the pharyngeal contraction waves. It is assessed by measuring the intrabolus pressure. Intrabolus pressure in the proximal pharyngoesophageal segment is measured at the time T_b (see Fig. 7–16). Intrabolus pressure in the UES and the more distal pharyngoesophageal segment is measured during the passage of the head (T_2) and tail (T_3) of the bolus through the open UES (see Fig. 7–17). The highest pressure measured at T_b (see Fig. 7–16), T_2 or T_3 (see Fig. 7–17) is considered to be the intrabolus pressure for a swallow. The average of five swallows is used to calculate the final intrabolus pressure. A patient is considered to have an elevated intrabolus pressure when the pressure measured with a 5-ml swallow is greater than the 95th percentile for 56 normal subjects (>16.3 mm Hg). A patient is classified as having low pharyngeal contraction amplitudes when the pressure measured with a 5-ml swallow is below the 5th percentile for 56 normal subjects (<27.7 mm Hg).

The UES is normally open and relaxed on arrival of a bolus, and this can be depicted manometrically by a subatmospheric drop in pressure, before any radiologic contrast material can be seen in the UES. Any impairment in UES relaxation and opening is evident by a failure of the intersphincteric pressure to fall during the opening phase of the swallow. In this situation, the intrabolus pressure is elevated as the fluid bolus meets the increased outflow resistance at the level of the UES. If, however, the glossopharyngeal contraction amplitudes are below normal, the intrabolus pressure will be within the normal range. In this situation, a myotomy can still be of benefit by reducing the active and passive tone of the muscles and thereby decreasing the resistance to flow through the pharyngoesophageal segment. As a consequence, it is easier for the weak glossopharyngeal contractions to overcome outflow resistance. For this reason, a poor pharyngeal peak contraction pressure is not a predictor of poor outcome. Selecting which patient will benefit from a myotomy in this situation is difficult because of the absence of an elevated bolus pressure. If pharyngeal contraction pressure is normal, it may help to plot the peak bolus pressure that occurs with progressive increases in the volume of the swallowed bolus (Fig. 7–18). In this situation, the intrabolus pressures at T_2 and T_3 (see Fig. 7–17) are higher, indicating that the patient's dysphagia is due to poor compliance in the cricopharyngeal and cervical esophageal muscle. The most important

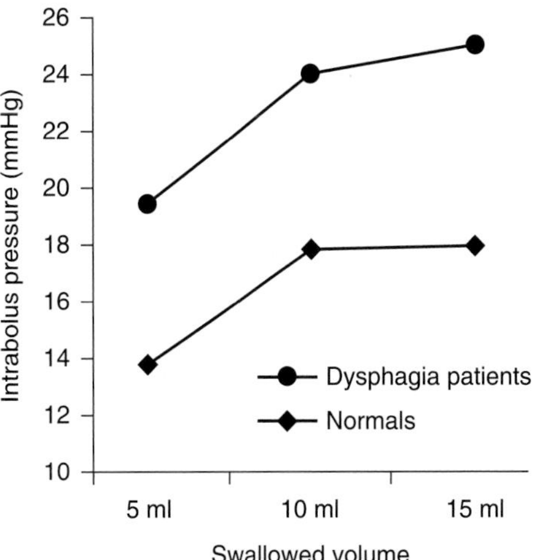

FIGURE 7–18 ■ Relationship of swallow volume to intrabolus pressure in patients who have lost compliance of the cricopharyngeal and cervical esophageal muscle. Higher pressure for increasing swallowed volume indicates that patients have sufficient pharyngeal muscle power to create an intrabolus pressure, and improvement of the compliance with a myotomy of the cricopharyngeal and cervical esophageal muscle should result in clinical improvement.

manometric marker in selecting patients for myotomy is the absence of the subatmospheric intrasphincteric pressure drop. When this is combined with an increased intrabolus pressure, the surgeon has the mechanical indicators that myotomy will result in improved swallowing.

ESOPHAGEAL PROVOCATIVE TESTS

Technique

The spontaneous occurrence of symptoms during a standard esophageal motility study is rare, especially in patients with noncardiac chest pain. Consequently, a number of provocative tests have been designed to identify the esophagus as the cause of these symptoms. Of these, the most commonly used are (1) the intraesophageal acid perfusion (Bernstein) test, (2) the edrophonium (Tensilon) test, and (3) the intraesophageal balloon distention test.

Acid Perfusion Test (Bernstein Test)

Introduced more than 40 years ago (Bernstein and Baker, 1958), this simple test aims to determine whether the patient's symptoms are reproduced by the infusion of acid into the esophagus. If results are positive, the test indicates that the esophagus is sensitive to acid and increased esophageal exposure to acid is assumed. As originally described, the distal esophagus is perfused with 0.1 normal HCl at 6 to 8 ml/minute, with the patient sitting upright. Ideally, a placebo is also infused; that is, acid or saline is perfused alternately without the patient knowing the identity of the perfusate. The patient is asked to report any symptom that develops during infusion. Consistent reproduction of the patient's usual symptoms only during acid perfusion and rapid abatement during saline perfusion or after antacid administration indicate a positive test. Development of symptoms during both the saline and acid perfusion or development of symptoms foreign to the patient's usual experience represent an equivocal test. Failure to develop any symptoms during a 30-minute acid perfusion indicates a normal test finding.

Various investigators have reported that 34% to 100% of patients with typical symptoms of GERD have a positive acid perfusion test result (Battle et al, 1973; Behar et al, 1976; Bennett and Atkinson, 1966; Benz et al, 1972). Failure to include certain components of gastric juice (pepsin, bile, pancreatic enzymes) in the perfusate may account for some of the normal results. A false-negative result can also occur in patients who have an insensitive esophagus and has been exemplified in patients with severe hemorrhagic esophagitis without pain. False-positive results are seen in 15% of asymptomatic subjects (Behar et al, 1976). Of concern is that symptomatic subjects whose pain is not caused by reflux may have a similar incidence of false-positive findings, resulting in an erroneous diagnosis. Patients with duodenal ulcer may have heartburn as well and often have symptoms during esophageal acid perfusion (deMoraes-Filho and Bettarello, 1974). This condition can cause diagnostic confusion if the ulcer is overlooked.

Edrophonium Test (Tensilon Test)

The edrophonium test is used to identify chest pain of esophageal origin in patients in whom cardiac disease has been excluded. The cholinesterase inhibitor edrophonium HCl (Tensilon) is injected intravenously at a dose of 80 μg/kg not to exceed a total dose of 10 mg. A syringe with 1 mg of the antidote atropine should always be at hand while the test is performed. The test is ideally placebo-controlled. The end point of the test is the patient's chest pain and the similarity of the pain to that which is spontaneously experienced.

A *positive* result is defined as replication of the patient's chest pain within 5 minutes of the edrophonium injection, but not after the placebo injection. The test is positive in 20% to 30% of patients with noncardiac chest pain but not in asymptomatic volunteers (Benjamin et al, 1983; Richter et al, 1985). In both, edrophonium causes a marked increase in amplitude and duration of esophageal contractions, but the end point of the test is the reproduction of the patient's typical chest pain rather than a specific change in esophageal motility. The disadvantages of the test are that it is helpful in only a small portion of patients with chest pain, carries a risk of side effects, and reproduces symptoms with an unphysiologic stimulus (Landon et al, 1981). The test should not be performed in patients with asthma, chronic obstructive airway disease, or cardiac arrhythmias.

Esophageal Balloon Distention Test

First described in 1955 as a diagnostic test to distinguish esophageal from cardiac chest pain (Kramer and Hollander, 1955), the balloon distention test has received interest as a useful esophageal provocative test (Barish et al, 1986; Costantini et al, 1992c; Richter et al, 1986). An inflatable balloon is positioned 10 cm above the LES and gradually inflated with air in 1-ml increments. The balloon must be completely deflated between two consecutive inflations to avoid esophageal accommodation. Esophageal motility is simultaneously monitored above and below the balloon.

The test result is considered positive when typical symptoms are reproduced with distention of the balloon to volumes less than those required to produce pain in normal subjects. One study has indicated that the test reproduces chest pain episodes in up to 48% of patients with noncardiac chest pain but not in volunteers (Richter et al, 1986). Although the test has a greater diagnostic yield than provocative drug studies, it is relatively invasive and provides no information on spontaneously occurring symptoms.

AMBULATORY 24-HOUR MOTILITY MONITORING OF THE DISTAL ESOPHAGUS

Technique

The intermittent and unpredictable occurrence of motor abnormalities and symptoms in patients with esophageal motility disorders limits the diagnostic value of standard manometry performed in a laboratory setting over a short time period. The new technique of prolonged esophageal manometry was developed to overcome these shortcomings. Because of the high sampling frequency required to evaluate esophageal motor activity (at least 4 Hz) (Bremner et al, 1992a; Castell et al, 1988), prolonged outpatient monitoring of esophageal motility became available only after the introduction of portable digital data recorders with a large storage capacity. Today, ambulatory manometry allows the evaluation of esophageal motor function based on more than 1000 contraction sequences monitored under a variety of physiologic conditions (i.e., upright activity, eating, and sleeping).

The technique was introduced in the mid-1980s, and first pioneering recorders stored the data on an analogic basis on a magnetic tape, from which analogic paper tracings were obtained (Janssens et al, 1986). Early solid-state digital dataloggers either had to perform on-line reduction of pressure data (Smout et al, 1989) or only allowed the recording of two pressure signals for a limited period of time (3 to 4 hours). In this latter situation, an intermittent recording (i.e., 128 seconds, every 17 minutes, or whenever the patient pressed an event marker) was necessary in order to monitor the patient over a complete circardian period (Eypasch et al, 1990b). Even though the intermittent recording showed good correlation and reliability with the continuous recording, the latter certainly represents a better choice. Further, in order to characterize the esophageal contraction sequence, the use of only two recording sites may be insufficient. The omission of a pharyngeal transducer prevents the ability to detect pharyngeal swallows, since external devices such as microphones are unreliable. Continuous hardware progress has now provided dataloggers with high storage capacity (4.0 megabytes), allowing 24-hour continuous recording of three esophageal and one pharyngeal pressure channels along with contemporary recording of two pH channels for complete foregut physiologic ambulatory monitoring (Fig. 7–19).

The test is performed on an outpatient basis. After the standard stationary manometry, a 7 French catheter with four electronic microtransducers (Sentron, Amsterdam, the Netherlands) is passed through the nose into the esophagus. The three distal transducers, 5 cm apart from each other, are positioned 5, 10, and 15 cm above the upper border of the LES. The most proximal transducer, 10 cm apart from the others, is located in the cricopharyngeal area, in order to record pharyngeal swallowing. The transducers are calibrated at 0 and 50 mm Hg by immersion in a water column before and after the test. To ensure test reliability, eventual drifts must not exceed 8 mm Hg.

The transducers are connected to a portable digital datalogger (Microdigitrapper 4.0, Medtronic, Minneapolis), and data are stored at an 8-Hz sampling rate. After placement of the catheter, patients are sent home and encouraged to perform normal daily activity. They are instructed to keep a detailed diary for the next 24 hours. It should indicate the time of meals, when they assume the supine position for sleep, when they arise in the morning, and when symptoms occur.

After the test, the raw data are transferred to a computer for further analysis. Approximately 1000 to 1400

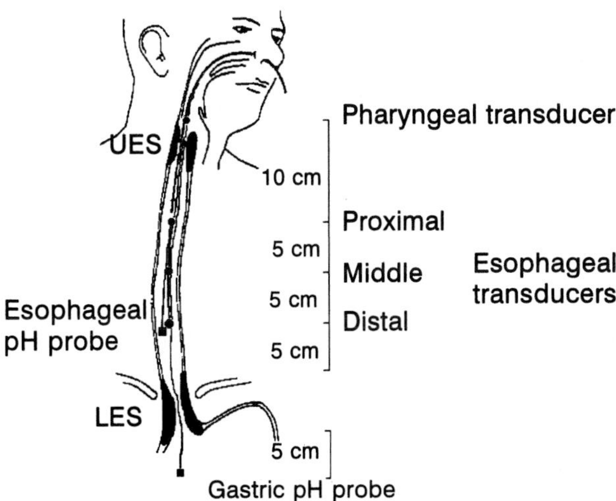

FIGURE 7–19 ■ Prolonged esophageal motility monitoring is performed with three electronic microtransducers positioned 5, 10, and 15 cm above the upper border of the lower esophageal sphincter (LES). An additional microtransducer is located in the pharynx, to detect pharyngeal swallows. Concomitant pH monitoring of the distal esophagus (electrode 5 cm above the LES) and of the stomach (electrode 5 cm below the LES) can be performed. This procedure allows a complete ambulatory foregut physiologic monitoring.

contractions are recorded by each pressure transducer over the 24-hour period, and a fully automated analysis of such a large amount of data is mandatory. We have developed and validated against manual analysis a software program for automated computer analysis of 24-hour esophageal motility monitoring. The program is commercially available from Medtronic (Minneapolis) (Bremner et al, 1993). In brief, the esophageal baseline is reset every 60 seconds according to the mode value for that time period. Contraction recognition is based on an algorithm that defines a *contraction* as a rise in pressure greater than a threshold value for a specified period of time. An amplitude threshold of 15 mm Hg and a duration threshold of 1.0 second showed the best sensitivity and specificity for contraction detection. Most of the artifacts (e.g., cough, sneeze) are usually rejected by these thresholds. Algorithms based on contraction slope and morphology are employed to differentiate artifacts and repetitive contractions. Recognized contractions are then related to each other in esophageal "sequences" or "waves," and are classified as (1) *peristaltic*, (2) *simultaneous* (if the propagation speed exceeds 20 cm/second), (3) *interrupted* (a sequence lacking a contraction in the proximal or middle esophageal channel, but reappearing in the last channel) or (4) *dropped* (a sequence in which the contractions are present only in the proximal and/or middle channel, but absent in the distal one). The esophageal sequences are also related to a pharyngeal swallow and further classified as *primary* or *secondary*.

The final report graphically displays amplitude, duration, propagation speed, and characteristics of the detected contractions against a background of normal, for the total period of the test and, separately, for predefined periods, that is, meal periods, upright and supine periods, and pain or GER-related periods. Further, since, in order

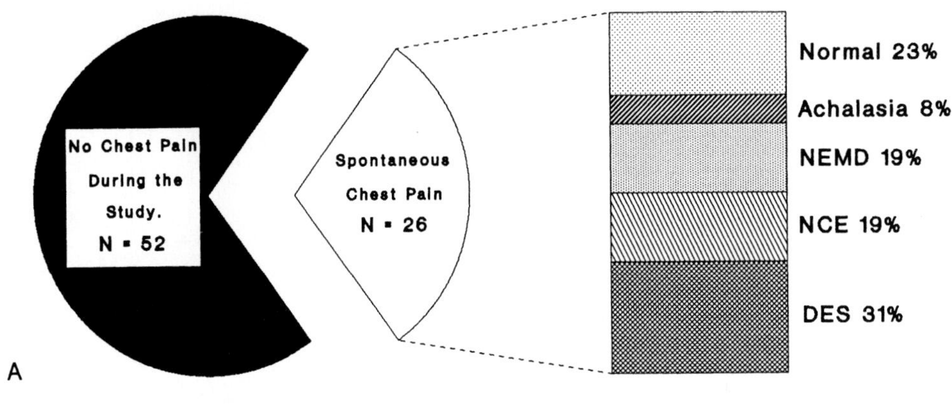

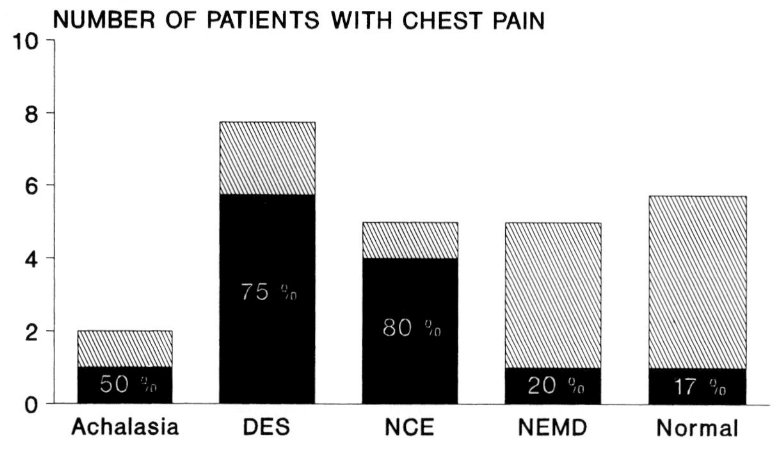

FIGURE 7–20 ■ *A*, Frequency of patients who experience at least one episode of chest pain during ambulatory 24-hour esophageal manometry and their underlying motor abnormality as diagnosed by 24-hour manometry. *B*, Number of patients who had abnormal esophageal motor activity associated with noncardiac chest pain that varied statistically outside their underlying motor activity during the symptom-free period. (DES, diffuse esophageal spasm; NCE, nutcracker esophagus; NEMD, nonspecific esophageal motor disorder.) (From Stein HJ, DeMeester TR, Eypasch EP, Klingman RR: Ambulatory 24-hour esophageal manometry in the evaluation of esophageal motor disorders and noncardiac chest pain. Surgery 110:753, 1991.)

to clear the esophagus of a liquid bolus, esophageal contractions must be peristaltic and have adequate amplitude (Kahrilas et al, 1988b), a classification of sequences as effective (peristaltic contractions with amplitude above 20, 25, and 30 mm Hg, respectively, at 15, 10, and 5 cm above the LES), possibly effective (peristaltic contractions with amplitude less than these values but higher than 15 mm Hg), and ineffective (simultaneous, interrupted, or dropped contractions) can be obtained for the overall and specific periods. This program allows a complete quantitative and qualitative evaluation of the patient's esophageal motility during an entire circadian cycle.

Clinical Applications

Noncardiac Chest Pain

Since its introduction in 1985, ambulatory-esophageal manometry has been primarily used to identify esophageal motility abnormalities as the cause of noncardiac chest pain (Stein and DeMeester, 1993). Initial experience often showed a direct correlation of esophageal motor abnormalities with spontaneously occurring chest pain episodes (Janssens et al, 1986; Maas et al, 1985). These patients were, however, highly selected and analysis techniques were inadequate due to limited experience with normal asymptomatic baseline recordings (Richter and Castell, 1989). Later studies in a larger number of unselected patients showed that many patients do not experience spontaneous chest pain episodes during the 24-hour monitoring period. In those who do, only a small number had motor abnormalities associated with the symptom (Breumelhof et al, 1990; Peters et al, 1988; Soffer et al, 1989).

In our experience, 33% of patients with a history of noncardiac chest pain had at least one pain episode during 24-hour esophageal motility monitoring (Stein et al, 1991c). When a spontaneous episode of chest pain occurred during the monitored period, motor abnormalities were rarely associated with the symptom in patients with normal motor activity or a nonspecific motor disorder during their symptom-free period. Short episodes of gastroesophageal reflux may have been responsible for the symptom in these patients (DeMeester et al, 1982). On the other hand, patients whose motor function during the asymptomatic period was consistent with nutcracker esophagus or diffuse esophageal spasm frequently showed an even more severe esophageal motor abnormality in association with spontaneous chest pain episodes as compared to their own asymptomatic baseline motor activity (Fig. 7–20).

Esophageal contractions of abnormal high amplitude or long duration have been suggested to be responsible for esophageal chest pain (Ferguson and Little, 1988; Hennington et al, 1984). Contrary to this belief, ambulatory motility monitoring demonstrated in our patients that amplitude and duration of esophageal contractions associated with chest pain episodes are similar to contractions during the asymptomatic recording periods. Rather, the abnormal motor activity associated with the pain episodes is characterized by an increased frequency of contractions immediately preceding and during the symptom.

In contrast to asymptomatic periods, these contractions are mainly simultaneous, double-peaked, and triple-peaked; they have a high amplitude or are of long duration. These observations suggest that, similar to that of the heart, esophageal blood supply may be interrupted during bursts of abnormal esophageal contractions, especially if the resting blood flow to the esophagus is already compromised, as shown for the hypertropic esophageal muscle in patients with severe esophageal motor disorders (MacKenzie et al, 1988). A burst of disorganized motor activity in this situation may give rise to ischemic pain. Consequently, chest pain caused by a burst of uncoordinated esophageal motor activity under ischemic conditions has been termed *esophageal claudication* (Stein et al, 1989).

Primary Esophageal Motor Disorders

Current identification and classification of esophageal motor disorders are based on an increased frequency of abnormal contractions following 10 wet swallows on stationary manometry. Ambulatory 24-hour esophageal manometry multiplies the number of esophageal contractions available for analysis and provides an opportunity to assess esophageal motor function in a variety of physiologic situations such as sleep and awake states and during meal periods. This method should increase the accuracy and dependability of the measurement compared with standard manometry.

Studies have been done in large series of consecutive patients that compared the diagnoses obtained by both stationary manometry and ambulatory motility monitoring. Surprisingly, there was little agreement between the two tests (Stein et al, 1991c). Ambulatory manometry frequently documented a more severe motor abnormality in patients thought to have normal esophageal motor function, a nonspecific motor disorder, or nutcracker esophagus on standard manometry (Fig. 7–21). This

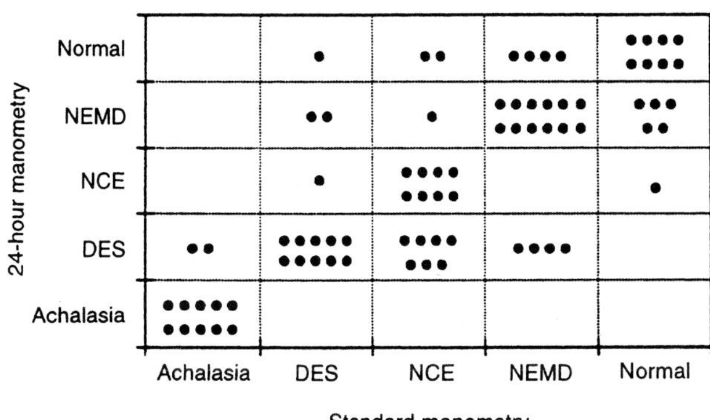

FIGURE 7–21 ■ Classification of esophageal motor disorders in 108 patients with dysphagia and/or noncardiac chest pain according to the findings on standard or ambulatory 24-hour manometry. (DES, diffuse esophageal spasm; NCE, nutcracker esophagus; NEMD, nonspecific esophageal motor disorder.) (From Stein HJ, DeMeester TR, Eypasch EP, Klingman RR: Ambulatory 24-hour esophageal manometry in the evaluation of esophageal motor disorders and noncardiac chest pain. Surgery 110:753, 1991.)

finding appears to be a result of the intermittent expression of esophageal motor abnormalities, which can be missed easily on standard manometry. Yet ambulatory manometry also frequently showed normal or only mildly disordered circadian motor function in patients thought to have a nonspecific disorder or nutcracker esophagus on standard manometry, suggesting that the unphysiologic conditions under which standard manometry is performed may trigger these abnormalities in patients known to have a low anxiety threshold (Clouse and Lustman, 1983).

A change in diagnosis was less prevalent in patients who met the criteria for diffuse esophageal spasm or achalasia on standard manometry. This finding would indicate that a failure of peristalsis on standard manometry is a reliable indicator for the presence of a severe motor disorder. These observations suggest that the current classification of esophageal motor disorders on standard manometry may not be a reliable guide for the clinical management of symptomatic patients.

Nonobstructive Dysphagia

In the absence of esophageal obstruction, dysphagia is a common symptom in patients with esophageal motor disorders. The underlying pathophysiologic abnormality responsible for the symptom is not always readily apparent on stationary manometry (Katz et al, 1987). Ambulatory 24-hour esophageal motility monitoring has shown that amplitude and duration of contractions in the esophageal body are not significantly different between volunteers, patients without dysphagia, and patients who have dysphagia but no evidence of obstruction on endoscopy or barium swallow (Stein et al, 1991b). In all groups, the frequency of esophageal contractions increased from the supine, to upright, to meal periods but was not different among the groups. In volunteers and patients without dysphagia, this finding was caused by an increase in the frequency of peristaltic contractions. This cause was not

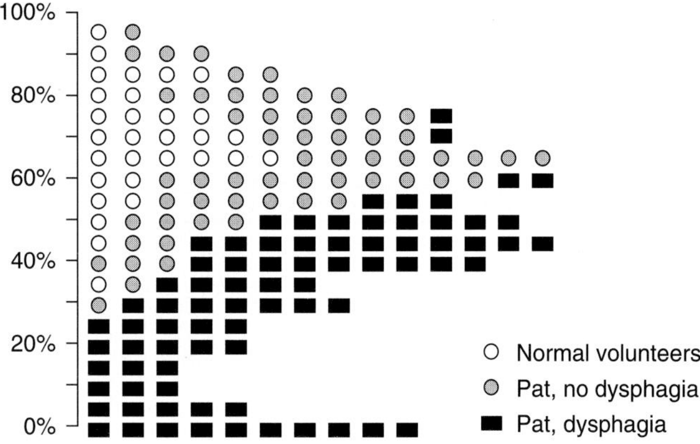

FIGURE 7–22 ■ Prevalence of "effective contractions," or peristaltic contractions with an amplitude above 30 mm Hg during meal periods in normal individuals, in patients without dysphagia, and in patients with nonobstructive dysphagia. (Pat, patient.)

evident in patients with dysphagia, who had a significantly decreased frequency of peristaltic contractions during meals compared with both other groups. Less than 60% of peristaltic contractions during meal periods were associated with a 92% prevalence of dysphagia, suggesting that dysphagia in patients with no esophageal obstruction may result from the inability to organize esophageal motor activity into peristaltic contractions during meal periods.

The prevalence of "effective contractions" (peristaltic contractions with an amplitude above 30 mm Hg during meals) during meal periods in normal individuals and patients with and without dysphagia is shown in Figure 7–22; 91% of the patients with dysphagia had 50% or fewer effective contractions during meals, whereas 84% of normal individuals and patients without dysphagia had more than 50% effective contractions during meal periods. When the percentage of effective contractions drops below 50, the patient is likely to experience dysphagia. Such patients may benefit from the use of prokinetic agents. When the esophageal motor activity is severely compromised because of a high prevalence of simultaneous contractions, patients usually receive little benefit from medical therapy. In these patients, a surgical myotomy of the esophageal body can improve the dysphagia, provided that the loss of contraction amplitude of the existing peristaltic waveforms caused by the myotomy has less effect on the swallowing function than the excessive simultaneous contraction had before the myotomy. Experience has shown that this situation is reached when the prevalence of effective contractions during meals drops below 30%.

Gastroesophageal Reflux Disease

Esophageal motor activity is the most important factor in the clearance of refluxed gastric contents. Simultaneous manometry and video fluoroscopy have shown that in the distal esophagus peristaltic contractions with a minimum amplitude of 30 mm Hg are required to completely occlude the esophageal lumen and propel a liquid barium bolus (Kahrilaset et al, 1988b). This finding is confirmed by studies using combined esophageal pH and motility monitoring, which showed that the duration of a spontaneously occurring reflux episode is directly related to the frequency of peristaltic esophageal contractions with sufficient amplitude after the onset of the reflux episode (Bumm et al, 1990) (Fig. 7–23). These studies suggest that ambulatory esophageal motility monitoring allows evaluation of esophageal clearance function by assessing the prevalence of efficient esophageal contractions, that is, peristaltic contractions with an amplitude above 30 mm Hg, over an entire circadian cycle (Figs. 7–24 and 7–25).

Application of ambulatory 24-hour esophageal motil-

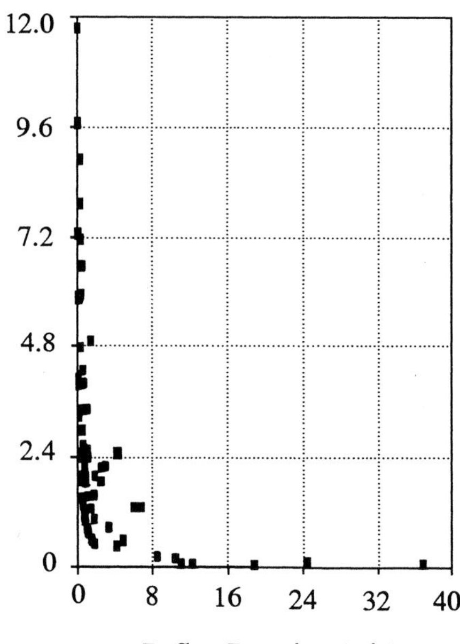

FIGURE 7–23 ■ Frequency of esophageal contractions per minute versus duration of single reflux episodes derived from seven healthy volunteers. Each square represents one reflux episode. Transformation of frequencies (*y* axis) into 1/frequency and linear regression of resulting data. (From Bumm R, Feussner H, Emde C: Interaction of gastroesophageal reflux and esophageal motility in healthy men undergoing combined 24-hour mano/pH-metry. In Little AG, Ferguson MK, Skinner DB [eds]: Diseases of the Esophagus. Mount Kisco, NY, Futura Publishing Company, 1990, p 101.)

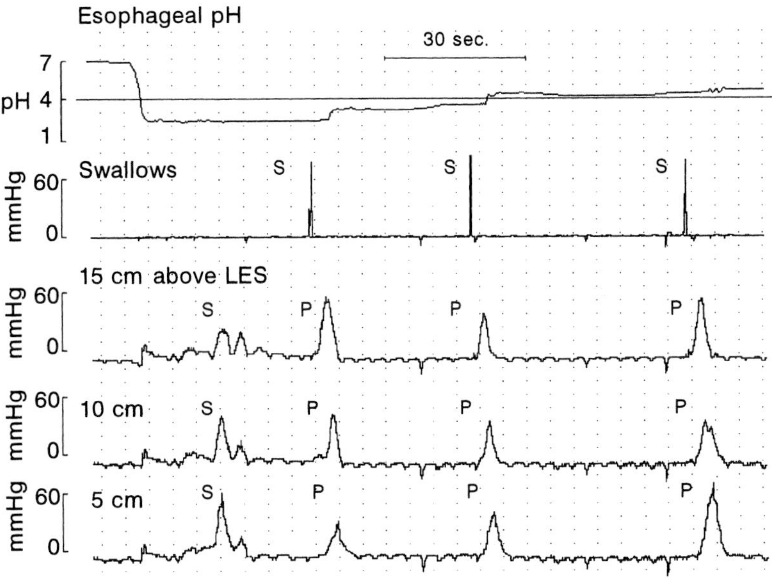

FIGURE 7–24 ■ Twenty-four hour ambulatory esophageal motility and pH record in a normal subject. A gastroesophageal reflux episode *(top tracing)* was rapidly cleared by two swallows (S, *second tracing*) that initiated effective contractions (P) in the esophageal body (primary peristalsis). Note that the first contraction sequence (S) after the occurrence of the reflux was not initiated by a swallow and represents a secondary contraction that appeared to be simultaneous. The combined esophageal motility and pH monitoring with swallowing detection revealed that secondary contractions actually play little role in esophageal clearance. (From Bremner RM, Costantini M, DeMeester TR, et al: Secondary peristalsis is rare and is not important in clearing the esophagus of refluxed gastric acid. Gastroenterology 102:A30, 1992.)

ity monitoring in a series of patients with increased esophageal acid exposure and various degrees of esophageal mucosal injury shows that esophageal contractility deteriorates with increasing severity of esophageal mucosal injury (Stein et al, 1990) (Fig. 7–26). This deterioration appears to occur secondary to persistent reflux across a mechanically defective LES and results in a marked increase in the frequency of inefficient esophageal contractions during the supine, upright, and meal periods, particularly in patients with a stricture or Barrett's esophagus. In this instance, the compromised clearance activity prolongs esophageal exposure to refluxed gastric juice, as also indicated by the increased frequency of reflux episodes lasting longer than 5 minutes in these patients. Thus, a vicious circle is established. Deteriorated contractility also affects propulsion of swallowed food, and once contractility is lost, it is not recovered with treatment, even after a successful antireflux operation (Fig. 7–27).

A surgical correction of the underlying defect (i.e., of the mechanically defective LES) early in the course of the disease is indicated. Once effective contractility has been lost, the surgical approach may have to be altered by a repair with minimal outflow obstruction (a partial fundoplication).

STANDARD ACID REFLUX TEST

The acid reflux test attempts to induce reflux by loading the stomach with acid and having the subject perform four maneuvers in four different positions (Skinner and Booth, 1970). It assesses LES competence rather than the degree of spontaneously occurring reflux.

Following manometry, a pH electrode is placed 5 cm above the upper border of the LES. The manometry catheter is then advanced temporarily into the stomach and 300 ml of 0.1 normal HCl is infused. In children the volume of acid load is reduced accordingly. The pH of

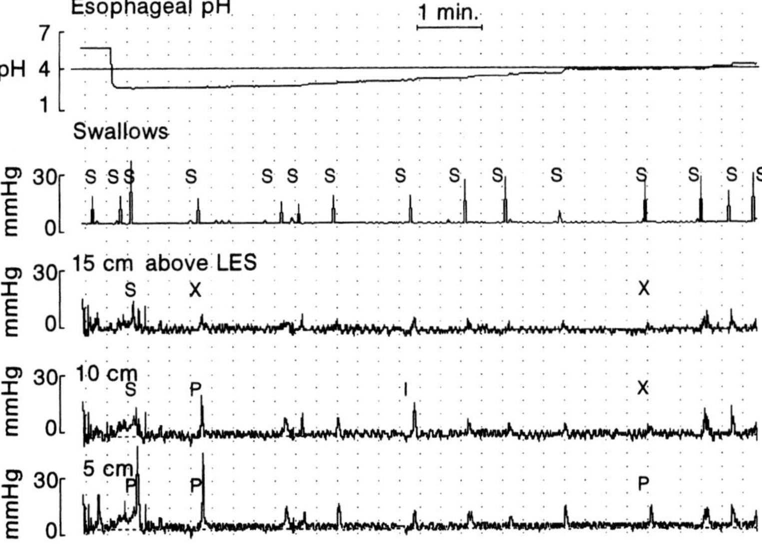

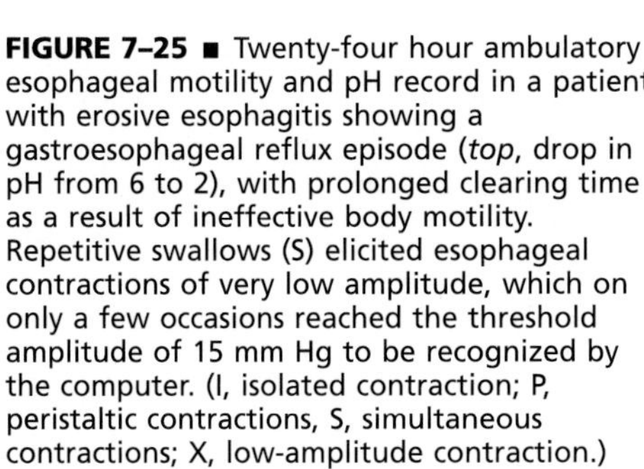

FIGURE 7–25 ■ Twenty-four hour ambulatory esophageal motility and pH record in a patient with erosive esophagitis showing a gastroesophageal reflux episode (*top*, drop in pH from 6 to 2), with prolonged clearing time as a result of ineffective body motility. Repetitive swallows (S) elicited esophageal contractions of very low amplitude, which on only a few occasions reached the threshold amplitude of 15 mm Hg to be recognized by the computer. (I, isolated contraction; P, peristaltic contractions, S, simultaneous contractions; X, low-amplitude contraction.)

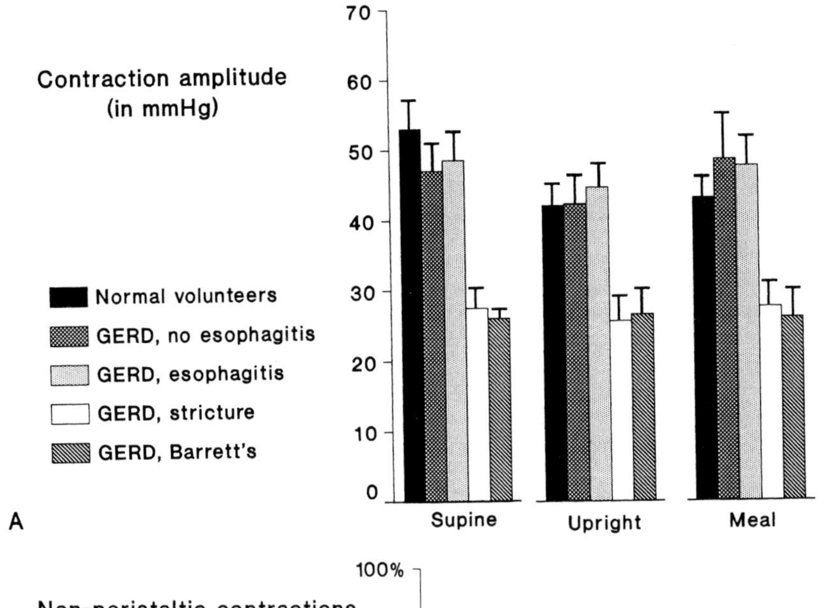

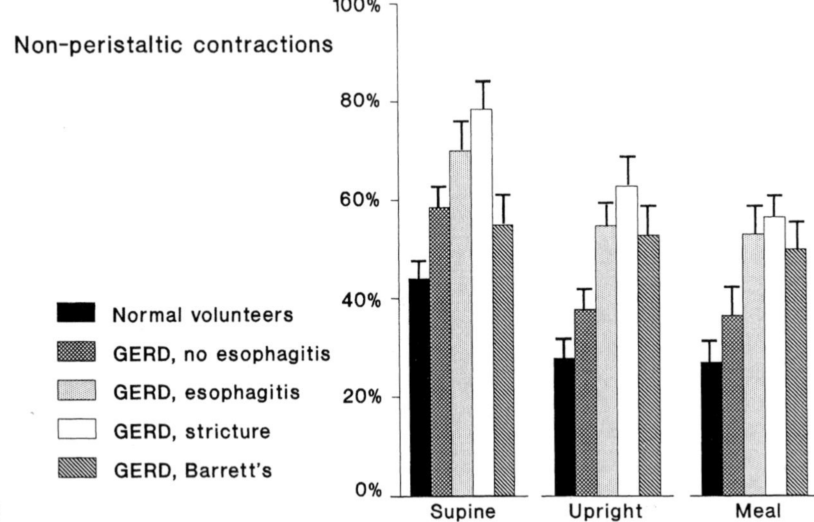

FIGURE 7–26 ■ *A*, Median contraction amplitude in the distal esophagus in normal volunteers and patient groups during the supine, upright, and meal periods. Stricture or Barrett's esophagus versus all other groups, $P < .01$. *B*, Percentage of nonperistaltic contractions in normal volunteers and patient groups during the supine, upright, and meal periods. Normal volunteers versus all other groups, $P < .05$; esophagitis or stricture versus no esophagitis, $P < .05$. (GERD, gastroesophageal reflux disease.) (From Stein HJ, Eypasch EP, DeMeester TR, et al: Circadian esophageal motor function in patients with gastroesophageal reflux disease. Surgery 108:769, 1990.)

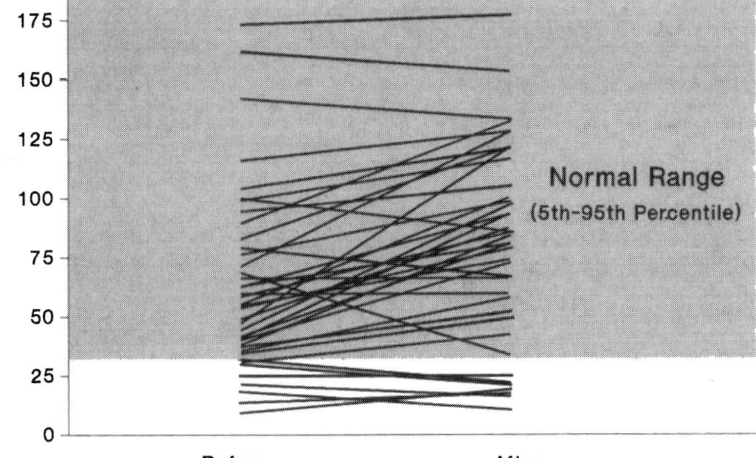

FIGURE 7–27 ■ Mean amplitude of contractions of the distal 15 cm of the esophagus in patients before and 42 months after Nissen fundoplication. No improvement was noted in patients with a preoperative mean contraction amplitude below the 10th percentile or 35 mm Hg. (From Stein HJ, Bremner RM, Jamieson J, DeMeester TR: Effect of Nissen fundoplication on esophageal motor function. Arch Surg 127:788, 1992.)

the esophagus is monitored while patients rest quietly in the supine position and then while performing four maneuvers: deep breathing, Valsalva, Mueller (inspiration against a closed glottis), and cough. These maneuvers are repeated in the right and left lateral decubitus position and with the head down 20 degrees, giving 16 possibilities for acid reflux to occur. A decrease in esophageal pH to less than 4 is considered evidence of reflux.

At the beginning of the test, before the patient is placed in the supine position, the distal esophagus must have a pH greater than 4. This requirement has necessitated that the patient stand erect and swallow repeatedly in order to clear the esophagus of acid. Patients who cannot clear the esophagus in the erect position after 20 effective swallows, monitored on a motility tracing, are considered to have an abnormal result in all positions and maneuvers and are scored as 16. The algorithm for performing the test is shown in Figure 7–28.

In healthy volunteers, more than two reflux episodes during the test rarely occur. Accordingly, 1 or 2 drops in pH during these 16 challenges to the cardia are considered normal, and 3 or more drops in pH are taken as evidence of mechanical incompetence of the cardia. Patients with severe reflux may be unable to clear acid from the esophagus after reflux has been documented (Booth et al, 1968).

When evaluated in a test population with an equal distribution of normal healthy subjects and patients with classic symptoms of GERD, the standard acid reflux test had a sensitivity (i.e., the ability to detect the disease when known to be present) of 59%; and a specificity (i.e., the ability to exclude the disease when known to be absent), of 98%. This finding gave a predictive value of a positive test of 96% and a negative test of 75% with an overall accuracy of 81% (Fuchs et al, 1987).

AMBULATORY 24-HOUR pH MONITORING OF THE DISTAL ESOPHAGUS

Prolonged esophageal pH monitoring was first described by Miller (1964) in a publication on gastric pH monitoring. Ten years later, it was used to quantitate the actual time the esophageal mucosa is exposed to gastric juice (Johnson and DeMeester, 1974). Subsequently, it was shown that the test also assessed the ability of the esophagus to clear the refluxed acid juice and documented the relationship between esophageal exposure to gastric juice and the symptoms experienced by the patient (DeMeester et al, 1980).

A small pH electrode is passed transnasally and placed 5 cm above the upper border of the LES, previously measured by manometry. Different probes are available, but bipolar glass electrodes are preferred for their greater reliability (McLaughlan et al, 1987) and the elimination of the need for an external reference electrode. The electrode is connected to an external portable solid-state datalogger, and pH values of the distal esophagus are continuously recorded at 4-second intervals for 24 hours, a complete circadian cycle. Precalibration and postcalibration of the system at pH 1 and 7 is important to exclude electrode drift over the period of the study (Emde et al, 1987). All medications interfering with gastric acid secretion must be discontinued at least 48 hours before the test begins. A washout period of at least 1 week, and in some situations up to 2 weeks, is necessary

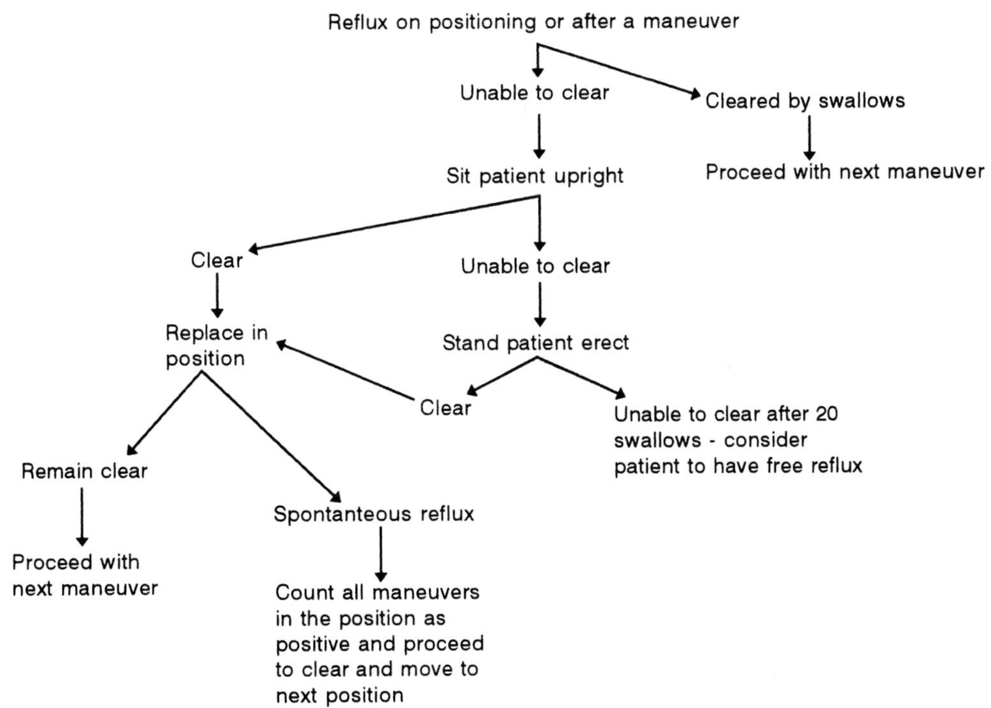

FIGURE 7–28 ■ Procedure to be followed after a reflux episode in the performance of the standard acid reflux test. (From Fuchs KH, DeMeester TR, Albertucci M: Specificity and sensitivity of objective diagnosis of gastroesophageal reflux disease. Surgery 102:575, 1987.)

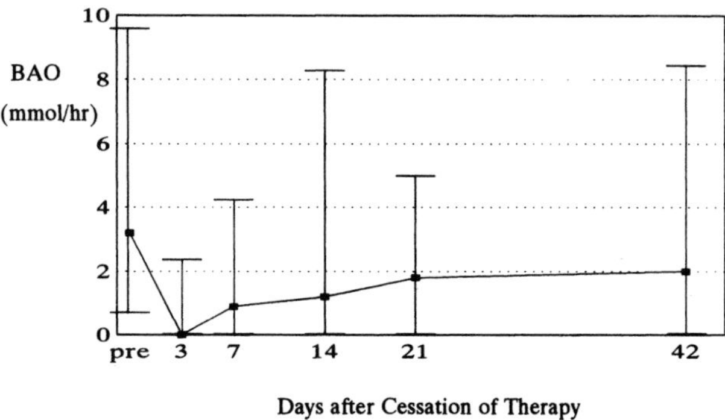

FIGURE 7–29 ■ Range and median of basal acid output (BAO) in 10 duodenal ulcer patients after a 4-week course of omeprazole (20 mg/day). Even after 6 weeks, there were patients with a basic acid output of 0. (From Marks IN, Young GO, Winter T, et al: South African Gastroenterology Society, Congress abstract, 1992.)

in patients treated with omeprazole because of its long-lasting action (Fig. 7–29).

The test is performed on an outpatient basis, preferably while the subject is attending normal activities. The patient is requested to remain in the upright position (or sitting) while awake during the day, lying down supine only at night while sleeping, and to ingest two meals at the usual time. The diet is standardized only in the absence of food or beverages with a pH value less than 5.0 and greater than 6.0. Only water is allowed between meals. Patients are also instructed to keep a detailed dairy of their symptoms during the study in order to correlate them with episodes of gastroesophageal reflux (GER). They are asked to record the time when retiring for the night and when rising in the morning. Figure 7–30 shows a typical esophageal pH-monitoring trace in a healthy subject and in a patient with GERD.

It is important to emphasize that 24-hour esophageal pH monitoring should not be considered a test for reflux but, instead, a measurement of the esophageal exposure to gastric juice (i.e., of the amount of time the esophageal pH is below a given threshold during the 24-hour period). This expression, however, does not reflect how the exposure has occurred; for example, it may have occurred in a few long or several short reflux episodes. Consequently, two other assessments are necessary: the frequency of the reflux episodes and their duration. For this reason, esophageal exposure to gastric juice is best assessed by the following measurements (Johnson and DeMeester, 1974):

1. Cumulative time the esophageal pH is below a chosen threshold expressed as the percent of the total, upright, and supine monitored time.
2. Frequency of reflux episodes below a chosen threshold expressed as number of episodes per 24 hours.
3. Duration of the episodes expressed as the number of episodes greater than 5 minutes per 24 hours.
4. The time in minutes of the longest episode recorded.

Normal values for these six components of the 24-hour record at each whole number pH threshold were derived from 50 asymptomatic control subjects. The upper limits of normal were established initially at the 95th percentile (DeMeester, 1989) and later using percentiles selected by receiver operator characteristic (ROC) analysis (Jamieson et al, 1992). Figure 7–31 shows the median and the 95th percentile of the normal values for each component. If the values of symptomatic patients are outside the 95th percentile of normal subjects, they are considered abnormal for the component measured. Most centers use pH 4 as the threshold. With this threshold, there is a uniformity of normal values for the six components from centers throughout the world (Emde et al, 1987; Richter et al, 1992). This finding indicates that esophageal acid exposure can be quantitated and that normal individuals have similar values despite nationality or dietary habits. The normal values for the six components obtained in 50 healthy volunteers are shown in Table 7–3.

To combine the result of the six components into one expression of the overall esophageal acid exposure below a pH threshold, a pH score can be calculated by using the standard deviation (SD) of the mean of each of the six components measured in the 50 normal subjects as a weighing factor (Johnson and DeMeester, 1986). By

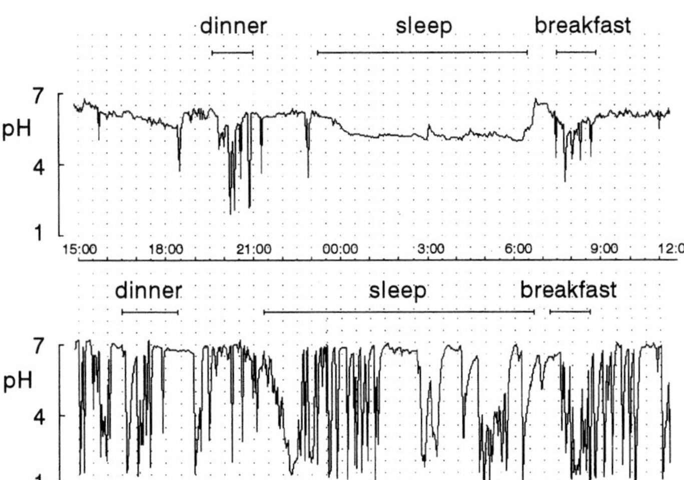

FIGURE 7–30 ■ Twenty-four hour pH monitoring of the distal esophagus in a healthy subject *(top)* and in a patient with esophagitis *(bottom)*. Physiologic gastroesophageal reflux episodes occur in a normal subject, mainly in the upright position and after meals. The patient's record shows the presence of an increased number of reflux episodes, both in the upright and supine position, some of them with prolonged clearing time.

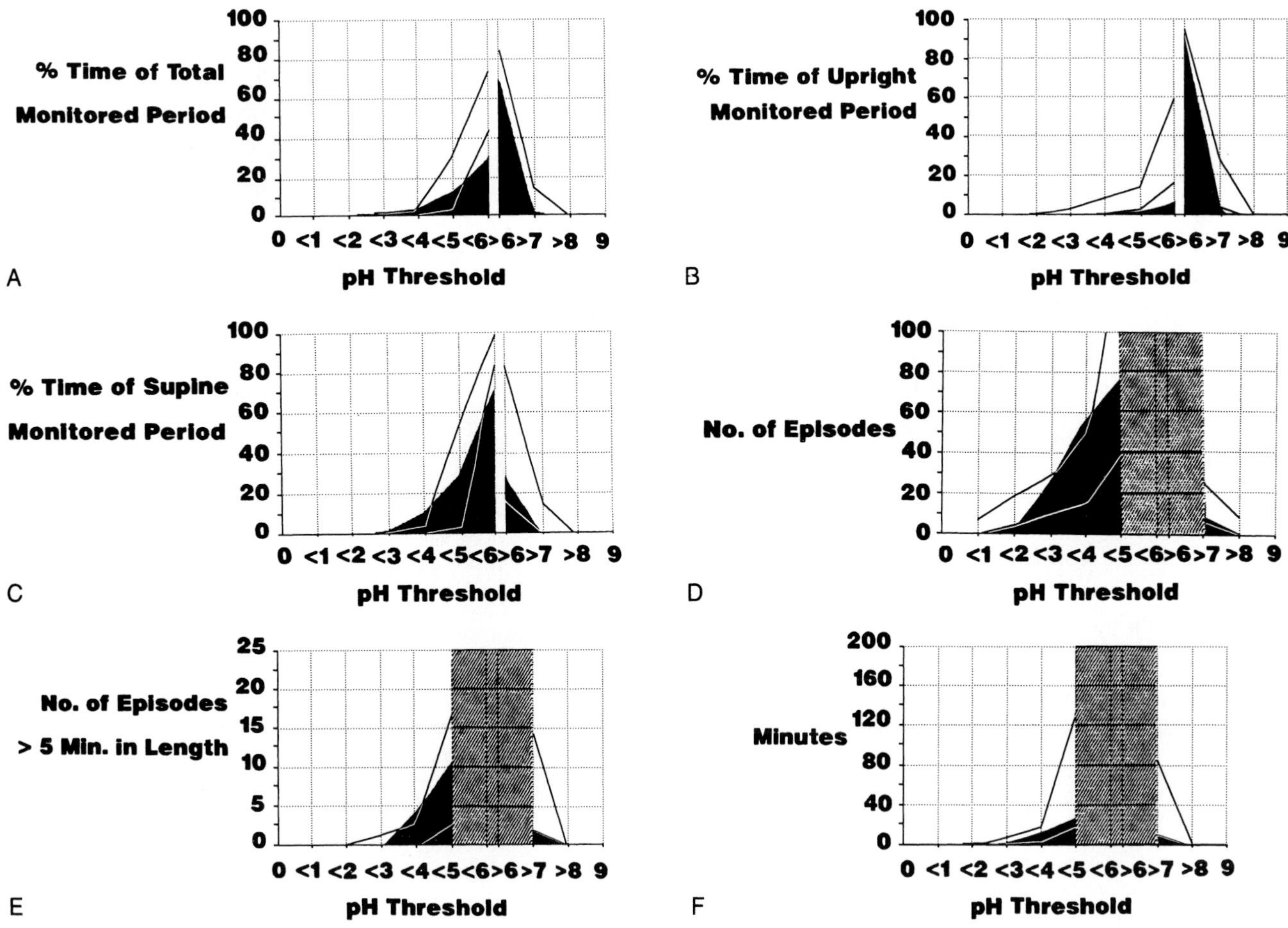

FIGURE 7–31 ■ *A–F,* Graphic display of the six components of the composite pH score showing the median and 95th percentile levels in 50 normal individuals using whole pH values above and below 6 as thresholds. The *black area* represents measurements made in the patient. The *lower black line* shows the median, and *upper black line*, the 95th percentile value for the 50 normal subjects. When the *black area* exceeds the 95th percentile line for a given pH threshold, the patient has an abnormal value for the component measured. *A,* Percent cumulative exposure for total time. *B,* Percent cumulative exposure for upright time. *C,* Percent cumulative exposure for supine time. *D,* Number of episodes in 24 hours. *E,* Number of episodes longer than five minutes. *F,* Duration of longest episode. (From DeMeester TR: Prolonged oesophageal pH monitoring. In Read NW [ed]: Gastrointestinal Motility: Which Test? Wrightson Biomedical, Petersfield, England, 1989, p 41.)

accepting an abstract zero level 2 SDs below the mean, we can treat the data measured in normal subjects as though they have a normal distribution. Thus, any measured patient value can be referenced to this zero point and, in turn, can be awarded points based on whether it is below or above the normal mean value for that component. The formula used for performing the calculation, illustrated in Figure 7–32, is as follows:

$$\text{component score} = \frac{\text{patient value} - \text{mean}}{\text{standard deviation}} + 1$$

This formula is used to score each of the six components of the 24-hour pH record obtained from the 50 normal subjects. The score for each component is added to obtain a composite score for each of the 50 normal subjects, and the upper level of a normal score is established at

TABLE 7–3 ■ **Normal Values for Ambulatory Esophageal pH Monitoring in 50 Healthy Volunteers**

	Mean	*Standard Deviation*	*Median*	*Minimum*	*Maximum*	*95th Percentile*
% Total time with pH < 4	1.5	1.4	1.2	0	6.0	4.5
% Upright time with pH < 4	2.2	2.3	1.6	0	9.3	8.4
% Supine time with pH < 4	0.6	1.0	0.1	0	4.0	3.5
Number of episodes	19.0	12.8	16.0	2.0	56.0	46.9
Number of episodes > 5 min	0.8	1.2	0	0	5.0	3.5
Longest episode (min)	6.7	7.9	4.0	0	46.0	19.8
Composite score	6.0	4.4	5.0	0.4	18.0	14.7

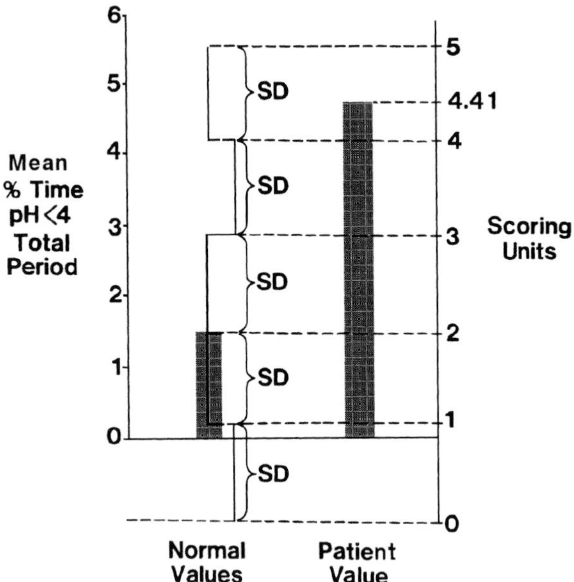

FIGURE 7–32 ■ Concept of using the standard deviation (SD) as the unit to score esophageal acid exposure (in this example, the percentage of total time the pH was below 4). Note the establishment of an abstract zero point 2 standard deviations below the mean value for percentage of time the pH was less than 4 in normal volunteers. This method allows scoring the measurement in patients as though the normal values were parametric. By this method, a patient who had a percentage of time with a pH less than 4 of 4.8% would have a score for this component of 4.41. (From Jamieson JR, Stein HJ, DeMeester TR, et al: Ambulatory 24-hour esophageal pH monitoring: Normal values, optimal thresholds, specificity sensitivity, and reproducibility. Am J Gastroenterol 87:1102–1111, 1992.)

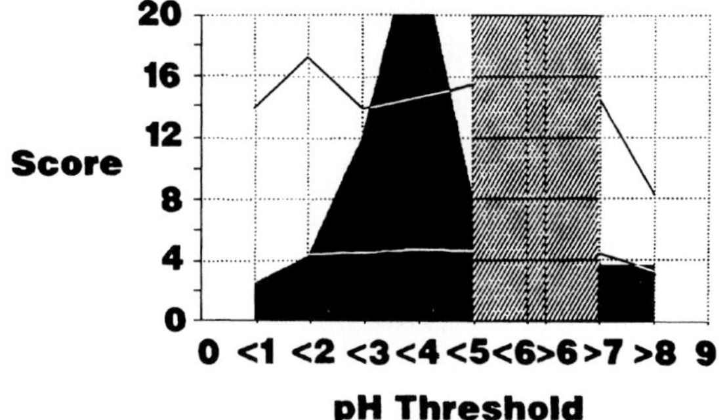

FIGURE 7–33 ■ Composite pH score used to express the overall results for esophageal pH monitoring for the pH thresholds shown. The *lower black line* represents median score; the *upper black line*, the 95th percentile of 50 normal subjects. The *black area* represents the score of a patient with increased esophageal acid exposure using the various pH thresholds as an indicator of reflux. A score for esophageal acid exposure of less than 4 is abnormal; for less than 3, it is increased but not above the 95th percentile line. (From DeMeester TR, Stein HJ: Gastroesophageal reflux disease. In Moody FG, Carey LC, Jones RC, et al [eds]: Surgical Treatment of Digestive Disease, 2nd ed. Chicago, Year Book Medical Publishers, 1989, p 72.)

the 95th percentile. The upper limits of normal for the composite score for each whole number pH threshold are shown in Table 7–4. The median and 95th percentile for the composite score for each whole number pH threshold can also be expressed graphically (Fig. 7–33). An IBM-compatible program to perform this function is available from Medtronic (Minneapolis).

ROC analysis, in which sensitivity is plotted against specificity for a given test, was applied to each of the six parameters and to the composite score, using pH 4 as the threshold. Both total percent time below pH 4 and the composite score were found to have optimal specificity and sensitivity (Jamieson, 1992). However, there was a difference in normal values between males and females

TABLE 7–4 ■ **Composite Score for Various pH Thresholds (95th Percentile)**

pH Threshold	*95th Percentile*
pH < 1	14.2
pH < 2	17.4
pH < 3	14.1
pH < 4	14.7
pH < 5	15.8
pH < 7	14.9
pH < 8	8.5

when only the percent total time the pH is below 4 was used. Consequently, the sex of the subject must be taken into account in borderline situations when the percent total time that pH below 4 is used to express esophageal acid exposure. The composite score value is applicable to both males and females.

The detection of increased esophageal exposure to acid gastric juice is more dependable than that of alkaline gastric juice. The latter is suggested by an alkaline exposure above pH 7 or 8. Increased exposure in this pH range can be caused by (1) abnormal calibration of the pH recorder, (2) presence of a dental infection that increases salivary pH, (3) presence of esophageal obstruction that results in static pools of saliva with an increase in pH secondary to bacterial overgrowth, or (4) presence of regurgitation of alkaline gastric juice into the esophagus (Stein et al, 1992a). Combined gastric and esophageal pH monitoring in this situation increases the reliability of the test in detecting alkaline reflux.

Analyzing the pH data of patients with GERD using the time of exposure to different pH intervals (e.g., pH 0 to 1, 1 to 2, 2 to 3), we have found that increased esophageal exposure to pH 0 to 2 and pH 7 to 8 was associated with mucosal injury (esophagitis, stricture, Barrett's esophagus) in 89% of patients (Bremner et al, 1992c). In a different group of patients (Zaninotto et al, 1992), the amount of exposure to pH 1.5 to 2.5 in the supine position allowed for discrimination of the severity of the mucosal damage in 75% of the patients. Therefore, 24-hour esophageal pH monitoring is useful not only in diagnosing the presence of GERD but also in predicting the presence of complications of the disease.

In patients with symptoms of chronic cough, hoarseness, or aspiration, placement of an additional pH electrode in the proximal part of the esophagus or pharynx can be helpful (Jacob et al, 1991). If reflux episodes reach to the proximal esophagus or pharynx and a temporary relationship between these reflux episodes and the onset of the symptom can be documented, GERD can be assumed to be the cause of the patient's complaint.

AMBULATORY 24-HOUR ESOPHAGEAL BILIRUBIN MONITORING

Reflux of alkaline duodenal contents into the stomach and up into the esophagus is increasingly recognized as an important pathophysiologic factor in GERD. About 25% of patients with GERD develop recurrent progressive disease manifested by advancing complications of erosive esophagitis to stricture, ulceration, and/or Barrett's esophagus while under medical therapy (Ollyo et al, 1993). Evidence is accumulating that the composition of the refluxed gastric juice plays an important role in the development of this progressive mucosal injury (Gillen et al, 1987; Iascone et al, 1983). Animal studies have shown marked augmentation of the acid-induced mucosal injury by the presence of components of duodenal juice (Attwood et al, 1992; Clark et al, 1994). Clinical observations have shown that the prevalence of complications (e.g., esophagitis, stricture, and Barrett's esophagus) in patients with GERD is related to an increased esophageal exposure to both acid and alkalinity, and the severity of these complications is greater in patients with acid-alkaline reflux than in patients with acid reflux alone (Stein et al, 1992a). Prolonged esophageal aspiration studies have shown an increase in bile acids in patients with severe esophagitis and Barrett's esophagus (Stein et al, 1994). These observations strongly suggest a noxious and synergistic role of components of duodenal juice in the refluxed gastric juice.

An ambulatory monitoring system allowing spectrophotometric measurement of luminal bilirubin concentration has been developed (Kauer et al, 1995a). With bilirubin used as a marker, the time of esophageal exposure to duodenal contents can be measured. In the absence of carotene and serum lipids, the bilirubin concentration in a solution can be measured directly by spectrophotometry on the basis of its specific absorption at a wavelength of 453 nm (Bechi et al, 1992). According to *Beer's law*, absorbance (A) is the logarithm of the ratio between the intensity of light transmitted (I°) through a solution containing an absorbing substance and the intensity of light transmitted (I) in the absence of the absorbing substance

$$A = \log (I°/I)$$

The apparatus used to measure the presence of bilirubin consists of a portable optoelectronic datalogger (80 C196KC, Intel, Santa Clara, Calif.) (1200 g), which can be strapped to the patient's side, and a fiberoptic probe, which can be passed transnasally and positioned anywhere in the lumen of the foregut (Bilitec 2000, Medtronic, Minneapolis). The spectrophotometric probes are 3 mm in diameter and 140 cm in length, and they contain 36 plastic optical fibers (each 250 μm diameter), which are bonded together and covered with biocompatible polyurethane. Two plugs connect 50% of the optic fibers to the transmitting light-emitting diodes (LEDs) and 50%

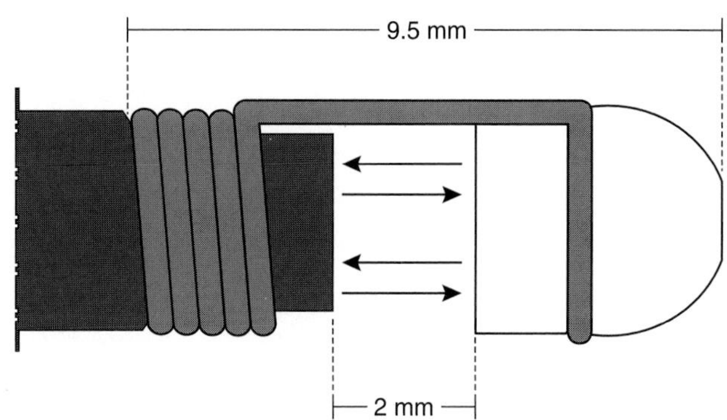

FIGURE 7–34 ■ Tip of the fiberoptic probe with a 2-mm space for sampling. Fluid can easily move into and out of the space, and the presence of bilirubin can be detected by its absorbance.

to the receiving photodiode. The tip of the probe contains a 2-mm space for sampling. Fluids and blenderized solids can flow easily through the space, and their bilirubin concentration can be measured. The probes are flexible, durable, easy to sterilize, and reusable.

The optoelectronic unit acts simultaneously as a light signal generator, a data processor, and a data storage device. The unit has two channels, allowing dual measurement with two probes if desired. The light source for each channel is provided by two LEDs (Fig. 7–34), emitting a 470-nm signal light (blue spectrum) and a 565-nm reference light (green spectrum). Reference and signal LEDs are stimulated alternatively, for a duration of 0.5 second. To avoid fluctuations in the source, the final 20 msec of each pulse is used for signal processing. Optical signals reflected back from the probe are converted to electrical impulses by a photodiode. This electrical signal is then amplified and processed within the datalogger. Absorbance readings are averaged every two cycles. The system is capable of recording 225 individual absorbance values per hour and allows up to 30 hours of continuous monitoring.

AMBULATORY 24-HOUR ESOPHAGEAL pH AND BILIRUBIN MONITORING

The fiberoptic probe to detect bilirubin is passed through the nose and positioned 5 cm above the upper border of the LES. Esophageal pH can also be recorded at the same time. Bilirubin absorbance is measured and recorded by the portable optoelectronic datalogger. Figure 7–35 shows the cumulative descending frequency distribution of 24-hour bilirubin exposure at distinct threshold values for absorbance in 25 normal subjects. An absorbance threshold of 0.2 is selected, because at this level bilirubin was detected in the esophagus in fewer than 5% of healthy subjects. The fiberoptic probe is calibrated in water before and after monitoring. Records with bilirubin absorbance drift greater than 0.15 are discarded.

Medications must be discontinued for 48 hours before testing, except for omeprazole, which must be discontinued at least 2 weeks earlier. With monitors in place, the patient is sent home and instructed to remain in the upright or sitting position until retiring for the night and

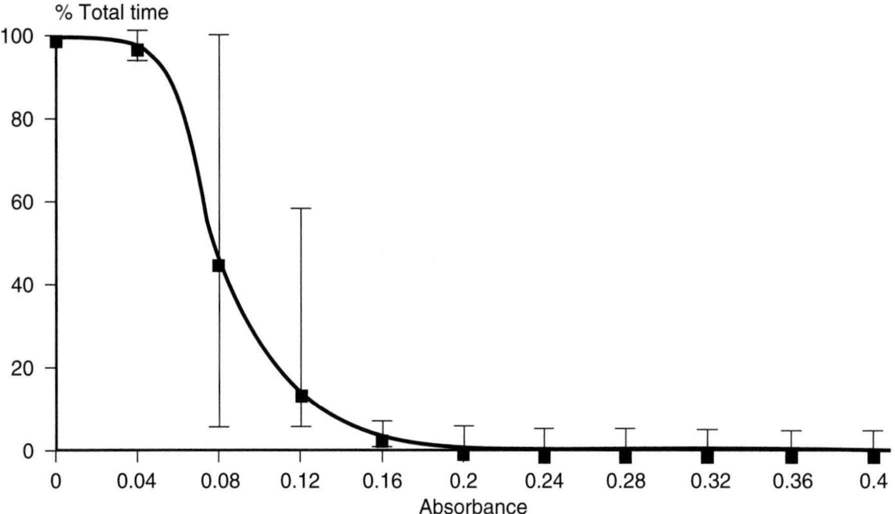

FIGURE 7–35 ■ Cumulative descending frequency distribution graph of the prevalence of total study time in which bilirubin was detected above distinct absorbance thresholds in 25 healthy subjects. Data are plotted as medians with the 25th and 75th percentiles. Based on this curve, the threshold absorbance of 0.2 was chosen as an indicator of the presence of bile in the esophageal lumen.

to follow a special diet, which involves restriction to three meals a day composed of food free of a high bilirubin absorbance (Kauer et al, 1995a). The patient keeps a diary of food and fluid intake, symptoms, and the time of the supine and upright positions. The bilirubin absorbance data are analyzed with a commercially available software program (Medtronic, Minneapolis).

Esophageal bilirubin exposure in 25 normal subjects, all of whom were asymptomatic and had normal 24-hour ambulatory esophageal pH studies to exclude the presence of pathologic acid reflux, is shown in Figure 7–36. The median percentage time of esophageal bilirubin exposure over a 24-hour period in healthy subjects was 0.1%, and the 95th percentile value was 2.9%. The upright and supine exposure values differed slightly, with a 95th percentile of 4.0% and 0.4%, respectively. Values above the 95th percentile level among healthy subjects for the total 24-hour period are used to identify increased esophageal exposure to duodenal juice in patients with foregut symptoms (Kauer et al, 1995b).

Figure 7–37 shows the composition of the reflux juice, gastric, gastroduodenal or duodenal juice, seen in 100 consecutive patients with GERD and its relationship to endoscopic evidence of mucosal damage (DeMeester et al, 1999). The reflux of duodenal juice is more common in patients with GERD than pH studies alone would suggest. The combined reflux of gastric and duodenal juice causes severe esophageal mucosal damage. The vast majority of duodenal reflux occurs at a pH of 4 to 7, at which bile acids, the major component of duodenal juice,

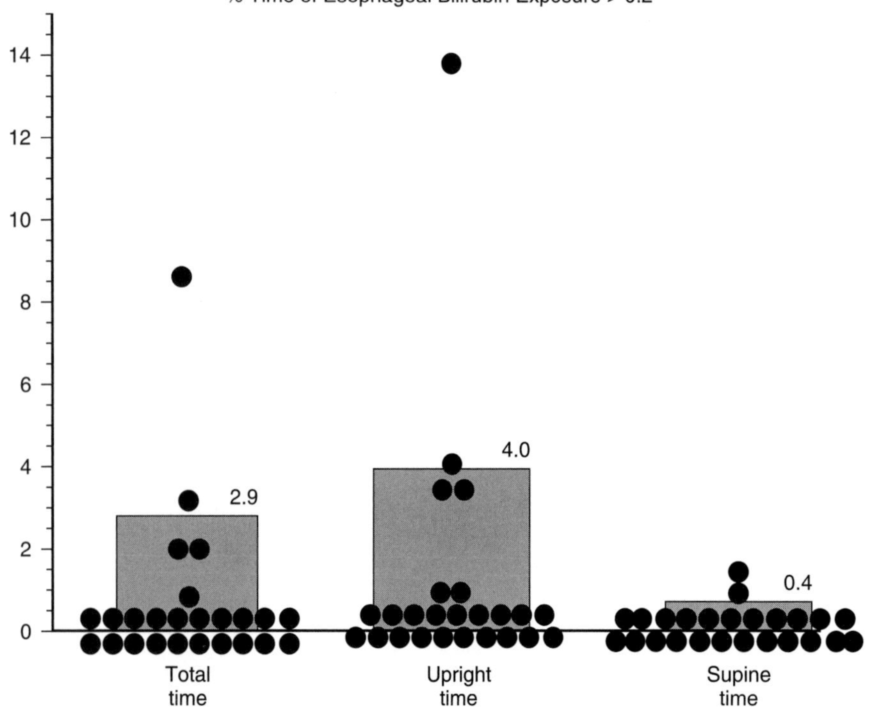

FIGURE 7–36 ■ Percentage of time of esophageal bilirubin exposure in 25 normal subjects for the total upright and supine time periods of a 24-hour study. The *shaded area* represents the normal range (95th percentile, upper limit of normal).

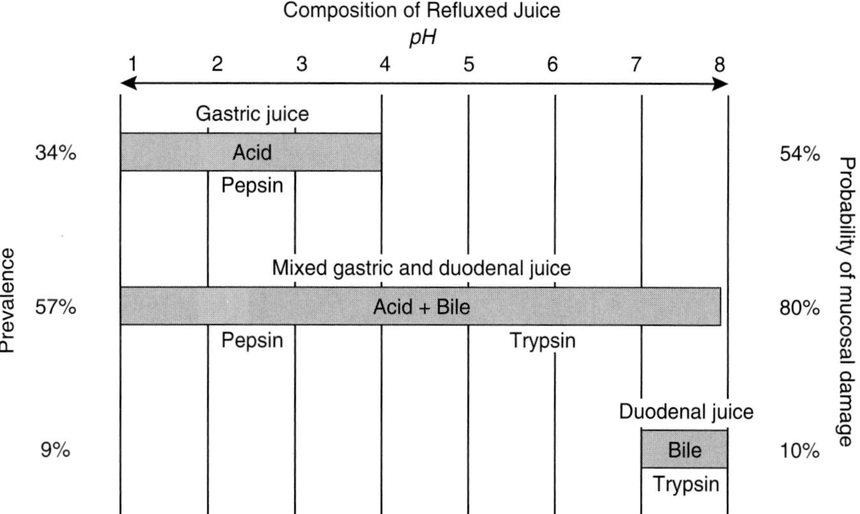

FIGURE 7–37 ■ Prevalence of gastric acid reflux, gastroduodenal reflux, and duodenal reflux into the esophagus and the probability of mucosal injury based on the monitoring of 100 consecutive patients with gastroesophageal reflux disease defined by an increased esophageal exposure to acid and/or bilirubin.

are capable of damaging the esophageal mucosa (Kauer et al, 1995b). Consequently, duodenal juice adds a noxious dimension to the refluxed gastric juice and potentiates the injurious effects of gastric juice on the esophageal mucosa (Fein et al, 1997).

AMBULATORY 24-HOUR GASTRIC pH MONITORING

Functional disorders of the esophagus are often not confined to the esophagus alone but are associated with functional disorders of the rest of the foregut (i.e., of the stomach and the duodenum). Abnormalities of the gastric reservoir or increased gastric acid secretion can be responsible for increased esophageal exposure to gastric juice. Reflux of alkaline duodenal juice, including bile salts and pancreatic enzymes, is involved in the pathogenesis of esophagitis and the complication of stricture and Barrett's esophagus.

Following the wide acceptance of 24-hour esophageal pH monitoring as the "gold standard" for assessing GER, much work has focused on 24-hour gastric pH monitoring as a clinical tool in the evaluation of gastroduodenal disorders. The interpretation of gastric pH recordings however, is more difficult than that of esophageal recordings. The difficulty is greater because the gastric pH environment is determined by a complex interplay of acid and mucous secretion; ingested food; swallowed saliva; regurgitated duodenal, pancreatic, and biliary secretions; and the effectiveness of the mixing and evacuation of the chyme. Consequently, after its clinical introduction in the 1980s, gastric pH monitoring was used primarily to study the effect, optimal dose, and timing of antisecretory drugs when the calculation of median pH over a given period of time was sufficient (Fimmel et al, 1985).

With the use of gastric pH monitoring for the diagnosis of gastroduodenal disorders, the simple measurements of median or mean pH proved unreliable. The diagnosis required a more sophisticated approach. For diagnosis, we developed a set of parameters describing the circadian gastric pH pattern based on (1) the percent of time spent at a pH band, that is, between whole number pH thresholds during the upright, supine, mealtime, and postprandial periods; (2) the number of times the pH moved from a lower band into a higher band; (3) the most common pH below 2 or the baseline pH; (4) the most common pH of the meal plateau; and (5) the pattern of pH decline from the plateau (Fuchs et al, 1991). This approach allows the quantitation of duodenogastric reflux and gastric acid secretion based on the circadian gastric pH record and may be helpful in the assessment of gastric emptying disorders.

Outpatient 24-hour gastric pH monitoring is performed using combined Ingold (Urdorf, Switzerland) glass electrodes with a built-in reference electrode. Antimony probes are less accurate in the gastric environment (McLaughlan et al, 1987). The probe is calibrated in standard buffer solutions at pH 7 and 1 before and after the study. Only recordings with an electrode drift of less than 0.2 pH units over the 24-hour monitoring period are accepted.

The electrode is passed transnasally and placed 5 cm below the lower border of the LES. The electrode is connected to a portable digital data recorder that stores pH readings every 4 seconds. After placement of the probes, the subjects are sent home and instructed to remain in the upright or sitting position until they retire for the night, to perform normal daily activities but to avoid strenuous exertion, and to follow a diet restricted to two meals composed of food with a pH between 5 and 7. Only water is permitted between meals. A diary is kept of food and fluid intake, symptoms experienced during the monitored period, the time the supine position is assumed in preparation for sleep, and the time of rising in the morning. All medications known to interfere with foregut motor or secretory function are stopped at least 48 hours prior to the study. As with esophageal pH monitoring, omeprazole is stopped 1 to 4 weeks before the study (see Fig. 7–29).

To quantitate reflux, the gastric pH record is divided into (1) the upright period, (2) the supine period, (3) the prandial pH plateau period, and (4) the postprandial pH decline period. For each of these periods, the following parameters are calculated:

1. The pH frequency distribution (the percentage time the gastric pH was at the pH intervals 0 to 1, 1 to 2, 2 to 3, 3 to 4, 4 to 5, 5 to 6, 6 to 7, and above 7).
2. The frequency of pH changes (the incidence of pH movements from a lower into a higher pH interval).
3. The duration of pH exposure expressed as the longest time the pH remained at a pH interval during the monitoring period.
4. Duration-frequency of pH exposure expressed as the number of times the pH remained at a pH interval for longer than 5 minutes.

Using discriminant analysis, we showed that a scoring system based on 16 of these parameters can completely differentiate the gastric pH profile of normal volunteers from patients with classic duodenogastric reflux disease. When applied prospectively, this scoring system was superior to DISIDA scanning with cholecystokinin (CCK) stimulation in the diagnosis of excessive duodenogastric reflux and detected the disease with a sensitivity of 90% and a specificity of 100% (Fuchs et al, 1991).

Ambulatory 24-hour gastric monitoring can also be used to evaluate the gastric secretory state of the patient. This monitoring is of particular value, since the role of gastric acid secretion in the pathogenesis of GERD is well documented (Boesby, 1977), and we have shown that 28% of patients with objectively proven GERD had gastric hypersecretion (Barlow et al, 1989). To do so, we plotted the frequency distribution and the cumulative frequency distribution graphs of the pH data of the patient against the range (5th to 95th percentiles) obtained in 50 healthy volunteers (Fig. 7–38). In our experience, this approach correlates well with the data obtained by traditional gastric secretion studies (Stein et al, 1992a).

Evaluation of gastric emptying on the basis of the postprandial alkalinization of the gastric pH record is a new concept that evolved from multiple-probe gastric pH monitoring during gastric emptying studies with radiolabeled meals. These studies demonstrated a good correlation between the emptying of oatmeal and the duration of the postprandial plateau and decline phases of the gastric pH record (Stein et al, 1992b). A prolonged postprandial decline of the pH in the corpus may, however, also be caused by excessive postprandial duodenogastric reflux or a decreased meal-induced stimulation of acid secretion.

To assess gastric emptying, the gastric pH record during and following a standardized dinner was assessed. A typical meal resulted in a rapid increase of the gastric pH from the interdigestive pH baseline (pH 1.1 to pH 1.6) to a pH between 4 and 7. This pH was maintained for approximately 10 to 20 minutes (plateau period). The plateau period was usually followed by a period of rapid decrease in the pH to approximately 1 pH unit above the baseline (Attwood et al, 1989). This period was followed by a period of slow decline to the interdigestive baseline pH. Gastric emptying studies with a radiolabeled solid and liquid meal have shown that the postprandial pH profile in the corpus correlates closely with emptying of the liquid component of the meal from the stomach (Fig. 7–39). A prolonged postprandial alkalinization of the pH in the corpus may indicate delayed gastric emptying of solids (Stein et al, 1992b) (Fig. 7–40).

COMPLETE FOREGUT OUTPATIENT PHYSIOLOGIC MONITORING

Many of the classic tests used to evaluate esophageal function described in this chapter have several shortcomings in the face of current technology. Standard manometry and provocative tests are performed in a laboratory environment, are unphysiologic, and restrict data sampling to short time periods. Consequently, the results of these tests are often inaccurate and symptoms are frequently misinterpreted as being psychogenic. Overall, the

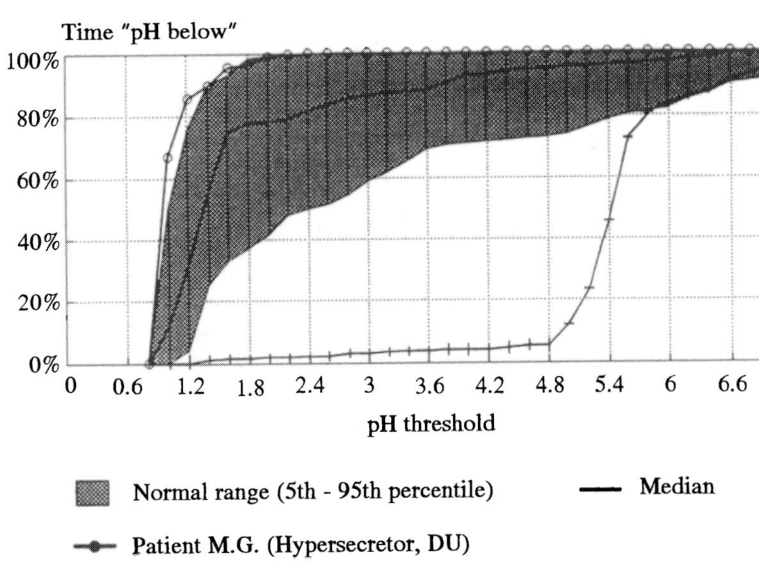

FIGURE 7–38 ■ Cumulative frequency distribution of gastric pH values during the supine period. The *shaded area* represents the 5th and 95th percentiles of 50 healthy volunteers; the *solid line* shows the median. Patient M. G. with a duodenal ulcer (DU) had a shift of the median values above the normal range, suggesting gastric acid hypersecretion. Patient B. C. had a shift of the median values below the normal range, indicating hypochlorhydria. (From Stein HJ, DeMeester TR, Hinder RA: Outpatient physiologic testing and surgical management of foregut motility disorders. Curr Probl Surg 24:418, 1992.)

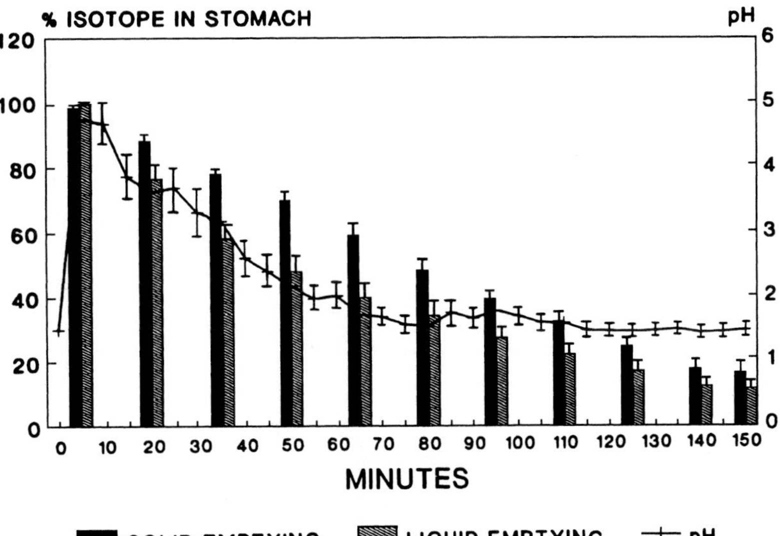

FIGURE 7–39 ■ Gastric emptying of a radiolabeled solid and liquid meal and simultaneously recorded pH values in the gastric corpus in 15 subjects. There is a close correlation between the emptying curve of the solid and liquid meal and the postprandial drop in pH measured by a pH electrode located 5 cm below the lower esophageal sphincter. (From Stein HJ, DeMeester TR, Hinder RA: Outpatient physiologic testing and surgical management of foregut motility disorders. Curr Probl Surg 24:418, 1992.)

shortcomings of these classic laboratory tests account, at least in part, for the unsatisfactory results of surgical or medical management of patients with complex functional esophageal disorders.

The development of miniaturized pH electrodes and electronic pressure transducers plus the introduction of portable digital data recorders with large storage capacity have made possible prolonged monitoring of luminal pH and motor activity of the foregut in an outpatient environment (Fig. 7–41). Ambulatory 24-hour monitoring of foregut pH and motility overcomes the limitations of the standard tests. It allows the recording of foregut function under physiologic conditions over a complete circadian cycle. This monitoring increases the probability of recording disordered motility and episodes of spontaneous GER or duodenogastric reflux. It allows quantitation of the observed abnormalities and their direct correlation with spontaneously occurring symptoms. With the use of modern solid-state recording technology and computerized reading, prolonged foregut monitoring over pe-

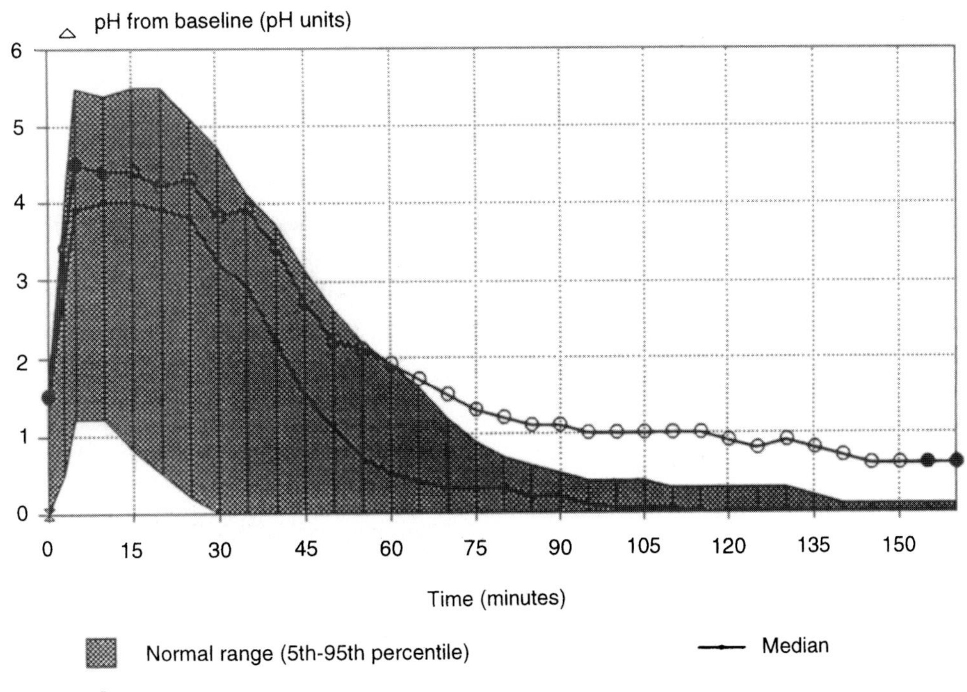

FIGURE 7–40 ■ Graphic report showing the time for the prandial plateau pH to return to preprandial gastric baseline pH measured as the difference in pH units from the preprandial baseline pH. Patient J. B. showed a markedly prolonged recovery time, suggesting delayed gastric emptying. (From Stein HJ, DeMeester TR, Hinder RA: Outpatient physiologic testing and surgical management of foregut motility disorders. Curr Probl Surg 24:418, 1992.)

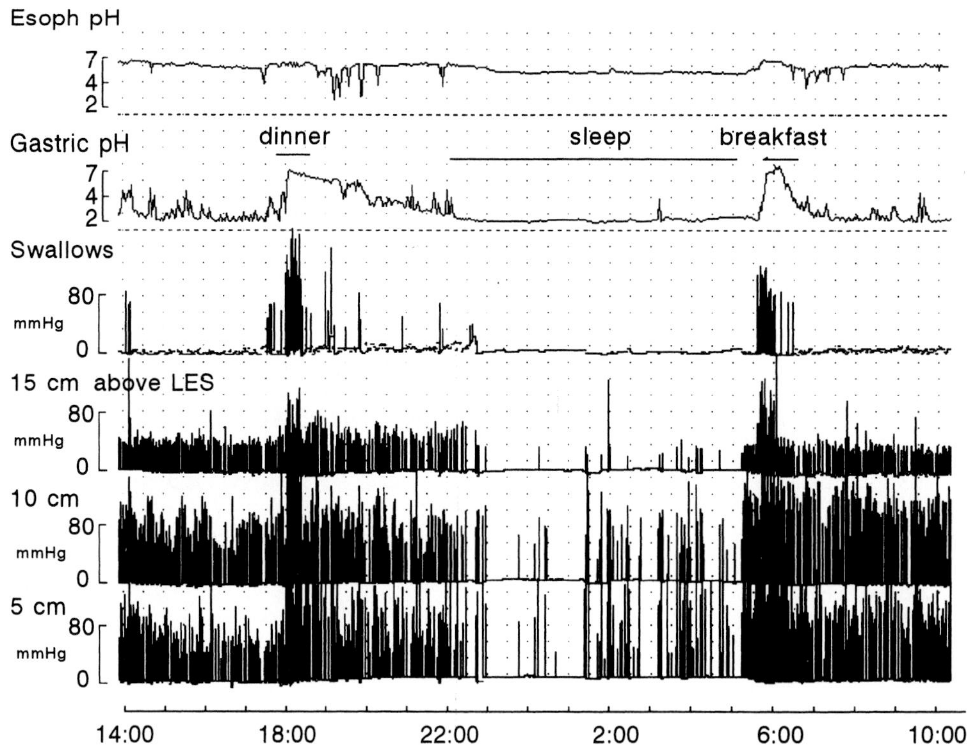

FIGURE 7–41 ■ Complete 24-hour foregut ambulatory monitoring in a healthy subject. From *top* to *bottom*: esophageal pH record, gastric pH record, compressed pharyngeal swallowing record, and compressed esophageal motility record at 15, 10, and 5 cm above the lower esophageal sphincter (LES). Increase in swallows and esophageal motility with meals is evident, together with the typical rise in gastric pH (prandial plateau), followed by slow return to the baseline (postprandial decline phase). During sleep, a marked reduction in swallowing and esophageal activity is normal.

riods of 24 hours has become safe to perform and easy to analyze. Broad clinical application of this new technology will replace the series of laboratory tests classically required to evaluate thoroughly foregut function. This new technology puts into the surgeons' hands tools to evaluate complex foregut problems within their own offices and places surgical therapy for functional abnormalities of the foregut on a more scientific basis.

■ *KEY REFERENCES*

Kahrilas PJ, Dodds WJ, Dent J, et al: Upper esophageal sphincter function during deglutition. Gastroenterology 95:52, 1988a.

In this carefully designed study, the function of the upper esophageal sphincter during deglutition has been evaluated with concurrent manometry and videofluorography. Most of the current concepts on pharyngoesophageal function, namely the correlation between the morphoanatomic and the manometric aspects, are based on this paper.

Kahrilas PJ, Dodds WJ, Hogan WJ: Effect of peristaltic dysfunction on esophageal volume clearance. Gastroenterology 94:73, 1988b.

The application of combined manometry and videofluorography to the study of the esophageal body led the authors to relate the efficacy of esophageal peristalsis to the amplitude and propagation characteristics of esophageal contractions. This study gave new and relevant insights on esophageal body function.

Stein HJ, DeMeester TR: Indications, technique and clinical use of ambulatory 24-hour esophageal motility monitoring in a surgical practice. Ann Surg 217:128, 1993.

This paper represents a comprehensive description of the new technique of 24-hour esophageal motility monitoring, with particular relevance to its application in the diagnostic evaluation of patients with esophageal motor disorders, GERD, noncardiac chest pain, and nonobstructive dysphagia.

Stein HJ, Barlow AP, DeMeester TR, et al: Complications of gastroesophageal reflux disease: Role of the lower esophageal sphincter, esophageal acid and acid/alkaline exposure and duodenogastric reflux. Ann Surg 216:35, 1992a.

In this paper, the authors assessed the importance of manometric evaluation of the lower esophageal sphincter and of results of the 24-hour pH monitoring of the distal esophagus and the stomach in discriminating patients with GERD of varying severity. The clinical application of these tests is carefully outlined.

Stein HJ, DeMeester TR, Hinder RA: Outpatient physiologic testing and surgical management of foregut motility disorders. Curr Probl Surg 24:418, 1992b.

This monograph describes the pathophysiology and the diagnostic and therapeutic aspects of foregut motility disorders in detail. Particular attention has been paid by the authors to describing the traditional and modern tests available for a careful diagnosis and correct treatment of functional disorders of the esophagus.

■ *REFERENCES*

Arndorfer RC, Stef JJ, Dodds WJ, et al: Improved infusion system for intraluminal esophageal manometry. Gastroenterology 73:23, 1977.

Asoh R, Goyal RK: Manometry and electromyography of the upper esophageal sphincter in the opossum. Gastroenterology 74:514, 1978.

Attwood SEA, Fok F, Hinder RA, et al: The interaction of gastric pH and gastric emptying in normal volunteers and patients with non-ulcer dyspepsia. Gastroenterology 96:A17, 1989.

Attwood SEA, Smyrk TC, DeMeester TR, et al: Duodenoesophageal reflux and development of esophageal adenocarcinoma in rats. Surgery 111:503–510, 1992.

Barish CF, Castell DO, Richter JE: Graded esophageal balloon distension: A new provocative test for noncardiac chest pain. Dig Dis Sci 31:1292, 1986.

Barlow AP, DeMeester TR, Ball CS, Eypasch EP: The significance of the gastric secretory state in gastroesophageal reflux disease. Arch Surg 124:937, 1989.

Battle WS, Nyhus LM, Bombeck CT: Gastroesophageal reflux: Diagnosis and treatment. Ann Surg 177:560, 1973.

Bechi P, Falciai R, Baldini F, et al: A new fiber optic sensor for ambulatory entero-gastric reflux detection. Proc SPIE 1648:130–135, 1992.

Behar J, Biancani P, Sheahan DG: Evaluation of esophageal tests in the diagnosis of reflux esophagitis. Gastroenterology 71:9, 1976.

Benjamin SB, Gerhardt DC, Castell DO: High amplitude, peristaltic esophageal contractions associated with chest pain and/or dysphagia. Gastroenterology 77:478, 1979.

Benjamin SB, Richter JE, Cordova CM, et al: Prospective manometric evaluation with pharmacologic provocation of patients with suspected esophageal motility dysfunction. Gastroenterology 84:893, 1983.

Bennett JR, Atkinson M: Oesophageal acid-perfusion in the diagnosis of precordial pain. Lancet 2:1150, 1966.

Benz LJ, Hootkin LA, Margulies S, et al: A comparison of clinical measurements of gastroesophageal reflux. Gastroenterology 62:1, 1972.

Bernstein LM, Baker LA: A clinical test for esophagitis. Gastroenterology 34:760, 1958.

Boesby S: Relationship between gastroesophageal reflux, basal gastroesophageal sphincter pressure, and gastric acid secretion. Scand J Gastroenterol 12:547, 1977.

Bombeck CT, Vas O, DeSalvo J, et al: Computerized axial manometry of the esophagus: A new method for the assessment of antireflux operation. Ann Surg 206:405, 1987.

Bonavina L, Evander A, DeMeester TR, et al: Length of the distal esophageal sphincter and competency of the cardia. Am J Surg 151:25, 1986.

Bondi JL, Godwin DH, Garrett JM: "Vigorous" achalasia: Its clinical interpretation and significance. Am J Gastroenterol 58:145, 1972.

Booth DJ, Kemmerer WT, Skinner DB: Acid clearing from the distal esophagus. Arch Surg 96:731, 1968.

Brasseur JG, Hsieh PY, Kern MK, Shaker R: Mathematical models of UES opening and transphincteric flow. Gastroenterology 110:A640, 1996.

Bremner RM, Costantini M, Nicholas K, et al: Optimal sampling frequencies for 24-hour ambulatory esophageal motility. Gastroenterology 102:A430, 1992a.

Bremner RM, Costantini M, DeMeester TR, et al: Secondary peristalsis is rare and is not important in clearing the esophagus of refluxed gastric acid. Gastroenterology 102:A430, 1992b.

Bremner RM, Crookes PF, DeMeester TR, et al: Concentration of refluxed acid and esophageal mucosal injury. Am J Surg 164:522, 1992c.

Bremner RM, Costantini M, Hoeft SF, et al: Manual verification of computer analysis of 24-hour esophageal motility. Biomed Instrum Technol 27:49, 1993.

Breumelhof R, Nadorp JHSM, Akkermans LMA, Smout AJPM: Analysis of 24-hour esophageal pressure and pH data in unselected patients with noncardiac chest pain. Gastroenterology 99:1257, 1990.

Bumm R, Feussner H, Emde C: Interaction of gastroesophageal reflux and esophageal motility in healthy men undergoing combined 24-hour mano/pH-metry. In Little AG, Ferguson MK, Skinner DB (eds): Diseases of the Esophagus. Mount Kisco, NY, Futura Publishing Company, 1990, p 101.

Cannon WB, Moser A: The movements of the food in the oesophagus. Am J Physiol 1:435, 1898.

Castell DO: Hypocontractile Esophagus: Ineffective Esophageal Motility (IEM) and Hypotensive LES. Esophageal Motility and pH Testing, 3rd ed. Sandhill Scientific, Inc, Highlands Ranch, Colo, 2000.

Castell JA, Richter JE, Castell DO: Comparison of effect of decreasing sampling rates on measurements of esophageal peristaltic amplitudes and durations. Gastroenterology 95:A859, 1988.

Castell JA, Dalton CB, Castell DO: Pharyngeal and upper esophageal sphincter manometry in humans. Am J Physiol 258:G173, 1990.

Clark GWB, Smyrk TC, Mirvish SS, et al: Effect of gastroduodenal juice and dietary fat on the development of Barrett's esophagus and esophageal neoplasia: An experimental rat model. Ann Surg Oncol 1:252–261, 1994.

Clouse RE, Lustman JJ: Psychiatric illness and contraction abnormalities of the esophagus. N Engl J Med 309:1337, 1983.

Code CF, Schlegel JF, Kelley ML Jr, et al: Hypertensive gastroesophageal sphincter. Mayo Clin Proc 35:391, 1960.

Cook IJ, Dodds WJ, Dantas RO, et al: Opening mechanisms of the human upper esophageal sphincter. Am J Physiol 257:G748, 1989.

Cook IJ, Gabb M, Panagopoulos V, et al: Zenker's diverticulum: A defect in upper esophageal sphincter compliance? Gastroenterology 96:A98, 1990.

Costantini M, Bremner RM, Cookes P, DeMeester TR: The slow motorized pull-through: An improved technique to evaluate the lower esophageal sphincter. Gastroenterology 102:A53, 1992a.

Costantini M, Bremner RM, Hoeft SF, et al: Normal esophageal motor function: A manometric study of 136 healthy subjects. Gastroenterology 103:1407, 1992b.

Costantini M, Sturniolo GC, Zaninotto G, et al: Altered esophageal pain threshold in irritable bowel syndrome. Dig Dis Sci 38:206, 1992c.

Dalton CB, Castell DO, Richter JE: The changing faces of the nutcracker esophagus. Am J Gastroenterol 83:623, 1988.

Dantas RO, Kern MK, Massey BT, et al: Effect of swallowed bolus variables on oral and pharyngeal phases of swallowing. Am J Physiol 258:G675, 1990a.

Dantas RO, Cook IJ, Dodds WJ, et al: Biomechanics of cricopharyngeal bars. Gastroenterology 99:1269, 1990b.

DeMeester TR: Prolonged oesophageal pH monitoring. In Read NW (ed): Gastrointestinal Motility: Which Test? Petersfield, England, Wrightson Biomedical, 1989, p 41.

DeMeester TR, Crookes PF: Benign and malignant disease of the esophagus. In Levine BA, Copeland III EM, Howard RJ, et al (eds): Current Practice of Surgery. New York, Churchill Livingstone, 1993, p 14.

DeMeester TR, Wang CI, Wernly JA, et al: Technique, indications, and clinical use of 24-hour esophageal pH monitoring. J Thorac Cardiovasc Surg 79:656, 1980.

DeMeester TR, O'Sullivan GC, Bermudez G, et al: Esophageal function in patients with angina-like chest pain and normal coronary angiograms. Ann Surg 196:488, 1982.

DeMeester TR, Bonavina L, Iascone C, et al: Chronic respiratory symptoms and occult gastroesophageal reflux. Ann Surg 211:337, 1990.

DeMeester TR, Peters JH, Bremner CG, Chandrasoma P: Biology of gastroesophageal reflux: Pathophysiology related to medical and surgical treatment. Ann Rev Med 50:469, 1999.

DeMeester TR, Stein HJ: Gastroesophageal reflux disease. In Moody FG, Carey LC, Jones RC, et al (eds): Surgical Treatment of Digestive Disease, 2nd ed. Chicago, Year Book Medical Publishers, 1989, p 72.

deMoraes-Filho JPP, Bettarello A: Lack of specificity of the acid perfusion test in duodenal ulcer patients. Am J Dig Dis 19:785, 1974.

Ekberg O: The normal movements of the hyoid bone during swallow. Invest Radiol 21:408, 1986.

Emde C, Garner A, Blum A: Technical aspects of intraluminal pH-metry in man: Current status and recommendations. Gut 23:1177, 1987.

Eypasch EP, Stein HJ, DeMeester TR, et al: The hypercontracting-hypertensive lower esophageal sphincter as a cause of dysphagia and chest pain. In Little AG, Ferguson MK, Skinner DB (eds): Diseases of the Esophagus, Vol II. Benign Diseases. Mount Kisco, NY, Futura Publishing Company, 1990a, p 351.

Eypasch EP, Stein HJ, DeMeester TR, et al: A new technique to define and clarify esophageal motor disorders. Am J Surg 159:144, 1990b.

Fein M, Ireland AP, Ritter MP, et al: Duodenogastric reflux potentiates the injurious effects of gastroesophageal reflux. J Gastrointest Surg 1:27–33, 1997.

Ferguson ME, Little AG: Angina-like chest pain associated with high amplitude peristaltic contractions of the esophagus. Surgery 104:713, 1988.

Fimmel CJ, Etienne A, Cilluffo TR, et al: Long-term ambulatory gastric pH monitoring: Validation of a new method and effect of H_2-antagonists. Gastroenterology 88:1842, 1985.

Fuchs KH, DeMeester TR, Albertucci M: Specificity and sensitivity of objective diagnosis of gastroesophageal reflux disease. Surgery 102:575, 1987.

Fuchs KH, DeMeester TR, Hinder RA, et al: Computerized identification of pathologic duodenogastric reflux using 24-hour gastric pH monitoring. Ann Surg 213:13, 1991.

Fyke FE, Code CF, Schlegel JF: The gastroesophageal sphincter in healthy human beings. Gastroenterologia 86:135, 1956.

Gillen P, Keeling P, Bryne PJ, Hennessy TPJ: Barrett's oesophagus: pH profile. Br J Surg 74:774–776, 1987.

Hellemans J, Pelemans W, Vantrappen G: Pharyngoesophageal swallowing disorders and the pharyngoesophageal sphincter. Med Clin North Am 65:1149, 1981.

Hinder RA: Outpatient physiologic testing and surgical management of foregut motility disorders. Curr Probl Surg 24:441, 1992.

Hollis JB, Castell DO: Effect of dry swallows and wet swallows of different volumes of esophageal peristalsis. J Appl Physiol 38:1161, 1975.

Iascone C, DeMeester TR, Little AG, Skinner DB: Barrett's esophagus: Functional assessment, proposed pathogenesis, and surgical therapy. Arch Surg 118:543–549, 1983.

Jacob P, Kahrilas PJ, Herzon G: Proximal esophageal pH-metry in patients with "reflux laryngitis." Gastroenterology 100:305, 1991.

Jamieson J, Stein HJ, DeMeester TR, et al: Ambulatory 24-hour esophageal pH monitoring: Normal values, optimal thresholds, specificity, sensitivity, and reproducibility. Am J Gastroenterol 87:1102, 1992.

Janssens J, Vantrappen G, Ghillebert G: 24-hour recording of esophageal pressure and pH in patients with noncardiac chest pain. Gastroenterology 90:1978, 1986.

Joelsson BE, DeMeester TR, Skinner DB, et al: The role of the esophageal body in the antireflux mechanism. Surgery 92:417, 1982.

Johnson LF, DeMeester TR: Twenty-four hour pH monitoring of the distal esophagus: A quantitative measure of gastroesophageal reflux. Am J Gastroenterol 62:325, 1974.

Johnson LF, DeMeester TR: Development of the 24-hour intraesophageal pH monitoring composite scoring system. J Clin Gastroenterol 8:52, 1986.

Kahrilas PJ, Dent J, Dodds WJ, et al: A method for continuous monitoring of the upper esophageal sphincter pressure. Dig Dis Sci 32:121, 1987.

Kahrilas PJ, Dodds WJ, Dent J, et al: Upper esophageal sphincter function during deglutition. Gastroenterology 95:52, 1988a.

Kahrilas PJ, Dodds WJ, Hogan WJ: Effect of peristaltic dysfunction in esophageal volume clearance. Gastroenterology 94:73, 1988b.

Katz PO, Dalton CB, Richter JE, et al: Esophageal testing of patients with noncardiac chest pain or dysphagia: Results of three years' experience with 1161 patients. Ann Intern Med 106:593, 1987.

Kauer WKH, Burdiles P, Ireland AP, et al: Does duodenal juice reflux into the esophagus of patients with complicated GERD? Evaluation of a fiberoptic sensor for bilirubin. Am J Surg 169:98–104, 1995a.

Kauer WKH, Peters JH, DeMeester TR, et al: Mixed reflux of gastric and duodenal juices is more harmful to the esophagus than gastric juice alone: The need for surgical therapy re-emphasized. Ann Surg 222:525–533, 1995b.

Kramer P, Hollander W: Comparison of experimental esophageal pain with clinical pain of angina pectoris and esophageal disease. Gastroenterology 29:719, 1955.

Kronecker H, Meltzer SJ: Der Schluckmechanismus, seine Erregung und seine Hemmung. Arch Ges Anat Physiol (suppl):328, 1883.

Landon RL, Ouyang A, Snape WJ, et al: Provocation of esophageal chest pain by ergonovine or edrophonium. Gastroenterology 81:10, 1981.

Lieberman DA: Medical therapy for chronic reflux esophagitis: Long-term follow-up. Arch Intern Med 147:1717, 1987.

Lydon SB, Dodds WJ, Hogan WJ, et al: The effect of manometric assembly diameter on intraluminal esophageal pressure recording. Dig Dis Sci 20:968, 1975.

Maas LC, Gordon RK, Penner D, et al: 24-hour ambulatory manometry in diagnosis of esophageal motor disorders causing chest pain. South Med J 78:810, 1985.

MacKenzie J, Belch J, Land D, et al: Oesophageal ischemia in motility disorders associated with chest pain. Lancet 2:592, 1988.

Marks IN, Young GO, Winter T, et al: South African Gastroenterology Society, Congress abstract, 1992.

Mason RJ, Bremner CG, DeMeester TR, et al: Pharyngeal swallowing disorders: Selection for the outcome after myotomy. Ann Surg 228:598, 1998.

McConnel FM, Cerenko D, Jackson RT, Hersh T: Clinical application of the manofluorogram. Laryngoscope 98:705, 1988a.

McConnel FM, Cerenko D, Mendelsohn MS: Manofluorographic analysis of swallowing. Otolaryngol Clin North Am 21:625, 1988b.

McConnel FM, Cerenko D, Hersh T, Weil LJ: Evaluation of pharyngeal dysphagia with manofluorography. Dysphagia 2:187, 1988c.

McLaughlan G, Rawlings JM, Lucas ML, et al: Electrodes for 24 hour pH monitoring: A comparative study. Gut 28:935, 1987.

Mellow MH: Return of esophageal peristalsis in idiopathic achalasia. Gastroenterology 70:1148, 1976.

Miller FA: Utilization of inlying pH-probe for evaluation of acid-peptic diathesis. Arch Surg 89:199, 1964.

Ollyo JB, Monnier P, Fontolliet C, Savary M: The natural history and incidence of reflux oesophagitis. Gullet 3:3–10, 1993.

Orringer MB, Dabich L, Zarafonetis CJD, et al: Gastroesophageal reflux in esophageal scleroderma: Diagnosis and implications. Ann Thorac Surg 22:120, 1976.

Palmer JB, Tanaka E, Siebens AA: Electromyography of the pharyngeal musculature: Technical considerations. Arch Phys Med Rehabil 70:283, 1989.

Peters L, Maas L, Petty D, et al: Spontaneous noncardiac chest pain: Evaluation by 24-hour ambulatory esophageal motility and pH monitoring. Gastroenterology 94:878, 1988.

Richter JE, Castell DO: Diffuse esophageal spasm: A reappraisal. Ann Intern Med 100:242, 1984.

Richter JE, Castell DO: 24-hour ambulatory oesophageal motility monitoring: How should motility data be analyzed? Gut 30:1040, 1989.

Richter JE, Hackshaw BT, Wu WC: Edrophonium: A useful provocative test for esophageal chest pain. Ann Intern Med 103:14, 1985.

Richter JE, Barish CF, Castell DO: Abnormal sensory perception in patients with esophageal chest pain. Gastroenterology 91:845, 1986.

Richter JE, Wu WC, Johns DM, et al: Esophageal manometry in 95 healthy adult volunteers: Variability of pressure with age and frequency of "abnormal" contractions. Dig Dis Sci 32:583, 1987.

Richter JE, Bradley LA, DeMeester TR, et al: Normal 24-hour ambulatory esophageal pH values: Influence of study center. pH electrode, age and gender. Dig Dis Sci 37:849, 1992.

Shaker R, Ren J, Xie P, et al: Characterization of the pharyngo-UES contractile reflex in humans. Am J Physiol 273:G854, 1997.

Shipp T, Deatsch WW, Robertson K: Pharyngoesophageal muscle activity during swallowing in man. Laryngoscope 80:1, 1970.

Skinner DB, Booth DJ: Assessment of distal esophageal function in patients with hiatal hernia and/or gastroesophageal reflux. Ann Surg 172:627, 1970.

Smout AJPM, Breedijk M, Van der Zouw C, Akkermans LMA: Physiological gastroesophageal reflux and esophageal motor activity studied with a new system for 24-hour recording and automated analysis. Dig Dis Sci 34:372, 1989.

Soffer EE, Scalabrini P, Wingate DL: Spontaneous noncardiac chest pain: Value of ambulatory esophageal pH and motility monitoring. Dig Dis Sci 34:1651, 1989.

Stein HJ, Barlow AP, DeMeester TR, et al: Complications of gastroesophageal reflux disease: Role of the lower esophageal sphincter, esophageal acid and acid/alkaline exposure and duodenogastric reflux. Ann Surg 216:35, 1992a.

Stein HJ, Bremner RM, Jamieson J, DeMeester TR: Effect of Nissen fundoplication on an esophageal motor function. Arch Surg 127:788, 1992c.

Stein HJ, DeMeester TR: Integrated ambulatory foregut monitoring in patients with functional foregut disorders. In Nyhus LM (ed): Surgery Annual. Part 1, Vol 24. Norwalk, CT, Appleton & Lange, 1992.

Stein HJ, DeMeester TR: Indications, technique, and clinical use of ambulatory 24-hour esophageal motility monitoring in a surgical practice. Ann Surg 217:128, 1993.

Stein HJ, DeMeester TR, Hinder RA: Outpatient physiologic testing and surgical management of foregut motility disorders. Curr Probl Surg 24:418, 1992b.

Stein HJ, DeMeester TR, Naspetti R, et al: Three-dimensional imaging of the lower esophageal sphincter in gastroesophageal reflux disease. Ann Surg 214:374, 1991a.

Stein HJ, DeMeester TR, Singh S: Circadian esophageal motor function in patients with non-obstructive dysphagia and normal esophageal acid exposure. Gastroenterology 100:168, 1991b.

Stein HJ, DeMeester TR, Eypasch EP, Klingman RR: Ambulatory 24-hour esophageal manometry in the evaluation of esophageal motor disorders and noncardiac chest pain. Surgery 110:753, 1991c.

Stein HJ, Eypasch EP, DeMeester TR: "Esophageal claudication" as the cause of chest pain in diffuse spasm and nutcracker esophagus? Gastroenterology 96:A491, 1989.

Stein HJ, Eypasch EP, DeMeester TR, et al: Circadian esophageal motor function in patients with gastroesophageal reflux disease. Surgery 108:769, 1990.

Stein HJ, Feussner H, Kauer W, et al: "Alkaline" gastroesophageal reflux: Assessment by ambulatory esophageal aspiration and pH monitoring. Am J Surg 167:163–168, 1994.

Tuttle SG, Grossman MI: Detection of gastroesophageal reflux by simultaneous measurement of intraluminal pressures and pH. Proc Soc Exp Biol Med 98:225, 1958.

Vantrappen G, Janssens J, Hellemans J, Coremans G: Achalasia, diffuse esophageal spasm, and related motility disorders. Gastroenterology 76:450, 1979.

Welch RW, Luckmann K, Ricks PM, et al: Manometry of the normal upper esophageal sphincter and its alterations in laryngectomy. J Clin Invest 63:1036, 1979.

Winans CS, Harris LD: Quantitation of lower esophageal sphincter competence. Gastroenterology 52:773, 1967.

Winkelstein A: Peptic esophagitis: A new clinical entity. JAMA 104:906, 1935.

Zaninotto G, DeMeester TR, Schwizer W, et al: The lower esophageal sphincter in health and disease. Am J Surg 155:104, 1988a.

Zaninotto G, DeMeester TR, Eypasch EP, et al: Advantages of computer assisted analysis of esophageal manometry. Gastroenterology 94:A514, 1988b.

Zaninotto G, Peserico A, Costantini M, et al: Oesophageal motility and lower esophageal competence in progressive systemic sclerosis and localized scleroderma. Scand J Gastroenterol 24:95, 1989.

Zaninotto G, DiMario F, Costantini M, et al: Oesophagitis and pH of the refluxate: An experimental and clinical study. Br J Surg 79:161, 1992.

Pediatric Disorders

CHAPTER 8

Congenital Anomalies

ESOPHAGEAL ATRESIA AND TRACHEOESOPHAGEAL FISTULA

Allan M. Goldstein
Daniel P. Doody
Patricia K. Donahoe

HISTORICAL NOTE

Thomas Gibson (1697) described a child who, upon swallowing, "was liked to be choked, and what should have gone down returned by the mouth and nose." In the 250 years following this first description of a patient with esophageal atresia and tracheoesophageal fistula, there were multiple failed attempts at operative treatment of this anomaly (Gross, 1953; Ladd, 1944). The futility encountered led many surgeons to conclude that children affected with this aberration were best left to die.

In 1939, Leven (Leven, 1941) and Ladd (Ladd, 1944) had performed staged repairs involving gastrostomy and cervical esophagostomy, fistula ligation, and subsequent creation of an antesternal neoesophagus with successful outcomes. In 1941, Haight (Haight and Towsley, 1943) used the left extrapleural approach to ligate the fistula and repair the esophagus primarily. Thus began the modern era of esophageal surgery in infants.

HISTORICAL READINGS

Gibson T: The Anatomy of Humane Bodies Epitomized. London, Awnsham & Churchill, 1697.

Gross R: Atresia of the esophagus. In Gross R (ed): The Surgery of Infancy and Childhood. Philadelphia, WB Saunders, 1953, p 75.

Haight C, Towsley H: Congenital atresia of the esophagus with tracheoesophageal fistula: Extrapleural ligation of fistula and end-to-end anastomosis of esophageal segments. Surg Gynecol Obstet 76:672–688, 1943.

Ladd W: The surgical treatment of esophageal atresia and tracheoesophageal fistulas. N Engl J Med 230:625–637, 1944.

Leven N: Congenital atresia of the esophagus with tracheoesophageal fistula: Report of successful extrapleural ligation of fistulous communication and cervical esophagostomy. J Thorac Surg 10:648–657, 1941.

EPIDEMIOLOGY

Esophageal atresia occurs in 1 to 2 of every 4000 live births, its incidence being slightly higher in males and in the children of older or diabetic mothers (Skandalakis et al, 1994). Various environmental influences have been implicated as causative, including (1) intrauterine exposure to contraceptive pills, progesterone, estrogen, or thalidomide and (2) the unique environment created by diabetes.

Although the anomaly is usually sporadic, the occurrence of familial esophageal atresia is well recognized. Children born to an affected parent have a 3% to 4% risk, children with one affected sibling have a 0.5% to 2% risk, and the risk rises to 20% when two siblings are affected (Pletcher et al, 1991). In addition, a number of chromosomal regions have been identified based on deletions, translocations, and duplications in affected cohorts (Spitz, 1996). The recent mouse knockout models described later lend further support to a genetic basis of this condition (Litingtung et al, 1998; Motoyama et al, 1998).

EMBRYOLOGY

A thorough understanding of the developmental pathways leading to normal foregut anatomy is essential in order to comprehend tracheoesophageal anomalies and to improve their management in these infants. Although early development of the human foregut and its separation into intestinal and respiratory components remains poorly understood, meticulous analysis of thin sections of staged human embryos from the Carnegie Embryological

Collection has been informative (O'Rahilly and Muller, 1984; Sutliff and Hutchins, 1994).

On day 26 of human gestation, 6 days following the initial appearance of the foregut, the lung bud can be seen as a ventral outgrowth from the foregut (Fig. 8–1*A*). As the lung bud grows ventrally and caudally into the surrounding mesenchyme, it descends in front of the esophagus, leaving a mesenchymal layer (the tracheoesophageal septum) between these two epithelial tubes. The most cranial aspect of the septum, the tracheoesophageal sulcus, remains fixed at the level of the first cervical vertebra (between somites 5 and 6) throughout development (Fig. 8–1*B*) (O'Rahilly and Muller, 1984; Sutliff and Hutchins, 1994).

In none of these observations of foregut morphogenesis was a common "esophagotrachea" identified. Therefore, the commonly postulated separation of a common channel into digestive and respiratory components by the ingrowth of lateral epithelial ridges may not apply to human embryonic development (Kluth et al, 1987). In addition, the tracheoesophageal sulcus, which marks the separation point of trachea from esophagus, does not extend rostrally, as previously thought. Instead, the sulcus remains fixed in position while the tracheal bifurcation descends.

The aberrations of normal morphogenesis that give rise to esophageal atresia and tracheoesophageal fistula remain uncertain. However, a recently discovered experimental animal model enhances our understanding of this process.

Intraperitoneal injection of pregnant rats with doxorubicin (Adriamycin) at 6 to 9 days of gestation (prior to lung bud formation on day 12) causes development of tracheoesophageal anomalies in 40% to 60% of offspring. Many of the newborn rats also have associated defects commonly seen in humans, including duodenal atresia, anorectal anomalies, and genitourinary defects (Diez-Pardo et al, 1996; Merei et al, 1997a, 1997b). The majority (90%) of affected offspring exhibit esophageal atresia with a distal fistula, whereas the remainder have atresia without a fistula or an N-type fistula (Diez-Pardo et al, 1996). These embryos lack a tracheal bud, and the foregut itself gives rise to both main bronchi, as is observed in the rare cases of tracheal agenesis (Faro et al, 1979). The abnormal foregut in the affected rats continues caudally to the stomach (Merei et al, 1997a, 1997b). The Adriamycin-induced abnormality also appears similar to the most severe (type IV) laryngotracheoesophageal cleft observed in children (Ryan et al, 1991; Simpson et al, 1996).

After Adriamycin treatment, histologic examination reveals that the upper foregut, proximal to the origin

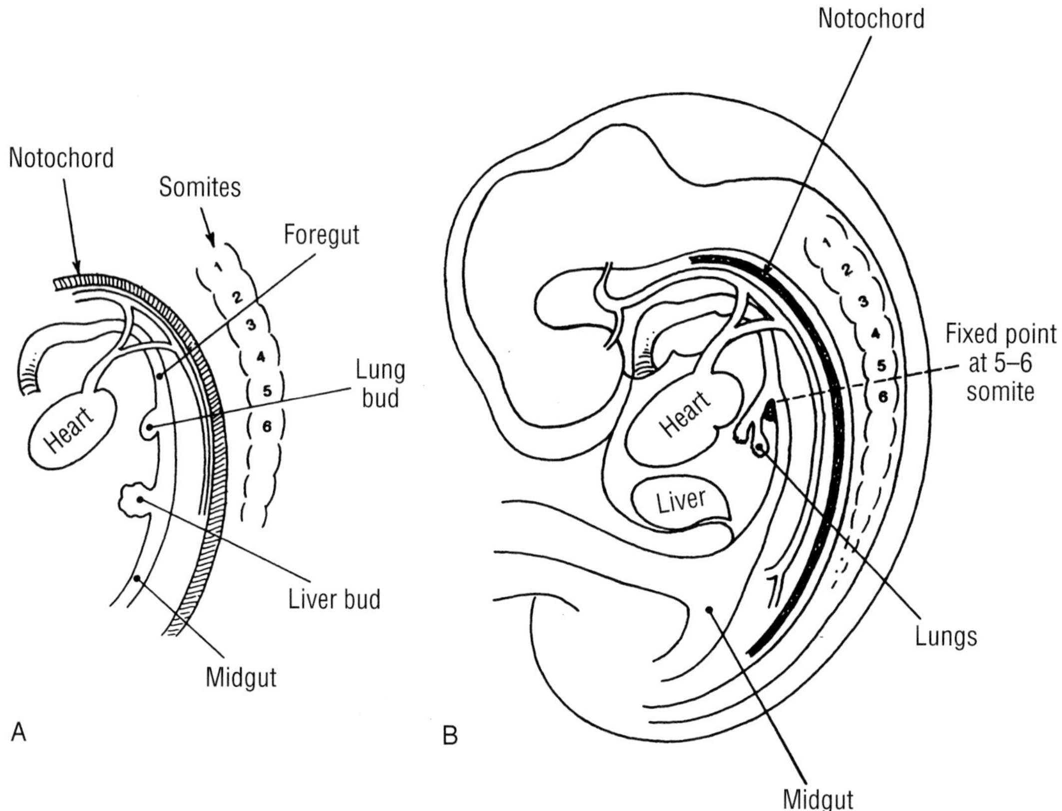

FIGURE 8–1 ■ Separation of pulmonary and intestinal tracts during development. Human embryos are depicted in the left lateral median plane. *A,* At Carnegie stage 12 (26 to 28 days after fertilization), the lung primordium buds from the foregut. *B,* At stage 13 (28 to 32 days after fertilization), the lung bud has started its caudal descent. The top of the tracheoesophageal septum (*shaded area* in *B*) is referred to as the tracheoesophageal sulcus. As the lung bud descends, this point remains fixed at the level of the fifth or sixth somite throughout development, corresponding to the level of the first cervical vertebra.

of the bronchi, develops tracheal elements with ciliated pseudostratified columnar epithelium and cartilage, thereby comprising, in essence, a common esophagotrachea. The lower foregut demonstrates a variable transition from tracheobronchial to esophageal histology (Merei et al, 1997a, 1997b). This pattern is similar to that in humans (Hokama et al, 1986) and may account for the patient with a tracheoesophageal anomaly and coexisting severe distal esophageal stenosis with associated cartilaginous remnants. The abnormal histopathology in both the upper and lower foregut in the rat model may, in addition, explain the frequent clinical findings of tracheomalacia and esophageal dysmotility in children with esophageal atresia. The additional contribution of abnormal sympathetic and parasympathetic innervation to the dysmotility characteristic of the syndrome is appreciated but not fully understood.

Adriamycin-induced failure of lung bud formation may represent a defect in normal interactions between the epithelium of the foregut and its surrounding mesenchyme. Two recent mouse knockout models lend support to this theory.

Sonic hedgehog (Shh), expressed in the ventral foregut endoderm and in the early lung bud, is an evolutionarily conserved, secreted molecule that signals via serine/threonine kinase receptors to activate downstream genes, essential to proper development and differentiation of numerous structures. Shh protein induces expression of *Gli*, a gene that encodes a transcription factor expressed in the mesenchyme surrounding the lung bud. Mice with mutations in either the *Shh* or *Gli* genes demonstrate foregut malformations strikingly similar to human esophageal atresia with tracheoesophageal fistula (Litingtung et al, 1998; Motoyama et al, 1998). Thus, these two genes may represent critical components of the epithelial-mesenchymal communication necessary for normal foregut morphogenesis. It would be interesting to investigate whether Adriamycin (an anthracycline anticancer agent which functions via such mechanisms as deoxyribonucleic acid [DNA] intercalation, inhibition of topoisomerase II, cell membrane binding, and free radical formation) interferes with this pathway. One might then devise pathways for pharmacologic rescue of these defects if discovered sufficiently early in gestation.

Current experimental data, both genetic and teratogenic, suggest a model for understanding the developmental etiology of esophageal atresia with tracheoesophageal fistula. Endoderm-mesoderm interactions are essential for signaling normal lung bud formation, initiating the development of the tracheobronchial tree from the esophagus. Failure of this critical early event, as occurs in the Adriamycin model, results in trachealization of the proximal foregut, with the main bronchi branching directly from this structure, and the foregut continues caudally to the stomach (Litingtung et al, 1998; Merei et al, 1997a, 1997b).

Although many questions remain unanswered, these novel experimental models are yielding a new conceptual framework upon which to advance our understanding of this fascinating anomaly. A full understanding of the genetics and pathways in which molecular defects occur can lead to improved prenatal and postnatal therapeutic strategies.

CLASSIFICATION

Numerous classification schemes describe the anatomic arrangements seen in esophageal atresia and these are variously referenced in the literature. We prefer to avoid using any classification by simply describing the anatomy of the esophagus and trachea. However, the more commonly used classifications of Ladd (Ladd, 1944) and Gross (Gross, 1953) are summarized in Table 8–1.

ASSOCIATED CONGENITAL ANOMALIES

Because the surgical and perioperative management of the tracheoesophageal disorder has improved dramatically in recent decades, the associated anomalies have become an increasingly important factor in the prognosis of these children. No longer are respiratory failure and sepsis primarily responsible for mortality; instead, the coexis-

TABLE 8–1 ■ **Types and Relative Frequencies of Tracheoesophageal Anomalies**

Description	*EA with Distal TEF*	*Isolated EA*	*"N-Type" TEF*	*EA with Proximal TEF*	*EA with Proximal and Distal TEF*
Gross Classification	C	A	E	B	D
Ladd Classification	III/IV*	I		II	V
Frequency (%)	86.5	7.7	4.2	0.8	0.7

*Type III if fistula enters above tracheal bifurcation; type IV if fistula enters at carina.
EA, esophageal atresia; TEF, tracheoesophageal fistula.

tence of severe congenital anomalies, particularly cardiac, has emerged as the major cause of death (Beasley and Myers, 1992).

Approximately 50% of all infants born with esophageal atresia, with or without tracheoesophageal fistula, can be expected to have additional anomalies, with a higher likelihood (58%) in infants with isolated atresia, compared with infants with an N-type fistula (27%) (Holder et al, 1964). A careful search for these associated anomalies is crucial to the comprehensive evaluation and ultimate prognosis of these infants as well as to the formulation of a logical approach to their care. The incidence of associated anomalies is several-fold higher among infants weighing less than 2000 g, making the care of these children particularly challenging.

Cardiac Anomalies

Although associated defects have been identified in nearly every organ system, the most frequently encountered anomalies involve the heart. Approximately 20% to 30% of infants with esophageal atresia also have an associated cardiovascular anomaly (Holder et al, 1964; Mee et al, 1992; Skandalakis et al, 1994; Waterston et al, 1962). The most common of the cardiovascular anomalies (Mee et al, 1992) are:

- Atrial and ventricular septal defects
- Patent ductus arteriosus
- Tetralogy of Fallot
- Aortic arch anomalies

The presence of coexisting complex congenital heart disease is a major factor accounting for mortality in these patients, reducing the usual survival from nearly 100% (Beasley and Myers, 1992) to 70% (Mee et al, 1992; Spitz, 1996).

Gastrointestinal Anomalies

Associated gastrointestinal anomalies occur in about 25% of patients with esophageal atresia, and most of these are easily repaired at the time of esophageal repair. The most common of these is anal atresia, accounting for 42% of all gastrointestinal anomalies in one series (Holder et al, 1964). Other defects include duodenal and ileal atresia, malrotation, Meckel's diverticulum, annular pancreas, and pyloric stenosis.

Urinary Tract Anomalies

Abnormalities of the urinary tract have been identified in 24% of patients (Beasley et al, 1992). Early identification of these anomalies in the neonate is essential in order to prevent potential renal damage. Anomalies frequently encountered include:

- Unilateral or bilateral renal agenesis or hypoplasia
- Multicystic kidney
- Horseshoe kidney
- Vesicoureteral reflux

Neurologic or Skeletal Anomalies

Ten percent of patients have neurologic or skeletal anomalies, including neural tube defects, hydrocephalus, scoliosis, and other anomalies affecting the vertebrae and extremities (Harris et al, 1995).

Multiple Congenital Anomalies

Quan and Smith (1973) gave the nonrandom occurrence of multiple congenital anomalies in association with esophageal atresia the acronym VATER to denote *v*ertebral anomalies, *a*nal atresia, *t*racheoesophageal fistula with *e*sophageal atresia, *r*enal defects, and *r*adial limb dysplasia. The acronym has been expanded to VACTERL to include *c*ardiac and *l*imb (especially radial ray) defects as well. The VACTERL association (defined as the coexistence of at least three of these anomalies) occurs in approximately 15% of children with esophageal atresia and contributes to an increased mortality rate, particularly as a result of the cardiac anomalies (Iuchtman et al, 1992; Poenaru et al, 1993).

A less common and more severe group of anomalies associated with esophageal atresia is known as CHARGE, which includes *c*oloboma, *h*eart disease, *a*tresia choanae, growth and developmental *r*etardation, genital hypoplasia, and *e*ar anomalies (deafness) (Kutiyanawala et al, 1992).

Infrequently, esophageal atresia is present in the Schisis association (omphalocele, neural tube defects, cleft lip/palate, genital hypoplasia), or in other complexes such as trisomy 18 or 21, Potter's syndrome, polysplenia, or Turner's syndrome (Poenaru et al, 1993; Spitz et al, 1994).

SYMPTOMS AND DIAGNOSIS

Esophageal Atresia with or without Tracheoesophageal Fistula

Suspicion of esophageal atresia often begins before birth, when a prenatal ultrasound study demonstrates polyhydramnios in association with a small or absent stomach (Stringer et al, 1995). Early diagnosis may lend itself to treatment strategies using minimally invasive delivery techniques.

Polyhydramnios presumably results from the inability of the fetus to swallow amniotic fluid through the atretic esophagus. Consequently, pure atresia nearly always leads to maternal polyhydramnios. In those infants with a distal fistula, however, amniotic fluid may pass into the trachea and, via the fistula, reach the stomach, thereby accounting for the absence of polyhydramnios in many of these cases. Prematurity is often associated with esophageal atresia, with 40% of newborns weighing less than 2500 g (Poenaru et al, 1993).

Within hours after birth, the infant demonstrates excessive drooling of saliva with pooling in the posterior pharynx. This is often followed by aspiration, with choking spells, respiratory distress, and cyanosis with the first feeding. If the aspiration is significant, apnea, bradycardia, and even death may ensue. The presence of a distal fistula often results in more severe respiratory distress as gastric secretions reflux into the tracheobronchial tree, causing pneumonitis and the potential for sepsis.

The infant displays excessive salivation from the nose and mouth as well as noisy breathing. The abdomen appears scaphoid in the presence of pure esophageal atresia. If a distal fistula is present, air can enter the stomach via the trachea and may distend the abdomen. A thorough assessment, including cardiac auscultation, evaluation of the extremities and spine, and digital rectal examination, commonly reveals associated anomalies.

A firm 10 French catheter passed gently through the mouth of the infant typically meets resistance at about 10 cm. A plain radiograph shows the catheter tip in the proximal esophageal pouch, giving a rough indication of the length of the esophageal gap. Dilute barium may help to demonstrate the proximal pouch, but it must be administered with caution to avoid further aspiration.

Isolated Tracheoesophageal Fistula

The rare tracheoesophageal fistula without esophageal atresia (3% to 5% of cases) produces subtle symptoms, thus necessitating a high index of suspicion. Isolated tracheoesophageal fistula is also referred to as *H-type* or, more descriptively, *N-type* or *diagonal*, fistula to describe the higher insertion of the fistula on the trachea. Coughing and choking occur with feeding, and reflux of gastric fluid into the trachea produces a tracheobronchial pneumonitis that is often bilateral and recurrent.

The barking cough typical of infants with tracheoesophageal fistula, with or without esophageal atresia, is secondary to associated tracheomalacia. The structure of the trachea can be abnormal, with staple-shaped cartilaginous rings and a widely redundant membranous mucosa, permitting apposition of the anterior and posterior walls and producing the barking cough (Qi et al, 1997). Abnormal tracheal development has been attributed to the loss of normal tracheobronchial pressure during lung development as pulmonary amniotic fluid is lost through the fistula into the esophagus (Davies and Cywes, 1978). Trachealization of the foregut during early development, however (see previous topic), more likely accounts for the abnormal structure and function of the trachea.

SURGERY

Preoperative Evaluation

Prior to operation for esophageal atresia or tracheoesophageal fistula, it is important that the surgeon carefully delineate the anatomy, search for associated anomalies, and treat comorbid conditions to optimize the infant's ability to tolerate definitive esophageal repair. A plain radiograph after passage of an esophageal tube can, with slight inflation, outline the size and shape of the proximal esophageal pouch. In exceptional cases, dilute barium may be used and may reveal a proximal fistula to the trachea. The barium should be promptly removed to prevent aspiration; water-soluble contrast is contraindicated.

Air in the abdomen confirms the presence of a distal fistula, whereas an absence of air suggests pure atresia. Coexisting duodenal atresia may explain air in the stomach but not in the bowel. Plain films may also reveal the presence of pneumonia, an abnormal cardiac contour suggesting congenital heart disease, or the existence of skeletal abnormalities. It is also mandatory to search for a right-sided aortic arch, the presence of which dictates a left-sided approach to avoid operative catastrophe.

The diagnosis of a fistula without esophageal atresia can be more challenging. Chest films may show aspiration pneumonitis with distention of the stomach. The diagnosis can occasionally be made with contrast esophagography with the patient in the prone position with the head slightly down. A tube is placed in the distal esophagus, and contrast is injected as the tube is gradually withdrawn. Often, bronchoscopy and esophagoscopy may be required for a definitive diagnosis to be made.

The routine search for associated anomalies must include an echocardiogram because of the high incidence of associated heart disease, a renal ultrasound study to detect kidney abnormalities, and a voiding cystourogram to detect vesicoureteral reflux (Beasley et al, 1992). Chromosomal analysis should be obtained in infants with multiple associated anomalies.

Infants with esophageal atresia and tracheoesophageal fistula are nursed in a semiupright sitting position to minimize reflux of gastric acid through the fistula and into the trachea. A soft sump catheter placed in the atretic esophageal pouch with frequent oropharyngeal suctioning can minimize aspirations. Infants with isolated esophageal atresia can be safely placed in the prone position, since their only risk is aspiration of saliva. Systemic antibiotics, usually ampicillin and gentamicin, should be administered empirically.

If pneumonitis is present and severe or if the infant has concomitant respiratory distress syndrome, endotracheal intubation and mechanical ventilation may be indicated. In this situation, prompt gastrostomy prevents continued reflux into the trachea and avoids massive gastric distention from passage of air through the fistula and into the stomach. Failure to vent the stomach effectively, as by inadvertent twisting or clamping of the gastrostomy tube, can result in gastric perforation. Unfortunately, the gastrostomy vent may make effective pulmonary ventilation difficult, particularly in infants who require high-pressure ventilation. This situation may force early thoracotomy for ligation of the fistula and, if tolerated, esophageal repair. Definitive repair need be delayed only in the rare infant who is severely unstable (Templeton et al, 1985).

Preoperative Management

Preoperative risk stratification schemes have been developed according to the severity of illness and the expected outcome of infants with esophageal atresia with or without tracheoesophageal fistula (Table 8–2). The risk factors thus identified are useful for assessing an infant's prognosis and for giving parents realistic expectations. Moreover, these stratification schemes can serve as guidelines for surgical management while also allowing the comparison of outcomes among institutions.

The Waterston prognostic classification (Waterston et

TABLE 8–2 ■ **Risk Stratification Schemes**

*Classification**	*Study, Years*	*No. of Patients*	*Subgroup Stratification*	*Survival (%)*
Waterston	1946–1959	218	A: wt > 5.5 lb	95
			B: wt 4–5.5 lb or wt > 5.5 lb with pneumonia or other anomaly	68
			C: wt < 4 lb or severe pneumonia or significant congenital anomaly	6
Randolph	1982–1988	37	1: physiologically stable	100
			2: physiologically unstable (major cardiac anomaly or severe pulmonary disease)	77
Poenaru	1969–1989	95	I: patients not in Class II	93
			II: life-threatening anomalies or major anomalies with preoperative ventilatory dependence	31
Spitz	1980–1994	393	I: wt > 1500 g	96
			II: wt < 1500 g or major congenital heart disease	60
			III: wt < 1500 g and major congenital heart disease	18

Data from Waterston et al, Lancet 1:819, 1962; Randolph et al, Ann Surg 209:526, 1989; Poenaru et al, Surgery 113:426, 1993; Spitz et al, J Pediatr Surg 29:723, 1994; Spitz, J Pediatr Surg 31:22, 1996.

al, 1962), devised in 1962, is primarily of historical interest. In that era, survival was adversely affected by severe pneumonia, significant associated anomalies, or low birth weight. Fortunately, neonatal care, especially since the 1960s, has greatly improved the outcome of these infants and rendered these criteria less necessary. As a result, a variety of more appropriate classification schemes have been proposed.

Randolph and colleagues (1989) found that the overall cardiopulmonary status of the infant, independent of birth weight or coexisting anomalies, is highly predictive of mortality and can serve to select those patients appropriate for early primary repair. All "physiologically stable" infants, defined as those with the absence of a major cardiac anomaly or severe pulmonary compromise, underwent primary esophageal repair with 100% survival. The remaining one third of infants were deemed "physiologically unstable," requiring initial gastrostomy with delayed primary or staged repair. This group experienced an overall survival of 77%. Their liberalized stratification scheme permitted a greater number of early primary repairs than would have been performed using Waterston's classification.

In the largest and most recent series, 393 infants were grouped on the basis of (1) birth weight greater than or less than 1500 g and (2) the presence or absence of major cardiac anomalies. As shown in Table 8–2, survival was directly related to these two risk factors (Spitz et al, 1994; Spitz, 1996). On the basis of these findings, further improvements in the survival of children with esophageal atresia would depend largely upon additional advances in the treatment of complex congenital heart disease and in the care of very-low-birth-weight infants.

Virtually all infants can undergo early primary esophageal repair with division of the fistula. The surgeon can usually perform the operation within the first 2 days of life to allow complete preoperative evaluation while maintaining aggressive pulmonary care, oropharyngeal and proximal pouch suctioning, and systemic antibiotics. Infants with severe pulmonary compromise who require mechanical ventilation may benefit from gastrostomy and, on rare occasions, emergent thoracotomy with fistula ligation, with esophageal repair delayed until the pulmonary status has sufficiently improved. Once the field is exposed for fistula ligation, however, it may be more prudent to complete the esophageal mobilization and anastomosis.

Patients with severe associated anomalies, profound prematurity, sepsis, or any other significant complicating medical condition may benefit from a period of support, including early gastrostomy to prevent further gastrotracheal reflux, systemic antibiotics, parenteral nutrition, pulmonary toilet, and management of serious coexisting conditions. Staged repair is sometimes necessary in the case of a long gap esophageal atresia (see later).

In deciding how to manage esophageal atresia in the setting of congenital heart disease, Mee and colleagues (1992) divided infants into two groups. For the infants who are not dependent on a patent ductus arteriosus for their pulmonary or systemic circulation, early esophageal repair can proceed. In duct-dependent infants, the infusion of prostaglandin E may allow for early esophageal repair. Infants who do not improve may benefit from initial corrective heart surgery. Division of the fistula and gastrostomy placement can be performed at the time of cardiac surgery when indicated. In these severely compromised infants, definitive esophageal repair should be delayed.

Operative Approach

We now focus on repair of the long gap esophageal atresia, since this operation requires multiple maneuvers for successful primary repair, including those maneuvers used when the esophageal gap is much shorter. A bronchoscopic study is routinely performed at the beginning of the procedure in order to:

- Locate the fistula
- Identify any undiagnosed upper fistulas
- Assess the presence and severity of tracheomalacia
- Position the endotracheal tube, if possible, distal to the fistula yet above the carina

With the chest, abdomen, neck, and upper arm included in the operative field (Fig. 8–2*A*), a posterolateral thoracotomy is made 1 cm below the tip of the scapula on the right side except in the case of a right-sided aortic arch. The incision should stay in the inframammary crease so as not to scar the breast.

The chest is entered via the fourth intercostal space, although the third may be better for a high proximal pouch. If necessary, the surgeon can retract the skin incision inferiorly so that the chest can also be entered at the fifth or sixth intercostal space (Fig. 8–2*A*) to help when the distal esophagus is being mobilized. We prefer a retropleural approach, as this limits any esophageal leak to the retropleural space. The surgeon carefully dissects the pleura away from the chest wall using moist pledgets, from the apex of the chest to several interspaces below the incision and posteriorly to the mediastinum.

The azygos vein is divided and the vagus nerve identified and preserved as it courses along the side of the esophageal pouches. The mediastinal pleura is retracted anteriorly until the trachea is exposed (Fig. 8–2*B*). The distal esophagus is then identified and circumscribed with a traction loop to inhibit the air leak through the fistula if this is impairing ventilatory support.

Dissection of the upper pouch is facilitated if the anesthetist inserts a Bakes dilator and pushes the proximal esophagus toward the operator. The surgeon dissects the upper pouch into the neck, taking care to identify any proximal fistula, which should be suspected if the upper pouch is very high and appears small and decompressed. If the esophageal gap is so large as to preclude approximation of the two segments, circular myotomies can be made in the proximal pouch to increase esophageal length (Fig. 8–2*C*). One to three myotomies can be made, each adding 1 cm of length to the esophagus (Eraklis et al, 1976; Livaditis, 1973). If a very high pouch is not easily accessible through the chest, the pouch can be delivered through a neck incision to facilitate performance of the myotomies (Hoffman and Moazam, 1984).

The fistula is then isolated and divided, and the tracheal side is closed with interrupted 5–0 absorbable suture. The distal esophagus is dissected sufficiently to allow approximation to the upper pouch. Despite the canonical belief that the lower segment should not be mobilized, we find that dissection even through the esophageal hiatus can be done without mishap and may permit an otherwise impossible primary anastomosis.

The proximal pouch is opened, and a single-layer end-to-end anastomosis is fashioned with interrupted 5–0 nonabsorbable sutures on the posterior wall with the knots tied on the outside (Fig. 8–2*C*). The break in the table is released at this point to minimize tension on the anastomosis. A feeding tube is then carefully passed across the anastomosis into the stomach and carefully fixed at the nose before the anterior closure is completed.

If the gap is extreme or if the infant is premature, a gastrostomy tube is placed prior to thoracotomy and a transanastomotic feeding tube is not used. The need for a gastrostomy tube is individualized according to the age and size of the patient as well as the length of the gap and degree of tension in the repair. A chest tube is placed near the repair but is sutured to the posterior chest wall to prevent direct contact with the anastomosis. Using these techniques, we have been able to close 6-cm defects primarily. Under conditions of extreme tension, we may paralyze the infant for a number of days to prevent excessive movement during the early healing phase.

Every attempt should be made to achieve primary repair because esophageal continuity is superior to any substitute yet devised. If primary repair is not possible, even with extreme tension, the distal esophagus is oversewn and sutured to the prevertebral fascia. Delayed primary repair usually can be accomplished after daily upper pouch dilatations for 1 to 2 months. In the unusual case when primary repair remains difficult despite all these techniques, esophageal replacement using colon interposition may be necessary (Hendren and Hendren, 1985). Other substitutes, such as a gastric tube (Anderson and Randolph, 1973) or a free vascularized jejunal interposition (Ring et al, 1982), can also be considered.

Complications

Although there has been dramatic improvement in the survival of infants born with esophageal atresia, a significant number of early or late complications are associated with tracheoesophageal defects and their repair (Table 8–3). Among the more common early postoperative complications is an esophageal anastomotic leak, which can occur in 15% to 20% of patients (Engum et al, 1995; Louhimo and Lindahl, 1983; McKinnon and Kosloske, 1990). Anastomotic leaks, which can result in sepsis and are associated with an increased risk for recurrent fistula and esophageal stenosis, should be suspected when frothy saliva appears in the chest tube.

The diagnosis is confirmed by oral administration of methylene blue, and the size and location of the leak are delineated by barium swallow. Conservative management is appropriate, because the majority of cases constitute small leaks that seal spontaneously with proximal esophageal suctioning, adequate drainage, antibiotics, and parenteral nutrition. Gastrostomy drainage and histamine H_2-blockers can hasten closure of the leak.

Major disruption of the esophageal or tracheal suture line is uncommon but should be suspected when the chest tube drainage is excessive or when a large air leak is present. In the absence of chest tubes, the presence of uncontrolled sepsis or tension pneumothorax suggests the diagnosis. In these situations, operative intervention is mandatory to prevent or control progression of mediastinitis or empyema. Primary suture repair is feasible if the dehiscence is early (<3 days). In rare instances, if the anastomosis cannot be repaired, closure of the distal

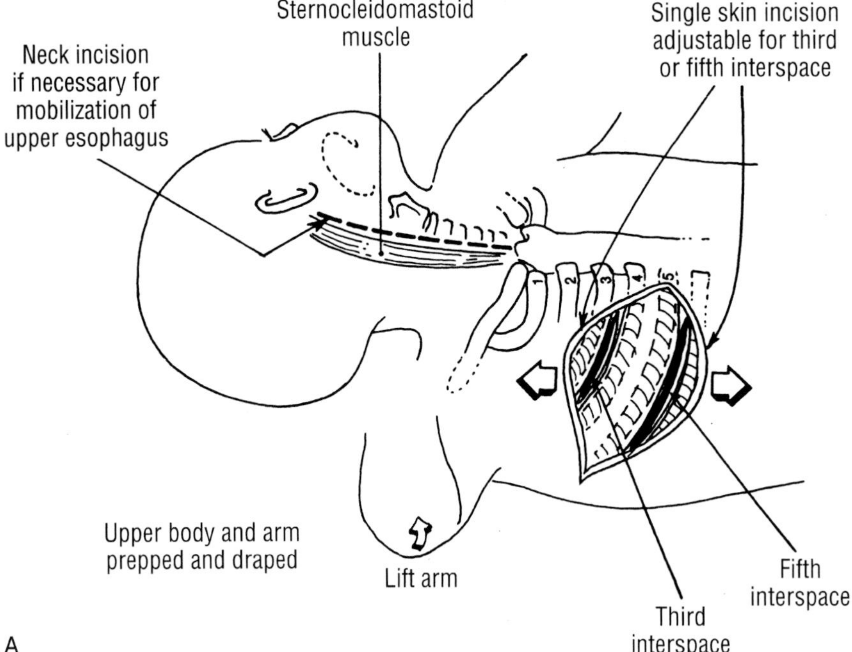

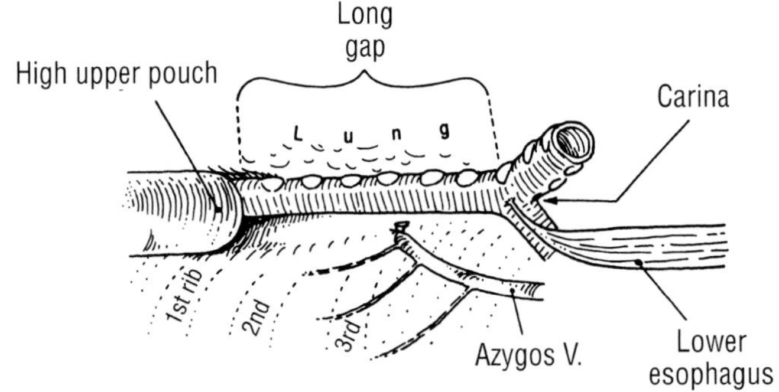

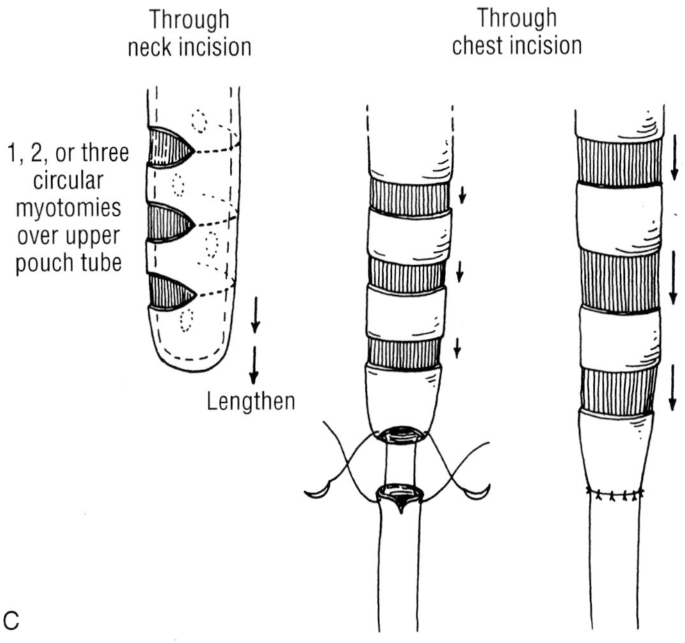

FIGURE 8–2 ■ Surgical repair of a long gap esophageal atresia. *A,* A right posterolateral thoracotomy incision is shown. Most esophageal atresias are repaired through the fourth intercostal space. In a long gap atresia, the proximal pouch may be very high, necessitating use of the third interspace, as shown. The surgeon can retract the same skin incision inferiorly to enter the fifth or sixth interspace in order to dissect the distal segment. Exposure of the trachea and both esophageal segments *(B)* allows assessment of the gap length. Circular myotomies *(C)* can be made in the proximal pouch to increase esophageal length. Myotomies extend through the muscular layers without injuring the submucosa, where the blood supply runs. Gentle traction on the esophagus further increases the length obtained. The distal esophagus can be mobilized down through the hiatus in the diaphragm if necessary. The surgeon performs a single one-layer anastomosis using 4–0 nonabsorbable suture, accepting tension to avoid having to resort to interposition grafts.

TABLE 8–3 ■ **Complications Associated with Esophageal Atresia and Its Repair**

Complication	*Incidence (%)**
Anastomotic leak	15–20
Recurrent fistula	3–10
Anastomotic stricture	10–35
Gastroesophageal reflux	55–82
Tracheomalacia	10–20

*See text for references.

esophagus with proximal cervical esophagostomy should be performed, with definitive repair delayed for several months.

Recurrent tracheoesophageal fistula occurs in 3% to 10% of infants (Ein et al, 1983; Engum et al, 1995; Louhimo and Lindahl, 1983; McKinnon and Kosloske, 1990) and usually presents a few months after repair. Typical symptoms include cyanosis, wheezing, coughing or choking during feeding, and recurrent pneumonias. This spectrum of symptoms is also seen with a variety of other complications, including a missed proximal fistula, anastomotic stricture, tracheomalacia, pharyngoesophageal dyskinesia, and gastroesophageal reflux. Barium swallow should therefore be performed in all children with these symptoms.

As with congenital fistulas, recurrent or missed fistulas can be difficult to diagnose and are potentially serious and life-threatening. Contrast studies with the patient in the prone position often confirm the definitive diagnosis. Bronchoscopy, if necessary, must be done with great care to avoid further disruption of the anastomosis. Operative intervention should follow, since spontaneous closure of these fistulas is unusual. Patients are explored via the neck for high fistulas (T1-T3, by far the most common) or via the chest for lower fistulas, which are extremely rare. Closure of both ends of the fistula must be accompanied by interposition of tissue flaps to prevent a second recurrence.

The most reliable tissue interposition for fistulas that can be reached from the neck is the distal-based medial head of the sternocleidomastoid muscle (Ryan et al, 1991). Other tissue flaps, such as pleural (Donahoe and Gee, 1984), pericardial (Wheatley and Coran, 1992), and intercostal muscle flaps (Soriano et al, 1987), have been used but are less reliable. We have unfurled the parietal pleura if the retropleural approach can be employed (Ryan et al, 1991).

Esophageal anastomotic stricture, which has been reported in up to 35% of patients (Engum et al, 1995), results from an anastomotic leak, gastroesophageal reflux, or primary repair performed under excessive tension, the latter being accepted in the interest of achieving a primary anastomosis. Many surgeons believe that most strictures are a result of persistent gastroesophageal reflux. The symptoms of esophageal stricture include dysphagia, aspiration, and, in later childhood, food impaction, all of which can also be secondary to abnormal motility without an associated stenosis.

Once a stenosis is identified by barium study, balloon dilatations can safely and effectively treat the problem (Hoffer et al, 1987). Concomitant severe gastroesophageal reflux is often revealed after the stricture is dilated and must be suspected in the setting of recurrent or refractory strictures. Antireflux surgery is required in such cases. Esophageal resection is rarely necessary for treatment of a refractory stricture.

Gastroesophageal reflux is a common late complication after esophageal atresia repair. The patient presents with heartburn, dysphagia, vomiting, chronic coughing, and recurrent respiratory infections. Esophageal manometry and pH monitoring demonstrate the presence of reflux in 55% to 82% of patients, even decades after their operation (Jolley et al, 1980; Orringer et al, 1977; Parker et al, 1979; Tovar et al, 1995). These esophageal function tests show disorganized peristalsis throughout the length of the esophagus, often associated with decreased lower esophageal sphincter (LES) tone (Orringer et al, 1977; Tovar et al, 1995). The presence of reflux in the setting of weak and uncoordinated peristalsis leaves these individuals unable to clear acid effectively from the distal esophagus and, therefore, at high risk for recurrent aspiration pneumonia.

The etiology of the esophageal dysfunction has been attributed to either a congenital defect in the development of esophageal innervation or excessive dissection of the lower esophageal pouch. However, intraoperative manometry shows motor incoordination of the esophagus even before surgical repair, supporting a congenital origin of the esophageal dysfunction (Romeo et al, 1987) and making it more acceptable to mobilize the lower pouch in order to achieve a primary anastomosis. The presence of reflux in infants with isolated fistulas, in whom no dissection of an esophageal pouch is necessary, further supports an intrinsic defect in esophageal motility (Parker et al, 1979). Whether surgical dissection exacerbates this defect or whether traction on the distal pouch alters LES function remains unknown. However, more aggressive dissection of the lower esophageal pouch to correct long gap esophageal atresia has not appeared to worsen the outcome of these infants.

The diagnosis of gastroesophageal reflux is confirmed by contrast study, with careful attention to other potential causes of the patient's symptoms. Medical treatment, consisting of acid reduction, thickened feeds, and positional measures, is indicated in patients with symptomatic reflux. Unfortunately, 15% to 45% of these patients do not respond to medical therapy and ultimately require an antireflux procedure because of refractory symptoms, repeated pneumonia or pneumonitis, or recurrent esophageal anastomotic strictures (Ashcraft et al, 1977; Engum et al, 1995; Jolley et al, 1980; Parker et al, 1979; Wheatley et al, 1993). Traditionally, the Nissen fundoplication has been used as the procedure of choice; however, several groups have noted an unacceptably high incidence of severe dysphagia and recurrent reflux following this operation in patients who have undergone prior repair of esophageal atresia (Lindahl et al, 1989; Wheatley et al, 1993), with a mean failure rate of 30% (Snyder et al, 1997). This high rate may result from esophageal motility that is too weak and disorganized to overcome the high resistance associated with a 360-degree wrap. Therefore, a loose wrap or a partial (Thal) fundoplication may be more appropriate in these patients (Ashcraft et al, 1977; Snyder et al, 1997).

Tracheomalacia describes a weakness of the trachea that permits easy apposition of the anterior and posterior walls during coughing or expiration. The condition appears in 15% of patients within days to months following esophageal atresia repair (Engum et al, 1995). Tracheomalacia is a consequence of abnormal foregut development, giving rise to a trachea with diminished structural integrity due to abnormal cartilaginous rings and a redundant posterior membranous wall (Wailoo and Emery, 1979). Moreover, this flaccid trachea is easily compressed between the aorta anteriorly and the dilated upper esophageal pouch posteriorly (Davies and Cywes, 1978). Symptoms may vary from mild expiratory stridor and a typical barking cough to recurrent pneumonias. Dying spells, characterized by cyanosis, apnea, and bradycardia, are the most serious problem and typically occur within minutes of a feeding. Because the symptoms may mimic those of gastroesophageal reflux, recurrent fistula, or anastomotic leak, bronchoscopy under light anesthesia, demonstrating collapse of the lumen during spontaneous breathing, is essential for making the diagnosis. A lateral chest radiograph showing tracheal collapse during expiration is suggestive. Simultaneous esophageal contrast studies also serve to exclude strictures, recurrent fistula formation, or leak as the etiologic mechanism.

Roughly 50% of patients with tracheomalacia require surgery, most commonly for dying spells, inability to extubate, or recurrent pneumonias. Milder symptoms usually improve significantly without surgery after about 1 year of life. The procedure of choice is aortopexy, performed through a left thoracotomy, with suturing of the aortic arch to the posterior surface of the sternum, thereby opening the tracheal lumen (Filler et al, 1992; Schwartz and Filler, 1980). In the rare instance when aortopexy cannot resolve the tracheal collapse, splinting of the airway is warranted (Vinograd et al, 1987). The use of bronchoscopically placed airway stents has been reported in children and may offer an alternative approach (Bousamra et al, 1996).

LARYNGOTRACHEOESOPHAGEAL CLEFT

The laryngotracheoesophageal cleft is a rare midline congenital anomaly characterized by an extensive opening between the posterior surface of the larynx and membranous trachea and the anterior surface of the esophagus. The embryologic basis of this anomaly is unknown, although 20% to 50% of cases occur in association with esophageal atresia and tracheoesophageal fistula (Donahoe and Hendren, 1972; DuBois et al, 1990; Wolfson et al, 1984), suggesting a common developmental origin. The anomaly may be recapitulated by the Adriamycin rat model (Merei et al, 1997a). A genetic basis is further supported by the description of a spontaneous mutation in the mouse that results in this disorder (Essien and Maderious, 1981). Unfortunately, the defective gene remains unknown. Children with a cleft should be evaluated thoroughly for cardiovascular, gastrointestinal, and genitourinary anomalies, which accompany this defect and are often severe (DuBois et al, 1990).

The clefts are classified into four subtypes according to length of the defect and degree of difficulty of repair and management (Pettersson, 1969; Ryan et al, 1991; Simpson et al, 1996):

Type I clefts are limited to the larynx and may extend to the cricoid cartilage.
Type II clefts extend through the cricoid to the cervical trachea.
Type III clefts extend to the carina.
Type IV clefts involve one or both mainstem bronchi.

Symptoms, the severity of which varies with the extent of the cleft, are similar to those encountered in patients with tracheoesophageal fistula. The diagnosis is suspected in infants having immediate and severe symptoms, including choking, respiratory distress, and cyanosis with feeding. Aspiration pneumonia, caused by an incompetent laryngeal mechanism, occurs frequently and may be severe. These infants also have a characteristic toneless cry, a result of the inability of the abnormal larynx to appose the vocal cords sufficiently to generate sound. Delayed diagnosis, which occurs all too often in this syndrome and is attributed to its rarity and subtle differences from the classic tracheoesophageal fistula, often leads to progressive and potentially irreversible respiratory compromise.

Contrast esophagography may suggest the diagnosis if rapid filling of the tracheobronchial tree is seen following a small dose (1 ml) of oral barium (Donahoe and Gee, 1984). If the bronchoscope falls posteriorly from the larynx into the upper esophagus during endoscopy, the diagnosis is confirmed (Donahoe and Gee, 1984; Simpson et al, 1996). The precise extent of the cleft, as well as accurate measurements of the airway and the extent of tracheal malformation, can be assessed at the first bronchoscopy.

At this time, the surgeon should design a customized bifurcated endotracheal tube or a short-neck, right-angle tracheostomy tube to be used during and after the repair (Simpson et al, 1996). As with infants with esophageal atresia and an associated fistula, these children should be nursed in an upright position to minimize reflux; to avert aspiration, they require continuous oropharyngeal sump suctioning.

At the time of diagnostic bronchoscopy, if the lesion is type IV and the stomach is small, we recommend transecting the stomach, with gastrostomy tubes placed proximally and distally to prevent further aspiration of gastric contents and to allow for enteral nutrition (Ryan et al, 1991; Simpson et al, 1996). This drastic step is required because, in our experience, microgastria does not improve with growth of the child, making severe reflux a constant and mortal threat to these children.

Operative Approach

Various techniques are described for repairing the cleft, depending on its distal extent.

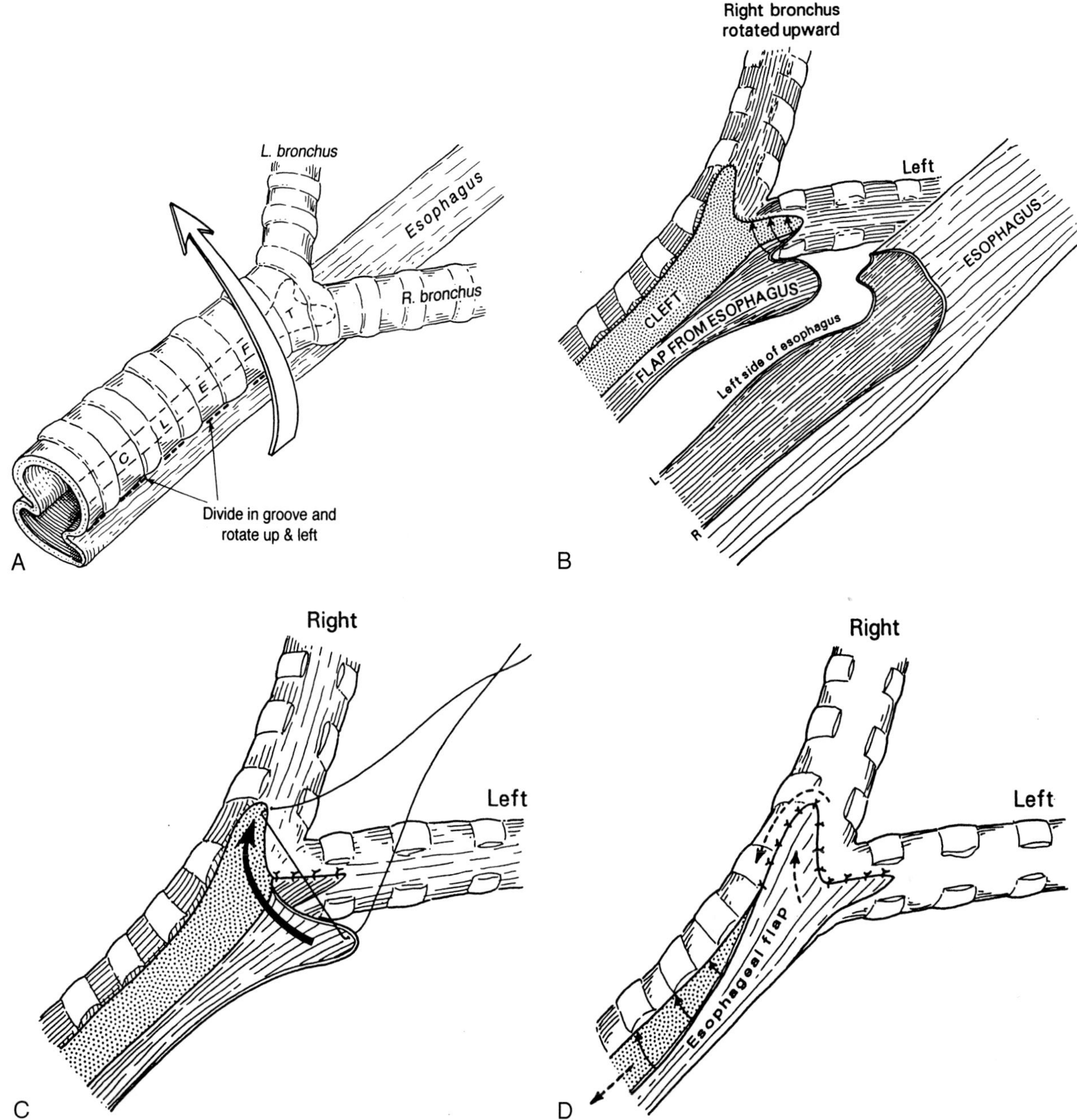

FIGURE 8–3 ■ Surgical repair of a type IV laryngotracheoesophageal cleft. The surgeon begins a type IV cleft repair *(A)*, most often done through the neck, by incising the right tracheoesophageal groove and rotating the trachea to the left. The surgeon incises the left side of the esophagus *(B)*, leaving a U-flap of esophageal wall, which is rotated to the right to close the bronchial and tracheal defects *(C)*. The membranous trachea and the narrowed esophagus are closed in a caudocranial direction, each in a single layer with the suture lines displaced to avoid fistula formation *(D)*.

Type I and II Clefts

Type I defects may be repaired endoscopically (DuBois et al, 1990), whereas *type II* defects call for posterior or lateral pharyngotomy. Although some espouse an anterior approach with division of the larynx and trachea in the midline, we avoid this approach because it requires another division of the cricoid, which is essential for stability of the upper airway.

Type III and IV Clefts

Surgery for patients with complete laryngotracheoesophageal clefts (types III and IV) is challenging and necessitates careful planning to protect a precarious airway. At the beginning of the operation, the airway may need to be secured by a custom-fitted bifurcated endotracheal tube positioned bronchoscopically from above and suspended anteriorly with a No. 3 ureteral catheter loop placed through the tracheostomy site (Ryan et al, 1991). A combined approach via a right posterolateral thoracotomy through the fourth intercostal space and a right cervical incision may be required. However, infants with the most severe type IV (and occasionally type III) clefts have a foreshortened trachea, allowing adequate exposure of the full extent of the cleft through the cervical incision

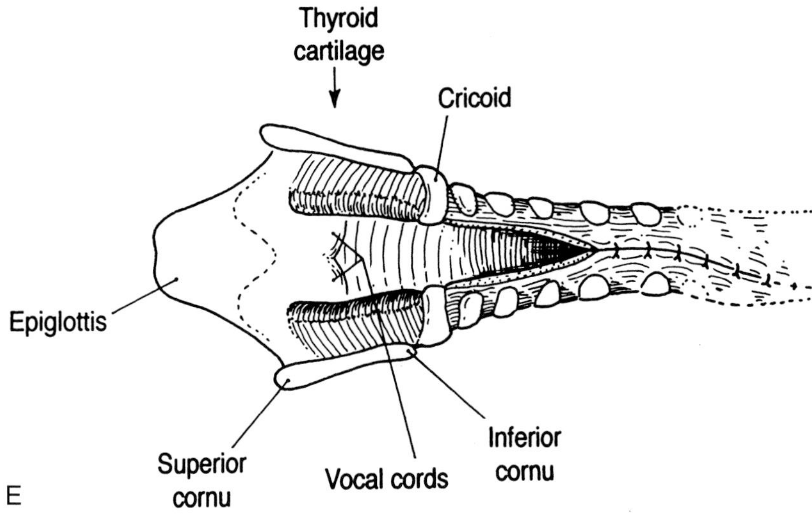

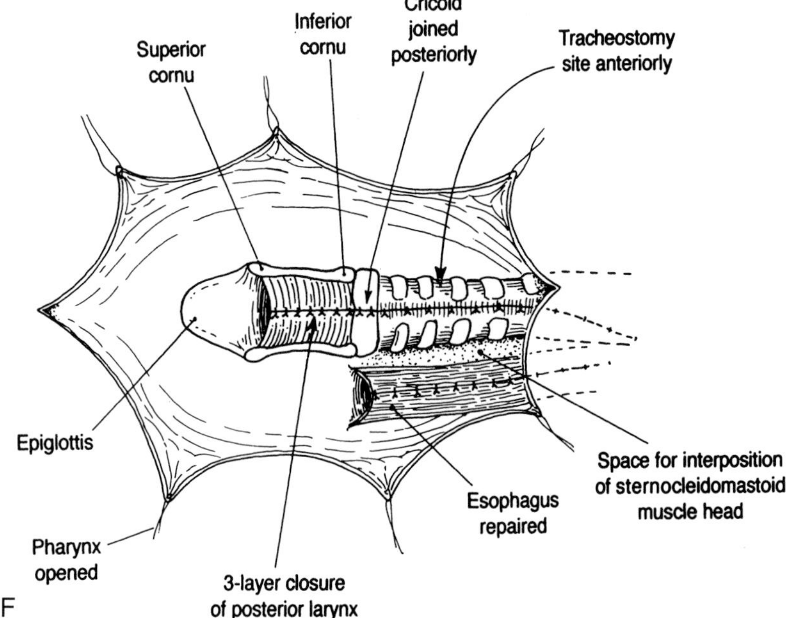

FIGURE 8–3 *Continued* ■ With the larynx rotated anteriorly and to the left, the laryngeal cleft *(E)* is repaired *(F)* in three layers. The medial head of the sternocleidomastoid muscle is interposed between the repairs and behind the tracheostomy site.

alone (Simpson et al, 1996). A partial upper sternotomy can be added if necessary.

The incision is made anterior to the right sternocleidomastoid muscle, and the pharynx, trachea, and esophagus are exposed. The surgeon then incises the right tracheoesophageal groove from the thoracic inlet to the carina, taking care to expose and protect the recurrent laryngeal nerve (Fig. 8–3*A*). From inside the cleft, the surgeon incises the left side of the esophagus approximately 5 to 7 mm below the tracheoesophageal groove (Fig. 8–3*B*), pushing aside the left periesophageal tissue to avoid injury to the left recurrent laryngeal nerve. The esophageal flap is rotated to the right (Fig. 8–3*C*) to create the neomembranous trachea. The surgeon closes the esophagus and trachea longitudinally, starting at the most distal extent of the defect (Fig. 8–3*D*) and continuing to the larynx.

The surgeon exposes the laryngeal defect by entering the pharynx laterally and continues the repair cephalad (Fig. 8–3*E*). The larynx is commonly more generous than expected. The edges of the membranous posterior defect of the larynx and upper trachea are freshened and then closed in two or three layers (Fig. 8–3*F*) from the third tracheal ring to the top of the larynx in interrupted fashion. This step accurately reconstructs the cricoid and larynx. To deter fistula formation, the head of the right sternocleidomastoid muscle is divided cephalad and rotated on its distal base for placement behind the tracheostomy site and between the two suture lines beneath the pharynx.

Complications

The postoperative course, particularly of infants with type IV clefts, is often complicated by severe tracheomalacia caused by malformed tracheal rings, redundant membranous mucosa, or prolonged endotracheal tube pressure in children receiving ventilation. The child with tracheomalacia requires prolonged mechanical ventilation to prevent the intermittent collapse of the trachea that occurs in the absence of positive pressure. We have been successful in discharging infants home with bifurcated tracheostomy tubes in place to prevent collapse of these "floppy" airways (Simpson et al, 1996).

Anastomotic leaks, recurrent tracheoesophageal fistulas, oropharyngeal dysfunction, and gastroesophageal reflux are all common postoperative complications. The long-term outlook for survivors of the type IV clefts remains unknown and depends largely on early diagnosis and correction of the defect, meticulous perioperative management of the infant, and continued growth and stabilization of the airway. The outlook for infants with type III defects without microgastria should be good and continues to improve as more experience is garnered.

Microgastria invariably accompanies type IV clefts. The divided or diverted stomach, contrary to early expectations, does not grow. Bypass with a long Roux-en-Y loop with or without an intussuscepting nipple or a Laurence pouch may be needed. Newer techniques of tissue engineering, it is hoped, may be used to enlarge the stomach or to stabilize or reconstruct the abnormal tracheal cartilages in order to reduce the prolonged morbidity imposed by severe tracheomalacia.

■ *REFERENCES*

Anderson KD, Randolph JG: The gastric tube for esophageal replacement in children. J Thorac Cardiovasc Surg 66:333–342, 1973.

Ashcraft KW, Goodwin C, Amoury RA, Holder TM: Early recognition and aggressive treatment of gastroesophageal reflux following repair of esophageal atresia. J Pediatr Surg 12:317–321, 1977.

Beasley S, Myers N: Trends in mortality in oesophageal atresia. Pediatr Surg Int 7:86–89, 1992.

Beasley S, Phelan E, Kelly J, et al: Urinary tract abnormalities in association with oesophageal atresia: Frequency, significance, and influence on management. Pediatr Surg Int 7:94–96, 1992.

Bousamra M 2nd, Tweddell JS, Wells RG, et al: Wire stent for tracheomalacia in a five-year-old girl. Ann Thorac Surg 61:1239–1240, 1996.

Davies MR, Cywes S: The flaccid trachea and tracheoesophageal congenital anomalies. J Pediatr Surg 13:363–367, 1978.

Diez-Pardo JA, Baoquan Q, Navarro C, Tovar JA: A new rodent experimental model of esophageal atresia and tracheoesophageal fistula: Preliminary report. J Pediatr Surg 31:498–502, 1996.

Donahoe PK, Gee PE: Complete laryngotracheoesophageal cleft: Management and repair. J Pediatr Surg 19:143–148, 1984.

Donahoe PK, Hendren WH: The surgical management of laryngotracheoesophageal cleft with tracheoesophageal fistula and esophageal atresia. Surgery 71:363–368, 1972.

DuBois JJ, Pokorny WJ, Harberg FJ, Smith RJ: Current management of laryngeal and laryngotracheoesophageal clefts. J Pediatr Surg 25:855–860, 1990.

Ein SH, Stringer DA, Stephens CA, et al: Recurrent tracheoesophageal fistulas—seventeen-year review. J Pediatr Surg 18:436–441, 1983.

Engum SA, Grosfeld JL, West KW, et al: Analysis of morbidity and mortality in 227 cases of esophageal atresia and/or tracheoesophageal fistula over two decades. Arch Surg 130:502–508, 1995; discussion, 508–509.

Eraklis AJ, Rossello PJ, Ballantine TV: Circular esophagomyotomy of upper pouch in primary repair of long-segment esophageal atresia. J Pediatr Surg 11:709–712, 1976.

Essien F, Maderious A: A genetic factor controlling morphogenesis of the laryngotracheoesophageal complex in the mouse. Teratology 24:235–239, 1981.

Faro RS, Goodwin CD, Organ CH Jr, et al: Tracheal agenesis. Ann Thorac Surg 28:295–299, 1979.

Filler RM, Messineo A, Vinograd I: Severe tracheomalacia associated with esophageal atresia: Results of surgical treatment. J Pediatr Surg 27:1136–1140, 1992; discussion, 1140–1141.

Gibson T: The Anatomy of Humane Bodies Epitomized. London, Awnsham & Churchill, 1697.

Gross R: Atresia of the esophagus. In Gross R (ed): The Surgery of Infancy and Childhood. Philadelphia, WB Saunders, 1953, p 75.

Haight C, Towsley H: Congenital atresia of the esophagus with tracheoesophageal fistula: Extrapleural ligation of fistula and end-to-end anastomosis of esophageal segments. Surg Gynecol Obstet 76:672–688, 1943.

Harris J, Kallen B, Robert E: Descriptive epidemiology of alimentary tract atresia. Teratology 52:15–29, 1995.

Hendren WH, Hendren WG: Colon interposition for esophagus in children. J Pediatr Surg 20:829–839, 1985.

Hoffer FA, Winter HS, Fellows KE, Folkman J: The treatment of postoperative and peptic esophageal strictures after esophageal atresia repair: A program including dilatation with balloon catheters. Pediatr Radiol 17:454–458, 1987.

Hoffman DG, Moazam F: Transcervical myotomy for wide-gap esophageal atresia. J Pediatr Surg 19:680–682, 1984.

Hokama A, Myers N, Kent M, et al: Esophageal atresia with tracheoesophageal fistula: A histopathological study. Pediatr Surg Int 1:117–121, 1986.

Holder T, Cloud D, Lewis E, Pilling G: Esophageal atresia and tracheoesophageal fistula: A survey of its members by the surgical section of the American Academy of Pediatrics. Pediatrics 34:542–549, 1964.

Iuchtman M, Brereton R, Spitz L, et al: Morbidity and mortality in 46 patients with the VACTERL association. Isr J Med Sci 28:281–284, 1992.

Jolley SG, Johnson DG, Roberts CC, et al: Patterns of gastroesophageal reflux in children following repair of esophageal atresia and distal tracheoesophageal fistula. J Pediatr Surg 15:857–862, 1980.

Kluth D, Steding G, Seidl W: The embryology of foregut malformations. J Pediatr Surg 22:389–393, 1987.

Kutiyanawala M, Wyse RK, Brereton RJ, et al: CHARGE and esophageal atresia. J Pediatr Surg 27:558–560, 1992.

Ladd W: The surgical treatment of esophageal atresia and tracheoesophageal fistulas. N Engl J Med 230:625–637, 1944.

Leven N: Congenital atresia of the esophagus with tracheoesophageal fistula: Report of successful extrapleural ligation of fistulous communication and cervical esophagostomy. J Thorac Surg 10:648–657, 1941.

Lindahl H, Rintala R, Louhimo I: Failure of the Nissen fundoplication to control gastroesophageal reflux in esophageal atresia patients. J Pediatr Surg 24:985–987, 1989.

Litingtung Y, Lei L, Westphal H, Chiang C: Sonic hedgehog is essential to foregut development [see comments]. Nat Genet 20:58–61, 1998.

Livaditis A: A method of overbridging large segmental gaps. Z Kinderchir 13:298, 1973.

Louhimo I, Lindahl H: Esophageal atresia: Primary results of 500 consecutively treated patients. J Pediatr Surg 18:217–229, 1983.

McKinnon LJ, Kosloske AM: Prediction and prevention of anastomotic complications of esophageal atresia and tracheoesophageal fistula. J Pediatr Surg 25:778–781, 1990.

Mee R, Beasley S, Auldist A, Myers N: Influence of congenital heart disease on management of oesophageal atresia. Pediatr Surg Int 7:90–93, 1992.

Merei J, Kotsios C, Hutson JM, Hasthorpe S: Histopathologic study of esophageal atresia and tracheoesophageal fistula in an animal model. J Pediatr Surg 32:12–14, 1997a.

Merei JM, Farmer P, Hasthorpe S, et al: Timing and embryology of esophageal atresia and tracheo-esophageal fistula. Anat Rec 249:240–248, 1997b.

Motoyama J, Liu J, Mo R, et al: Essential function of Gli2 and Gli3 in the formation of lung, trachea and oesophagus [see comments]. Nat Genet 20:54–57, 1998.

O'Rahilly R, Muller F: Chevalier Jackson lecture. Respiratory and alimentary relations in staged human embryos: New embryological data and congenital anomalies. Ann Otol Rhinol Laryngol 93(5 Pt 1):421–429, 1984.

Orringer MB, Kirsh MM, Sloan H: Long-term esophageal function following repair of esophageal atresia. Ann Surg 186:436–443, 1977.

Parker AF, Christie DL, Cahill JL: Incidence and significance of gastroesophageal reflux following repair of esophageal atresia and tracheoesophageal fistula and the need for anti-reflux procedures. J Pediatr Surg 14:5–8, 1979.

Pettersson G: Laryngotracheoesophageal cleft. Z Kinderchir 7:43–49, 1969.

Pletcher BA, Friedes JS, Breg WR, Touloukian RJ: Familial occurrence of esophageal atresia with and without tracheoesophageal fistula: Report of two unusual kindreds. Am J Med Genet 39:380–384, 1991.

Poenaru D, Laberge JM, Neilson IR, Guttman FM: A new prognostic classification for esophageal atresia. Surgery 113:426–432, 1993.

Qi BQ, Merei J, Farmer P, et al: Tracheomalacia with esophageal atresia and tracheoesophageal fistula in fetal rats. J Pediatr Surg 32:1575–1579, 1997.

Quan L, Smith DW: The VATER association: *V*ertebral defects, *A*nal atresia, *T-E* fistula with esophageal atresia, *R*adial and renal dysplasia: A spectrum of associated defects. J Pediatr 82:104–107, 1973.

Randolph JG, Newman KD, Anderson KD: Current results in repair of esophageal atresia with tracheoesophageal fistula using physiologic status as a guide to therapy. Ann Surg 209:526–530, 1989; discussion, 530–531.

Ring WS, Varco RL, L'Heureux PR, Foker JE: Esophageal replacement with jejunum in children: An 18- to 33-year follow-up. J Thorac Cardiovasc Surg 83:918–927, 1982.

Romeo G, Zuccarello B, Proietto F, Romeo C: Disorders of the esophageal motor activity in atresia of the esophagus. J Pediatr Surg 22:120–124, 1987.

Ryan DP, Muehrcke DD, Doody DP, et al: Laryngotracheoesophageal cleft (type IV): Management and repair of lesions beyond the carina. J Pediatr Surg 26:962–969, 1991; discussion, 969–970.

Schwartz MZ, Filler RM: Tracheal compression as a cause of apnea following repair of tracheoesophageal fistula: Treatment by aortopexy. J Pediatr Surg 15:842–848, 1980.

Simpson BB, Ryan DP, Donahoe PK, et al: Type IV laryngotracheoesophageal clefts: Surgical management for long-term survival. J Pediatr Surg 31:1128–1133, 1996.

Skandalakis J, Gray S, Ricketts R: The esophagus. In Skandalakis J, Gray S (eds): Embryology for Surgeons. Baltimore, Williams & Wilkins, 1994, pp 65–112.

Snyder CL, Ramachandran V, Kennedy AP, et al: Efficacy of partial wrap fundoplication for gastroesophageal reflux after repair of esophageal atresia. J Pediatr Surg 32:1089–1091, 1997; discussion, 1092.

Soriano A, Hernandez-Siverio N, Carrillo A, et al: Intercostal pedicled flap in esophageal atresia. J Pediatr Surg 22:115–116, 1987.

Spitz L: Esophageal atresia: Past, present, and future. J Pediatr Surg 31:19–25, 1996.

Spitz L, Kiely EM, Morecroft JA, Drake DP: Oesophageal atresia: At-risk groups for the 1990s. J Pediatr Surg 29:723–725, 1994.

Stringer MD, McKenna KM, Goldstein RB, et al: Prenatal diagnosis of esophageal atresia. J Pediatr Surg 30:1258–1263, 1995.

Sutliff KS, Hutchins GM: Septation of the respiratory and digestive tracts in human embryos: Crucial role of the tracheoesophageal sulcus. Anat Rec 238:237–247, 1994.

Templeton JM Jr, Templeton JJ, Schnaufer L, et al: Management of esophageal atresia and tracheoesophageal fistula in the neonate with severe respiratory distress syndrome. J Pediatr Surg 20:394–397, 1985.

Tovar JA, Diez Pardo JA, Murcia J, et al: Ambulatory 24-hour manometric and pH metric evidence of permanent impairment of clearance capacity in patients with esophageal atresia. J Pediatr Surg 30:1224–1231, 1995.

Vinograd I, Filler RM, Bahoric A: Long-term functional results of prosthetic airway splinting in tracheomalacia and bronchomalacia. J Pediatr Surg 22:38–41, 1987.

Wailoo MP, Emery JL: The trachea in children with tracheo-oesophageal fistula. Histopathology 3:329–338, 1979.

Waterston D, Bonham Carter R, Aberdeen E: Oesophageal atresia: Tracheo-oesophageal fistula: A study of survival in 218 infants. Lancet 1:819–822, 1962.

Wheatley MJ, Coran AG: Pericardial flap interposition for the definitive management of recurrent tracheoesophageal fistula. J Pediatr Surg 27:1122–1115, 1992; discussion, 1125–1126.

Wheatley MJ, Coran AG, Wesley JR: Efficacy of the Nissen fundoplication in the management of gastroesophageal reflux following esophageal atresia repair. J Pediatr Surg 28:53–55, 1993.

Wolfson PJ, Schloss MD, Guttman FM, Nguyen L: Laryngotracheoesophageal cleft: An easily missed malformation. Arch Surg 119:228–230, 1984.

OTHER CONGENITAL DISORDERS IN CHILDREN

Dorry L. Segev
Patricia K. Donahoe
Daniel P. Doody

Esophageal Cysts and Duplications

HISTORICAL NOTE

An esophageal cyst, or *duplication*, was first recognized by Blasius in 1674 (Blasius, 1674). More than a century later, Roth (1881) described a mediastinal cyst adherent to the vertebral column, now known as a neurenteric cyst. A cyst within the spinal canal itself was first reported in 1928 (Kubie and Fulton, 1928). Only one year later, a cyst was successfully removed in a two-stage procedure because of its large size (Mixter and Clifford, 1929). In 1931, the first one-stage resection of an esophageal cyst was performed (Sauerbruch and Fick, 1931).

■ *HISTORICAL READINGS*

Blasius G: Observata anatomica in homine, simia, equo. Amstelodam, Gaasbeeck, 1674.
Kubie LS, Fulton JF: A clinical and pathological study of two teratomatous cysts of the spinal cord, containing mucous and ciliated cells. Surg Gynecol Obstet 47:297, 1928.
Mixter CG, Clifford SH: Congenital mediastinal cysts of gastrogenic and bronchogenic origin. Ann Surg 90:714, 1929.
Roth M: Ueber Missbildungen im Bereich des Ductus omphalomesentericus. Arch Pathol Anat 86:25, 1881.
Sauerbruch F, Fick W: Operative Beseitigung einer kongenitalen Cyste der Speiserohre. Zentralbl Chir 58:2938, 1931.

DEFINITION

Enteric cysts above the diaphragm account for 18% of all intestinal cysts (Grosfeld et al, 1970). Only 12% of patients from a large series of mediastinal masses were reported to have esophageal cysts (Haller et al, 1969). However, it has been estimated that in children at least 30% of mediastinal masses are of foregut origin and eventually develop into (1) esophageal, (2) neurenteric, (3) bronchogenic, or (4) isolated cysts (O'Neill et al, 1979). Of interest, esophageal cysts have been described in association with esophageal atresia (Hemalatha et al, 1987). Although these cysts are commonly considered benign, neoplastic degeneration has been reported (Lee et al, 1998; Orr and Edwards, 1975).

Because of their appearance, Ladd and Scott (1944) proposed that all cysts located near the esophagus be known as *esophageal duplication*. Unfortunately, this term does not allow for explanation of embryologic or pathologic findings. Since 1944, various characteristics of these cysts have been considered in designing an appropriate classification scheme.

Esophageal cysts have been described in all locations along the esophagus (Cohen et al, 1982; Plachta, 1962), including those that originate below the diaphragm and ascend from the abdomen (Ruffin and Hansen, 1989). They are less common in the cervical region (Borcar and Hughes, 1988). Esophageal cysts can be intramural or completely separate from the esophagus. Although they infrequently communicate with the esophageal lumen, common openings between the cyst and the esophagus are reported (Pokorny and Goldstein, 1984), and in rare instances complete esophageal duplications with entrance *and* exit openings have been described (Blasius, 1674; Butler and Ende, 1950). Thoracic cysts originating from the primitive foregut can communicate with hollow abdominal viscera, such as the intestine, biliary tree, or even the pancreatic duct (Davis and Barnes, 1952; Fitzgibbons et al, 1980).

Most *duplication cysts* are *solitary*, although *multiple cysts* have been described (Harmand et al, 1981; Robison et al, 1987). In particular, the posterior esophageal cysts may be multiple (Superina et al, 1984). Thick, viscous fluid fills most esophageal cysts, although necrotic debris, inflammatory cells, or old blood can accompany ulceration, infection, or hemorrhage. Aside from the likelihood of finding gastric cells in cysts with hemorrhage and ulceration, the contents of a cyst seem to provide little insight into its embryologic derivation (Bower et al, 1978). Similarly, the variety of mucosa found in an esophageal cyst is less helpful in categorizing the cyst, because the types of epithelial cells that have been reported in these cysts (squamous, columnar, cuboid, pseudostratified, ciliated) are seen at different stages of embryonic esophageal development (Johns, 1952; Johnson, 1910). Two exceptions are the presence of cartilage, which usually suggests a tracheobronchial foregut duplication, and gastric mucosa, which occurs more commonly (although *not* exclusively) in cysts that originate in the abdominal esophagus (Arbona et al, 1984).

Because the nomenclature of esophageal cysts and duplications has been confusing, Fallon and associates (1954) grouped these cysts into categories based on histologic and embryologic features.

Intramural esophageal cysts, also termed *true duplications of the esophagus* or *archenteric cysts*, are found within the esophageal wall. Lined with squamous or columnar epithelium, they are thought to be aberrations in primitive esophageal vacuolation.

Enteric cysts, in contrast, contain epithelia from assorted embryonic tissues and well-developed muscular layers in the cyst wall.

Tracheobronchial foregut duplications are anteriorly located cysts that most likely arise from a portion of the primitive lung bud that has incompletely separated from the primitive foregut. These cysts are typically lined with a ciliated columnar or respiratory epithelium.

Posterior cysts, commonly adjoined to the spinal column, are believed to arise embryologically from anomalous adhesions between the endoderm of the developing foregut and the mesoderm of the notochord or the ectoderm of the primitive neural tube. These cysts have been called a variety of names (enterogenous cysts, esophageal duplications, gastrocystomas, neurenteric cysts), although *dorsal enteric cysts* may be the best terminology to encompass their varied manifestations despite their common embryologic origin. These cysts are usually located in the posterior mediastinum and can be attached to anterior vertebral bodies. They range from simple posterior cysts without vertebral attachments to fistulas from the esophagus to the dorsal thoracic skin through the vertebral column and spinal canal (Kirwan et al, 1973). Dorsal enteric cysts may be associated with intra-abdominal intestinal duplication cysts (Bentley and Smith, 1960), with abnormalities of the vertebral bodies, or with the presence of intraspinal enterogenous cysts.

Neurenteric cysts are the subset of dorsal enteric cysts that attach to the dura through a defect in a vertebra (Holcomb et al, 1989). At least 50% of dorsal enteric cysts are associated with vertebral anomalies such as spina bifida occulta or anterior hemivertebrae (Fallon et al, 1954). These vertebral defects are typically seen in the cervical or upper thoracic spine as the defect occurs as an early embryologic event, adhering to the ascending notochord while the foregut is forming from the endoderm of the two-layered embryonic disk.

BASIC SCIENCE

Kirwan and colleagues (1973) suggested that errors in vacuolation might contribute to the formation of intramural esophageal cysts. During the 4th week of development, the primordial esophageal lumen is filled with mucosa. Vacuoles within the epithelial cells begin to form in the 6th week, and the lumen is gradually re-established as these vacuoles slowly coalesce. If this process is disrupted, epithelial cells similar to those that line intramural cysts are left within the esophageal wall.

Other authors implicate improper budding in the development of certain cysts. Remnants of cells left after ventral tracheobronchial budding from the primitive foregut can cause formation of cysts (Simpson and Campbell, 1991), stenoses of the esophagus, or a combination of stenosis and cystic duplication (Narasimharao and Mitra, 1987; Snyder et al, 1996). Errors in budding can be as remarkable as a bronchus and a lobe of lung parenchyma arising from the esophagus (Gans and Potts, 1951).

The development of dorsal enteric cysts has been linked to the *endoderm-ectoderm adhesion theory* (Fig. 8–4). Adhesions occur at an early embryonic stage between the ectoderm (or mesodermal notochord) and the endoderm as it is forming the primitive foregut. Discordant longitudinal growth of the neural tube and the foregut creates a shear force, which may detach the developing enteric cells (Beardmore and Wiglesworth, 1958; Prop et al, 1967).

The *split-notochord theory* advocates the presence of an abnormal fissure between the endoderm and the ectoderm, allowing the formation of an enterogenous diverticulum in the space created by the notochordal cleft. This diverticulum of endoderm, as the primitive foregut precursor, expands posteriorly to fill this abnormal space (McLetchie et al, 1954). The endodermal intrusion leaves the notochord split, can prevent the formation of the anterior vertebral body, and may affect the neural tube as it becomes the spinal cord.

Whichever theory is correct, the various clinical manifestations include (1) simple intramural esophageal cysts, (2) extraesophageal cysts with or without vertebral anomalies, (3) cysts that extend through vertebral anomalies to the spinal cord, and (4) fistulas between the esophagus and the dorsal thoracic skin (Beardmore and Wiglesworth, 1958; Bentley and Smith, 1960; Fallon et al, 1954; Kirwan et al, 1973). Tracts between posterior esophageal cysts and dorsal skin are commonly obliterated but may be found as persistent fibrous strands.

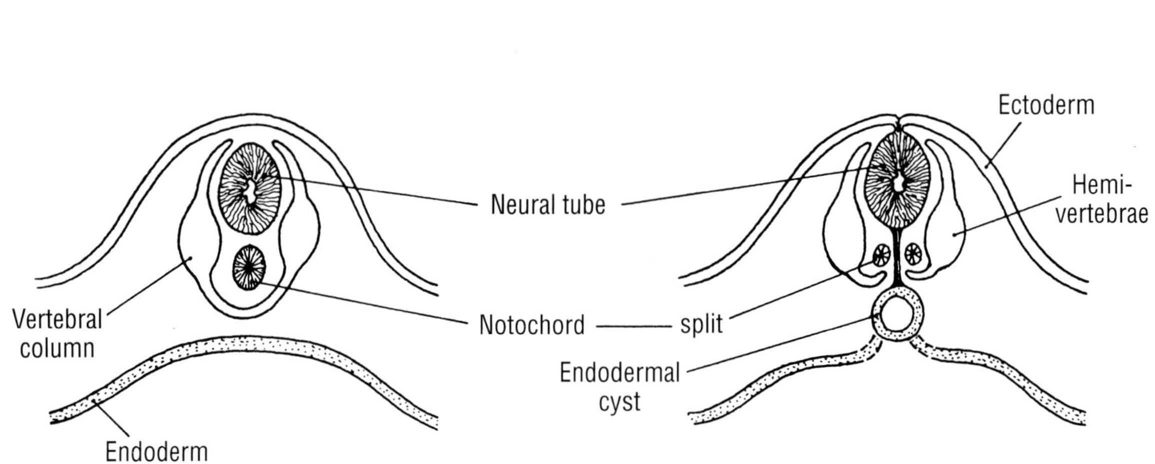

FIGURE 8–4 ■ Development of dorsal enteric cysts.

DIAGNOSIS

Clinical Features

One third or more of patients with esophageal cysts remain asymptomatic throughout childhood, and the cyst is incidentally discovered on chest x-rays taken for other reasons. Most other patients present with a minimal to moderate amount of dysphagia, although complete dysphagia is possible. Very large esophageal cysts have been reported to cause superior vena cava syndrome (Helund and Bisset, 1989) or, in the case of large distal cysts, to present as abdominal masses (Ruffin and Hansen, 1989). More common, however, would be a symptom attributable to gastric epithelium within the cyst, such as esophageal perforation, hemorrhage, or pain from ulceration (Beardmore and Wiglesworth, 1958; Ladd and Scott, 1944).

Additionally, some patients with neurenteric cysts can present with neurologic symptoms. Pain is common, and spinal cord compression with associated weakness and even paralysis can be seen with intraspinal lesions (Holmes et al, 1978; Piramoon and Abbassioun, 1974).

The most dramatic presentations, however, derive from compromised ventilation in young patients. Symptoms can arise from (1) reduction in ventilatory volume alone, (2) mechanical compression of the trachea (Sethi et al, 1974), or (3) extrinsic pressure of the large bronchi causing emphysema (air trapping and atelectasis) or consolidation (complete collapse) (Rogers and Osmer, 1964; Weichert et al, 1970). Respiratory distress is not uncommon in this age group and may be life threatening (Haller et al, 1975). More common but less dramatic forms of respiratory compromise include stridor, persistent cough, or recurrent pneumonia in patients with smaller esophageal cysts (Grosfeld et al, 1970).

Differential Diagnosis

Esophageal cysts are typically located retropleurally in the posterior mediastinum, although bronchogenic cysts, ganglioneuromas, neuroblastomas, neurofibromas, anterior meningoceles, pulmonary sequestrations, and hemangiomas can also be found posteriorly (Pokorny and Goldstein, 1984). In addition, cystic hygromas, substernal goiters, and enlarged lymph nodes can present as mediastinal masses, although these are usually found in the superior mediastinum, an uncommon location for esophageal cysts.

Investigative Techniques

An esophageal cyst should be suspected if a chest film reveals a large mass on one side of the chest. The cyst, typically, is a sharply defined, spherical or tubular mass that commonly displaces the trachea or the esophagus. A propensity for the right hemithorax is presumably a result of changes during intestinal rotation (Beardmore and Wiglesworth, 1958; Pokorny and Goldstein, 1984). Chest radiographs may also occasionally demonstrate vertebral anomalies, such as bifid vertebrae in the lower cervical or upper thoracic spine, suggesting the need for further workup of neurenteric findings, including evaluation of the spinal canal with magnetic resonance imaging (MRI).

A contrast esophagogram may demonstrate a smooth filling defect distorting the lumen or even displacing the esophagus. Filling of cysts with contrast is uncommon because they rarely communicate with the lumen of the esophagus, although large distal cysts have been described in communication with a visceral structure (usually the stomach) below the diaphragm (Grosfeld et al, 1970).

For radiographically obscure lesions, some have advocated transthoracic sonography to confirm the cystic nature of these lesions and to differentiate these lesions from solid tumors of the posterior mediastinum (Fitch et al, 1986), although computed tomographic (CT) imaging has largely superseded ultrasonography to better delineate posterior mediastinal lesions. Other authors also recommend abdominal sonography to rule out associated intestinal duplications (Grosfeld et al, 1970), although plain abdominal films may detect the same. Technetium radionuclide scanning in patients who present with symptoms of ulceration, such as anemia or frank hemorrhage, can reveal gastric mucosa in the cysts.

Esophagoscopy is of little value in differentiating esophageal cysts from other posterior mediastinal lesions because the esophageal mucosa near the cyst is normal. Esophagoscopy may be of value immediately preoperatively to determine whether a cyst-esophageal connection is present. Although bronchoscopy is a typical modality for evaluating airway obstruction, Haller and coauthors (1975) reported precipitation of ventilation problems by airway instrumentation in the setting of a duplication cyst.

CT scanning can clarify obscure masses as well as define their relation to surrounding structures and evaluate for associated vertebral defects (Weiss et al, 1983). When available, however, and especially in the setting of a suspected neurenteric component to the cyst, MRI is the most accurate in detecting vertebral and intraspinal abnormalities and thus is the diagnostic study of choice (Lupetin and Dash, 1987; Rafal and Markisz, 1991). It is important to remember that intraspinal neurenteric cysts can occur, particularly in patients with vertebral anomalies or neurologic abnormalities (Superina et al, 1984).

MANAGEMENT

Operative Technique

With the propensity for infection, hemorrhage, and possible neoplastic change, prudent management of esophageal cysts must eventually include surgical excision. For most patients, since growth is slow and neoplastic change is rare, surgery can be elective. The rare exception is the patient who presents with severe respiratory compromise from rapid expansion of a cyst that may be initially treated with percutaneous aspiration for decompression until the patient is stable enough for planned surgical excision.

When reviewing the radiographic studies and during intraoperative exploration, the surgeon should remember that multiple intramural cysts are not unusual (Robison et al, 1987). A limited posterolateral thoracotomy, based on the rostrad or caudal location of the cyst, provides adequate exposure. It may be necessary to enter a second separate interspace using the same skin incision for longer or multiple cysts. The use of video-assisted thoracoscopy has been described for small cysts (Lewis et al, 1992). For large distal cysts that extend beyond the diaphragm, an additional abdominal incision may be required.

Because it is the gastric mucosa in esophageal cysts that causes most of the associated morbidity, including necrosis, hemorrhage, and ulceration with symptomatic pain and possible perforation, it is essential to remove the cyst mucosa during the surgical excision. Dividing the overlying esophageal musculature and carefully dissecting out the cyst extramucosally can enucleate intramural cysts. If the lumen of the esophagus is not violated surgically, the integrity of the wall and its function should remain intact (Waterston, 1972).

Although they are uncommon, communications between the cyst and the esophageal lumen can be closed with a fine monofilament suture. The muscular wall should be reapproximated in a manner that does not compromise the lumen. In the rare case that the esophageal mucosa is violated or lumen narrowed, a protective gastrostomy has been used during healing and can be helpful if postoperative esophageal dilatations are necessary.

Enteric cysts are usually completely separate from the true esophageal wall and most often are connected by a fibrous band with either a free subpleural cyst or one attached to an anterior vertebral body. These cysts can be easier to resect, although adherence to important structures or a rich blood supply can complicate the repair. Again, if necessary, shelling out the mucosa and repairing the subsequent defect would probably accomplish the same ends as excision, alleviating symptoms and future risks posed by the cyst. If a concomitant intraspinal cyst is found, priority should be given to resection of the spinal component to prevent acute neurologic complications during resection of the intrathoracic component (Superina et al, 1984).

Results

Short-term results are excellent in children as well as adults, with appropriate relief of initial symptoms. Although adequate follow-up in children has not been reported, studies in adults teach us that late reflux, esophagitis, and Barrett's esophagus are more common than previously anticipated (Salo and Ala-Kulju, 1987), thereby stressing the importance of long-term follow-up in all patients after excision of an esophageal cyst.

Congenital Stenosis and Webs

HISTORICAL NOTE

Early reports of esophageal stenosis of a congenital nature described "webs" (thin membranes) treated by dilatation (Clark, 1911; Mosher, 1917). The first large series and review of the literature was in 1928 and consisted of 50 cases (Beatty, 1928). Tracheobronchial remnants were described in case reports as early as 1936 (Frey and Duschl, 1936) and hypertrophic stenosis was best originally described 23 years later (Bonilla and Bowers, 1959). At about that time, Dunbar reported a case of congenital stenosis with tracheoesophageal fistula, an uncommon association (Dunbar, 1958). Although dilatation is the common therapy, resection has been historically described as well (Gross, 1948; Tuttle and Day, 1950).

■ *HISTORICAL READINGS*

Beatty CC: Congenital stenosis of the esophagus. Br J Child Dis 25:237, 1928.

Bonilla KB, Bowers WF: Congenital esophageal stenosis: Pathologic studies following resection. Am J Surg 97:772, 1959.

Clark JP: Congenital web of the esophagus: Report of a case. Laryngoscope 21:810, 1911.

Dunbar JS: Congenital oesophageal stenosis. Pediatr Clin North Am 5:433, 1958.

Frey EK, Duschl L: Der Kardiospasmus. Ergeb Chir Orthop 29:637, 1936.

Gross RE: Treatment of short stricture of the esophagus by partial esophagectomy and end-to-end esophageal reconstruction. Surgery 23:735, 1948.

Mosher HP: Webs and pouches of the oesophagus: Their diagnosis, and treatment. Surg Gynecol Obstet 25:175, 1917.

Tuttle WM, Day JC: The treatment of short esophageal strictures by resection and end-to-end anastomosis. J Thorac Cardiovasc Surg 19:534, 1950.

DEFINITION

Congenital esophageal stenosis has been defined as "intrinsic stenosis of the esophagus, present at birth, which is caused by congenital malformation of the esophageal wall architecture" (Nihoul-Fékété et al, 1987). Although easily confused with inflammatory esophageal strictures, such as those from reflux disease, true congenital stenosis is uncommon. The reported incidence is between 1:25,000 and 1:50,000 births (Nihoul-Fékété et al, 1987; Valerio et al, 1977), with a poorly understood higher incidence in Japan (Nishima et al, 1981). A review in 1995 found only 500 cases described in the world literature (Murphy et al, 1995).

A 17% to 33% reported incidence of associated anomalies includes esophageal or intestinal atresia, midgut malrotation, anorectal malformations, cardiac anomalies, hypospadias, chromosomal abnormalities, and malformations of the head, face, and limbs (Nihoul-Fékété et al, 1987; Nishima et al, 1981).

Amidst a number of confusing classification schemes, Nihoul-Fékété and coworkers (1987) described three mechanisms representing most clearly the morphologic and possibly embryologic spectrum of this disease:

1. *Fibromuscular thickening.* Also referred to as *idiopathic muscular hypertrophy* or *fibromuscular stenosis*, this is a diffuse fibrosis of the wall in the setting of segmental hypertrophy of the muscularis and submucosa. Most hypertrophic segments are found in the distal esophagus, with the remaining few found in the middle third (Todani et al, 1984). These lesions are long and tapering, with considerable variation in the degree of stenosis. Of the

different types of stenosis, this type is most commonly associated with esophageal atresia.

2. *Tracheobronchial remnants,* or rests, are composed of cartilage, respiratory mucous glands, or ciliated epithelium that produces a rigid, discrete stenosis most commonly in the distal third of the esophagus (Frey and Duschl, 1936; Kumar, 1962). Associated inflammation and fibrosis around very small islands of tissue can produce surprisingly marked obstruction. Tracheobronchial remnants can be associated with esophageal atresia and tracheoesophageal fistula (Goldman and Ban, 1972; Nishima et al, 1981; Yeung et al, 1992).

3. A *congenital membranous web* (or *diaphragm*), the rarest type of congenital stenosis, is a thin, diaphragm-like lesion with an eccentric opening that has been reported in all levels of the esophagus (Clark, 1911; Mosher, 1917; Murphy et al, 1995; Todani et al, 1984). The membrane is usually covered on both sides by squamous epithelium. Some have considered these to represent missed variations of esophageal atresia (Kluth, 1976), although webs are not commonly associated with congenital lesions, as are the other types of congenital esophageal stenoses (Nihoul-Fékété et al, 1987).

BASIC SCIENCE

Fibromuscular Thickening

Although fibromuscular thickening is the most common cause of congenital stenosis, embryologic or pathogenic factors remain unknown (Nihoul-Fékété et al, 1987). Histologic findings are well described and include normal squamous epithelium overlying fibrous connective tissue and proliferation of smooth muscle fibers in the submucosa. Of interest, but not yet helpful in understanding the embryology, is the recognition that these lesions are histologically quite similar to hypertrophic pyloric stenosis (Todani et al, 1984).

Tracheobronchial Remnants

Tracheobronchial remnants are perhaps the best understood type of congenital esophageal stenosis, believed to result from incomplete separation of the primitive foregut from the respiratory tract around the 25th embryonic day (Yeung et al, 1992). The separation of pulmonary and esophageal primordia was originally explained as proliferation of the lateral ridges of the foregut into lung diverticulum and esophagus. Others describe the initial event as induction and growth of a lung bud on the ventral surface of the foregut.

Regardless, tracheobronchial tissue can be sequestered in the esophageal wall and then carried caudally by normal development of the esophagus, coming to reside in its typical distal location because of faster growth in the esophagus in comparison to the bronchial tree (Yeung et al, 1992). Although less commonly described, larger rests of cells can even organize into anomalous lobes of lung arising from the esophagus.

Finally, the syndrome of atresia and remnants can be described by the presence of mesenchyme that induces tracheobronchial differentiation along a short segment of foregut, thereby locally preventing normal esophageal development and narrowing the resulting lumen.

Congenital Webs

Congenital webs are generally thought to occur by failure of complete vacuolization of a mucosa-filled primordial esophageal lumen between the 6th and 10th weeks of development, as previously described for esophageal cysts (Kirwan et al, 1973). Although vacuolization occurs until the 10th week, the separation of the primordial pulmonary and esophageal structures occurs in week 5 (Scherer and Grosfeld, 1986). This timing helps account for the lack of association between webs and other congenital lesions such as atresias as well as the fact that they can occur at any level of the esophagus (Longstreth et al, 1979; Nihoul-Fékété et al, 1987).

DIAGNOSIS

Clinical Features

Congenital esophageal stenosis usually presents in infancy with progressive dysphagia and vomiting after the introduction of semisolid or solid foods, which typically occurs around the age of 6 months (Ohkawa et al, 1975). On rare occasion, a patient who presents with a lodged foreign body, after careful examination upon removal of the object, may be shown to have an esophageal stenosis (Bluestone et al, 1969).

The degree of obstruction and location within the esophagus produce an equally varied spectrum of clinical symptoms. Mild stenoses can remain undiagnosed for years; interestingly, a careful history even with presentation in adulthood can retrospectively reveal earlier swallowing difficulties (Longstreth et al, 1979). More severe stenoses can present with regurgitation and subsequent respiratory distress in the newborn (Nihoul-Fékété et al, 1987). Almost complete obstruction can resemble esophageal atresia. Proximal stenosis can cause inability to swallow food, whereas more distal lesions can cause regurgitation and, in more serious cases, aspiration with recurrent pneumonias (Adler, 1963).

Differential Diagnosis

Esophageal stenosis caused by caustic ingestion, esophagitis, chronic foreign body entrapment, and Barrett's esophagus can resemble congenital lesions. Patients with acquired stenoses, however, usually present with associated signs, symptoms, and a history related to the mechanism of injury. More difficult diagnoses involve distinguishing congenital esophageal stenosis from reflux esophagitis and esophageal narrowing from distal esophageal inflammation (Briceno et al, 1981) or distinguishing near-complete web from esophageal atresia. Achalasia and extrinsic compression from mediastinal masses should always be considered as well.

Investigative Techniques

Although a congenital cause is occasionally difficult to demonstrate, barium esophagogram and endoscopy provide reliable information regarding the location and the severity of esophageal stenoses. In the distal esophagus, a long and tapered narrowing suggests fibromuscular thickening, whereas a more discrete and abrupt narrowing suggests tracheobronchial remnants, although the latter is commonly interpreted as a reflux-related stricture. Webs or fibromuscular hypertrophy can present as lesions in the middle or even upper third of the esophagus (Grabowski and Andrews, 1996).

Esophagoscopy demonstrates normal-appearing mucosa overlying a narrow lumen. Esophageal biopsy can confirm the absence of significant esophagitis or gastric metaplasia and help reaffirm the congenital nature of a lesion (Bluestone et al, 1969). With both studies, dilatation of the esophagus proximal to the stenosis can introduce the question of achalasia, especially with the dysmotility that can be caused by dilatation itself. Esophageal manometry and pH monitoring can help to distinguish these clinical entities (Neilson et al, 1991).

MANAGEMENT

The goal of any treatment of congenital esophageal stenosis is twofold:

1. Symptoms should be relieved.
2. The antireflux mechanism should be maintained to avoid long-term complications.

Dilatation by bougienage, surgical resection, and myotomy has been performed with varying degrees of success in patients with the different types of congenital stenosis.

Dilatation

As early as the first reported series in 1953, therapeutic regimens for esophageal stenosis have begun with dilatation (Gross, 1953). A series of vigorous antegrade and retrograde dilatations with mercury-weighted tapered Maloney or Avaray bougies is usually performed. Use of Gruntzig balloon catheter dilatations under fluoroscopic or direct endoscopic guidance has also been reported, with success rates close to 95% in some children (Goldthorn et al, 1984; Lindor et al, 1985). Most children undergo at least one attempt at nonoperative management before surgical options are explored, and many patients are adequately treated in this fashion periodically, with results meeting both goals of treatment.

The ideal candidate for dilatation is a patient with a thin esophageal web or mild fibromuscular thickening, although successful treatment of all types of congenital esophageal stenoses has been reported. Success rates following dilatation of congenital webs are increased by endoscopic cautery resection, although the addition of cautery resection is associated with a higher morbidity risk (Huchzermeyer et al, 1979).

Complications of dilatation include esophageal leak and failure of therapy. Long-term results are promising, but many patients require an indefinite series of intermittent dilatations (Bluestone et al, 1969).

Resection

When dilatation fails to provide measurable improvement in symptoms with maintenance of esophageal function, resection and primary anastomosis should be considered with earlier rather than delayed operative treatment (Morger et al, 1991). Resection is almost always required if tracheobronchial remnants are suspected by tight unyielding strictures that have not responded to repeated dilatations (Fonkalsrud, 1972).

It is important to identify clearly the location and severity of the stenosis preoperatively. A right thoracotomy provides adequate access to the middle third of the esophagus, whereas a left thoracotomy is preferred for more distal lesions. Occasionally, laparotomy is needed to access the abdominal portion of the esophagus. Because it can be difficult to define the extent of the stenosis intraoperatively, a balloon catheter passed beyond the point of stenosis and then pulled back against the stenosis with an inflated balloon may assist in this endeavor (Ohi and Tseng, 1996). Additionally, advancing an esophageal dilator to the point of resistance can aid in identifying the proximal extent of the stenosis.

In most cases, segmental resection and end-to-end esophageal anastomosis can be accomplished with careful attention to preserving the vagal nerves. Uncommonly, long fibromuscular stenoses that do not respond to dilatation may require resection and subsequent esophageal replacement.

Resections of lesions near the gastroesophageal junction cause significant reflux if they are not treated with a concomitant antireflux procedure. Nihoul-Fékété and coauthors (1987) reported success with a modified Hill gastropexy and a Nissen fundoplication, with or without pyloroplasty. Other authors have recommended Collis gastroplasty with the Nissen fundoplication instead (Chahine et al, 1995).

Complications of surgical resection include esophageal leak with mediastinitis and significant reflux, as mentioned earlier.

Myotomy

Many long, tapered fibromuscular lesions can be treated with dilatation; surgical resection of those lesions that do not respond to dilatations would require esophageal replacement for anastomotic reconstruction. As an alternative, some authors have suggested myotomy similar to that used to treat hypertrophic pyloric stenosis or achalasia (Todani et al, 1984) as primary treatment. Given the paucity of follow-up reports, myotomy remains an attractive although untested therapy for these lesions.

Esophageal Diverticula

HISTORICAL NOTE

The relatively uncommon reports of congenital diverticula occurring in the esophagus began in 1908 (Lewis and Thyng, 1908), and the clinical picture of congenital esophageal diverticula was described two decades later by Jackson and Shallow (Jackson and Shallow, 1926).

DeBakey and coworkers (1952) later successfully repaired a congenital diverticulum with a single-stage operation.

■ *HISTORICAL READINGS*

DeBakey ME, Heancy JP, Creech O: Surgical considerations in diverticula of the esophagus. JAMA 150:1076, 1952.
Jackson C, Shallow TA: Diverticula of the esophagus: Pulsion, traction, malignant, and congenital. Ann Surg 83:1, 1926.
Lewis FT, Thyng FW: Regular occurrence of intestinal diverticula in embryos of pig, rabbit and man. Am J Anat 7:505, 1908.

DEFINITION

Both forms of acquired diverticula of the esophagus (pulsion and traction) result from herniation of the submucosa and mucosa through a defect in the muscularis. A *true* congenital diverticulum, in contrast, contains all layers of the esophagus (mucosa, submucosa, muscularis) within the outpouching (Brintnall and Kridelbaugh, 1950). Congenital occurrences of these diverticula are extremely rare and lack detail in the literature. They occur mostly in the cervical region of the esophagus around the pharyngoesophageal junction, as do most acquired lesions, but have been reported in the mid-esophagus.

An anatomic study of these lesions in 1908 proposed an embryologic defect during early foregut formation as the mechanism of diverticula, although the cause of this susceptibility remains unclear (Lewis and Thyng, 1908). Since then, a question has arisen regarding the possible overlap of esophageal cysts with luminal communication and congenital diverticula, although few cysts contain all layers of the esophageal wall, as do true diverticula.

DIAGNOSIS

Newborns with esophageal diverticula typically present with excessive mucous secretions in a pattern that can simulate esophageal atresia. If the diverticulum is large enough and fills while the infant is feeding, respiratory obstruction can be the presenting picture, with a significant danger of aspiration if spillover occurs suddenly. In some cases, foul-smelling breath gives a clue to the diagnosis. A nasogastric tube may not pass, coiling in the diverticulum, but in most cases the tube passes beyond the lesion with surprising ease.

A contrast study usually confirms the diagnosis, although it may require the careful injection of contrast during withdrawal of an intraesophageal tube. The most superior lesions can be difficult to assess by contrast radiography, and esophagoscopy may be required.

MANAGEMENT

Surgical excision is the treatment of choice, although long-term follow-up is unavailable. A three-layer closure is preferred after careful dissection and excision of the diverticulum. Satisfactory mucosal closure in a transverse direction, followed by a multiple layered muscular repair, reduces the risk of recurrence.

■ *REFERENCES*

Adler RH: Congenital esophageal webs. J Thorac Cardiovasc Surg 45:175, 1963.
Arbona JL, Figueroa JG, Mayoral J: Congenital esophageal cysts: Case report and review of the literature. Am J Gastroenterol 79:177, 1984.
Beardmore HE, Wiglesworth FW: Vertebral anomalies and alimentary duplications. Pediatr Clin North Am 5:457, 1958.
Beatty CC: Congenital stenosis of the esophagus. Br J Child Dis 25:237, 1928.
Bentley JFR, Smith JR: Developmental posterior enteric remnants and spinal malformation. Arch Dis Child 35:76, 1960.
Blasius G: Observata anatomica in homine, simia, equo. Amstelodam, Gaasbeeck, 1674.
Bluestone CD, Kerry R, Sieber WK: Congenital esophageal stenosis. Laryngoscope 79:1095, 1969.
Bonilla KB, Bowers WF: Congenital esophageal stenosis: Pathologic studies following resection. Am J Surg 97:772, 1959.
Borcar J, Hughes CF: Duplication of the cervical oesophagus in adults. Aust N Z J Surg 58:746, 1988.
Bower RJ, Sieber WK, Kiesewetter WB: Alimentary tract duplication in children. Ann Surg 188:669, 1978.
Briceno LI, Grases PJ, Gallego S: Tracheobronchial and pancreatic remnants causing esophageal stenosis. J Pediatr Surg 16:731, 1981.
Brintnall ES, Kridelbaugh WW: Congenital diverticulum of posterior hypopharynx simulating atresia of the esophagus. Ann Surg 131:564, 1950.
Butler C, Ende M: Double esophagus with carcinoma in one: Report of a case with autopsy. Arch Pathol 49:605, 1950.
Chahine AA, Campbell AB, Hoffman MA: Management of congenital distal esophageal stenosis with combined Collis gastroplasty-Nissen fundoplication. Pediatr Surg Int 10:23, 1995.
Clark JP: Congenital web of the esophagus: Report of a case. Laryngoscope 21:810, 1911.
Cohen SR, Geller KA, Birns JW, et al: Foregut cysts in infants and children: Diagnosis and management. Ann Otol Rhinol Laryngol 91:622, 1982.
Davis JE, Barnes WA: Intrathoracic duplications of the alimentary tract communicating with the small intestine. Ann Surg 136:287, 1952.
DeBakey ME, Heancy JP, Creech O: Surgical considerations in diverticula of the esophagus. JAMA 150:1076, 1952.
Dunbar JS: Congenital oesophageal stenosis. Pediatr Clin North Am 5:433, 1958.
Fallon M, Gordon ARG, Lendrum AC: Mediastinal cysts of the foregut origin associated with vertebral abnormalities. Br J Surg 41:520, 1954.
Fitch SJ, Tonkin ILD, Tonkin AK: Imaging of foregut duplication cysts. RadioGraphics 6:189, 1986.
Fitzgibbons RJ Jr, Nugent FW, Ellis FH Jr, et al: Unusual thoracoabdominal duplication associated with pancreaticopleural fistula. Gastroenterology 79:344, 1980.
Fonkalsrud EW: Esophageal stenosis due to tracheobronchial remnants. Am J Surg 124:101, 1972.
Frey EK, Duschl L: Der Kardiospasmus. Ergeb Chir Orthop 29:637, 1936.
Gans SL, Potts WJ: Anomalous lobe of lung arising from the esophagus. J Thorac Surg 21:313, 1951.
Goldman RL, Ban JL: Chondroepithelial choristoma (tracheobronchial rest) of the esophagus associated with esophageal atresia: Report of an unusual case. J Thorac Cardiovasc Surg 63:318, 1972.
Goldthorn JF, Ball WS, Wilkinson LG, et al: Esophageal strictures in children: Treatment by serial balloon catheter dilation. Radiology 153:655, 1984.
Grabowski ST, Andrews DA: Upper esophageal stenosis: Two case reports. J Pediatr Surg 31:1438, 1996.
Grosfeld JL, O'Neill JA, Clatworthy WH: Enteric duplications in infancy and childhood: An 18-year review. Ann Surg 172:83, 1970.
Gross RE: The Surgery of Infancy and Childhood. Philadelphia, WB Saunders, 1953.
Gross RE: Treatment of short stricture of the esophagus by partial esophagectomy and end-to-end esophageal reconstruction. Surgery 23:735, 1948.
Haller JA, Mazur DO, Morgan WW: Diagnosis and management of mediastinal masses in children. J Thorac Cardiovasc Surg 58:385, 1969.

Haller JA, Shermeta DW, Donahoo JS, White JJ: Life-threatening respiratory distress from mediastinal masses in infants. Ann Thorac Surg 19:364, 1975.

Harmand D, Grosdidir J, Hoeffel JC: Multiple bronchogenic cysts of the esophagus. Am J Gastroenterol 75:321, 1981.

Helund GL, Bissett GS II: Esophageal duplication cyst and aberrant right subclavian artery mimicking a symptomatic vascular ring. Pediatr Radiol 19:543, 1989.

Hemalatha V, Batcup G, Brereton RJ, et al: Esophageal atresia associated with esophageal duplication cyst. J Pediatr Surg 22:984, 1987.

Holcomb GW, Gheissari A, O'Neill JA, et al: Surgical management of alimentary tract duplications. Ann Surg 209:167, 1989.

Holmes GL, Trader S, Ignatiadis P: Intraspinal enterogenous cysts. Am J Dis Child 132:906, 1978.

Huchzermeyer H, Burdelski M, Hruby M: Endoscopic therapy of a congenital oesophageal stricture. Endoscopy 4:259, 1979.

Jackson C, Shallow TA: Diverticula of the esophagus: Pulsion, traction, malignant, and congenital. Ann Surg 83:1, 1926.

Johns BAE: Developmental changes in the oesophageal epithelium in man. J Anat 86:29, 1952.

Johnson FP: The development of the mucous membrane of the oesophagus, stomach, and small intestine in the human embryo. Am J Anat 10:521, 1910.

Kirwan WO, Walbaum PR, McCormack RJM: Cystic intrathoracic derivatives of the foregut and their complications. Thorax 28:424, 1973.

Kluth D: Atlas of esophageal atresia. J Pediatr Surg 11:901, 1976.

Kubie LS, Fulton JF: A clinical and pathological study of two teratomatous cysts of the spinal cord, containing mucous and ciliated cells. Surg Gynecol Obstet 47:297, 1928.

Kumar R: A case of congenital oesophageal stricture due to a cartilaginous ring. Br J Surg 49:533, 1962.

Ladd WE, Scott HW: Esophageal duplications or mediastinal cysts of enteric origin. Surgery 16:815, 1944.

Lee MY, Jensen E, Kwak S, Larson RA: Metastatic adenocarcinoma arising in a congenital foregut cyst of the esophagus: A case report with review of the literature. Am J Clin Oncol 21:64–6, 1998.

Lewis FT, Thyng FW: Regular occurrence of intestinal diverticula in embryos of pig, rabbit and man. Am J Anat 7:505, 1908.

Lewis RJ, Caccavale RJ, Sisler GE: Imaged thoracoscopic surgery: A new thoracic technique for resection of mediastinal cysts. Ann Thorac Surg 53:318, 1992.

Lindor KD, Ott BJ, Hughes RW: Balloon dilatation of upper digestive tract strictures. Gastroenterology 89:545, 1985.

Longstreth GF, Wolochow DA, Tu RT: Double congenital midesophageal webs in adults. Dig Dis Sci 24:162, 1979.

Lupetin AR, Dash N: MRI appearance of esophageal duplication cyst. Gastrointest Radiol 12:7, 1987.

McLetchie NGB, Purves JK, Saunders RL deCH: The genesis of gastric and certain intestinal diverticula and enterogenous cysts. Surg Gynecol Obstet 99:135, 1954.

Mixter CG, Clifford SH: Congenital mediastinal cysts of gastrogenic and bronchogenic origin. Ann Surg 90:714, 1929.

Morger R, Muller M, Sennhauser F, Waibel P: Congenital esophagostenosis. Eur J Pediatr Surg 1:142, 1991.

Mosher HP: Webs and pouches of the oesophagus: Their diagnosis, and treatment. Surg Gynecol Obstet 25:175, 1917.

Murphy SG, Yazbeck S, Russo P: Isolated congenital esophageal stenosis. J Pediatr Surg 30:1238, 1995.

Narasimharao KL, Mitra SK: Esophageal atresia associated with esophageal duplication cyst. J Pediatr Surg 22:984, 1987.

Neilson IR, Croitoru DP, Guttman FM, et al: Distal congenital esophageal stenosis associated with esophageal atresia. J Pediatr Surg 26:478, 1991.

Nihoul-Fékété C, De Backer A, Lortat-Jacob S, Pellerin D: Congenital esophageal stenosis: A review of 20 cases. Pediatr Surg Int 2:86, 1987.

Nishima T, Tsuchida Y, Saito S: Congenital esophageal stenosis due to tracheobronchial remnants and its associated anomalies. J Pediatr Surg 16:190, 1981.

O'Neill JA, Holcomb GW, Neblett WW: Recent experience with esophageal atresia. Ann Surg 114:48, 1979.

Ohi R, Tseng SW: Congenital oesophageal stenosis. In Puri P (ed): Newborn Surgery. Oxford, Butterworth-Heinemann, 1996.

Ohkawa H, Takahashi H, Saito H: Lower esophageal stenosis in association with tracheobronchial remnants. J Pediatr Surg 10:453, 1975.

Orr MM, Edwards AJ: Neoplastic change in duplications of the alimentary tract. Br J Surg 62:269, 1975.

Piramoon AM, Abbassioun KK: Mediastinal enterogenic cyst with spinal cord compression. J Pediatr Surg 9:543, 1974.

Plachta A: Benign tumors of the esophagus: Review of the literature and report of 99 cases. Am J Gastroenterol 38:639, 1962.

Pokorny WJ, Goldstein IR: Enteric thoracoabdominal duplications in children. J Thorac Cardiovasc Surg 87:821, 1984.

Prop N, Frensdorf EL, van de Stadt FR: A postvertebral entodermal cyst associated with axial deformities: A case showing the "entodermal-ectodermal adhesion syndrome." Pediatrics 39:555, 1967.

Rafal RB, Markisz JA: Magnetic resonance imaging of an esophageal duplication cyst. Am J Gastroenterol 86:1809, 1991.

Robison, RJ, Pavlina PM, Scherer LR, Grosfeld JL: Multiple esophageal duplication cysts. J Thorac Cardiovasc Surg 94:144, 1987.

Rogers LF, Osmer JC: Bronchogenic cyst: A review of 46 cases. Am J Roentgenol 91:273, 1964.

Roth M: Ueber Missbildungen im Bereich des Ductus omphalomesentericus. Arch Pathol Anat 86:25, 1881.

Ruffin WK, Hansen DE: An esophageal duplication cyst presenting as an abdominal mass. Am J Gastroenterol 84:571, 1989.

Salo JA, Ala-Kulju KV: Congenital esophageal cysts in adults. Ann Thorac Surg 44:135, 1987.

Sauerbruch F, Fick W: Operative Beseitigung einer kongenitalen Cyste der Speiserohre. Zentralbl Chir 58:2938, 1931.

Scherer LR, Grosfeld JL: Congenital esophageal stenosis, esophageal duplication, neurenteric cyst, and esophageal diverticulum. In Ashcraft KW, Holder TM (eds): Pediatric Esophageal Surgery. Orlando, FL, Grune & Stratton, 1986, p 53.

Sethi G, Marsden J, Johnson D: Duplication cysts of the esophagus. South Med J 67:616, 1974.

Simpson I, Campbell PE: Mediastinal masses in childhood: A review from a paediatric pathologist's point of view. Prog Pediatr Surg 27:92, 1991.

Snyder CL, Bickler SW, Gittes GK, et al: Esophageal duplication cyst with esophageal web and tracheoesophageal fistula. J Pediatr Surg 31:968, 1996.

Superina RA, Ein SH, Humphreys RP: Cystic duplications of the esophagus and neurenteric cysts. J Pediatr Surg 19:527, 1984.

Todani T, Watanabe Y, Mizuguchi T, et al: Congenital oesophageal stenosis due to fibromuscular thickening. Z Kinderchir 39:11, 1984.

Tuttle WM, Day JC: The treatment of short esophageal strictures by resection and end-to-end anastomosis. J Thorac Cardiovasc Surg 19:534, 1950.

Valerio D, Jones PF, Stewart AM: Congenital oesophageal stenosis. Arch Dis Child 52:414, 1977.

Waterston D: Oesophageal diseases in infancy and childhood, excluding oesophagotracheal fistula. In Smith RA, Smith RE (eds): Surgery of the Oesophagus: The Coventry Conference. East Norwalk, CT, Appleton & Lange, 1972, p 81.

Weichert RF, Lindsey ES, Pearce CW, Waring WW: Bronchogenic cyst with unilateral obstructive emphysema. J Thorac Cardiovasc Surg 59:287, 1970.

Weiss LM, Fagelman D, Warhit JM: CT demonstration of an esophageal duplication cyst. J Comput Assist Tomogr 7:716, 1983.

Yeung CK, Spitz L, Brereton RJ, et al: Congenital esophageal stenosis due to tracheobronchial remnants: A rare but important association with esophageal atresia. J Pediatr Surg 27:852, 1992.

CHAPTER **9**

Vascular Rings

William G. Williams
John C. Mullen

DEFINITION

The term *vascular ring* was introduced by Dr. Robert Gross (1946) to describe mediastinal vascular anomalies causing tracheal or esophageal compression. For the most part, vascular rings are a result of abnormal development of the primitive aortic arches. In a true vascular ring, the ligamentum arteriosum and/or the vessels form a true ring or circle around the trachea and esophagus, leading to the compression. Other vascular anomalies of the brachiocephalic trunk, although not forming a true ring, may compress the trachea or esophagus, creating a "pseudo" vascular ring. The term vascular ring has been used loosely to encompass these lesions as well. Surgical procedures in the chest may also produce iatrogenic vascular rings.

HISTORICAL NOTE

In 1735, Hunauld reported the autopsy finding of anomalous origin of a right subclavian artery from the descending aorta. In 1737, Hommel described a persistent double aortic arch. Vascular compression of the esophagus by an anomalous retroesophageal right subclavian artery was first described by Bayford (1794). He called the finding a lusus naturae, or "prank of nature," and coined the term *dysphagia lusoria.*

Gross (1946) performed the first successful operation for a vascular ring in 1945 by dividing a double aortic arch in a 1-year-old boy. A classification of vascular rings was devised by Edwards (1948) based upon a hypothetical embryologic development of a double aortic arch system.

■ *HISTORICAL READINGS*

Bayford DV: An account of a singular case of obstructed deglutition. Mem Med Soc London 2:275, 1794.

Edwards JE: Anomalies of the derivation of the aortic arch system. Med Clin North Am 32:925, 1948.

Gross RE: Surgical treatment of dysphagia lusoria in the adult. Ann Surg 124:532, 1946.

BASIC SCIENCE

Embryology and Pathology

The formation of the vascular ring depends on preservation or deletion of specific segments of six pairs of aortic arches, which arise sequentially from the truncus arteriosus and join paired dorsal aortas (Edwards, 1948). Various anomalies can be visualized by using Edwards' scheme of an ascending aorta, right and left aortic arches, a descending aorta on either the right or the left, and bilateral ductus arteriosi. Involution of the right fourth arch and persistence of the left fourth arch at 38 days in utero lead to normal left aortic arch anatomy. Involution of the ring at only one point allows 36 possible configurations, although not all have appeared in humans (Blake and Manion, 1962). Associated cardiac defects may be encountered, especially in patients with a right aortic arch, where tetralogy of Fallot is frequently coexistent.

Classification

Four groups are commonly identified: double aortic arch, right aortic arch with left ligamentum arteriosum, left aortic arch plus aberrant right subclavian artery or right descending aorta and pulmonary artery sling. The most

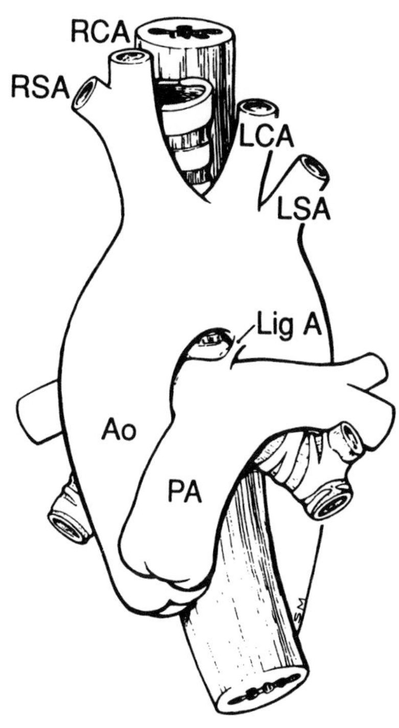

FIGURE 9–1 ■ The normal anatomy is displayed, showing the intimate relationship between the aortic arch, great vessels, trachea, and esophagus. (Ao, aorta; Lig A, ligamentum arteriosum; LCA, left carotid artery; LSA, left subclavian artery; PA, pulmonary artery; RCA, right carotid artery; RSA, right subclavian artery.)

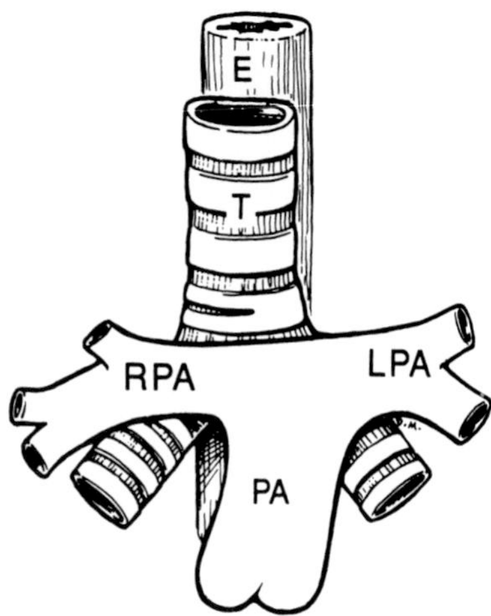

FIGURE 9–2 ■ The normal anatomy is displayed, showing the close relationship between the main pulmonary artery (PA), right pulmonary artery (RPA) and left pulmonary artery (LPA), trachea (T), and esophagus (E).

common anomaly resulting in a vascular ring is the double aortic arch. The initial classification of Edwards (1948) was enlarged upon by others (Keith et al, 1978) to include rare anomalies associated with right aortic arch.

Pathophysiology

The intimate relationship of the aortic arch, great vessels, trachea, and esophagus is depicted in Figures 9–1 and 9–2. A vascular ring can compress the trachea, esophagus, or both. Compression of the trachea and/or bronchi limits flow in both inspiration and expiration. In addition, chronic or severe compression results in tracheomalacia in the compressed segment, producing an unstable airway even after release of the compression (Wiatrak et al, 1991).

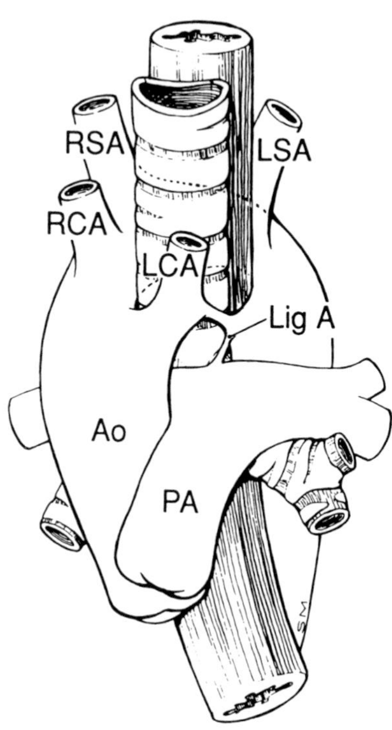

FIGURE 9–3 ■ A double aortic arch with atretic anterior arch (the usual finding) is depicted. Surgical repair would require division of the atretic arch between the left carotid artery (LCA) and descending aorta. (Ao, aorta; Lig A, ligamentum arteriosum; LSA, left subclavian artery; PA, pulmonary artery; RCA, right carotid artery; RSA, right subclavian artery.)

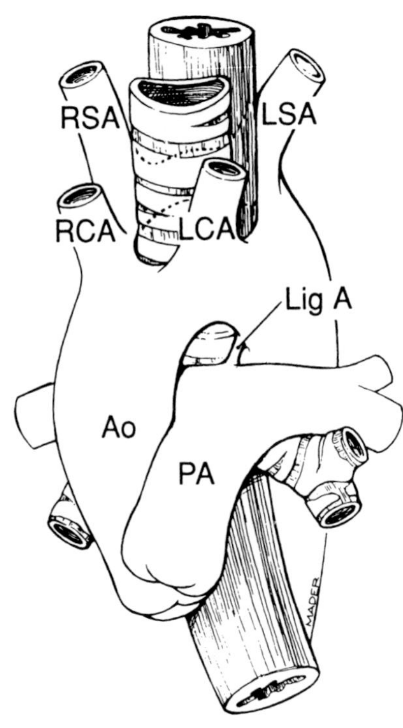

FIGURE 9–4 ■ A double aortic arch with smaller posterior arch is shown. The smaller arch would require division between the right subclavian artery (RSA) and the left subclavian artery (LSA). (Ao, aorta; Lig A, ligamentum arteriosum; LCA, left carotid artery; PA, pulmonary artery.)

Double aortic arch and aortic variants form true vascular rings completely encircling the trachea and esophagus (Figs. 9–3 and 9–4). In a *pulmonary artery sling*, the left pulmonary artery arises aberrantly from the right pulmonary artery and runs between the esophagus and trachea (Fig. 9–5), usually compressing the distal trachea and mainstem bronchi (most often the right mainstem bronchus). This lesion does not form a true vascular ring. Sade and colleagues (1975) reported that approximately 30% to 50% of infants with a pulmonary artery sling have associated complete tracheal rings (Fig. 9–6). The absence of the membranous portion of the trachea results in severe hypoplasia of the trachea, which often extends through the entire length of the trachea and into the bronchi, with abnormal bronchial branching and bronchiomalacia. This entity is also called a "stovepipe," "O ring," or "napkin ring" trachea. The association has been referred to as "the ring-sling complex" (Berdon, 1984).

Innominate artery compression (IAC) occurs when the innominate artery arises further to the left on the aortic arch than usual, causing compression of the trachea and buckling of the cartilages. However, the innominate artery normally arises from the left of the median plane, and the cause of the tracheal compression is unknown.

CLASSIFICATION OF VASCULAR RINGS

True Rings

- Double aortic arch
- Aortic arch variants
  - Right aortic arch with left ligamentum
  - Left aortic arch with aberrant right subclavian artery
  - Left aortic arch with right descending aorta in the presence of a right ligamentum or patent ductus or an aberrant right subclavian artery

Pseudorings

- Pulmonary artery sling
- Innominate artery compression
- Other vascular compressions
  - Enlarged left atrium
  - Postreconstruction of aorta

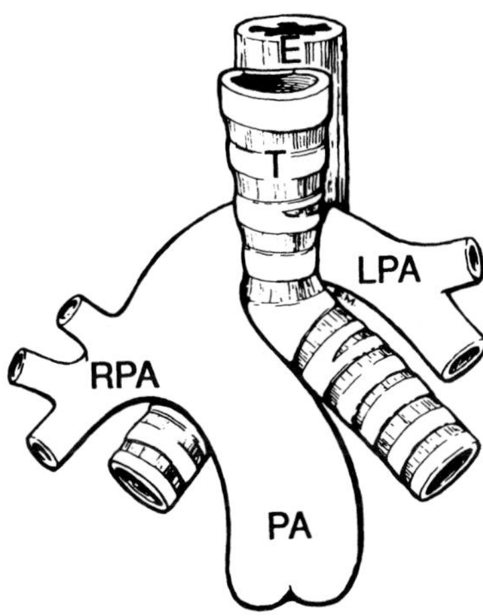

FIGURE 9–6 ■ A pulmonary artery sling with associated tracheal stenosis is depicted. This lesion has sometimes been referred to as the *ring-sling complex*. (E, esophagus; LPA, left pulmonary artery; PA, pulmonary artery; RPA, right pulmonary artery; T, trachea.)

DIAGNOSIS

Clinical Features

Compression of the esophagus or trachea may result in variable degrees of airway obstruction or dysphagia or both. Generally, airway obstruction with stridor on inspiration and expiration is both more severe and more life-threatening in infants than in older patients. Adults may present with respiratory obstruction, manifested by gasping while speaking in short phrases, or inability to complete a sentence in normal conversation. A harsh, brassy cough (often described as similar to a seal's bark) is common in the older patient, and obstruction is usually worse with an upper respiratory infection. Occasionally, patients may present with recurrent upper respiratory infection.

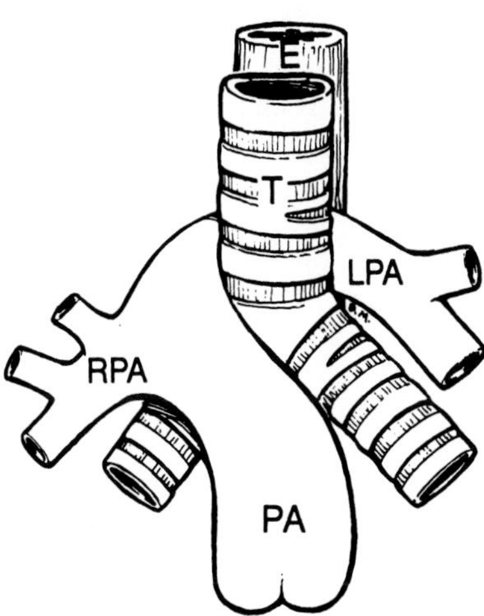

FIGURE 9–5 ■ A typical pulmonary artery sling is shown. The left pulmonary artery (LPA) arises aberrantly from the right pulmonary artery (RPA) and courses between the trachea (T) and the esophagus (E).

Dysphagia in infants is usually overshadowed by the associated respiratory obstruction. Prolonged difficult feeding with wheezing, regurgitation, aspiration, or even sudden collapse and death may occur. In older patients, difficulty in swallowing solid food may be evident. Stasis and regurgitation may lead to symptoms from associated esophagitis.

Natural History

Most patients with vascular rings present during infancy. Symptoms in the first few days or weeks of life indicate an urgent situation requiring prompt diagnosis and treatment. The group of patients with a pulmonary artery sling usually present with severe respiratory distress by 1 year of age (77%) (Sade et al, 1975). Some patients are mildly symptomatic or asymptomatic into childhood before dysphagia or stridor develops, often during an intracurrent infection. Some children with mild symptoms show marked improvement as they grow (Godtfredsen et al, 1977).

The critical factor in causing symptoms is the degree of compression rather than simply the presence of a vascular ring. For example, approximately 1% of the general population have an aberrant subclavian artery and generally remain asymptomatic, never requiring treatment.

IAC produces noisy respiration, often exacerbated by feeding. Apneic spells are common and may lead to cyanosis and even sudden death. Mustard and associates (1969) reported 285 cases of IAC, but only 14% required surgical intervention, with reflex apnea (respiratory arrest following stimulation of the compressed area of the trachea) being the major indication for operation. Dysphagia does not occur with IAC because the esophagus is not obstructed. Reflex apnea may result from tracheal irritation by a bolus of food, causing further compression. Recurrent pneumonia and atelectasis may also occur. Vascular rings are not necessarily inconsistent with prolonged survival, and many patients are totally asymptomatic (Dupuis et al, 1988).

Differential Diagnosis

Vascular rings should be suspected in any child with stridor, dysphagia, recurrent respiratory infections, difficulty feeding, or failure to thrive. In patients with suspected innominate artery compression, it is important to rule out other causes of apneic spells. Sleep studies, investigation for gastroesophageal reflux, and a complete neurologic examination should be performed.

Investigative Techniques

Investigation should start with a careful history and physical examination. Approximately 10% to 20% of patients with vascular rings have associated cardiac or noncardiac anomalies. These may have an important impact on treatment and outcome.

A plain chest x-ray (Fig. 9–7) and barium swallow (Fig. 9–8) can establish the diagnosis of vascular ring in most situations. The combination of posterior compression of the esophagus on barium swallow (what we call a *ball bearing esophagus*) and anterior tracheal compression is almost pathognomonic for a vascular ring. Barium swallow is the best single diagnostic test for patients with complete vascular rings (Backer et al, 1989).

For double aortic arch and aortic arch anomalies, the dominant arch is usually right-sided (see Fig. 9–3). The barium esophagogram shows bilateral compression on anteroposterior views and a posterior indentation on the lateral view because of the dominant right aortic arch. The diagnosis can be confirmed by two-dimensional echocardiography in almost all patients. Angiography is rarely required. Computed tomography (CT) (Fig. 9–9) and nuclear magnetic resonance imaging (MRI) can also be used for diagnosis but are more expensive and yield similar information. Bronchoscopy may be hazardous by stimulating tracheal inflammation in an anatomically narrow airway and is usually unnecessary for the diagnosis of aortic arch anomalies.

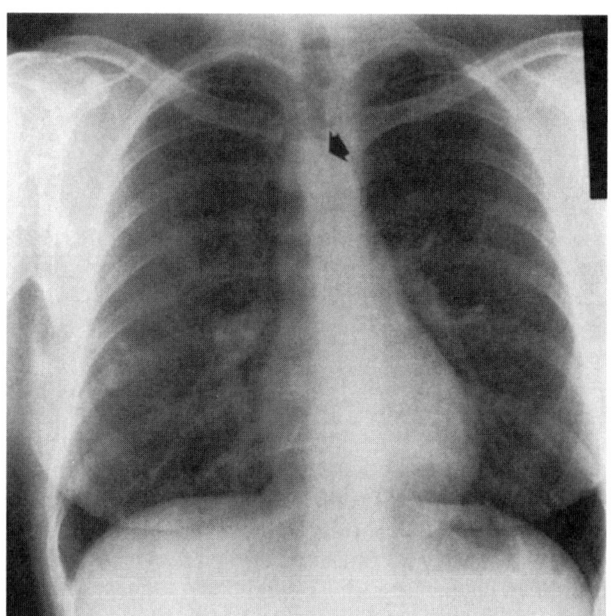

FIGURE 9–7 ■ A chest x-ray shows compression and displacement of the trachea *(arrow)*, which are often seen with a vascular ring.

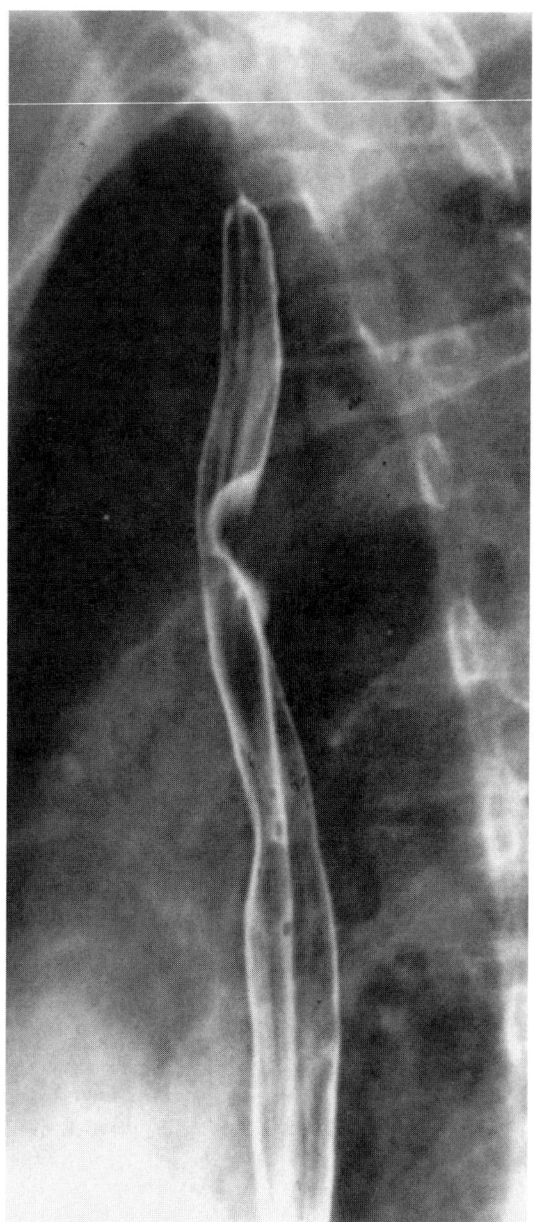

FIGURE 9–8 ■ A barium swallow displays a characteristic posterior compression of the esophagus (a "ball bearing" esophagus), which is almost pathognomonic of a vascular ring.

In patients with a pulmonary artery sling, the mainstay of the diagnosis has been the barium esophagogram. A lateral finding described no other vascular lesions (Capitanio et al, 1971). Chest x-ray and two-dimensional echocardiography should be supplemented by pulmonary arteriography to delineate the size and distribution of the aberrant left pulmonary artery. An angiogram, CT scans, or MRI can also be used to confirm the diagnosis (Backer

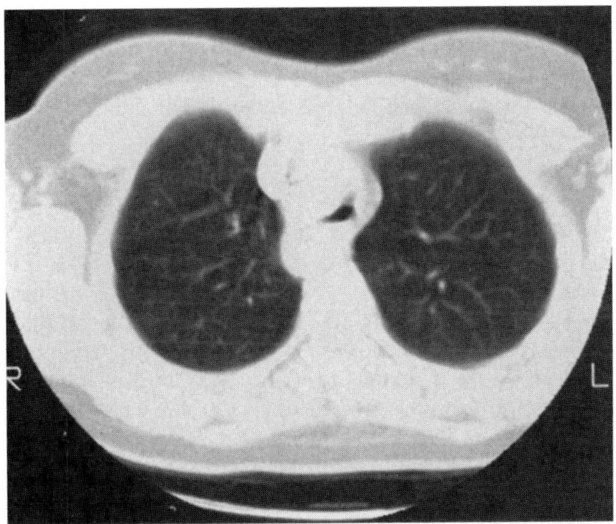

FIGURE 9–9 ■ CT scan shows compression of the trachea and left mainstem bronchus. Tracheal or bronchial compression is frequently encountered with vascular rings.

et al, 1989). Bronchoscopy is important for detection of associated tracheal stenosis or complete tracheal rings.

For innominate artery compression, bronchoscopy is the investigation of choice (Filston et al, 1987). The degree of obstruction is determined and the diagnosis is confirmed by levering a bronchoscope anteriorly to occlude the innominate (right subclavian) pulse. Rigid bronchoscopy during repair is also useful to confirm relief of the compression while the artery is suspended anteriorly.

MRI is being employed more frequently as a noninvasive alternative to aortography. With the rapid evolution of this technology and experience in interpreting the scans, MRI may soon supersede aortography as the diagnostic modality of choice for patients with vascular rings (Gomes, 1989; Gomes et al, 1987).

MANAGEMENT

General Principles

Although some vascular rings improve as the child grows, the long-term prognosis of medical therapy is poor in symptomatic patients. Surgical intervention is indicated in any symptomatic patient or for complications of the anomalies. Initiation of early and appropriate surgical therapy is important to prevent mortality and avoid serious complications that may arise from hypoxic and apneic spells. Significant obstruction that produces severe symptoms requires prompt relief.

The principles of surgical therapy involve adequate exposure, division of the ring, adequate mobilization of normal structures to provide relief of the constriction, and preservation of circulation to the aortic branches. Most of these lesions can be approached through a left thoracotomy. Prior to division of any artery (such as in a double aortic arch with equal arches), the artery in question can be test occluding and proximal and distal pressures can be measured.

Operative Technique

Double Aortic Arch

Double aortic arch anomalies can almost always be repaired through a left posterolateral third (in infants), fourth (in children), or fifth (in adults) intercostal incision.

The dissection is similar to that for ligation of a patent ductus. It is important to dissect all of the vascular structures carefully in anatomic planes, protecting adjacent vital structures such as the vagus, recurrent laryngeal, and phrenic nerves and the thoracic duct. Each vessel should be identified once the dissection is complete.

In most patients with double aortic arch, the posterior rightward artery is usually dominant (see Fig. 9–3). The anterior structure, often a fibrous cord, is divided. In addition, the ligamentum arteriosum (which rarely is patent) must also be divided. There may be a prominent bulge at the site of origin of the obstruction from the descending aorta (Kommerell's diverticulum). This diverticulum can be side-clamped and partially excised, and its base can be oversewn flush with the wall of the descending aorta. The anterior surface of the trachea should be cleared of any remaining adhesions and allowed to bow anteriorly.

In Backer's series (1989) of 61 double aortic arches, the right-sided (posterior) arch was dominant in 73%, the left-sided (anterior) arch was dominant in 20% (see Fig. 9–4), and the arches were equal in 7% of patients. With a dominant right arch, segments of the left arch were atretic in 40% of the patients. With a dominant left arch, segments of the right arch were atretic in 33% of patients, occurring most frequently in the posterior or distal end of the lesser arch.

When the two aortic arches are of equal size, we prefer to divide the posterior arch, thereby allowing the aorta and trachea to lie in normal position. Confirmation of adequate size of the remaining arch should be established by measuring proximal and distal aortic pressures while test occluding the arches sequentially prior to division of the arch. Rarely, a right descending aorta is encountered, in which case the right arch is anterior.

Right Aortic Arch and Left Ligamentum

The most common arch anomaly apart from double aortic arch is a right-sided arch with left ligamentum (Fig. 9–10) with or without an aberrant left subclavian artery. It is often referred to as *Neuhauser's anomaly* after the radiologist who first described it (Neuhauser, 1946). Dissection is similar to that required for a double aortic arch. The ligamentum is divided, and the trachea and esophagus are dissected free of adhesive bands. If an aberrant left subclavian artery is present, it does not need to be divided. Only in the extremely rare situation in which an aberrant left subclavian artery passes anterior to the trachea should consideration be given to dividing the artery. Felson and Palayew (1963) reported a 56% incidence of retroesophageal left subclavian artery and a 44% incidence of mirror-image left innominate artery (see Fig. 9–5). If there is mirror-image branching with the ligamentum arising from the innominate artery instead of

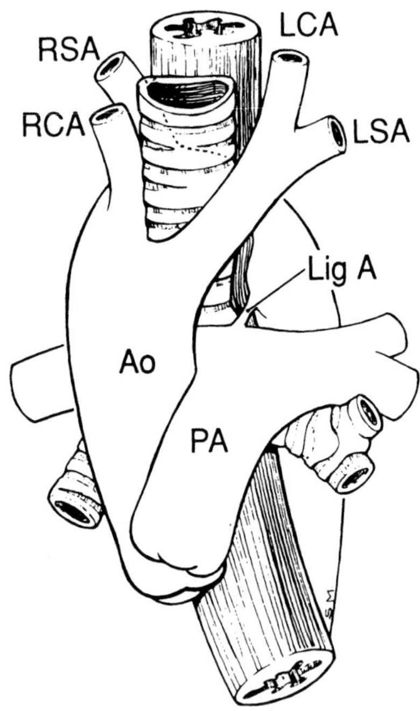

FIGURE 9–10 ■ A right aortic arch with left-sided ligamentum and mirror-image innominate artery is displayed (Neuhauser's anomaly). Surgical repair would require dividing the ligamentum arteriosum and dissecting free any adhesive bands surrounding the trachea and esophagus. (Ao, aorta; Lig A, ligamentum arteriosum; LCA, left carotid artery; LSA, left subclavian artery; PA, pulmonary artery; RCA, right carotid artery; RSA, right subclavian artery.)

the aorta, a complete ring will not be formed and there will be no symptoms (D'Cruz et al, 1966).

Pulmonary Artery Sling

The pulmonary artery sling (see Figs. 9–5 and 9–6) is best approached through a median sternotomy. We prefer using normothermic cardiopulmonary bypass with a single cannula in the right atrium and ascending aorta to facilitate the repair. The left pulmonary artery is dissected from its origin in the proximal right pulmonary artery and is mobilized behind the esophagus and trachea into the hilum. It is then divided from the right pulmonary artery, with its anterior surface carefully marked for subsequent reimplantation. The left pulmonary artery is withdrawn from its aberrant course and repositioned in an anatomically normal course, with the surgeon bringing it through a large incision in the pericardium posterior to the phrenic nerve. Care must be taken to avoid rotation of the artery. An ellipse of the main pulmonary artery is excised, and a long oblique anastomosis is then made to the side of the main pulmonary artery (we prefer an absorbable suture). The base of its origin from the right pulmonary artery is oversewn transversely to prevent kinking.

In patients with associated tracheal stenosis from hypoplasia and complete tracheal ring (see Fig. 9–6), an anterior tracheoplasty with autologous pericardium across the entire level of the obstruction is performed at the same operation (Idriss et al, 1984). Hickey and Wood (1987) and Pawade and colleagues (1992) reported single-stage correction by left pulmonary artery reimplantation and tracheal resection using cardiopulmonary bypass with good results. Jonas and associates (1989) reported resection of the trachea posterior to the aberrant left pulmonary artery but leaving the left pulmonary artery in situ (no vascular anastomosis).

Innominate Artery Compression

The general anesthetic for this procedure is given through a rigid bronchoscope to allow visualization of the obstruction. In boys, a short second interspace incision anteriorly from the sternal edge, either on the right or the left, may be used. In girls, we employ a submammary anterior fifth interspace incision on the right. The thymus is cleared from the base of the innominate artery.

Two strong sutures are placed as figure-of-eight adventitial sutures. Each suture is then brought through a separate part of the sternum and used to pull the innominate artery and aorta anteriorly. The innominate artery is not dissected free from the trachea but is suspended, thereby exerting traction through its adventitial attachments to open up the collapsed tracheal cartilages. Visual confirmation of the relief of tracheal compression is obtained via the bronchoscope. The two sutures are then tied to each other under tension. Occasionally, more than two pairs of sutures may be required to suspend a length of vessel sufficiently to relieve the obstruction.

Indications for Right Thoracotomy

Although almost all double aortic arches and arch anomalies may be relieved through a left thoracotomy, occasionally a right thoracotomy is required (McFaul et al, 1981). The presence of a left aortic arch with retroesophageal right-sided descending aorta is a rare arch anomaly, first reported by Paul (1948), and may require right thoracotomy. The vascular ring is normally completed by a right-sided ligamentum arteriosum. Most patients with this anomaly have had minimal symptoms (de Balsac, 1960).

A rare lesion for which right thoracotomy is beneficial is a double aortic arch with an atretic right posterior segment. Associated cardiac disease is probably more common with this entity. These patients, almost always infants, require careful investigation, which should probably include angiography. A right thoracotomy or median sternotomy is the approach of choice for division and anastomosis of an anomalous right subclavian artery (Wychulis et al, 1971). Innominate artery compression may be approached through a right or left thoracotomy, but we favor a right thoracotomy.

Perioperative Care

Timely intervention is important in preventing serious complications and may be especially urgent in the infant. Careful respiratory care is essential, with administration of high humidity for loosening secretions, oxygen as needed, chest physiotherapy, and nasopharyngeal suctioning. Early extubation is preferable to limit tracheal edema and avoid aggravating the already narrowed airway.

Generally, complications are minimal. When the dominant aortic arch is right-sided, the persistent displacement of the trachea and esophagus anteriorly may require a longer time (weeks or months) for the airway to stabilize. With severe chronic compression, tracheomalacia is usual and postoperative stridor may persist for some weeks. Continued postextubation observation is important to detect signs of significant airway obstruction. Tracheostomy is almost never required. Children with pulmonary artery sling and associated tracheal stenosis from complete tracheal rings have higher morbidity and mortality rates from persistent airway obstruction (Pawade, 1992).

In the series by Chun and colleagues (1992) of 39 patients with congenital vascular rings, postoperative complications occurred in 33% of patients. The complications included bleeding (8%), respiratory arrest with reintubation (5%), pneumonia (13%), sepsis (3%), chylothorax (10%), and pneumothorax (3%). Two of the four patients with chylothorax required thoracic duct ligation, and the other two were managed with chest tube drainage and dietary restriction. Chylothorax is not uncommon because of the necessary dissection in the posterior mediastinum, and it may lead to substantial morbidity and a prolonged hospital course. It is very easy for a lymph leak to develop because of the proximity of the thoracic duct and abundant lymphatic channels. At the time of the initial operation, a careful check for both hemostasis and lymph leakage should be carried out prior to chest closure to minimize the incidence of these complications.

Early and Late Results

Results in terms of both survival and relief of symptoms are good with isolated vascular rings. In Backer's series (1989) of 204 children, the operative mortality rate was 4.9% and the incidence of late death was 3.4%. None of the children in whom the vascular ring was an isolated finding died. Follow-up data in 159 patients (mean follow-up, 8.5 months) revealed that 92% were symptom-free and 8% had residual respiratory problems.

Postoperative morbidity is often related to the secondary tracheomalacia (Roesler et al, 1983). Symptoms and signs of tracheoesophageal compression improve significantly after surgery but may continue (especially residual noisy breathing) for a few months to several years, diminishing as the child grows. With associated cardiac anomalies, the long-term outcome is related to the severity of the cardiac defect.

Unresolved Issues and Future Trends

Innominiate artery compression is not a true vascular ring, and some doubt its validity. Nevertheless, it can and does produce significant life-threatening compression. It is easily, predictably, and safely relieved by suspending the base of the innominate artery against the sternum.

Adequate relief of tracheomalacic segments continues to be a vexing problem and the major source of morbidity and mortality. Ongoing research in treatment of tracheal stenosis and tracheomalacia will aid in treatment of these conditions. Tracheal or bronchial stenting inserted through the trachea may be a valuable tool for those children who have not improved after surgical relief of compression.

In many cases, vascular rings may be suitable for management by thoracoscopic technology. Improved technology in thoracoscopic vascular staplers makes this treatment a real possibility. Vascular rings involving only a ligamentum, as opposed to patent ductus, may be readily divisible by this approach. Analysis of the risks and benefits of thoracoscopic versus open operations will guide the choice of approach as instruments and expertise evolve.

CONCLUSION

Vascular rings result from abnormal development of the embryonic aortic arch complex and may compress the trachea or esophagus. Presenting symptoms are either dysphagia or stridor, respiratory distress, apnea, or recurrent upper respiratory infections. Some patients may remain asymptomatic for prolonged periods.

Vascular rings are an uncommon but important cause of tracheal and esophageal compression. They may be life-threatening and can be cured by early appropriate surgery.

Double aortic arch is the most common cause of compression. The anatomy of other anomalies of the aortic arch may be extremely varied and can best be understood by studying the hypothetical double arch theory, as first proposed by Edwards.

Double aortic arch and right aortic arch with left ligamentum are diagnosed by barium swallow (anterior bowing of the posterior esophageal wall). The presence of a pulmonary artery sling is suggested by barium swallow (posterior bowing of the anterior esophageal wall) and is confirmed by bronchoscopy and CT or angiography. Innominate artery compression is diagnosed by bronchoscopy and negative neurologic findings.

Left thoracotomy provides excellent exposure for most vascular rings. A pulmonary artery sling is best treated by a median sternotomy, usually with the aid of cardiopulmonary bypass. The displaced innominate artery may be more easily treated by a right thoracotomy. The double aortic arch with atretic posterior segment and the left aortic arch with retroesophageal right-sided descending aorta are also more easily treated by a right thoracotomy.

When symptomatic, vascular rings should be repaired, since the risk is small and long-term results are excellent. Respiratory distress from tracheomalacic segments constitutes the greatest risk for morbidity and mortality.

COMMENTS AND CONTROVERSIES

The management of the malacic segment of compressed trachea and bronchus after division of vascular rings is somewhat controversial. Many surgeons follow the principle espoused by Gross of meticulously dividing all adhesions of the airway to vascular structures. This leaves the malacic segment unsuspended. Residual respiratory symptoms may persist for many months because the cartilage does not become firm quickly after relief of pulsatile compression. Drs. Williams and Mullen support Gross's policy for rings but favor Mustard's strategy of leaving adhesions intact to facilitate suspending the airway in an open position after arteriopexy, when the innominate artery is fixed to the sternum. This technique can also be helpful when a ring is opened. Its anterior or posterior component, or both, can be sutured to the spine and chest wall to facilitate suspension in an open position.

Maturation of malacic cartilage is slow but complete in many patients with "innominate compression" of the trachea. Suspension should be reserved for the minority with severe symptoms, as emphasized by Sloan in his pithy editorial comment accompanying Mustard's landmark article on this subject (Mustard, 1969).

MARTIN McKNEALLY (TORONTO)

■ KEY REFERENCES

Backer CL, Ilbawi MN, Idriss FS, DeLeon SY: Vascular anomalies causing tracheoesophageal compression: Review of experience in children. J Thorac Cardiovasc Surg 97:725, 1989.

An important review of 204 children operated on between 1947 and 1987 at the Children's Memorial Hospital in Chicago.

Chun K, Colombani PM, Dudgeon DL, Haller JA: Diagnosis and management of congenital vascular rings: A 22-year experience. Ann Thorac Surg 53:597, 1992.

A review of 39 children operated on between 1968 and 1990 at The Johns Hopkins University School of Medicine in Baltimore.

Edwards JE: Anomalies of the derivation of the aortic arch system. Med Clin North Am 32:925, 1948.

First description of the hypothetical double aortic arch that forms the basis of classification of vascular rings.

Gross RE: Arterial malformations which cause compression of the trachea or esophagus. Circulation 11:124, 1955.

A classic review of vascular rings in 70 children by the initial surgeon attempting repair of these anomalies.

Sade RM, Rosenthal A, Fellows K, Castenada AR: Pulmonary artery slings. J Thorac Cardiovasc Surg 69:333, 1975.

Excellent review of embryology, natural history, and surgical correction of pulmonary artery sling.

■ REFERENCES

Berdon WE, Baker DM, Wung JT et al: Complete cartilage and tracheal stenosis associated with anomalous left pulmonary artery: The ring-sling complex. Radiology 152:57, 1984.

Blake HA, Manion WC: Thoracic arterial arch anomalies. Circulation 26:251, 1962.

Capitanio MA, Ramos R, Kirkpatrick JA: Pulmonary slings: Roentgen observations. Am J Roentgenol Radium Ther Nucl Med 112:28, 1971.

D'Cruz IA, Cantez T, Namin EP, Licata R, Hastreiter AR: Right sided aorta. Br Heart J 28:722, 1966.

de Balsac RH: Left aortic arch (posterior or circumflex type) with right descending aorta. Am J Cardiol 5:546, 1960.

Dupuis C, Vaksmann G, Pernot C, et al: Asymptomatic form of left pulmonary artery sling. Am J Cardiol 61:177, 1988.

Felson B, Palayew MJ: The two types of right aortic arch. Radiology 81:745, 1963.

Filston HC, Ferguson TB Jr, Oldham HN: Airway obstruction by vascular anomalies: Importance of telescopic bronchoscopy. Ann Surg 205:541, 1987.

Godtfredsen J, Wennenvold A, Efsen F, Lauridsen PP: Natural history of vascular rings with clinical manifestations: A follow-up study of eleven unoperated cases. Scand J Thorac Cardiovasc Surg 11:75, 1977.

Gomes AS: MR imaging of congenital anomalies of the thoracic aorta and pulmonary arteries. Radiol Clin North Am 27:1171, 1989.

Gomes AS, Lois JF, George B, et al: Congenital abnormalities of the aortic arch: MRI imaging. Radiology 165:691, 1987.

Gross RE: Surgical treatment of dysphagia lusoria in the adult. Ann Surg 124:532, 1946.

Hickey M St J, Wood AE: Pulmonary artery sling with tracheal stenosis. Ann Thorac Surg 44:416, 1987.

Idriss FS, DeLeon SY, Ilbawi MN, et al: Tracheoplasty with pericardial patch for extensive tracheal stenosis in infants and children. J Thorac Cardiovasc Surg 88:527, 1984.

Jonas RA, Spevak PT, McGill T, Castenada AR: Pulmonary artery sling: Primary repair by tracheal resection in infancy. J Thorac Cardiovasc Surg 97:548, 1989.

Keith JD, Rowe RD, Vlad P: Heart Disease in Infancy and Childhood, 3rd ed. New York, Macmillan, 1978.

McFaul R, Millard P, Nowicki E: Vascular rings necessitating right thoracotomy. J Thorac Cardiovasc Surg 82:306, 1981.

Mustard WT, Bayliss CE, Fearon B, et al: Tracheal compression by the innominate artery in children. Ann Thorac Surg 8:312, 1969.

Neuhauser EBD: Roentgen diagrams of double aortic arch and other anomalies of great vessels. Am J Roentgenol Radiat Ther 56:1, 1946.

Paul RN: A new anomaly of the aorta: Left aortic arch with right descending aorta. J Pediatr 32:19, 1948.

Pawade A, de Leval MR, Elliott MJ, Stark J: Pulmonary artery sling. Ann Thorac Surg 54:967, 1992.

Roesler M, deLeval M, Chrispin A, Stark J: Surgical management of vascular ring. Ann Surg 197:139, 1983.

Wiatrak BJ, Myer CM, Cotton RT: Atypical tracheobronchial vascular compression. Am J Otolaryngol 12:347, 1991.

Wychulis AR, Kincaid OW, Weidman WH, Danielson GK: Congenital vascular ring: Surgical considerations and results of operation. Mayo Clin Proc 46:182, 1971.

Hiatal Hernia, Gastroesophageal Reflux, and Other Conditions

CHAPTER 10

Pathophysiology of Hiatal Hernia and Gastroesophageal Reflux

F. Griffith Pearson

This chapter provides background information that lends understanding to the clinical presentations of hiatal hernia and gastroesophageal reflux and to the rationale for management.

DEFINITION

It is important to emphasize that normal individuals experience some gastroesophageal reflux on a regular basis (DeMeester et al, 1980). The range of *physiologic* reflux may vary among races and among regions of the world.

Pathologic reflux may result in progressive inflammatory changes in the wall of the esophagus as well as injury above the level of the cricopharyngeal sphincter in cases of regurgitation with overspill and aspiration.

Incarceration, on the other hand, produces a series of mechanical problems that relate to a progressively enlarging and irreducible hiatal hernia. Complications of incarceration include the following:

1. Retention of food and fluid in the intrathoracic gastric pouch.
2. Peptic ulcer in the intrathoracic gastric pouch (with penetration, perforation, or massive bleeding).
3. Vascular congestion of incarcerated mucosa, resulting in iron deficiency anemia.
4. Volvulus with lower esophageal or gastric outlet obstruction.
5. Occasional strangulation with gangrene.

The complications of hiatal hernia and gastroesophageal reflux are summarized later.

HISTORICAL NOTE

Historically, the association between hiatal hernia and gastroesophageal reflux was first noted in England by Allison (1946, 1951). In his classic and beautifully written papers, Allison (1951) clearly describes the common symptoms of gastroesophageal reflux, noting the inflammatory esophagitis, including erosive ulceration and stricture, that sometimes ensues. He subsequently reported on a group of patients with a columnar-lined segment of distal esophagus. Allison and Johnstone (1953) correctly speculated that this condition might be the result of the replacement of denuded squamous epithelium (due to reflux and ulceration) with adjacent columnar epithelium.

Barrett (1950) described "chronic peptic ulcer of the esophagus and esophagitis" on the basis of postmortem observations and concluded that all of these patients had gastric ulceration in a pouch of intrathoracic stomach due to a congenitally short esophagus. Allison and Johnstone (1953) clearly distinguished between superficial ulceration due to reflux esophagitis in squamous epithelium and the less common condition of chronic peptic ulcer in a columnar-lined segment. Allison observed that these chronic ulcers were in the segment of columnar-lined esophagus, and it was Allison who coined the term *Barrett's ulcer*.

Allison and Johnstone (1953) postulated that columnar-lined esophagus might be of acquired rather than congenital origin:

Is healing of the ulcer (in squamous epithelium) in an acid medium more likely to be by the overgrowth of gastric rather than squamous epithelium? If this were so, it might be that some examples of the gastric mucosa in the esophagus were acquired rather than congenital.

For the next 20 years, popular opinion held that the hiatal hernia was the primary cause of gastroesophageal reflux and resulted in loss of competence of the "valve-like mechanism" at the esophagogastric junction. Cohen and Harris (1971) were the first to influence and radically alter this opinion, particularly among gastroenterologists. Their observations led to the opinion that the actual hiatal hernia had little to do with the control of reflux. They attributed the antireflux barrier (competence) primarily to the lower esophageal sphincter (LES).

This concept was held with stubborn conviction by many physicians for the next 20 years (Dent et al, 1980; Dodds et al, 1982). It is only since the mid-1980s that gastroenterologists have again acknowledged the common association between sliding hiatal hernia and pathologic reflux. Endoscopic and radiographic studies show that between 50% and 90% of patients with reflux disease have an associated hiatal hernia (Berstad et al, 1986; Kaul et al, 1986; Ott et al, 1985; Sontag et al, 1991).

A review of the appropriate pathophysiology includes both the complications of gastroesophageal reflux and the sequelae of mechanical problems related to the hiatal hernia itself.

GASTROESOPHAGEAL REFLUX: COMPLICATIONS

Peptic Esophagitis

1. Mucosal inflammation/ulceration
2. Peptic stricture
3. Acquired short esophagus
4. Acquired columnar-lined esophagus
   a. Barrett's ulcer
   b. Dysplasia/adenocarcinoma

Motor Dysfunction

1. Impaired peristalsis
2. Impaired LES pressure
3. Pharyngoesophageal sphincter dysfunction

Aspiration of Refluxate

1. Pharyngitis/laryngitis
2. Tracheobronchitis
3. Pneumonia/bronchiectasis/pulmonary fibrosis
4. Asthma

Incarceration

1. Gastric obstruction, partial or complete
2. Chronic iron deficiency anemia
3. Gastric pouch ulcer
4. Space occupation/dyspnea
5. Strangulated intrathoracic stomach

■ *HISTORICAL READINGS*

Allison PR: Reflux esophagitis, sliding hiatal hernia, and the anatomy of repair. Surg Gynecol Obstet 92:149, 1951.

Allison PR: Peptic ulcer of the esophagus. J Thorac Surg 15:308, 1946.

Allison PR, Johnstone AS: The esophagus lined with gastric membrane. Thorax 8:87, 1953.

Barrett NR: Chronic peptic ulcer of the esophagus and esophagitis. Br J Surg 38:175, 1950.

Cohen S, Harris LD: Does hiatus hernia affect competence of the gastroesophageal sphincter? N Engl J Med 284:1053, 1971.

GASTROESOPHAGEAL REFLUX

Inflammation

The extent of inflammatory change in the wall of the exposed distal esophagus is dependent on the following:

1. The strength and content of the refluxate (acid, bile, and duodenal and pancreatic enzymes).
2. The effectiveness of esophageal clearance mechanisms.
3. The effectiveness of gastric emptying.
4. Neutralizing factors such as saliva.

The degrees of inflammation, or *esophagitis*, were staged by Skinner and Belsey (1967):

- *Stage 1*, mucosal reddening, without ulceration
- *Stage 2*, linear erosions in squamous epithelium (adjacent to the squamocolumnar interface)
- *Stage 3*, confluent superficial erosions, becoming circumferential
- *Stage 4*, peptic stricture, acquired columnar-lined esophagus

Mucosal reddening without ulceration is an equivocal observation; changes in the intensity of endoscopic illumination may modify the interpretation. The histologic changes seen in a mucosal biopsy sample provide a more objective assessment of this early stage.

Linear erosions due to gastroesophageal reflux are typical in appearance and location. They are disposed in a vertical, linear configuration and are most pronounced in the squamous epithelium immediately proximal to the squamocolumnar junction. These gross changes rarely extend more than 4 to 5 cm above the squamocolumnar interface. These linear ulcers have a narrow red margin, and there usually is a thin coating of pale whitish exudate centrally.

Confluent ulceration is commonly circumferential in the patient with a peptic stricture. Like ulcerative esophagitis, the peptic stricture is inevitably most pronounced just at, and above, the squamocolumnar junction.

The inflammatory change may extend deep to the ulcerated epithelium and involve the submucosa, muscular wall, and periesophageal areolar tissue. When this occurs, the distal esophagus becomes palpably and visibly thickened. These changes are evident to the experienced surgeon.

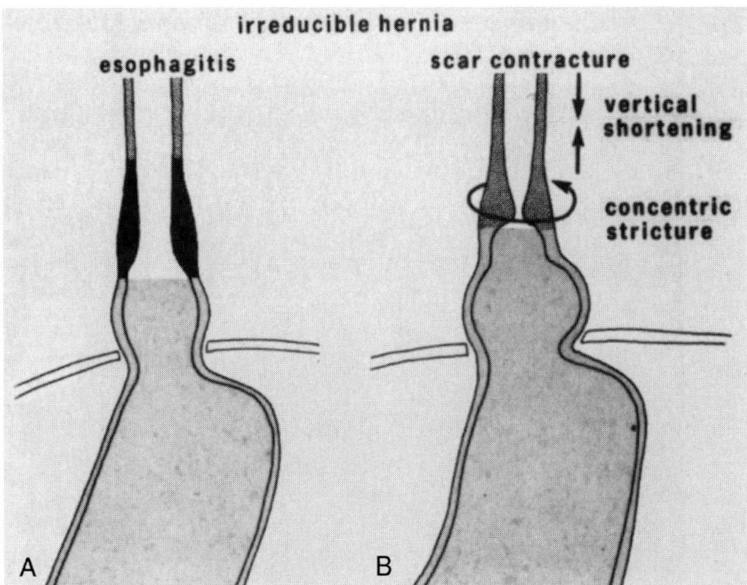

FIGURE 10–1 ■ Diagram illustrating changes due to scarring in patients with panmural peptic esophagitis. *A*, A segment of panmural inflammation (in black) is seen in the distal esophagus extending upward from the squamocolumnar interface. *B*, During the healing phase, scar contraction in this segment results in stenosis due to concentric contraction and in vertical shortening due to longitudinal contraction.

During the healing phase, inflammatory granulation tissue is replaced by scar and collagen. Concentric scar contracture results in stenosis, and vertical scar contracture may produce actual shortening of the esophagus (Fig. 10–1). In extreme cases, the scar may involve periesophageal areolar tissues, and the operating surgeon finds the distal esophagus embedded and adherent in the posterior mediastinum. Esophageal shortening and stenosis are illustrated in Figures 10–2 to 10–4. The histologic appearance of panmural esophagitis with extreme scarring, including the external surface of the distal esophagus, is illustrated in Figure 10–5.

Acquired columnar-lined esophagus is widely accepted as a reflux-related condition that represents a late stage of damage due to reflux esophagitis. Aspects of acquired columnar-lined esophagus are described in detail in Chapters 17 (Pathophysiology), 45, and 46. The mechanism of columnar lining, in my opinion, is one of replacement rather than of metaplasia. As previously stated, the most severe changes due to peptic ulceration occur at the squamocolumnar interface in the squamous epithelium. In cases of ulcerative esophagitis, the entire region is repeatedly bathed in an acid medium (acid, bile, and other digestive juices), and it is logical to assume that only columnar epithelium would grow again in this environment.

The earliest configuration of replacement often is a tongue-like vertical projection of columnar epithelium that extends proximal from the squamocolumnar junction upward in the adjacent squamous mucosa. Experienced endoscopists recognize these flame-shaped projections as the earliest abnormality consistent with columnar replacement. Such changes have been referred to as *short-segment Barrett's esophagus*.

As columnar replacement extends, it may become confluent and ultimately ascend to a very high level (e.g., the aortic arch). During the evolution of this columnar replacement, islands of squamous epithelium may remain behind. Savary and Miller (1977) believe that these squamous islands may form the setting and subsequent site for the development of a peptic ulcer (Barrett's ulcer) in the columnar-lined esophagus. The pathologic changes that occur during the development of acquired columnar-lined esophagus are illustrated diagrammatically in Figures 10–6 to 10–11.

A peptic ulcer in the columnar-lined segment (Barrett's ulcer) has an appearance that is distinctly different from that of the superficial peptic erosions that occur in squamous epithelium. Peptic ulceration in columnar epithelium resembles a gastric or duodenal ulcer, with raised margins and a deep central crater (Fig. 10–12). Such ulcers may occur at any level, including the squamocolumnar junction (junctional ulcer). They may perforate the full thickness of the wall (often producing chest or back pain), bleed massively, or penetrate the pleural or pericardial spaces.

The portion of the distal esophagus that becomes lined with columnar epithelium is no longer susceptible to the same reflux damage that occurs in squamous epithelium. Ongoing esophagitis, therefore, produces esophagitis only in squamous epithelium above the columnar-lined segment. This may lead to peptic strictures in the mid or upper esophagus (Fig. 10–13).

The complications of the development of metaplasia, dysplasia, and adenocarcinoma in acquired columnar-lined esophagus are discussed in Chapters 17 (both subsections), 45, and 46.

Aspiration

If the refluxate rises above the level of the cricopharyngeal sphincter, inflammatory injury may occur in the hypopharynx, larynx, and tracheobronchial tree. Hypopharyngeal inflammation may lead to intermittent sore throat that often is of an obscure origin to the patient. Inflammation and irritation of the larynx may produce hoarseness, and chronic changes in the posterior glottic mucosa have been described that appear secondary to

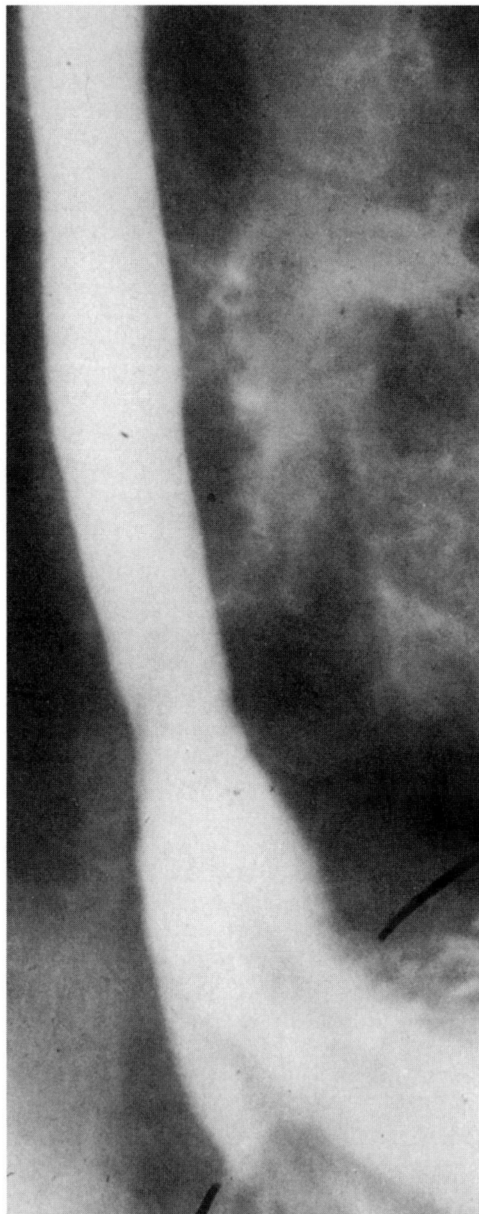

FIGURE 10–2 ■ A barium swallow illustrating a sliding hiatal hernia, which is irreducible in the upright position. An early mild narrowing is evident at the esophagogastric junction. The intrathoracic esophagus runs a straight course through the posterior mediastinum. In the upright position, there is no reduction of the herniated stomach, which is clearly not incarcerated.

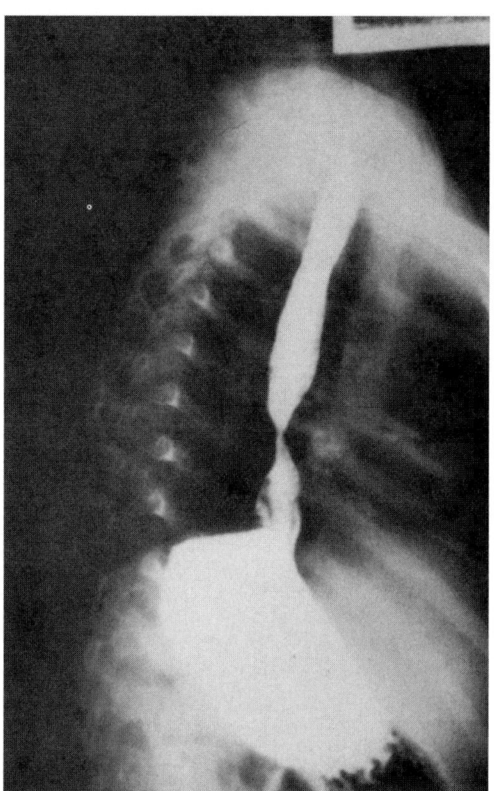

FIGURE 10–3 ■ Photograph illustrating the appearance of the barium swallow in a patient with early acquired shortening and a short, tight peptic stricture. As in Figure 10–2, neither the hernia nor the region of the stenosis changes position with the patient upright.

repeated aspiration of gastroesophageal refluxate. Aspiration into the trachea can produce tracheobronchitis, aspiration pneumonitis, pneumonia, and, on occasion, lung abscess and bronchiectasis (Figs. 10–14 and 10–15).

Aspiration into the tracheobronchial tree may trigger episodes of asthma. This commonly occurs in patients with pre-existing true asthma, who experience exacerbations due to aspiration, usually at night, and to nocturnal regurgitation.

Secondary Motor Defects

Controversy persists regarding the mechanisms of changes that occur in the function of the smooth muscle

Text continued on page 231

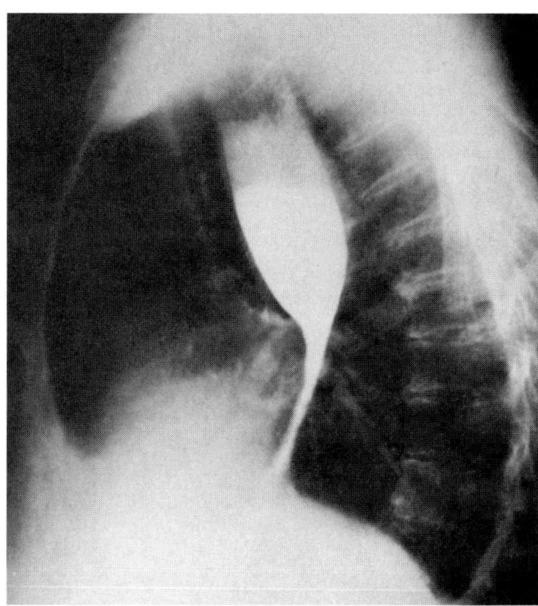

FIGURE 10–4 ■ Photograph showing the barium study in a patient with severe, long-standing peptic stenosis. The top of the stricture lies almost in the midthorax. The proximal esophagus is markedly dilated and contains retained food and fluid.

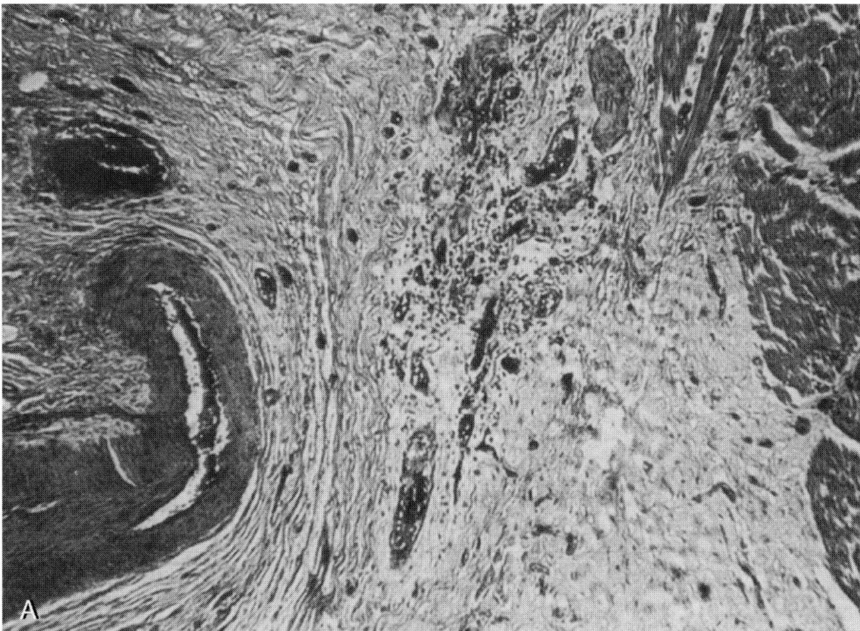

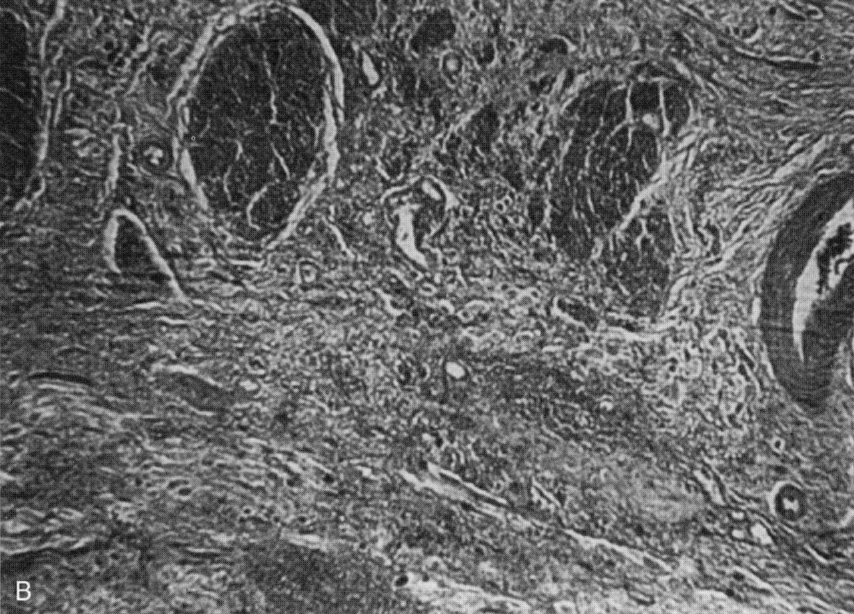

FIGURE 10–5 ■ *A*, Photomicrograph of histology in a patient with severe, panmural esophagitis. The section is taken from the external surface of the esophagus and shows highly vascular inflammatory scar tissue surrounding the muscular wall *(left)*. The longitudinal muscle remains intact and is seen as a thin margin *(right)*. *B*, Photomicrograph showing histology of the esophageal wall in an area of severe panmural esophagitis. The circular muscle is reasonably preserved, although it is infiltrated with some scar and inflammatory tissue *(top half)*. The longitudinal muscle is markedly infiltrated with inflammatory scan and partially replaced *(bottom half)*.

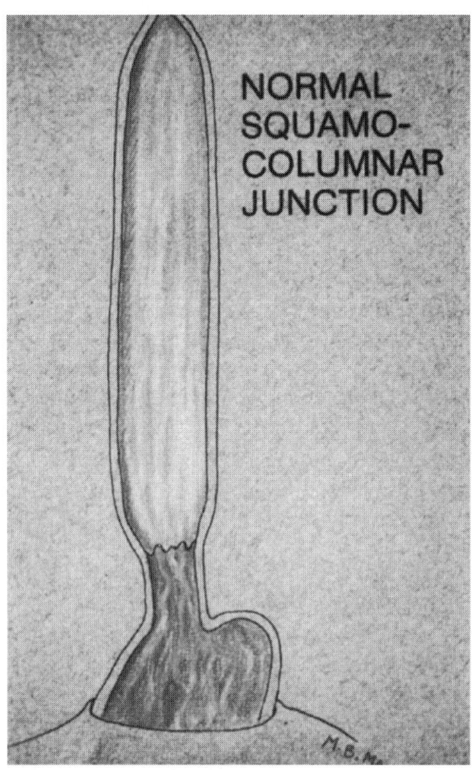

FIGURE 10–6 ■ Diagram illustrating the normal location and configuration of the squamocolumnar mucosal interface. This junction usually lies a little above the level of the anatomic esophagogastric junction and is slightly irregular.

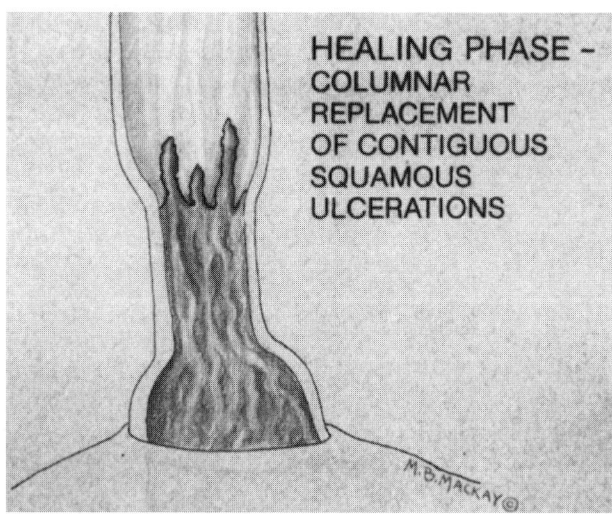

FIGURE 10–8 ■ Diagram illustrating the same case shown in Figure 10–2. With healing, the linear ulcers, which were contiguous with the columnar border, have become replaced with columnar epithelium.

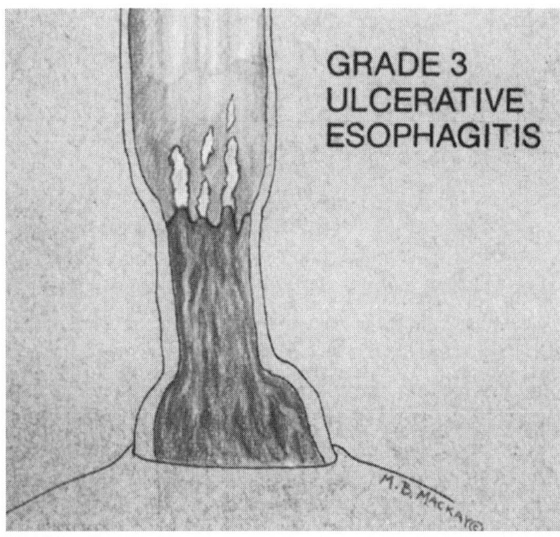

FIGURE 10–7 ■ Diagram illustrating stage 2 linear, ulcerative peptic esophagitis. Linear areas of superficial ulceration involve the distal squamous epithelium. The most severe changes occur just above the squamocolumnar interface, and some of these ulcers are contiguous with the adjacent columnar mucosa.

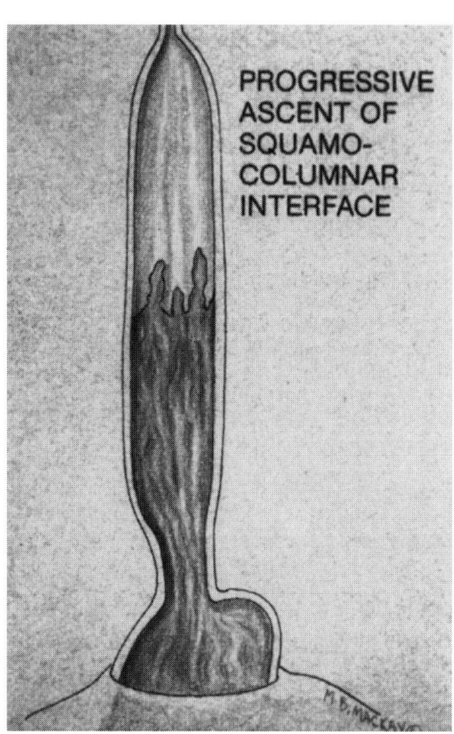

FIGURE 10–9 ■ Diagram illustrating an extensive segment of acquired columnar-lined esophagus in which the squamocolumnar junction now lies in the midthoracic esophagus near the level of the aortic arch.

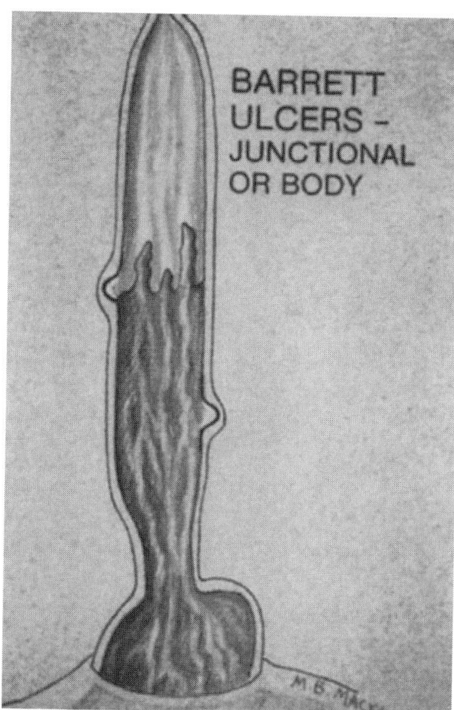

FIGURE 10–10 ■ Diagram illustrating the locations of peptic ulcers (Barrett's ulcers) in columnar-lined esophagus. These ulcers have raised margins and a deep, penetrating base (unlike the superficial erosions of esophagitis in squamous epithelium). They may occur anywhere in the body of the columnar-lined segment. They are referred to as *junctional* ulcers when they occur at the squamocolumnar interface, which is the most common site.

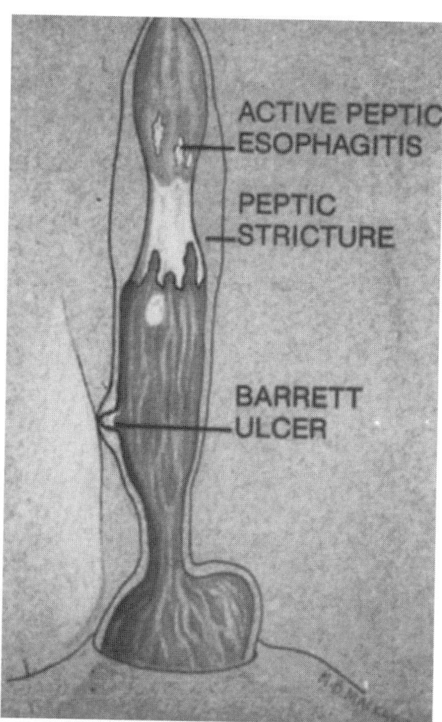

FIGURE 10–11 ■ Diagram illustrating a long segment of acquired columnar-lined esophagus. The columnar-lined segment is protected against the inflammatory changes of reflux, but ongoing inflammation may occur in the adjacent squamous epithelium, even at this high level. The diagram depicts a high peptic stricture with adjacent active ulcerative esophagitis.

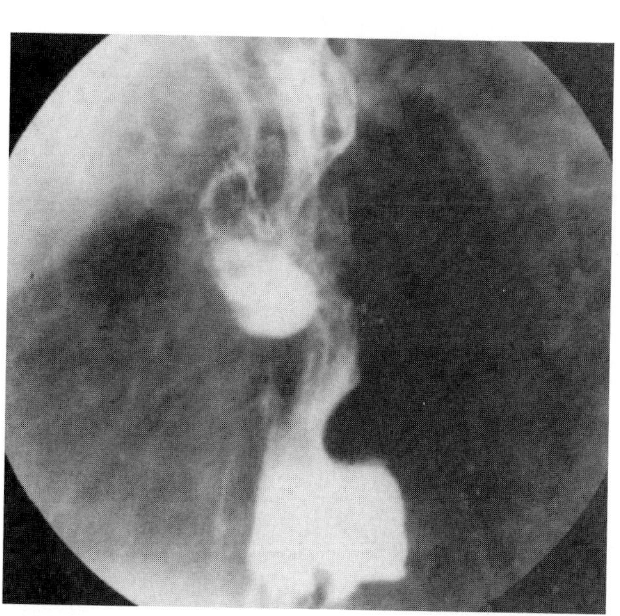

FIGURE 10–12 ■ Photograph of a barium examination showing a very large Barrett's ulcer. This ulcer was in the distal third of the esophagus in a patient with an acquired columnar lining extending to the level of the aortic arch. The deep penetrating ulcer caused pain, and the patient presented acutely with massive, upper gastrointestinal bleeding.

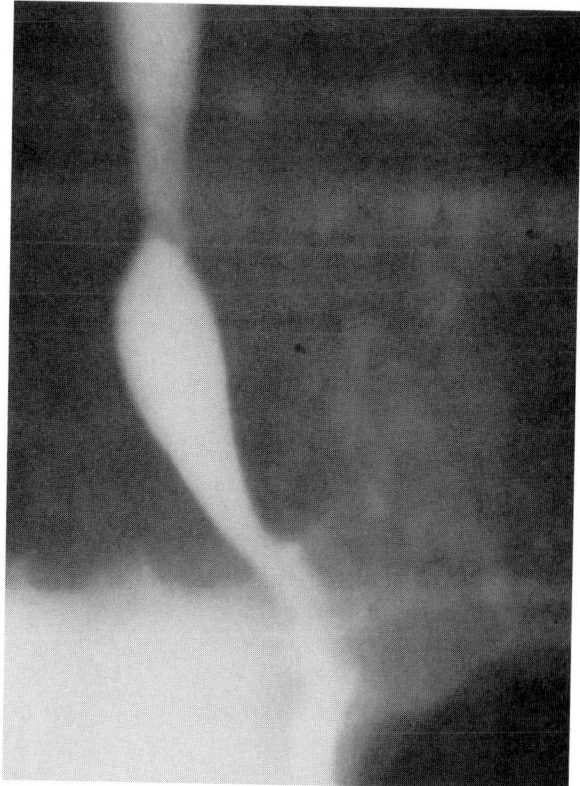

FIGURE 10–13 ■ Photograph illustrating the appearance of a peptic stricture in the middle third of the esophagus, lying above a long segment of acquired columnar lining.

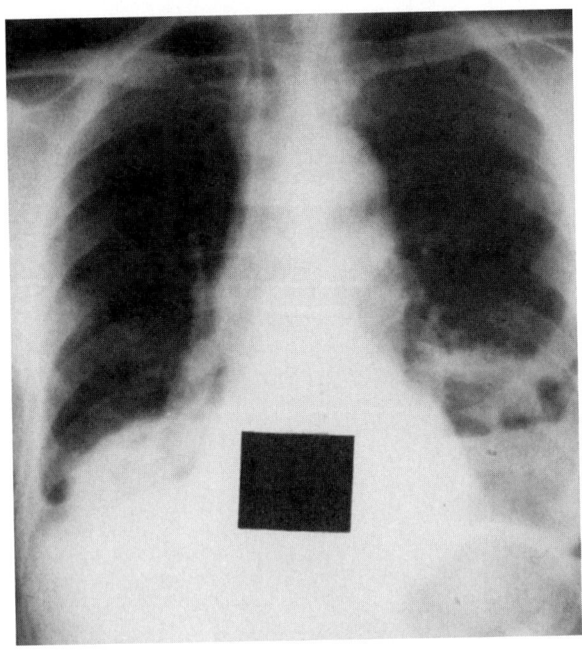

FIGURE 10–14 ■ Plain chest film illustrating bilateral chronic basal pneumonia. A lung biopsy revealed exogenous lipoid pneumonia. It was subsequently established that this patient had experienced years of nocturnal reflux and regularly took large amounts of mineral oil for his chronic constipation before retiring at night.

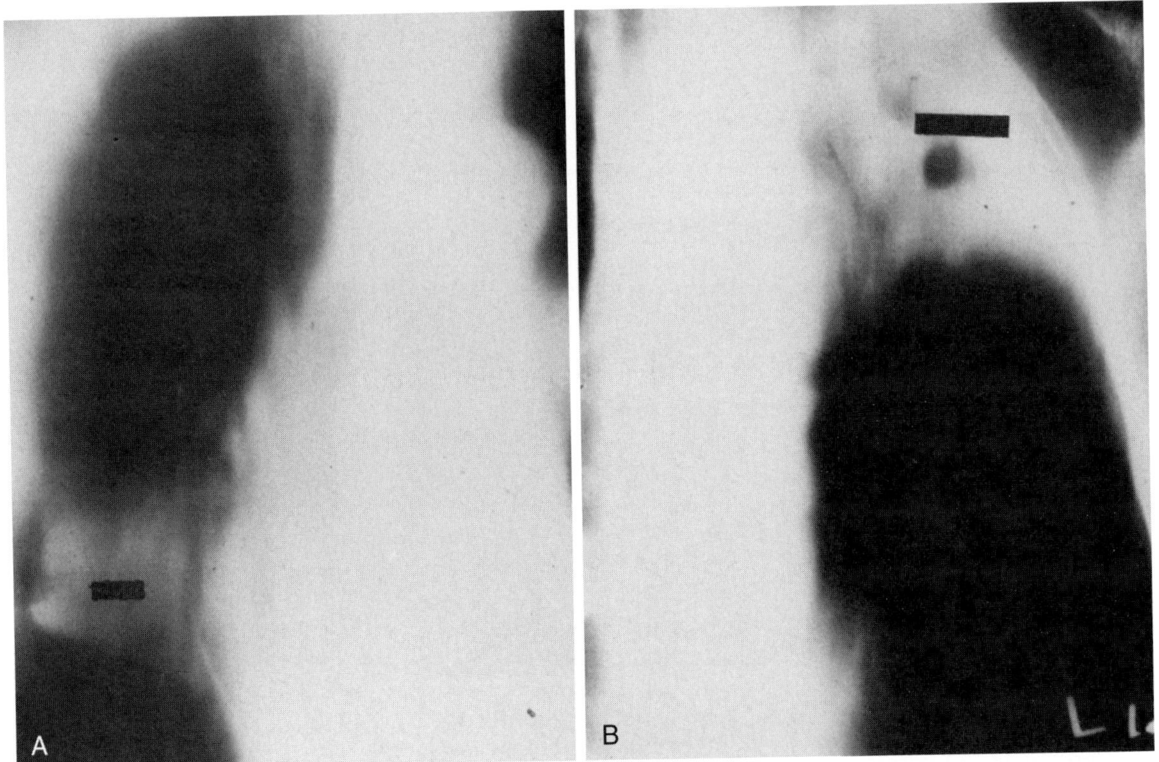

FIGURE 10–15 ■ *A*, A patient presenting with consolidation in the right middle lobe. The appearance was highly suggestive of malignancy, and a middle lobectomy was performed; however, the pathology was found to be exogenous lipoid pneumonia. This patient had a long-standing history of constipation and mineral oil ingestion, associated with free nocturnal reflux. *B*, Despite advice to the contrary, he continued to take mineral oil before going to bed at night, and 2 years later presented with another focus of oil pneumonia in the left upper lobe.

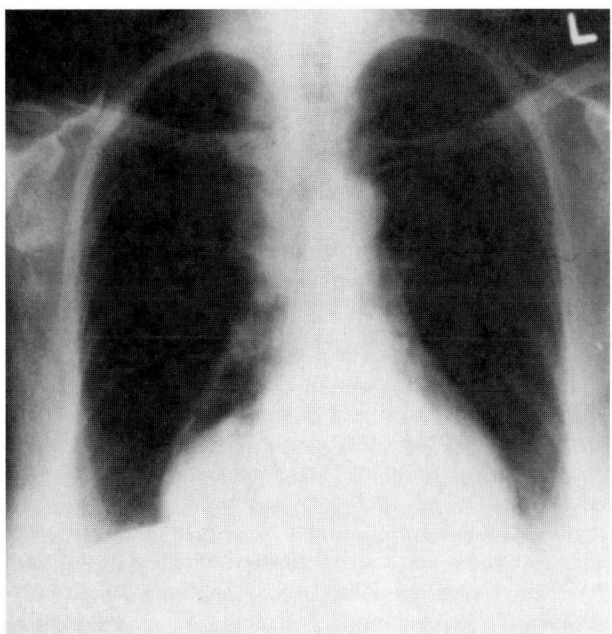

FIGURE 10–16 ■ Chest radiograph showing a large incarcerated hiatal hernia with organoaxial volvulus. The greater curvature side of the stomach now presents to the right of the lower right heart border, which is easily seen in the chest film.

of the distal esophagus and the LES. There is definitive evidence for a significant association of gastroesophageal reflux with diminished pressure in the distal esophageal sphincter (Feldman, 1993; Sloan et al, 1992). Changes have also been observed in peristaltic function. The amplitude of peristaltic contraction may be reduced, particularly in the distal thoracic esophagus. The rate of progression of the peristaltic wave is also slowed. This deterioration in smooth muscle function, both in peristalsis and in the high-pressure zone, is attributed by some to the effects of damage caused by reflux inflammatory change.

A number of studies document the fact that these muscular changes are most pronounced in the more severe stages of reflux esophagitis (DeMeester et al, 1980). Others, on the contrary, suggest that the muscular changes are the primary cause of reflux and that their origin remains obscure (Singh et al, 1992). In either event, a number of studies document that deterioration in both sphincter pressure and the effectiveness of peristalsis does *not* significantly reverse with either medical treatment, including omeprazole (Losec), or successful antireflux surgery (Singh et al, 1992; Sloan et al, 1992).

INCARCERATED HIATAL HERNIA

The detailed pathophysiology and management of incarcerated sliding hiatal hernia are outlined in Chapter 16.

Almost all hiatal hernias are of the sliding axial type. As the size of the herniated stomach increases, the greater curvature rolls up along the left side of the esophagogastric junction. This is understandable, because the greater curvature has a long and free margin whereas the lesser curvature is short and is tethered at the pyloric end. As the intrathoracic stomach enlarges, the greater curvature side of the stomach rotates in the posterior mediastinum and undergoes organoaxial volvulus. The greater curvature side of the stomach now lies on the right side of the inferoposterior mediastinum and is visible on a plain chest film (Fig. 10–16). Once these large hernias reach a sufficient dimension, they become trapped and incarcerated above the diaphragm and do not slide back through the relatively narrow diaphragmatic hiatus even with the patient in the upright position (Fig. 10–17). It is at

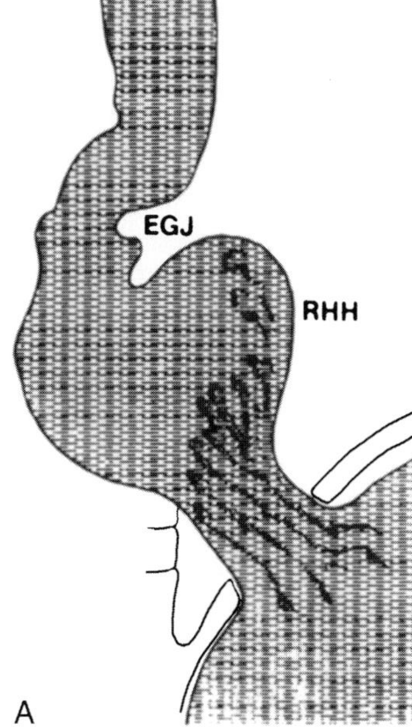

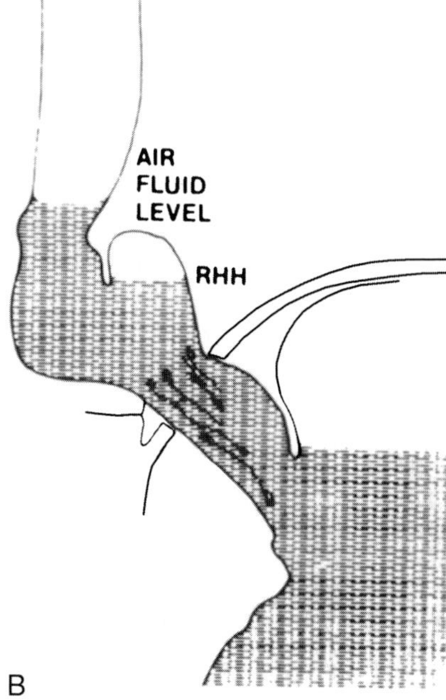

FIGURE 10–17 ■ Diagram illustrating a large, rolling hiatal hernia. *A*, The patient is prone. The hernia (RHH) and the esophagogastric junction (EGJ) are marked. *B*, The patient is upright, and the hernia will not reduce. The stomach remains above the diaphragm, with an air-fluid level in both the stomach and the distal esophagus indicating some degree of trapping or retention.

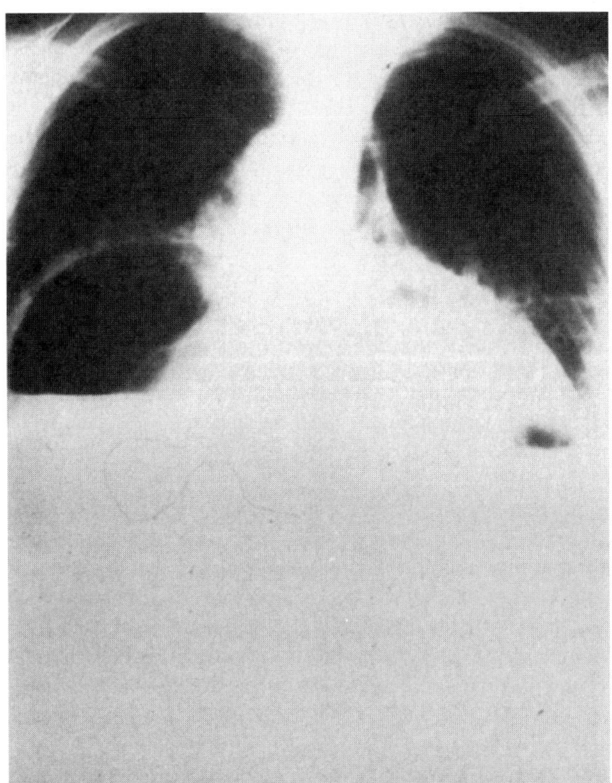

FIGURE 10–18 ■ Grossly distended intrathoracic stomach with organoxial volvulus and trapping of air and fluid in an elderly woman. The distended intrathoracic stomach, occupying almost half of the thoracic cavity on both sides, was responsible for significant exertional dyspnea in the patient.

this stage of incarceration that a number of mechanical complications may occur:

1. *Vascular congestion* may result in bleeding from the incarcerated gastric mucosa. This frequently is subtle and occult, and the patient may initially present with symptoms due to an iron deficiency anemia of obscure origin (dyspnea, palpitations). Gastric ulceration in the intrathoracic pouch probably is the result of ischemia and may result in perforation or massive bleeding. A penetrating intrathoracic gastric ulcer can be responsible for severe and intractable pain.
2. The incarcerated stomach involves varying degrees of *obstruction*. It is common to have some retention of swallowed liquid and solid food, resulting in the complaints of postprandial fullness and retrosternal pressure or discomfort. The incarcerated pouch, filled with air and fluid, may be visible on a plain chest film. On occasion, the organoaxial volvulus is sufficient to produce torsion and complete obstruction of the stomach. The obstruction usually occurs at the pyloric end of the stomach but may occur at the level of the esophagogastric junction. In extreme cases, vascular strangulation with necrosis of the stomach occurs.
3. Certain giant hernias may impair *pulmonary function* as a result of simple space occupation. If the twisted, distended stomach is sufficiently large, it may produce disabling dyspnea and loss of exercise tolerance (Fig. 10–18).

COMMENTS AND CONTROVERSIES

There is ongoing controversy regarding the relative role of the LES and the anatomic presence of a hiatal hernia as positive factors in the creation of pathologic gastroesophageal reflux. A majority of experienced surgeons (with whom I agree) believe that a sliding hiatal hernia creates conditions that predispose to failure of esophagogastric competence. First and foremost, the LES is displaced from the abdomen and surrounded by an environment that is repeatedly exposed to negative pressure. I believe it is likely that the sliding hiatal hernia is of key importance in the induction of reflux. When the esophagogastric junction lies in the chest, the LES is unsupported by positive abdominal pressure and the angle of His is lost. With the development of pathologic reflux and inflammation, there is the potential for a vicious circle of progressive deterioration in both LES sphincter pressure and peristaltic esophageal clearance.

There is continued confusion regarding the origin of acquired columnar-lined esophagus. All agree that most cases are acquired and reflux-related. Some have suggested that this metaplastic change is similar to that which occurs in the ciliated epithelium of the tracheobronchial tree during exposure to cigarette smoke (conversion to squamous epithelium). For a number of reasons, I believe that this perceived mechanism is incorrect. Savary and Miller (1977) have clearly shown with serial endoscopy (documented with photography) that columnar epithelium precisely replaces lost tissue in areas of linear peptic ulceration that abut the squamocolumnar junction. Although islands of squamous epithelium may remain in the columnar-lined segment (presumably they were never lost because of full-thickness ulceration), no islands of columnar epithelium are seen lying above the squamocolumnar interface and totally surrounded by squamous mucosa. One would expect this latter phenomenon to occur if metaplasia of squamous epithelium were the explanation for conversion to an acquired columnar lining.

Another feature of the pathophysiology of reflux esophagitis that is not widely appreciated and has never been clearly documented quantitatively is the phenomenon of "vertical shortening." In extreme, advanced cases, such shortening is evident in the barium study and to the surgeon at the operation. However, shortening is difficult to judge from an abdominal approach and cannot be precisely evaluated with a transthoracic approach in a patient who is anesthetized and paralyzed. Gozzetti and associates (1987) reported efforts to quantify this abnormality. I believe that acquired shortening is of critical importance in the appropriate selection of surgery for patients undergoing antireflux reconstruction.

F. G. P.

■ REFERENCES

Allison PR: Peptic ulcer of the esophagus. J Thorac Surg 15:308, 1946.

Allison PR: Reflux esophagitis, sliding hiatal hernia, and the anatomy of repair. Surg Gynecol Obstet 92:149, 1951.

Allison PR, Johnstone AS: The esophagus lined with gastric membrane. Thorax 8:87, 1953.

Barrett NR: Chronic peptic ulcer of the esophagus and esophagitis. Br J Surg 38:175, 1950.

Berstad A, Weberg R, Fryshov Larsen I, et al: Relationship of hiatus hernia to reflux esophagitis: A prospective study of coincidence, using endoscopy. Scand J Gastroenterol 21:55, 1986.

Cohen S, Harris LD: Does hiatus hernia affect competence of the gastroesophageal sphincter? N Engl J Med 284: 1053, 1971.

DeMeester TR, Wang CI, Wernly JA, et al: Technique, indications and clinical use of 24-hour esophageal pH monitoring. J Thorac Cardiovasc Surg 79:656, 1980.

Dent J, Dodds W J, Friedman RH, et al: Mechanism of gastroesophageal reflux in recumbent asymptomatic human subjects. J Clin Invest 65:256, 1980.

Dodds W J, Dent J, Hogan WJ, et al: Mechanisms of gastroesophageal reflux in patients with reflux esophagitis. N Engl J Med 307:1547, 1982.

Feldman M: Hiatal hernia and gastroesophageal reflux: Another attempt to resolve the controversy. Gastroenterology 105:951, 1993.

Gozzetti G, Mattloll S, Pilotti V, et al: Brachiesofago acquisito. In Magistrelli P, Masett R (eds): Proceedings of the 4th Congress Surgery of Digestive System, June 4–6, 1987, CIC Edizioni Internazionali.

Kaul B, Petersen H, Myrvoid HE, et al: Hiatus hernia in gastroesophageal reflux disease. Scand J Gastroenterol 21:31, 1986.

Ott DJ, Gelfand DW, Chen YM, et al: Predictive relationship of hiatal hernia to reflux esophagitis. Gastrointest Radiol 10:317, 1985.

Savary M, Miller G: L'Oesophage: In Gassman SA (ed): Manuel et Atlas d'Endoscopie. Soleure, Switzerland, 1977.

Singh P, Adamopoulos A, Taylor RH, Colin-Jones DG: Esophageal motor function before and after healing of esophagitis. Gut 33:1590, 1992.

Skinner DB, Belsey RHR: Surgical management of esophageal reflux and hiatus hernia. J Thorac Cardiovasc Surg 53:33, 1967.

Sloan S, Rademaker AW, Kahrilas PJ: Determinants of gastroesophageal junction incompetence: Hiatal hernia, lower esophageal sphincter, or both? Ann Intern Med 117: 12:977, 1992.

Sontag SJ, Schnell TG, Miller TQ, et al: The importance of hiatal hernia in reflux esophagitis compared with lower esophageal sphincter pressure or smoking. J Clin Gastroenterol 13:628, 1991.

CHAPTER **11**

Medical Treatment of Gastroesophageal Reflux Disease

Stuart Jon Spechler

Gastroesophageal reflux disease (GERD) results when the backflow of gastric material into the esophagus or oropharynx causes symptoms, tissue injury, or both. GERD is one of the most common chronic disorders of the gastrointestinal tract (Kahrilas, 1996; Orlando, 1995), and surveys suggest that approximately 20% of adult Americans experience GERD symptoms, such as heartburn and acid regurgitation, at least once each week (Locke et al, 1997; Nebel et al, 1976).

GERD can cause erosions and ulcerations in the squamous epithelium that normally lines the distal esophagus. Esophageal ulcerations can stimulate fibrous tissue deposition with esophageal stricture formation, and the ulcerated squamous epithelium can be replaced by a metaplastic, intestinal-type mucosa (a condition called *Barrett's esophagus*) that predisposes to malignancy. GERD has recently been shown to be a strong risk factor for esophageal adenocarcinoma (Lagergren et al, 1999), a tumor that has nearly quadrupled in frequency in the United States over the past two decades (Richter, 2000).

In addition to the classic manifestations of heartburn and regurgitation, GERD has a number of "atypical" manifestations. For example, acid reflux can cause chest pain that mimics ischemic heart disease (Devesa et al, 1998). In some patients, refluxed gastric material reaches the oropharynx and causes globus, sore throat, burning tongue, dental erosions, and sinusitis (Jailwala and Shaker, 2000). Aspiration of refluxed material into the airway can cause laryngitis and pulmonary problems such as chronic cough and asthma (Harding and Richter, 1997; Koufman, 1991; Ormseth and Wong, 1999).

The development of GERD is a multifactorial process that involves dysfunction of mechanisms that normally prevent excessive gastroesophageal reflux and of mechanisms that normally clear noxious material rapidly from the esophagus (Dodds et al, 1981). These mechanisms are reviewed next.

THE ANTIREFLUX BARRIER

Ordinarily, ambient pressure in the abdomen is higher than that in the chest; consequently, gastroesophageal reflux would occur continuously in the absence of effective antireflux mechanisms (Dodds et al, 1981). Two major elements comprise the normal antireflux barrier: (1) the lower esophageal sphincter (LES), and (2) the crural diaphragm (Mittal and Balaban, 1997).

Lower Esophageal Sphincter

The LES is a segment of specialized, circular, smooth muscle in the wall of the distal esophagus that prevents reflux by maintaining a resting pressure about 10 to 30 mm Hg higher than that in the stomach (Holloway and Dent, 1990). Although the muscle of the LES is morphologically indistinguishable from the muscle of the adjacent esophageal body, LES muscle exhibits a number of distinctive functional characteristics. Unlike muscle of the esophageal body, for example, strips of LES muscle develop spontaneous tension on stretching, and transmural electrical stimulation causes LES muscle strips to relax. With swallowing, the LES normally relaxes for 5 to 8 seconds to allow the swallowed bolus to enter the stomach.

In the 1940s and 1950s, Allison (1951) and others proposed that reflux esophagitis was due primarily to herniation of the stomach into the chest through the esophageal hiatus in the diaphragm (hiatal hernia). The notion that GERD was caused by hiatal hernia prevailed until the 1960s, when researchers (Palmer, 1968) observed the following:

1. Most patients with hiatal hernia had no signs or symptoms of GERD.
2. Some patients with reflux esophagitis had no hiatal hernia.
3. Hiatal hernia repair did not often alleviate reflux esophagitis.

In the early 1970s, investigators at Boston University reported that patients with GERD had feeble LES resting pressures irrespective of the presence of hiatal hernia (Cohen and Harris, 1971). These investigators downplayed the role of hiatal hernia in GERD and popularized the concept that the disorder was caused by an LES that was intrinsically too weak to prevent reflux. Subsequently, it was found that many patients with GERD had normal resting LES pressure values, an observation that cast doubt on the concept that the LES was the primary antireflux barrier (Behar et al, 1976).

In the 1980s, Dodds and his colleagues showed that episodic collapse of LES pressure, a phenomenon called *transient LES relaxation* (TLESR), was the major mechanism of reflux both in normal individuals and in patients with GERD (Dent et al, 1980; Dodds et al, 1982). When LES pressure falls to zero during a TLESR, the sphincter no longer functions as an antireflux barrier. Unlike the brief, appropriate LES relaxations that accompany primary (swallow-induced) peristalsis, TLESRs are not preceded by swallowing, and they last from 10 to 45 seconds (Mittal et al, 1995); in addition, they are associated with relaxation of the crural diaphragm, a phenomenon that also favors gastroesophageal reflux (see later).

The TLESR is part of the normal belch reflex that is triggered by gaseous distention of the stomach (Mittal et al, 1995). In this situation, the TLESR allows gas to escape from the gastric fundus. The nucleus tractus solitarius in the medulla is involved in the reflex, both in integrating sensory information from the stomach and in controlling the neural circuits that trigger the TLESR (Blackshaw et al, 1999).

Medullary neurons with γ-aminobutyric acid B ($GABA_B$) receptors appear to inhibit TLESRs and, accordingly, the $GABA_B$ agonist baclofen has been shown to decrease the frequency of TLESRs in normal subjects (Lidums et al, 2000). Cholinergic blockade with atropine also inhibits TLESRs through a central mechanism (Fang et al, 1999). The sphincter relaxation that characterizes a TLESR is mediated by the activation of cholecystokinin-A (CCK-A) receptors in LES muscle, an effect that can be blocked by the administration of the CCK-A receptor antagonist loxiglumide (Boulant et al, 1997). These observations suggest potential roles for $GABA_B$ agonists, centrally acting anticholinergics, and CCK-A receptor antagonists in the treatment of GERD. Controlled trials are necessary to confirm the therapeutic value of such agents.

Brief episodes of gastroesophageal reflux occur every day in normal individuals, and most of these episodes are the result of TLESRs. In patients with severe GERD, approximately 70% of reflux episodes are the result of TLESRs; the remaining reflux episodes are associated with a variety of events, including (1) periods of feeble basal LES pressure, (2) swallow-induced LES relaxation, and (3) sudden elevations in abdominal pressure (Holloway and Dent, 1990). TLESRs occur approximately two to six times per hour in normal subjects and three to eight times per hour in patients with GERD. Approximately 40% to 50% of TLESRs in normal subjects are accompanied by acid reflux, whereas acid reflux is observed in 60% to 70% of TLESRs in patients with GERD.

Crural Diaphragm

The esophagus passes from the chest into the abdomen through the diaphragmatic hiatus, a tunnel-like opening in the right crus of the diaphragm. By encircling the distal esophagus, the crural muscle can function as an external sphincter that buttresses the LES and prevents gastroesophageal reflux. During inspiration, when the abdominothoracic pressure gradient increases in order to favor reflux, the diaphragmatic crurae contract and pinch the distal esophagus. The pinching effect of the crurae helps to prevent reflux during inspiration and during the sudden increases in abdominal pressure that accompany events such as coughing, sneezing, and straining.

TLESRs are often accompanied by relaxation of the crurae, and studies in dogs have shown that gastroesophageal reflux does not occur during a TLESR unless the episode is attended by neural inhibition of the crural diaphragm (Martin et al, 1992).

Anatomic Features of the Gastroesophageal Junction

In addition to the LES and crural diaphragm, certain anatomic features of the gastroesophageal junction appear to contribute to the antireflux barrier. For example, the acute angle formed by the junction of esophagus and stomach (the angle of His) may function as a one-way flap valve that prevents reflux. Also, a segment of the distal esophagus ordinarily is located within the abdomen, where it is subject to high ambient pressure that tends to force the walls together, thereby preventing reflux (O'Sullivan et al, 1982).

Disruption of the Antireflux Barrier by Hiatal Hernia

Hiatal hernia frequently accompanies severe GERD. It has been known for decades that large hiatal hernias are associated with low LES pressure (Sloan et al, 1992), but only recently has the mechanism underlying this association been elucidated (Kahrilas et al, 1999). During a standard esophageal motility study, esophageal pressures are measured by transducers that are placed in the lumen of the esophagus. The *LES pressure* measured during such a study reflects pressure on the transducer that is generated by both the LES muscle (intrinsic sphincter) and the crural diaphragm (extrinsic sphincter). A better term for this value would be *gastroesophageal junction pressure*, but the term LES pressure is conventional.

With a large hiatal hernia, the LES muscle is displaced up into the chest, dissociated from the crural diaphragm. The intrinsic pressure generated by the sphincter muscle of the esophagus may be normal; however, when separated from the crural diaphragm, which ordinarily contributes to the pressure at the gastroesophageal junction, the measured LES pressure value appears to be low.

When a large hiatal hernia dissociates the function of the internal and external sphincters of the distal esophagus, reflux may occur during the elevations in abdominal pressure caused by events such as inspiration, coughing, and straining. In this situation, the crurae can no longer buttress the LES by pinching the distal esophagus. Instead, contraction of the crurae creates an intrathoracic pouch of stomach whose contents are readily available for reflux. In contrast to normal individuals, furthermore, patients with large hiatal hernias exhibit an increased frequency of TLESRs, induced by gastric distention (Kahrilas et al, 2000). All of these mechanisms appear to contribute to GERD in the patients with a large hiatal hernia.

GASTRIC CONTENTS AND GASTRIC EMPTYING

To cause damage to the esophageal mucosa, the refluxed gastric contents must be caustic. Caustic agents that might be present in the gastric juice include acid and pepsin, produced by the stomach, and pancreaticobiliary products (e.g., bile salts, lysolecithin, and pancreatic digestive enzymes), which can enter the stomach in a retrograde fashion (from the duodenum through the pylorus).

In the era before potent antisecretory medications, such as proton-pump inhibitors (PPIs), physicians debated the relative contributions of the different gastric contents to the pathogenesis of reflux esophagitis. The modern clinical observation that aggressive acid inhibition with PPIs almost always results in the healing of reflux esophagitis suggests that refluxed material other than acid and pepsin contributes little to esophageal damage in GERD (DeVault, 1999). Some experts have proposed that the reflux of bile may play a carcinogenic role in Barrett's esophagus and that non–acid reflux may contribute to some of the extraesophageal manifestations of GERD (DeMeester and DeMeester, 2000). Few data, however, directly support these allegations.

Using sensitive radionuclide tests, McCallum (1990) noted delayed gastric emptying has been found in more than 50% of patients with GERD. With delayed gastric emptying, gastric material available for reflux lingers in and distends the stomach. Gastric distention has at least two undesirable effects for patients with GERD:

1. Gastric distention stimulates gastric acid secretion.
2. Gastric distention is a potent trigger for TLESRs, which allow the acid to flow back into the esophagus.

ESOPHAGEAL CLEARANCE MECHANISMS

To cause injury to the esophagus, caustic refluxed material must be in contact with the mucosa for a sufficient duration. Duration of contact is a function of esophageal clearance mechanisms, which include (1) gravity, (2) peristalsis, (3) salivation, and (4) bicarbonate secretion by the submucosal glands of the esophagus.

When a bolus of acid enters the esophagus, most of the material is cleared by the combined effects of gravity and peristalsis (DeMeester and DeMeester, 2000). The small quantity of residual acidic material that escapes clearance by gravity and peristalsis may cause mucosal damage if it is not neutralized by swallowed saliva (which is highly alkaline) and, to a lesser extent, by bicarbonate secreted into the lumen by the submucosal glands of the esophagus (Helm et al, 1984; Meyers and Orlando, 1992).

GERD often is associated with impaired esophageal acid clearance. Manometric studies have shown that 25% to 48% of patients with reflux esophagitis exhibit abnormalities in peristalsis (e.g., failed or hypotensive peristalsis) that can interfere with esophageal emptying (Kahrilas et al, 1986, 1988). Reflux that occurs during sleep can be particularly damaging to the esophagus for several reasons related to esophageal clearance. In recumbency, gravity retards the clearance of refluxed material. Swallowing and salivation virtually cease during sleep; therefore, there is no primary peristalsis and little saliva available to clear acid from the esophagus.

Cigarette smoking has been shown to increase esophageal acid exposure by increasing the frequency of acid reflux events and by decreasing salivary flow (Kahrilas and Gupta, 1989, 1990). Large hiatal hernias also can impair esophageal clearance because esophageal material that is emptied into the hernia sac often returns to the esophagus (retrograde flow), either during the LES relaxations that normally accompany swallowing or during contractions of stomach muscle that push the gastric contents in both antegrade and retrograde directions (Sloan and Kahrilas, 1991).

ESOPHAGEAL MUCOSAL RESISTANCE

Compared with the stomach and duodenum, the esophagus is highly susceptible to acid-peptic injury (Orlando, 1996). Gastric and duodenal epithelial cells are shielded from luminal acid by a prominent coat of mucus and by a layer of unstirred water that is rich in bicarbonate.

In contrast, the stratified squamous epithelium of the esophagus has only a rudimentary cover of mucus and acid-buffering fluid that provides little protection from attack by hydrogen (H^+) ions. In the stomach and duodenum, minor peptic lesions are repaired quickly through a process called *rapid restitution*, in which epithelial defects left by cells that have succumbed to peptic injury are sealed promptly by the migration of adjacent, healthy cells. Also, acid-induced gastroduodenal damage results in the formation of a protective cap of mucus, cellular debris, and bicarbonate ions that clings to the injured epithelium, like a bandage, to facilitate the healing process. The squamous epithelium of the esophagus lacks the capacity for both rapid restitution and mucus cap formation. Consequently, exposure of the acid-damaged esophagus even to small amounts of refluxed acid can perpetuate and extend the initial peptic injury.

Despite its relative vulnerability, the esophagus has some capacity to resist acid-peptic attack (Orlando, 2000). To penetrate the esophageal epithelium, H^+ ions must pass either through the cell membrane or through intercellular spaces where ion movement is restricted by tight junctions and by intercellular material such as lipid and mucin. Both the squamous cell membranes and their intercellular junctional complexes pose substantial barriers to the passage of H^+ ions. Nevertheless, exposure to relatively high concentrations of acid can overwhelm these barriers. H^+ ions that enter the epithelial cells are buffered by intracellular proteins, phosphate, and bicarbonate. Also, squamous cell membranes have ion transport systems that can extrude H^+ ions out of the cell. These transport systems include a Na^+/H^+ exchanger and a Cl^-/HCO_3^- exchange mechanism. Finally, the esophageal blood supply provides postepithelial protection by removing noxious substances that are extruded from the epithelial cells (e.g., CO_2 and H^+ ions) and by supplying bicarbonate that is used for buffering acid in the intercellular space.

Ambulatory esophageal pH monitoring studies have shown that normal individuals experience brief episodes of acid reflux each day (Orlando, 1996). Apparently, the normal epithelial defenses are sufficient to prevent these brief episodes from causing esophageal injury. Most patients with reflux esophagitis have an abnormally prolonged duration of esophageal acid exposure that overwhelms the normal epithelial defenses. However, some patients have reflux esophagitis even though 24-hour pH monitoring studies demonstrate a normal daily duration of acid reflux (Mattioli et al, 1989). These patients may have yet uncharacterized defects in their epithelial protective factors.

NONSTEROIDAL ANTI-INFLAMMATORY DRUGS

Epidemiologic studies suggest that the ingestion of aspirin and other nonsteroidal anti-inflammatory drugs (NSAIDs) can contribute to GERD (Lanas and Hirschowitz, 1991). Patients with esophageal strictures appear to be especially susceptible to NSAID-induced esophageal injury (Wilkins et al, 1984). Many NSAID preparations are caustic to the mucosa, and severe local injury can result when a stricture or motility abnormality impedes passage of the NSAID tablet into the stomach. In a recent study, furthermore, the NSAID ibuprofen was shown to significantly increase gastroesophageal acid reflux in patients who had symptomatic GERD (Cryer and Spechler, 2000).

HELICOBACTER PYLORI

A number of reports have suggested that gastric infection with *H. pylori* may help to protect the esophagus from the development of GERD and its complications (O'Connor, 1999). For example, one large prospective study of consecutive patients in a general endoscopy unit found that *H. pylori* infection was significantly less common in patients with reflux esophagitis than in control patients without reflux disease (Werdmuller and Loffeld, 1997). Labenz and colleagues (1997) found that patients with duodenal ulcers whose *H. pylori* infections were eradicated with antibiotics developed reflux esophagitis twice as often as patients whose infections persisted. Furthermore, the eradication of *H. pylori* infection has been found to render PPIs less effective in elevating the gastric pH in some patients (Labenz et al, 1996); in one study, patients who had reflux esophagitis and *H. pylori* infection responded significantly better to PPI therapy than did their uninfected counterparts (Holtmann et al, 1999). Graham and others (1998) have proposed that *H. pylori* infections that cause pangastritis also cause a decrease in gastric acid production that protects against GERD. At present, the role of *H. pylori* infection in GERD is disputed.

ENDOSCOPY

For patients with GERD, an endoscopic examination of the esophagus can answer the following four clinical questions listed below:

Clinical Question	Implications of a "Yes" Answer
Is there reflux esophagitis?	Establishes a diagnosis of GERD
Is the esophagitis severe?	Potent antisecretory therapy (e.g., a PPI) will be needed
Is there an esophageal stricture?	Esophageal dilatation may be needed
Is there Barrett's esophagus?	Regular endoscopic surveillance should be advised

The clinician should appreciate that endoscopy does not always answer the question, "Does the patient have GERD?" The endoscopic finding of reflux esophagitis establishes a diagnosis of GERD, but *normal endoscopic findings do not eliminate GERD as a cause of symptoms.* Gastroesophageal reflux can cause disabling symptoms without causing visible esophageal damage (Richter et al, 2000). Endoscopic examination reveals esophagitis in only approximately 50% of patients who complain of frequent heartburn, and a number of studies suggest that heartburn severity is not a reliable index of esophagitis (Johnson et al, 1986; Knill-Jones, 1984; Spechler, 1992). Furthermore, the esophagus typically appears normal endoscopically in patients who have only extraesophageal symptoms of GERD (Koufman, 1991). Patients with classic heartburn who respond readily to conventional antireflux therapy can be assumed to have GERD, and endoscopy is not necessary simply to confirm that diagnosis. Without endoscopic examination, however, it is not possible to answer all of the four clinical questions listed earlier.

The Practice Parameters Committee of the American College of Gastroenterology (1999) has recommended the following guideline on when to perform endoscopic evaluation for patients with GERD:

> If the patient's history is typical for uncomplicated GERD, an initial trial of empirical therapy (including lifestyle modification) is appropriate. Patients in whom empirical therapy is unsuccessful or who have symptoms suggesting complicated disease should have further diagnostic testing. Selected individuals who have long-standing symptoms or who require continuous therapy may need endoscopic screening for Barrett's esophagus.

In another publication dealing specifically with Barrett's esophagus (1999), this same committee recommended the following:

> Patients with long-standing GERD symptoms, particularly those ≥50 years of age, should have upper endoscopy to detect Barrett's esophagus.

Symptoms that might suggest complicated disease requiring early endoscopic evaluation (without an empirical trial of therapy) include fever, anorexia, weight loss, dysphagia, odynophagia, and bleeding. Although these proposed approaches to patient management seem reasonable, it is important to recognize that they are merely committee recommendations whose efficacy has not been established by formal clinical investigation. Also, there is no clear consensus regarding which is the most appropriate medication to use for initial empirical therapy of GERD (i.e., a histamine H_2-receptor blocker or a PPI).

MANAGEMENT

When planning a management strategy for patients with GERD, we must appreciate that the efficacy of any antireflux therapy is inversely related to the severity of the underlying reflux esophagitis; that is, the worse the esophagitis, the poorer the healing rate (DeVault and Castell, 1995; Kahrilas, 1996). A treatment that is highly effective for mild esophagitis may be virtually useless for patients with severe disease (Wesdorp et al, 1993). This part of the text outlines a stepwise approach to the therapy of GERD. However, for patients with severe, ulcerative reflux esophagitis, it is appropriate to begin therapy immediately with potent acid suppression (i.e., by administering a PPI) rather than proceeding stepwise through trials of agents unlikely to effect healing. Conversely, it may not be appropriate to begin the treatment of very mild GERD with a PPI.

Life-style Modifications

It is traditional to recommend that the management of GERD begin with the following life-style modifications aimed at decreasing esophageal acid exposure:

1. *Elevate the head of the bed on 4- to 6-inch blocks.* This step exploits the effect of gravity on esophageal clearance.
2. *Advise weight loss for obese patients.* In theory, obesity may increase abdominal pressure and thereby promote reflux.
3. *Avoid recumbency for 3 hours after meals.* TLESRs associated with gastroesophageal reflux occur most commonly after meals, and recumbency delays esophageal clearance of the refluxed material.
4. *Avoid bedtime snacks.* Eating before bed may trigger TLESRs and may stimulate nocturnal acid secretion, thereby promoting nocturnal reflux that can be especially damaging to the esophagus.
5. *Avoid fatty foods, chocolate, peppermint, onions, and garlic.* These foods may decrease LES pressure and may delay gastric emptying, thereby promoting acid reflux.
6. *Avoid cigarettes and alcohol.* These agents may decrease LES pressure. Cigarette smoking also may decrease salivation, which is important for esophageal acid clearance.
7. *Avoid drugs that decrease LES pressure and delay gastric emptying.* This category includes calcium channel blockers and drugs that have anticholinergic effects.
8. *Avoid NSAIDs.*

Data that support the efficacy of these life-style modifications in controlling GERD are limited, and it is unclear how many patients who are prescribed such modifications actually implement the measures.

Antacids and Alginic Acid

Antacids and alginic acid can temporarily relieve episodic heartburn (Graham and Patterson, 1983; Sampliner et al, 1999; Wesdorp et al, 1993). However, few data are available on the utility of these agents for healing of reflux esophagitis or for long-term management of GERD symptoms.

Histamine H_2-Receptor Blocking Agents

For patients with mild GERD who respond well to life-style modifications, medications may not be necessary, and antacids can be used to relieve occasional episodes of heartburn. For patients with persistent symptoms, H_2-receptor blocking agents can be prescribed. Four agents are available in the United States (cimetidine, ranitidine, famotidine, and nizatidine), and all are similar in efficacy and side effect profiles.

When administered in conventional doses, these agents are safe medications that can be expected to relieve GERD symptoms and heal esophagitis within 12 weeks in approximately half to two thirds of all patients (Chiba et al, 1997; DeVault and Castell, 1995; Graham and Patterson, 1983; Kitchin and Castell, 1991; Sontag, 1990; Wesdorp et al, 1993). H_2-blockers are most useful for patients with GERD of mild to moderate severity in whom high rates of healing can be anticipated; however, healing rates with H_2-blockers are poor for patients with severe reflux esophagitis (Wesdorp et al, 1993). High doses of H_2-receptor blockers (up to eight times the conventional dose) have been used effectively to treat esophagitis in resistant cases (Collen et al, 1990; Collen and Johnson, 1992), but this approach generally is not recommended.

Few data document the long-term efficacy of H_2-blockers used in any dosage, and tolerance to these agents is known to develop (Smit et al, 1996). For patients with severe GERD, it seems preferable to use a more potent inhibitor of gastric acid secretion (i.e., a PPI) than to use high-dose H_2-blocker therapy.

Prokinetic Agents

In theory, prokinetic agents may be able to decrease gastroesophageal reflux by increasing LES pressure and by enhancing gastric emptying (McCallum, 1990). Only two prokinetics have been used widely in the United States: metoclopramide and cisapride.

Metoclopramide, a dopamine antagonist, has some therapeutic efficacy in patients with mild GERD. The use of metoclopramide is limited by its frequent side effects, such as agitation, restlessness, somnolence, and extrapyramidal symptoms that occur in up to 30% of patients.

Cisapride, a serotonin-4 (5-HT_4) receptor agonist, appears to work as a prokinetic agent by increasing the availability of acetylcholine released from enteric neurons. A number of studies have shown therapeutic efficacy for cisapride in patients with mild GERD. However, as of July 14, 2000, Janssen Pharmaceutica discontinued the marketing of cisapride because the drug was found to cause lethal cardiac arrhythmias in patients with a number of predisposing conditions. Consequently, cisapride is no longer available for the treatment of GERD.

Sucralfate

Sucralfate is an exceptionally safe medication that has some demonstrated efficacy in the treatment of mild reflux esophagitis (Hameeteman, 1991; Orlando, 1991). Relatively little published information is available on the use of sucralfate in GERD, however, and the drug has never achieved popularity as an antireflux therapeutic agent.

Proton-Pump Inhibitors

The PPIs omeprazole, lansoprazole, rabeprazole, and pantoprazole have been shown to be extremely effective agents for the treatment of GERD. Like the four H_2-receptor blockers, the four available PPIs are similar in efficacy and side effect profiles. A fifth agent, esomeprazole, is expected to be available soon.

Preliminary studies suggest that when used in conventional dosage, esomeprazole may bring about marginally higher rates of healing of reflux esophagitis compared with the use of other PPIs (Kahrilas et al, 2000). In patients with mild to moderately severe reflux esophagitis treated with PPIs in conventional dosages, healing rates of 80% to 100% can be expected within 8 to 12 weeks (Chiba et al, 1997; DeVault and Castell, 1995; Sontag, 1990); however, very severe (grade 4) reflux esophagitis may persist despite conventional-dose PPI therapy in up to 40% of cases (Kahrilas et al, 2000). In most such resistant cases, the esophagitis usually can be healed by increasing the dose of the PPI (Hetzel et al, 1988; Holloway et al, 1996; Klinkenberg-Knol et al, 1994, 2000). Recent studies also have shown that aggressive acid suppression with PPIs improves dysphagia and decreases the need for esophageal dilatation in patients with peptic esophageal strictures (Marks et al, 1994; Smith et al, 1994).

For patients with severe GERD who respond to PPIs, GERD usually returns shortly after the drug is discontinued, and maintenance therapy is required (Dent et al, 1994). For most patients, the dose of PPI necessary to maintain remission is at least the dose required to heal the acute esophagitis. This phenomenon is illustrated in Figure 11–1 which shows the results of a study on maintenance therapies for GERD (Dent et al, 1994).

One hundred fifty-nine patients with reflux esophagitis who healed within 8 weeks of treatment with omeprazole 20 mg once a day were randomly assigned to receive long-term maintenance therapy with daily omeprazole (20 mg once a day), weekend omeprazole (20 mg on 3 consecutive days of the week), or daily ranitidine (150 mg twice a day). At 12 months, actuarial analysis revealed an 89% rate of sustained remission for patients treated with daily omeprazole in contrast to rates of only 32% and 25% for patients receiving weekend omeprazole and daily ranitidine, respectively ($P < .001$). For patients with severe GERD, furthermore, the PPI maintenance dose requirement often increases with time. One long-term study of patients who had severe GERD treated with a maintenance dose of omeprazole (20 mg/day) found that relapses occurred frequently (at the rate of 1 per 9.4 treatment-years) and that patients often required increasing doses of omeprazole (up to 120 mg/day) to maintain GERD in remission (Klinkenberg-Knol et al, 2000).

The profound acid suppression that can be achieved with the use of PPIs has raised theoretical concerns regarding their long-term safety. Protracted acid suppression can elevate the serum level of gastrin, a hormone that exerts trophic effects on the stomach and colon and that has the potential to result in colonization of the stomach with bacteria that can convert dietary nitrates to carcinogenic nitrosamines. These effects, conceivably, might contribute to the development of gastric and colonic neoplasms. Furthermore, some data suggest that sustained acid suppression with PPIs might hasten the development of gastric atrophy in patients who are infected with *H. pylori* (Kuipers et al, 1996) and that chronic PPI therapy might interfere with vitamin B_{12} absorption (Schenk et al, 1996).

Despite these theoretical concerns, there have been no reports of tumors or nutritional deficiencies clearly attributable to the use of PPIs after more than a decade of extensive clinical experience with these agents (DeVault et al, 1999).

Antireflux Surgery

There are a number of different antireflux operations (e.g., Nissen, Belsey, Toupet fundoplication), but all share some fundamental features (Dunnington and DeMeester, 1993; Hinder et al, 1999; Peters et al, 1995). In each of these procedures, the surgeon creates an intra-abdominal segment of esophagus, reduces the hiatal hernia, approximates the diaphragmatic crurae, and wraps a portion of

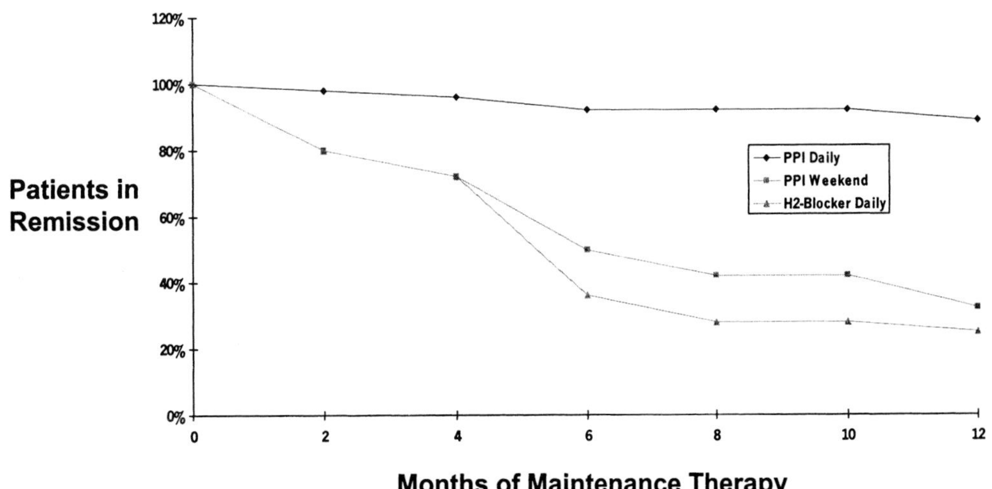

FIGURE 11–1 ■ Maintenance therapy for patients with reflux esophagitis. (Data from Dent J, Yeomans ND, Mackinnon M, et al: Omeprazole v ranitidine for prevention of relapse in reflux oesophagitis. Gut 35:590–598, 1994.)

the gastric fundus around the distal esophagus (fundoplication). These maneuvers create a barrier to gastroesophageal reflux through a number of potential mechanisms (Jamieson, 1987; Rydberg et al, 1999).

The surgery narrows the angle of His, which may create an antireflux flap-valve effect. Restoration of the distal esophagus to the positive-pressure environment of the abdomen also may prevent reflux. Reduction of the hiatal hernia and approximation of the diaphragmatic crurae may enable the crural diaphragm to buttress the LES and to pinch the distal esophagus during inspiration, thereby restoring a normal antireflux mechanism. The fundoplication itself may act as a one-way valve and also may prevent the distention of the gastric fundus, a state that can trigger TLESRs.

A number of reports have described excellent results for fundoplication, with more than 85% of patients experiencing relief of their signs and symptoms of GERD (Dunnington and DeMeester, 1993; Hinder et al, 1999; Peters et al, 1995). However, few studies on this issue have been prospective and randomized. A large Department of Veterans Affairs Cooperative Study conducted in the late 1980s prospectively compared the efficacy of available medical and surgical therapies for GERD (Spechler, 1992). All 247 study subjects had GERD complicated by Barrett's esophagus, esophageal ulceration, esophageal stricture, or severe erosive esophagitis. Antireflux life-style modifications were prescribed for all patients regardless of treatment group. Patients were randomly assigned to receive one of three types of treatment:

1. *Continuous medical therapy* included antacid tablets and ranitidine taken on a daily basis regardless of symptoms; metoclopramide and sucralfate were added in a stepwise fashion for patients who remained symptomatic.
2. *Symptomatic medical therapy* included drugs used only for control of symptoms. Therapy began with antacid tablets, and ranitidine, metoclopramide, and sucralfate were added in a stepwise fashion for symptoms that could not be controlled with antacids alone.
3. *Surgical therapy* consisted of a Nissen fundoplication.

All three therapies resulted in significant improvements in the symptoms and endoscopic signs of GERD for up to 2 years. However, surgical therapy produced significantly better results than both medical therapies administered for the 2-year duration of the study. Overall satisfaction with therapy also was higher for the surgical patients. This prospective, randomized study clearly demonstrated that surgical therapy was superior to medical therapy (without PPIs) for the short-term treatment of GERD.

Today, antireflux surgery can be performed laparoscopically, and a number of reports have described the short-term results of laparoscopic fundoplication (Anvari et al, 1995; Hinder et al, 1994, 1999; Jamieson et al, 1994; Peters et al, 1995). The technique of laparoscopic Nissen fundoplication is virtually identical to that of the open procedure, and the mortality rate is between 0.2% and 0.4% (Jamieson et al, 1994; Rantanen et al, 1999). The laparoscopic approach has become popular, not because it is safer or because it produces a better functional result than the open procedure, but because of proposed advantages in the degree of postoperative discomfort, duration of hospital stay, and cosmetic outcome (Collard et al, 1994).

Two randomized trials of laparoscopic and open Nissen fundoplication have found no significant differences in the functional results of the two procedures, such as relief of GERD symptoms and reduction in esophageal acid exposure (Bais et al, 2000; Laine et al, 1997). However, one of those studies was terminated prematurely because an interim analysis showed an excess of adverse outcomes in the group treated laparoscopically (Bais et al, 2000). Furthermore, at least one study has shown that the primary factor involved in overall patient satisfaction with antireflux surgery is relief of GERD symptoms, not the operative approach (Rattner and Brooks, 1995). These observations suggest that the availability of laparoscopic surgery should not be a major factor in the physician's decision regarding the advisability of fundoplication. The primary decision for the clinician is whether or not the patient should have an antireflux operation, not how the operation should be performed.

One of the most crucial and controversial issues concerning the role of antireflux surgery in the treatment of GERD relates to the long-term outcome of the procedure. Relatively few reports deal with the late results of fundoplication, and those that do describe contradictory findings. Some investigators have reported success rates that exceed 90% at 10 to 20 years after open fundoplication (DeMeester et al, 1986; Grande et al, 1994); others have described breakdown of the operation and the return of reflux esophagitis in more than 50% of cases within 6 years (Brand et al, 1979). Furthermore, the conclusions of long-term studies on fundoplication often have been based on subjective results alone, and few reports have included objective evidence for control of GERD (e.g., results of endoscopic examinations and 24-hour esophageal pH monitoring studies) (Luostarinen et al, 1993). Fundoplication has been performed laparoscopically only since 1991, and long-term results of laparoscopic antireflux surgery are thus not yet available.

Recently, the preliminary results of a follow-up study on the patients who participated in the Veterans Affairs Cooperative Study on reflux disease were reported in abstract form (Spechler et al, 2000a, 2000b). The follow-up study is unique in providing data on the long-term outcome of a well-defined cohort of patients who had participated in a prospective, randomized trial of medical and surgical treatments for GERD.

Using a professional search agency, the investigators determined the whereabouts of 239 (97%) of the original 247 study patients. One hundred twenty-nine of the 160 known survivors agreed to participate in the follow-up study, which included a GERD history, GERD symptom scoring, endoscopic examination, and completion of the Short Form (SF)-36 Survey on general health and well-being. Seventy-nine patients died: 33 (40%) of the 82 surgical patients and 46 (28%) of the 165 medical patients. Survival over a period of 140 months was significantly shorter in the surgical group (P = .047; RR, 1.57, 95% confidence interval 1.01 to 2.46).

During the follow-up period of 10 to 13 years, surgical patients were much less likely to take antireflux medications regularly, and when antireflux medications were discontinued, their GERD symptoms were significantly less severe than those of the medical patients. However, 62% of the surgical patients took antireflux medications on a regular basis, and there were no significant differences between the groups in the rates of neoplastic and peptic complications of GERD, overall physical and mental well-being scores, and overall satisfaction with antireflux therapy. For reasons that are not clear, antireflux surgery was associated with a significant decrease in long-term survival.

Endoscopic Antireflux Procedures

Two new endoscopic therapies for GERD have now been approved by the Food and Drug Administration (FDA):

1. The Bard endoscopic suturing system uses an endoscopic sewing machine device to plicate the gastroesophageal junction from the mucosal side.
2. The Stretta radiofrequency energy system delivers radiofrequency (microwave) energy that creates thermal lesions in the LES muscle.

Although these devices have been FDA-approved and are being sold to physicians for clinical application, there have been no controlled trials demonstrating the efficacy of the procedures. The small clinical studies (the largest has only 64 patients) available on these procedures have been reported only in abstract form (DiBaise et al, 2000; Filipi et al, 2000; Kim et al, 2000; Triadafilopoulos et al, 2000). Consequently, the efficacy of these endoscopic techniques is not known. Furthermore, it is not clear how the procedures create an antireflux barrier (if, in fact, they do), and the safety of the techniques is questionable, even though no serious complications were observed in the small clinical studies.

Before recommending any invasive antireflux procedure, the clinician should consider that GERD is a rare cause of mortality (Spechler, 2000). Despite the rising incidence of esophageal adenocarcinoma, GERD is a benign condition in the majority of affected patients. Esophageal cancer is an uncommon cause of death, even for patients with severe GERD, and the Veterans Affairs Cooperative Study found no significant difference in the rate of esophageal cancer development between groups of medically and surgically treated patients (Spechler et al, 2000a, 2000b). Indeed, long-term survival for the surgical patients was shorter than that for the medical group.

Rather than preventing deaths from cancer, the use of the invasive therapy, unexpectedly, was associated with a higher long-term mortality rate. In light of these findings, the new endoscopic antireflux procedures should not be recommended with the promise that they can prevent esophageal adenocarcinoma. The wise clinician will await the results of controlled, clinical trials before recommending invasive and potentially hazardous therapies for the treatment of a benign condition that is easily controlled with safe medications.

COMMENTS AND CONTROVERSIES

This chapter begins with a concise but thorough presentation on the currently perceived mechanisms responsible for reflux disease and sets the stage for the presentation of a stepwise approach to management.

During the past few years, it has been repeatedly demonstrated that only therapy with one of the PPIs provides likely and more realistic control of the advanced stages of reflux esophagitis—confluent ulceration, peptic stricture, and extensive columnar replacement (Barrett's esophagus). Thus, it is recommended that therapy start with PPI drugs in these complicated cases. The author appropriately notes the dearth of long-term follow-up data, even for medical and surgical management in regular use throughout many years. Even less frequent are efforts to evaluate therapy with randomized trials.

At the conclusion of this chapter, Dr. Spechler emphasizes the benign nature of almost all cases of reflux disease. Although the incidence of adenocarcinoma of the distal esophagus has increased 4-fold during the past decade, it is still a very rare malignancy, and the incidence of adenocarcinoma development in an area of columnar replacement (Barrett's esophagus) is currently reported to be 0.5 per 100 cases per year. Importantly, Dr. Spechler points out that there has been no evidence, until now, to indicate that either medical or surgical management of reflux is capable of reducing the risk of malignancy.

F.G.P.

REFERENCES

Allison PR: Reflux esophagitis, sliding hiatal hernia, and the anatomy of repair. Surg Gynecol Obstet 92:419–431, 1951.

Anvari M, Allen C, Borm A: Laparoscopic Nissen fundoplication is a satisfactory alternative to long-term omeprazole therapy. Br J Surg 82:938–942, 1995.

Bais JE, Bartelsman JRWM, Bonjer HJ, et al, and the Netherlands Antireflux Surgery Study Group: Laparoscopic or conventional Nissen fundoplication for gastro-oesophageal reflux disease: Randomised clinical trial. Lancet 355:170–174, 2000.

Behar J, Biancani P, Sheahan DG: Evaluation of esophageal tests in the diagnosis of reflux esophagitis. Gastroenterology 71:9–15, 1976.

Blackshaw LA, Staunton E, Lehmann A, Dent J: Inhibition of transient LES relaxations and reflux in ferrets by GABA receptor agonists. Am J Physiol 277:G867–G874, 1999.

Boulant J, Mathieu S, D'Amato M, et al: Cholecystokinin in transient lower oesophageal sphincter relaxation due to gastric distention in humans. Gut 40:575–581, 1997.

Brand DL, Eastwood IR, Martin D, et al: Esophageal symptoms, manometry, and histology before and after antireflux surgery: A long-term follow-up study. Gastroenterology 76:1393–1401, 1979.

Chiba N, De Gara CJ, Wilkinson JM, Hunt RH: Speed of healing and symptom relief in grade II to IV gastroesophageal reflux disease: A meta-analysis. Gastroenterology 112:1798–1810, 1997.

Cohen S, Harris LD: Does hiatus hernia affect competence of the gastroesophageal sphincter? N Engl J Med 284:1053–1056, 1971.

Collard JM, de Gheldere CA, De Kock M, et al: Laparoscopic antireflux surgery: What is real progress? Ann Surg 220:146–154, 1994.

Collen MJ, Johnson DA: Correlation between basal acid output and daily ranitidine dose required for therapy in Barrett's esophagus. Dig Dis Sci 37:570–576, 1992.

Collen MJ, Lewis JH, Benjamin SB: Gastric acid hypersecretion in refractory gastroesophageal reflux disease. Gastroenterology 98:654–661, 1990.

Cryer B, Spechler SJ: Effects of nonsteroidal anti-inflammatory drugs

(NSAIDs) on acid reflux in patients with gastroesophageal reflux disease (GERD). Gastroenterology 118:A862, 2000.

DeMeester SR, DeMeester TR: Columnar mucosa and intestinal metaplasia of the esophagus: Fifty years of controversy. Ann Surg 231:303–321, 2000.

DeMeester TR, Bonavina L, Albertucci M: Nissen fundoplication for gastroesophageal reflux disease: Evaluation of primary repair in 100 consecutive patients. Ann Surg 204:9–20, 1986.

Dent J, Dodds WJ, Friedman RH, et al: Mechanism of gastroesophageal reflux in recumbent asymptomatic human subjects. J Clin Invest 65:256–267, 1980.

Dent J, Yeomans ND, Mackinnon M, et al: Omeprazole v ranitidine for prevention of relapse in reflux oesophagitis. Gut 35:590–598, 1994.

DeVault KR: Overview of medical therapy for gastroesophageal reflux disease. Gastrointest Clin North Am 28:831–845, 1999.

DeVault KR, Castell DO: Guidelines for the diagnosis and treatment of gastroesophageal reflux disease. Arch Intern Med 155:2165–2173, 1995.

DeVault KR, Castell DO, and The Practice Parameters Committee of the American College of Gastroenterology: Updated guidelines for the diagnosis and treatment of gastroesophageal reflux disease. Am J Gastroenterol 94:1434–1442, 1999.

Devesa SS, Blot WJ, Fraumeni JF Jr: Changing patterns in the incidence of esophageal and gastric carcinoma in the United States. Cancer 15;83:2049–2053, 1998.

DiBaise JK, Akromis I, Quigley EM: Efficacy of radiofrequency energy delivery to the lower esophageal sphincter in the treatment of GERD. Gastrointest Endosc 51:AB96, 2000.

Dodds WJ, Dent J, Hogan WJ, et al: Mechanisms of gastroesophageal reflux in patients with reflux esophagitis. N Engl J Med 307:1547–1552, 1982.

Dodds WJ, Hogan WJ, Helm JF, Dent JF: Pathogenesis of reflux esophagitis. Gastroenterology 81:376–394, 1981.

Dunnington GL, DeMeester TR: The outcome effect of adherence to operative principles of Nissen fundoplication by multiple surgeons. Am J Surg 166:654–657, 1993.

Fang JC, Sarosiek I, Yamamoto Y, et al: Cholinergic blockade inhibits gastro-oesophageal reflux and transient lower oesophageal sphincter relaxation through a central mechanism. Gut 44:603–607, 1999.

Filipi CJ, Edmundowicz SA, Gostout CH, et al: Transoral endoscopic suturing for gastroesophageal reflux disease: A multicenter trial. Gastrointest Endosc 51:AB143, 2000.

Graham DY, Patterson DJ: Double-blind comparison of liquid antacid and placebo in the treatment of symptomatic reflux esophagitis. Dig Dis Sci 28:559–563, 1983.

Graham DY, Yamaoka Y: *H. pylori* and cagA: Relationships with gastric cancer, duodenal ulcer, and reflux esophagitis and its complications. Helicobacter 3:145–150, 1998.

Grande L, Toledo-Pimentel V, Manterola C, et al: Value of Nissen fundoplication in patients with gastro-oesophageal reflux judged by long-term symptom control. Br J Surg 81:548–550, 1994.

Hameeteman W: Clinical studies of sucralfate in reflux esophagitis: The European experience. J Clin Gastroenterol 13(Suppl 2):S16–S20, 1991.

Harding SM, Richter JE: The role of gastroesophageal reflux in chronic cough and asthma. Chest 111:1389–1402, 1997.

Helm JF, Dodds WJ, Pele LR, et al: Effect of esophageal emptying and saliva on clearance of acid from the esophagus. N Engl J Med 310:284–288, 1984.

Hetzel DJ, Dent J, Reed WD, et al: Healing and relapse of severe peptic esophagitis after treatment with omeprazole. Gastroenterology 95:903–912, 1988.

Hinder RA, Filipi CJ, Wetscher G, et al: Laparoscopic Nissen fundoplication is an effective treatment for gastroesophageal reflux disease. Ann Surg 220:472–481, 1994.

Hinder RA, Libbey JS, Gorecki P, Bammer T: Antireflux surgery: Indications, preoperative evaluation, and outcome. Gastroenterol Clin North Am 28:987–1005, 1999.

Holloway RH, Dent J: Pathophysiology of gastroesophageal reflux: Lower esophageal sphincter dysfunction in gastroesophageal reflux disease. Gastroenterol Clin North Am 19:517–535, 1990.

Holloway RH, Dent J, Narielvala F, Mackinnon AM: Relation between oesophageal acid exposure and healing of oesophagitis with omeprazole in patients with severe reflux oesophagitis. Gut 38:649–654, 1996.

Holtmann G, Cain C, Malfertheiner P: Gastric *Helicobacter pylori* infection accelerates healing of reflux esophagitis during treatment with the proton pump inhibitor pantoprazole. Gastroenterology 117:11–18, 1999.

Jailwala JA, Shaker R: Oral and pharyngeal complications of gastroesophageal reflux disease: Globus, dental erosions, and chronic sinusitis. J Clin Gastroenterol 30(3 Suppl):S35–S38, 2000.

Jamieson GG: Anti-reflux operations: How do they work? Br J Surg 74:155–156, 1987.

Jamieson GG, Watson DI, Britten-Jones R, et al: Laparoscopic Nissen fundoplication. Ann Surg 220:137–145, 1994.

Johansson KE, Ask P, Boeryd B, et al: Oesophagitis, signs of reflux, and gastric acid secretion in patients with symptoms of gastro-oesophageal reflux disease. Scand J Gastroenterol 21:837–847, 1986.

Kahrilas PJ: Gastroesophageal reflux disease. JAMA 276:983–988, 1996.

Kahrilas PJ, Dodds WJ, Hogan WJ: Effect of peristaltic dysfunction on esophageal volume clearance. Gastroenterology 94:73–80, 1988.

Kahrilas PJ, Dodds WJ, Hogan WJ, et al: Esophageal peristaltic dysfunction in peptic esophagitis. Gastroenterology 91:897–904, 1986.

Kahrilas PJ, Falk G, Whipple J, et al: Comparison of esomeprazole, a novel PPI, vs. omeprazole in GERD patients with erosive esophagitis. Gastroenterology 118:A193, 2000.

Kahrilas PJ, Gupta RR: Mechanisms of acid reflux associated with cigarette smoking. Gut 31:4–10, 1990.

Kahrilas PJ, Gupta RR: The effect of cigarette smoking on salivation and esophageal acid clearance. J Lab Clin Med 114:431–438, 1989.

Kahrilas PJ, Lin S, Chen J, Manka M: The effect of hiatus hernia on gastro-oesophageal junction pressure. Gut 44:476–482, 1999.

Kahrilas PJ, Shi G, Manka M, Joehl RJ: Increased frequency of transient lower esophageal sphincter relaxation induced by gastric distention in reflux patients with hiatal hernia. Gastroenterology 118:688–695, 2000.

Kim MS, Dent J, Holloway RH, Utley DS: Radiofrequency energy delivery to the gastric cardia inhibits triggering of transient lower esophageal sphincter relaxation in a canine model. Gastroenterology 118:A860, 2000.

Kitchin LI, Castell DO: Rationale and efficacy of conservative therapy for gastroesophageal reflux disease. Arch Intern Med 151:448–454, 1991.

Klinkenberg-Knol EC, Festen HPM, Jansen JBMJ, et al: Long-term treatment with omeprazole for refractory reflux esophagitis: Efficacy and safety. Ann Intern Med 121:161–167, 1994.

Klinkenberg-Knol EC, Nelis F, Dent J, et al, and the Long-Term Study Group: Long-term omeprazole treatment in resistant gastroesophageal reflux disease: Efficacy, safety, and influence on gastric mucosa. Gastroenterology 118:661–669, 2000.

Knill-Jones RP, Card WI, Crean GP, et al: The symptoms of gastro-oesophageal reflux and oesophagitis. Scand J Gastroenterol 19(Suppl 106):72–76, 1984.

Koufman JA: The otolaryngologic manifestations of gastroesophageal reflux disease (GERD): A clinical investigation of 225 patients using ambulatory 24-hour pH monitoring and an experimental investigation of the role of acid and pepsin in the development of laryngeal injury. Laryngoscope 101:1–64, 1991.

Kuipers EJ, Lundell L, Klinkenberg-Knol EC, et al: Atrophic gastritis and *Helicobacter pylori* infection in patients with reflux esophagitis treated with omeprazole or fundoplication. N Engl J Med 334:1018–1022, 1996.

Labenz J, Blum AL, Bayerdörffer E, et al: Curing *Helicobacter pylori* infection in patients with duodenal ulcer may provoke reflux esophagitis. Gastroenterology 112:1442–1447, 1997.

Labenz J, Tillenburg B, Peitz U, et al: *Helicobacter pylori* augments the pH-increasing effect of omeprazole in patients with duodenal ulcer. Gastroenterology 110:725–732, 1996.

Lagergren J, Bergström R, Lindgren A, Nyrén O: Symptomatic gastroesophageal reflux as a risk factor for esophageal adenocarcinoma. N Engl J Med 340:825–831, 1999.

Laine S, Rantala A, Gullichsen R, Ovaska J: Laparoscopic vs. conventional Nissen fundoplication: A prospective randomized study. Surg Endosc 11:441–444, 1997.

Lanas A, Hirschowitz BI: Significant role of aspirin use in patients with esophagitis. J Clin Gastroenterol 13:622–627, 1991.

Lidums I, Lehmann A, Checklin H, et al: Control of transient lower esophageal sphincter relaxations and reflux by the $GABA_B$ agonist baclofen in normal subjects.

Locke GR III, Talley NJ, Fett SL, et al: Prevalence and clinical spectrum of gastroesophageal reflux: A population-based study in Olmsted County, Minnesota. Gastroenterology 112:1448–1456, 1997.

Luostarinen M, Isolauri J, Laitinen J, et al: Fate of Nissen fundoplication after 20 years: A clinical, enodscopical, and functional analysis. Gut 34:1015–1020, 1993.

Marks RD, Richter JE, Rizzo H, et al: Omeprazole versus H_2-receptor antagonists in treating patients with peptic stricture and esophagitis. Gastroenterology 106:907–915, 1994.

Martin CJ, Dodds WJ, Liem HH, et al: Diaphragmatic contribution to gastroesophageal competence and reflux in dogs. Am J Physiol 263:G551–G557, 1992.

Mattioli S, Pilotti V, Spangaro M, et al: Reliability of 24-hour home esophageal pH monitoring in diagnosis of gastroesophageal reflux. Dig Dis Sci 34:71–78, 1989.

McCallum RW: Gastric emptying in gastroesophageal reflux and the therapeutic role of prokinetic agents. Gastroenterol Clin North Am 19:551–564, 1990.

Meyers RL, Orlando RC: In vivo bicarbonate secretion by human esophagus. Gastroenterology 103:1174–1178, 1992.

Mittal RK, Balaban DH: The esophagogastric junction. N Engl J Med 336:924–932, 1997.

Mittal RK, Holloway RH, Penagini R, et al: Transient lower esophageal sphincter relaxation. Gastroenterology 109:601–610, 1995.

Nebel OT, Fornes MF, Castell DO: Symptomatic gastroesophageal reflux: Incidence and precipitating factors. Dig Dis 21:953–956, 1976.

O'Connor HJ: *Helicobacter pylori* and gastro-oesophageal reflux disease: Clinical implications and management. Aliment Pharmacol Ther 13:117–127, 1999.

Orlando RC: Mechanisms of reflux-induced epithelial injuries in the esophagus. Am J Med 108:104S–108S, 2000.

Orlando RC: Reflux esophagitis: An overview. Scand J Gastroenterol 210:36–37, 1995.

Orlando RC: Sucralfate therapy and reflux esophagitis: An overview. Am J Med 91(Suppl 2A):123S–124S, 1991.

Orlando RC: Why is the high grade inhibition of gastric acid secretion afforded by proton pump inhibitors often required for healing of reflux esophagitis? An epithelial perspective. Am J Gastroenterol 91:1692–1696, 1996.

Ormseth EJ, Wong RKH: Reflux laryngitis: Pathophysiology, diagnosis and management. Am J Gastroenterol 94:2812–2817, 1999.

O'Sullivan GC, DeMeester TR, Joelsson BE, et al: Interaction of lower esophageal sphincter pressure and length of sphincter in the abdomen as determinants of gastroesophageal competence. Am J Surg 143:40–46, 1982.

Palmer ED: The hiatus hernia-esophagitis-esophageal stricture complex: Twenty year prospective study. Am J Med 44:566–579, 1968.

Peters JH, Heimbucher J, Kauer WK, et al: Clinical and physiologic comparison of laparoscopic and open Nissen fundoplication. J Am Coll Surg 180:385–393, 1995.

Rantanen TK, Salo JA, Sipponen JT: Fatal and life-threatening complications in antireflux surgery: Analysis of 5,502 operations. Br J Surg 86:1573–1577, 1999.

Rattner DW, Brooks DC: Patient satisfaction following laparoscopic and open antireflux surgery. Arch Surg 130:289–294, 1995.

Richter JE: Chest pain and gastroesophageal reflux disease. J Clin Gastroenterol 30(3 Suppl):S39–S41, 2000.

Richter JE, Peura D, Benjamin SB, et al: Efficacy of omeprazole for the treatment of symptomatic acid reflux disease without esophagitis. Arch Intern Med 160:1810–1816, 2000.

Rydberg L, Ruth M, Lundell L: Mechanism of action of antireflux procedures. Br J Surg 86:405–410, 1999.

Sampliner RE, and The Practice Parameters Committee of the American College of Gastroenterology: Updated guidelines for the diagnosis and treatment of gastroesophageal reflux disease. Am J Gastroenterol 94:1434–1442, 1999.

Schenk BE, Festen HP, Kuipers EJ, et al: Effect of short- and long-term treatment with omeprazole on the absorption and serum levels of cobalamin. Aliment Pharmacol Ther 10:541–545, 1996.

Sloan S, Kahrilas PJ: Impairment of esophageal emptying with hiatal hernia. Gastroenterology 100:596–605, 1991.

Sloan S, Rademaker AW, Kahrilas PJ: Determinants of gastoesophageal junction incompetence: Hiatal hernia, lower esophageal sphincter, or both? Ann Intern Med 117:977–982, 1992.

Smit MJ, Leurs R, Alewijnse AE, et al: Inverse agonism of histamine H_2 antagonist accounts for upregulation of sponteanously active histamine H2 receptors. Proc Natl Acad Sci U S A 93:6802–6807, 1996.

Smith PM, Kerr GD, Cockel R, et al: A comparison of omeprazole and ranitidine in the prevention of recurrence of benign esophageal stricture. Gastroenterology 107:1312–1318, 1994.

Sontag SJ: The medical management of reflux esophagitis: Role of antacids and acid inhibition. Gastroenterol Clin North Am 19:683–712, 1990.

Spechler SJ: Barrett's esophagus: An overrated cancer risk factor. Gastroenterology 119:587–589, 2000;

Spechler SJ: Comparison of medical and surgical therapy for complicated gastroesophageal reflux disease in veterans. N Engl J Med 326:786–792, 1992.

Spechler SJ: Epidemiology and natural history of gastro-oesophageal reflux disease. Digestion 51(Suppl 1):24–29, 1992.

Spechler SJ, Lee E, Ahnen D, et al: Long-term outcome of medical and surgical therapies for GERD: Effects on survival. Gastroenterology 118:A489, 2000.

Spechler SJ, Lee E, Ahnen D, et al: Long-term outcome of medical and surgical therapies for GERD: Effects on GERD symptoms and signs. Gastroenterology 118:A193, 2000.

Triadafilopoulos G, Utley DS, DiBaise J, et al: Radiofrequency energy application to the gastroesophageal junction for the treatment of gastroesophageal reflux disease. Gastrointest Endosc 51:AB223, 2000.

Werdmuller BFM, Loffeld RJLF: *Helicobacter pylori* infection has no role in the pathogenesis of reflux esophagitis. Dig Dis Sci 42:103–105, 1997.

Wesdorp ICE, Dekker W, Festen HPM: Efficacy of famotidine 20 mg twice a day versus 40 mg twice a day in the treatment of erosive or ulcerative reflux esophagitis. Dig Dis Sci 12:2287–2293, 1993.

Wilkins WE, Ridley MG, Pozniak AL: Benign stricture of the oesophagus: Role of nonsteroidal anti-inflammatory drugs. Gut 25:478–480, 1984.

CHAPTER **12**

Indications for Surgical Referral for Hiatal Hernia and Gastroesophageal Reflux: A Gastroenterologist's Viewpoint

Joel E. Richter

Gastroesophageal reflux disease (GERD) is the most common disease of humans, affecting approximately 20% of the American population (Locke et al, 1997). It frequently leads to complications such as esophagitis, peptic strictures, and ulcers, Barrett's esophagus, and aspiration associated with asthma or ear, nose, and throat complaints. Surgery offers the opportunity to cure the disease by reducing the hiatal hernia back into the abdomen and improving lower esophageal sphincter (LES) function with a fundoplication. Antireflux surgery can now be done laparoscopically with a minimal hospital stay and rapid return to work in 5 to 10 days. Therefore, there is increasing enthusiasm among patients and the surgical community for wider use of antireflux surgery.

At the same time that antireflux surgery has become less invasive, there have been major advances in the medical treatment of GERD. These advances were heralded by the introduction in the United States of the first proton pump inhibitor (PPI), omeprazole, in 1989 (Sontag et al, 1992). This class of drugs blocks the final common pathway of acid secretion, the H^+,K^+-adenosine triphosphatase (ATPase) pump, thereby markedly inhibiting acid secretion by as much as 80% to 90% in the basal and postprandial states (Maton, 1991). Before the PPIs, the histamine (H_2)-antagonists decreased acid secretion by only 30% to 50% (Maton, 1991). Therefore, symptoms were relieved in only the milder forms of GERD, and the more severe grades of esophagitis were difficult to heal (Sontag, 1990).

Currently, four PPIs are on the market: omeprazole (Prilosec), lansoprazole (Prevacid), rabeprazole (Aciphex), and pantoprazole (Protonix). Throughout the world, numerous studies have consistently shown healing rates of 80% to 90% for all grades of esophagitis treated with PPIs over 8 to 12 weeks; complete symptom relief has paralleled the healing of esophagitis (Sontag, 1990).

Some have suggested, therefore, that 10% to 20% of patients with GERD have "intractable" GERD despite PPI therapy (Attwood et al, 1989). However, the lack of response is actually an artifact of the drug study design, in which patients are treated with a specific dose of the PPI and not allowed to increase the dose as needed. Clinical experience and dose-ranging studies consistently show that nearly all patients with GERD experience relief of symptoms and healing of esophagitis if acid is adequately controlled by medical therapy (Bianchi et al, 1997). Therefore, over the years I have evolved a "golden rule" in the treatment of patients with GERD. That is, lack of improvement with PPIs suggests the strong likelihood that a disease other than GERD is causing the patient's symptoms or esophagitis (Table 12–1). On the other hand, patients who respond well to PPIs are also the ones who do well with antireflux surgery after appropriate physiologic studies and operation by a skilled surgeon.

With this as a background, let us review the changes in the indications for antireflux surgery from the era of the H_2-antagonists to the present PPI era from the viewpoint of a gastroenterologist and esophagologist who has studied this disease and has treated patients for 20 years. Finally, I review my approach to helping the patient make an informed decision about the choice between maintenance medical therapy and surgery for GERD.

INDICATIONS FOR ANTIREFLUX SURGERY

The Histamine (H_2)-Antagonist Era

Table 12–2 summarizes the common indications for antireflux surgery during the 1970s and 1980s, when the primary medical treatment for GERD consisted of H_2-antagonists and promotility drugs. By far, the most common indication for surgery was symptoms and/or esophagitis that was intractable to medical therapy. Two

TABLE 12–1 ■ **Common Reasons for Treatment Failures in Gastrointestinal Reflux Disease**

Incorrect diagnosis
Inadequate acid suppression (much less common with use of proton pump inhibitors)
Noncompliance with drug regimen (cost versus psychosocial issues)
Pill-induced injury
Hypersecretor of acid (Zollinger-Ellison syndrome)
Delayed gastric emptying
Bile reflux (?)

TABLE 12–2 ■ **Common Indications for Antireflux Surgery in the Era of the Histamine (H_2)-Antagonists**

GERD not responsive to medical therapy—"intractable" GERD
Difficult-to-manage peptic strictures
Nonhealing esophageal ulcers
Barrett's esophagus

GERD, gastroesophageal reflux disease.

head-to-head comparison studies during this period showed the superiority of surgery to antacids, H_2-antagonists, metoclopramide, and/or sucralfate (Behar et al, 1975; Spechler, 1992). The introduction of the PPIs has totally changed this scenario. In fact, direct comparison studies now find equal efficacy for the PPIs and surgery in the relief of symptoms and healing of esophagitis in the long term (Lundel et al, 1998).

Before the availability of the PPIs, difficult-to-manage esophageal strictures and nonhealing ulcers were other indications for antireflux surgery. The H_2-antagonists do not decrease the need for esophageal dilatation in patients with peptic strictures (Ferguson et al, 1979). Omeprazole and lansoprazole, however, dramatically reduce the need for stricture dilatation and are cost effective in managing this disease compared with the use of H_2-antagonists (Marks et al, 1994; Smith et al, 1994). Furthermore, the number of esophageal dilatations has dramatically decreased in both Canada and the United States; this change seems to parallel the introduction of the PPIs (Dunne et al, 1997; Ugheoke et al, 1999).

Today, the patient with a difficult-to-manage stricture, especially if esophagitis is present, should be carefully evaluated for the possibility of pill-induced injury. Medications to be identified include doxycycline, quinidine, iron tablets, vitamin C, and especially aspirin and nonsteroidal anti-inflammatory drugs (NSAIDs). Alternatively, the esophagus may be irreversibly damaged with diffuse muscle scarring as a result of chronic GERD. These patients are characterized by needing frequent dilatations and having poor motility or even aperistalsis on esophageal manometry (Zaninotto et al, 1989). Esophageal resection, rather than antireflux surgery, is the treatment of choice for this group with difficult-to-manage esophageal strictures.

Proton pump inhibitors can heal all acid-related ulcers. Thus, persistence of an ulcerative esophagitis should raise concern about other diagnoses. Ambulatory pH testing with PPI therapy can be helpful in proving that acid reflux is adequately controlled. Here again, the major culprit is likely to be pill-induced injury, but other causes should be considered, including bullous skin diseases (phemphigus vulgaris) or cancer, especially in a patient with Barrett's esophagus.

Overall, the findings of Barrett's esophagus in a patient with known GERD should not alter the approach to medical or surgical therapy. Patients with Barrett's esophagus usually have more severe disease, however, and consequently often require more intensive medical therapy. Treatment with H_2-antagonists was often unsuccessful, resulting in the need for surgery. With the advent of the PPIs, reflux symptoms, esophagitis, and previously difficult-to-heal esophageal ulcers can now be medically treated, although twice-daily or thrice-daily dosing with the PPIs is frequently required (Sampliner, 1997).

Some have suggested that antireflux surgery can promote the regression of Barrett's esophagus. In six reported series, a total of 190 patients were followed over 4 to 6 years (Table 12–3) (Martinez de Haro et al, 1992; Ortiz et al, 1996; Sagar et al, 1995; Skinner et al, 1983; Wellinger et al, 1988; Williamson et al, 1990). Complete regression of Barrett's esophagus occurred in only six patients, with all but one coming from one series (Sagar et al, 1995). An additional 31 patients showed some decrease in the length of Barrett's epithelium, although only six patients had a decrease in length of more than 1 cm. Therefore, antireflux surgery is an acceptable alternative to maintenance PPI therapy for patients with Barrett's esophagus; however, the metaplastic epithelium rarely regresses, and these patients still need careful endoscopic surveillance for adenocarcinoma.

The Proton Pump Inhibitor Era

Table 12–4 summarizes the most common indications for antireflux surgery since the widespread use and acceptance of the PPIs. True intractable GERD cases are rare; PPI failure suggests that GERD is the wrong diagnosis, that noncompliance with drug therapy may be the problem, or that the patient cannot metabolize the drug and obtain adequate blood levels, which is unusual. A favor-

TABLE 12–3 ■ **Antireflux Surgery and Its Influence on Barrett's Esophagus (BE)**

Authors	*No. of Patients*	*Years of Follow-up*	*No. of Patients in Whom BE Decreases in Length*	*No. of Patients in Whom BE Disappears*	*No. of Patients Who Develop Esophageal Cancer*
Skinner et al, 1983	10	4	1	1	0
Wellinger et al, 1988	39	5.4	0	0	2
Williamson et al, 1990	37	4.2	4	0	3
Martinez de Haro et al, 1992	16	6.6	0	0	0
Sagar et al, 1995	56	5.5	24	5	1
Ortiz et al, 1996	32	5	8	0	0
Total	190		37	6	6

TABLE 12–4 ■ Common Indications for Antireflux Surgery in the Era of the Proton Pump Inhibitors (PPIs)

Option for healthy patient with GERD well controlled with PPIs
Cost
Compliance
Fear of unknown long-term side effects
Atypical symptoms of GERD relieved with PPIs
Chest pain
Pulmonary—asthma, aspiration pneumonia
Ear, nose, and throat—hoarseness, cough, vocal cord lesions
Volume regurgitation and aspiration symptoms not controlled with PPIs
Barrett's esophagus to decrease risk of dysplasia or cancer (?)

GERD, gastroesophageal reflux disease.

able response to PPIs helps identify patients who do best after antireflux surgery. Furthermore, everyone who treats these patients must realize that no particular expertise is required for prescribing PPIs, morbidity associated with their use has proved trivial to nonexistent (i.e., rare side effects and no carcinoid tumors in humans after follow-up for 12 to 15 years), and their use has no irreversible attributes (Kahrilas, 1999; Klinkenberg-Knol et al, 1994).

Unfortunately, the same cannot be said about antireflux surgery. Postoperative dysphagia, excessive flatus, and gas bloat are frequent postoperative complications. Mortality is rare but has occurred in up to 0.2% in large series (Perdikis et al, 1997). Recurrent symptoms and esophagitis have occurred in 10% to 30% of patients after follow-up for 5 to 20 years (DeMeester et al, 1986; Low et al, 1989; Rantanen et al, 1999). Furthermore, the best surgical results are presented from academic centers with highly trained esophageal surgeons, whereas the majority of antireflux operations are being done by general surgeons in community hospitals. Both sides of these arguments deserve discussion with our patients, as do concerns about cost, compliance with drug regimens, and fears about long-term safety issues with the PPIs, because we have safety data for only up to 15 years.

Cost is frequently argued as a factor favoring antireflux surgery in the long-term management of the disease in the healthy adult who will have to suffer with it for 20 to 50 years. Considering the current cost of PPIs ($2 to $3 per pill), the cost of maintenance medical treatment will approach the initial cost of antireflux surgery ($10,000 to $15,000) in 5 to 10 years (Laycock et al, 1995). However, these analyses are far more complicated than they appear initially.

There are numerous hidden costs for both medical and surgical therapy. For example, patients who do poorly with medical therapy require further diagnostic tests and physician visits. In addition, many patients treated medically require double and triple doses of PPIs to control symptoms and to keep their esophagitis healed (Klinkenberg-Knol et al, 1994). On the other hand, most patients who have antireflux surgery should have a thorough preoperative evaluation that medical patients do not require for long-term medical therapy (i.e., barium esophagram, esophageal manometry, 24-hour pH testing, and gastric function studies). Some patients do not respond to antireflux surgery, whereas others have the previously discussed complications. If the success of surgery is less than lifelong, additional medical or surgical therapy is necessary.

Finally, none of these scenarios consider the impact of generic and over-the-counter PPIs, which will rapidly become a reality when the patent for omeprazole expires in the year 2002. For example, even some of the most favorable models for surgery find the PPIs to be the preferred cost-effective approach when the price of medication falls below $30 per month (Heudebert et al, 1997). Overall, cost comparisons of long-term medical versus surgical therapy for GERD are far too complicated and rapidly evolving to make a comprehensive statement in favor of either therapy. In reality, many of our patients decide for or against antireflux surgery on the basis of the cost that they personally incur because of their insurance or health care plan and their level of satisfaction with medical treatment in terms of symptom relief, quality of life, and convenience of their medical regimen.

Since the mid-1980s, increasing attention has focused on the atypical or supraesophageal presentations of GERD, including chest pain, asthma, aspiration pneumonia, and a variety of ear, nose, and throat symptoms and signs (e.g., hoarseness, globus, cough, vocal cord granulomas, and even laryngeal cancer) (Richter, 1997). These patients may be difficult to identify, because 20% to 40% have "silent" gastroesophageal reflux (GER), without classic symptoms of heartburn and acid regurgitation, and barium radiographs and endoscopy may be normal. Prolonged 24-hour pH testing is the best method for identifying the coexistence of GER with these atypical complaints, but the pattern of reflux or symptom correlation scores do not guarantee causality because these patients may have multiple potential trigger factors for the atypical symptoms aside from acid reflux.

The patients with atypical symptoms do not predictably respond to PPI therapy; therefore, it should not be surprising that antireflux surgery is less successful in patients with atypical symptoms than in patients with typical heartburn. For example, of 150 consecutive patients undergoing laprosocopic antireflux surgery, 35 (23%) had primarily atypical symptoms (So et al, 1998). Surgery relieved heartburn in 93% of patients, whereas only 56% of patients had relief of their atypical complaints. The only useful preoperative predictors of relief of atypical symptoms were the response to aggressive acid suppression with PPIs and the presence of hypopharyngeal reflux on pH testing in patients with laryngeal complaints. Therefore, we should inform patients considering antireflux surgery for atypical symptoms that their complaints may be no better after surgery than they are while taking high doses of PPIs.

Despite the use of PPIs, some patients continue to have volume reflux with aspiration symptoms after meals and at night. Many of these patients complain that the "fire is gone," but they still have intermittent reflux of fluid with a bitter taste into their mouths. These patients are usually found to have low LES pressures and sometimes coexisting gastroparesis, resulting in constant volume reflux unless the stomach is completely emptied.

Only antireflux surgery to reconstruct the weak LES sphincter can alleviate these complaints.

Although antireflux surgery does not predictably promote regression of Barrett's esophagus, can it decrease the risk of dysplasia or cancer? Two studies tantalize us concerning this intriguing question.

The Dartmouth group observed 15 patients after surgery for up to 9 years during which time none developed dysplasia or adenocarcinoma (Katz et al, 1998). In contrast, 26 of 82 (31%) medically treated patients with Barrett's esophagus developed dysplastic lesions over the same follow-up period, including three cancers, four high-grade dysplasias, and nine low-grade dysplasias. This protective association persisted in a multivariant analysis after adjustments for age, sex, smoking history, and presence of a hiatal hernia.

The Mayo Clinic group published their results of antireflux surgery in 113 patients with Barrett's esophagus followed for an average of 6.5 years (range, 4 months to 18 years) (McDonald et al, 1996). Three patients subsequently had adenocarcinoma of the esophagus at 13, 25, and 39 months after surgery; two of these died of their cancer. The authors suggested that these cancers may have been prevalent cancers missed in evaluations before surgery, with no true incidence cancers developing after 4 years or more of follow-up. On the other hand, the reports summarized in Table 12–3 identified six patients who developed adenocarcinoma despite effective antireflux surgery. This cancer incidence is (Martinez de Haro et al, 1992; Ortiz et al, 1996; Sagar et al, 1995; Skinner et al, 1983; Wellinger et al, 1988; Williamson et al, 1990) 1 per 162 patient-years of follow-up, similar to the incidence found in medically treated patients (Drewitz et al, 1995).

How might antireflux surgery be protective against esophageal cancer? Both acid reflux and bile reflux occur in increasing amounts across the spectrum of GERD, especially in patients with Barrett's esophagus (Vaezi and Richter, 1996). Proponents of the "dangers of bile reflux" argue that medical treatment reduces only the acid component of reflux, whereas the barrier created by antireflux surgery prevents reflux of both acid and duodenal contents (Attwood et al, 1989, 1993). Two studies (Champion et al, 1994; Marshall et al, 1998), however, found that omeprazole is equally effective in decreasing both acid and bile reflux, the latter measured by the new Bilitec system (Vaezi et al, 1994). This protective effect of PPIs probably results from two mechanisms: reducing the gastric volume available for reflux into the esophagus and raising intragastric pH, causing the harmful conjugated bile acids to precipitate out of solution.

At this time, I believe that the protective effects of antireflux surgery in Barrett's esophagus are only speculative, but this area deserves close observation and studies in which the two cohort groups are equally matched for risk factors and followed over extended periods of time. Until that time, the dangers of bile reflux seem a needless scare tactic to promote surgery while attempting to counterbalance the widespread use of PPIs, when in reality the number of antireflux operations has markedly increased rather than decreased.

MEDICAL VERSUS SURGICAL TREATMENT OF CHRONIC GASTROINTESTINAL REFLUX DISEASE

At the Cleveland Clinic, all patients being considered for antireflux surgery are jointly evaluated by both the gastroenterology and surgery departments. If GER is causing the patients' symptoms, I am convinced that all of these patients can obtain symptomatic relief and healing of esophagitis with the currently available treatments. There are benefits and risks to both medical and surgical treatment, however, and long-term issues are unresolved for both therapies.

Medical treatment, especially with PPIs, can effectively treat all forms of GERD, and the efficacy of these medications has not waned over time in studies up to 12 years. However, many patients require daily lifelong medications that are expensive and whose long-term risks are not known. Surgery offers a unique opportunity to "cure" this chronic disease, depending on the diagnosis being correct and an experienced surgeon. Paradoxically, the best surgical candidates are the patients who respond completely to PPIs and I would encourage my surgical colleagues not to break the golden rule. On the downside, postoperative complications are common and the long-term durability of both open and laparoscopic antireflux surgery is unknown.

This issue of surgical durability versus long-term safety of PPIs is especially crucial for young people with chronic GERD. I take the approach of openly discussing both options with my patients and allowing them to make informed decisions. In this way, the patients are proactive in their treatment, happy with the results, and not surprised, disappointed, or angry if complications occur.

■ *REFERENCES*

Attwood SEA, Ball CS, Barlow AP, et al: Role of intragastric and intraesophageal alkalization in the genesis of the complications in Barrett's columnar lined oesophagus. Gut 34:11–15, 1993.

Attwood SEA, DeMeester TR, Brenner CG, et al: Alkaline gastroesophageal reflux: Implications in the development of complications in Barrett's columnar lined lower esophagus. Surgery 106:764–770, 1989.

Behar J, Sheahan DG, Biancani P, et al: Medical and surgical treatment of reflux esophagitis: A 38-month report of a prospective clinical trial. N Engl J Med 293:263–268, 1975.

Bianchi Poiro G, Pace F, Peracchia A, et al: Short-term treatment of refractory reflux esophagitis with different doses of omeprazole or ranitidine. J Clin Gastroenterol 15:192–198, 1997.

Champion G, Richter JE. Vaezi MF, et al: Duodenogastroesophageal reflux: Relationship to pH and importance in Barrett's esophagus. Gastroenterology 107:747–754, 1994.

DeMeester TR, Bonavina L, Albertucci M: Nissen fundoplication for gastroesophageal reflux disease: Evaluation or primary repair in 100 consecutive patients. Ann Surg 204:9–20, 1986.

Drewitz DJ, Sampliner RE, Garewal HS: The incidence of adenocarcinoma in Barrett's esophagus: A prospective study of 170 patients followed 4.8 years. Am J Gastroenterol 90:1567–1571, 1995.

Dunne D, Mercer D, Paterson WG: Decreasing frequency of esophageal dilation for peptic stricture correlates with omeprazole use. Can J Gastroenterol 11(Suppl A):43 A, 1997

Ferguson R, Dronfield MW, Atkinson M: Cimetidine in the treatment of reflux esophagitis with peptic stricture. Br Med J 2:472–474, 1979.

Heudebert GR, Marks R, Wilcox CM, Center RM: Choice of long-term strategy for the management of patients with severe esophagitis: A cost-utility analysis. Gastroenterology 112:1078–1086, 1997.

Kahrilas PJ: Laparoscopic anti-reflux surgery: Silver bullet or the emperor's new clothes? Am J Gastroenterol 94:1721–1722, 1999.

Katz D, Rothstein R, Schned A, et al: The development of dysphagia and adenocarcinoma during endoscopic surveillance of Barrett's esophagus. Am J Gastroenterol 93:536–541, 1998.

Klinkenberg-Knol EC, Fester HPM, Janssen JBMJ, et al: Long-term treatment with omeprazole for refractory reflux esophagitis: Efficacy and safety. Ann Intern Med 121:161–167, 1994.

Laycock WS, Oddsdottir M, Franco A, et al: Laparoscopic Nissen fundoplication is less expensive than open Belsey Mark IV. Surg Endosc 9:426–429, 1995.

Locke GR, Talley NJ, Felts SL, et al: Prevalence and clinical spectrum of gastroesophageal reflux disease: A population-based study in Olmsted County, Minnesota. Gastroenterology 112:1448–1456, 1997.

Low DE, Anderson RP, Lives R, et al: Fifteen to twenty year results after the Hill antireflux operation. J Thorac Cardiovasc Surg 98:444–450, 1989.

Lundel L, Dalenback J, Hattlebakk J, et al: Omeprazole or antireflux surgery in the long-term management of gastroesophageal reflux disease: Results of a multicenter, randomized clinical trial. Gastroenterology 114:A207, 1998.

Marks RD, Richter JE, Rizzo J, et al: Omeprazole vs H_2-receptor antagonists in treating patients with peptic stricture and esophagitis. Gastroenterology 106:907–914, 1994.

Marshall REK, Anggiansah A, Manifold DK, et al: Effect of omeprazole 20 mg twice daily on duodenogastric and gastroesophageal bile reflux in Barrett's esophagus. Gut 43:603–606, 1998.

Martinez de Haro LF, Ortiz A, Parrilla P, et al: Long-term results of Nissen fundoplication in reflux esophagitis without stricture. Dig Dis Sci 37:523–527, 1992.

Maton PN: Drug therapy: Omeprazole. N Engl J Med 324:965–971, 1991.

McDonald ML, Trastek VK, Allen MS, et al: Barrett's esophagus: Does an antireflux procedure reduce the need for endoscopic surveillance? J Thorac Cardiovasc Surg 111:1135–1140, 1996.

Ortiz A, Martinez de Haro LF, Parrilla P, et al: Conservative treatment vs antireflux surgery in Barrett's oesophagus: Long-term results of a prospective study. Br J Surg 83:274–278, 1996.

Perdikis G, Hinder RA, Lund RJ, et al: Laparoscopic Nissen fundoplication: Where do we stand? Surg Laparosc Endosc 7:17–21, 1997.

Rantanen TK, Halone TV, Luostarinen ME, et al: The long-term results of open antireflux surgery in a community-based health care center. Am J Gastroenterol 94:1777–1781, 1999.

Richter JE: Extraesophageal presentations of gastroesophageal reflux disease. Semin Gastrointest Dis 8:75–89, 1997.

Sagar PM, Ackroyd R, Hosie KB, et al: Regression and progression of Barrett's oesophagus after antireflux surgery. Br J Surg 82:806–810, 1995.

Sampliner RE: New treatment for Barrett's esophagus. Semin Gastrointest Dis 8:68–74, 1997.

Skinner DB, Walther BC, Riddell RH, et al: Barrett's esophagus, comparison of benign and malignant cases. Ann Surg 198:554–566, 1983.

Smith PL, Kerr GD, Cockel R, et al: A comparison of omeprazole and ranitidine in the prevention of recurrence of benign esophageal stricture. Gastroenterology 107:1312–1318, 1994.

So JBY, Zeitel SM, Rattner DW: Outcomes of atypical symptoms attributed to gastroesophageal reflux treated by laparoscopic fundoplication. Surgery 124:28–32, 1998.

Sontag SJ: The medical management of reflux esophagitis: Role of antacids and acid inhibition. Gastroenterol Clin North Am 19:683–712, 1990.

Sontag SJ, Hirschowitz BI, Holt S, et al: Two doses of omeprazole versus placebo in symptomatic erosive esophagitis: The US multicenter study. Gastroenterology 102:109–118, 1992.

Spechler JJ for the Department of Veteran Affairs Gastroesophageal Reflux Disease Study Group: Comparison of medical and surgical therapy for complicated gastroesophageal reflux disease. N Engl J Med 326:786–792, 1992.

Ugheoke E, Schaberg JW, Philip S, et al: Peptic esophageal strictures in the era of proton pump inhibitors: Where have they all gone? Gastrointest Endosc 49:AB202, 1999.

Vaezi MF, Richter JE: Role of acid and duodenogastroesophageal reflux in gastroesophageal reflux disease. Gastroenterology 111:1192–1199, 1996.

Vaezi MF, LaCamera RG, Richter JE: Validation studies of Bilitec 2000: An ambulatory duodenogastric reflux monitoring system. Am J Physiol 30:G1050–G1057, 1994.

Wellinger J, Ollyo JB, Savary M, et al: Le traitement chirugical de l'endobrachyesophagus. Helv Chir Acta 55:695–698, 1988.

Williamson WA, Ellis FH, Gibbs SP, et al: Effective anti-reflux operation on Barrett's mucosa. Ann Thorac Surg 49:537–542, 1990.

Zaninotto G, DeMeester TR, Bremner CG, et al: Esophageal function in patients with reflux induced strictures and its relevance to surgical treatment. Ann Thorac Surg 47:362–370, 1989.

CHAPTER **13**

Indications for Surgery for Hiatal Hernia and Gastroesophageal Reflux: The Surgeon's Perspective

Robert J. Ginsberg

F. Griffith Pearson

The selection of patients for the surgical management of gastroesophageal reflux disease and hiatal hernia continues to generate controversy and challenge. Although both conditions are extremely common, relatively few patients become disabled or have complications that warrant the consideration of surgical management. Furthermore, unlike most operations, the successful correction of hiatal hernia and reflux requires the restoration or preservation of a number of highly sophisticated physiologic functions: a successful operation preserves or restores normal deglutition and prevents pathologic reflux while maintaining the physiologic functions of eructation, vomiting when necessary, and normal gastric emptying. These are challenging and often difficult requirements.

In patients selected for surgical management, the surgeon must consider abnormalities of esophageal motility, gastric function, and local anatomy before choosing the procedure that best meets the requirements for the individual patient. Unfortunately, there is no single operation that can correct all of the various presentations of hiatal hernia and reflux.

Most important, surgery is rarely *mandatory* in patients with benign reflux disease. In most cases, the decision to proceed with surgery is shared by the surgeon and the patient. The patient should be clearly informed in regard to the nature and anticipated results of a surgical repair. It is the patient who ultimately makes the choice between continued medical therapy or surgery for a condition that rarely results in severe or life-threatening complications.

Most recently, there has been an alarming rise in the incidence of adenocarcinoma of the lower esophagus and gastrointestinal junction. The relationship to reflux disease and the development of a columnar-lined esophagus appears to have been confirmed. It has been suggested that antireflux procedures may indeed prevent the progression of the metaplastic columnar-lined epithelium to frank dysplasia, but this has yet to be confirmed.

BASIC SCIENCE

For a detailed discussion of the pertinent anatomy and physiology of the esophagus, see Chapters 2 and 3.

In addition to the patience and persistence required to elicit an accurate description of symptoms, the surgeon who treats a patient with esophageal disease must be knowledgeable about local anatomy, esophageal and gastric function, and all aspects of interventional investigation and therapy. This requires expertise in endoscopy, which should not be abrogated to gastroenterologists, who ultimately hold no direct responsibility for surgical management and results. The surgeon who does not perform upper gastrointestinal endoscopy is at a great disadvantage. The old adage "diagnosis precedes treatment" applies aptly to reflux disease. A surgeon who has performed the endoscopic evaluation learns from errors in endoscopic interpretation. For these reasons, it is best that the surgeon be intimately familiar with the esophageal function laboratory.

HISTORICAL NOTES

Allison (1951) wrote the first clear description of the anatomy, pathophysiology, and surgical correction of hiatal hernia and gastroesophageal reflux. In this classic and beautifully descriptive paper, he described the complications of erosive peptic esophagitis, peptic stricture, columnar replacement (Barrett's esophagus), aspiration, and the incarceration associated with large paraesophageal hernias. He designed a repair that was an attempt to restore the normal anatomy of the esophagogastric junction using a left transthoracic exposure and an incision in the left hemidiaphragm to afford access to the upper abdomen. Twenty-five years later, Allison (1973) had the intellectual honesty and integrity to report the long-term follow-up of his cases: an unacceptable 50% recurrence rate.

Belsey (1995), with his inimitable writing skill, provides a brief history of antireflux surgery that highlights the early years, during which he was a major contributor in the field. He knew almost all of the pioneers: Allison, Barrett, Nissen, Dor, Toupet, Lortat-Jacob, Harrington, Hill, and Collis. Belsey trained and profoundly influenced a large number of young surgeons from North America,

Europe, and the United Kingdom, who subsequently made significant, original contributions in the field.

Since Allison's historic paper in 1951, the indications for surgery have undergone major cycles of enthusiasm and restraint. During the 1950s and 1960s, just the finding of a hiatus hernia was an indication for repair in the opinion of many surgeons. During the subsequent two decades, however, there was a progressive decrease in the number of operations for hiatal hernia and related complications. Medical management was greatly advanced with the introduction of histamine (H_2) blockers and proton-pump inhibitors (PPIs). Patients were increasingly under the control of gastroenterologists, many of whom were understandably skeptical of surgical referral because of a significant reported incidence of poor results, often at the hands of the "occasional" operator. The introduction of laparoscopic fundoplication (Dallemagne, 1991), however, resulted in a substantial and still increasing incidence of referral for surgery. Antireflux surgery is again one of the most common operations performed in the Americas and Europe.

Surgeons have now added another indication, not yet proven scientifically, for the use of antireflux procedures—the prevention of metaplastic and dysplastic changes in the lower esophagus and possibly, therefore, the prevention of the development of carcinoma of the esophagus in patients with reflux.

■ *HISTORICAL READINGS*

Allison PR: Reflux esophagitis, sliding hiatal hernia, and the anatomy of repair. Surg Gynecol Obstet 92:149, 1951.

Allison PR: Hiatus hernia: A 20-year retrospective survey. Ann Surg 178:273–276, 1973.

Dallemagne B, Weerts JM, Jehaes C, et al: Laparoscopic Nissen fundoplication: Preliminary report. Surg Laparosc Endosc 1:138–143, 1991.

INDICATIONS FOR SURGERY

There are relatively few *absolute* indications for the surgical management of hiatal hernia or reflux disease. In most instances, the surgeon is confronted by patients with reflux symptoms that interfere with a comfortable lifestyle. In such cases, the indications for surgery are *relative* because the unoperated condition rarely results in serious morbidity or catastrophe. The patient must choose between unpleasant symptoms and a surgical procedure that cannot be guaranteed to be 100% effective.

Absolute Indications

In rare circumstances, surgery is urgent and mandatory for the management of catastrophic, sometimes life-threatening complications of hiatal hernia or reflux disease. These conditions are listed in the following box.

ABSOLUTE INDICATIONS FOR SURGERY

Perforation

Barrett's ulcer
Peptic ulcer in intrathoracic stomach
Iatrogenic (i.e., instrumental)

Uncontrolled Bleeding

Barrett's ulcer
Peptic ulcer in intrathoracic stomach

Unrelieved Obstruction

Organoaxial volvulus
Extreme peptic stenosis

Gastric Necrosis

Organoaxial volvulus and strangulation

Unmanageable Aspiration

Recurrent laryngotracheitis, bronchitis

Malignancy

Proven or suspected malignancy in columnar-lined esophagus

Perforation

On rare occasion, a peptic ulcer that arises in a columnar-lined segment of esophagus or in the incarcerated intrathoracic gastric pouch perforates the pleural space, pericardial space, bronchial tree, or aorta (Allen et al, 1993; Bremner, 1987; Cappell et al, 1989; Diehl et al, 1988; Geha et al, 2000; Gerstenberger et al, 1986; Katyal et al, 1993; Limburg et al, 1989; Ozdemir et al, 1973; Pearson et al, 1987; Skinner and Belsey, 1967). Intrathoracic perforation from the stomach or esophagus obviously is a life-threatening emergency, and there is no standard method of surgical management. Each case is individualized and requires adequate drainage and control of further spillage of gastric or esophageal content.

Esophageal perforation may complicate endoscopy, particularly rigid esophagoscopy or instrumental dilatation of peptic stricture. The indications for surgery are similar to those for any instrumental perforation of the thoracic esophagus (see Chapter 38). In selected cases, it may be possible to combine an antireflux reconstruction with repair of the perforation.

Uncontrolled Bleeding

Barrett's ulcer or gastric pouch ulcer occasionally results in massive and uncontrollable upper gastrointestinal hemorrhage (Bremner, 1987; Geha et al, 2000; Ozdemir et al, 1973; Pearson et al, 1987; Skinner and Belsey, 1967). In the rare instances when bleeding cannot be managed conservatively or endoscopically, surgical intervention is indicated. The underlying condition should be dealt with during the same operation, whenever possible.

Severe or Total Obstruction

When a sufficient extent of stomach herniates into the posterior mediastinum (massive incarcerated type III or IV hernia or paraesophageal hernia type II), organoaxial volvulus inevitably occurs. Occasionally, volvulus is associated with complete obstruction at the esophagogastric junction, which cannot be relieved with passage of a nasogastric tube or an esophagoscope. An urgent operation with reduction of the giant hernia may be necessary (Allen et al, 1993; Carter et al, 1980; Geha et al, 2000; Maziak et al, 1998; Pearson et al, 1983).

Extreme degrees of peptic stricture may result in esophageal obstruction that is close to complete. Although it is exceedingly uncommon, occasionally a patient is unable to maintain satisfactory nutrition as a result of severe peptic stenosis. If the obstruction cannot be managed with dilatation, an urgent operation may be the only solution. In such cases, resection of the distal esophagus and replacement may be necessary (Carter et al, 1980). Strictures of this advanced degree are rarely seen since the advent of more effective medical management with H_2 blockade and PPIs.

Gastric Necrosis

With a giant incarcerated hernia, organoaxial volvulus occasionally results in strangulation, with impairment of circulation and gastric necrosis or gangrene. In such cases, emergency surgery and resection are necessary along with immediate or delayed reconstruction (Allen et al, 1993; Carter et al, 1980; Geha et al, 2000; Semb et al, 1977).

Malignancy

Proven or suspected malignancy in an acquired columnar-lined esophagus is an absolute indication for operation in patients at suitable risk for such major surgery. Whether antireflux surgery prevents the development of a metaplasia (Barrett's esophagus) or dysplasia when columnar-lined esophagus is already present has yet to be proved. Certainly, this approach warrants further scientific investigation. The management of dysplasia and malignancy in columnar-lined esophagus is discussed in detail in both parts of Chapter 17.

On occasion, patients with severe ulcerative peptic esophagitis may present with an appearance on endoscopy that is indistinguishable from malignancy. In such cases, the surgeon may elect to operate on the patient to establish the correct diagnosis even when biopsy and brush cytologic findings are negative or equivocal.

Relative Indications

The term *relative indications* implies that there is an element of choice in the decision for surgery that is shared by the physician and the patient. Relative indications can be subdivided into three categories:

1. Complications caused by the mechanical problem of incarceration and irreducibility of the hernia.
2. Complications caused by gastroesophageal reflux.
3. Problems caused by disabling symptoms due to otherwise uncomplicated reflux.

These indications are summarized in the following box.

RELATIVE INDICATIONS FOR SURGERY

Paraesophageal Hiatal Hernia

Incarceration
Chronic iron deficiency anemia
Volvulus, intermittent obstruction
Space occupation
Chronic gastric ulcer

Complications of Reflux

Ulcerative peptic esophagitis
Peptic stricture
Chronic ulcer (Barrett's) in columnar-lined esophagus
Chronic aspiration

Disabling Symptoms: Uncomplicated Reflux

Inadequate medical control

Paraesophageal Hiatal Hernia

In most instances, a *paraesophageal hernia* is an advanced sliding rather than a true, or pure, paraesophageal hernia. As a sliding hernia progressively enlarges, it becomes a "rolling hiatal hernia" (a term coined by Belsey [Skinner and Belsey, 1967]) and may ultimately progress to massive herniation and organoaxial volvulus. There is no medical therapy for this anatomic derangement.

Controversy continues as to whether all patients with paraesophageal hernias should be offered surgical correction because of the potential for late and hazardous complications, including massive bleeding, torsion and strangulation, and unmanageable peptic ulceration. There have been no prospective epidemiologic studies that convincingly provided an answer to this question. Retrospective analysis suggests that in a significant number of patients with such hernias, major and often emergency complications develop and demand surgical correction (Allen et al, 1993; Geha et al, 2000; Hill, 1973; Ozdemir et al, 1973; Skinner and Belsey, 1967).

Incarceration

When volvulus has occurred, almost all patients report symptoms if a careful history is obtained. In a retrospective study, Allen and associates (1993) reported that of 147 such patients, all except 5 were asymptomatic. Symptoms are commonly due to retention of swallowed air, fluid, and food in the incarcerated intrathoracic pouch. This results in varying degrees of postprandial discomfort, which range from mild fullness to severe precordial pain and pressure with nausea and retching (Pearson et al, 1983). If symptoms are sufficiently distressing, nothing short of surgical reduction of the trapped intrathoracic stomach resolves the problem.

Chronic Iron Deficiency Anemia

A relatively common complication of paraesophageal hernias is persistent or recurrent iron deficiency anemia. The bleeding is almost always occult, and such patients may present with a chronic iron deficiency anemia and complaints of pallor, dyspnea on exertion, and palpitations (Allen et al, 1993; Geha et al, 2000; Maziak et al, 1998; Ozdemir et al, 1973; Pearson et al, 1983; Skinner and Belsey, 1967). The blood loss is attributed to congestion of the gastric mucosa in the incarcerated pouch and to superficial ulceration, which is observed in the gastric mucosa at the level of the diaphragmatic hiatus. If the anemia cannot be satisfactorily controlled with iron replacement therapy, surgical correction of the hernia provides a dependable solution.

Volvulus: Intermittent Obstruction

Some patients experience episodes of complete esophageal obstruction as a result of reversible degrees of organoaxial volvulus. The obstruction usually occurs at the esophagogastric junction and may be relieved spontaneously or through the passage of a nasogastric tube (Pearson et al, 1983). Recurrent episodes of complete obstruction may prompt the recommendation for repair.

Space Occupation

When a hernia is sufficiently large, the intrathoracic pouch may actually compromise the mechanics of respiration. This occurs only with massive herniation and volvulus. The stomach may be chronically distended with retained air and fluid and fill a significant portion of each lower hemithorax in addition to the posterior mediastinum. Obviously, nothing short of surgical reduction of the hernia can correct this complication (Allen et al, 1993; Geha et al, 2000; Pearson et al, 1983).

Persistent Gastric Ulceration

The incarcerated intrathoracic pouch may be the site of a chronic gastric ulcer that is unmanageable with medical therapy (Ozdemier et al, 1973; Pearson et al, 1983; Skinner and Belsey, 1967). These ulcers often are large, painful, and penetrating and ultimately may result in perforation or uncontrolled bleeding. They usually respond to reflux control after surgical correction of the underlying hernia.

Complications of Gastroesophageal Reflux

Ulcerative Peptic Esophagitis

If gross ulcerative esophagitis persists despite medical therapy, surgical correction of the gastroesophageal reflux should be seriously considered. Although medical therapy with acid-suppressing drugs promotes healing of ulcerative peptic esophagitis in a high proportion of cases, cessation of drug therapy frequently results in a florid recurrence of symptoms. Not all patients are compliant with long-term drug therapy; for some, there is a problem with cost. In patients at an appropriate risk, surgical correction is an appropriate alternative to medical therapy in selected circumstances. In patients who do not respond to the most intensive medical therapy, surgical correction of reflux is clearly advised.

Peptic Stricture

Although peptic stricture may be treated with interval dilatation combined with acid suppression and other medical measures, the problem may continue to recur despite therapy. In such circumstances, it is reasonable to recommend antireflux surgery because in most instances effective prevention of reflux ultimately results in resolution of the stricture. The management of peptic stricture is detailed in Chapter 15.

Chronic Peptic Ulcer in Columnar-Lined Esophagus: Barrett's Ulcer

Although most peptic ulcers heal with medical therapy, which includes the powerful acid suppressant PPIs, in some instances a chronic ulcer may persist or recur. It has been clearly documented that surgical correction of reflux results in prompt healing of such ulcers (Pearson et al, 1987).

Columnar-Lined Esophagus: Barrett's Esophagus

In the absence of symptoms, acquired columnar-lined esophagus is not considered an indication for surgery. Unmanageable symptoms, Barrett's ulcer, or associated peptic esophagitis and stricture may be strong indications for surgery.

The problem of dysplasia and malignant transformation in the columnar epithelium of Barrett's esophagus is an increasingly prominent finding (see Chapter 17).

Chronic Aspiration

In some patients, chronic or recurrent aspiration of gastric content is not predictably manageable with any form of medical therapy. Conservative management includes elevation of the head of the bed, avoidance of food immediately before retiring, and acid suppression with PPIs. Unmanageable aspiration is a clear indication for surgical correction.

Determining that gastroesophageal reflux and aspiration are the cause of respiratory symptoms may be difficult. Patients with unexplained cough, episodic asthma and bronchitis, and recurrent pneumonitis may be difficult to evaluate in the absence of a clear history of regurgitation with aspiration. Aspiration commonly occurs with the patient lying down and asleep at night. In some instances, patient awareness is minimal or absent.

Disabling Symptoms: Uncomplicated Reflux

In the absence of complications that warrant surgery, there is nothing more problematic than the selection of management for the patient with recurrent or unremitting "but tolerable" symptoms. When fully informed of the risks and benefits, the patient should make the decision for a surgical option.

CHOICE OF OPERATION

Since the first edition of this textbook in 1995, laparoscopic antireflux surgery has become widely practiced and is increasingly accepted as the preferable technique for an increasing proportion of surgical cases. Furthermore, the popularity of minimally invasive and, therefore, less morbid operations has resulted in many more patients undergoing surgery: Both the patients and their referring physicians and gastroenterologists have become more amenable to surgical correction. Laparoscopic management of the most technically difficult problems is reported with increasing frequency: short esophagus with laparoscopic gastroplasty, giant paraesophageal hernia, and reoperation for failed prior repair.

Whether the access is laparoscopic or "open," surgery for hiatal hernia and reflux is extremely demanding if predictably acceptable results are to be obtained. Because the lower esophagus straddles the diaphragm, it is not surprising that open surgery has been accomplished through thoracic, abdominal, and thoracoabdominal approaches. The practicing esophageal surgeon should be familiar with all of these options to manage the varying and individual problems confronted.

Furthermore, the best type of antireflux procedure continues to generate debate. In general, all antireflux operations are characterized by the following elements:

1. Replacement of an intra-abdominal segment of esophagus
2. Prevention of recurrent herniation of the gastroesophageal junction into the chest, and
3. Creation of an antireflux valvular mechanism that allows normal swallowing, belching, and vomiting but prevents abnormal spontaneous reflux of gastric content.

In most instances, the valvular mechanism is created by a partial or total fundoplication of some kind. Partial fundoplication includes the Belsey, Dor, and Toupet repairs. Total fundoplication is accomplished with the Nissen and Nissen-Rosetti procedures. The Hill repair has several unique features, although Hill's "posterior gastropexy" is somewhat like a snug fundoplication. The Belsey, Dor, Toupet, Hill, and Nissen repairs are described in Chapters 20 to 23.

For each of these approaches and antireflux techniques, technical precision is necessary if *repeatedly* good results are to be obtained. There is no perfect single operation. Despite more than 50 years of surgical effort, failure is all too common, especially in inexperienced hands.

Before selecting the correct surgical procedure for the patient, the surgeon must consider whether significant esophageal shortening has occurred. This is usually related to the changes that occur with reflux esophagitis, panmural inflammation of the esophageal wall, and ultimate stricture and shortening. Barrett's esophagus is commonly associated with some degree of shortening (Gastal et al, 1999). Giant paraesophageal hernia (types III and IV) may be associated with such shortening (Maziak et al, 1998). When significant esophageal shortening occurs, an intraoperative decision must be made as to whether complete mobilization of the esophagus develops sufficient esophageal length for a tension-free repair. If not, an esophageal lengthening procedure is recommended. Acquired short esophagus and the indications for gastroplasty are considered in Chapters 15 and 24.

The surgeon should always assess esophageal motor function. Repairs that necessitate total fundoplication should be avoided if severe esophageal dysmotility is present. In such instances, even a "loose" total fundoplication can produce an antireflux valve that is "too strong" and lead to esophageal obstruction. A partial fundoplication creates a somewhat "weaker," but, it is hoped, adequate, valve that better serves the patient with absent or significantly impaired peristalsis. Defective peristalsis may occur secondary to panmural reflux damage or primary motor disorders such as scleroderma and achalasia. The influence of dysmotility on the selection of operation is reviewed, and recommendations are presented by Ritter and associates (1998).

■ *REFERENCES*

Allen MS, Trastek VF, Deschamps C, et al: Intrathoracic stomach. J Thorac Cardiovasc Surg 105:253–259, 1993.

Allison PR: Reflux esophagitis, sliding hiatal hernia, and the anatomy of repair. Surg Gynecol Obstet 92:149, 1951.

Allison PR: Hiatus hernia: A 20-year retrospective survey. Ann Surg 178:273–276, 1973.

Belsey RHR: History of Antireflux surgery. In Thoracic Surgery. London/New York, Churchill Livingston, 1995, pp 209–213,

Bremner CG: Barrett's esophagus. Int Trends Gen Thorac Surg 3:227, 1987.

Cappell MS, Sciales C, Biempica L: Esophageal perforation at a Barrett's ulcer. J Clin Gastroenterol 11:663, 1989.

Carter R, Brewer LA, Hinshaw DB: Acute gastric volvulus: A study of 25 cases. Am J Surg 140:99, 1980.

Dallemagne B, Weerts JM, Jehaes C, et al: Laparoscopic Nissen fundoplication: Preliminary report. Surg Laparosc Endosc 1:138–143, 1991.

Diehl JT, Thomas L, Bloom MB, et al: Tracheoesophageal fistula associated with Barrett's ulcer: The importance of reflux control. Ann Thorac Surg 45:449, 1988.

Gastal OL, Hagen JA, Peters JH, et al: Short esophagus: Predictors and clinical implications. Arch Surg 134:633–636, 1999.

Geha AS, Malek G, Massad MD, et al: A 32 year experience in 100 patients with giant paraesophageal hernia: The case for abdominal approach and selective antireflux repair. Surgery 128:623–630, 2000.

Gerstenberger PD, Pellegrini CA, Tieney LM: Barrett's ulcer of the esophagus: Previously unrecognized cause of acquired esophagorespiratory fistula. Am J Med 81:713, 1986.

Hill LD: Incarcerated paraesophageal hernia. Am J Surg 126:286–292, 1973.

Katyal D, Jewell LD, Yakimets WW: Aortoesophageal fistula secondary to benign Barrett's ulcer: A rare cause of massive gastrointestinal hemorrhage. Can J Surg 36:480, 1993.

Limburg AJ, Jesselink EJ, Kleibeuker JH: Barrett's ulcer: Cause of spontaneous esophageal perforation. Gut 30:404, 1989.

Maziak DE, Todd TRJ, Pearson FG: Massive hiatus hernia: Evaluation and surgical management. J Thorac Cardiovasc Surg 115:53–60, 1998.

Ozdemir IA, Burke WA, Ikins PM: Paraesophageal hernia: A life-threatening disease. Ann Thorac Surg 16:547, 1973.

Pearson FG, Cooper JD, Ilves R, et al: Massive hiatal hernia with incarceration: A report of 53 cases. Ann Thorac Surg 35:45, 1983.

Pearson FG, Cooper JD, Patterson GA, Prakash D: Peptic ulcer in columnar-lined esophagus. Ann Thorac Surg 43:241, 1987.

Ritter MP, Peters JH, DeMeester TR, et al: Treatment of advanced gastroesophageal reflux disease with Collis gastroplasty and Belsey partial fundoplication. Arch Surg 133:523–529, 1998.

Semb BKH, Halvorsen JF, Fossdal JE: Acute gastric volvulus with necrosis of the stomach and the left lower pulmonary lobe. Acta Chir Scand 143:256, 1977.

Skinner DB, Belsey RHR: Surgical management of esophageal reflux and hiatus hernia. J Thorac Cardiovasc Surg 53:33, 1967.

CHAPTER **14**

Gastroesophageal Reflux in Infants and Children

David P. Campbell
Darroch W. O. Moores

Over the past 3 decades, gastroesophageal reflux disease (GERD) and its complications have been recognized with increasing frequency in infants and children. Our understanding of the pathophysiology, diagnostic techniques, and treatment of this disorder has increased significantly during this period. Antireflux surgery has, in fact, become one of the most commonly performed operations in the pediatric age group.

HISTORICAL NOTE

By 1950, the knowledge that GERD could lead to peptic esophagitis and peptic stricture was well recognized in the adult population but poorly understood in infants and children. Neuhauser and Berenberg (1950) used the term *chalasia* to describe incompetence of the lower esophageal sphincter (LES) in infants in the absence of hiatus hernia. In 1950, Carré and Astley (Carré, 1979; Carré and Astley, 1960) recognized the clinical significance of hiatal hernia in association with GERD in the pediatric population. Carré and Astley noted that in many children with repeated vomiting and severe reflux there existed some degree of "partial thoracic stomach." These small hiatal hernias were diagnosed radiologically and were attributed to structural congenital abnormalities. The patients that Carré and Astley identified were children with the most severe reflux disease. Vomiting was the earliest symptom in almost all patients; 80% had hematemesis, and peptic stricture was found in 5%. Despite the severity of the disease, 60% to 65% of children studied by Carré became asymptomatic by 2 years of age.

As our understanding of GERD and techniques of diagnosis have improved, the term *chalasia* has been dropped. We have come to understand that GERD with or without hiatal hernia is a distinct pathologic process. The process can be completely benign or may lead to profound, even life-threatening complications.

HISTORICAL READINGS

Carré IJ: A historical review of the clinical consequences of hiatal hernia (partial thoracic stomach) and gastroesophageal reflux. In Gellis S (ed): Gastroesophageal Reflux: Report of the 76th Ross Conference on Pediatric Research. Columbus, OH, Ross Laboratories, 1979, p 1.

Carré IJ, Astley R: The fate of the partial thoracic stomach ("hiatus hernia") in children. Arch Dis Child 35:484, 1960.

Neuhauser EBD, Berenberg W: Cardioesophageal relaxation (chalasia) as a cause of vomiting in infants. Pediatrics 5:414, 1950.

BASIC SCIENCE: PATHOPHYSIOLOGY

Normal esophageal function is dependent on complex neurogenic and hormonal interaction. The LES, or high-pressure zone, functions as a pressure barrier to prevent gastric contents from refluxing back into the esophagus. It is not a distinct muscle but an extension of the esophageal circular muscle at the junction between the esophagus and the gastric cardia. The LES does not remain in a constant state of contraction but relaxes physiologically in response to swallowing, burping, and vomiting.

Zaninotto and associates (1988) found that patients with a chronic LES pressure below 5 mm Hg or those with short LES length are at high risk for pathologic reflux. Werlin and associates (1980) simultaneously monitored distal esophageal pH, upper esophageal sphincter (UES) pressure, LES pressure, intragastric pressure, and intraesophageal pressure at several sites in the esophagus. They found that in *children* with GERD, only 12% of reflux episodes occurred while there was a reduction in resting lower esophageal pressure. The majority of reflux episodes (54%) occurred during transient increases in intra-abdominal pressure above the level of the resting LES pressure. These transient spikes in intragastric pressure occurred mainly while patients were awake and performing normal activities. Thirty-four percent of reflux episodes occurred during transient, spontaneous, complete relaxation of the LES. Spontaneous relaxations of the LES were brief, not associated with esophageal peristalsis, and presumed not to be the result of swallowing.

It has been postulated by Dent (1981, 1988), Farrell (1974), Lipshutz (1974), and their coworkers that abnormal hormonal and neurogenic control mechanisms lead to spontaneous LES pressure drifts unassociated with swallowing that predispose the individual to pathologic reflux. Relaxation of the LES in response to gastric distention seems to be mediated via vagosympathetic reflexes initiated by stimulation of mechanoreceptors in the gastric wall. Hillemeier and colleagues (1981) demonstrated that *newborn infants* with GERD tend to have delayed gastric emptying. Delayed gastric emptying increases intragastric pressure.

Transient inappropriate episodes of LES relaxation or pressure drifts, with or without gastric distention, are currently thought to be the major mechanism permitting reflux to occur (Cucchiara et al, 1993; Dent et al, 1981;

Werlin et al, 1980). It is not clear whether these transient sphincter relaxation episodes are more frequent or last longer in patients with reflux disease.

The ability of the esophagus to clear refluxed material is vitally important to mucosal integrity. Poor clearance exposes the esophageal mucosa to gastric contents for prolonged periods of time, causing damage to the esophageal mucosa and esophagitis. Esophagitis further impairs the LES mechanism, both decreasing tone and impairing peristalsis.

Boix-Ochoa and Canals (1976) performed 4028 esophageal manometric studies in 680 infants and newborns ranging in age from 1 day to 6 months. They found the LES to be hypotensive in newborns, with maturation occurring by the seventh week of life. In contrast, a study of 97 infants by Moroz and associates (1976) demonstrated that in control subjects without GERD the LES was well developed by 2 weeks of life and that children younger than 1 year of age had a mean LES pressure significantly greater than the mean LES pressure in children older than 1 year of age. Hollwarth and Uray (1985) demonstrated normal LES pressure in newborns. They postulated that the findings of Boix-Ochoa were the result of inferior manometric equipment lacking high-pressure pumps and constant perfusion systems.

Ott and coworkers (1985) found that the length of the LES is approximately 1 cm in infants and increases to 2 to 4 cm by adolescence. DeMeester and colleagues (1979) demonstrated that a normal length of intra-abdominal esophagus is important for gastroesophageal competence. As the infant grows, the intra-abdominal segment increases in length to help establish an effective antireflux barrier.

At birth, infants tend to have an obtuse angle of His, in keeping with the short length of the intra-abdominal esophageal segment (Fig. 14–1). With increased intra-abdominal pressure, an obtuse angle of His converts the upper stomach into a funnel, directing the intragastric contents into the esophagus. As the length of the intra-abdominal segment of esophagus increases, the angle of His becomes more acute and becomes a more effective antireflux barrier. Secretin, prostaglandin, cholecystokinin, glucagon, vasopressin, and gastric inhibitory peptide all cause a decrease in LES pressure and presumably favor GERD (Boix-Ochoa, 1986).

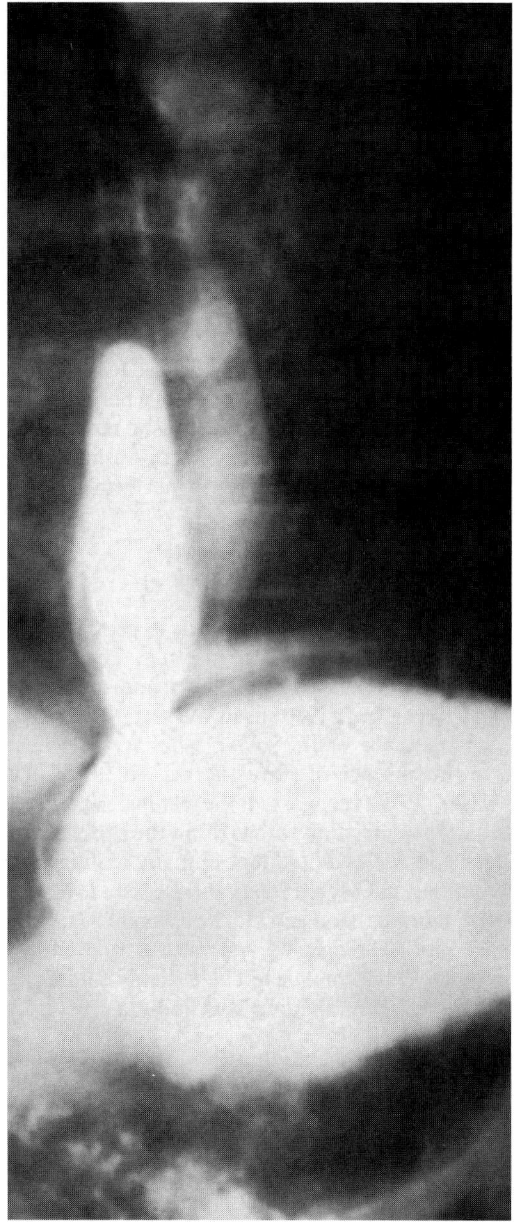

FIGURE 14–1 ■ Free gastroesophageal reflux in a 6-month-old child. The patient has a short intra-abdominal esophageal segment. The angle of His tends to be somewhat obtuse.

Response to GERD differs from patient to patient. Some individuals remain unaffected, but others experience severe complications. The chemical makeup of the refluxate, emptying proficiency, mucosal defense barriers, mucosal healing processes, and acid-base sensitivity determine responses to GERD. Esophageal dysmotility occurs in 35% of infants with symptomatic GERD (Fonkalsrud et al, 1987). Clearance of the refluxate by the esophagus is reduced when the efficiency of peristalsis is diminished. Whether this dysmotility is the cause or effect of reflux is unknown.

When gastric juice bathes the esophageal mucosa, neural stimulation triggers voluntary and involuntary activity to promote clearance of the refluxate. The ability to appreciate reflux episodes, particularly those that may be subclinical, is determined in part by the sensitivity of the esophagus to gastric juice (Orr et al, 1983). Some patients develop complications without experiencing symptoms. Such a situation may be encountered when the pH of the refluxate remains between 4 and 7 or when the esophagus is relatively insensitive to acid (Vandenplas and Loeb, 1991; VanTrappen et al, 1987).

The degree of injury to the esophageal mucosa depends partially on mucosal resistance to the toxic effects of the refluxate. The mucosal barrier is incompletely understood, and resistance appears to vary from patient to patient. Similarly, healing of the mucosal injury is an intrinsic attribute. The inflammatory process that initially ensues as a result of mucosal injury is unique to the individual, as is the reparative process, which includes the degree of scarring and the cellular pathologic changes.

Both acid and alkaline reflux can inflict mucosal injury (Vandenplas and Loeb, 1991). A pH below 4 or greater than 7 leads to damage, but a pH outside the normal range is not the sole cause of injury. Pepsin, trypsin, lipase, bile salts, and carboxypeptidase, key constituents in gastric and duodenogastric refluxate, may produce epithelial changes in the esophageal mucosa (DeMeester, 1987). The overall effect upon the esophageal mucosa is determined by the composition of the esophageal refluxate and the exposure time.

DIAGNOSIS

Clinical Features

Regurgitation of gastric contents in the newborn is a common physiologic event. Therefore, spitting up or vomiting during the first year of life is quite common. These physiologic reflux episodes are brief and occur approximately five times in the first hour after each meal. By 1 to 2 hours after feeding, these episodes return to a baseline frequency close to zero. Although all infants have some degree of GERD in the newborn period, the vast majority experience resolution of symptoms between the ages of 9 and 24 months (Hillemeier, 1996).

The clinical manifestations of GERD in infants include regurgitation, failure to thrive, apnea spells, nonspecific irritability, episodic bradycardia, ruminative behavior, stridor, cough, and lower respiratory symptoms. Newborns and infants with complications of GERD present primarily with failure to thrive and bronchopulmonary problems. Some degree of esophagitis is also common in infants with GERD (61% to 82%) (Black et al, 1990; Shub et al, 1985), but it is not usually the primary manifestation. Older children manifest GERD symptoms similar to adults. These include retrosternal burning, which is worsened by ingestion of spicy or fatty foods and relieved by antacids.

The relationship between GERD and bronchopulmonary manifestations (possibly including sudden infant death syndrome [SIDS]) has been well described (Darling et al, 1978; Herbst et al, 1978; see Gastro-oesophageal, 1988; Leape et al, 1977). Respiratory complications constitute the major indication for antireflux surgery for pediatric patients in North America. Boyle and associates (1985) demonstrated a clear relationship between GERD and bronchospasm. Control of GERD is particularly important in patients with *chronic* respiratory disease such as cystic fibrosis and bronchopulmonary dysplasia (Scott et al, 1985; Vinocur et al, 1985).

Investigative Techniques

No single test is diagnostic of GERD. A variety of studies are available that collectively identify patients who have pathologic GERD. Standardization and modification of currently available tests continue to improve accuracy in diagnosis and treatment.

Barium Esophagogram

A barium esophagogram is nonspecific, but when performed by an experienced pediatric radiologist, it is the best initial screening study. It is helpful in identifying anatomic abnormalities, mucosal lesions, and gross motility disorders. When it is performed as an initial study, much useful information can be gained, but it should not be relied upon as the only diagnostic study.

Endoscopy

The availability of small fiberoptic endoscopes has resulted in many infants and children with symptoms of GERD undergoing endoscopy. Endoscopy makes the exact diagnosis of mucosal pathology possible. The grade and degree of esophagitis can be recognized and confirmed with biopsy. Eosinophilic infiltrates have been found to be specific indicators of GERD in infants (Winter et al, 1982). The absence of esophagitis does not rule out significant GERD, however, because inflammatory mucosal changes do not occur in all individuals with pathologic reflux disease.

Manometry

Manometry is helpful in recognizing motility disorders, locating and assessing the tone of the LES, and measuring the length of the intra-abdominal segment of the esophagus. It does not, however, diagnose GERD. Because manometric studies are difficult to perform in infants and young children and have proved to be of little clinical value, they remain primarily a research tool.

Scintigraphy

Scintiscanning can be used to document GERD and delayed gastric emptying (DiLorenzo et al, 1987). It provides information about esophageal bolus transit time, the degree of retention, and alterations in esophageal clearance. Scintiscans can also detect pulmonary aspiration after GERD but are a less sensitive indicator of aspiration. If reflux-induced aspiration is suspected, this test may be confirmatory if results are positive. The greatest problem with the gastroesophageal scintiscan is that it does not correlate closely with pH studies. It is therefore not a practical test for quantitating GERD (Vandenplas et al, 1992), although it is very useful in the diagnosis of delayed gastric emptying.

pH Monitoring

Long-term pH monitoring is the most sensitive and specific test for diagnosis of GERD and is considered the diagnostic standard. This test has undergone extensive development and standardization in both adult and pediatric populations (Davidson, 1985; DeMeester et al, 1980; Johnson and DeMeester, 1974; Jolley et al, 1978). pH monitoring is the only technique that can detect and quantify both acid and alkaline GERD and identify the patients most at risk for complications from reflux. Long-term pH monitoring can be used both for diagnosis and for monitoring the patient's response to therapy.

Normal esophageal pH ranges from 5.0 to 6.8 (Johnson and DeMeester, 1974). Acid reflux is characterized by a fall in lower esophageal pH below 4.0, whereas alkaline reflux is characterized by a distal esophageal pH above 7.0. Patterns of normal pH values have been

TABLE 14–1 ■ Normal Values for Ambulatory pH Monitoring in Infants

Observation	*Infants Younger than 15 days*	*Infants 3.5 to 4.4 mo*
Acid reflux	1.20 ± 0.91	4.18 ± 2.60
Total percentage of time pH is less than 4.0		
Reflux episodes per 24 hr	7.73 ± 6.51	19.98 ± 16.10
Reflux episodes are greater than 5 min per 24 hr	0.6 ± 1.2	3.24 ± 2.41
Longest episode (min)	3.86 ± 1.9	11.8 ± 7.8
Alkaline reflux	1.3 ± 2.6	
Percentage of time pH is greater than 7.0		
Number of episodes per 24 hr	10.4	

Data from Vandenplas Y, Loeb H: Alkaline gastroesophageal reflux in infancy. J Pediatr Gastroenterol Nutr 12:448, 1991; and Vandenplas Y, Sacre-Smits L: Continuous 24-hour esophageal pH monitoring in 285 asymptomatic infants 0–15 months old. J Pediatr Gastroenterol Nutr 6:220, 1987.

established but continue to be refined as methodology is improved and new pathophysiologic functions are uncovered (Table 14–1).

For optimal results, a pH study should include awake and sleeping periods, feeding and fasting intervals, and positional changes. Although shorter studies have been evaluated extensively, 24-hour studies produce the most reliable data. A pH study involves transnasal placement of a pH probe in the distal esophagus. A variety of probes exist with multichannel monitoring capability. Sondheimer (1980) reported the ideal probe position to be at a distance above the LES that is 13% of the entire length of the esophagus. The probe is positioned with fluoroscopy or radiography. The ability to detect reflux diminishes the higher the probe is placed above the LES, hence the need for proper placement of the probe using fluoroscopy or radiography.

Optimal monitoring is accomplished with a portable recorder, which allows normal activity and feeding. Twenty-four-hour esophageal monitoring is 100% accurate in the diagnosis of reflux when the pH is below 4.0 for more than 5% of the total time monitored (Fonkalsrud and Ament, 1996).

MANAGEMENT

The general principles of treatment of GERD focus on decreasing the volume and toxicity of the refluxate. Most infants and children, but particularly infants, can be treated conservatively. Antireflux therapy starts with conservative measures to prevent reflux and proceeds through pharmacologic agents to surgery. Surgical management is reserved for serious complications and cases of reflux that cannot be managed medically.

Treatment of GERD should be based on the collective findings during evaluation. Selection of the appropriate mode of therapy depends on the predisposing factors, including:

- Esophageal motility disorders
- Poor esophageal clearance
- Delayed gastric emptying
- Concurrent illnesses

The neurologically impaired infant or child with GERD represents a unique group. These patients often have concomitant esophageal and gastric motility disorders that predispose them to reflux. Their ability to appreciate and register symptoms is often impaired. Some of the neuroleptic agents taken by such patients exacerbate the reflux by reducing LES tone. Chronic seizure activity, irritability, retching, and abdominal muscle spasms add to the problem because of elevation of intra-abdominal pressure. The complications most commonly encountered in this neurologic group include malnutrition, aspiration, severe esophagitis, recurrent pneumonia, and vomiting.

Conservative, nonoperative measures often fail to resolve the problem. Surgical intervention is effective and involves low morbidity and mortality. Early surgical management should be considered for this exceptional group.

Medical Management

Conservative treatment of reflux is effective in most pediatric patients. From 85% to 95% respond satisfactorily to selected measures with complete or adequate control of symptoms or complications (Boix-Ochoa et al, 1985). The three pillars of nonoperative therapy for symptomatic GERD in infants and children are positional maneuvers, feeding changes, and medications (Fonkalsrud and Ament, 1996) (see "Medical Management" Box).

Most patients younger than age 2 years are well managed with medical therapy, and relatively few require surgical intervention. Beyond this age, however, children tend to be less responsive to medical management. If reflux continues beyond age 2, it often becomes a chronic problem during childhood and adolescence (Orenstein, 1991).

Position

The prone position is the best one for reducing or preventing reflux in infants. From a study of 90 infants who had documented abnormal GERD, Orenstein (1990) concluded that there was no significant difference in reflux between the flat prone position and the head-elevated prone position, in which children were kept prone on a mattress inclined 30 degrees. In an elegant and important previous study, Orenstein and coworkers (1983) had shown that the traditionally recommended

MEDICAL MANAGEMENT OF GASTROESOPHAGEAL REFLUX

Postural alterations—prone (upright) position
Dietary changes—small frequent feedings
Medications
  Histamine (H_2)-blockers
  Antacids
  Prokinetics

seated position in an infant seat was associated with more GERD than the horizontal prone position in children younger than 6 months (Orenstein et al, 1983). The prone position was also superior when infants were held in a harness in a head-elevated prone position versus in an infant seat (Orenstein and Whitington, 1983).

In addition to decreasing reflux, the prone position has been shown to improve gastric emptying (Yu, 1975), decrease aspiration (Hewitt, 1976), and decrease energy expenditure (Masterson et al, 1987). However, the increased risk of SIDS for infants placed in the prone position has led to negative enthusiasm for its use at the present time.

Diet

Small, frequent feedings of formula thickened with rice cereal have long been recommended as treatment for GERD and have been demonstrated by pH studies to decrease reflux (Orenstein et al, 1987). Older children should fast for several hours before bed and should avoid foods such as chocolate and coffee, which diminish LES tone. Foods that promote gastric acidity, such as fatty foods, citric acid, carbonated beverages, and tomatoes, should also be avoided. Obesity and tight abdominal clothing should be discouraged.

Drug Therapy

Prokinetics. Prokinetic drugs augment LES tone and decrease gastric emptying time. Extensive experience with the use of these drugs supports their role in the treatment of GERD.

Bethanechol (a muscarinic agonist), the first prokinetic agent used in children (Moroz et al, 1976), stimulates motor activity in the upper intestinal tract. LES pressure is increased and esophageal clearance may be enhanced with oral bethanechol. Bethanechol, however, has not been shown conclusively to alter the degree of reflux. The relative lack of success with bethanechol may be due to the fact that most infants with GERD do not have reduced basal LES pressure (Hillemeier, 1996).

Metoclopramide (Reglan) is a dopamine antagonist with cholinomimetic agonist effects. It improves esophageal and gastric motor activity and increases LES pressure. Several studies have confirmed its usefulness in GERD, although some reports have shown mixed results (Hyams et al, 1986; Machida et al, 1988; McCallum et al, 1983; Rozen et al, 1984; Tolia et al, 1989). The main disadvantage of metoclopramide is that it crosses the blood-brain barrier, leading to extrapyramidal side effects such as dystonias, dyskinesias, and parkinsonian symptoms (De Silva et al, 1973).

Cisapride (Propulsid) is an indirect cholinergic agonist with muscarinic effects. Cisapride enhances gastrointestinal motility, improves antroduodenal coordination, increases LES pressure, and increases esophageal contractility. Although several studies have confirmed the value of the drug in the treatment of GERD, cisapride has been reported to cause cardiac arrhythmias in infants, particularly premature neonates. The arrhythmias are more noticeable with high doses of cisapride and when cisapride inactivation is impaired by drugs such as macrolide antibiotics and azole antifungals. Cisapride should thus be used with caution in infants and young children (Lander and Desai, 1998; Ward et al, 1999). In fact, cisapride has recently been removed from the market.

Histamine (H_2)-Blockers and Antacids. Antacids are clearly useful in reducing the acidity of gastric content; however, dosing frequency and taste make compliance with antacid therapy difficult in the pediatric age group. The primary role of antacids is as a supplement to histamine antagonist (H_2-blocker) therapy or for children who require only intermittent therapy for relief of symptoms.

H_2-blockers are the mainstay of medical treatment in children with GERD. Cimetidine (Lambert et al, 1992), ranitidine (Sutphen and Dillard, 1989), and famotidine (Sontag, 1990) all have been used successfully.

Omeprazole, an agent that blocks the proton pump, results in complete blockage of acid secretion and is more effective than the H_2-blockers in controlling acid secretion (Hetzel et al, 1988; Klinkenberg-Knol et al, 1987). Omeprazole has been effective in otherwise intractable esophagitis in adults (Hetzel et al, 1988; Klinkenberg-Knol et al, 1987). It has not been used extensively in children because the safety and dosage in young infants are not well established (Faubion and Zein, 1998).

Sucralfate, a basic aluminum salt of a sulfated sucrose, is effective in the treatment of peptic esophagitis in children (Arguelles-Martin et al, 1989). Although it is not considered an antacid, in an acid environment sucralfate forms a sticky paste-like substance (Nagashima and Yoshida, 1979) that has a relative affinity for ulcerated tissue (Nakazawa et al, 1981). This substance acts as a barrier to diffusion of acid, pepsin, and bile salts (Brogden et al, 1984). It is most effective when given in suspension form for the treatment of reflux esophagitis.

Surgery

Indications

For most patients, a trial of medical management should be employed. If improvement or resolution of symptoms occurs, continued conservative therapy is justified. In infants, because there is a strong propensity for spontaneous resolution of GERD with maturation of the LES, surgical treatment should be employed only after a thorough trial of medical management has failed. An acceptable time frame of 6 to 12 months of conservative management should be tried unless exceptional circumstances require earlier intervention. Patients with life-threatening complications or those less likely to respond to conservative management such as neurologically impaired infants should be considered for early surgical treatment.

There appears to be an indirect association of SIDS with GERD, but direct evidence incriminating GERD as a cause of SIDS has been inconclusive (Jeffery et al, 1983). Near-miss SIDS, in association with confirmed GERD, is considered an absolute indication for an antireflux procedure (Kiely, 1990; Ramenofsky, 1986) (see "Indications for Surgery" Box). There is still no clearly documented evidence to support the existence of a true clinical syndrome of reflux-related apnea and bradycardia

INDICATIONS FOR SURGERY IN INFANTS AND CHILDREN WITH DOCUMENTED GASTROESOPHAGEAL REFLUX

Near-miss sudden infant death syndrome (SIDS)
Failure to thrive
Respiratory complications
Severe intractable esophagitis
Peptic esophageal stricture
Barrett's esophagus
Failure to respond to medical therapy

spells despite widely held belief in its existence (Andze et al, 1991; Jolley et al, 1990; Kahn et al, 1990; Padman and Quijano, 1989).

Reports comparing medical and surgical management of infants with SIDS have implied that surgery can make a difference. Several authors have shown resolution of symptoms in surgically treated patients while medically treated patients continue to experience complications (Leape and Ramenofsky, 1980; Ribet et al, 1989; Sacre and Vandenplas, 1989; St. Cyr et al, 1989). Other groups have shown that such patients improve with medical therapy and time (Andze et al, 1991; Boyle, 1989). The authors think that absolute confirmation of the relationship between reflux and apnea is not required when apneic episodes and documented pathologic GERD coexist. These infants should be seriously considered for early surgical intervention.

The presence of a peptic esophageal stricture in the pediatric age group indicates pathologic reflux that is unlikely to respond to long-term medical measures. This complication occurs in 2.3% to 15% of patients with symptomatic reflux (Hicks et al, 1980; Ohhama et al, 1990; O'Neill et al, 1982). Children with peptic stricture may have no symptoms of reflux disease before presenting with dysphagia. The majority of children with this complication are younger than 5 years of age (Nihoul-Fekete et al, 1979), and a high percentage have undergone repair of esophageal atresia. Anastomotic strictures after surgery for esophageal atresia have a reported incidence of 14% to 27% (Hicks et al, 1980; Holder et al, 1964; O'Neill et al, 1982). In our experience, most of these strictures are related to reflux. If dilatation and medical therapy cannot resolve the stricture, the most effective method for permanent and prompt cure is operative intervention with an antireflux procedure and intraoperative dilatation. Most cases of reflux-related strictures respond to this form of management, and esophageal dilatations are seldom needed postoperatively. Resection of peptic strictures is rarely indicated.

Barrett's esophagus is believed to be a complication of reflux esophagitis and is closely associated with longstanding severe esophagitis. Dahms and Rothstein (1984) reported the prevalence of Barrett's esophagus in children with GERD to be 13%. In adults, the most serious complication of Barrett's esophagus is adenocarcinoma of the esophagus. The estimated incidence of adenocarcinoma development in Barrett's esophagus is between 1 carcinoma in 52 patient-years and 1 in 441 patient-years (Cameron et al, 1985; Hameeteman et al, 1989; Spechler et al, 1984). This risk is particularly worrisome in patients in the pediatric age group, for such children have many years of life remaining. One may speculate that chronic reflux esophagitis with Barrett's esophagus in infants and children would increase their susceptibility to carcinoma. The authors strongly recommend that patients in the pediatric age group with a diagnosis of Barrett's esophagus undergo surgery to control reflux and be followed by long-term endoscopic surveillance for any early detection of malignant change.

Reflux-related respiratory complications, such as recurrent pneumonia, aspiration, and asthma, warrant consideration for early surgery, especially in children and adolescents. A trial of medical management is justified, but surgery is indicated if prompt improvement is not seen or if symptoms worsen.

Infants and young children who experience severe regurgitation and repeated vomiting may quickly become malnourished with failure to thrive. Such malnourishment occurs more commonly in young infants and in neurologically disabled children. A prolonged course of conservative management may worsen the problem or may permit the development of significant complications. Lack of response to adequate medical therapy within a 4-week period in this unique group of patients justifies consideration of surgery.

Antireflux Procedures

Antireflux procedures have been devised to restructure and augment the LES mechanisms. The primary objectives are to tighten the esophageal hiatus, lengthen the intra-abdominal esophagus, and augment the LES. Many antireflux procedures exist. Each has its proponents, and each has been reported to give good results. The more popular techniques in the pediatric age group include the following:

- Nissen procedure(Nissen, 1961)
- Thal procedure (Ashcraft et al, 1981; Thal, 1968)
- Boix-Ochoa procedure (Boix-Ochoa, 1986)
- Toupet procedure (Toupet, 1963)

Nissen Procedure. The transabdominal Nissen procedure remains the most popular antireflux operation. The antireflux procedure used by the authors is a modification of the Nissen procedure.

The intra-abdominal segment of the esophagus is mobilized to add intra-abdominal length as it traverses the crural tunnel. Several short gastric vessels are divided to provide adequate gastric fundus for fundoplication. The esophageal hiatus is tightened by posterior approximation of the esophageal crura (Fig. 14–2*A*). The mobilized gastric fundus is passed behind the intra-abdominal esophagus (see Fig. 14–2*A*). The vagus nerves are carefully preserved for inclusion within the wrap.

The gastric fundus is loosely wrapped circumferentially around the esophagus to create a 1- to 3-cm fundoplication (depending upon the size of the child). The fundoplication sutures are placed from gastric fundus, to the lateral esophageal wall at 9 o'clock, to gastric fundus

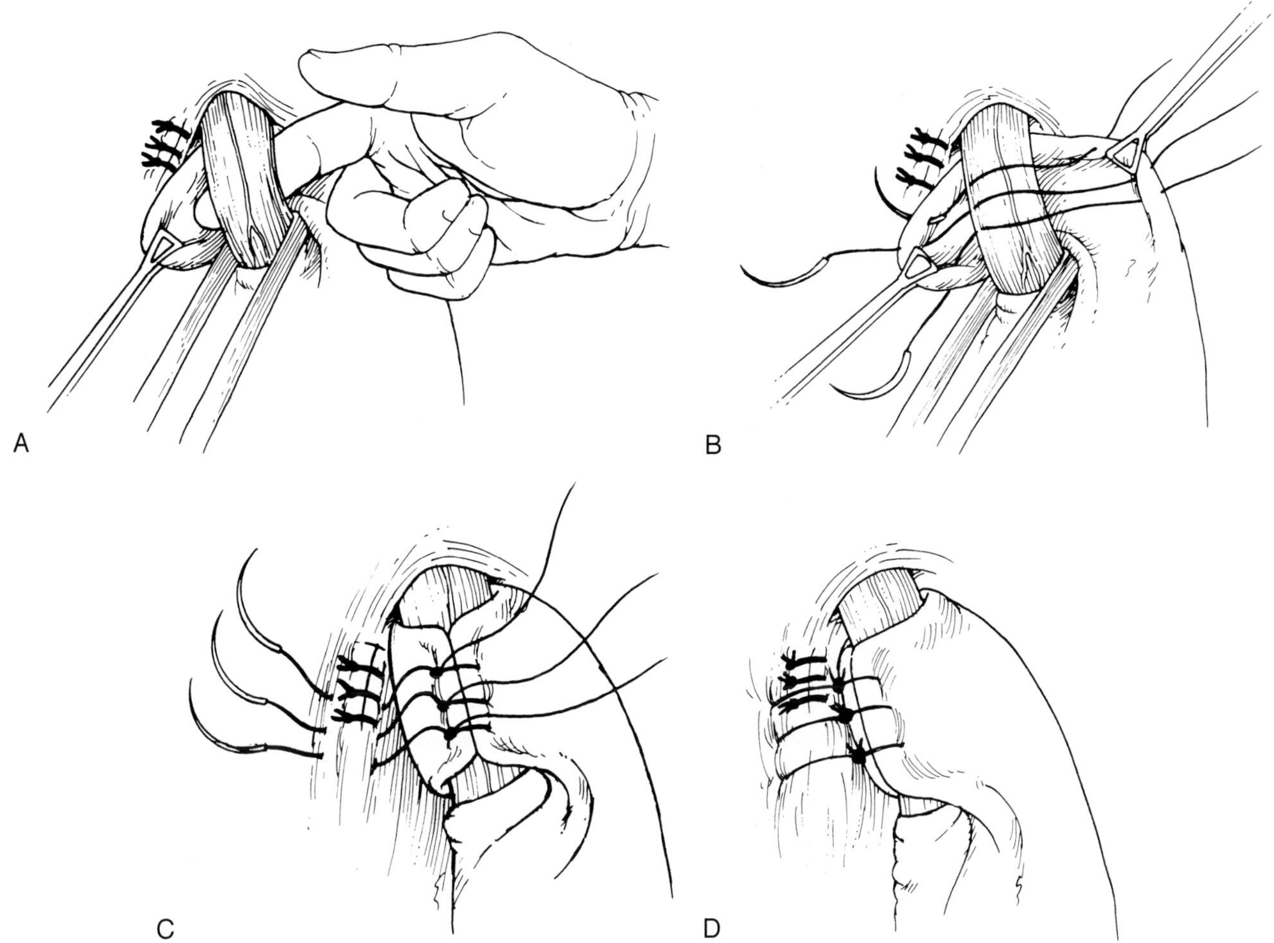

FIGURE 14–2 ■ *A–D*, Nissen fundoplication showing recommended reinforcement by anchoring fundoplication sutures to closed crura to prevent postoperative herniation.

(Fig. 14–2*B*). The fundoplication sutures are then passed through the approximated crura. When these sutures are pulled through and tied, the fundoplication is securely anchored within the abdomen (Fig. 14–2*C*, *D*). We feel that fixation of the fundoplication in this manner is crucial to prevent postoperative herniation (Fig. 14–3). A 360-degree fundoplication of this type assists in preserving intra-abdominal esophageal length and adds an external force to the LES during gastric distention to prevent GERD.

A gastrostomy may be performed to facilitate postoperative feedings and to function as an anterior gastropexy as a further security for the position of the repair.

Thal Fundoplication. The Thal fundoplication, as advocated by Ashcraft and colleagues (1981), has been used effectively. The primary difference between the Nissen and Thal fundoplications is the use of an anterior 180- to 270-degree fundoplication in the Thal rather than the 360-degree wrap used in the Nissen. The Thal procedure rarely causes gas bloat and permits burping and physiologic vomiting if necessary.

Boix-Ochoa Partial Fundoplication. The Boix-Ochoa (Boix-Ochoa, 1986) procedure creates a partial fundoplication. The gastric fundus is affixed to the diaphragm and the lesser gastric curvature to the anterior abdominal wall. This technique is based on the concept that the LES is "displaced" and, consequently, incapable of normal physiologic function. By simple repositioning of the structures important to the LES complex with no significant alterations, such as the 360-degree wrap, Boix-Ochoa thought that competence could be achieved in addition to allowing further maturation of the LES mechanism. Physiologic vomiting is preserved. This procedure is rarely used in the United States.

Toupet Procedure. The Toupet procedure (Toupet, 1963) is a posterior fundoplication in which the gastric fundus is brought behind the intra-abdominal esophagus and sewn to each limb of the hiatal crura. The remainder of the transposed fundus is secured to each side of the esophagus, thus producing a 180-degree to 270-degree wrap. The ability to belch or vomit is retained with this procedure, thereby decreasing the incidence of gas bloat syndrome in contrast to the Nissen fundoplication.

Laparoscopic Fundoplication. The laparoscopic approach to fundoplication in infants and children is now a widely accepted procedure. Several large series have

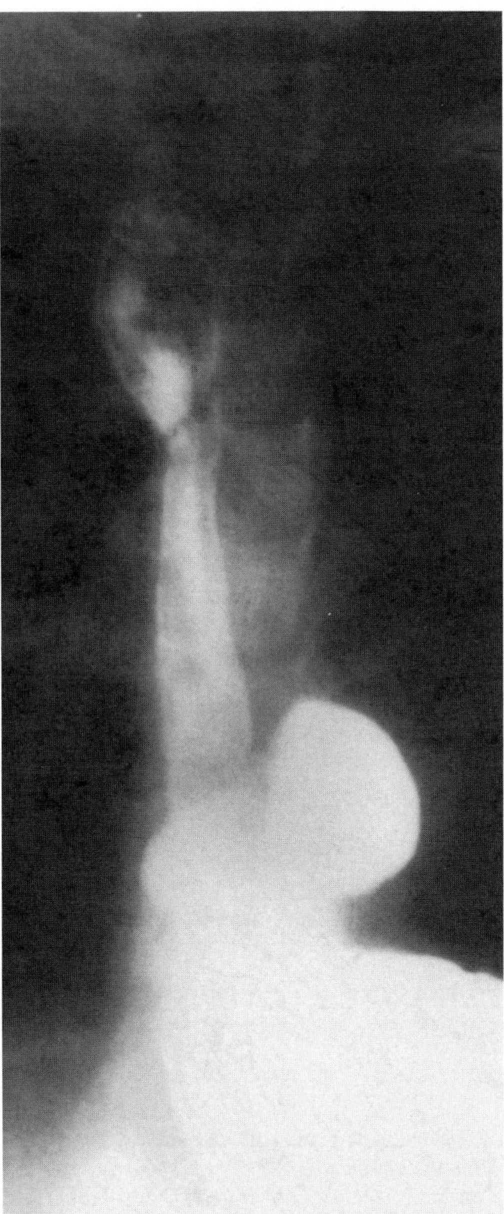

FIGURE 14–3 ■ Radiograph of wrap herniation through the esophageal hiatus.

been reported (Georgeson, 1998; Rothenberg, 1998) with results comparable to those achieved with the open procedures. Nissen, Toupet, and Thal fundoplications have been performed by laparoscopy. The advantages attributed to the laparoscopic approach include a shorter recovery period, lower complication and failure rates, and shorter hospital stays (Georgeson, 1998; Rothenberg, 1998). Long-term results, however, are not yet available.

Heineke-Mikulicz Pyloroplasty. A Heineke-Mikulicz pyloroplasty is sometimes indicated as an adjunct to an antireflux procedure. If gastric-emptying studies show significant gastric hypomotility with slow emptying, a pyloroplasty should be considered. This addition to the antireflux procedure may be necessary in 10% to 12.5% of patients with symptomatic reflux and in 18% to 21.8% of patients with neurologic impairment in whom gastric dysmotility is more frequent (Fonkalsrud et al, 1987, 1989; Papaila et al, 1989).

Perioperative Care

Perioperative management of infants and children undergoing antireflux surgery follows general surgical principles. The anesthesiologist involved should be experienced in pediatric anesthesia. Broad-spectrum prophylactic antibiotics to avoid wound infection are used.

A nasogastric tube is used during the intraoperative period. The tube is removed when bowel function has returned, usually within 24 hours. Feeding is begun with clear liquids and advanced to full feeding as tolerated. A gastrostomy is utilized in neurologically impaired and malnourished children. Feeding through the gastrostomy tube is begun when bowel function has resumed. The gastrostomy tube is removed when the child is able to sustain adequate nutrition with oral intake. In a significant number of neurologically impaired children, the gastrostomy is permanent.

Postoperative Complications

Complications seen with the Nissen technique are often related to construction of an overly tight or lengthy wrap that produces an overcompetent LES. This construction may result in inability to burp or to experience physiologic vomiting. Swallowed air that cannot be burped or passed causes gas bloat syndrome (Boyle, 1989) (see “Complications” Box).

Controversy exists regarding the degree of tightness required by the wrap and crural approximation to prevent reflux while preserving normal swallowing and eructation. The wrap should be no longer than 2 to 3 cm in the pediatric age group. We suggest that postfundoplication symptoms are best avoided by the construction of such a loose and short wrap.

Patients with associated congenital abnormalities, especially those who are neurologically impaired, tend to have more complications and poorer results after antireflux surgery. This group constitutes 35% to 70% of patients undergoing such surgery. Morbidity rates ranging from 5% to 26% have been cited (Pearl et al, 1990; Tuggle et al, 1988; Vane et al, 1985). Mortality is also higher than in neurologically normal children but is usually attributable to the underlying disease and not directly related to the surgery (Tuggle et al, 1988; Turnage et al, 1989; Vane et al, 1985; Wilkinson et al, 1981).

COMPLICATIONS OF OPERATIVE TREATMENT OF GASTROESOPHAGEAL REFLUX

Gas bloat
Prolapse/wrap herniation
Dysphagia
Pulmonary
Wound infection
Intestinal obstruction

The complications encountered in neurologically impaired children are in general similar to those found in neurologically normal children. Wrap herniation, however, is more common (see Fig. 14–3) (Alrabeeah et al, 1988; Pearl et al, 1990; Wilkinson et al, 1981).

In these neurologically impaired patients, seizures and prolonged retching, which greatly elevate intra-abdominal pressure, are quite common and are thought to be the main cause of wrap herniation. Usually, only a portion of the wrap herniates or prolapses, resulting in a paraesophageal hernia. Reoperation to prevent gastric necrosis is usually indicated. Reflux does not usually recur with these paraesophageal hernias. If the entire wrap herniates through the esophageal hiatus into the mediastinum, GERD may recur, often associated with dysphagia. This complication almost always necessitates surgical repair.

Results

Success in correcting GERD and its associated complications has been reported in 88% to 98% of infants and children undergoing antireflux surgery (Boix-Ochoa and Cassasa, 1989; Fonkalsrud et al, 1985, 1987; Henderson and Marryatt, 1985; St. Cyr et al, 1986; Turnage et al, 1989). In the largest pediatric series reported to date, Fonkalsrud and associates (1998) reported good to excellent results in 95% of neurologically normal children and 84.6% of neurologically impaired children undergoing antireflux surgery. Their combined hospital study included 7467 patients. Sixty-four percent of their patients underwent a Nissen fundoplication, 34% a Thal procedure, and 1.5% a Toupet procedure. Major complications occurred in 4.2% of the neurologically normal patients and 12.8% of the neurologically impaired patients. The most frequent complications noted were recurrent reflux secondary to wrap disruption (7.1%), respiratory problems (4.4%), gas bloat syndrome (3.6%), and intestinal obstruction (2.6%). Postoperative mortality was 0.07% in the neurologically normal children and 0.8% in the neurologically impaired children.

Our smaller series of 127 children who underwent fundoplication for GERD between 1985 and 1994 mirrors Fonkalsrud and associates' much larger series as far as results, morbidity, and mortality are concerned.

In summary, GERD is a common and potentially life-threatening problem in the pediatric age group. Early recognition and treatment require a high level of awareness among physicians dealing with this group of patients. Each patient should be evaluated carefully and appropriate therapy instituted. Most patients in this age group can be successfully managed by conservative means. One must not lose track of the fact that GERD in infants usually resolves spontaneously with growth and development. Children with persistent GERD, and especially those with serious complications, should be considered for surgical intervention. Neurologically impaired children represent a special group in whom surgery should be considered early.

Many surgical procedures have been described to deal with GERD. Modification of the Nissen procedure, as described in this chapter, is a rapid, safe, and technically easy procedure. It is associated with excellent results and few postoperative complications.

COMMENTS AND CONTROVERSIES

This concise but thoroughly updated chapter again emphasizes some of the idiosyncrasies in presentation, evaluation, and management of reflux disease in the pediatric population, which are distinctly different from those of the adult condition.

Recurrent vomiting, failure to "thrive," and recurrent respiratory illness are presentations that are easily overlooked as reflux-related problems in neonates and infants during the first year or two of life. In these early years, however, medical management tides over the majority of patients because the condition subsides with maturation of the antireflux mechanism in many or most such cases. When reflux control is not satisfactory, however, there is still limited reported experience with the proton pump inhibiting drugs, and prokinetic agents result in more undue side effects in infants.

The authors clearly define the indications for antireflux surgery and emphasize the importance of recognition and early surgical intervention in the neurologically impaired. Unrecognized, advanced complications of reflux and aspiration are much commoner in this group. Diagnosis can be difficult and may be missed using standard pH probe protocols. The newer application of "electrical impedance manometry" appears significantly more sensitive than pH evaluation in a reported study of 22 infants (69 ± 38 days).

REFERENCE

Wenzl TG, Silny J, Schenke S, et al: Gastroesophageal reflux and respiratory phenomena in infants: Status of the intraluminal impedance technique. J Pediatr Gastroenterol Nutr 28:423–428, 1999.

F. G. P.

KEY REFERENCES

Boix-Ochoa J, Cassasa JM: Surgical treatment of gastroesophageal reflux in children. Surg Annu 21:97, 1989.

This article is a comprehensive review of the surgical options available for the management of gastroesophageal reflux disease. Boix-Ochoa writes with the experience of having surgically treated one of the largest pediatric patient populations in the world who have had this problem.

DeMeester TR: Definition, detection and pathophysiology of gastroesophageal reflux disease. In DeMeester TR, Matthews HR (eds): International Trends in General Thoracic Surgery, Vol 3. Benign Esophageal Disease. St. Louis, CV Mosby, 1987. Discussion by DF Evans, p 99.

This chapter is a state-of-the-art review of the pathophysiology of gastroesophageal reflux disease.

Fonkalsrud EW, Ament ME: Gastrointestinal reflux in children. Curr Probl Surg 33(1):1, 1996.

A comprehensive review of the medical and surgical aspects of gastroesophageal reflux is presented.

Fonkalsrud EW, Ashcraft KW, Coran AG, et al.: Surgical treatment of gastroesophageal reflux in children: A combined hospital study of 7467 patients. Pediatrics 101:419, 1998.

The largest reported series of children who have undergone a fundoplication for treatment of gastroesophageal reflux.

Hillemeier AC: Gastroesophageal reflux. Diagnostic and therapeutic approaches. Pediatr Clin North Am 43(1):197, 1996.

A comprehensive review of the diagnostic and therapeutic approaches to gastroesophageal reflux.

■ REFERENCES

Alrabeeah A, Giacomantonio M, Gillis DA: Paraesophageal hernia after Nissen fundoplication: A real complication in pediatric patients. J Pediatr Surg 23:766, 1988.

Andze GO, Brandt ML, St. Vil D, et al: Diagnosis and treatment of gastroesophageal reflux in 500 children with respiratory symptoms: The value of pH monitoring. J Pediatr Surg 26:295, 1991.

Arguelles-Martin F, Gonzalez-Fernandez F, Gentles MG: Sucralfate versus cimetidine in the treatment of reflux esophagitis in children. Am J Med 86(Suppl 6A):73, 1989.

Ashcraft KW, Holder TM, Amoury RA: Treatment of gastroesophageal reflux in children by Thal fundoplication. J Thorac Cardiovasc Surg 82:706, 1981.

Black DD, Haggitt RC, Orenstein SR, et al: Esophagitis in infants: Morphometric histological diagnosis and correlation with measures of gastroesophageal reflux. Gastroenterology 98:1408, 1990.

Boix-Ochoa J: Gastroesophageal reflux. In Welch KJ (ed): Pediatric Surgery, 4th ed. Chicago, Year Book Medical Publishers, 1986, p 712.

Boix-Ochoa J, Canals J: Maturation of the lower esophagus. J Pediatr Surg 11:749, 1976.

Boix-Ochoa J, Cassasa JM: Surgical treatment of gastroesophageal reflux in children. Surg Annu 21:97, 1989.

Boix-Ochoa J, Cassasa JM, Vernet JMG: Gastroesophageal reflux in pediatrics: Experience in 2,000 cases. In DeMeester TR, Skinner DB (eds): Esophageal Disorders: Pathophysiology and Therapy. New York, Raven Press, 1985, p 459.

Boyle JT: Gastroesophageal reflux in the pediatric patient. Gastroenterol Clin North Am 18:315, 1989.

Boyle JT, Tuchman DN, Altschuler SM, et al: Mechanisms for the association of gastroesophageal reflux and bronchospasm. Am Rev Respir Dis 131(Suppl):S16–S20, 1985.

Brogden RN, Heel RC, Speight TM, et al: Sucralfate: A review of its pharmacodynamic properties and therapeutic use in peptic ulcer disease. Drugs 27:194, 1984.

Cameron AJ, Ott BJ, Payne WS: The incidence of adenocarcinoma in columnar-lined (Barrett's) esophagus. N Engl J Med 313:857, 1985.

Carré IJ: A historical review of the clinical consequences of hiatal hernia (partial thoracic stomach) and gastroesophageal reflux. In Gellis S (ed): Gastroesophageal Reflux: Report of the 76th Ross Conference on Pediatric Research. Columbus, OH, Ross Laboratories, 1979, p 459.

Carré IJ, Astley R: The fate of the partial thoracic stomach ("hiatus hernia") in children. Arch Dis Child 35:484, 1960.

Cucchiara S, Bortolotti M, Minella R, et al: Fasting and postprandial mechanisms of gastroesophageal reflux in children with gastroesophageal reflux disease. Dig Dis Sci 38(1):86, 1993.

Dahms BB, Rothstein FC: Barrett's esophagus in children: A consequence of chronic gastroesophageal reflux. Gastroenterology 86:318, 1984.

Darling DB, McCauley RGK, Leonidas JC, et al: Gastroesophageal reflux in infants and children: Correlation of radiological severity and pulmonary pathology. Radiology 127:735, 1978.

Davidson GP: Annotation: Usefulness of oesophageal pH monitoring. Aust Paediatr J 21:243, 1985.

DeMeester TR: Definition, detection and pathophysiology of gastroesophageal reflux disease. In DeMeester TR, Matthews HR (eds): International Trends in General Thoracic Surgery, Vol 3. Benign Esophageal Disease. St. Louis, CV Mosby, 1987. Discussion by DF Evans, p 99.

DeMeester TR, Wernly JA, Bryant GH, et al: Clinical and in vitro analysis of determinants of gastroesophageal competence. Am J Surg 137:39, 1979.

DeMeester TR, Wang CI, Wernly JA, et al: Technique, indications, and clinical use of 24 hour esophageal pH monitoring. J Thorac Cardiovasc Surg 79:656, 1980.

Dent J, Davidson GP, Barnes BE, et al: The mechanism of gastrooesophageal reflux in children. Aust Paediatr J 17:125, 1981.

Dent J, Holloway RH, Tooulis J, et al: Mechanisms of lower esophageal sphincter incompetence in patients with symptomatic gastroesophageal reflux. Gut 29:1020, 1988.

De Silva KL, Muller PJ, Pearce J: Acute drug-induced extrapyramidal syndromes. Practitioner 211:316, 1973.

DiLorenzo C, Piepsz A, Ham H, et al: Gastric emptying with gastrooesophageal reflux. Arch Dis Child 62:449, 1987.

Farrell RL, Castell DO, McGuigan JE: Measurements and comparisons of lower esophageal sphincter pressures and serum gastrin levels in patients with gastroesophageal reflux. Gastroenterology 67:415, 1974.

Faubion WA Jr, Zein NN: Gastroesophageal reflux in infants and children. Mayo Clin Proc 73:166, 1998.

Fonkalsrud EW, Ament ME: Gastrointestinal reflux in children. Curr Probl Surg 33(1):1, 1996.

Fonkalsrud EW, Ament ME, Berquist W: Surgical management of the gastroesophageal reflux syndrome in childhood. Surgery 97:42, 1985.

Fonkalsrud EW, Ashcraft KW, Coran AG, et al: Surgical treatment of gastroesophageal reflux in children: A combined hospital study of 7467 patients. Pediatrics 101:419, 1998.

Fonkalsrud EW, Berquist W, Vargas J, et al: Surgical treatment of the gastroesophageal reflux syndrome in infants and children. Am J Surg 154:11, 1987.

Fonkalsrud EW, Foglia RP, Ament ME, et al: Operative treatment for the gastroesophageal reflux syndrome in children. J Pediatr Surg 24:525, 1989.

Gastro-oesophageal reflux and apparent life-threatening events in infancy (review). Lancet 2:261, 1988.

Georgeson KE: Laparoscopic fundoplication and gastrostomy. Semin Laparosc Surg 5:25, 1998.

Hameeteman W, Tytgat GNJ, Houthoff HJ, et al: Barrett's esophagus: Development of dysplasia and adenocarcinoma. Gastroenterology 96:1249, 1989.

Henderson RD, Marryatt GV: Transabdominal total fundoplication gastroplasty to control reflux: A preliminary report. Can J Surg 28:127, 1985.

Herbst JJ, Book LS, Bray PF: Gastroesophageal reflux in the "near miss" sudden infant death syndrome. J Pediatr 92:73, 1978.

Hetzel DJ, Dent J, Reed WD, et al: Healing and relapse of severe peptic esophagitis after treatment with omeprazole. Gastroenterology 95:902, 1988.

Hewitt VM: Effect of posture on the presence of fat in tracheal aspirate in neonates. Aust Paediat J 12:267, 1976.

Hicks LM, Christie DL, Hall DG, et al: Surgical treatment of esophageal stricture secondary to gastroesophageal reflux. J Pediatr Surg 15:863, 1980.

Hillemeier AC: Gastroesophageal reflux. Diagnostic and therapeutic approaches. Pediatr Clin North Am 43(1):197, 1996.

Hillemeier AC, Lange R, McCallum R, et al: Delayed gastric emptying in infants with gastroesophageal reflux. J Pediatr 98:190, 1981.

Holder TM, Cloud DT, Lewis JE Jr, et al: Esophageal atresia and tracheoesophageal fistula: A survey of its members by the Surgical Section of the American Academy of Pediatrics. Pediatrics 34:542, 1964.

Hollwarth M, Uray E: Physiology and pathophysiology of the esophagus in childhood. In Wurnig P (ed): Progress in Pediatric Surgery, Vol 18. Berlin-Heidelberg, Springer-Verlag, 1985, p 1.

Hyams JS, Leichtner AM, Zamett LO, et al: Effect of metoclopramide on prolonged intraesophageal pH testing in infants with gastroesophageal reflux. J Pediatr Gastroenterol Nutr 5:716, 1986.

Jeffery HE, Rahilly P, Read DJC: Multiple causes of asphyxia in infants at high risk for sudden infant death. Arch Dis Child 58:92, 1983.

Johnson LF, DeMeester TR: Twenty-four-hour pH monitoring of the distal esophagus: A quantitative measure of gastroesophageal reflux. Am J Gastroenterol 83:325, 1974.

Jolley SG, Johnson DG, Herbst JJ, et al: An assessment of gastroesophageal reflux in children by extended pH monitoring of the distal esophagus. Surgery 84:16, 1978.

Jolley SG, Halpern CT, Sterling CE, et al: The relationship of respiratory complications from gastroesophageal reflux to prematurity in infants. J Pediatr Surg 25:755, 1990.

Kahn A, Rebuffat E, Sottiaux M, et al: Sleep apneas and acid esophageal reflux in control infants and in infants with an apparent life threatening event. Biol Neonate 57:144, 1990.

Kiely EM: Surgery for gastro-oesophageal reflux. Arch Dis Child 65:1291, 1990.

Klinkenberg-Knol EC, Jansen JMB, Festen HPM, et al: Doubleblind multicentre comparison of omeprazole and ranitidine in the treatment of reflux oesophagitis. Lancet 1:349, 1987.

Lambert J, Mobassaleh M, Grand RJ: Efficacy of cimetidine for gastric acid suppression in pediatric patients. J Pediatr 120:474, 1992.

Lander A, Desai A: The risks and benefits of cisapride in premature neonates, infants, and children. Arch Dis Child 79:469, 1998.

Leape LL, Ramenofsky ML: Surgical treatment of gastroesophageal reflux in children. Am J Dis Child 134:935, 1980.

Leape LL, Holder TM, Franklin JD, et al: Respiratory arrest in infants secondary to gastroesophageal reflux. Pediatrics 60:924, 1977.

Lipshutz WH, Gaskins RD, Lukash WM, et al: Hypogastrinemia in patients with lower esophageal sphincter incompetence. Gastroenterology 67:423, 1974.

Machida HM, Forbes DA, Gall DG, et al: Metoclopramide in gastroesophageal reflux of infancy. J Pediatr 112:483, 1988.

Masterson J, Zucker C, Schulze K: Prone and supine positioning effects on energy expenditure and behavior of low birth weight neonates. Pediatrics 80:689, 1987.

McCallum RW, Fink SM, Lerner E, et al: Effects of metoclopramide and bethanechol on delayed gastric emptying present in gastroesophageal reflux patients. Gastroenterology 84:1573, 1983.

Moroz SP, Espinoza J, Cumming WA, et al: Lower esophageal sphincter function in children with and without gastroesophageal reflux. Gastroenterology 71:236, 1976.

Nagashima R, Yoshida N: Sucralfate: A basic aluminum salt of sucrose sulfate. I. Behaviors in gastroduodenal pH. Arzneimittelforschung 29:1668, 1979.

Nakazawa S, Nagashima R, Samloff IM: Selective binding of sucralfate to gastric ulcer in man. Dig Dis Sci 26:297, 1981.

Neuhauser EBD, Berenberg W: Cardioesophageal relaxation (chalasia) as a cause of vomiting in infants. Pediatrics 5:414, 1950.

Nihoul-Fékété C, Mitrofanoff P, Lortat-Jacob S: Les sténoses peptiques de l'oesophage chez l'enfant. Ann Pediatr 26:692, 1979.

Nissen R: Gastropexy and "fundoplication" in surgical treatment of hiatal hernia. Am J Dig Dis New Ser 6:954, 1961.

Ohhama Y, Tsunoda A, Nishi T, et al: Surgical treatment of reflux stricture of the esophagus. J Pediatr Surg 25:758, 1990.

O'Neill JA Jr, Betts J, Ziegler MM, et al: Surgical management of reflux strictures of the esophagus in childhood. Ann Surg 196:453, 1982.

Orenstein SR: Prone positioning in infant gastroesophageal reflux: Is elevation of the head worth the trouble? J Pediatr 117:184, 1990.

Orenstein SR: Gastroesophageal reflux. Curr Probl Pediatr May/Jun:193, 1991.

Orenstein SR, Whitington PF: Positioning for prevention of infant gastroesophageal reflux. J Pediatr 103:534, 1983.

Orenstein SR, Whitington PF, Orenstein DM: The infant seat as treatment for gastroesophageal reflux. N Engl J Med 309:760, 1983.

Orenstein SR, Magill HL, Brooks P: Thickening of infant feedings for therapy of gastroesophageal reflux. J Pediatr 110:181, 1987.

Orr WC, Robinson MG, Johnson LF: Esophageal mucosal sensitivity in asymptomatic controls. Gastroenterology 84:1266, 1983.

Ott DJ, Katz PO, Wu WC: Anti-reflux barrier. In Castell DO, Wu WC, Ott DJ (eds): Gastroesophageal Reflux Disease: Pathogenesis, Diagnosis, Therapy. Mount Kisco, NY, Futura, 1985, p 35.

Padman R, Quijano R: Gastroesophageal reflux and recurrent/chronic pulmonary disease in infants and children. Del Med J 61:547, 1989.

Papaila JG, Wilmot D, Grosfeld JL, et al: Increased incidence of delayed gastric emptying in children with gastroesophageal reflux. Arch Surg 124:933, 1989.

Pearl RH, Robie DK, Ein SH, et al: Complications of gastroesophageal antireflux surgery in neurologically impaired versus neurologically normal children. J Pediatr Surg 25:1169, 1990.

Ramenofsky ML: Gastroesophageal reflux in infants: Controversies in diagnosis and therapy. Curr Surg 43:282, 1986.

Ribet M, Pruvot FR, Mensier E, et al: Gastro-oesophageal reflux and respiratory disorders treated by Hill's procedure. Eur J Cardiothorac Surg 3:414, 1989.

Rothenberg SS: Experience with 220 consecutive laparoscopic Nissen fundoplications in infants and children. J Pediatr Surg 33:274, 1998.

Rozen P, Hallak A, Gelfond M, et al: A comparison of the lower esophageal sphincter response of reflux patients to metoclopramide or domperidone. Gastroenterology 86:1225, 1984.

Sacre L, Vandenplas Y: Gastroesophageal reflux associated with respiratory abnormalities during sleep. J Pediatr Gastroenterol Nutr 9:28, 1989.

Scott RB, O'Loughlin EV, Gall DG: Gastroesophageal reflux in patients with cystic fibrosis. J Pediatr 106:223, 1985.

Shub MD, Ulshen MH, Hargrove CB, et al: Esophagitis: A frequent consequence of gastroesophageal reflux in infancy. J Pediatr 107:881, 1985.

Sondheimer JM: Continuous monitoring of distal esophageal pH: A diagnostic test for gastroesophageal reflux in infants. J Pediatr 96:804, 1980.

Sontag SJ: The medical management of reflux esophagitis: Role of antacids and acid inhibition. Gastroenterol Clin North Am 19:683, 1990.

Spechler SJ, Robbins AH, Rubins HB, et al: Adenocarcinoma and Barrett's esophagus: An overrated risk? Gastroenterology 87:927, 1984.

St. Cyr JA, Ferrara TB, Thompson T, et al: Treatment of pulmonary manifestations of gastroesophageal reflux in children two years of age or less. Am J Surg 157:400, 1989.

St. Cyr JA, Ferrara TB, Thompson TR, et al: Nissen fundoplication for gastroesophageal reflux in infants. J Thorac Cardiovasc Surg 92:661, 1986.

Sutphen JL, Dillard VL: Effect of ranitidine on twenty-four-hour gastric acidity in infants. J Pediatr 114:472, 1989.

Thal AP: A unified approach to surgical problems of the esophagogastric junction. Ann Surg 168:542, 1968.

Tolia V, Calhoun J, Kuhns L, et al: Randomized, prospective doubleblind trial of metoclopramide and placebo for gastroesophageal reflux in infants. J Pediatr 115:141, 1989.

Toupet A: La technique d'oesophago-gastropastie avec phréno-gastropexie appliquée dans la cure radicale des hernies hiatales et comme complément de l'operation de Heller dans les cardiospasms. Med Acad Chir 89:394, 1963.

Tuggle DW, Tunell WP, Hoelzer DJ, et al: The efficacy of Thal fundoplication in the treatment of gastroesophageal reflux: The influence of central nervous system impairment. J Pediatr Surg 23:638, 1988.

Turnage RH, Oldham KT, Coran AG, et al: Late results of fundoplication for gastroesophageal reflux in infants and children. Surgery 105:457, 1989.

Vandenplas Y, Derde MP, Piepsz A: Evaluation of reflux episodes during simultaneous esophageal pH monitoring and gastroesophageal reflux scintigraphy in children. J Pediatr Gastroenterol Nutr 14:256, 1992.

Vandenplas Y, Loeb H: Alkaline gastroesophageal reflux in infancy. J Pediatr Gastroenterol Nutr 12:448, 1991.

Vandenplas Y, Sacre-Smits L: Continuous 24-hour esophageal pH monitoring in 285 asymptomatic infants 0–15 months old. J Pediatr Gastroenterol Nutr 6:220, 1987.

Vane DW, Harmel RP Jr, King DR, et al: The effectiveness of Nissen fundoplication in neurologically impaired children with gastroesophageal reflux. Surgery 98:662, 1985.

VanTrappen G, Janssens J, Ghillebert G: The irritable oesophagus: A frequent cause of angina-like pain. Lancet 1:1232, 1987.

Vinocur CD, Marmon L, Schidlow DV, et al: Gastroesophageal reflux in the infant with cystic fibrosis. Am J Surg 149:182, 1985.

Ward RM, Lemons JA, Molteni RA: Cisapride: A survey of the frequency of use and adverse events in premature newborns. Pediatrics 103:469, 1999.

Werlin SL, Dodds WJ, Hogan WJ, et al: Mechanisms of gastroesophageal reflux in children. J Pediatr 97:244, 1980.

Wilkinson JD, Dudgeon DL, Sondheimer JM: A comparison of medical and surgical treatment of gastroesophageal reflux in severely retarded children. J Pediatr 99:202, 1981.

Winter HS, Madara JL, Stafford RJ, et al: Intraepithelial eosinophils: A new diagnostic criterion for reflux esophagitis. Gastroenterology 83:818, 1982.

Yu VYH: Effect of body position on gastric emptying in the neonate. Arch Dis Child 50:500, 1975.

Zaninotto G, DeMeester TR, Schwizer W, et al: The lower esophageal sphincter in health and disease. Am J Surg 155:104, 1988.

CHAPTER **15**

Peptic Esophagitis, Stricture, and Short Esophagus

F. Griffith Pearson

DEFINITION

Peptic esophagitis is an inflammatory change in the esophageal wall caused by the erosive effects of acid-pepsin and other digestive secretions that reflux abnormally from the stomach into the esophageal lumen. (The pathophysiology of gastroesophageal reflux is presented in detail in Chapter 10.) The gross injury from reflux esophagitis, identifiable at endoscopy, includes erosive ulceration of the distal squamous epithelium, which is always most pronounced immediately above the squamocolumnar interface. Confluent and circumferential ulceration may result in peptic stricture, panmural inflammatory changes, and scarring in the distal esophagus with acquired esophageal shortening. The ulcerated squamous mucosa may be replaced by columnar epithelium.

These features of severe, advanced peptic esophagitis commonly occur together and warrant specific consideration during surgical management.

HISTORICAL NOTE

As long ago as 1831, Fletcher published a paper on esophageal strictures and the danger of the bougie in which he described blind bougienage for dilatation of esophageal strictures. Some of these stenoses were almost certainly of reflux origin.

In 1935, Winkelstein described five patients with erosive esophagitis, which was associated with duodenal ulcer in three of the five. He speculated that the ulcerative changes in the esophagus might be the result of reflux from the stomach. This paper was presented at an annual meeting of the American Medical Association. Chevalier Jackson (1935), commenting on the paper, stated that such cases were associated with hiatal hernia. It remained, however, for Allison, in 1948, to clearly describe erosive esophagitis in the lower esophagus, associated with hiatal hernia and resulting in peptic stricture in some cases. He clearly attributed the etiology to gastroesophageal reflux. In 1968, Meunier-Kuhn and Gaillard reported observations dating from 1950 in a group of patients with peptic esophagitis and stenosis.

Lortat-Jacob (1957) was the first to describe the phenomenon of acquired esophageal shortening. He described the pathophysiology of reflux esophagitis leading to a stenosis and, in some cases, to acquired esophageal shortening due to scar contracture in the wall. He coined the term "endo-brachyesophagus" for this condition. In the same year in England, Leigh Collis (1957) reported his initial experience with a new operation, gastroplasty, which was combined with hiatal hernia repair for the management of patients with peptic stricture and acquired short esophagus.

The historical background of the techniques of dilatation of peptic strictures is provided in Chapter 19.

■ *HISTORICAL READINGS*

Allison PR: Peptic ulcer of the esophagus. Thorax 3:20, 1948.

Collis JL: An operation for hiatus hernia with short esophagus. J Thorac Cardiovasc Surg 34:768, 1957.

Fletcher R: On strictures of the esophagus and the danger of the bougie herein. Med Chir Notes 26, 1831.

Jackson C: In discussion of Winkelstein A: Peptic esophagitis: A new clinical entity. JAMA 104:906, 1935.

Lortat-Jacob JL: L'endo-brachyesophage. Ann Chir 11:1247, 1957.

Meunier-Kuhn P, Gaillard J: La Pathologie de Reflux Gastro-oesophagien. (Esophagite et Stenose Peptique). Paris, Arnette Editions, 1968.

Winkelstein A: Peptic esophagitis: A new clinical entity. JAMA 104:906, 1935.

CLINICAL PRESENTATION

The signal symptom of peptic stricture is dysphagia. A sense of obstruction is commonly localized at the anatomic level of the stricture, which is usually located at the distal end of the esophagus. Such patients register "sticking" at the lower retrosternal level. It is not unusual, however, for patients with distal obstruction to register their dysphagia at a higher level, in the region of the cricopharyngeal sphincter. The reverse of this misleading sensory aberration does not occur; patients with high levels of obstruction never sense the location of the dysphagia at a lower level.

Certain features of the dysphagia caused by peptic esophagitis and stricture support the diagnosis and distinguish the complaint from other causes, such as neoplasm. A peptic stricture may occur at any age from infancy on, and there is almost always an antecedent history of symptomatic gastroesophageal reflux. In some older patients, however, there are no symptoms of prior reflux, even in the presence of active and gross peptic ulceration of esophageal mucosa. In these cases, dysphagia may be the initial symptom of severe reflux diseases with stenosis. The onset and progression of dysphagia due to peptic stricture tends to be gradual, and patients frequently present with a history of difficulty in swallowing dating back several years. By contrast, the patient with malignancy is usually over 50 years of age and has a brief history of rapidly and inexorably progressive dysphagia, which is frequently associated with weight loss. Weight loss is uncommon in patients with peptic stricture.

The diagnosis is usually established from information obtained by contrast radiographs and endoscopy. The radiologic distinction between benign peptic stricture and malignancy is clearly defined in the first part of Chapter 5. At endoscopy, the classical appearance is that of a concentric stenosis, usually short in length, sited just proximal to the squamocolumnar junction. The stricture is often associated with active peptic esophagitis in the adjacent squamous epithelium. A sliding hiatal hernia is present in 85% of cases (Savary and Ollyo, 1986). On occasion, the associated proximal esophagitis is absent as a result of spontaneous remission or effective medical therapy.

The severity of stricture varies from weblike obstruction to segments measuring 3 cm in length or more (Figs. 15–1 to 15–3). The cicatricial changes responsible for stenosis may be restricted to the submucosa or may extend through the full thickness of the esophageal wall to involve the surrounding areolar tissue. Long, fibrous strictures (3 cm or longer) are relatively uncommon and have been seen even less frequently since the introduction of proton-pump inhibitors (PPIs). The association of columnar-lined esophagus and peptic stricture was documented in 150 of 300 consecutive cases of acquired columnar-lined esophagus (Savary and Ollyo, 1986).

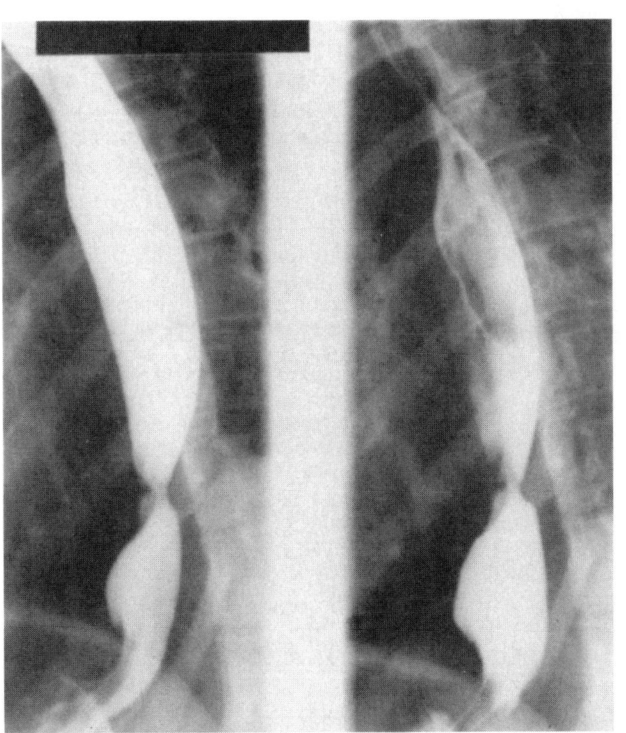

FIGURE 15–1 ■ Barium radiograph illustrating a short peptic stricture (<1 cm in length) at the esophagogastric junction, which lies several centimeters above the diaphragmatic hiatus. A sliding hiatal hernia is irreducible in the upright position, which indicates some degree of esophageal shortening. The proximal esophagus is mildly dilated, which is consistent with the early changes of obstruction. These short strictures are usually easily dilated by indirect bougienage.

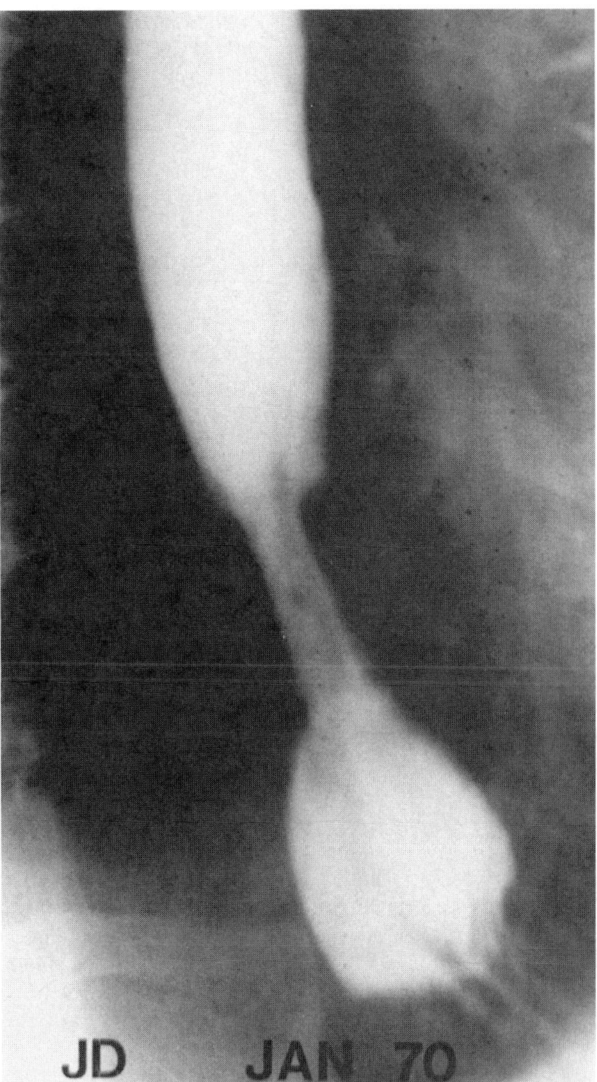

FIGURE 15–2 ■ Barium radiograph illustrating a moderate stricture in the distal esophagus above an irreducible, sliding hiatal hernia. The stricture is just under 2 cm in length. The margins of the stenotic segment are smooth from top to bottom, which is consistent with the benign nature of the obstruction. Many such strictures can be dilated by indirect bougienage, although some may require endoscopic placement of a guidewire and bougienage over the indwelling wire. This stricture lies at the junction of the middle and lower thirds of the esophagus and again is associated with significant acquired shortening of the esophagus.

Some specific variants of peptic stricture warrant description:

1. Short, web-like stenoses at the squamocolumnar interface called Schatzki rings (Fig. 15–4).
2. Peptic stenosis that occurs following periods of nasogastric intubation (Fig. 15–5).
3. Strictures in patients with columnar-lined esophagus (Fig. 15–6).
4. Peptic strictures that develop in the acquired short esophagus as a late sequel of corrosive injury (Fig. 15–7).
5. Peptic strictures that occur at and above the eso-

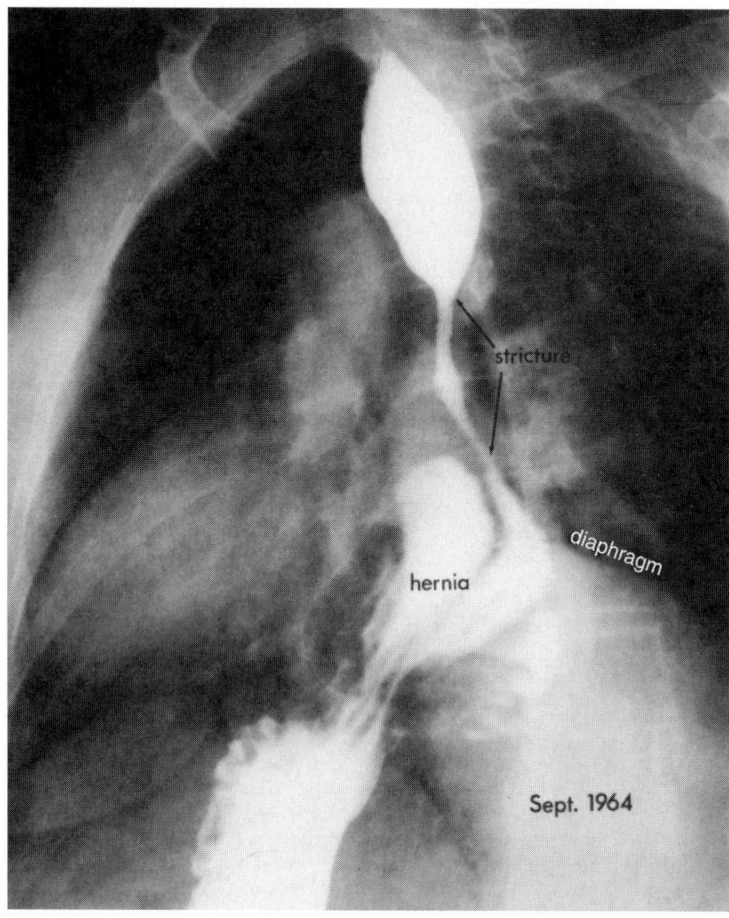

FIGURE 15–3 ■ Barium radiograph illustrating a long, severe fibrous stricture, which lies above an incarcerated, rolling-type hiatal hernia. This stricture lies in the middle third of the mediastinum, and the upper end of the stricture lies above the level of the main carina. The stricture is almost 4 cm in length. Dilatation of such strictures is difficult and potentially dangerous and should be done with fluoroscopic control over an endoscopically placed guidewire. Fortunately, strictures of this severity are relatively uncommon.

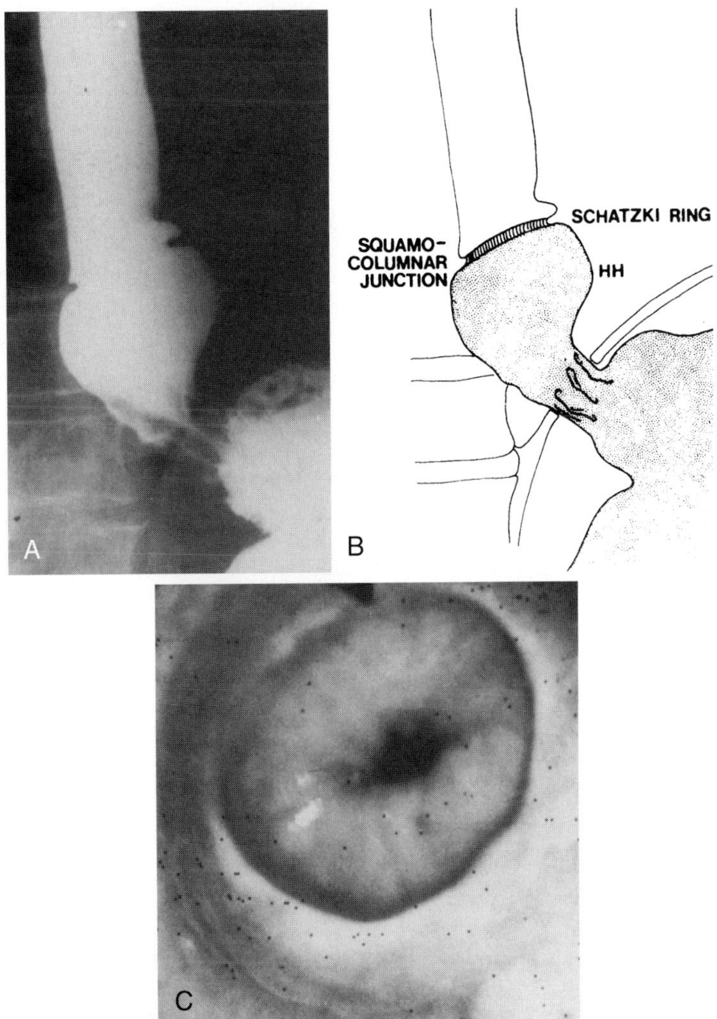

FIGURE 15–4 ■ Illustrations of Schatzki rings. These are acquired lesions, almost always seen in adults, and are due to a web-like circular scar lying in the submucosa at the squamocolumnar interface. They always appear to be associated with a sliding hiatal hernia and are almost certainly peptic in origin. The degree of narrowing in a Schatzki ring progresses spontaneously in about half the cases. Spontaneous resolution never occurs. *A*, Barium radiograph illustrating the typical appearance of a Schatzki ring. There is a small sliding hiatal hernia, and the weblike indentation at the esophagogastric junction is demonstrable only when the esophagus is fully distended with barium. *B*, A diagrammatic illustration of the anatomy shown in the barium radiograph in *A*. *C*, Endoscopic photograph of a Schatzki ring. A symmetrical, weblike ring is clearly seen. As in the barium radiograph, this ring is visible only when the distal esophagus is fully distended with air during endoscopy; otherwise, it is almost never noted. In the photograph, the ring lies above a small sliding hiatal hernia and the diaphragmatic hiatus is seen in the center of the pouch of gastric mucosa.

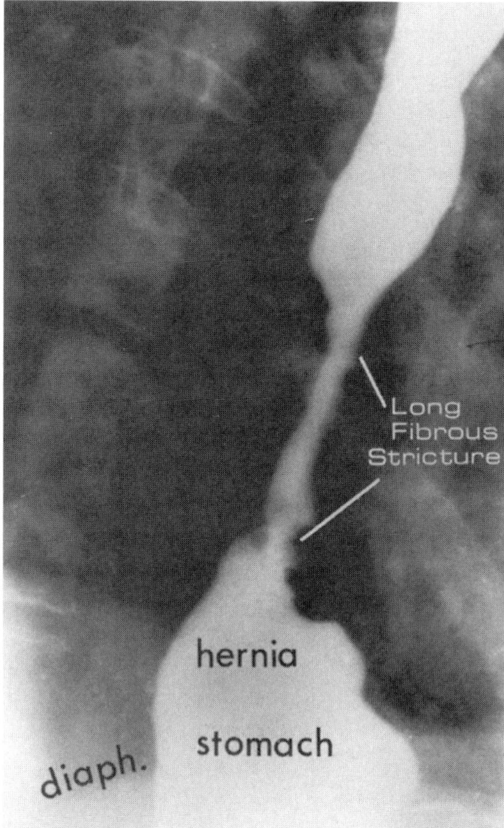

FIGURE 15–5 ■ Barium radiograph showing a long and severe fibrous stricture, which was due to a period of nasogastric intubation required in the management of ileus occurring as a complication of abdominal surgery. These strictures may develop quickly, are often long and severe, as seen in this patient, and may be difficult to dilate and manage. Most appear to be associated with a preexisting hiatal hernia.

phagogastric anastomosis following esophagectomy with gastric replacement and esophagogastrostomy (Fig. 15–8).

6. Strictures associated with an underlying primary motor disorder such as scleroderma, achalasia (postmyotomy) (Fig. 15–9), or congenital tracheoesophageal fistula.

7. Double peptic strictures, which represent approximately 1% of cases or less (Savary and Ollyo, 1986) (Fig. 15–10).

On occasion, the appearance of ulcerative inflammation associated with peptic stricture may be difficult to distinguish from that of an esophageal neoplasm. In every case, endoscopic biopsy and/or brush cytology is advisable to rule out the possibility of malignancy.

ACQUIRED SHORT ESOPHAGUS

The phenomenon of acquired shortening of the esophagus is still not widely appreciated and is difficult to document in quantitative fashion. In advanced cases, such shortening is obvious from an appraisal of the barium radiograph and a high mediastinal location of the esophagogastric (EG) junction at endoscopy, and it is clearly evident at operation. The presence of lesser degrees of acquired shortening is less obvious. The presence of acquired shortening has significant implications for surgical management.

The possibility that some degree of acquired shortening is present should be considered in any patient with

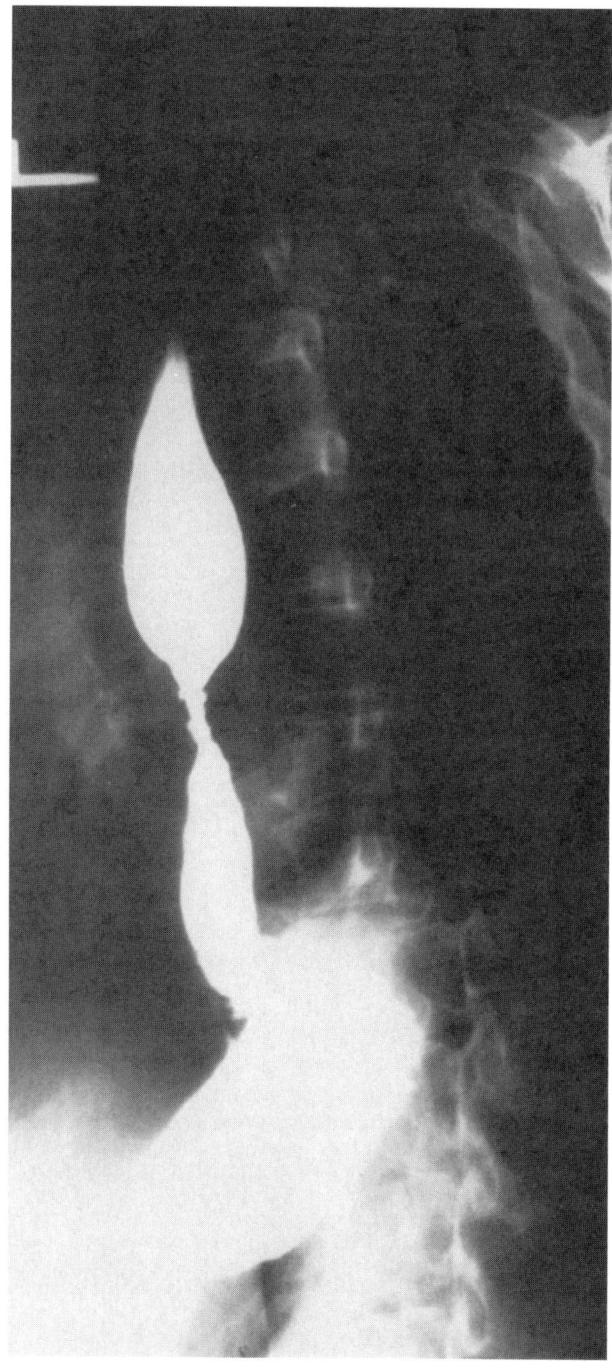

FIGURE 15–6 ■ Barium radiograph illustrating a moderate peptic stricture at the squamocolumnar interface in a patient with a long segment of acquired columnar-lined esophagus. In the radiograph, a moderately large sliding hiatal hernia is seen. There is a segment of columnar-lined distal esophagus about 5 cm in length, and, as always, the peptic stricture is situated in the distal squamous epithelium above the acquired columnar lining. The esophagus above the stricture is mildly dilated owing to obstruction and was the site of active ulcerative peptic esophagitis noted at endoscopy.

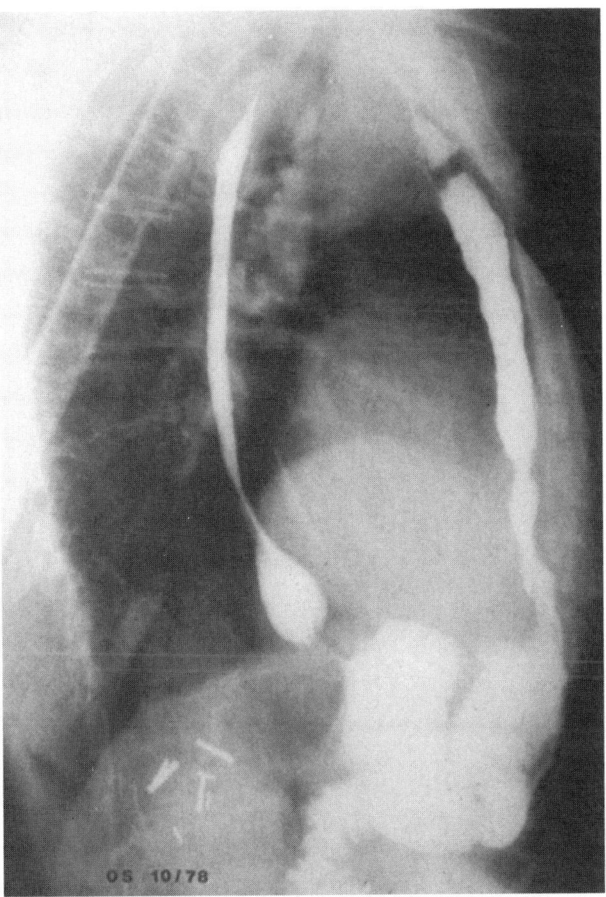

FIGURE 15–7 ■ Barium radiograph, lateral projection, illustrating a long corrosive stricture of the esophagus (due to lye ingestion during childhood) in a 52-year-old woman. At the time of this x-ray, the patient had experienced worsening dysphagia, which was due to ulcerative esophagitis and peptic stricture in the already scarred distal esophagus. A small sliding hernia is evident. Many such patients develop late reflux, which is probably a complication of esophageal scarring and shortening over time. In this patient, the problem was managed by a substernal bypass using a nonreversed gastric tube, which is also filled with barium in the radiograph.

gross inflammatory reflux changes observed at endoscopy. These changes include the sequelae of gross ulcerative peptic esophagitis, such as stricture and acquired columnar replacement, or Barrett's esophagus. The diagnosis of shortening is further supported by an appraisal of the barium radiograph. In such cases, the EG junction lies above the diaphragmatic hiatus and is irreducible in the upright position. There is loss of the normal angle of His. A detailed evaluation and description of these changes is provided in a review by Gozzetti and co-workers (1987). Measurements obtained at endoscopy may also identify shortening: if the EG junction lies more than 4 to 5 cm above the level of the diaphragmatic hiatus at endoscopy, shortening is suggested (Gastal et al, 1999; Horvath et al, 2000).

During esophageal manometry, the distance between the cricopharyngeal sphincter and the lower esophageal sphincter (LES) is accurately measurable and was first reported in a group of adults by Castell and colleagues in 1989 (Li Qun et al, 1989). The distance is referred to as *esophageal length* (EL). Subsequent reports identify that patients with acquired short esophagus have a mean esophageal length that is significantly reduced below normal values (Gastal et al, 1999; Maziak et al, 1998; Mittal et al, 2000).

Gross esophageal shortening is readily evident intraoperatively; following mobilization of the lower esophagus, it is difficult or impossible to restore the EG junction below the hiatus. Lesser degrees of shortening may be identified only after completion of the repair, as evidenced by tension on the mediastinal esophagus. With

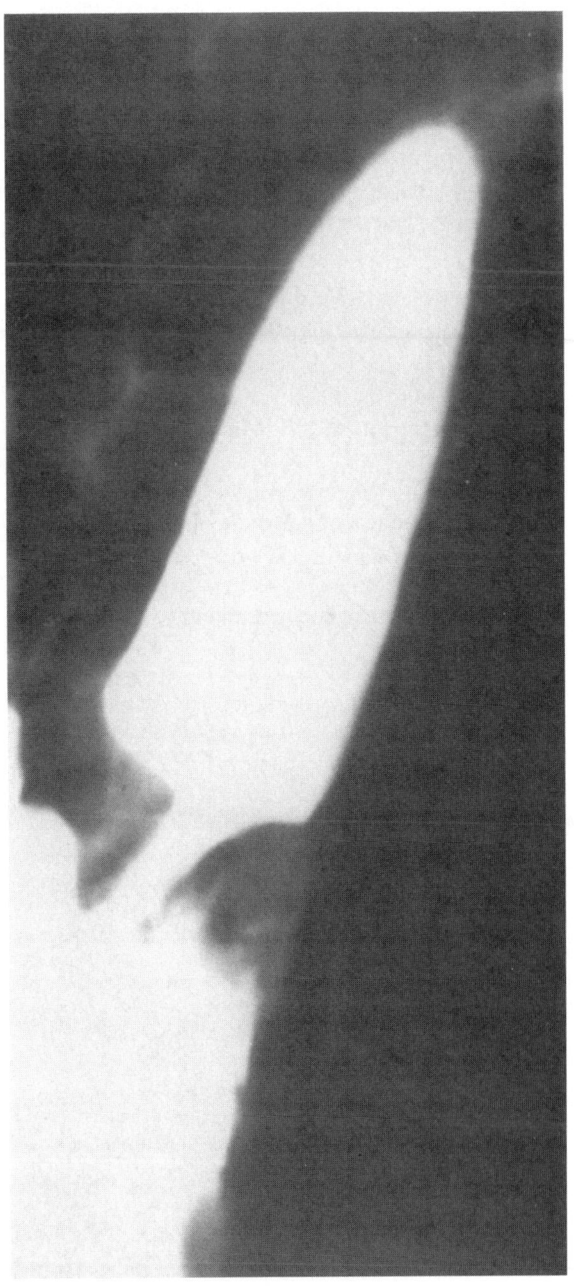

FIGURE 15–8 ■ Barium radiograph illustrating a short, tight stricture due to reflux esophagitis following esophagogastrostomy with intrathoracic anastomosis for the management of esophageal cancer. Dysphagia and stricture occurred within 18 months of the initial surgery.

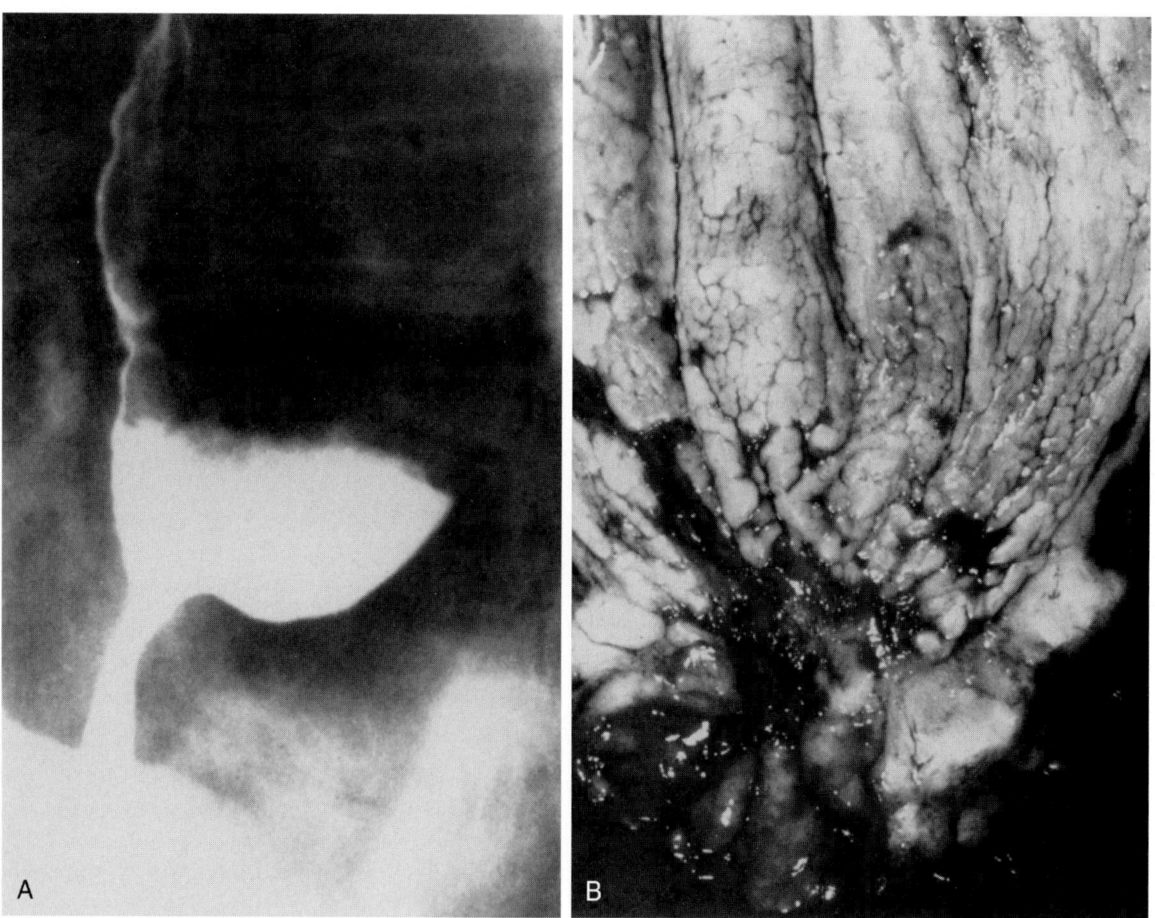

FIGURE 15–9 ■ *A,* A tight stricture in the distal esophagus, just above the diaphragmatic hiatus, with a grossly dilated and obstructed proximal esophagus. This patient had undergone an esophagomyotomy for achalasia 18 years previously. The stricture was due to the complications of ulcerative reflux esophagitis, which can be seen in the squamous epithelium just above the squamocolumnar junction in the opened resected specimen *(B).*

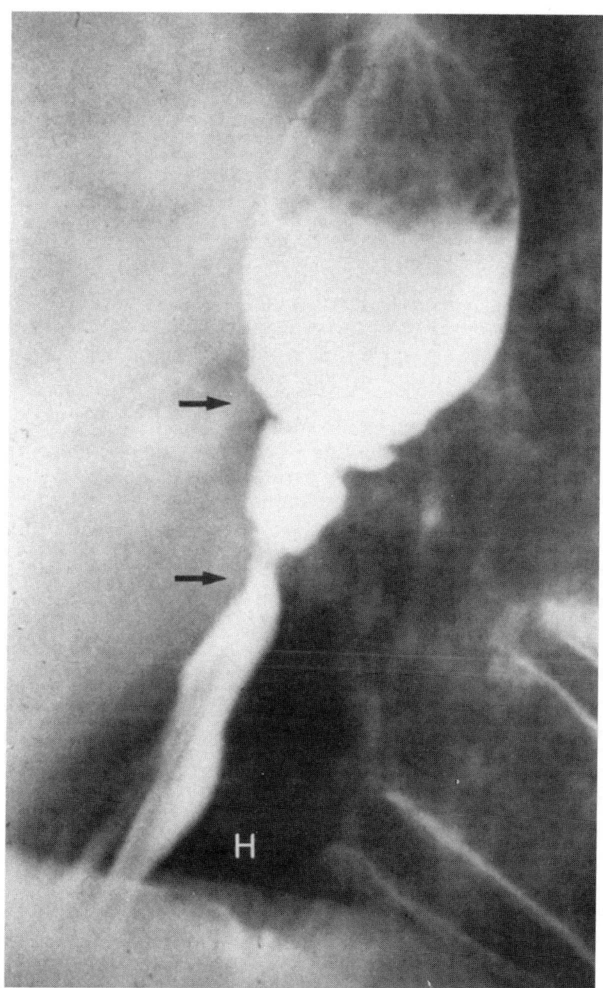

FIGURE 15–10 ■ Barium radiograph illustrating a double peptic stricture *(arrows)*. A short weblike stricture *(top arrow)* is seen superiorly, just below a moderately dilated and obstructed esophagus. Within a few centimeters there is another short stricture *(bottom arrow)*, which lies above a moderate-size sliding hiatal hernia (H). At endoscopy, the uppermost stricture was situated, as usual, at the squamocolumnar interface. The more distal stricture *(bottom arrow)* had developed in a ring of squamous epithelium, which appeared to be left behind during the original process of acquired columnar replacement. These strictures represent about 1% of the strictures seen in a large review by Savary and Miller (see Manuel et Atlas, 1977).

open repairs, this tension is more easily recognized from a thoracic rather than abdominal exposure.

Subtle degrees of shortening are undoubtedly more difficult to assess during laparoscopic repair; the diaphragm and esophageal hiatus may be abnormally elevated and distorted by the intra-abdominal gas pressures. Only since 1996 has the presence of acquired short esophagus been reported by laparoscopic surgeons (Gastal et al, 1999; Horvath et al, 2000; Johnson et al, 1998; Luketich et al, 2000; Mittal et al, 2000; Swanström et al, 1996). With a laparoscopic exposure, short esophagus is judged to be present if the EG junction does not lie 2 or more cm below the hiatus following division and mobilization of the hiatal attachments. Swanstrom and coworkers measured the length of intra-abdominal esophagus by placing the opened jaws of a standard laparoscopic dissector (which measures 3 cm) between the EG junction and the inferior border of the diaphragmatic hiatus. Intraoperative endoscopy is used to accurately locate the position of the EG junction when necessary (Horvath et al, 2000).

After this dissection, the esophagus is considered short if the Penrose drain lies within the diaphragmatic hiatus when the esophagus is under no tension (Johnson et al, 1998). Mittal and co-workers (2000) measured the distance between the EG junction and the anterior "arch" of the diaphragmatic hiatus by a metal probe. The EG junction is located by palpation of the end of an indwelling gastroscope with the tip of the metal probe.

These same authors have all noted that the complications of peptic stricture, Barrett's esophagus, and massive paraesophageal hernias are important risk factors for the presence of acquired shortening. Reoperation for failed, prior antireflux surgery is another common risk factor (Horvath et al, 2000; Johnson et al, 1998; Luketich et al, 2000; Pearson et al, 1987; Rice, 2000).

MANAGEMENT

Medical Therapy and Interval Dilatation

Medical therapy alone cannot resolve the problem of stricture and obstruction; the presence of stenosis calls for some form of dilatation. In a double-blind, randomized, crossover study comparing treatment with cimetidine versus placebo in a group of patients with peptic strictures, stenosis did not resolve in either group (Ferguson et al, 1979). To date, there have been no similar randomized studies to evaluate the effectiveness of proton-pump inhibitor therapy.

A combination of good medical therapy and interval dilatation is effective in many patients and is often the only applicable therapy for patients considered unfit for surgical intervention. Techniques of dilatation are described in detail in Chapter 19 and vary with the requirements and clinical course in individual patients. Peptic stricture is most common in older people, and many elderly patients are managed satisfactorily in this way.

Severe confluent ulcerative esophagitis heals in most patients with medical therapy, which includes proton-pump inhibitors in adequate dosage. With the advent of proton-pump inhibitors, many patients with gross esophagitis but without an associated peptic stricture are well managed by long-term medical treatment (Klinkenberg-Knol, 1994).

Surgical Management

With current techniques, almost all peptic strictures can be dilated (see Chapter 19). In our reported experience, more than 95% of peptic strictures seen during a 20-year review (1964 to 1984) could be dilated to a satisfactory diameter (Pearson et al, 1987). If the stricture is dilatable, an operation that adequately prevents further reflux results in permanent resolution of the inflammation and stenosis in a majority of patients (Collis, 1961; Henderson, 1977; Hill et al, 1970; Larrain et al, 1970; Pearson et al, 1971 and 1987; Orringer, 1978; Orringer et al, 1976; Urschel et al, 1973).

The choice of operation for control of reflux in patients with peptic esophagitis, dilatable stricture, and acquired shortening remains controversial. Options are summarized in Table 15–1.

Dilatable Peptic Strictures

In patients with dilatable peptic strictures, any of the procedures listed in Table 15–1 may result in a successful outcome as long as further reflux is adequately controlled.

Standard Antireflux Repairs

The most commonly used standard operations for the control of reflux are the Nissen fundoplication and the Belsey Mark IV, Dor, Toupet, and Hill repairs. To restore competence, the Belsey, Dor, Toupet, and Nissen repairs depend on securing 2 to 4 cm of the distal esophagus on the abdominal side of the hiatus. The Hill repair, however, involves creating a tube, or narrowed segment of stomach, which extends for several centimeters distal to the anatomic EG junction; this repair thus does not depend on restoring a 2- to 4-cm length of distal esophagus to an intra-abdominal location. In the absence of acquired esophageal shortening, any of these standard repairs can provide a good result. If there is sufficient esophageal shortening, however, simple hernia repair more frequently fails because the EG junction cannot be secured in the abdomen without undue tension.

Several authors have reported an unacceptably high incidence of recurrent reflux in patients with peptic strictures managed by the Belsey Mark IV repair (Donnelly et al, 1973; Orringer et al, 1972; Pearson et al, 1987). The Nissen, Belsey, Dor, and Toupet procedures are not designed to withstand significant tension. The Hill repair, however, creates the antireflux "valve" at and below the level of the EG junction and anchors the junction to the stout median arcuate ligament. Several publications have reported a high proportion of good results in patients with peptic stricture managed by a Hill repair (Hill et al, 1970; Larrain et al, 1970, 1975; Lowe and Hill, 1989).

It is our experience that most patients with peptic stricture, extensive ulcerative esophagitis (even without stricture), and massive type III paraesophageal hernias) suffer some degree of acquired shortening (Maziak et al, 1998; Pearson et al, 1987). Optimal results of surgery can be obtained if such shortening is assumed to exist and is considered in the selection of the antireflux repair.

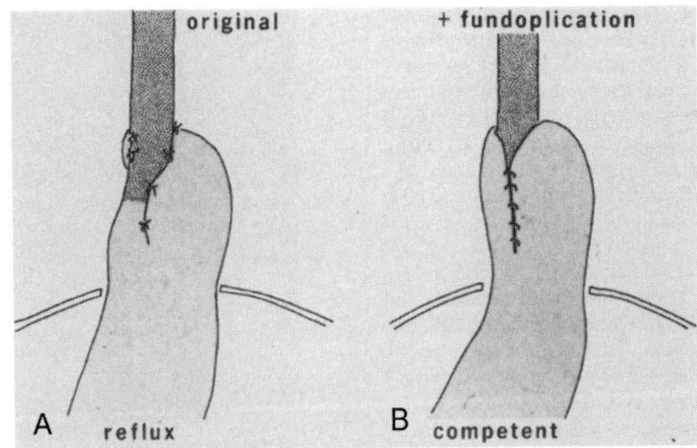

FIGURE 15–11 ■ *A*, Diagram illustrating the Thal procedure. The obstructing peptic stricture has been incised vertically, the stenosis thus opened, and the defect in the esophageal wall patched with the serosa of the gastric fundus. A partial fundoplication is performed around the distal esophagus in the thorax in order to avoid reflux. *B*, A modification of the Thal esophagogastroplasty, in which a complete fundoplication of the Nissen type is added. Hollenbeck and Woodward (1975) found that reconstruction could provide more dependable reflux control.

TABLE 15–1 ■ **Surgical Management of Peptic Stricture**

Required Repair	*Operation*
Dilatable stricture	
Standard antireflux repair	Belsey, Nissen, Hill, Dor
Gastroplasty and antireflux repair	Collis and Belsey Collis and Nissen "Uncut gastroplasty"
Intrathoracic reconstructions	Thal procedure Woodward-Thal operation Intrathoracic Nissen fundoplication
Acid suppression and bile diversion	
Esophagectomy and bowel interposition	
Nondilatable stricture	
Esophagoplasty	Thal procedure Woodward-Thal operation
Esophagectomy and interposition	Stomach Jejunum Colon

Intrathoracic Antireflux Repairs

In patients with stricture and acquired shortening, another option is an intrathoracic antireflux reconstruction, which leaves a part of the upper stomach lying above the diaphragm.

The first of these intrathoracic reconstructions was described by Thal (1968). Thal's "esophagogastroplasty" involves incision of the stricture and patching of the incisional defect with the gastric wall (Fig. 15–11*A*). Reflux control is obtained by the addition of a partial intrathoracic fundoplication. Hollenbeck and Woodward (1975) found that this reconstruction failed to control subsequent reflux in many cases. They modified Thal's intrathoracic esophagogastroplasty by adding a complete, Nissen-type fundoplication (Fig. 15–11*B*). This modification provides good reflux control in most cases, with healing of esophagitis and resolution of stenosis.

Another option in patients with dilatable strictures and short esophagus is stricture dilatation with supradiaphragmatic Nissen fundoplication alone. This operation was first described by Krupp and Rosetti (1966) and was subsequently reported by others (Harrison and Gompels, 1971; Maher et al, 1984; Naef and Savary, 1972; Nicholson and Nohl-Oser, 1976); Maher's group clearly demonstrated the effectiveness of reflux control in a majority (82%) of their patients managed in this way.

Intrathoracic reconstruction, however, may be associated with symptoms caused by postprandial retention of air and fluid in the intrathoracic stomach and to a troublesome incidence of gastric ulceration in the intrathoracic segment, resulting in perforation or massive hemorrhage (Franklin, 1972; Mansour et al, 1981; Richardson et al, 1982; Skinner and Belsey, 1967).

Esophageal Lengthening Procedures (Gastroplasty)

The addition of a lengthening gastroplasty was first described in 1957 by Collis for the management of patients with peptic stricture and obvious acquired short esophagus. Subsequent modifications in the technique of *open* gastroplasty have been reported by Pearson and associates (1971), Langer (1973), Demos and colleagues (1975), Henderson (1977), Orringer (1978), Steichen (1986), and Moores (2000). *Laparoscopic* gastroplasty techniques have recently been devised and reported by Swanström (1996), Johnson and co-workers (1998), Luketich (2000), and Mittal and colleagues (2000). Common to all of these modifications was Collis' original concept of lengthening the esophagus by creating a tube of stomach in continuity with the distal esophagus (gastroplasty), followed by an antireflux reconstruction, below the diaphragm at the distal end of the gastric tube. The addition of gastroplasty obviates tension on the repair in patients with acquired shortening.

The indications, surgical technique, and results of gastroplasty are reported in detail in both parts of Chapter 24.

Acid Suppression and Bile Diversion

Acid suppression and bile diversion are achieved by the combination of antrectomy and Roux-en-Y gastrojejunostomy. This procedure was first reported for the management of gastroesophageal reflux by Wells and Johnston (1955). If acid, bile, and upper gastrointestinal digestive enzymes are adequately suppressed, peptic esophagitis and dilatable strictures should resolve, as occurs following an effective antireflux reconstruction at the EG junction.

This procedure is applicable when an antireflux hiatal repair is not deemed feasible; for example, patients in whom prior surgery at the EG junction has created a technical obstacle to an adequate antireflux reconstruction. Such patients include those who have had one or more prior antireflux procedures that have failed and those with an underlying primary motor disorder who have undergone surgery and subsequently developed reflux esophagitis and stricture. The latter problem occurs most commonly in patients who have undergone myotomy for achalasia or diffuse esophageal spasm. Scleroderma, which may ablate the distal esophageal sphincter, also predisposes to disabling esophagitis and stricture in some cases. In all of these patients with primary motor disorders, there is loss of effective peristalsis in the body of the esophagus, which compounds the severity of reflux and damage because of the profound impairment in esophageal clearance.

When peptic esophagitis and stricture are associated with aperistalsis in the esophageal body and virtually complete ablation of the distal esophageal sphincter, no conservative antireflux repair is available that can predictably restore a competent antireflux mechanism without significant risk of producing disabling degrees of obstruction and dysphagia. In such cases, if the stricture is dilatable, prevention of further reflux by antrectomy and Roux-en-Y gastrojejunostomy may provide an effective solution. Furthermore, this procedure is technically easier and is associated with a lower morbidity and mortality than esophageal resection and interposition. Favorable experience with acid suppression and bile diversion has been reported by Payne (1970), Ellis (1986), and Gayet and Fekete (1991). The addition of antrectomy and Roux-en-Y diversion to an antireflux operation is described in Chapter 27.

Esophagectomy and Bowel Interposition

Another option for patients in whom a local antireflux reconstruction is not feasible is esophagectomy and reconstruction. The most common indication for this more radical surgery is peptic esophagitis and stricture complicating an underlying primary motor disorder, such as achalasia, diffuse spasm, or scleroderma. A small number of patients presenting with one or more failed antireflux repairs may be better managed by local esophagectomy than any further attempt at conservative repair (Little et al, 1986; Malthaner et al, 1994; Orringer and Stirling, 1989; Skinner et al, 1985).

In patients with an associated primary motor disorder such as achalasia or diffuse spasm, the entire thoracic esophagus is malfunctioning, aperistaltic, and often grossly dilated. In such cases a thoracic esophagectomy and interposition with cervical anastomosis is recommended (Malthaner et al, 1994; Orringer and Stirling, 1989). Most surgeons prefer replacement with stomach, although some prefer an interposed segment of colon. Techniques of gastric substitution are described in detail in the first part of Chapter 55. The techniques and complications of colon replacement are detailed in Chapters 65 and 66. A detailed review of esophageal replacement for reflux disease is provided in Chapter 28.

In patients with peptic strictures that are not associated with a motor disorder and in whom there is peristaltic function remaining in much of the thoracic esophagus, a local resection of the distal esophagus is preferable (Allison, 1970; Belsey, 1965; Merendino and Dillard, 1955; Polk and Richardson, 1981). Either colon (Belsey, 1965) (Fig. 15–12) or jejunum (Allison, 1970; Merendino and Dillard, 1955; Polk and Richardson, 1981) (Fig. 15–13) may be used as a substitute. Stomach is not recommended as a replacement in patients managed by distal esophagectomy because there is ample evidence that recurrent reflux and stenosis at the intrathoracic esophagogastric anastomosis occurs in an unacceptably high proportion of such patients.

Nondilatable Strictures

The nondilatable peptic stricture has become an uncommon problem with the advent of current techniques of

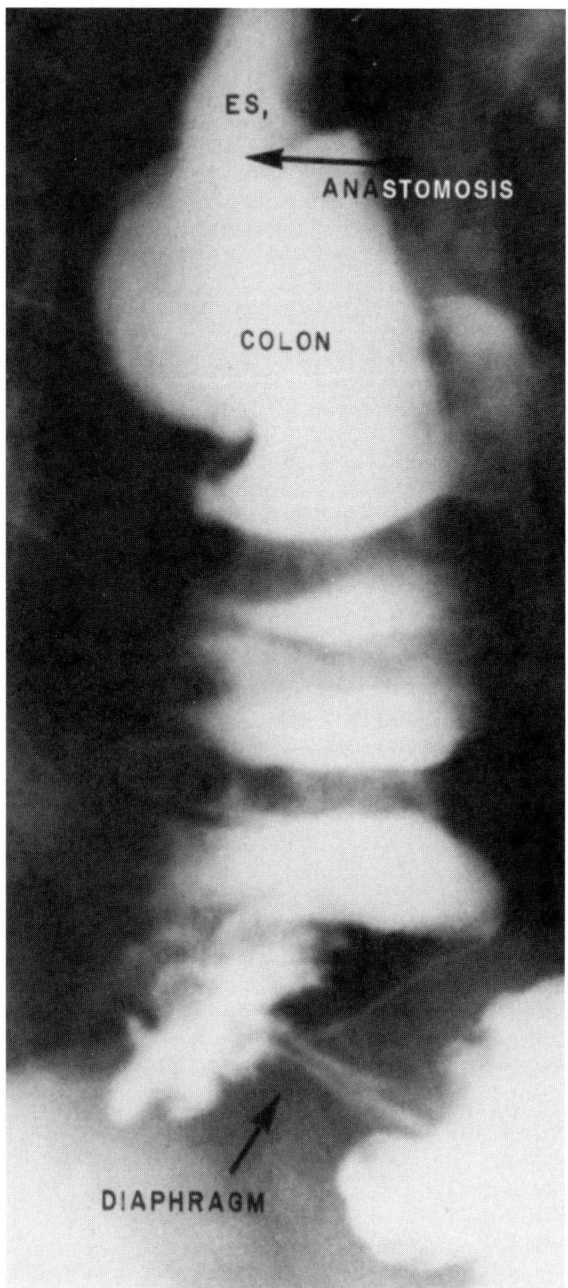

FIGURE 15–12 ■ Barium radiograph illustrating replacement of the resected distal esophagus using a short segment of pedicled left colon. This operation was performed for a nondilatable peptic stricture in a patient who still retained peristaltic function in the proximal half of the remaining esophagus. This type of reconstruction was popularized by Belsey (see J Thorac Cardiovasc Surg 49:33, 1965).

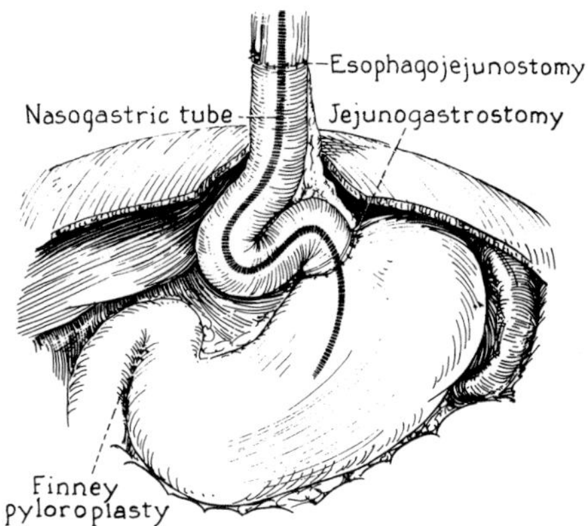

FIGURE 15–13 ■ Diagram illustrating the original operation of esophageal replacement using a short pedicled transplant of upper jejunum (see Merendino and Dillard, Ann Surg 142:486, 1955). Jejunal replacement is another option in the management of undilatable peptic strictures.

esophageal dilatation. There is, however, an occasional patient with a long, fibrous stricture in which the full thickness of the esophageal wall, including the muscular coats, has been largely replaced by fibrous scar. Despite dilatation and reflux control, such strictures recur rapidly and repeatedly. Another category of nondilatable stricture is that in which perforation of the stricture occurs during either preoperative or intraoperative dilatation. In many of these patients, an attempt at local repair of the perforation results in worsening of the stenosis. In patients considered at suitable risk, the preferable solution may be resection and bowel interposition.

Another option in the patient with nondilatable stricture or in the patient who sustains a split in the stricture at the time of dilatation is some form of esophagoplasty, such as the Thal procedure (Thal, 1968) or Woodward's modification of Thal's operation (Hollenbeck and Woodward, 1975). These operations leave a pouch of intrathoracic stomach, and I think that the alternative of local resection and bowel interposition is likely to provide better functional results. However, in an emergency in a patient with perforated peptic stricture, an intrathoracic esophagoplasty of the Thal type may be the simplest and safest operation to resolve a difficult problem.

Acid suppression and bile diversion by antrectomy and Roux-en-Y gastrojejunostomy has no role in the management of patients with nondilatable strictures. Reflux control alone cannot solve this problem.

COMMENTS AND CONTROVERSIES

It is very difficult to categorize the management of peptic strictures, as there is no clear definition of the indications for therapy beyond medical management and interval dilatation. The decision for surgery is modified by the physical status, age, and attitude of the individual patient. In considering therapy, it is essential to remember that these strictures are benign lesions and do not interfere with either the general nutrition or longevity of most sufferers.

The problem of acquired esophageal shortening is one that is still not widely perceived or considered in surgical management except in more obvious cases. It is our experience that subtle degrees of shortening are present in a majority of patients suffering from recurrent ulcerative peptic esophagitis, peptic stricture, or acquired columnar-lined esophagus (Pearson et al, 1987). Our observations are supported by DeMeester and colleagues, who documented a significant incidence of short esophagus in the presence of peptic stricture and Barrett's esophagus (Gas-

tal et al, 1999). Subtle degrees of shortening are likely to adversely influence recurrence rates if standard repairs are used. I do not hesitate to add gastroplasty to the repair if there is any question of acquired shortening (Fig. 15–14). Observations supporting this position are detailed in the first part of Chapter 24. Major obstacles to a critical evaluation of reported outcomes are the current lack of standardization of the pathology of peptic esophagitis, the technical features of operative management, and the objective measurement of results.

Intrathoracic antireflux reconstruction (Thal, Thal-Woodward, intrathoracic Nissen procedures) should not be used as an elective option in the management of peptic stricture with short esophagus. The "intrathoracic stomach" created by these operations may result in symptoms and complications akin to those observed in cases of incarcerated sliding hiatal hernia. Such sequelae include trapping of swallowed food, fluid, and air; progression of gastric herniation; and development of peptic ulcer in the intrathoracic gastric pouch, with complications of pain and penetration, massive bleeding, or intrathoracic perforation.

The role of proton-pump inhibitors, combined with interval dilatation in the management of peptic stricture, remains unclear. There is no doubt that these drugs are, by far, the most effective medical agents for reversal of severe peptic esophagitis. In some patients, of course, bile reflux may be a major cause of reflux esophagitis, and acid suppression will not provide effective treatment (Pellegrini et al, 1978).

In patients selected for resection and bowel interposition, the presence or absence of an associated primary motor disorder warrants emphasis. Resection of most of the esophagus with cervical reconstruction is desirable in patients with a grossly dilated, aperistaltic esophagus, a condition most commonly seen when reflux esophagitis complicates achalasia. The role of antrectomy and Roux-en-Y bile diversion in this same group of patients has not been broadly explored. The latter operation may prove to have wider application with further experience. It is undoubtedly a simpler and safer procedure than resection and interposition.

F. G. P.

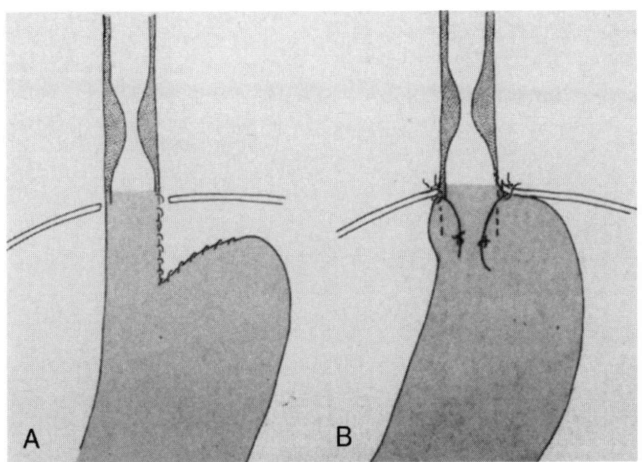

FIGURE 15–14 ■ Diagram illustrating a technique of management for a dilatable stricture with acquired esophageal shortening. *A*, A gastric tube of the Collis type (Collis, 1957) is created in continuity with the distal esophagus, extending for 4 to 5 cm. *B*, A Belsey-type fundoplication has been performed around the gastroplasty tube. The stricture and esophagogastric junction remain in the intrathoracic position. The addition of gastroplasty obviates tension on the repair for patients with acquired shortening (see Pearson et al, J Thorac Cardiovasc Surg 61:50, 1971).

■ REFERENCES

Allison PR: Peptic esophagitis and esophageal strictures. Lancet 2:199, 1970.

Allison PR: Peptic ulcer of the esophagus. Thorax 3:20, 1948.

Belsey R: Reconstruction of the esophagus with left colon. J Thorac Cardiovasc Surg 49:33, 1965.

Collis JL: An operation for hiatus hernia with short esophagus. J Thorac Cardiovasc Surg 34:768, 1957.

Collis JL: Gastroplasty. Thorax 16:197, 1961.

Demos NJ: Stapled, uncut gastroplasty for hiatal hernia: 12-year follow-up. Ann Thorac Surg 38:4, 393, 1984.

Demos NJ, Smith S, Williams D: A gastroplasty for short esophagus and reflux esophagitis: Experimental and clinical studies. Ann Surg 181:178, 1975.

Donnelly RJ, Deverall PB, Watson DA: Hiatus hernia with and without esophageal stricture: Experience with the Belsey Mark IV repair. Ann Thorac Surg 16:301, 1973.

Ellis FH: Reoperative achalasia surgery. J Thorac Cardiovasc Surg 92:859, 1986.

Ferguson R, Dronfield WA, Atkinson M: Cimetidine in treatment of reflux esophagitis with peptic stricture. Br Med J 2:472, 1979.

Fletcher R: On strictures of the esophagus and the danger of the bougie herein. Med Chir Notes 26, 1831.

Franklin RH: Management of strictures due to reflux esophagitis. Proc R Soc Med 65:37, 1972.

Gastal OL, Hagen JA, Peters JH, et al: Short esophagus: Predictors and clinical implications. Arch Surg 134:633, 1999.

Gayet B, Fekete H: Surgical management of failed esophagomyotomy. Hepatogastroenterology 38:488, 1991.

Gozzetti G, Mattioli S, Pilotti V, et al: Il brachiesofago acquisito. In Magistrelli P, Masetti R (eds): Proceedings of the 4th Congress on Surgery of the Digestive Tract, Rome, June 4–6, 1987. CIC Edizioni Internazionali, Rome, 1987.

Harrison GK, Gompels BM: Treatment of reflux strictures of the esophagus by the Nissen-Rosetti operation. Thorax 26:77, 1971.

Henderson RD: Reflux control following gastroplasty. Ann Thorac Surg 24:206, 1977.

Hill LD, Gelfand M, Bauermeister D: Simplified management of reflux esophagitis with stricture. Ann Surg 172:638, 1970.

Hollenbeck JI, Woodward ER: Treatment of peptic esophageal stricture with combined fundic patch fundoplication. Ann Surg 182:472, 1975.

Horvath KD, Swanstrom LL, Jobe BA: The short esophagus: Pathophysiology, incidence, presentation and treatment in the era of laparoscopic surgery. Ann Surg 232:630, 2000.

Jackson C: In discussion of Winkelstein A: Peptic esophagitis: A new clinical entity. JAMA 104:906, 1935.

Johnson AB, Oddsdottir M, Hunter JG: Laparoscopic Collis gastroplasty and Nissen fundoplication: A new technique for the management of esophageal foreshortening. Surg Endosc 12:1055, 1998.

Klinkenberg-Knol EC: Long treatment with omeprazole for refractory reflux esophagitis: Efficacy and safety. Ann Intern Med 121:3, 1994.

Krupp S, Rosetti M: Surgical treatment of hiatal hernias by fundoplication and gastroplasty. Ann Surg 164:927, 1966.

Langer B: Modified gastroplasty: A simple operation for reflux esophagitis with moderate degrees of shortening. Can J Surg 16:1, 1973.

Larrain A, Csendes A, Pope CE: Surgical correction of reflux esophagitis with stricture. Ann Surg 172:638, 1970.

Larrain A, Csendes A, Pope CE: Surgical correction of reflux: An effective therapy for esophageal strictures. Gastroenterology 69:578, 1975.

Li Qun, Castell JA, Castell DO: Manometric determination of esophageal length. Am J Gastroenterol 89:722, 1989.

Little AG, Ferguson MK, Skinner DB: Reoperation for failed antireflux operations. J Thorac Cardiovasc Surg 91:511, 1986.

Lortat-Jacob JL: L'endo-brachyesophage. Ann Chir 11:1247, 1957.

Lowe D, Hill LD: Hill repair: Long-term results. J Thorac Cardiovasc Surg 98:444, 1989.

Luketich JD, Grondin SC, Pearson FG: Minimally invasive approaches to shortening of the esophagus: Laparoscopic Collis-Nissen gastroplasty. Semin Thorac Cardiovasc Surg 12:173, 2000.

Maher JW, Hocking MP, Woodward ER: Supra-diaphragmatic fundoplications: Long-term follow-up and analysis of complications. Am J Surg 147:181, 1984.

Malthaner R, Todd TR, Miller J, et al: Long-term results in surgically managed achalasia. Ann Thorac Surg 58:1343, 1994.

Mansour KA, Burton HG, Miller JI, et al: Complications of intrathoracic Nissen fundoplication. Ann Thorac Surg 32:173, 1981.

Maziak DE, Todd TR, Pearson FG: Massive hiatus hernia: Evaluation and surgical management. J Thorac Cardiovasc Surg 115:53, 1998.

Merendino KA, Dillard DH: The concept of sphincter substitution by an interposed jejunal segment for anatomic and physiologic abnormalities at the esophagogastric junction. Ann Surg 142:486, 1955.

Meunier-Kuhn P, Gaillard J: La Pathologie de Reflux Gastro-oesophagien (Esophagite et Stenose Peptique). Paris, Arnette Editions, 1968.

Mittal SK, Awad ZT, Tasset M, et al: The preoperative predictability of the short esophagus in patients with stricture or paraesophageal hernia. Surg Endosc 14:464, 2000.

Moores DWO: Transabdominal Nissen fundoplication and gastroplasty. In Cox JL, Sundt TM (eds): Operative Techniques in Cardiac and Thoracic Surgery. Philadelphia, WB Saunders, 1997, pp 61–72.

Naef AP, Savary M: Conservative operations for peptic esophagitis with stenosis in columnar-lined lower esophagus. Ann Thorac Surg 13:543, 1972.

Nicholson DAS, Nohl-Oser HC: Hiatus hernia: A comparison between two methods of fundoplication by evaluation of the long-term results. J Thorac Cardiovasc Surg 72:938, 1976.

Orringer MB: Combined Collis gastroplasty–Nissen fundoplication operation for reflux esophagitis. Surg Rounds 1:10, 1978.

Orringer MB, Skinner DB, Belsey RH: Long-term result of the Mark IV operation for hiatal hernia. J Thorac Cardiovasc Surg 63:25, 1972.

Orringer MB, Sloan H: Collis-Belsey reconstruction of the esophagogastric junction. J Thorac Cardiovasc Surg 71:295, 1976.

Orringer MB, Stirling MC: Esophageal resection for achalasia: Indications and results. Ann Thorac Surg 47:338, 1989.

Payne WS: Surgical treatment of reflux esophagitis and stricture associated with permanent incompetence of the cardia. Mayo Clin Proc 45:553, 1970.

Pearson FG, Cooper JD, Patterson GA, et al: Gastroplasty and fundoplication for complex reflux problems. Ann Surg 206:473, 1987.

Pearson FG, Langer B, Henderson RD: Gastroplasty and Belsey hiatus hernia repair. J Thorac Cardiovasc Surg 61:50, 1971.

Pellegrini CA, DeMeester TR, Wernly JA, et al: Alkaline gastroesophageal reflux. Am J Surg 135:177, 1978.

Polk HC Jr, Richardson JD: Non-functional esophagogastric junction: Treatment jejunal interposition. In Stipa S, Belsey RHR (eds): Esophagus. In Sereno Symposium, vol 43. Orlando, FL, 1981, Academic Press, p 188.

Rice TW: Why antireflux surgery fails. Dig Dis 18:43–47, 2000.

Richardson JD, Larson GM, Polk HC: Intra-thoracic fundoplication for shortened esophagus: Treacherous solution to a challenging problem. Am J Surg 143:29, 1982.

Savary M, Miller G: L'oesophage. In Gassmann SA (ed): Manuel et Atlas d'Endoscopie. Soleure, Switzerland, 1977.

Savary M, Ollyo J: L'esophagite par reflux et ses complications. In Encyclopadie Medico-Chirurgicale, Paris, 1986, p 20822.

Skinner DB, Belsey RH: Surgical management of esophageal reflux and hiatus hernia: Long-term results with 1030 patients. J Thorac Cardiovasc Surg 53:33, 1967.

Skinner DB, Klementschitsch P, Little AG, et al: Assessment of failed antireflux repairs. In DeMeester TR, Skinner DB (eds): Esophageal Disorders: Pathophysiology and Therapy. New York, Raven Press, 1985, p 303.

Steichen FM: Abdominal approach to the Collis gastroplasty and Nissen fundoplication. Surg Gynecol Obstet 162:273, 1986.

Swanström LL, Marcus DR, Galloway GQ: Laparoscopic Collis gastroplasty is the treatment of choice for the shortened esophagus. Am J Surg 171:477, 1996.

Thal AP: A unified approach to surgical problems of the esophagogastric junction. Ann Surg 168:542, 1968.

Urschel HC, Razzuk MA, Wood RE, et al: An improved surgical technique for the complicated hiatal hernia with gastroesophageal reflux. Ann Thorac Surg 15:443, 1973.

Wells C, Johnston JH: Hiatus hernia: Surgical relief of reflux esophagitis. Lancet 268:937, 1955.

Winkelstein A: Peptic esophagitis: A new clinical entity. JAMA 104:906, 1935.

CHAPTER **16**

Massive (Paraesophageal) Hiatal Hernia

Clement A. Hiebert

DEFINITION

A small sliding hiatal hernia is an affair of the cardia, a common condition occasionally requiring operation for reflux esphagitis or because of irksome symptoms unrelieved by medicines and diet. In stark contrast is the massive incarcerated hiatal hernia, a true coelomic rupture, a viscus throttled and positioned for bleeding, obstruction, and strangulation. Paradoxically, this stealthy intruder of the lower mediastinum may lie undetected for years before the fulminant event. Early symptoms are meager and, at least in the era before laparoscopic repair, a surgeon would see fewer than 5 cases of massive herniation for every hundred patients referred. As a consequence, knowledge of the development and treatment of massive hernias has lagged behind our understanding of the smaller and much more common sliding hernias associated with gastroesophageal reflux.

The difficulty in identifying the problem is further confused by inexact nomenclature: "parahiatal," "paraesophageal," "rolling," and "type II" are terms applied to what in popular jargon was once called an "upside down" stomach—less elegant, perhaps, but in the end descriptive. The so-called parahiatal hernia, in which the thoracic pouch of stomach protrudes through a separate opening in the hiatal musculature, exists, but is a rara avis. The same probably holds for the paraesophageal variant, in which the massive herniation of the gastric body occurs in front of a gastroesophageal junction that supposedly remains anchored at or just below the hiatus. Pearson (1971) and Maziak (1998) and their associates consider the pure paraesophageal hernia a rare sighting and show that massive adult hernias are virtually always end-stage sliding hernias. Support for this thesis comes from endoscopic measurements, the operative findings in 91 of 94 consecutive patients, and manometric definition of the interval between upper and lower esophageal sphincters (Pearson, 1993).

The term *type II hernia* is Belsey's nomenclature for the condition and is a reminder of his astute and early comprehension of the difference between small hernias (type I) that are associated with reflux and large ones (type II) that are often silent but always ominous (Belsey, 1952; Skinner and Belsey, 1988).

HISTORICAL NOTE

The history of surgery for massive hiatal hernia is inextricably bound with the development of operations for small sliding hernias. Before Allison's (1951) classic thesis depicting hiatal hernia as a problem of gastroesophageal reflux, it was assumed in every instance that the patient's symptoms derived from a pinched-off pouch of thoracic stomach. Sporadic accounts of strangulations aside (Blades, 1956; Branson, 1955; Sellors, 1955), the fact that small hernias were usually more symptomatic than larger ones was confusing and spawned a variety of operations (Harrington, 1948; Sweet, 1952) with improvement that was either slight or short-lived. Belsey was the first to appreciate this spectrum of hernia from patulous cardia (Hiebert and Belsey, 1961) and severe reflux on the one hand to massive asymptomatic rupture with life-threatening consequences on the other (Belsey, 1952, 1977; Skinner and Belsey, 1967) (Table 16–1).

HISTORICAL READINGS

Allison PR: Reflux esophagitis, sliding hiatal hernia, and the anatomy of repair. Surg Gynecol Obstet 92:419, 1951.

Belsey RHR: Hiatus hernia. In Modern Trends in Gastroenterology. London, Butterworth, 1952.

Pearson FG, Cooper JD, Ilves R, Todd TRJ, Jamieson WRE: Massive hiatal hernia with incarceration: A report of 53 cases. Ann Thorac Surg 35:45, 1983.

Sellors TH, Papp C: Strangulated diaphragmatic hernia with torsion of the stomach. Br J Surg 43:289, 1955.

Skinner DB, Belsey RHR: Surgical management of esophageal reflux and hiatus hernia. J Thorac Cardiovasc Surg 53:33, 1967.

BASIC SCIENCE

Pathophysiology

The small and reflux prone sliding hernia is shy and may slip into the mediastinum only with bending over or when coaxed into view by a diligent radiologist. A massive hernia, by contrast, stays put regardless of the patient's position; catching one on film is simple (Fig. 16–1). In both instances, the hernia presents anteriorly but may enlarge on the left or right to the disadvantage of the ipsilateral lung.

In a sizable minority of patients, the hiatus widens and the endoabdominal fascia yields as the mobile greater curvature of the stomach body noses into the sac in front of the gastroesophageal junction. Hill (1968, 1973) has described posterior tethers on the perimeter of the bare area of the stomach, anchors that lengthen pari passu with the stretching of the hiatus and ballooning of the crowded sac. Localizing the cardia in relation to the hiatus is a difficult assignment with the stomach twisted

TABLE 16–1 ■ Spectrum of the Hiatal Hernia and Reflux Problem

	Patulous Cardia	*Sliding Hiatal Hernia*	*Early Incarceration (Rolling Phase)*	*End-Stage Incarceration*
Schematic				
Radiologic picture	GE junction widened but undisplaced	GE junction above diaphragm	GE junction near hiatus; one third or more of stomach in chest	GE junction near hiatus; most of stomach in chest (spleen and colon may also migrate)
Dominant symptoms	Posturally aggravated Heartburn/regurgitation Epigastric/substernal pain		Early satiety, fullness, postprandial pain Variable reflux symptoms	Obstruction Chronic bleeding More severe postprandial pain
Complications	Esophagitis, stricture, bleeding, aspiration		Ulceration of stomach Chronic bleeding	Acute obstruction Strangulation Ulceration and acute hemorrhage Perforation, aspiration
Indications for operation	Failed medical therapy Presence of complications		Presence of one third or more of stomach above diaphragm with or without symptoms	Urgent operation usually indicated

GE, gastroesophageal.

and filled with radiocontrast material. This more visible gastric herniation represents rotation of the stomach on an axis running from the gastroesophageal junction to the duodenum (Fig. 16–2). The rolling up of the greater curvature causes its former anterior surface to face posteriorly. To complicate matters further, omentum, transverse colon, and spleen may join the migration. The upside-down stomach is now cocked for volvulus and strangulation.

DIAGNOSIS

Clinical Features

Early Symptoms

It is unsettling that the symptoms of an uncomplicated massive incarcerated hernia are neither severe enough to take patients to the physician early nor specific enough to generate a concerned response when such patients do go. Complaints include heartburn, burping, mild dysphagia, queasiness, fullness, early satiety, and breathlessness with meals. Ulceration, gastritis, or microcytic anemia may be the first indication of massive incarceration in 30% to 40% of patients (Table 16–2). An even more subtle clue is the waning of reflux symptoms as a small sliding hernia is transformed into a large rupture with compression and/or angulation of the lower esophagus. Diminishing symptoms of reflux can also precede the development of dysphagia by several weeks when a malignant growth gradually blocks the esophagogastric junction (Hiebert, personal observation).

Symptoms of Advanced Rupture

Ulceration is thought to be secondary to stasis and excessive gastrin production. Erosions, often small and multiple, commonly appear at the point of greatest narrowing where the stomach passes through the hiatus. Single ulcers in the stomach or duodenum are not uncommon. I have encountered one patient with chronic obstruction, volvulus of the herniated stomach, and a perforated duodenal ulcer.

Symptoms of Terminal Complications

When patients with a massive incarceration develop acute chest symptoms, they are likely to be observed in the cardiac intensive care unit, where myocardial infarction, pneumonia, pneumothorax, dissecting aneurysm, other

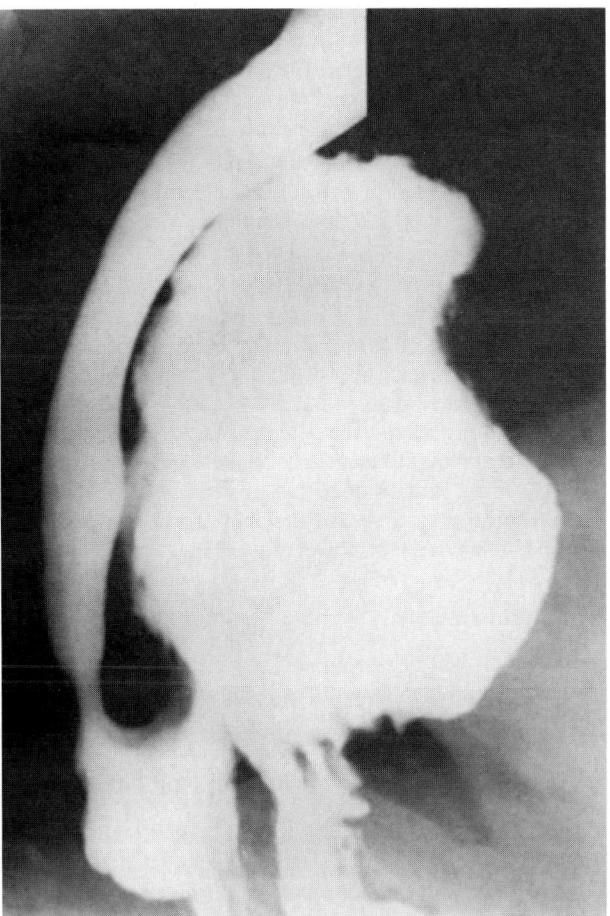

FIGURE 16–1 ■ Barium esophagogram showing a massive incarcerated end-stage hiatal hernia. The esophagogastric junction has been displaced several centimeters above the diaphragm.

intrathoracic catastrophes causing severe pain, hypotension, and hypercarbia are sorted out. Boerhaave syndrome has been reported as a complication (Hines and Faegenburg, 1980). Obstruction may be so complete, in fact, that the patient retches but produces nothing but saliva. Torsion and strangulation make for acute and severe chest and abdominal pain; large amounts of fluid may be lost consequent to perforation into either the mediastinum or abdomen.

Skinner and Belsey (1967) documented a group of 21 patients with massive hernias whose meager symptoms were treated medically or not at all. Six of these patients eventually died of acute and catastrophic complications, including ulceration, gangrene, perforation, hemorrhage, aspiration, and compression atelectasis.

Objective Findings

Postprandial symptoms noted previously in association with a retrocardiac air-fluid level on a lateral chest radiograph strongly suggests the diagnosis, but the thoracic stomach filled with air may be mistaken for a cyst or bulla. A radiocontrast study in the unobstructed patient affords helpful information about the hernia and its ability to empty (see Figs. 16–1 and 16–2).

If the patient is having elective surgery, preliminary flexible esophagoscopy is done to:

- Provide indirect information about the competency of the gastroesophageal junction
- Confirm the location of the gastroesophageal junction and hence the diagnosis
- Rule out other causes of dysphagia

Because of angulation and torsion, it is not regularly possible to view the gastric antrum, and one must be cautious about forceful advancement of any instrument or tube.

What, if any, is the role of 24-hour pH testing and manometry in the preoperative evaluation of a patient with a type II hernia? Fuller and coworkers (1996) found increased exposure of the esophagus to acid in 11 of 15 such patients (69%) and manometric evidence of a mechanically defective "sphincter" in 12 of the group (75%). The authors concluded that gastroesophageal reflux is often part of the massive hernia syndrome but stopped short of recommending manometry and pH testing as a routinely useful test.

MANAGEMENT

Although medicines may alleviate symptoms derived from wrong-way traffic at the esohagogastric junction, the condition of massive incarcerated hernia is a matter of geometry and the treatment is surgical. Because life-threatening complications can develop very swiftly even in an symptomatic patient, the presence of a massive hiatal hernia is itself an indication for repair. Exceptions include individuals with (1) insurmountable risks atten-

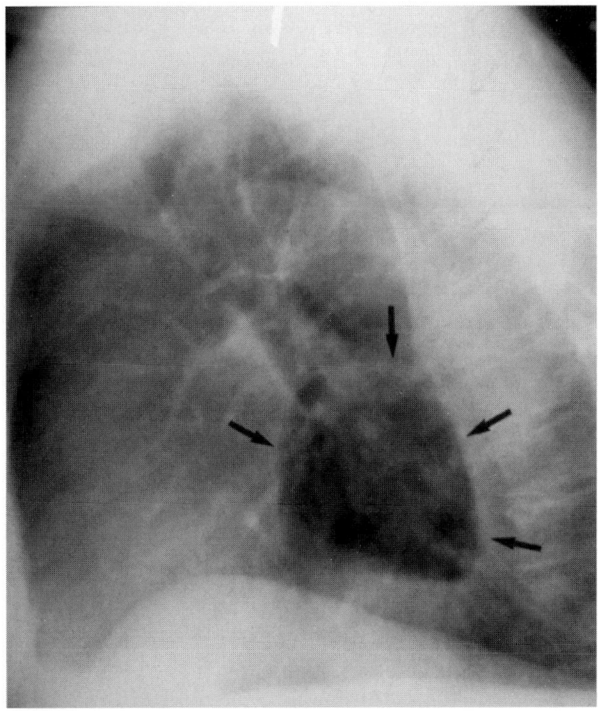

FIGURE 16–2 ■ Chest radiograph indicating a posterior mediastinal air shadow (*arrows*) that is pathognomonic of a large incarcerated hiatal hernia.

TABLE 16–2 ■ **Signs and Symptoms in 94 Consecutive Patients with Paraesophageal Herniation**

Sign and Symptom	Patients No.	Patients (%)	Duration (Avg. No. of Months)	Signs and Symptoms	Patients No.	Patients (%)	Duration (Avg. No. of Months)
Heartburn	29	(31)	13.6	Regurgitation	3	(3)	8.0
Reflux	75	(80)	11.2	Burping	15	(16)	13.4
Nausea	29	(31)	9.8	Dysphagia	45	(48)	7.9
Vomiting	11	(12)	4.8	Odynophagia	0	(0)	0
Hematemesis	7	(7)	3.7	Anemia	36	(38)	2.9
Postprandial fullness	14	(15)	11	Melena	15	(16)	1
Cough	5	(5)	9.6	Pain—postprandial	53	(56)	8.4
Aspiration	27	(29)	9.5	Pain—spontaneous	14	(15)	5.3
Shortness of breath: continual	3	(3)	3.3	Pain—pseudoangina	4	(4)	13.0
Shortness of breath: postprandial	3	(3)	10.5	Weight loss	5	(5)	1.5
Dyspnea	1	(1)	10	Gastrointestinal bleed	11	(12)	0

Data from Maziak DE, Todd RJ, Pearson FG: Massive hiatus hernia: Evaluation and surgical management. J Thorac Cardiovasc Surg 115:53, 1998.

dant to old age, (2) severe chronic obstructive pulmonary disease, (3) generalized atherosclerotic complications, and (4) terminal decrepitude. Elective herniorrhaphy carries a low risk with excellent prospects for full recovery, in contrast to a 40% or higher operative risk when acute complications have developed (Hoffman, 1968; Ozdemir et al, 1973).

Preoperative Preparation

Preoperative preparation may include antibiotics, hydration, blood replacement, and insertion of a no. 18 sump nasogastric tube. Owing to angulation of the stomach beyond the gastroesophageal junction, preoperative gastric decompression is not always possible. In any event, the anesthetist must be alert to the risk of unheralded aspiration both during induction and as the surgeon manipulates the hernia. Hill (1973) notes the serious implications of being unable to pass a nasogastric tube. In a series of ten patients being prepared for emergency operation for paraesophageal hernia, decompression was possible in six patients, all of whom recovered. Of the remaining four who patients unable to undergo decompression, two died during induction of anesthesia and two survived after a prolonged and complicated course.

Surgical Technique

Repairing a massive hiatal hernia may be accomplished through an upper midline abdominal incision, a left sixth or seventh interspace thoracotomy, or through a laparoscope. Each of these approaches has advantages and shortcomings (see chapters on technique). Some selected points and personal preferences are considered:

- Open repair: uncovering the hernia
- Delivery of viscera
- Excising the hernia sac
- Narrowing the hiatal arch
- Lengthening the esophagus
- Creating a competent esophagogastric junction
- Correcting life-threatening disease
- Relocating the organs

Open Repair: Uncovering the Hernia

When the thoracic route has been chosen, it is tempting to initiate the dissection at or below the esophagogastric junction by skiving off the overlying fat, fascia, and fine vessels. A better approach is to (1) encircle the naked esophagus with a Penrose drain *cephalad to the hernia sac* for later traction, and (2) open the ballooned out hernia sac close to the hiatal rim. The layer represents the fusion of pleura, endothoracic fascia, and peritoneum. With traction above and below the hernia mass, one can assess its geometry, divide intervening tissue, and return incarcerated viscera to the abdomen.

Delivery of Viscera

Should delivery of viscera prove difficult, the hiatal equivalent of an episiotomy may be done, or one may evacuate the distended and sometimes ischemic stomach using a trochar and sump suction. Babcock and similar forceps are used sparingly lest the thin gastric wall be rent asunder.

Excising the Hernial Sac

Remember the vagi when excising the hernia sac. Near the esophagogastric junction the left nerve swings away from the esophagus and is incorporated in the hernia sac. It tends to become lost and is easily mistaken for a band of connective tissue.

Narrowing the Hiatal Arch

With the stomach, colon, spleen, and omentum sorted out and returned to the abdomen, the surgeon tentatively narrows the hiatal arch by placing No. 0, nonabsorbable, pledgeted, matressed sutures between the two halves of the right crus. The remodeled hiatus should loosely accommodate the index finger up to the proximal interphalangeal joint. If a fundoplication is to be done, a No. 52 Maloney bougie should be passed first. Crural sutures must be cut out and replaced if the crus approximation leaves an opening that is either too snug or too loose. Large defects nay be closed lateral to the esophagus. Marlex mesh? We have never found it to be necessary.

Lengthening the Esophagus

As already noted, a paraesophageal hernia almost certainly represents the end stage of a sliding hernia and is virtually always associated with *reflux* and some degree of acquired *shortening of the esophagus*. There are two primary ways of lengthening the esophagus so that the effective sphincter lies without tension in the abdomen. The simple option is to clear the esophagus of its mediastinal attachments to the level of the aortic arch. More complicated, but also more effective, is the Pearson gastroplasty. This ingenious combination of the Collis and Belsey hiatal hernia repairs has recently been revisited by Maziak and colleagues (1998) (see also Chapter 24).

Creating a Competent Esophagogastric Junction

Whether repair is through the chest or abdomen, is the addition of an antireflux wrap a requirement or an embellishment? Ellis and colleagues (1986) and Williamson's group (1993) are among those who suggest that the extra sutures be taken only when the patient's history of pH studies is consistent with gastroesophageal reflux—the "if it's not broken, don't fix it" view. There are, however, increasing objective and clinical reports showing gastroesophageal reflux accompanies almost all paraesophageal hernia: Fuller (1996) and Altorki (1998) and their coworkers agree.

Even if one were to accept as ideal the reserving of an antireflux operation for proven reflux, confirming data may be unavailable, sometimes because the route of manometry catheter and pH probe is obstructed; at other times, the urgency of the operation may not justify such a delay. Besides, the first steps of an antireflux operation have already been taken, namely, reduction of the hernia, excision of the sac, narrowing the hiatus, and slackening the esophagus. The best opportunity to forestall reflux symptoms is to take the requisite fundoplicating sutures then and there.

Correcting Life-Threatening Disease

Sometimes a bleeding ulcer, closing a perforation, or resecting a questionable viable segment of stomach or other viscus must be done

Relocating and Fixing the Organs in Place

If the *thoracic approach* is used and there is any question about the matter, the diaphragm should be opened to check on the position of the reduced organs. Swapping a volvulus in the chest for a new obstruction in the abdomen is less than ideal. When the *abdominal approach* is employed, the lesser curvature of the stomach may be anchored to the preaortic fascia (Hill, 1973). A gastrostomy tube is occasionally used as an additional tether to the anterior abdominal wall, but its efficacy is not known.

Laparoscopic Repair of Paraesophageal Hernias

"Superbly convenient for the patient." Thus Kiviluoto (1994) explains the phenomenal flight of patients to surgeons handy with the laparoscope, surgeons whose wands and sleight of hand wizardry seem to offer relief without medicine, cure without pain. What began a decade ago as scattered reports of minimal access repairs has become a growth industry not seen since the early days of coronary bypass surgery. Lacking anything like a follow-up measured in years with which to compare the new and traditional approaches, one is forced, with notable exceptions, to settle for duration of operations (long), hospital stays (short), and observing how soon patients resume normal activity.

Willekes and colleagues (1996) reported 30 patients operated on by a single surgeon for elective laparoscopic repair of pure type II paraesophageal hernias. Satisfactory results were reported for all cases, and there were no deaths. Of the 30 patients, 28 were discharged by day 3 and 14 had resumed normal activity within 1 week after surgery. Johnson and colleagues (1998) described the use of a stapled laparoscopic Collis gastroplasty in nine individuals with shortened esophagus out of 220 patients who underwent minimal access antireflux procedures between 1966 and 1997. All patients were reported to be "improved."

Naunheim and coauthors (1996) presented 66 patients (10 with type II or III hernias) who underwent laparoscopic fundoplication. Conversion to open repair was required in six patients because of bleeding (two), poor exposure of the gastroesophageal junction (three), and gastric laceration in one patient. Complications included the need for dilation (11%), deep venous thrombosis in one patient, ileus in two, recurrent reflux in one patient and dysphagia requiring reoperation in one patient. Follow-up ranged from 6 to 30 months. It is the consensus of the cited authors and others that, so far, at least, *results of laparoscopic repair* of paraesophageal hernias compare favorable with the early results of open repair. Durability of the repair and definition of what constitutes a successful outcome remain debatable issues.

■ KEY REFERENCES

Allison PR: Reflux esophagitis, sliding hiatus hernia, and the anatomy of repair. Surg Gynecol Obstet 92:419, 1951.

The classic paper on gastroesophageal reflux defines the principal anatomic feature of sliding and rolling hernias. Although the Allison repair has been supplanted by more durable techniques and many of Allison's concepts have been refined, this treatise remains unsurpassed both for the novelty of ideas and the lucid—indeed, lyrical—exposition.

Maziak DE, Todd RJ, Pearson FG: Massive hiatus hernia: Evaluation and surgical management. J Thorac Cardiovasc Surg 115:53, 1998.

This article further elucidates the clinical features of massive herniation. Contrary to popular concepts, all but three of their 94 consecutive patients represented advanced degrees of sliding hiatal hernia. The term "paraesophageal" is a misnomer; the gastroesophageal junction also slides.

Rattner DW, Brooks DC: Patient satisfaction following laparoscopic and open antireflux surgery. Arch Surg 130:289, 1995.

A prospective nonrandomized study of 86 patients with reflux complications. The patients themselves elected to have either an open (12) or laparoscopic (74) fundoplication operations. Laparoscopic operations cost less, led to faster recovery, but did not result in higher patient satisfaction compared with the open surgery. The most important factor in patient satisfaction was abolition of preoperative symptoms, not the type of repair or approach used.

Skinner DB, Belsey RHR: Surgical management of esophageal reflux and hiatus hernia. J Thorac Cardiovasc Surg 53:33, 1967.

This article is a treasure trove of insights based on Belsey's extensive experience with 1030 patients with hiatal hernia. Of the many lessons, none is better illustrated than Belsey's remarkable restraint in deferring publication of the results of the Mark IV operation until more than two decades had passed.

Urschel HC: Invited commentary on paper by Belsey R: Mark IV repair of hiatal hernia by the transthoracic approach. World J Surg 1:4765, 1977.

Williamson WA, Ellis FH, Streitz JM Jr., Shahian DM: Paraesophageal hiatal hernia: Is an antireflux procedure necessary? Ann Thorac Surg 56:447, 1993.

The Ellis position is thoughtfully presented; in a word, why perform an antireflux operation for a massive hernia that is not associated with gastroesophageal reflux? The debate is joined by Skinner, Pearson, and Hiebert, who have countering views.

■ *REFERENCES*

Allison PR: Reflux esophagitis, sliding hiatal hernia, and the anatomy of repair. Surg Gynecol Obstet 92:419, 1951.

Altorki NK, Yankelevitz D, Skinner DB: Massive hiatal hernias: The anatomic basis of repair. J Thorac Cardiovasc Surg 115(4):828–835, 1998.

Belsey RHR: Hiatus hernia. In Modern Trends in Gastroenterology. London, Butterworth, 1952.

Belsey RHR: Mark IV repair of hiatal hernia by the transthoracic approach. World J Surg 1:475, 1977.

Blades B, Hall ER: Consequences of neglected hiatal hernias. Ann Surg 143:822, 1956.

Branson K: Case of incarcerated diaphragmatic hernia. Ann Surg 143:273, 1955.

Ellis FH, Crozier RE, Shea JA: Paraesophageal hiatus hernia. Arch Surg 121:416, 1986.

Fuller CB, Hagen JA, DeMeester TR, et al: The role of fundoplication in the treatment of type II paraesophageal hernia. J Thorac Cardiovasc Surg 111:655, 1996.

Harrington SW: Various types of diaphragmatic hernia treated surgically: Report of 430 cases. Surg Gynecol Obstet 86:735, 1948.

Hiebert CA, Belsey RHB: Incompetency of the gastric cardia without radiologic evidence of hiatal hernia: The diagnosis and management of 71 cases. J Thorac Cardiovasc Surg 43:352, 1961.

Hill LD: Incarcerated paraesophageal hernia. Am J Surg 126:286, 1973.

Hill LD, Tobias JA: Paraesophageal hernia. Arch Surg 96:735, 1968.

Hines GL, Faegenburg D: Boerhaave's syndrome with paraesophageal hiatus hernia. N Y State J Med 80:1924, 1980.

Hoffman E: Strangulated diaphragmatic hernia. Thorax 23:541, 1968.

Johnson AB, Oddsdottir M, Hunter JG: Laparoscopic Collis gastroplasty and Nissen fundoplication: A new technique for the management of esophageal foreshortening. Surg Endosc 12:1055–1060, 1998.

Kiviluoto T, Luukkonen P, Salo J: Laparoscopic gastro-oesophageal antireflux surgery. Ann Chir Gynaecol 83:101–106, 1994.

Nauenheim KS, Landreneau RJ, Andrus CH, et al: Laparoscopic fundoplication: A natural extension for the thoracic surgeon. Ann Thorac Surg 61:1062, 1996.

Ozdemir IA, Burke WA, Ikins PM: Paraesophageal hernia: A life-threatening disease. Ann Thorac Surg 16:547, 1973.

Pearson FG, Cooper JD, Ilves R, Todd TRJ, Jamieson WRE: Massive hiatal hernia with incarceration: A report of 53 cases. Ann Thorac Surg 35:45, 1983.

Pearson FG, Langer B, Henderson RD: Gastroplasty and Belsey hiatus hernia repair. J Thorac Cardiovasc Surg 651:50, 1971.

Polk HC: A rational approach to the management of hiatal hernia. South Med J 60:257, 1967.

Sellors TH, Papp C: Strangulated diaphragmatic hernia with torsion of the stomach. Br J Surg 43:289, 1955.

Skinner DB, Belsey RHR: Management of Esophageal Disease. Philadelphia, WB Saunders, 1988.

Skinner DB, Belsey RHR: Surgical management of esophageal reflux and hiatus hernia. J Thorac Cardiovasc Surg 53:33, 1967.

Sweet RH: Esophageal hiatus hernia of the diaphragm. Ann Surg 135:1, 1952.

Urschel HC, Razzuk MA: "Collis-Belsey" fundoplication for uncomplicated hiatal hernia gastroesophageal reflux. Ann Thorac Surg 27:564, 1979.

Walther B, DeMeester TR, Lafontaine E, et al: Effect of paraesophageal hernia on sphincter function and its implication on surgical therapy. Am J Surg 147:111, 1984.

Wichterman K, Geha AS, Cahow CE, Baue AE: Giant paraesophageal hiatus hernia with intrathoracic stomach and colon: The case for early repair. Surgery 86:497, 1979.

Willekes CL, Edoga JK, Frezza EE: Laparoscopic repair of paraesophageal hernia. Ann Surg 225:31–38, 1997.

CHAPTER **17**

The Columnar-Lined Esophagus

PATHOPHYSIOLOGY OF THE COLUMNAR-LINED ESOPHAGUS

Stuart Jon Spechler

In *Barrett's esophagus*, an intestinal, columnar epithelium replaces the stratified squamous epithelium that normally lines the distal esophagus (Spechler and Goyal, 1996). The condition develops through the process of *metaplasia*, in which one kind of fully differentiated (adult) cell replaces another kind of adult cell (Spechler, 1993). In a number of organs, metaplasia results when tissue is exposed chronically to noxious substances (Madri, 1990). These substances injure mature cells and simultaneously promote the aberrant differentiation of immature, proliferating cells (Madri, 1990). The metaplastic cells spawned by this process often are more resistant to injury by the offending substances than are the native cells, and therefore metaplasia has been viewed teleologically as an attempt to protect vulnerable tissues from a hostile environment. For reasons that are not clear, however, metaplastic cells may be predisposed to develop genetic alterations that lead to malignancy. Indeed, the incomplete intestinal metaplasia that characterizes Barrett's esophagus is a strong risk factor for esophageal adenocarcinoma (Spechler and Goyal, 1996).

In most organs that exhibit epithelial metaplasia, stratified squamous epithelium replaces an inflamed columnar mucosa (Madri, 1990). For example, squamous metaplasia is seen commonly as a response to chronic inflammation of columnar epithelia in the respiratory tract, the uterine cervix, the gallbladder, and the excretory ducts of the salivary glands. In contrast, epithelial metaplasia in the esophagus (Barrett's esophagus) involves the replacement of damaged squamous mucosa by columnar (intestinal-type) epithelium. For patients with Barrett's esophagus, chronic gastroesophageal reflux is the factor that both injures the squamous cells and promotes mucosal repair through columnar metaplasia. The intestinal metaplasia that characterizes Barrett's esophagus may be more resistant to reflux-induced injury than the native esophageal squamous mucosa, but the metaplastic cells are predisposed to malignancy (Spechler and Goyal, 1996). Carcinomas develop in Barrett's esophagus at the rate of approximately 0.5% per year, a rate more than 30-fold higher than that for the general population of the United States (Shaheen et al, 2000; Spechler, 2000).

PATHOGENESIS OF INTESTINAL METAPLASIA

Intestinal metaplasia is associated with adenocarcinoma both in the esophagus and in the stomach (Spechler and Goyal, 1996; Stemmermann, 1994). For patients with long segments of intestinal metaplasia in the esophagus (traditional, long-segment Barrett's esophagus), endoscopic surveillance is advised to detect esophageal neoplasia in an early, curable stage (Sampliner and The Practice Parameters Committee of the American College of Gastroenterology, 1998). However, short segments of intestinal metaplasia are far more common than are long segments.

Approximately 15% of patients in general endoscopy units have been found to have short segments of intestinal metaplasia in the region of the gastroesophageal junction (GEJ) (Spechler, 1997). A number of terms have been proposed for this condition (Table 17–1), whose pathogenesis and importance are hotly disputed. For patients who have short segments of intestinal metaplasia at the GEJ, it is difficult to determine whether the metaplastic cells arose from the distal esophagus or from the proximal stomach (the gastric cardia). For clinicians, this issue has practical significance only if there are important pathogenetic and clinical features that depend on the site of origin of the metaplasia. If intestinal metaplasia has the same pathogenesis and predisposition to cancer regardless of location, debates over terminology (e.g., *short-segment Barrett's esophagus* versus *intestinal metaplasia of the gastric cardia*) can be considered trivial, semantic arguments. However, if there are substantial clinical differences between esophageal and gastric intestinal metaplasia, it is important for clinicians to distinguish between the conditions. Much evidence suggests that there are indeed fundamental differences between the gastric and esophageal forms of intestinal metaplasia (Spechler, 1999).

In the body and antrum of the stomach, *Helicobacter*

TABLE 17–1 ■ **Proposed Names for Intestinal Metaplasia in the Gastroesophageal Junction Region**

Short-segment Barrett's esophagus
Ultra–short-segment Barrett's esophagus
No-segment Barrett's esophagus
Columnar-lined esophagus with metaplasia
Metaplasia at the gastroesophageal junction
Metaplasia of the gastric cardia

pylori infection is strongly associated with the development of intestinal metaplasia and cancer (Asaka et al, 1997; Stemmermann, 1994). The International Agency for Research on Cancer considers *H. pylori* to be a *group I carcinogen* (a definite cause of gastric cancer in humans) (Parsonnet, 1996), and the demonstration that infection with *H. pylori* causes intestinal metaplasia and gastric cancer in Mongolian gerbils provides strong experimental evidence for a pathogenetic role for *H. pylori* in these conditions (Watanabe et al, 1998). Correa (1995) and others have proposed that the chronic gastritis induced by *H. pylori* eventually results in metaplasia and adenocarcinoma. Strains of *H. pylori* that have cytotoxin-associated gene A (CagA) can cause a particularly severe form of gastritis that is especially predisposed to progress to cancer (Parsonnet et al, 1997; Spechler, 2000).

In the esophagus, *gastroesophageal reflux disease* (GERD) is an important risk factor for esophageal adenocarcinoma (Lagergren et al, 1999), presumably because GERD causes reflux esophagitis and intestinal metaplasia (Barrett's esophagus). As in the stomach, the development of intestinal metaplasia precedes the development of neoplasia in the esophagus. However, infection with *H. pylori* does not appear to play a direct role in the pathogenesis of esophageal inflammation and metaplasia.

A number of studies on this issue have found no positive association between gastric infection with *H. pylori* and either reflux esophagitis or Barrett's esophagus (Abbas et al, 1995; Liston et al, 1996; Loffeld et al, 1992; O'Connor and Cunnane, 1994; Ricaurte et al, 1996; Rosioru et al, 1993; Talley et al, 1988; Ursua et al, 1991). Reports have suggested that gastric infection with *H. pylori* may actually *protect* the esophagus by preventing the development of reflux esophagitis and Barrett's esophagus (Labenz et al, 1997; Werdmuller and Loffeld, 1997). In addition, some authors have found a significant negative association between esophageal adenocarcinoma and *H. pylori* infections, particularly for infections with CagA-positive strains (Chow et al, 1998; Vicari et al, 1998; Weston et al, 1998). For example, Vicari and associates (1998) found CagA positivity in 11 of 26 (42%) control subjects who were infected with *H. pylori* but in none of 7 infected patients who had dysplasia or adenocarcinoma in Barrett's esophagus. Graham and Yamaoka (1998) proposed that *H. pylori* infections that cause severe pangastritis also cause a decrease in gastric acid production that may protect against GERD.

Regardless of the mechanisms involved, *H. pylori* infection has been shown to be a risk factor for intestinal metaplasia in the stomach but not in the esophagus, whereas GERD is the major risk factor for intestinal metaplasia in the esophagus.

In addition to pathogenetic differences, certain morphologic, histochemical, and clinical features of intestinal metaplasia in the esophagus appear to differ from those of intestinal metaplasia in the stomach. Several schemes have been proposed for the classification of gastric intestinal metaplasia (Filipe et al, 1985; Jass and Felipe, 1981; Matsukura et al, 1980). These schemes focus on the "completeness" of the metaplasia (i.e., how strongly the epithelium resembles that of the normal small intestine) and, if the metaplasia is incomplete, on whether the mucus-secreting cells contain colonic-type sulfomucins that stain with high-iron diamine.

Complete, or *type I*, intestinal metaplasia consists in large part of the following:

1. Absorptive cells that do not secrete mucus and that have a well-defined brush border containing distinctive small intestinal enzymes, such as alkaline phosphatase, aminopeptidase, and disaccharidases.
2. Numerous goblet cells containing sialomucins that stain with Alcian blue.
3. Occasional Paneth cells.

Incomplete forms of intestinal metaplasia consist of few or no absorptive cells and generally are devoid of Paneth cells. The predominant cell type is a columnar "intermediate" cell that secretes mucus (Fig. 17–1). Incomplete forms also contain numerous goblet cells that secrete sialomucins, sulfomucins, or both.

The intestinal metaplasia is categorized as *type II* if the intermediate cells secrete neutral mucins (as do normal gastric surface cells) and acid sialomucins and as *type III* if the intermediate cells secrete mostly acid sulfomucins. Type I is the predominant form found in the stomach (Cassaro et al, 2000; Craanen et al, 1992; Filipe et al, 1985). Type III is the least common form in the stomach but is the form most strongly associated with gastric cancer (Cassaro et al, 2000; Filipe et al, 1994; Stemmermann, 1994; Tosi et al, 1993).

Although the intestinal metaplasia found in Barrett's esophagus can be morphologically indistinguishable from that in the stomach, it has not been a common practice

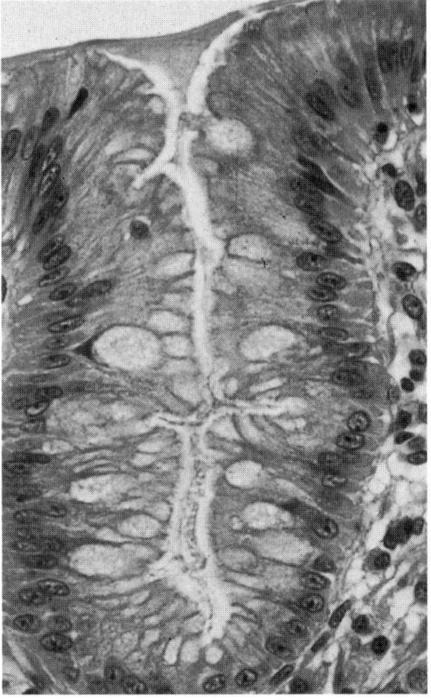

FIGURE 17–1 ■ High-magnification photomicrograph of incomplete intestinal metaplasia (specialized intestinal metaplasia) in Barrett's esophagus. There are gastric surface-type cells, intestinal-type goblet cells, and cells that resemble intestinal absorptive cells with a rudimentary brush border. (From the Clinical Teaching Project of the American Gastroenterological Association, Bethesda, MD.)

for investigators to characterize intestinal metaplasia in the esophagus according to type. However, studies that have focused on the morphology and mucin histochemistry of Barrett's esophagus suggest that the characteristic specialized intestinal metaplasia is usually incomplete (predominantly type III) (Glickman et al, 2000; Jass, 1981; Trier, 1985; Zwas et al, 1981). In addition, specialized intestinal metaplasia has been found to react with a monoclonal antibody (called $7E_{12}H_{12}$ or mAb DAS-1) raised against colonic epithelial cells (Das et al, 1994).

Morphologic studies of Barrett's esophagus using scanning electron microscopy have revealed distinctive features in esophageal intestinal metaplasia. In biopsy specimens taken from the squamocolumnar junction (SCJ) of patients with Barrett's esophagus, Shields and associates (1993) found a peculiar hybrid cell that had both microvilli (a feature of columnar cells) and intercellular ridges (a feature of squamous cells) on its surface.

More evidence that there are fundamental differences between esophageal and gastric intestinal metaplasia comes from studies showing that the cytokeratin staining pattern of intestinal metaplasia in the esophagus may differ from that in the stomach. Cytokeratins are a family of at least 20 structural proteins that are found in the cytoplasm of epithelial cells. Ormsby and colleagues (1999) identified unique patterns of staining for two cytokeratins (cytokeratins 7 and 20) in biopsy specimens of intestinal metaplasia from the esophagus and stomach. Salo and associates (1996) found that intestinal metaplasia in Barrett's esophagus showed immunoreactivity for cytokeratin 13 (a cytokeratin normally found in squamous epithelium), and Boch and colleagues (1997) found immunoreactivity for both squamous and glandular cytokeratin markers in esophageal columnar epithelium that exhibited the phenomenon of multilayering. These observations suggest that esophageal columnar metaplasia might arise from squamous precursor cells that are not present in the stomach.

All of these data suggest that there are important differences between the intestinal metaplasia found in the stomach and that found in the esophagus. If one accepts this premise, it is important for investigators who take biopsy specimens in the region of the GEJ to determine whether those specimens are taken from the distal esophagus or the gastric cardia.

Figure 17–2 shows endoscopically recognizable landmarks that can be used to identify structures at the GEJ. The SCJ (or *Z-line*) is the visible line formed by the juxtaposition of pale, glossy squamous epithelium and red, velvet-like columnar mucosa. The GEJ is the imaginary line at which the esophagus ends and the stomach begins anatomically. The GEJ has been defined by endoscopists, somewhat arbitrarily, as the level of the most proximal extent of the gastric folds (McClave et al, 1987).

In normal individuals, the proximal extent of the gastric folds generally corresponds to the point at which the tubular esophagus flares to become the sack-shaped stomach in the region of the lower esophageal sphincter (LES). In patients with hiatal hernias whose LES is weak and in whom there may be no clear-cut flare at the GEJ, the proximal margin of the gastric folds is determined when the distal esophagus is minimally inflated with air

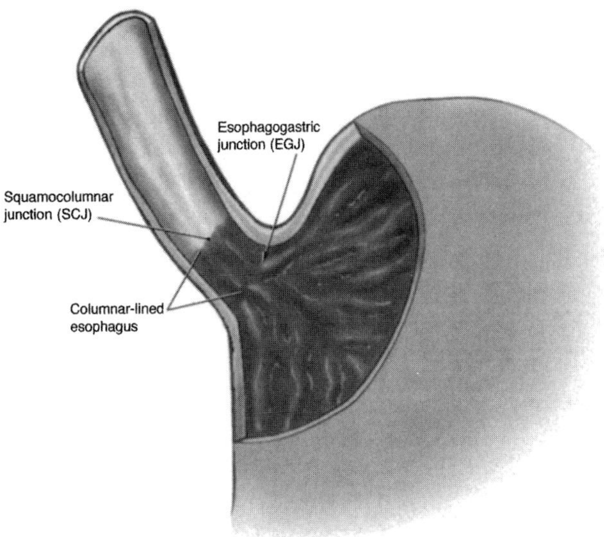

FIGURE 17–2 ■ Landmarks at the gastroesophageal junction (GEJ) region. The squamocolumnar junction (SCJ, or Z-line) is the visible line formed by the juxtaposition of squamous and columnar epithelia. The GEJ is the imaginary line at which the esophagus ends and the stomach begins. The GEJ corresponds to the most proximal extent of the gastric folds and marks the proximal extent of the gastric cardia. When the SCJ is located proximal to the GEJ, there is a columnar-lined segment of esophagus. (From Spechler SJ: The role of gastric carditis in metaplasia and neoplasia at the gastroesophageal junction. Gastroenterology 117:218–228, 1999.)

because overinflation obscures this landmark (Sharma et al, 1998). When the SCJ is located proximal to the GEJ (see Fig. 17–2), there is a columnar-lined segment of esophagus.

GASTROESOPHAGEAL REFLUX DISEASE IN PATIENTS WITH BARRETT'S ESOPHAGUS

Patients with traditional Barrett's esophagus have a number of physiologic abnormalities that predispose them to severe GERD. Some patients exhibit hypersecretion of gastric acid and may require high doses of antisecretory drugs to bring about esophageal healing (Collen et al, 1990; Mulholland et al, 1989). Some patients have duodenogastric reflux, and as a consequence bile may be present in the stomach (Gillen et al, 1988; Vaezi and Richter, 1997). With these abnormalities, the gastric contents available for reflux may be exceptionally caustic, containing high concentrations of acid and bile.

Manometric study of the Barrett esophagus often reveals extreme hypotension of the LES, an important barrier to gastroesophageal reflux, so these patients are exceptionally predisposed to reflux (Iascone et al, 1983; Lidums and Holloway, 1997). Poor esophageal contractility also has been described, a phenomenon that may delay the clearance of noxious material from the esophagus (Lidums and Holloway, 1997; Zaninotto et al, 1989). Some patients have diminished esophageal pain sensitivity, and consequently the reflux of caustic material into the Barrett esophagus may not be heralded by heartburn

(Johnson et al, 1987). Without heartburn, patients may have no warning that they are experiencing gastroesophageal reflux and little incentive to comply with antireflux therapy.

Finally, decreased salivary secretion of epidermal growth factor, a peptide that enhances the healing of peptic ulceration, has been reported in some patients with Barrett's esophagus (Gray et al, 1991). Decreased salivary secretion of this growth factor might delay the healing of the reflux-damaged esophagus.

These data suggest that patients with Barrett's esophagus may be exceptionally predisposed to the gastroesophageal reflux of unusually caustic material. Such reflux might not elicit pain, the esophagus may be unable to effectively clear the noxious material, and healing of the resulting esophageal injury may be delayed. In consideration of this substantial predisposition to reflux esophagitis, it is not surprising that patients with traditional Barrett's esophagus often have severe GERD complicated by esophageal ulceration, stricture, and bleeding.

These physiologic abnormalities, which predispose to severe GERD, have not been described in patients with short-segment disease. Indeed, many patients with short segments of intestinal metaplasia in the distal esophagus have no signs or symptoms of GERD (Spechler and Goyla, 1996). Some data suggest that the length of metaplastic mucosa in Barrett's esophagus may be related to the duration of esophageal acid exposure, as measured by 24-hour pH monitoring (Fass et al, 2000; Oberg et al, 1999). Thus, patients with short-segment Barrett's esophagus may have 24-hour esophageal acid exposure values that are normal or only minimally increased.

Given the propensity for severe GERD in patients with traditional Barrett's esophagus, it seems reasonable to assume that metaplasia should progress in extent over the years as columnar epithelium replaces more and more squamous epithelium that is damaged by ongoing reflux. For reasons that are not understood, however, such progression is observed infrequently. A study by Cameron and Lomboy (1992) suggests that Barrett's esophagus develops to its full extent relatively quickly in most cases. These investigators reviewed Mayo Clinic records of 377 patients found to have Barrett's esophagus between 1976 and 1989. When these patients were grouped according to age, the length of esophagus lined by columnar epithelium did not differ significantly among the various age groups (i.e., 20 year-old patients had a segment of columnar-lined esophagus similar in length to that of the 80-year-old patients). Furthermore, no significant change in the extent of metaplastic epithelium was found among 101 patients who underwent follow-up endoscopic examinations performed after a mean interval of 3.2 years.

GASTROESOPHAGEAL REFLUX DISEASE THERAPY FOR PATIENTS WITH BARRETT'S ESOPHAGUS

In some tissues, metaplasia can be reversed by controlling the factor that caused the chronic inflammation that initiated the metaplasia (Spechler, 1993). Unfortunately, control of GERD (the factor causing the chronic inflammation and metaplasia in Barrett's esophagus) rarely, if ever, results in complete reversal of the metaplastic epithelium (Sampliner, 1997). Partial regression of Barrett's esophagus, evidenced by the development of islands of squamous epithelium within the metaplastic columnar lining, is commonly observed in patients treated with proton-pump inhibitors (PPIs) (Sampliner, 1997). However, the importance of this phenomenon is not known.

In one prospective study, Sharma and associates (1998) obtained 39 biopsy specimens from squamous islands that had developed in 22 patients with Barrett's esophagus, most of whom had been treated on a long-term basis with PPIs. Intestinal metaplasia underlying the squamous epithelium was found in 15 of the 39 specimens (39%). Furthermore, Garewal and colleagues (1999) found abnormalities in Ki-67 staining and p53 expression frequently in biopsy specimens of squamous islands from patients who had been treated with PPIs. These findings suggest that the partial regression of metaplasia induced by PPI therapy might have little effect in decreasing the risk of cancer.

Some have proposed that aggressive control of acid reflux might prevent the progression from metaplasia to neoplasia in Barrett's esophagus (Castell and Katz, 1997). This contention is based on circumstantial evidence and conjecture. GERD appears to cause Barrett's esophagus, and GERD is clearly a strong risk factor for esophageal adenocarcinoma. It is not known whether GERD predisposes to malignancy by causing the initial metaplasia, by promoting the transition from metaplasia to neoplasia, or both. Although it seems reasonable to assume that chronic reflux esophagitis might predispose to cancer by increasing the turnover and proliferation of metaplastic epithelial cells, no study has established that the healing of reflux esophagitis with antireflux therapy reduces the risk of cancer in Barrett's esophagus.

Experimental data indirectly support the notion that control of acid reflux might prevent the development of neoplasia in Barrett's esophagus. For example, Fitzgerald and associates (1996) demonstrated that biopsy specimens of Barrett's esophagus maintained in organ culture exhibit cellular hyperproliferation when exposed to short pulses of acid (1 hour in duration). These findings suggest that the short pulses of esophageal acid exposure that occur frequently in patients with Barrett's esophagus might induce cellular hyperproliferation and thereby promote carcinogenesis.

In another investigation, the effects of acid suppression on the expression of proliferating cell nuclear antigen (PCNA, a marker of cellular proliferation) and villin (a marker of cellular differentiation) by specialized intestinal metaplasia in Barrett's esophagus were studied in 42 patients (Ouatu-Lascar et al, 1999). In biopsy specimens obtained at the baseline endoscopy, the investigators found a strong negative correlation between the expression of villin and PCNA in Barrett's esophagus. This indicates that cellular proliferation decreases as the degree of differentiation increases. After the baseline endoscopy, all patients were treated with PPIs at a dose that eliminated GERD symptoms. Esophageal pH monitoring for 24 hours revealed that this dose of PPI normalized esophageal acid exposure in 26 of the 42 patients, whereas the other 16 had abnormal acid reflux even though the antisecretory therapy had abolished their symptoms. Six months later, follow-up endoscopic biopsies showed that PCNA expression had decreased and villin expression had increased significantly in the patients with normal acid exposure but not in the patients with persistent abnormal acid reflux. These findings suggest that aggressive antisecretory therapy might prevent carcinogenesis by decreasing proliferation and increasing cellular differentiation in Barrett's esophagus.

Most patients treated with PPIs at conventional dosages do not exhibit complete suppression of gastric acid secretion. Indeed, approximately 70% of individuals who take a PPI twice a day experience nocturnal gastric acid breakthrough (gastric pH < 4 for more than 1 hour at night), and brief episodes of acid reflux occur frequently during these breakthrough periods in GERD patients (Katz et al, 1998; Peghini et al, 1998). For patients with Barrett's esophagus, furthermore, pathologic levels of acid reflux frequently persist, even during therapy with PPIs at doses that completely eliminate GERD symptoms (Katzka and Castell, 1994; Ouatu-Lascar et al, 1999; Ouatu-Lascar and Triadafilopoulos, 1998). These data suggest that most patients with Barrett's esophagus who are treated with PPIs at conventional dosages still experience episodes of acid reflux that might promote proliferation of the metaplastic cells.

For some patients who take a PPI twice daily, nocturnal acid breakthrough can be abolished by adding a histamine H_2-receptor blocker at bedtime (Peghini et al, 1998). Thus, with polypharmacy, it may be possible to eliminate acid reflux in most patients with Barrett's esophagus. It is not clear that this approach is desirable, however, for the following reasons (Spechler, 2000):

1. Complete elimination of acid reflux is not necessary to achieve healing of reflux esophagitis. Indeed, most patients who are treated with a PPI at a conventional dosage exhibit complete healing of their symptoms and signs of GERD (Castell et al, 1996).
2. The evidence suggesting that complete elimination of acid reflux reduces the risk of cancer in Barrett's esophagus is indirect and weak. It may not be appropriate to extrapolate the results of studies performed ex vivo to the clinical situation, and it has not been shown that PCNA and villin expression are useful prognostic factors. Furthermore, some data suggest that elimination of acid reflux may not be desirable. In an experimental model of esophageal adenocarcinoma involving rats treated with a carcinogen, for example, exposure of the esophagus to acidic gastric juice protected against the development of cancer (Ireland et al, 1996).
3. Complete elimination of acid reflux would entail considerable inconvenience and expense because of the high doses of the multiple medications that would be required and the esophageal pH monitoring studies necessary to document the efficacy of therapy in controlling acid reflux.

Pending the results of further studies, it seems prudent to recommend that patients with Barrett's esophagus receive antireflux therapy according to the general guidelines established for the medical treatment of GERD (DeVault et al, 1999). These guidelines do not mandate the complete abolition of acid secretion and recommend only that medications be administered in the dosages necessary to eliminate the symptoms and endoscopic signs of GERD.

COMMENTS AND CONTROVERSIES

The author is internationally recognized as one of the preeminent authorities on this condition, and he has studied and reported his observations and conjectures as one of the pioneers in North America. His interest and productivity continue, and this chapter is a thoughtful and practical analysis of background information and of the current state of reported knowledge and opinion.

Dr. Spechler emphasizes the fact that Barrett's esophagus, or acquired columnar replacement, is in most instances seen in advanced stages of reflux disease. He states that Barrett's esophagus predisposes to severe reflux, which may imply that the abnormal epithelium is the primary culprit. It is almost certain that Barrett's esophagus is the result of severe peptic ulceration of the squamous mucosa of the distal esophagus, which "heals" through replacement with the contiguous, or adjacent, columnar epithelium. It also is my opinion that islands of squamous epithelium seen within the columnar-lined segment are remnants of the original squamous mucosa that were spared during the earlier peptic ulceration (and therefore not replaced by columnar cells) and do not represent areas of regression of the columnar abnormality.

Dr. Spechler notes the excitement and concern regarding the premalignant potential of this transformed epithelium. Again, however, he notes that adenocarcinoma developing in an area of Barrett's esophagus is a relatively rare event and reports the incidence of this malignant change at 0.5 case per 100 patients per year. He further states that, until now, there had been no evidence that either medical or surgical antireflux therapy could reduce this incidence. These data also define the practicality of endoscopic surveillance in the early detection of these malignancies. No matter how accurate the endoscopy, the yield will be very small—and represents considerable effort and expense.

Research at a molecular level is directed at the detection of premalignant change at a much earlier stage in the sequence of transformation.

F. G. P.

REFERENCES

Abbas Z, Hussainy AS, Ibrahim F, et al: Barrett's oesophagus and *Helicobacter pylori*. J Gastroenterol Hepatol 10:331–333, 1995.

Asaka M, Takeda H, Sugiyama T, Kato M: What role does *Helicobacter pylori* play in gastric cancer? Gastroenterology 113:556–560, 1997.

Boch JA, Shields HM, Antonioli DA, et al: Distribution of cytokeratin markers in Barrett's specialized columnar epithelium. Gastroenterology 112:760–765, 1997.

Cameron AJ, Lomboy CT: Barrett's esophagus: Age, prevalence, and extent of columnar epithelium. Gastroenterology 103:1241–1245, 1992.

Cassaro M, Rugge M, Gutierrez O, et al: Topographic patterns of intestinal metaplasia and gastric cancer. Am J Gastroenterol 95:1431–1438, 2000.

Castell DO, Katz PO: Acid control and regression of Barrett's esophagus:

Is the glass half full or half empty? Am J Gastroenterol 92:2329, 1997.

Castell DO, Richter JE, Robinson M, et al, and the Lansoprazole Group: Efficacy and safety of lansoprazole in the treatment of erosive reflux esophagitis. Am J Gastroenterol 91:1749–1757, 1996.

Chow WH, Blaser MJ, Blot WJ, et al: An inverse relation between cagA+ strains of *Helicobacter pylori* infection and risk of esophageal and gastric cardia adenocarcinoma. Cancer Res 58:588–590, 1998.

Collen MJ, Lewis JH, Benjamin SB: Gastric acid hypersecretion in refractory gastroesophageal reflux disease. Gastroenterology 98:654–661, 1990.

Correa P: *Helicobacter pylori* and gastric carcinogenesis. Am J Surg Pathol 19 (Suppl 1):S37–S43, 1995.

Craanen ME, Blok P, Dekker W, et al: Subtypes of intestinal metaplasia and *Helicobacter pylori*. Gut 33:597–600, 1992.

Das KM, Prasad I, Garla S, Amenta PS: Detection of a shared colon epithelial epitope on Barrett epithelium by a novel monoclonal antibody. Ann Intern Med 120:753–756, 1994.

DeVault KR, Castell DO, and The Practice Parameters Committee of the American College of Gastroenterology: Updated guidelines for the diagnosis and treatment of gastroesophageal reflux disease. Am J Gastroenterol 94:1434–1442, 1999.

Fass R, Sampliner RE, Spechler SJ, and the GERD Cooperative Study Group: The relationship between esophageal acid exposure and Barrett's esophagus length and dysplasia. Gastroenterology 118:A685, 2000.

Filipe MI, Munoz N, Matko I, et al: Intestinal metaplasia types and the risk of gastric cancer: A cohort study in Slovenia. Int J Cancer 57:324–329, 1994.

Filipe MI, Potet F, Bogomoletz WV, et al: Incomplete sulphomucin-secreting intestinal metaplasia for gastric cancer: Preliminary data from a prospective study from three centers. Gut 26:1319–1326, 1985.

Fitzgerald RC, Omary MB, Triadafilopoulos G: Dynamic effects of acid on Barrett's esophagus: An ex vivo proliferation and differentiation model. J Clin Invest 98:2120–2128, 1996.

Garewal H, Ramsey L, Sharma P, et al: Biomarker studies in reversed Barrett's esophagus. Am J Gastroenterol 94:2829–2833, 1999.

Gillen P, Keeling P, Byrne PJ, et al: Implication of duodenogastric reflux in the pathogenesis of Barrett's oesophagus. Br J Surg 75:540–543, 1988.

Glickman JN, Wang H, Das KM, et al: Phenotype of Barrett's esophagus and intestinal metaplasia of the distal esophagus and gastroesophageal junction: An immunohistochemical study of cytokeratins 7 and 20, Das-1 and 45 MI. Am J Surg Pathol 25:87–94, 2001.

Graham DY, Yamaoka Y: *H. pylori* and cagA: Relationships with gastric cancer, duodenal ulcer, and reflux esophagitis and its complications. Helicobacter 3:145–150, 1998.

Gray MR, Donnelly RJ, Kingsnorth AN: Role of salivary epidermal growth factor in the pathogenesis of Barrett's columnar lined oesophagus. Br J Surg 78:1461–1466, 1991.

Iascone C, DeMeester TR, Little AG, Skinner DB: Barrett's esophagus: Functional assessment, proposed pathogenesis, and surgical therapy. Arch Surg 118:543–549, 1983.

Ireland AP, Peters JH, Smyrk TC, et al: Gastric juice protects against the development of esophageal adenocarcinoma in the rat. Ann Surg 224:358–371, 1996.

Jass JR: Mucin histochemistry of the columnar epithelium of the oesophagus: A retrospective study. J Clin Pathol 34:866–870, 1981.

Jass JR, Filipe MI: The mucin profiles of normal gastric mucosa, intestinal metaplasia and its variants and gastric carcinoma. Histochem J 13:931–939, 1981.

Johnson DA, Winters C, Spurling TJ, et al: Esophageal acid sensitivity in Barrett's esophagus. J Clin Gastroenterol 9:23–27, 1987.

Katz PO, Anderson C, Khoury R, Castell DO: Gastro-oesophageal reflux associated with nocturnal gastric acid breakthrough on proton pump inhibitors. Aliment Pharmacol Ther 12:1231–1234, 1998.

Katzka DA, Castell DO: Successful elimination of reflux symptoms does not insure adequate control of acid reflux in patients with Barrett's esophagus. Am J Gastroenterol 89:989–991, 1994.

Labenz J, Blum AL, Bayerdörffer E, et al: Curing *Helicobacter pylori* infection in patients with duodenal ulcer may provoke reflux esophagitis. Gastroenterology 112:1442–1447, 1997.

Lagergren J, Bergström R, Lindgren A, Nyrén O: Symptomatic gastroesophageal reflux as a risk factor for esophageal adenocarcinoma. N Engl J Med 340:825–831, 1999.

Lidums I, Holloway R: Motility abnormalities in the columnar-lined esophagus. Gastroenterol Clin North Am 26:519–531, 1997.

Liston R, Pitt MA, Banerjee AK: Reflux oesophagitis and *Helicobacter pylori* infection in elderly patients. Postgrad Med J 72:221–223, 1996.

Loffeld RJLF, Ten Tije BJ, Arends JW: Prevalence and significance of *Helicobacter pylori* in patients with Barrett's esophagus. Am J Gastroenterol 87:1598–1600, 1992.

Madri JA: Inflammation and healing. In Kissane JM (ed): Anderson's Pathology, Vol 1, 9th ed. St. Louis, Mosby–Year Book, 1990, pp 67–110.

Matsukura N, Suzuki K, Kawachi T, et al: Distribution of marker enzymes and mucin in intestinal metaplasia in human stomach and relation to complete and incomplete types of intestinal metaplasia to minute gastric carcinomas. J Natl Cancer Inst 65:231–240, 1980.

McClave SA, Boyce HW Jr, Gottfried MR: Early diagnosis of columnar-lined esophagus: A new endoscopic criterion. Gastrointest Endosc 33:413–416, 1987.

Mulholland MW, Reid BJ, Levine DS, Rubin CE: Elevated gastric acid secretion in patients with Barrett's metaplastic epithelium. Dig Dis Sci 34:1329–1335, 1989.

Öberg S, DeMeester TR, Peters JH, et al: The extent of Barrett's esophagus depends on the status of the lower esophageal sphincter and degree of esophageal acid exposure. J Thorac Cardiovasc Surg 117:572–580, 1999.

O'Connor HJ, Cunnane K: *Helicobacter pylori* and gastro-oesophageal reflux disease: A prospective study. Ir J Med Sci 163:369–373, 1994.

Ormsby AH, Goldblum JR, Rice TW, et al: Cytokeratin subsets can reliably distinguish Barrett's esophagus from intestinal metaplasia of the stomach. Hum Pathol 30:288–294, 1999.

Ouatu-Lascar R, Fitzgerald RC, Triadafilopoulos G: Differentiation and proliferation in Barrett's esophagus and the effects of acid suppression. Gastroenterology 117:327–335, 1999.

Ouatu-Lascar R, Triadafilopoulos G: Complete elimination of reflux symptoms does not guarantee normalization of intraesophageal acid reflux in patients with Barrett's esophagus. Am J Gastroenterol 93:711–716, 1998.

Parsonnet J: *Helicobacter pylori* in the stomach: A paradox unmasked. N Engl J Med 335:278–280, 1996.

Parsonnet J, Friedman GD, Orentreich N, Vogelman H: Risk for gastric cancer in people with CagA positive or CagA negative *Helicobacter pylori* infection. Gut 40:297–301, 1997.

Peghini PL, Katz PO, Bracy NA, Castell DO: Nocturnal recovery of gastric acid secretion with twice-daily dosing of proton pump inhibitors. Am J Gastroenterol 93:763–767, 1998.

Peghini PL, Katz PO, Castell DO: Ranitidine controls nocturnal gastric acid breakthrough on omeprazole: A controlled study in normal subjects. Gastroenterology 115:1335–1339, 1998.

Ricaurte O, Fléjou JF, Vissuzaine C, et al: *Helicobacter pylori* infection in patients with Barrett's oesophagus: A prospective immunohistochemical study. J Clin Pathol 49:176–177, 1996.

Rosioru C, Glassman MS, Halata MS, Schwarz SM: Esophagitis and *Helicobacter pylori* in children: Incidence and therapeutic implications. Am J Gastroenterol 88:510–513, 1993.

Salo JA, Kivilaakso EO, Kiviluoto TA, Virtanen IO: Cytokeratin profile suggests metaplastic epithelial transformation in Barrett's oesophagus. Ann Med 28:305–309, 1996.

Sampliner RE: New treatments for Barrett's esophagus. Semin Gastrointest Dis 8:68–74, 1997.

Sampliner RE and The Practice Parameters Committee of the American College of Gastroenterology: Practice guidelines on the diagnosis, surveillance, and therapy of Barrett's esophagus. Am J Gastroenterol 93:1028–1032, 1998.

Shaheen NJ, Crosby MA, Bozymski EM, Sandler RS: Is there publication bias in the reporting of cancer risk in Barrett's esophagus? Gastroenterology 119:333–338, 2000.

Sharma P, Morales TG, Bhattacharyya A, et al: Squamous islands in Barrett's esophagus: What lies underneath? Am J Gastroenterol 93:332–335, 1998.

Sharma P, Morales TG, Sampliner RE: Short segment Barrett's esophagus: The need for standardization of the definition and of endoscopic criteria. Am J Gastroenterol 93:1033–1036, 1998.

Shields HM, Zwas F, Antonioli DA, et al: Detection by scanning electron microscopy of a distinctive esophageal surface cell at the junction of squamous and Barrett's epithelium. Dig Dis Sci 38:97–108, 1993.
Spechler SJ: Barrett's esophagus: An overrated cancer risk factor. Gastroenterology 119:587–589, 2000.
Spechler SJ: Laser photoablation of Barrett's epithelium: Burning issues about burning tissues. Gastroenterology 104:1855–1858, 1993.
Spechler SJ: Medical treatment of Barrett's esophagus. J Gastrointest Surg 4:119–121, 2000.
Spechler SJ: The columnar lined oesophagus: A riddle wrapped in a mystery inside an enigma. Gut 41:710–711, 1997.
Spechler SJ: The role of gastric carditis in metaplasia and neoplasia at the gastroesophageal junction. Gastroenterology 117:218–228, 1999.
Spechler SJ, Fischbach L, Feldman M: Clinical aspects of genetic variability in *Helicobacter pylori.* JAMA 283:1264–1266, 2000.
Spechler SJ, Goyal RK: The columnar lined esophagus, intestinal metaplasia, and Norman Barrett. Gastroenterology 1996; 110:614–621.
Stemmermann GN: Intestinal metaplasia of the stomach: A status report. Cancer 74:556–564, 1994.
Talley NJ, Cameron AJ, Shorter RG, et al: *Campylobacter pylori* and Barrett's esophagus. Mayo Clin Proc 63:1176–1180, 1988.
Tosi P, Filipe MI, Luzi P, et al: Gastric intestinal metaplasia type III cases are classified as low-grade dysplasia on the basis of morphometry. J Pathol 169:73–78, 1993.
Trier JS: Morphology of the columnar cell-lined (Barrett's) esophagus. In Spechler SJ, Goyal RK (eds): Barrett's Esophagus: Pathophysiology, Diagnosis, and Management. New York, Elsevier Science, 1985, pp 19–28.
Ursua I, Ramos R, Val-Bernal JF: *Helicobacter pylori* in Barrett's esophagus. Histol Histopathol 6:403–408, 1991.
Vaezi MF, Richter JE: Bile reflux in columnar-lined esophagus. Gastroenterol Clin North Am 26:565–582, 1997.
Vicari JJ, Peek RM, Falk GW, et al: The seroprevalence of cagA-positive *Helicobacter pylori* strains in the spectrum of gastroesophageal reflux disease. Gastroenterology 115:50–57, 1998.
Watanabe T, Tada M, Nagai H, et al: *Helicobacter pylori* infection induces gastric cancer in Mongolian gerbils. Gastroenterology 115:642–648, 1998.
Werdmuller BFM, Loffeld RJLF: *Helicobacter pylori* infection has no role in the pathogenesis of reflux esophagitis. Dig Dis Sci 42:103–105, 1997.
Weston AP, Badr AS, Topalovski M, et al: Prospective evaluation of the association of gastric *H. pylori* infection with Barrett's dysplasia and Barrett's adenocarcinoma. Gastroenterology 114:A703, 1998.
Zaninotto G, DeMeester TR, Bremner CG, et al: Esophageal function in patients with reflux-induced strictures and its relevance to surgical treatment. Ann Thorac Surg 47:362–370, 1989.
Zwas F, Shields HM, Doos WG, et al: Scanning electron microscopy of Barrett's epithelium and its correlation with light microscopy and mucin stains. Gastroenterology 90:1932–1941, 1986.

INDICATIONS FOR SURGERY OF THE COLUMNAR-LINED ESOPHAGUS

Thomas W. Rice

The columnar-lined, or Barrett, esophagus represents the most advanced and difficult form of gastroesophageal reflux disease (GERD) to treat. The treatment of GERD in patients with columnar-lined esophagus does not restore normal squamous epithelium, may not prevent complications, and does not eliminate the need for continued endoscopic surveillance for cancer.

Patients with a columnar lining have very disturbed esophageal physiology. Lower esophageal sphincter (LES) pressures are lowest in these patients; the mean LES pressure was 5 mm Hg in patients with a columnar-lined esophagus, 9 mm Hg in patients with uncomplicated GERD, and 17 mm Hg in control subjects (Iascone et al, 1983). Patients with columnar-lined esophagus frequently have low-amplitude (Kahrilas et al, 1986) and nonperistaltic (Lidums and Holloway, 1997) esophageal contractions. Slow esophageal transit results in poor clearance of refluxed gastric contents (Karvelis et al, 1987).

Acid and bile reflux is most severe in patients with a columnar-lined esophagus. Esophageal pH was less than 4 during 28% of the study period in patients with columnar lining, 14% in patients with uncomplicated GERD, and 3% in control subjects (Iascone et al, 1983). Similar 24-hour pH abnormalities were reported in studies by Gillen (1987), Robertson (1987), and Fiorucci and their associates (1989).

Reflux patterns differ from those of other categories of GERD: Nocturnal reflux occurs more frequently in patients with columnar lining (Robertson et al, 1987). Twenty-four-hour bile monitoring by the Bilitec 2000 probe (Medtronic Synectics, Minneapolis) detected esophageal bile during 43% of the recording period in patients with columnar lining, during 12% of the period in patients with uncomplicated GERD, and during 2% of the period in control subjects (Champion et al, 1994).

Patients with columnar lining have the most abnormal anatomy of the esophagogastric junction. A hiatal hernia of 2 cm or greater was detected in 96% of patients with columnar lining and 42% of control subjects with or without esophagitis (Cameron, 1999). The diaphragmatic hiatus is larger in patients with columnar lining than in patients with hiatal hernia alone: 3.5 versus 2.2 cm (Cameron, 1999). Esophageal injury sufficient to cause replacement of the mucosal lining of the esophagus also results in edema, spasm, and eventual fibrosis of the mucosa, submucosa, and muscularis propria.

A columnar-lined esophagus is frequently associated with peptic esophageal stricture, esophageal shortening, or both. Columnar lining has been reported in 44% of patients with esophageal strictures (Spechler et al, 1983). In a study by Kim and associates (1998), however, the prevalence of columnar lining was nearly equal in patients with and without strictures: 25% of patients with strictures and 24% of patients without strictures. Long-segment (>3 cm) columnar lining is predictive of a short esophagus (Gastal et al, 1999). A short esophagus is strongly suspected on the basis of a history of peptic stricture or dilation and a large or irreducible hiatal hernia. All of these factors are often reported in patients with a columnar-lined esophagus.

The patient with a columnar-lined esophagus represents the utmost challenge to the esophageal surgeon. Standard repairs are subject to extremely high late failure rates (up to 64% at 100 months) when physiologic assessment is used instead of symptom control (Csendes et al, 1998). A 15% to 21% failure rate of antireflux operations has prompted some surgeons to consider esophageal lengthening (Collis gastroplasty) and total fundoplication (Nissen) as mandatory in these patients (Chen et al, 1999). Thoughtful consideration of the indications for surgical management of the columnar esophagus is important for successful surgical treatment in these most demanding of GERD patients. The presence of a columnar-lined esophagus is not in itself an indication for surgery.

INDICATIONS FOR ESOPHAGEAL REPAIR

Symptom Control

The principal objective of medical treatment for GERD is the control of acid reflux and regurgitation. Potent acid suppression with proton-pump inhibitors (PPIs) also decreases the volume of gastric secretion, reducing these typical symptoms in many patients. However, the relief of symptoms does not ensure the normalization of physiologic testing and does not eliminate reflux (Katzka et al, 1994; Ortiz et al, 1999; Ouatu-Lascar and Triadafilopoulos, 1998). To further complicate this treatment strategy, the patient with a columnar-lined esophagus may be relatively asymptomatic (Fass et al, 1997; Johnson et al, 1987).

Reconstructing the esophageal hiatus and LES and restoring the intra-abdominal length of the esophagus eliminate reflux and relieve typical symptoms. One of the few predictors of successful surgical outcome is control of typical symptoms with PPIs (Campos et al, 1999; So et al, 1998). The inability to control acid reflux with adequate medication suggests that GERD may not be the primary source of symptoms. The surgeon should be cautious with the patient with unmanageable acid reflux who seeks urgent surgery because symptoms are refractory to all medical therapy.

In patients with a columnar-lined esophagus, control with medical therapy alone is more difficult for regurgitation than for acid reflux (Sampliner et al, 1994). An excellent indication for surgery is persistent regurgitation despite good control of acid regurgitation with PPIs. For these patients, an effective LES is needed to control volume regurgitation.

Another important indication for surgery develops when patients who have had good symptom control with PPIs require escalating doses or multiple changes in PPIs because symptoms have become intractable. Some patients experience disabling side effects with these medications and may require surgery for symptom relief. The young patient whose symptoms are well controlled with medication but who has a lifelong requirement for PPIs may be a candidate for surgery. The cost of long-term medical therapy for severe esophagitis eventually equals the cost of surgery. The time at which these costs are equal is extremely variable and has been estimated to be between 1.4 and 10 years of medical therapy (Heudebert et al, 1997; Van Den Boom et al, 1996). In patients with a columnar-lined esophagus, however, the frequent need for complex surgical repairs, the higher failure rates of surgery, and the need for more aggressive medical therapy may greatly alter the break-even point and thus the indication for surgery.

Surgical results for atypical symptoms, such as chest pain, chronic cough, asthma, hoarseness, globus sensation, halitosis, laryngitis, sore throat, or enamel loss, cannot be predicted, and patients have about a 50% chance of relief (So et al, 1997). These symptoms alone, particularly if they do not respond to PPIs, are not indications for surgery.

Complications

Ulcer

Barrett's (1950) initial description of the entity that bears his name focused on peptic ulceration arising in the columnar-lined esophagus. He noted that these ulcers were large, deeply penetrating, often circumferential, and difficult to treat. During surveillance, 46% of patients acquired an esophageal ulcer complicating a columnar-lined esophagus, and 24% had an episode of gastrointestinal bleeding (Murphy et al, 1998). However, only 2% of acute gastrointestinal bleeding is due to esophageal ulcers, and the minority of patients (40%) have esophagitis (Wolfsen and Wang, 1992). In surgical series, true Barrett's ulcers are seen in fewer than 15% of patients with a columnar-lined esophagus (Williamson et al, 1991).

The addition of PPIs to medical therapy has improved the treatment of esophageal ulcers that complicate a columnar-lined esophagus; however, healing is slow and not always complete (Komorowski et al, 1996). In patients who do not respond to therapy, the use of gastroplasty and fundoplication has successfully healed recalcitrant ulcers and arrested acute bleeding (Pearson et al, 1987; Williamson et al, 1992). Primary suture repair and fundoplication are not advised for perforation complicating Barrett's esophagus (Guillem et al, 2000).

Stricture

The complaint of dysphagia in a patient with a columnar-lined esophagus necessitates a comprehensive endoscopic examination and vigorous biopsy protocol to exclude malignant degeneration. Peptic strictures are a common complication and have been reported in one third to one half of these patients (Naef and Savary, 1972; Williamson et al, 1991).

Medical therapy that includes PPIs and aggressive and repeated dilatation is the treatment of choice for strictures complicating benign columnar-lined esophagus. If therapy fails, exacerbating factors such as pill-induced injury, scleroderma, and motility disorders must be excluded. Surgery is indicated when medical therapy fails, when esophagitis does not heal, when strictures recur after adequate dilatation and medical therapy, and when patients are not candidates for long-term medical therapy. A shortened esophagus is a certainty in these patients, necessitating a complex repair with both gastroplasty and fundoplication. The surgical outcome is significantly poorer than that in the patient with uncomplicated disease.

Metaplasia-Dysplasia-Carcinoma Sequence

The length of columnar lining increases minimally during surveillance (Cameron et al, 1992). An early report suggested that, in some patients, the columnar lining was completely reversible with surgery (Brand et al, 1980). However, antireflux therapy rarely produces significant regression; in 75% of patients, the length of columnar lining is unchanged after surgery (DeMeester and DeMeester, 2000). Because surgery does not influence the length of columnar lining, the possibility of regression is not an indication for surgery.

The progression of metaplasia to dysplasia and carcinoma may be prevented with antireflux surgery. The reversion of low-grade dysplasia to metaplasia has been reported in two surgical series (DeMeester et al, 1998; Low et al, 1999). However, differenting acute inflammation from low-grade dysplasia may be difficult; the reported regression, instead, may be the elimination of inflammatory changes through effective surgical treatment of GERD.

The rate of progression of metaplasia to dysplasia and carcinoma may be diminished more by surgery than by medical therapy. The projected dysplasia and cancer-free survival rate at 9 years was 100% for 15 surgical patients compared with 58% for 82 medical patients (Katz et al, 1998). However, Ortiz and associates (1996) reported similar rates of malignancy regardless of therapy. For patients receiving medical therapy, cancer was projected for one patient for each 127 patient-years follow-up and one for each 160 patient-years after surgery. In this report, the study populations were small, there were few events, and the only surgical patient who developed carcinoma had an operation that was not successful.

Late occurrence of cancer after surgery is usually associated with the recurrence of GERD, confirmed by 24-hour pH monitoring (DeMeester and DeMeester, 2000). The early development of high-grade dysplasia or cancer after successful surgery may be the result of irreversible activation of the dysplasia-carcinoma process just before surgery. Of 113 patients, 2 patients developed adenocarcinoma and 1 developed high-grade dysplasia within 39 months of surgery, suggesting undetected dysplasia or carcinoma at the time of surgery (McDonald et al, 1996).

Although suggestive, the evidence that successful surgery induces quiescence in the columnar-lined esophagus is not confirmed. The prevention of dysplasia and carcinoma, albeit a potential benefit of surgery, is not an indication for surgery.

INDICATIONS FOR RESECTION

Penetrating ulcers and undilatable strictures are principal indications for resection of the nonmalignant columnar-lined esophagus (Altorki et al, 1990). Multiple failed operations that result in an end-stage, nonfunctioning esophagus warrant resection and reconstruction. The need for long-term surveillance in the young patient is never an indication for resection unless periodic endoscopy and biopsy are not available.

High-grade dysplasia is intraepithelial carcinoma in which cytologically malignant cells are present in the epithelium without invasion of the basement membrane. The difficulty in differentiating high-grade dysplasia from intramucosal carcinoma and the occurrence of intramucosal carcinoma or more invasive carcinomas in 43% of patients undergoing resection for high-grade dysplasia (Pelligrini and Pohl, 2000) has caused most surgeons to consider the detection of high-grade dysplasia as an indication for resection. Surgery must be accomplished with an operative mortality rate of less than 5% and a low morbidity rate (Rice et al, in press). Once invasion of the basement membrane is confirmed, there is no controversy concerning the need for resection.

CONCLUSION

Development of a columnar-lined esophagus is an irreversible complication of GERD. Patients are at an increased risk for complications and for development of carcinoma. Surgery in these patients is more complex and less successful than surgery in patients with uncomplicated GERD. Antireflux surgery is indicated in patients with symptoms or complications not controlled by aggressive medical therapy. Regression of columnar lining or prevention of carcinoma is not ensured by surgical repair. Resection is indicated in the patient with an end-stage esophagus, a perforated ulcer, an undilatable stricture, high-grade dysplasia, or invasive carcinoma.

COMMENTS AND CONTROVERSIES

The author stresses the critically important fact that columnar-lined esophagus is one of the most advanced stages of reflux disease and is characterized by greater severity of both acid and bile reflux, a higher incidence of ulcerative peptic esophagitis, stricture and acquired short esophagus, greater loss of LES pressure and of amplitudes of peristaltic pressures in the esophageal body, and association with anatomically larger hiatus hernia and widening of the diaphragmatic hiatus. These changes influence the selection of the antireflux operation and impair the quality of results. These observations are strongly supported by a prospective evaluation of 376 patients with reflux disease in whom the incidence of erosive esophagitis and stricture was significantly higher (P $<$ .0001) in the group with Barrett's esophagus (Csendes et al, 2000). Barrett's esophagus also occurs in an older age group.

The indications for surgery are concisely presented—and I am in agreement with all of them. Importantly, the finding of a columnar-lined esophagus, in the absence of symptoms or severe dysplasia, is not an indication for surgery.

Controversy and confusion persist regarding the type of antireflux repair that will provide optimal results in these patients. There is increasing recognition, however, that classic Barrett's esophagus (>3 cm) is very frequently associated with acquired esophageal shortening, which warrants mobilization of the mediastinal esophagus with or without a lengthening gastroplasty (Gastal et al, 1999). Whenever adequate esophageal length is equivocal after an intraoperative evaluation, I advise the addition of a gastroplasty.

Many surgeons recommend a partial fundoplication when the peristaltic amplitudes are unduly low (<45–50 mm Hg) in the body of the esophagus, although Chen and colleagues (1999) reported very favorable outcomes in 45 patients with Barrett's esophagus who were managed by gastroplasty and Nissen-type fundoplication and followed for an average of 3 years.

Csendes reported an unacceptably high failure rate for fundoplication in his patients and recommends the addition of acid suppression (antrectomy) and bile diversion (Roux-en-Y gastrojejunostomy) in patients with symptomatic, long-segment Barrett's esophagus (see Chapter 27).

A higher than usual incidence of failure can be anticipated in these patients after a laparoscopic fundoplication alone. However, there have been reports of the successful addition of a lengthening gastroplasty using laparoscopic or combined thoracoscopic/laparoscopic procedures (Johnson et al, 1998; Luketich et al, 2000; Swanström, 1996).

REFERENCES

Chen LQ, Nastos D, Hu CY et al: Results of the Collis-Nissen gastroplasty in patients with Barrett's esophagus. Ann Thorac Surg 68:1014–1020, 1999.

Csendes A, Smok G, Burdiles P, et al: Prevalence of Barrett's esophagus by endoscopy and histologic studies. Dis Esophagus 13:5–11, 2000.

Gastal OL, Hagen JA, Peters JH, et al: Short esophagus: Analysis of predictors and clinical implications. Arch Surg 134:633–636, 1999.

Johnson AB, Oddsdottir M, Hunter J: Laparascopic Collis gastroplasty and Nissen fundoplication: A new technique for the management of esophageal foreshortening. Surg Endosc 12:1055–1060, 1998.

Lutetich JD, Grondin SC, Pearson FG: Minimally invasive approaches to shortening of the esophagus: Laparoscopic Collis-Nissen gastroplasty. Semin Thorac Cardiovasc Surg 12:173–178, 2000.

Swanström LL: Laparoscopic Collis gastroplasty. Am J Surg 171:477–481, 1996.

F. G. P.

■ *REFERENCES*

Altorki NK, Skinner DB, Segalin A, et al: Indications for esophagectomy in nonmalignant Barrett's esophagus: A 10-year experience. Ann Thorac Surg 49:724, 1990.

Barrett NR: Chronic peptic ulcer of the oesophagus and 'oesophagitis.' Br J Surg 38:175, 1950.

Brand DL, Ylvisaker JT, Gelfand M, et al: Regression of columnar esophageal (Barrett's) epithelium after anti-reflux surgery. N Engl J Med 302:844, 1980.

Cameron AJ: Barrett's esophagus: Prevalence and size of hiatal hernia. Am J Gastroenterol 94:2054, 1999.

Cameron AJ, Lomboy C: Barrett's esophagus: Age, prevalence and extent of columnar epithelium. Gastroenterology 103:1241,1992

Campos GMR, Peters JH, DeMeester TR, et al: Multivariable analysis of factors predicting outcome after laparoscopic Nissen fundoplication. J Gastrointest Surg 3:292, 1999.

Champion G, Richter JL, Vaezi MF, et al: Duodenogastric reflux: Relationship to pH and importance in Barrett's esophagus. Gastroenterology 107:747, 1994.

Chen LQ, Nastos D, Hu C, et al: Results of the Collis-Nissen gastroplasty in patients with Barrett's esophagus. Ann Thorac Surg 68:1014, 1999.

Csendes A, Braghetto I, Burdiles P, et al: Long-term results of classic antireflux surgery in 152 patients with Barrett's esophagus: Clinical, radiologic, endoscopic, manometric, and acid reflux test analysis before and late after operation. Surgery 123:645, 1998.

DeMeester SR, Campos GM, DeMeester TR, et al: The importance of an antireflux procedure on intestinal metaplasia of the cardia. Ann Surg 228:547, 1998.

DeMeester SR, DeMeester TR: Columnar mucosa and intestinal metaplasia of the esophagus: 50 years of controversy. Ann Surg 231:303, 2000.

Fass R, Yalam JM, Camargo L, et al: Increased esophageal chemoreceptor sensitivity to acid in patients after successful reversal of Barrett's esophagus. Dig Dis Sci 42:1853, 1997.

Fiorucci S, Santucci L, Farroni F, et al: Effect of omeprazole on gastroesophageal reflux in Barrett's esophagus. Am J Gastroenterol 84:1263, 1989.

Gastal OL, Hagen JA, Peters JH, et al: Short esophagus: Analysis of predictors and clinical implications. Arch Surg 134:633, 1999.

Gillen P, Keeling P, Byrne PJ, et al: Barrett's esophagus: pH profile. Br J Surg 74:774, 1987.

Guillem PG, Porte HL, Saudemont A, et al: Perforation of Barrett's ulcer: A challenge in esophageal surgery. Ann Thorac Surg 69:1707, 2000.

Heudebert GR, Marks R, Wilcox CM, et al: Choice of long-term strategy for the management of patients with severe esophagitis: A cost-utility analysis. Gastroenterology 112:1078, 1997.

Iascone C, DeMeester TR, Little AG, et al: Barrett's esophagus: Functional assessment, proposed pathogenesis, and surgical therapy. Arch Surg 118:543, 1983.

Johnson DA, Winters C, Sperling TJ, et al: Esophageal acid sensitivity in Barrett's esophagus. J Clin Gastroenterol 9:23, 1987.

Kahrilas PJ, Dodds WJ, Hogan WJ, et al: Esophageal peristaltic dysfunction in peptic esophagitis. Gastroenterology 91:897, 1986.

Karevelis KC, Drane WE, Johnson DA, et al: Barrett's esophagus: Decreased esophageal clearance shown by radionuclide esophageal scintigraphy. Radiology 162:97, 1987.

Katz D, Rothstein R, Schmed A, et al: The development of dysplasia and adenocarcinoma during endoscopic surveillance of Barrett's esophagus. Am J Gastroenterol 93:536, 1998.

Katzka DA, Castell DO: Successful elimination of reflux symptoms does not insure adequate control of acid reflux in patients with Barrett's esophagus. Am J Gastroenterol 89:989, 1994.

Kim SL, Wo JM, Hunter JG, et al: The prevalence of intestinal metaplasia in patients with and without peptic strictures. Am J Gastroenterol 93:53, 1998.

Komorowski RA, Hogan WJ, Chausow DD: Barrett's ulcer: The clinical significance today. Am J Gastroenterol 91:2310, 1996.

Lidums I, Holloway R: Motility abnormalities in the columnar lined esophagus. Gastroenterol Clin North Am 26:519, 1997.

Low DS, Levine DS, Dail DH, et al: Histology and anatomic changes in Barrett's esophagus after antireflux surgery. Am J Gastroenterol 94:80, 1999.

McDonald ML, Trastek VF, Allen MS, et al: Barrett's esophagus: Does an antireflux procedure reduce the need for endoscopic surveillance? J Thorac Cardiovasc Surg 111:1135, 1996.

Murphy PP, Ballinger PJ, Massey BT, et al: Discrete ulcers in Barrett's esophagus: Relationship to acute gastrointestinal bleeding. Endoscopy 30:367, 1998.

Naef AP, Savary M: Conservative operations for peptic esophagitis with stenosis in columnar-lined lower esophagus. Ann Thorac Surg 13:543, 1972.

Ortiz A, Martinez de Haro LF, Parrilla P, et al: 24-h pH monitoring is necessary to assess acid reflux suppression in patients with Barrett's oesophagus undergoing treatment with proton pump inhibitors. Br J Surg 86:1472, 1999.

Ouatu-Lascar R, Triadafilopoulos G: Complete elimination of reflux symptoms does not guarantee normalization of intraesophageal acid reflux in patients with Barrett's esophagus. Gastroenterology 93:711, 1998.

Pearson FG, Cooper JD, Patterson GA, et al: Peptic ulcer in acquired columnar-lined esophagus: Results of surgical treatment. Ann Thorac Surg 43:241, 1987.

Pelligrini CA, Pohl D: High-grade dysplasia in Barrett's esophagus: Surveillance or operation. J Gastrointest Surg 4:131, 2000.

Rice TW, Blackstone EH, Goldblum JR, et al: Superficial adenocarcinoma of the esophagus. J Thorac Cardiovasc Surg, in press.

Robertson D, Aldersley M, Shepherd H, et al: Patterns of acid reflux in complicated acid esophagitis. Gut 28:1484, 1987.

Sampliner RE: Effect of up to 3 years of high-dose lansoprazole on Barrett's esophagus. Am J Gastroenterol 89:1844, 1994.

So JB, Zeitels SM, Rattner DW: Outcomes of atypical symptoms attributed to gastroesophageal reflux treated by laparoscopic fundoplication. Surgery 124:28, 1998.

Spechler SJ, Sperber H, Doos WG, et al: The prevalence of Barrett's esophagus in patients with chronic peptic esophageal strictures. Dig Dis Sci 28:769, 1983.

Van Den Boom G, Go PM, Hameeteman W, et al: Cost effectiveness of medical versus surgical treatment in patients with severe or refractory gastroesophageal reflux disease in the Netherlands. Scand J Gastroenterol 31:1, 1996.

Williamson WA, Ellis FH Jr, Gibb SP, et al: Barrett's ulcer: A surgical disease? J Thorac Cardiovasc Surg 103:2, 1992.

Wolfsen HC, Wang KK: Etiology and course of acute bleeding esophageal ulcers. J Clin Gastroenterol 14:342, 1992.

CHAPTER **18**

Rings and Webs

Earle W. Wilkins, Jr.

The grouping of esophageal rings and webs in a single discussion occurred initially at the first triennial International Symposium on Medical and Surgical Problems of the Esophagus (Rome, 1980). Despite our careful attempt (Wilkins and Dreyfuss, 1981) to dispel "needless confusion concerning the subject of rings and webs" with a differential description and classification, confusion clearly does persist. In this chapter, therefore, the term *ring* is limited exclusively to the lower esophageal ring, better known by its eponym *Schatzki's ring*. The subject of Schatzki's ring and esophageal webs is separated into two distinct discussions.

Lower Esophageal Ring

DEFINITION

The ring is "a diaphragm-like narrowing in the lower esophagus" (Schatzki and Gary, 1953), a concentric symmetric narrowing representing an area of decreased or restricted distensibility. It lies precisely at the squamocolumnar mucosal junction of esophagus and stomach. It consists of a double-backed mucosa, esophageal above and gastric below, with elements of muscularis mucosae and variable amounts of connective tissue between but never true esophageal muscle. It is accompanied by a small axial hiatal hernia.

HISTORICAL NOTE

Templeton (1944), in his textbook *X-ray Examination of the Stomach*, mentioned an asymptomatic diaphragmatic narrowing in the lower esophagus.

The gastroenterologists Ingelfinger and Kramer (1953) recognized a ring in the lower esophagus but called it a "contractile ring." In response, the radiologists Schatzki and Gary in the same year (1953) reported their interpretation of the ring as a morphologic constant rather than as a physiologic variable, which the term *contractile* implied. Although both pairs of authors located the ring in the lower esophagus in their respective titles, Wilkins and Bartlett (1963) located the ring at the precise squamocolumnar junction of esophagus and stomach in a series of four transthoracic, transesophagogastric mucosal excisions of the complete ring.

Finally, a scholarly progress report in radiology was presented by Friedland (1978) in which he recognized the Schatzki ring "as an organic stricture at the mucosal junction, due to reflux." This finding was but one in his "historical review of the changing concepts of lower esophageal anatomy: 430 B.C.–1977."

HISTORICAL READINGS

Friedland GW: Progress in radiology: Historical review of the changing concepts of lower esophageal anatomy: 430 B.C.–1977. Am J Roentgenol 131:373, 1978.

Ingelfinger FJ, Kramer P: Dysphagia produced by a contractile ring in the lower esophagus. Gastroenterology 23:419, 1953.

Schatzki R, Gary JE: Dysphagia due to diaphragm-like localized narrowing in the lower esophagus ("lower esophageal ring"). Am J Roentgenol Radium Ther Nucl Med 70:911, 1953.

Templeton FE: X-ray Examination of the Stomach: A Description of the Roentgenology, Anatomy, Physiology, and Pathology of the Esophagus, Stomach, and Duodenum. Chicago, University of Chicago Press, 1944.

Wilkins EW Jr, Bartlett MK: Surgical treatment of the lower esophageal ring. N Engl J Med 268:461, 1963.

BASIC SCIENCE

Morphology

The morphology of the lower esophageal ring is best presented in a series of illustrations showing it in a barium esophagogram (Fig. 18–1) (a transesophagogastric exposure) at operation (Fig. 18–2), an intact mucosal ring specimen (Fig. 18–3), the microscopic histology (Fig. 18–4), and an autopsy photograph (Fig. 18–5). Emphasis is placed on the mucosal anatomy of the ring, the absence of evidence of esophagitis, the presence of variable amounts of submucosal fibrosis, and the absence of esophageal muscle within the substance of the ring (other than strands of muscularis mucosae). Particular attention is drawn to Schatzki's autopsy case (Fig. 18–5*D* and *E*) in which the morphology of the ring is clearly demonstrated both grossly and microscopically.

Pathogenesis

The cause of the lower esophageal ring is not entirely clear. Because of its association with a sliding hiatal hernia, most authors ascribe its cause to gastroesophageal reflux. Yet there is no visible mucosal evidence of esophagitis and never ulceration. Postlethwait (1986a) concluded: "on the basis of the pathologic changes, we believe these patients develop a unique, localized manifestation of reflux esophagitis which produces a Schatzki's ring." This seems a reasonable assessment.

I subscribe to a theory that overcontractility of circular esophageal musculature at the level of the inferior esophageal sphincter, combined with the sliding gastric mucosa of the hiatal hernia, results in persisting apposition (buckling) back to back of the two mucosal layers.

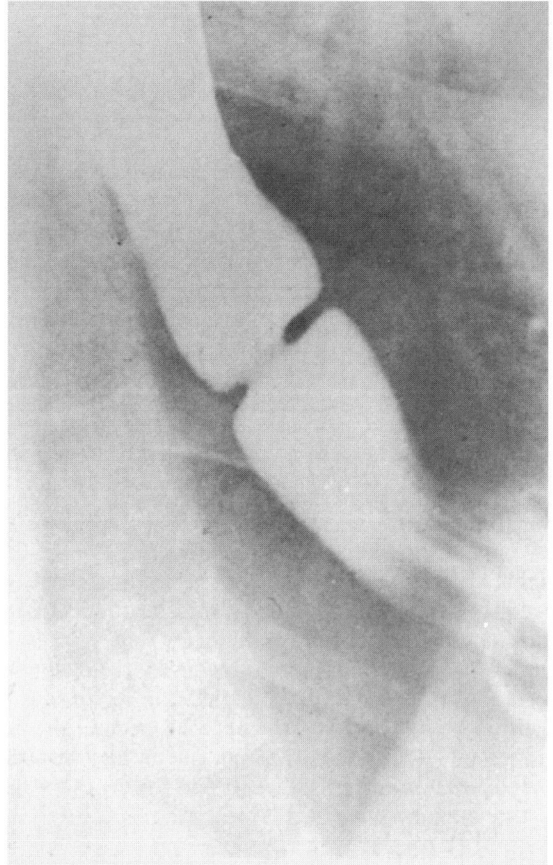

FIGURE 18–1 ■ A classical lower esophageal (Schatzki's) ring demonstrated by barium esophagogram. (From Wilkins EW Jr: Surgery for Schatzki's ring. In Jamieson GG [ed]: Surgery of Oesophagus. Melbourne, Churchill Livingstone, 1988, p 365.)

DIAGNOSIS

Clinical Features

The presenting symptom of the patient with a lower esophageal ring is dysphagia. It is almost exclusively confined to solid food; it is not uncommonly sudden and total. The term *episodic aphagia* is descriptive. The obstruction results most commonly from an incompletely masticated piece of meat, often beef or chicken, which impacts the nondistensible ring. The acute obstruction is accompanied by lower retrosternal distress, pressure, ache, or frank pain. This symptom is followed by salivation and the secretion by the esophagus of copious, thick, tenacious mucus. Further passage of food or liquid from the esophagus into the stomach is not possible.

The patient can do little to relieve the obstruction. Forced vomiting may produce upward dislodgment of the bolus but risks the possibility of esophageal rupture. Spontaneous passage of the bolus into the stomach, if it is to occur at all, usually does so within a few minutes.

Schatzki (1963), in a long-term follow-up of patients with both symptomatic and asymptomatic (those found on x-ray examination for other upper gastrointestinal problems) rings related obstruction to the diameter of the ring. Of 332 patients studied, 108 had dysphagia (32%); of these, all but 4 patients had rings with a diameter of 20 mm or less. All 40 patients with rings of 12 mm or less had dysphagia. Of 158 patients with ring diameters 12 to 20 mm, 64 had dysphagia (40%). It was Schatzki's impression that the caliber of the lower esophageal ring diminished very slowly with time.

Postlethwait (1986a) called attention to the fact that patients with larger-diameter rings may have associated symptomatic gastroesophageal reflux. In 107 patients studied, reflux was present in 8 of 34 with ring diameters 4 to 12 mm (23%), 24 of 45 with rings 13 to 20 mm (53%), and 13 of 28 with rings 21 to 25 mm (46%).

Investigative Techniques

The diagnosis of a lower esophageal ring is made by barium radiography (see Fig. 18–1). As Schatzki originally noted, the esophagus above and stomach below must be distended with barium to permit actual visualization. The experienced radiologist searches for the ring with the patient prone, turned slightly on the right side; as the bolus of barium approaches the distal esophagus, the patient is instructed to take a deep breath while the fluoroscopist takes a spot film as the transmitting barium distends the esophagogastric junction. The ring can be missed during the upright barium swallow but is rarely missed on a cineradiographic examination. The diagnosis may be suspected in the otherwise symptomless patient when ingested food impacts just above the esophagogastric junction. In this circumstance, the ring is not discernible radiographically until the impacted food is dislodged and extracted.

The exact nature of the Schatzki ring can be visualized directly by flexible fiberoptic esophagogastroscopy. The open rigid esophagoscope, which is preferable for removal of the foreign body (food), does not usually permit proper observation of the ring. Whether every patient with a Schatzki's ring should undergo esophagoscopy after radiographic confirmation is a subject of debate. I side with the optional approach, that is, esophagoscopy when the diagnosis is at all doubtful.

MANAGEMENT

The patient with an asymptomatic lower esophageal ring does not require treatment. Conservatism is the cornerstone of therapy for the symptomatic ring.

Therapy

Emergency Treatment

Papain, in a 2.5% aqueous solution, is useful for proteolytic digestion of impacted protein food. It is administered orally in 5 ml swallows every 30 minutes for four doses. Aspiration of accumulating proximal fluid with a large-bore stomach tube may be necessary to permit effective enzymatic action. More prolonged use of papain is to be avoided because of possible irritation of oral, pharyngeal, or esophageal mucosa. The intravenous (IV) administration of an analgesic, such as meperidine (Demerol) in a small dose, has in some cases permitted spontaneous downward dislodgment of the bolus.

Esophagoscopic retrieval is the standard emergency

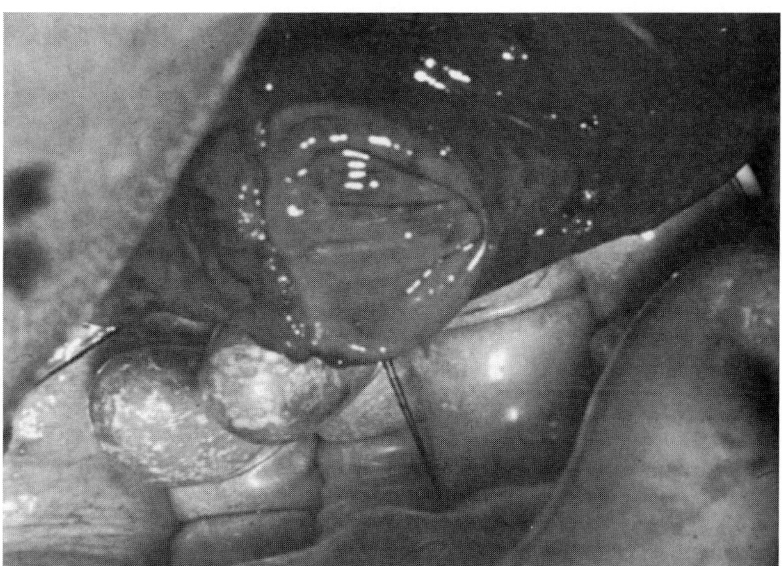

FIGURE 18–2 ■ The ring exposed by a vertical transesophagogastric incision. *Right*, Esophageal mucosa. *Left*, Gastric mucosa. The now flattened ring runs top to bottom. (From Wilkins EW Jr: Surgery for Schatzki's ring. In Jamieson GG [ed]: Surgery of Oesophagus. Melbourne, Churchill Livingstone, 1988, p 365.)

method of management. General anesthesia with endotracheal protection of the airway may be desirable in certain patients. The rigid esophagoscope facilitates extraction of the food. The flexible instrument may then be used for thorough evaluation of the interior of the esophagus, although care must be exercised if the foreign body has been lodged an unusually long period of time. In this case, I prefer a check-up radiographic study after removal of the food to be certain of the integrity of the esophageal wall.

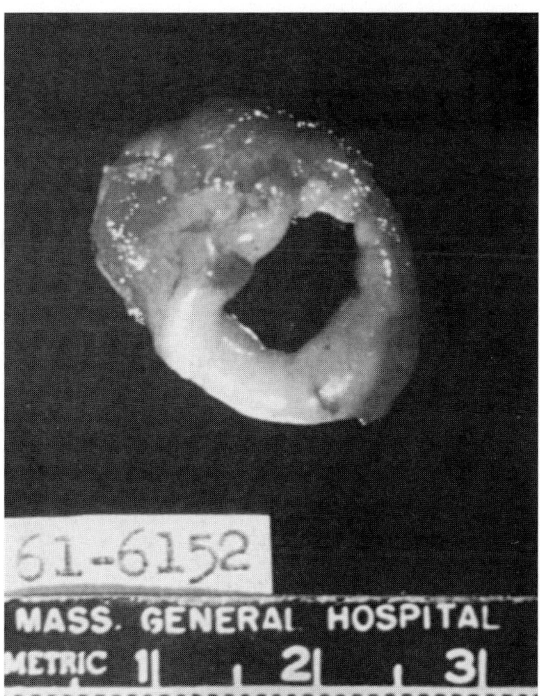

FIGURE 18–3 ■ An excised intact mucosal ring, as seen from the esophageal mucosa side. The maximal diameter is 9 mm (a 1961 pathologic specimen). (From Wilkins EW Jr: Surgery for Schatzki's ring. In Jamieson GG [ed]: Surgery of Oesophagus. Melbourne, Churchill Livingstone, 1988, p 365.)

Definitive Treatment

Surgery is not necessary for the usual patient with a lower esophageal ring. Mucosal excision, as I employed early in investigating the precise nature of the ring, is to be avoided. Such a procedure is frequently complicated by the formation of a dense inflammatory stricture (Ottinger and Wilkins, 1980).

Peroral dilatation or rupture of the ring with the tapered Maloney mercury bougie is now accepted as standard therapy. A bougie approximating 50 French is essential. Symptomatic relief persists for a variable period of time, often 6 to 18 months. Sequential office bougienage may then be carried out for further dilatation when symptoms recur.

Surgical intervention should be reserved for failure of bougienage or for the occasional patient with associated and intractable reflux. When it is necessary, repair of the accompanying hiatus hernia is carried out with peroral bougienage under direct vision or with transgastric retrograde finger fracture.

In the modern era of laparoscopic surgery, an appropriate combination of surgical techniques would be peroral bougienage and a laparoscopic Nissen antireflux procedure.

Results

An unexplainably high rate of recurrence has followed all of the antireflux procedures when carried out in the presence of Schatzki's ring. Ottinger and Wilkins (1980), in a review of 36 patients undergoing surgery for relief of the symptoms produced by Schatzki's ring, found an absolute 40% failure in providing persistent relief of dysphagia. In these Massachusetts General Hospital patients, the type of antireflux repair, whether transthoracic Belsey, transabdominal Hill, or Nissen, seemed not to be a factor. Of the greatest concern was the finding that 8 of the 14 patients in whom therapy had been unsuccessful had developed a true fibrous stricture of the esophagus, a complication much harder to treat than a simple recur-

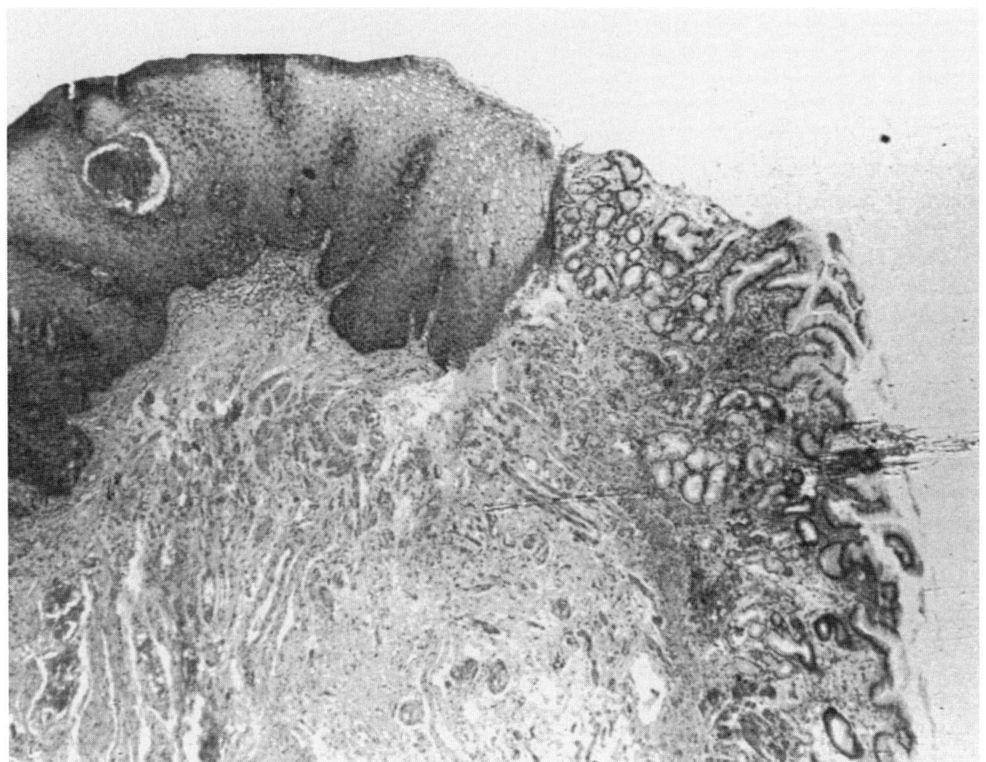

FIGURE 18–4 ■ Histologic examination of the ring shows squamous esophageal mucosa *(left)* and columnar gastric mucosa *(right)*. The actual juncture lies at the apex of the ring with strands of muscularis mucosae and some fibrosis beneath. There is no active inflammation. The fibrosis can be nicely defined by a Masson trichrome stain. (From Wilkins EW Jr: Surgery for Schatzki's ring. In Jamieson GG [ed]: Surgery of Oesophagus. Melbourne, Churchill Livingstone, 1988, p 365.)

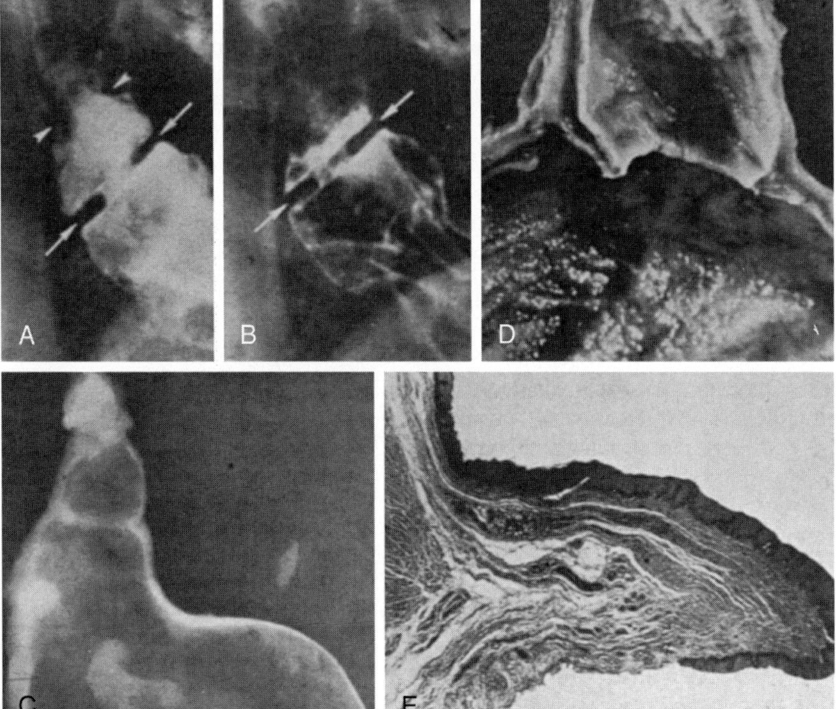

FIGURE 18–5 ■ Schatzki's 1963 evidence of the nature of the lower esophageal ring. *A* and *B*, Ring demonstrated by barium radiography. *C*, Postmortem barium distention of stomach and lower esophagus defining the transverse line of the ring. *D*, Hemisected fixed postmortem specimen showing the shelf-like ring. *E*, Histologic features. (From McMahon HE, Schatzki R, Gary JE: Pathology of a lower esophageal ring: Report of a case with autopsy, observed for nine years. N Engl J Med 259:1, 1958.)

rence of the ring. Postlethwait (1986a) too has noted adverse results from a direct surgical attack on Schatzki's ring.

Table 18–1 presents results comparing method of management in a series of 38 personally managed patients with lower esophageal rings. Adequate management of Schatzki's ring consists of peroral bougienage directed at relief of the dysphagia, with antireflux procedures used only for patients with uncontrolled reflux symptoms or with ineffective bougienage.

The management of Schatzki's ring, once the diagnosis is appropriately confirmed, is office bougienage. Excision of the ring is never indicated. If surgery is necessary, a total fundoplication with transgastric finger fracture is logical, or the combination of peroral bougienage and laparoscopic Nissen operation.

TABLE 18–1 ■ **Results of Antireflux Procedures**

Type of Therapy	*No. of Patients*	*No. of Patients Obtaining Relief (%)*
Mucosal excision of ring	4	2 (50)
Finger fracture and Belsey repair	9	5 (55)
Periodic office bougienage	25	22 (90)

The Esophageal Web

DEFINITION

Of the various interpretive definitions of an esophageal web, that of Postlethwait (1986b) seems the most comprehensive: "A very sharply localized narrowing due to a thin membranous intraluminal extension of the esophageal wall, usually only involving the mucosa and part of the submucosa." This wording specifically differentiates the web from congenital atresia or an acquired stricture. I would add the restriction that the mucosa involved is squamous, both above and beneath the web. This restriction thereby distinguishes a web from the lower esophageal (Schatzki's) ring. Needless confusion is avoided by excluding the lower esophageal ring from the classification of acquired webs, as listed by some authors.

An esophageal web is *not* involved in any esophageal motility disorder. What may appear on contrast esophagograms as web-like structures, as for instance in spiral staircase esophageal peristalsis, prove on endoscopic visualization to have no mucosal abnormality.

HISTORICAL NOTE

It is not possible with esophageal webs to pinpoint one time or one person when the management of the problem really began. Among the names Plummer, Vinson, Paterson, and Brown Kelly associated with sideropenic cervical esophageal web, it is the last who presented the most interesting early observations.

In a 1919 report, Brown Kelly described patients with dysphagia, not uncommon in middle-aged women, with "pale, waxy" oropharyngeal mucosa, smooth tongues, and cracking at the corners of the mouth in whom he attributed an accompanying anemia to the "insufficient dietary." Making the correct observation but the incorrect deduction, on direct inspection of one patient, he observed "a circular membranous web . . . reducing the lumen of the entrance to the oesophagus to about 5 mm." In careful endoscopy of the hypopharynx, he also stumbled on the still current therapy when his rigid esophagoscope "slipped onwards into the oesophagus," producing one of the early dilating ruptures of a web.

Waldenström and Kjellberg (1939) have been credited with the first report of the actual association of the cervical esophageal web with sideropenic anemia. It is now common knowledge that correction of the anemia is basic to permanent control of the dysphagia.

Shamma'a and Benedict (1958) were the first to attempt a classification of esophageal webs in a medical progress article reporting 58 cases. Their classification was fourfold:

1. Upper webs with and without anemia—48 patients (46 female, 2 male).
2. Webs of the middle third of the esophagus—4 patients (1 female, 3 male).
3. Lower esophageal webs—4 patients (2 female, 2 male).
4. Webs with mucous membrane pemphigus—2 patients (both male).

It seems clear, in retrospect, that the lower esophageal "webs" were indeed Schatzki's rings; however, this series also shows clearly the predominance of webs in the cervical esophagus, mainly in middle-aged women.

■ *HISTORICAL READINGS*

Brown Kelly A: Spasm at the entrance of the oesophagus. J Laryngol Rhinol Otol 34:285, 1919.

Shamma'a MH, Benedict EB: Esophageal webs: A report of 58 cases and an attempt at classification. N Engl J Med 259:378, 1958.

Waldenström J, Kjellberg SR: The roentgenological diagnosis of sideropenic dysphagia (Plummer-Vinson's syndrome). Acta Radiol 20:618, 1939.

BASIC SCIENCE

Morphology

The term *diaphanous* has been used to describe the esophageal web (Devitt, 1988), because it consists of mucosa only and in its thinness is usually quite translucent. The web is actually a thin partition of the esophagus; the partition may be a shelf-like protrusion of mucosa, from one side or segment of the perimeter (usually the anterior), or it may be a circumferential infolding of esophageal mucosa. Histologic study at autopsy (Fig. 18–6) demonstrates the transverse fold of normal mucosa and submucosa only, with squamous epithelium covering its entire surface. There is slight tenting of the muscularis mucosae. Inflammatory changes and scarring are absent in this specimen but have occasionally been reported in biopsy material.

Classification and Etiology

As Adler (1963) has described, "an attempt to formulate a meaningful analysis of the literature on esophageal

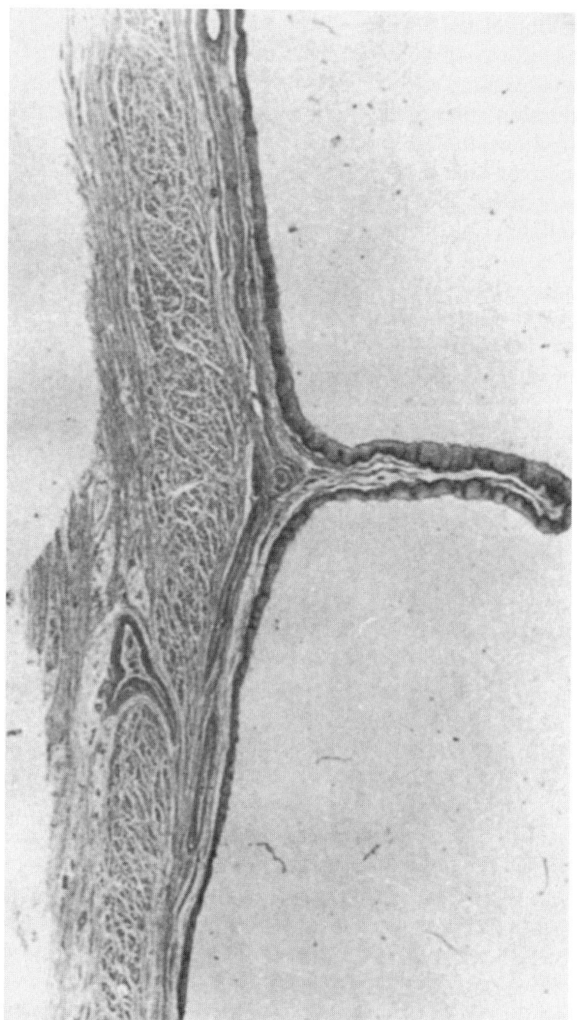

FIGURE 18–6 ■ Histologic examination of a typical web with squamous mucosa covering both its superior and inferior surfaces. There is little areolar tissue between and slight tenting of the muscularis mucosae at its base. (From Chisholm M, Ardran G, Callender S, Wright R: A follow-up study of patients with post-cricoid webs. Q J Med 40:409, 1971, with permission.)

webs is frustrating." The word *web* is loosely used; alternative descriptive phrases (e.g., congenital stenosis, band, stricture) are confusing, and descriptive data are incomplete. One text (Fallis et al, 1991) does not list the subject. Current usage, however, permits a simplified categorization of congenital and acquired webs.

Congenital Webs

The congenital web may occur at any level of the esophagus, usually in the middle or lower third. This web is apparently not a commonly diagnosed lesion, with Postlethwait (1986b) having reported only 20 in a literature review from 1922 to 1975. Ladd (1950) described the developmental abnormality as a "failure of coalescence of esophageal vacuoles which normally lead to complete luminal patency" between days 25 to 31 of embryologic development.

The congenital web is more likely to be circumferential with a central or eccentric orifice and may be thick and tough rather than of the thin, diaphanous character. In the newborn, the web may actually be imperforate. If the diagnosis of a congenital web is to be made later than childhood, even in late life, symptoms must have been present since the age of eating solid food, and causes of acquired webs must be absent.

Acquired Webs

The acquired web is more common than the congenital web and usually is found in the proximal esophagus. At one time, this web was most frequently associated with iron-deficiency (sideropenic) anemia known by its eponyms, Plummer-Vinson (United States) or Paterson-Kelly (United Kingdom) syndromes. It is also seen in patients with pemphigoid, ulcerative colitis, and the rare hereditary epidermolysis bullosa (Stewart et al, 1991). Although the acquired web is usually of the thin, translucent variety projecting from the anterior wall, webs associated with sideropenic anemia may reveal histologic evidence of atrophy, desquamation, or even hyperkeratosis, leukoplakia, and chronic inflammation. Simson and colleagues (1985) have described web-like "mucosal bridges" of the esophagus in *Candida* infection of the esophagus.

Waring and coworkers (1997) have described a case involving a cervical web caused by an inlet patch of ectopic gastric mucosa. In this 55-year-old woman with chronic progressive dysphagia, barium studies demonstrated a circumferential cervical web and endoscopy, a small patch of columnar epithelium adjacent to the web.

Care must be taken to avoid confusion with the entity of acquired stricture in the squamous epithelium proximal to a high level of Barrett esophagus.

Longstreth and Sitzer (1997) have described patients with multiple webs: seven in all, ages 34 to 61 (five men, two women), with no apparent relation to skin disorders, ingestion of caustic substance, or gastroesophageal reflux. Because of the ages of onset, the webs did not appear to be congenital.

DIAGNOSIS

Clinical Features

The principal and presenting symptom of the esophageal web is dysphagia. Its onset varies with the type: the congenital in the neonatal or early childhood periods and the acquired in later decades of life. The severity of dysphagia is in direct relationship to the percentage of lumen obstructed by the web.

Congenital Webs

In those webs with minor degrees of occlusion of the esophageal lumen, dysphagia may not develop until the child is fed solid foods. Some children may actually continue growth without diagnosis or treatment, adjusting naturally to the minor degree of obstruction. Adler (1963) reported two cases of "congenital web" in women aged 75 and 76 years in whom dysphagia had been lifelong since childhood, for which no other cause, such as sideropenic anemia, was elicited. These cases are obviously extreme examples of the minimally symptomatic congenital web.

On the other hand, the neonate with major luminal obstruction may have regurgitation of undigested bile-free feeding very early. This condition indeed may be life-threatening with the possibility of aspiration and consequent airways problems that mandate prompt treatment. In these cases, early diagnosis is accomplished by a diatrizoate meglumine (Gastrografin) swallow after tube evacuation of esophageal contents and, if necessary, after esophagoscopy. If the tube is used to empty the esophagus, the contrast material can be administered immediately by this route.

Acquired Webs

Most acquired or adult webs are indeed asymptomatic. They may be idiopathic with no apparent cause and are uniformly located in the cervical esophagus. They are often discovered as incidental findings during upper gastrointestinal radiographic studies for other problems.

Clements and coauthors (1974) emphasized the need to differentiate webs from normal folds lying in relation to the pharyngoesophageal juncture, "the post-cricoid impression," and "the cricopharyngeal indentation" (Fig. 18–7). The true cervical esophageal web is an anterior, thin, mucosal defect with an eccentric posterior lumen (Fig. 18–8). In a random survey of 100 hospitalized patients, they found eight such webs, with only two causing dysphagia. Asymptomatic cervical webs may not be uncommon. They also discovered a postcricoid impression in 71 patients, 13 with some degree of dysphagia. In contrast, there was just one instance of dysphagia in 18 patients showing a cricopharyngeal indentation.

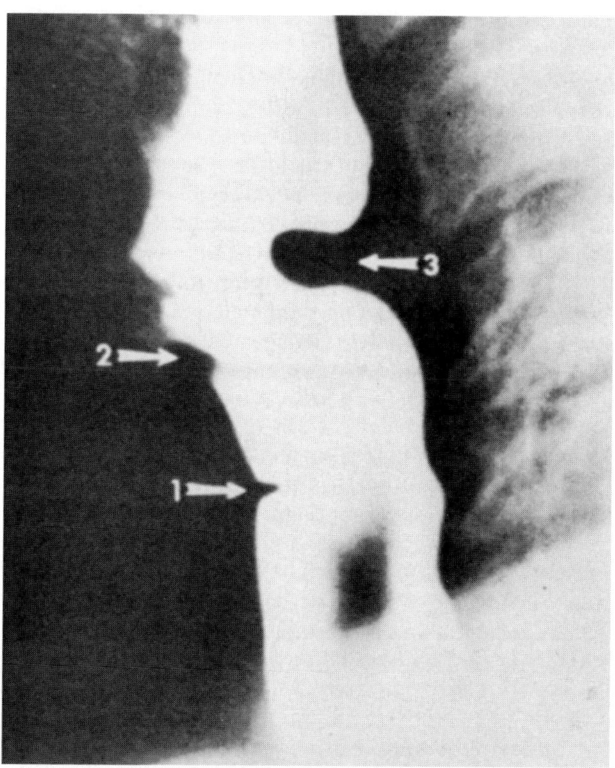

FIGURE 18–7 ■ The Clements differentiation of barium contrast radiographic structures in the cervical esophagus: a small anterior web (1), the postcricoid impression (2), and the cricopharyngeal indentation (3). (From Clements JL Jr, Cox GW, Torres WE, Weens HS: Cervical esophageal webs: A Roentgen-anatomic correlation. Observations on the pharyngoesophagus. Am J Roentgenol 121:221, 1974.)

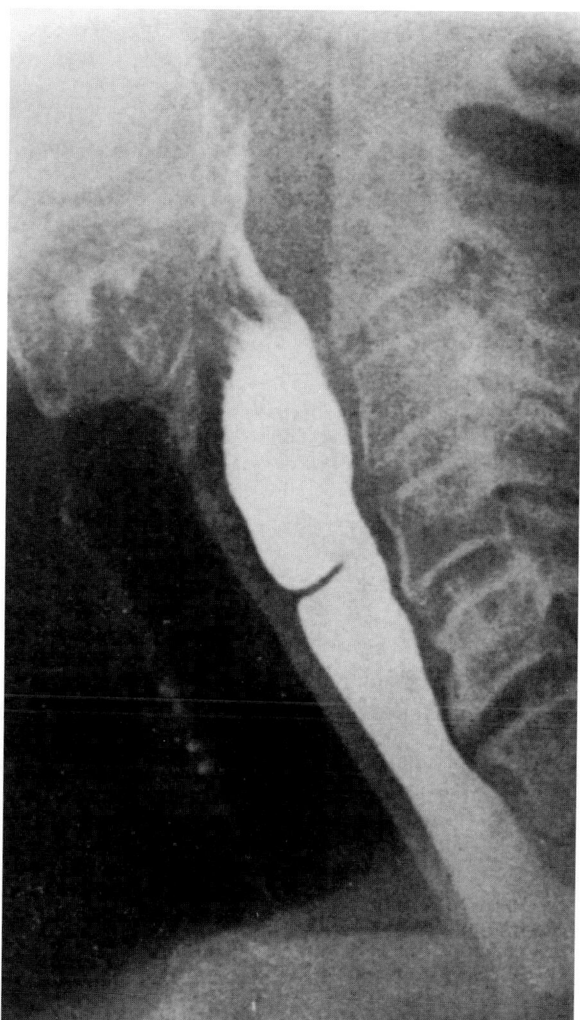

FIGURE 18–8 ■ A true cervical anterior esophageal web with its eccentrically placed posterior lumen.

Nosher and associates (1975), in reviewing 1000 consecutive cinefluorographic examinations of the cervical esophagus and pharyngoesophageal junction, found 55 patients with webs (5.5%), 17 males and 38 females. There were nine patients with multiple webs, eight patients with two webs, and one patient with three webs. Almost all patients were over age 50 years. Eleven patients had dysphagia, but the authors concluded it was related to the web in only six (11%). Comparing the 55 patients having webs with their control patients (those without webs), the authors found no difference in gender, although the patients were "generally older" in age, had the same incidence of iron-deficiency anemia, and were lacking the clinical criteria of the Plummer-Vinson syndrome. The authors concluded that "most cervical and hypopharyngeal webs are of no clinical significance."

"Significant" webs occur only in pemphigoid, epidermolysis bullosa, and the Plummer-Vinson syndrome.

Low and Hill (1988), in reviewing 12 patients undergoing diverticulectomy and cricopharyngeal myotomy for a Zenker's diverticulum, found six (50%) with a cervical esophageal web, five with the web located anteriorly, and one with the web nearly circumferential. They reported that "the association of Zenker's diverticulum and esophageal web is new." Wilkins and Dreyfuss (1981), reflecting their experience with Sweet dating back to 1945, reported that

> a web may occur just distal to the inferior aspect of the mouth of a pulsion diverticulum. This often is detectable only at time of surgical correction. If the diverticulum is excised, the interior of the cervical esophagus must be inspected directly; if the hypopharynx is not opened, a Maloney mercury bougie should be passed during the operative procedure.

The diagnosis of an acquired esophageal web is facilitated by cineradiography. Confirmatory visualization by endoscopy may not be easy. The blind passage of the flexible fiberoptic esophagoscope almost invariably takes the instrument past the web. Devitt (1988) concluded "the rigid oesophagoscope is better suited to examination of the upper oesophagus, the examiner never passing the instrument blind." The endoscopist must always keep in mind, especially in patients with a Plummer-Vinson syndrome and web, that a mucosal carcinoma may be lurking in the area.

MANAGEMENT

Procedures

The treatment of congenital or acquired esophageal webs depends on the physical nature of the web. If it is a thin, membranous, diaphanous web, inadvertent or intentional rupture with the esophagoscope may be all that is required. Recurrence of dysphagia may then be treated by Maloney mercury bougienage. The area of the web should always be inspected on one occasion, however, and bougienage should not be carried out on the basis of the radiograph alone. Webs beyond the cervical region may be dilated or ruptured by the esophagoscope or even biopsied piecemeal, usually with the flexible instrument. Laser lysis (Krevsky and Pusateri, 1989), although still an unproved method, may well be the approach of the future.

A more likely, and possibly more proved clinically, mode of therapy for esophageal webs is balloon dilatation. Huynh and colleagues (1995) described treatment of symptomatic webs with fluoroscopically guided balloon dilators. The basic technique involves passage of a fixed-caliber angioplasty balloon catheter over the guidewire and inflation of the balloon with water-soluble contrast material under carefully monitored pressure. Treatment was successful in all nine patients so treated with no complications.

For the unusual thick web or one that cannot be dilated, transcervical or transthoracic excision may be necessary. This excision is accomplished through a longitudinal esophagotomy with circumferential excision of the web and closure with interrupted sutures (Ikard and Rosen, 1977). The closure is anatomic, that is, circumferential of the mucosa from which the web has been excised and longitudinal of the esophagotomy.

There is never an indication for esophageal resection in the treatment of true esophageal webs. Webb and coauthors (1984) have reported perforation during bougienage, always a threat in any esophageal dilatation; in general, however, complications of the treatment of esophageal webs are unusual (Devitt, 1988).

Results

Follow-up studies of the management of esophageal webs were not reported in the medical literature searched (1981 to 1998). In general, however, the treatment—whether by endoscopic or surgical methods—is most satisfactory. Recurrent dysphagia is uncommon. When it occurs, repeated bougienage should be adequate therapy. In patients with sideropenic cervical esophageal webs, now rather uncommon with treatment of iron-deficiency anemia, dilatation of the web with simultaneous correction of the anemia is curative.

COMMENTS AND CONTROVERSIES

It is interesting that each of the three primary layers of the esophagus is associated with a morphologically distinct indentation, web, or ring. Muscle constitutes the cricopharyngeal bar, squamous mucosa is the substance of a cervical web, and a fibrous circle of submucosa makes a lower esophageal ring. Although barium profiles and textbooks may suggest a family resemblance, Dr. Wilkins has established webs and rings as separate entities with dissimilar morphology, location, and (probable) etiology. Ostensibly, hypertrophic cricopharyngeal muscle bolted the "family" some years before and is mentioned only because mistaking the muscle bar for a mucosal web may confound treatment. Webs split; muscle stretches.

We know more about the cure than about the cause of these constrictions. Reflux has had its day in the sun, but I agree with Earle Wilkins that the association is likely spurious and that correction of an associated hernia should be done for relief of reflux symptoms rather than relief of cervical esophageal dysphagia.

Are rings and webs to remain curiosities, forever swept aside by more complex issues facing the esophageal surgeon? Why does the presence of a Schatzki ring diminish the likelihood of a favorable outcome of hiatal repair? Is the combination of a web, ring, or cricopharyngeal muscle band with a hiatal hernia the sign of a blighted foregut? Why are webs characteristically in the upper thoracic or cervical esophagus? Have foods laced with vitamins relegated the Plummer-Vinson syndrome to the pages of history? Might a Heimlich maneuver safely dislodge a bolus caught on a lower esophageal ring?

Webs, rings, and bars are the nearly forgotten cousins in the family of esophageal obstructions. This chapter reintroduces them clearly and concisely.

C. A. H.

■ KEY REFERENCES

Brown Kelly A: Spasm at the entrance of the oesophagus. J Laryngol Rhinol Otol 34:285, 1919.

This article is an early clinical description of what is now termed the Plummer-Vinson or Brown Kelly-Paterson syndrome, including the dysphagia, atrophic mucosa, smooth tongue, and cracking at the corners of the mouth.

Nosher JL, Campbell WL, Seaman WB: The clinical significance of cervical esophageal and hypopharyngeal webs. Radiology 117:45, 1975.

These radiologists defined the frequency of cervical esophageal webs (5.5%) and the infrequency of dysphagia related thereto (11%).

Ottinger LW, Wilkins EW Jr: Late results in patients with Schatzki rings undergoing destruction of the rings and hiatus herniorrhaphy. Am J Surg 139:591, 1980.

The authors evaluate the late results of management of the lower esophageal ring by destruction of the ring and repair of its accompanying hiatal hernia. The article warns against the standard use of such an aggressive approach. Management by periodic dilatation is preferred.

Schatzki R, Gary JE: Dysphagia due to diaphragm-like localized narrowing in the lower esophagus ("lower esophageal ring"). Am J Roentgenol Radium Therapy Nuclear Med 70:911, 1953.

This truly original radiologic description is of a lower esophageal ring that has come to be known by the first author's name, Schatzki's ring.

Wilkins EW Jr, Bartlett MK: Surgical treatment of the lower esophageal ring. N Engl J Med 268:461, 1963.

In this discussion of the surgical treatment of the lower esophageal ring, the location of the ring at the esophagogastric mucosal junction is firmly established.

■ REFERENCES

Adler RH: Congenital esophageal webs. J Thorac Cardiovasc Surg 45:175, 1963.

Chisholm M, Ardran G, Callender S, Wright R: A follow-up study of patients with post-cricoid webs. Q J Med 40:409, 1971.

Clements JL Jr, Cox GW, Torres WE, Weens HS: Cervical esophageal webs: A Roentgen-anatomic correlation. Observations on the pharyngoesophagus. Am J Roentgenol 121:221, 1974.

Devitt PG: Oesophageal webs. In Jamieson GG (ed): Surgery of the Oesophagus, Melbourne, Churchill Livingstone, 1988, pp 515–518.

Fallis JC, Filler RM, Lemoine G: Pediatric Thoracic Surgery. Elsevier Science Publishing, New York, 1991.

Friedland GW: Progress in radiology: Historical review of the changing concepts of lower esophageal anatomy: 430 B.C.–1977. Am J Roentgenol 131:373, 1978.

Huynh PT, deLange EE, Shaffer HA Jr: Symptomatic webs of the upper esophagus: Treatment with fluoroscopically guided balloon dilation. Radiology 196:789, 1995.

Ikard RW, Rosen HE: Midesophageal web in adults. Ann Thorac Surg 24:355, 1977.

Ingelfinger FJ, Kramer P: Dysphagia produced by a contractile ring in the lower esophagus. Gastroenterology 23:419, 1953.

Krevsky B, Pusateri JP Jr: Laser lysis of an esophageal web. Gastrointest Endosc 35:451, 1989.

Ladd WE: Congenital anomalies of the esophagus. Pediatrics 6:9, 1950.

Longstreth GF, Sitzer ME: Multiple esophageal webs: Treatment and follow-up of seven patients. J Clin Gastroenterol 24:199, 1997.

Low DE, Hill LD: Cervical esophageal web in association with Zenker's diverticulum. Am J Surg 156:34, 1988.

McMahon HE, Schatzki R, Gary JE: Pathology of a lower esophageal ring: report of a case with autopsy, observed for nine years. N Engl J Med 259:1, 1958.

Postlethwait RW: Complications of gastroesophageal reflux. In Postlethwait RW (ed): Surgery of the Esophagus, 2nd ed. Norwalk, CT, Appleton-Century-Crofts, 1986a, p 284.

Postlethwait RW: Other congenital anomalies. In Postlethwait RW (ed): Surgery of the Esophagus, 2nd ed. Norwalk, CT, Appleton-Century-Crofts, 1986b, p 39.

Schatzki R: The lower esophageal ring: Long-term follow-up of symptomatic and asymptomatic rings. Am J Roentgenol Radium Ther Nuclear Med 90:805, 1963.

Shamma'a MH, Benedict EB: Esophageal webs: A report of 58 cases and an attempt at classification. N Engl J Med 259:378, 1958.

Simson JNL, Kindel RB, Isaacs PET, Jourdan MN: Mucosal bridges of the oesophagus in candida oesophagitis. Br J Surg 72:209, 1985.

Stewart MI, Woodley DT, Brissaman RA: Epidermolysis bullosa acquisita and associated symptomatic esophageal webs. Arch Dermatol 127:373, 1991.

Templeton FE: X-ray Examination of the Stomach: A Description of the Roentgenology, Anatomy, Physiology, and Pathology of the Esophagus, Stomach, and Duodenum. Chicago, University of Chicago Press, 1944.

Waldenström J, Kjellberg SR: The roentgenologic diagnosis of sideropenic dysphagia (Plummer-Vinson's syndrome). Acta Radiol 20:618, 1939.

Waring JP, Wo JM: Cervical esophageal web caused by an inlet patch of gastric mucosa. South Med J 90:554, 1997.

Webb WA, McDaniel L, Jones L: Endoscopic evaluation of dysphagia in two hundred ninety-three patients with benign disease. Surg Gynecol Obstet 158:152, 1984.

Wilkins EW Jr: Surgery for Schatzki's ring. In Jamieson GG (ed): Surgery of Oesophagus. Melbourne, Churchill Livingstone, 1988, p 365.

Wilkins EW Jr, Dreyfuss JR: Esophageal rings and webs. In Stipa S, Belsey RHR, Moraldi A (eds): Medical and Surgical Problems of the Esophagus. London, Academic Press, 1981, p 224.

CHAPTER 19

Dilation of Peptic Esophageal Strictures

Thomas W. Rice

A peptic esophageal stricture is the result of excessive and uncontrolled reflux of upper gastrointestinal contents into the esophagus. The amount and composition of refluxed material and the extent of exposure of the esophagus to this material determine the magnitude of damage. Multiple factors control these elements of injury.

Peptic esophageal strictures represent very disturbed esophageal physiology. Lower esophageal sphincter (LES) pressures are lowest in patients with peptic esophageal strictures. Ahtaridis and associates (1979) reported a mean LES pressure of 4.9 mm Hg in patients with peptic strictures, of 7.5 mm Hg in patients with uncomplicated gastroesophageal reflux disease (GERD), and of 20 mm Hg in control subjects. There was no overlap of LES pressures between the patients with peptic stricture and the control subjects. Impaired esophageal motility causes inadequate clearance of the refluxed material, which permits prolonged esophageal exposure and heightens injury. In the same report (Ahtaridis et al, 1979), 64% of patients with peptic strictures had motility disorders compared with only 32% of patients without strictures. Simultaneous or nonpropulsive contractions are most common.

In the extreme, aperistalsis has been reported and may be reversible with adequate control of reflux (Moses, 1987). Abnormal distal gastrointestinal motility may result in excessive intragastric pressures and increased volumes of refluxed material; however, there is only indirect evidence that delayed gastric emptying promotes the development of peptic strictures (Azpiroz, 1987; Richter, 1999).

Insufficient esophageal mucosal protection may magnify the injury caused by refluxed material. Although these protective mechanisms are poorly understood, the amount and quality of neutralizing saliva and esophageal secretions may be important in the prevention of reflux injury. The nature and volume of refluxed material are primary determinants of injury. Undoubtedly, acid is the principal agent. Acid combined with alkaline duodenal contents may cause more injury to the esophageal mucosa than acid alone (Vaezi et al, 1995). Although speculation continues regarding alkaline and enzymatic esophageal injury, some experimental data suggest that nonacid injury alone may play a minimal role in peptic esophagitis (Gotley et al, 1992; Penagini et al, 1988b).

Hiatal hernia is the main structural defect that facilitates reflux and promotes peptic strictures. The prevalence of hiatal hernia increases with the severity of GERD. Hiatal hernias have been reported in 42% of patients with reflux, 63% of patients with esophagitis, and 85% of patients with peptic strictures (Berstad et al, 1986; Hiatt, 1977).

At esophagoscopy, peptic mucosal injury is easily visualized and graded but the damage reaches beyond the mucosa. Peptic stricture is usually the end-stage finding in any rating scheme of esophagitis, but changes in peptic injury deep to the mucosa are themselves progressive and can be graded (Watson, 1987). Early injury is confined to the submucosa and characterized by edema, inflammation, spasm, and the deposition of immature collagen (type III). The resultant grade 1 stricture is “soft” and dilates easily. A grade 2 stricture occurs with maturation of the collagen (type I) in the submucosa, is hard (firm and annular), and requires significant force to dilate. With continued reflux, inflammation and fibrosis advance to involve the entire esophageal wall and periesophageal tissue. This process generally occurs over a substantial length of the esophagus and produces vertical contracture and significant shortening of the esophagus. The result of panmural scarring and cicatricial contracture is a grade 3 peptic stricture.

Dysphagia is the chief complaint of patients with peptic esophageal stricture, but this symptom is not exclusive to reflux injury. Attempts must be made to exclude all other causes of esophageal stricture. Once confirmed, the mainstay of symptomatic control of peptic esophageal stricture is dilation. Long-term management requires the prevention of progressive damage by addressing the multiple factors that cause reflux and by eliminating further reflux injury. Once reflux is controlled, further dilation usually is needed to treat submucosal, muscular, and periesophageal peptic damage.

HISTORICAL NOTE

Esophageal dilation, or *bougienage*, was first used to dislodge impacted food and to push it distal into the stomach. *Bougienage* is derived from the Arabic *Boujiyah*, which is an Algerian city that was a medieval center of the wax trade. Fabricius ab Acquapendente (1537–1619) is credited with the use of a wax taper to disimpact a foreign body lodged in the esophagus (Earlam and Cunha-Melo, 1981). Early esophageal bougies were constructed of various materials, including leather, quills, bone, baleen, iron, and lead. They were used mostly for disimpaction. Caustic strictures, however, were also dilated with these early instruments. By the early 19th century, the shortcomings of blind bougienage of esophageal strictures were recognized (Fletcher, 1831). In the United States, Hildreth (1821) performed the first successful dilation of an esophageal stricture. He used a self-designed bougie constructed of iron wire and plaster to repeatedly treat a 61-year-old man with an esophageal stricture.

By the late 1800s, retrograde dilation of esophageal strictures was a common practice (Woolsey, 1895). Although this procedure required a gastrostomy, it was thought that the retrograde introduction of a dilator was better tolerated, and the cardioesophagogastric junction provided a safe funnel for guidance to the stricture. The passage of a string per os and retrieval in a gastrostomy allowed for "cutting" of the stricture with a sawing motion of the string. This practice was called *bow stringing* and was enhanced by the use of silk thread or piano wire. A dilator may also be tied to the string and then pulled through the stricture; this was the earliest form of *guided dilation* (Plummer, 1910; Tucker, 1924). Because it required permanent gastrostomy, retrograde dilation was reserved for severe, recalcitrant strictures and the technique fell into disfavor. Vinson (1939) wrote, "Gastrostomy is seldom necessary in the management of benign stricture of the esophagus and adds to the risk of treatment."

Although great attention was given to instrument design and the technique of bougienage, the next important breakthrough in dilation came from an entirely unrelated area. Soon after the discovery of the x-ray by Röntgen in 1895, contrast materials were being used for radiographic visualization of the esophagus. Dawson (1907) was the first to radiographically diagnose an esophageal stricture. The importance of x-rays was immediately realized by Dawson, as depicted in his description of visualization of his first patient's stricture:

> The stricture was evidently a considerable one opposite the fifth dorsal vertebra and the esophagus was dilated above it. The illustration explains why a bougie would sometimes get through the stricture and at other times not, for it would only get through if it happened to hit the aperture in the centre of the sac.

The *esophagram* was an important advance in the treatment of peptic esophageal strictures. In addition to aiding in diagnosis, it provided visualization, control, assessment, and long-term follow-up of dilation.

The *esophagoscope*, which was introduced in the 1800s, had limited use because of poor illumination. In the early 1900s, *rigid esophagoscopy* with blind passage of bougies was frequently used. The advantages in the treatment of peptic stricture with visualization of the upper aspect of the stricture and observation of the entry of the dilator into the stricture outweighed the risk of anesthesia. The introduction of *flexible endoscopy* in the 1970s provided the full potential of esophagoscopy in the diagnosis and treatment of peptic strictures. The use of flexible guidewires under endoscopic direction allowed guided dilation in the outpatient setting (Lilly and McCaffrey, 1971). Plastic guided bougies have become the mainstay in the dilation of peptic strictures (Celestin and Campbell, 1981; Monnier et al, 1985).

Although pneumatic dilation had been used to treat achalasia and strictures, its use in the treatment of peptic esophageal strictures was not fully appreciated until the introduction of percutaneous transluminal angioplasty. Adoption of this technology advanced the development of instrumentation that was acceptable for the dilation of peptic strictures. London and colleagues reported the successful balloon dilation of peptic strictures in 1981.

■ *HISTORICAL READINGS*

Dawson B: Roentgen rays as an aid to the diagnosis of stricture of the oesophagus. Lancet 2:1144, 1907.

Fletcher R: On strictures of the esophagus and the danger of the bougie herein. In Medico-Chirurgical Notes and Illustrations. Part I. London, Longman, 1831.

Hildreth CT: Stricture of the esophagus. N Engl J Med Surg 10:235, 1821.

Plummer HS: The value of silk thread as a guide in esophageal technique. Surg Gynecol Obstet 10:519, 1910.

Tucker G: Cicatricial stenosis of the esophagus, with particular reference to treatment by continuous string, retrograde bouginage with the author's bougie. Ann Otol Rhinol Laryngol 33:1180, 1924.

Vinson PP: Management of benign stricture of the esophagus. JAMA 113:2128, 1939.

Woolsey G: The treatment of cicatricial stricture of the oesophagus by retrograde dilatation. Ann Surg 21:253, 1895.

BASIC SCIENCE

Types of Dilators

There are two basic types of esophageal dilators.

The esophageal bougie is a tapered, flexible, yet semi-rigid sound. Esophageal bougies apply both a radial splitting force and a longitudinal stretching force during dilation. The longitudinal force may contribute to perforation during dilation.

The balloon dilator results in only a radial force when applied correctly. This radial force is evenly applied along the length of the stricture and has no longitudinal component. It has been proposed that balloon dilation may result in fewer perforations (Kollath et al, 1984), but this theory has not been substantiated by clinical experience.

Physics of Dilation

The dilation of a peptic esophageal stricture requires the application of sufficient force to split the encasing fibrotic tissue in the submucosa and muscularis, allowing expansion of the esophageal lumen while maintaining mucosal integrity. The mucosal contribution to the strength of the esophagus is minimal at small bougie diameters but becomes significant when the outer esophageal diameter is doubled (Goyal et al, 1971). This finding suggests that initial increments of pressure are absorbed by the muscular layers, which eventually split with progressive dilation. At higher pressures, the strength of the mucosa must prevent rupture. Excessive force causes perforation of the esophagus. Cadaver studies show that the mean pressure required to pneumatically rupture the normal esophagus is approximately 260 mm Hg (Burt, 1931). However, the diseased esophagus with an abnormally thickened and inflamed wall may require pressures much higher than this for successful dilation without perforation.

For pneumatic dilation of patients with achalasia, Van Trappen and Hellemans (1980) suggested pressures of 300 to 500 mm Hg, depending on the dilating apparatus. This pressure is known to cause a muscular tear but generally does not rupture the esophagus. Pressures between 25 and 830 mm Hg were measured during the dilation of peptic strictures (Kozarck et al, 1981). Pressures generated during dilation were considerably higher in untreated patients and generally lower in patients undergoing chronic bougienage. As expected, maximal pressure increased with larger-diameter dilators. Pressures generated during dilation in patients with peptic esophageal strictures tended to remain stable or to decrease after multiple dilations with the same bougie.

Results of Dilation

The maximal diameter of a stricture does not occur immediately after dilation. During the 4 to 7 days after dilation, there is an average increase in diameter of 1.2 mm (Bennett et al, 1985). This increase is thought to be secondary to the relief of muscular spasm and the reabsorption of hematoma and edema. The postdilation diameter of the stricture is always less than the diameter of the last bougie passed; differences vary from 1 to 11 mm. This variation is caused by spasm and rigidity of the damaged esophageal wall.

Peptic strictures generally recur and reach predilation severity by 12 weeks after dilation (Penagini et al, 1988a). In that study, dysphagia decreased by 4 days after dilation, remained improved until 6 weeks after dilation, and returned to predilation intensity by 12 weeks. Stricture diameter, however, was not predictive of dysphagia during this time. Heartburn did not worsen after dilation. No differences were seen in pH monitoring results before or after dilation in the group as a whole. In one third of the group (three patients), however, an increase in reflux after dilation was measured on 24-hour pH monitoring. These patients had absent LES pressures (0 to 2 mm Hg) and low-amplitude pressure waves in the esophageal body (0 to 36 mm Hg).

An objective outcome rather than relief of dysphagia should be used to define the end point for dilation of peptic strictures. The passage of a 12-mm barium pill as the objective for dilation reduced both stricture recurrence and the need for subsequent dilation (Saeed et al, 1997).

After dilation, esophageal transit decreases markedly; this effect lasts for 3 weeks (Kjellén, 1989). Improvement in esophageal transit was not predictive of outcome; symptomatic relief was predicted by postdilation stricture diameter measured radiographically.

After the initial dilation, some patients require further dilation. Composition of the study group, length of follow-up, and aggressiveness of dilation and reflux control determine the percentage of dilation failures. Need for repeated dilations ranged from 22% to 65% in various studies (Glick, 1982; Lanza and Graham, 1978; Ogilvie et al, 1980; Patterson et al, 1983). After two or more dilations, the likelihood of further dilation has been reported to be between 86% and 94% (Glick, 1982). In this study, the interval between dilations varied but approximated 1 month after eight dilations.

Unsuccessful dilation is difficult to explain or predict. At least 75% of patients require more than one dilation if reflux is inadequately managed (Farup et al, 1998). In these patients, most restricturing occurred during the first 6 months after dilation. Predictors of rapid restricturing were small diameter of stricture at initial endoscopy, a long history of symptomatic GERD, and a short period of dysphagia before dilation. The number or frequency of dilations was not predictive of outcome in patients treated with histamine H_2-blockers or surgery (Jaffray and Anderson, 1998). Patients without symptoms of heartburn or those who reported weight loss are more likely to require repeat dilation (Agnew et al, 1996).

In a study of 195 patients, male gender was predictive of poor outcome (Hands et al, 1989). Women constituted 58% of the patients and were significantly older than the men in the group. Although 54% of both groups required more than one dilation, men required many more dilations over a longer period of time. Both stricture length and diameter were reported as independent predictors of persistent dysphagia after dilation (Bonavina et al, 1990). Patients with strictures longer than 2 cm or narrower than 9 mm before dilation had poor long-term outcome with bougienage.

DIAGNOSIS

Clinical Features

Dysphagia is the primary presenting symptom of patients with peptic strictures. In general, with mechanical obstruction, difficulty swallowing is not perceived until the esophageal lumen is approximately one-half the normal diameter (20 to 25 mm). Because the obstruction is structural, dysphagia associated with peptic stricture is constant and reproducible. Patients first complain of solid dysphagia with sticky, spongy foods such as beef, chicken, fish, and fresh bread. The onset and progression are insidious; patients learn to avoid these foods before seeking medical advice. Liquids are not a problem until the stricture is advanced or food is impacted. When food impaction occurs, attempts to dislodge the bolus, such as dry swallowing or drinking water, are usually unsuccessful. Regurgitation is often required before swallowing can resume.

Differential Diagnosis

Dysphagia due to peptic stricture must be differentiated from an esophageal motor disorder. With functional disorders, dysphagia is typically intermittent. Liquids are poorly handled in oropharyngeal dysphagia. Symptoms include drooling, gagging, aspiration, choking, and nasal regurgitation. Motor disorders of the esophageal body are equally symptomatic with liquids and solids. Food impaction does not generally result in regurgitation, and swallowing water may clear the obstructing bolus.

A careful history may elicit other symptoms of reflux in patients with peptic strictures. Most of these patients present de novo with dysphagia. It is uncommon to see a patient develop a symptomatic stricture during the treatment and follow-up of GERD. Watson (1987) reported that 68% of his patients with peptic esophageal strictures had no antecedent diagnosis of GERD; however, on subsequent questioning, 76% had symptoms of reflux. Not all patients with gastroesophageal reflux who complain of dysphagia have a peptic stricture. Of 100 patients with reflux, 53 patients complained of dysphagia; only 2 were found to have peptic stricture (DeMeester et al, 1976).

In complex cases, the association of motility disorder with reflux disease is not predictive of dysphagia. Bombeck and associates (1972) reported on 19 patients with reflux; dysphagia was present in 7 of 14 without motility disorders and 2 of 5 with motility disorders.

Dysphagia may be multifactorial. In the absence of a peptic stricture or motility disorder, patients with severe reflux may still complain of dysphagia. In a surgical series, Kiroff and coworkers (1984) reported that 12 of 43 patients without strictures and motor disorders had dysphagia. After surgical management, 10 of these patients had no further symptoms.

Dysphagia is not an exclusive symptom of peptic strictures; other causes, both benign and malignant, must be considered. The epidemic of adenocarcinoma in middle-aged men with columnar-lined esophagus has made the onset of dysphagia in a patient with chronic reflux a worrisome presentation. In this setting, reflux and dysphagia are no longer synonymous with peptic stricture (Table 19–1).

TABLE 19–1 ■ Causes of Esophageal Strictures

CONGENITAL
Esophageal atresia
Tracheoesophageal fistula
Webs
ACQUIRED
Infections
Fungal
Moniliasis
Histoplasmosis
Viral
Herpes
Cytomegalovirus
Bacterial and mycobacterial
Syphilis
Tuberculosis
Granulomatous
Sarcoidosis
Crohn's disease
Dermatosis
Pemphigoid
Behçet's syndrome
Gastroesophageal reflux
Primary
Scleroderma
Drug-induced
Aspirin
Nonsteroidal anti-inflammatory drugs
Clinitest
Vitamin C
Quinidine
Progesterone
Theophylline
Anticholinergic medications
Tetracycline
Potassium supplements
Caustic ingestion
Iatrogenic
Sclerotherapy
Postoperative (anastomotic)
Radiation
Postinstrumentation
Malignant
Primary
Secondary

Investigative Technique

Barium esophagography confirms the clinical suspicion of an esophageal stricture and provides a hard copy documentation of the stricture (Fig. 19–1). Both the length and diameter of the stricture are measured. Strictures longer than 2 cm and tighter than 10 mm are considered severe, may be difficult to dilate, and tend to recur. Examination may be conducted with barium-soaked marshmallows or a barium pill to detect early strictures, which are difficult to recognize unless there is complete esophageal distention. Video study of solid-bolus passage also may demonstrate an unsuspected motility disorder. Double-contrast studies allow an assessment of mucosal damage. The presence of a columnar-lined esophagus may be suspected on the basis of a barium esophagram. Barrett's mucosa has been reported in 44% of patients with peptic esophageal strictures (Spechler et al, 1983). Because most peptic strictures arise at the squamocolumnar junction, the occurrence of the stricture well above the esophagogastric junction is predictive of a columnar-lined esophagus. Associated abnormalities, such as hiatal hernia, Schatzki's ring, and esophageal ulcer, may be seen.

Finally, barium upper gastrointestinal study allows an examination of the stomach and duodenum distal to the stricture. Differentiation of benign from malignant strictures with the use of barium esophagography is possible, but the study lacks both sensitivity and specificity. The accuracy of barium esophagography was reported to be 59% in the diagnosis of malignant strictures and 89% in the diagnosis of benign strictures (Eastman et al, 1978).

Most important, barium esophagography provides a guide for esophagoscopy, the crucial invasive investigation in the diagnosis of peptic esophageal strictures (Fig. 19–2). Diagnosis can be obtained at endoscopy in 90% to 95% of patients (Eastman et al, 1978; Webb et al, 1984). Cytologic brushing of the stricture must be added to random biopsy to reach this level of diagnostic accu-

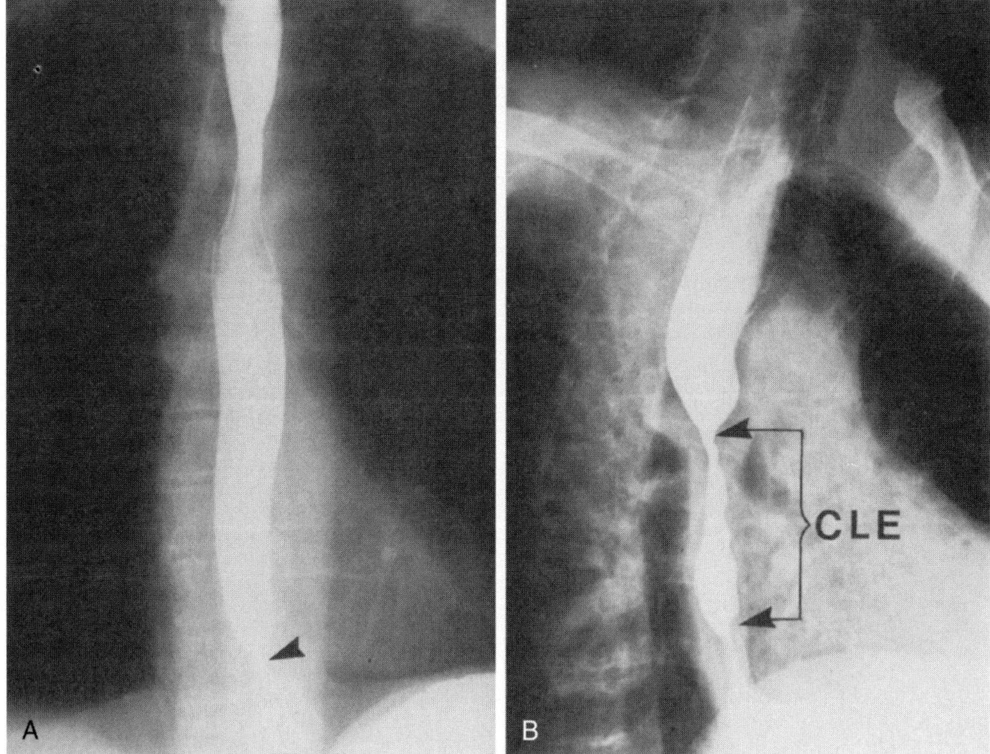

FIGURE 19–1 ■ *A,* Barium esophagram of a typical peptic stricture *(arrow)* shows a smooth, short, symmetric esophageal narrowing with no mucosal destruction, situated immediately above a hiatal hernia. *B,* Barium esophagram of a peptic stricture in a columnar-lined esophagus. The stricture occurs at the squamocolumnar junction *(upper arrow)*, well above the esophagogastric junction *(lower arrow)*, which is localized by the hiatal hernia. The intervening columnar epithelium (CLE) is free of mucosal defects.

racy. Endoscopy, biopsy, and dilation can be safely performed at one sitting (Barkin et al, 1981). After dilation, careful endoscopic examination of the stricture and the distal gastrointestinal tract is required.

On completion of the dilation procedure, manometric studies of the esophagus should be considered. A peptic esophageal stricture may be associated with motility disorders of the esophagus, most notably scleroderma, which greatly affects the management of the associated stricture.

MANAGEMENT

There is no perfect dilator or dilating procedure for the management of peptic esophageal strictures. Successful dilation requires versatility in technique and instrumentation. A common means of dilation had been the passage of dilators via a rigid esophagoscope with the patient under general anesthesia. The routine use of this technique has become obsolete, and it is reserved for special situations such as an uncooperative patient, high cervical esophageal strictures, or dilations that have been unsuccessful with the patient under local anesthesia and sedation. The avoidance of general anesthesia and unguided dilation has reduced the morbidity and mortality rates associated with esophageal dilation.

Most dilations may be conducted with an awake patient in the outpatient setting. Preparation is crucial for a good outcome. The patient is instructed to ingest only clear fluids the day before the procedure and nothing after midnight. Dilations that are performed early in the day allow adequate observation time. In addition, if complications arise, further investigations and management may be optimally performed. To ensure full cooperation, the patient should receive complete instructions before the procedure. Fluoroscopy should be available but is not crucial for every dilation.

Medication with a narcotic analgesic and a minor tranquilizer (50 to 75 mg of meperidine and 2 to 4 mg of midazolam intravenously) provides sufficient sedation, making the patient comfortable and cooperative but not stuporous and combative. Topical anesthesia (4% viscous xylocaine gargle or 1% topical spray) is optional. If performed at the time of endoscopy, dilation can be conducted with the patient in the left lateral decubitus position. Otherwise, the patient may be sitting or in either lateral decubitus position.

To minimize complications, a guided system should be used during the first session of dilation. The patient should recover in a monitored setting. Once the sedation has been adequately reversed, the patient should be questioned concerning odynophagia, dysphagia, and chest pain. If any of these are present or if they occur within the next 24 to 48 hours, the physician who performed the dilation should be contacted immediately.

Finally, the patient is given an appointment for follow-

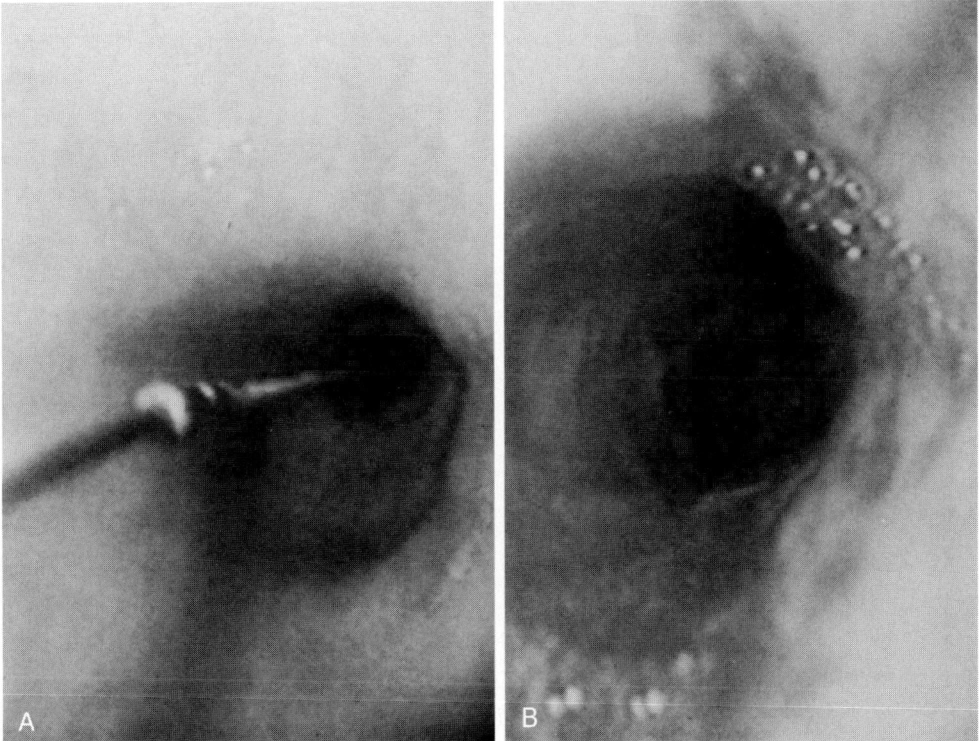

FIGURE 19–2 ■ *A,* Endoscopic appearance of a peptic stricture. The stricture occurs at the squamocolumnar junction. There is associated esophagitis but no other mucosal abnormalities. The stricture is symmetric and smooth. After brushing and biopsy, the guidewire of the Savary-Gillard system is passed, under visual control, through the stricture to facilitate the first guided dilation of this peptic stricture. *B,* The stricture after dilation.

up and, possibly, a subsequent dilation, usually within 4 to 6 weeks. If the dilation was difficult or if a satisfactory bougie size was not reached, a follow-up visit and possible repeated dilation may be required much sooner, sometimes within 7 to 14 days.

The goal of dilation is to sufficiently increase the diameter of the esophageal lumen to eliminate dysphagia. In difficult cases, the dilation achieved should be confirmed with radiographic passage of a barium pill. For most dilators, the circumference, not the diameter, of the dilator is gauged in French units. One French unit is equal to 1 mm of circumference (the circumference of a 40 French dilator is 40 mm). Diameter of the dilator is approximately one-third the French size. Most patients with peptic esophageal strictures are relieved of their symptoms by dilation to 40 French or higher. To minimize perforation and other complications, some suggest the passage of no more than three dilators (sequentially sized) after resistance is felt. The symmetric, circumferential, and panmural nature of the peptic injury and the associated periesophageal inflammation make this guideline not as important as in malignant strictures.

Most guided bougies have a tip of constant initial diameter, the same for a range of dilators, and expand gradually to the maximal dilator size. In the dilation of peptic strictures, it is acceptable to select a dilator in the range of 40 to 50 French and to start the dilation by first carefully engaging the tip of the bougie in the stricture. Slow passage of the bougie with constant pressure allows the stricture to be gently and gradually dilated until resistance is felt and dilation is stopped. This technique avoids multiple passes of progressively larger dilators and, if performed carefully, is not associated with increased complications.

The choice of dilator is dependent on characteristics of the stricture, operator preference, availability, and the patient's dilation history. A facility with a variety of dilators allows for optimal management of peptic strictures.

Nonguided Dilators

Gum Elastic Dilators

Gum elastic bougies are designed to be passed under direct vision through a rigid esophagoscope. The maximum size of the dilator is therefore limited by the internal diameter of the scope. The gum elastic tip of a Jackson bougie (Fig. 19–3) is mounted on a firm slender wire shaft that does not obstruct the operator's vision when passed down the dilating esophagoscope. The tip is constructed by coating molded woven silk with vegetable oil.

Although rigid, these dilators are plastic, and their flexibility can be increased by warming the dilating tips; heating to the point of sterilization melts them. These dilators are used infrequently because of the limited availability of both the dilators and special dilating esophagoscopes (which allow the passage of larger dilators) and the problems of unguided dilatation in an anesthetized patient.

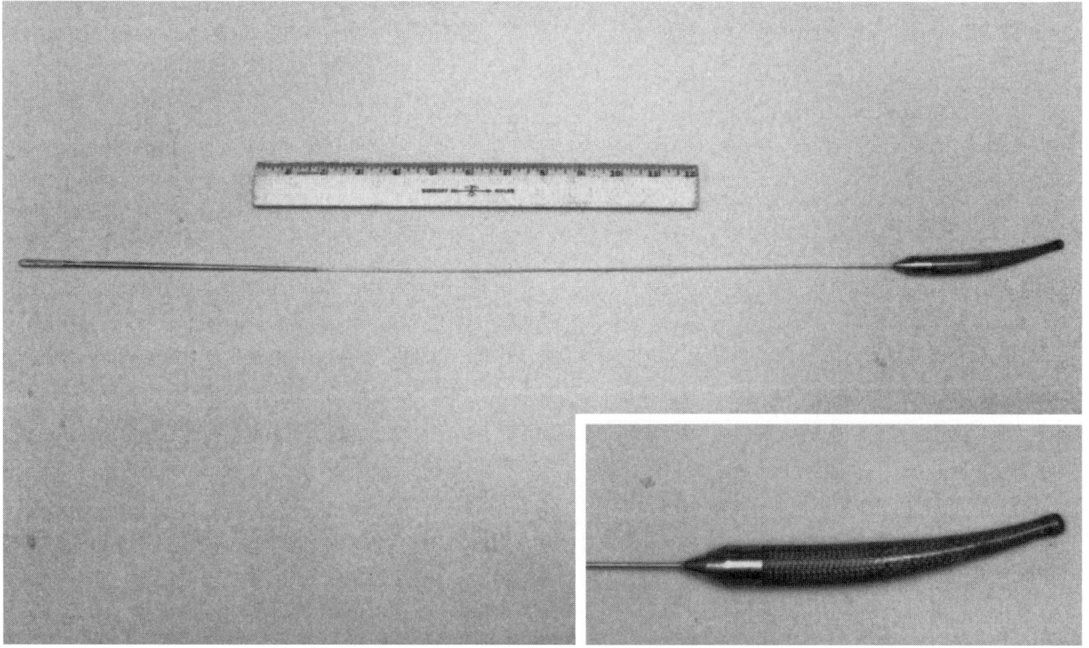

FIGURE 19–3 ■ Jackson bougie. *Inset,* Gum elastic tip of this bougie.

Mercury-Weighted Dilators

Mercury-weighted bougies are constructed of rubber and are filled with mercury. This combination provides stiffness and flexibility. The weight of the mercury does not generally aid in the passage of the dilator. Blunt-tipped Hurst dilators have been replaced by tapered Maloney dilators (Fig. 19–4). These dilators are available in 2-French increments from 12 to 60 French. Coiling due to their extreme flexibility is a major problem with smaller dilators, but for bougies of more than 40 French, coiling is not a significant problem. Although not useful in tight, long, tortuous, or eccentric strictures, these bougies are excellent for repeat dilations after the initial guided session and for chronic self-bougienage (Grobe et al, 1984; Kim et al, 1990). Mercury-weighted bougies are cost-effective and least demanding of hospital resources.

Guided Dilators

Eder-Puestow Dilator

The Eder-Puestow dilator is a flexible guided system that uses metal olives of progressively larger diameters (Fig. 19–5). After each passage, the tip must be disassembled and the next olive fixed in place. The dilator is extremely useful in tight, tortuous strictures where its "positive" feel is cited as a major benefit. However, the necessary manipulation of the tip with each passage (there are 12 different olive sizes), the excessive damage of guidewires, and an increased incidence of oral and pharyngeal trauma are major disadvantages (Hine et al, 1984).

The Key Med dilator was a variation of this system. It had two plastic oblong dilators that replaced the metal olives. These systems are not used today and are mentioned only for historical interest.

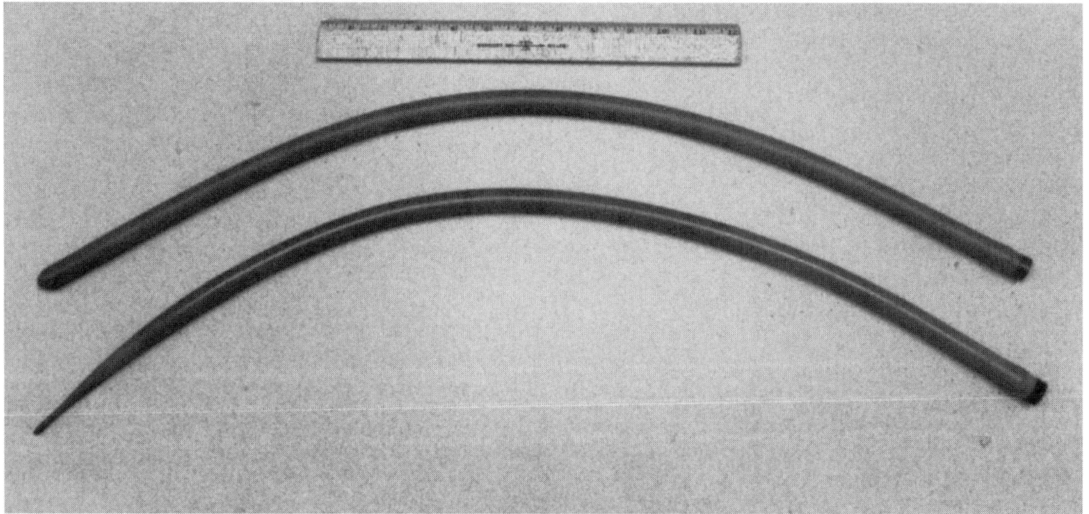

FIGURE 19–4 ■ Mercury-weighted bougies. *Top,* A 48 French Hurst bougie. *Bottom,* A 48 French Maloney bougie.

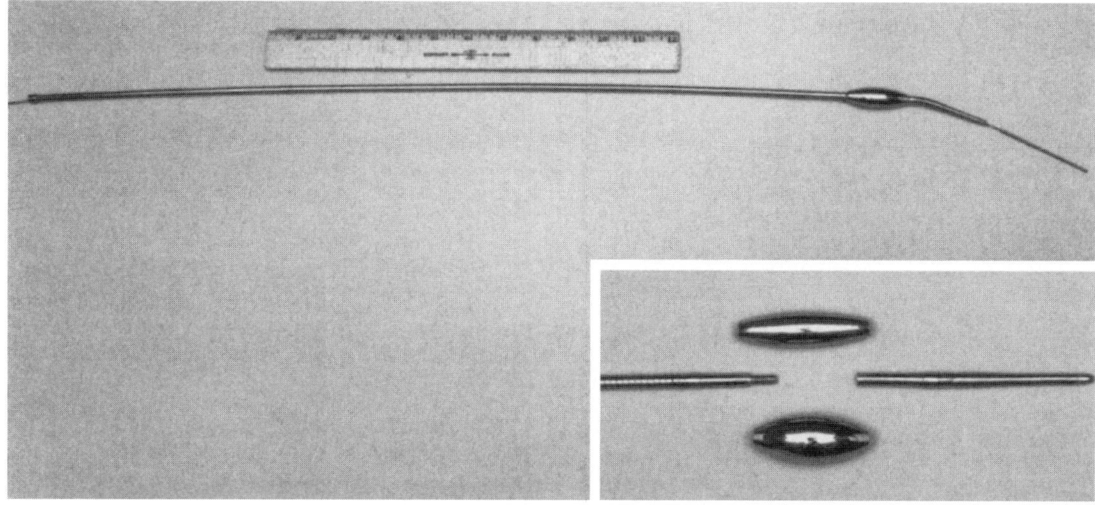

FIGURE 19–5 ■ The Eder-Puestow dilator. *Inset,* The repeated assembly of the three-piece distal tip allows the passage of progressively larger metal olives.

Savary-Gilliard Dilator

The Savary-Gilliard dilator is a bougie of polyvinyl chloride with a central channel for passage over a guidewire (Fig. 19–6). The spring tip of the guidewire is constructed of wound wire with progressively wider winding as the distal tip is approached. The graduated flexibility of this device prevents acute angulation at the junction of the rigid guide and the flexible tip. This acute angulation was a problem of the Eder-Puestow and other guidewires and was responsible for some of the guidewire perforations of the esophagus (Sanderson and Trotter, 1980).

The Savary guidewire is extremely long, which is a prerequisite for passage through the suction channel of a flexible esophagoscope. The dilators are gauged by diameter measured in millimeters and range from 5 to 20 mm. These guided dilators can be used for tight, tortuous strictures, and their plastic construction avoids oropharyngeal injury. Multiple passes of progressively larger dilators may be required.

The Celestin system is a similar plastic guided dilator that was designed to dilate strictures with no more than two passes of bougies. It uses two stepped dilators that increase in diameter by 2-mm increments along the length of the dilator. The first dilator covers the range of 4 to 12 mm; the second, 4 to 18 mm.

The Buess dilator is a similar stepped system, designed to pass over a flexible 9-mm esophagoscope.

Balloon Dilators

Balloon dilators are guided and may be placed either endoscopically or over a guidewire (Fig. 19–7). The posi-

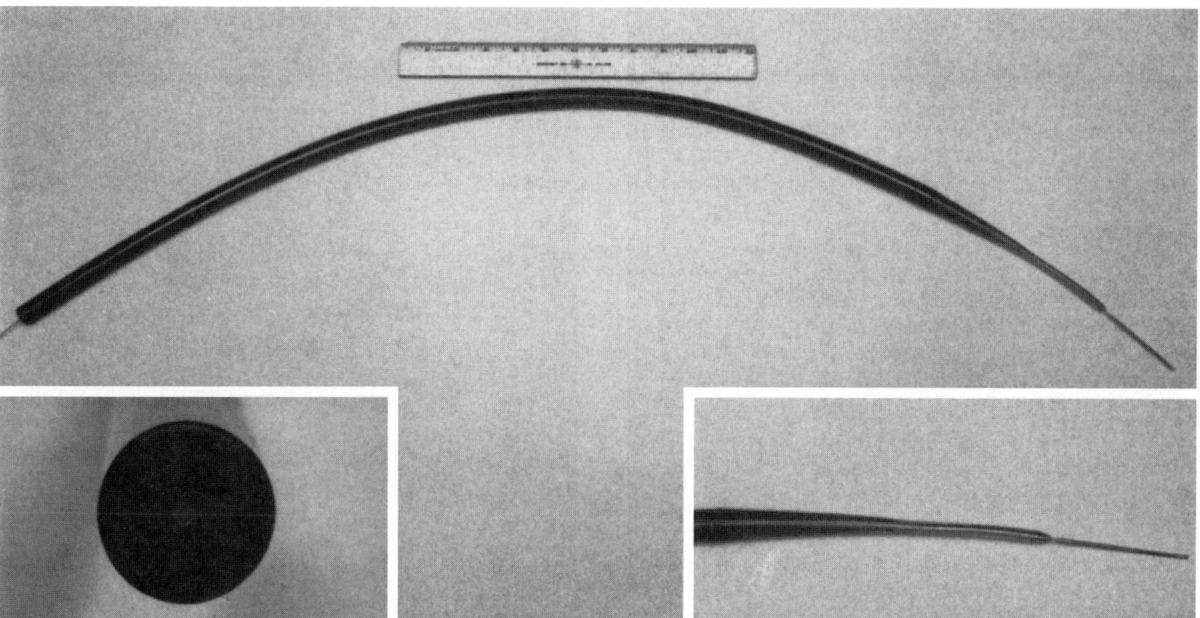

FIGURE 19–6 ■ Savary-Gilliard dilator. *Left inset,* The nontapered end of the dilator with the central channel for passage over the guidewire. *Right inset,* The dilator is passed over the flexible guidewire.

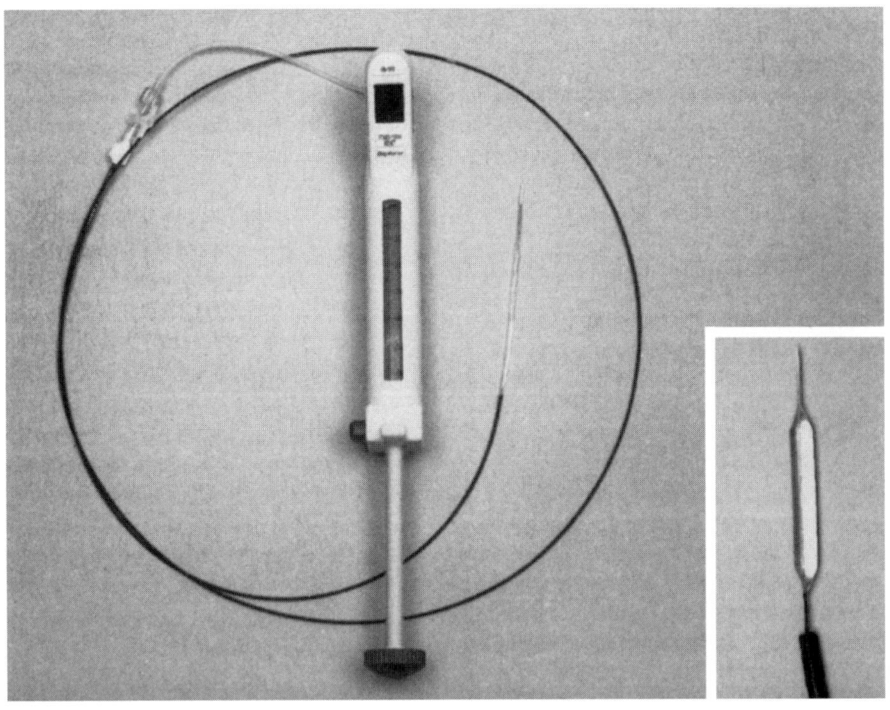

FIGURE 19–7 ■ The balloon dilator. *Inset,* The balloon dilator is passed through the suction channel of the flexible endoscope.

tion of the balloon must be confirmed endoscopically or fluoroscopically before or during dilation. These dilators are well tolerated by patients and are useful for narrow strictures. The dilators tend to migrate out of short strictures. In severe cases, the radial force exerted by the balloon is insufficient to dilate the stricture. This results in only an hourglass deformity of the balloon and failure to dilate the stricture. Compared with other dilators, the fragility of the balloon dilator is a major disadvantage of this system.

Complications

Esophageal perforation is the most feared complication of esophageal dilation. Despite meticulous technique and correct use of the appropriate dilators, perforation is a potential complication. Unguided dilation of a complex stricture is the procedure most likely to be complicated by perforation (Hernandez et al, 2000).

Perforation is not limited to the difficult dilation and may occur during the routine dilation of a simple peptic stricture with a guided dilator, but this occurrence is uncommon. Perforation may occur when strictures secondary to disease processes that do not cause panmural and circumferential involvement are mistaken for peptic strictures. This situation is seen in (1) undiagnosed malignancies; (2) nasogastric tube strictures, in which inflammation is limited to superficial esophageal layers (mucosa and submucosa) with minimal muscular or periesophageal inflammation; and (3) caustic strictures, which have minimal acute inflammation and dense fibrosis and scarring that replace the esophageal wall. The misdiagnosis of a peptic stricture in any of these three situations may result in unexpected esophageal perforations during dilatation.

Prompt recognition and treatment of perforation minimize further complications and death. Perforation should be suspected in a patient who complains of excessive and prolonged pain after dilation. Subcutaneous emphysema and a pneumothorax may be detected on physical examination. A chest radiograph obtained on an urgent basis demonstrates a hydropneumothorax and possibly mediastinal and subcutaneous emphysema. Early surgical intervention is required with lavage and débridement of the mediastinum and pleural cavity, repair of the perforation, and surgical management of the stricture and its underlying cause. Rarely, there may be a contained leak (intramural dissection) with free, preferential drainage into the esophagus, which may be managed nonsurgically.

Other, less frequent complications of dilation include bacteremia, cerebral abscess, septic arthritis, bacterial endocarditis, bleeding, and equipment failure (Tulman and Boyce, 1981). From 15% to 20% of dilations of benign strictures are complicated by bacteremia (Nelson et al, 1998; Zuccaro et al, 1998). Oral organisms, most commonly *Streptococcus viridans,* are the frequent pathogens, and antibiotic prophylaxis must be provided to patients at risk of endocarditis and those with implanted devices.

CONCLUSION

The quest for the perfect dilator continues. No such instrument exists, and the most appropriate dilator available at the time must be used. The patient, the stricture, the operator's experience, the dilating technique, and the facility are more important in determining outcome than the dilating system. The theoretical advantage of a radial force with no longitudinal component that is offered by balloon dilatation has not reduced complications and may be responsible for potentially inferior results (Cox et al, 1988; Shemesh and Czerniak, 1990). However, randomized prospective studies found rigid bougies and balloon dilators to be equally effective in the treatment of benign esophageal strictures (Saeed et al, 1995; Scolapio et al, 1999).

The use of meticulous dilating technique minimizes complications and improves long-term results. Guided dilatation should be used whenever possible. Fluoroscopy may be helpful in difficult dilations (Bailey and Goldner, 1990); it is a cumbersome and time-consuming procedure, however, and is not necessary for every dilation (Pereira-Lima et al, 1999). Endoscopy is a prerequisite in the diagnosis of peptic esophageal stricture. The combination of endoscopy, biopsy, brushing, and dilation is safe (Barkin et al, 1981). Endoscopic guidance of the initial dilation is the standard of care. Unguided dilation at subsequent dilation is a safe and practical practice.

Long-term management of these patients is crucial. Rarely, a patient requires only one dilation and no treatment of gastroesophageal reflux. Most patients require aggressive management of the stricture and reflux. Initial medical management is indicated in all patients and allows assessment of the severity of reflux and the tempo of stricturing. Proton-pump inhibitors are superior to histamine H_2-blockers in the prevention of restricturing (Barbezat et al, 1999; Silvis et al, 1996; Stal et al, 1998; Swarbrick et al, 1996). Failure of adequate medical management, complications of the disease or treatment, or the development of precancerous or cancerous changes warrants surgery.

COMMENTS AND CONTROVERSIES

Dr. Rice provides a thorough review of the history and status of methods of dilation for peptic esophageal strictures. I would like to add some observations from my experience and understanding of stricture management.

The author correctly notes that peptic strictures are less easily perforated than are some others, such as mature caustic strictures, in which there is no wall thickening due to active inflammation—only thin, avascular scar. Then, such scar is disrupted by the dilation; it requires little more to breach the full thickness of the esophageal wall, with free perforation into the mediastinum or pleural space. Some postnasogastric tube strictures are similar to those caused by caustic injury: after extubation and recovery, there may be no ongoing reflux esophagitis, and the ring of acute peptic injury heals and becomes a pale, avascular scar, without surrounding inflammation. These thin-walled strictures can usually be anticipated on the basis of their appearance at endoscopy: the overlying mucosa is intact, uninflamed, and pale. Such strictures may split and perforate from the single passage of a mercury-weighted Maloney bougie in the diameter range of 46 to 50 (or greater) French.

Chronic but active peptic strictures, with ongoing reflux, can be safely dilated with Maloney boogies in the range of 46 to 50 French, when the bougienage is performed with mild sedation and topical anesthesia and the patient is positioned with his or her trunk in a semiupright position. The esophageal wall in these cases is significantly thickened, and even when there is no mucosa, due to active peptic ulceration, the underlying scar does not split through the full thickness of the wall. It is essential, however, to ascertain that one is dealing with an active peptic stricture with preliminary endoscopy before proceeding with this type of indirect dilation. When these principles have been followed, I have not seen a perforation occur due to indirect Maloney bougienage in patients with active peptic stenosis.

With new cases after endoscopic evaluation, the surgeon may initiate the dilation with the larger Maloney dilators. If the 46 to 50 French bougie does not advance fully through the stricture, with the use of gentle forward pressure added to the weight of the bougie when the patient is upright, the surgeon may revert to the use of a smaller-diameter bougie. If the smaller-diameter bougies fail to pass (they are less effective because of reduced weight and undue flexibility), Savary dilators may be used, passed over an endoscopically positioned guidewire. If the stricture cannot be dilated with the Savary method, it may be necessary to undertake direct bougienage with a rigid esophagoscope and the patient under general anesthesia. This is rarely necessary but does occur with very tight, long fibrous strictures. Small-diameter (12 to 14 French) gum elastic esophageal dilators may be necessary to initiate the dilation in such cases.

As Dr. Rice notes, it is difficult to judge the interval required before bringing the patient back for a repeated dilation. I usually advise the patient to call and schedule a repeated dilation with a significant return or worsening of dysphagia. If reflux can be adequately controlled by medical or surgical therapy, the interval between dilations becomes progressively longer in almost all cases.

F. G. P.

KEY REFERENCES

Barkin JS, Taub S, Rogers AI: The safety of combined endoscopy, biopsy and dilation in esophageal strictures. Am J Gastroenterol 76:23, 1981.

This article documents the safety of combined endoscopy, biopsy, and dilation, now a standard of practice in the management of peptic esophageal strictures.

Earlam R, Cunha-Melo JR: Benign oesophageal strictures: Historical and technical aspects of dilatation. Br J Surg 68:829, 1981.

The authors provide an overview of the history and techniques of dilation.

Glick ME: Clinical course of esophageal stricture managed by bougienage. Dig Dis Sci 27:884, 1982.

An excellent retrospective study of dilation for the management of peptic esophageal strictures.

Hands LJ, Papavramidis S, Bishop H, et al: The natural history of peptic oesophageal strictures treated by dilatation and antireflux therapy alone. Ann R Coll Surg Engl 71:306, 1989.

The natural history of dilation and of the medical treatment of peptic esophageal stricture is presented in an excellent study.

REFERENCES

Agnew SR, Pandya SP, Reynolds RP, et al: Predictors of frequent esophageal dilations of benign peptic strictures. Dig Dis Sci 41:931, 1996.

Ahtaridis G, Snape WJ Jr, Cohen S: Clinical and manometric findings in benign peptic strictures. Dig Dis Sci 24:858, 1979.

Azpiroz F: Gastroesophageal reflux: The role of delayed gastric emptying and duodenogastric reflux. In DeMeester TR, Matthews HR (eds): International Trends in General Thoracic Surgery: Benign Esophageal Disease. St. Louis, CV Mosby, 1987, p 16.

Bailey AD, Goldner F: Can clinicians accurately assess esophageal dilation without fluoroscopy? Gastrointest Endosc 36:373, 1990.

Barbezat GO, Schlup M, Lubcke R: Omeprazole therapy decreases the need for dilatation of peptic oesophageal strictures. Aliment Pharmacol Ther 13:1041, 1999.

Barkin JS, Taub S, Rogers AI: The safety of combined endoscopy, biopsy and dilation in esophageal strictures. Am J Gastroenterol 76:23, 1981.

Bennett JR, Sutton DR, Price JF, Dyet JF: Effects of bougie dilatation on esophageal stricture size. In DeMeester TR, Skinner DB (eds): Esophageal Disorders: Pathophysiology and Therapy. New York, Raven Press, 1985, p 221.

Berstad A, Weberg R, Froyshov I, et al: Relationship of hiatus hernia to reflux esophagitis: A prospective study of incidence using endoscopy. Scand J Gastroenterol 21:55, 1986.

Bombeck CT, Battle WS, Nyhus LM: Spasm in the differential diagnosis of gastroesophageal reflux. Arch Surg 104:477, 1972.

Bonavina L, Norberto L, Cusumano A et al: Reflux-induced esophageal strictures: Factors influencing long-term results of dilatation. In Little AG, Ferguson MK, Skinner DB (eds): Diseases of the Esophagus. Mount Kisco, NY, Futura, 1990, p 247.

Burt CA: Pneumatic rupture of the intestinal canal with experimental data showing mechanism of perforation and the pressure required. Arch Surg 22:875, 1931.

Celestin LR, Campbell WB: A new and safe system for oesophageal dilatation. Lancet 1:74, 1981.

Cox JGC, Winter RK, Maslin SC et al: Balloon or bougie for dilatation of benign oesophageal stricture? An interim report of a randomized controlled trial. Gut 29:1741, 1988.

Dawson B: Roentgen rays as an aid to the diagnosis of stricture of the oesophagus. Lancet 2:1144, 1907.

DeMeester TR, Johnson LF, Joseph GJ, et al: Patterns of gastroesophageal reflux in health and disease. Ann Surg 184:459, 1976.

Earlam R, Cunha-Melo JR: Benign oesophageal strictures: Historical and technical aspects of dilatation. Br J Surg 68:829, 1981.

Eastman MC, Gear MWL, Nicol A: An assessment of the accuracy of modern endoscopic diagnosis of oesophageal stricture. Br J Surg 65:182, 1978.

Farup PG, Modalsli B, Tholfsen J: The natural restricturing process after dilation of peptic esophageal strictures. Dis Esophagus 11:116, 1998.

Fletcher R: On strictures of the esophagus and the danger of the bougie herein. In Medico-Chirurgical Notes and Illustrations: Part I. London, Longman, 1831.

Glick ME: Clinical course of esophageal stricture managed by bougienage. Dig Dis Sci 27:884, 1982.

Gotley DC, Appleton GV, Cooper MJ: Bile acids and trypsin are unimportant in alkaline esophageal reflux. J Clin Gastroenterol 14:2, 1992.

Goyal RK, Biancani P, Phillips A et al: Mechanical properties of the esophageal wall. J Clin Invest 50:1456, 1971.

Grobe JL, Kozarek RA, Sanowski RA: Self-bougienage in the treatment of benign esophageal stricture. J Clin Gastroenterol 6:109, 1984.

Hands LJ, Papavramidis S, Bishop H, et al: The natural history of peptic oesophageal strictures treated by dilatation and antireflux therapy alone. Ann R Coll Surg Engl 71:306, 1989.

Hernandez LJ, Jacobson JW, Harris MS: Comparison among the perforation rates of Maloney, balloon and Savary dilation of esophageal strictures. Gastrointest Endosc 51:460, 2000.

Hiatt GA: The roles of esophagoscopy vs radiography in diagnosing benign peptic esophageal strictures. Gastrointest Endosc 23:194, 1977.

Hildreth CT: Stricture of the esophagus. N Engl J Med Surg 10:235, 1821.

Hine KR, Hawkey CJ, Atkinson M, Holmes GKT: Comparison of the Eder-Pnestow and Celestin techniques for dilating benign oesophageal strictures. Gut 25:1100, 1984.

Jaffray B, Anderson JR: A patient's perspective on the management of peptic esophageal stricture: Experience and results in 113 consecutive cases. Dis Esophagus 11:109, 1998.

Kim CH, Groskreutz JL, Gehrking CGC: Recurrent benign esophageal strictures treated with self-bougienage: Report of seven cases. Mayo Clin Proc 65:799, 1990.

Kiroff GK, Maddern GJ, Jamieson GG: A study of factors responsible for the efficacy of fundoplication in the treatment of gastrooesophageal reflux. Aust N Z J Surg 54:109, 1984.

Kjellén G: Assessment of benign esophageal stricture dilated by balloon using liquid scintigraphy. Dysphagia 4:155, 1989.

Kollath J, Starck E, Vittorio P: Dilatation of esophageal stenosis by balloon catheter. Cardiovasc Interv Radiol 7:35, 1984.

Kozarck RA, Phelps JE, Partyka EK, Sanowski RA: Intraluminal pressure generated during esophageal bougienage. Gastroenterology 81:833, 1981.

Lanza FL, Graham DY: Bougienage is effective therapy for most benign esophageal strictures. JAMA 249:844, 1978.

Lilly J, McCaffery TD: Esophageal stricture dilatation: A new method adapted to the fiberoptic esophagoscope. Am J Dig Dis 16:1137, 1971.

London RL, Trotman BW, DiMarino HA, et al: Dilatation of severe esophageal strictures by an inflatable balloon catheter. Gastroenterology 80:173, 1981.

Monnier P, Hsieh V, Savary M: Endoscopic treatment ofesophageal stenosis using Savary-Gilliard bougies: Technical innovations. Acta Endosc 15:119, 1985.

Moses FM: Reversible aperistalsis as a complication of gastroesophageal reflux disease. Am J Gastroenterol 82:272,1987.

Nelson DB, Sanderson SJ, Azar MM: Bacteremia with esophageal dilation. Gastrointest Endosc 48:641, 1998.

Ogilvie AL, Ferguson R, Atkinson M: Outlook with conservative treatment of peptic oesophageal stricture. Gut 21:23, 1980.

Patterson DJ, Graham DY, Smith JL et al: Natural history of benign esophageal stricture treated by dilatation. Gastroenterology 85:346, 1983.

Penagini R, Al Dabbagh M, Misiewicz JJ, et al: Effects of dilatation on peptic esophageal strictures on gastroesophageal reflux, dysphagia, and stricture diameter. Dig Dis Sci 33:389, 1988a.

Penagini R, Yuen H, Misiewicz JJ, Bianchi PA: Alkaline intra-oesophageal pH and gastro-oesophageal reflux in patients with peptic oesophagitis. Scand J Gastroenterol 23:675, 1988b.

Pereira-Lima JC, Ramires RP, Zamin I Jr, et al: Endoscopic dilation of benign esophageal strictures: Report on 1043 procedures. Am J Gastroenterol 94:1497, 1999.

Plummer HS: The value of silk thread as a guide in esophageal technique. Surg Gynecol Obstet 10:519, 1910.

Richter JE: Peptic strictures of the esophagus. Gastroenterol Clin North Am 28:875,1999.

Saeed ZA, Winchester CB, Ferro PS, et al: Prospective randomized comparison of polyvinyl bougies and through-the-scope balloons for dilation of peptic strictures of the esophagus. Gastrointest Endosc 41:189, 1995.

Saeed ZA, Ramierz FC, Hepps KS, et al: An objective end point for dilation improves outcome of peptic esophageal strictures: A prospective randomized trial. Gastrointest Endosc 45:354, 1997.

Sanderson CJ, Trotter GA: Eder-Puestow oesophageal dilatation: A new hazard. Br J Surg 67:300, 1980.

Scolapio JS, Pasha TM, Gostout CJ, et al: A randomized prospective study comparing rigid to balloon dilators for benign esophageal strictures and rings. Gastrointest Endosc 50:13, 1999.

Shemesh ES, Czerniak A: Comparison between Savary-Gilliard and balloon dilatation of benign esophageal strictures. World J Surg 14:518, 1990.

Silvis SE, Farahmand M, Johnson JA, et al: A randomized blinded comparison of omeprazole and ranitidine in the treatment of chronic esophageal stricture secondary to acid peptic esophagitis. Gastrointest Endosc 43:216, 1996.

Spechler SJ, Sperber H, Doos S, et al: The prevalence of Barrett's esophagus in patients with chronic peptic esophageal strictures. Dig Dis Sci 28:769, 1983.

Stal JM, Gregor JC, Preiksaitis HG, et al: A cost-utility analysis comparing omeprazole with ranitidine in the maintenance therapy of peptic esophageal stricture. Can J Gastroenterol 12:43, 1998.

Swarbrick ET, Gough AL, Foster CS, et al: Prevention of recurrence of oesophageal stricture, a comparison of lansoprazole and high-dose ranitidine. Eur J Gastroenterol Hepatol 8:431, 1996.

Tucker G: Cicatricial stenosis of the esophagus, with particular reference to treatment by continuous string, retrograde bouginage with the author's bougie. Ann Otol Rhinol Laryngol 33:1180, 1924.

Tulman AB, Boyce HW Jr: Complications of esophageal dilation and guidelines for their prevention. Gastrointest Endosc 27:229, 1981.
Watson A: Reflux stricture of the esophagus. Br J Surg 74:443, 1987.
Webb WA, McDaniel L, Jones L: The use of endoscopy in assessment and treatment of peptic strictures of the esophagus. Am Surg 50:476, 1984.
Vaezi M, Singh S, Richter JE: Role of acid and duodenogastric reflux in esophageal mucosal injury: A review of animal and human studies. Gastroenterology 108:1897, 1995.
Van Trappen G, Hellemans J: Treatment of achalasia and related motor disorders. Gastroenterology 79:144, 1980.
Vinson PP: Management of benign stricture of the esophagus. JAMA 113:2128, 1939.
Woolsey G: The treatment of cicatricial stricture of the oesophagus by retrograde dilatation. Ann Surg 21:253, 1895.
Zuccaro G Jr, Richter JE, Rice TW, et al: Viridans streptococcal bacteremia after esophageal stricture dilation. Gastrointest Endosc 48:641, 1998.

CHAPTER **20**

Open Nissen Fundoplication

OPEN NISSEN FUNDOPLICATION REPAIR

F. Henry Ellis, Jr.

The Nissen fundoplication is the most commonly used operation for the relief of gastroesophageal reflux disease (GERD), particularly by surgeons in North America. Dissatisfaction with long-term results of previous anatomically designed operations led to the realization by surgeons that GERD was the result of a physiologic abnormality secondary to hypotension of the lower esophageal sphincter (LES) and not the result of an anatomic abnormality, such as a sliding esophageal hiatus hernia. Thus, it became clear that the prerequisite of a successful antireflux procedure was to restore normal function rather than to simply restore normal anatomy.

In a review of the origins of the Nissen fundoplication and other antireflux procedures, however, it is interesting to note that, with few exceptions, the surgeons responsible for the development of these procedures based their techniques more on anatomic than on physiologic grounds. Belsey's operation, for example, was designed to reestablish an intra-abdominal esophagus, whereas the Hill posterior gastropexy took advantage of what Hill thought were the strongest structures available—namely, the phrenoesophageal ligament along the lesser curvature of the stomach and the arcuate ligament crossing the aorta, just cephalad to the celiac axis. Only later did it become evident that these two operations, as well as the Nissen procedure, owed their effectiveness to varying degrees of esophageal encirclement by the adjacent gastric fundus.

Because there are many variations of the Nissen fundoplication, it is hoped that a preliminary discussion of its historical and experimental background provides a better understanding of the surgical procedure, the technique of which is described in this chapter.

HISTORICAL NOTE

In December 1955, Rudolph Nissen (1956) of Basel, Switzerland, operated on a 49-year-old woman with a long history of GERD without radiographic evidence of a hiatal hernia. He used a technique that he had used nearly 20 years earlier to minimize postoperative reflux after resection of a peptic ulcer in the region of the cardia. This technique involved envelopment of the lower esophagus with the gastric fundus by suture approximation of anterior and posterior fundal folds anterior to the esophagus, within which a large intraesophageal bougie had been positioned.

Since this original description, the Nissen fundoplication has been modified in many ways. Nissen (1961) combined his operation with anterior gastropexy, only to discontinue that modification. Subsequently, Nissen and Rossetti (1965) suggested that only the anterior wall of the stomach be wrapped around the lower esophagus. In none of these techniques did Nissen recommend division of the short gastric vessels. Other modifications have included narrowing of the esophageal hiatus posterior to the esophagus, anchoring of the fundoplication to the preaortic fascia, and the addition of highly selective vagotomy.

The degree of the fundal wrap has been varied to encircle less than 360 degrees of the esophageal tube to avoid the "gas bloat" syndrome, with the anterior portion of the esophagus being wrapped by Dor and associates (1962) and the posterior portion of the esophagus being wrapped by Toupet (1963) and Guarner and colleagues (1980). For a similar reason, Donahue and associates (1985) proposed the creation of a loose wrap. The wrap initially performed by Nissen extended over 4 to 6 cm of the esophagus, but a shorter wrap was recommended by DeMeester and associates (1986) to avoid some of the potential complications of the operation.

■ *HISTORICAL READINGS*

DeMeester TR, Bonavina L, Albertucci M: Nissen fundoplication for gastroesophageal reflux disease: Evaluation of primary repair in 100 consecutive patients. Ann Surg 204:9, 1986.

Donahue PE, Samuelson S, Nyhus LM, Bombeck CT: The floppy Nissen fundoplication: Effective long-term control of pathologic reflux. Arch Surg 120:663, 1985.

Dor J, Humbert P, Dor V, Figarella J: L'intérêt de la technique de Nissen modifée la prevention du reflux après cardiomyotomie extra muquesuse de Heller. Mem Acad Chir 88:877, 1962.

Guarner V, Martinez N, Gavino JF: Ten year evaluation of posterior fundoplasty in the treatment of gastroesophageal reflux: Long-term and comparative study of 135 patients. Am J Surg 139:200, 1980.

Nissen R: Eine einfache Operation zur Beeinflussung der Refluxoesophagitis. Schweiz Med Wochenschr 86:590, 1956.

Nissen R: Gastropexy and "fundoplication" in surgical treatment of hiatal hernia. Am J Dig Dis 6:954, 1961.

Nissen R, Rossetti M: Surgery of hiatal and other diaphragmatic hernias. J Int Coll Surg 43:663, 1965.

Toupet A: Technique d'oesophago-gastroplastie avec phreno-gastropexie appliquée dans la cure radicale des hernia hiatales et comme complement de l'operation de Heller dans les cardiospasmus. Mem Acad Chir 89:394, 1963.

EXPERIMENTAL BACKGROUND

That the Nissen total fundoplication is more effective in the prevention of gastroesophageal reflux (GER) than other antireflux procedures is well documented experimentally. The results of Bombeck and associates (1971), working with dogs, and of Butterfield (1971), working with cadaver specimens, support this view, as do the results of the in vitro studies of Alday and Goldsmith (1973). In a series of experiments reported by Leonardi and associates (1977a) that involve in vivo studies in cats, the Nissen procedure proved superior to the Hill and Belsey operations on the basis of postoperative manometry and pH testing. Leonardi and associates (1977b) also showed that a complete wrap was preferable to a partial wrap for the restoration of normal LES function. The superiority of the Nissen 360-degree wrap compared with partial wraps was confirmed in the comparative clinical study of DeMeester and coworkers (1974).

The precise mechanism by which these antireflux procedures prevent GER remains controversial. Siewert and associates (1973) postulated that the smooth muscle of the gastric fundus that composes the wrap acts in a manner similar to the smooth muscle of the normal LES, thus accounting for its effectiveness. The anatomic studies of Liebermann-Meffert (1975) support this concept.

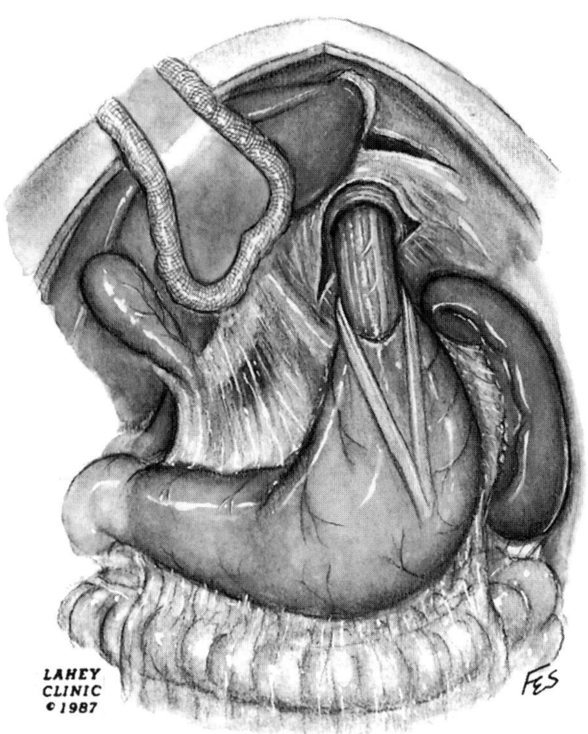

FIGURE 20–1 ■ After mobilization, the intrathoracic esophagus is partially delivered into the abdomen and encircled with a Penrose drain. (From Ellis FH Jr: Nissen fundoplication. In Braasch JW, Sedgwick CE, Veidenheimer MC, Ellis FH Jr [eds]: Atlas of Abdominal Surgery. Philadelphia, WB Saunders, 1991, p 14.)

TECHNICAL CONSIDERATIONS

Transabdominal Approach

Details of the surgical technique have been given by Ellis (1990, 1997) and are summarized here. An abdominal approach is preferred, with a thoracic incision used in patients with presumed esophageal shortening and in patients who have previously undergone a left thoracotomy. An upper midline incision is made from the xiphoid to a point just below the umbilicus, skirting to the left of that structure. The incision is continued cephalad on the left side of the xiphoid to provide optimal exposure of the esophageal hiatus.

The left lobe of the liver is mobilized by division of the triangular ligament, permitting retraction of the liver to provide exposure of esophageal hiatus. The hernia, if present, is reduced, and the phrenoesophageal membrane is incised to expose the anterior aspect of the distal esophagus and to permit its accurate mobilization. The esophagus is freed from its hiatal attachments, with care taken to preserve the vagus nerves. It then is encircled with a Penrose drain, and esophageal mobilization is continued until approximately 3 to 5 cm of distal esophagus lies free in the abdomen (Fig. 20–1).

To provide a loose wrap of gastric fundus around the distal esophagus, the surgeon must mobilize the upper stomach completely. This part of the procedure is initiated by division of the short gastric vessels and is facilitated by the placement of a moist pack behind the spleen, thus relieving tension on the short gastric vessels during their control and division. The importance of this maneuver in the prevention of a wrap that is too tight was emphasized by Hunter and associates (1996), who reported a higher incidence of postoperative dysphagia after a Nissen-Rossetti procedure in which these vessels are not divided.

The vessels are successively clamped, divided, and tied, starting distally and moving proximally along the greater curvature of stomach (Fig. 20–2*A*). One or two posterior gastric vessels—specifically, the posterior gastric artery arising from the splenic artery and a left inferior phrenic arterial branch—must also be divided to permit complete mobilization of the gastric fundus (Fig. 20–2*B*). The importance of recognizing the posterior gastric artery as a branch of the splenic artery in permitting complete mobilization of the gastric fundus has been emphasized by others (Wald and Polk, 1983). The gastrohepatic omentum is left undisturbed. Its division with subsequent traction on the stomach may cause incorrect placement of the wrap around the proximal stomach instead of around the distal esophagus.

With the right hand, the surgeon passes the freed gastric fundus behind the esophagus, where it is grasped with a Babcock clamp to the right of this organ (Fig. 20–3*A*). A large-bore indwelling (48 to 50 French) Maloney dilator is introduced transorally by the anesthesiologist and passed into the stomach. All subsequent parts of the wrapping procedure are conducted with this in place as a stent to permit the performance of a loose wrap. Heavy nonabsorbable interrupted sutures are used to approximate the seromuscular walls of adjacent gastric fundus anterior to the esophagus, with a small bite of an esophageal wall caught in one or both sutures. Two sutures of this type are placed, permitting encirclement of the distal 1 to 1.5 cm of esophagus with a loose gastric wrap (Fig. 20–3*B*).

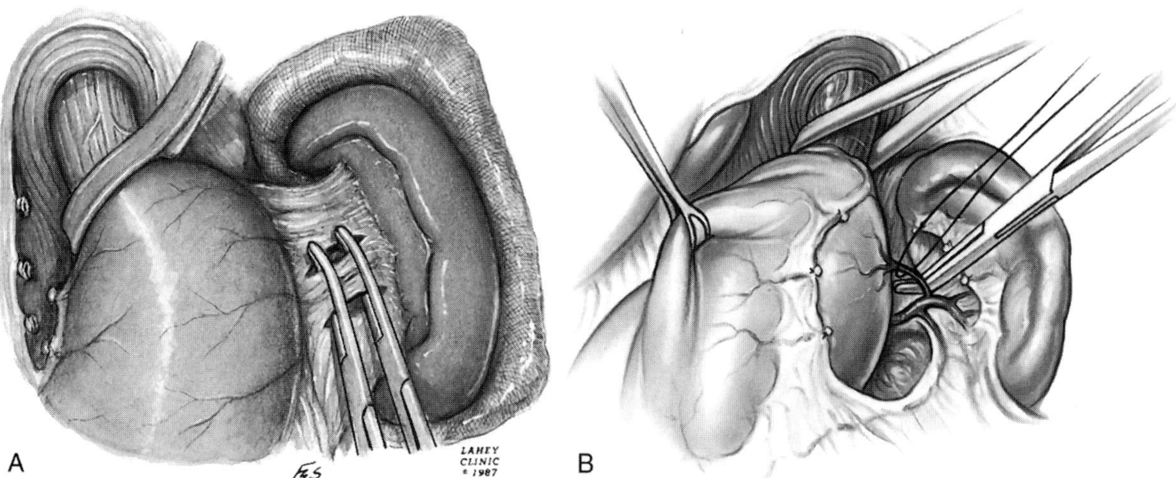

FIGURE 20–2 ■ Mobilization of the gastric fundus requires ligation and division of the short gastric vessels. *A,* The placement of a moist pack behind the spleen relieves tension on these vessels, facilitating their safe division. *B,* To complete its mobilization so as to permit performance of a loose "floppy" wrap, the posterior gastric artery arising from the splenic artery also usually requires ligation and division. (*A* from Ellis FH Jr: Nissen fundoplication. In Braasch JW, Sedgwick CE, Veidenheimer MC, Ellis FH Jr [eds]: Atlas of Abdominal Surgery. Philadelphia, WB Saunders, 1991, p 14. *B,* from Ellis FH Jr: The Nissen fundoplication. In Cox JL, Sundt TS III [eds]: Operative Techniques in Cardiac & Thoracic Surgery, Vol 2. Philadelphia, WB Saunders, 1997, p 37.)

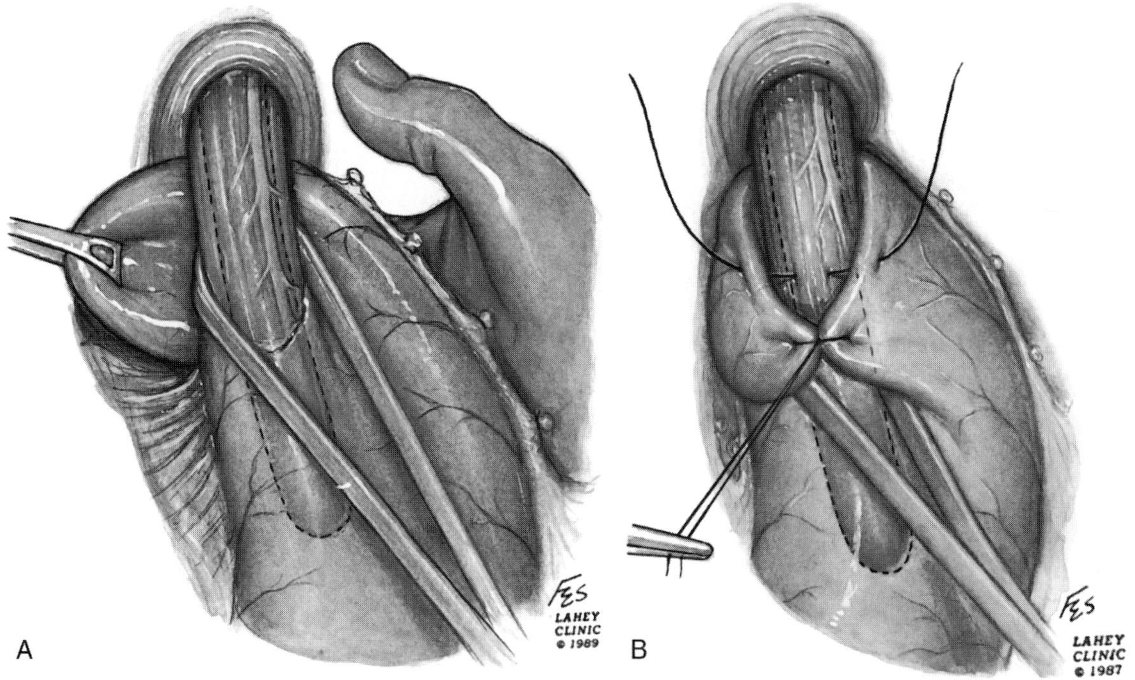

FIGURE 20–3 ■ *A,* After the short and posterior gastric vessels are divided, the mobilized gastric fundus is passed behind the esophagus and grasped with a Babcock clamp. *B,* Heavy nonabsorbable sutures are used to approximate the seromuscular walls of the adjacent fundus anterior to the esophagus, with a small bite of esophageal wall caught in the suture. (From Ellis FH Jr: Nissen fundoplication. In Braasch JW, Sedgwick CE, Veidenheimer MC, Ellis FH Jr [eds]: Atlas of Abdominal Surgery. Philadelphia, WB Saunders, 1991, pp 15–16.)

Fine nonabsorbable sutures are then placed between the heavy sutures, and the collar of the wrap is applied to the esophageal wall with similar sutures to complete the fundoplication (Fig. 20–4*A*). The esophagus is elevated to expose the esophageal hiatus, and the hiatus is narrowed by the placement of two or three loosely tied nonabsorbable interrupted heavy sutures in the diaphragmatic crura posterior to the esophagus (Fig. 20–4*B*). Because this maneuver simply prevents migration of the fundoplicated esophagus into the chest, the degree of hiatal narrowing should be slight so as not to compress the esophagus. The abdomen is then closed in the usual manner. Oral feedings are resumed with the recurrence of bowel sounds, and hospitalization rarely exceeds 4 to 5 days.

Transthoracic Approach

Although the abdominal approach is preferred when a Nissen fundoplication is performed, under certain circumstances a transthoracic approach is appropriate. I use this approach to effect safe mobilization of the distal esophagus when the patient has previously undergone a left thoracotomy. It should also be the preferred approach if there is radiographic and/or endoscopic evidence of esophageal shortening that might require an esophageal lengthening procedure such as a Collis gastroplasty to allow intra-abdominal placement of the wrap. A Nissen fundoplication should never be left within the chest because of the complications that may ensue (Richardson et al, 1982).

The surgical approach involves a left thoracotomy through the bed of the nonresected eighth rib, the angle of which may be divided for additional exposure. The mediastinal pleura is opened, and the esophagus is encircled with a Penrose drain (Fig. 20–5*A*). It is important at this point in the procedure to determine whether the length of the esophagus is sufficient to permit a fundoplication around its distal 1 to 2 cm and its placement in an intra-abdominal position. If that cannot be achieved, then an esophageal lengthening procedure, such as a Collis gastroplasty, must be performed before proceeding with the Nissen wrap. The procedure to be described assumes that there is sufficient length of esophagus to allow intra-abdominal positioning of the wrapped distal esophagus.

After mobilization of the distal esophagus, the pleura and peritoneum overlying the esophagogastric junctional area are incised to permit access to the peritoneal cavity and to the gastric fundus (Fig. 20–5*B*). Mobilization of the gastric fundus is facilitated by tension on a Babcock clamp placed at the apex of the crural sling, followed by ligation and division of several short gastric vessels (Fig. 20–6*A*). After division of the short gastric vessels, the gastric fundus is elevated to expose the posterior gastric artery, which is then ligated and divided as described for the transabdominal approach. A large (48 to 50 French) Maloney dilator is positioned across the esophagogastric junction area, and the completely mobilized and redun-

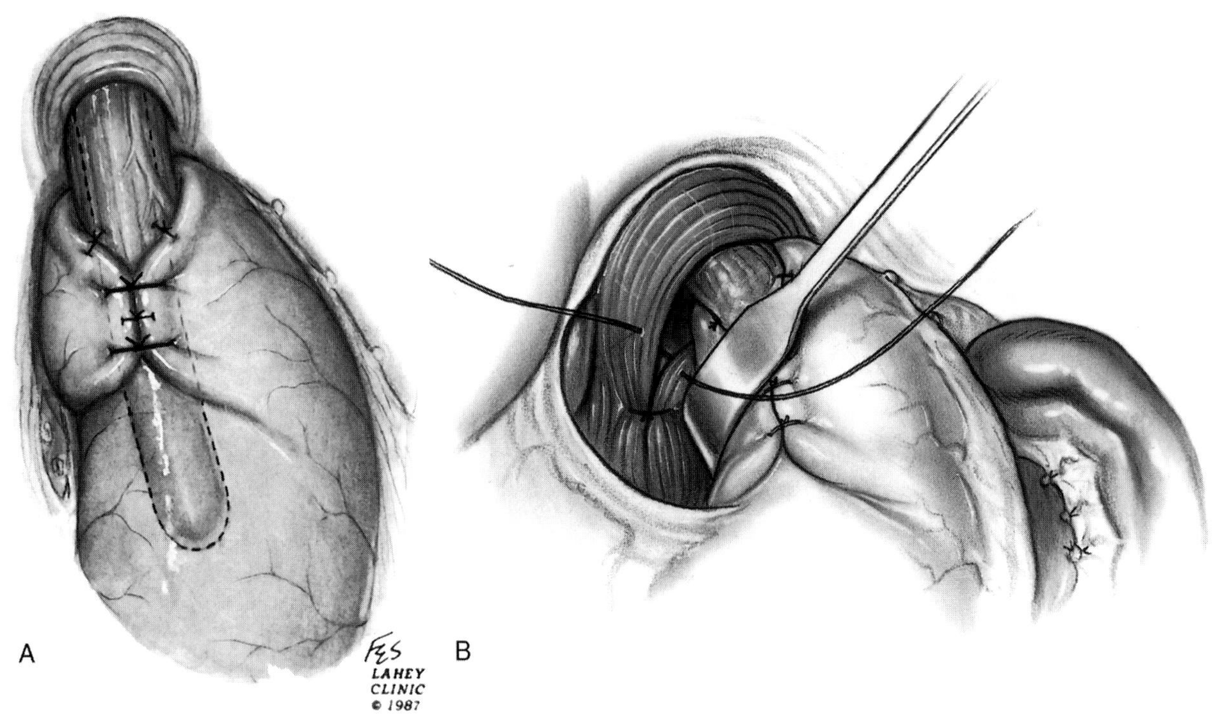

FIGURE 20–4 ■ *A,* Completed fundoplication with reinforcing sutures of nonabsorbable material that anchor the esophagus; the vagus nerves are carefully preserved. *B,* The wrapped esophagus with the indwelling probe still in place is elevated to permit approximation of the hiatal crura posteriorly with two or more nonabsorbable sutures. (*A* from Ellis FH Jr: Nissen fundoplication. In Braasch JW, Sedgwick CE, Veidenheimer MC, Ellis FH Jr [eds]: Atlas of Abdominal Surgery. Philadelphia, WB Saunders, 1991, p 16. *B* from Ellis FH Jr: The Nissen fundoplication. In Cox JL, Sundt TS III [eds]: Operative Techniques in Cardiac & Thoracic Surgery, Vol 2. Philadelphia, WB Saunders, 1997, p 37.)

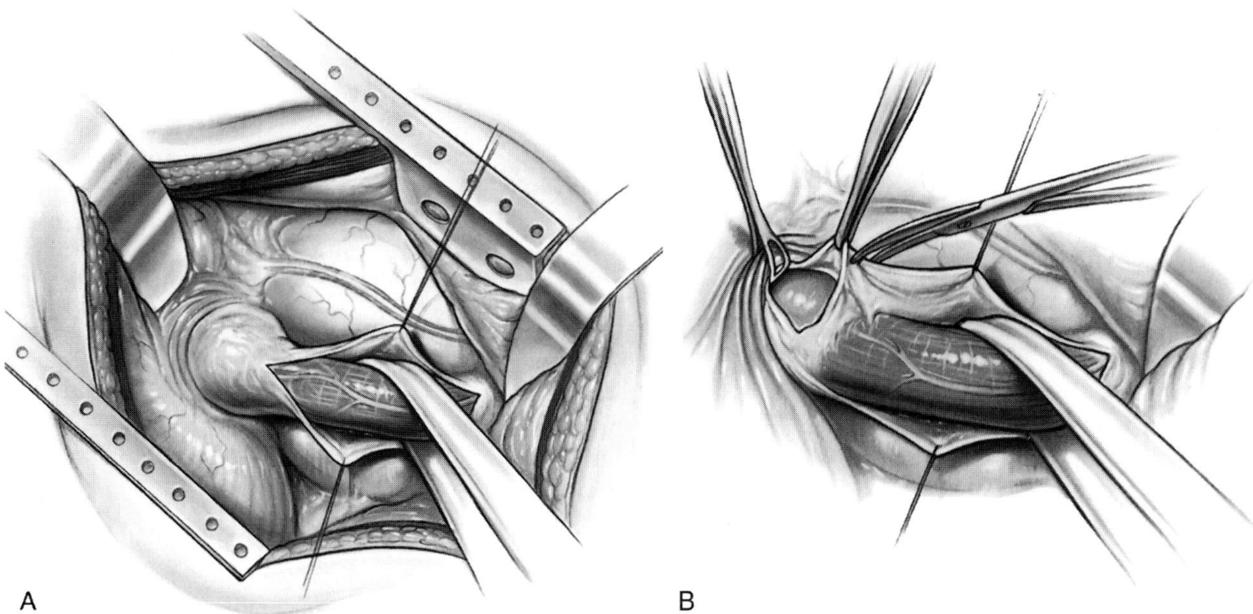

FIGURE 20–5 ■ *A,* Transthoracic exposure of esophagus and cardia. *B,* Opening of hernial sac to provide entry to the abdominal cavity. (From Ellis FH Jr: The Nissen fundoplication. In Cox JL, Sundt TS III [eds]: Operative Techniques in Cardiac & Thoracic Surgery, Vol 2. Philadelphia, WB Saunders, 1997, p 37.)

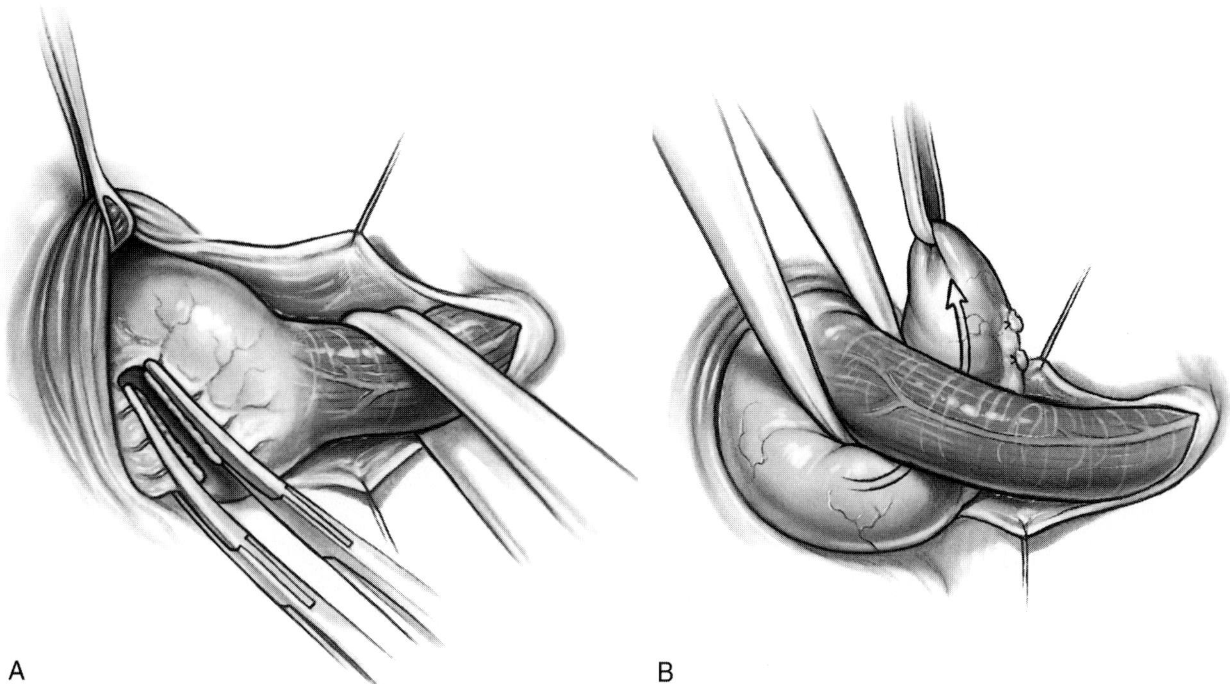

FIGURE 20–6 ■ *A,* Short gastric arteries are clamped and divided. *B,* Partial encirclement of distal 1.5 to 2 cm of the esophagus by the completely mobilized gastric fundus. (From Ellis FH Jr: The Nissen fundoplication. In Cox JL, Sundt TS III [eds]: Operative Techniques in Cardiac & Thoracic Surgery, Vol 2. Philadelphia, WB Saunders, 1997, p 37.)

dant gastric fundus is passed behind the esophagus (Fig. 20–6*B*).

The fundoplication is performed by placing nonabsorbable sutures in the adjacent seromuscular walls of the fundus that completely surround the distal 1.5 to 2 cm of the esophagus, incorporating a superficial bite of the esophageal muscular wall, with care being taken to avoid injury to the vagus nerve. Reinforcing interrupted fine silk sutures are then placed between the esophagus and the encircling gastric fundus (Fig. 20–7*A*). The wrapped distal esophagus is placed in an intra-abdominal position, and the hiatal orifice is narrowed by the placement of two or more nonabsorbable sutures in the crura, posterior to the esophagus (Fig. 20–7*B*).

DISCUSSION

To achieve good results and to avoid complications after the Nissen fundoplication, it is important that patients be properly selected. This selection requires objective confirmation of the presence of GER before the initiation of an antireflux operation. Often, in controversial cases, it is necessary to carry out esophageal manometry, and particularly 24-hour pH monitoring, to document the presence of GER. The use of esophageal manometry also provides the physician with the information necessary to avoid the pitfall of operating on a patient with a motility disorder of the esophageal body, such as achalasia. Clearly, such a mistaken diagnosis leads to postoperative dysphagia, because a total wrap in the presence of an aperistaltic esophagus may prevent the easy passage of food into the stomach after surgery.

Numerous reports have been published regarding the clinical results of open Nissen fundoplication, with hospital mortality rates approaching zero and 80% to 90% of patients experiencing good to excellent results overall. Undoubtedly, the largest reported series of Nissen fundoplications is that of Rossetti and Hell (1977). Some of these procedures were Rossetti's modification of the original Nissen operation, which differs from the one described in this chapter.

Long-term follow-up of 590 patients with uncomplicated GER disclosed that 87.5% were free of symptoms. The report of DeMeester and colleagues (1986) is a more objective evaluation of the surgical procedure as described in this chapter and involved 100 consecutive patients with GER without stricture or motility abnormalities. The operation was 91% effective in controlling symptoms of reflux during a follow-up period of up to 10 years. In my experience with 241 fundoplications, of which 157 were of the type described in this chapter, reflux symptoms were relieved permanently in more than 90% of patients (Ellis and Crozier, 1984). One fourth of the procedures were reoperations, and these patients experienced less satisfactory results than did patients after primary procedures. Even more significant is a study of a long-term randomized comparison of the results of medical therapy with patients after a Nissen fundoplication, which disclosed that surgery was significantly more effective than medical therapy in the relief of symptoms and endoscopic signs of esophagitis (Spechler, 1992).

Although these reports are generally extremely favorable, the procedure is subject to complications if patients are not properly selected and if technical details are not handled in a meticulous manner. Although it is difficult to determine the percentage of patients who require reoperations after a failed Nissen procedure, the rate has been estimated to range from 4% to 6% (Jamieson, 1993).

The major symptoms described by patients with poor results after the Nissen fundoplication are recurrent GER, dysphagia, and gas bloat syndrome. These complications can be avoided or minimized by using a floppy wrap such as that just described. In addition, a number of less frequently observed events have been reported, including

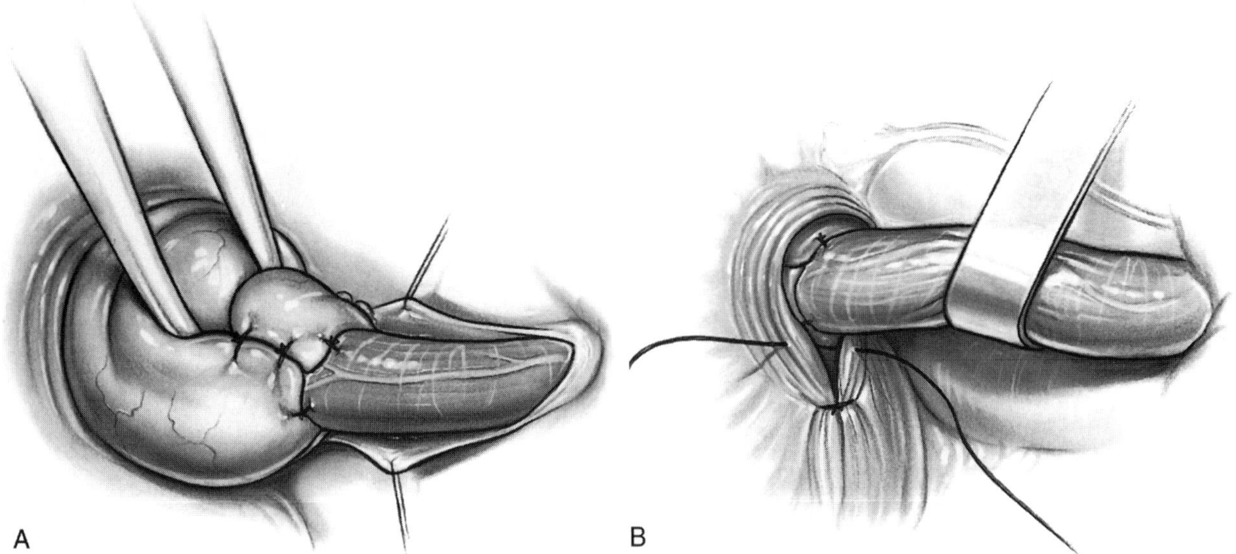

FIGURE 20–7 ■ *A,* Completed fundoplication. *B,* Wrapped distal esophagus placed intra-abdominally and hiatal crura approximated posteriorly with nonabsorbable sutures. (From Ellis FH Jr: The Nissen fundoplication. In Cox JL, Sundt TS III [eds]: Operative Techniques in Cardiac & Thoracic Surgery, Vol 2. Philadelphia, WB Saunders, 1997, p 37.)

paraesophageal hiatal hernia (Balison et al, 1973), gastric ulceration (Bremner, 1979; Herrington et al, 1982), gastric obstruction resulting from a slipped Nissen fundoplication (Olsen et al, 1977), and perforation of the wrap with fistula formation (Burnett et al, 1977).

With Gibb and Heatley (Ellis et al, 1996), I reviewed 101 reoperations performed on my service from 1970 to 1994; only 8 operations involved patients on whom I originally operated. Two thirds of the patients experienced failure for technical reasons. A wrap that was too tight was the most common technical mishap and led to postoperative dysphagia in 11 patients, recurrent reflux in 6, and the gas bloat syndrome in 4. Seventeen patients had persistent reflux due to an inadequate wrap. A paraesophageal hiatus hernia developed in 13 patients because of failure to narrow the esophageal hiatus posterior to the esophagus after performance of the wrap. A "slipped" Nissen was diagnosed in 12 patients, a complication that, in my opinion, is due to wrapping the stomach rather than the esophagus, usually occurring in a patient with a short esophagus hiatus hernia, rather than true slippage of the original wrap. Two patients experienced perforation at the time of the wrap. The remaining third of the operations failed because of an incorrect diagnosis or inappropriate application of the procedure.

Regurgitation due to a motility disorder was misinterpreted as GER in 22 patients: 16 of these patients had achalasia, 3 patients had diffuse esophageal spasm, and an additional 3 patients had scleroderma. Inappropriate use of the wrap in patients with a panmural fibrous stricture or a wrap left in the chest after surgery in patients with a shortened esophagus accounted for 10 additional complications of the Nissen fundoplication. Four antireflux procedures failed for unclassifiable reasons.

To avoid the need for a reoperation after a Nissen fundoplication, patients should be selected carefully and certain technical aspects of the operation must be observed. When these recommendations are followed, satisfactory and permanent relief of symptoms of GER can be achieved in more than 90% of patients. Postoperative symptoms of persistent or recurrent reflux, dysphagia, and gas bloat syndrome are extremely rare, and few patients should require a second operation.

COMMENTS AND CONTROVERSIES

Surgeons aspiring to duplicate Ellis' enviable results are advised to select patients carefully, to operate meticulously, and to stifle the temptation, common to residents and established surgeons alike, to improve on the basic design. Inability to belch or vomit, dysphagia, gastric ulcer, impaired gastric emptying, persistent or recurrent symptoms, and slippage of the repair are among the array of problems that may foil even the best of surgeons. The most notorious of these problems is postoperative bloating.

The Nissen repair requires following a fine line between a repair that obstructs and one that gapes. This is especially true when esophageal peristalsis is less than ideal. Concern for these factors has led surgeons to vary the caliber of the esophageal bougie, to adjust the length and tension of the wrap, to include or exclude tethering sutures into the esophageal muscle, and to experiment with leaving the vagus nerves in or out of the encirclement.

As if this were not confusing enough, the performance of "a Nissen" can mean either using the anterior or the posterior wall for the fundoplication or even looping a finger-sized diverticulum of stomach around the neoesophagus created in the "Collis-Nissen" procedure.

Less painful options are available, and it is important for those of us who still place a premium on full exposure to look carefully at the surgical prescription of surgeons like Ellis.

F. G. P.

KEY REFERENCES

DeMeester TR, Bonavina L, Albertucci M: Nissen fundoplication for gastroesophageal reflux disease: Evaluation of primary repair in 100 consecutive patients. Ann Surg 204:9, 1986.

The excellent clinical results after the Nissen procedure with a short 360-degree wrap in 100 consecutive patients are well documented in this article by DeMeester's group.

DeMeester TR, Johnson FF, Kent AH: Evaluation of current operations for the prevention of gastroesophageal reflux. Ann Surg 180:511, 1974.

In this article, the superiority of the Nissen procedure over other antireflux operations is clearly demonstrated for the first time.

Ellis FH Jr: Nissen fundoplication. In Braasch JW, Sedwick CE, Veidenheimer MC, Ellis FH Jr (eds): Atlas of Abdominal Surgery. Philadelphia, WB Saunders, 1990, p 11.

The technique of open Nissen fundoplication is fully described and clearly illustrated in this chapter.

Rossetti M, Hell K: Fundoplication for the treatment of gastroesophageal reflux in hiatal hernia. World J Surg 1:439, 1977.

This article from Basel, the site of origin of the Nissen procedure, reviews the largest reported series of patients operated on with Rossetti's modification of Nissen's original procedure using only the anterior gastric wall for the wrap.

Siewert R, Jennewein HM, Waldeck F, et al: Experimentelle und klinische Untersuchungen zum Wirkungsmechanismus der Fundoplication. Langenbecks Arch Chir 333:5, 1973.

This article contains a well-conceived and experimentally documented explanation for the mechanism of action of fundoplication.

REFERENCES

Alday ES, Goldsmith HS: Efficacy of fundoplication in preventing gastric reflux. Am J Surg 126:322, 1973.

Balison JR, Macgregor AM, Woodward ER: Postoperative diaphragmatic herniation following transthoracic fundoplication: A note of warning. Arch Surg 106:164, 1973.

Bombeck CT, Coelho RG, Castro VA, et al: An experimental comparison of procedures for the operative correction of gastroesophageal reflux. Bull Soc Int Chir 30:435, 1971.

Bremner CG: Gastric ulceration after a fundoplication operation for gastroesophageal reflux. Surg Gynecol Obstet 148:62, 1979.

Burnett HF, Read RC, Morris WD, Campbell GS: Management of complications of fundoplication and Barrett's esophagus. Surgery 82:521, 1977.

Butterfield WC: Current hiatal hernia repairs: Similarities, mechanisms, and extended indications: An autopsy study. Surgery 69:910, 1971.

DeMeester TR, Bonavina L, Albertucci M: Nissen fundoplication for gastroesophageal reflux disease: Evaluation of primary repair in 100 consecutive patients. Ann Surg 204:9, 1986.

Donahue PE, Samuelson S, Nyhus LM, Bombeck CT: The floppy Nissen fundoplication: Effective long-term control of pathologic reflux. Arch Surg 120:663, 1985.

Dor J, Humbert P, Dor V, Figarella J: L'intérêt de la technique de Nissen modifée la prevention du reflux après cardiomyotomie extra muquesuse de Heller. Mem Acad Chir 88:877, 1962.

Ellis FH Jr: The Nissen fundoplication. Oper Tech Card Thorac Surg 2:37, 1997.

Ellis FH Jr, Crozier RE: Reflux control by fundoplication: A clinical and manometric assessment of the Nissen operation. Ann Thorac Surg 38:387, 1984.

Ellis FH Jr, Gibb SP, Heatley GJ: Reoperation after failed antireflux surgery: Review of 101 cases. Eur J Cardiothorac Surg 10:225, 1996.

Guarner V, Martinez N, Gavino JF: Ten year evaluation of posterior fundoplasty in the treatment of gastroesophageal reflux: Long-term and comparative study of 135 patients. Am J Surg 139:200, 1980.

Herrington JL Jr, Meacham PW, Hunter RM: Gastric ulceration after fundic wrapping: Vagal nerve entrapment, a possible factor. Ann Surg 195:574, 1982.

Hunter JG, Swanstrom L, Waring JP: Dysphagia after laparoscopic antireflux surgery: The impact of operative technique. Ann Surg 224:51, 1996.

Jamieson GG: The results of anti-reflux surgery and reoperative anti-reflux surgery. Gullet 3:41, 1993.

Leonardi HK, Ellis FH Jr, Cormack J, Gorrilla M: Experimental fundoplication: Comparison of results of different techniques. Surgery 82:514, 1977b.

Leonardi HK, Lee ME, El-Kurd MF, Ellis FH Jr: An experimental study of the effectiveness of various antireflux operations. Ann Thorac Surg 24:215, 1977a.

Liebermann-Meffert D: Architecture of the musculature at the gastroesophageal junction and in the fundus. Chir Gastroenterol 9:425, 1975.

Nissen R: Eine einfache Operation zur Beeinflussung der Refluxoesophagitis. Schweiz Med Wochenschr 86:590, 1956.

Nissen R: Gastropexy and "fundoplication" in surgical treatment of hiatal hernia. Am J Dig Dis 6:954, 1961.

Nissen R, Rossetti M: Surgery of hiatal and other diaphragmatic hernias. J Int Coll Surg 43:663, 1965.

Olsen RC, Read RC, Morris WD, Campbell GS: Management of complications of fundoplication and Barrett's esophagus. Surgery 82:521, 1977.

Richardson JD, Larson GM, Polk HC: Intrathoracic fundoplication for shortened esophagus: Treacherous solution to a challenging problem. Am J Surg 143:29, 1982.

Spechler SJ: Comparison of medical and surgical therapy for complicated gastroesophageal reflux disease in veterans. The Department of Veterans Affairs Gastroesophageal Reflux Disease Study Group. N Engl J Med 326:786, 1992.

Toupet A: Technique d'oesophagogastroplastie avec phrenogastropexie appliquée dans la cure radicale des hernia hiatales et comme complement de l'operation de Heller dans les cardiospasmus. Mem Acad Chir 89:374, 1963.

Wald H, Polk HCJ: Anatomic variations in hiatal and upper gastric areas and their relationship to difficulties experienced at operations for reflux esophagitis. Ann Surg 1971:389, 1983.

LAPAROSCOPIC NISSEN FUNDOPLICATION REPAIR

Tom R. DeMeester

Sheryl Lewin

It is estimated that before the development of laparoscopic antireflux surgery, fewer than 10,000 antireflux procedures were performed annually in the United States. With the advent of laparoscopic surgery, the number of procedures per year has exceeded 50,000 and is increasing annually. Why has this occurred? There are four reasons for this change.

First, GERD is a very common disease. The prevalence of the disease in Western countries is 5%, with approximately 10% of the general population in Western countries experiencing daily heartburn. As a consequence, GERD is the most common upper gastrointestinal disorder in Western society. Typical symptoms of the disease, namely heartburn and regurgitation, account for 1.3 million outpatient visits to medical care facilities annually. Obviously, a disease so prevalent is apt to provide a demand for any new or improved therapy whether it is medical or surgical.

Second, GERD can be a debilitating disease. The disease encompasses a spectrum that ranges from early disease manifested by intermittent annoying symptoms with normal endoscopic and manometric findings to late disease manifested by life-disrupting symptoms often associated with severe esophagitis, luminal stricture, Barrett's metaplasia, anatomic deformities of the cardia, and gross abnormalities on manometry. Intermittent medical therapy is effective only for early, uncomplicated disease. More than half of patients with GERD require chronic lifelong medication that results in minimal alterations in the natural history of the disease. For example, nearly three fourths of the patients diagnosed as having esophagitis still have significant complications related to GERD more than 10 years after the diagnosis (McDougall et al, 1996). On the other hand, antireflux surgery has been shown to be curative, to relieve patients of their need for chronic medication, and to heal even the most severe esophagitis (DeMeester et al, 1986; Spechler, 1992). Consequently, it is the only known therapy that changes the natural history of GERD. As patients become aware of this fact, a greater number are choosing surgical therapy.

Third, the invention of the video laparoscope has made surgery more acceptable to the patient. The impact of its acceptance has forever changed the face of antireflux surgery. A rather complex surgical procedure can now be performed with laparoscopic access, with minimal disruption of the patient's life and a marked reduction in the pain associated with major surgery. The advent of laparoscopic technology with its low morbidity rates and short hospital stay has catalyzed renewed interest by patients in the surgical treatment of reflux disease. Early clinical studies of laparoscopic Nissen fundoplication have documented that the procedure can be performed with outcomes similar to the 90% rate achieved with the open procedure (Hunter et al, 1994, 1996; Peters et al, 1995, 1998; Weerts et al, 1993). As a result, laparoscopic Nissen fundoplication has become the standard surgical procedure for patients with early and uncomplicated GERD. This popularity has significantly increased the number of patients referred for surgical therapy.

Fourth, the public has become aware of the link between chronic GERD and esophageal cancer. This has created the desire for patients with the disease to correct rather than manage the problem. This along with a desire to be free from the dependency on medication for symptom relief has led patients to seek a surgical solution.

TECHNIQUE OF LAPAROSCOPIC NISSEN FUNDOPLICATION

The important technical elements of laparoscopic antireflux repair are (1) insertion of the laparoscopic ports, (2) the hiatal dissection, (3) the crural closure, (4) fundic mobilization, (5) configuration of the geometry of the fundoplication, and (6) fixation of the fundoplication.

Insertion of the Laparoscopic Ports

We prefer to use the open technique to insert the camera port and to establish the pneumoperitoneum. We accomplish this by making a small 1.5-cm incision three fingerbreadths above the umbilicus just to the left of the midline. Two small S retractors are used to dissect through the subcutaneous fat down to the anterior fascia of the left rectus abdominis muscle. The anterior rectus fascia is cut transversely with a cautery, and the muscle is retracted laterally to expose the posterior rectus fascia. This fascia is cut similarly with the cautery and lifted up with an S retractor to tent up the parietal peritoneum. The peritoneum is grasped with a tonsil clamp and cut with scissors to allow entry into the peritoneal cavity. The S retractor is placed into the peritoneal cavity and lifted upward to allow a suture to be placed through fascia at each end of the incision.

The camera port is placed through the incision into the peritoneal cavity and secured in place with the sutures. A pneumoperitoneum is created using carbon dioxide gas to a maximum pressure of 16 mm Hg. Under videoscopic visualization, two dissection ports, a subxiphoid liver retraction port, and a left flank gastric retraction port are placed as illustrated (Fig. 20–8). The surgeon stands between the patient's legs with the camera assistant on the surgeon's left and the retraction assistant on the surgeon's right.

Hiatal Dissection

The key to the hiatal dissection is identification of the right crus and taking down the fibrous attachments between the gastric fundus and the lateral surface of the left crus. Metzenbaum-type scissors and fine grasping forceps are preferred for this dissection. A Babcock retractor is placed through the left flank port and is used to retract the stomach by grasping it just below the cardioesophageal fat pad. In all except the most obese patients, there is a thin gastrohepatic ligament overlying the caudate lobe of the liver.

The dissection is begun with an incision in the gastrohepatic ligament above and, on occasion, below the he-

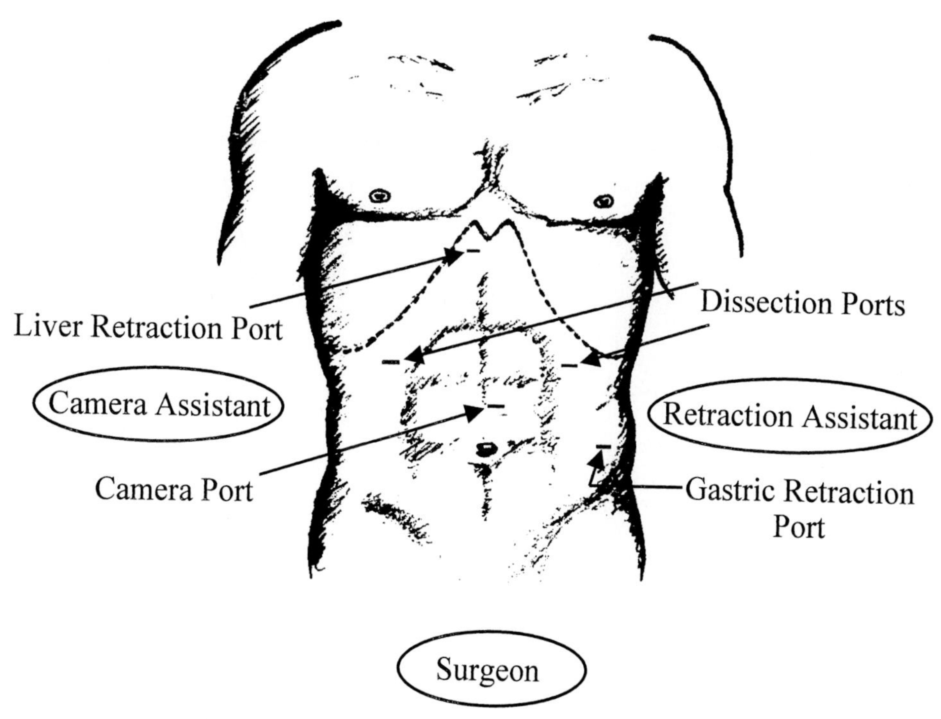

FIGURE 20–8 ■ Position of the operative team and port insertion sites during the performance of a laparoscopic Nissen fundoplication.

patic branch of the anterior vagal nerve and a small arterial branch of the left gastric artery that goes to the left hepatic lobe. This nerve is routinely spared, because taking it predisposes the patient to gallstones. A large left hepatic artery that arises from the left gastric artery is present in up to 25% of patients; it should be identified and avoided.

After incision of the gastrohepatic ligament, the lateral surface of the right crus is evident. The fatty peritoneum that overlies the anterior aspect of the right crus is incised with scissors and electrocautery, and the right crus is dissected as much as possible in the anterior and posterior direction. The medial surface of the right crus can usually be identified by careful inspection. It leads into the mediastinum and is entered by blunt dissection using both instruments. During this dissection, the esophagus becomes evident (Fig. 20–9). The right crus is retracted laterally, and the tissues to the right of the esophagus are dissected. No attempt is made at this point to dissect behind the gastroesophageal junction.

Meticulous hemostasis is critical. Blood and fluid tend to pool in the hiatus and are difficult to remove. Irrigation should be kept to a minimum. Care must be taken to not injure the phrenic vein as it courses above the hiatus. A large hiatal hernia often makes this portion of the procedure easier because it accentuates the diaphragmatic crura. On the other hand, dissection of a large mediastinal hernia sac can be difficult.

After dissection of the right crus, attention is turned toward the anterior crural confluence. With use of the left hand grasper, the esophagus is swept downward and to the right, separating it from the left crus. Care must be taken in performance of this maneuver not to get under the anterior vagal nerve. The anterior crural tissues are held up with the left hand grasper and divided with the cautery to expose the left crus (Fig. 20–10). The anterior margin of the left crus is dissected inferiorly as far as possible. This involves taking down the angle of His and the attachments of the fundus of the stomach to

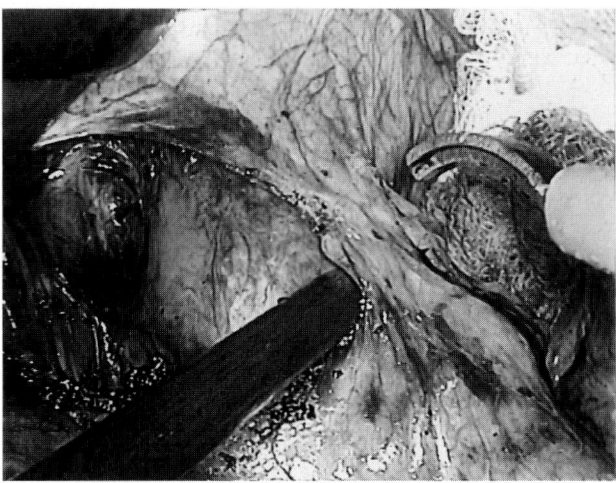

FIGURE 20–10 ■ Intraoperative photograph showing the exposure of the left crus by lifting the tissues anterior to the esophagus upward and dividing them without harming the esophagus or the anterior nerve.

the left diaphragm and the lateral surface of the left crus. A complete dissection of the lateral and inferior aspect of the left crus and fundus of the stomach is the key maneuver to allow circumferential mobilization of the esophagus (Fig. 20–11). Failure to do so results in difficulty encircling the esophagus. Repositioning of the Babcock retractor toward the fundic side of the stomach facilitates gastric retraction for this portion of the procedure.

If the crura have been completely exposed, dissection to create a window posterior to the esophagus is not difficult. With a Babcock clamp used through the left flank port, the esophagus is retracted anteriorly and inferiorly. The posterior vagus nerve is lifted with the esophagus. The posterior esophageal dissection is accomplished from the patient's right side. The medial surface and anterior margin of the left crus are identified, and the

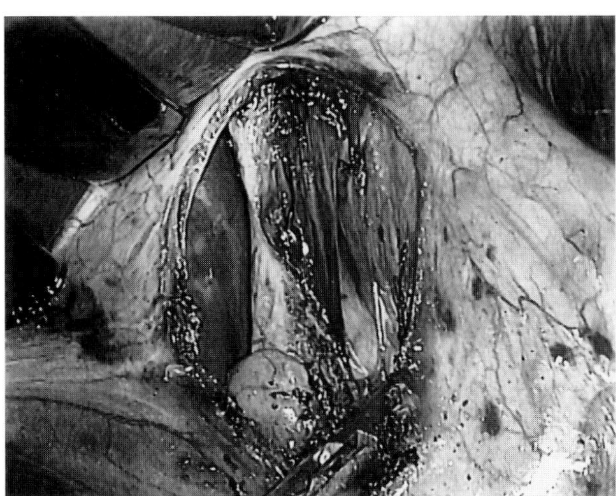

FIGURE 20–9 ■ Intraoperative photograph showing the dissection of the gastrohepatic omentum. A window is created above the hepatic branch of the vagus nerve. The medial surface of the right crus is separated by blunt dissection from the esophageal body.

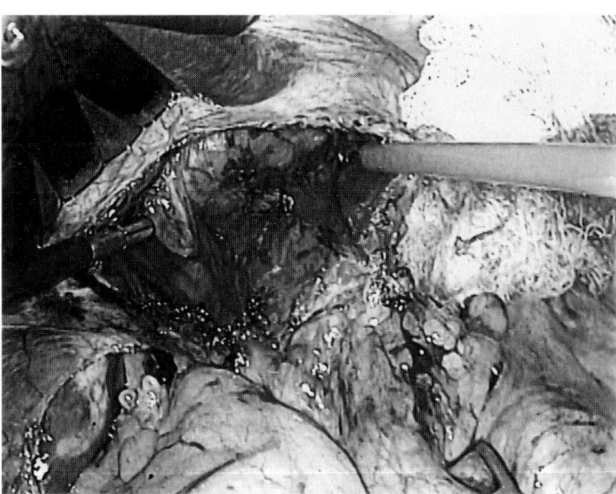

FIGURE 20–11 ■ Intraoperative photograph showing complete dissection of the right and left crura with the esophagus lying in the middle of the dissected esophageal hiatus.

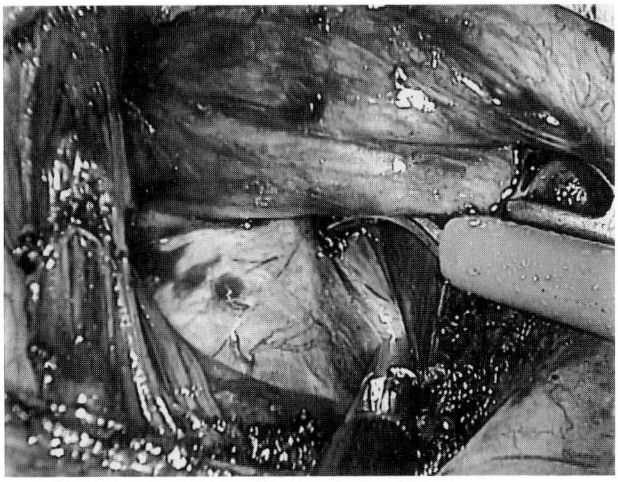

FIGURE 20–12 ■ Intraoperative photograph showing the posterior esophageal dissection. The esophagus and posterior vagal nerve are lifted with the scissors and pushed to the left by the surgeon's right hand. In this case, the instrument is a scissors. The dissection is made with the instrument in the surgeon's left hand, in this case a grasper, caudal to the anterior border of the left crus.

dissection is kept caudad to it (Fig. 20–12). The tendency to dissect into the mediastinum and into the left pleural space should be avoided.

This dissection may be unduly difficult in the presence of severe esophagitis, transmural inflammation, esophageal shortening, or a large posterior fat pad. If so, it should be abandoned and the hiatus approached from the left side after division of the short gastric vessels. After posterior dissection, the grasper in the surgeon's left hand is passed behind the esophagus and over the left crus. A Penrose drain is grasped, pulled around the esophagus, and used as an esophageal retractor for the remainder of the procedure (Fig. 20–13). The crura are further dissected inferiorly to expose the decussation of the right with the left anterior to the aorta. This enlarges the space behind the gastroesophageal junction.

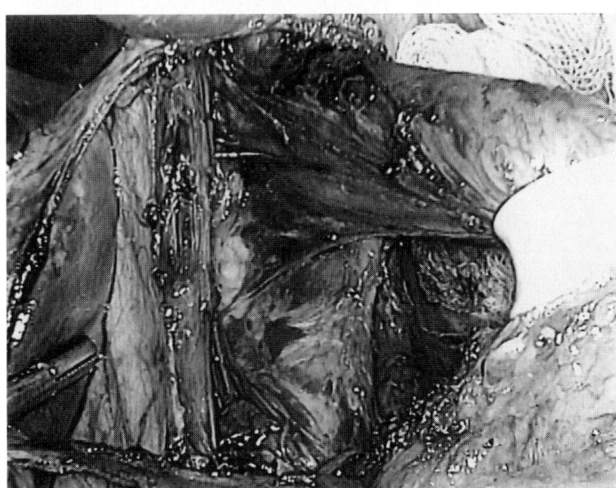

FIGURE 20–13 ■ Intraoperative photograph showing the completed dissection of the crura. The esophagus and posterior vagal nerve are retracted with a Penrose drain.

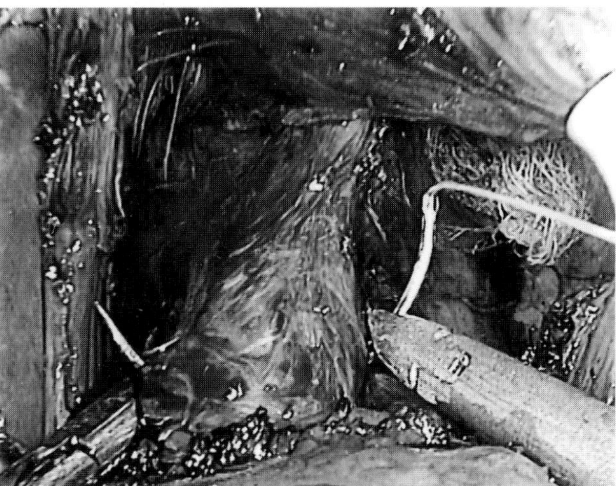

FIGURE 20–14 ■ Intraoperative photograph showing the placement of a needle (CT1) through the base of the left crus. The grasper in the surgeon's left hand is placed above the aorta to guide the tip of the needle to avoid the aorta.

Crural Closure

The esophagus is retracted anteriorly and to the left, and the crura are approximated with three or four interrupted figure-eight sutures, starting just above the aortic decussation. Only permanent suture material should be used. We prefer a large needle (CT1) passed down the left upper 10-mm dissection port to facilitate a durable crural closure. A grasper in the surgeon's left hand is placed above the aorta and serves as a guide to the tip of the needle to avoid the aorta (Fig. 20–14). We prefer to tie the knots extracorporeally, using a standard knot pusher. The figure-eight suture approximates the crura with minimal tension and prevents the suture from cutting through the muscle (Fig. 20–15).

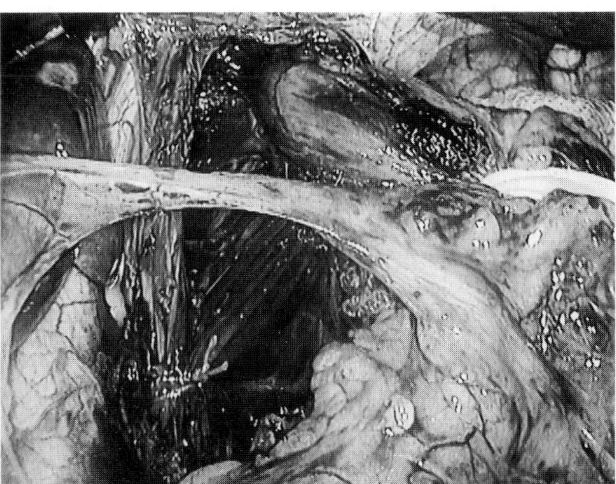

FIGURE 20–15 ■ Intraoperative photograph showing the compilation of the first figure-eight crural stitch. Approximately three or four additional figure-eight sutures are placed to finish the crural closure. The last suture is placed as the last step in the procedure, when the fundoplication has been constructed and the bougie has been removed.

At this time, the crura are only partially closed, leaving considerable space for the passage of the bougie to size the fundoplication. The remainder of the crural closure is performed as the last step of the procedure when the fundoplication has been constructed and the bougie removed. At that time, one or two additional figure-eight sutures are placed to bring the crura closely around the esophagus.

Fundic Mobilization

Complete fundic mobilization allows construction of a fundoplication free of lateral tension and without torsion of the cardia. The liver retractor is removed, letting the liver return to its normal position. Babcock clamps are placed through the liver retraction port and the left flank port to suspend the gastrosplenic mesentery during division of the short gastric vessels. A 5-cm length of the gastrosplenic omentum is suspended in a clothesline fashion between both Babcock clamps at a point approximately one third the distance down the greater curvature of the stomach (Fig. 20–16). A clear spot in the omentum is opened, and the short gastric vessels are sequentially divided with a harmonic scalpel (Ethicon Endosurgery, Cincinnati) (Fig. 20–17). To facilitate division of the vessels, a slight medial-to-lateral orientation of the omentum is preferred.

After entrance is made into the lesser sac, the gastrosplenic omentum is retracted to the left with the Babcock clamp through the left flank port and the stomach to the right with the Babcock forceps through the liver retraction port. Eventually, the Babcock clamp through the left flank port can be released from the gastrosplenic omentum and used to retract the body of stomach to the right. This gives access to the short gastric vessels close to the cephalad tip of the spleen and the posterior short gastric vessels above the pancreas (Fig. 20–18). The dissection requires division of these vessels and the fibroareolar tissue between the posterior wall of the stomach and the pancreas until the Penrose drain encircling the esophagus and the inferior closure of the crura are seen. With caution and meticulous dissection, the fundus can be completely mobilized in virtually all patients.

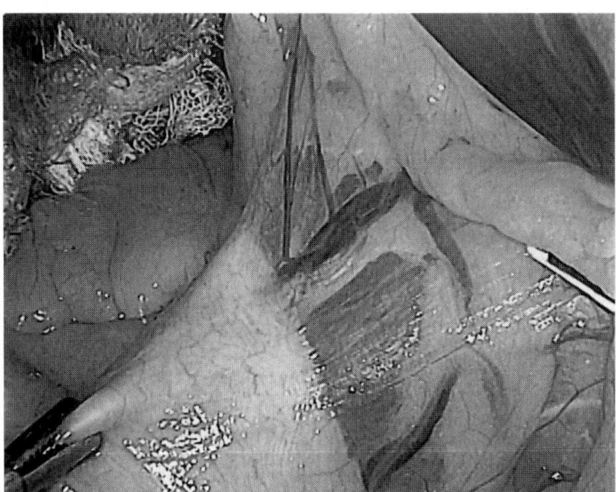

FIGURE 20–16 ■ Intraoperative photograph showing suspension of the gastrosplenic omentum in a clothesline manner in preparation for entrance into the lesser sac.

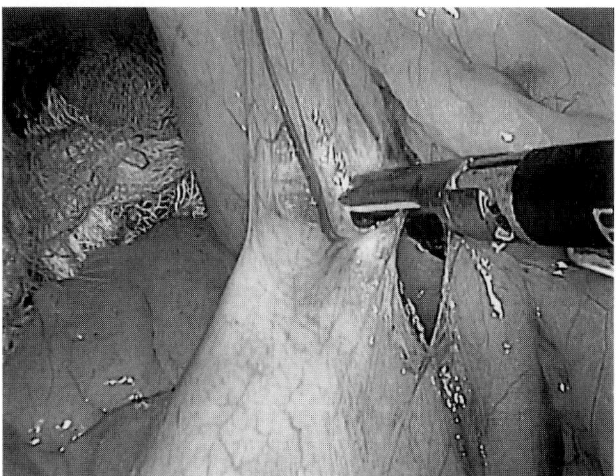

FIGURE 20–17 ■ Intraoperative photograph showing the division of the short gastric vessels with the harmonic scalpel. Each vessel is taken sequentially in a march up to the cardia. This provides full mobilization of the fundus and access to the lesser sac for division of the posterior short gastric vessels.

Configuration of the Geometry of the Fundoplication

The fundoplication is created with particular attention to the finished geometry of the repair. In detail, sufficient posterior fundic wall is passed posterior to the esophagus between the esophagus and the posterior vagus nerve. This ensures that the fundoplication has been positioned at the proper level and prevents the fundoplication from slipping down over the stomach. The anterior fundic wall is passed anterior to the esophagus. The appropriate amount of fundus is used so that the fundoplication is

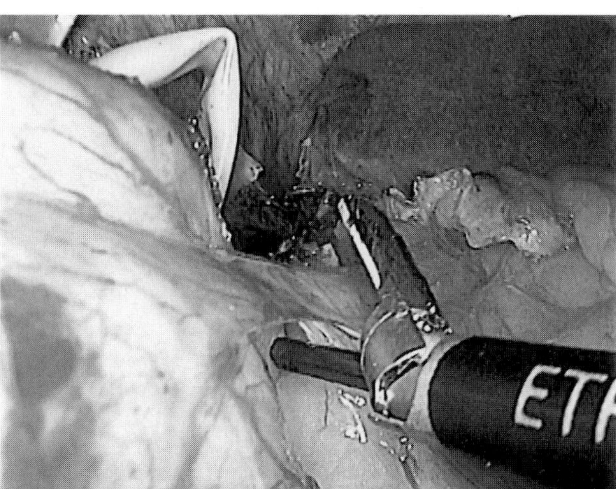

FIGURE 20–18 ■ Intraoperative photograph showing the fundus of the stomach retracted to the right after division of the short gastric vessels. This exposes the posterior fundic wall, the posterior short gastric vessels, and the fibroareolar attachments between the stomach and the pancreas. These are divided with the harmonic scalpel.

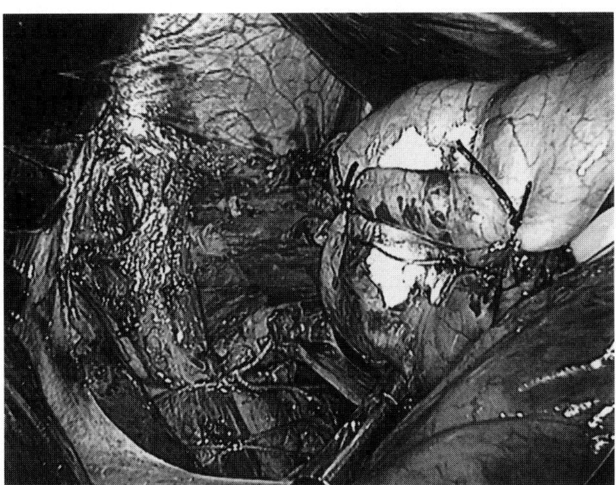

FIGURE 20–19 ■ Intraoperative photograph showing the proper configuration of the completed Nissen fundoplication. Note that (1) the esophagus is enveloped by the anterior and posterior fundic wall, (2) the fundoplication is properly placed by passage of the posterior fundic wall between the posterior vagus nerve and the esophagus, and (3) the closure of the lips of the fundoplication lies in the 10 o'clock position.

not too loose or too tight and the lips of the fundoplication meet at a right anterior lateral position, or at about 10 o'clock (Fig. 20–19). The stumps of the short gastric vessels along the greater curvature should lie against the left lateral surface of the esophagus while the remainder of the greater curvature lies in its normal plane (Fig. 20–20).

The passage of the posterior fundic wall between the posterior vagus nerve and the esophagus can best be accomplished by placing a second Penrose drain around the esophageal body, with exclusion of the posterior vagus nerve. To ensure use of the precise area of the posterior fundus to pull behind the esophagus, a marking suture is placed about 4 cm down from the gastroesophageal junction and 4 cm in from the edge of the greater curvature on the posterior fundic wall. A grasper held in the surgeon's left hand is passed between the esophagus and the posterior vagus nerve to the left side to pick up the marking suture. The surgeon pulls the suture through the window between the posterior vagus nerve and the esophagus, dragging the posterior fundic wall behind it.

The lip of the posterior fundic wall attached to the marking stitch is finally secured with a Babcock clamp through the right dissection port. The anterior wall of the fundus is brought over the anterior wall of the esophagus with a Babcock clamp through the patient's left dissection port, above the Penrose drain retracted with a Babcock clamp placed through the gastric retraction port. Both posterior and anterior fundic lips are manipulated so that the esophagus is enveloped without twisting the fundus.

The most common error in construction of the fundoplication is to grasp the anterior fundic wall of the stomach and pull it behind the esophagus. This results in twisting of the gastric fundus around the esophagus. Instead, the esophagus should be enveloped by the anterior and posterior fundic wall like a "hot dog in a bun" (Fig. 20–21). The laparoscope exaggerates the size of the posterior window. Consequently, the space between the posterior vagus nerve and the esophageal body may be smaller than thought; if it is too small, it can cause obstruction of the fundic venous drainage. If the posterior lip of the fundoplication has a bluish discoloration before the insertion of the bougie to size the fundoplication, the stomach should be returned to its original position and the posterior window enlarged.

Fixation of the Fundoplication

A 60-French bougie is passed through the esophagus and into the stomach. The fundoplication is constructed

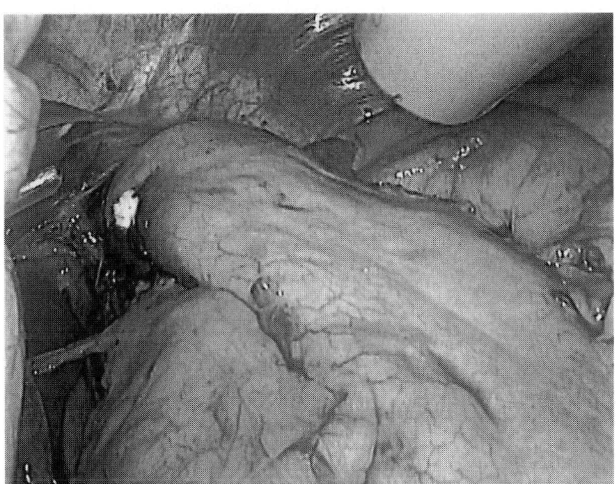

FIGURE 20–20 ■ Intraoperative photograph. After a fundoplication, the stomach remains in its proper plane, with the stumps of the short gastric vessels along the greater curvature.

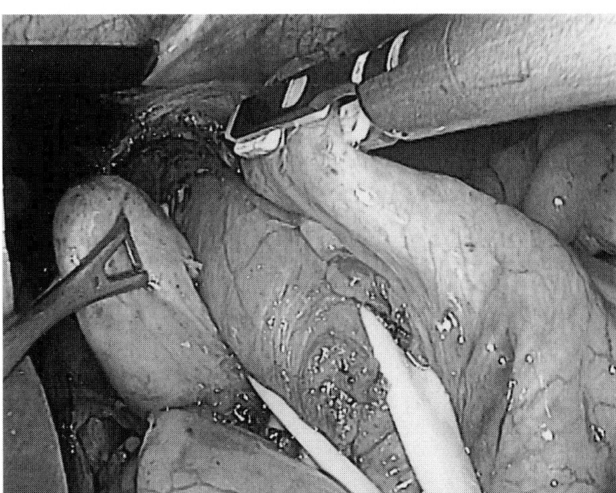

FIGURE 20–21 ■ Intraoperative photograph showing the lips of the anterior and posterior fundic wall held with Babcock clamps, and a 60 French bougie within the esophagus. There is no twisting of the fundus around the esophagus; rather, the esophagus is enveloped by the anterior and posterior fundic walls like a "hot dog in a bun."

around the bougie to size its diameter properly. The anterior and posterior lips of the fundoplication are sutured together at what is judged to be the proper tightness with a 2–0 polypropylene (Prolene) "holding stitch" (Fig. 20–22). The fundoplication is then inspected as to size, position on the esophagus, and orientation of the lips. If it is acceptable, it is permanently secured; if it is not acceptable, the holding stitch is removed and replaced repeatedly until the fundoplication passes inspection.

The fundoplication is permanently secured with a single U stitch of 2–0 polypropylene buttressed with felt pledgets on the outside of each lip. The limbs of the polypropylene U suture are about 1 cm apart and incorporate the muscular wall of the esophagus. An anchoring stitch of 2–0 silk is placed above and below the tied U stitch to ensure that the fundoplication is about 1.5 cm long (Fig. 20–23*A–D*). The fundoplication is inspected with the bougie in place to ensure it is not too tight or too loose (Fig. 20–24).

The holding stitch is removed, and the bougie is withdrawn. The remainder of the crura is closed, with the crura brought close around the esophageal body. A nasogastric tube is passed into the stomach. If it is difficult to pass through the newly constructed fundoplication, the patient undergoes endoscopy to exclude the possibility of a mechanical obstruction. Before removal of the ports, the abdomen is irrigated and hemostasis is ensured.

OUTCOME

We reviewed a series of 100 patients who had undergone fundoplication performed for the primary symptoms of heartburn, regurgitation, and dysphagia (Peters et al, 1998). In all of the patients, the diagnosis of GERD was confirmed with measurement of increased esophageal acid exposure on 24-hour pH monitoring. We used both subjective and objective (i.e., symptomatic and functional) measures to analyze the outcome of the procedure. The symptomatic outcome was assessed by a physician other than the responsible surgeon and was considered as follows:

- "Excellent" if the patient was asymptomatic
- "Good" if symptoms were relieved but minor gastrointestinal complaints, such as bloating or flatulence, persisted
- "Fair" if symptoms were improved but medication was necessary for complete relief
- "Poor" if there was no improvement in symptoms

Particular attention was paid to determine whether the primary symptom responsible for surgical referral was relieved.

In addition, the patients were asked to make their own assessment of the outcome of the procedure by judging whether they were cured, improved, or worsened by the procedure and whether they would undergo surgery again under similar circumstances. These results were obtained through telephone or personal interview with use of a standardized questionnaire. Patients who had preoperative erosive esophagitis underwent endoscopy again to determine whether the esophagitis had healed. Postoperative physiologic studies were performed in unselected patients who volunteered to undergo these studies, which consisted of 24-hour esophageal pH monitoring and manometry of the LES.

All of the patients were admitted the day of surgery. For two of the patients in the series, it was decided to switch to open laparotomy because of difficulty in fundic mobilization and short gastric division. There were no deaths. Significant complications occurred in four patients and consisted of gastrointestinal bleeding, a partial splenic infarct, heparin-induced hemothorax, and pneumonia in one patient each. The mean hospital stay was 3.1 ± 0.2 days, decreasing from a mean of 4.3 days in the first 10 patients to 2.0 days in the last 10 patients.

Ninety-five patients were followed for a median of 21 months after surgery (range, 8 months to 5 years). Follow-up was more than 4 years in 5 patients, 3 to 4 years in 13, 2 to 3 years in 22, 1 to 2 years in 56, and less than 1 year in 4. All patients had daily symptoms before surgery. The primary symptom responsible for surgery was relieved in 91 (96%) of the 95 patients. Four patients continued to have heartburn, and none had persistent regurgitation or dysphagia.

When all gastrointestinal symptoms were considered, 67 patients were asymptomatic. Twenty-three patients reported, when asked, that they had occasional symptoms of bloating, flatulence, or early satiety, but the symptoms were not sufficient to require further therapy. Three reported improvement but had persistent symptoms that required additional therapy (heartburn in two patients and crampy abdominal pain in one patient). For two patients, the procedure was considered a failure—one patient whose heartburn improved but postoperative regurgitation and dysphagia developed, and one patient in whom daily dysphagia developed that persisted for more than 3 months after fundoplication.

When asked whether the operation cured, improved, or worsened their symptoms, 99% of patients (94 of 95) reported being cured or improved. Some form of antire-

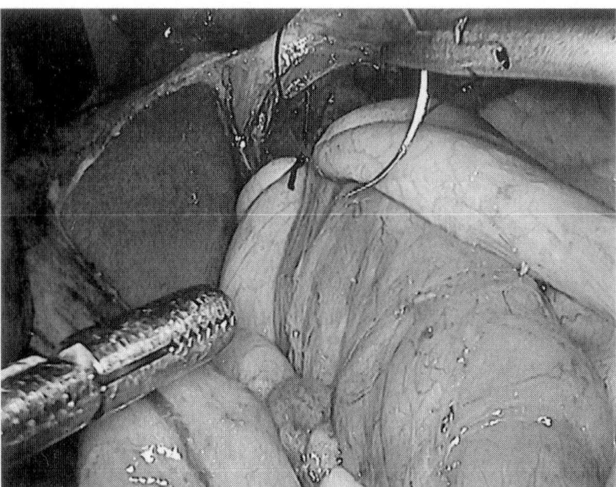

FIGURE 20–22 ■ Intraoperative photograph showing the bougie in the esophagus and the anterior and posterior fundic lips held in place with a holding stitch. This allows proper placement and tightness of the fundoplication before its fixation.

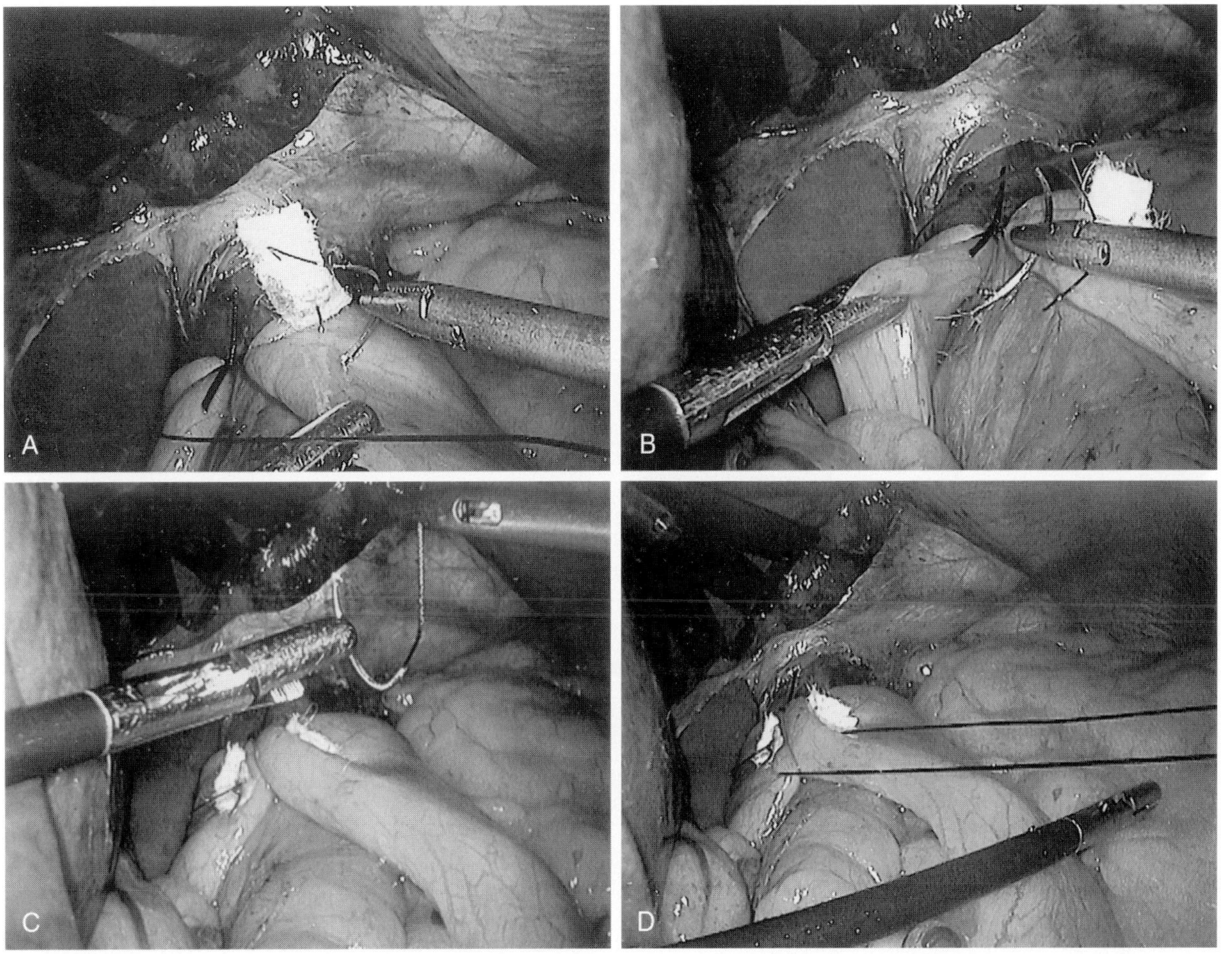

FIGURE 20–23 ■ Intraoperative photograph showing fixation of the fundoplication with a pledgeted 2-0 polypropylene (Prolene) U stitch. The limbs of the U stitch are about 1 cm apart *(A)* and incorporate the muscular wall of the esophagus *(B)*. When the anterior and posterior fundic lips are tied, they are buttressed together by the pledgets *(C)*. An anchoring stitch of 2-0 silk is placed above and below the tied U stitch to ensure the fundoplication is about 1½ cm long *(D)*.

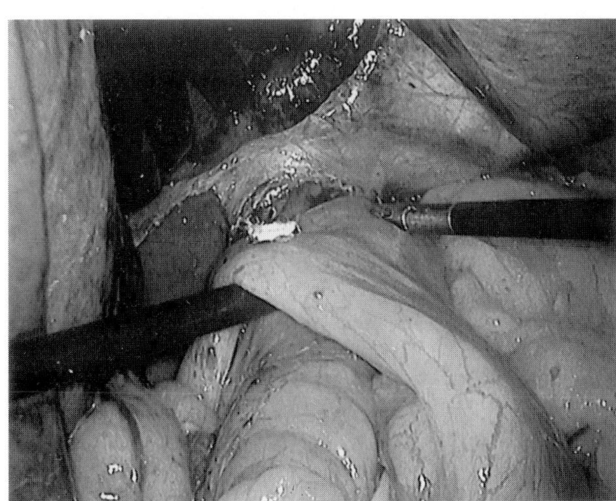

FIGURE 20–24 ■ Intraoperative photograph showing inspection of the completed fundoplication to ensure that it is properly placed around the esophagus, properly oriented in the 10 o'clock position, and not too tight in the circumference.

flux medication was taken by 90% of patients before surgery, and after surgery, only four patients required any form of acid suppression or prokinetic therapy.

The most frequent side effects of the surgery were temporary difficulty in swallowing, which lasted less than 3 months and occurred in 47 patients. Increased flatus occurred in 45, and occasional bloating or early satiety occurred in 42. Twenty-four patients reported the inability to vomit, although none of these experienced discomfort as a result. Most patients (76) were able to belch after fundoplication. Seven patients had dysphagia more than 3 months after surgery; in five patients, it was occasional; in one, weekly; and in one, daily. By 13 months after surgery, dysphagia had resolved in all except one patient. All of the patients who had preoperative dysphagia reported relief of the symptom after surgery.

Forty-six patients had erosive esophagitis before surgery; 38 were grade II and 8 were grade III. Of these, 30 returned for follow-up endoscopy, and esophagitis was completely resolved in 28 (93%). Two patients had persistent esophagitis; one of these patients returned for postoperative pH studies and had persistent increased esophageal acid exposure.

LES characteristics were significantly improved, compared with preoperative values ($P < .001$) in 27 patients who volunteered for a follow-up study. The Nissen fundoplication restored LES pressure, overall length, and abdominal length to normal (Fig. 20–25). Esophageal acid exposure returned to normal in 26 of 28 patients (Fig. 20–26). The two for whom exposure did not return to normal had markedly reduced exposure. Mean composite acid scores decreased from 50 to less than 5 (normal, < 14.8, $P < .05$), and the mean percentage of time the esophagus was exposed to pH less than 4 also was reduced below the normal range of less than 4.3% ($P < .05$).

CURRENT STATUS OF LAPAROSCOPIC NISSEN FUNDOPLICATION

On the basis of our experience and that reported by Weerts and associates (1993), Hunter and colleagues (1996), and Hinder and coworkers (1994), laparoscopic Nissen fundoplication can be considered an effective procedure. The therapeutic benefit can be accomplished in a single surgical intervention with minimal discomfort to the patient and little disruption of his or her life. Although the invasive nature of surgery is associated with risk, complications after laparoscopic fundoplication are uncommon and tend to be minor.

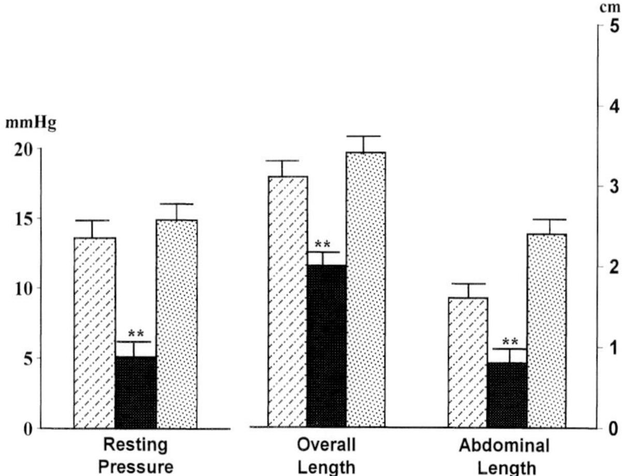

FIGURE 20–25 ■ Lower esophageal sphincter characteristics in 35 normal volunteers *(left)*, 100 patients before surgery *(middle)*, and 26 patients after surgery *(right)*. ** $P < .001$ versus other groups.

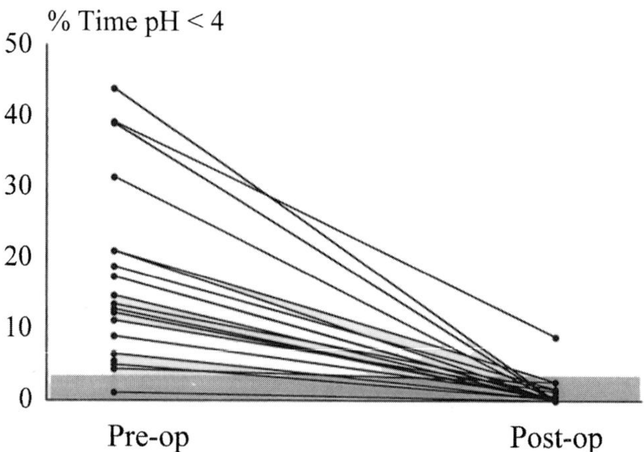

FIGURE 20–26 ■ Preoperative and postoperative 24-hour pH scores in 26 patients. *Shaded area* represents normal range.

The challenge is to reestablish the gastroesophageal barriers without inducing dysphagia. Dysphagia that exists before surgery usually improves after laparoscopic fundoplication (Bremner et al, 1994; Hunter et al, 1996; Jamieson et al, 1994). Some temporary dysphagia is common after surgery (perhaps even desirable!) and generally resolves within 3 months. Dysphagia that persists beyond 3 months has been reported in up to 10% of patients. In our experience, dysphagia (i.e., occasional difficulty swallowing solids) was present in 7% of our patients at 3 months, 5% at 6 months, 2% at 12 months, and in one patient at 24 months after surgery. Others have observed a similar improvement in postoperative dysphagia with time (Jamieson et al, 1994).

It should be emphasized that induced dysphagia is usually mild, need not require dilatation, and is temporary. It can be induced by technical misjudgments, but this explanation does not hold in all instances. In experienced hands, its prevalence should be less than 3% at 1 year (DeMeester et al, 1986).

It is our firm belief that the widespread application of laparoscopic Nissen fundoplication in patients without objective documentation of increased esophageal acid exposure on 24-hour esophageal pH monitoring and the identification of deficits in esophageal length or function leads to poor results in a significant number of patients. Physiologic assessment before antireflux surgery is particularly important due to the lessened threshold for surgical referral brought about by the rising popularity and enthusiasm for a minimally invasive surgical approach. Patients with GERD who have a relatively early form of the disease and can be managed with intermittent acid suppression therapy do not require antireflux surgery. When chronic daily acid suppression therapy is necessary, particularly if proton-pump inhibitors or dose escalation is required to control symptoms, antireflux surgery should be discussed as an option.

Traditionally, the presence of esophagitis has been the primary criterion by which to identify patients with severe disease who are candidates for surgical therapy. Although this remained true in the early years of laparoscopic fundoplication, the excellent outcome achieved with the procedure has encouraged reevaluation of these guidelines. Many now consider antireflux surgery in patients who do not have esophagitis but are dependent on proton-pump inhibitors to remain symptom-free. This is particularly true in patients younger than 50 years and those at risk for severe disease. Studies of the natural history of GERD have suggested that approximately 25% of patients fall into this category (Ollyo et al, 1993).

High-risk features include supine reflux (Fein et al, 1997), a structurally defective LES (Kuster et al, 1994), reflux of a mixture of gastric and duodenal juice (Kauer et al, 1995b; Vaezi and Richter, 1996), and the presence of severe esophagitis (Hetzel et al, 1988), stricture, or Barrett's esophagus at the initial endoscopy (Stein et al, 1993). In these patients, the need for long-term medical therapy is the rule and their medical management is likely to be problematic. We believe that these patients should be identified early and given the option of laparoscopic fundoplication if their physiology and anatomy permit (Kauer et al, 1995a).

The advent of the laparoscopic approach provides an ideal opportunity for standardization of the technique of Nissen fundoplication because it markedly limits the technical variability that can occur with the open procedure (Dunnington et al, 1993). When the technical aspects of the procedure are agreed on, the referring physician can have greater confidence in a predictable outcome from an experienced surgeon. Studies have suggested that the learning curve for laparoscopic Nissen fundoplication is in the range of 35 to 50 procedures (Watson et al, 1996). At the present rate of surgical referral, most surgeons encounter only a handful of patients with GER each year. This makes it difficult to develop technical expertise.

Although the advent of laparoscopic fundoplication has increased both patient and physician acceptance of antireflux surgery, most of these procedures are concentrated in centers with demonstrable interest in the surgical treatment of GER. The teaming of a gastroenterologist with a gastrointestinal surgeon allows both to increase their experience of using surgery to treat this disease. In so doing, they bring a balanced approach that becomes an important community resource.

■ *REFERENCES*

Bremner RM, DeMeester TR, Crookes PF, et al: The effect of symptoms and non-specific motility abnormalities on surgical therapy for gastroesophageal reflux disease. J Thorac Cardiovas Surg 107:1244–1250, 1994.

DeMeester TR, Bonavina L, Albertucci M: Nissen fundoplication for gastroesophageal reflux disease: Evaluation of primary repair in 100 consecutive patients. Ann Surg 204:9–20, 1986.

Dunnington GL, DeMeester TR, and the Department of Veterans Affairs Gastroesophageal Reflux Disease Study Group: Outcome effect of adherence to operative principles of Nissen fundoplication by multiple surgeons. Am J Surg 166:654–659, 1993.

Fein M, Hagen JA, Ritter MP, et al: Isolated upright gastroesophageal reflux is not a contraindication for antireflux surgery. Surgery 122:829–835, 1997.

Hetzel DJ, Dent J, Reed WD, et al: Healing and relapse of severe peptic esophagitis after treatment with omeprazole. Gastroenterology 95:903, 1988.

Hinder RA, Filipi CJ, Wetscher G, et al: Laparoscopic Nissen fundoplication is an effective treatment for gastroesophageal reflux disease. Ann Surg 220:472–483, 1994.

Hunter JG, Swanstrom L, Waring JP: Dysphagia after laparoscopic antireflux surgery: The impact of operative technique. Ann Surg 224:51–57, 1996.

Hunter JG, Trus TL, Branum GD, et al: A physiologic approach to laparoscopic fundoplication for gastroesophageal reflux disease. Ann Surg 223:673–687, 1996.

Jamieson GG, Watson DI, Britten-Jones R, et al: Laparoscopic Nissen fundoplication. Ann Surg 220:137–145, 1994.

Kauer WKH, Peters JH, DeMeester TR, et al: A tailored approach to antireflux surgery. J Thoracic Cardiovasc Surg 110:141–147, 1995a.

Kauer WKH, Peters JH, DeMeester TR: Mixed reflux of gastric juice is more harmful to the esophagus than gastric juice alone: The need for surgical therapy reemphasized. Ann Surg 222:525–533, 1995b.

Kuster E, Ros E, Toledo-Pimentel V, et al: Predictive factors of the long term outcome in gastroesophageal reflux disease: Six year follow up of 107 patients. Gut 35:8–14, 1994.

McDougall N, Johnston B, Kee F, et al: Natural history of reflux oesophagitis: A 10 year follow up of its effect on patient symptomatology and quality of life. Gut 38:481–486, 1996.

Ollyo JB, Monnier P, Fontolliet C, Savary M: The natural history and incidence of reflux oesophagitis. Gullet 3:3–10, 1993.

Peters JH, DeMeester TR, Crookes P, et al: The treatment of gastroesophageal reflux disease with laparoscopic Nissen fundoplication. Ann Surg 228:40–50, 1998.

Peters JH, Heimbucher J, Kauer WKH, et al: Clinical and physiologic comparison of laparoscopic and open Nissen. J Am Coll Surg 180:385–393, 1995.

Spechler S: Comparison of medical and surgical therapy for complicated gastroesophageal reflux disease study group. Department of Veterans Affairs Gastroesophageal Reflux Disease Study Group. N Engl J Med 326:786–792, 1992.

Stein JH, Hoeft S, DeMeester TR: Functional foregut abnormalities in Barrett's esophagus. J Thorac Cardiovasc Surg 105:107–111, 1993.

Vaezi MF, Richter JE: Role of acid and duodenogastroesophageal reflux in gastroesophageal reflux disease. Gastroenterology 111:1192–1199, 1996.

Watson D, Balgrie RJ, Jamieson GG: A learning curve for laparoscopic fundoplication: Definable, avoidable or a waste of time? Ann Surg 224:198–203, 1996.

Weerts JM, Dallemagne B, Hamoir E, et al: Laparoscopic Nissen fundoplication: Detailed analysis of 132 patients. Surg Laparosc Endosc 3:359–364, 1993.

CHAPTER **21**

Belsey Mark IV Repair

Clement A. Hiebert

Toni Lerut

To appreciate the full significance of Ronald Belsey's contribution to the surgery of hiatus hernia, it is necessary to revisit the orthodoxy of the first half of the 20th century, a time when surgeons viewed hiatal hernia as a rupture to be repaired, a rim to be snugged, an organ to be tethered. How large the hernia must be to qualify for fixing and whether the approach to it should be through the chest or abdomen were topics of vigorous debate. Philip Allison (1951), soon to be named regius professor of surgery at Oxford, ended the era of protrusion surgery by showing that the symptoms of an ordinary sliding hernia derive not from a throttled pouch of stomach but from wrong-way traffic at the lower end of the esophagus. The culprit was the valve, and symptoms were the lament of esophageal mucosa washed in acid.

Allison's thesis proved correct, even though the operation that bears his name failed the test of his own follow-up clinic (Allison, 1973). It remained for Belsey in Bristol and Nissen in Basel to more or less simultaneously develop reliable operations to curb gastroesophageal reflux. Nissen's discovery was serendipitous; Belsey's, the product of a decade of correlating patients' complaints with the findings on the operating table and in the endoscopy and follow-up clinics (Belsey, 1952; Hiebert, 1991; Nissen, 1956, 1961, 1970). Together with the more recently described repairs of Hill (see Chapter 22) and Dor and Toupet (see Chapter 23), the four procedures constitute the principal repertoire of a surgeon whose goal is to relieve gastroesophageal reflux.

In this chapter, we examine an amalgam of details of the Mark IV operation from a more than 30-year perspective of two former Frenchay Hospital registrars who learned the operation from its inventor.

HISTORICAL NOTE

Belsey's preoccupation with developing a physiologic rather than an anatomic repair began in 1942 (Hiebert, 1991). Using a rigid 50-cm esophagoscope and examining the minimally sedated patient in the seated position, Belsey came to appreciate that competency of the esophagogastric junction depended on its lying well below the diaphragm. If the junction became displaced to a level at or above the hiatal arch, the esophagogastric opening was seen to gape, allowing a tide of gastric mucus to flow into the terminal esophagus with each deep inspiration. He called the parent condition a "patulous cardia" and set as his operative goal the repositioning of the esophagogastric junction several centimeters below the diaphragm.

The *Mark I* operation was essentially a variant of the anatomic restoration urged by Allison. *Mark II* and *Mark III* operations represented degrees of trial and error fundoplication to provide a serosal covered muscular collar more suitable than the naked esophagus for anchoring sutures. A bonus of this crescentic overlay of stomach was its restraining influence on any tendency of the intra-abdominal esophagus to dilate. Belsey waited a half dozen years before he was sufficiently satisfied with the durability of the operation to publish the results of repair in 71 patients with isolated primary gastroesophageal reflux (Hiebert and Belsey, 1961) and a full 12 years before collaborating with Skinner in reporting the results of operating on 632 patients with hiatal hernia and/or reflux (Skinner and Belsey, 1967). Belsey called his invention the *Mark IV* operation to remind his students that this statement was neither his first on the subject, nor was it necessarily his last.

■ *HISTORICAL READINGS*

Belsey R: Diaphragmatic hernia. In Modern Trends in Gastroenterology. London, Butterworths, 1952, p 128.

Hiebert CA, Belsey R: Incompetency of the gastric cardia without radiologic evidence of hiatal hernia. J Thorac Cardiovasc Surg 53:33, 1961.

Skinner DB, Belsey RH: Surgical management of esophageal reflux and hiatus hernia: Long-term results with 1,030 patients. J Thorac Cardiovasc Surg 53:33, 1967.

ADVANTAGES OF THE MARK IV REPAIR

The advantages of the Mark IV repair are numerous:

1. When correctly done, the operation provides a barrier to reflux but leaves other gullet functions undisturbed. More than 75% of patients retain the capacity for normal swallowing, belching, and vomiting. (See Results.)
2. A tension-free return of the terminal esophagus to the abdomen requires the gullet to be freed up, often to the level of the aortic arch. This requirement is especially important when the esophagus has been shortened by transmural esophagitis.
3. The mediastinum may be approached directly when it is socked in with fibrous tissue owing to previous esophageal surgery.
4. Surgery in an obese patient is more easily accomplished through the chest.
5. If primary reduction and repair cannot be done without tension, especially in a child with a stricture, the

incision may be extended across the costal arch and the left colon may be substituted for the stenosed esophagus.

6. The transthoracic Mark IV technique is an essential component of Pearson's ingenious solution to the short esophagus. The *Pearson gastroplasty*, incorrectly referred to as the *Collis-Belsey operation*, is the subject of Chapter 24.

7. In a patient with scleroderma, or following an esophageal myotomy for achalsia or other motility disorder, the anti-reflux barrier can be restored and tailored to less than robust esophageal propulsion (see Chapters 32 and 34).

8. Enlargement of the spleen or liver may occasionally militate against an abdominal repair.

9. A thoracic approach allows the surgeon to manage coexisting disease in the left chest wall, lung, esophagus, or upper abdomen.

10. The operating time is short, usually an hour.

DISADVANTAGES OF THE MARK IV REPAIR

There are some disadvantages to the Mark IV procedure:

1. The operation is conceptually more complex than than a Nissen repair and is more difficult to teach.

2. *The location, depth, and spacing of each suture are crucial to a favorable result* (i.e., eliminating abnormal reflux while maintaining agreeable swallowing, ability to belch, and vomiting when circumstances require).

3. A laparoscopic Mark IV procedure is not possible.

4. Orringer and colleagues (1972 noted that the Mark IV is "a fairly easy operation to do but a difficult one to do well." For example, the naked esophagus is unreliable holding ground for sutures that are placed too superficially or are tied too tightly. Baue (1980) proposed using sutures with pledgets to overcome this concern.

5. Post-thoracotomy wound pain used to be a concern, but not since institution of a strict policy of separating ribs no more than 3 to 5 cm (measured!).

OBTAINING GOOD RESULTS

As with all hiatal hernia repairs, good results with the Mark IV repair depend on: (1) proper selection of patients, (2) optimal preoperative and postoperative care, (3) a meticulous operation, and (4) relating long-term results to what was done (Belsey, 1977).

Proper Patient Selection

Proper selection of patients means answering a number of questions, such as:

- Has the diagnosis been confirmed?
- Is the hernia or patulous cardia the undoubted source of the patient's complaint?
- Are there overlapping symptoms of coronary artery disease?
- How serious is the reflux?
- Is there evidence for aspiration, esophagitis, columnar lined esophagus, or microcytic anemia?
- Do the complaints justify the small but significant risk of a less than perfect outcome?
- Is the patient otherwise fit?
- What is the cost of long-term medical management vis-à-vis operation?

Optimal Preoperative Care

Optimal preoperative care includes ensuring that the heart and lungs are at their best:

- Has the chest physiotherapist cleared the airway?
- Is a bronchoscopy in order?
- Has pulmonary inflammation been controlled?
- Has the patient been told where the incision will be and instructed in the use of coughing, postural drainage, and breathing exercises?
- Is the anesthesiologist aware of the potential for regurgitation and aspiration during induction?
- Is the anesthesiologist adept at inserting a bronchial blocker or double lumen tube so that, if desired, the lung may be deflated to improve exposure without additional separation of the ribs?

A Meticulous Operation

The *physiologic* goal of the Mark IV operation is elimination of gastroesophageal reflux while preserving the other functions of the gullet. The *anatomic goal* is to return a 4- to 5-cm segment of terminal esophagus to the abdomen and to fix it in place (DeMeester et al, 1979).

The operation has four parts: (1) exposure, (2) mobilization, (3) crus approximation, and (4) fundoplication (Figs. 21–1 to 21–8). Certain points require emphasis, noted are follows.

Exposure

Make the incision in the left sixth or seventh interspace; use the higher level in obese patients. The incision should

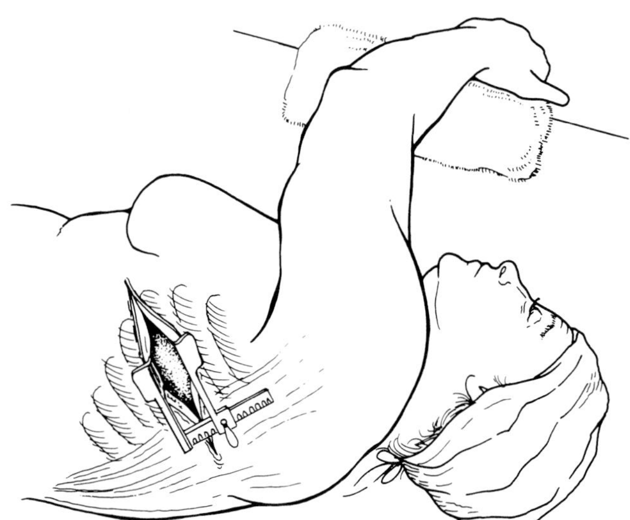

FIGURE 21–1 ■ Adequate exposure of the lower esophagus and hiatus is afforded by a left sixth or seventh interspace incision. The higher incision is employed if the patient is obese. Postoperative chest pain is minimal if the retractor blades are separated no more than a measured 3 to 5 cm.

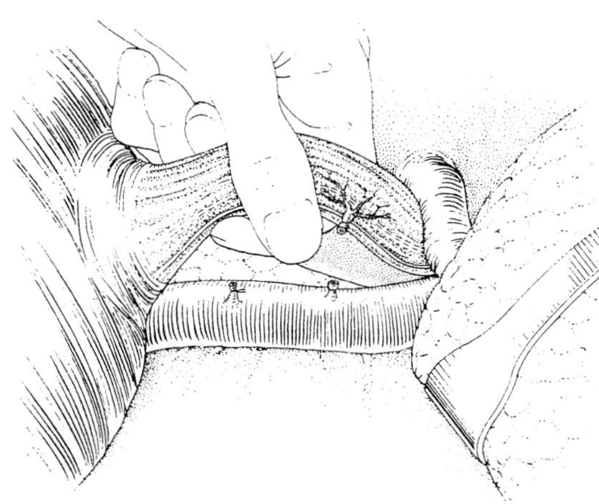

FIGURE 21–2 ■ The inferior pulmonary ligament (not shown) is divided. With incision of the mediastinal pleura medial to the aorta, the esophagus is easily divested of areolar and vascular attachments. A finger around the esophagus ensures that both vagus nerves will be included in encircling soft rubber drain. (From Hiebert CA: Antireflux surgery by the thoracic approach. In Rob & Smith's Operative Surgery. Jamieson GJ, Debas HT [eds]: Surgery of the Upper Gastrointestinal Tract, 5th ed. Chapman & Hall, London, 1994, p 301.)

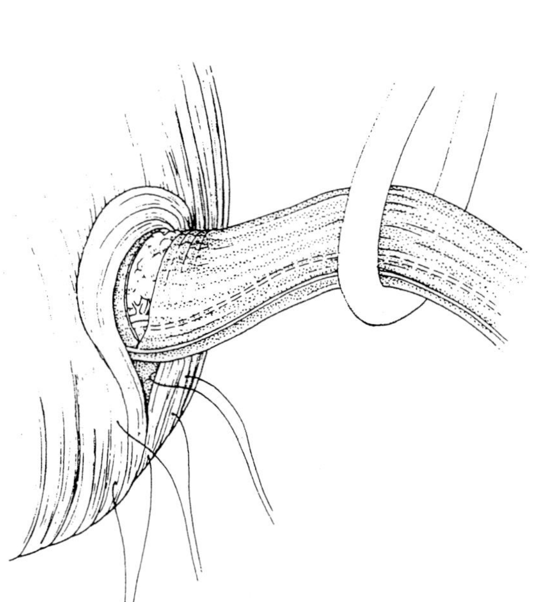

FIGURE 21–3 ■ A patulous cardia's attachments to the diaphragm have been partially cleared. The two halves of the right crus are to be joined with No. 0 nonabsorbable sutures and left unknotted until later. (The uppermost posterior suture will ultimately include a bite of the esophageal muscle layer to discourage early herniation of fat.) (From Hiebert CA: Antireflux surgery by the thoracic approach. In Rob & Smith's Operative Surgery. Jamieson GJ, Debas HT [eds]: Surgery of the Upper Gastrointestinal Tract, 5th ed. London, Chapman & Hall, 1994, p 301.)

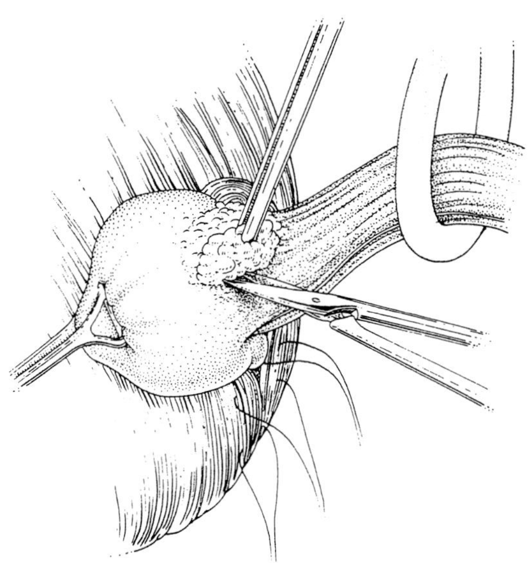

FIGURE 21–4 ■ Removal of the vascular pad of fat that overlies the anterior aspect of the esophagogastric junction is done to encourage union of the raw surfaces, soon to be joined in the first of two fundoplicating layers. (From Hiebert CA: Antireflux surgery by the thoracic approach. In Rob & Smith's Operative Surgery. Jamieson GJ, Debas HT [eds]: Surgery of the Upper Gastrointestinal Tract, 5th ed. London, Chapman & Hall, 1994, p 301.)

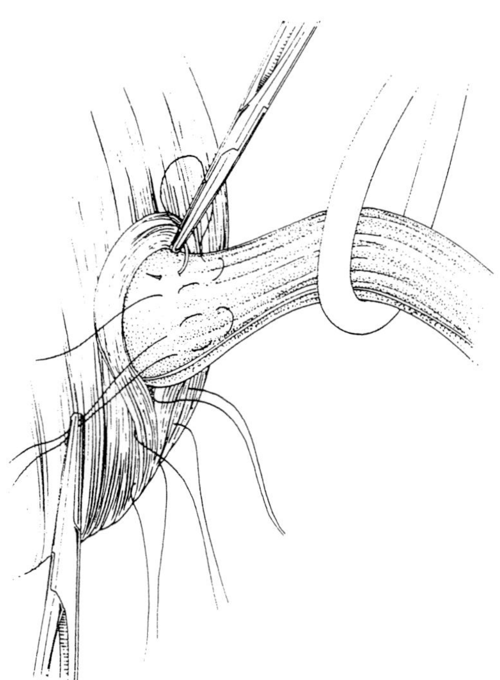

FIGURE 21–5 ■ Fundoplication is begun by placing mattressed sutures between stomach fundus and adjacent esophagus to initiate a crescentic fold spanning the anterior interval of the two vagus nerves. The nerves may be pushed aside, but should not be snared. (From Hiebert CA: Antireflux surgery by the thoracic approach. In Rob & Smith's Operative Surgery: Jamieson GJ, Debas HT [eds]: Surgery of the Upper Gastrointestinal Tract, 5th ed. London, Chapman & Hall, 1994, p 301.)

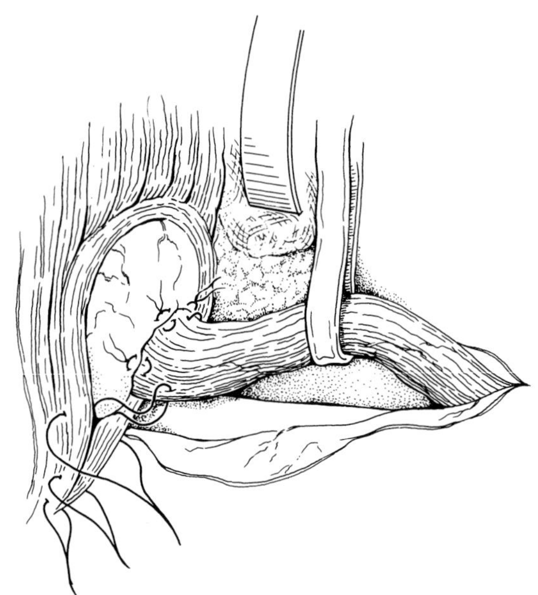

FIGURE 21–6 ■ The first layer of fundoplicating sutures are knotted, and the crescentic fold tends to drop out of sight. As with all other sutures, they must not be snugged so tightly as to invite necrosis. In placing these sutures, the surgeon must avoid bites that are too superficial and invite recurrence or bites too deep that may invite fistula formation. (From Hiebert CA: Antireflux surgery by the thoracic approach. In Rob & Smith's Operative Surgery. Jamieson GJ, Debas HT [eds]: Surgery of the Upper Gastrointestinal Tract, 5th ed. London, Chapman & Hall, 1994, p 301.)

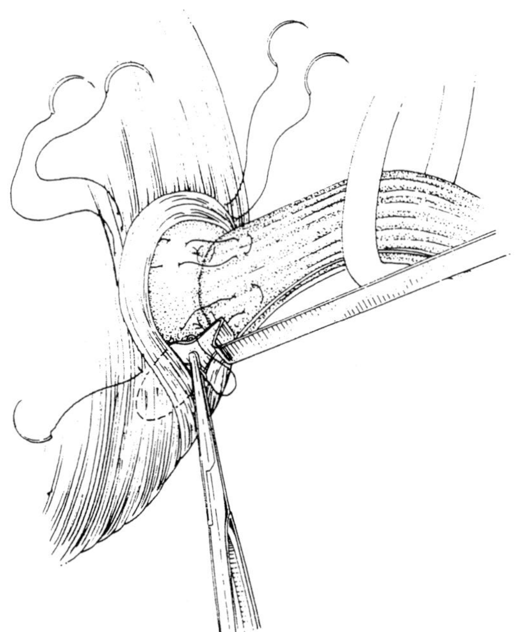

FIGURE 21–7 ■ A second row of three sutures is placed: a modified teaspoon is used to keep the needle from piercing the abdominal organs. The surgeon tucks the reconstructed cardia below the diaphragm by gently pushing on the cardia while drawing up the three suture pairs. (From Hiebert CA: Antireflux surgery by the thoracic approach. In Rob & Smith's Operative Surgery. Jamieson GJ, Debas HT [eds]: Surgery of the Upper Gastrointestinal Tract, 5th ed. London, Chapman & Hall, 1994, p 301.)

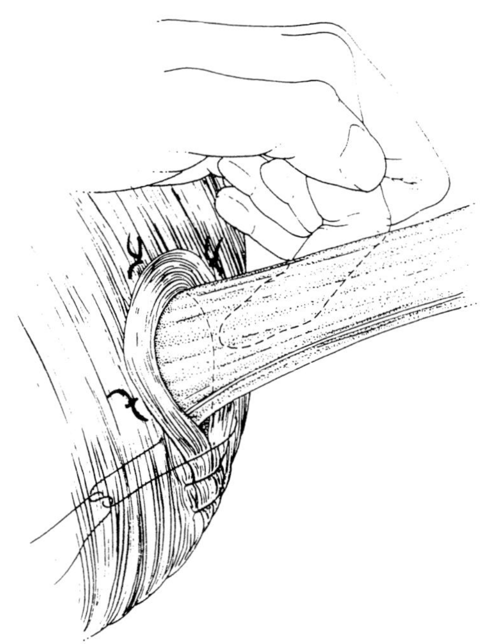

FIGURE 21–8 ■ The fundoplication must lie below the diaphragm without tension, and it should be possible to insert the index finger to the distal interphalangeal joint into the posteromedial hiatal gap. The closure must not be tight. (From Hiebert CA: Antireflux surgery by the thoracic approach. In Rob & Smith's Operative Surgery. Jamieson GJ, Debas HT [eds]: Surgery of the Upper Gastrointestinal Tract, 5th ed. London, Chapman & Hall, 1994, p 301.)

be directly over the appropriate interspace because the serratus anterior muscle arises from the lower ribs and precludes adjusting exposure via the standard posterolateral thoracotomy employed for ribs five and above.

The Mark IV operation can be done through minimally separated ribs. *It is unnecessary to have the (measured) interval between the blades of the retractor greater than 5 cm.* (For much of the operation, 3 cm is adequate.) Wound discomfort has virtually ceased to be a problem since the program of limited retraction was instituted more than two decades ago.

Mobilization

With the left lung collapsed or retracted, the inferior pulmonary ligament is ligated and divided, and the esophagus together with both vagus nerves is freed of mediastinal connections. Adequate mobilization means carrying the dissection up to the level of the aortic arch. Respect the diaphanous right pleura; it is at the most dependent level of the wound, and opening it allows unseen blood to accumulate in the right chest. The diaphragmatic end of the original longitudinal pleural incision is continued transversely to expose the muscular margin of the hiatus in front and the two halves of the right crus of the diaphragm behind.

Peritoneal entry is made at the anteromedial aspect where, upon cutting of the phrenoesophageal ligament, the sudden bulging of extraperitoneal fat may be mistaken for omentum. But the peritoneum is deeper still; after incising it close to the hiatal rim, the surgeon continues the cut laterally to the first short gastric artery and medially until a thickened band of fibrofatty tissue is encountered. Ligation and division of this band open the lesser sac and expose the caudate lobe of the liver posteromedially. Skinner and Belsey (1988) has cautioned that inattention to this step may result in bleeding from an ascending communication of the left gastric and phrenic arteries.

Near the hiatus, each vagus nerve is gently dissected from the esophagus to provide space for the fundoplicating sutures. Occasionally, one or two of the upper short gastric vessels are taken to achieve full mobilization of the cardia. Finally, the pad of fat in front of the gastroesophageal junction is excised by ligating and dividing its multiple fine vascular attachments. The goal is to promote adhesion between the soon to be juxtaposed stomach and esophagus.

Crus Approximation

Crus approximation is an essential component of the Mark IV operation. A firm posterior buttress, not a narrow hiatus, is the goal. The near edge of the right crus is less well defined than its opposite member. Sharp separation of pericardium from the diaphragm gains exposure; however, to locate with certainty the essential pillar through which sutures are to be taken, it is helpful to palpate the inner half of the crus while tugging on a Babcock clamp applied to the central tendon of the diaphragm. This maneuver identifies the sturdy inner portion of the right crus and elevates it away from the vena cava. By contrast, the lateral half of the hiatal arch is stout, visible, and ideal for suturing. The spleen lies immediately beneath and is easily palpated.

Three to five No. 0 sutures of linen or silk are placed from behind forward at approximately 1 cm. The sutures are temporarily snugged but are not tied until later. One of us (C.A.H.) places the uppermost suture only through the medial half of the crus until after the hernia is reduced. This suture is then passed through posterior esophageal muscle before the final bite of the lateral half of the crus is taken. The strategy is to discourage early herniation at the notch between the esophagus and the reunited halves of the crus.

Fundoplication

Fundoplication is started by placing the first of two mattressed rows of 2–0 silk or linen sutures between stomach and adjacent esophagus to create a crescentic fold encompassing an estimated 240 degrees of the circumference of the esophagus. The previously mobilized lower vagal trunks are gently moved aside if necessary. Proper passage of the atraumatic needles through the submucosa of the esophagus and stomach is important. Bites that are too superficial predispose to recurrence, and sutures passed through the mucosa invite fistula formation. A critical point of technique is to avoid drawing the first throw of any knot too tight. *Suture tension is determined by vision, not feel.* Umbilicated tissue is best regarded as strangulated tissue. Use of polytetrafluoroethylene (Teflon) felt washers is suggested by Baue (1990).

A second row of three mattressed sutures is placed 1.5 to 2.0 cm from the junction created by the first row and is passed through the diaphragm from below upward. A modified teaspoon serves as a retractor to avoid hapless puncturing of abdominal viscera. Spearing of subserosal gastric vessels happens occasionally, and any resulting hematoma is controlled by traction on and occasionally by ligation of the appropriate suture pair. The surgeon achieves reduction of the hernia by gentle downward pressure, using the fingers or a sponge stick. With the hernia reduced, the fundoplicating and posterior crural sutures are tentatively snugged. An index finger in the posteromedial hiatal gap should slip effortlessly to the distal interphalangeal joint. Better that the hiatal opening be too loose than too tight; if there is any doubt about adequacy of the opening, the uppermost crural suture should be withdrawn or replaced.

The esophagus must not be taut. With increasing experience, the surgeon is usually spared the uncomfortable decision whether to mobilize the esophagus still further, dismantle the repair and perform a Pearson gastroplasty, or let the repair stand and accept a 50/50 risk of a less than ideal result (Pearson and Henderson, 1976).

The typical appearance of a properly constructed Mark IV operation is shown in Figure 21–9.

Optimal Postoperative Care

Optimal postoperative care begins in the recovery room, where retching or vomiting can be the undoing of a fresh repair. The surgeon should anticipate possible emetogenic side effects of an analgesic drug by including the pro-

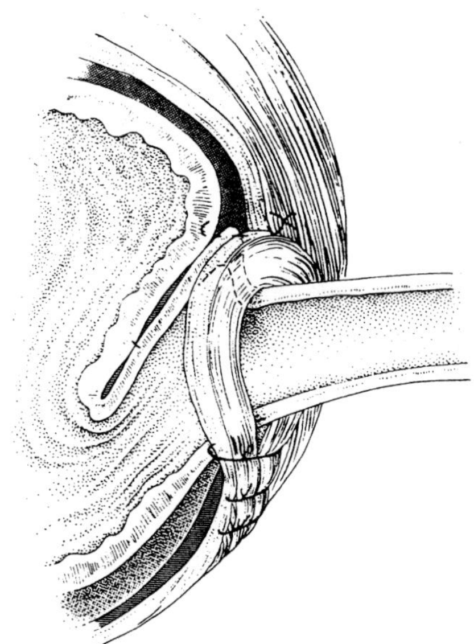

FIGURE 21–9 ■ A 3- to 4-cm length of intra-abdominal esophagus is depicted in sagittal section. A crescent of stomach folded on the esophagus over an estimated 240 degrees of the esophageal circumference to discourage dilatation of the terminal esophagus as well as to provide better holding ground than that afforded by the naked esophagus. (From Hiebert CA: Antireflux surgery by the thoracic approach. In Rob & Smith's Operative Surgery. Jamieson GJ, Debas HT [eds]: Surgery of the Upper Gastrointestinal Tract, 5th ed. London, Chapman & Hall, 1994, p 301.)

TABLE 21–1 ■ **Follow-up and Outcome: 1524 Mark IV Operations at Various Centers**

	No. of Patients	*Follow-up (%)*	*Period of Follow-up*	*Results: Good to Excellent (%)**
Hiebert & Belsey (1961)	71	95	2 mo–8 yr	87
Orringer, Belsey, & Skinner (1972)	892	86	3–15 yr	84
Hiebert & O'Mara (1979) (2nd series)	209	95	1–20 yr	80*
Lerut et al (1990)	147	100	1–13 yr	78†
Fenton et al (1997)	276	53	2 mo–16 yr	95‡

*Ten percent of failures occurred in 2nd decade of follow-up.
†Figure includes complications unrelated to gastroesophageal reflux.
‡"Failure" defined in this Atlanta series as the need for reoperation or dilatation.

posed postoperative narcotic in the premedication for endoscopy.

Postoperative gastric distention is another source of stress on sutured tissues. Although the limited fundoplication of the Mark IV allows belching after tissue swelling subsides, temporary use of a nasogastric tube is advisable. The time to insert it is after fundoplicating sutures are in place but before they are knotted. Safe passage of the well-lubricated tube is facilitated by the surgeon's fingers guiding the tube from outside of the esophagus.

Although many patients tolerate early ingestion of oral fluids, delayed gastric emptying sometimes occurs. Rather than allow gastric distention to spoil convalescence, it seems prudent to postpone eating and drinking until peristalsis has returned and only then to proceed with limited amounts of water, flat ginger ale, broth, and gelatin dessert. Fruit juices may not be tolerated until later.

Discharge instructions to the patient include the advice to remain on a soft diet for 3 weeks and to chew food for twice as long as previously. Patients are urged not to lift children, pets, or objects weighing more than 20 kg because an occasional patient may associate the onset of recurrent symptoms with heavy lifting during the first weeks after surgery.

Results

A summary of the results of 1.248 standard Mark IV operations reported from Bristol, Leuven, Atlanta, Ann Arbor, and Portland, Maine, are given in Tables 21–1 and 21–2. Eighty-four percent of patients had good to excellent results. The clinical criterion was overall satisfaction—the equivalent of an affirmative response to the question, "Would you have had the operation if you had known what to expect?" Not surprisingly, in the updated Bristol series reported by Orringer and coauthors (1972), Belsey's *personal* operative record of 94% good to excellent results in 423 patients remains the "24-karat gold standard." In reaching for the elusive goal of perfection, it is important to relate the details of patient selection, perioperative care, and technical aspects of the operation to what the patient has to say on follow-up visits.

Hiebert and O'Mara (1979) reviewed 209 patients who had undergone the unmodified Mark IV operation with 95% follow-up to 18 years. Review of original data shows

TABLE 21–2 ■ **Comparison of Belsey Mark IV and Laparoscopic Nissen Repairs**

	Belsey Mark IV	*Nissen*
Technical difficulty	Moderate	Moderate
Valve competence	Patient usually able to belch and to vomit as necessary; reflux curbed in about 85% of patients	Excellent reflux control but at expense of gas bloat
Impedance	Agreeable swallowing	Dysphagia more likely
Complications	Intraoperative complications rare; operative death rate <1%	Intraoperative complications uncommon but may be serious; operative deaths less than 1%
Operating time	±60 min	160 min ± 59
Wound concerns	Seven-inch intercostal incision; minimal discomfort if ribs are separated 2 inches or less	Four or five half-inch incisions allegedly make for least possible wound pain
Time in hospital	4–6 days	2.6±1.2 days
Resumption of full activity	6 wk	1 wk
Early results	85% good to excellent	95% (128/135) good to excellent
Best use	A very serviceable operation for reflux control, especially when esophageal peristalsis is of low amplitude or is ineffective	In setting of normal esophageal motility

Modified from Landreneau RJ, Weichmenn RJ, Hazelrigg SR, et al: Success of laparoscopic fundoplication for gastroesophageal reflux disease. Ann Thorac Surg 66:1886, 1998.

that in only eight of the group (3.3%) was there less than a five-year follow-up. Eighty-four percent of patients were sufficiently satisfied with the surgical results that they would go through it again in the light of their experience. Only 5% felt the result to be unsatisfactory. As for specific esophageal functions, 78% found swallowing to be agreeable, 86% could belch, and 78% could vomit when required.

Lerut (1990) reports using the Mark IV operation in 177 patients with 100% follow-up ranging from 1 to 13 years (mean, 4.4 years). Fifty-five percent of the group had associated pathology in the gullet or upper abdomen; 17 patients (11.6%) had symptoms suggesting reflux, and two more individuals without symptoms had evidence of recurrence. A total of 13 patients (8.8%) had either gas bloat (5), dysphagia (5), or other gastrointestinal side effects (3). Post-thoracotomy pain requiring treatment was seen in 13 patients (8.8%).

LAPAROSCOPIC AND OTHER TECHNIQUES

Surgeons wishing to compare the Mark IV repair with the other techniques will find that the literature contains a bewildering array of variables, haphazard reporting, and unanswered questions, such as:

1. *Which patients were included?* Is the author speaking of small uncomplicated sliding hernias, or are patients with severe grades of esophagitis included? It makes a difference. The recurrence rate of the Mark IV operation for patients with mural fibrosis and esophageal shortening is 50% or greater, according to Skinner and Belsey (1988).

2. *Are patients with additional esophageal or upper abdominal disease included?*

3. *Are there enough patients to justify the conclusions?* "Don't publish results until you have operated on a hundred patients," advises Belsey.

4. *Was the follow-up period sufficient?* Hiebert and O'Mara (1979) found that 50% of recurrent symptoms appeared during the first postoperative year, but 10% of component failures were not manifest until the second decade (Fig. 21–10). Skinner and Belsey (1988) recommend a minimum follow-up period of 5 years.

Lacking long-term data to show that the operation is both effective and durable, proponents of the laparoscopic Nissen repair have trumpeted the short hospital stay of their patients and their quick return to the workplace as good omens. The extrapolation of preliminary results of a new hiatal hernia repair to the long term, however, recalls Allison's humbling presentation of his life's work before the American Surgical Association in Los Angeles (1973). In a 3- to 20-year retrospective survey of 553 patients treated with the once promising technique that bore his name, the recurrence rate was 49% for and type I hernias and 33% for type II. *Of the recurrences, 32% took place 5 years after the operation.*

Belsey waited 6 years before he was satisfied with the durability of the Mark IV operation to certify its usefulness in restoring competency to the esophagogastric junction in the isolated condition of patulous cardia (Hiebert and Belsey, 1961) and a full 12 years before his landmark presentation with Skinner (1967). Belsey's restraint in deferring publication until 1000 patients had been and treated was remarkable. We shall not see the likes of this again.

5. *Who was the surgeon?* Orringer observes, with colleagues Belsey and Skinner (1972), the failure rate of Mark IV operations performed by a senior surgeon to be 5.9% as compared with 14.6% for those performed by house staff. "Unfortunately for surgical training programs," notes Orringer ruefully, "this difference is highly significant ($P = .001$)."

COMMENTS AND CONTROVERSIES

Acceptance of the value to the patient of any surgical procedure is determined by (1) immediate and permanent symptomatic relief; (2) acceptable risk; and (3) freedom from subsequent relapse and long-term complications. For the surgeon, there are additional criteria: patient symptomatic satisfaction, certainly, but in addition, objective confirmation of the lasting correction of the basic physio-

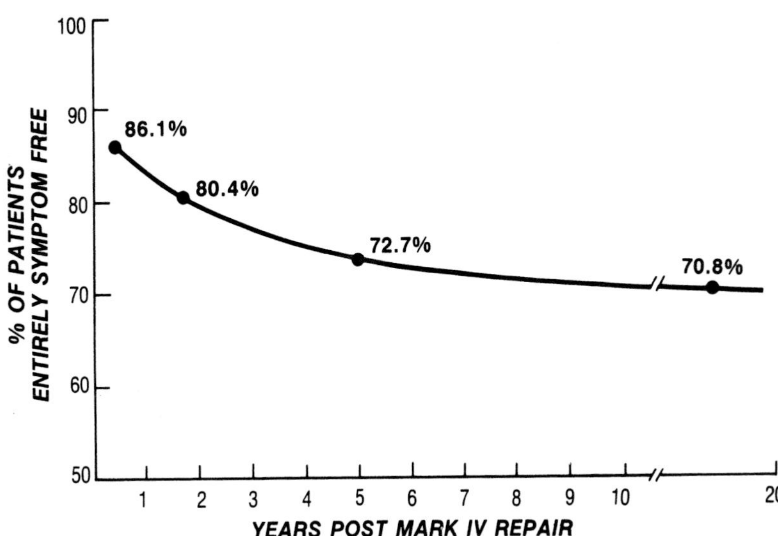

FIGURE 21–10 ■ Follow-up of 209 patients who underwent surgery with the Mark IV technique. Ten percent of component failures were not noticed until the 2nd decade. (From Hiebert CA, O'Mara CB: The Belsey operation for hiatal hernia: A twenty-year experience. Am J Surg 137:532, 1979.)

pathology or anatomic defect responsible for the patient's presenting symptoms. Hence there is a necessity for long-term routine follow-up consultations. If sufficiently self-critical, surgeons may be satisfied with their personal concept of the late results, assuming that they are dedicated to the "follow-up philosophy." Not all surgeons are so dedicated.

Surgeons intimately involved in a specialist discipline are inevitably involved in teaching programs. The fruits of these programs should be as important to them as the success of their personal activities. If a technique cannot be communicated to other surgeons, experienced or in training, a fundamental error exists in that technique. There is no place for "secret" operations that can be performed successfully only by an individual surgeon. Objective corroboration of the advantages, or defects, of any surgical technique from other centers is an essential element in the assessment of the value of that technique. I therefore welcome this review of the Mark IV procedure by Hiebert and Lerut.

R. H. R. Belsey

■ KEY REFERENCES

Belsey R: Mark IV repair of hiatal hernia by the transthoracic approach. World J Surg 1:475, 1977.

These notes by the inventor of the Mark IV repair are "presented in the hope that they will help the budding exponent of this technique to avoid some of the errors that have caused confusion and disappointment in the past . . . short of a practical demonstration of the technique, [the author] has done his best."

DeMeester TR, Wernly JA, Bryant GH, et al: Clinical and in vitro analysis of determinants of gastroesophageal competence. Am J Surg 137:39, 1979.

This report gives experimental confirmation of the Belsey principle that competency of the gastroesophageal function depends on a 4- to 5-cm length of subdiaphragmatic esophagus.

Hiebert CA: Surgical management of esophageal reflux and hiatal hernia: Classics in thoracic surgery. Ann Thorac Surg 52:159, 1991.

This article contains an invited commentary by Belsey's first overseas senior registrar, 25 years after publication of Skinner and Belsey's landmark paper on the use of the Mark IV operation in the management of patients with gastroesophageal reflux.

Skinner DB, Belsey RHR: Surgical management of esophageal reflux and hiatus hernia. J Thorac Cardiovasc Surg 53:33, 1967.

Whether judged by fresh insights, number of cases, or length of follow-up, the Skinner–Belsey report was a winner 33 years ago and remains so today.

■ REFERENCES

Allison PR: Reflux esophagitis, sliding hiatal hernia, and the anatomy of repair. Surg Gynecol Obstet 92:419, 1951.

Allison PR: Hiatus hernia: A 20-year retrospective survey. Ann Surg 178:273, 1973.

Baue AR: The Belsey Mark V procedure. Ann Thorac Surg 29:265, 1980.

Belsey R: Diaphragmatic hernia. In Modern Trends in Gastroenterology. London, Butterworths, 1952, p 163.

Fenton KN, Miller JM Jr, Lee RB, Mansour KA: Belsey Mark IV antireflux procedure for complicated gastroesophageal reflux disease. Ann Thorac Surg 64:790, 1997.

Hiebert CA: Antireflux surgery by the thoracic approach. In Rob & Smith's Operative Surgery. Jamieson GJ, Debas HT (eds): Surgery of the Upper Gastrointestinal Tract, 5th ed. London, Chapman & Hall, 1994, p. 301.

Hiebert CA, Belsey R: Incompetency of the gastric cardia without radiologic evidence of hiatal hernia. J Thorac Cardiovasc Surg 53:33, 1961.

Hiebert CA, O'Mara CS: The Belsey operation for hiatal hernia: A twenty-year experience. Am J Surg 137:532, 1979.

Landreneau RJ, Weichmann RS, Hazelrigg et al: Gastroesophageal reflux disease. Ann Thorac Surg 66:1886, 1998.

Lerut T, Coosemans W, Christiaens R, Gruwez JA: The Belsey Mark IV antireflux procedure: Reflections on indications and long-term results. Acta Gastroenterol Belg 13:585, 1990.

Nissen R: Eine einfache Operation zur Beinflussung der Refluxoesophagitis. Schweiz Med Wochenschr 86:590, 1956.

Nissen R: Reminiscences—reflux esophagitis and hiatal hernia. Rev Surg 307:14, 1970.

Nissen R: Gastropexy and fundoplication in surgical treatment of hiatus hernia. Am J Dig Dis 6:954, 1961.

Orringer MB, Belsey RHR, Skinner DB: Long-term results of the Mark IV operation for hiatal hernia and analyses of recurrences and their treatment. J Thorac Cardiovasc Surg 63:25, 1972.

Pearson FG, Henderson RD: Long-term follow-up of peptic strictures managed by dilatation, modified Collis gastroplasty, and Belsey hiatus hernia repair. Surgery 80:396, 1976.

Skinner DB, Belsey RH: Surgical management of esophageal reflux and hiatus hernia: Long-term results with 1,030 patients. J Thorac Cardiovasc Surg 53:33, 1967.

Skinner DB, Belsey RHR: Management of Esophageal Disease. Philadelphia, WB Saunders, 1988.

CHAPTER **22**

The Hill Repair

Lucius D. Hill*
Ralph W. Aye
Claes Nilsson

DEFINITION

The Hill repair can be described as the restoration of the gastroesophageal junction (GEJ) with posterior anchoring and reconstruction of the flap-valve mechanism of the gastroesophageal valve (GEV), calibration of the cardia, and intraoperative measurement of the lower esophageal sphincter (LES) pressure. Clinical and experimental evidence has shown that gastroesophageal reflux results from the loss of competence of the gastroesophageal antireflux barrier.

HISTORICAL NOTE

Over the course of time, several factors have been suggested to explain the antireflux barrier. They include the LES, the diaphragm, the phrenoesophageal membrane, the GEV, and the intra-abdominal location of the GEJ (Lyons et al, 1956). The importance of a physiologic flap-valve mechanism was not sufficiently recognized until the last decade (1990s), however, despite previous reports describing such a mechanism (Barrett, 1954; Braune, 1878; Collis et al, 1954; von Gubaroff, 1886).

*Deceased.

In 1977, Hill reported a procedure consisting of calibration of the lower esophageal sphincter and posterior fixation of the GEJ to the median arcuate ligament. This procedure became known as the *Hill repair* (Hill, 1977; Kraemer et al, 1992).

■ *HISTORICAL READINGS*

Hill LD: Progress in the surgical management of hiatal hernia. World J Surg 1:425, 1977.

Kraemer SJM, Hill LD, Low DE: The Hill repair: Reconstruction of the gastroesophageal junction and the flap valve for gastroesophageal reflux. In Nyhus LM, Baker R (eds): Mastery of Surgery, 2nd ed. Boston, Little, Brown, 1992, p 534.

ANATOMY AND PHYSIOLOGY

In order to correct the failed antireflux barrier, the surgeon must understand the components of the barrier. The pertinent anatomy is illustrated in Figure 22–1. The antireflux barrier consists of the LES, the GEV, the diaphragm, posterior fixation of the GEJ, and esophageal clearance. In 1956, Fyke and associates produced manometric evidence of a lower esophageal sphincter (Fyke et

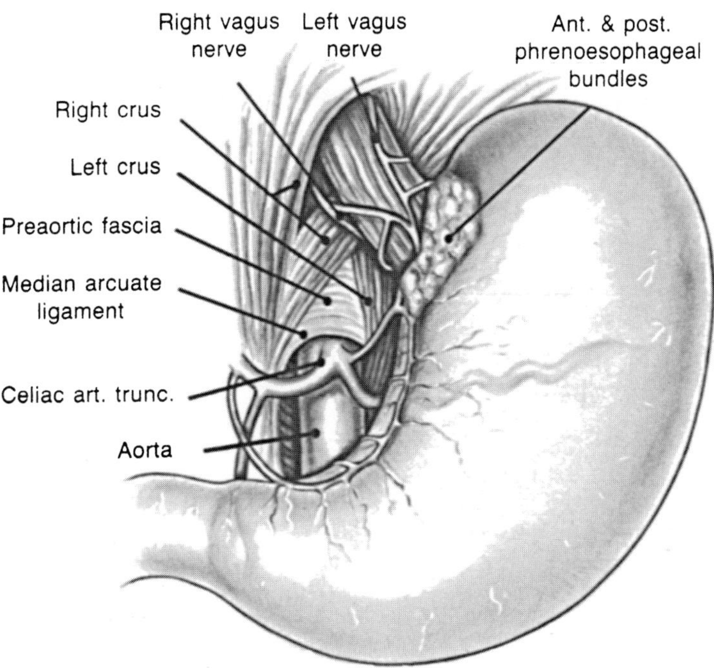

FIGURE 22–1 ■ Anatomic overview and relationship of the structures at the gastroesophageal junction.

al, 1956). All attention was then focused on the LES as the sole barrier to reflux. The GEV mechanism has been largely ignored. With development of the fiberoptic endoscope and the ability to view the GEJ with retroflexion of the scope, it became clear to us that the GEV is an important component of the antireflux barrier.

In cadaver and clinical experiments, we have shown that the GEV is an important component of the antireflux barrier. The GEV is a musculomucosal fold created by the angle of entry of the esophagus into the stomach. It extends 3 to 4 cm along the lesser curve of the stomach. Our studies led to the development of the following grading system (Fig. 22–2):

Grade I: GEV is normal, with a musculomucosal fold that hugs the scope through all phases of respiration, opens during swallowing, and then closes promptly without allowing reflux.
Grade II: GEV is a less well-defined fold, slightly shorter, which opens during swallowing and thereafter closes promptly.
Grade III: GEV opens frequently, remains open for varying lengths of time, and may be associated with an intermittent hiatal hernia.
Grade IV: No GEV is evident. The GEJ is wide open and is always associated with a hiatal hernia.

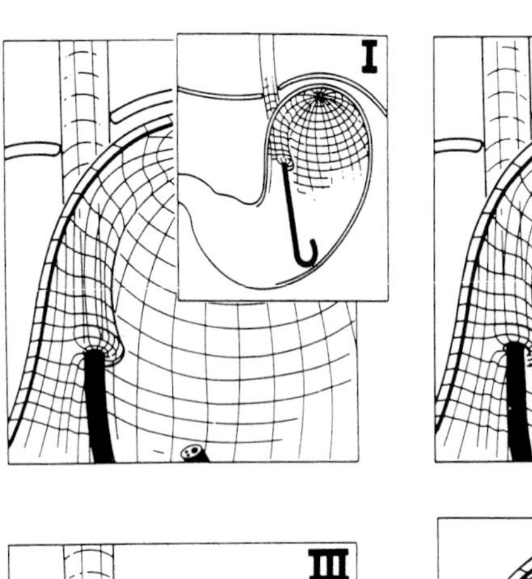

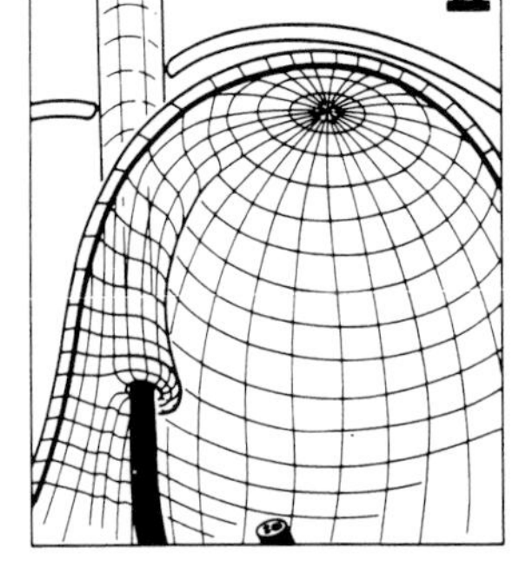

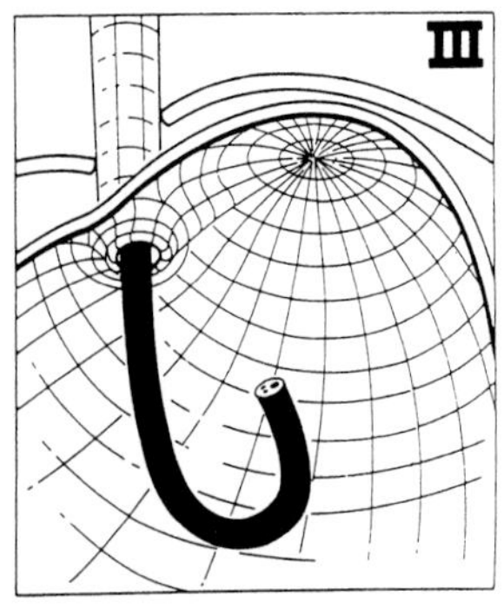

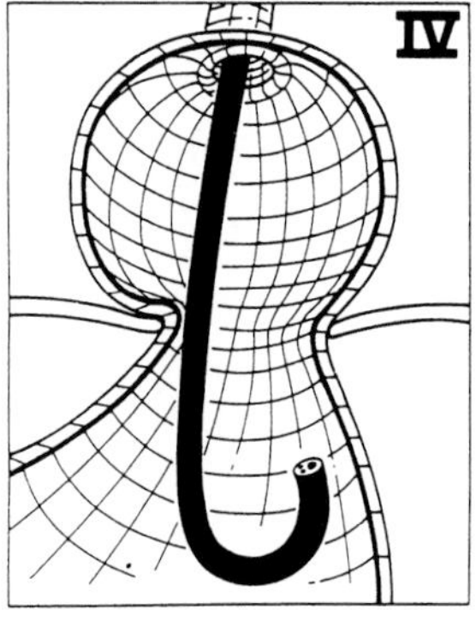

FIGURE 22–2 ■ Grading of the gastroesophageal valve (GEV). *Grade I,* Well-defined GEV, created through the oblique angle in which the esophagus enters the stomach. A mucosal fold is opposed in the endoscope through all phases of respiration and Valsalva maneuver. *Grade II,* Well-defined mucosal fold, which opens occasionally and closes promptly. *Grade III,* Poorly defined mucosal fold, which opens frequently and closes slowly or incompletely. *Grade IV,* No defined mucosal fold; open orifice, accompanied by a hiatal hernia.

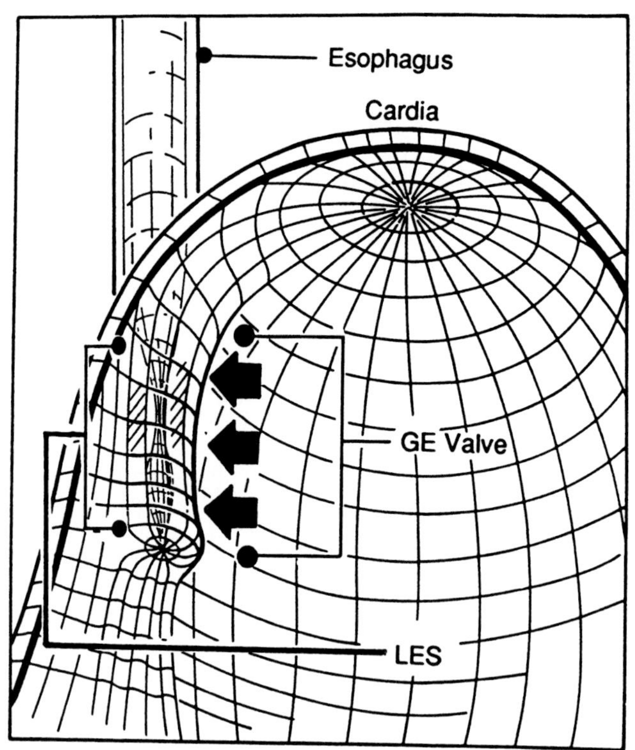

FIGURE 22–3 ■ The gastroesophageal flap valve mechanism and the high-pressure zone *(diagonal lines)* in relation to the gastroesophageal junction in a computer-generated view. *Arrows* indicate pressure vectors. GE, gastroesophageal; LES, lower esophageal sphincter.

Figure 22–3 is a composite drawing of the GEJ. The sphincter resides in the valve and increases its efficiency.

This anatomic and physiologic concept is illustrated in *Gray's Anatomy* (Gray et al, 1995), and our observations have been confirmed by Contractor and associates (1999) in Saudi Arabia. Öberg and coworkers (1999) have graded the efficiency of the GEV and concluded that it is useful in the understanding and management of gastroesophageal reflux disease (GERD) (Fig. 22–4). We believe it is important that any surgical procedure aim at restoring the GEV. This valve is a 180-degree mucosal fold that is a highly competent antireflux mechanism. Antireflux procedures that create a 360-degree valve or fold cause "gas bloat."

In addition to restoration of the valve, calibration of the LES is important and can be done with intraoperative measurements of the sphincter pressure during surgery. The relationship of the LES to the valve is shown in Figure 22–3. This computer-generated view shows that the sphincter resides inside the valve and helps the valve discriminate between gas, liquids, and solids. While the LES does the discriminatory work, the valve does the "heavy" work in preventing reflux. Increased intragastric pressure serves to compress and close the valve against the lesser curve side of the hiatus. The barrier can withstand enormous pressures that would overwhelm a weak sphincter if it were the sole barrier to reflux.

Posterior fixation of the GEV is also an important issue. The esophagus is normally fixed posteriorly by a

Endoscopic Grading of the Gastroesophageal Valve in Patients with Symptoms of Gastroesophageal Reflux Disease. Stefan Öberg, MD, Jeffrey H. Peters, MD, Reginald Lord, MD, Jan Johansson, MD, Steven R. DeMeester, Peter F. Crookes, MD, Jeffrey A. Hagen, Tom R. DeMeester, MD, Department of Surgery, University of Southern California, Los Angeles

Endoscopic grading of the geometry of the gastroesophageal valve (Hill grading) has been suggested to be a better predictor of the reflux status than the LES pressure. The aim of this study was to test the usefulness of the Hill grading system in the evaluation of patients with symptoms of GERD.

Two hundred and sixty-eight consecutive patients with symptoms suggestive of GERD underwent upper gastrointestinal endoscopy, esophageal manometry, and 24-hour pH monitoring between August 1996 and April 1998. The geometry of the gastroesophageal valve was graded endoscopically, from I–IV, according to criteria published by Hill. Esophageal acid exposure, LES characteristics, and degree of esophageal mucosal injury were assessed in patients with varying Hill grades.

	Hill Grade I	*Hill Grade II*	*Hill Grade III*	*Hill Grade IV*
No.	43	57	71	97
% Esophagitis	0.0 (0/43)	10.5 (10/57)*	26.8 (19/71)*	46.4 (45/97)†
% Barrett's esophagus	0.0 (0/43)	24.0 (8/57)*	15.5 (11/71)*	32.0 (31/97)†
% Increased acid exposure	11.6 (5/43)	49.1 (28/57)*	54.9 (39/71)*	75.3 (73/97)†
% Defective LES	20.9 (9/43)	56.1 (3257)*	60.6 (43/71)*	87.6 (86/97)†

$P < .05$ vs. Hill grade I

$P < .05$ vs. Hill grades I, II, and IV.

Increased esophageal acid exposure and mucosal injury [were] uncommon in patients with Hill grade I. LES length and pressure decreased with increasing Hill grade. The presence of a grade IV valve predicted increased esophageal acid exposure in 75% of the patients. The predictive value of Hill grading was similar to LES pressure and length but not as good as the presence of esophagitis (88%) or Barrett's esophagus (82%).

The endoscopic appearance of the gastroesophageal valve is a useful predictor of the presence of GERD. It may be used as a complement to esophageal manometry and pH monitoring in the evaluation of patients with symptoms of GERD.

GERD, gastroesophageal reflux disease; LES, lower esophageal sphincter.

FIGURE 22–4 ■ Report from the Peters and DeMeester group using the grading system. (Modified from Öberg S, Peters JH, Lord R, et al: Endoscopic grading of the gastroesophageal valve in patients with symptoms of GERD. Surg Endosc 13:1184–1188, 1999.)

layer of fibroareolar tissue extending from the median arcuate ligament up to the aortic arch. This fixation is lost when a hiatal hernia develops and the GEJ ascends into the posterior mediastinum (Fig. 22–5). The esophagus can no longer generate propulsive waves that are necessary for esophageal clearance because it no longer has a fulcrum from which to work. The posterior attachment of the GEJ (by the dorsal mesentery to the preaortic fascia) is key to restoration of the normal barrier to reflux. In cadavers, with division of the posterior attachments, the GEJ can slide into the chest, thereby losing an effective barrier. This condition can be seen with a retroflexed endoscope in humans. When the GEJ ascends into the posterior mediastinum, the valve disappears and the sphincter is open. Reattachment of the GEJ is thus important for restoration of esophageal function.

Closure of the enlarged diaphragmatic opening is important to prevent recurrence of hiatal hernia. The diaphragm should be closed loosely about the esophagus so that at least one finger can be placed alongside the esophagus with a nasogastric tube in the lumen. In the laparoscopic repair, a bougie is used because the surgeon cannot palpate the opening. Fixation of the cardia to the rim of the diaphragm is important both to accentuate the valve and to close the opening into the posterior mediastinum and thereby prevent paraesophageal herniation into the posterior mediastinum.

One may summarize the goals of surgery as follows:

1. Restoration of the GEV.
2. Calibration of the LES to the proper range.
3. Posterior fixation of the GEJ to restore esophageal peristalsis and clearance.

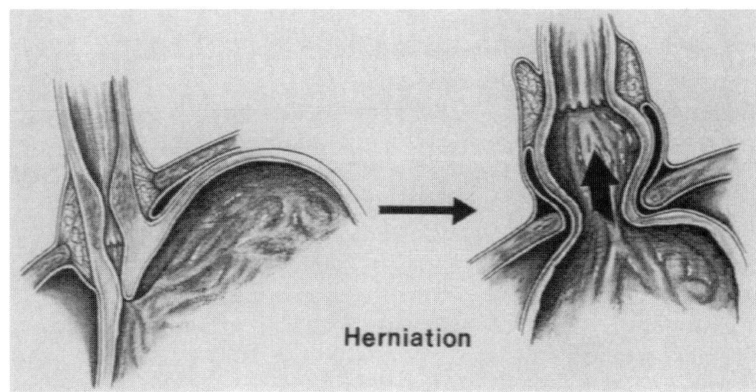

FIGURE 22–5 ■ Development of a hiatal hernia (an axial hiatal hernia is depicted) is associated with loss of the posterior fixation of the gastroesophageal junction, leading to the loss of the angle of His, which in turn causes a loss of the gastroesophageal valve.

4. Reduction of the hiatal hernia.
5. Closure of the diaphragm.

PREOPERATIVE EVALUATION

Preoperative evaluation of the symptoms of GERD should identify the presence and severity of reflux and its potential complications as well as exclude or document coexistent problems. Upper gastrointestinal radiographs, although the most common initial examination, are somewhat insensitive to reflux. Radiographs, however, can demonstrate stenosis along with its level and extent, ulceration, and the type of hiatal hernia present.

Other, more objective tests include esophageal manometry with pH studies. These tests are important to establish the level of acid in the stomach, the volume of acid that is refluxing into the esophagus, and the pressure of the LES. Such studies can be used postoperatively to test the success of the operation. In our laboratory, a sphincter pressure of less than 10 mm Hg raises the question of sphincter incompetence. A sphincter pressure in the range of 30 mm Hg or more suggests the possibility of a hypertensive sphincter. In addition, manometric testing can demonstrate the motility of the esophagus and the presence of high-pressure simultaneous waves, which should raise the suspicion of diffuse esophageal spasm.

In our experience, 24-hour pH monitoring is reserved when endoscopy and esophageal manometry have not clarified the problem; pH testing also identifies a subpopulation of patients with reflux who show a greater propensity for reflux in the upright position with little or no reflux in the supine position.

Preoperative endoscopy, with or without biopsy, provides valuable information regarding the presence of esophagitis, ulceration, and Barrett's esophagus and serves to rule out carcinoma. Grading of the valve as previously described yields valuable information.

Radionuclide studies are an additional valuable test for the detection of reflux, especially in patients who cannot tolerate or who refuse intubation for pH and manometric studies. Russell and Velasco (1988) clearly demonstrated that radionuclide studies can show reflux and can help distinguish early achalasia from diffuse spasm and other motility disorders. They also serve to detect delayed gastric emptying.

MANAGEMENT

Operative Technique

The Hill repair is performed both by the conventional *open technique* and *laparoscopically*.

The Hill repair is unique because of the addition of the crucial surgical maneuver that anchors the GEJ to the preaortic fascia (Larrain, 1971; Larrain et al, 1992). This anchor gives the esophagus a fulcrum from which it can generate propulsive peristaltic waves to propel a bolus aborally. The esophagus is not placed under tension but rather is fixed posteriorly, where it is normally positioned. The esophagus resumes normal motility and clearance from this restored point of fixation.

The restored GEV, like the natural valve, is a 180-degree valve. (In contrast, in the Nissen repair, a 360-degree valve is created [Matikainen and Kaukinen, 1984; Lundell et al, 1991].) The 180-degree valve allows important functions, such as belching, and thus avoids gas bloat, through simple depression of the fundus through the diaphragm, leading to a more obtuse angle of His and allowing air to be vented (see Fig. 22–3).

In 1978, Hill first reported on the use of intraoperative manometry with a modified nasogastric tube (Island Scientific, Bainbridge Island, Wash.) to verify objectively whether an adequate pressure barrier has been created (Hill, 1978). Since then, the method has been further simplified to allow the surgeon to calibrate the antireflux pressure barrier by loosening or tightening the "calibrating repair stitches" during the repair and thus to provide objective information.

The Hill repair is performed through a midline incision (Fig. 22–6). The xiphoid process may be removed to enhance exposure. For maximum exposure, the use of a table-mounted, self-retaining "upper hand" retractor (V. Mueller) or a similar (e.g., Rochard [Aesculap]) retractor is invaluable. An additional Balfour retractor may improve the exposure.

The abdomen is thoroughly explored, with careful attention given to the pyloroduodenal region to exclude peptic ulcer disease. Pyloric stenosis should be treated with appropriate surgery when significant obstruction is present. The attachment of the left lobe of the liver is released by division of the anterior and posterior leaves of the triangular ligament parallel to the liver edge. Care is taken not to injure the phrenic vein. The left lobe of the liver is retracted inferiorly, to the patient's right. After dividing the peritoneum of the lesser sac vertically, the surgeon incises the phrenoesophageal membrane at its diaphragmatic origin, over the esophageal hiatus, to expose the underlying esophagus and herniated stomach. This membrane is divided high on the diaphragm to preserve the phrenoesophageal bundles (Fig. 22–7), which are of major importance for the subsequent repair.

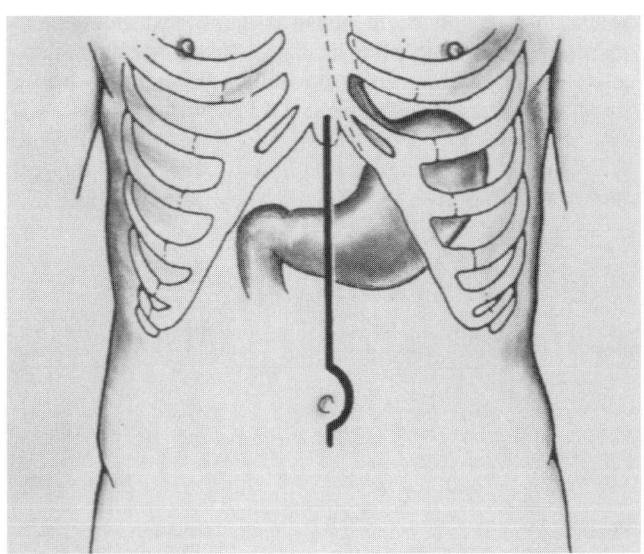

FIGURE 22–6 ■ The upper median abdominal incision is preferred. To enhance exposure, the surgeon may remove the xiphoid process.

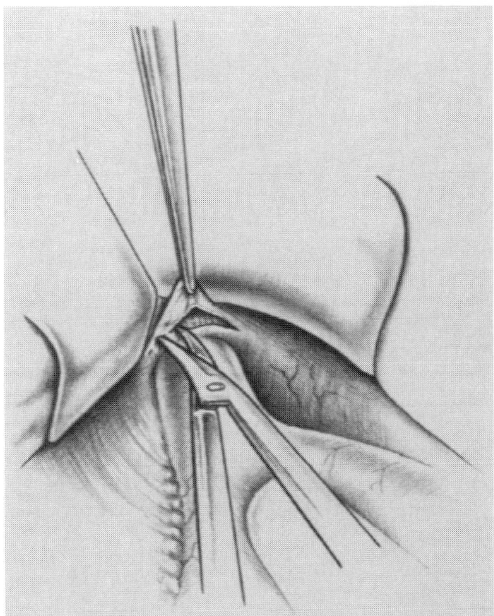

FIGURE 22–7 ■ Dissection of the pre-esophageal peritoneum is carried out as high as possible on its diaphragmatic attachments in order to retain the phrenoesophageal bundles as much as possible.

The esophageal hiatus is now clearly visible. Careful dissection of the posterior aspect of the esophagus (Fig. 22–8) with division of any adhesions, while gentle traction is exerted simultaneously on the stomach, exposes the crura and allows return of the herniated stomach to the abdominal cavity. Great care should be taken to preserve the vagus nerves. A 3- to 4-cm length of intra-abdominal esophagus is regularly obtained.

An accessory hepatic artery arising from the left gastric artery is often encountered in the gastrohepatic ligament and is usually divided and ligated (Fig. 22–9). The dissection is carried through the superior portion of the gastrohepatic ligament, exposing the caudate lobe of the liver.

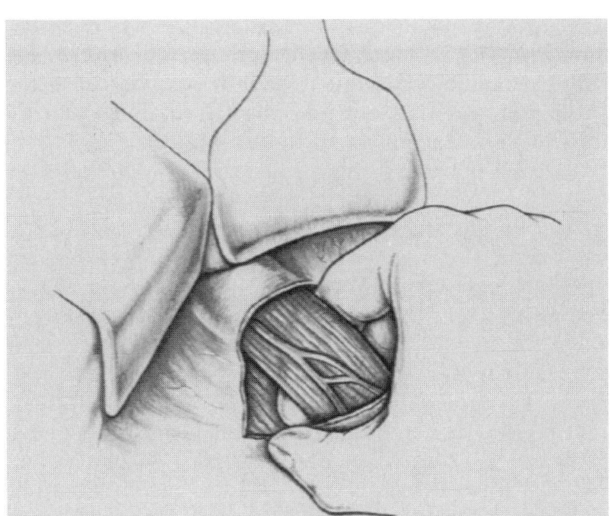

FIGURE 22–8 ■ The surgeon performs blunt and/or sharp mobilization of the esophagus in order to divide the posterior attachments of the gastroesophageal junction.

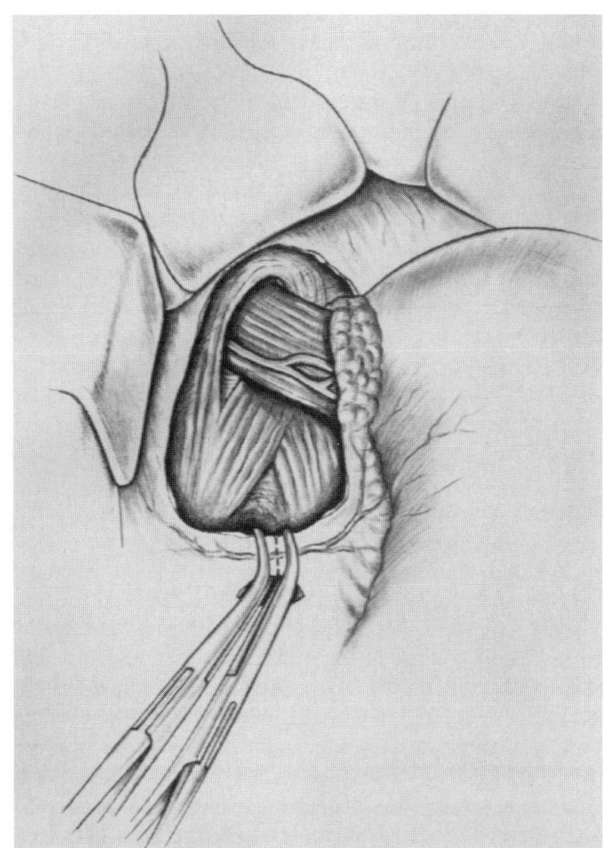

FIGURE 22–9 ■ The dissection is carried through the superior portion of the gastrohepatic ligament, where an accessory gastrohepatic artery (arising from the left gastric artery) is usually encountered, which may be ligated and divided as shown.

These maneuvers expose the right crus and the preaortic fascia and give access to the median arcuate ligament.

The gastric fundus is partially mobilized by division of the phrenogastric and superior portions of the gastrolienal ligaments. The tip of the spleen is exposed. This procedure may require careful ligation of one or two superior short gastric vessels (Fig. 22–10). Inspection of the cardiac region of the stomach now reveals an anterior and posterior bundle of fascial condensation. These bundles, the gastric portions of the severe phrenoesophageal ligament, are important structures in the procedure. If care has been taken earlier to divide the phrenoesophageal ligament close to the diaphragmatic origin, the ligament will be substantial.

The surgeon opens the esophageal hiatus by dividing the areolar tissue above the aorta. A finger is placed beneath the preaortic fascia, lifting it off the aorta (Fig. 22–11). It is not necessary to dissect out the median arcuate ligament. Use of the preaortic fascia is preferable for fixation.

The safest approach to the preaortic fascia requires exposure of the esophageal hiatus, division of the fibroareolar tissue ventral to the aorta, and passage of the index finger down behind the preaortic fascia. The celiac artery is easily palpable at the tip of the finger. Elevating the preaortic fascia and the crura of the diaphragm with

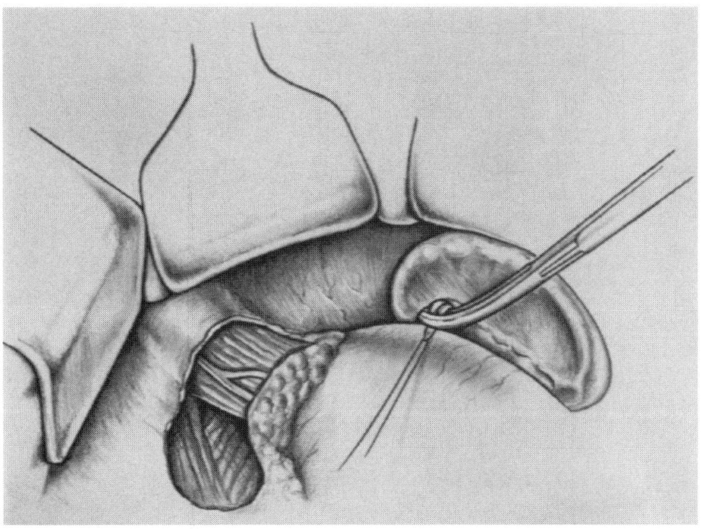

FIGURE 22–10 ■ Sometimes the surgeon must divide some superior short gastric vessels in order to partially free the gastroesophageal junction and the fundus.

the finger enables the surgeon to place a long Babcock clamp on the preaortic fascia and the confluence of both crura above the celiac axis (Fig. 21–12). Lifting on this Babcock clamp then allows the surgeon to pass the crural stitches safely along the side of the clamp without injury to the aorta.

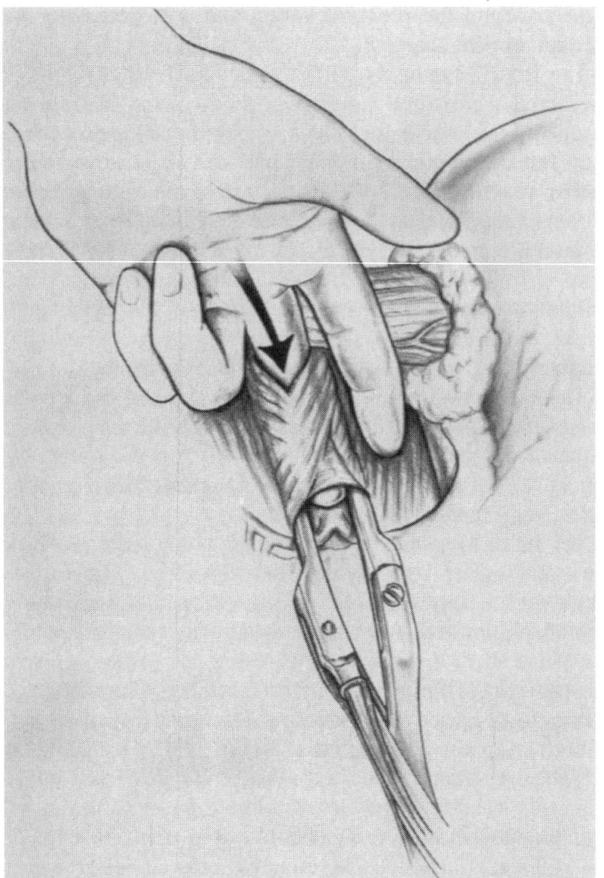

FIGURE 22–11 ■ A safe approach to the preaortic fascia includes division of the fibroareolar tissue ventral to the aorta and passage of a finger down behind the preaortic fascia. Placement of a Goodell dilator underneath the dissected median arcuate ligament is shown here.

If the median arcuate ligament is used for esophageal fixation, the free edge of the ligament is identified and retracted, and a Goodell cervical dilator is passed underneath this free edge in the cephalad direction (see Fig. 22–11). As the dilator is passed, little or no resistance should be encountered if the instrument is in the correct tissue plane. To avoid damage to the aorta or the celiac artery, the surgeon should never force passage of the instrument.

The crura of the esophageal hiatus are loosely approximated with at least two heavy through-and-through nonabsorbable sutures, which should include fascia and peritoneum as well as muscle. We prefer to use size 0 sutures with small polytetrafluoroethylene (polytef, Teflon) pledgets (5 × 5 mm). The crura are approximated posterior to the esophagus. At completion, passage of an index finger alongside the esophagus with its indwelling nasogastric tube should be easily possible. If the hiatus is still too loose, a third or fourth suture should be added (Fig. 22–13). After hiatal closure, the anterior and posterior phrenoesophageal bundles are exposed and elevated with Babcock clamps. The anterior and posterior divisions of the vagus nerves must be visualized to avoid their subsequent damage or inclusion by sutures.

A strong nonabsorbable suture with one polytef pledget is then placed close to the cephalad end of the anterior bundle and the angle of His. A deep bite is taken that includes the seromuscular layers of the stomach. This suture is passed cephalad through the posterior phrenoesophageal bundle and preaortic fascia, just cranial to the median arcuate ligament. If the Babcock clamp has been carefully positioned and retracted, there is no risk to the aorta, because elevation separates the ligament and the aorta by 2 to 3 cm. The needle is passed alongside the Babcock clamp (Fig. 22–14), and a second polytef pledget is then threaded. The suture is not tied until all other stitches have been placed, a practice that preserves good exposure throughout the procedure. Polytef pledgets are routinely used for the diaphragm stitches and the three upper repair stitches.

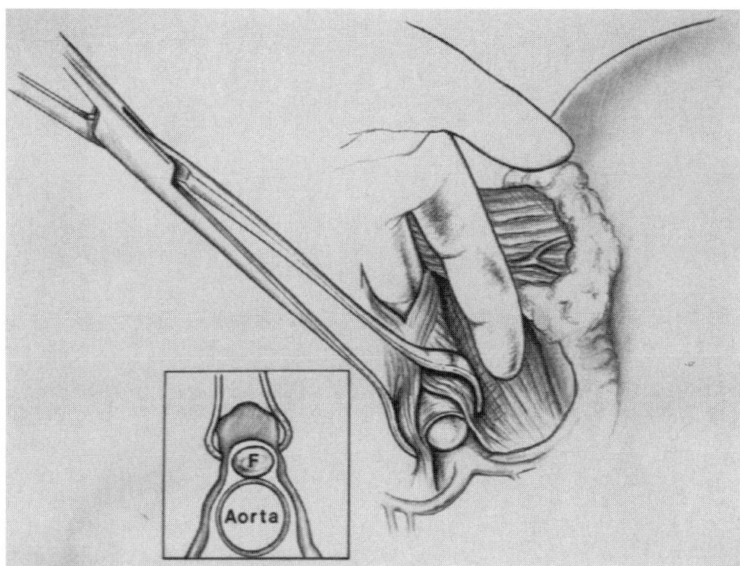

FIGURE 22–12 ■ The safest and most commonly used approach to the preaortic fascia involves lifting it off the aorta with a finger (F) and grasping it with a long Babcock clamp above the celiac axis.

Four more sutures are placed in like manner caudad to the initial suture (Fig. 22–15). Care is taken to ensure that both vagus nerves lie within the approximated bundles. At this point, the three upper sutures are tied with a single throw, and each is secured with a long clamp to prevent slipping of the knot. This maneuver approximates the phrenoesophageal bundles and tightens the "collar sling" musculature, which accentuates the angle of His, recreates the GEV, and augments the LES pressure.

During this stage, calibration of the LES is necessary to provide a barrier to reflux that is adequate but not excessive. Intraoperative manometry with a perfused catheter system is valuable in this calibration, which is most easily accomplished with the use of a modified nasogastric tube attached to a pressure monitor. The manometric measurements can be recorded effectively with a regular manometry recorder or with arterial line pressure transducers and the cardiac monitoring equipment that is present in any operating room. Adjusting suture tension creates an intraluminal pressure of between 35 and 40 mm Hg. The pressure should not exceed this level, because higher pressures would cause dysphagia; an intraoperative pressure lower than 25 mm Hg may allow reflux. When the desired suture tension has been

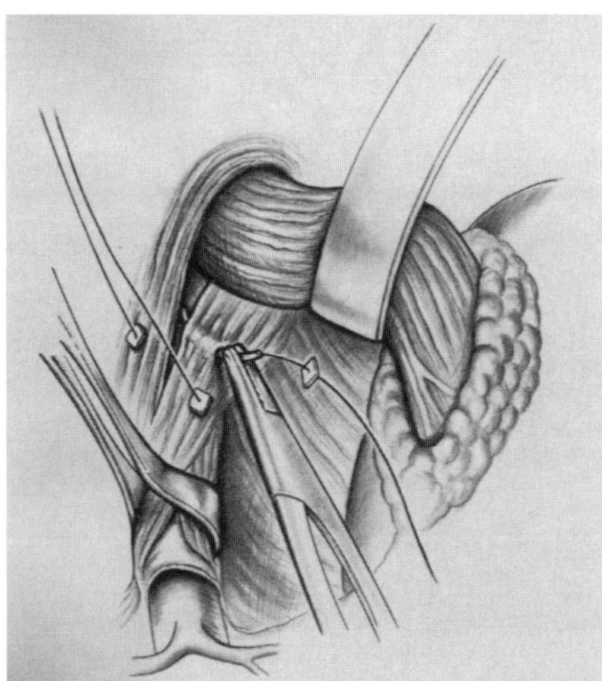

FIGURE 22–13 ■ The right crus is closed with interrupted sutures with small polytetrafluoroethylene (Teflon) pledgets.

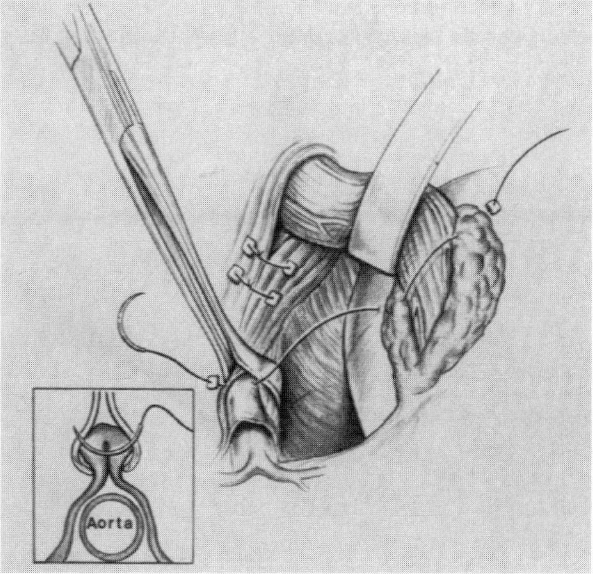

FIGURE 22–14 ■ A nonabsorbable 0 suture with polytetrafluoroethylene (Teflon) pledget is placed close to the angle of His deep into the anterior bundle to include the seromuscular layers of the stomach. It is then passed through the posterior bundle in the same way and through the preaortic fascia as shown while the surgeon lifts it off the aorta with the Babcock clamp. Note how the needle is passed alongside the clamp *(inset)* for additional safety.

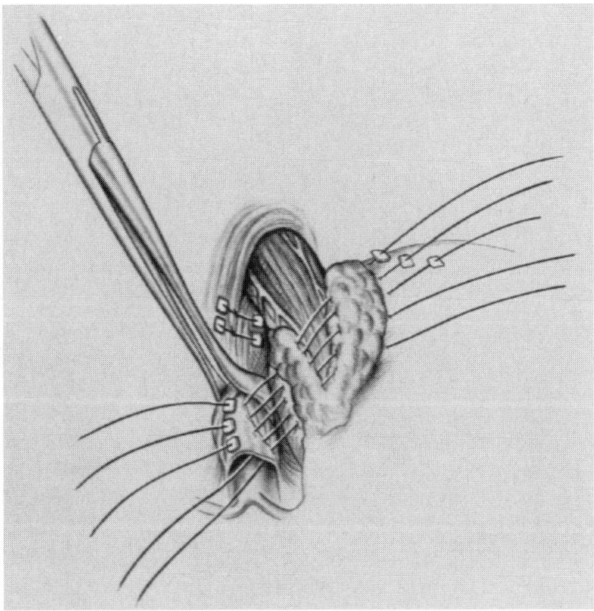

FIGURE 22–15 ■ Completed repair before the surgeon ties the sutures with a single throw to perform intraoperative manometry. The vagus nerves must be carefully avoided.

achieved, the knots are completed and the remaining sutures are tied down.

Figure 22–16 shows the completed in situ repair with the accentuated flap-valve mechanism in relief. The completed repair is firmly anchored in the abdomen and provides a 3- to 4-cm segment of intra-abdominal esophagus. The restored flap valve can be palpated through the stomach wall against the nasogastric tube. The valve can be further strengthened by placement of three to five additional stitches (using nonabsorbable 2–0 sutures) from the gastric fundus to the diaphragm (see Fig. 22–16). This step further accentuates the angle of His and secures the GEJ in its abdominal location.

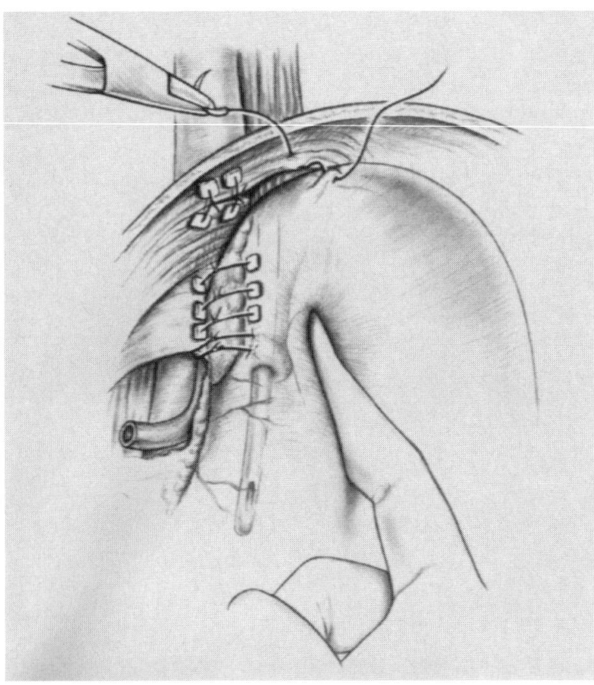

FIGURE 22–16 ■ Completed Hill repair. Both the accentuated fold and the tightness of the valve can be palpated through the stomach wall, which should allow the tip of the index finger to pass alongside the Hill tube. Additional nonabsorbable sutures (2–0) from the fundus to the hiatus further reinforce the angle of His and secure the gastroesophageal junction against the danger of ever herniating again.

Operation for Recurrence

The presence of adhesions, the loss of normal tissue planes, and the increased risk of causing damage to the esophagus, stomach, and spleen make reoperation technically very difficult. Such surgery should not be undertaken by the occasional or inexperienced surgeon.

Intraoperative manometry is especially important in patients undergoing reoperation. The tissues used for the repair in such cases are often less pliable, attenuated, or even absent, making it difficult to ensure the quality of the repair. Hill and associates (1979, 1981) believe it crucial to use intraoperative manometry as an objective and reliable tool for the calibration of the antireflux barrier to better ensure an adequate and lasting repair. The polytef pledgets are important in these repairs because they promote fibrous ingrowth around the polytef, thereby augmenting and protecting the repair. In a 15-year period, we have seen only one complication involving a polytef pledget; in the case involved, we removed a pledget from the base of an esophageal ulcer, which healed rapidly. The phrenoesophageal bundles must be carefully preserved when the previous repair is taken down.

We have used a modification of the Hill repair following failed prior antireflux operations. After the failed repair is taken down, an elliptical incision is made around the esophageal hiatus 1.5 cm from the inner edge, beginning at one side of the crus and ending at the other (Fig. 22–17). This creates a viable muscular and tendinous sling that ascends from one side of the crus, encircles the esophagus in the angle of His, and descends to the other side of the crus. The pedicles are not dissected so that the blood supply is preserved. When the surgeon places tension on the anterior part of this muscular sling by pulling it caudad with a soft (Babcock) clamp, the angle of His is restored, reinforcing the GEV (Fig. 22–18). This procedure creates a competent GEJ, as intraoperative manometry and endoscopy have shown. The enlarged hiatus is then closed securely with heavy nonabsorbable mattress sutures protected with polytef pledgets. A primary tension-free closure is attempted. Remaining crural defects can be closed with a nonabsorbable mesh graft (see Fig. 21–18). It should be easy for the surgeon to pass an index finger alongside the esophagus.

Following closure of the hiatus, the Hill repair is performed as described previously. The muscular sling or diaphragm graft is then folded once anteriorly to shorten it to the desired length and is fixed to the crus with several nonabsorbable 2–0 sutures in a adequate position that will ensure stable fixation (see Fig. 22–18). We secure the fundus to the sling with 2–0 nonabsorbable

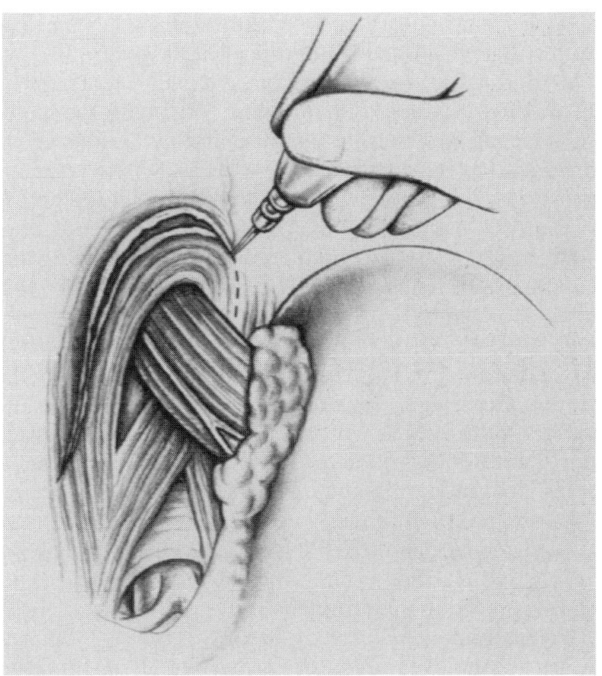

FIGURE 22–17 ■ Dissection of the diaphragm is carefully performed, in this case with the use of electrocautery.

sutures and stitch the top of the gastric fundus to the diaphragm with three to five stitches. This maneuver further lengthens the valve and secures the esophageal hiatus (Fig. 22–19).

Figure 22–20 shows the completed Hill repair with the addition of the diaphragm graft. This procedure is reserved for complicated reoperation procedures only. The short-term results are promising.

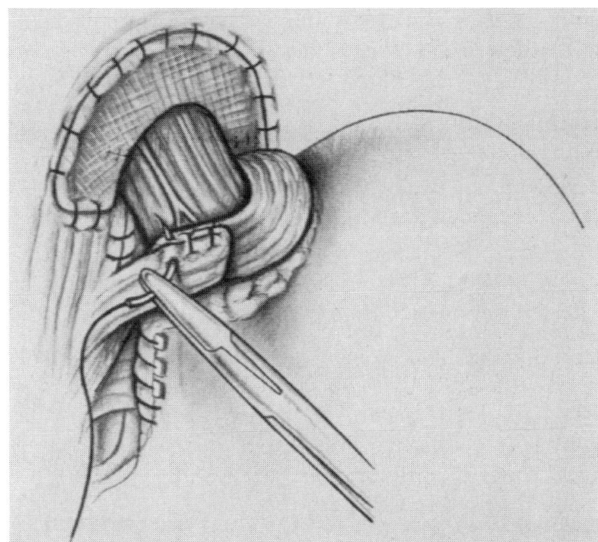

FIGURE 22–18 ■ The surgeon can easily improve the angle of His by applying traction to the diaphragmatic sling, first with a clamp and then by suturing it down after folding the excess tissue. The diaphragmatic hiatus is closed with mattress sutures and an additional nonabsorbable mesh graft.

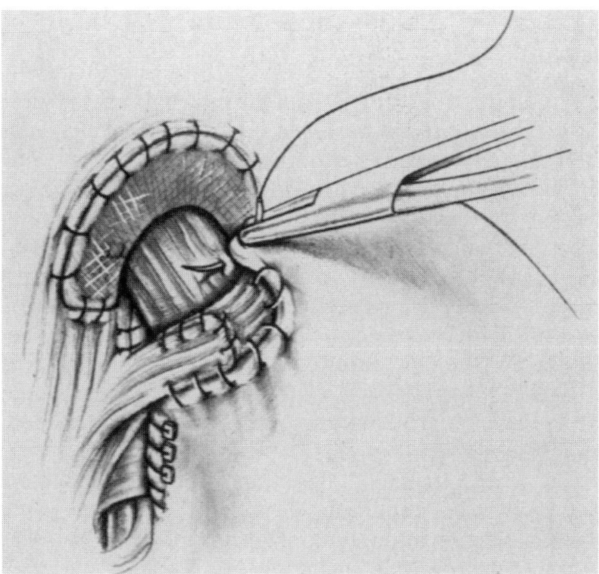

FIGURE 22–19 ■ The surgeon sutures the fundus of the stomach to the diaphragm graft to lengthen the valve.

Stricture

Hill and colleagues reported experience with peptic stricture in 1970 and in 1986 (Mercer and Hill, 1986). An effective antireflux procedure allows healing of most peptic strictures, making resection unnecessary. A single dilatation is a reasonable approach in the primary treatment of an esophageal stricture. Generally, this procedure should be performed after a careful evaluation. Our experience with 190 patients with stricture shows that multiple dilatations damage the esophagus and impair esophageal motility (Mercer and Hill, 1986). Resection is reserved for patients (1) who have undergone multiple dilatations, (2) in whom multiple antireflux procedures have failed, (3) in whom dilatation has caused injuries of the esophagus, or (4) who have associated diseases, such as severe scleroderma.

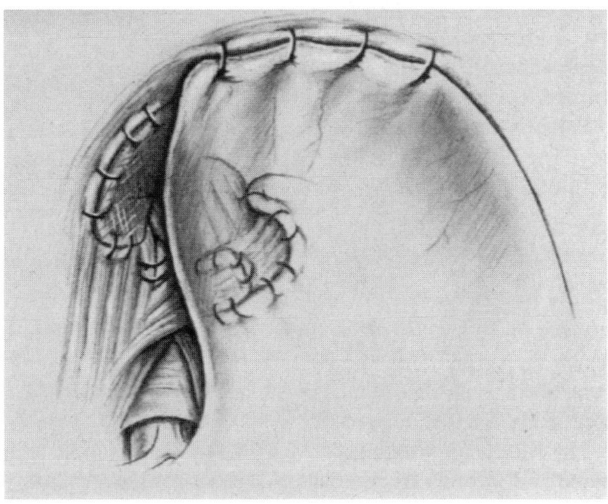

FIGURE 22–20 ■ Final aspect of the Hill repair with diaphragm graft and additional fundodiaphragmatic sutures to further secure the esophageal hiatus.

Surgical Technique: Laparoscopic Hill Repair

Laparoscopic Hill repair was performed in 33 pigs before we utilized it in humans. More than 600 laparoscopic Hill repairs have been performed since 1992.

The surgeon stands between the patient's legs with the assistant to the surgeon's right and the camera operator to the surgeon's left. Pneumoperitoneum is instituted by placement of the Veress needle just below the left costal margin, roughly 5 cm from the xiphoid in order to avoid the liver and the spleen. Five ports are usually used, but a sixth port may be required to retract the omentum in markedly obese patients. All ports are 5 mm except for the assistant's port and the surgeon's right-sided port, which are 10 mm (Fig. 22–21).

The liver retractor is placed, and the left lobe of the liver is retracted cephalad. The phrenoesophageal membrane is divided, and the esophagus is dissected out. The laparoscopic repair is essentially the same as the open repair. In blunt dissection, the confluence of both crura is often exposed, and following the left crus superiorly opens a retroesophageal space that allows exposure of the posterior wall of the stomach. The final part of this dissection includes defining the most caudal portion of the preaortic fascia marked at the level of emergence of the celiac axis. Both vagus nerves are carefully identified and avoided.

Next, the diaphragmatic hiatus is closed, with two to three sutures closing the opening loosely about the esophagus. Sutures are then taken in the anterior and posterior phrenoesophageal bundles. As in the open repair, these sutures are carried through the preaortic fascia, which the surgeon lifts off the aorta initially with a Babcock clamp and then by pulling upward on the first sutures that are placed in the preaortic fascia.

With the four sutures in place, a 43 French clean hollow dilator (Cook, Bloomington, Ind.) with the modified nasogastric (NG) tube through the middle (positioned so that the manometric port is 5–7 cm beyond the tip of the dilator) is positioned across the GEJ. The top two sutures are tied with a single throw in the knot and clamped. The dilator is pulled back, drawing the manometric port across the GEJ, and a manometric reading is obtained as in the open repair. When a pressure range of 25 to 35 mm Hg is reached, the sutures are all tied and a final manometric reading is obtained. If the reading is too high, the sutures are loosened; if it is too low, the sutures are tightened. Sutures are then placed from the anterior fundus to the diaphragm to prevent a paraesophageal hernia and to further augment the valve.

At this point, an endoscope is inserted and the valve is visualized. A grade I GEV must have been developed. If the valve has not been sufficiently developed by the surgical procedure, additional sutures are taken.

The wound is inspected for any bleeding, and the trocars are removed under direct vision. All 10-mm port sites are closed with a fascia-closing device, and subcuticular sutures are used for the skin.

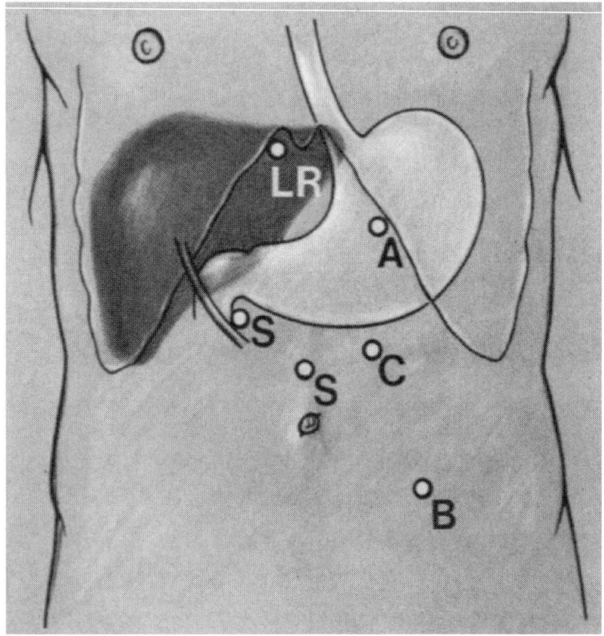

FIGURE 22–21 ■ The placement of the ports is shown for a laparoscopic Hill repair, with the surgeon standing at the right side of the patient. A, Assistant's work post; B, Babcock clamp; C, camera/laparoscope; LR, liver retractor; S, surgeon's work probe.

Postoperative Care

After a laparoscopic Hill repair, the NG tube is attached to low intermittent suction until the residue obtained after a 4-hour period with a tube clamped is less than 200 ml. This process usually takes 24 to 36 hours. Once the NG tube has been removed, clear liquids are started; if they are tolerated, diet is progressed to full liquid or pureed foods.

After a laparoscopic procedure is completed, the NG tube is removed immediately, and liquids are started the night of the procedure.

Patients are discharged with a soft diet and the caution that some dysphagia for solids is not uncommon during the first few weeks after surgery.

Results

Results of surgery are rated as follows:

Excellent: no significant symptoms
Good: heartburn requiring occasional medication
Fair: significant heartburn requiring medication on a regular basis
Poor: unimproved or worsened

Our (Hill and Aye) total experience, updated in 1999, consists of 2390 cases, of which 1880 involved open repairs followed for up to 33 years and 510 involved laparoscopic repairs. This experience represents the largest series of antireflux operations with long-term follow-up reported in the literature.

Open Hill Repair

An ongoing multi-institution review of the Hill repair has included 2253 open operations; 1784 were initial operations for reflux disease, and 469 were performed for failed antireflux surgery. The latter cases primarily involved patients with failed Nissen repairs who were referred from other institutions. The multi-institution study has shown that the Hill repair can be done with good to excellent results in other institutions. The centers include the University of Virginia, the University of Kansas, Massachusetts General Hospital, and Queens University in Canada. The results in these centers were categorized as good to excellent in 90% of cases, which were followed for an average of 12 years.

From an earlier group of 370 cases (Low et al, 1989), 140 cases were available for follow-up at 15 to 20 years. Among the cases involving only primary repairs, good to excellent results were obtained in 90% of cases followed for an average of 18 years.

We were interested to determine whether technologic and other advances have influenced outcome. We analyzed 200 cases from our experience before we began to use intraoperative manometry and 200 cases in which intraoperative manometry was used. The results in the premanometry cases showed 87% good to excellent results. Analysis of the 200 later cases, with use of calibration and intraoperative manometry, showed 95.6% good to excellent results over 5 years.

CONCLUSION

In our opinion, the Hill repair is the only antireflux operation that anchors the GEJ in its normal intra-abdominal position. Recurrent hernia is very rare. When the GEJ slides above the diaphragm, the esophagus "accordions" onto itself and cannot function normally. Restoration of normal esophageal length reestablishes normal mechanics and motility (Aye et al, 1997).

Endoscopic visualization of valve as well as intraoperative measurement of sphincter pressure has improved results over time.

The Hill repair is technically feasible as a laparoscopic procedure, providing a safe and effective antireflux repair. Our laparoscopic results are comparable to those obtained with the open technique.

COMMENTS AND CONTROVERSIES

Since the early 1960s, the Hill operation has been one of the internationally recognized repairs for hiatal hernia and gastroesophageal reflux disease. Like the Belsey Mark IV repair, the Hill operation is technically demanding and relatively hard to "teach." It is, therefore, difficult for the inexperienced or occasional surgeon to reproduce the results reported by the originators of either repair. The Hill procedure is further complicated by the recommendation that optimal results require intraoperative manometry to effectively create the antireflux mechanism. Few surgeons are familiar with this technology in the operating room, and this feature may have discouraged a more widespread adoption of the technique.

The results reported from Hill's personal series (Low et al, 1989) are very good: 90% good to excellent outcomes with the use of a Visick-type grading scale. Furthermore, these favorable results were largely sustained over very long periods of follow-up. Unfortunately, there is a relative paucity of reports of the results of the Hill repair from other surgical centers. The authors provide some results from a "multi-institutional review" in this chapter, but this work has not yet been published and referenced.

Although Hill and his colleagues do not believe that acquired esophageal shortening occurs, most surgeons reporting experience with antireflux surgery recognize acquired short esophagus as a significant complication of reflux disease in a varying proportion of cases. It is due to postinflammatory scarring of the esophageal wall. I believe that, on occasion, all of the standard repairs may fail when performed in the presence of significant esophageal shortening unless some accommodation, such as a lengthening gastroplasty, is added. Having made this statement, I believe that the Hill repair is more likely to remain intact in the presence of shortening than the other standard repairs, which use either a complete (Nissen) or partial (Belsey, Dor, Toupet) fundoplication. Why so? First, in the Hill repair, the sutures that anchor the esophagogastric junction to the median arcuate ligament secure purchase in stouter tissues than alternative operations and can better withstand some degree of tension. Second, Hill's procedure is the only antireflux operation that does not require maintenance of a 3- to 4-cm length of distal esophagus within the abdomen. The "valve" constructed by the Hill operation has its upper end situated at the esophagogastric junction and is extended for 3 to 4 cm inferiorly down the lesser curvature side of the stomach. In some ways, the Hill operation is anatomically similar to a gastroplasty in both location and function.

There is no doubt that the Hill repair is amenable to a laparoscopic approach. Hill and his associates have yet to report the results of their large laparoscopic experience in detail.

F. G. P.

REFERENCES

Aye RW, Mazza DE, Hill LD: Laparoscopic Hill repair in patients with abnormal motility. Am J Surg 173:379, 1997.

Barrett NJ: Hiatus hernia: A review of some controversial points. Br J Surg 42:231, 1954.

Braune W: Topographisch-anatomischer-Atlas nach Durchshnitten an gefrorenen Cadavern, Limited Edition. Leipzig, 1878, p 113.

Collis JL, Kelly TD, Wiley AM: Anatomy of the crura of the diaphragm and surgery of hiatus hernia. Thorax 9:175, 1954.

Contractor QQ, Akhtar SS, Contractor TQ: Endoscopic esophagitis and gastroesophageal flap valve. Clin Gastroenterol 28:233, 1999.

Fyke RE, Code CF, Schlegel JF: The gastroesophageal sphincter in healthy human beings. Gastroenterologia 86:135, 1956.

Gray H, et al: Alimentary system. In Williams P, Dyson M, Bannister LH, et al (eds): Gray's Anatomy: The Anatomical Basis of Medicine and Surgery, 38th ed. Edinburgh, Churchill Livingstone, 1995, p 1757.

Hill LD: Intraoperative measurement of lower esophageal sphincter pressure. J Thorac Cardiovasc Surg 75:3, 1978.

Hill LD: Progress in the surgical management of hiatal hernia. World J Surg 1:425, 1977.

Hill LD, Gelfand M, Bauermeister D: Simplified management of reflux esophagitis with stricture. Ann Surg 172:638, 1970.

Hill LD, Ilves R, Stevenson JK, Pearson JM: Reoperation for disruption and recurrence after Nissen fundoplication. Arch Surg 114:542, 1979.

Hill LD, Velasco M, Russell COH, Ilves R: Results of Hill antireflux operation before and after intraoperative manometry. Gastroenterology 80:1176, 1981.

Kraemer SJM, Hill LD, Low DE: The Hill repair: Reconstruction of the gastroesophageal junction and the flap valve for gastroesophageal reflux. In Nyhus LM, Baker R (eds): Mastery of Surgery, 2nd ed. Boston, Little, Brown, 1992, p 534.

Larrain A: Technical considerations in posterior gastropexy. Surg Gynecol Obstet 132:299, 1971.

Larrain A, Carvajal C, Hill LD, Kraemer SJM: Posterior gastropexy with cardial calibration: A laparoscopic antireflux procedure (Abstract). Submitted. 1992.

Low DE, Anderson RP, Ilves R, et al: Fifteen- to twenty-year results after the Hill antireflux operation. J Thorac Cardiovasc Surg 98:444, 1989.

Lundell L, Abrahamsson H, Ruth M, et al: Lower esophageal sphincter characteristics and esophageal acid exposure following partial or 360-degree fundoplication: Results of a prospective, randomized clinical study. World J Surg 15:115, 1991.

Lyons WS, Ellis FH Jr, Olsen AM: The gastroesophageal "sphinctermechanism": A review. Mayo Clin Proc 31:605, 1956.

Matikainen M, Kaukinen L: The mechanism of Nissen fundoplication. Acta Chir Scand 150:653, 1984.

Mercer CD, Hill LD: Surgical management of peptic esophageal stricture: Twenty-year experience. J Thorac Cardiovasc Surg 91:371, 1986.

Öberg S, Peters JH, Lord R, et al: Endoscopic grading of the gastroesophageal valve in patients with symptoms of GERD. Surg Endosc 13:1184, 1999.

Pope CE: Complications of gastroesophageal reflux. In Hill L, McCallum R, Mercer CD (eds): The Esophagus: Medical and Surgical Management. Philadelphia, WB Saunders, 1988, p 60.

Reid BJ, Haggitt RC, Rubin CE: Barrett's esophagus and esophageal adenocarcinoma. In Hill L, McCallum R, Mercer CD (eds): The Esophagus: Medical and Surgical Management. Philadelphia, WB Saunders, 1988, p 157.

Russell COH, Velasco N: Symptoms of esophageal disease. In Hill L, McCallum R, Mercer CD (eds): The Esophagus: Medical and Surgical Management. Philadelphia, WB Saunders, 1988, p 33.

Vansant JH, Baker JW, Ross DG: Modification of the Hill technique for repair of hiatal hernia. Surg Gynecol Obstet 143:637, 1976.

Von Gubaroff A: Ueber den Verschluss des menschlichen Magens an der Cardai. Arch Anat Physiol 395, 1886.

CHAPTER **23**

Dor and Toupet Repairs

OPEN TECHNIQUE FOR DOR AND TOUPET REPAIRS

Sandro Mattioli

The Dor and the Toupet antireflux procedures consist of a 180-degree anterior and a 180-degree posterior gastric fundoplication. These partial fundoplications are particularly indicated in cases of impairment of the esophageal body motility. In the past, these techniques were known in Europe and in the Latin countries. Today, because of the continuous exchange of information among the international scientific community, the increased knowledge of pathophysiology of functional surgery of the esophagus and the general adoption of laparoscopic techniques, the Dor and the Toupet operations have spread in popularity. In laparoscopic antireflux repair, the risk of overcompetence of the wrap is reduced with these procedures.

HISTORICAL NOTE

Both techniques were developed and presented in France in the early 1960s by Jacques Dor, professor of thoracic surgery of the University of Marçeilles, and André Toupet, surgeon of the City Hospitals of Paris.

Dor and Toupet, conceived very similar principles almost contemporaneously. Although the two techniques are different, both were developed in order to avoid the frequent failures reported following the Lortat-Jacob and Allison procedures, and to reduce the incidence of dysphagia (10%) reported by Nissen and Rossetti (1959), using a total 360-degree fundoplication. Interestingly, both Dor and Toupet initially proposed their repair for the prevention of reflux following the Heller myotomy for achalasia. Subsequently, both techniques were utilized as operations for the control of primary gastroesophageal reflux.

HISTORICAL READINGS

Dor J, Humbert P, Dor V, et al: L'intérêt de la technique de Nissen modifiée dans la prevention de reflux après cardiomyotomie extramuqueuse de Heller. Mem Acad Chir (Paris) 88:877, 1962.

Dor J, Humbert P, Paoli JM, et al: Traitement du reflux par la technique dite de Heller-Nissen modifiée. Presse Med 75:2563, 1967.

Nissen R, Rossetti M: Gastropexy and fundoplication in hiatal hernia and reflux oesophagitis. Med World Lond 91:20, 1959.

Toupet A: Technique d'oesophagoplastie avec phréno-gastropexie appliquée dans la cure radicale des hernies hiatales et comme complément de l'opération de Heller dans les cardiospasmes. Mem Acad Chir 89:394–399, 1963.

MANAGEMENT

Principles

The principles of the Dor and Toupet operations are (1) restoration of an abdominal segment of esophagus, (2) accentuation of the angle of His, (3) creation of a long anterior or posterior mucosal valve at the gastroesophageal junction, and (4) gastropexy to the right crus. Both fundoplications are partial in order to avoid overcompetence and to obviate the complications of dysphagia and the inability to belch and vomit normally when necessary.

Operative Technique

Some steps are common to both the Dor and the Toupet repairs: (1) the position of the patient on the table, (2) the anatomic dissection of the diaphragmatic hiatus, and (3) mobilization of the gastroesophageal junction.

The patient is placed on the operating table in the supine position, with a small bolster under the chest, below the inferior angle of the scapula. An upper midline, supraumbilical incision is made, beginning at the xiphoid process. The subcostal margins are retracted with a broad-bladed "third-hand" retractor.

The left triangular ligament of the liver and the gastrohepatic omentum are divided; the left and the quadrate hepatic lobes are gently displaced. The phrenoesophageal membrane is incised circumferentially for the full 360 degrees. The distal esophagus and diaphragmatic crura are isolated, and the hernial sac is completely resected.

Care is taken to avoid injury to the trunk and to the hepatic branches of the vagus nerves. The stomach is gently pulled down by the first assistant to expose at least 5 cm of esophagus below the hiatus.

A hiatal repair, or closure was not included in the original procedures.

Dor Gastroplasty

The steps are as follows:

1. The right margin of the gastric fundus is sutured to the left margin of the esophagus with five or six interrupted 3–0 nonabsorbable sutures, extending upward from the angle of His for at least 5 cm. After the last two sutures are tied, the ends are not cut, since they

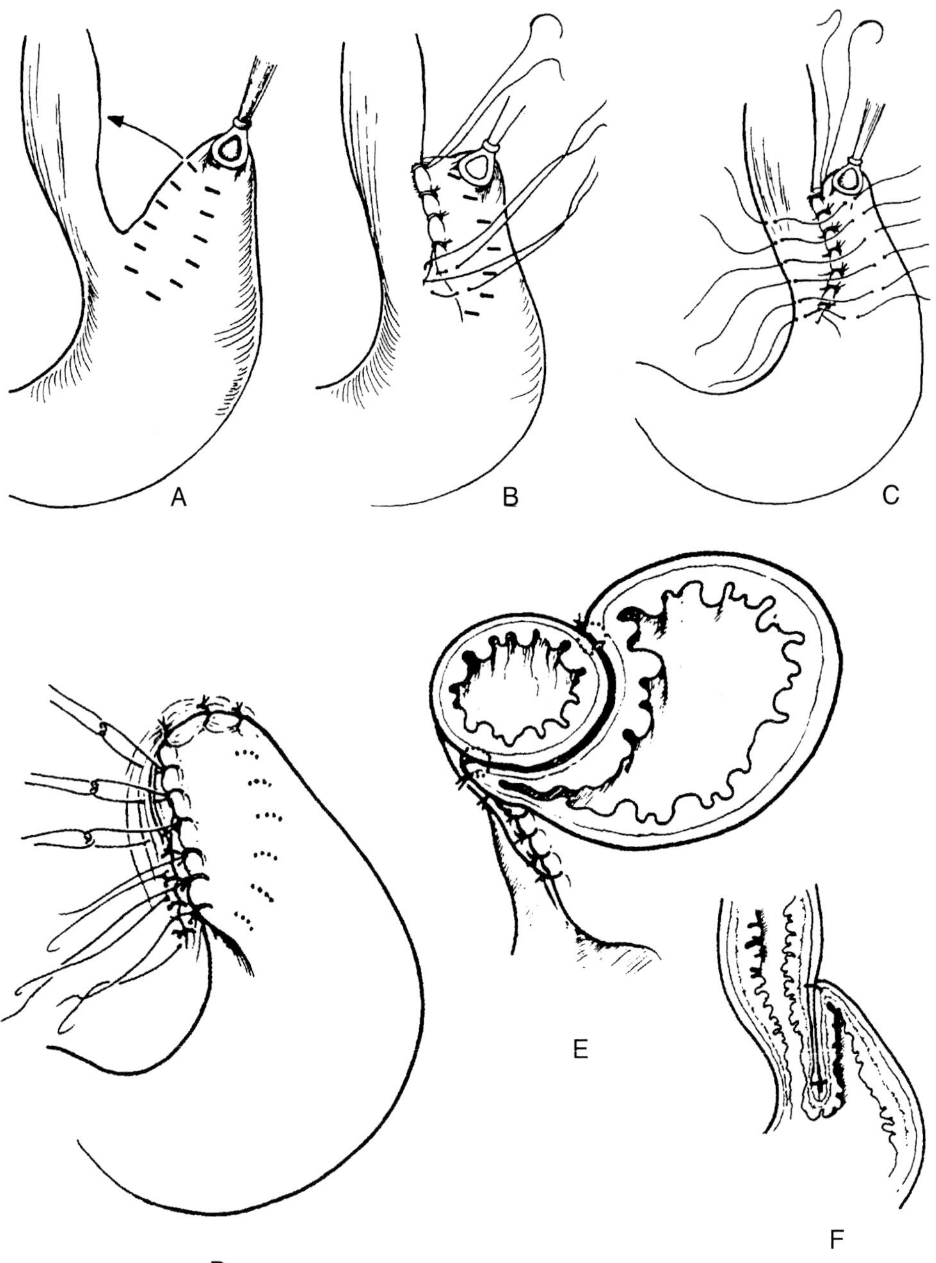

FIGURE 23–1 ■ Dor procedure. *A* and *B*, The right margin of the gastric fundus is sutured to the left margin of the esophagus. *C*, The anterior aspect of the fundus is sutured to the right margin of the esophagus. *D*, The stitches of the second row are sutured to the right crura. Transverse *(E)* and sagittal *(F)* sections of the hemifundoplication.

will be used to fix the gastroplasty to the left margin of the hiatus (Fig. 23–1*A* and *B*).

2. The gastric fundus is folded over the anterior aspect of the esophagus. A suture is positioned between the gastric fundus and the anterior aspect of the esophagus at the superior margin of the gastroplasty.
3. The folded fundus is then secured to the right margin of the esophagus with five or six sutures (Fig. 23–1*C*). Two or three sutures, 1 cm apart, are placed below the esophagogastric junction between the lesser gastric curvature and the plicated gastric fundus.
4. The sutures of the fundoplication, beginning with the top two of the first series and all of the second series, are secured with large bites to the diaphragmatic ring, from left to right and top to bottom.
5. At the end of the procedure, the 5-cm-long partial fundoplication is fixed below the diaphragm and the hiatus is closed anteriorly and laterally to the right (Fig. 23–1*D*).

The restoration of at least 5 cm of esophagus in the abdomen, without tension, and fixation of the gastric fundus (gastropexy) to the diaphragmatic crura are fundamental features of the Dor repair. If the effort to pull down the esophagus into the abdomen is difficult, as a result of acquired shortening of the esophagus secondary to panmural esophagitis, an alternative antireflux technique should be used. The short gastric vessels need to be divided only in the rare circumstance that the apical suture is under excessive tension. My associates and I believe that mobilization of the gastric fundus by dividing the short gastric vessels reduces the effectiveness of the fundoplication. Using intraoperative manometry, we observed that the division of the short gastric vessels diminished the level of pressure created by the fundoplication and reduced the effectiveness of the repair (unpublished data).

Other surgeons have developed techniques similar to the Dor repair or have modified the original operation. Thal (1968), proposed a transabdominal anterior fundoplication for hiatal hernia with reflux esophagitis but without stricture. The technique proposed by Schobinger (1969) differs from the original Dor repair in a few details; that is, two sutures between the lesser gastric curvature and the right diaphragmatic crus fix the gastroesophageal junction in the abdomen. After plication to the anterior aspect of the esophagus, the gastric fundus is fixed to the diaphragm and to the diaphragmatic crura rather than to the right esophageal margin.

For achalasia, Pinotti and coworkers (1974) proposed a modification to the Dor gastroplasty designed to improve the antireflux effectiveness. After the myotomy, the anterior fundoplication is tailored with three series of sutures. The first one is between the posterior aspect of the gastric fundus and the posterior aspect of the esophagus. The remaining two series are sutured as in the Dor technique. The Pinotti technique results in a more extensive fundoplication. Gavriliu (1976) added a pyloroplasty to the Heller-Dor procedure, and Gallone and colleagues (1982) added a proximal gastric vagotomy.

The Thal technique was adopted in pediatric patients by Ashcraft with a few modifications. The Thal-Ashcraft anterior fundoplication is performed through a transverse upper abdominal incision (Ashcraft et al, 1981; Ashcraft and Holder, 1993). Ashcraft proposed two different running suture techniques for the fundoplication. Boix-Ochoa (1987) uses the anterior fundoplication in pediatric patients. His technique differs from the Dor repair in that the gastric fundus is suspended to the diaphragm.

Toupet Gastroplasty

The gastroesophageal junction is circumferentially isolated, and at least 4 cm of tubular esophagus is placed below the diaphragmatic orifice without tension. Steps are as follows:

1. The gastric fundus is passed behind the esophagus and the posterior vagus nerve; the anterior aspect of the fundus now faces the posterior aspect of the lower esophagus.
2. The right side of the fundus is sutured to the right margin of the esophagus with four 3–0 nonabsorbable sutures; the lowest stitch is applied to the lesser curvature, just below the esophagogastric junction (Fig. 23–2*A*).
3. The right posterior aspect of the fundus is sutured to the right limb of the diaphragmatic pillar with four to five stitches. The highest suture includes esophagus, fundus, and diaphragmatic ring; the lowest includes the folded fundus and the arcuate ligament.
4. A similar row of stitches secures the left-posterior gastric fundus to the left limb of the diaphragmatic pillar

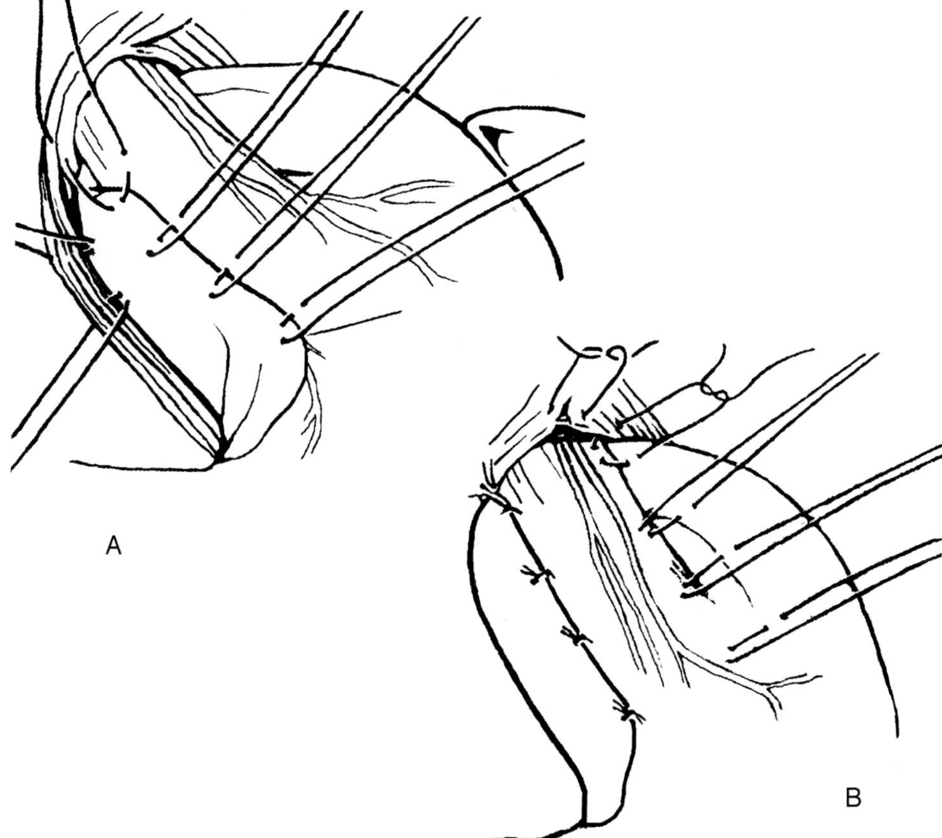

FIGURE 23–2 ■ Toupet procedure. *A*, The right edge of the fundus is sutured to the right margin of the esophagus. The fundus is sutured to the right branch of the diaphragmatic pillar with two stitches. *B*, A few stitches secure the left posterior gastric fundus to the left branch of the diaphragmatic pillar; the left anterior edge of the gastric fundus is sutured to the left margin of the esophagus.

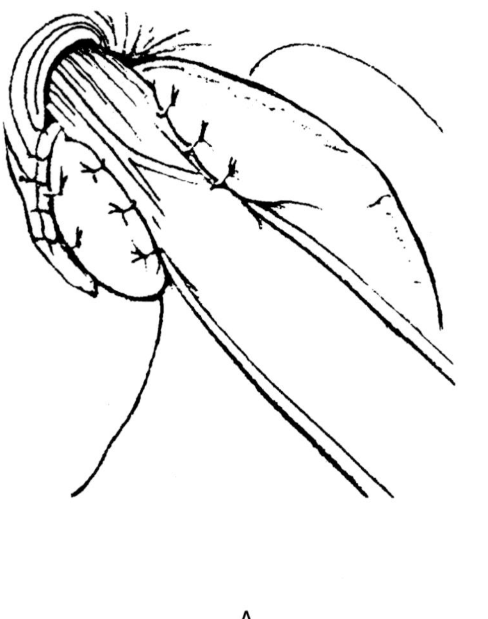

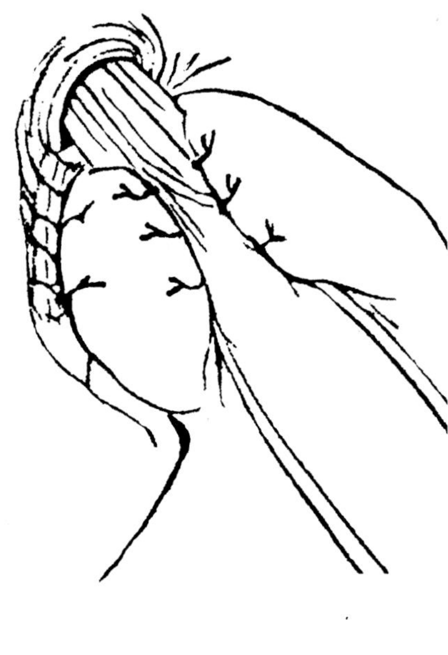

FIGURE 23–3 ■ Toupet repair according to Ténière. *A*, Separate closure of the diaphragmatic hiatus and 180-degree gastric wrap around the esophagus. *B*, Separate closure of the diaphragmatic hiatus and 270-degree gastric wrap around the esophagus.

from the bottom to the top. Both rows of sutures should be free of tension.

5. Finally, the left-anterior margin of the gastric fundus is symmetrically sutured (four or five sutures) to the left margin of the esophagus (Fig. 23–2*B*). If the hiatal orifice is still too wide, one or two stitches can be placed across the hiatus, anterior to the esophagus.

A few variants to the original technique, described here, have been proposed. In the method of Vayre and colleagues (1970), the gastric fundus is passed behind the esophagus and the right-posterior fundus is fixed to the right pillar of the diaphragm with four nonabsorbable sutures. The anterior aspect of the fundus is sutured to the left margin of the lower esophagus; the left-anterior portion of fundus is sutured to the diaphragmatic dome.

The modern version of the Toupet's procedure (Ténière et al, 1994) differs from the original: Ténière uses separate closure of the diaphragmatic hiatus and increases the gastric wrap around the esophagus to 270 degrees (Fig. 23–3*A* and *B*).

These modifications originate from experiences subsequent to the original report of Toupet; it was demonstrated that any fundoplication can slip into the chest when the hiatus is not properly closed (Ténière, 1994) and that the degree of competence of the fundoplication is related to the extent of envelopment around the esophagus (DeMeester et al, 1974).

Laparoscopy

Today, laparoscopic antireflux procedures are routinely performed in many centers in the world; the detailed description of instrumentation, techniques, and approaches are available from many sources. In this chapter, we briefly illustrate our current technique.

The principles and the steps of the open procedures are the same for the laparoscopic techniques. The patient position on the table, and the approach to the supramesocolic abdominal cavity, however, are different. Minor modifications in the isolation of the diaphragmatic hiatus and of the gastroesophageal junction are advisable in order to proceed safely; the esophagus is not directly dissected because of the higher risk of perforation. The dissection starts from the diaphragmatic hiatus, once the right plain is entered. The phrenoesophageal membrane is dissected and mobilization of the esophagus is started.

Surgical Team and Trocar Position

The patient's position and the surgical team and the site of insertion of the trocars are shown in Figure 23–4. The surgeon stands between the legs of the patient, and two assistants are on the left and on the right side. The surgeon operates through port No. 3 (5 mm) and port No. 4 (10 mm). The first assistant on the right operates

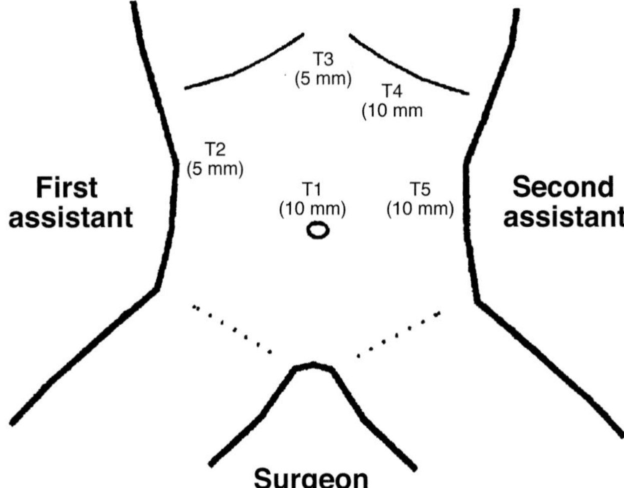

FIGURE 23–4 ■ Position of surgical team and trocars for laparoscopic procedures.

the video camera (port No. 1, 10 mm) and the liver retractor (port No. 2, 5 mm). The second assistant holds the stomach through port No. 5 (10 mm).

Exposure of the Proximal Stomach and Distal Esophagus

After the five ports have been inserted and the pneumoperitoneum is established, the patient is placed in reverse Trendelenburg position. The left lobe of the liver is displaced up and forward to the right side. Division of the triangular ligament is not mandatory. The second assistant holds the stomach with the Babcock forceps as close to the angle of His as possible and exerts traction downward and to the left.

Isolation of the Diaphragmatic Crura

The gastrohepatic omentum is divided in its upper portion. The lower branches of the vagus nerves to the hepatic hilum are preserved in order to avoid impaired gallbladder motility and to reduce the risk of wrapping the gastric fundus around stomach instead of esophagus. Care is taken to identify the presence of an accessory hepatic artery, which is clipped and divided. The diaphragmatic ring is localized and isolated from top to bottom until both branches of the right pillar are cleared. The phrenoesophageal membrane is opened posteriorly, and the mediastinal tissue is seen between the two branches of the diaphragmatic pillar. Through this plane the esophagus is localized and elevated. Clearance of the left diaphragmatic branch is continued upward.

Isolation of the Lower Esophagus

The stomach is pulled inferiorly, and the hernia, if present, is reduced. The phrenoesophageal membrane is opened circumferentially. The esophagus is dissected from the mediastinal bed, and the hernial sac is reduced completely. The anterior and posterior vagus nerves are localized but not isolated.

Closure of the Diaphragmatic Hiatus

The anesthetist introduces a Maloney bougie (56 to 58 French) into the stomach. The surgeon lifts the gastroesophageal junction upward by inserting a Babcock forceps (port No. 5) behind the esophagus while Dor fundoplication is performed.

When the gastric fundus is to be passed behind the esophagus, as for the Toupet fundoplication, it is easier to encircle the esophagus with a Penrose drain, which is held by the second assistant. The surgeon narrows the hiatus by placing two or three nonabsorbable, interrupted sutures through the diaphragmatic crura, tying them loosely. It is mandatory to secure a good bite of tissue with the diagonal stitch, which is placed higher on the left limb and lower through the right limb.

Dor and Toupet Fundoplications

The laparoscopic surgical technique is similar to that described for the open procedures. Even though it takes more time, the same number of sutures are used for the two rows in order to evenly distribute the tension on the repair.

We perform the Toupet procedure using a modification of the original technique, which consists of routine repair of the diaphragmatic crura and 270-degree posterior fundoplication.

RESULTS

It has been repeatedly stated that the ability of the lower esophageal sphincter (LES) to protect the esophageal mucosa from exposure to gastric juice depends on its resting pressure and on its length. Normally, the LES lies two thirds below and one third above the diaphragmatic hiatus. Incompetence of the cardia can occur when one or more of these components fail (Lundell et al, 1991).

Length and pressure of the distal high pressure zone (HPZ) are cofactors of cardial competence (DeMeester et al, 1974). The aim of both Dor and Toupet repairs is to achieve a competent antireflux barrier by the combination of a moderate increase of pressure in the LES region and a long intra-abdominal segment of esophagus to which the pressure is applied.

Table 23–1 summarizes the long-term manometric characteristics of the Dor and Toupet repairs reported by different authors in patients operated on for gastroesophageal reflux and for cases of achalasia managed by the Heller-Dor operation. A meaningful comparison between these results is of uncertain validity because the authors do not report normal values for their manometric system. There is no obvious difference in results between the series of cases operated on for gastroesophageal reflux in which the LES is left intact and the series of patients with achalasia managed by a Heller-Dor operation. The Heller-Dor operation is a good model to evaluate the manometric effect of the 180-degree anterior fundoplication because the LES is completely abolished by a complete myotomy.

The LES pressures created by the Dor fundoplication are relatively low—certainly lower than the pressures created by the Nissen or Belsey repairs (DeMeester et al, 1974). The length of the high pressure zone varies between 2 and 4 cm. According to Mir and coauthors, (1986) and Bonavina and colleagues (1992), about 0.5 cm of the superior part of the gastroplasty is positioned above the respiratory inversion point. In our series of 60 patients, distal HPZ mean pressure is 8.00 ± 3.86 mm Hg and length is 5 ± 0.9 cm. The entire fundoplication lies below the diaphragm in 96.7%. The adaptive response of the Dor fundoplication to an increase in abdominal pressure induced by the Valsalva maneuver is shown in Figure 23–5.

In 52.2%, the increase of pressure in the fundoplication and in the abdomen is equivalent to a $\Delta HPZ/\Delta GP$ ratio of 1. In 47.8% of cases, the increase in intragastric pressure is greater than the increase in pressure in the fundoplication $\Delta HPZ/\Delta GP < 1$. There is no relationship between the grade of adaptive response to the intra-abdominal pressure increases and reflux esophagitis (see Fig. 23–5). This observation is consistent with that reported by Behar and associates (1974), who observed increases of the HPZ pressure with ratios less than 1 in

TABLE 23–1 ■ **Dor and Toupet Fundoplications: Distal High-Pressure Zone (HPZ) Pressure and Length After Long-Term Follow-up (>3 Years)**

Author	*Year*	*No. of Cases*	*Surgical Procedure*	*Distal HPZ Pressure* Mean (mm Hg)	*Distal HPZ Length* Mean (cm)
Mussa et al	1986	32	Dor	7.5	—*
Mir et al	1986	67	Dor	3.66	3.32
Csendes et al	1988	42	Heller-Dor	10.5	2
Bonavina et al	1992	193	Heller-Dor	9.7	2.7
Juan et al	1992	86	Dor	11.7	2.2
Guarner et al	1980	135	Toupet	16	5.4†
Thor and Silander	1989	19	Toupet	16.9	—*
Lundell et al	1991	33	Toupet	13	2
Kabbej et al	1992	251	Toupet	17‡	5†
Michot et al	1992	45	Toupet	23.9‡	4.1†
Ottignon et al	1994	28	Toupet	17.4‡	—*

*Data not reported.
†Total high-pressure zone length.
‡Data reported in cm H_2O.

response to gastric pressure increases in patients undergoing successfully operation with a Belsey Mark IV procedure. From manometric study of the Toupet repair, Galmiche and coauthors (1983) reported postoperative failure of the 180-degree posterior fundoplication when the preoperative LES pressure was below 10 cm H_2O.

Michot and coworkers (1992) confirmed these data, suggesting that the Toupet procedure might be insufficient in patients with a low preoperative LES resting pressure. By increasing the intent of fundoplication around the esophagus, an effective sphincteric pressure can be restored in all patients, with satisfactory early clinical results and no digestive symptoms beyond the postoperative 3rd month. Michot suggests that the 180-degree posterior fundoplication is adequate in patients with a preoperative LES pressure above 10 cm H_2O. In patients with a preoperative LES pressure below 10 cm H_2O, a 270-degree fundoplication results in correction of gastroesophageal reflux without postoperative symptoms.

The early results of the open Dor and Toupet repairs for primary gastroesophageal reflux disease (GERD) are reported in Table 23–2. Mortality and morbidity rates for

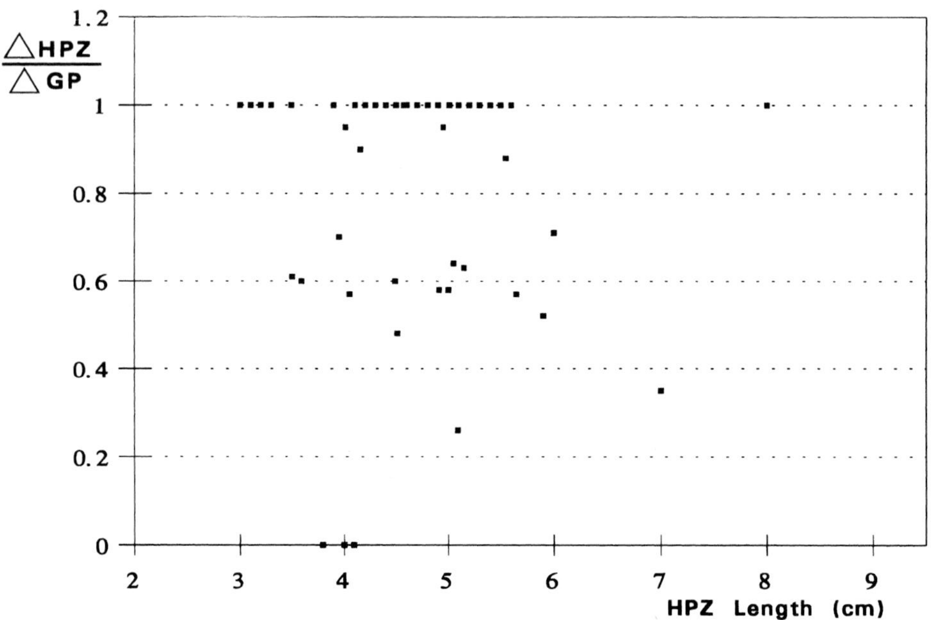

FIGURE 23–5 ■ Effect of the Valsalva maneuver on the high-pressure zone (HPZ) in 46 patients undergoing the Heller-Dor procedure obtained by station pull-through technique. ΔHPZ/ΔGP, differences between pressures recorded in the HPZ and in the stomach (GP) during the Muller maneuver and in resting condition. Increases in gastric pressure (GP) caused by the Muller maneuver were associated with equal or minor increases in HPZ (ΔHPZ/ΔGP ≤ Δ1) of five patients with reflux esophagitis. In three patients, ΔHPZ/ΔGP = 1; in two patients, ΔHPZ/ΔGP = 0.58 and 0.52.

TABLE 23–2 ■ **Dor and Toupet Open Fundoplications: Early Results***

Author	*Year*	*No. of Cases*	*Surgical Procedure*	*Postperative Deaths (%)*	*Surgical Complications*† (%)*	*Dysphagia (%)*	*Abdominal Discomfort (%)*	*Gas Bloat Syndrome (%)*
Dodat et al	1978	51§	Dor	3.9	17.6	—‡	—‡	—‡
Anselmetti et al	1980	22	Dor	0	4.5	4.5	23	—‡
Mir et al	1986	67	Dor	1.5	—‡	3	15	1.5‡
Mussa et al	1986	32	Dor	0	—‡	0	0	0
Zaragosi Moliner et al	1989	146	Dor	0	—‡	—‡	—‡	—‡
Lefebvre et al	1989	37§	Dor	0	16	27	—‡	—‡
Juan et al	1992	86	Dor	0	8	70	0	0
Ashcraft and Holder	1993	1,150§	Dor	0.09	0.7	—‡	—‡	1
Guarner et al	1980	135	Toupet	0	0	2.9	0	—‡
Galmiche et al	1983	25	Toupet	0	0	—‡	—‡	—‡
Gutierrez et al	1988	90	Toupet	0	0	—‡	—‡	—‡
Thor and Silander	1989	19	Toupet	0	21	—‡	—‡	—‡
Segol et al	1989	18	Toupet	0	5.5	0	0	0
Vara-Thorbeck et al	1989	99	Toupet	0	0	—‡	—‡	—‡
Lundell et al	1991	33	Toupet	0	0	10	15	—‡
Kabbej et al	1992	251	Toupet	0	15.5	18	9	0.3
Michot et al	1992	45	Toupet	0	0	13.3	—‡	—‡
Bensoussan et al	1994	112§	Toupet	0	28.5	7	1.7	—‡
Ottignon et al	1994	28	Toupet	0	7	38	15	—‡

*First 30 days after surgical treatment.
†Surgical complications included incisional hernia, wound infection, leakage, bowel obstruction, thomboembolism, pleuritis, bronchopneumonia, and splenectomy.
‡Data not reported.
§Pediatric patients.

a Dor repair are low. Postoperative dysphagia and the gas bloat syndrome are infrequent except in one series (Juan et al, 1992). Some abdominal discomfort, localized below the left costal margin, may appear after larger meals during the first 3 to 4 months after the operation. This symptom is probably the result of the distention of the gastric fundus.

With the Toupet repair, mortality in the reported series is nil and morbidity varies from 0 to 28.5%. The highest morbidity (28.5%) was reported by Bensoussan and associates (1994) in a group of 112 children with a mean age of 39 months (range, 2 months to 19 years); of these patients, 30% were neurologically impaired.

Temporary dysphagia is infrequent and disappears spontaneously in most cases in the first postoperative months. Other postoperative symptoms such as abdominal discomfort and gas bloat syndrome are very infrequent in reported case series.

Long-term results of Dor and Toupet repairs are shown in Table 23–3. With the Dor repair, it appears that the incidence of recurrent hernia or reflux doubles in the presence of reflux complications such as stenosis or severe esophagitis (Juan et al, 1992). With the Toupet repair, satisfactory results are obtained in 83.3% to 96.5% of cases except in two series: 56.5% (Galmiche et al, 1983) and 56% (Ottignon et al, 1994).

Early and intermediate-term results of laparoscopic Dor and Toupet procedures are reported in Tables 23–4 and 23–5. The Dor antireflux procedure is most frequently used with the Heller myotomy. A few case series regard the surgical treatment of primary gastroesophageal reflux. Early results are probably influenced by the learning curve. Clinical results after a mean follow-up of 12 to 22 months appear in the whole satisfactory.

COMMENTS AND CONTROVERSIES

Experimental (Alday and Goldsmith, 1973; Leonardi et al, 1977) and clinical (DeMeester et al, 1974) studies support the concept that 360-degree fundoplication is more effective than partial fundoplications in restoring LES pressure and preventing reflux. The Dor and the Toupet repairs constitute a 180- to 270-degree wrap of the gastric fundus around the anterior or posterior aspects of the distal esophagus. The resting LES pressure obtained with these procedures is lower than that obtained with the full fundoplication.

The Dor and Toupet repairs were conceived as additions to the Heller myotomy for the treatment of achalasia. In the aperistaltic patient, an efficient—but not too efficient—fundoplication acts to prevent or diminish postoperative gastroesophageal reflux following myotomy. Compared to total 360° fundoplication, relatively weak pressure is applied over a long segment of abdominal esophagus.

Today, the Dor technique is almost always used in association with the Heller myotomy. In the treatment of achalasia, the Dor anterior fundoplication has an additional advantage over the posterior fundoplication: It protects the exposed outer surface of the esophageal mucosa created after myotomy. Leakage due to inadvertent mucosal

TABLE 23–3 ■ **Dor and Toupet Open Fundoplications: Late Results**

Author	*Year*	*No. of Cases*	*Surgical Procedure*	*Follow-up (Months)*	*Satisfactory Results (%)*	*Poor Results (%)*
Dodat et al	1978	51*	Dor	†	82.3	7.7
Anselmetti et al	1980	22	Dor	48	86.3	13.7
Aulagnier	1980	59	Dor	†	89.9	10.1
Maillet	1980	*	Dor	†	91	9
Mir et al	1986	67	Dor	42	94	6
Mussa et al	1986	32	Dor	38	83.7	16.3
Zaragosi Moliner et al	1989	146	Dor	†	92	8
Lefebvre et al	1989	37*	Dor	74	92	8
Juan et al	1992	86	Dor	120	88	12
Ashcraft and Holder	1993	362*	Dor	12–96	95	5
Guarner et al	1980	135	Toupet	60–120	90.3	9.7
Galmiche et al	1983	25	Toupet	21	56.5	43.5
Gutierrez et al	1988	90	Toupet	12–108	95	5
Thor and Silander	1989	19	Toupet	60	95	5
Segol et al	1989	18	Toupet	24	83.3	16.7
Vara-Thorbeck et al	1989	99	Toupet	60	94	6
Kabbej et al	1992	251	Toupet	32	96.5	3.5
Bensoussan et al	1994	112*	Toupet	48	90.5	9.5
Ottignon et al	1994	28	Toupet	28	56	44

*Pediatric patients.
†Data not reported.

TABLE 23–4 ■ **Dor and Toupet Laparoscopic Fundoplications: Early Results**

Author	*Year*	*No. of Cases*	*Surgical Procedure*	*Mean Operative Time (Hours)*	*Postoperative Deaths (%)*	*Laparotomic Conversion (%)*	*Surgical Complications* (%)*	*Mean Hospital Stay (Days)*	*Dysphagia (%)*	*Abdominal Discomfort (%)*
Kleimann and Halbfass	1998	25	Dor	—†	0	—†	—†	—†	0	—†
Watson et al	1999	54	Dor	1	0	7.4	20.3	3	1.8	—†
Jobe et al	1997	100	Toupet	3.2	0	0	10	2.8	20	6
Wetscher et al	1997	32	Toupet	2.5	0	0	15.6	3	3.1	—†
Lefebvre et al	1998	100	Toupet	—†	0	1	4	4	—†	—†

*Esophageal perforation, delayed small-bowel perforation, gastric perforation, intra-abdominal hematoma, opening of the pleura, deep venous thrombosis, adult respiratory distress syndrome, delayed gastric emptying, pleural effusion and pneumonia, acute paraesophageal herniation, severe postoperative dysphagia, urinary retention, respiratory atelectasis, and pneumothorax.
†Data not reported.

TABLE 23–5 ■ **Dor and Toupet Laparoscopic Fundoplications: Intermediate-Term Results**

Author	*Year*	*No. of Cases*	*Surgical Procedure*	*Follow-up (Months)*	*Satisfactory Results (%)*	*Poor Results (%)*
Kleimann and Halbfass	1998	25	Dor	16.7	94	6
Watson et al	1999	54	Dor	6	90	10
Jobe et al	1997	100	Toupet	22	71	29
Wetscher et al	1997	32	Toupet	15	96.9	3.1
Lund et al	1997	46	Toupet	6	91	9
Lefebvre et al	1998	100	Toupet	12	93	7

perforation, or late postoperative dysphagia due to scar, is avoided or greatly diminished by the anterior Dor fundoplication.

My associates and I have performed 72 Heller-Dor operations with no operative mortality. Postoperative complications occurred in 5.5% of patients (two incidental splenectomies, one bronchopneumonia, and one abscess between myotomy and fundoplication). We monitored 69 patients with radiology, manometry, and endoscopy over a mean period of 86.9 months (range, 12 to 180 months). Results were excellent in 66.7% of patients, good in 20.3%, and poor in 13% (of whom 10.2% had postoperative reflux esophagitis) (Mattioli et al, 1996). Conversely, there is little evidence that the Dor repair provides good control for GERD, especially if LES pressure is very low and if the GERD is long-standing and complicated by severe esophagitis.

Only in very selected cases, such as in patients with hiatal incompetence as a result of caustic injury, in esophageal scleroderma, or after "redo" antireflux surgery do we use this operation for the surgical treatment of GERD.

In cases of primary GERD associated with severe impairment of esophageal body motility, the Toupet procedure can be a very reasonable option. It may be the elective procedure if the laparoscopic approach is chosen.

S. M.

■ REFERENCES

Alday ES, Goldsmith HS: Efficacy of fundoplication in preventing gastric reflux. Am J Surg 126:322, 1973.

Anselmetti G, Grassamp G, Fusaro M, et al: L'ernia iatale da scivolamento trattata secondo la tecnica di Dor. Min Chir 35:363, 1980.

Ashcraft KW, Holder TM: Pediatric Surgery, 2nd ed. Philadelphia, WB Saunders, 1993.

Ashcraft KW, Holder TM, Amoury RA: Treatment of gastroesophageal reflux in children by Thal fundoplication. J Thorac Cardiovasc Surg 82:706, 1981.

Aulagnier G, Tissot E, Lombard-Platet R, et al: Résultats éloingés du traitement chirurgical des hernies hiatales par glissement. Lyon Chir 76:16, 1980.

Behar J, Biancani P, Spiro HM, et al: Effect of an anterior fundoplication on lower esophageal sphincter competence. Gastroenterology 67:209, 1974.

Bensoussan AL, Yazbeck S, Arceller-Blanchard A: Results and complications of Toupet partial posterior wrap: 10 years' experience. J Pediatr Surg 29:1215, 1994.

Boix-Ochoa J: Children and reflux. In DeMeester TR, Matthews HR (eds): International Trends in General Thoracic Surgery: Benign Esophageal Disease. St. Louis, CV Mosby, 1987.

Bonavina L, Nosadini A, Bardini R, et al: Primary treatment or esophageal achalasia: Long-term results of myotomy and Dor fundoplication. Arch Surg 127:222, 1992.

Csendes A, Braghetto I, Mascaro J et al: Late subjective and objective evaluation of the results of esophagomyotomy in 100 patients with achalasia of the esophagus. Surgery 104:469, 1988.

DeMeester TR, Johnson LF, Kent AH: Evaluation of current operations for the prevention of gastroesophageal reflux. Ann Surg 180:511, 1974.

Dodat H, Chappus JP, Allantaz F et al: Pour un traitement chirurgical précoce raisone des hernies hiatales du nourrisson. Chir Pédiatr 19:153, 1978.

Dor J, Humbert P, Dor V, et al: L'intétét de la technique de Nissen modifiée dans la prevention de reflux après cardiomyotomie extramuqueuse de Heller. Mem Acad Chir (Paris) 88:877, 1962.

Dor J, Humbert P, Paoli JM, et al: Traitement du reflux par la technique dite de Helle-Nissen modifiée. Presse Med 75:2563, 1967.

Gallone L, Peri G, Galliera M: Proximal gastric vagotomy and anterior fundoplication as complementary procedures to Heller's operation for achalasia. Surg Gynecol Obstet 155:337, 1982.

Galmiche JP, Téniére P, Ducrotte P, et al: Treatment of acid gastroesophageal reflux by posterior hemifundoplication. Clinical and pH metric results. Gastroenterol Clin Biol 7:385, 1983.

Gavriliu D: Operation for functional obstruction of the cardia. Curr Probl Surg 12:19, 1976.

Gozzetti G, Mattioli S, Spangaro M, et al: Results of surgical therapy of achalasia with three different techniques. In Sievert JR, Hölscher AH (eds): Disease of the Esophagus. Berlin, Springer-Verlag, 1988.

Guarner V, Martinez N, Gavino JF: Ten year evaluation of posterior fundoplasty in the treatment of gastroesophageal reflux. Am J Surg 139:200, 1980.

Gutierrez AG, Del Portal DA, Molina JB, et al: Toupet's valvuloplasty for sliding hiatal hernia and incompetent inferior esophageal sphincter. Zentralbl Chir 113:772, 1988.

Jobe BA, Wallace J, Hansen PD, et al: Evaluation of laparoscopic Toupet fundoplication as a primary repair for all patients with medically resistant gastroesophageal reflux. Surg Endosc 11:1080, 1997.

Juan M, Ponce J, Garrigues V, et al: Long-term efficacy of 180R anterior fundoplication for severe gastro-oesophageal reflux disease. J Gastroenterol Hepatol 4:215, 1992.

Kabbej M, Cargill G, Fékété F: Reflux gastro-oesophagien trait par hémifundoplicatur postérieure. Presse Méd 21:1369, 1992.

Kleimann E, Halbfass HJ: Laparoscopic anti-reflux surgery in gastroesophageal reflux. Langenbecks Arch Chir Suppl Kongressbd 115:1520, 1998.

Lefebvre F, Bouche-Pillon MA, Lefort G, et al: Traitement chirurgical du reflux gastro-oesophagien de l'enfant par hémivalve antédeure. Chir Pediatr 30:229, 1989.

Lefebvre JC, Belva P, Takieddine M, et al: Laparoscopic Toupet fundoplication: Prospective study of 100 cases. Results at one year and literature review. Acta Chir Belg 98:1, 1998.

Leonardi HJ, Lee ME, Fathi El-Kurd M, et al: An experimental study on the effectiveness of various antireflux operations. Ann Thorac Surg 24:215, 1977.

Lund RJ, Wetcher GJ, Raiser F, et al: Laparoscopic Toupet fundoplication for gastroesophageal reflux disease with poor esophageal body motility. J Gastrointest Surg 1:301, 1997.

Lundell L, Abrahamsson H, Ruth M, et al: Lower esophageal sphincter characteristics and esophageal acid exposure following partial or 360° fundoplication: Results of a prospective, randomized, clinical study. World J Surg 15:115, 1991.

Maillet P: Hernies hiatales de l'adulte: Étude critique des techniques chirurgicales. In Mouiel J (ed): Actualités Digestives Médico-Chirurgicales. Paris, Masson, 1980.

Maillet P, Micol P, Parsat JPH, et al: Les résultats du traitment chirurgical du méga-oesophage (72 observations). Ann Chir 27:579, 1973.

Mattioli S, Di Simone M, Bassi F, et al: Surgery for esophageal achalasia: Long-term results with three different techniques. Hepatogastroenterology 43:492, 1996.

Mattioli S, Pilotti V, Felice V, et al: Intraoperative study on the relationship between the lower esophageal sphincter pressure and the muscular components of the gastro-esophageal junction in achalasic patients. Ann Surg 218:635, 1993.

Michot F, Le Blanc I, Denis P, et al: Surgical treatment of gastroesophageal reflux—180° or 270° fundoplication results on the basis of preoperative sphincter pressure: Prospective study in 45 patients. Dig Surg 9:241, 1992.

Mir J, Ponce J, Juan M, et al: The effect of 180° anterior fundoplication on gastroesophageal reflux. Am J Gastroenterol 81:172, 1986.

Mussa A, Giugno G, Festa V, et al: Correzione chirurgica secondo la tecnica di Dor modificata dell'ernia iatale con reflusso gastroesofageo. Min Chir 41:1555, 1986.

Nissen R, Rosetti M: Gastropexy and fundoplicatio in hiatal hernia and reflux oesophagitis. Med World London 91:20, 1959.

Ottignon Y, Pelissier EP, Mantion G, et al: Reflux gastro-oesophagien. Comparaison des résultats cliques, pH-métriques des procédés de Nissen et de Toupet. Gastroenterol Clin Biol 18:920, 1994.

Pinotti HW, Gama-Rodrigues JJ, Ellenbogen G, et al: Novas bases para o tratamento cirùrgico do megaesôfago: esofagocardiomiotomia com esofagofundogastropexia. Rev Assoc Med Brasil 20:331, 1974.

Schobinger RA: Dextrorotation et fixation sous-phrénique préoesopha-

gienne du fundus gastrique avec fixation du cardia dans le traitement de la hernie hiatale. Heir Chir Acta 2:3, 1969.
Segol PH, Hay JM, Pottier D: Traitment chirurgical du reflux gastro-oesophagien: quelle intervention choisir: Nissen, Toupet ou Lortat-Jacob? Gastroenterol Clin Biol 13:873, 1989.
Téniére P, Scotté M, Le Blanc I, et al: Reflux gastro-oesophagien de l'adulte. In Laffonnt A, Durieux F (eds): Editions Techniques, Techniques Chirurgicales–Appareil Digestif. Paris, Encyclopedie Medico-Chirurgicale, 1994, p 40.
Thal AP: A unified approach to surgical problems of the eosophagogastric junction. Ann Surg 168:542, 1968.
Thor KBA, Silander T: A long-term randomized prospective trial of the Nissen procedure versus a modified Toupet technique. Ann Surg 210:719, 1989.
Toupet A: Technique d'oesophagoplastie avec phréno-gastropexie apliquée dans la cure radicale des hernies hiatales et comme complément de l'opération de Heller dans less cardiospasmes. Mem Acad Chir 89:394–399, 1963.
Vara-Thorbeck R, Morales OI, Gurrero JA, et al: Evaluation of Toupet antireflux operation, by means of gastroesophageal scintiscan. Zentralbl Chir 114:722, 1989.
Vayre P, Hureau J, Roux M: La cure chirurgicale des hérnies hiatales de l'adulte. Ann Chir 24:627, 1970.
Watson DI, Jamieson GG, Pike GK, et al: Prospective randomized double-blind trial between laparoscopic Nissen fundoplication and anterior partial fundoplication. Br J Surg 86:123, 1999.
Wetscher GJ, Glaser K, Wieschemeyer T, et al: Tailored antireflux surgery for gastroesophageal reflux disease: Effectiveness and risk of postoperative dysphagia. Worl J Surg 21:605, 1997.
Zaragosi Moliner J, Zaragosi Esparza A, Zaragosi Esparza JL: Eclectic surgery of gastroesophageal reflux–hiatal hernia. Rev Esp Enferm Apar Dig 76:567, 1989.

LAPAROSCOPIC TOUPET FUNDOPLICATION

Lee L. Swanström

HISTORICAL NOTE

The introduction of laparoscopic Nissen fundoplication in 1991 by Dallemagne and associates initiated a renaissance in the surgical treatment of reflux disease and swallowing disorders. With the resulting rapid increase in patient referrals, many investigators began adapting other (non-Nissen) procedures to the laparoscopic approach. These included laparoscopic versions of the Belsey, Hill, Dor, and Toupet procedures. These repairs were chosen either for specific clinical indications or because of traditional institutional bias.

Partial fundoplications, most notably the modified Toupet repair, were particularly attractive to surgeons based on the desire to provide their "minimally accessed" patients with a "minimally morbid" procedure (Coster et al, 1997). There was a general feeling that the short surgical recovery of laparoscopic repairs would make patients less likely to accept the side effects associated with the Nissen such as dysphagia, inability to belch or vomit, and "gas bloat" syndrome (Swanström and Wayne, 1994). There is certainly sound evidence from the open experience with the Toupet repair to support these hopes. Both long-term outcome studies, and comparative studies with the Nissen repair, show that the Toupet procedure provides excellent symptomatic results with a low incidence of postoperative side effects (Boutelier and Jonsell, 1992; Lundell et al, 1991; Thor and Silander, 1989).

Since the laparoscopic Toupet procedure was first reported by Cuschieri and colleagues (1993), substantial numbers of cases have been performed worldwide. The reported follow-up data give a better understanding of the role of Toupet repairs in the treatment of reflux disease.

■ *HISTORICAL READINGS*

Cuschieri A, Hunter J, Wolfe B, et al: Multicenter prospective evaluation of laparoscopic antireflux surgery. Surg Endosc 7:505–510, 1993.
Toupet A: Technique d'oesophago-gastroplastie avec phrenogastropexie appliquée dans lla cure radicale des hernies hiatales et comme complement de l'operation d'Heller dans les cardiospasmes. Mem Acad Chir 89:394–395, 1963.

The laparoscopic Toupet repair has become a fairly standardized procedure but is somewhat different than originally described by Andre Toupet (1963). Adopting the modifications described by Boutelier and Jonsell (1992) the most common current repair is a 270-degree posterior wrap that is fixed to both the right and left crura. Standard 5 port laparoscopic access is used. Traditionally the hiatus is left open or only loosely closed although other variations of the wrap, such as that of Lind and colleagues (1965), close the hiatus in a standard fashion. The sides of the fundus are sutured to the esophagus at the 10 o'clock and 2 o'clock positions to achieve a partial wrap 3 to 4 cm long (Fig. 23–6).

INDICATIONS AND DIAGNOSIS

Indications for the Toupet repair are summarized in Table 23–6. The traditional indication for the Toupet fundoplication is a transabdominal antireflux procedure for patients with esophageal motility disorders. This can be as an adjunct to the primary surgical treatment of the disorder (e.g., after an esophagomyotomy for a named motility disorder) or as a temporizing, nonobstructive treatment for reflux patients with nonspecific peristaltic dysfunction. Use of the Toupet as an antireflux procedure for

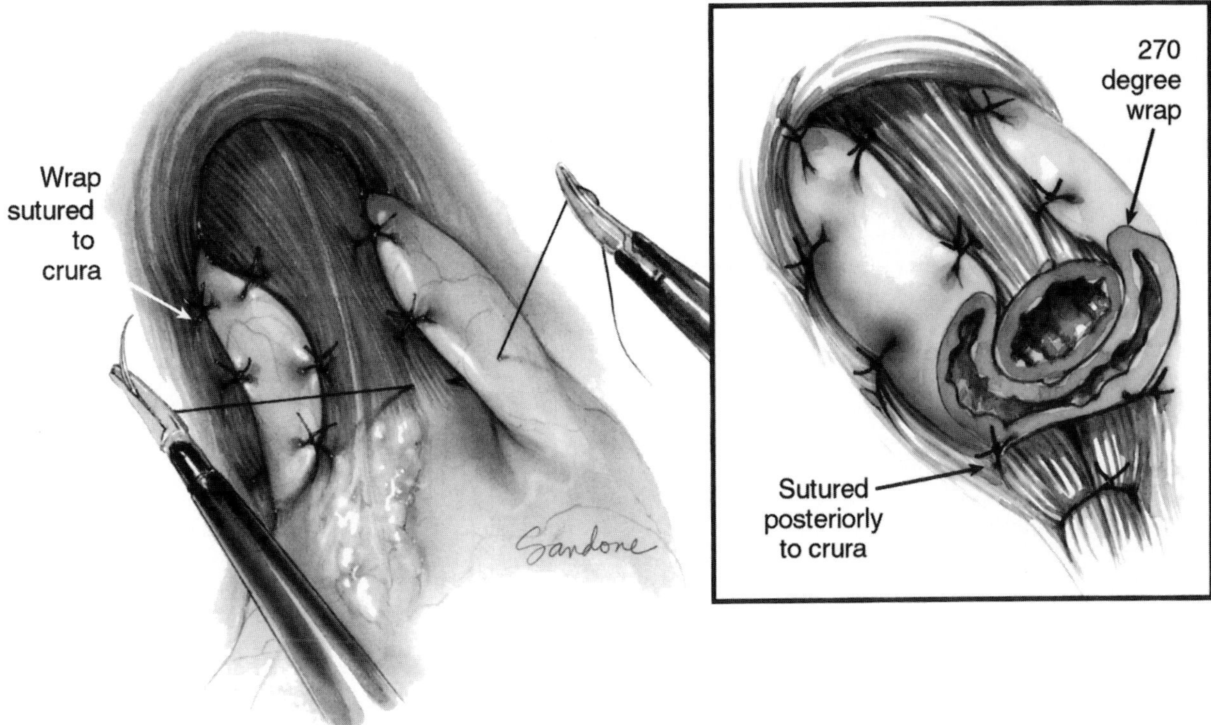

FIGURE 23–6 ■ Current configuration of the modified laparoscopic Toupet repair. *Inset,* a 270-degree posterior wrap sewn posteriorly to the loosely closed crura. (© Corinne Sandone.)

patients with normal motility has been practiced at some institutions but remains controversial.

In addition to these general indications are rare specific instances of reflux disease that are ideally suited for a Toupet repair. These include patients with psychological issues who would be unlikely to tolerate even the transient side effects of a standard fundoplication or patients with an inadequate amount of fundus to achieve a tension-free, 360-degree wrap (Swanström and Hunter, 1994).

Contraindications include the inability to undergo general anesthesia, inability to give informed consent, and any condition that might make laparoscopy dangerous, such as a hostile abdomen from previous upper abdominal surgeries or the inability to tolerate a carbon dioxide pneumoperitoneum due to profound pulmonary carbon dioxide retention. Pregnancy, morbid obesity, and a shortened esophagus represent relative contraindications, and such cases should be assessed on an individual basis.

Preoperative workup for a patient undergoing laparoscopic Toupet repair is the same as for any patient being evaluated for antireflux surgery (Waring et al, 1995). Particular attention should be paid to the preoperative motility test because the procedure is typically done for patients with a motility disorder and the type and severity of the disorder may be relevant in planning the surgical approach. Anatomic factors that might complicate the surgery (e.g., shortened esophagus, esophageal diverticulum, paraesophageal hernia) should be assessed by a barium swallow or an upper endoscopy.

Finally, a 24-hour pH study should be obtained in all patients, especially for patients with atypical symptoms, to help arrive at the correct diagnosis (Jamieson et al, 1992). Even in patients with typical symptoms, we find that a preoperative 24-hour pH test provides important preoperative information that may alter the surgical approach. This is particularly true when the preoperative 24-hour pH test documents an extremely high DeMeester score because the partial fundoplication alone is more likely to fail over the long term (Horvath et al, 1999). Such patients may, in fact, be candidates for an adjuvant procedure such as a vagotomy or a gastric emptying procedure (Csendes et al, 1997).

A final reason to perform 24-hour pH testing in all

TABLE 23–6 ■ **Indications for the Laparoscopic Toupet Fundoplication**

General Indications

- Documented gastroesophageal reflux
- Adequate esophageal length
- Ability to tolerate general anesthesia

Indications for Toupet versus Nissen Repair

- Poor esophageal body motility (peristaltic amplitudes < 30 mm Hg, $> 50\%$ dropped or simultaneous waves)
- Following Heller's myotomy
- Severe aerophagia
- Inadequate gastric fundus for a full wrap
  - Tubular stomach
  - Previous gastric surgery
  - Previous splenorrhaphy

patients is to obtain a baseline value that will allow future objective follow-up testing for patients who experience postoperative problems.

SURGICAL TECHNIQUE

After appropriate consent is obtained, the patient is admitted, an intravenous line is started, preoperative antibiotics are given, and deep venous thrombosis prophylaxis is initiated. General anesthesia is initiated, and an oral gastric tube is placed. The patient is positioned with both arms outstretched on well-padded armboards at less than a 90-degree angle. A split-leg table is used to allow the cameraperson to sit comfortably between the table legs during the procedure. The surgeon stands on the patient's left, and the assistant stands on the patient's right (Fig. 23–7). All port sites are pre-infiltrated with bupivacaine.

The initial port site, for the laparoscope, is placed 15 cm below the xiphoid process and 2.5 cm to left of the midline. Depending on the diameter of the 45-degree angled laparoscope available, this port will be either 5 mm or 10 mm. A quick visual exploration is made to ensure that no adhesions or other pathologic process would complicate placement of the additional access ports. Depending on the size of instrumentation available, most access ports can be 5 mm in diameter. Typical port placement is shown in Figure 27–8. The left lobe of the liver is elevated with an atraumatic retractor, which is then secured to a table-mounted instrument holder.

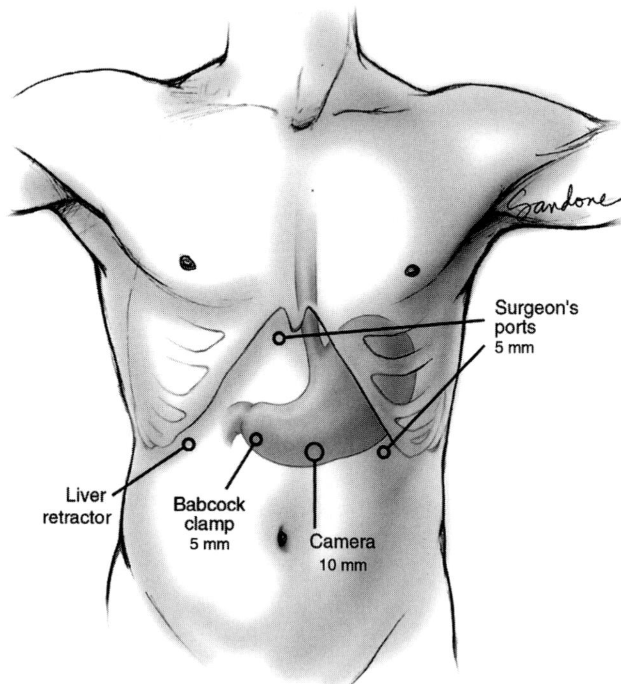

FIGURE 23–8 ■ Optimal port placement is crucial for efficient laparoscopic antireflux surgery. Shown are the typical placements for a laparoscopic Toupet fundoplication. (© Corinne Sandone.)

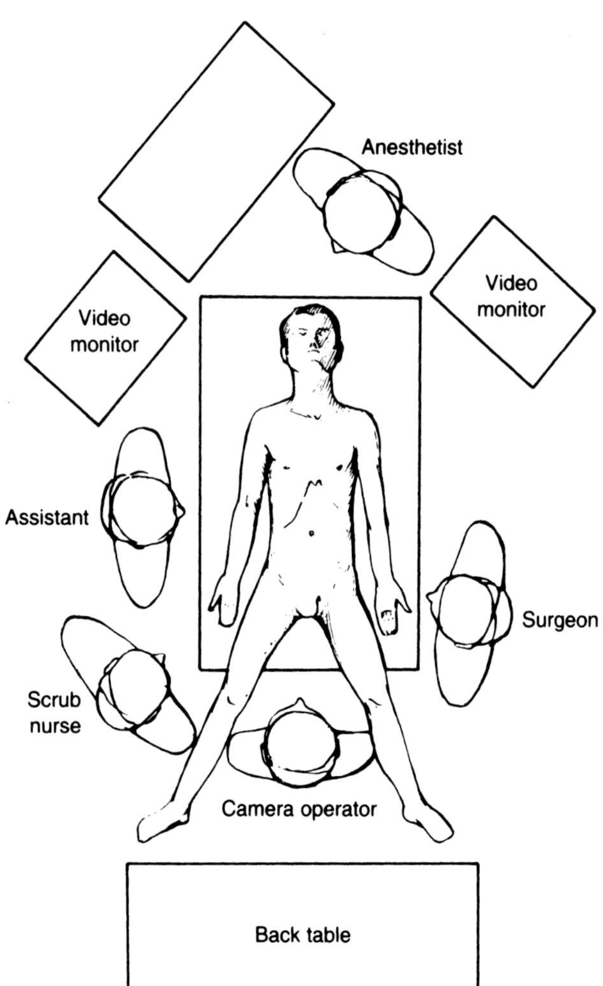

FIGURE 23–7 ■ Room setup and patient position for the laparoscopic Toupet procedure. (© Corinne Sandone.)

The assistant retracts the stomach downward using an atraumatic grasper, and the surgeon divides the hepatogastric ligament using either bipolar shears or the ultrasonic coagulating shears. Fifteen percent of patients have a left hepatic arterial branch coming from the left gastric artery and running through the hepatogastric ligament. This accessory artery is spared if it is greater than 2 or 3 mm, since in rare instances division can lead to hepatic ischemia. The phrenoesophageal ligament is divided after the right crus has been identified. Both the right and left crural limbs are dissected free anteriorly and posteriorly to the point where they fuse. The mediastinal esophagus is freed with blunt and sharp dissection to obtain 3 to 4 cm of tension-free intra-abdominal esophageal length.

The short gastric vessels along the upper third of the gastric fundus are divided with the ultrasonic coagulating shears or with clip ligation and division. This allows the fundus to be rotated medially, allowing direct access to the retrogastric attachments, which are then divided. The retroesophageal window is created carefully behind the posterior vagus nerve under the direct vision achieved with the angled laparoscope. The posterior wall of the fundus is grasped near the short gastric vessels and brought beneath the esophagus.

Using the fundus as an esophageal retractor, the assistant exposes the posterior hiatus to allow the crural

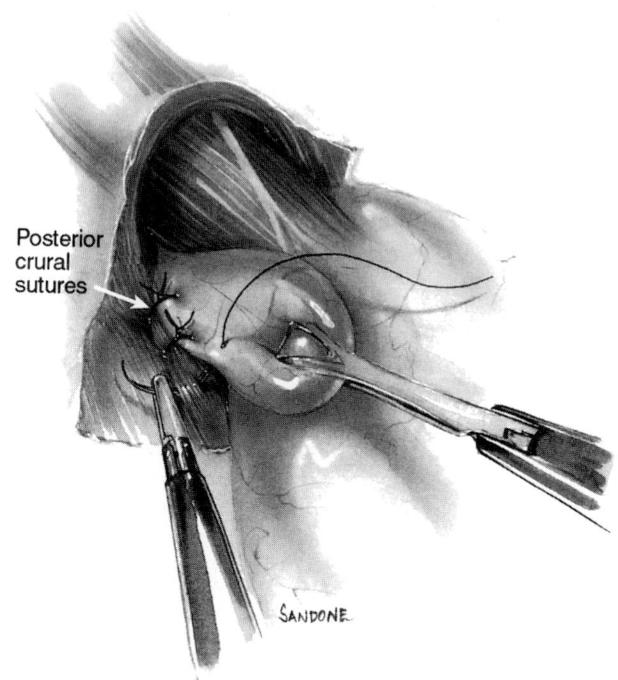

FIGURE 23–9 ■ Visualization for the placement of the posterior crural sutures is obtained by using the fundal wrap as an esophageal retractor and by the use of a 45-degree angled laparoscope. (© Corinne Sandone.)

stitches to be placed (Fig. 23–9). Starting caudally, each suture includes both the posterior wrap and crura.

Unlike the originally described Toupet repair, which bridged the hiatus with the gastric fundus, we prefer to reapproximate the right and left crura with the posterior sutures. The crural closure must be loose, however, to prevent resistance to esophageal emptying. Subsequent sutures are placed from the right and left fundal wrap to the corresponding crura.

Finally, three or four interrupted sutures are placed from the esophagus to the left and right wrap at the 10 o'clock and 2 o'clock positions to create a wrap 3 to 4 cm long. This is done with a 56 French bougie in place to accurately gauge the 270 degrees of the fundoplication (see Fig. 23–6*A*). All sutures should be of permanent materials, and intracorporeal tying techniques are preferred because they are less traumatic to the tissues (Swanstrom and Pennings, 1995). The abdomen is then deinsuflated, and all 10-mm fascial defects are closed. A nasogastric tube is not routinely left in place.

Postoperatively, the patient takes nothing by mouth until nausea-free and then is advanced to a full liquid diet as tolerated. Antiemetic agents are liberally used to prevent postoperative retching or vomiting, which may cause wrap herniation. The patient is typically allowed to go home on postoperative day 1. Heavy lifting is restricted for 2 weeks after surgery. The patient is told to expect dysphagia for 2 to 4 weeks and to avoid bread and meats during this time.

RESULTS

Since first described by Cuchieri and colleagues (1993), the laparoscopic Toupet has been shown to be a safe procedure with low operative morbidity. Reported operative complications include esophageal or gastric perforation, vagal nerve injury and sequelae due to trocar insertion. Large series have reported perioperative morbidity rates between 10% and 15% (Bell et al, 1996; Coster et al, 1997; Jobe et al, 1997; McKernan and Champion, 1995; Mosnier et al, 1995). Postoperative success rates vary according to the indications for the surgery.

Oddly enough, patients with profound esophageal motility disorders seem to have better success than do those with normal motility. For instance, the Toupet procedure has gained wide popularity as an adjunct antireflux procedure following a laparoscopic Heller myotomy based both on theoretical considerations and on reported good results, (Swanstrom and Pennings, 1995). Whether it is a better antireflux procedure than the traditional Dor following a Heller myotomy is not known. Similar good results have been reported in series using both types of laparoscopic partial fundoplications following esophagomyotomy (Anselmino et al, 1997; Delgado et al, 1996; Vogt et al, 1997). Only one study has directly compared the two procedures (Raiser et al, 1996). This study showed improved reflux control after myotomy with the Toupet repair compared with the Dor procedure. The study was, however, retrospective and the numbers were barely significant.

The ability to perform antireflux surgery laparoscopically has created new expectations among surgeons and their patients (Rattner and Brooks, 1995). Surgeons are often concerned that their patients and their referral physicians will not tolerate the transient side effects associated with the Nissen procedure. In an effort to minimize postoperative dysphagia and the inability to belch or vomit, these practitioners have advocated routine use of the Toupet procedure as a more physiologic alternative to the Nissen repair in all patients with gastroesophageal reflux disease (GERD) (Bell et al, 1996; Coster et al, 1997; McKernan, 1994). Early results from these centers have shown encouragingly low rates of postoperative side effects and good control of reflux symptoms. Others, however, have shown unacceptable rates of postoperative reflux, which is frequently asymptomatic. Bell and coworkers (1999) documented a 50% symptomatic failure rate in 82 laparoscopic Toupet patients operated on for severe GERD at a 30-month follow-up. Our group has shown a 49% failure rate by 24-hour pH testing at a mean follow-up of 2 years (Jobe et al, 1997). This is in spite of documentation of an adequate Toupet fundoplication in the majority of patients (Horvath et al, 1999) (Table 23–7). The weakness of the Toupet repair, at least in patients with normal esophageal motility, seems to be its generally less competent reverse flow (Richardson et al, 1997).

Most surgeons, therefore, reserve the use of the Toupet fundoplication for patients with GERD and disordered esophageal motility (DeMeester and Stein, 1992; Hunter et al, 1996a, 1996b; Kauer, 1995; Peters and DeMeester, 1995). This group of patients presents a particularly difficult therapeutic dilemma. Reflux tends to be particularly severe in patients with delayed esophageal clearance, yet these patients cannot tolerate a "heavy-duty" antireflux procedure without unacceptable rates of postoperative

TABLE 23–7 ■ **Results of the Laparoscopic Toupet Procedure in 100 Consecutive Patients Studied Prospectively (Follow-up at 22 Months)**

SYMPTOM FOLLOW-UP	
Dysphagia	9% (1% dilatation)
Heartburn	20% (17% on medication, 3% surgery revised to a Nissen)
OBJECTIVE FOLLOW-UP	
Endoscopy	18% esophagitis
Manometry	23 mm Hg mean postoperative pressure (130% increase)
24 hr pH	51% abnormal findings (50% asymptomatic)

Data from Jobe BA, Wallace J, Hansen PD, Swanstrom LL: Evaluation of laparoscopic Toupet fundoplication as a primary repair for all patients with medically resistant gastroesophageal reflux. Surg Endosc 11:1080–1083, 1997.

dysphagia (Lund et al, 1997; Stein et al, 1992). Many groups, therefore, choose the Toupet fundoplication for patients accepting a higher postoperative reflux rate as the price of an acceptable postoperative dysphagia rate. Some investigators have theorized that a short floppy Nissen would be tolerated in patients with poor esophageal motility and report limited clinical data to support that position (Donahue et al, 1985; Eypasch et al, 1997; Topart et al, 1992). There are, however, no definitive outcome studies that show acceptable postoperative dysphagia rates with the Nissen repair in this complex patient group. The current "gold standard" for laparoscopic fundoplications is the "tailored" approach, which calls for a short floppy Nissen repair for patients with normal motility and a partial fundoplication, most commonly the Toupet, for all patients with markedly decreased esophageal body motility (Hunter et al, 1996b).

FUTURE TRENDS

The almost universal acceptance of the laparoscopic approach for Heller's myotomy and fundoplication has created a renewed, and sometimes increased, interest in the Toupet repair. Several clinical questions, however, need to be answered. Although it is generally accepted that a partial fundoplication should accompany a Heller myotomy, it has never been documented whether the Dor or the Toupet fundoplication provides better reflux protection with the least degree of esophageal outflow obstruction. Obviously, this question can be answered only by a well-constructed, prospective clinical study.

The true effectiveness of the laparoscopic Toupet procedure as an antireflux surgical procedure also needs to be documented over the long term. Outcome studies with limited short-term follow-up and subjective postoperative assessment are common and frequently favorable in their assessment of the technique. These studies are flawed, as they are weighted toward assessment of the short-term transient side effects common with any antireflux surgery, such as dysphagia and inability to belch. Because of its unique characteristics, the Toupet repair has always fared well in such assessments. Proof of long-term success in controlling reflux is much more difficult. Objective postoperative testing is needed, since as many as 50% of patients with postoperative reflux are asymptomatic (Jobe et al, 1997). It is also difficult to recruit and monitor patients for the 5- to 10-year follow-up that is needed. At least two studies with objective follow-up in the short term have indicated higher rates of failure with the laparoscopic Toupet repair when compared to the Nissen (Bell et al, 1999; Horvath et al, 1999). These authors concluded that in spite of lower postoperative side effects, laparoscopic Toupet should be reserved for patients with significant esophageal motility disorders. Even this dogma deserves to be questioned: Is the Toupet really superior to a complete fundoplication in patients with esophageal motor dysfunction? A few studies have indicated that a short floppy Nissen wrap is well tolerated in these patients (Bremner et al, 1994). Considering the diminished reflux control of the Toupet, this is certainly an outcome study worth initiating.

CONCLUSION

The laparoscopic Toupet repair was first described in 1993 and has achieved wide acceptance as the procedure of choice in patients with poor esophageal motility and GERD. It has also been widely adopted as an adjuvant procedure following a laparoscopic Heller myotomy. It is certainly associated with a low incidence of annoying postoperative side effects, including dysphagia and the inability to belch, which makes it very suited to patients undergoing a minimally invasive surgical procedure. It is, however, associated with lower long-term success rates in controlling reflux. Therefore, surgeons should carefully consider the relative benefits and disadvantages of the laparoscopic Toupet before selecting it for their patients.

■ *REFERENCES*

Anselmino M, Zaninotto G, Constantini M, et al: Collis gastroplasty plus fundoplication is more effective than bouginage plus acid suppressive therapy in the treatment of reflux induced strictures of the esophagus. J Gastrointest Surg. 1, 1–10, 1997.

Bell RCW, Hanna P, Mills MR, Bowrey D: Patterns of success and failure with laparoscopic Toupet fundoplication. Surg Endosc 13:1189–1194, 1999.

Bell RC, Hanna P, Powers B, et al: Clinical and manometric results of laparoscopic partial (Toupet) and complete (Rosetti-Nissen) fundoplication. Surg Endosc 10:724–728, 1996.

Boutelier P, Jonsell G: An alternative fundoplicative maneuver for gastroesophageal reflux. Am J Surg 143:260–264, 1992.

Bremner RM, DeMeester TR, Crookes P, et al: The effect of symptoms and nonspecific motility abnormalities on outcomes of surgical therapy for gastroesophageal reflux disease. J Thorac Cardiovasc Surg 107:1244–1250, 1994.

Coster DD, Bower WH, Wilson VT, et al: Laparoscopic partial fundoplication vs. laparoscopic Nissen-Rosetti fundoplication. Surg Endosc 11:625–631, 1997.

Csendes A, Braghetto I, Burdiles P, et al: A new physiologic approach for the surgical treatment of patients with Barrett's esophagus: Technical considerations and results in 65 patients. Ann Surg 226:123–133, 1997.

Cuschieri A, Hunter J, Wolfe B, et al: Multicenter prospective evaluation of laparoscopic antireflux surgery. Surg Endosc 7:505–510, 1993.

Dallemagne B, Weerts JM, Jehaes C: Laparoscopic Nissen fundoplication: Preliminary report. Surg Laparosc Endosc 1:138–143, 1991.

Delgado F, Bolufer JM, Martinez-Abad M, et al: Laparoscopic treatment of esophageal achalasia. Surg Laparose Endosc 6:83–90, 1996.

DeMeester TR, Stein HJ: Surgery for esophageal motor disorders. In Castell DO (ed): The Esophagus. Boston, Little, Brown, 1992, pp 401–439.

Donahue PE, Samuelson S, Nulus LM, Bombeck CT: The floppy Nissen fundoplication effective long-term control of pathologic reflux. Arch Surg 120:663–667, 1985.

Eypasch E, Neugebauer E, Fischer R, Troidl H: Laparoscopic antireflux surgery for gastroesophageal reflux disease: Results of a consensus development conference. Surg Endosc 11:413–426, 1997.

Horvath KD, Jobe BA, Herron DM, Swanström LL: Laparoscopic Toupet fundoplication is an inadequate procedure for patients with severe reflux disease. J Gastrointest Surg 3:583–591, 1999.

Hunter JG, Swanström LL, Waring JP: Dysphagia after laparoscopic anti-reflux surgery: The impact of operative technique. Ann Surg 224:51–57, 1996a.

Hunter JG, Trus TL, Branum GD: A physiologic approach to laparoscopic fundoplication for gastroesophageal reflux disease. Ann Surg 223:673–685, 1996.

Jamieson JR, Stein HJ, DeMeester TR, et al: Ambulatory 24-hour esophageal pH monitoring: Normal values, optimal thresholds, specificity, sensitivity and reproducibility. Am J Gastroenterol 87:1102–1111, 1992.

Jobe BA, Wallace J, Hansen PD, Swanström LL: Evaluation of laparoscopic Toupet fundoplication as a primary repair for all patients with medically resistant gastroesophageal reflux. Surg Endosc 11:1080–1083, 1997.

Kauer WK: A tailored approach to antireflux surgery. J Thorac Cardiovasc Surg 110:141–146, 1995.

Lind JF, Burns CM, MacDougall JT: "Physiologic" repair for hiatus hernia: Manometric study. Arch Surg 91:233–234, 1965.

Lund RJ, Wetcher GF, Raiser F, et al: Laparoscopic Toupet fundoplication for gastroesophageal reflux disease with poor esophageal body motility. Gastrointest Surg 1:301–308, 1997.

Lundell L, Abrahamsson H, Ruth M, et al: Lower esophageal sphincter characteristics and esophageal acid exposure following partial or 360-degree fundoplication: The results of a prospective, randomized, clinical study. World J Surg 15:115–120, 1991.

McKernan JB: Laparoscopic repair of gastroesophageal reflux disease: Toupet partial fundoplication versus Nissen fundoplication. Surg Endosc 8:851–856, 1994.

McKernan JB, Champion JK: Laparoscopic antireflux surgery. Am Surg 61:530–536, 1995.

Mosnier H, Leport J, Aubert A, et al: A 270-degree laparoscopic posterior fundoplasty in the treatment of gastroesophageal reflux. J Am Coll Surg 181:1088–1094, 1995.

Peters JH, DeMeester TR: Indications, principles of procedure selection, and techniques of laparoscopic Nissen fundoplication. Semin Laparosc Surg 2:27–44, 1995.

Raiser F, Perdikis G, Hinder RA, et al: Heller myotomy via minimal access surgery: An evaluation of antireflux procedures. Arch Surg 131:598, 1996.

Rattner DW, Brooks DC: Patient satisfaction following laparoscopic and open antireflux surgery. Arch Surg 130:289–292, 1995.

Richardson WS, Trus TL, Thompson S, Hunter J: Nissen and Toupet fundoplications effectively inhibit gastroesophageal reflux irrespective of natural anatomy and function. Surg Endosc 11:261–263, 1997.

Stein HJ, Bremner RM, Jamieson J, DeMeester TR: Effect of Nissen fundoplication on esophageal motor function. Arch Surg 127:788–791, 1992.

Swanström L, Hunter J: Techniques of laparoscopic partial fundoplications. In DeMeester TR, Peters JH (eds): Minimally Invasive Foregut Surgery. St. Louis, Quality Medical Publishing, 1994.

Swanström L, Pennings J: Laparoscopic esophagomyotomy for achalasia. Surg Endosc 9:286–292, 1995.

Swanström L, Wayne R: Spectrum of gastrointestinal symptoms after laparoscopic fundoplications. Am J Surg 167:538–541, 1994.

Thor KBA, Silander T: A long-term randomized prospective trial of the Nissen procedure versus a modified Toupet technique. Ann Surg 210:719–724, 1989.

Topart P, Deschamps C, Taillefer R, Duranceau A: Long-term effect of total fundoplication on the myotomized esophagus. Ann Thorac Surg 54:1046–1052, 1992.

Toupet A: Technique d'oesophago-gastroplastie avec phrenogastropexie appliquée dams la cure radicale des hernies hiatales et comme complement de l'operation d'Heller dans les cardiospasmes. Mem Acad Chir 89:394–395, 1963.

Vogt D, Curet M, Pitcher D, et al: Successful treatment of esophageal achalasia with laparoscopic Heller myotomy and Toupet fundoplication. Am J Surg 174:709–714, 1997.

Waring JP, Hunter J, Oddsdottir M, et al: The preoperative evaluation of patients considered for laparoscopic antireflux surgery. Am J Gastroenterol 90:35–38, 1995.

CHAPTER **24**

Gastroplasty

OPEN GASTROPLASTY

F. Griffith Pearson

DEFINITION

Gastroplasty is an esophageal "lengthening" technique that is designed to obviate tension on an antireflux repair in patients with acquired esophageal shortening. A tube of stomach is fashioned from the lesser curvature side of the cardia in continuity with the distal esophagus. At completion, the distal end of this "gastroplasty tube" is dealt with as if it were the esophagogastric junction. The esophagus has therefore been "lengthened," and the potential for tension on the subsequent antireflux repair is avoided. This technique of "gastroplasty" should not be confused with the various operations for the management of morbid obesity.

HISTORICAL NOTE

The operation of gastroplasty was first described by Leigh Collis in 1957 (Fig. 24–1). He combined gastroplasty with his technique of hiatal hernia repair. The operation was "designed to help patients with hiatus hernia associated with *short esophagus*." In 1961, Collis reported on observations from experience with 32 patients.

I visited Mr. Collis in Birmingham in 1960 and observed some of his patients managed by this technique. We began to add gastroplasty to the antireflux repair in selected patients beginning in the early part of 1960 and reported preliminary experience in 1971 (Pearson et al, 1971). We modified Collis' original operation as follows: Exposure was restricted to a left thoracotomy rather than a left thoracoabdominal incision. The gastroplasty tube was fashioned so that the tube diameter remained constant from top to bottom (Fig. 24–2). A Belsey Mark IV repair, rather than Collis' original repair, was done (see Fig. 24–2).

Subsequent modifications, by other surgeons, include the technique of "uncut gastroplasty" (Demos 1975, 1984; Langer, 1973), the use of a Nissen type fundoplication rather than a Belsey Mark IV procedure (Henderson, 1977; Orringer and Sloan, 1977), and a transabdominal technique requiring the use of the smallest diameter end-to-end anastomosis (EEA) stapler (Steichen, 1986).

■ *HISTORICAL READINGS*

Collis JL: Gastroplasty. Thorax 16:197, 1961.

Demos NJ, Smith N, Williams D: A gastroplasty for short esophagus and reflux esophagitis. Ann Surg 181:178–181, 1975.

Demos NJ: Stapled uncut gastroplasty for hiatal hernia: 12 year follow-up. Ann Thorac Surg 38:393–398, 1984.

Henderson RD: Reflux control following gastroplasty. Ann Thorac Surg 24:206, 1977.

Langer B: Modified gastroplasty: A simple operation for reflux esophagitis with moderate degrees of shortening. Can J Surg 16:1, 1973.

Orringer MB, Sloan H: Complications and failings of combined Collis-Belsey operation. J Thorac Cardiovasc Surg 74:726, 1977.

Pearson FG, Langer R, Henderson RD: Gastroplasty and Belsey hiatus hernia repair. J Thorac Cardiovasc Surg 61:50, 1971.

Steichen FM: Abdominal approach to the Collis gastroplasty and Nissen fundoplication. Surg Gynecol Obstet 162:372–374, 1986.

INDICATIONS

Gastroplasty is indicated as an addition to any antireflux operation (hiatal hernia repair) when it is anticipated that the repair alone would result in an unacceptable level of tension on the reconstruction. All of the commonly used standard repairs restore a segment of distal esophagus to an intra-abdominal position (Nissen, Belsey, and Hill). In fact, the normal esophagogastric junction lies within the channel of the diaphragmatic hiatus (Fig. 24–3). All of these standard repairs exaggerate the length of the intra-abdominal segment of esophagus and are assumed to be under some degree of tension. An exception may be the Hill repair, in which the reconstruction (posterior gastropexy) begins at the esophagogastric junction and extends distally along the lesser curvature side of the stomach.

The primary indication for the addition of gastroplasty is acquired shortening caused by mural scarring, with vertical scar contracture secondary to peptic esophagitis. This complication occurs as a feature of the most advanced stages of reflux esophagitis, which include confluent ulceration, peptic stricture, acquired columnar-lined esophagus (Gastal et al, 1999; Pearson et al, 1987), and massive, paraesophageal hernia (types III and IV) (Horvath et al, 2000; Maziak et al, 1998; Pearson et al, 1983). Gross degrees of shortening are easily recognized on the barium radiograph, at endoscopy, and by the surgeon at the time of the operation. Subtle degrees of shortening, however, may be difficult to appreciate. The diagnosis of acquired short esophagus is made from observations obtained through contrast radiographs, esophagoscopy, specific measurements during esophageal

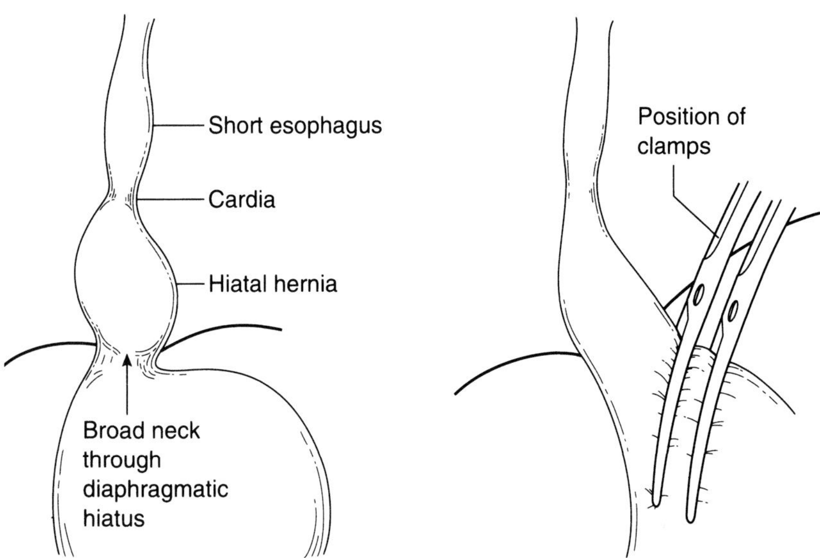

FIGURE 24–1 ■ Diagrammatic representation of the original Collis gastroplasty. (Adapted from Collis JL: Gastroplasty. Thorax 16:197, 1961.)

manometry, and intraoperative findings at surgery (Gastal et al, 1999; Horvath et al, 2000; Maziak et al, 1998).

Contrast Radiography

As the esophagus shortens, the angle of His is lost and the sliding hernia becomes irreducible, even in the upright position (Fig. 24–4). In patients with extreme esophageal shortening, the cardia and top of the stomach may be pulled well up into the posterior mediastinum.

Esophagoscopy

The distance from the upper teeth, or gum, to the esophagogastric junction can be determined accurately during flexible esophagoscopy. If the esophagogastric junction lies at a high level, in the posterior mediastinum above the diaphragmatic hiatus (≥5 cm), shortening is considered a likely possibility. At esophagoscopy, the finding of severe, gross peptic esophagitis (confluent ulceration, peptic stricture, or acquired columnar-lined esophagus) should alert the surgeon to the possibility of significant acquired shortening caused by transmural inflammation and scar contracture.

Esophageal Manometry

The distance between the cricopharyngeal sphincter and the lower esophageal sphincter (LES) can be measured

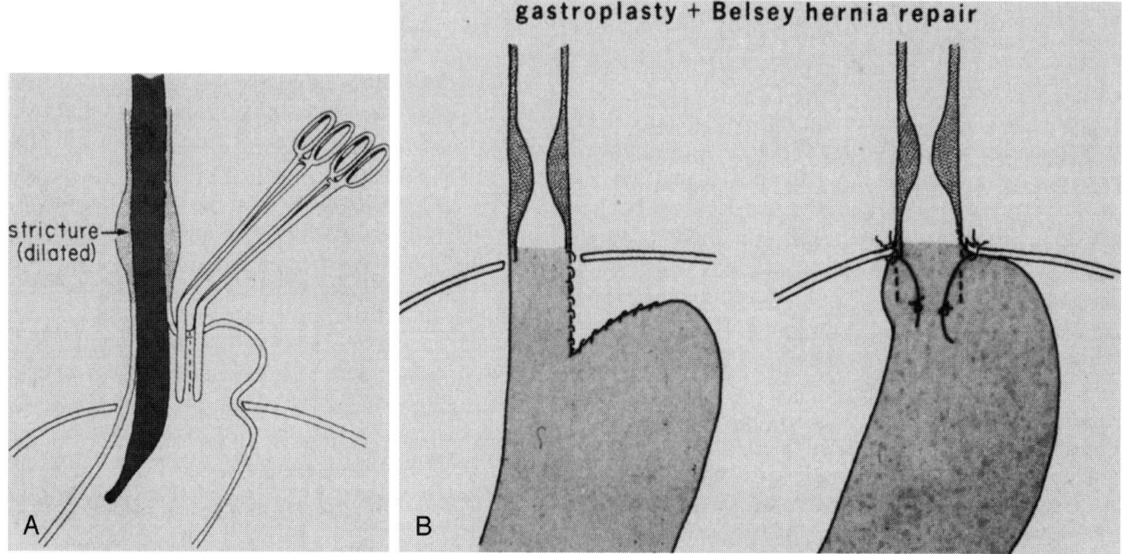

FIGURE 24–2 ■ *A*, Diagrammatic illustration of the Pearson technique of gastroplasty and Belsey partial fundoplication. The peptic stricture has been dilated to a 48 French Maloney bougie, and a gastric tube will be created from the lesser curvature side of the stomach in continuity with distal esophagus and of an approximate esophageal diameter. In this diagram, the stomach will be divided between angulated clamps. In most cases today, the gastrointestinal anastomosis stapler is used. *B*, Diagram illustrating closure of the esophageal and gastric sides of the divided stomach, followed by a Belsey-type partial fundoplication. Most of the gastric tube lies below the diaphragmatic hiatus.

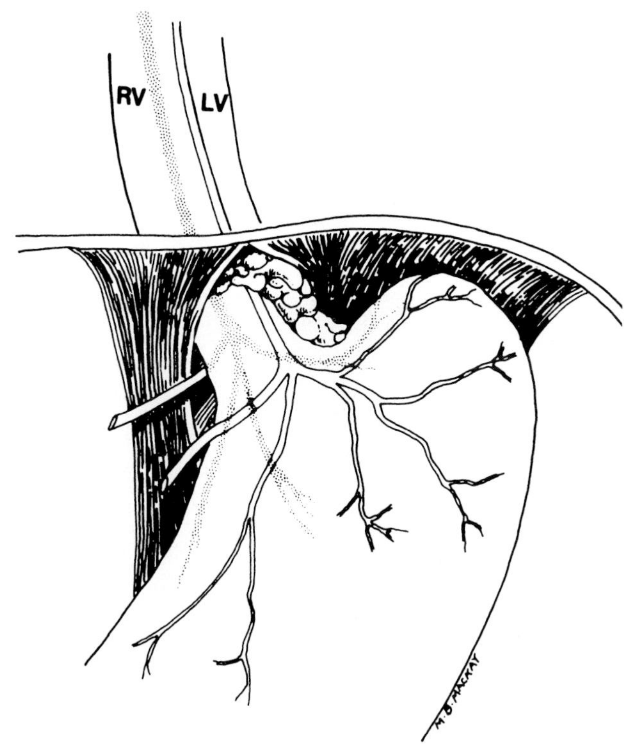

FIGURE 24–3 ■ Diagram showing the normal anatomy at the esophagogastric junction. The distal esophagus actually lies within the tunnel of the diaphragmatic hiatus. There is no significant length of esophagus that is completely intra-abdominal. (LV, left vagus nerve; RV, right vagus nerve.)

during manometry. This distance varies between individuals and depends on height and body configuration. Nevertheless, in most normal adults, the mean distance between these two sphincters is 22 cm: 21.5 cm in females and 22.5 cm in males (measured from the upper border of the LES to the lower border of the cricopharyngeal sphincter). Significantly shorter distances are a further indication of the possibility of acquired shortening (Gastal et al, 1999; Maziak et al, 1998; Mittal et al, 2000).

Intraoperative Findings

The presence of acute and chronic panmural esophagitis suggests shortening: edema and thickening of the esophageal wall, chronic periesophageal lymphadenopathy, and in some cases actual scarring in the periesophageal areolar tissues, which embeds the esophagus in the posterior mediastinum. After circumferential mobilization of the distal esophagus, it may become apparent that the location of the esophagogastric junction lies well above the diaphragmatic hiatus. A precise judgment of acquired shortening is gained only with experience. Because I have used both approaches over the years, I am certain that the judgment of acquired shortening is more easily made from the thoracic exposure than from the abdominal side.

Controversial Indications

Reoperation for Failed Previous Antireflux Surgery

In any patient who has undergone one or more prior antireflux operations, the tissues that are involved in the subsequent repair are relatively damaged. The reported results of reoperation are significantly less favorable, and any maneuver that reduces tension on the repair seems desirable.

Massive Hiatal Hernia and Intrathoracic Stomach

Giant hernias are almost always the result of a sliding hiatal hernia. They occur in older people, whose tissues are often relatively atrophic. The diaphragmatic hiatus is enormously widened, and the crural margins are thinned and frail. Eighty-five percent of these patients have a definite history of gastroesophageal reflux and may have had scarring and some vertical shortening during the evolution of the massive hernia (Maziak et al, 1998; Pearson et al, 1983). I have noted a high incidence of tension on the repair when a standard Belsey Mark IV operation was used in patients with this type of giant hernia. Belsey reported a high recurrence rate in this group of patients with his Mark IV repair (Orringer et al, 1972). These observations do not pertain in patients with a true paraesophageal hernia, in which the esophagogastric junction remains tethered in the normal, intra-abdominal location. In a report of our Toronto experience (Maziak et al, 1998), only 3 of 94 cases were true paraesophageal hernias (type II).

Some surgeons recommend the addition of gastroplasty in patients with gross obesity, chronic cough, or asthma. They contend that there is an increased strain on the repair and a higher risk of recurrence in patients with these conditions (Urschel, 1978).

SURGICAL TECHNIQUE

Next, the technical details of the operation of modified gastroplasty combined with a Belsey Mark IV fundoplication (Pearson et al, 1971) are illustrated. Today, this

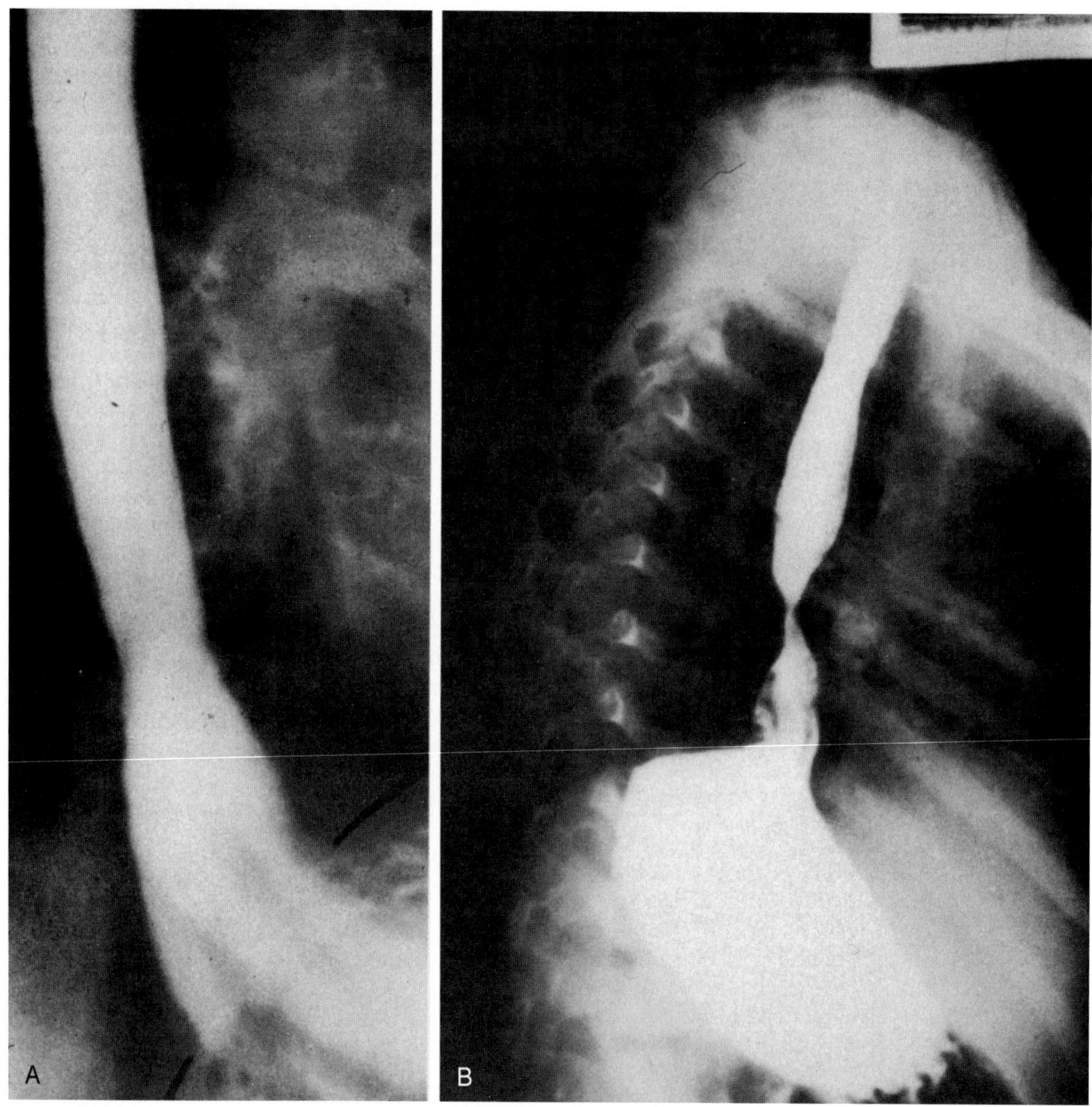

FIGURE 24–4 ■ *A*, Barium swallow illustrating acquired esophageal shortening in a patient with a sliding hiatal hernia. The angle of His is lost, and the appearance suggests that a funnel of stomach has been pulled up into the posterior mediastinum as a result of esophageal shortening. *B*, Barium swallow illustrating a short peptic stricture at the esophagogastric junction, which appears elevated and fixed in the posterior mediastinum.

technique of gastroplasty is much more frequently combined with a 360-degree Nissen-type fundoplication. Creation of the gastroplasty by a transthoracic route is identical. The addition of a Nissen fundoplication—the "Collis-Nissen" procedure—is clearly illustrated in a publication by Moores (1997). In this same report, Moores also illustrates his preferred technique with an abdominal exposure for the Collis-Nissen operation.

Modified Collis Gastroplasty and Belsey Fundoplication

Anesthesia

Split-lung ventilation is desirable so that the left lung can be collapsed during the operation. Either a double-lumen tube or a bronchial blocker may be used.

Incision

The patient is positioned for a full posterolateral thoracotomy. The operating table can be angulated or "broken" at its midpoint, which elevates the left hemithorax for improved exposure. The operating table is tilted with the patient in the reverse Trendelenburg position, which allows the abdominal contents to fall away from the left hemidiaphragm and improves exposure.

Exposure is obtained with a left posterolateral thoracotomy through the sixth intercostal space (Fig. 24–5). The anterior end of the incision is carried almost to the left costal margin so that it ends within a few centimeters of the diaphragmatic origin. This provides optimal exposure for subsequent dissection at the diaphragmatic hiatus and for application of the gastrointestinal anastomosis (GIA) stapler when the gastric tube is constructed.

The ribs are spread as gently as possible and are not

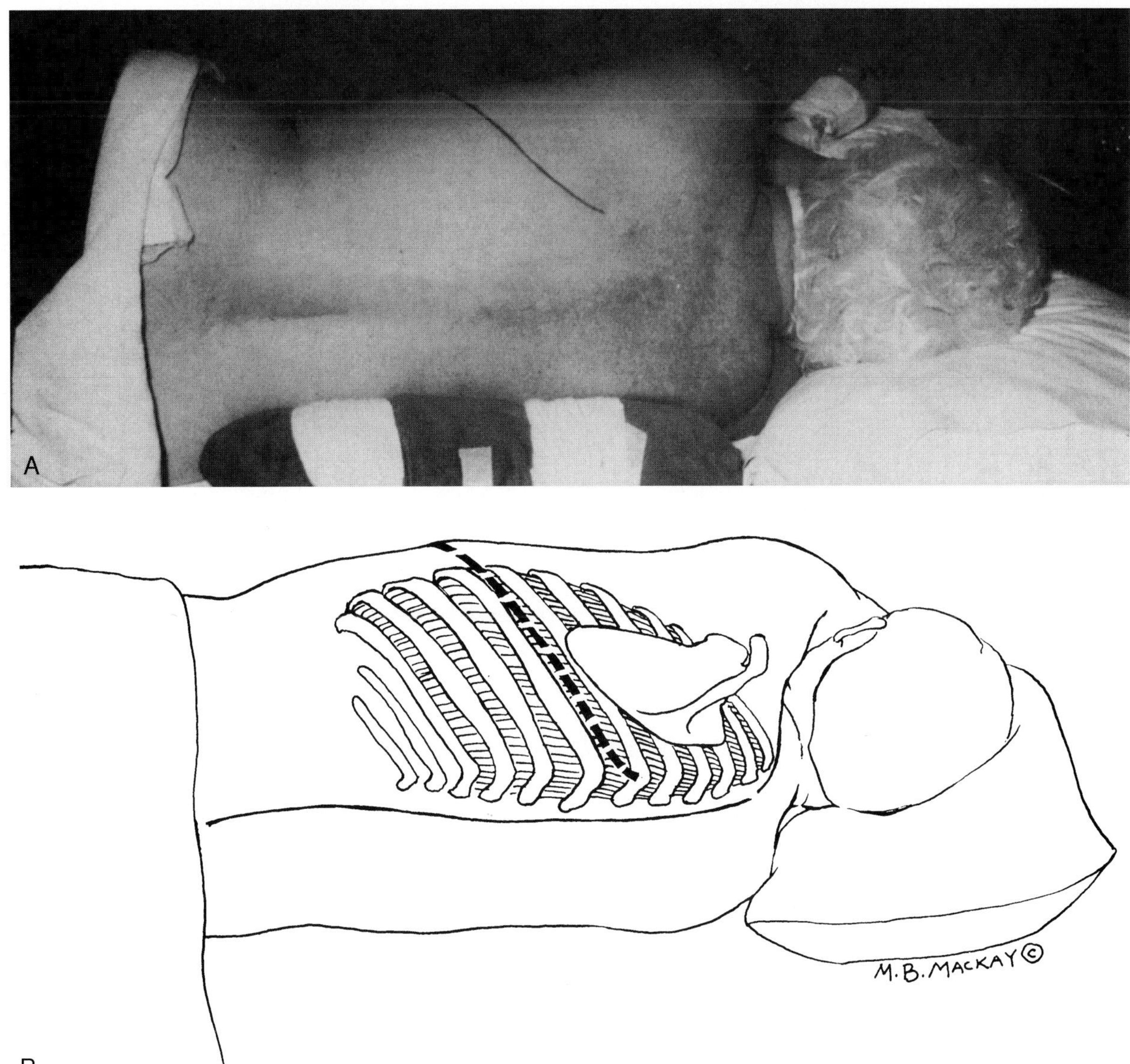

FIGURE 24–5 ■ *A*, Intraoperative photograph illustrating the location of the sixth interspace, left posterolateral thoracotomy. *B*, Diagrammatic illustration of the incision shown in *A*.

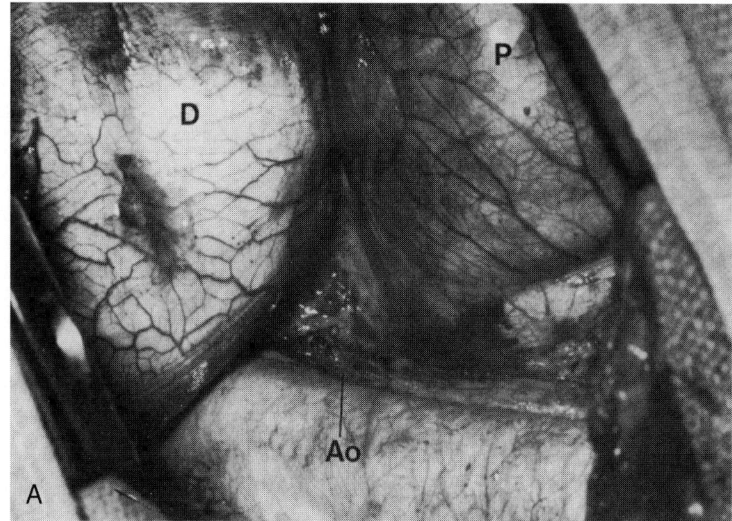

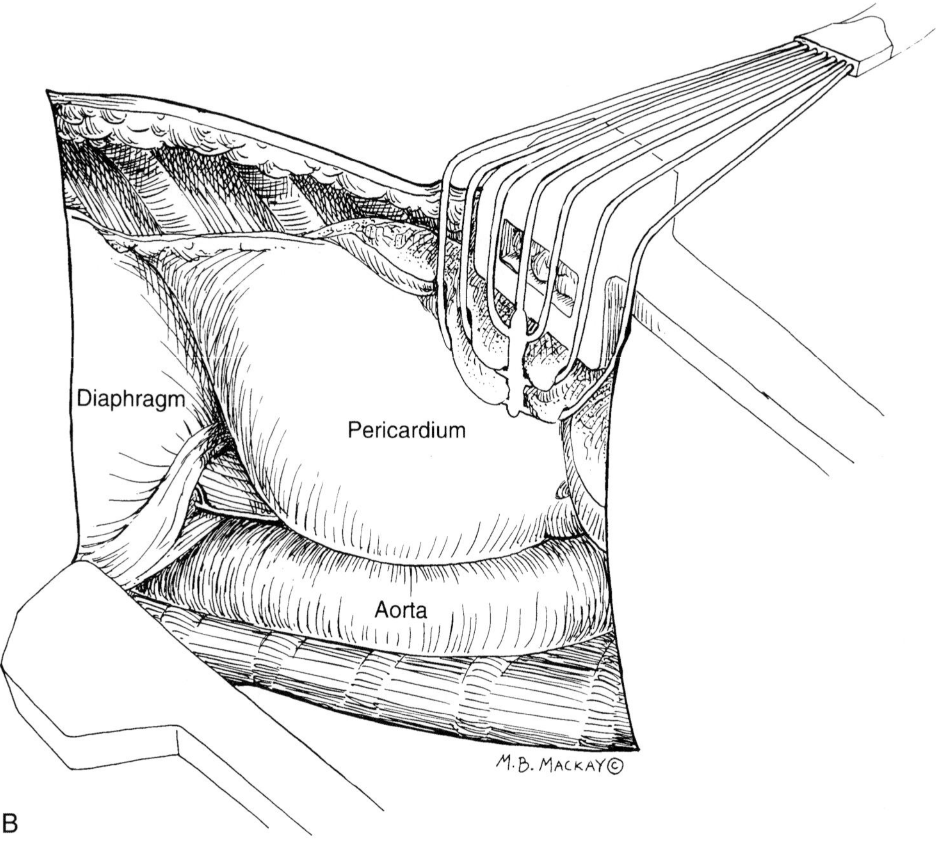

FIGURE 24–6 ■ Intraoperative photograph (*A*) and diagram (*B*) illustrating the exposure obtained through the sixth left intercostal space, with the lung collapsed or retracted. The esophagus will be exposed in the posterior mediastinum above the diaphragm, anterior to the aorta, and lateral to the pericardium. (Ao, aorta; D, diaphragm; P, pericardium.)

separated more than 5 to 7 cm to diminish postoperative incisional pain.

The inferior pulmonary ligament is divided, the left lung is retracted anterosuperiorly, and the posterior mediastinum is clearly exposed (Fig. 24–6).

The esophagus is then mobilized circumferentially from the inferior pulmonary vein above to the diaphragmatic hiatus below. During mobilization, both vagus nerves are palpated, identified, and carried with the esophagus. The right vagus nerve lies just to the right of the anterior border of the descending aorta and is easily separated from the mobilized esophagus unless the surgeon deliberately seeks it and includes it in the mobilization (Fig. 24–7). Also during mobilization, the mediastinal pleura over the right lung is visualized and the surgeon takes care to avoid opening it. The right mediastinal pleura is displaced by blunt dissection from the margins of the diaphragmatic hiatus below and from the right wall of the esophagus behind the pulmonary hilum above. The mobilized esophagus is then elevated and placed on tension with a Penrose drain (Fig. 24–8).

The hiatal margins are freed circumferentially, and the anterior peritoneal sac of the hernia is opened into the greater sac of the peritoneal cavity. The lesser sac is opened posteriorly. The upper end of the gastrohepatic omentum, which often contains a sizable artery, is identified and divided between clamps (Fig. 24–9). Division of this part of the lesser omentum allows the entire cardia of the stomach to rise freely into the left hemithorax. Mobilization of the greater curvature side of the stomach does *not* require division of any short gastric vessels.

There is always a collection of fat between the upper and lower limbs of the phrenoesophageal membrane, which envelops the esophagogastric junction (Fig. 24–10). This "fat pad" is meticulously dissected from most of the circumference of the esophagogastric junction. During dissection, the left vagus nerve is elevated from the muscular wall of the esophagus and carried with the fat pad (see Fig. 24–10*C* and *D*). Fat is cleared from the entire anterior surface of the esophagogastric junction and the adjacent lesser curvature side of the stomach.

This dissection is tedious and requires precise coagulation, or ligation, of the many small vessels between the fat pad and the stomach. The technique is similar to that used during highly selective vagotomy. Removal of this fat pad is a part of the technique of a standard Belsey Mark IV repair and makes it possible to construct the gastric tube through an area of stomach that is free of any fatty covering. However, clearance of a greater circumference of esophagogastric junction is required if gastroplasty is to be added to the repair.

At this stage, a 48 French Maloney dilator is passed through the mouth by the anesthetist. The bougie is advanced so that the distal end lies well within the stomach (Fig. 24–11). In most instances, a gastric tube 4 to 5 cm in length is sufficient to obviate unwanted tension on the repair. The objective is to create a gastric tube of uniform diameter, from top to bottom, over the

Text continued on page 384

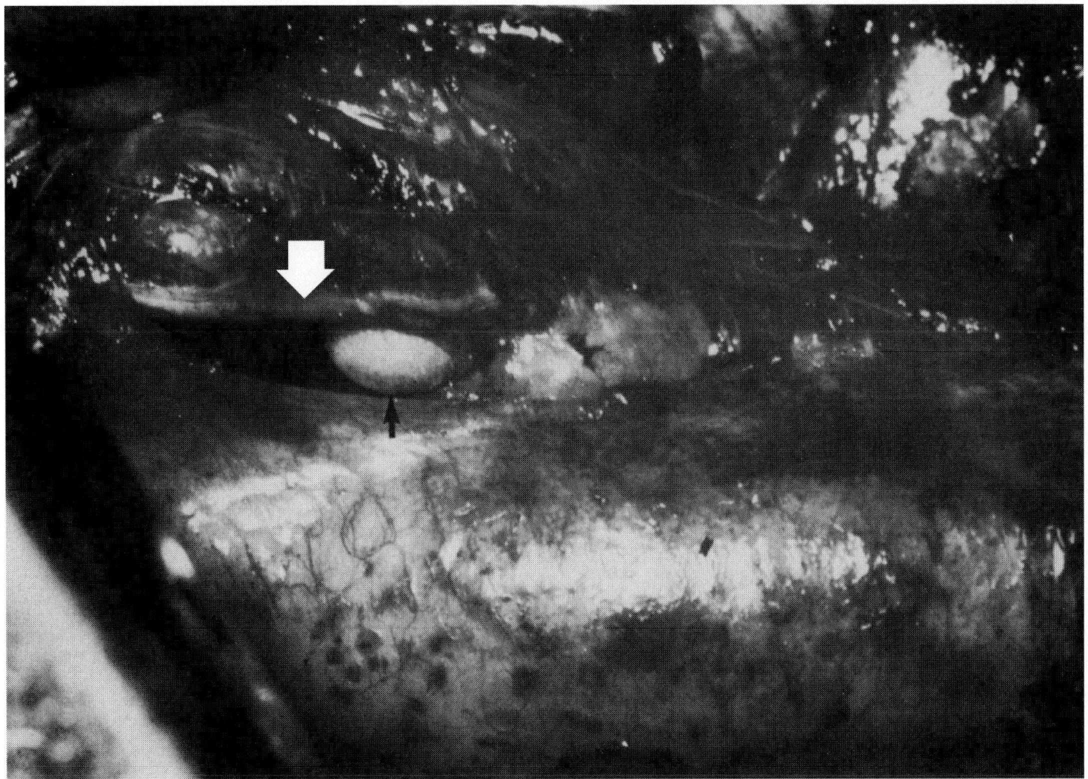

FIGURE 24–7 ■ Intraoperative photograph following mobilization of the distal intrathoracic esophagus. The tip of the surgeon's index finger is seen coming around the distal esophagus (*small arrow*) and displays the right posterior vagus nerve (*large arrow*). Both nerves are identified and mobilized with the distal thoracic esophagus.

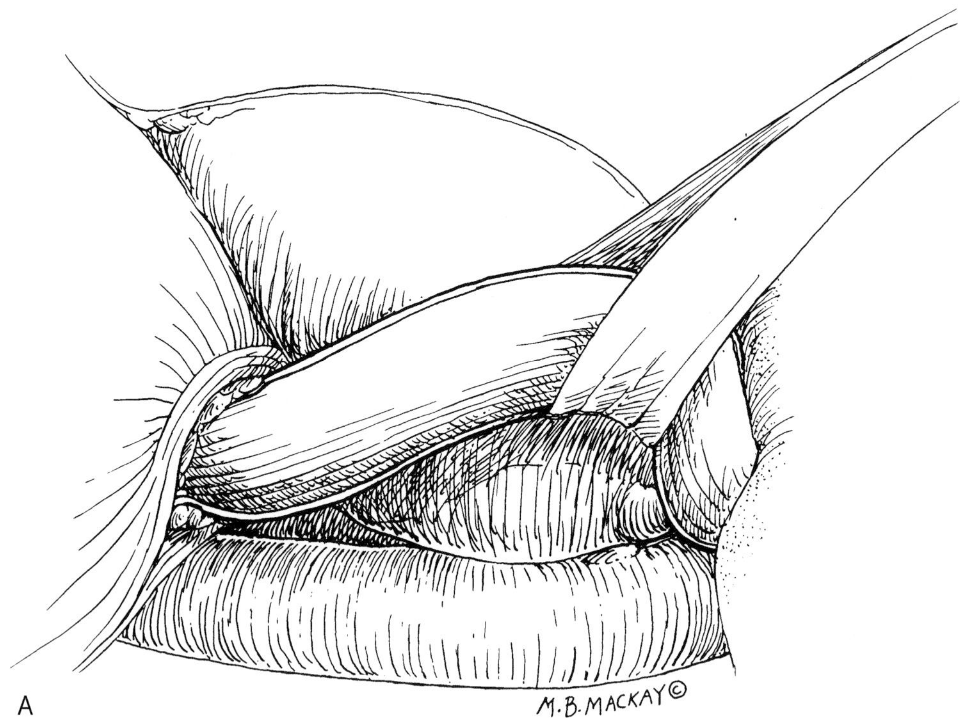

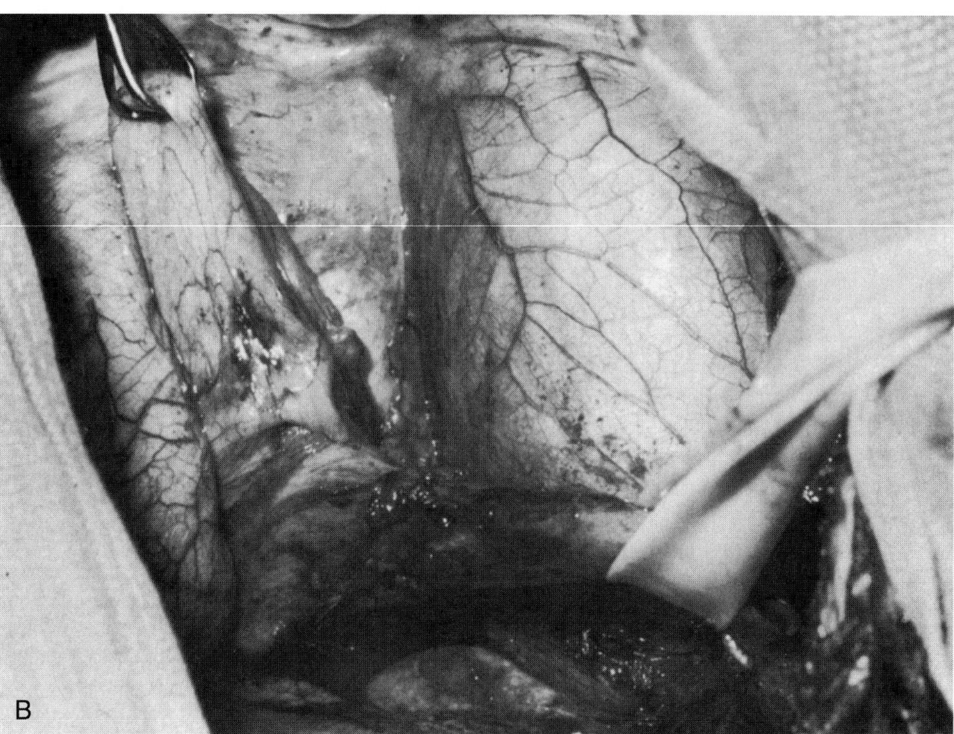

FIGURE 24–8 ■ Diagram (*A*) and photograph (*B*) illustrating mobilization of the distal esophagus and hiatus. In the diagram, the esophagus has been mobilized circumferentially from the level of the pulmonary hilum above to the diaphragmatic hiatus below. The esophagus is elevated with a Penrose drain, and both vagus nerves are carried with the mobilized esophagus. In the photograph, the hiatal margins at the diaphragm have been freed circumferentially and the gastric fundus has been drawn up into the left hemithorax and held with a Babcock clamp.

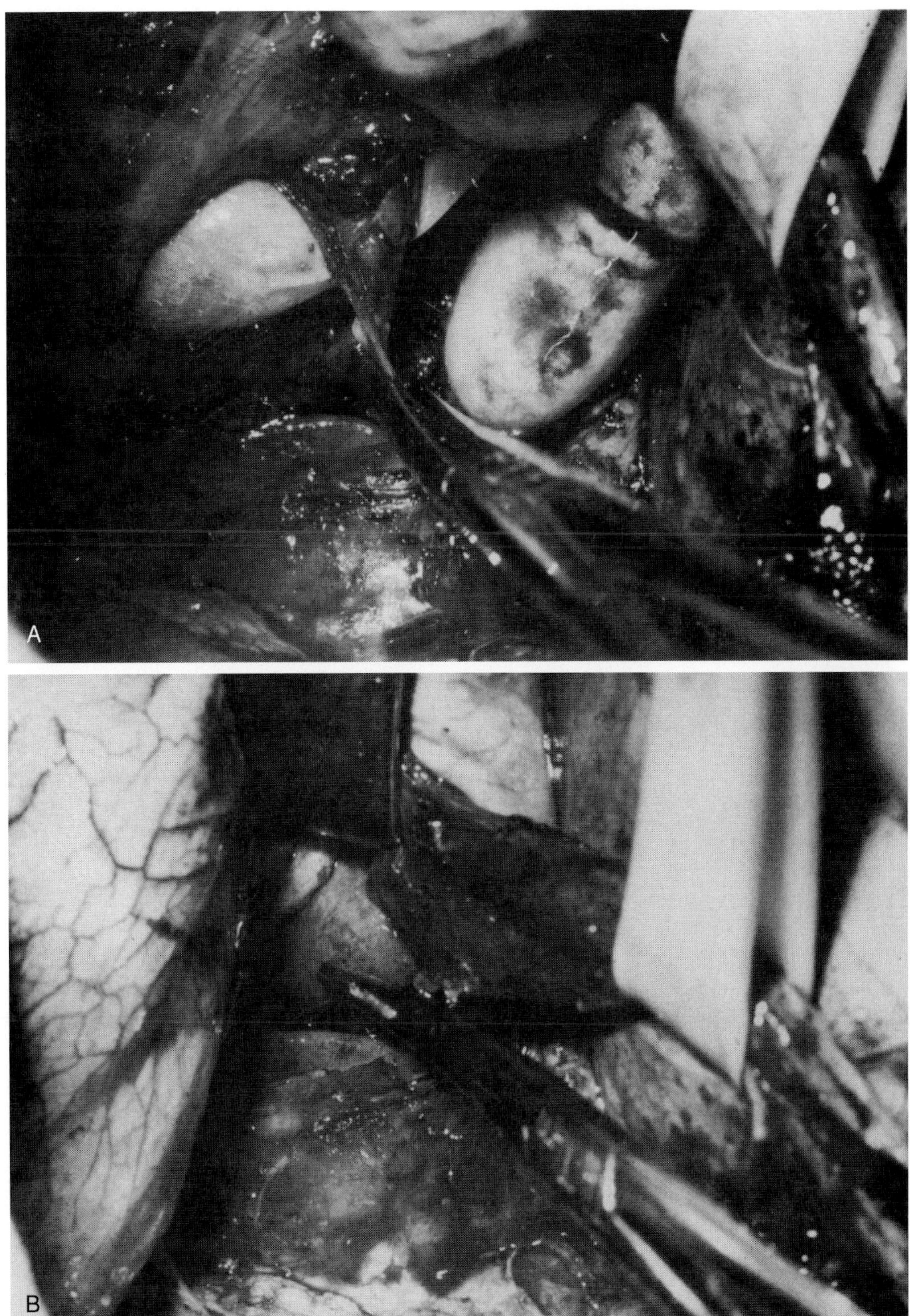

FIGURE 24–9 ■ Operative photographs illustrating the display and division of the upper end of the gastrohepatic omentum. *A*, The operator's middle finger lies behind the upper slip of the gastrohepatic omentum, and a clamp is applied on the abdominal side, posteriorly. *B*, The omental slip has been divided between two clamps, and the gastric cardia has been elevated into the thorax.

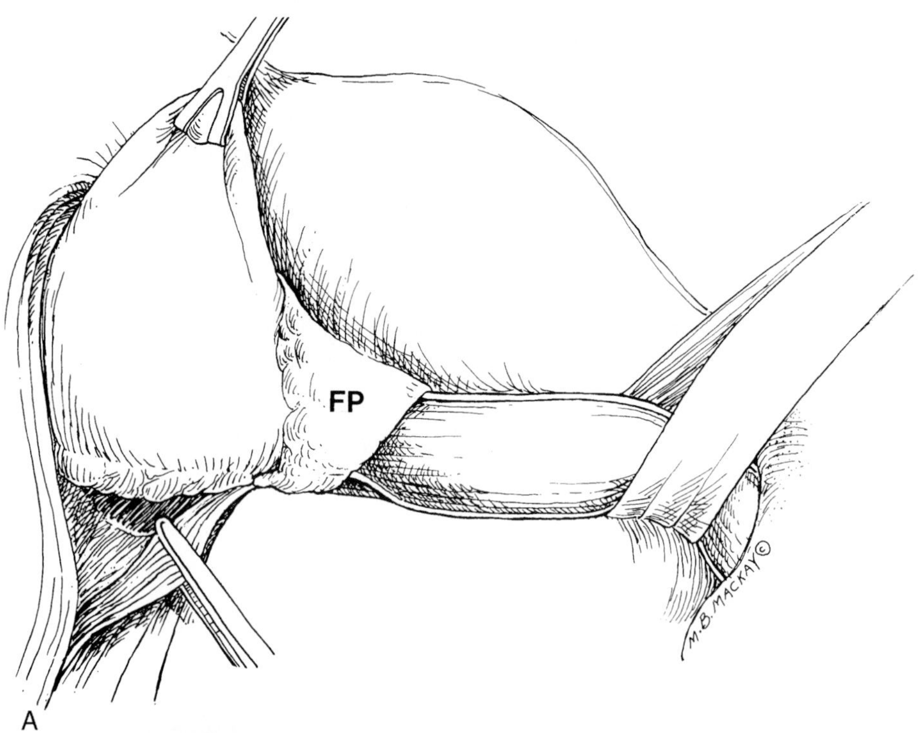

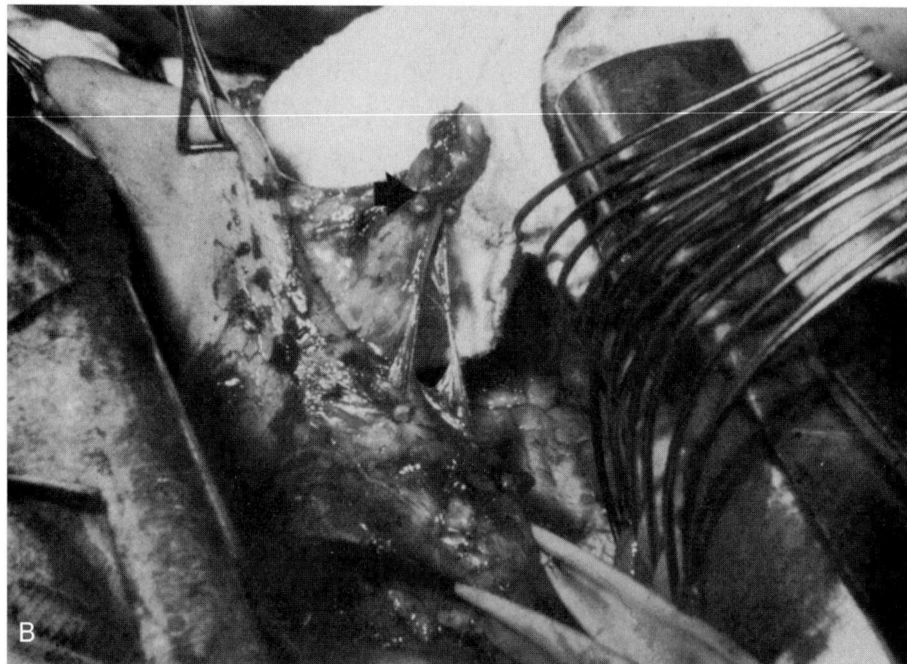

FIGURE 24–10 ■ *A*, Diagram illustrating the ever-present fat pad (FP) lying at the esophagogastric junction. *B*, Fat pad (*arrow*) has been partially freed from the anterior and left lateral aspect of the esophagogastric junction.

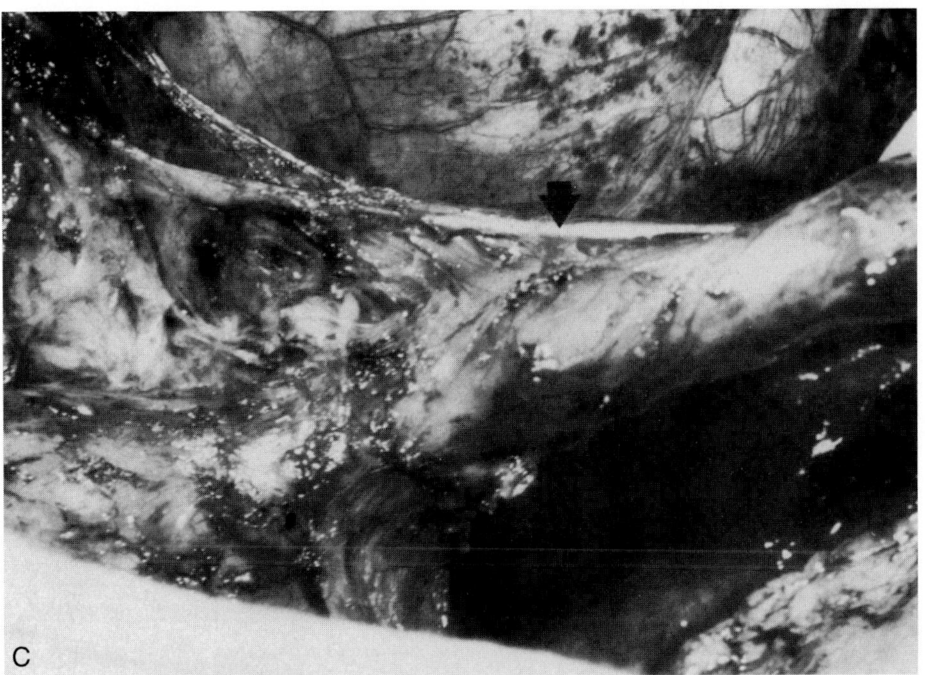

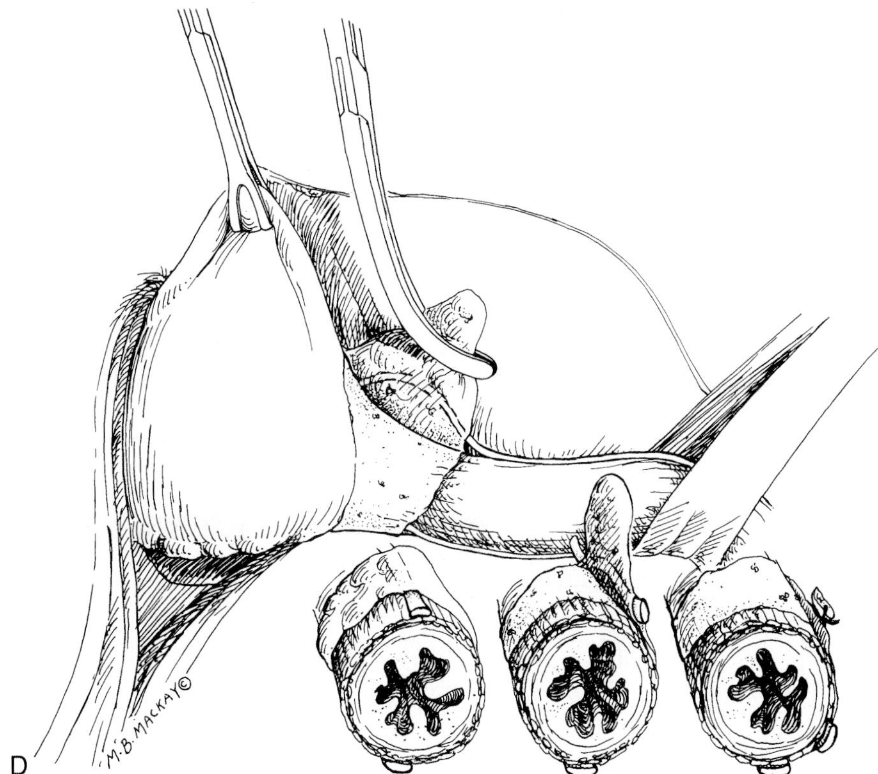

Figure 24–10 ■ *Continued. C,* The left vagus nerve is displayed. It has been freed from the esophagogastric junction and courses through the mobilized fat pad (*arrow*). *D,* Diagram illustrating mobilization of the esophagogastric fat pad along with the left vagus nerve.

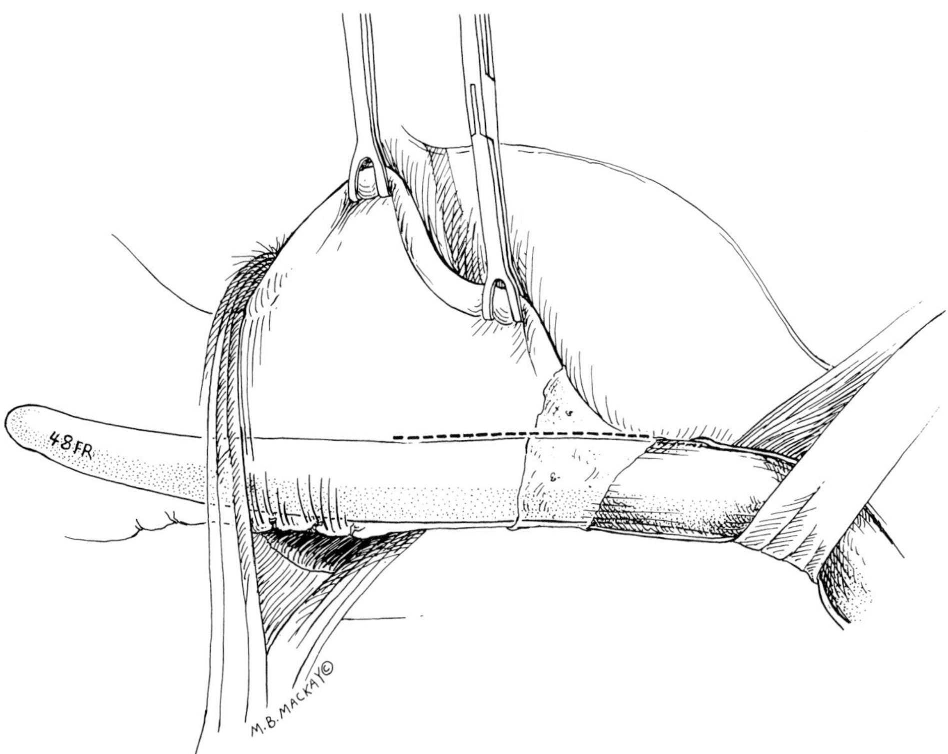

FIGURE 24–11 ■ A 48 French Maloney bougie has been passed from above, across the esophagogastric junction, and well down into the stomach. The proposed gastric tube will be created along the dotted line for a distance of approximately 5 cm.

indwelling 48 French bougie (see Fig. 24–11). The stomach is divided with a GIA stapler (Fig. 24–12).

The margins of the newly created gastric tube are reinforced and oversewn with a running suture of 3–0 chromic catgut. On the esophageal side of the gastroplasty, the staple line is oversewn, but not inverted, to ensure maintenance of the luminal diameter created by the indwelling, 48-French Maloney bougie (Fig. 24–13*A*). The gastric side of the suture line is inverted with a running chromic catgut suture, which will bury the "dog-ear" of stomach at the distal end of the gastric suture line (see Fig. 24–13*B*).

A 270-degree (Belsey type) fundoplication is now completed with three tiers of 3–0 silk sutures. Each tier is spaced approximately 1.5 cm apart, which creates a fundoplication that is approximately 4.5 cm in length. The first tier of fundoplicating sutures is illustrated in Figure 24–14. Sutures are placed in the identical manner as for a Belsey Mark IV repair. In a Belsey repair, however, only two tiers of fundoplicating sutures are used and a shorter fundoplication is done. The third, and final, tier of fundoplicating sutures is illustrated in Figure 24–15.

Interrupted sutures of 1–0 silk are then placed through the crural margins of the hiatus posteriorly but are not tied at this stage of the operation (Fig. 24–16). The sutures in the right limb of the crus are more widely spaced than are those in the left limb (see Fig. 24–16*A*). The most anterior crural suture on the right side should include a margin of the stout, tendinous diaphragmatic band that is found at the anterior end of the right crus.

A spoon is placed through the anterior aspect of the hiatus to facilitate passage of the last tier of fundoplicating sutures (Fig. 24–17). These sutures are directed through the hiatus to the abdominal side and then passed through the diaphragm and brought out on the thoracic side. In Figure 23–17, both ends of the fundoplicating sutures on the right side have been passed in this fashion but not tied. This suture is passed through the diaphragm just to the right side of the anterior "apex" of the hiatus. The middle suture is in the process of placement just to the left of the apex of the hiatus, and the third suture has yet to be passed (see Fig. 24–17). These three sutures are separated along the diaphragmatic margin by the same distances that separate them on the circumference of the gastric tube or esophageal wall.

When the last tier of fundoplicating sutures is pulled taut, the entire fundoplication is reduced below the diaphragm (Fig. 24–18). When these sutures are tied, a length of esophagus (gastric tube) of approximately 5 cm in length is secured in the abdomen below the hiatus. No tension is created on the intrathoracic esophagus or repair.

The final step in repair is closure of the diaphragmatic hiatus posteriorly (Fig. 24–19*A* and *B*). The hiatus is not closed tightly and should allow passage of the index finger alongside the esophagus and through the hiatus, without an undue sense of constriction (see Fig. 24–19*C*).

The pleural space is drained with a single 28 French intercostal tube, and the incision is closed.

Modified Collis Gastroplasty and Nissen Fundoplication

Today, a 360-degree Nissen fundoplication is the most frequently used fundoplication that is added to a lengthening gastroplasty. A Nissen reconstruction is conceptually simple and is technically easier to do than the Belsey

Text continued on page 392

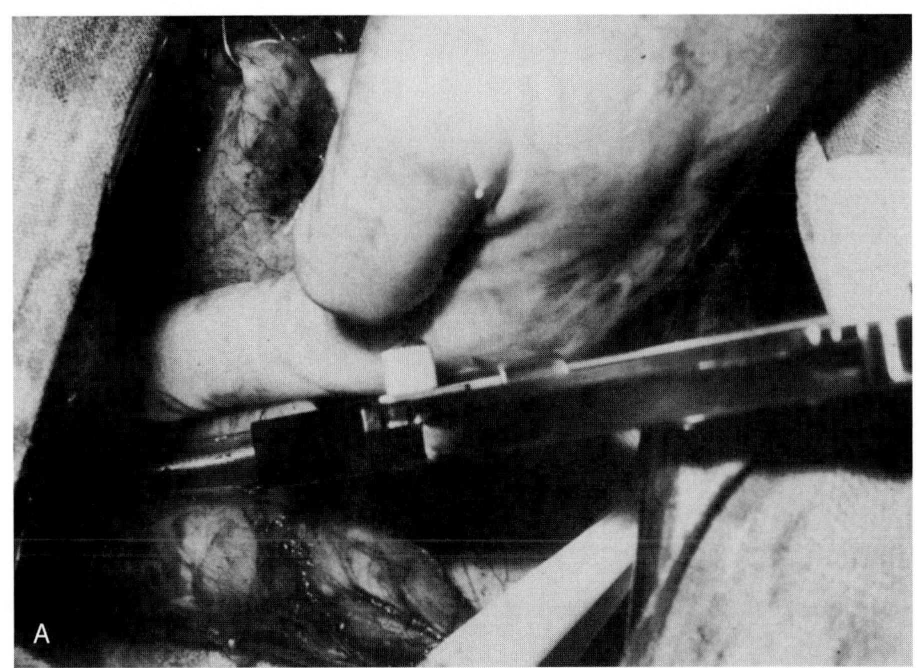

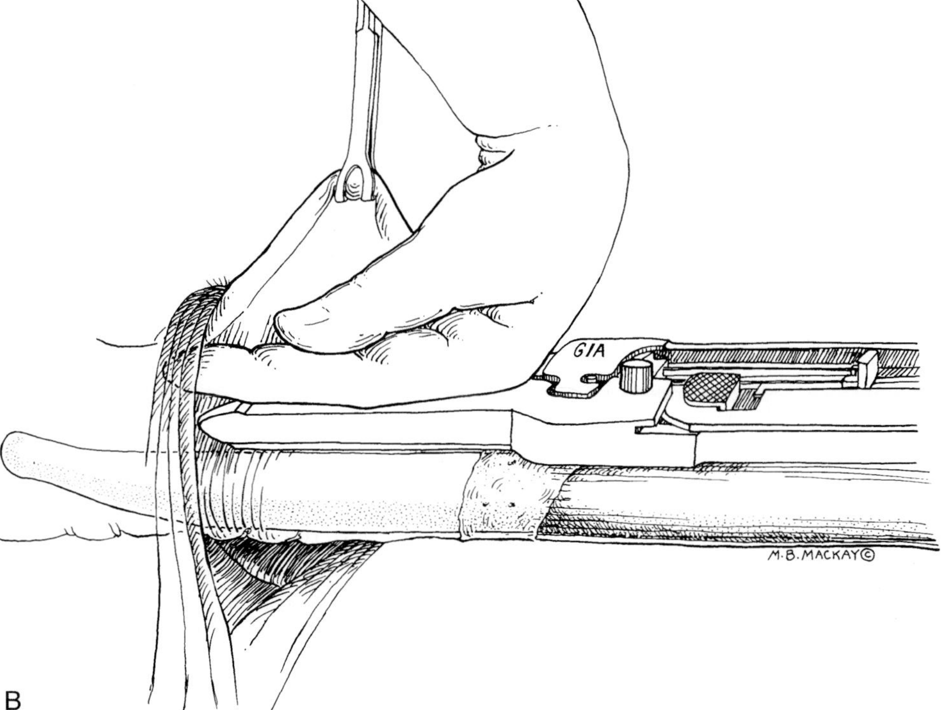

FIGURE 24–12 ■ Photograph (*A*) and diagram (*B*) illustrating the technique for creating the gastric tube using the gastrointestinal anastomosis (GIA) stapler.

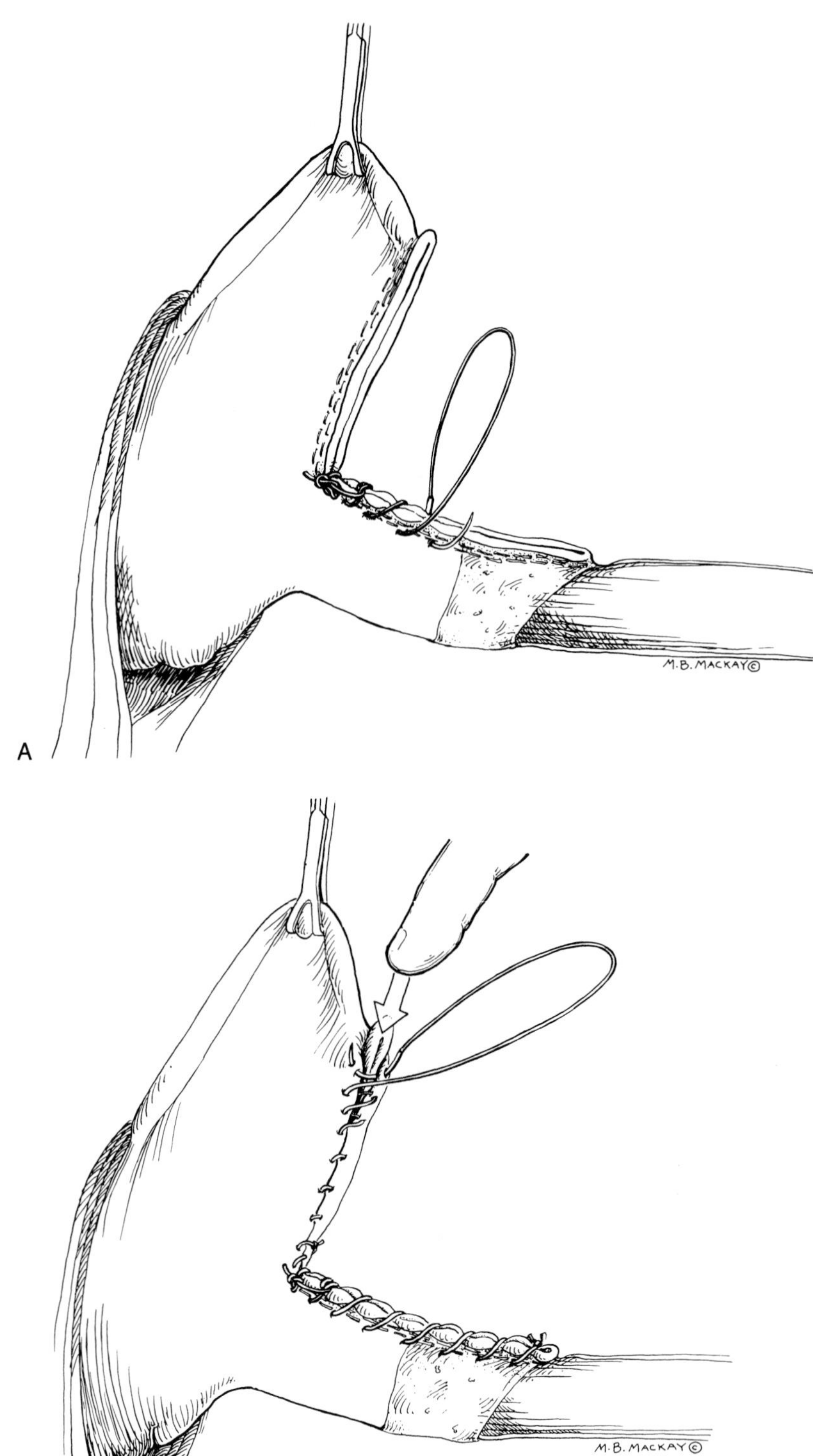

FIGURE 24–13 ■ The gastric tube is oversewn. *A*, The esophageal side of the tube is oversewn with a 3–0 chromic catgut, without inversion, which might prejudice the diameter of the lumen. *B*, The gastric side is oversewn and inverted. This eliminates the dog-ear of stomach at the distal end of the gastric staple line.

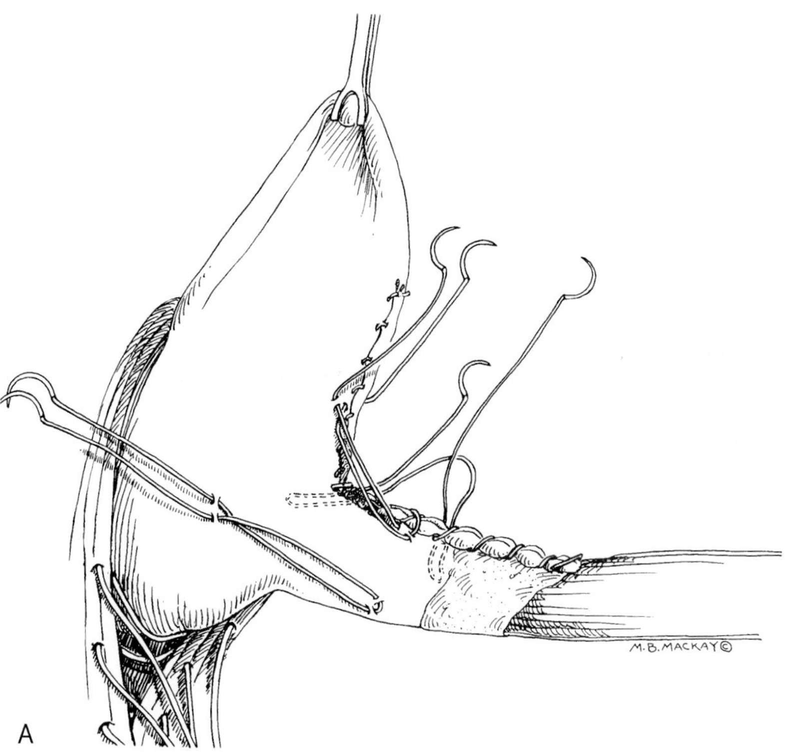

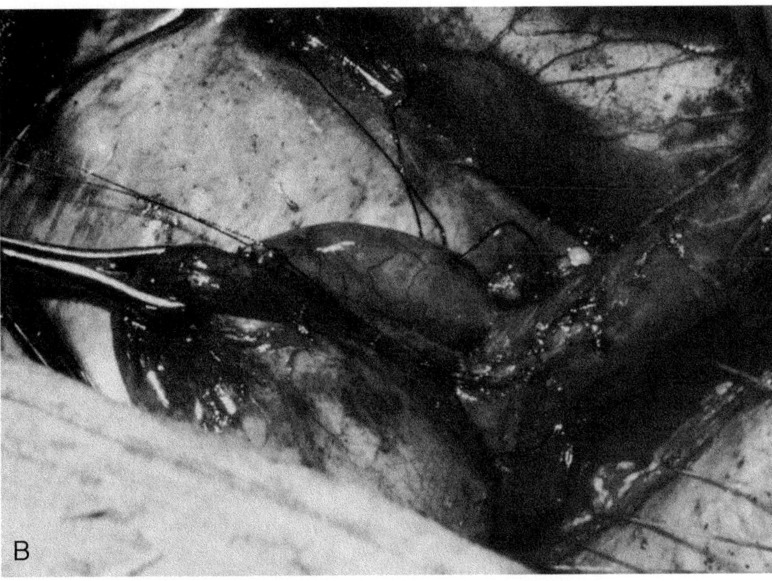

FIGURE 24–14 ■ Diagram (*A*) and photograph (*B*) illustrating placement of the first tier of three fundoplicating sutures. The position of these sutures encircles 270 degrees of the circumference of the gastric tube. Mattress-type sutures are placed using 3–0 silk with double-ended needles.

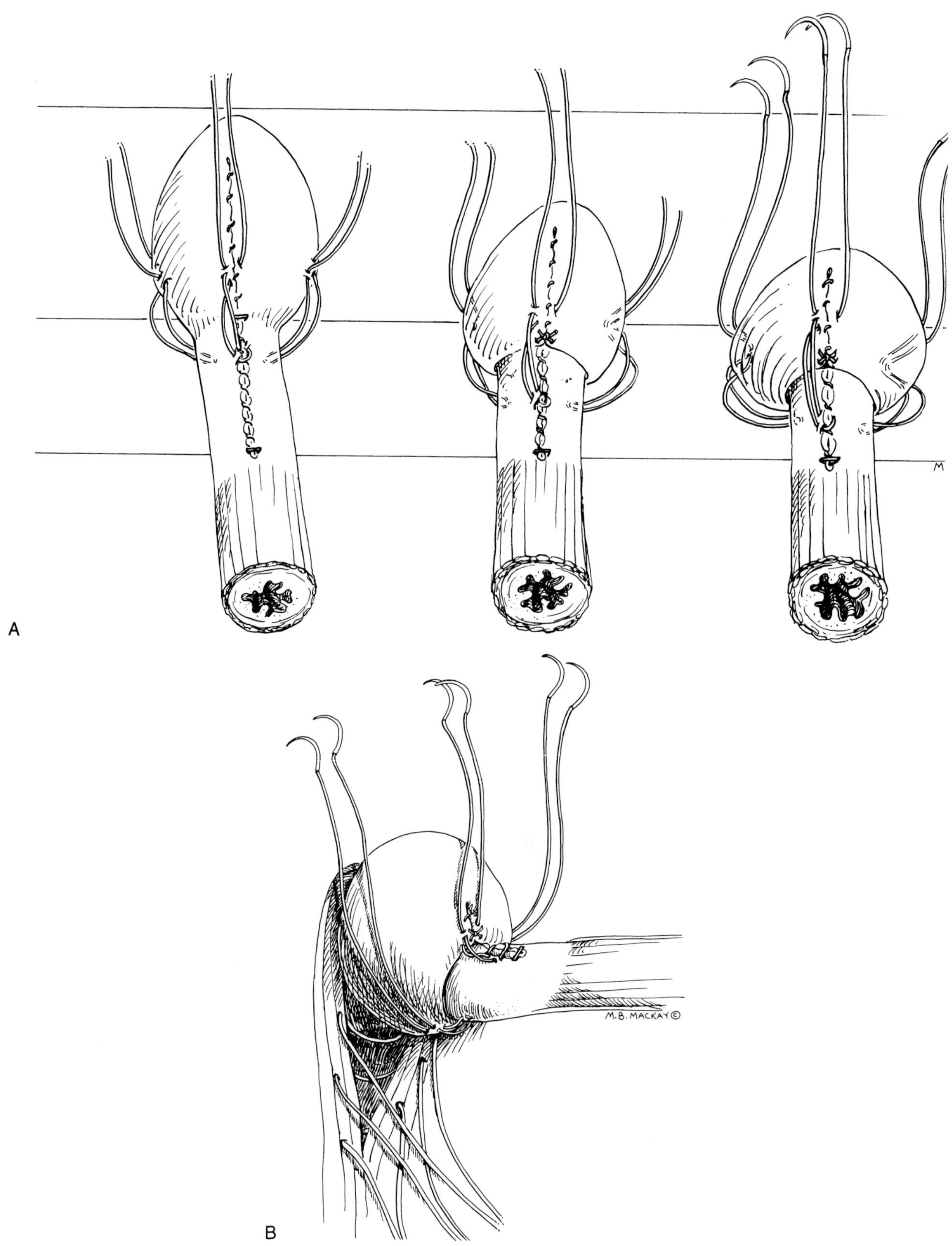

FIGURE 24–15 ■ *A* and *B*, Diagrams illustrating the sequence of suturing for the 270-degree, that is, partial, fundoplication. In all, three tiers of fundoplicating sutures are placed; each tier is positioned about 1.5 cm above the other.

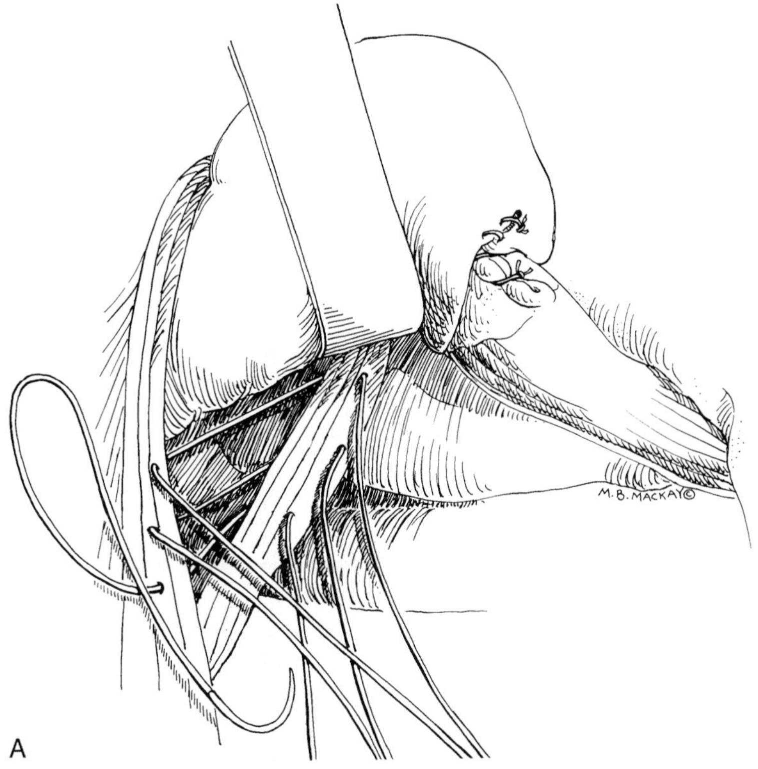

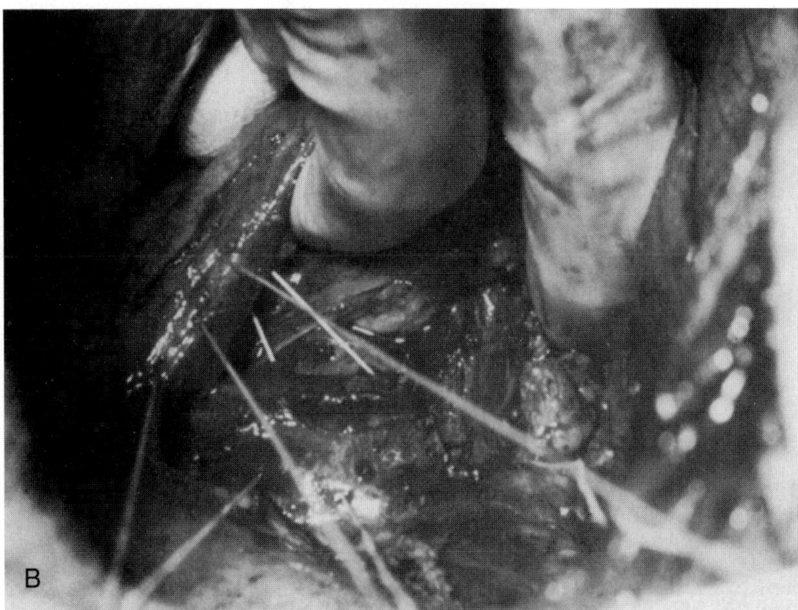

FIGURE 24–16 ■ Diagram (*A*) and photograph (*B*) showing placement of the sutures for posterior closure of the diaphragmatic hiatus. Interrupted sutures of 1–0 silk are used. The sutures are left untied at this stage in the operation. Three or four sutures usually suffice.

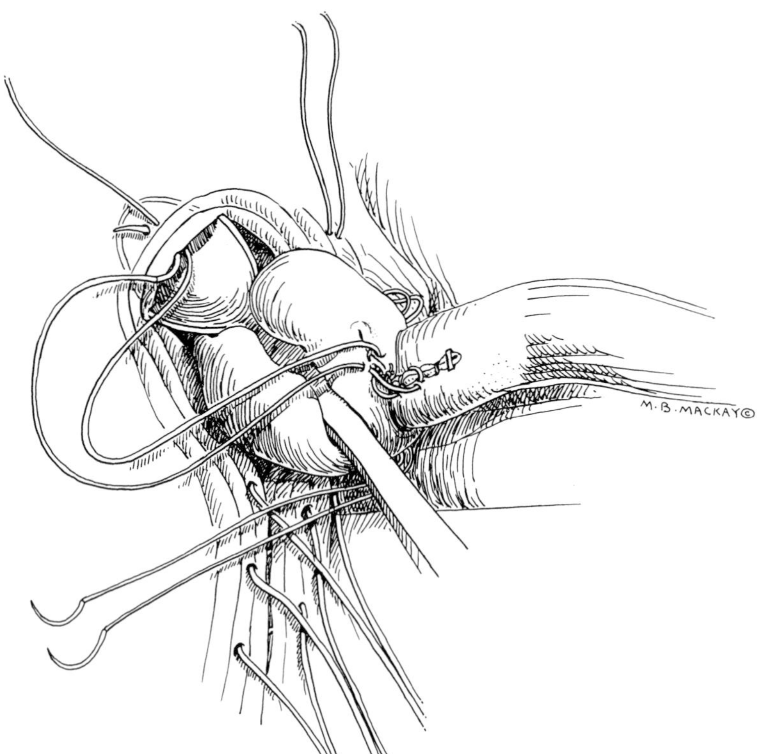

FIGURE 24–17 ■ Diagram illustrating the use of a spoon to facilitate passage of the last tier of fundoplicating sutures through the diaphragmatic hiatus and then back from the abdominal to the thoracic side of the diaphragmatic margin.

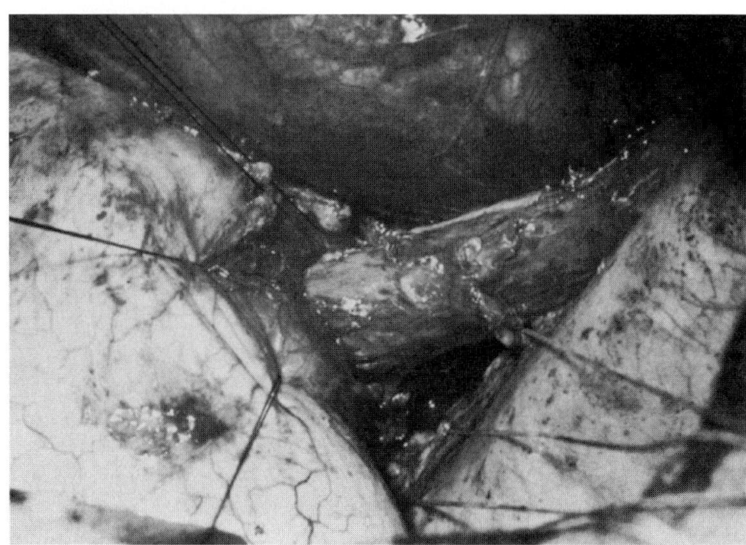

FIGURE 24–18 ■ Operative photograph in which the last three fundoplicating sutures have been pulled taut, with reduction of the hernia and a 4- to 5-cm segment of esophagus and gastric tube. These sutures are then tied to secure the fundoplication and intra-abdominal segment, without tension on the intrathoracic esophagus.

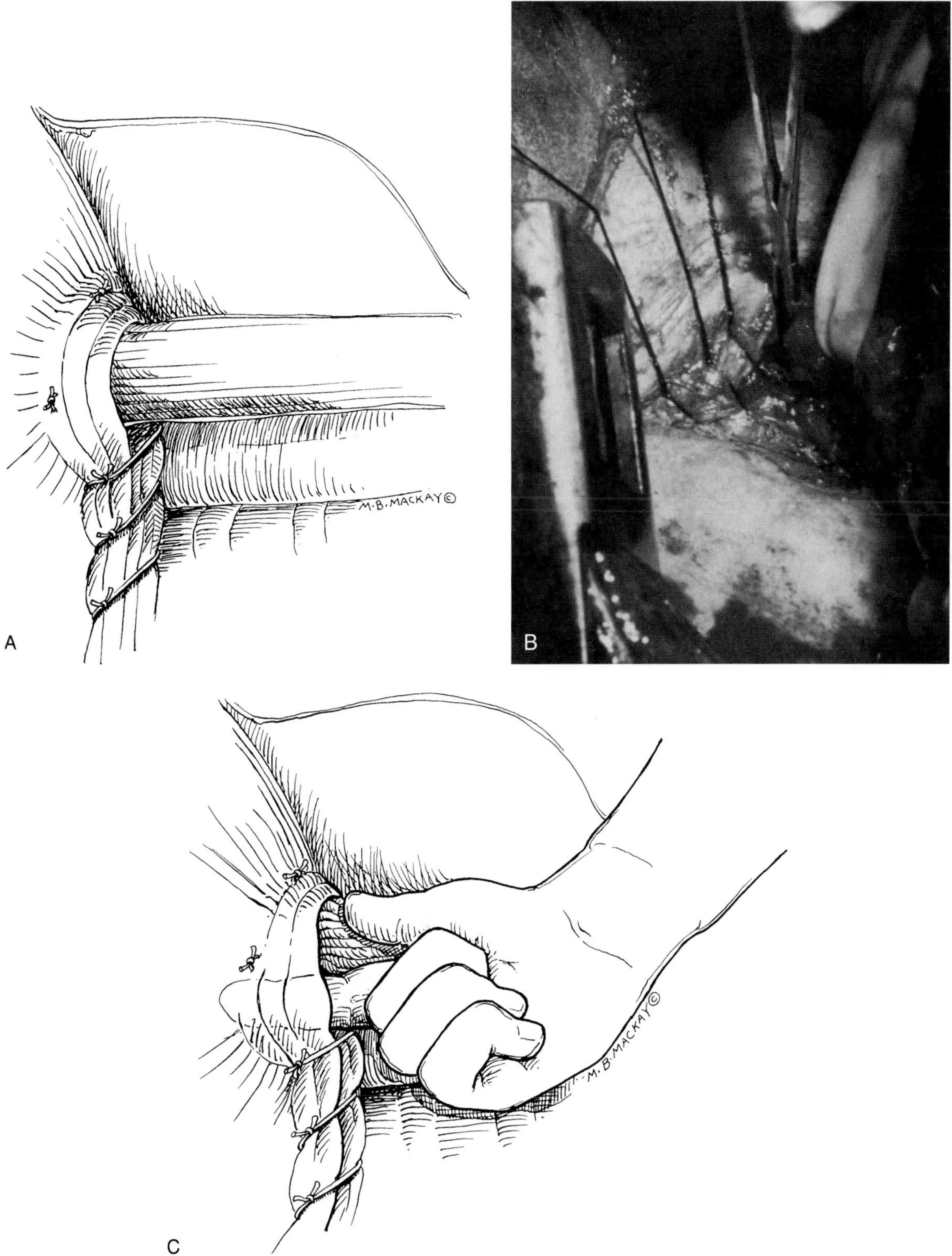

FIGURE 24–19 ■ Diagram (*A*) and photograph (*B*) illustrating closure of the diaphragmatic hiatus posteriorly. The sutures are tied at this stage in the operation, without undue compression of the soft crural muscle. The hiatus (*C*) is closed relatively loosely and should allow easy passage of a finger alongside the esophagus in the newly created hiatus.

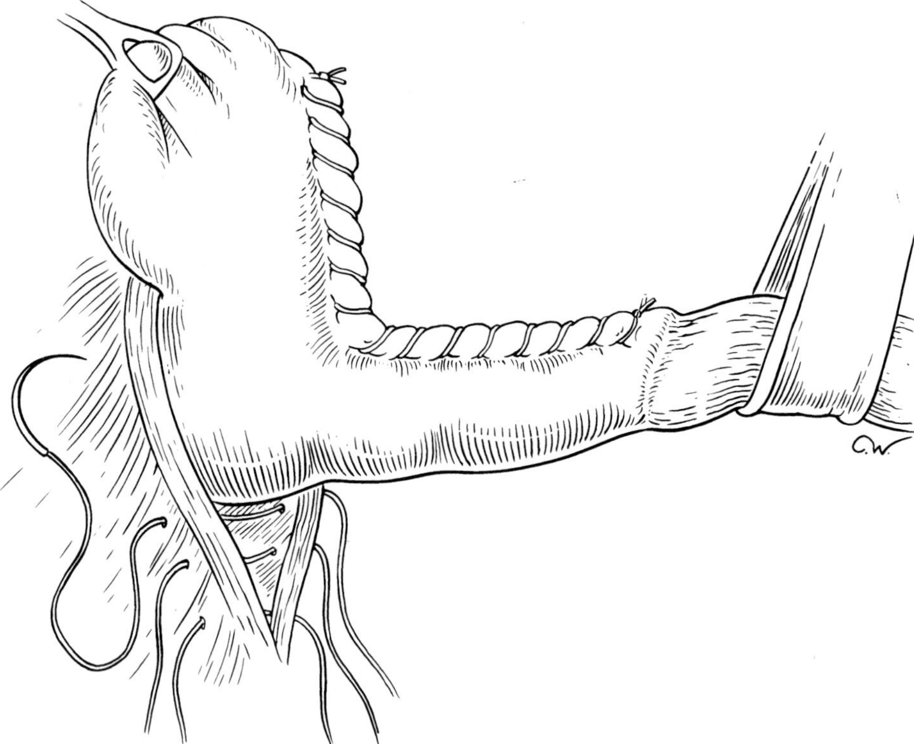

FIGURE 24–20 ■ Once the staple line has been oversewn, large nonabsorbable suture such as No. 1 Ethibond is placed through the crurae posterior to the stomach. Good thick bites of the hiatal margin (~2 cm deep) should be obtained. These sutures are left untied at this time. (From Moores DWO: The Collis-Nissen procedure. In Cox JL, Sundt TS III [eds]: Operative Techniques in Cardiac & Thoracic Surgery: A Comparative Atlas, Vol 2. Philadelphia, WB Saunders, 1997, pp 61–72.)

Mark IV procedure. A complete fundoplication affords more certain control of reflux than a partial wrap. However, a 360-degree wrap may be associated with adverse functional side effects from creation of an unphysiologic or "overcorrected" valve, which totally prevents reflux but also precludes belching and vomiting when necessary. These undesirable side effects can be reduced, or avoided, by creation of a short (2 cm or less), *loose* gastric wrap.

The technique of gastroplasty is identical regardless of the extent of the subsequent fundoplication (see Figs. 24–5 to 24–13). The illustrations that follow were prepared by Moores for publication in his *Operative Tech-*

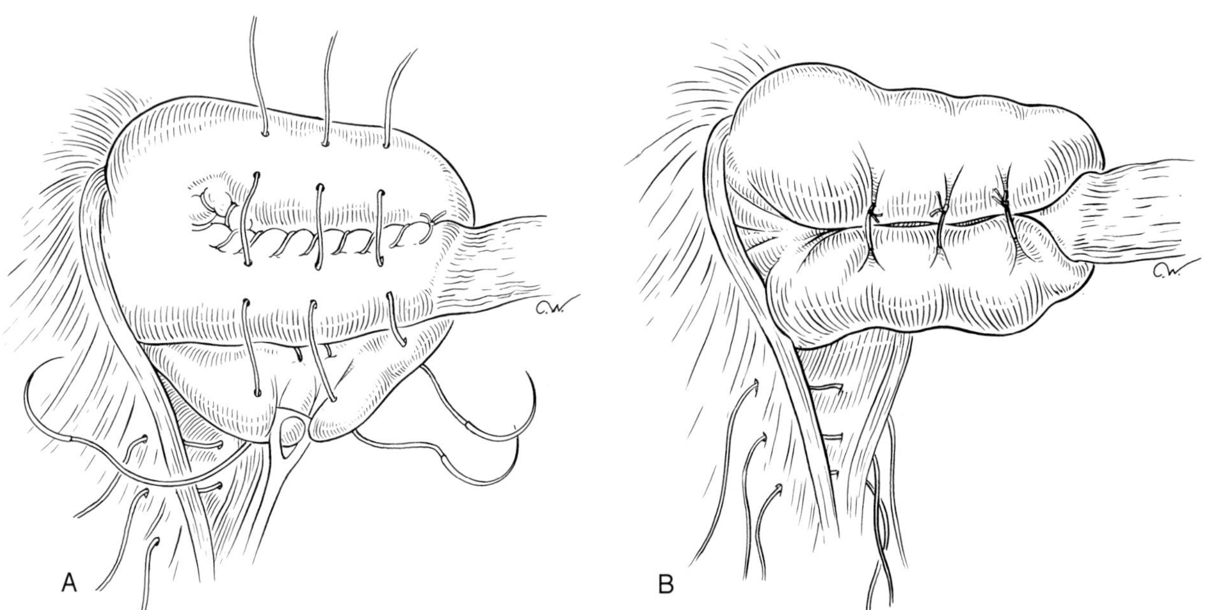

FIGURE 24–21 ■ *A*, Once the crural sutures have been placed, a 360-degree loose Nissen fundoplication is carried out over a 2-cm length with interrupted 0 Ethibond suture from gastric fundus to gastroplasty tube to gastric fundus. *B*, Three interrupted sutures are placed 1 cm apart, creating a 2-cm-long complete Nissen fundoplication. (From Moores DWO: The Collis-Nissen procedure. In Cox JL, Sundt TS III [eds]: Operative Techniques in Cardiac & Thoracic Surgery: A Comparative Atlas, Vol 2. Philadelphia, WB Saunders, 1997, pp 61–72.)

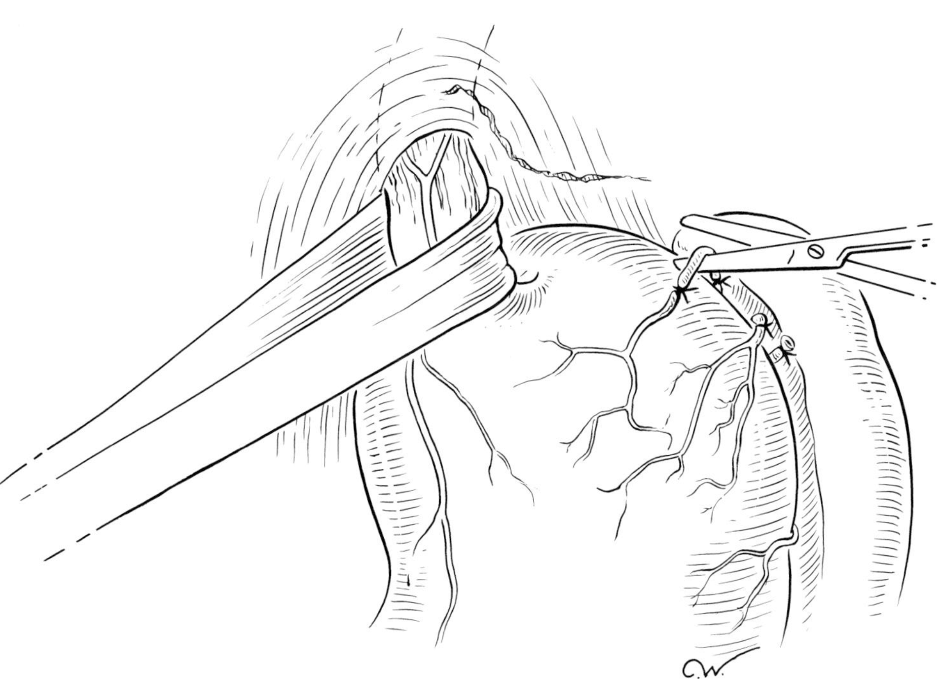

FIGURE 24–22 ■ The intra-abdominal portion of the esophagus is mobilized, and a Penrose drain is placed around the intra-abdominal esophagus incorporating the anterior and posterior vagus nerves within the Penrose drain. Multiple short gastric vessels are then divided in the gastrosplenic omentum all the way down to the bare area of the greater curve, which is the junction point between the blood supply from the left and right gastroepiploic arcades. The esophageal fat pad is then removed as described previously. (From Moores DWO: The Collis-Nissen procedure. In Cox JL, Sundt TS III [eds]: Operative Techniques in Cardiac & Thoracic Surgery: A Comparative Atlas, Vol 2. Philadelphia, WB Saunders, 1997, pp 61–72.)

niques in Cardiac and Thoracic Surgery: A Comparative Atlas (1997).

Once the gastroplasty staple line is oversewn, the crural sutures are placed but not tied. Nonabsorbable 1–0 suture material is used (Fig. 24–20).

A 360-degree loose Nissen fundoplication is done using three 0 nonabsorbable sutures, which are placed as illustrated in Figure 24–21*A* and tied to provide a 2-cm-long fundoplication (Fig. 24–21*B*).

The crural sutures are then tied, as shown in Figure 24–19.

Transabdominal Gastroplasty and Nissen Fundoplication

In 1986, Steichen described a transabdominal approach for gastroplasty using a small-diameter EEA stapler, followed by a linear stapler, to fashion the gastric tube. In this report, Steichen clearly illustrated the proposed technique but did not report any clinical experience. Later, Moores (1997) reported on 44 patients managed by Steichen's proposed transabdominal approach.

Exposure is obtained through a midline upper abdominal incision, extending from the xiphoid process to the umbilicus.

The procedure is clearly outlined in Figures 24–22 to 24–30.

PERIOPERATIVE AND POSTOPERATIVE CARE

Prophylactic antibiotics are given perioperatively. Cefazolin (Ancef), 1 g intravenously, is administered at the time of induction of anesthesia, and a second dose is given in the recovery room approximately 4 hours later. The intercostal tube is attached to suction drainage and can usually be removed after 24 hours. Nasogastric suction is *not* used. Ileus has proved to be a very rare complication of this transthoracic repair.

Clear fluids are usually begun within 24 hours, and if they are well tolerated, the patient's intake is rapidly advanced to a solid diet. Most patients can manage a soft diet and are discharged by the fourth or fifth postoperative day.

Postoperative Dilatation of Peptic Strictures

The need for postoperative dilatation varies and depends on the severity of the associated stricture. Short, mild strictures are easily dilated by passage of a 50 French Maloney bougie before the operation and rarely require dilatation after repair. In those patients with moderate degrees of stricture, however, postoperative dilatation may be necessary. Interval postoperative dilatation is inevitably required in patients with severe, long, fibrous strictures. Dilatations can usually be performed with indirect bougienage with Maloney dilators in the outpatient clinic under topical anesthesia. In the most severe cases, interval dilatation is necessary for periods up to 1 year while we wait for the resolution of inflammation and scar contracture. A detailed description of the techniques of dilatation of peptic stricture is provided in Chapter 19.

Postoperative Follow-up

Antireflux surgery is used in patients of all ages for the management of a benign disorder that produces derangements of important and sophisticated physiologic functions, such as the ability to swallow normally, to vent gas from the stomach, to vomit when necessary, and to prevent pathologic reflux of gastric contents into the esophagus. These functions should be maintained, or restored, without new or additional side effects being created, such

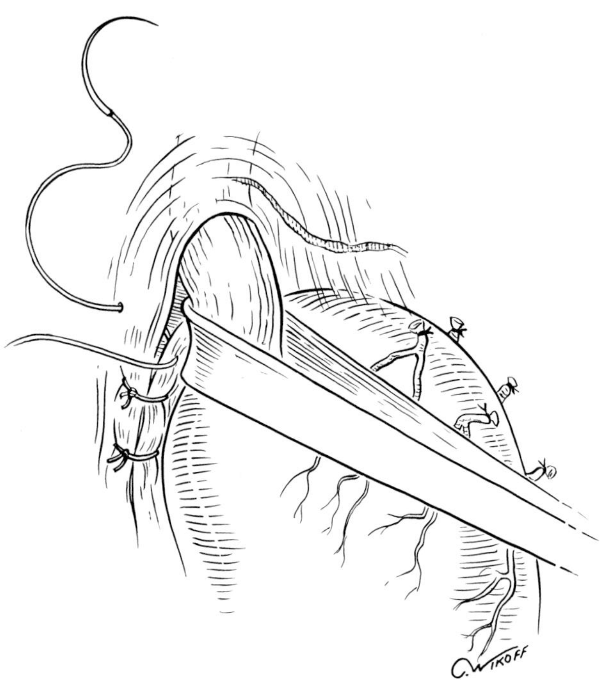

FIGURE 24–23 ■ The Penrose drain is used to retract the esophagus and gastroesophageal junction toward the patient's left side. At this point the hiatus is repaired with large nonabsorbable suture such as No. 1 Ethibond. Again large bites of the crurae (~2 cm deep) are taken, incorporating the peritoneum overlying the muscle of the crurae. These sutures may be tied or left untied at this time. (From Moores DWO: The Collis-Nissen procedure. In Cox JL, Sundt TS III [eds]: Operative Techniques in Cardiac & Thoracic Surgery: A Comparative Atlas, Vol 2. Philadelphia, WB Saunders, 1997, pp 61–72.)

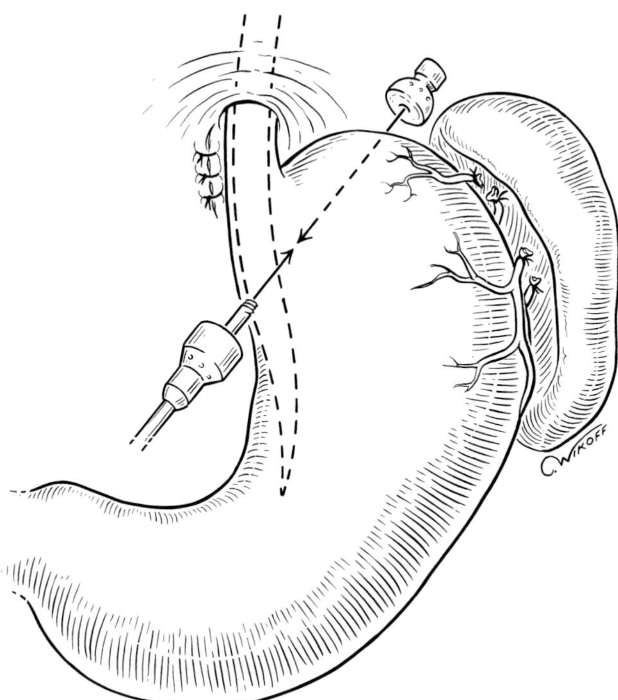

FIGURE 24–24 ■ The anesthesiologist then passes a Maloney bougie (52 French) through the esophagus into the stomach. (From Moores DWO: The Collis-Nissen procedure. In Cox JL, Sundt TS III [eds]: Operative Techniques in Cardiac & Thoracic Surgery: A Comparative Atlas, Vol 2. Philadelphia, WB Saunders, 1997, pp 61–72.)

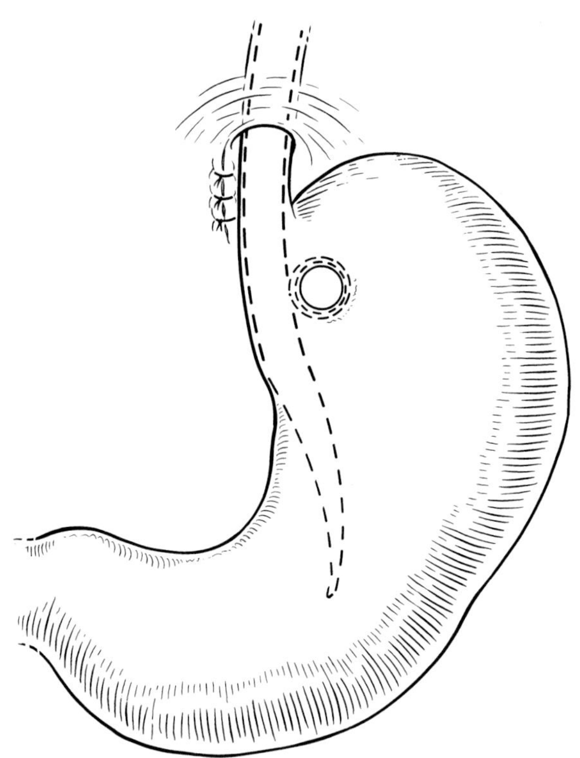

FIGURE 24–25 ■ A 25-mm circular stapler is then used to create a secure buttonhole in the stomach approximately 3 cm distal to the gastroesophageal junction. (From Moores DWO: The Collis-Nissen procedure. In Cox JL, Sundt TS III [eds]: Operative Techniques in Cardiac & Thoracic Surgery: A Comparative Atlas, Vol 2. Philadelphia, WB Saunders, 1997, pp 61–72.)

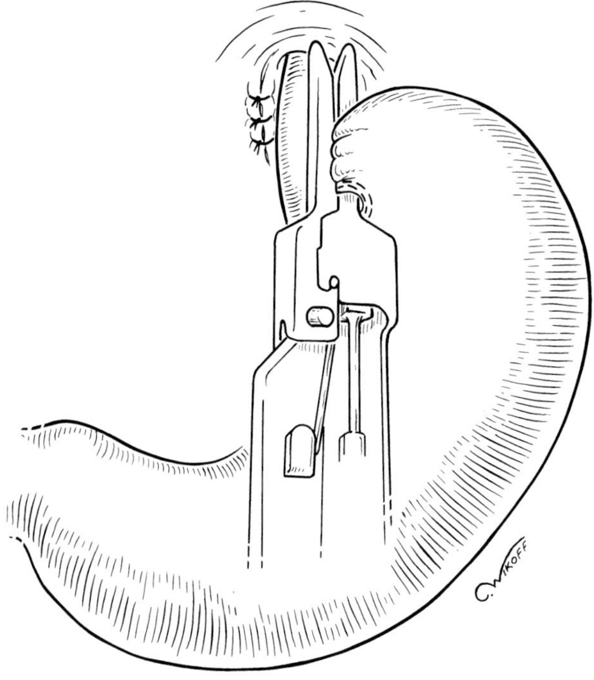

FIGURE 24–26 ■ A 5-cm linear stapler (e.g., gastrointestinal anastomosis) is then placed through the buttonhole and applied tight against the Maloney bougie and fired, creating a 5-cm-long Collis gastroplasty. (From Moores DWO: The Collis-Nissen procedure. In Cox JL, Sundt TS III [eds]: Operative Techniques in Cardiac & Thoracic Surgery: A Comparative Atlas, Vol 2. Philadelphia, WB Saunders, 1997, pp 61–72.)

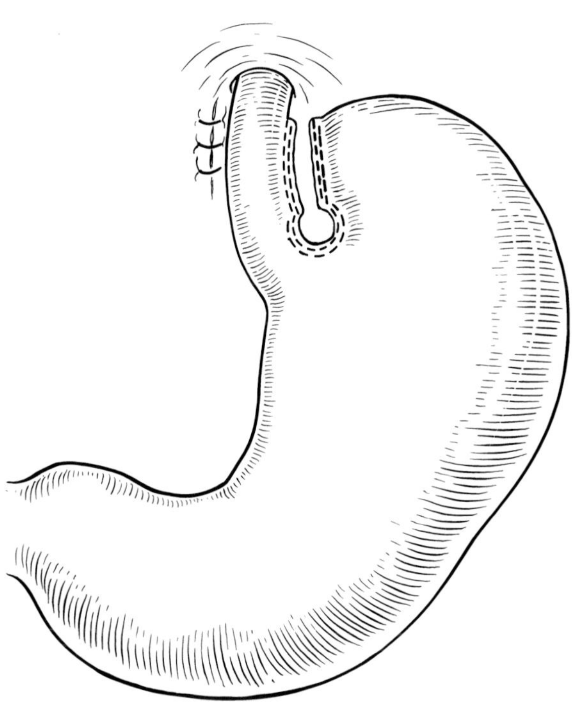

FIGURE 24–27 ■ Once the gastroplasty has been performed, the esophagus is effectively lengthened by 5 cm. (From Moores DWO: The Collis-Nissen procedure. In Cox JL, Sundt TS III [eds]: Operative Techniques in Cardiac & Thoracic Surgery: A Comparative Atlas, Vol 2. Philadelphia, WB Saunders, 1997, pp 61–72.)

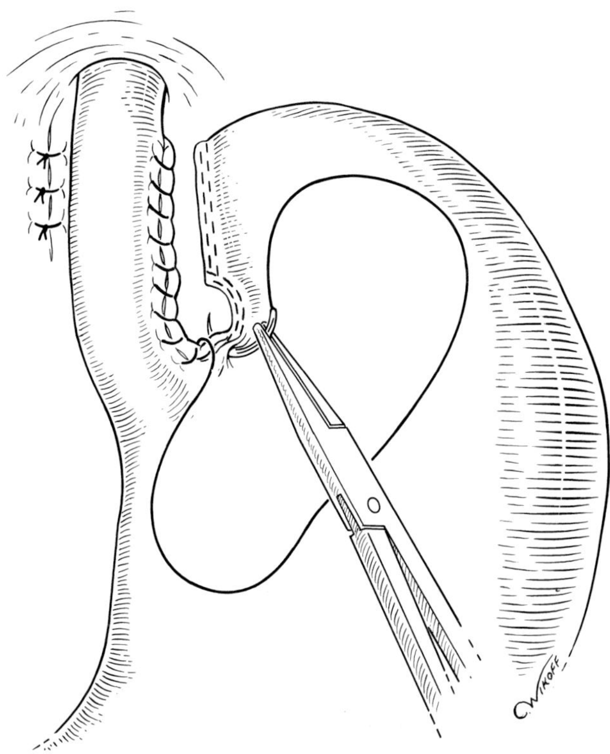

FIGURE 24–28 ■ The gastroplasty tube is then oversewn with running absorbable suture such as 3–0 polyglactin (Vicryl). Again, the gastroplasty tube is not turned in but is simply oversewn. (From Moores DWO: The Collis-Nissen procedure. In Cox JL, Sundt TS III [eds]: Operative Techniques in Cardiac & Thoracic Surgery: A Comparative Atlas, Vol 2. Philadelphia, WB Saunders, 1997, pp 61–72.)

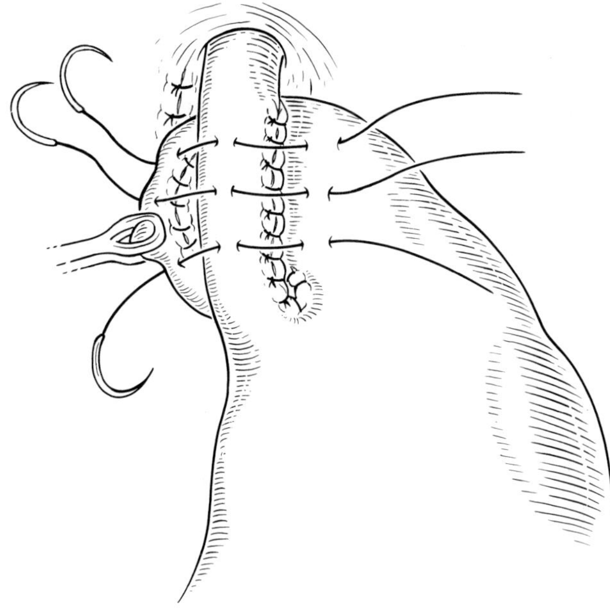

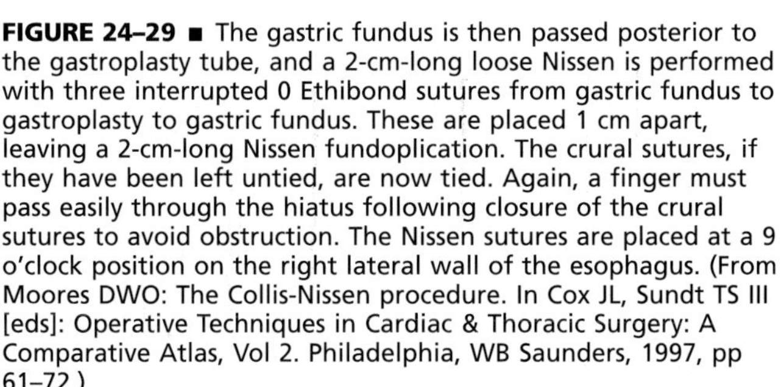

FIGURE 24–29 ■ The gastric fundus is then passed posterior to the gastroplasty tube, and a 2-cm-long loose Nissen is performed with three interrupted 0 Ethibond sutures from gastric fundus to gastroplasty to gastric fundus. These are placed 1 cm apart, leaving a 2-cm-long Nissen fundoplication. The crural sutures, if they have been left untied, are now tied. Again, a finger must pass easily through the hiatus following closure of the crural sutures to avoid obstruction. The Nissen sutures are placed at a 9 o'clock position on the right lateral wall of the esophagus. (From Moores DWO: The Collis-Nissen procedure. In Cox JL, Sundt TS III [eds]: Operative Techniques in Cardiac & Thoracic Surgery: A Comparative Atlas, Vol 2. Philadelphia, WB Saunders, 1997, pp 61–72.)

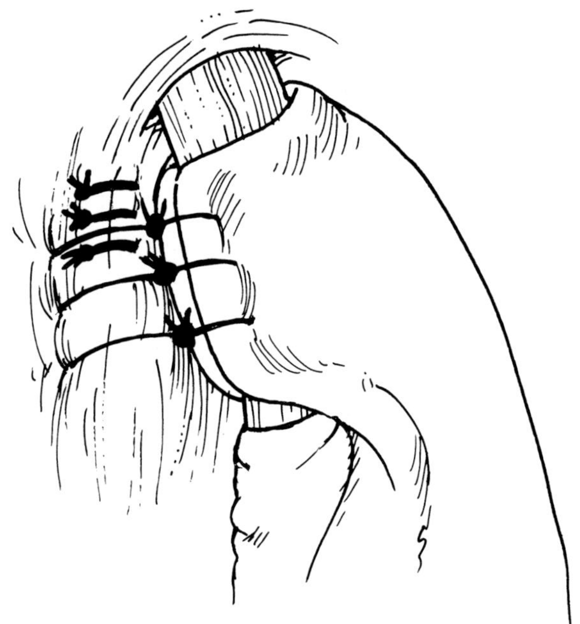

FIGURE 24–30 ■ Once tied, the sutures are passed through the already closed crurae to fix the wrap within the abdomen, thereby reducing the possibility of herniation by the wrap into the chest. (From Moores DWO: The Collis-Nissen procedure. In Cox JL, Sundt TS III [eds]: Operative Techniques in Cardiac & Thoracic Surgery: A Comparative Atlas, Vol 2. Philadelphia, WB Saunders, 1997, pp 61–72.)

as the inability to belch or to vomit when necessary, dysphagia, secondary effects caused by vagal nerve injury, and incisional pain or hernia. Furthermore, surgery should carry a minimal risk of operative death or serious morbidity. With few exceptions, the complications of hiatal hernia and reflux do not influence the patient's longevity or seriously impair general health.

Whenever possible, and within the limits of cost and geography, these patients should be observed for the rest of their lives. Our follow-up protocol consists of these recommendations:

An early postoperative visit is advised at 6 weeks. The patient is then seen at annual intervals for the next 5 years and every 2 years thereafter as long as the patient is able to comply. The visits consist of a personal interview by the surgical staff or resident, completion of a standard questionnaire, and an appropriate examination, including a chest radiograph. A barium swallow is performed to evaluate the repair at 1, 5, 10, and 15 years. Contrast studies of the esophagus and stomach, esophageal manometry, 24-hour pH studies, and endoscopy may be done at any time during follow-up for the investigation of significant symptoms.

The position of the gastric tube and repair may be identified in plain chest radiographs if the reconstruction is marked by the placement of small metal clips at the time of the operation. We place a clip at the top and bottom of the gastric tube and two small parallel clips on the top side of the diaphragmatic hiatus. These are easily seen in the posteroanterior and lateral chest films (Fig. 24–31). As long as there is no change in the position of these clips, we can assume that there has been no anatomic recurrence of the hiatal hernia.

LONG-TERM RESULTS

In 1987, we reported long-term results obtained in a consecutive series of 430 patients with complex reflux problems who were managed by a modified Collis gastroplasty and partial fundoplication (Pearson et al, 1987). The results were stratified by category: short esophagus with peptic stricture (138) or gross ulcerative esophagitis (77), reoperation following one or more previous unsuccessful repairs (118), peptic stricture (25) or esophagitis (12) associated with a primary motor disorder, and massive incarcerated hernia or intrathoracic stomach (54). These results are summarized in Table 24–1.

It is apparent that gastroplasty and fundoplication provide a high proportion of good results in patients with acquired, short esophagus caused by peptic esophagitis. Equally good results were obtained in patients with massive, incarcerated hiatal hernias. The incidence of unsatisfactory results was significantly higher in patients who required reoperation after a previous unsuccessful antireflux repair. The poorest results in this series occurred in patients who presented with peptic stricture and reflux esophagitis associated with an underlying primary motor disorder, such as achalasia, diffuse spasm, or scleroderma. The worst results occurred in patients with achalasia.

The long-term results of gastroplasty combined with a complete (Nissen type) fundoplication have been reported in detail by Henderson and Marryatt in 1985 and Stirling and Orringer in 1989. Both publications report favorable results. More recent reports indicate favorable and relatively long-term results after the Collis-Nissen operation for peptic stricture (Beggs et al, 1995; Richard-

TABLE 24–1 ■ **Results by Category**

	No. of Cases	*Results*		
		Good	*Fair*	*Poor*
Short esophagus caused by stricture (138) or esophagitis (77) (excluding reoperations and motor disorders)	215	93% (199)	4% (10)	3% (6)
Reoperations: 1 or more previous unsuccessful antireflux operations	118	80% (93)	12% (15)	8% (10)
Peptic stricture (25) or esophagitis (12) associated with a primary motor disorder	37	54% (19)	24% (10)	22% (8)
Intrathoracic stomach	54	91% (40)	9% (5)	0% (0)

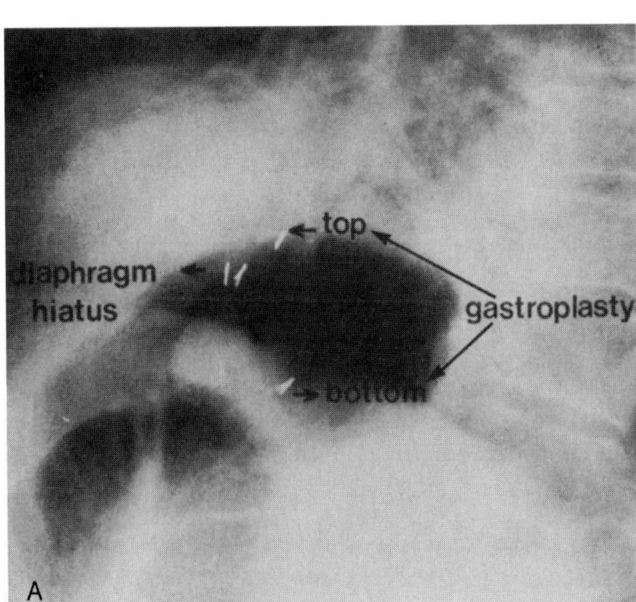

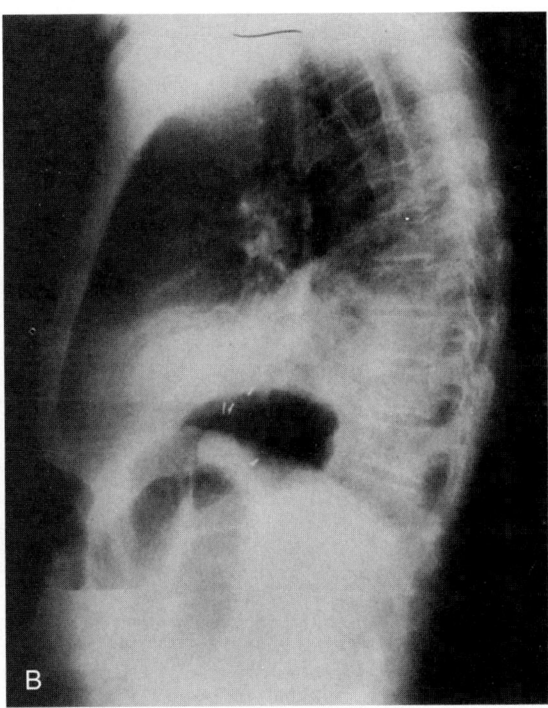

FIGURE 24–31 ■ *A* and *B*, Lateral chest radiograph illustrating small metal clips placed at operation. Single clips mark the top and bottom of the gastroplasty tube; double clips mark the edge of the diaphragmatic hiatus. The position of these clips is easily seen in the follow-up chest x-ray. If their position is unchanged, there is no anatomic recurrence of hiatal hernia.

son and Richardson, 1998), for Barrett's esophagus (Chen et al, 1999), and for reoperation after failed antireflux surgery (Deschamps et al, 1997).

In 1999, Demos reported his long-term follow-up in 153 patients managed by his original technique of "uncut gastroplasty and Nissen fundoplication," again with a series of excellent results. Pera and associates, in 1995, reported favorable short-term results with the "uncut Collis-Nissen" operation. Jobe and co-workers (1998) have reported the short-term functional results of their technique of laparoscopic Collis gastroplasty.

It is difficult, however, to make meaningful comparisons between the results in these reported series. There is variation in the indications for adding gastroplasty, the mix of patients, the length of follow-up, the method of results reporting, and the details of the operative technique. These problems beset the evaluation of all reports on the outcomes of antireflux surgery.

COMMENTS AND CONTROVERSIES

The addition of gastroplasty in patients with acquired esophageal shortening affords reflux control that is at least as favorable as that reported with standard repairs, such as the Nissen, Belsey Mark IV, and Hill operations. The reported morbidity and mortality rates are no greater, and functional results are good in most cases. An anatomic recurrence of the hernia is rare because of the absence of tension on the reconstruction.

Before 1998 or so, like most of my thoracic surgical colleagues, I contended that the addition of gastroplasty would not prove safe and effective using laparoscopic techniques. I no longer think so. Although there are very few centers with significant experience at the present time, these groups have clearly demonstrated the capability to add a gastroplasty using current, minimally invasive methods. Swanström was the first surgeon to report clinical experience with his original technique of laparoscopic fundoplication, combined with a gastroplasty, created using a combined thoracoscopic and laparoscopic exposure (Swanström et al, 1966). In 1998, Hunter described his experience with a laparoscopic and purely abdominal approach for adding a gastroplasty (Johnson et al, 1998). Hunter employed a laparoscopic modification of the Steichen procedure that uses a circular stapler (Steichen, 1986). Luketich has since reported his experience with a very similar technique of laparoscopic gastroplasty for short esophagus (Luketich et al, 2000a).

Some years may elapse before these skills, along with the necessary experience and technology, are widely practiced. In time, however, I believe it highly likely that minimally invasive methods will be commonly employed for complex antireflux operations such as gastroplasty, and even reoperation for failed prior repairs.

F. G. P.

■ REFERENCES

Beggs FD, Salama FD, Knowles KR: Management of benign esophageal stricture by total fundoplication gastroplasty. J R Coll Surg Edinb 40:305–307, 1995.

Chen LQ, Nastos D, Hu CY, et al: Results of the Collis Nissen gastroplasty in patients with Barrett's esophagus. Ann Thorac Surg 68:1014–1020, 1999.

Collis JL: An operation for hiatus hernia with short esophagus. J Thorac Cardiovasc Surg 34:768, 1957.
Collis JL: Gastroplasty. Thorax 16:197, 1961.
Demos NJ: Stapled uncut gastroplasty for hiatal hernia: 12 year follow-up. Ann Thorac Surg 38:393–398, 1984.
Demos NJ: The stapled uncut gastroplasty for hiatal hernia 24 years' follow-up. Dis Esophagus 12:14–21, 1999.
Demos NJ, Smith N, Williams D: A gastroplasty for short esophagus and reflux esophagitis. Ann Surg 181:178–181, 1975.
Deschamps C, Trastek VF, Allen MS, et al: Long term results after reoperation for failed antireflux procedures. J Thorac Cardiovasc Surg 113:545–550, 1997.
Gastal OL, Hagen JA, Peters JH, et al: Short esophagus: Predictors and clinical implications. Arch Surg 134:633–636, 1999.
Henderson RD: Reflux control following gastroplasty. Ann Thorac Surg 24:206, 1977.
Henderson RD, Marryatt GV: Total fundoplication gastroplasty (Nissen gastroplasty): Five-year review. Ann Thorac Surg 39:74, 1985.
Horvath KD, Swanstrom LL, Jobe BA: The short esophagus: Pathophysiology, incidence presentation and treatment in the era of laparoscopic surgery. Ann Surg 232:630–640, 2000.
Jobe RA, Horvath KD, Swanström LL: Postoperative function following laparoscopic Collis gastroplasty for shortened esophagus. Arch Surg 133:867–874, 1998.
Johnson AB, Oddsdottir M, Hunter JG: Laparoscopic Collis gastroplasty and Nissen fundoplication: A new technique for the management of esophageal foreshortening. Surg Endosc 12:1055–1060, 1998.
Langer B: Modified gastroplasty: A simple operation for reflux esophagitis with moderate degrees of shortening. Can J Surg 16:1, 1973.
Luketich JD, Grondin SC, Pearson FG: Minimally invasive approaches to acquired shortening of the esophagus: Laparoscopic Collis-Nissen gastroplasty. Semin Thorac Cardiovasc Surg 12:173–178, 2000a.
Luketich JD, Raja S, Fernando HC: Laparoscopic repair of giant para-esophageal hernia: 100 consecutive cases [Abstract]. In Proceedings of the American Surgical Association, Philadelphia, March 2000b, pp 98–99.
Maziak DE, Todd TR, Pearson FG: Massive hiatus hernia: Evaluation and surgical management. J Thorac Cardiovasc Surg 115:53–62, 1998.
Mittal SK, Awad ZT, Tasset M, et al: The preoperative predictability of the short esophagus in patients with stricture or paraesophageal hernia. Surg Endosc 14:464–468, 2000.
Moores DWO: The Collis-Nissen procedure. In Cox JL, Sundt TS III (eds): Operative Techniques in Cardiac & Thoracic Surgery: A Comparative Atlas. Philadelphia, WB Saunders, 1997, pp 61–72.
Orringer M, Skinner D, Belsey R: Long term result of the Mark IV operation for hiatal hernia: An analysis of recurrences and their treatment. J Thorac Cardiovasc Surg 74:226, 1972.
Orringer MB, Sloan H: Complications and failings of combined Collis-Belsey operation. J Thorac Cardiovasc Surg 74:726, 1977.
Pearson FG, Cooper JD, Ilves R, et al: Massive hiatal hernia with incarceration: A report of 53 cases. Ann Thorac Surg 35:45, 1983.
Pearson FG, Cooper J, Patterson G, et al: Gastroplasty and fundoplication for complex reflux problems. Ann Surg 206:473, 1987.
Pearson FG, Langer R, Henderson RD: Gastroplasty and Belsey hiatus hernia repair. J Thorac Cardiovasc Surg 61:50, 1971.
Pera M, Deschamps C Taillefer R, Duranceau A: Uncut Collis-Nissen gastroplasty: Early functional results. Ann Thorac Surg 60:915–920, 1995.
Richardson JD, Richardson RL: Collis-Nissen gastroplasty for shortened esophagus: Long term evaluation. Ann Surg 227:735–740, 1998.
Steichen FM: Abdominal approach to the Collis gastroplasty and Nissen fundoplication. Surg Gynecol Obstet 162:273–274, 1996.
Stirling MC, Orringer MB: Continued assessment of the combined Collis-Nissen operation. Ann Thorac Surg 47:224, 1989.
Swanström LL, Marcus DR, Galloway GQ: Laparoscopic Collis gastroplasty is the treatment of choice for the shortened esophagus. Am J Surg 171:477–481, 1996.
Urschel H: Discussion of Pearson FG, Cooper J, Nelems J: Gastroplasty in the management of complex reflux problems. J Thorac Cardiovasc Surg 76:665, 1978.

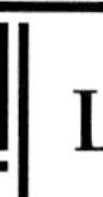

LAPAROSCOPIC GASTROPLASTY

Lee L. Swanström

HISTORICAL BACKGROUND

Successful antireflux surgery depends on proper positioning of the fundal wrap and in making the reconstruction tension-free. These basic surgical precepts are equally true for laparoscopic and open fundoplications. Violation of either of these principles inevitably results in higher rates of postoperative dysphagia or subsequent herniation, slippage, or disruption of the repair (DeMeester et al, 1986).

Axial shortening of the esophagus secondary to chronic acid injury can make either of these goals impossible to achieve without resorting to additional surgical maneuvers. Several surgical approaches have been described for treating the shortened esophagus using open operative techniques:

- Intrathoracic fundoplication
- Circular myotomy
- Esophagectomy

Each of these options is considered less than satisfactory because of high patient morbidity or poor outcomes (Allen and Matthews, 1993; Mansour, 1981). Since it was first described in 1957, the Collis gastroplasty—with an associated partial or total fundoplication—has achieved primary status as treatment of choice for the short esophagus because of its demonstrated efficacy and low morbidity (Collis, 1957; Pearson et al, 1987).

Laparoscopic fundoplication was introduced in 1991, and its popularity has subsequently stimulated new interest in the evaluation and treatment of esophageal reflux disease. Until recently, however, the issue of the short esophagus encountered during laparoscopic antireflux surgery either was not considered, was ignored, or was treated as a contraindication to the laparoscopic approach (Hinder et al, 1994; Peters et al, 1995). The problem was compounded by the fact that many procedures were being performed by surgeons having little experience with open techniques of antireflux surgery, and, perhaps, by the lack of tactile feedback inherent with the laparoscopic approach. Ignoring or missing the shortened esophagus may also account for early reports of a higher incidence of complications (dysphagia and wrap herniation) in some laparoscopic series (Collet and Cadiere, 1995; Watson et al, 1995). Because of the significant patient benefits of the laparoscopic approach, and the resulting increase in surgical referrals, it was inevitable that the issue of the short esophagus would be addressed. Currently, much more attention is being paid to the diagnosis and laparoscopic treatment of this clinical entity.

■ HISTORICAL READINGS

Collis JL: An operation for hiatus hernia with short oesophagus. Thorax 12:181–182, 1957.

DeMeester TR, Bonavina L, Alberucci M: Nissen fundoplication for gastroesophageal reflux disease: Evaluation of primary repair in 100 consecutive patients. Ann Surg 204:9–20, 1986.

Swanström LL: Laparoscopic Collis gastroplasty is the treatment of choice for the shortened esophagus. Am J Surg 171:477–481, 1996.

DIAGNOSIS

Accurate preoperative selection of patients who will require a lengthening procedure is difficult. Not infrequently the patient may have a preoperative study showing a gastroesophageal junction displaced within the mediastinum, only to find that it easily reduces with moderate dissection intraoperatively. Conversely, one occasionally finds an esophagus so lacking in elasticity that even with a small hiatal hernia it cannot be mobilized enough during surgery to achieve the 2 to 3 cm of tension-free intra-abdominal length needed to effectively perform an antireflux procedure.

Tests such as barium swallow, cine esophagography, and upper gastrointestinal endoscopy help to locate the position of the lower esophageal sphincter (LES) but are less specific than intraoperative evaluation in determining need for a Collis procedure. Of tests available, cine esophagograms have probably the highest predictive value when an upright study shows that the gastroesophageal junction does not reduce during swallowing (Peters and DeMeester, 1995). Other investigators have looked at manometric measurements compared with normal nomograms to predict patients with an intrinsically shortened esophagus, using either the esophageal length, determined by measuring the length between the upper esophageal sphincter and the LES or by the difference between the respiratory inversion point and the LES (Gastal et al, 1999; Jobe et al, 1999). Such tests, however, have yet to be widely validated.

Although no single test can reliably identify all patients with refractory esophageal shortening preoperatively, there are some well-described risk factors (Table 24–2). If the patient has two or more of these preoperative findings, he or she is definitely at high risk of requiring an extensive esophageal mobilization or a lengthening procedure. Ultimately, the definitive determination of the need for a Collis procedure can be made only at surgery after full mobilization of the gastroesophageal junction and distal esophagus.

TABLE 24–2 ■ **Risk Factors for Intrinsic Shortening of the Esophagus**

Finding	*Examination*
Gastroesophageal junction > 5 cm above the hiatus	Barium swallow, EGD
Nonreducible hiatal hernia in the upright position	Cine-esophagram
Giant, type III paraesophageal hernia	Barium swallow
Savary grade III esophagitis	EGD
Esophageal stricture	
Barrett's esophagus	EGD with biopsy
Previous fundoplication that failed because of mediastinal herniation, disruption, or "slipping"	EGD, barium swallow

EGD, esophagogastroduodenoscopy.

MANAGEMENT

The esophageal surgeon must have a strategic plan in place for dealing with the short esophagus, whether suspected preoperatively or determined at surgery. The choice of treatment may be (1) to perform an open transthoracic approach on all patients at risk, (2) to start the procedure laparoscopically and convert it to an open (laparotomy or thoracotomy) procedure if transhiatal mobilization fails, or (3) to perform a laparoscopic Collis gastroplasty, followed by a fundoplication.

In our experience, 14% or more of patients have some indication of a short esophagus preoperatively; more than half of these, however, have responded to simple laparoscopic esophageal mobilization without the need for a gastroplasty (Swanstrom, 1996). It follows that choosing an open approach preoperatively would unnecessarily subject a large number of patients to the morbidity of a thoracotomy. Because of this, and because of the extremely low morbidity of laparoscopy, we believe that all patients, even those with a suspected short esophagus, deserve an initial laparoscopic approach with an attempt to mobilize and reduce the gastroesophageal junction. If a gastroplasty is needed, the surgeon can convert to an open operation or, preferably, can perform a laparoscopic lengthening procedure.

Laparoscopic Management

Two laparoscopic versions of the Collis gastroplasty procedure have been described. We developed a combined thoracoscopic/laparoscopic approach in 1993 that is similar to the traditional transthoracic stapled Collis gastroplasty and have used it clinically over the past 5 years (Swanström, 1996). Johnson and colleagues (1998) from Atlanta have reported an alternative, totally laparoscopic technique fashioned after the open transabdominal procedure described by Steichen (1986).

Technique

Both techniques begin with the standard approach to laparoscopic antireflux surgery (Hunter et al, 1996). Patients are placed on a split-legged table and positioned with the arms extended laterally. The patient is in reverse

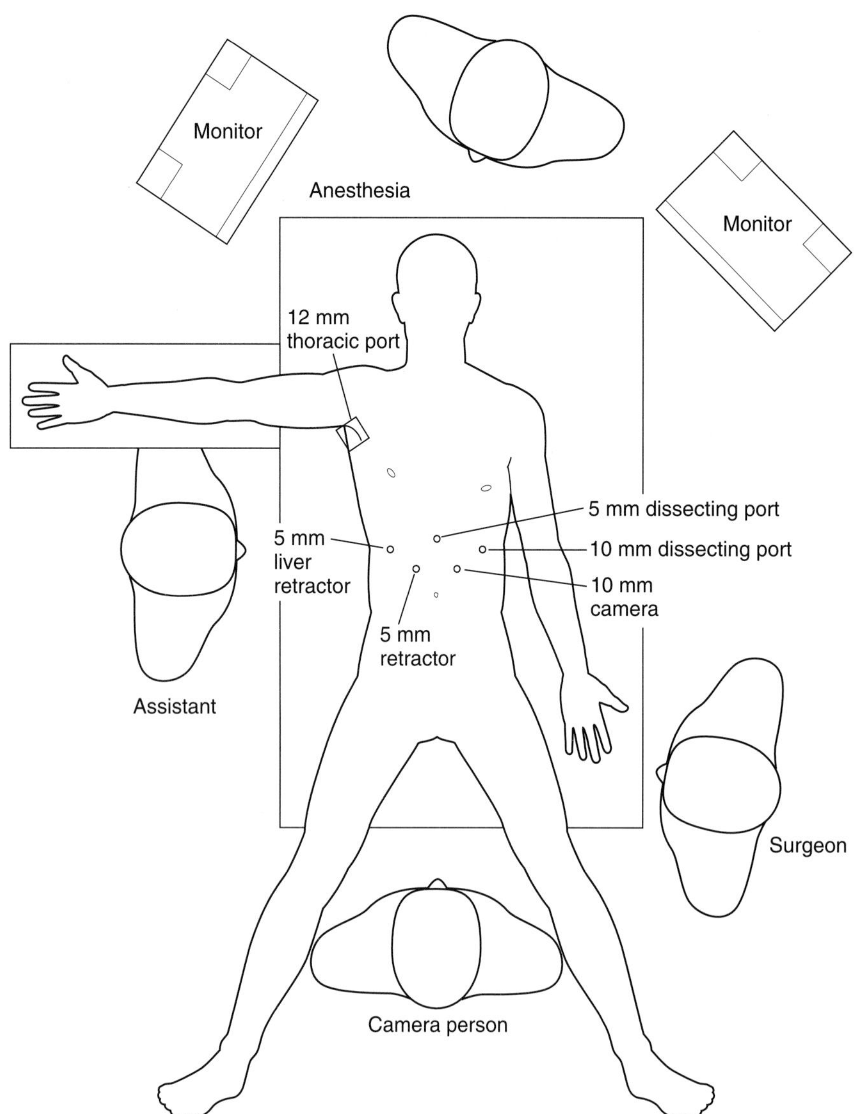

FIGURE 24–32 ■ Patient position and port placement for the gastric and esophageal mobilization and fundoplication portions of an endoscopic Collis procedure.

Trendelenburg position. A five-port technique is used for access. A 45-degree scope is used to allow all dissection to be done under direct vision (Fig. 24–32).

After atraumatic elevation of the left lobe of the liver, the hepatogastric ligament and phrenoesophageal ligament are divided with bipolar scissors to completely free both limbs of the right crus. The surgeon extensively mobilizes the gastric fundus by dividing the short gastric vessels of the upper one third of the fundus and by completely freeing all retrogastric attachments. For speed and safety reasons, the surgeon usually uses ultrasonic coagulating shears to perform this mobilization.

In patients with a large paraesophageal hernia, the mediastinal hernia sac should be reduced and excised from its attachment to the gastroesophageal junction. Transhiatal dissection of the distal esophagus is performed under direct visualization. The surgeon can use either the bipolar scissors or the ultrasonic coagulating shears, always being careful to avoid injury to the vagus nerves. It is possible to perform extensive dissection of the distal esophagus (as much as 10 to 15 cm) by inserting the angled scope across the hiatus, along with the dissecting instruments, while the assistant retracts the epiphrenic fat pad caudad (Swanström, 1996). If, despite this step, the surgeon is unable to achieve the required tension-free 2 to 3 cm of intra-abdominal esophageal length, a Collis procedure should be performed.

Laparoscopic/Thoracoscopic Approach

All patients at risk for shortened esophagus are prepared with the right axilla exposed and with a small flat pad placed beneath the right scapula. Usual precautions should be taken to pad and secure the arm on the armrest to prevent nerve injury. If the need to perform a Collis procedure is encountered unexpectedly during a routine laparoscopic fundoplication, the drapes can be split and the axilla prepared and redraped at that time. A double-lumen endotracheal tube is not needed for this procedure because the surgeon performs thoracoscopy using positive-pressure carbon dioxide pneumothorax, which partially collapses the right lung and allows visualization. Additional invasive monitoring (arterial lines or even Swan-Ganz monitoring) may be advisable for patients

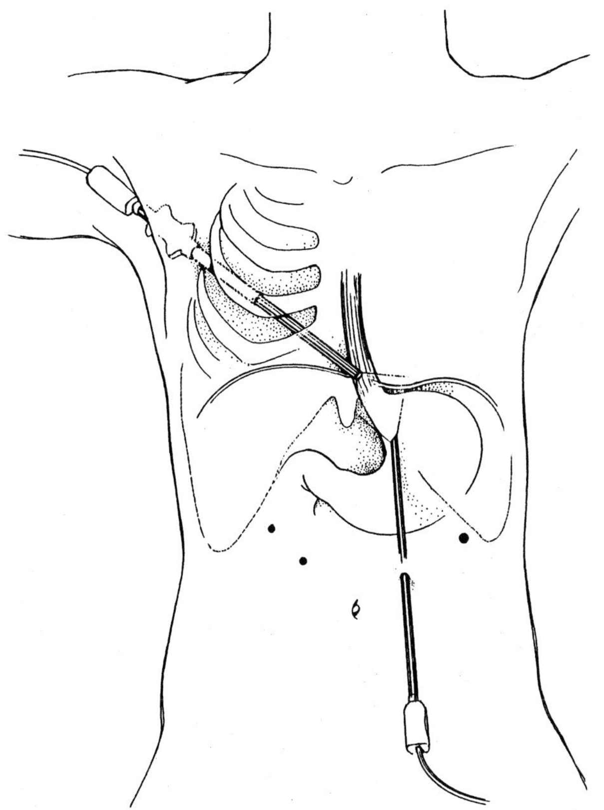

FIGURE 24–33 ■ The endoscopic staples are inserted through a 12-mm thoracic port and advanced across the mediastinum while it is visualized laparoscopically.

with underlying cardiopulmonary disease. A second camera, light source, and 0-degree laparoscope are required.

A single 12-mm trocar is placed by direct cutdown in the anterior axillary line in the third or fourth intercostal space. A standard laparoscopic port, instead of a valveless thoracic port, should be used to allow thoracic insufflation. Once it has been ensured that the pleural space is clear, carbon dioxide insufflation is started through the thoracic port at no more than 10 mm Hg pressure. This is usually well tolerated by the patient, although the anesthetist needs to be prepared to adjust ventilator support to compensate for increased carbon dioxide absorption and higher peak inspiratory pressures.

Thoracoscopy is performed to ensure that the lung has collapsed and that there are no pleural adhesions that might restrict passage of the endoscopic stapling device. If adhesions are encountered or if the lung does not collapse, a second 5-mm port can be placed to help mobilize or retract the lung.

If the pleural space is free, the 0-degree thoracoscope is advanced to the posterior inferior diaphragmatic sulcus. At this point, the light from the thoracoscope is visible through the right mediastinal pleura, which is being visualized with the intra-abdominal angled laparoscope.

Having established the correct trajectory, the surgeon withdraws the thoracoscope while holding the thoracic port firmly in position. A 35-mm endoscopic stapler with a standard gastrointestinal cartridge, is then advanced carefully along the previously established pathway until it is seen laparoscopically indenting the mediastinal pleura. An incision is made in the pleura, and the stapler is advanced into the abdominal cavity (Fig. 24–33). A 45 French bougie is passed into the stomach after removal of the oral gastric tube. The previously mobilized greater curvature of the stomach is rotated anteriorly and fed into the opened stapler (Fig. 24–34).

After it is ensured that the anterior vagus has not been caught in the staple line, the stapler is pressed against the bougie and closed. A single firing of the stapler results in a 3.5-cm gastroplasty. It is rarely, but occasionally, necessary to perform a second firing to achieve even greater length. The resulting gastric tube will be larger than the 45 French bougie because of the width of the staple cartridge. The stapler is removed, leaving the thoracic port closed and in place. No attempt is made to close the small hole in the right pleura. Posterior crural closure is performed in the standard manner, and a partial or complete fundoplication is created around the neoesophagus with a 56 French bougie in place (Fig. 24–35). Either a partial (Toupet) or complete wrap (Nissen) is performed, depending on the preoperative motility status. Partial fundoplication is reserved for patients with significantly impaired esophageal peristalsis, as determined by preoperative motility testing.

After the fundoplication is completed, a 5-mm drain

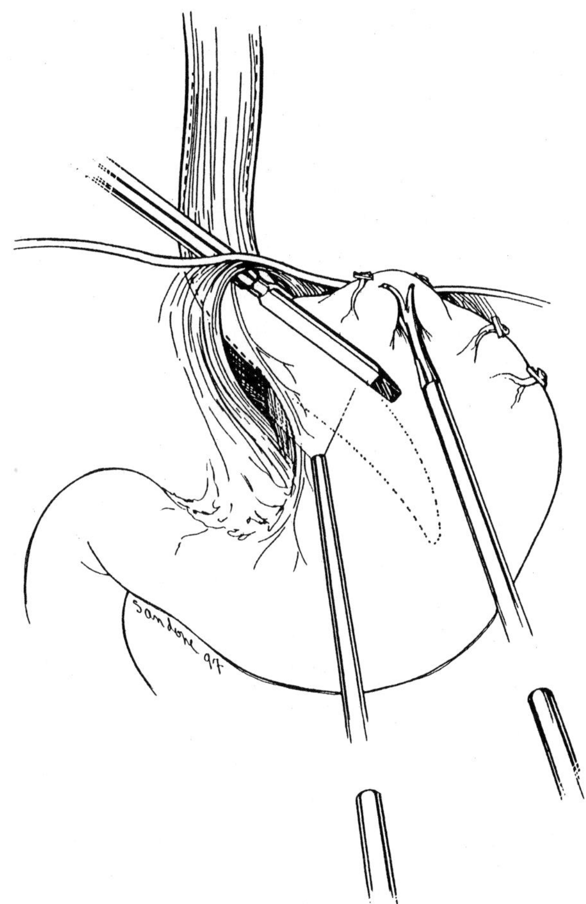

FIGURE 24–34 ■ With a 45 French bougie in place, the anteriorly rotated stomach is fed into the stapler.

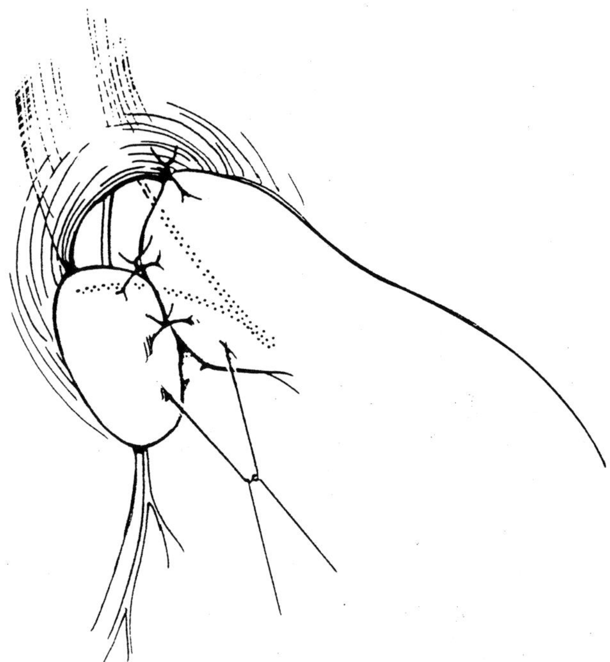

FIGURE 24–35 ■ A partial or total fundoplication (shown) is created around the intra-abdominal neoesophagus with a large bougie in place (56 French).

is placed laparoscopically across the hiatus and brought out through one of the 5-mm trocars. The pneumoperitoneum is evacuated, 10-mm fascial defects are closed, and the skin is closed in the usual fashion. The pneumothorax is evacuated as the thoracic port is removed and while the anesthetist fully expands the right lung. A chest tube is not required unless there was injury to the lung during retraction or lysis of pleural adhesions. A nasogastric tube is not used.

Postsurgical Care

Patients take nothing by mouth until a meglumine diatrizoate (Gastrografin) esophagogram is obtained on postoperative day 1. If no leak is seen, clear liquids are started and the diet advanced to full liquids as tolerated by the patient. Most patients are able to go home on postoperative day 2 and are discharged with liquid pain medications. Patients are kept on a full liquid diet for 2 weeks.

Alternative Technique

In 1998, Hunter's group at Emory described a totally laparoscopic technique for performing a Collis gastroplasty (Johnson et al, 1998). As described in the previous technique, complete gastric mobilization is performed and distal esophageal dissection is carried out in attempt to avoid a lengthening procedure. If gastroplasty is required, a 3-cm subxiphoid incision is made to allow insertion of the anvil of a 25-mm circular stapler. A 45 French bougie is passed through the esophagus into the stomach, and a Keith needle is used to pass a strong nylon suture through both walls of the stomach from anterior to posterior, adjacent to the bougie and 3 cm below the angle of His (Fig. 24–36). The suture is used to pull the spike of the stapler anvil through the stomach from posterior to anterior. The handle of the circular stapler is inserted through the subxiphoid incision and connected to the anvil. Firing the circular stapler creates a full-thickness hole in the stomach. An endoscopic stapler with a standard tissue cartridge can then be passed through one of the lower trocar sites, inserted through the gastric hole, and fired parallel to the bougie (Fig. 24–37). Once again, because of the width of the stapler cartridge, the resulting neoesophagus will be of a caliber to permit easy passage of a 56 to 58 French bougie. A standard antireflux procedure can then be performed with the same postoperative care as described for the previous technique.

An advantage of this approach is that the procedure can be performed totally laparoscopically without violating the right pleural space and without the need to prepare and drape the right axilla. A disadvantage is the need to create an open incision in the subxiphoid area, which makes it difficult to maintain subsequent pneumoperitoneum and results in some increased pain and scarring as well as an increased cost for the additional stapling devices. Theoretically, there may also be an increased risk of leaks from the intersecting staple lines. Both techniques, however, accomplish the goal of allowing a fundoplication to be performed without tension around an intra-abdominal segment of esophagus.

RESULTS

Laparoscopic Collis gastroplasty, fortunately, has rarely been needed in our experience. In three larger series of laparoscopic fundoplications, shortened esophagus requiring conversion to an open procedure or gastroplasty was reportedly encountered in 3% to 4% of the procedures (Falk, 1998; Jobe et al, 1998, Johnson, 1998). A report from a center with an aggressive policy of using an open transthoracic approach in all patients with suspected esophageal shortening gastroplasty was used in 14% of the cases (Peters and DeMeester, 1995). When needed, however, endoscopic gastroplasty and fundoplication provides good to excellent symptomatic results in a majority of patients.

Morbidity associated with the procedure in these small case series has been extremely low (Table 24–3). This compares favorably with the 2% to 11% morbidity rates reported in open series (Pearson et al, 1987; Stirling, 1989). Postoperative results are good in 89% to 100% of patients when symptoms alone are considered. When objective testing is performed, however, higher rates of persistently abnormal 24-hour pH testing have been described. Our own study reported a 50% incidence of abnormal 24-hour pH testing with a 36% rate of postoperative esophagitis. Symptomatically, manometrically, and endoscopically there was no evidence of failure of the antireflux mechanism and the cause was believed to be the presence of the ectopic gastric mucosa created by the gastroplasty (Jobe et al, 1998).

FUTURE TRENDS

Debate continues over the true incidence of intrinsically short esophagus in the reflux population and how it

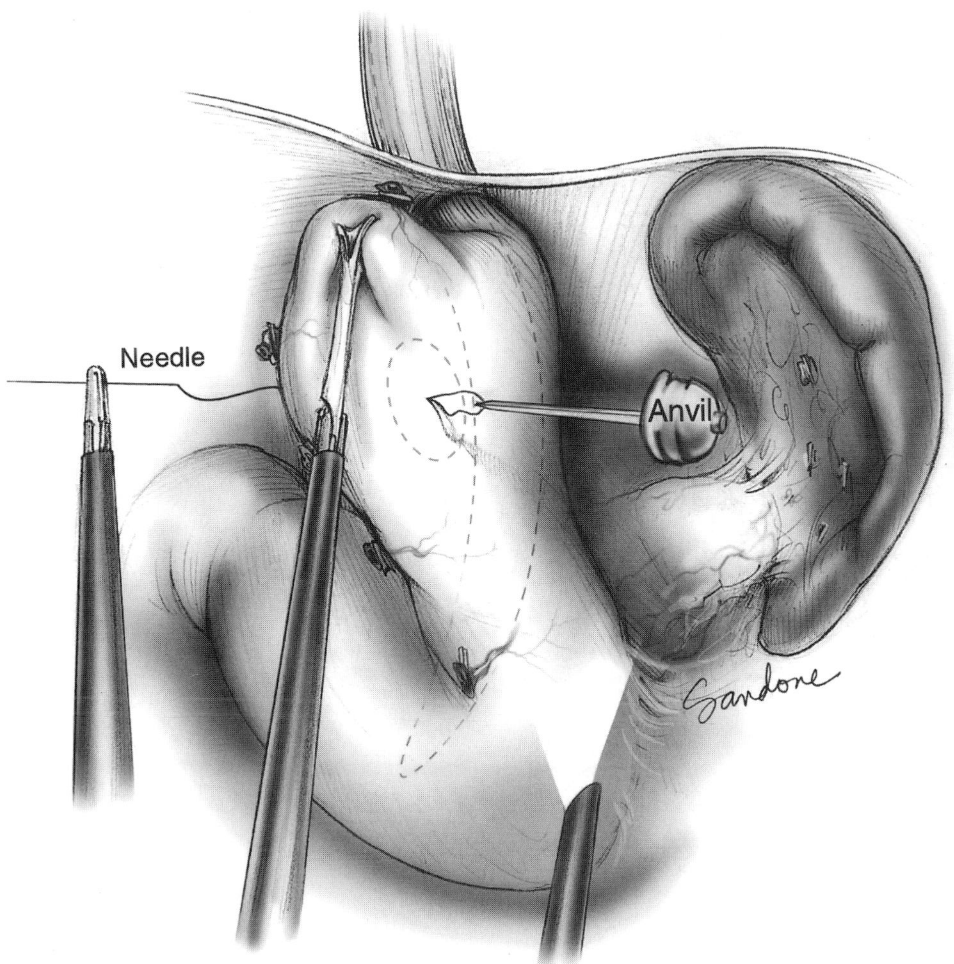

FIGURE 24–36 ■ A straight needle is used to penetrate the stomach to allow a 25-mm circular stapler anvil to be pulled through.

should be treated. Early in the laparoscopic antireflux experience, the finding was ignored or treated as a contraindication to surgery. Now it is generally acknowledged to exist, but it remains frustratingly unpredictable in occurrence. The incidence may also be decreasing with improved medical treatment and earlier referral for laparoscopic treatment.

Our group and others continue to try to define accurate and objective preoperative criteria to allow surgeons and patients to be better prepared for the presence of acquired short esophagus. There is no consensus on how the short esophagus is best handled. Options include (1) an initial open approach (with the risk of subjecting many patients to an unneeded thoracotomy), (2) conversion from a laparoscopic to an open procedure (with the risk of disappointing a patient expecting a minimally invasive procedure), and (3) an endoscopic gastroplasty. Obviously, more outcome data need to be accumulated to determine which approach is most effective, most cost-effective, and most patient-friendly.

One may question whether the endoscopic Collis gastroplasty is as effective as the traditional open approach, specifically, whether a transabdominal approach provides adequate esophageal exposure compared with a left thoracotomy. We believe that the open and endoscopic approaches are equivalent. Although we have chosen to

TABLE 24–3 ■ **Results of Endoscopic Techniques of Collis Gastroplasty**

Series	*No. of Patients*	*% Incidence*	*Technique*	*Operating Room Time (min)*	*Complication*	*Success*
Falk, 1998	3	NA	Laparoscopy/stapled	140–240	0	100
Johnson, 1998	9	4 (9/220)	Laparoscopy/stapled	210–394	0	89
Swanström*	24	5 (24/480)	Laparoscopy/thoracoscopy	180–390	0	100

*Clinical experience from February 1995 to March 1999.

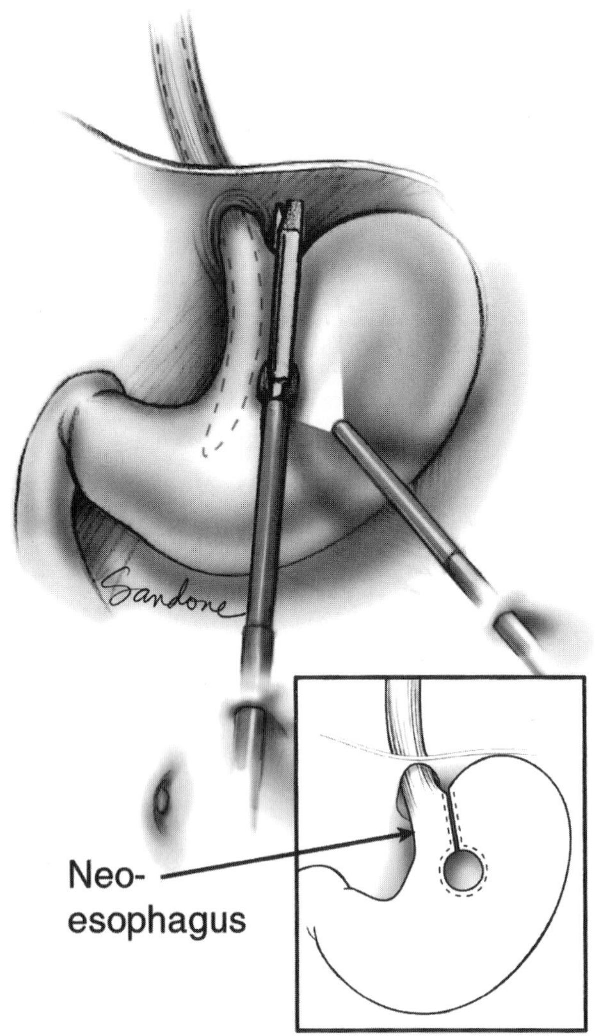

FIGURE 24–37 ■ After a circular hole is made in the stomach by firing the circular stapler, a standard linear cutting endoscopic stapler (shown) can be fired parallel to a 45 French bougie, creating the neoesophagus (*inset*).

limit mediastinal esophageal mobilization to 15 cm, this is because of concerns about devascularizing the esophagus and not a limitation of the transhiatal approach. Experience with laparoscopic transhiatal esophagectomy has shown that full mobilization of the thoracic esophagus is possible (Swanström and Hansen, 1997). The endoscopic staplers have been shown to be effective and no leaks have been reported, even though the staple line was not oversewn, as was often done in open gastroplasties.

Few outcome data are available to support the preference of one endoscopic technique over the other. We have found the thoracoscopic approach to be less awkward, less expensive, and easier to perform than the laparoscopic Collis. Mean operative times are also less, but this may be because of greater experience with the thoracoscopic procedure. Concern has been expressed regarding the need to open the right mediastinal pleura (Falk, 1998). We have found that the controlled carbon dioxide pneumothorax, which is also encountered during routine laparoscopic fundoplications, is known to be a benign condition and has not presented a problem to date (Marcus et al, 1996). The approach that we have developed relies on access through the right side of the chest. This is needed to achieve proper parallel placement of the stapler alongside the esophagus, which enters the abdomen from a right-to-left direction (see Fig. 24–34). The newer articulating staplers may allow the option of a left-sided chest approach.

Finally, there remains the finding of the high rate (50%) of abnormal postoperative 24-hour pH tests after the gastroplasty (Jobe et al, 1998). This phenomenon has also been reported after open Collis gastroplasty by several investigators who noted that between 30% and 56% of patients have abnormal postoperative findings (Anselmino et al, 1997; Martin et al, 1992). It is especially of concern that many of these patients are totally symptom-free. Future areas of study should obviously address this finding with the idea of developing surgical methods to decrease acid secretion from the neoesophagus to prevent complications such as strictures or even adenocarcinoma (Maziak, 1995). A potential method may be to include an extensive superselective esophageal vagotomy or, alternatively, to initiate postoperative maintenance medical therapy on a routine basis. Certainly, it is logical to obtain postoperative 24-hour pH studies or an upper endoscopy on all patients who have undergone a Collis gastroplasty.

CONCLUSION

Failure to recognize the shortened esophagus during laparoscopic fundoplication and to treat it appropriately results in misplaced fundoplications or repairs under tension with subsequent high failure rates from wrap herniation or disruption. Unfortunately, there are no definitive preoperative tests to indicate patients who would require a surgical lengthening procedure, and the diagnosis can be made only at the time of surgery. Surgeons must therefore be continuously aware of the possibility of this entity and should have a treatment strategy prepared to deal with it. This strategy might be to electively perform open surgery on a large number of "at-risk" patients, to convert to an open procedure if the esophagus cannot be mobilized, or to perform an endoscopic Collis gastroplasty using the techniques described earlier. For surgeons with a high volume of antireflux surgical procedures, it is in the patient's best interest for the surgeon to master the techniques of laparoscopic Collis gastroplasty so that a minimally invasive approach can be ensured despite the operative findings. The addition of gastroplasty, however, should be performed only when absolutely necessary. In our experience, patients with this nonphysiologic reconstruction will frequently require chronic medical therapy despite effective symptomatic control of reflux (Jobe et al, 1998).

COMMENTS AND CONTROVERSIES

As the author notes, the presence of acquired esophageal shortening is a complication of reflux esophagitis that should modify the surgical option selected for an antireflux repair. During the present era of laparoscopic antireflux surgery, this complication is more fre-

quently overlooked than recognized, which often results in a less favorable or failed outcome. Dr. Swanström is a pioneer in the development of thoracoscopic and laparoscopic techniques for adding a gastroplasty to an antireflux operation. Since his initial publication in 1996, an increasing number of reports have described the problem of acquired short esophagus and its management by a laparoscopic gastroplasty or lengthening procedure. I have no doubt but that further time and experience will increase the frequency of recognition of shortening and the addition of gastroplasty in laparoscopic or thoracoscopic management.

There is an important emphasis by the author on the criteria for adding a lengthening procedure to the repair following mobilization of the esophagogastric junction and the adjacent mediastinal esophagus. These observations are made from the abdominal side of the diaphragmatic hiatus, under the potentially modified conditions of a peritoneal space inflated with gas. In theory, this environment may underestimate the incidence of more subtle degrees of acquired shortening. It can be argued that tension on the complete repair is more accurately evaluated from the thoracic side of the hiatus. This latter concern, and opinion, is expressed in the reports by Maziak and associates (1998) and Gastal and colleagues (1999).

The high incidence of abnormal reflux after laparoscopic/thoracoscopic gastroplasty, observed by Swanström and reported by Orringer in the past, following the "Collis-Belsey" operation may relate to the relatively large-diameter gastroplasty tube that they use. Dr. Swanström has described the creation of a tube that can easily accommodate a 54 or 56 French bougie. Orringer commonly employed a 56 or even a 60 French bougie. In 1977, we reported observations on the levels of pressure developed in the reconstructed LES after Collis gastroplasty and Belsey repair using intraoperative manometry in some 60 clinical cases. The larger the bougie over which the gastroplasty tube was fashioned, the lower the reconstructed LES pressure obtained. For many years now, we have found that fashioning the gastric tube snugly over a 48 French Maloney bougie provides adequate and lasting reflux control, without troublesome dysphagia, in about 90% of a selected group of patients with complex reflux in whom a gastroplasty was used because of obvious, or presumed, short esophagus.

I have little doubt that time, experience, and new technology will soon see laparoscopic and thoracoscopic techniques replace almost all open antireflux procedures. Dr. Swanström is one of the pioneers leading the way in this field.

REFERENCES

Cooper JD, Gill SS, Nelems JM, Pearson FG: Intraoperative and postoperative manometric findings with Collis gastroplasty and Belsey hiatal hernia repair for gastroesophageal reflux. J Thorac Cardiovasc Surg 74:744–751, 1977.

Orringer MG, Sloan H: Complications and failings of the combined Collis-Belsey operation. J Thorac Cardiovasc Surg 74:726–735, 1977.

F. G. P.

■ *REFERENCES*

Allen SM, Matthews HR: Circular myotomy and Belsey repair for acquired shortening of the oesophagus. Eur J Cardiothorac Surg 7:645–647, 1993.

Anselmino M, Zaninotto G, Constantini M, et al: Collis gastroplasty plus fundoplication is more effective than bouginage plus acid suppressive therapy in the treatment of reflux induced strictures of the esophagus [Abstract]. J Gastrointest Surg 1:000–005, 1997.

Collet D, Cadiere GB: Conversions and complications of laparoscopic treatment of GERD. Am J Surg 169:622–626, 1995.

Collis JL: An operation for hiatus hernia with short oesophagus. Thorax 12:181–182, 1957.

Cooper JD, Gill SS, Nelems JM, Pearson FG: Intraoperative and postoperative manometric findings with Collis gastroplasty and Belsey hiatal hernia repair for gastroesophageal reflux. J Thorac Cardiovasc Surg 74:744–751, 1977.

DeMeester TR, Bonavina L, Alberucci M: Nissen fundoplication for gastroesophageal reflux disease: Evaluation of primary repair in 100 consecutive patients. Ann Surg 204:9–20, 1986.

Falk GL: Laparoscopic cut Collis gastroplasty: A novel technique. Dis Esophagus 11:260–262, 1998.

Gastal OL, Hagan JA, Peters JH, et al: Short esophagus: Analysis of predictors and clinical implications. Arch Surg 134:633–636; discussion, 637–638, 1999.

Hinder RA, Filipi CJ, Wescher G, et al: Laparoscopic Nissen fundoplication is an effective treatment for gastroesophageal reflux disease. Ann Surg 220:472–481, 1994.

Horvath KD, Swanström LL, Jobe B: The short esophagus: Pathophysiology, incidence, presentation and treatment in the era of laparoscopic anti-reflux surgery. Ann Surg 232:630–640, 2000.

Hunter JG, Trus TL, Branum GD: A physiologic approach to laparoscopic fundoplication for gastroesophageal reflux disease. Ann Surg 223:673–685, 1996.

Jobe BA, Horvath KD, Swanström LL: Postoperative function following laparoscopic Collis gastroplasty for shortened esophagus. Arch Surg 133:867–874, 1998.

Johnson AB: Laparoscopic Collis gastroplasty and Nissen fundoplication: A new technique for the management of esophageal foreshortening. Surg Endosc 12:1055–1060, 1998.

Mansour KA: Complications of intrathoracic Nissen fundoplication. Ann Thorac Surg 32:173–178, 1981.

Marcus DR, Lau W, Swanström LL: Carbon dioxide pneumothorax in laparoscopic surgery. Am J Surg 171:464–466, 1996.

Martin CJ, Cox MR, Cade RJ: Collis-Nissen gastroplasty fundoplication for complicated gastro-oesophageal reflux disease. Aust N Z J Surg 62:126–129, 1992.

Maziak DE: Adenocarcinoma of the neo-esophagus after Collis gastroplasty. Ann Thorac Surg 60:1795–1797, 1995.

Maziak DE, Todd TR, Miller L, Pearson FG: Massive hiatus hernia: Evaluation and management. J Thorac Cardiovasc Surg 115:53–62, 1998.

Orringer MG, Sloan H: Complications and failings of the combined Collis-Belsey operation. J Thorac Cardiovasc Surg 74:726–735, 1977.

Pearson FG, Cooper JD, Patterson GA, et al: Gastroplasty and fundoplication for complex reflux problems: Long-term results. Ann Surg 206:473–481, 1987.

Peters JH, DeMeester TR: Indications, principles of procedure selection and techniques of laparoscopic Nissen fundoplication. Semin Laparosc Surg 2:27–44, 1995.

Peters JH, Heimbucher J, Auer WK, et al: Clinical and physiologic comparison of laparoscopic and open Nissen fundoplication. J Am Coll Surg 180:385–393, 1995.

Steichen FM: Abdominal approach to the Collis gastroplasty and Nissen fundoplication. Surg Gynecol Obstet 162:272–274, 1986.

Stirling MC: Continued assessment of the combined Collis-Nissen operation. Ann Thorac Surg 47:224–230, 1989.

Swanström LL: Laparoscopic Collis gastroplasty is the treatment of choice for the shortened esophagus. Am J Surg 171:477–481, 1996.

Swanström LL, Hansen P: Laparoscopic total esophagectomy. Arch Surg 1:1–2, 1997.

Watson DI, Jamieson GG, Devitt PG, et al: Changing strategies in the performance of laparoscopic Nissen fundoplication as a result of experience with 230 operations. Surg Endosc 9:961–966, 1995.

CHAPTER **25**

Laparoscopic Antireflux Surgery

OVERVIEW AND CURRENT STATUS OF LAPAROSCOPIC ANTIREFLUX SURGERY

Thomas W. Rice

Treatment of gastroesophageal reflux disease (GERD) evolves with the introductions of new drug therapies and advancements in surgical techniques. Initial unbridled enthusiasm for each new therapy has been tempered by clinical studies that identify deficiencies. The appropriateness and benefit of each new therapy are determined only after time and close scrutiny. It has taken 10 years after the first report of laparoscopic antireflux surgery (Dallemagne et al, 1991) to clarify the use and results of laparoscopy in the treatment of GERD.

PRINCIPLES OF ANTIREFLUX SURGERY AND LAPAROSCOPY

The principles of antireflux surgery, regardless of the approach, are (1) restoration of the intra-abdominal esophagus, (2) reconstruction of the diaphragmatic hiatus, and (3) reinforcement of the lower esophageal sphincter (LES) by fundoplication. However, it is necessary to consider the individual needs of each patient and the best-suited surgical approach. Both the principles that apply to laparoscopy and the care that is necessary for successful laparoscopic antireflux surgery are discussed.

Restoring an Adequate Length of Intra-abdominal Esophagus

Circumferential mobilization of the thoracic esophagus deep into the posterior mediastinum re-establishes the normal intra-abdominal esophageal length in most patients with uncomplicated GERD and a reducible hiatal hernia. A critical component of the reflux barrier, an adequate intra-abdominal esophagus, ensures a tension-free repair. At thoracotomy, extensive thoracic esophageal mobilization is necessary to accomplish antireflux surgery. Freeing of the esophagus to the aortic arch is recommended for successful thoracic repair (Skinner and Belsey, 1988a). During open abdominal antireflux surgery 4 to 6 cm of esophagus should be mobilized by transhiatal dissection (Rosetti and Nadjafi, 1988; Skinner and Belsey, 1998b). Laparoscopy may not allow adequate esophageal mobilization. Pneumoperitoneum effaces the diaphragmatic hiatus, artificially and temporarily increasing the length of intra-abdominal esophagus (Awad et al, 1999). Aggressive thoracic esophageal mobilization, particularly if there is reflux-induced paraesophageal inflammation, can result in pleural damage and pneumothorax. This complication may require conversion to open surgery. A major cause of mortality and serious morbidity of laparoscopic esophageal mobilization is esophageal and gastric perforation. When it occurs, it is frequently not recognized at the initial operation (Rantanen et al, 1999b; Schauer et al, 1996; Swanström and Pennings, 1995). Laparoscopic antireflux surgery may be associated with more life-threatening complications than open surgery (Rantanen et al, 1999b). To avoid the complications of pneumothorax, perforation, and open surgery, the surgeon may accept inadequate esophageal mobilization. If laparoscopic mobilization of the esophagus is limited to its abdominal portion as defined by the left and right crura (Hinder and Filipi, 1995), there will be inadequate intra-abdominal length. This results in repairs under tension and subsequent late failure.

Despite adequate mobilization, there may be insufficient intra-abdominal esophagus. This condition is known as "short esophagus." Short esophagus is suspected if there is extensive reflux injury reflected by peptic stricture, history of stricture and dilatation, long-segment Barrett's esophagus, large hiatal hernia (>4 cm at esophagoscopy), irreducible hiatal hernia (at barium esophagram), or paraesophageal hernia (Gastal et al, 1999; Hunter et al, 1999; Maziak et al, 1998). Laparoscopic assessment alone may fail to define the extent of shortening (Awad et al, 1999). One author maintains that 200 to 400 antireflux procedures are required for a surgeon to become experienced enough to recognize and successfully lengthen the short esophagus (Waring, 1999).

Esophageal lengthening (Collis gastroplasty) combined with an antireflux procedure has been successfully used to manage short esophagus during open surgery. Techniques for laparoscopic esophageal lengthening have been described (Johnson et al, 1998; Luketich et al, 2000; Swanström et al, 1996). In a report of a follow-up of 15 patients who underwent laparoscopic esophageal lengthening, 36% demonstrated persistent esophagitis and 43% had aperistalsis of the distal esophagus (Jobe et al, 1998). These initial results are discouraging. Presently, many surgeons believe that thoracotomy, conventional Collis gastroplasty, and fundoplication must be considered in all patients with suspected short esophagus who cannot

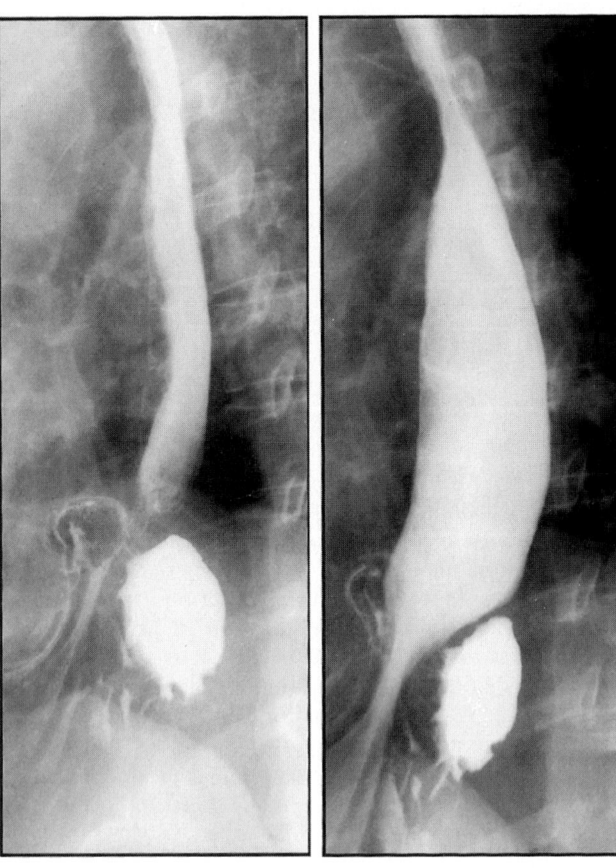

FIGURE 25–1 ■ *Left,* Nissen fundoplication in an unrecognized short esophagus. This barium esophagram demonstrates the three means of failure of antireflux surgery. The total fundoplication has "unwrapped" (pulled apart), "slipped" (passed from the distal esophagus onto the stomach), and "reherniated" (migrated into the thoracic cavity). *Right,* Free reflux to the level of the carina is easily induced.

be treated adequately by laparoscopy (Kauer et al, 1995; Little, 1995).

Inadequate mobilization or failure to lengthen the short esophagus produces tension on the repair and is a principal factor in slippage of the wrap onto the stomach (slipped Nissen) or herniation of the fundoplication into the thoracic cavity (Fig. 25–1). These problems result in poor control of reflux or the onset of new or additional symptoms such as dysphagia, postprandial discomfort, or pain.

Reconstruction of the Diaphragmatic Hiatus

The extrinsic LES mechanism is composed of the striated muscle of the esophageal diaphragmatic hiatus. The cru-

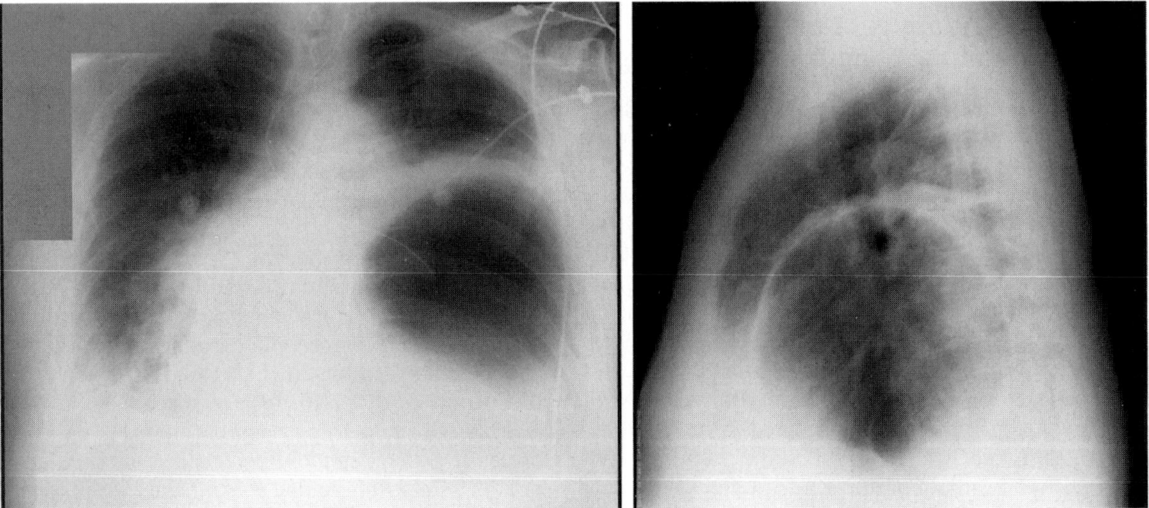

FIGURE 25–2 ■ Herniation of the stomach into the left pleural space. Incomplete approximation of the crura, attempted prosthetic reconstruction of the diaphragmatic hiatus, and entry into the left pleural space during laparoscopic repair of a type III (mixed) hiatal hernia permitted massive herniation of the stomach into the left chest. The patient was transferred to our service 5 days after failed laparoscopic antireflux surgery. At urgent operation, infarction of the distal esophagus and proximal stomach necessitated emergency esophagogastrectomy.

ral musculature exerts a pinchcock effect that reinforces the intrinsic LES (Kahrilas et al, 1999; Mittal and Balaban, 1997). Reconstruction of the esophageal hiatus is a principal component of antireflux surgery that was neglected by some surgeons in the laparoscopic era (Watson and Jamieson, 1998). In early follow-up, development of a paraesophageal hernia complicated 10% of laparoscopic antireflux surgery where the hiatus had not been reconstructed (Watson et al., 1995) (Fig. 25–2).

Difficulty in closure of the hiatus at laparoscopy prompted some surgeons to propose prosthetic closure for reinforcement of the hiatus. This technique abolishes the dynamic nature of the hiatus and destroys the extrinsic sphincter mechanism. Strategies for reconstruction of the large hiatus should be considered before surgery. This problem should be anticipated in patients with large hiatal hernias, paraesophageal hernias, and Barrett's esophagus (Cameron, 1999). I believe that hiatal reconstruction without prosthetic material can be obtained in all patients but may require an open approach.

Reinforcement of the Lower Esophageal Sphincter

Nissen fundoplication produces an excellent reflux barrier. It is superior to partial fundoplication in the control of acid reflux and in the healing of reflux esophagitis (Alexiou et al, 1999). Although partial fundoplication produces less dysphagia, gas bloat, and postprandial symptoms, it may provide inadequate reflux control and may predispose to late failure (Bell et al, 1999; Horvath et al, 1999). Many postoperative swallowing problems result from a fundoplication that is too tight or too long (Fig. 25–3). Dysphagia and fundoplication side effects are excessive if short gastric vessels are not divided and the fundus is not mobilized (Rosetti modification) (Bell et al, 1999; Dallemange et al, 1995, Hunter et al, 1996). A carefully constructed Nissen fundoplication, one that is short, loose, untethered, and centered over the distal esophagus, minimizes these complications. A partial fundoplication should not be used in uncomplicated GERD with the intent of minimizing dysphagia or postprandial symptoms.

In the patient with an amotile esophagus, Nissen fundoplication is associated with dysphagia and a partial fundoplication is mandatory. However, most motility disorders are not absolute and lay within the spectrum between the uncomplicated patient with normal peristalsis and the aperistaltic patient. This problem is best defined by esophageal manometry, which demonstrates either aperistalsis or low amplitude peristalsis (averaging < 20 mm Hg) or poorly conducted contractions in the distal esophagus. Although there are reports of freedom from dysphagia in patients with esophageal motility abnormalities who receive a Nissen fundoplication, such results are not universally reported. Partial fundoplication should be selectively applied to patients with motility disorders and only after an analysis of esophageal motility based on barium esophagram and esophageal manometry (Wetscher et al, 1997). In these patients complete control of reflux may not be possible because defective motility of the esophagus dictates less than a complete 360-degree fundoplication. Compromise procedures such as partial fundoplication and esophageal lengthening may be required to avoid dysphagia, at the cost of persistent but reduced reflux. Chronic medication with proton pump inhibitors may be required.

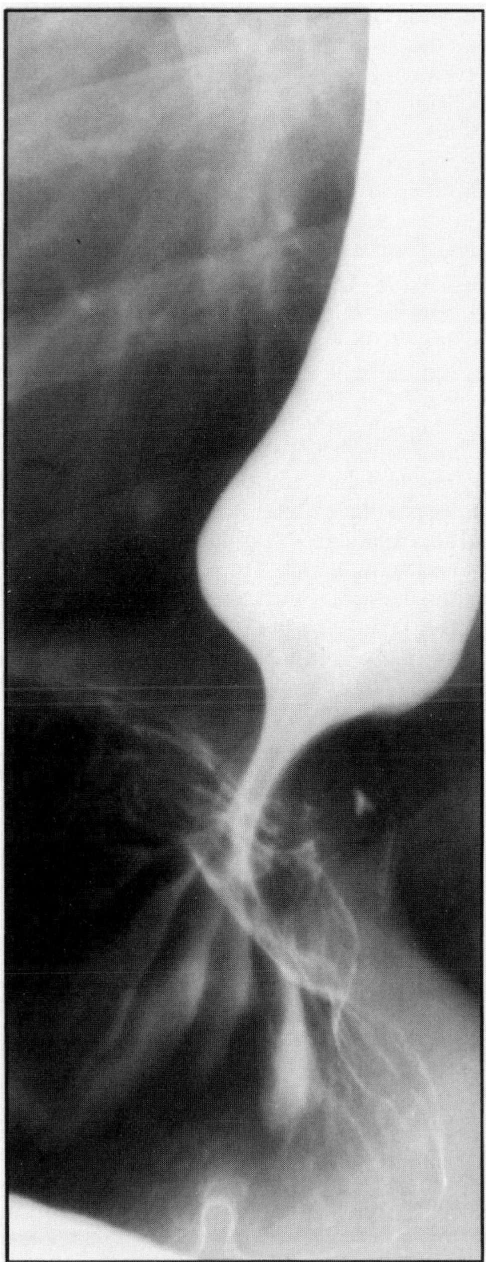

FIGURE 25–3 ■ Tight Nissen fundoplication. A short, tight laparoscopic total fundoplication was the result of incomplete mobilization of the gastric fundus (Rosetti modification).

THE SURGEON AND LAPAROSCOPIC ANTIREFLUX SURGERY

Laparoscopic antireflux surgery is most successful in a center that specializes in the treatment of GERD. In experienced hands, results are superior and provide better symptom relief, improved healing of esophagitis, and freedom from reoperation (Luostarinen and Isolauri, 1999; Watson et al, 1996). To minimize both conversion to open surgery and failure of laparoscopic antireflux surgery, a center needs experience with at least 50 laparoscopic repairs. The individual surgeon should have performed 20 laparoscopic repairs (Voitk et al, 1999; Watson et al, 1996).

Laparoscopic antireflux surgery, a reparative procedure, is not a natural extension of laparoscopic cholecystectomy, an extirpative procedure. Different dissecting skills and the mastery of intracorporeal suturing and knot tying are necessary for laparoscopic antireflux surgery. Despite previous laparoscopic or esophageal surgical experience, there is a steep and long learning curve for laparoscopic antireflux surgery. Failure rate for laparoscopic surgery, defined as conversion to open surgery, was 26% for one surgeon's first 20 operations and 11% after 20 operations (Voitk et al, 1999). This phenomenon can be modified but not eliminated if an experienced surgeon assists the trainee. The rate of failure was 55% without an experienced assistant and 21% if there was experienced help.

Occasional surgical treatment of GERD should be discouraged. In a 12-year period, 39 of 45 patients treated at a nonspecialized unit with open antireflux surgery were available for follow-up at a mean of 78 months (Rantanen et al, 1999a). Although 85% had no, or mild, reflux symptoms, symptoms of dysphagia (31%), flatulence (67%), and bloating (46%) predominated after repair. Thirty-seven percent had a defective fundoplication. At endoscopic assessment, 29% had erosive esophagitis, 13% required H_2-blockers or omeprazole for symptom control, and 13% required reoperation.

THE PATIENT AND LAPAROSCOPIC ANTIREFLUX SURGERY

The ideal patient for laparoscopic surgical correction of GERD has typical symptoms, heartburn that is easily controlled with proton pump inhibitors, a small reducible hiatal hernia, a hypotensive LES, adequate peristalsis of the esophageal body, and pathologic reflux documented by 24-hour pH monitoring. *Uncomplicated* GERD is simply and reliably treated by laparoscopic Nissen fundoplication.

Patients with a high potential for surgical failure (despite a technically correct operation) are identified through a careful history. The presence of typical symptoms of reflux, regurgitation, and dysphagia and the ability to control these symptoms with acid suppression therapy are the best predictors of successful laparoscopic antireflux surgery (Campos et al, 1999; So et al, 1998). Unrelenting symptoms despite adequate medical therapy, atypical symptoms (e.g., pain, odynophagia, bloating, hoarseness, cough, sore throat, asthma), dysphagia requiring dilation, and an urgency for immediate surgical relief of symptoms are clues that *complicated* GERD or a disease other than GERD is the cause of the patient's symptoms.

The existence of acid reflux and its relationship to symptoms must be documented. Although 24-hour esophageal pH monitoring is not the "perfect" gold standard for GERD, it is the most reliable test available. Abnormal 24-hour esophageal pH testing (esophageal pH score and percent time pH below 4) is the only investigation that predicts successful antireflux surgery (Campos et al, 1999). Lack of pathologic reflux after an adequate period of interrupted medical therapy, although not an absolute exclusion of GERD, should precipitate careful review of the patient's symptoms. If symptoms persist despite normalization of 24-hour esophageal pH studies by medication, the search for another cause of symptoms should ensue.

Incomplete evaluation of anatomy and physiology of the antireflux mechanism may result in inadequate or inappropriate surgical therapy of GERD. Assessment of every potential surgical candidate should include barium esophagram, esophagogastroduodenoscopy with biopsy, and esophageal manometry. Significant bloating and belching should prompt the investigation of gastric emptying.

The patient's clinical status must be optimum. Weight loss, smoking cessation, and treatment of reversible airway obstruction, bronchitis, and constipation are necessary preoperative measures. The patient's expectations after laparoscopic repair are for early return to work and resumption of preoperative activities. These expectations may foster failure of laparoscopic antireflux surgery. "Stressors of the diaphragm" (Soper and Dunnegan, 1999), activities that increase intra-abdominal pressure either early in the postoperative course (e.g., vomiting and constipation) and or long-term (e.g., weight training), must be avoided (Dickerman et al, 1997).

RESULTS

It is difficult to assess outcomes of laparoscopic antireflux surgery because follow-up is short, postoperative reports are selective, and criteria for outcome assessment are not uniform (Hogan and Shaker, 2000). Discrepancies between reported success and clinical reality are reflected in the increased number of publications that outline failed laparoscopic antireflux surgery (Rice, 2000). As it is currently practiced, laparoscopic antireflux surgery has not yet reached marketing expectations (Kahrilas, 1999).

Laparoscopy does not reduce operative time and may increase it (Nilsson et al, 2000). Laparoscopy reduces the physiologic insult to patients, as measured by immune function, pulmonary function, and so on. It may reduce postoperative pain. The need for narcotic analgesics may be higher initially but rapidly decreases in the first 24 hours so that overall requirements may be similar to open surgery (Dick et al, 1998). Because of advanced technology, operative costs are higher than those of open antireflux surgery; however, laparoscopy shortens hospital stay and therefore reduces the overall costs of hospitalization (Blomqvist et al, 1998; Frantzides and Carlson, 1995; Rattner and Brooks, 1995). Operative deaths are uncommon. A 0.2% mortality rate was reported in a review of multiple publications of laparoscopic antireflux surgery (Perdikis et al, 1997). Postoperative complications are reduced. Return to work is not necessarily hastened (Nilsson et al, 2000).

Symptom control is an important outcome of antireflux surgery; however, normalization of esophageal acid exposure should be the ultimate goal (Fig. 25–4). Al-

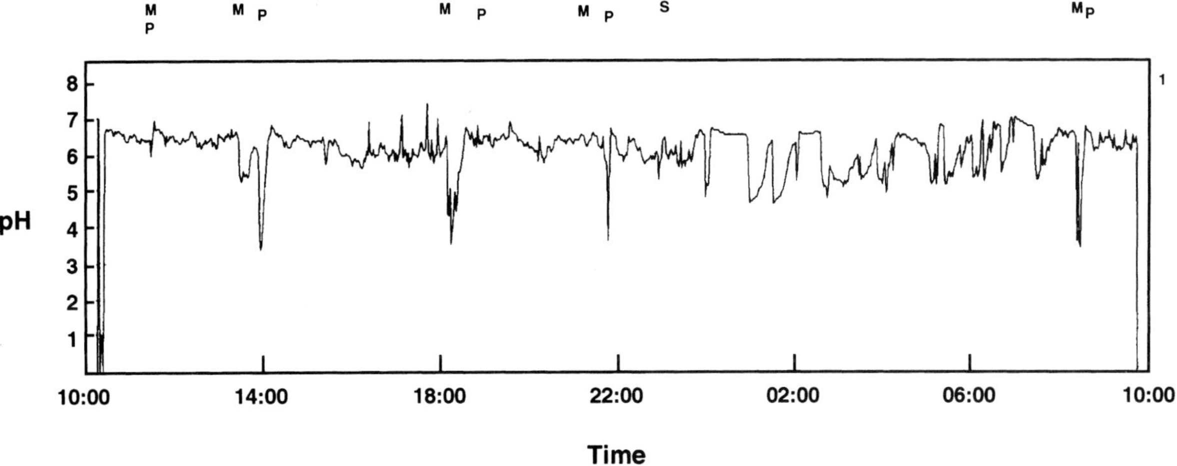

FIGURE 25–4 ■ Twenty-four-hour pH monitoring 12 weeks after laparoscopic Nissen fundoplication demonstrates the abnormal physiology of a successful total fundoplication. There is insignificant postprandial upright reflux (upright time pH $<$ 4 = 0.7%; normal, up to 8%; total time = 0.4%; normal, up to 5%); and no supine reflux (normal, up to 3%). (M, meal; P, postprandial.)

though 93% of patients reported symptom improvement after laparoscopic antireflux surgery, only 82% of patients undergoing postoperative 24-hour pH monitoring had normal acid exposure (Eubanks et al, 2000). Postoperative heartburn is the only symptom predictive of abnormal acid exposure. Ninety percent of patients were free of heartburn, but 18% had abnormal acid exposure. Of symptomatic patients, 60% had normal acid exposure.

Unfortunately, dysphagia and abdominal complaints are frequent after laparoscopic antireflux surgery (Figs. 25–5 and 25–6). Excessive dysphagia in patients treated with laparoscopic antireflux surgery caused the early closure of a trial comparing laparoscopic with open surgery (Bais et al, 2000). One of the first reports of long-term outcome (follow-up complete in 59% of 291 patients at 5 to 8 years after laparoscopic Nissen fundoplications) reported dysphagia in 27.5% of patients, abdominal bloating in 20.5%, and diarrhea in 12.3% (Bammer et al, 2001). These symptoms required additional diagnostic procedures in 21% of patients, and esophageal dilation was necessary in 7%. Despite a 96.5% satisfaction with surgical results, 6.4% reported regurgitation and 5.8% had heartburn. Continuous proton pump inhibitor therapy was necessary in 14% of patients. Like open surgery, the need for postoperative medical therapy may eliminate any cost advantage of laparoscopic antireflux surgery (Lundell et al, 2001). Although quality of life is improved in patients treated with laparoscopic antireflux surgery, it does not reach that equal to the healthy population because of functional dyspepsia that persists despite surgery (Kamolz et al, 2000; Rattner, 2000; Slim et al, 2000; Velanovich, 1999).

CONCLUSION

Potential benefits of laparoscopic antireflux surgery can be offset or overwhelmed by poor patient selection, surgical inexperience, and problems unique to this approach. Successful antireflux surgery is measured by long-term control of reflux, maintenance of normal swallowing, and prevention of postfundoplication symptoms and not by the number or length of incisions. Unfortunately, failed antireflux surgery has increased and has not been eliminated by laparoscopic antireflux surgery. The attraction of minimally invasive techniques and the insistence of patients for laparoscopic antireflux surgery exerts an inordinate pressure on the surgeon to select a laparoscopic solution to the patient's symptoms. This causes inappropriately selected patients to undergo inadequately performed operations by inexperienced surgeons. Laparoscopic antireflux surgery is an excellent operation that produces superb results given the right parameters.

A multidisciplinary team with an experienced surgeon working at a specialty center can provide the best results. Antireflux failure can be avoided by careful patient evaluation, selection, and preparation. Establishing reasonable expectations of outcome and anticipating significant but potentially reversible postoperative complications are part of patient education. The principles of antireflux surgery must be followed. Lessons learned at open surgery must be remembered and implemented for an effective laparoscopic repair.

The patient with Barrett's esophagus, a large hiatal hernia, an irreducible hiatal hernia, a short esophagus, excessively enlarged esophageal hiatus, and ineffective esophageal peristalsis should be identified before surgery. Surgical approach and operation must be tailored to the patient. In patients with complicated GERD, a compromise operation (partial fundoplication and Collis gastroplasty) may be necessary to ensure adequate swallowing and minimize side effects. This may, however, result in less effective control of reflux.

COMMENTS AND CONTROVERSIES

Dr. Rice, Head of the Section of General Thoracic Surgery, has developed an extensive personal experience with laparoscopic antireflux surgery during the past decade. Before this laparoscopic era, he was fully familiar and

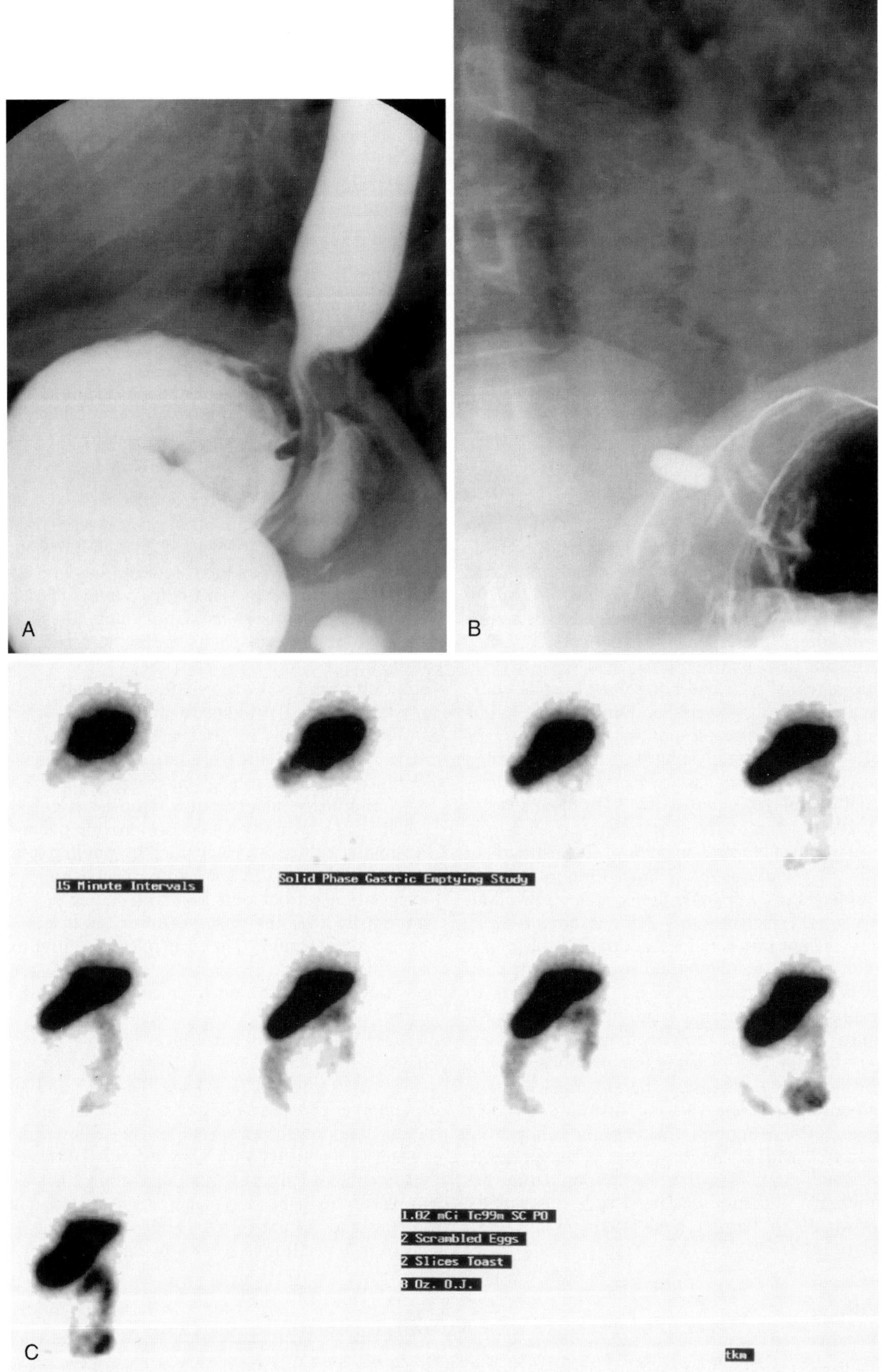

FIGURE 25–5 ■ Dysphagia and early satiety after laparoscopic Nissen fundoplication. *A,* A long, tight "twisted" total fundoplication was constructed about the distal esophagus and proximal stomach. *B,* Prolonged obstruction of passage of a barium tablet above the fundoplication reproduced the patient's symptoms of dysphagia. *C,* Vagal dysfunction resulted in functional gastric outlet obstruction. Essentially no solid gastric emptying was seen in this nuclear medicine study imaged at 15-minute intervals. Gastric emptying half-time was calculated to be more than 600 minutes (normal <90 minutes).

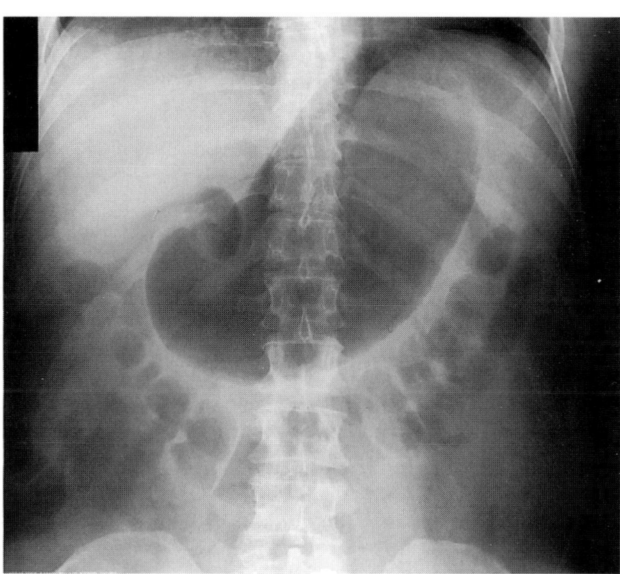

FIGURE 25–6 ■ Disabling gas bloat complicating a technically successful partial (Toupet) fundoplication in this habitual air swallower with classic gastroesophageal reflux disease and normal gastric emptying. Failure of conservative measures necessitated takedown of the repair.

clinically active with the various open techniques for the surgical management of hiatus hernia and reflux. This background gives him a broad perspective from which to evaluate the current role and future potential of minimally invasive, video-assisted antireflux surgery.

He emphasizes that the preoperative evaluation, the indications for operation, and the principles of reconstruction for surgery of hiatal hernia and reflux are no different for laparoscopic operations than for their open counterparts. In properly selected patients, the laparoscopic approach reduces postoperative pain and significantly reduces hospital stay. Dr. Rice records ample documentation for the "long learning curve" required to become proficient with laparoscopic repairs.

Early follow-up studies suggest that the outcomes are comparable to those achieved by open repair. There is, however, almost no information on long-term outcomes. A report by Bammer and associates (2001) identifies a less favorable long-term outcome than was suggested by early follow-up study in the same group of patients.

Dr. Rice implies that the only clear indication for laparoscopic correction is in the patient with uncomplicated reflux disease. Considering the current level of capability and knowledge available to a majority of practitioners in this field, his statement appears safe, practical, and reasonable. He notes that it has taken 10 years to achieve this level of confidence and expertise.

I believe, however, that the experience reported from a very small number of centers of excellence in North America and Europe has already demonstrated clearly that even the most complex problems are becoming regularly and predictably manageable using laparoscopic and thoracoscopic approaches. The mediastinal esophagus can be mobilized through the hiatus to, and above the level of, the pulmonary hilus. A lengthening gastroplasty can be added using techniques developed by Swanström (Swanström et al, 1996), Hunter (Johnson et al, 1998), or Luketich (Luketich et al, 2000). Giant paraesophageal hernia is successfully operated on with excellent early results (Luketich et al, 2000). Reoperation is being regularly undertaken at a few of these same centers (Hunter et al, 1999) (see Chapter 29).

F. G. P.

REFERENCES

Alexiou C, Salama FD, Beggs D, et al: Comparison of long-term results of total fundoplication gastroplasty and Belsey Mark IV antireflux operations in relation to the severity of oesophagitis. Eur J Cardiothorac Surg 15:320, 1999.

Awad ZT, Dickason TJ, Filipi CJ, et al: A combined laparoscopic-endoscopic method of assessment to prevent complications of short esophagus. Surg Endosc 13:626, 1999.

Bais JE, Bartelsman JF, Bonjer HJ, et al: Laparoscopic or conventional Nissen fundoplication for gastro-oesophageal reflux disease: Randomized clinical trial. The Netherlands Antireflux Surgery Group. Lancet 355:170, 2000.

Bammer T, Hinder RA, Klaus A, et al: Five-to-eight year outcome of the first laparoscopic Nissen fundoplications. J Gastrointest Surg 5:42, 2001.

Bell RC, Hanna P, Mills MR, et al: Patterns of success and failure with laparoscopic Toupet fundoplication. Surg Endosc 13:1189, 1999.

Blomqvist AM, Lonroth H, Dalenback J, et al: Laparoscopic or open fundoplication? A complete cost analysis. Surg Endosc 12:1209, 1998.

Cameron AJ: Barrett's esophagus: Prevalence and size of hiatal hernia. Am J Gastroenterol 94:2054, 1999.

Campos GMR, Peters JH, DeMeester TR, et al: Multivariable analysis of factors predicting outcome after laparoscopic Nissen fundoplication. J Gastrointest Surg 3:292, 1999.

Dallemagne B, Weerts JM, Jehaes C, et al: Laparoscopic Nissen fundoplication: Preliminary report. Surg Laparosc Endosc 1:138, 1991.

Dallemagne B, Weerts JM, Jehaes C, et al: Causes of failure of laparoscopic antireflux operations. Surg Endosc 10:305, 1995.

Dick AC, Coulter P, Hainsworth, et al: A comparative study of the analgesia requirements following laparoscopic and open fundoplication in children. J Laparoendosc Adv Surg Tech A 8:425, 1998.

Dickerman RD, McConathy WJ, Smith AB: Can pressure overload cause sliding hiatal hernia? A case report and review of the literature. J Clin Gastroenterol 25:352, 1997.

Eubanks TR, Omelanczuk P, Richards C, et al: Outcomes of laparoscopic antireflux procedures. Am J Surg 179:391, 2000.

Frantzides CT, Carlson MA: Laparoscopic versus conventional fundoplication. J Laparoendosc Surg 5:137, 1995.

Gastal OL, Hagen JA, Peters JH, et al: Short esophagus: Analysis of predictors and clinical implications. Arch Surg 134:633, 1999.

Hinder RA, Filipi CJ: Benign esophageal disease. In Bailey RW, Flowers JL (eds): Complications of Laparoscopic Surgery. St. Louis, Quality Medical Publishing, 1995, p 244.

Hogan WJ, Shaker R: Life after antireflux surgery. Am J Med 108:181S, 2000.

Horvath KD, Jobe BA, Herron DM, et al: Laparoscopic Toupet fundoplication is an inadequate procedure in patients with severe reflux disease. J Gastrointest Surg 3:583, 1999.

Hunter JG, Smith CD, Branum GD, et al: Laparoscopic fundoplication failures: Patterns of failure and response to fundoplication revision. Ann Surg 230:595, 1999.

Hunter JG, Swanstrom L, Waring JP: Dysphagia after laparoscopic antireflux surgery: The impact of operative technique. Ann Surg 224:51, 1996.

Jobe BA, Horvath KD, Swanstrom LL: Postoperative function following laparoscopic Collis gastroplasty for shortened esophagus. Arch Surg 133:867, 1998.

Johnson AB, Oddsdottir M, Hunter JG: Laparoscopic Collis gastroplasty and Nissen fundoplication: A new technique for the management of esophageal foreshortening. Surg Endosc 12:1055, 1998.

Kahrilas PJ: Laparoscopic antireflux surgery: Silver bullet or emperor's new clothes? Am J Gastroenterol 94:1721, 1999.

Kahrilas PJ, Lin S, Chen J, et al: The effect of hiatus hernia on gastro-oesophageal junction pressure. Gut 44:476, 1999.

Kamolz T, Bammer T, Wykypiel H Jr, et al: Quality of life and surgical outcome after laparoscopic Nissen and Toupet fundoplication: One-year follow-up. Endoscopy 32:363, 2000.

Kauer WKH, Peters JH, DeMeester TR, et al: A tailored approach to antireflux surgery. J Thorac Cardiovasc Surg 110:141, 1995.

Little AG: Gastro-oesophageal reflux and oesophageal motility disease: Who should perform antireflux surgery? Ann Chir Gynaecol 84:103, 1995.

Luketich JD, Grondin SC, Pearson FG: Minimally invasive approaches to acquired shortening of the esophagus: Laparoscopic Collis-Nissen gastroplasty. Semin Thorac Cardiovasc Surg 12:173, 2000.

Lundell L, Miettinen P, Myrvold HE, et al: Continued (5-year) follow-up of a randomized study comparing antireflux surgery and omeprazole in gastroesophageal reflux disease. J Am Coll Surg 192:172, 2001.

Luostarinen ME, Isolauri JO: Surgical experience improves long-term results of Nissen fundoplication. Scand J Gastroenterol 34:117, 1999.

Maziak DE, Todd TRJ, Pearson FG: Massive hiatal hernia: Evaluation and surgical management. J Thorac Cardiovasc Surg 115:53, 1998.

Mittal RK, Balaban DH: The esophagogastric junction. N Engl J Med 336:924, 1997.

Nilsson G, Larsson S, Johnsson F: Randomized clinical trial of laparoscopic versus open fundoplication: Blind evaluation of recovery and discharge period. Br J Surg 87:873, 2000.

Perdikis G, Hinder RA, Lund RJ, et al: Laparoscopic Nissen fundoplication: Where do we stand? Surg Laparosc Endosc 7:17, 1997.

Rantanen TK, Halme TV, Luostarinen ME, et al: The long-term results of open antireflux surgery in a community-based health care center. Am J Gastroenterol 94:1777, 1999a.

Rantanen TK, Salo JA, Sipponen JT: Fatal and life-threatening complications in antireflux surgery: Analysis of 5502 operations. Br J Surg 86:1573, 1999b.

Rattner DW: Measuring improved quality of life after laparoscopic Nissen fundoplication. Surgery 127:258, 2000.

Rattner DW, Brooks DC: Patient satisfaction following laparoscopic and open antireflux surgery. Arch Surg 130:289, 1995.

Rice TW: Why antireflux surgery fails. Dig Dis 18:43, 2000.

Rossetti ME, Nadjafi SA: Fundoplication. In Jamieson GG (ed): Surgery of the Oesophagus. Edinburgh, Churchill Livingstone, 1988, p 247.

Schauer PR, Meyers WC, Eubanks S, et al: Mechanisms of gastric and esophageal perforations during laparoscopic Nissen fundoplication. Ann Surg 223:43, 1996.

Skinner DB, Belsey RHR: Surgical treatment-thoracic approach. In Skinner DB, Belsey RHR (eds): Management of Esophageal Disease. Philadelphia: WB Saunders, 1988a, p 576.

Skinner DB, Belsey RHR: Techniques of antireflux procedures: Abdominal repairs. In Skinner DB, Belsey RHR (eds): Management of Esophageal Disease. Philadelphia: WB Saunders, 1988b, p 558.

Slim K, Bousquet J, Kwiatkowski F, et al: Quality of life before and after laparoscopic fundoplication. Am J Surg 180:41, 2000.

So JB, Zeitels SM, Rattner DW: Outcomes of atypical symptoms attributed to gastroesophageal reflux treated by laparoscopic fundoplication. Surgery 124:28, 1998.

Soper NJ, Dunnegan D: Anatomic fundoplication failure after laparoscopic antireflux surgery. Ann Surg 229:669, 1999.

Swanström LL, Marcus DR, Galloway GQ: Laparoscopic Collis gastroplasty is the treatment of choice for the shortened esophagus. Am J Surg 171:477, 1996.

Swanström LL, Pennings JL: Safe laparoscopic dissection of the gastroesophageal junction. Am J Surg 169:507, 1995.

Velanovich V: Comparison of symptomatic and quality of life outcomes of laparoscopic versus open antireflux surgery. Surgery 126:782, 1999.

Voitk A, Joffe J, Alvarez C, et al: Factors contributing to laparoscopic failure during the learning curve for laparoscopic Nissen fundoplication in a community hospital. J Laparoendosc Adv Surg Tech A 9:243, 1999.

Waring JP: Management of postfundoplication complications. Semin Gastrointest Dis 10:121, 1999.

Watson DI, Baigrie RJ, Jamieson GG: A learning curve for laparoscopic fundoplication: Definable, avoidable, or a waste of time? Ann Surg 224:198, 1996.

Watson DI, Jamieson GG: Antireflux surgery in the laparoscopic era. Br J Surg 85:1173, 1998.

Watson DI, Jamieson GG, Devitt PG, et al: Paraoesophageal hiatus hernia: An important complication of laparoscopic Nissen fundoplication. Br J Surg 82:521, 1995.

Wetscher GJ, Glaser K, Wiesschemeyer T, et al: Tailored antireflux surgery for gastroesophageal reflux disease: Effectiveness and risk of postoperative dysphagia. World J Surg 21:605, 1997.

ANALYSIS OF COMPLICATIONS IN LAPAROSCOPIC ANTIREFLUX SURGERY

Stephen B. Archer
John G. Hunter

DEFINITION

Complications arising specifically from laparoscopic hiatal hernia repair and laparoscopic operations for gastroesophageal reflux disease may be divided into intraoperative and postoperative categories. Postoperative complications are further divided into those that occur early after operation and those that occur later. The latter group are often failures of the repair. As is true of most other intraoperative complications, deficiencies in the surgeon's knowledge of the relevant anatomy or deficiencies in operative technique are often the cause of problems that occur during the laparoscopic procedure. Some late fundoplication failures, however, result from declining esophageal motility (Hinder et al, 1997), deterioration or dislodgment of the repair (Hunter et al, 1999), or progression of the advanced esophageal disease.

HISTORICAL BACKGROUND

Most complications associated with laparoscopic repair of hiatal hernia and antireflux operations have been described in the literature of open antireflux operations. There are a few new complications, unique to laparoscopic surgery, such as acidemia associated with carbon dioxide pneumoperitoneum. As well, twisted or grossly misplaced fundoplication ("two-compartment stomach") was not described before the advent of laparoscopic fundoplication (Hunter et al, 1996a). These problems are discussed in greater detail later.

Long-term follow-up (10 years or more) is lacking for laparoscopic fundoplication; however, the intermediate follow-up (2 to 5 years) indicates that results compare favorably with those for open antireflux surgery. Fundoplication performed through a laparotomy incision or a thoracotomy fails in 9% to 30% of patients (DeMeester et al, 1986; Shirazzi et al, 1987). Laparoscopic Nissen fundoplication has a reported failure rate between 2% and 17% (Cuschieri et al, 1995; Hunter et al, 1999; Peters et al, 1995). Symptom relief for both open and laparoscopic fundoplication is scored as "good" or "excellent" for over 90% of patients (Hunter et al, 1996b; Urschel, 1993; Weerts et al, 1993).

Because the natural history of mixed paraesophageal hernias (type III hiatal hernias) sometimes progresses to life-threatening complications, and often is associated with gastroesophageal reflux symptoms (Walther et al, 1984), many surgeons contend that repair is indicated in all cases. Complications resulting from the open repair of paraesophageal hernia occurred in 2% to 27% of patients (Harriss et al, 1992; Williamson et al, 1993). Although laparoscopic paraesophageal hernia repair is feasible and effective, it is often a challenging operation, requiring excellent laparoscopic skills.

Complications of laparoscopic paraesophageal hernia repairs are more common than those seen with repair of type I hiatal hernias, as is discussed later.

■ *HISTORICAL READINGS*

Cuschieri A, Hunter JG, Wolfe B, et al: Multicenter prospective evaluation of laparoscopic antireflux surgery. Surg Endosc 7:505, 1995.

Hunter JG, Trus TL, Branum GD, et al: A physiologic approach to laparoscopic fundoplication for gastroesophageal reflux disease. Ann Surg 223:673, 1996b.

Peters JH, Heimbucher J, Kauer WK, et al: Clinical and physiologic comparison of laparoscopic and open Nissen fundoplication. J Am Coll Surg 180:385, 1995.

INTRAOPERATIVE COMPLICATIONS

Complications occurring during laparoscopic antireflux operations (Table 25–1) are often dealt with satisfactorily if they are discovered during the operation. The same cannot always be said for complications that are recognized after the operation. Although often listed as a complication, conversion to an open technique is often a sign of sound judgment rather than a complication. Conversion to open repair is reported in 2% to 4% of cases (Collet and Cadière, 1995; Hinder et al, 1994).

Reasons to convert to an open repair, other than to address an intraoperative problem, include a large left lobe of the liver that precludes safe retraction, obesity that prevents the laparoscopic instruments from reaching the hiatus, and impenetrable adhesions from previous operations. Intolerance to pneumoperitoneum is almost never seen in the population of patients undergoing antireflux operations; however, it is occasionally necessary to reduce pneumoperitoneum pressure, use abdominal lifting devices, or use nitrous oxide to relieve acidosis and reduce postoperative pain.

TABLE 25–1 ■ **Intraoperative Complications of Laparoscopic Antireflux Operations**

Esophageal/gastric perforation
Bleeding
Pneumothorax
Vagal injury
Inadequate esophageal length
Massive subcutaneous emphysema
Improperly placed fundoplication
Cardiac arrhythmia
Hypotension
Hypoxia and/or hypercarbia

Visceral Perforation

Perforation of the esophagus or stomach during laparoscopic foregut operation results from one of several mechanisms. A retrospective review of 1620 operations performed at several high volume centers identified 13 esophagogastric perforations (0.8%) resulting from the passage of dilators (11 patients) and nasogastric tubes (2 patients) (Lowham et al, 1996). Weerts and co-workers (1993) report an incidence of intraoperative perforation of 2% to 3%.

Most perforations occur in and around the gastroesophageal junction, within the field of surgical dissection (Fig. 25–7; see Color Plate). These injuries are entirely avoidable if the following techniques are observed:

1. Complete the esophageal dissection before passing the bougie.
2. Make sure that the esophagus and gastroesophageal junction are not angulated while the bougie is being passed.

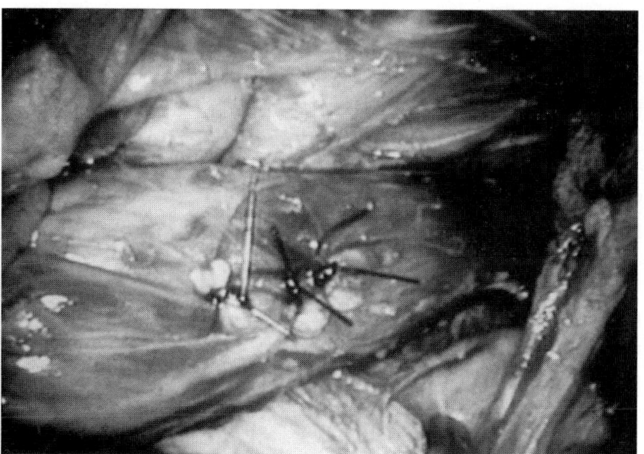

FIGURE 25–7 ■ Repair of an esophageal perforation at the level of the gastroesophageal junction accomplished laparoscopically. (See also Color Plate.)

3. Observe the smooth passage of the bougie into the stomach.

Preventing angulation of the gastroesophageal junction is accomplished by gentle traction with a Penrose drain that has been passed around the circumferentially dissected distal esophagus. When any tube is being passed through the esophageal lumen (especially through a diseased and strictured esophagus), the surgeon must exercise particular care. It is dangerous to assume that the anesthesiologist can safely pass the bougie without supervision and direction from the surgeon. Communication between anesthetist and surgeon is the key to safe bougienage. Occasionally, in patients with peptic strictures or with an inexperienced anesthetist, it is wise for the surgeon to break scrub and personally pass the dilator.

Perforation may occur if the esophagus is improperly dissected (Schauer et al, 1996). Rather than dissect the esophagus, one should expose it by dissecting the crura. This exposes the esophagus. The esophagus itself should need little direct dissection and should not be grasped with any instrument. Electrocautery can arc to the esophagus, causing perforation. Ultrasonic dissectors, although incapable of arcing because they do not generate heat by electrical current, become hot as they are applied. Their use should also be avoided adjacent to the esophagus. The areolar peritoneal reflections along the crura can easily be separated by blunt dissection if the proper plane is entered. Exposing the right and left crura incrementally is safer than persisting on either side exclusively.

For proper dissection, an angled laparoscope must be employed; visualizing instruments passing behind the esophagus is nearly impossible using a 0-degree scope. It was reported that the majority of esophageal perforations occurred during the surgeon's first 10 laparoscopic foregut procedures (Schauer et al, 1996). Proper instruction preoperatively and proper mentoring intraoperatively are essential in advanced laparoscopic operations to prevent avoidable injuries.

Finally, esophageal perforation can occur secondary to sutures in the repair pulling out. These injuries may be the most dangerous type of perforation, because they are discovered after the operation is completed. This mechanism may be the result of a repair that is under tension or one in which the sutures are tied down too tightly. Some advocate using pledgets to avoid any "cutting" effect of the sutures on the stomach wall. We believe that intracorporeal knot tying reduces the risk of tissue "sawing" by decreasing the need to pull a great length of suture through tissue. Proper dissection of the stomach's greater curve (division of the short gastric vessels) and full dissection of the posterior aspects of the stomach avoid tension on the completed fundoplication.

If an esophageal perforation does occur, it should be repaired immediately using a single layer of permanent sutures. The fundoplication should bolster the repair if possible. Testing the repair with air insufflation, or with methylene blue administration through a nasogastric tube (our preference), helps ensure the adequacy of the closure. No drains are necessary if the injury is recognized and properly repaired. Injuries that are recognized later should be managed like any iatrogenic esophageal perforation. Treatment should include débridement, closure, buttressing, and placement of drains. The longer the injury goes unrecognized, the greater the morbidity and mortality. This is especially true if the perforation occurs in the chest.

Because most mechanisms of visceral perforation are related to the limitations of the laparoscopic technique, and because repair may tax the skills of the occasional laparoscopic surgeon, conversion to laparotomy may be preferable in selected cases.

Hemorrhage

Bleeding requiring transfusion or conversion to an open operation is rare. However, bleeding within the operative field may lead to other complications, because it decreases visibility. Hemoglobin absorbs light, diminishing reflection, thereby causing the operative field to dim. For this reason, we keep the operative field very dry by using suction and 4 × 4-inch sponges that are passed through a 10-mm trocar. Although the incidence of splenectomy in reports of open antireflux operation is between 2% and 5% (Donahue et al, 1985), it occurs in fewer than 1 in 1000 laparoscopic procedures (Cuschieri et al, 1993; Jamieson et al, 1994).

Blood vessels encountered during a laparoscopic Nissen fundoplication that could cause serious hemorrhage include the short gastric arteries, the left gastric artery, the phrenic arteries and veins, and the left hepatic vein, which can course close to the phrenohepatic membrane superior to the caudate lobe of the liver. The phrenic artery on the left side may be injured while dividing the short gastric vessels at the superior pole of the spleen. This is especially true if bleeding has already occurred in the area. Vena cava injury leading to death has occurred when the surgeons confused the anatomic landmarks (Swanström LL, personal communication, 1999).

The aorta lies posterior to the left crus. Injuries to the aorta can occur when closing the crura if one takes too deep a bite of the left crus or if the angle of the needle passing through the left crus is too posterior. This can result in pseudoaneurysm or laceration with life-threatening hemorrhage. Laceration of the liver parenchyma during insertion of trocars in the upper abdomen or during placement of the liver retractor may also result in bothersome bleeding. Fatty livers are prone to fragmentation when compressed and may require laparotomy and partial hepatectomy to control bleeding.

Whereas use of the ultrasonic scalpel has decreased operative time and costs significantly, operative blood loss in a prospective, randomized trial was not different when it was compared with use of hemostatic clips (Laycock et al, 1996). If one uses clips to control bleeding, further use of the ultrasonic scalpel in the same area is difficult.

Pneumothorax

Although pneumothoraces do occur during laparoscopic antireflux operations, they do not usually persist postoperatively and if promptly recognized are not problematic intraoperatively. The left pleural space is more often entered than the right. Pneumothoraces occur more frequently when dissecting high in the mediastinum to mobilize a shortened esophagus or when reducing a large hiatal hernia.

Pneumothorax occurring on the left side can be diagnosed intraoperatively by observing the left diaphragm tenting downward during inspiration. A right pneumothorax is more difficult to diagnose this way, because the liver is retracted up and against the right diaphragm. When pneumothorax occurs, the anesthesiologist may notice an increase in airway pressures on the ventilator or a decrease in oxygen saturation. Most frequently, however, respiratory physiology is undisturbed.

Pneumothoraces may be dealt with at the end of the laparoscopic procedure. During the operation, a red rubber catheter or a length of endotracheal suction tubing with additional holes cut in it is placed across the esophageal hiatus and into the open pleural cavity. At the end of the operation, the tail of the tube is brought out a trocar site and placed in a bowl containing water. The anesthesiologist expands the lungs, pushing all residual gas out the water seal. The tube is withdrawn as vital capacity volumes are administered until the tube is completely out. Chest tubes placed during the operation vent the insufflating gas from the abdomen via the pleural vent. They are not indicated. When subcutaneous emphysema occurs, it usually abates without treatment within 1 or 2 days.

Vagus Nerve Injury

Injuries to the left or right vagal trunks are the result of injudicious dissection. The hepatic branch of the right vagus nerve lies in the phrenohepatic membrane. It is usually well visualized, because there is little or no fat in this structure, even in obese patients. Dissection of the right diaphragmatic crura should start above this nerve, because injury to it carries the theoretical risk of gallbladder dysfunction. While repairing large paraesophageal hernias, however, it is sometimes necessary to divide this nerve to visualize the entirety of the hiatus and right crus of the diaphragm.

Division of both vagal trunks can lead to the well-known postvagotomy syndrome (Fig. 25–8). Inexplicable postfundoplication diarrhea and dyspepsia have sometimes been attributed to vagal nerve injury. However, gastric emptying scans done on patients with documented preservation of the vagal nerve (by pancreatic polypeptide response to insulin hypoglycemia) demonstrate that at least some dyspeptic syndromes may be caused by increased rates of postfundoplication gastric emptying (Vu et al, 1999). Conversely, this phenomenon can be of help to patients with delayed gastric emptying before operation (Viljakka et al, 1999). Dissection of the vagus nerves away from the esophagus to prevent postvagotomy syndrome does not change postoperative subjective outcomes, tests of acid reflux, or gastric emptying and is therefore not necessary (Peillon et al, 1994).

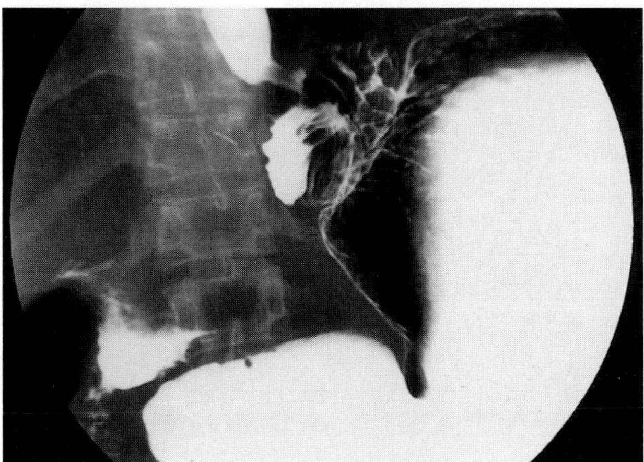

FIGURE 25–8 ■ This barium swallow depicts two complications: a slipped Nissen and a dilated stomach secondary to truncal vagal injury.

Patients with documented vagus nerve injury who become symptomatic, often present with nausea, retching, bloating, or diarrhea. These patients should undergo a gastric emptying scan and, if positive, are managed by a drainage procedure, such as a pyloroplasty. Vagus nerve injuries recognized in the operating room, however, do not require an immediate drainage procedure, because only a small minority of such patients become symptomatic (Burden and O'Leary, 1991). Avoiding the vagus nerve is accomplished by avoiding dissection of the esophagus itself, by concentrating on exposure of the esophagus by crural dissection, and by avoiding placing sutures into the nerve during creation of the fundoplication. One can often "feel" the left vagus nerve on the anterior surface of the esophagus by gently rolling a blunt instrument over it.

POSTOPERATIVE COMPLICATIONS

If the fundoplication itself is constructed incorrectly, the patient usually becomes symptomatic after the operation. Construction of a floppy laparoscopic fundoplication is initially more difficult than one done open, because tactile sensation is greatly reduced and depth perception is only inferred on a two-dimensional screen.

Two of the six commonly recognized failure patterns are unique to laparoscopy (Hunter et al, 1999). They are the twisted fundoplication and the two-compartment stomach. The other four have been described for open fundoplications as well. Slipped fundoplications, herniated fundoplications, disrupted fundoplications, and those that are too tight or too long can all lead to symptomatic failures requiring reoperation. Table 25–2 lists the causes of failures in patients who underwent redo antireflux operations at Emory University. In patients whose initial fundoplication was done open, the most common cause of subsequent failure was disruption of the fundoplication (51%). By contrast, in the laparoscopic group operated, the most common anatomic failure pattern was transdiaphragmatic herniation of the intact fundoplication (84%). Patients referred from other institutions had a wider variety of anatomic problems. The reasons for some of these different failure patterns are not clear. To decrease the frequency of herniation, we have been adding a laparoscopic Collis gastroplasty (Johnson et al, 1998) when esophageal mobilization does not return more than 2 cm of distal esophagus to the abdomen without tension. In addition, snug crural closure helps maintain the stomach below the diaphragm in most cases. Fewer herniations have been seen since

TABLE 25–2 ■ **The Causes of Failure of Fundoplications Performed Open Compared with Those Performed Laparoscopically**

Cause of Failure	***Open Fundoplication (n = 29)***	***Laparoscopic Fundoplication (n = 71)***	
		Emory (31)	*Referred (40)*
Transdiaphragmatic fundoplication herniation	5 (22%)	26 (84%)	10 (25%)
Fundoplication disruption	15 (51%)	1 (3%)	0
Slipped/misplaced fundoplication	5 (22%)	1 (3%)	12 (30%)
Fundoplication too tight/too long	3 (13%)	1 (3%)	2 (5%)
Achalasia	1 (4%)	0	4 (10%)
Fundoplication twisted*	0	2 (6%)	12 (30%)

*Includes "two-compartment stomach" in four patients.
(Courtesy of John G. Hunter, M.D.)

instituting the practice of more complete esophageal mobilization and a snug crural closure.

Although patients undergoing a second operation for reflux are usually improved by their second procedure, the symptomatic failure rate of "redo" surgery (11%) is significantly higher than for the first operation (3.6%).

Depending on the anatomic problem, patients may present with recurrent reflux, bloating, vomiting, chest pain, dysphagia, or a combination of symptoms. A barium contrast swallow is the most useful radiologic test to help with the diagnosis and to plan reoperation. Endoscopy should also be carried out to detect pathology in the esophageal and gastric mucosa and to evaluate the integrity of the fundoplication (O'Hanrahan et al, 1990).

Symptoms of recurrent reflux should alert one to the possibility of a disrupted, herniated, or a slipped fundoplication (see Fig. 25–8). Acute disruption may be the result of gross gastric dilatation or retching. Postoperative nausea should be aggressively treated to avoid this. With a slipped Nissen the wrap is intact but encircles the cardia of the stomach rather than the distal esophagus. This defect may occur if the fundoplication is positioned around the stomach at the initial procedure, or can be the result of postoperative displacement from forces such as retching or coughing. Whether slipped or misplaced, reoperation is usually necessary to relieve adverse symptoms.

A herniated fundoplication may occur acutely, often as a result of postoperative retching (Fig. 25–9). Acute herniation requires immediate reoperation. Some herniated fundoplications cause few symptoms and may be detected only by routine follow-up endoscopy or radiography. Attempting a standard antireflux operation in a patient with a foreshortened esophagus is one of the more common reasons for acute herniation of the fundoplication. Fourteen to 20 percent of patients presenting for laparoscopic antireflux operations have preoperative evidence of a shortened esophagus: that is, the gastroesophageal junction lies 5 cm or more above the diaphragm (Johnson et al, 1998; Swanström et al, 1996). Although esophageal mobilization adequately lengthens the esophagus in most of these patients, 4% to 8% of patients require an esophageal lengthening procedure (gastroplasty) in addition to fundoplication to avoid undue tension on the repair. This may be carried out laparoscopically (Johnson et al, 1998) or via thoracoscopy (Swanstrom et al, 1996).

If the Penrose drain encircling the distal esophagus migrates above the hiatus after maximal mediastinal dissection, the patient should undergo a laparoscopic Collis gastroplasty. In appropriately selected patients, no difference in postoperative symptom scores is found between patients undergoing laparoscopic gastroplasty in addition to fundoplication and those undergoing fundoplication only (Johnson et al, 1998).

Fundoplications that are too tight are infrequent since the introduction of the loose or "floppy" Nissen fundoplication (Donahue et al, 1985). If the fundoplication is too tight or too long, patients typically present with dysphagia or bloating. Although many patients have edema-related dysphagia early after fundoplication, only about 4% will have long-term dysphagia (see Fig. 25–9). Not all such cases are amenable to reoperation, because no mechanical abnormality can be found in some individuals

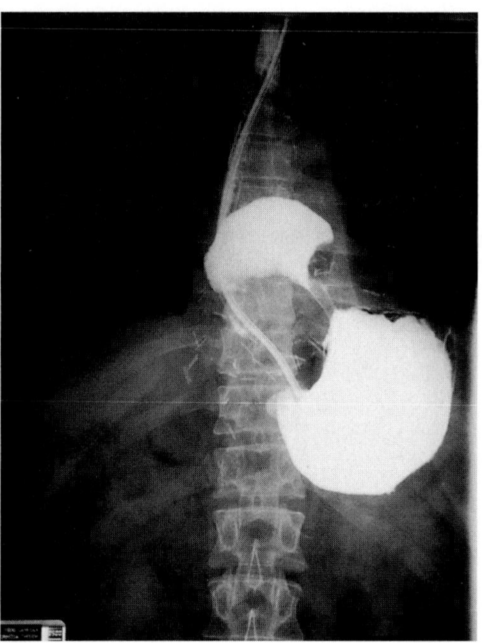

FIGURE 25–9 ■ Barium swallow demonstrates an acute paraesophageal hernia that occurred during recovery after the patient retched.

in this group of challenging patients (Wo et al, 1996). In a small group of patients, intense fibrosis in the field of dissection creates extrinsic compression (hiatal stenosis) about the gastroesophageal junction. Consistency in creating the floppy Nissen fundoplication is, at present, learned only by experience. To ensure a loose fundoplication, one should be able to easily slide a blunt laparoscopic grasping instrument between the esophagus and the fundoplication while the 60 French bougie is still in place in the esophagus.

A twisted or "spiral fundoplication" occurs when the fundus is not fully mobilized and is then pulled around the esophagus under tension (Fig. 25–10; see Color Plate). The reconstruction twists as the fundoplication unwinds (Hunter et al, 1996a). These patients present with dysphagia.

The two-compartment stomach (Fig. 25–11) occurs when the body rather than the fundus of the stomach is used to create the antireflux reconstruction. The gastric antrum becomes separated from the fundus by the newly created, but misplaced antireflux valve (Jamieson et al, 1994). The fundus fills with food but empties poorly. Patients complain of postprandial pain and are unable to vomit, because the valve remains competent.

Other postoperative complications associated with laparoscopic antireflux operations are relatively rare. These include chylous ascites secondary to injury to the cisterna chyli or the thoracic duct (Slim et al, 1997), cardiac tamponade (Farlo et al, 1998), and bleeding ulceration (Cuito-Garcia et al, 1998).

Some postoperative problems such as gas-bloat syndrome, inability to belch, and diarrhea have similar incidences in patients treated laparoscopically to those treated with open operation. Conversely, pulmonary complications such as atelectasis and wound infections are less common in the laparoscopic group (Rieger et al, 1994).

COMPLICATIONS OF LAPAROSCOPIC PARAESOPHAGEAL HERNIA

Although many of the complications associated with laparoscopic repair of the large type II, III, and IV paraesophageal hernias are similar to those after repair of smaller hernias, differences are worthy of separate discussion. The operation is usually technically more demanding than a standard antireflux procedure and requires a more detailed knowledge of the anatomy of the esophageal hiatus. Furthermore, the population of patients undergoing repair of paraesophageal hernias is generally older and has more comorbidity than those undergoing the usual antireflux repair.

Recurrent hiatal herniation is considered a failed result by most surgeons. The true incidence of failure, however, is elusive because many recurrences are asymptomatic. The surgeon may be alerted to the possibility of a failed repair when the patient describes the onset of reflux symptoms. Alternatively, recurrent herniation may produce symptoms of incarceration such as pain, bleeding, and sepsis. Barium esophagography confirms the diagnosis (Dallemagne et al, 1996).

A report on 55 laparoscopic paraesophageal hernia repairs identified total excision of the anterior and posterior hernia sacs as a key element of success (Edye et al, 1998). In this series, five early recurrences (within 6 months) in 25 patients were attributed to failure to remove both peritoneal linings of the hernia sac around the gastroesophageal junction. Unless this is done, the esophagus is tethered to the mediastinum and tends to prolapse through the hiatal repair up into the mediastinum. As in most studies, recurrences usually occurred within the first year after operation.

An analysis of 76 patients who underwent paraesophageal hernia repair at two different institutions reported a complication rate of 17% (Trus et al, 1997). The reopera-

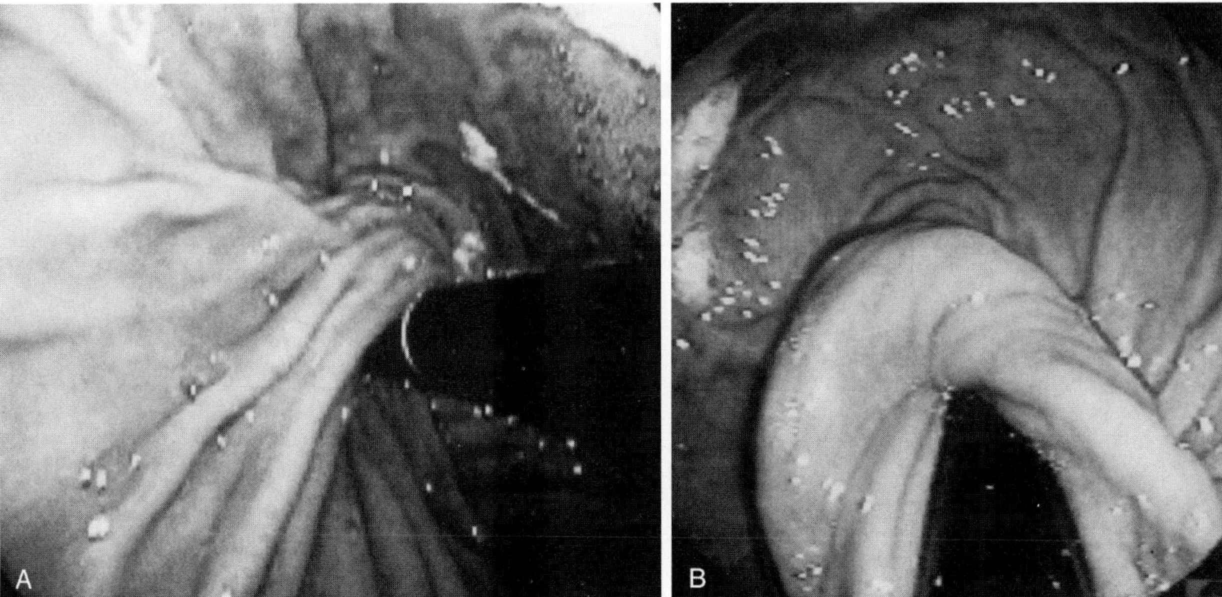

FIGURE 25–10 ■ *A,* Retroflexed endoscopic view of a twisted fundoplication. *B,* Retroflexed endoscopic view of a well-placed fundoplication. (See also Color Plate.)

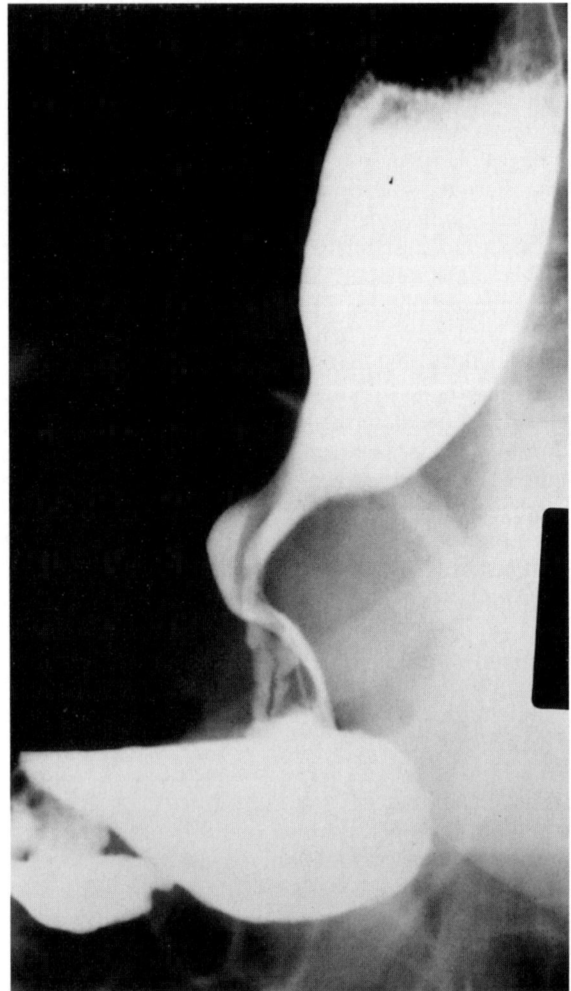

FIGURE 25–11 ■ This barium swallow depicts a two-compartment stomach. This is the result of placing the fundal wrap around the stomach instead of around the gastroesophageal junction.

tion rate was 14% (8% within 30 days). Perforations during the operation were the most common complication and occurred in eight patients. Three were caused by gastric laceration, two were from esophageal laceration, and three were injuries sustained during dilation. All were recognized and repaired during the operation, except one that was not recognized until the following day with routine barium swallow. The vagus nerve was injured in 3 patients, all of whom required a further operation for gastric atony. Three patients presented with delayed perforations (two gastric, one esophageal), and all required open repair. Two patients had pulmonary complications that resolved before discharge.

Based on this reported experience the following recommendations were made to avoid intraoperative mishaps and postoperative complications in patients with large paraesophageal hernias:

1. Handle incarcerated stomachs gently.
2. Start the dissection along the left crus. It is easier to identify than the right crus once the fundus is reduced.
3. Stay cephalad to the fat along the lesser curvature of the stomach. This avoids injury to the large vessels in the gastrohepatic omentum.
4. Use an esophageal lengthening procedure (Collis gastroplasty) in those cases when it appears difficult to obtain a tension-free repair after adequate mobilization of the esophagus.
5. Close the hiatal defect behind the esophagus. The geometry is more favorable for securing adequate esophageal length. Do not place mesh near the esophagus.
6. Communicate with the anesthesia team during passage of dilators.
7. Insufflation pressures must occasionally be lowered to 10 mm Hg to avoid hypercarbia and hypotension when dissecting in the mediastinum of elderly, frail patients. Lowering insufflation pressures is also an aid in approximating the crura in larger defects.
8. In these giant hernias, the vagus nerves are often located well away from the esophageal wall and are more prone to injury.
9. An irreducible hernia is often an indication for open repair.

Repair of paraesophageal hernias, even more than in smaller sliding hiatal hernias, requires advanced laparoscopic skills and experienced judgment.

CONCLUSION

Intraoperative complications associated with laparoscopic antireflux operations are best avoided by a thorough familiarity with the anatomy of the esophageal hiatus, careful technique, and judgment born of experience. Proper training in the placement of operative ports, dissection strategies, and repair techniques and mentoring during the early learning period are of essential importance to obtaining optimal results and minimizing complications.

COMMENTS AND CONTROVERSIES

As the authors identify, many of the complications that occur during and after laparoscopic repair are the same as those reported after open operation:

1. *"Overcorrection," by creating too tight or too long a fundoplication (this problem does not apply to repairs using a partial, rather than complete, fundoplication). Either of these technical errors may result in significant, persistent dysphagia or an inability to belch or vomit.*
2. *"Slipped Nissen fundoplication," owing to upward migration of the distal esophagus and esophagogastric junction above the fundoplication itself. This problem commonly results in both dysphagia and recurrent reflux.*
3. *Recurrent herniation of the esophagogastric junction and fundoplication through the diaphragmatic hiatus into the posterior mediastinum. The fundoplication itself may or may not become disrupted, or "undone," in these cases. When the fundoplication remains intact, adequate reflux control may be retained and the patient may remain asymptomatic. In other cases, however, recurrent herniation may result in symptoms of incarceration, obstruction, and recurrent reflux. I believe that a common cause of*

recurrent herniation, particularly the high incidence reported in cases after repair of large paraesophageal hernias, is the result of unrecognized esophageal shortening leading to undue tension on the laparoscopic repair. Furthermore, the hiatal barrier is less secure, because these massive hernias are almost always associated with a grossly dilated hiatus, which has flimsy, thinned muscular margins.

4. Complications that are peculiar to, or more frequently associated with laparoscopic repairs include a higher incidence of perforation of the esophageal or gastric wall, a pneumothorax on either side, and intraoperative respiratory depression resulting from insufflation of the peritoneal space with gas under pressure, with or without a pneumothorax.

5. The failure rate, or incidence of poor results, caused by dysphagia, gas bloat, or recurrent reflux, is not significantly different from the results reported following open operation. The incidence of reported reoperation, however, is significantly higher after laparoscopic repair, at least up until the present time.

F. G. P.

REFERENCES

Burden WR, O'Leary JP: The vagus nerve, gastric secretions, and their relationship to peptic ulcer disease. Arch Surg 126:259–264, 1991.

Collet D, Cadière GB: Conversions and complications of laparoscopic treatment of gastroesophageal reflux disease. Am J Surg 169:622–626, 1995.

Cuito-Garcia J, Rodriguez-Diaz M, Salas J, et al: Postoperative ulcer and hemorrhage: An uncommon complication of laparoscopic Nissen fundoplication. Surg Laparosc Endosc 8:219–222, 1998.

Cuschieri A, Hunter JG, Wolfe B, et al: Multicenter prospective evaluation of laparoscopic antireflux surgery. Surg Endosc 7:505, 1993.

Dallemagne B, Weerts JM, Jehaes C, Markiewicz S: Causes of failures of laparoscopic antireflux operations. Surg Endosc 10:305–310, 1996.

DeMeester TR, Bonavina L, Albertucci M: Nissen fundoplication for gastroesophageal reflux disease: Evaluation of primary repair in 100 consecutive patients. Ann Surg 204:9, 1986.

Donahue PE, Samelson S, Nyhus LM, et al: The floppy Nissen fundoplication: Effective long-term control of pathologic reflux. Arch Surg 120:663, 1985.

Edye M, Canin-Endres J, Salky B: Durability of laparoscopic repair of paraesophageal hernia. Ann Surg 228:528–535, 1998.

Farlo J, Thawgathurai D, Mikhail M, et al: Cardiac tamponade during laparoscopic Nissen fundoplication. Eur J Anaesthesiol 15:246–247, 1998.

Harriss DR, Graham TR, Galea M, et al: Paraesophageal hiatal hernias: When to operate. J R Coll Surg Edinb 37:97, 1992.

Hinder RA, Filipi CJ, Wetscher G, et al: Laparoscopic Nissen fundoplication is an effective treatment for gastroesophageal reflux disease. Ann Surg 220:472, 1994.

Hinder RA, Klingler PJ, Perdikis G, Smith SL: Management of the failed antireflux operation. Surg Clin North Am 77:1083, 1997.

Hunter JG, Smith CD, Branum GD, et al: Laparoscopic fundoplication failures: Patterns of failure and response to fundoplication revision. Ann Surg 230:595–604, 1999.

Hunter JG, Swanstrom L, Waring JP: Dysphagia after laparoscopic antireflux surgery. Ann Surg 224:51, 1996a.

Hunter JG, Trus TL, Branum GD, et al: A physiologic approach to laparoscopic fundoplication for gastroesophageal reflux disease. Ann Surg 223:673, 1996b.

Jamieson GG, Watson DI, Britten-Jones R, et al: Laparoscopic Nissen fundoplication. Ann Surg 220:137, 1994.

Johnson AB, Oddsdottir M, Hunter JG: Laparoscopic Collis gastroplasty and Nissen fundoplication: A new technique for the management of esophageal foreshortening. Surg Endosc 12:1055, 1998.

Laycock WS, Trus TL, Hunter JG: New technology for the division of short gastric vessels during laparoscopic Nissen fundoplication: A prospective randomized trial. Surg Endosc 10:71–73, 1996.

Lowham AS, Filipi CJ, Hinder RA, et al: Mechanisms and avoidance of esophageal perforation by anesthesia personnel during laparoscopic foregut surgery. Surg Endosc 10:979–982, 1996.

O'Hanrahan T, Marples M, Bancewicz J: Recurrent reflux and wrap disruption after Nissen fundoplication: Detection, incidence and timing. Br J Surg 77:545, 1990.

Peillon C, Manouvrier JL, Labreche J, et al: Should the vagus nerves be isolated from the fundoplication wrap? A prospective study. Arch Surg 129:814–818, 1994.

Peters JH, Heimbucher J, Kauer WK, et al: Clinical and physiologic comparison of laparoscopic and open Nissen fundoplication. J Am Coll Surg 180:385, 1995.

Rieger NA, Jamieson GG, Britten-Jones R, Tew S: Reoperation after failed antireflux surgery. Br J Surg 81:1159–1161, 1994.

Schauer PR, Meyers WC, Eubanks S, et al: Mechanisms of gastric and esophageal perforations during laparoscopic Nissen fundoplication. Ann Surg 223:43–52, 1996.

Shirazzi SS, Schulze K, Soper RT: Long-term follow-up for treatment of complicated chronic reflux oesophagitis. Arch Surg 122:548, 1987.

Slim K, Pezet D, Chipponi J: Development of chylous ascites after laparoscopic Nissen fundoplication. Eur J Surg 163:793–794, 1997.

Swanström LL, Marcus DR, Galloway GQ: Laparoscopic Collis gastroplasty is the treatment of choice for the shortened esophagus. Am J Surg 171:477, 1996.

Trus TL, Swanström LL, Hunter JG: Complications of laparoscopic paraesophageal hernia repair. J Gastrointest Surg 1(3):221, 1997.

Urschel JD: Complications of antireflux procedures. Ann Thorac Surg 57:129, 1993.

Viljakka M, Saali K, Koskinin M, et al: Antireflux surgery enhances gastric emptying. Arch Surg 134:18–21, 1999.

Vu MK, Straathof JW, Schaar PJ, et al: Motor and sensory function of the proximal stomach in reflux disease and after laparoscopic Nissen fundoplication. Am J Gastroenterol 94:1481–1489, 1999.

Walther B, DeMeester TR, Lafontaine E, et al: Effect of paraesophageal hernia on sphincter function and its implication on surgical therapy. Am J Surg 147:111, 1984.

Weerts JM, Dallemagne B, Hammoir E, et al: Laparoscopic Nissen fundoplication: Detailed analysis of 132 patients. Surg Lap Endosc 3:359, 1993.

Williamson WA, Ellis FH Jr, Streitz JM, et al: Paraesophageal hiatal hernia: Is an antireflux procedure necessary? Ann Thorac Surg 56:447, 1993.

Wo JM, Trus TL, Richardson WS, et al: Evaluation and management of postfundoplication dysphagia. Am J Gastroenterol 91:2318–2322, 1996.

RANDOMIZED CONTROLLED TRIALS FOR ANTIREFLUX SURGERY

David I. Watson
Glyn G. Jamieson

The recent development of laparoscopic antireflux surgery has focused debate between protagonists of various surgical techniques for the treatment of gastroesophageal reflux (Table 25–3). Although a total fundoplication remains the technique advocated by a majority of surgeons, the role of division of the short gastric blood vessels, as well as the place of partial fundoplication variants and other techniques, remains controversial (Aye et al, 1994; Coster et al, 1997; Patti et al, 1997; Watson et al, 1995). Some surgeons advocate selective use of a partial fundoplication for patients with esophageal dysmotility (Hunter et al, 1996; Kauer et al, 1995). Others advocate routine application of a particular partial fundoplication technique (Coster et al, 1997; Watson et al, 1995). Some of these issues have been investigated within prospective randomized trials, although many controversial issues are yet to be evaluated critically. It is opportune, therefore, to review the evidence available from prospective randomized trials that have evaluated antireflux surgery and to consider areas of controversy that require further objective evaluation.

OPEN NISSEN FUNDOPLICATION

Fundoplication was first described by Nissen in 1956. His original operation achieved good control of pathologic reflux for the majority of patients (Rossetti and Hell, 1977), although an incidence of adverse outcomes subsequently led to modifications to his original technique. Shortening the fundoplication length to 1 to 2 cm, dividing the short gastric vessels to achieve full mobilization of the gastric fundus, calibration of a loose fundoplication over a large intraesophageal bougie, and modification of the complete fundoplication to a partial fundoplication have all been advocated (DeMeester et al, 1986; Hill, 1967; Toupet, 1963), although not all of these modifications have been evaluated within prospective randomized trials.

TABLE 25–3 ■ **Controversies in Laparoscopic Antireflux Surgery**

- Should the short gastric vessels be divided during laparoscopic Nissen fundoplication?
- When should one undertake a partial fundoplication?
- Which partial fundoplication is appropriate?
- Should the hiatus be repaired selectively or routinely?
- Should the choice of procedure be tailored to certain preoperative findings?
- How common is the short esophagus and how should it be dealt with?

TABLE 25–4 ■ **Expected Outcomes After Open Nissen Fundoplication**

Short Term	
Complication rate	10%–20%
Incidental splenectomy	1%–3%
Mortality	<0%–1%
Length of hospital stay	10–14 days
Long Term	
Control of reflux at 5 years+	90%
Good or excellent long-term outcome	90%
Long-term troublesome dysphagia	5%

After 4 decades of experience with open antireflux procedures, long-term outcomes have been well described. These results provide a baseline against which laparoscopic techniques should be evaluated. Long-term success is achieved for the majority of patients. Rossetti and Hell (1977) reported that 87.5% of patients followed for more than 10 years after a 360-degree fundoplication without short gastric vessel division were free of reflux symptoms and adverse sequelae. Similarly, DeMeester and colleagues (1986) reported a 91% success rate for a total fundoplication procedure at an average follow-up of 45 months. Other studies report long-term success rates of 85% to 90% after open antireflux surgery (Johansson et al, 1993; Lundell et al, 1996) (Table 25–4).

Adverse outcomes after open surgery were not uncommon, and these included persistent dysphagia and the gas-bloat syndrome (DeMeester et al, 1986; Johansson et al, 1993). The assessment of dysphagia symptoms, however, can be difficult because variable methods of clinical assessment and scoring have been used in the various studies reported. This makes comparisons of outcomes from different studies unreliable. However, it is likely that the incidence of persistent long-term troublesome dysphagia is approximately 5% after Nissen fundoplication (DeMeester et al, 1986; Hill et al, 1994; Johannson et al, 1993; Lundell et al, 1996). The results of uncontrolled studies have suggested that using a posterior partial fundoplication technique may reduce the incidence of this problem.

RANDOMIZED TRIALS FOR OPEN FUNDOPLICATION

Despite the large number of publications describing fundoplication outcomes from the era of open surgery, only a limited number of randomized trials were conducted, and many of these enrolled only small numbers of patients (Table 25–5). Three trials compared a total fundoplication with a posterior partial fundoplication (Lundell et al, 1991, 1996; Thor and Silander, 1989; Walker et al, 1992), and one compared a total fundoplication with Hill and Belsey procedures (DeMeester et al, 1974). None of these studies demonstrated a statistically significant increase in the likelihood or severity of dysphagia after Nissen fundoplication, compared with a posterior partial fundoplication procedure. Only the study reported by Lundell and associates (1996), which enrolled 137 patients, entered a sufficient number of patients to allow one to draw statistically valid conclusions.

Other small studies have compared Nissen fundoplication with the Angelchik prosthesis and the ligamentum teres cardiopexy, demonstrating advantages for Nissen fundoplication (Hill et al, 1994; Janssen et al, 1993); and there have been three studies, all of them larger, that compared medication with surgical therapy (Behar et al, 1975; Ortiz et al, 1996; Spechler, 1992).

Nissen Versus Partial Fundoplication

DeMeester et al (1974)

This trial has the distinction of being the first randomized study ever reported in the field of surgery for reflux disease. The trial randomized 45 patients to undergo one of three operations (Nissen fundoplication, 15; Hill repair, 15; and Belsey repair, 15). Follow-up to 6 months was reported. The dysphagia rate 6 months after surgery was similar for all three procedures. Reflux recurred early in 1 patient after the Hill procedure and in two after a Belsey procedure. No patients in the Nissen group developed recurrent reflux. Patients remained in hospital for 20 days after the transthoracic Belsey repair, and for 12 days after the other two procedures.

Because of the small number of patients enrolled in this study, it is difficult to draw any firm conclusions about the relative advantages of the different approaches. Those surgeons who think that early dysphagia is more common with laparoscopic than open surgery could read this paper with profit, because early dysphagia was recorded in 13/15, 13/15, and 6/15, respectively, for the Nissen, Hill, and Belsey procedures.

TABLE 25–5 ■ **Randomized Trials from the Open Antireflux Surgery Era**

Trial	*No. of Patients Entered*
Nissen vs. Hill vs. Toupet (DeMeester et al, 1974)	45
Nissen vs. posterior partial fundoplication (Lundell et al, 1991, 1996; Rydberg et al, 1999a; Thor and Silander, 1989; Walker et al, 1992)	137, 33, 52
Nissen vs. Angelchik prosthesis (Hill et al, 1994; Kmiot et al, 1991)	61, 50
Nissen vs. ligamentum teres cardiopexy (Janssen et al, 1993)	20
Nissen vs. medication (Spechler, 1992)	247
Nissen with vs. without division of short gastric vessels (Luostarinen et al, 1995, 1996, 1999)	50

Thor and Silander (1989)

The Thor and Silander study enrolled 31 patients, who were randomized to undergo either a Nissen fundoplication (12 patients) or a Toupet posterior 180- to 200-degree partial fundoplication (19 patients). The Nissen wrap was 4 cm in length, and it was calibrated over a 40 French bougie. The esophageal hiatus was not repaired, the hepatic branch of the vagus nerve was divided, and the short gastric vessels were not divided. Follow-up was for 5 years. A good or excellent outcome was achieved in 8/12 of the Nissen group and 18/19 of the Toupet group. However, because of the small number of patients enrolled, this difference did not reach statistical significance ($P = .06$, Fisher's exact test; calculated from the data reported in the publication).

The incidence of postoperative complications was similar, as was the control of reflux at 5 years. Four of the 12 Nissen patients experienced persistent dysphagia, compared with 2 of the 19 Toupet patients ($P = .18$, Fisher's exact test). The resting lower esophageal sphincter pressure (LES) measured by postoperative manometry was higher after Nissen fundoplication (19.5 versus 16.9 mm Hg). Three of the patients who underwent Nissen fundoplication underwent further surgery for dysphagia. In each instance this was for the development of a "slipped" Nissen. No reoperations were required in the Toupet group.

This study did not enroll enough patients to demonstrate statistically significant differences between the clinical outcomes after the two procedures. The fundoplication technique used differs from current practice in which the fundoplication is shortened to 1 to 2 cm, and a larger calibrating bougie is now used by most surgeons (DeMeester et al, 1986; Jamieson et al, 1994). Also, there was a very high incidence of reoperation for the "slipped Nissen" phenomenon, with the 25% reoperation rate for this problem being far in excess of the low rate reported in other studies (DeMeester et al, 1986; Lundell et al, 1996; Luostarinen et al, 1995; Walker et al, 1992).

Walker et al (1992)

The Walker study compared a Nissen fundoplication performed with selective division of the short gastric vessels with a 300-degree posterior partial fundoplication (Lind). Because only 26 patients were enrolled in each group, the same statistical criticisms that applied to the study from Thor and Silander (1989) can also be made of this study. The Nissen fundoplication was 3 cm in length, and it was calibrated over a 40-cm bougie. New dysphagia was seen postoperatively at 6 weeks in 8 of the Nissen group and 6 of the Lind group ($P = .75$, Fisher's exact test; calculated from the data). Persistent late dysphagia occurred more often after posterior partial fundoplication

(4 patients) than Nissen fundoplication (2 patients, *P* = .67). The incidence of early and late gas-bloat syndromes was identical, as was the rate of postoperative complications. No advantages for the posterior partial fundoplication technique were demonstrated by this study.

Lundell et al (1991, 1996); Rydberg (1999a, 1999b)

This study has been reported in four separate publications (Lundell et al, 1991; 1996; Rydberg 1999a, 1999b). The first report described 6-month postoperative outcomes in 71 patients (38 Nissen fundoplications without dividing short gastric vessels versus 33 Toupet partial fundoplications) (Lundell et al, 1991). Resting LES pressure was higher in the Nissen group (20 versus 14 mm Hg). No differences were seen for any clinical outcome except for dysphagia at 3 months. Dysphagia was experienced in 15 (39%) of the Nissen group and 3 (9%) of the Toupet group at 3 months (*P* = .005). At 6 months, the incidence of dysphagia had fallen to 4 (10%) and 2 (6%), respectively, (*P* = .68). Heartburn was well controlled in 37 (97%) of the Nissen patients and 31 (94%) of the Toupet patients. Belching was said to be normal in 34 (89%) and 30 (91%), respectively. The incidences of gas-bloat symptoms and flatulence after the two procedures were also similar. The initial results of this trial demonstrated no important outcome differences at 6 months.

A subsequent report described outcomes after 3 to 5 years of follow-up in 137 patients (65 Nissen, 72 Toupet) (Lundell et al, 1996). Three patients underwent splenectomy during their initial Toupet fundoplication, versus no patients in the Nissen group. Dysphagia at 5 years was more likely after partial than Nissen fundoplication (16% versus 10%, *P* = NS), although in all instances the symptom was reported to be mild. Flatulence was more common after Nissen fundoplication at 2 and 3 years but not at other earlier or later time intervals. Recurrence of reflux occurred in 6% of the Toupet group and 5% of the Nissen group.

Reoperation was more common in the Nissen group than in the Toupet group, although this did not reach statistical significance (5/65 versus 1/71; *P* = .10, Fisher's exact test). One patient in the Toupet group underwent further surgery for severe gas bloat symptoms. Five of the Nissen group underwent reoperation for a postoperative paraesophageal hiatal hernia. Hiatal repair was performed infrequently in this trial, and in only one of the five patients who developed a postoperative hernia.

The authors concluded that Toupet partial fundoplication performed better, owing to the lower reoperation rate and the lower incidence of late flatulence. However, the dysphagia rate was not improved after partial fundoplication and it is possible that the reoperation rate could have been greatly reduced in the Nissen group if the hiatus had been routinely repaired at the original procedure.

A reanalysis of the data from this trial (Rydberg et al, 1999a) has sought to answer the question of whether a tailored approach to antireflux surgery should be applied. The authors were unable to demonstrate any disadvantages for the Nissen procedure in those patients who had abnormal peristalsis demonstrated by preoperative esophageal manometry, compared with the group undergoing partial fundoplication.

A further subgroup of 24 patients from the original trial underwent manometric studies 4 years after their original surgery. This demonstrated higher basal LES tone after Nissen fundoplication. In addition, esophagogastric common cavity phenomena, which reflect the patient's ability to belch gas from the gastric lumen, were sought. These were more common after a posterior partial fundoplication, suggesting a more physiologic manometric pattern after this particular operation. However, whether this finding is clinically important remains to be determined.

Pooling of Data

Bringing the data together, in a sort of "mini meta-analysis" (Table 25–6), appears to support the view that the only differences in outcome, between the total fundoplication and the posterior fundoplication, are in the gas-related problems. Although this pooled analysis is only at short-term follow-up, the longer-term data of Lundell and associates suggest these results may be representative of the longer term also (Lundell et al, 1996; Rydberg et al, 1999a).

Medical Versus Surgical Therapy

Behar et al (1975)

The Behar study is old, and enrolled only small numbers (15 and 16 in the surgical and medical groups, respectively). It was noteworthy because the good to excellent results were 73% for surgery (reported as an anterior fundoplication–Belsey Mark IV operation) versus 19% in the medical group, and yet it was largely ignored by the medical community.

Ortiz et al (1996)

The Ortiz study involved 59 patients randomly assigned at the more severe end of the reflux spectrum with Barrett's esophagus. Twenty-seven patients had the best medical treatment available, and 32 patients underwent antireflux surgery (short Nissen fundoplication). Satisfactory symptomatic control was achieved in 24 patients and 29 patients, respectively. However, there was significantly better control of esophageal inflammation and stenosis in

TABLE 25–6 ■ **Pooled Data from Randomized Trials of Total Versus Posterior Partial Fundoplication—Analysis at More Than 12 Months of Follow-Up**

Factor	*Total Fundoplication*	*Posterior Fundoplication*
Number of patients	103	117
Dysphagia	23%	17%
Gas-related problems	16%	1%*
Recurrent reflux	4%	4%

*$P < .001$.

the surgical group (54% and 47% in the medical group versus 5% and 15% in the surgical group). Because proton pump inhibitors were only used in the last couple of years of the study, it also becomes of historical rather than current relevance.

Spechler et al (1992)

Spechler and associates (1992) reported a study that compared operative with nonoperative therapy for reflux. In this study, performed in veterans hospitals in the United States, 247 patients (243 men and 4 women) were randomized to one of three groups: continuous medical therapy with an H_2-blocker, medical therapy for symptoms only, or open Nissen fundoplication. Forty patients withdrew from the trial after randomization, 24 of these from the surgery group; 176 were followed for at least 1 year, and 106, for 2 years. Seven patients' symptoms persisted on medical therapy to the extent that they were reallocated to a surgical procedure. Overall patient satisfaction was highest in the surgical group at both the 1- and 2-year follow-up intervals. However, neither the surgical approach nor the medical treatment used in the trials in this study would now be regarded as optimal management for reflux disease in the new era of laparoscopic surgery and proton pump inhibitor medications.

Overview of Randomized Studies Comparing Medical with Surgical Treatment

It is clear that surgery produced better results in the era before the introduction of proton pump inhibitors. The early results of a large randomized Swedish study comparing the two treatments using omeprazole are yet to be published. However, early reports suggest that the gap between medical and surgical therapy has closed somewhat. Of course, it remains a truism that surgery remains the only treatment that cures reflux.

Other Trials

Other small studies have compared the Nissen fundoplication with the Angelchik prosthesis (Eyre-Brook et al, 1993; Hill et al, 1994; Kmiot et al, 1991) and the Nissen fundoplication with the ligamentum teres repair (Janssen et al, 1993). Although these studies only enrolled a small number of patients, because of the magnitude of the differences identified, they did reveal distinct advantages for the Nissen procedure in terms of the rates of surgical revision and the incidence of recurrent reflux. A further trial has evaluated the issue of division of the short gastric vessels (Luostarinen et al, 1995, 1996; Luostarinen and Isolauri, 1999).

Two other small studies have looked at the relationship of the vagus nerves to the fundoplication (Peillon et al, 1994) and compared a fundoplication to a Roux-en-Y gastrectomy in patients with severe disease (Washer et al, 1984).

Hill et al (1994)

Sixty-one patients were randomly assigned to undergo either a Nissen fundoplication without division of the short gastric vessels or the placement of an Angelchik antireflux prosthesis. Follow-up was over a 7-year period, with a good long-term result obtained in 17/22 from the Angelchik group and 20/25 of the Nissen group. Two of the Angelchik prostheses were removed for persistent dysphagia and one more because of postoperative infection. Five patients also had persistent dysphagia after placement of the Angelchik prosthesis. No Nissen fundoplications required surgical revision. One patient required endoscopic dilatation for dysphagia after Nissen fundoplication. Although long-term outcomes were similar, the Angelchik prosthesis was associated with a higher likelihood of surgical revision.

Kmiot et al (1991)

The Kmiot trial enrolled 50 patients to undergo either a Nissen fundoplication or placement of the Angelchik prosthesis (25 in each group). The incidence of persistent dysphagia was greater after placement of the Angelchik prosthesis (20% versus 0%), and 3 patients required removal of the prosthesis for this problem. The overall outcome, measured by Visick grading, was poorer after placement of the Angelchik prosthesis at short-term follow-up. The authors chose to stop this trial at an early stage because of the high incidence of problems associated with the Angelchik prosthesis.

Eyre-Brook et al (1993)

Eyre-Brook and colleagues reported results of a trial randomizing the Angelchik prosthesis against a floppy Nissen fundoplication at 4 to 6 years after surgery. They reported a good to excellent result in 21 of 25 patients in the Angelchik group and in 18 of 23 after fundoplication. It is a little unclear from the paper how many prostheses were removed—possibly three.

This paper also reports a further consecutive series of 119 patients having an Angelchik prosthesis placed, with good results in 85% of the patients. Although the authors are generally supportive of the prosthesis, there were seven migrations of the prosthesis (mainly above the diaphragm) with 5 of the patients having had to undergo reoperation. They report a zero rate of gas bloating in their Angelchik group, which suggests they are referring to severe forms of the problem because unoperated patients have gas bloating rates of approximately 50% (Watson et al, 1997, 1999a).

Overview of the Angelchik Prosthesis

The most interesting fact about this prosthesis is that it controlled reflux and induced a rethinking about the pathophysiology of reflux. It may work by preventing proximal gastric distention, which in turn mitigates against transient LES relaxation, or effacement and weakening of the LES, or both mechanisms. Whether the prosthesis would have established a place had laparoscopic fundoplication not appeared is a moot point, but this would probably have not occurred because of the occasional problems of dysphagia and migration.

Janssen et al (1993)

Janssen and associates randomly assigned 20 patients to undergo either Nissen fundoplication (10 patients) or ligamentum teres cardiopexy (10 patients). Although both procedures effectively corrected reflux for the first 3 months after surgery, by 12 months, 6 of the 10 patients who underwent the ligamentum teres repair required further surgery for recurrent reflux, compared with only one in the Nissen group ($P = .05$).

Results of postoperative ambulatory pH monitoring were very poor in the patients undergoing the ligamentum teres repair, with a mean acid exposure time of 24.0% versus 3.8% for the Nissen procedure ($P < .05$). Despite the small number of patients in this trial, the results of the ligamentum teres repair were so poor that continued use of this procedure by either laparoscopic or open techniques cannot be justified.

Luostarinen et al (1995, 1996); Luostarinen and Isolauri (1999)

Luostarinen and colleagues reported the results of a small trial of division versus no division of the short gastric vessels during open total fundoplication. Twenty patients were entered into this trial. No significant advantages for division of the short gastric vessels were demonstrated, although the number of patients randomized was too small in this initial report to adequately address any potential differences in postoperative dysphagia rates. Interestingly, there was a trend (nonstatistically significant) toward a slower rate of transit of a radiolabeled liquid bolus through the esophagus after full mobilization of the gastric fundus, the opposite to what would be expected if fundal mobilization was associated with less postoperative dysphagia.

A subsequent report (Luostarinen and Isolauri, 1999) of 50 patients from the same trial, followed for a median of 3 years, demonstrated equivalent prevention of esophagitis. There was, however, a trend toward a higher incidence of disruption of the fundoplication (five patients vs. two), and reflux symptoms (six patients versus one) when the short gastric vessels were divided. Furthermore, 9 of 26 (35%) patients who underwent vessel division developed a recurrent sliding hiatus hernia, compared with only 1 of 24 (4%) patients whose vessels were kept intact ($P = .02$). The likelihood of long-term dysphagia or gas-related symptoms was not influenced by mobilizing the gastric fundus.

Peillon et al (1994)

In this study, 42 patients had a 270-degree posterior partial fundoplication, with one group randomized to have both the anterior and posterior vagus nerves dissected and excluded from their wrap and the other group to have the vagus nerves included within their wrap. No significant differences between the groups were found (including a relatively simple assessment of gastric emptying).

Washer et al (1984)

This study randomized patients with "severe reflux esophagitis" to receive either a total fundoplication or an antrectomy with Roux-en-Y duodenal diversion. Severe esophagitis is not defined by the authors, although they also state that "most patients had preoperative stricture dilatation." At an average of 5 years' follow-up, good to excellent results were achieved in 91% of 22 patients having an antrectomy and Roux-en-Y anastomosis, compared with 65% of 20 patients having a fundoplication. It is a pity that so many terms are undefined in this study, because the differences are significant and striking. Nevertheless, most surgeons think that gastrectomies of any ilk add a disease dimension in their own right, and so remain unconvinced of the utility of this approach—at least in first-time operations for reflux disease.

EARLY RESULTS AND COMPLICATIONS AFTER LAPAROSCOPIC FUNDOPLICATION

Initial reports of case series of laparoscopic Nissen fundoplication with follow-up of 3 months or less first appeared in the published literature in 1991 and 1992 (Dallemagne et al, 1991; Geagea, 1991). Although these studies confirmed the technical feasibility of laparoscopic antireflux surgery, the lack of adequate follow-up data and the small patient numbers precluded adequate assessment of the merits of the procedures described. The first large study was published by Cuschieri and colleagues in 1993, who reported promising results from a multicenter series of 116 patients. Further large single-center experiences describing series of more than 100 patients have been reported since (Anvari et al, 1995; Gotley et al, 1996; Hinder et al, 1994; Jamieson et al, 1994; Trus et al, 1996), with follow-up intervals of 2 to 3 years described in some later studies (Coster et al, 1997; Hunter et al, 1996; Trus et al, 1996; Watson et al, 1996).

Mean or median operating times vary from 30 to 185 minutes in these studies. Reported complication rates range from 2% to 26% (Gotley et al, 1996; Hallerback et al, 1994; Hinder et al, 1994; Watson et al, 1996), and surgical revision has been needed in a small group of patients in most series. Variation in these rates may be influenced by the effect of the institutional learning curve, technical factors associated with the choice of surgical technique, and different criteria used for the recognition and classification of complications in different reports.

Laparoscopic Nissen fundoplication is reported to control reflux symptoms in 91% to 100% of patients followed up to 2 years (Trus et al, 1996; Watson et al, 1996), results that mirror previous experience with open antireflux surgery (DeMeester et al, 1986; Rossetti and Hell, 1977). Postoperative hospital stays have been short in all published reports, with mean/median stays ranging from 2 to 5 days (Gotley et al, 1996; Watson et al, 1996). Overall results from these initial case series suggest that laparoscopic antireflux surgery is effective, and that it results in an overall reduction in the short-term morbidity associated with surgery for reflux. However, several complications unique to the laparoscopic approach have now been described (Watson and Jamieson, 1998) (Table 25–7).

LAPAROSCOPIC VERSUS OPEN SURGERY

Although laparoscopic approaches may reduce short-term surgical morbidity, initially it was considered unreason-

TABLE 25–7 ■ **Unique or Common Complications After Laparoscopic Antireflux Surgery**

Pneumothorax	Esophageal perforation
Pneumomediastinum	Gastric perforation
Pulmonary embolism	Duodenal perforation
Injury to major vessels	Bowel perforation
Paraesophageal hiatal hernia	Cardiac laceration
Hiatal stenosis	Pleuropericarditis
Mesenteric thrombosis	

Modified from Watson DI, Jamieson GG: Antireflux surgery in the laparoscopic era (Review). Br J Surg 85:1173–1184, 1998.

able to expect better long-term outcomes than those following equivalent open procedures. It is even possible that technique modifications introduced to facilitate various laparoscopic approaches could result in poorer long-term outcomes, although until the results of long-term studies become available the true outcome of laparoscopic antireflux surgery, and its status compared with open antireflux surgery, remains to some extent unknown. Nevertheless, the view of the anatomy of the hiatus is undoubtedly superior with the laparoscopic approach and the intriguing prospect remains that more exact placement of sutures and modifications to surgical technique may yet lead to better results with laparoscopic surgery than open surgery.

Nonrandomized comparisons between open and laparoscopic fundoplication have generally shown that laparoscopic surgery requires more operating time than the equivalent open surgical procedure (Peters et al, 1995; Rattner and Brooks, 1995), that the incidence of postoperative complications is reduced, the length of postoperative hospital stay is shortened by 3 to 7 days, patients return to full physical function between 6 to 27 days quicker, and overall hospital costs are reduced after laparoscopic antireflux surgery. The efficacy of reflux control appears to be similar between the two approaches.

Randomized Comparisons

The early results of five randomized controlled trials that have compared a laparoscopic Nissen fundoplication with its open surgical equivalent have been reported (Franzen et al, 1996; Heikkinen et al, 1999; Laine et al, 1997; Perttila et al, 1999; Watson et al, 1994) (two of these studies have been reported in abstract only). The results of all trials confirm advantages for the laparoscopic approach, albeit less dramatic than the advantages expected from the results of nonrandomized studies.

Watson et al (1994)

In a study from Sheffield, England, that initially enrolled 42 patients to undergo a Nissen fundoplication without division of the short gastric blood vessels, equivalent short-term efficacy and clinical outcomes were demonstrated and a quicker postoperative recovery was evident. The median postoperative stay was shortened by 1 day (3 versus 4), and the convalescent period was shortened from 8 to 2 weeks. However, operating time was longer (79 versus 43 minutes). The overall incidence of complications was also reduced. This suggests that the overall morbidity of antireflux surgery is reduced by the laparoscopic approach. The outcome for the group of patients undergoing attempted laparoscopic surgery was similar to the outcome from the early uncontrolled series.

It was somewhat surprising that the postoperative hospital stay was shortened by only 1 day, owing entirely to a shorter hospital stay after open fundoplication. This suggests that a significant proportion of the reduction in hospital stay was independent of the particular technique performed and not solely because of the introduction of the laparoscopic approach. On the other hand, the greatly reduced time taken to return to normal physical activity suggests that there may be significant community advantages for the laparoscopic approach. The results and conclusions from this trial are similar to the other four prospective randomized trials of laparoscopic versus open Nissen fundoplication.

Franzen et al (1996)

This study has been published in abstract form only. It describes similar advantages for laparoscopic fundoplication, after an initial analysis of 36 patients who underwent antireflux surgery. A 1-day reduction in hospital stay because of earlier discharge after open surgery also was reported in this trial.

Laine et al (1997)

Laine and co-workers reported the outcome of 110 patients randomized to undergo laparoscopic or open Nissen fundoplication, the majority without division of the short gastric vessels. Hospital stay was halved from 6.4 to 3.2 days, and patients returned to work quicker (37 versus 15 days). Operating time was prolonged 31 minutes from 57 to 88 minutes, an increase that is similar to that reported in the other trials. Control of reflux symptoms was similarly effective in both of these studies, although outcomes beyond 12 months after surgery have not been reported.

Perttila et al (1999)

This small study randomized 20 patients to undergo laparoscopic or open Nissen fundoplication. The stated aim of the study was to assess immune responses associated with the different surgical procedures. No differences were seen between the groups undergoing laparoscopic and open procedures, although this may reflect the small number of patients enrolled. Operating time was significantly longer after laparoscopic fundoplication (92 versus 46 minutes), but hospital stay was shorter (2.9 versus 5.8 days mean).

Heikkinen et al (1999)

Forty-two patients were enrolled in this trial of open (20) versus laparoscopic (22) Nissen fundoplication. Unfortunately the operation performed laparoscopically was usually different from that performed in the open surgical group. The short gastric vessels were divided in only 1 patient at laparoscopic fundoplication, compared with 17 at open surgery, and the esophageal hiatus was repaired in 20 patients laparoscopically compared with 9 patients at open surgery, even though the authors stated that the vessels were only divided when a loose fundoplication could not be constructed and the hiatus was narrowed only if it was considered to be enlarged. Hence, the results should be interpreted carefully, because the operations performed for each group were not equivalent. Follow-up in this trial was limited to the first 3 months after surgery. The stated aim was to the compare the cost of the different surgical techniques. Operating time was lengthened by laparoscopic surgery (98 versus 74 minutes), hospital stay was shorter (3 versus 5.5 days), and convalescence was quicker (14 versus 31 days). Laparoscopic surgery achieved a 5% reduction in overall hospital costs. Clinical efficacy was not reported.

Overview of Laparoscopic Versus Open Fundoplication

The overall results of these five randomized trials confirm that laparoscopic antireflux surgery has short-term advantages over the open approach. Short-term control of reflux is similar to that after open surgery. Nevertheless, longer-term outcomes of trials are needed before improved efficacy can be claimed with certainty.

OTHER RANDOMIZED TRIALS

Five randomized trials examining technical aspects of laparoscopic antireflux surgery have been published.

Technique for Division of the Short Gastric Vessels

Two of these studies have compared different techniques for dividing the short gastric vessels during laparoscopic Nissen fundoplication. Laycock and associates (1996) randomized 20 patients to have these vessels divided between metal clips or by Ultrasonic Shears (Ultracision, Smithfield, RI). A time saving was demonstrated by use of the Ultrasonic Shears. Swanström and Pennings (1995) randomized 31 patients in a similar study that also demonstrated a time saving of 10 minutes for the Ultrasonic Shear technique. Neither of these studies enrolled a large group of patients or attempted to assess outcome differences between different antireflux procedures.

Division Versus Nondivision of the Short Gastric Vessels

Until recently, this issue was rarely discussed. However, after anecdotal reports of increased problems with postoperative dysphagia after laparoscopic Nissen fundoplication without division of the short gastric vessels, this aspect of surgical technique has become a much debated topic. Routine division of the short gastric vessels during fundoplication, to achieve full fundal mobilization and thereby ensure a loose fundoplication, is now thought by some to be an essential step during laparoscopic Nissen fundoplication. This opinion has been popularized by the publication of studies that have compared experience with division of the short gastric vessels with historical experience with a Nissen fundoplication performed without dividing these vessels (DeMeester et al, 1986; Donahue and Bombeck, 1977; Donahue et al, 1985). However, other uncontrolled studies of Nissen fundoplication either with or without division of the short gastric vessels confuse the issue further, because good results have been reported whether these vessels were divided or not (Donahue et al, 1985; Johansson et al, 1993; Rossetti and Hell, 1977). This suggests that conclusions drawn from historical studies should be regarded as tentative at best and therefore valuable primarily to enable hypotheses to be constructed that might be tested in randomized trials.

Only two randomized studies looking at this issue have been published (Luostarinen et al, 1996; Luostarinen and Isolauri, 1999; Watson et al, 1997). The study from the open era from Luostarinen and associates (1995, 1996, 1999) has been discussed previously. The other study comprised patients undergoing laparoscopic surgery.

Watson et al (1997)

This trial enrolled 102 patients undergoing a laparoscopic Nissen fundoplication to have a procedure either with or without division of the short gastric blood vessels. No difference in overall outcome was demonstrated at short-term follow-up of 6 months, with the exception of a longer operating time if the vessels were divided. Dividing the vessels was associated with a prolongation of operating time by approximately 40 minutes, resulting in increased expense and technical difficulty. After short-term clinical follow-up at 6 months and objective investigation 3 to 4 months after surgery, this trial failed to show any reduction in the incidence or severity of dysphagia after division of short gastric vessels during laparoscopic Nissen fundoplication.

Although some minor differences in individual dysphagia scores were apparent (but not statistically significant), when all criteria used for dysphagia assessment were considered together, the overall results revealed no trend toward an improved outcome in either group, nor any significant difference in LES pressure, esophageal emptying time, or barium meal radiographic outcome. It might be argued that a trend of difference was established between the groups for certain parameters measured at 6 months, favoring division of short gastric vessels—dysphagia for lumpy solids (33% versus 29%), LES pressure (24.5 versus 20.9), LES residual relaxation pressure (13.3 versus 11.0 mm Hg)—and that these figures may have reached significance in a larger study. However, the other dysphagia scores and patient satisfaction with the overall outcome were comparable between the two groups, and esophageal emptying was quicker in the "nondivision" group. Longer-term follow-up is needed to assess the durability of each type of operation and the incidence of recurrent reflux.

This trial demonstrated similar results to those reported by Luostarinen and associates (1995, 1996); that is, there was no advantage for patients who undergo division of the short gastric vessels. On the other hand, a study of similar size to that of Watson and colleagues (1997) has been conducted by Lundell and his colleagues in Sweden. The results have so far appeared only in abstract (Dalenback et al, 1998). These authors found a significantly greater incidence of dysphagia in the group without division of short gastric vessels.

Overview of Division of Short Gastric Vessels Versus No Division of Short Gastric Vessels

Data available to us are combined in Table 25–8. Once again the data are of relatively short-term outcomes, but there are no significant differences between the outcomes. At present it remains for the "dividers" to prove that the extra time taken to divide the short gastric vessels is justified by improved outcomes.

Nissen Versus Partial Fundoplication

Analysis of the previously reported trials of Nissen fundoplication versus a posterior partial fundoplication during the open surgical era suggested that there is no significant advantage for either technique. However, these studies did not evaluate the alternative technique of anterior partial fundoplication. Two trials have evaluated the efficacy of an anterior and a posterior partial fundoplication.

Laws et al (1997)

Laws and co-workers reported a trial in which 39 patients were randomized to undergo either a laparoscopic Nissen fundoplication or a laparoscopic Toupet fundoplication. No significant short-term outcome differences were demonstrated between the two procedures, supporting the results of the previous Nissen versus posterior partial fundoplication trials from the open surgical era. However, this study used only a small number of patients so that in statistical terms its power was low to have a reasonable chance of demonstrating any significant differences.

Watson et al (1999a)

This is the first prospective randomized trial to compare a Nissen fundoplication with an anterior partial fundoplication technique. Both procedures were performed laparoscopically. The study enrolled 107 patients to undergo either a Nissen or anterior partial fundoplication. The partial fundoplication variant entailed a 180-degree fundoplication that was anchored to the right hiatal pillar and the esophageal wall. Outcomes after 6 months postoperative follow-up have been published as a full paper (Watson et al, 1999a), with 2-year outcomes reported in a published abstract (Watson et al, 1999b). No overall outcome differences between the two procedures were demonstrated at 1 and 3 months' follow-up. At 6 months, however, patients undergoing laparoscopic anterior partial fundoplication were less likely to experience dysphagia for solid food, were less likely to be troubled by excessive passage of flatus, and were more likely to be able to belch normally (Table 25–9). Overall satisfaction and outcome scores were better after anterior fundoplication at 6 months, and patients were more likely to express a willingness to undergo the same procedure again, if confronted with similar preoperative circumstances. These differences have continued to be evident 2 years after surgery, and control of reflux symptoms has been similar after partial fundoplication. Endoscopic and ambulatory pH monitoring study outcomes were also similar between the two study groups.

Despite the encouraging early outcome after anterior partial fundoplication, this trial has not fully resolved the question as to whether which procedure would be the most appropriate in the long term. The durability of anterior fundoplication remains unproved for now. However, if durability proves to be as good as the Nissen fundoplication, the results of this study would support a preference for partial fundoplication because of the advantages of less dysphagia, improved ability to belch, and less adverse side effects. It is possible, however, that the long-term incidence of recurrent reflux after anterior fundoplication may be higher than that seen after Nissen fundoplication, in which case a risk versus benefit assessment must be made for each individual, balancing the risk of recurrent reflux against the risk of other adverse outcomes. Long-term follow-up is needed to clarify this issue.

TABLE 25–8 ■ **Overview of Data from Trials of Division of Short Gastric Vessels During Total Fundoplication**

	Total Fundoplication with Division of Vessels	*Total Fundoplication Without Division of Vessels*
Number of patients	129	124
Dysphagia	19%	28%
Gas-related problems	47%	53%
Recurrent reflux	8%	8%

TABLE 25–9 ■ **Anterior Partial Fundoplication Versus Total Fundoplication**

	6-Month Follow-Up		*2-Year Follow-Up*	
Factor	*Total*	*Anterior Partial*	*Total*	*Anterior Partial*
Number of patients	53	54	40	42
Dysphagia	40%	15%*	19%	19%
Gas-related problems	49%	28%*	33%	12%
Heartburn	9%	9%	3%	7%

$^{*}P < .005$.

SYNTHESIS OF THE RESULTS FROM PROSPECTIVE RANDOMIZED TRIALS

The results of trials from both the laparoscopic and open surgical eras can be assessed together to facilitate the development of evidence-based guidelines for antireflux surgery (Table 25–10). Some of these will meet with wide acceptance because they support the current body of thought of the international surgical community. However, others are controversial, because they do not support the opinions of the majority of experts in the field. Nevertheless, in the hierarchy of evidence, the results of

TABLE 25–10 ■ Evidence from Prospective Randomized Trials for Antireflux Surgery

1. Laparoscopic Nissen fundoplication is associated with fewer complications overall and a shorter convalescence than open Nissen fundoplication.*
2. The Nissen fundoplication has a lower complication and reoperation rate than the Angelchik prosthesis.*
3. The Nissen fundoplication controls reflux better than the ligamentum teres cardiopexy.
4. Whether both vagus nerves are included or excluded from the wrap makes no difference.
5. Division of the short gastric blood vessels does not improve the outcome after Nissen fundoplication.*
6. Dysphagia and recurrent reflux after posterior partial fundoplication and Nissen fundoplication are similar:
   In unselected patients*
   In patients with poor esophageal motility
7. The incidence of dysphagia and "gas-related" complications is reduced after anterior partial fundoplication.
8. Partial fundoplications are associated with less gas-related problems than total fundoplication.*

*Statement is supported by evidence from more than one randomized trial.

prospective randomized trials take precedence over the opinion of experts and it should be recognized that expert opinion from previous surgical eras, although highly regarded at the time, has sometimes been shown to be erroneous when better evidence becomes available. With this in mind, even the opinions drawn from the outcomes of currently reported prospective randomized trials may later prove to be in error as further trial data become available. Nevertheless, this level of evidence is a better starting point than relying on expert opinion alone.

Little argument can be met with the conclusion that the Nissen fundoplication outperforms the Angelchik prosthesis and the ligamentum teres cardiopexy and that the latter procedures should be consigned to surgical history. Furthermore, most surgeons performing surgery for reflux agree that the laparoscopic approach has been one of the most important advances in surgical technique for antireflux surgery in recent times. Controversy, however, is raised by any conclusions drawn about division of the short gastric blood vessels and the place of partial fundoplications in the surgeon's armamentarium. The only published trials that have investigated division of the short gastric vessels support the position that this maneuver is not necessary for the creation of a satisfactory Nissen fundoplication. However, as results of further trials are published, the role of vessel division will be clearer.

It is perhaps surprising that the three studies of posterior versus Nissen fundoplication have demonstrated no real advantages for the posterior partial fundoplication technique (with the exception of gas related problems), because these trials are often used to support the positions of either selective or routine use of the posterior fundoplication technique. Nevertheless, a critical analysis of the trials reported to date provides little supporting evidence for the proponents of these procedures. On the other hand an anterior partial fundoplication technique appears to be a more promising alternative, and it may provide a more physiologic restoration of the antireflux barrier. However, with only one relatively small trial reported so far, more studies are needed.

The large caseload of many surgical units now performing laparoscopic surgery for gastroesophageal reflux provides a unique opportunity to conduct additional trials of surgical techniques so that we can further refine and develop better techniques for surgery for gastroesophageal reflux. Because the current evidence base for surgical techniques is small, enrolling patients in well-conducted trials is both feasible, desirable, and ethical.

COMMENTS AND CONTROVERSIES

Watson and Jamieson have prepared a comprehensive review of reported trials, for both open and laparoscopic antireflux surgery and included a very useful "mini meta-analysis" for each of the two groups. Importantly, they emphasize the relative inadequacy of many of these trials, owing to small numbers of cases and very short follow-up. For example, the influential paper of 25 years ago by DeMeester and associates (1974) reported results from a prospective study of three antireflux techniques (Belsey, Hill, and Nissen operations), with only 15 patients in each group and a follow-up of 6 months.

The reported results of trials comparing open and laparoscopic techniques do, however, persuasively demonstrate that laparoscopic antireflux operations are associated with a reduced length of stay, an earlier return to normal activity and employment, and no greater an incidence of complications than that from open operations. The control of reflux and other associated symptoms appears to be comparable to the results obtained with open operation. There are few reports, however, that detail long-term follow-up data in the laparoscopic group. This is understandable, because laparoscopic repairs were not done at all before 1991 (Dallemagne et al, 1991).

In almost every one of these trials there is no clear definition of the severity or stage of esophagitis and its complications, with the exception of the presence or absence of defective esophageal motility and clearance. The complication of acquired esophageal shortening is not addressed in any of the reports and was not considered by any of the laparoscopic surgeons before 1996 (Swanstrom et al, 1996). The benefits of a partial, rather than complete, fundoplication in patients with poor motility and clearance in the distal esophagus remain somewhat equivocal from a review of these trials.

REFERENCES

Dallemagne B, Weerts JM, Jehaes C, et al: Laparoscopic Nissen fundoplication: Preliminary report. Surg Laparosc Endosc 1:138–143, 1991.

DeMeester TR, Johnson LF, Kent AH: Evaluation of current operations for the prevention of gastroesophageal reflux. Ann Surg 180:511–525, 1974.

Swanström LL, Marcus DR, Galloway GQ: Laparoscopic Collis' gastroplasty is the treatment of choice for the shortened esophagus. Am J Surg 171:477, 1996.

F. G. P.

■ REFERENCES

Anvari M, Allen C, Borm A: Laparoscopic Nissen fundoplication is a satisfactory alternative to long-term omeprazole therapy. Br J Surg 82:938–942, 1995.

Aye RW, Hill LD, Kraemer SJM, Snopkowski P: Early results with the laparoscopic Hill repair. Am J Surg 167:542–546, 1994.

Behar J, Sheahan DG, Biancani P, et al: Medical and surgical management of reflux esophagitis. N Engl J Med 293:263–268, 1975.

Coster DD, Bower WH, Wilson VT, et al: Laparoscopic partial fundoplication vs laparoscopic Nissen-Rosetti fundoplication. Surg Endosc 11:625–631, 1997.

Cuschieri A, Hunter J, Wolfe B, et al: Multicentre evaluation of laparoscopic antireflux surgery: Preliminary report. Surg Endosc 7:505–510, 1993.

Dalenback J, Lonroth H, Blomqvist A, et al: Improved functional outcome after laparoscopic fundoplication by complete gastric fundus mobilization (Abstract). Gastroenterology 114:A1384, 1998.

Dallemagne B, Weerts JM, Jehaes C, et al: Laparoscopic Nissen fundoplication: Preliminary report. Surg Laparosc Endosc 1:138–143, 1991.

DeMeester TR, Bonavina L, Albertucci M: Nissen fundoplication for gastroesophageal reflux disease: Evaluation of primary repair in 100 consecutive patients. Ann Surg 204:9–20, 1986.

DeMeester TR, Johnson LF, Kent AH: Evaluation of current operations for the prevention of gastroesophageal reflux. Ann Surg 180:511–525, 1974.

Donahue PE, Bombeck CT: The modified Nissen fundoplication—reflux prevention without gas bloat. Chir Gastroent 11:15–27, 1977.

Donahue PE, Samelson S, Nyhus LM, Bombeck T: The floppy Nissen fundoplication: Effective long-term control of pathological reflux. Arch Surg 120:663–668, 1985.

Eyre-Brook IA, Codling BW, Gear MWL: Results of a prospective randomized trial of the Angelchik prosthesis and a consecutive series of 119 patients. Br J Surg 80:602–604, 1993.

Franzen T, Anderberg B, Tibbling L, Johansson KE: A report from a randomized study of open and laparoscopic 360° fundoplication (Abstract). Surg Endosc 10:582, 1996.

Geagea T: Laparoscopic Nissen's fundoplication: Preliminary report on ten cases. Surg Endosc 5:170–173, 1991.

Gotley DC, Smithers BM, Rhodes M, et al: Laparoscopic Nissen fundoplication—200 consecutive cases. Gut 38:487–491, 1996.

Hallerback B, Glise H, Johansson B, Radmark T: Laparoscopic Rossetti fundoplication. Surg Endosc 8:1417–1422, 1994.

Heikkinen T-J, Haukipuro K, Koivukangas P, et al: Comparison of costs between laparoscopic and open Nissen fundoplication: A prospective randomized study with a 3-month follow-up. J Am Coll Surg 188:368–376, 1999.

Hill ADK, Walsh TN, Bolger CM, et al: Randomized controlled trial comparing Nissen fundoplication and the Angelchik prosthesis. Br J Surg 81:72–74, 1994.

Hill LD: An effective operation for hiatal hernia: An eight year appraisal. Ann Surg 166:681–692, 1967.

Hinder RA, Filipi CJ, Wetscher G, et al: Laparoscopic Nissen fundoplication is an effective treatment for gastroesophageal reflux disease. Ann Surg 220:472–483, 1994.

Hunter JG, Trus TL, Barum GD, Waring JP: A physiologic approach to laparoscopic fundoplication for gastroesophageal reflux disease. Ann Surg 223:673–687, 1996.

Jamieson GG, Watson DI, Britten-Jones R, et al: Laparoscopic Nissen fundoplication. Ann Surg 220:137–145, 1994.

Janssen IM, Gouma DJ, Klementschitsch P, et al: Prospective randomised comparison of Teres cardiopexy and Nissen fundoplication in the surgical therapy of gastro-oesophageal reflux disease. Br J Surg 80:875–878, 1993.

Johansson J, Johnsson F, Joelsson B, et al: Outcome 5 years after 360° fundoplication for gastro-oesophageal reflux disease. Br J Surg 80:46–49, 1993.

Kauer WKH, Peters JH, DeMeester TR, et al: A tailored approach to antireflux surgery. J Thorac Cardiovasc Surg 110:141–147, 1995.

Kmiot WA, Kirby RM, Akinola D, Temple JG: Prospective randomized trial of Nissen fundoplication and the Angelchik prosthesis. Br J Surg 78:1181–1184, 1991.

Laine S, Rantala A, Gullichsen R, Ovaska J: Laparoscopic vs conventional Nissen fundoplication: A prospective randomized study. Surg Endosc 11:441–444, 1997.

Laws HL, Clements RH, Swillies CM: A randomized, prospective comparison of the Nissen versus the Toupet fundoplication for gastroesophageal reflux disease. Ann Surg 225:647–654, 1997.

Laycock WS, Trus TL, Hunter JG: New technology for the division of short gastric vessels during laparoscopic Nissen fundoplication. Surg Endosc 10:71–73, 1996.

Lundell L, Abrahamsson H, Ruth M, et al: Lower esophageal sphincter characteristics and esophageal acid exposure following partial or 3600 fundoplication: Results of a prospective, randomized clinical study. World J Surg 15:115–121, 1991.

Lundell L, Abrahamsson H, Ruth M, et al: Long-term results of a prospective randomized comparison of total fundic wrap (Nissen-Rossetti) or semifundoplication (Toupet) for gastro-oesophageal reflux. Br J Surg 83:830–835, 1996.

Luostarinen ME, Isolauri JO: Randomized trial to study the effect of fundic mobilization on long-term results of Nissen fundoplication. Br J Surg 86:614–618, 1999.

Luostarinen MES, Koskinen MO, Isolauri JO: Effect of fundal mobilisation in Nissen-Rossetti fundoplication on oesophageal transit and dysphagia. Eur J Surg 162:37–42, 1996.

Luostarinen M, Koskinen M, Reinikainen P, et al: Two antireflux operations: Floppy versus standard Nissen fundoplication. Ann Med 27:199–205, 1995.

Ortiz A, Martinez de Haro LF, Parrilla P, et al: Conservative treatment versus antireflux surgery in Barrett's oesophagus: Long-term results of a prospective study. Br J Surg 83:274–278, 1996.

Patti MG, De Bellis M, De Pinto M, et al: Partial fundoplication for gastroesophageal reflux. Surg Endosc 11:445–448, 1997.

Peillon C, Manouvrier J-L, Labreche J, et al: Should the vagus nerves be isolated from the fundoplication wrap? A prospective study. Arch Surg 129:814–818, 1994.

Perttila J, Salo M, Ovaska J, et al: Immune response after laparoscopic and conventional Nissen fundoplication. Eur J Surg 165:21–28, 1999.

Peters JH, Heimbucher J, Kauer WKH, et al: Clinical and physiological comparison of laparoscopic and open Nissen fundoplication. J Am Coll Surg 180:385–393, 1995.

Rattner DW, Brooks DC: Patient satisfaction following laparoscopic and open antireflux surgery. Arch Surg 130:289–294, 1995.

Rossetti M, Hell K: Fundoplication for the treatment of gastroesophageal reflux in hiatal hernia. World J Surg 1:439–444, 1977.

Rydberg L, Ruth M, Abrahamsson H, Lundell L: Tailoring antireflux surgery: A randomized clinical trial. World J Surg 23:612–618, 1999a.

Rydberg L, Ruth M, Lundell L: Mechanism of action of antireflux procedures. Br J Surg 86:405–410, 1999b.

Spechler SJ: Comparison of medical and surgical therapy for complicated gastroesophageal reflux disease in veterans. N Engl J Med 326:786–792, 1992.

Swanström LL, Marcus DR, Galloway GQ: Laparoscopic Collis' gastroplasty is the treatment of choice for the shortened esophagus. Am J Surg 171:477, 1996.

Swanström LL, Pennings JL: Laparoscopic control of short gastric vessels. J Am Coll Surg 181:347–351, 1995.

Thor KBA, Silander T: A long-term randomized prospective trial of the Nissen procedure versus a modified Toupet technique. Ann Surg 210:719–724, 1989.

Toupet A: Technique d'oesophago-gastroplastie avec phrenogastropexie appliquée dans la cure radicale des herniés hiatales et comme complement de l'operation d'Heller dans les cardiospasmes. Med Acad Chir 89:394, 1963.

Trus TL, Laycock WS, Branum G, et al: Intermediate follow-up of laparoscopic antireflux surgery. Am J Surg 171:32–35, 1996.

Walker SJ, Holt S, Sanderson CJ, Stoddard CJ: Comparison of Nissen total and Lind partial transabdominal fundoplication in the treatment of gastro-oesophageal reflux. Br J Surg 79:410–414, 1992.

Washer GF, Gear MWL, Dowling BL, et al: Randomized prospective trial of Roux-en-Y duodenal diversion versus fundoplication for severe reflux oesophagitis. Br J Surg 71:181–184, 1984.

Watson A, Spychal RT, Brown MG, et al: Laparoscopic "physiological" antireflux procedure: Preliminary results of a prospective symptomatic and objective study. Br J Surg 82:651–656, 1995.

Watson DI, Gourlay R, Globe J, et al: Prospective randomised trial of laparoscopic versus open Nissen fundoplication (Abstract). Gut 35(Suppl 2):S15, 1994.

Watson DI, Jamieson GG: Antireflux surgery in the laparoscopic era (Review). Br J Surg 85:1173–1184, 1998.

Watson DI, Jamieson GG, Baigrie RJ, et al: Laparoscopic surgery for gastro-oesophageal reflux: Beyond the learning curve. Br J Surg 83:1284–1287, 1996.

Watson DI, Jamieson GG, Pike GK, et al: A prospective randomised double blind trial between laparoscopic Nissen fundoplication and anterior partial fundoplication. Br J Surg 86:123–130, 1999a.

Watson DI, Jamieson GG, Pike GK, et al: Laparoscopic vs. anterior fundoplication: A randomised double blind controlled trial (Abstract). Aust N Z J Surg 69(Suppl):A57, 1999b.

Watson DI, Pike GK, Baigrie RJ, et al: Prospective double blind randomised trial of laparoscopic Nissen fundoplication with division and without division of short gastric vessels. Ann Surg 226:642–652, 1997.

CHAPTER **26**

Vagotomy, Antrectomy, and Roux-en-Y Diversion

F. Henry Ellis, Jr.

Selection of proper surgical therapy for the patient with complex problems arising from gastroesophageal reflux disease (GERD) is controversial. A variety of surgical options are available when medical therapy fails, including variations on the classic antireflux procedures such as the Collis-Nissen, Collis-Belsey, and Thal-Nissen procedures. Resection with intestinal interposition or resection alone, preferably of the transhiatal type, may be employed in the presence of an undilatable esophageal stricture.

Although not widely used in North America, the procedure of acid suppression and alkaline diversion by vagotomy, antrectomy, and Roux-en-Y diversion, accompanied by resection of an esophageal stricture if present, has been performed by European, Scandinavian, and British surgeons. The origins of the procedure, the technique of its performance, its indications, and the reported and personal results of its use are detailed in this chapter.

HISTORICAL NOTE

More than 40 years ago, dissatisfaction with available methods of surgical management for the complications of reflux esophagitis, particularly those with short esophagus and stricture, led me to seek a solution in the experimental laboratory. Esophagogastrectomy with esophagogastrostomy was then the most frequently performed operation for complications of GERD, but this procedure merely set the stage for continuation of the damaging effects of acid gastric reflux on the esophageal mucosa with recurrence of the complications of GERD.

It was postulated that a localized resection of the stricture, if present, coupled with bilateral vagotomy would relieve the obstruction and eliminate the cephalic phase of gastric acid secretion. With the addition of antrectomy, the gastric phase of acid secretion would be eliminated, and the poor results that followed esophagogastrectomy and esophagogastrostomy alone would be avoided. Restoration of alimentary tract continuity by a Billroth I gastroduodenostomy was part of the original experimental procedure (Ellis, 1956a). The postoperative esophageal findings in nine dogs so treated were compared with those after esophagogastrectomy and esophagogastrostomy plus pyloromyotomy in a control group of eight dogs. Esophagitis developed in only one dog in the experimental group compared with five dogs in the control group.

The technique of the operation as applied to humans, employing a thoracoabdominal incision, was described in detail in a later publication (Ellis, 1956b), and its early results in nine patients were favorably reported the same year by Ellis and colleagues (1956). A longer follow-up on these and other patients operated on subsequently was reported 2 years later (Ellis et al, 1958). Twenty-four patients were available for evaluation, 22 of whom (92%) were considered to have had either an excellent or good result in terms of relief of preoperative symptoms of reflux and/or dysphagia. These results were in marked contrast to those of a group of 32 patients treated by resection with either esophagogastrostomy or esophagojejunostomy, subtotal gastric resection, or a miscellaneous group of procedures, only 69% of whom were considered to have been improved.

Longer follow-up on these original 24 patients and an additional 12 patients, of whom 34 were available for follow-up 6 months to 8 years (mean, 4.9 years) postoperatively, was reported by Payne and colleagues (1964) and revealed that 21% were classified as having had a poor overall result. Three patients had developed strictures, and regurgitation was a chief complaint of all but one of the patients with a poor result.

These findings pinpointed the necessity of diverting the alkaline secretions; subsequently, a Roux-en-Y alkaline diversion procedure was employed to re-establish gastrointestinal continuity after antrectomy in place of the originally proposed gastroduodenostomy. This operation has remained the procedure of choice for these complicated cases during subsequent years.

■ *HISTORICAL READINGS*

Ellis FH Jr: Experimental aspects of surgical treatment of reflux esophagitis and esophageal stricture. Ann Surg 143:465, 1956a.

Ellis FH Jr: Physiologic operation for ulceration and stricture of terminal esophagus. Mayo Clin Proc 31:615, 1956b.

Ellis FH Jr, Anderson HA, Clagett OT: Surgical management of complications of reflux esophagitis. Arch Surg 73:578, 1956.

Ellis FH Jr, Anderson HA, Clagett OT: Treatment of short esophagus with stricture by esophagogastrectomy and antral excision. Ann Surg 148:526, 1958.

Payne WS, Anderson HA, Ellis FH Jr: Reappraisal of esophagogastrectomy and antral excision in the treatment of short esophagus. Surgery 55:344, 1964.

SURGICAL TECHNIQUE

The surgical approach for vagotomy, antrectomy, and Roux-en-Y diversion depends on whether resection of the distal esophagus and cardia is required because of an undilatable stricture or ulcerative esophagitis with hemorrhage. When a localized resection of the involved area (cardiectomy) must be performed, a thoracic approach is required (Fig. 26–1). A left posterolateral thoracotomy entering the chest through the bed of the nonresected seventh or eighth rib is the preferred approach (Fig. 26–1*A*).

After the mediastinal pleura is opened and distal esophagus is mobilized, the hiatal attachments are divided to permit freeing of the proximal stomach by division of some of the short gastric and posterior gastric vessels (Fig. 26–1*B*). Use of a stapling device applied to the stomach just distal to the cardia permits division of the stomach at an appropriate level. Continuity is restored after resecting the esophagus proximal to the diseased area by advancing part of the gastric greater curvature, after freeing its vascular connections and dividing the vagus nerves, and performing an end-to-side esophagogastrostomy (Fig. 26–1*C*). An open anastomosis with an inner layer of running catgut and an outer layer of interrupted nonabsorbable sutures is preferred. A nasogastric tube is passed transnasally across the anastomosis into the intrathoracic stomach for decompression.

Although the thoracic incision may be extended as a thoracoabdominal incision, permitting performance of the intra-abdominal portion of the procedure without repositioning the patients, I prefer a separate abdominal incision to avoid some of the potential complications of transecting the costal arch as well as to avoid the necessity of partial denervation of the diaphragm by such an approach. Accordingly, the thoracotomy is closed with intercostal tube drainage in the usual fashion, and the patient is repositioned in a supine position for an upper midline incision to provide adequate exposure of the upper abdomen (Fig. 26–2*A*). When cardiectomy is not needed, the entire diaphragmatic operative procedure is performed through an upper midline incision (see Fig. 26–2*A*).

Exposure of the upper stomach and hiatus is provided by mobilization of the left lobe of the liver (Fig. 26–2*B*). If the esophagogastric junction has not been resected, both vagus nerves are isolated and divided, and the operation proceeds as an antrectomy with partial division of the stomach beginning at the greater gastric curvature and extended cephalad along the lesser gastric curvature, where a stapler is used. The stapled lesser curvature portion of the stomach is oversewn with interrupted nonabsorbable sutures, and the antrectomy is completed by ligation of the right gastroepiploic and right gastric arteries. The duodenum is divided with a stapler, and the stapled end is oversewn with interrupted nonabsorbable

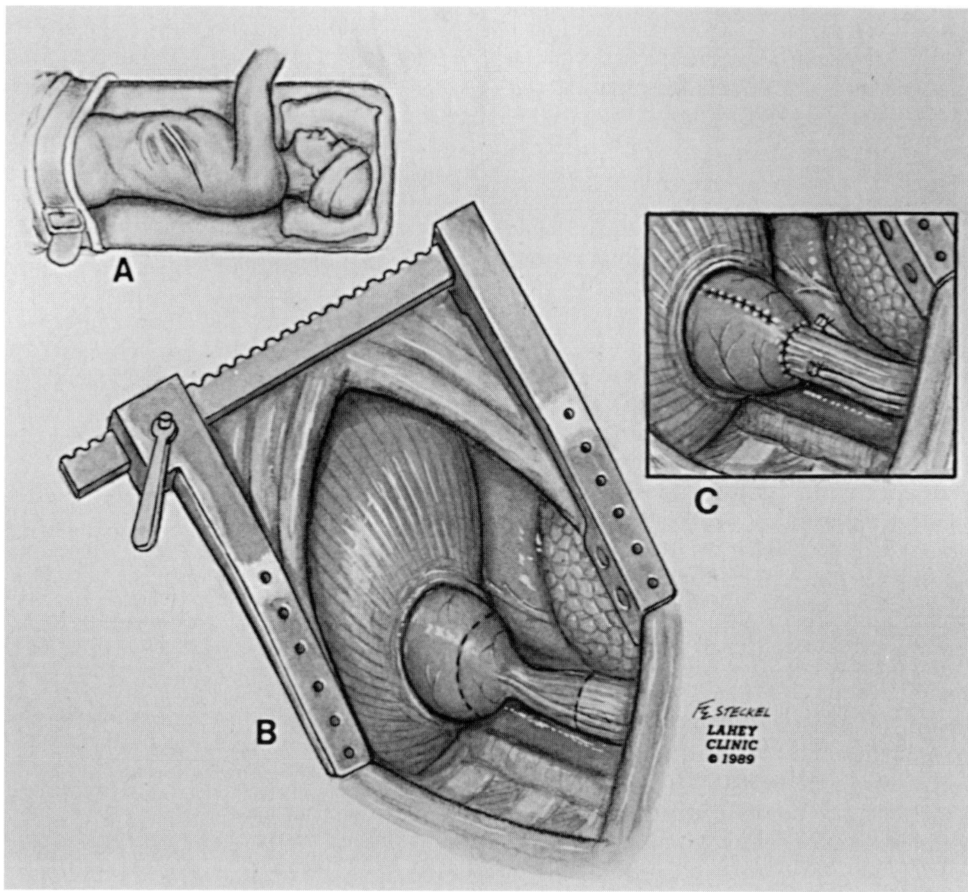

FIGURE 26–1 ■ Operative technique of cardiectomy. *A*, Location of incision; *B*, operative exposure indicating area to be resected; *C*, completed anastomosis. (From Ellis FH Jr, Gibb SP: Acid-suppression and alkaline-diversion; A safe and effective operation for patients with complex benign esophageal diseases requiring reoperation. In Little AG, Ferguson MN, Skinner DB [eds]: Diseases of the Esophagus, Benign Disease, Vol II. Armonk, NY, Futura Publishing, 1990, p 394.)

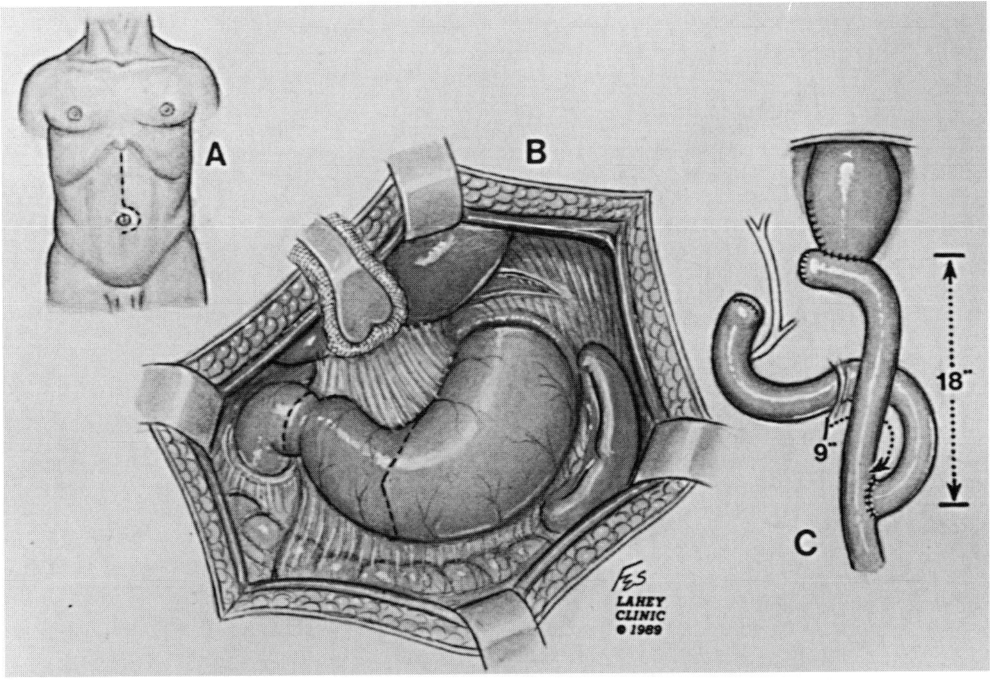

FIGURE 26–2 ■ Operative technique of antrectomy and Roux-en-Y gastrojejunostomy. *A*, Location of incision; *B*, operative exposure indicating area to be resected; *C*, completed anastomosis. (From Ellis FH Jr, Gibb SP: Acid-suppression and alkaline-diversion: A safe and effective operation for patients with complex benign esophageal disease requiring reoperation. In Little AG, Ferguson MN, Skinner DB [eds]: Diseases of the Esophagus, Benign Disease, Vol II. Armonk, NY, Futura Publishing, 1990, p 395.)

sutures. The left gastric artery should remain intact, as this artery will constitute the major gastric blood supply when the fundus has been mobilized by division of the short gastric vessels when cardiectomy is required.

The colon is then elevated. The ligament of Treitz is identified, and a point on the jejunum 9 inches from the ligament is selected for division of the jejunum using the GIA stapler (U.S. Surgical Corp., Norwalk, CT). A retrocolic gastrojejunostomy is then performed to the distal divided jejunum in an end-to-side fashion, the previously stapled jejunal end being oversewn with interrupted nonabsorbable sutures (Fig. 26–2*C*). A running inner layer of catgut and an outer layer of interrupted nonabsorbable sutures are used to perform the gastrojejunostomy. The proximal divided jejunum is then anastomosed to the jejunal limb 18 inches distal to the gastrojejunostomy (see Fig. 26–2*C*). The area is then peritonealized to prevent development of an internal hernia, and the abdomen is closed in the usual fashion after placement of Penrose drains near the duodenal stump through a separate stab wound.

REPORTED RESULTS

Enthusiasm for this approach to the management of selected patients with complications of GERD is apparent from the reports summarized in Table 26–1, a preponderance of which originated in Europe, Scandinavia, and Great Britain. Relatively few of the operations involved resection of a stricture, suggesting that the populations of patients in these reports may have been at a less advanced stage of disease than those in my series, reported in the following section.

Wells and Johnston (1955) were the first to report the clinical results of vagotomy, gastrectomy, and Roux-en-Y gastrojejunostomy without an esophageal resection. Twelve patients with hiatal hernia and reflux esophagitis treated in this way experienced good results, although the follow-up was short.

Holt and Large (1961) from the United States reported the use of this procedure in 11 patients in 1961. A report on 10 of these patients 8 to 12 years after operation, 6 of whom required resection of the strictured area, described successful results in all patients (Weaver et al, 1970). Subsequently, there have been other similar reports, usually on small numbers of patients, most of whom did not exhibit an advanced stage of GERD and did not require resection of a stricture.

The largest experience with antrectomy and Roux-en-Y diversion is that of Fékété and Pateron (1992), who reported an 80% improvement rate in 83 patients, none of whom required cardiectomy, after a median follow-up of 6 years.

PERSONAL EXPERIENCE

Patients

From January 1970 to January 1996, 37 patients, some of whom have been reported previously (Ellis and Gibb, 1994), underwent vagotomy, antrectomy, and Roux-en-Y diversion. The patients' ages ranged from 26 to 75 years with a median of 54 years. Seventeen patients were men,

TABLE 26–1 ■ **Acid Suppression and Alkaline Diversion: Results of Operation**

Authors	*Country*	*No. of Patients*	*Resection*	*Results (%)*	
				Improved	*Poor*
Wells and Johnston (1955)	England	12	0	100	0
Holt and Large (1961)	United States	(11)†	NS‡		
Weaver et al* (1970)	United States	10	6	100	0
Payne (1970)	United States	15	6	73	27
Royston et al (1975)	England	8	0	88	12
Herrington and Mody (1976)	United States	6	0	100	0
Payne (1984)	United States	13	3	85	15
Matikainen (1984)	Finland	6	0	83	17
DeMiguel (1985)	Spain	7	0	100	0
Washer et al (1986)	England	57	0	86	14
Hesselink et al (1988)	Holland	22	0	86	14
Rossetti et al (1990)	Switzerland	43	0	83	17
Salo et al (1991)	Finland	11	0	100	0
Fékété and Pateron (1992)	France	83	0	80	20
Panis and Fékété (1994)	France	29	0	83	17
Deschamps et al (1997)	United States	17	0	NS‡	NS‡
Total		339	15	89.1	10.9

*Late follow-up of cases originally reported by Holt and Large (1961).
†Not included in total.
‡Not stated.

and 20 were women. Pertinent associated disorders were achalasia in 19 patients and scleroderma in 3, one of whom also had Barrett's esophagus, as did three other patients. Two patients had an esophageal ulcer, and one had a gastric ulcer. The indication for a reconstructive esophageal procedure was severe GERD in 31 patients, 23 of whom also had a stricture. Five patients underwent operation for post-Nissen dysphagia, and one patient underwent operation for persistent achalasia after two previous myotomies.

Thirty-three of these patients had undergone a total of 68 previous operative procedures on the distal esophagus and stomach (Table 26–2). Of the four of these patients who had not undergone previous surgery, three had scleroderma with undilatable strictures and the fourth a long history of severe GERD with a long peptic esophageal stricture associated with Barrett's esophagus unresponsive to bougienage. The most common previous procedure was fundoplication, usually of the Nissen variety. Esophagomyotomy, usually of the modified Heller type, was the next most common previous operation. Two of the 23 esophagomyotomies were of the extended variety, for suspected but unproven diffuse esophageal spasm.

Thirty patients required a limited esophagogastrectomy and esophagogastrostomy. Two patients with an esophageal stricture underwent cardioplasty to relieve the obstruction, a modification preferred by others (Braghetto et al, 1998) for some patients with stricture, and only one patient required freeing of the esophagus at the hiatus. Only four patients required no operative procedure on the distal esophagus and cardia. Two separate incisions, one thoracic and one abdominal, was the preferred approach used in 31 patients, and these were performed in two stages in 4 patients. Five patients had a thoracoabdominal incision, and one patient, who had previously undergone an esophagogastrectomy, required only an abdominal incision.

TABLE 26–2 ■ **Previous Operations of 33 Patients Undergoing Vagotomy, Antrectomy, and Roux-en-Y Diversion**

Procedure	*No. of Patients*	
Fundoplication	23	
Nissen		13
Belsey		3
Collis-Nissen		3
Thal-Nissen		1
Collis-Belsey		1
Hill		1
Angelchik		1
Esophagomyotomy	23	
Repair of diaphragmatic hernia	4	
Limited esophagogastrectomy	4	
Closure of esophageal perforation	3	
Subtotal gastrectomy	3	
Miscellaneous	8	
Total	68	

Results

No hospital deaths occurred. Nine postoperative complications occurred (24%), including five major complications. In one patient with Raynaud's disease secondary to scleroderma, two gangrenous toes developed, necessitating amputation. An empyema in one patient required decortication. Gastrointestinal leaks developed in two patients, one from the duodenal stump and the other from the gastric wall; these leaks were contained, and they healed spontaneously.

The most serious complication occurred in a patient who had previously undergone an operative procedure on the cardia for removal of a leiomyoma and who developed ischemic contraction and near obliteration of the gastric remnant after surgery. The patient required gastrectomy and a subsequent colon interposition. In retrospect, although the gastric remnant was clearly viable after antrectomy, its blood supply must have been impaired at the earlier operation, resulting in this unusual postoperative complication.

Two patients had urinary tract infections. One of these patients required bronchoscopy, and the other patient experienced chemical pancreatitis that subsided without therapy.

Clinical evaluation after hospital discharge was available for 34 patients. For one patient, the postoperative time interval has been too short to be meaningful. Two patients were lost to follow-up. Results were classified as "excellent" if the patient was virtually asymptomatic, "good" when only occasional symptoms were present, and "fair" if symptoms persisted but to a lesser degree than preoperatively. If the patient's condition remained unchanged or was worsened by operation, the result was classified as "poor."

The follow-up interval ranged from 1 month to 20 years, with a median of 4½ years. Twenty-nine patients (85%) were considered to have been improved (Table 26–3). Of the five patients classified as having poor results, one patient has already been described (the patient requiring gastrectomy and colon interposition). Two patients had recurrent dysphagia, and two other patients complained of nausea and vomiting with inability to maintain weight. One patient temporarily experienced dumping, and another patient experienced occasional diarrhea. Nocturnal aspiration has not occurred. No patient developed the "afferent loop" syndrome related to delayed Roux loop transit time, a recognized complication of the Roux-en-Y duodenal diversion procedure (Miedema et al, 1992).

CURRENT INDICATIONS

It is difficult to establish rigid criteria for vagotomy, antrectomy, and Roux-en-Y diversion in patients with complex esophageal disorders secondary to GERD. Most of these patients have had one or more previous operative procedures; thus, each case becomes a unique problem in evaluation and judgment. Even so, some general categories might qualify as indications for the operation.

Certainly, patients with an undilatable stricture require resection. Patients with megaesophagus, fortunately rarely seen today, in whom an esophagomyotomy has failed to provide adequate emptying of the esophagus, have another indication for the procedure. If two previous myotomies for achalasia of less advanced degree have failed, a more radical procedure, such as the one described, is appropriate. Similarly, two failed antireflux procedures (e.g., the Nissen procedure) demand a more radical approach. Failure of the Collis-Nissen operation also demands a radical approach, and the operation described has functioned well under these circumstances.

Rarely is the operation indicated as a primary reoperative procedure, a more conservative approach being justified prior to its implementation. One exception might be patients with a stricture secondary to scleroderma, a notably difficult problem to treat by conventional techniques.

TABLE 26–3 ■ Results of Acid Suppression/Alkaline Diversion Procedure in 34 Patients

Result	*Number of Patients*	*Percent*
Improved	29	85
Excellent	16	
Good	9	
Fair	4	
Poor	5	15
Total	34	

Acknowledgments

Supported in part by the Thelma and Jerry Sturgios Esophageal Research Fund.

■ KEY REFERENCES

Ellis FH Jr, Gibb SP: Vagotomy, antrectomy, and Roux-en-Y diversion for complex reoperative gastroesophageal reflux disease. Ann Surg 220:536–543, 1994.

This report details the authors' experience with the acid suppression/alkaline diversion procedure, combined when necessary with limited esophagogastrectomy in the presence of an undilatable stricture.

Fékété F, Pateron D: What is the place of antrectomy with Roux-en-Y in the treatment of reflux disease? Experience with 83 total duodenal diversions. World J Surg 16:349–354, 1992.

This report is the largest published experience employing the acid suppression/alkaline diversion concept in the management of complex cases of GERD.

Wells C, Johnston JH: Hiatus hernia: Surgical relief of reflux esophagitis. Lancet 1:937, 1955.

This article is the first published report of the use of vagotomy, antrectomy, and Roux-en-Y diversion in patients with severe reflux esophagitis.

■ REFERENCES

Braghetto I, Korn O, Csendes A, Frias JC: Esophagocardioplasty, vagotomy-antrectomy and Roux-en-Y gastrojejunostomy: Indication in cases with severe esophageal motor disfunction. Dis Esophagus 11:58–61, 1998.

DeMiguel J: Tratamiento de ciertas estrecheces pépticas del esófago mediante vagotomia, gastrectomía parcial y anastomosis gastroyeyunal en "Y" de Roux [English abstract]. Rev Esp Enferm Apar Dig 67:511, 1985.

Deschamps C, Trastek VF, Allen MS, et al: Long-term results after reoperation for failed antireflux procedures. J Thorac Cardiovasc Surg 113:545–551, 1997.

Ellis FH Jr, Gibb SP: Vagotomy, antrectomy, and Roux-en-Y diversion for complex reoperative gastroesophageal reflux disease. Ann Surg 220:536–543, 1994.

Herrington JL Jr, Mody B: Total duodenal diversion for treatment of reflux esophagitis uncontrolled by repeated antireflux procedures. Ann Surg 183:636–644, 1976.

Hesselink EJ, Slooff MJH, Bleichrodt RP, et al: Gastrectomy and Roux-en-Y duodenal diversion as treatment for severe reflux esophagitis. In Siewert JR, Hölsck AH (eds): Diseases of the Esophagus. Berlin, Springer-Verlag, 1988, p 1248.

Holt CJ, Large AM: Surgical management of reflux esophagitis. Ann Surg 153:555–562, 1961.

Matikainen M: Antrectomy: Roux-en-Y reconstruction and vagotomy for recurrent reflux oesophagitis. Acta Chir Scand 150:643–645, 1984.

Miedema BW, Kelly KA, Camilleri M, et al: Human gastric and jejunal transit and motility after Roux gastrojejunostomy. Gastroenterology 103:1133–1143, 1992.

Panis Y, Fékété F: La diversion duodénale totale dans les réinterventions pour reflux gastro-oesophagien: Indications et résultats chez vingt-neuf patients. Ann Chir 48:27–30, 1994.

Payne WS: Surgical treatment of reflux esophagitis and stricture associated with permanent incompetence of the cardia. Mayo Clin Proc 45:553–562, 1970.

Payne WS: Surgical management of reflux-induced oesophageal stenoses: Results in 101 patients. Br J Surg 71:971–973, 1984.

Rossetti M, Hitz P, von Aarburg R: Die distale Y-Gastrektomie bei komplexem und Rezidivreflux. Helv Chir Acta 56:935–938, 1990.

Royston CM, Dowling BL, Spencer J: Antrectomy with Roux-en-Y anastomosis in the treatment of peptic oesophagitis with stricture. Br J Surg 62:605–607, 1975.

Salo JA, Ala-Kulju KV, Heikkinen LO, Kivilaakso EO: Treatment of severe peptic esophageal stricture with Roux-en-Y partial gastrectomy, vagotomy, and endoscopic dilation: A follow-up study. J Thorac Cardiovasc Surg 101:649–653, 1991.

Washer GF, Gear MW, Dowling BL, et al: Duodenal diversion with vagotomy and antrectomy for severe or recurrent reflux oesophagitis and stricture: An alternative to operation at the hiatus. Ann R Coll Surg Engl 68:222–226, 1986.

Weaver AW, Large AM, Walt AJ: Surgical management of severe reflux esophagitis: Eight to seventeen year follow-up study. Am J Surg 119:15–18, 1970.

CHAPTER 27

Combined Operations

Attila Csendes
Italo Braghetto
Owen Korn
Patricio Burdiles
Jorge Rojas

PATHOPHYSIOLOGY

The competence of the antireflux mechanism is improved by most of the surgical procedures designed to control reflux. The Nissen-Rossetti and Hill-Larrain techniques increase the abdominal length of the esophagus and elevate the lower esophageal sphincter pressure (Csendes and Larraín, 1972; Rosetti and Hell, 1977). Similar results are obtained after the Belsey procedure (Skinner and Belsey, 1967). Other, less commonly employed techniques (Narbona, Toupet, Dor, and Angelchik) have similar objectives.

None of these antireflux operations influences other important mechanisms responsible for the pathogenesis of reflux esophagitis. Csendes and colleagues have developed a combined operation for reflux control in patients with uncomplicated reflux esophagitis, which consists of (1) highly selective vagotomy (HSV) (Csendes et al, 1981), (2) calibration of the cardia (Csendes, 1987), and (3) posterior gastropexy (Csendes et al, 1972).

Highly Selective Vagotomy

HSV decreases the volume and potency of gastric acid that may reflux into the esophagus. The procedure also enhances gastric emptying of fluids.

A prospective study demonstrated a significant decrease of gastric acid secretion (both basal and stimulated) when HSV was performed in patients with reflux esophagitis (Oster et al, 1982). Boesby (1977) also showed that the duration of the fall in esophageal pH below 4, as well as the number of reflux episodes correlated with the volume of basal acid secretion, was reduced after HSV. Furthermore, gastric emptying of fluid is improved after HSV, whereas emptying time for solids remains unchanged (Wilbur and Kelly, 1973).

In patients who undergo Nissen-Rossetti procedures, the addition of HSV has the favorable effect of raising intragastric pressure through loss of the capacity for accommodation after distention and loss of receptive relaxation (Staadas and Aune, 1970; Wilbur and Kelly, 1973). The creation of a cuff around the distal abdominal esophagus promotes an increase in intragastric pressure surrounding the distal esophagus and lower esophageal sphincter, thereby improving competence (Wilbur and Kelly, 1973).

HSV has no deleterious effect on the lower esophageal sphincter. The extensive extrinsic denervation and dissection of the distal esophagus do not appear to alter the dynamics of gastroesophageal sphincter pressure. Several studies have demonstrated the following features of this procedure:

1. Resting gastroesophageal sphincter pressure is not changed after HSV (Csendes et al, 1978b, 1978c, 1979b).
2. The length and location of the gastroesophageal sphincter are not changed after HSV (Braash et al, 1980; Csendes et al, 1979b).
3. Gastroesophageal reflux does not increase after HSV alone (Csendes et al, 1978c).
4. No significant changes occur in esophageal sphincter pressure in spite of an increase in basal serum gastrin levels (Csendes et al, 1978b, 1979a).
5. The response of this sphincter to cholinergic stimulation is not changed after HSV (Csendes et al, 1979b).
6. Sphincter relaxation, the increase in sphincter pressure after step-by-step increase in intragastric pressure, and the amplitude of the peristaltic waves of the distal esophagus are not changed after HSV (Csendes et al, 1978c, 1979a).

Calibration of the Cardia, or 360-Degree Fundoplication

The procedure for calibration of the cardia was created to decrease the dilated diameter of the distal esophagus and the esophagogastric junction, or cardia. In a prospective study, we measured the external circumference of the esophagogastric junction in 20 patients who had duodenal ulcer without reflux and who underwent HSV (control group) and in 40 patients with reflux esophagitis (Csendes et al, 1981). In the control group, the mean circumference of the cardia was 6 cm (Fig. 27–1), whereas in patients with reflux esophagitis, the mean circumferences was 9.5 cm ($P < .001$). There was a direct correlation between the severity of esophagitis and the enlargement of the circumference of the cardia (Fig. 27–2). We have submitted for publication the report of a

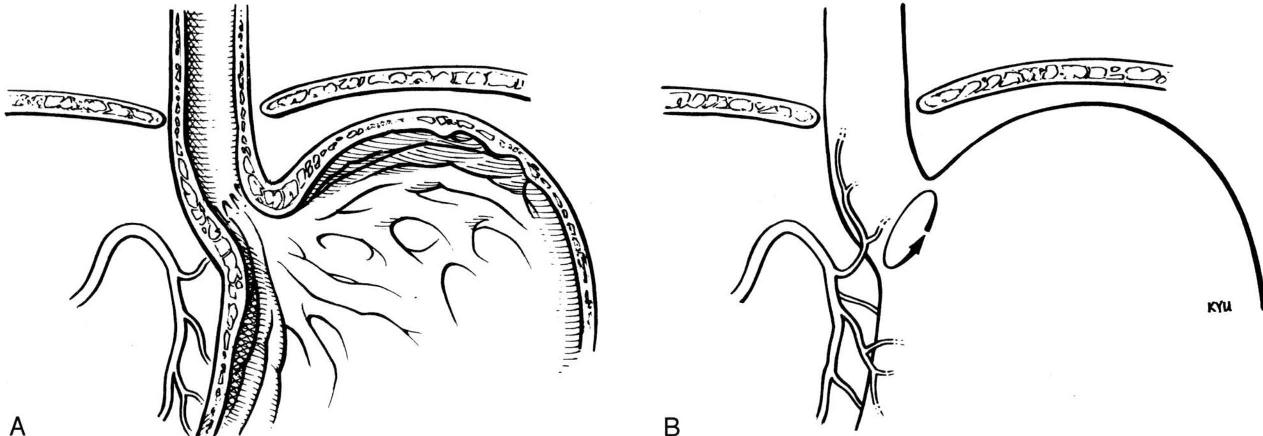

FIGURE 27–1 ■ Internal (*A*) and external (*B*) appearances of the normal esophagogastric junction, with a circumference of 6 cm.

study in which we measured the perimeter of the cardia in control patients with reflux esophagitis but without Barrett's esophagus and in patients with short-segment or long-segment Barrett's esophagus (Fig. 27–3) (Korn et al, 2000). The two latter groups had a significantly greater cardial perimeter and a more dilated gastroesophageal junction than the control group.

These clinical findings were confirmed by DeMeester's group in an experimental study demonstrating that the competence of the cardia depends on both the length of the lower esophageal sphincter and the diameter of the cardia (Bonavina et al, 1986; DeMeester et al, 1979). With a cardia 1 cm in diameter, a sphincter 2 cm long may be 100% competent, whereas a 3-cm cardia requires a 5-cm sphincter to achieve competence. A Nissen 360-degree fundoplication is easily performed and achieves these objectives. The objective of the Nissen operation is to increase the length of the abdominal esophagus, decrease the diameter of the abdominal esophagus and cardia, and enhance the intragastric pressure at the level of the gastric cuff around the abdominal esophagus and lower esophageal sphincter.

Posterior Gastropexy

The addition of a posterior gastropexy increases the length of the distal esophagus as well as the abdominal portion of the lower esophageal sphincter. Posterior gastropexy is not used when a Nissen fundoplication is performed.

OPERATIVE TECHNIQUE

Antireflux Procedure

The major steps of the antireflux procedure we employ in patients with mild and moderate esophagitis are:

1. HSV.
2. Closure of the diaphragmatic crus (right crus of the diaphragm) behind the esophagus.
3. Either calibration of the cardia over a 30 French catheter (1 cm diameter) or a Nissen-type 360-degree fundoplication.
4. Posterior gastropexy, securing the repair to the median arcuate ligament, if calibration of the cardia is performed.

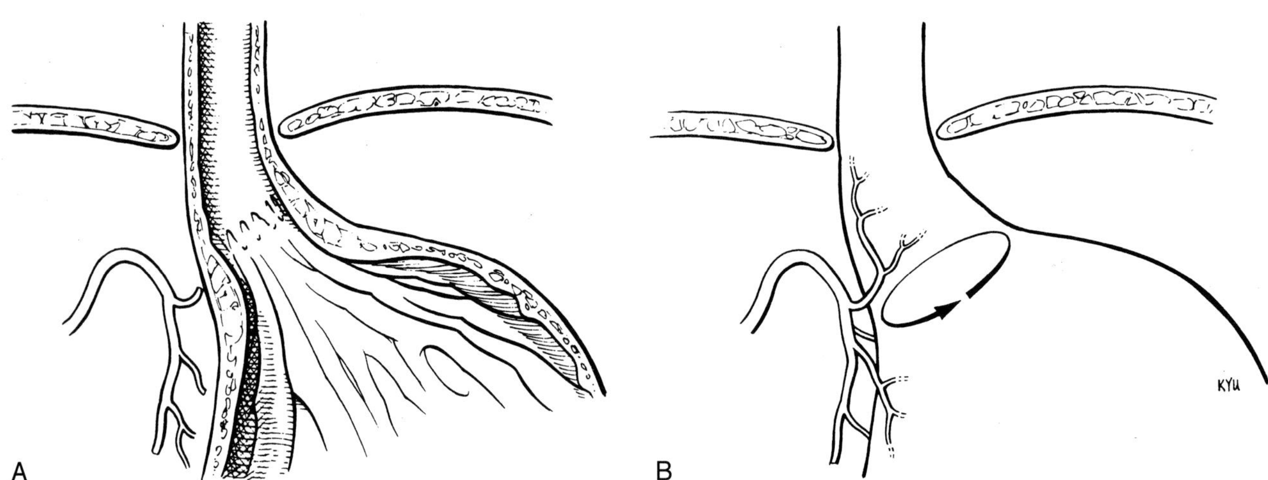

FIGURE 27–2 ■ Internal (*A*) and external (*B*) appearances of the esophagogastric junction in a patient with severe gastroesophageal reflux and Barrett's esophagus, with a dilated cardia with a circumference of 14 cm.

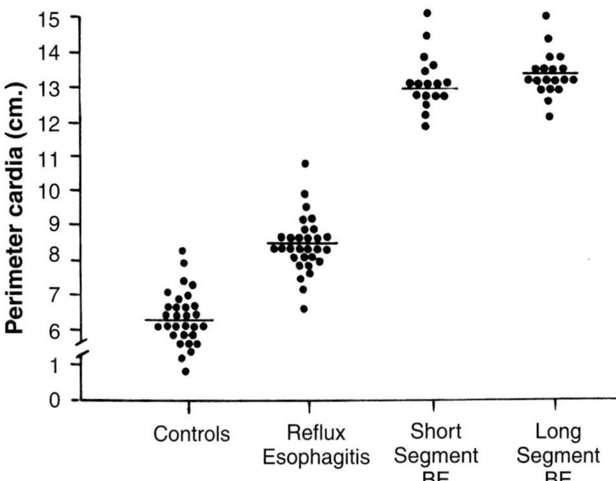

FIGURE 27–3 ■ Perimeter of the gastroesophageal junction or cardia in controls and in patients with reflux esophagitis, short-segment and long-segment Barrett's esophagus (BE).

5. Anterior fundophrenopexy to avoid a late, iatrogenic anterior paraesophageal hernia.

Highly Selective Vagotomy

HSV facilitates the technical performance of the operation. Any surgeon who has performed HSV for duodenal ulcer will appreciate this point. In patients with reflux esophagitis, increased fibrolipomatous tissue usually surrounds the esophagogastric junction. Furthermore, in patients with long-standing and severe esophagitis, the distal esophagus can develop a columnar lining (Barrett's esophagus), and transmural inflammation may alter the external surface of the esophageal wall so that it resembles gastric serosa. Our experience of several hundred HSV operations for duodenal ulcer has shown that with this procedure, surgical exposure of the abdominal esophagus, the esophagogastric junction, the lesser curvature of the stomach, and the angle of His is uniformly excellent. This exposure sets the stage for the performance of a very precise antireflux operation and has the physiologic advantages already described.

The patient is placed in a tilted position with the chest elevated relative to the feet (Grassi's position). A median supraumbilical incision is performed. A rib-elevating (sternal) retractor is always used; this provides excellent exposure of the supramesocolic space. HSV is performed as described previously (Amdrup, 1977; Csendes et al, 1979c). The dissection begins at the angle of His and is extended distally to the proximal branch of the "crow's foot" of the anterior and posterior hypogastric nerves of Latarjet, which are sectioned (Figs. 27–4 and 27–5; see Fig. 27–3). Dissection continues proximally from the lesser curvature until the distal 6 to 7 cm of the esophagus is isolated (Fig. 27–6). This isolation leads to displacement of the vagal trunks and the nerves of Latarjet along with the lesser omentum. The lesser curve is closed by interrupted sutures of 3–0 silk (Fig. 27–7).

Closure of the Hiatus

We do not consider closure of the hiatus to be an important step in controlling reflux. To avoid a postopera-

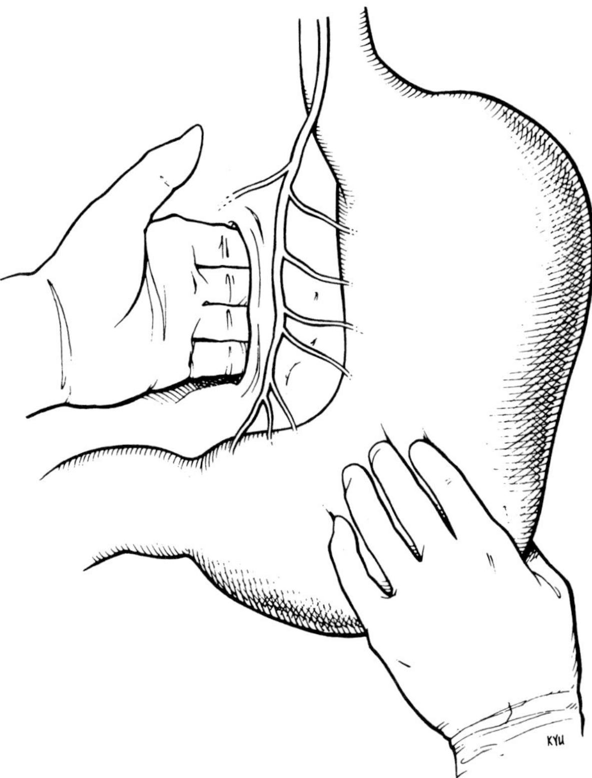

FIGURE 27–4 ■ Division of the lesser omentum, with introduction of the surgeon's left hand in order to apply traction to the hypogastric nerves of Latarjet while the assistant's right hand pulls down on the stomach.

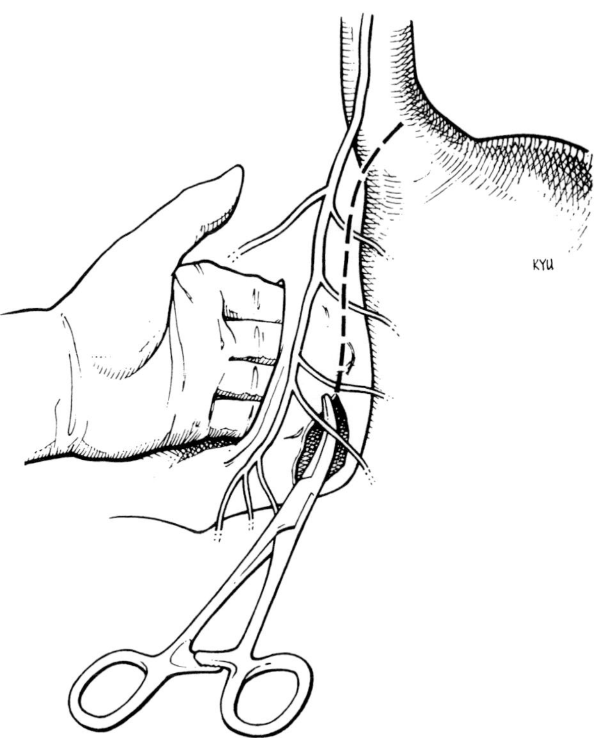

FIGURE 27–5 ■ Section of the proximal branch of the "crow's foot" at the start of the highly selective vagotomy.

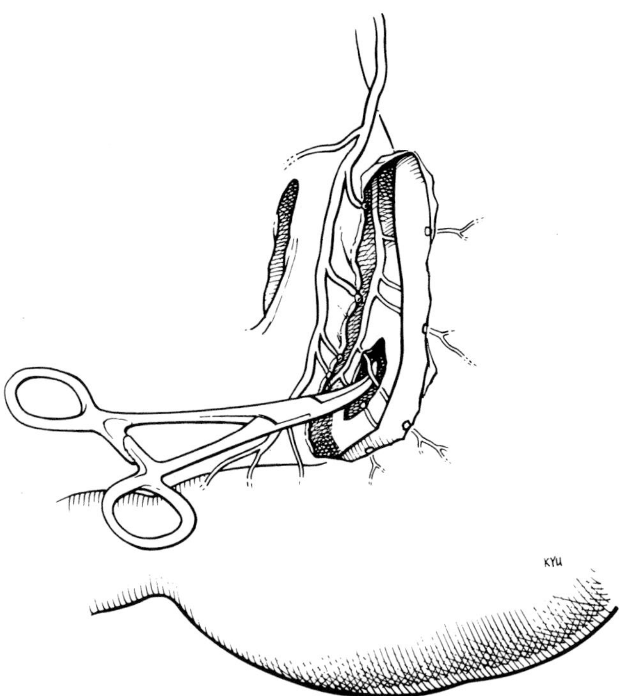

FIGURE 27–6 ■ Division of the posterior leaf of the lesser omentum in order to complete the highly selective vagotomy on the lesser curve.

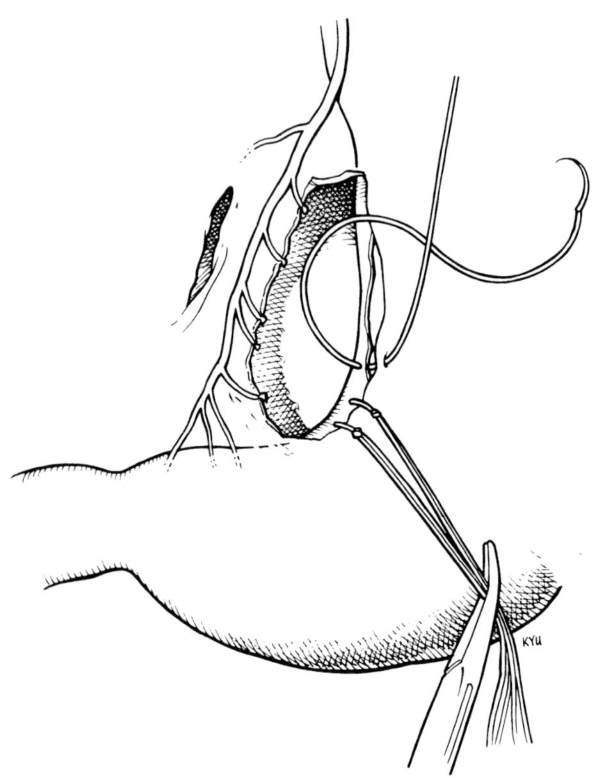

FIGURE 27–7 ■ Suture and closure of the lesser curve in order to avoid necrosis.

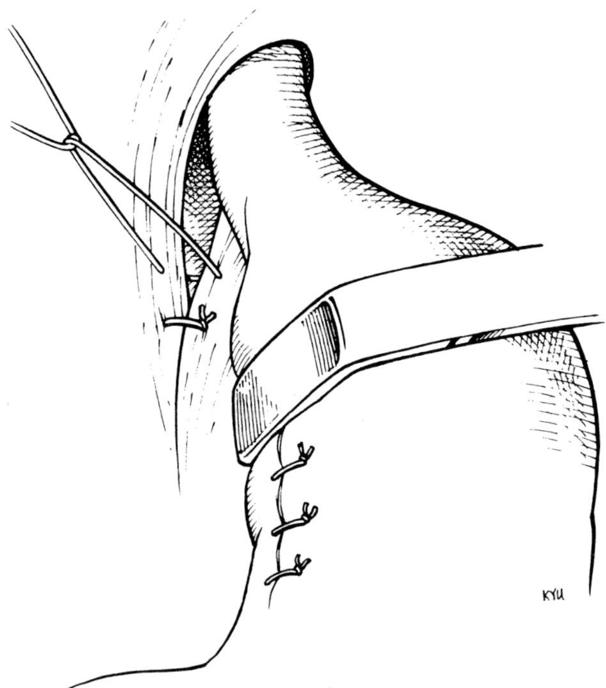

FIGURE 27–8 ■ Closure of the hiatus behind the esophagus.

tive hiatal hernia due to the extensive periesophageal and perihiatal dissection, however, we always close the hiatus with two sutures placed posteriorly. The esophagus is retracted anteriorly and to the left with a narrow Deaver ("baby Deaver") retractor. This allows visualization of the right and left portions of the right crus of the diaphragm, which are then approximated with two nonabsorbable sutures (Fig. 27–8). In the patient with a large hiatal hernia (seen in 20% of our cases), the hiatus is closed with two additional sutures placed anteriorly.

Calibration of the Cardia

Calibration of the cardia, an essential step in the antireflux procedure, is performed to narrow the dilated distal esophagus and esophagogastric junction or cardia. There is a direct correlation between the severity of esophagitis and the increased circumference of the cardia. We use a 30 French Hurst bougie (10 mm), which narrows the cardia to a diameter of 10 mm (less than the normal diameter, which is approximately 15 to 20 mm). The fatty tissue at the gastroesophageal junction is removed (Fig. 27–9).

For calibration of the cardia, a strong nonabsorbable suture is placed in the anterior surface of the stomach, 1 to 2 cm distal to the gastroesophageal junction on the lesser curve side. The site is perpendicular to the midpoint of the cardia. The suture is placed at the anatomic border of the cardia without including esophagus (Fig. 27–10). To avoid ulceration, perforation, and leak at this level, the suture must secure only seromuscular layers and should not include the mucosa. The calibrating suture includes the gastroesophageal muscular junction and some part of the gastric sling fibers.

The stomach is now easily rotated to the patient's left

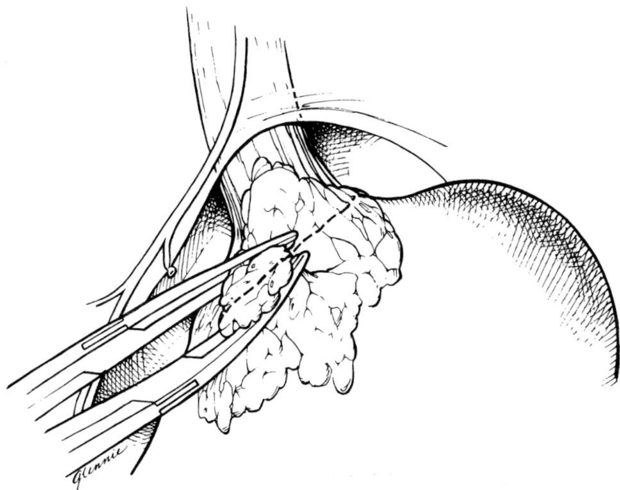

FIGURE 27–9 ■ Resection of the fatty tissue surrounding the gastroesophageal junction.

for exposure of the posterior gastric wall. A suture is placed so that its position is exactly symmetric with the position of the calibrating suture on the anterior wall. Therefore, it enters at the posterior, muscular gastroesophageal junction and exits 2 cm distally on the posterior surface of the stomach. Two or three similar sutures are then placed, extending to the left toward the angle of His. Thus, three or four sutures are inserted for calibration.

The sutures are then crossed, and the surgeon evaluates calibration of the cardia by pushing the 30 French Hurst bougie into the stomach (Fig. 27–11). The surgeon invaginates the greater curvature of the stomach, using a finger to follow the tip of the bougie. The bougie is now withdrawn into the esophagus. A muscular ring should be palpable at the cardia. The bougie passes easily, but the surgeon should be able to feel the cardia closing completely when the tip of the bougie is pulled into the esophagus. Thus, the opening of the cardia and distal esophagus has been converted into a long channel.

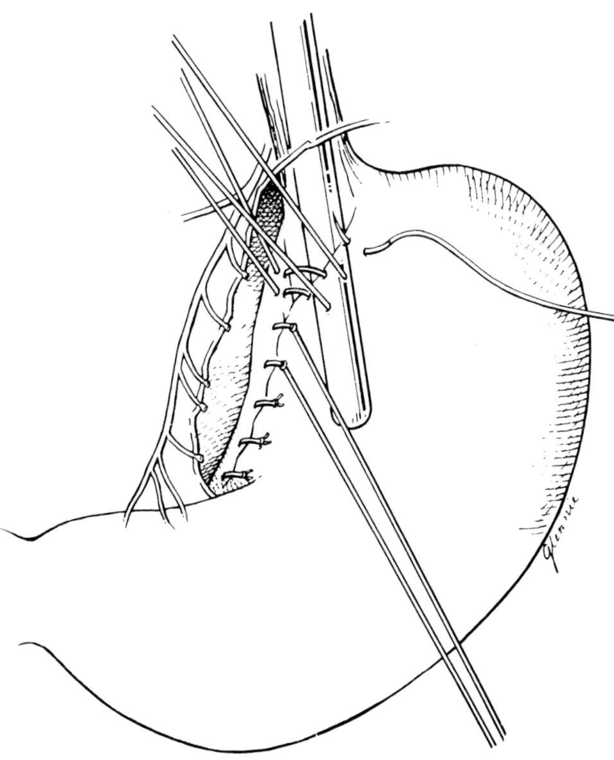

FIGURE 27–10 ■ Sutures for calibration of the cardia, including its anterior and posterior portions.

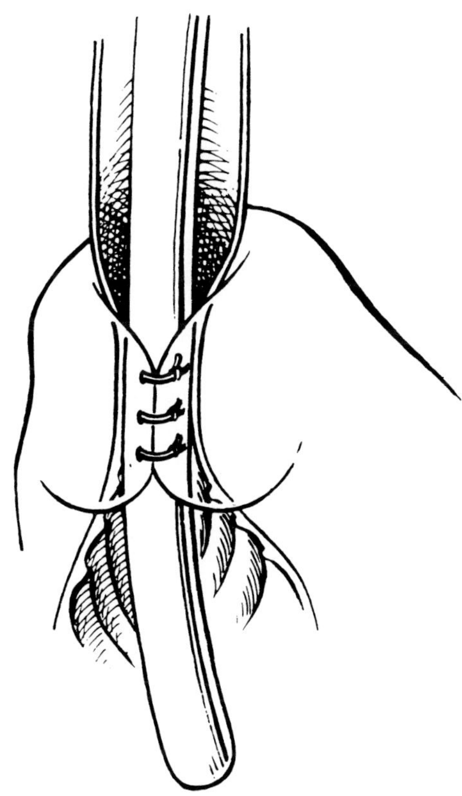

FIGURE 27–11 ■ Calibration of the cardia with a Hurst bougie (30 French).

Posterior Gastropexy

Posterior gastropexy is similar to the Hill repair (Hill, 1967) and creates a long segment of intra-abdominal esophagus. It is not necessary, however, to dissect out the median arcuate ligament; rather, this ligament can be picked up together with the crus of the diaphragm with the use of a special Babcock clamp.

The surgeon begins the posterior gastropexy by placing two seromuscular nonabsorbable sutures in the anterior and posterior surfaces of the stomach near the lesser curvature, just below the cardia (Fig. 27–12). The median arcuate ligament is identified in front of the aorta, just proximal to the celiac axis and below the junction of both crura (Fig. 27–13). With the second and third fingers of the right hand, the assistant pulls the celiac trunk distally, and a large Babcock clamp is used to firmly grasp the preaortic fascia, including the median arcuate ligament. Without further dissection, each of the two sutures is passed through this fibromuscular tissue by lifting of

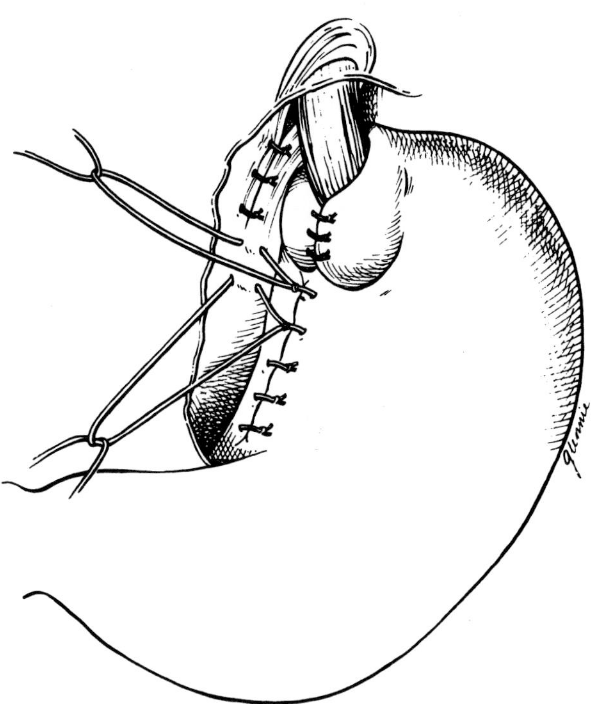

FIGURE 27–12 ■ Sutures for posterior gastropexy.

the clamp upward, permitting the sutures to pass easily without damage to the aorta.

Anterior Fundophrenopexy

We have noted that an anterior paraesophageal hernia occurred in up to 5% of patients 3 to 5 years after antireflux surgery (Csendes et al, 1985). To avoid this complication, two sutures must be placed in the anterior surface of the stomach to secure it to the diaphragm (Fig. 27–14).

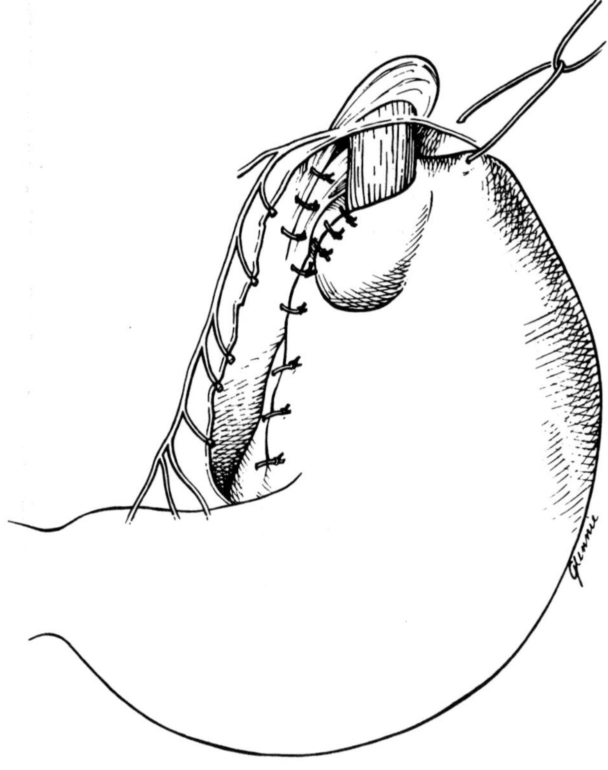

FIGURE 27–14 ■ Completed operation, including the sutures for the fundophrenopexy.

Calibration is again checked with the Hurst bougie, which has remained in the stomach during these maneuvers. The bougie is now withdrawn, and a soft nasogastric tube (14 French) is passed into the stomach. No abdomi-

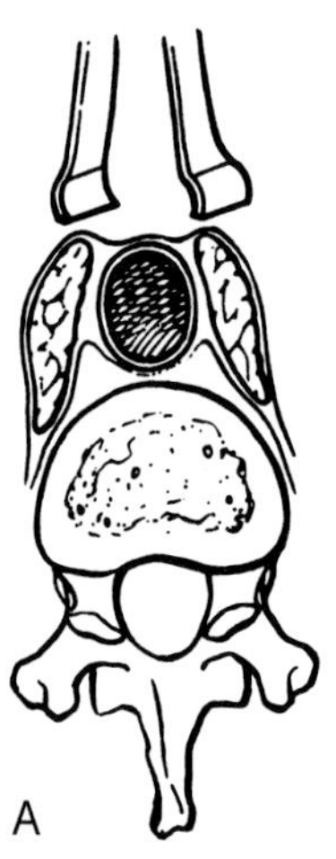

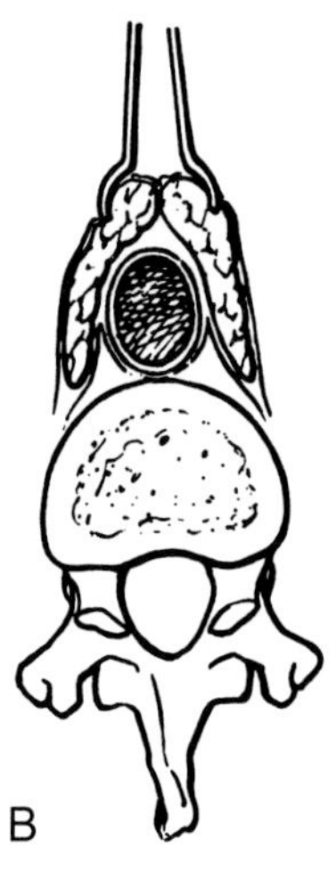

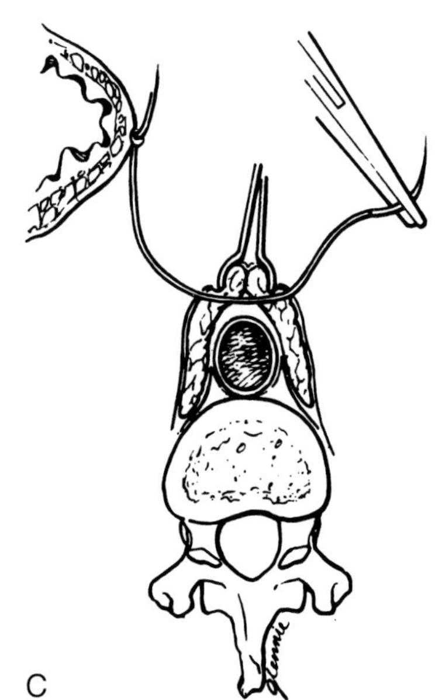

FIGURE 27–13 ■ *A–C,* Sutures for posterior gastropexy, which include the crural decussation and the median arcuate ligament in front of the aorta.

nal drainage is used. The nasogastric tube is removed 24 hours later, and oral feeding is begun on the second day after surgery. Patients are discharged from the hospital 5 days after surgery.

Fundoplication

The main steps of the fundoplication operation are:

1. HSV.
2. Closure of the limbs of the right crus of the diaphragm.
3. A 360-degree, loose fundoplication.
4. Anterior fundophrenopexy.

Steps 1, 2, and 4 are performed exactly as already described for the combined operation. The 360-degree fundoplication, or any variation thereof, is extremely easy to perform after completion of the HSV, which allows clear identification and dissection of the distal esophagus, the esophagogastric junction, and the lesser and greater curvatures. The gastric fundus is easily rotated behind the abdominal esophagus. Following section of two or three short vessels, four nonabsorbable sutures are placed in such a way that the more proximal and the more distal of sutures include esophageal muscular wall, to avoid complications of the fundoplication such as intussusception, or the "slipped Nissen."

A 30 French bougie is kept in place during this operation. The purpose of the fundoplication is to create a long intra-abdominal segment of esophagus and a "cuff" that exerts pressure against the abdominal portion of the sphincter. The bougie is then withdrawn, and a nasogastric tube is left in place as described previously.

Results

The results in a group of 215 patients who underwent antireflux surgery have been reported elsewhere (Csendes et al, 1989). Table 27–1 shows the early postoperative results of antireflux techniques employed in patients with uncomplicated reflux esophagitis operated on between 1980 and 1995. A total of 535 patients with mild and moderate esophagitis underwent operation during a period of 15 years.

No operative mortality occurred, and early postoperative complications were low in incidence. The late results in 180 patients followed up for 5 or more years after surgery, and covering the years 1980 to 1991, are shown in Table 27–2. Excellent or good results were observed in 85%. Table 27–3 shows the early and late results in 152 patients with severe esophagitis and complicated Barrett's esophagus who underwent surgery between 1980 and 1992 (Csendes et al, 1998).

TABLE 27–1 ■ **Early Results of Open Antireflux Surgery (1980–1995) for Esophagitis (Grades 0 to III) in 535 Patients**

Postoperative Results	*Highly Selective Vagotomy + Fundoplication (n = 210)*	*Highly Selective Vagotomy + Posterior Gastropexy and Cardial Calibration (n = 325)*
Well patients	201 (95.7%)	308 (94.8%)
Morbidity	9 (4.3%)	17 (5.2%)
Mortality	0	0
		$P > .05$

TABLE 27–2 ■ **Late Results of Antireflux Surgery (1980–1991): Five or More Years After Operation for Esophagitis (Visick Grades I–IV) in 180 Patients**

Grade	*No.*	*Percent (%)*	
I (excellent)	128	71	
II (well)	25	14	
III (fair)	12	7	} 15
IV (surgical failure and/or reoperation)	15	8	

LAPAROSCOPIC ANTIREFLUX SURGERY

The principles that have been used for classic open antireflux surgery can be employed for an adequate laparoscopic antireflux surgery (Awad et al, 1997). In 85 patients, we have performed a 360-degree Nissen fundoplication, employing the "right posterior" approach instead of the "left approach" used by others (Csendes et al, 1996). The principles of this operation are as follows.

Dissection of the esophagogastric junction and abdominal esophagus is performed, in similar fashion as for HSV but without a complete, standard HSV (Figs. 27–15 and 27–16). This requires beginning dissection in the midportion of the lesser curvature, dissecting the anterior and posterior attachments of the lesser omentum along the lesser curvature of the stomach but without the necessity of dividing the branches of the "crow's foot." Next, a 4- to 5-cm length of the abdominal esophagus is dissected. The surgeon then divides two or three short gastric vessels through a right posterior approach, entering the lesser sac and exposing the posterior surface of the stomach. This approach makes it extremely easy to identify and section the short gastric vessels, obviating

TABLE 27–3 ■ **Early and Late Results of Classic Antireflux Surgery in Patients with Barrett's Esophagus (Cardial Calibration or Fundoplication)**

	Patients (n = 152)	
	No.	*Percent (%)*
Operative mortality	1	0.7
Postoperative morbidity	12	7.9
Follow-up (months)	106	
Lost to follow-up	10	6.6
True follow-up	141	93.4
Visick I and II status	58	41
Visick III and IV status	83	59
Subsequent dysplasia	15	10.6
Years after operation	8.5	
Subsequent adenocarcinoma	6	4
Years after operation	7	

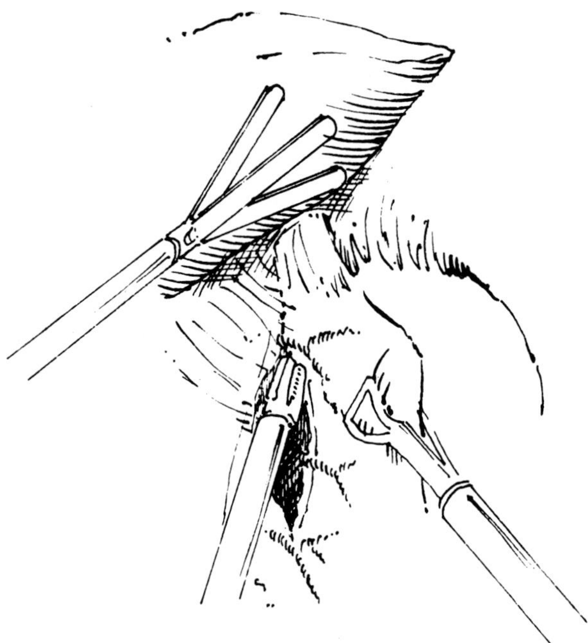

FIGURE 27–15 ■ Section of the lesser omentum in order to reach the esophagogastric junction by the right and posterior approach.

tension on the fundoplication. Then, the crus of the diaphragm is closed with nonabsorbable sutures (Fig. 27–17).

The fundoplication is performed exactly as described for the open route: 360-degree total fundoplication, 4 cm in length, with four nonabsorbable sutures while a 30 French bougie and a nasogastric tube are in place (Figs. 27–18 and 27–19). An anterior fundophrenopexy is always performed to avoid a subsequent anterior paraesophageal hernia. Patients usually leave the hospital after 72 hours. The results of the laparoscopic operation are shown in Table 27–4.

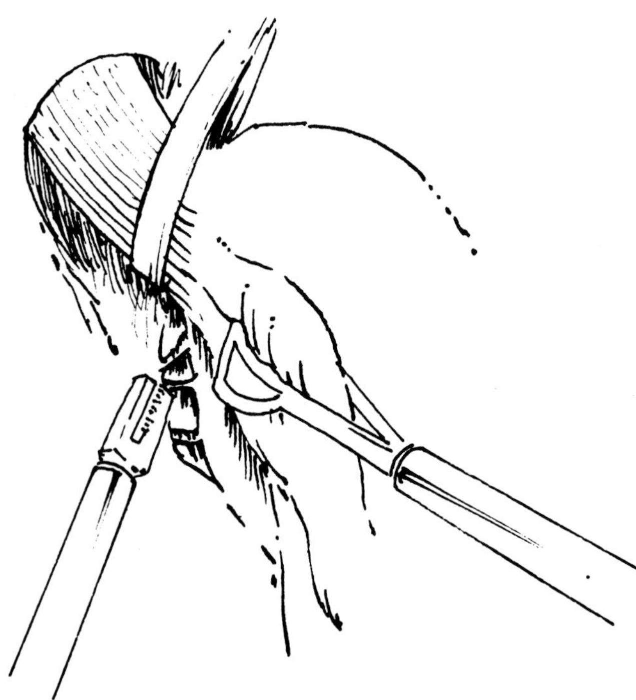

FIGURE 27–16 ■ Section of short vessels by the right posterior approach.

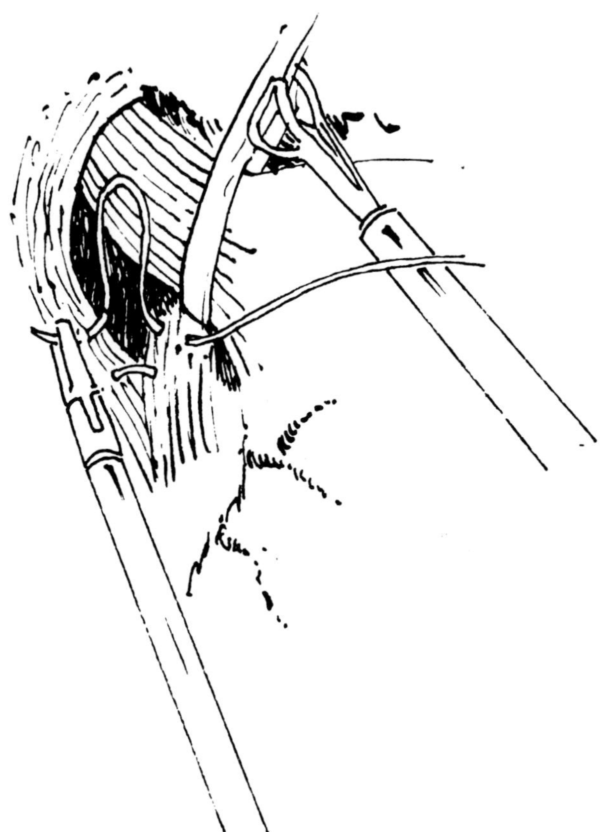

FIGURE 27–17 ■ Closure of the diaphragmatic crus.

TRUNCAL VAGOTOMY WITH PYLOROPLASTY

It is surprising, and inappropriate, that many surgeons have evaluated patients subjected to HSV and patients subjected to truncal vagotomy plus pyloroplasty as a single group. We must stress that in cases with reflux esophagitis, HSV is a completely different operation from truncal vagotomy and pyloroplasty, a technique advo-

TABLE 27–4 ■ **Early and Late Results of Laparoscopic Nissen Fundoplication by the "Right and Posterior" Approach**

	Patients (n = 85)	
	No.	*Percent (%)*
Operative mortality	0	
Postoperative morbidity	1	1.2
Follow-up (months)	36	
Visick I and II status	78	91.8
Visick III and IV status	7	8.2

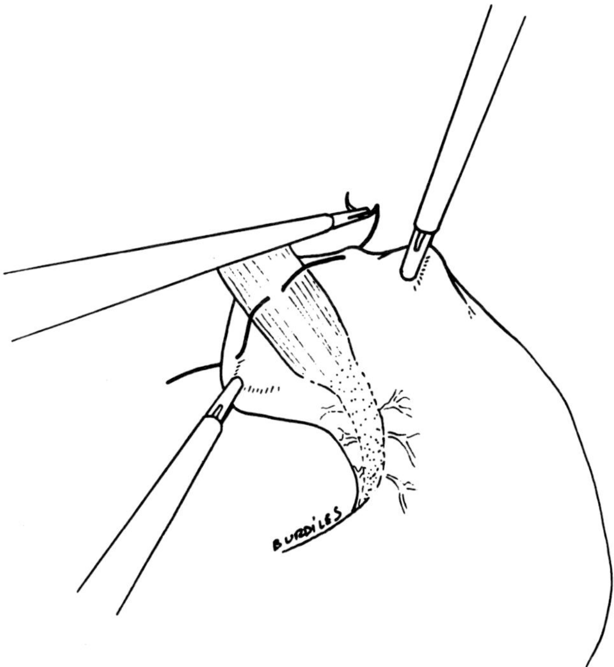

FIGURE 27–18 ■ Performance of 360-degree fundoplication by suturing the proximal stitch into the esophagus.

cated in the 1960s by some surgeons as a "balanced operation" for reflux esophagitis (Clarke et al, 1964; Harrington, 1962; Pearson et al, 1969).

Some researchers have added truncal vagotomy in patients with an associated duodenal ulcer (past or present) and in patients with peptic strictures or severe esophagitis (Casten, 1967; Mustard, 1970). This operation, however, profoundly impairs the antral pump, the pyloric sphincter, and gastric emptying. In addition, it promotes a great increase in duodenogastric alkaline reflux. Truncal vagotomy also raises the incidence of gallstone formation after surgery (Csendes et al, 1978a). We strongly advise against its use in patients with reflux esophagitis, and we have never used it in such cases.

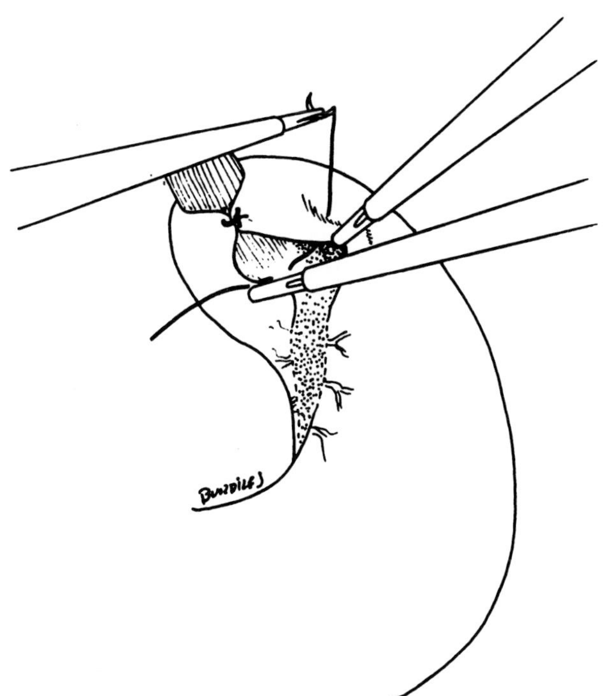

FIGURE 27–19 ■ Completion of fundoplication.

ACID SUPPRESSION AND BILE DIVERSION OPERATION

Classically, pathologic reflux esophagitis is considered a consequence of excessive and prolonged contact of esophageal mucosa with acid and pepsin refluxed from the stomach (Vaezi et al, 1995). There are, however, reports of reflux esophagitis occurring in the absence of acid reflux, for instance, after total gastrectomy and in patients with achlorhydria. The esophagitis in these cases appears to be due to the injurious effect of biliopancreatic components in refluxed material (Hellsinger, 1959; Palmer, 1960). In experimental models, the addition of bile salts to gastric refluxed can potentiate the deleterious effect of acid and pepsin to the esophageal mucosa, even in the presence of a pH below 4 (Harmon et al, 1981; Lillemoe et al, 1983). The presence of bile salts together with acid in the refluxate has been reported in humans, supporting the hypothesis that acid reflux may consist of a mixture of gastric and duodenal content, keeping the pH less than 4 (Gotley et al, 1988, 1991).

Experimental studies have clearly shown that enteroesophageal or duodenoesophageal reflux can induce the following conditions (Attwood et al, 1992):

- Severe epithelial damage with ulceration
- Intestinal metaplasia
- Adenocarcinoma of the distal esophagus

In an effort to demonstrate the presence of duodenal reflux into the esophagus, several researchers performed 24-hour ambulatory esophageal pH studies. Excessive exposure to pH greater than 7 was demonstrated in patients with severe esophagitis and Barrett's esophagus, suggesting that the high pH was due to duodenoesophageal reflux (Pellegrini et al, 1978; Stein, 1992, 1993). It has also been demonstrated that in more than 95% of cases, the finding of a pH greater than 7 in the esophagus is due to (1) retention of food, (2) inadequate calibration of the antimony electrode, (3) dental sepsis, (4) retention of saliva with deficient esophageal peristalsis, or (5) a combination of these factors (Devault et al, 1993; Singh et al, 1993). Such elevations of pH, therefore, do not reflect a precise measure of duodenoesophageal reflux.

Bechi and colleagues (1993) developed a portable spectrophotometer that detects bilirubin—a direct index of duodenogastroesophageal reflux. This new method demonstrated that duodenoesophageal reflux is a significant finding in patients with Barrett's esophagus, in contrast to patients with acid reflux esophagitis and to control patients (Kauer et al, 1995).

The DeMeester group propose the following five pathophysiologic features in patients with Barrett's esophagus (Oberg et al, 1998; Stein et al, 1993):

- An incompetent lower esophageal sphincter
- Impaired esophageal peristalsis

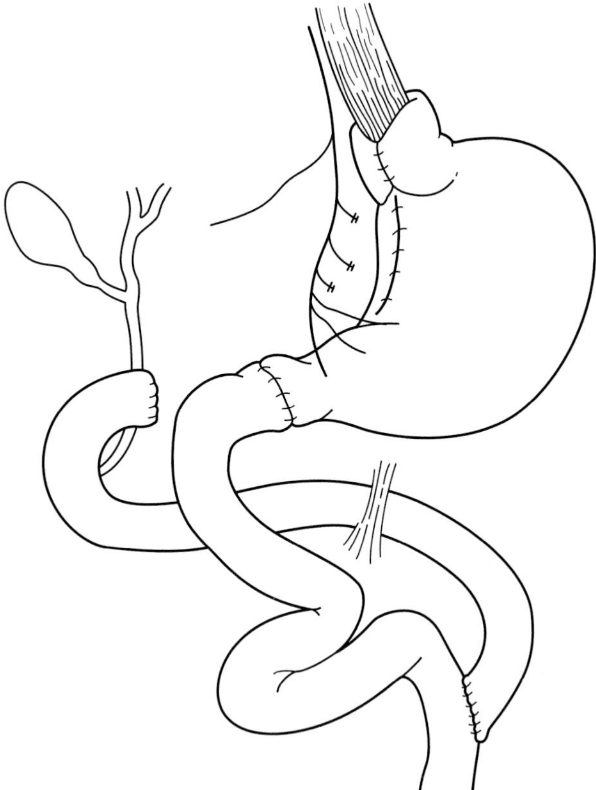

FIGURE 27–20 ■ Acid suppression and bile diversion by means of selective vagotomy and duodenojejunal terminal anastomosis to a 50-cm-long Roux-en-Y limb.

- Pathologic acid reflux
- Acid hypersecretion in some cases
- Excessive duodenoesophageal reflux

We have added a sixth constant finding—the presence of a dilated cardia or esophagogastric junction (Csendes, 1981; Korn and Csendes, 1999).

Results

When evaluating the results of surgery in patients with Barrett's esophagus, we have made two important observations. First, a majority of surgeons make no distinction between the results in patients with and without Barrett's esophagus. Since 1990, only 9 of more than 200 papers reviewed have reported the results of surgical treatment in patients with Barrett's esophagus as a separate or distinct group. Second, in the majority of the surgical reports, long-term follow-up is missing. If all patients are considered together in one group, the poor results in patients with Barrett's esophagus may be "buffered" by the good results obtained in patients without Barrett's esophagus.

We have observed an unacceptable incidence of poor late results in our patients with Barrett's esophagus managed with our standard antireflux operations (Csendes et al, 1998). Because the presence of duodenal reflux is a key factor in the pathogenesis of Barrett's esophagus, we have proposed two alternative operations in patients who have Barrett's esophagus and intestinal metaplasia, both procedures utilizing the principle of *bile diversion*. Our purpose was to improve the results in patients with Barrett's esophagus by performing a *combined procedure* with the following components:

- Antireflux surgery (either fundoplication of calibration of the cardia)
- Decrease or ablation of acid secretion by HSV or selective vagotomy with antrectomy
- Elimination of duodenal reflux by Roux-en-Y diversion, using a 50-cm jejunal loop

Two different types of surgery were performed:

1. Duodenal switch procedure plus HSV and antireflux surgery (Fig. 27–20).
2. Selective or truncal vagotomy, partial distal gastrectomy, antireflux surgery, and Roux-en-Y anastomosis with a 50-cm limb (Fig. 27–21).

The *duodenal switch procedure* consists of the following steps (Csendes et al, 1997):

1. HSV to decrease acid secretion and avoid anastomotic ulcer at the duodenojejunal anastomosis.
2. Antireflux surgery, as either a 360-degree total fun-

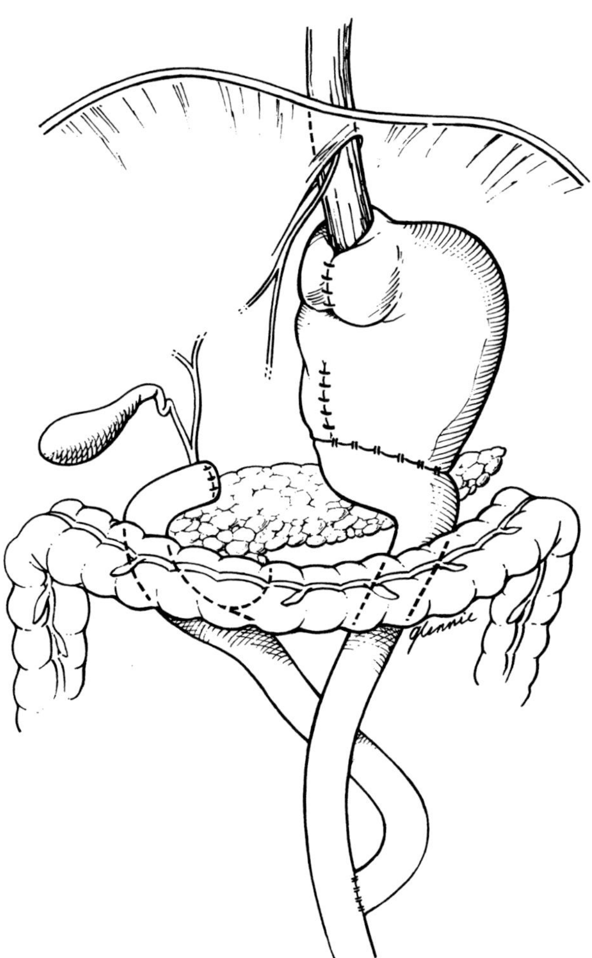

FIGURE 27–21 ■ Schematic representation of the suppression-diversion operation.

TABLE 27–5 ■ **Clinical Results of Bile Diversion Operation**

	Duodenal Switch Procedure (n = 75)	*Vagotomy Partial Gastrectomy and Roux-en-Y Anastomosis (n = 170)*
Operative mortality (%)	0	2 (1.2%)
Postoperative morbidity (%)	12	47
Follow-up (%)	95	92
Months of follow-up	55	74
Visick I and II status (%)	75	93.6
Visick III and IV status (%)	25	6.4
Appearance of dysplasia (%)	0	0
Appearance of adenocarcinoma (%)	0	0

doplication or "calibration" of the cardia plus posterior gastropexy.

3. Duodenal switch operation—performance of a duodenojejunal terminoterminal anastomosis using a 50-cm-long Roux-en-Y jejunal limb.

4. Closure of the crura of the diaphragm and anterior fundophrenopexy.

The steps of the *acid suppression and bile diversion procedure* are as follows:

1. Selective or truncal vagotomy to decrease gastric acid secretion.

2. Antireflux surgery, as either a 360-degree total fundoplication or "calibration" of the cardia plus posterior gastropexy.

3. Distal partial gastrectomy to abolish gastrin release and gastric acid secretion and to avoid acid reflux.

4. Gastrojejunoanastomosis with a 50-cm-long Roux-en-Y jejunal limb (see Fig. 27–21).

5. Closure of the crura of the diaphragm and anterior fundophrenopexy.

Selective vagotomy is performed in the same way as HSV, with division of both nerves of Latarjet. Completion of this vagotomy is similar to that in HSV, with exposure of at least 5 cm of the distal esophagus. Two or three short gastric vessels are divided to allow mobilization of the gastric fundus for performance of a proper antireflux surgery without tension.

Partial distal gastrectomy is performed with the use of mechanical staplers, preserving the gastroepiploic vessels along the greater curvature. Care is taken to avoid a dependent sump by including sufficient greater curvature in the gastric resection (Ferguson et al, 1990). The duodenum is divided and then is closed 1 to 2 cm distal to the pylorus with a stapler. The terminolateral gastrojejunostomy is performed with the use of manual sutures in an antiperistaltic fashion (Schirmer, 1994).

Our clinical results are summarized in Table 27–5. The duodenal switch procedure resulted in no mortality, whereas vagotomy and partial gastrectomy were associated with a mortality rate of 1.2%. At late follow-up, the results were significantly better after vagotomy and partial gastrectomy than after the duodenal switch procedure.

This difference can be explained by the observations summarized in Table 27–6, which shows the results of acid and duodenal reflux evaluations before and after surgery. Duodenal reflux is completely eliminated after both procedures by the long Roux-en-Y diversion. There is, however, much more acid reflux after the duodenal switch procedure than after vagotomy and partial gastrectomy. The latter procedure can completely suppress gastric acid secretion.

A beneficial effect of duodenal diversion was regression of low-grade dysplasia in more than 50% of the cases. This regression was observed after both procedures, and no progression or new dysplasia developed in any of the patients. This result appears to confirm the importance of duodenal reflux in the development of these preneoplastic histologic changes in patients with intestinal metaplasia in the distal esophageal mucosa.

COMMENTS AND CONTROVERSIES

The experience reported by Csendes and his colleagues in this chapter is unique. The senior author, Attila Csendes, has been clinically active in the field of antireflux surgery for more than 3 decades. He was among the earliest surgeons to adopt the Hill repair and to subsequently modify management with the addition of HSV. It is clear from this chapter that he has continued to select and adapt his surgical management over the years, as he has evaluated long-term follow-up results. Very few surgeons have so regularly reported such well-studied observations with long-term follow-up.

From a practical perspective, the Visick grading of reported results provides the most reasonable evaluation for long-term application. Economic factors and patient compliance are barriers to repeated and long-term evaluation with invasive studies such as 24-hour pH testing, manometry, and routine endoscopy. Patient satisfaction,

TABLE 27–6 ■ **Acid and Duodenal Reflux Before and After Surgery**

	Duodenal Switch Procedure		*Vagotomy (Partial) Gastrectomy and Roux-en-Y Anastomosis*	
	Preoperative	*Postoperative*	*Preoperative*	*Postoperative*
24-hr pH studies (% of time with pH less than 4 in 24 hr)	24.8 ± 1.9	4.8 ± 5.7	34.3 ± 19	1.1 ± 0.3
Bilitec studies (% of time with bilirubin with absorbance rate >0.2 in 24 hr)	23.5 ± 17	0.7 ± 0.7	27.8 ± 14	0.5 ± 0.3

after all, should remain the standard for evaluating results after surgery for symptomatic, benign esophageal disease.

These authors report very unfavorable long-term results for their "standard antireflux operations" in patients with Barrett's esophagus; results in only 41% of cases can be rated as Visick grade I or II. I believe that a proportion of these poor results may be the result of failure to recognize the complication of acquired short esophagus in many patients with advanced reflux esophagitis, which certainly includes the group with acquired columnar epithelial replacement, or Barrett's esophagus. The authors of this chapter make no mention of this complication. Any local reconstruction may fail, if significant acquired shortening is not considered in the repair, by some tension-reducing modification, such as a lengthening gastroplasty.

I am certain that the operation consisting of acid suppression and bile diversion is very effective in relieving the symptoms of acid and alkaline reflux. At present, however, I recommend that this more complex procedure be reserved for relatively few, well-selected complex cases in which the anatomy at the level of the esophagogastric junction is judged to preclude a local antireflux reconstruction. Such cases include patients who have undergone previous (usually multiple) failed operations. Nevertheless, the very favorable results reported by Csendes and his colleagues are a strong testimonial to the effectiveness of this combined operation for symptom control. Their relatively preliminary data also suggest that this operation is capable of preventing the progression of dysplasia and reducing the incidence of subsequent adenocarcinoma at the esophagogastric junction.

F. G. P.

■ KEY REFERENCES

Csendes A, Braghetto I, Burdiles P, et al: Long term results of classic antireflux surgery in 152 patients with Barrett's esophagus: Clinical, radiologic, endoscopic, manometric, and acid reflux test analysis before and late after operation. Surgery 123:645, 1998.

Csendes A, Braghetto I, Korn O, Cortés C: Late subjective and objective evaluations of antireflux surgery in patients with reflux esophagitis: Analysis of 215 patients. Surgery 105:374, 1989.

■ REFERENCES

Amdrup E: Parietal cell (highly selective) vagotomy for duodenal ulcer. In Dudley H, Rob C, Smith R (eds): Operative Surgery Abdomen, 3rd ed. London, Butterworth, 1977, p 137.

Attwood SEA, Smyrk TC, DeMeester TR, et al: Duodenoesophageal reflux and the development of adenocarcinoma in rats. Surgery 111:503, 1992.

Awad W, Csendes A, Braghetto I, et al: Laparoscopic highly selective vagotomy: Technical considerations and preliminary results in 119 patients with duodenal ulcer or gastroesophageal reflux disease. World J Surg 21:261, 1997.

Bechi P, Paucciani F, Baldini F, et al: Long-term ambulatory enterogastric reflux monitoring: Validation of a new fiberoptic technique. Dig Dis Sci 38:1297, 1993.

Boesby S: Relationship between gastroesophageal acid reflux, basal gastroesophageal sphincter pressure and gastric acid secretion. Scand J Gastroenterol 12:547, 1977.

Bonavina L, Evander A, DeMeester TR, et al: Length of the distal esophageal sphincter and competence of the cardia. Ann Surg 151:25, 1986.

Braash IT, Sala LE, Ellis EM: Parietal cell vagotomy: Its effect in lower esophageal sphincter function. Arch Surg 115:699, 1980.

Casten DF: Peptic esophagitis, hiatus hernia and duodenal ulcer: A unified concept. Am J Surg 113:638, 1967.

Clarke ID, Border HE, Winner RB: Treatment of hiatus hernia by hiatus herniorrhaphy, vagotomy and drainage procedure. Am J Surg 107:253, 1964.

Csendes A: A modified posterior cardio-gastropexy for surgical treatment of gastroesophageal reflux with the adding of highly selective vagotomy and bougie calibration. In Belsey R, Moraldi A (eds): Medical and Surgical Problems of the Esophagus. San Diego, Academic Press, 1981, p 91.

Csendes A: Highly selective vagotomy, posterior gastropexy and calibration of the cardia for reflux esophagitis. In Siewart JR, Holscher AH (eds): Diseases of the Esophagus. New York, Springer-Verlag, 1987, p 1272.

Csendes A, Braghetto I, Burdiles P, et al: A new physiological approach for the surgical treatment of patients with Barrett's esophagus. Ann Surg 226:123, 1997.

Csendes A, Braghetto I, Burdiles P, et al: Long term results of classic antireflux surgery in 152 patients with Barrett's esophagus: Clinical, radiologic, endoscopic, manometric and acid reflux test before and late after operation. Surgery 123:645, 1998.

Csendes A, Braghetto I, Korn O, et al: Late subjective and objective evaluations of antireflux surgery in patients with reflux esophagitis: Analysis of 215 patients. Surgery 105:374, 1989.

Csendes A, Braghetto I, Velasco N: A comparison of three surgical techniques for the treatment of reflux esophagitis: A prospective study. In DeMeester TR, Skinner DB (eds): Esophageal Disorders: Pathophysiology and Therapy. New York, Raven Press, 1985, p 177.

Csendes A, Burdiles P, Díaz JC, et al: Subjective and objective evaluation of the results of laparoscopic antireflux surgery in patients with gastroesophageal reflux. Rev Méd Chile 124:1077, 1996.

Csendes A, Larach J, Godoy M: Incidence of gallstone development after selective hepatic vagotomy. Acta Chir Scand 144:289, 1978a.

Csendes A, Larraín A: Effect of posterior gastropexy on gastroesophageal sphincter pressure and symptomatic reflux in patients with hiatal hernia. Gastroenterology 63:19, 1972.

Csendes A, Miranda M, Espinoza M, Braghetto I: Perimeter and location of the muscular gastroesophageal junction or 'cardia' in control subjects and in patients with reflux esophagitis or achalasia. Scand J Gastroenterol 16:951, 1981.

Csendes A, Oster MI, Brandsborg O: Gastroesophageal sphincter pressure and serum gastrin in relation to food intake before and after vagotomy. Scand J Gastroenterol 13:437, 1978b.

Csendes A, Oster MI, Brandsborg O, et al: Effect of vagotomy on human gastroesophageal sphincter pressure in the resting state and following increase in intraabdominal pressure. Surgery 85:419, 1979a.

Csendes A, Oster MI, Moller IT, et al: Effect of extrinsic denervation of the lower end of the esophageal sphincter in man. Surg Gynecol Obstet 148:375, 1979b.

Csendes A, Oster MI, Moller IT, et al: Gastroesophageal reflux in duodenal ulcer patients before and after vagotomy. Ann Surg 188:804, 1978c.

Csendes A, Velasco N, Amat J: Highly selective vagotomy: Preoperative studies and mortality. Rev Chil Cir 31:165, 1979c.

DeMeester TR, Wernley JA, Bryant GH, et al: Clinical and in-vitro analysis of determinants of gastroesophageal competence. Am J Surg 157:39, 1979.

Devault KR, Georgeson S, Castell DO: Salivary stimulation mimics esophageal exposure to refluxed duodenal content. Am J Gastroenterol 88:1040, 1993.

Ferguson GH, Rose M, Maclennan I, et al: Vomiting after Roux-en-Y biliary diversion: Relationship to surgical technique. Br J Surg 77:548, 1990.

Gotley DC, Morgan AP, Ball D, et al: Composition of gastroesophageal refluxate. Gut 32:1093, 1991.

Gotley DC, Morgan AP, Cooper MJ: Bile acid concentrations in the refluxate of patients with reflux oesophagitis. Br J Surg 75:587, 1988.

Harmon JW, Johnson LF, Maydonivitch CL: Effects of acid and bile salts on the rabbit esophageal mucosa. Dig Dis Sci 26:65, 1981.

Harrington JL: Treatment of esophageal hiatal hernia. Arch Surg 84:370, 1962.

Hellsinger H: Oesophagitis following total gastrectomy: A follow-up study on 9 patients 5 years or more after operation. Acta Chir Scand 118:190, 1959.

Hill LD: An effective operation for hiatal hernia: An eight-year appraisal. Ann Surg 166:681, 1967.

Kauer WKH, Burdiles P, Ireland AP, et al: Does duodenal juice reflux into the esophagus of patients with complicated GERD? Evaluation of a fiberoptic sensor for bilirubin. Am J Surg 169:98, 1995.

Korn O, Csendes A, Burdiles P, et al: Anatomic dilatation of the cardia and competence of the lower esophageal sphincter: A clinical and experimental study. J Gastrointest Surg 4:398, 2000.

Lillemoe KD, Johnson LE, Harmon JW: Alkaline esophagitis: A comparison of the ability of components of gastroduodenal contents to injure rabbit mucosa. Gastroenterology 85:621, 1983.

Mustard RA: A survey of techniques and results of a hiatus hernia repair. Surg Gynecol Obstet 230:131, 1970.

Oberg S, Clark GWB, DeMeester TR: Barrett's esophagus: Update of pathophysiology and management. Hepatogastroenterology 45:1348, 1998.

Oster MI, Csendes A, Fünch-Jensen P, Amdrup E: PVC and modified Hill procedure as surgical treatment of reflux esophagitis: Results in 108 patients. World J Surg 6:412, 1982.

Palmer DE: Subacute erosive ("peptic") esophagitis associated with achlorhydria. N Engl J Med 262:927. 1960.

Pearson FG, Stone RM, Parrish RM: Role of vagotomy and pyloroplasty in the therapy of symptomatic hiatus hernia. Am J Surg 117:130, 1969.

Pellegrini CA, DeMeester TR, Wernly JA, et al: Alkaline gastroesophageal reflux. Am J Surg 75:177, 1978.

Rossetti M, Hell K: Fundoplication for the treatment of gastroesophageal reflux in hiatal hernia. World J Surg 1:439, 1977.

Schirmer BD: Gastric atony and the Roux syndrome. Gastroenterol Clin North Am 23:327, 1994.

Singh S, Bradley LA, Richter JE: Determinants of esophageal 'alkaline' pH environment in controls and patients with GER disease. Gut 34:309, 1993.

Skinner D, Belsey R: Surgical management of esophageal reflux and hiatus hernia: Long term results with 1030 patients. J Thorac Cardiovasc Surg 53:33, 1967.

Staadas J, Aune S: Intragastric pressure volume relationship before and after vagotomy. Acta Clin Scand 136:611, 1970.

Stein HJ, DeMeester TR, Hinder RA: Outpatient physiological testing and surgical management of foregut motor disorders. Curr Probl Surg 24:418, 1992.

Stein HJ, Haeft S, DeMeester T: Functional, foregut abnormalities in Barrett's esophagus. J Thorac Cardiovasc Surg 105:107, 1993.

Vaezi MF, Singh S, Richter JE: Role of acid and duodenogastric reflux in esophageal mucosal injury: A review of animal and human studies. Gastroenterology 108:1897, 1995.

Wilbur BG, Kelly KA: Effect of proximal gastric and truncal vagotomy on canine gastric activity, motility and emptying. Ann Surg 178:295, 1973.

CHAPTER **28**

Esophagectomy for Benign Disease

Pasquale Ferraro
André Duranceau

HISTORICAL NOTE

Esophagotomy for the removal of impacted foreign bodies has been recorded in France as early as 1701. Although the first partial resection of the cervical esophagus was reported by Czerny of Heidelberg in 1877, early attempts at resection of the intrathoracic esophagus in the late 19th century proved to be fatal because the principles of positive-pressure ventilation had yet to be developed. Denk of Vienna (1913) demonstrated in cadavers the possibility of avoiding an open thoracotomy and removing the entire esophagus through a blunt transhiatal route. It was also in 1913 that the first successful transthoracic esophagectomy for a squamous cell cancer of the middle third was performed by Franz Torek of New York. The patient, refusing to undergo alimentary tract reconstruction, survived more than 13 years. Attempts at transthoracic esophagectomies by Meyer (1909), Lilienthal (1921), and Hedblom (1922), however, reported high rates of mortality caused by anesthetic problems, anastomotic dehiscence, and pleural sepsis. In 1933, a successful transhiatal esophagectomy was carried out by Grey Turner in Newcastle, England.

Dilatation and bougienage of esophageal strictures have been commonly practiced for centuries. Relieving the obstruction of undilatable strictures, however, remained problematic, and by the early 1900s physicians were suggesting routes to bypass the diseased esophagus. Antethoracic esophagoplasties using skin tubes or jejunum were thus developed by Wullstein (1904) and Bircher (1907). Unfortunately, these surgical procedures required multiple stages, were highly morbid, and produced less than satisfactory results. Once again, transthoracic procedures aimed at bypassing or resecting the strictures awaited the advent of secure ventilatory support. By 1946, Reinhoff, in Baltimore, reported three successful cases of partial esophagectomy and transthoracic reconstruction.

With esophagectomy being possible through both the transhiatal and transthoracic routes, surgeons turned their attention to methods of reconstruction to restore continuity of the alimentary tract. Antethoracic skin tubes, popular at the turn of the 20th century, were discarded as a number of different conduits became available. Techniques were developed with replacement organs, such as the jejunum (Roux, 1907), the transverse colon (Kelling, 1911), and the whole stomach (Kirschner, 1920). By the mid-1940s, alimentary tract continuity could be safely re-established with seemingly acceptable functional results. Later, the development of microvascular surgery permitted the use of free jejunal grafts to bridge the gap between conventional conduits, or as substitutes when no other organ was available for reconstruction.

The second half of the 20th century saw pioneers such as Ivor Lewis (London), Richard Sweet (Boston), and Ronald Belsey (Bristol) further define the indications and perfect the techniques of esophageal resection and reconstruction.

■ *HISTORICAL READINGS*

Bircher E: Ein Beitrag zur plastischen Bildung eines neuen Oesophagus. Zentralbl Chir 34:1479, 1907.

Czerny V: Neue Operationen. Zentralbl Chir 4:433–434, 1877.

Denk W: Zur Radikaloperation des Oesophagus-karzinom. Zentralbl Chir 40:1065–1068, 1913.

Hedblom C: Combined transpleural and transperitoneal resection of the thoracic esophagus and cardia for carcinoma. Surg Gynecol Obstet 35:284–287, 1922.

Kelling G: Oesophagoplastik mit Hilfe des Querkolon. Zentralbl Chir 38:1209–1212, 1911.

Kirschner M: Ein neues Verfahren der Oesophagoplastik. Arch Klin Chir 114:606–663, 1920.

Lilienthal H: Carcinoma of the thoracic oesophagus: Successful resection. Ann Surg 74:116–120, 1921.

Meyer W: Oesophagogastrostomy after intrathoracic resection of the oesophagus. Ann Surg 50:175–189, 1909.

Rienhoff WF: Intrathoracic esophagojejunostomy for lesions of the upper third of the esophagus. South Med J 39:928–940, 1946.

Roux C: L'oesphago-jejuno-gastrostomie, nouvelle operation pour le rétrécissement infranchissable de l'oesophage. Semana Med 27:37–40, 1907.

Torek F: The first successful case of resection of the thoracic portion of the oesophagus for carcinoma. Surg Gynecol Obstet 16:614–617, 1913.

Turner GG: Excision of the thoracic oesophagus for carcinoma with construction of an extra-thoracic gullet. Lancet 2:1315–1316, 1933.

Wullstein L: Ueber antethorakale Oesophago-jejunostomie und Operationen nach gleichen Prinzip. Dtsch Med Wochenschr 31:734–736, 1904.

GASTROESOPHAGEAL REFLUX DISEASE

Failed control of pathologic gastroesophageal reflux may lead to irreversible esophageal damage and progressive loss of function. Severe intractable symptoms and incapacitating dysphagia develop, and with end-stage disease, stricture formation or Barrett's esophagus is commonly found. When both medical management and repeated antireflux operations have failed, resection of the diseased esophagus may become the only valid alternative. Esophagectomy for complications of gastroesophageal reflux disease (GERD), fortunately, is a rare occurrence, even in centers with an interest in complex esophageal disorders. Careful preoperative evaluation and patient selection are essential to obtain satisfactory long-term functional results with acceptable rates of morbidity and mortality.

Indications for esophagectomy in this group of patients are usually related to the presence of a nondilatable peptic stricture, complications of Barrett's esophagus such as hemorrhage or perforation, or previous multiple, failed antireflux operations (Table 28–1). Dysplasia in a columnar-lined mucosa as a premalignant condition is not discussed here.

Stricture formation in the distal esophagus results from the inflammatory reaction induced by prolonged exposure to acid, bile, and pancreatoduodenal secretions. With time, the mucosa develops erosion and ulcerations and the submucosa is the site of intense inflammation and fibrosis. Scarring eventually extends through the muscular layers, invading the whole thickness of the esophageal wall as well as the periesophageal soft tissues (Ismail-Beigi et al, 1970). Luminal narrowing invariably develops, and as the normal anatomy of the muscle layers is obliterated, associated loss of motor function ensues.

Once a common finding, the incidence of peptic strictures has decreased significantly with the advent of more effective medical therapy to control gastric acid production. In Skinner and Belsey's series of more than 2000 adult patients undergoing antireflux surgery, strictures were found in 15.2% of cases (Skinner and Belsey, 1967). Stricture formation is estimated to occur in 1% to 5% of patients presenting with esophagitis (Ben Rejeb et al, 1992; Loof et al, 1993). Usually, symptoms of gastroesophageal reflux can be elicited in more than 75% of patients found to have strictures (Bonavina et al, 1995; Patterson et al, 1983). The development of a stricture is associated with heartburn, slow progressive dysphagia, and epigastric pain. Secondary disorders of peristalsis, common in patients with severe reflux, also contribute to the patients' symptomatology, as reported by Singh and associates (1992) and Dakkak and colleagues (1993). Although uncommon in more recent years, mucosal ulceration with chronic blood loss leading to anemia and malnutrition are still noted in the occasional patient.

Anatomically, peptic strictures are found at the squamocolumnar junction in the distal esophagus. In patients with a shortened esophagus, a large type I hiatal hernia, or Barrett's esophagus, the stricture may be situated as high as the level of the aortic arch. As described by Sandry (1972), peptic strictures are invariably accompanied by some degree of acquired shortening. Further, as the luminal narrowing progresses, the stricture acts as a protective barrier and limits reflux and secondary esophagitis more proximally. In late stages, as the proximal esophagitis heals, a long fibrotic stricture may take on the appearance of a malignant lesion.

TABLE 28–1 ■ Indications for Esophagectomy in Gastroesophageal Reflux Disease

Nondilatable peptic stricture
Complications of Barrett's esophagus (perforation, bleeding)
Multiple previous, failed antireflux operations

Patients presenting with a stricture require a thorough evaluation to confirm the clinical diagnosis, to help establish the cause of the stricture, and to exclude an underlying malignancy. In addition, important issues concerning patient management and preoperative decision making depend on results of the investigation. On upper gastrointestinal barium studies, peptic strictures show a smooth, tapered conical outline with possible ulcerations or craters. The studies are also helpful in defining the site of the stricture, the degree of luminal narrowing, and the presence of a hiatal hernia or shortened esophagus. Under no circumstances, however, can a malignant stenotic lesion be excluded with certainty on the basis of a contrast study alone.

Endoscopic examination of a stricture is invaluable in obtaining a histologic diagnosis, in assessing for the presence of esophagitis and Barrett's esophagus, and in ruling out cancer with four-quadrant biopsies and brush cytology. Furthermore, endoscopy is useful in establishing the need for dilatation and the feasibility of obtaining a sufficient lumen to permit adequate oral intake. To select the most appropriate therapy, the patient workup must be completed with a functional evaluation, including a motility and 24-hour pH monitoring study as well as a radionuclide gastric emptying study.

Medical therapy, including dietary modifications, weight loss, and smoking cessation, plays an important role in all patients with a peptic stricture. Esophageal dilatation is also used as an initial form of therapy in all cases because it is relatively safe and effective. The success of nonsurgical therapy, however, is variable and difficult to assess, as reported by Ferguson (1994). Outcome is dependent on the length of follow-up, the criteria used to define success, and the associated therapy. Overall, dilatation combined with acid suppression is adequate therapy in 75% of patients and carries a 2% to 3% complication rate (Kadakia et al, 1993; Ogilvie et al, 1980; Patterson et al, 1983; Stoddard and Simms, 1984; Yamamoto et al, 1992).

Generally, with ongoing medical therapy, a single dilation is sufficient to relieve dysphagia in 20% to 30% of patients.

Patients with a peptic stricture who are not candidates for medical therapy and dilation or who do not respond to conservative measures should be considered for surgery unless their overall condition or cardiopulmonary status contraindicates general anesthesia. Specific indications are thus as follows:

1. Recurrent strictures after successful dilatation.
2. Persistent esophagitis despite maximal medical therapy.
3. The need for prolonged treatment in a young patient.

4. Presence of a large hiatal hernia with esophageal shortening.
5. Barrett's esophagus.

Certain issues, however, remain controversial, such as the definition of prolonged treatment and the indications for surgery in nonmalignant Barrett's esophagus.

Surgical options for peptic strictures are numerous and include:

1. Fundoplication (total or partial).
2. Elongation gastroplasty with fundoplication.
3. Stricturoplasty (Thal) with fundoplication.
4. Acid suppression and bile diversion.
5. Esophageal resection and reconstruction.

Results of surgery in this setting have been difficult to interpret because the definition of success varies greatly and few authors present long-term follow-up data.

In the presence of a stricture and a shortened esophagus, or columnar-lined Barrett's esophagus, we believe that the addition of an elongation gastroplasty to the fundoplication is necessary in all cases to ensure satisfactory results. With this procedure, success rates of 75% to 100% have been reported by Pearson and co-workers (1987), Stirling and Orringer (1989), Henderson and colleagues (1990), and our group (Chen et al, 1999).

The decision to proceed with an esophagectomy for a benign peptic stricture is a difficult one. Commonly recognized indications include:

1. An undilatable stricture.
2. An esophageal perforation during dilatation.
3. A stricture in the presence of severe dysplasia in a columnar-lined mucosa.
4. A stricture with a possible underlying malignancy.

In a subset of patients, failed multiple previous antireflux operations also constitute an indication for resection.

An "undilatable" stricture is generally defined as (1) failure to pass any dilatator because of luminal narrowing or tortuosity, (2) failure to relieve dysphagia, (3) increasing frequency of dilatation at short intervals, and (4) previous perforation or rupture during dilatation (Fig. 28–1). In the management of benign strictures, as reported by Mansour and colleagues (1981), the presence of an undilatable stricture represented the indication for resection in 68% of patients. Similarly, in a report by Little and associates (1988), 18 of 50 patients with operated nonmalignant strictures required esophageal resection for undilatable strictures, Barrett's ulcer, or mucosal dysplasia. Esophagectomy for undilatable strictures was necessary in 22% of patients with benign strictures from reflux disease, as noted by Bonavina and colleagues (1995).

Orringer (2000) has presented the most extensive experience of esophageal resections for strictures with a series of 75 patients. End-stage GERD with strictures was the indication for surgery in 56% of the 75 cases.

Esophagectomy for complications of GERD other than strictures include hemorrhage and perforations. With the advent of more effective medical therapy, these complications have, fortunately, become increasingly rare. In patients with columnar-lined Barrett's mucosa, however, penetrating ulcers are found in 10% to 15% of cases. These ulcers, similar to gastric ulcers, are well circumscribed and penetrate the columnar mucosa posteriorly. Associated symptoms include dysphagia and, occasionally, pain radiating to the back. Perforation into the mediastinum, pleural space, airway, or pericardium is possible (Altorki et al, 1990; Andersson and Nilsson, 1985). Although massive bleeding does occur from a Barrett ulcer, patients usually present with chronic iron deficiency anemia.

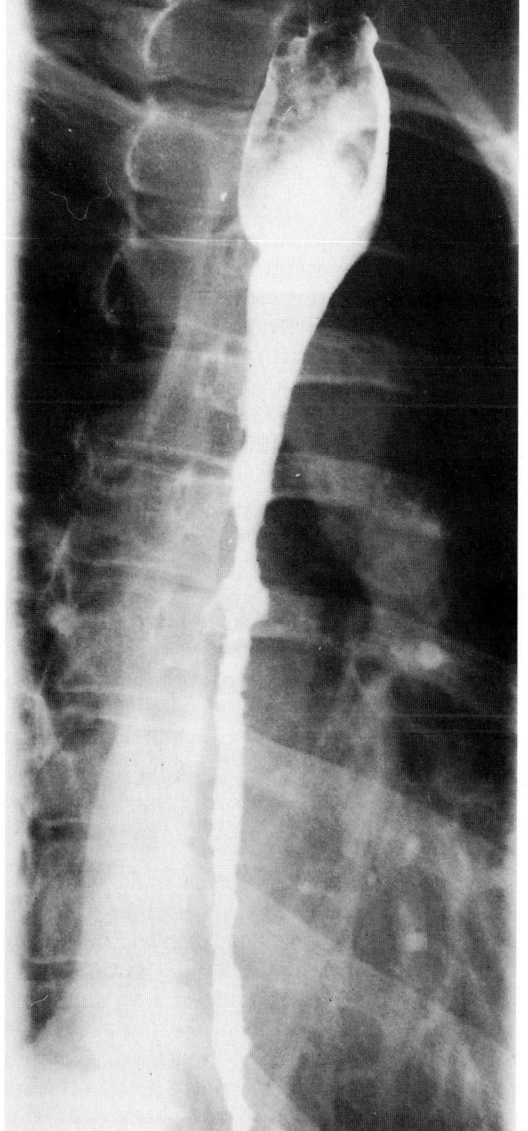

FIGURE 28–1 ■ Extensive nondilatable esophageal stricture requiring resection.

Management of Barrett's ulcer includes standard medical therapy using histamine H_2-blocker and proton-pump inhibitors for periods of 8 to 12 weeks. As reported by Williamson and associates (1992), although recurrence is common, as many as 85% of patients respond to an aggressive medical regimen. Ulcers that fail to heal or that recur despite adequate therapy should be considered for antireflux surgery.

Patients who present with a complicated Barrett ulcer generally require esophageal resection and reconstruction. In a study by Altorki and associates (1990), a penetrating ulcer was the most common indication for resection in nonmalignant Barrett's esophagus. Perforations were found in four patients with ulcers, and hematemesis requiring transfusions occurred in one patient. In our experience, complications of Barrett's esophagus, including deep penetrating ulcers, bleeding ulcers, perforations, and the association of strictures and ulcers, led to an esophagectomy in 10 patients from a group of 50 patients requiring resection for benign disease (Salamao et al, 1996).

Previous unsuccessful antireflux procedures also constitute a common indication for esophagectomy for benign disease. In patients who have undergone two or more previous attempts to control reflux disease, resection and reconstruction should be considered seriously. Repeated surgical procedures are associated with tissue damage, loss of function, and reduced blood supply leading to ischemic necrosis. Conserving a devitalized and dysfunctional esophagus invariably leads to progressive dysphagia, pain, and weight loss.

The proper selection of patients for esophageal resection in this setting is difficult. A number of reports have shown that after two previous antireflux procedures, results with a third intervention are satisfactory in only 50% to 60% of patients (Little et al, 1986; Pearson et al, 1987; Skinner, 1992; Stirling and Orringer, 1986). The need for esophagectomy, however, should not be based solely on the number of previous operations. The type of procedure as well as anatomic factors, such as the presence of esophageal shortening or fibrotic strictures, are usually of far greater significance. Specific indications for esophagectomy in these patients, as suggested by DeMeester's group, include (1) presence of severe dysphagia, (2) an undilatable stricture, and (3) esophageal organ failure, as defined by manometric criteria (Gadenstätter et al, 1998). "Organ failure" in that study was defined as the presence of more than 40% simultaneous waveforms, contractile amplitudes below the 5th percentile of normal (<25 mm Hg), or both. One should be cautious, however, with the definition and interpretation of organ failure. As noted by Orringer (1985) and Pearson and associates (1987), the severe functional abnormalities found in long-standing GERD generally do not contraindicate an antireflux procedure.

In a review of 23 esophageal resections after a failed antireflux procedure, Stirling and Orringer (1986) reported highly satisfactory results with a 0% operative mortality and a 22% complication rate. The functional outcome was considered good or excellent in 65% of patients. In a similar group of 17 patients requiring an esophagectomy, Gadenstätter and associates (1998) recorded no operative mortalities, a 24% complication rate, and good to excellent functional results in 81% of patients.

Furthermore, in the course of a repeated operation for reflux control, dissection and mobilization of the proximal stomach and distal esophagus may reveal obvious signs of ischemia and tissue necrosis. These findings should preclude any attempt at antireflux surgery and should establish the need for resection and reconstruction. Adequate preoperative preparation and judicious decision making during surgery are thus essential to ensure satisfactory results.

FUNCTIONAL MOTOR DISORDERS

Esophageal resection and reconstruction for motility disorders are seldom required. Esophagectomy may be indicated in patients with end-stage disease after previously failed esophageal procedures or in patients presenting with major complications of a motor disorder, such as perforation, bleeding, or malignancy. Patient evaluation must be thorough and objective, and sound preoperative decision making is essential in obtaining acceptable results.

Achalasia, a primary motor disorder, is characterized by the absence of peristalsis in the body of the esophagus and failure or incomplete relaxation of the lower esophageal sphincter (LES) in response to swallowing. In its idiopathic form, achalasia is a rare disease, with an estimated incidence of 0.5 to 1 per 100,000 population per year in the United States and Europe (Howard et al, 1992; Sonnenberg et al, 1993). Megaesophagus associated with Chagas' disease, a much more common secondary form of achalasia, is found in South America, with an incidence of 1% to 2% (Pinotti and Bettarello, 1988).

The exact cause of achalasia remains unknown, although a number of theories exist. As described by Cassella and colleagues (1964, 1965), the characteristic pathologic features or changes found in the body as well as the distal esophagus favor a neurogenic pathophysiology. These changes include an absence or deficiency of ganglionic cells in the myenteric plexus of Auerbach and abnormalities in the dorsal vagal nucleus and vagal nerves.

Histologic examination reveals hypertrophy and interstitial fibrosis of the smooth muscle layer, mononuclear cell infiltration, and diffuse squamous cell hyperplasia at the level of the mucosa (Goldblum et al, 1994). In Chagas' disease, achalasia results from the destruction of Auerbach's plexus by the protozoan *Trypanosoma cruzi*. In a manner similar to idiopathic achalasia, the absence of ganglion cells leads to the loss of peristalsis and coordination and to the progressive distention and distortion of the esophagus.

The onset of clinical manifestations in patients with achalasia is usually insidious and generally occurs in the third to fifth decade with no preference for gender. The predominant symptoms include progressive dysphagia, regurgitation, chest pain, and weight loss. Pulmonary complications related to chronic aspiration such as recurrent pneumonia and bronchiectasis have been reported to occur in 10% to 33% of patients in older series (Ellis and Olsen, 1969). Patients with long-standing achalasia are also at increased risk for development of esophageal carcinoma. The prevalence has been found to be as high as 30% in patients dying of achalasia as reported by Ellis (1960). In a later study by Meijssen and associates (1992), the risk of carcinoma development has been found to be 33 times greater than the risk in the general population. In South America, Ximenes and colleagues (1987) reported a 2.9% incidence of carcinoma in patients with achalasia. The tumors—squamous cell carcinoma of the middle third—are thought to develop in areas of chronic esophagitis and metaplasia secondary to the stasis of food and fluid. Patients present with symptoms that are often difficult to distinguish from the underlying disease, thus accounting for the delayed diagnosis and poor prognosis.

Because there is no known cure for achalasia, therapy is aimed at palliating symptoms by relieving the obstruction in the distal esophagus. Treatment options include drugs, botulinum toxin injections, forceful esophageal dilatation, and distal esophagomyotomy.

The effectiveness of both dilatation and esophagomyotomy with satisfactory functional results and acceptable morbidity has been shown over the years. In a review by Ferguson (1991) of 899 patients with achalasia treated with dilatation from 1980 to 1990, results were satisfactory in 71% of patients, with a rate of perforation of 1.4% and mortality of 0.3%. Repeated therapy in this group, however, was required in 16.6% of patients. In the same review, Ferguson found excellent results in 89% of the 1199 patients treated surgically, with a mortality of 0.3%. In the esophagomyotomy group, 10% of patients presented symptomatic gastroesophageal reflux and 2.9% required reoperation.

Long-term follow-up of treated achalasia patients revealed symptoms of dysphagia or reflux in 20% to 30% of cases (Malthaner et al, 1994). Recurrent dysphagia may occur as a result of an inadequate distal esophagomyotomy or a healed myotomy, a peptic stricture resulting from chronic reflux, or the use of a total fundoplication at the time of the myotomy (Topart et al, 1992). Also, the presence of a megaesophagus (>8 cm in diameter) with a redundant supradiaphragmatic segment can lead to incapacitating symptoms, even in the myotomized patient (Fig. 28–2).

Management of patients with recurrent symptoms after a previous myotomy represents a major challenge for the esophageal surgeon. Reoperation for achalasia is possible through a variety of procedures, including:

1. Another myotomy with or without an antireflux procedure.
2. Revision of a previous antireflux procedure.
3. Fundoplication with or without a gastroplasty.
4. A Thal-Hatafuku procedure (Hatafuku et al, 1972).
5. Vagotomy and antrectomy.
6. Segmental esophageal resection and reconstruction.
7. Esophagectomy with esophagogastrostomy.

In the presence of recurrent or persistent dysphagia resulting from an incomplete myotomy, a second distal esophagomyotomy is appropriate in most patients in the absence of a megaesophagus or reflux-induced peptic stricture, as suggested by Peters and DeMeester (1995), Ellis and associates (1986), and Fekete and colleagues (1982). The mobilization of the distal esophagus and hiatus required during these reoperations renders some form of antireflux procedure necessary. Results with the repeated myotomies, however, have been satisfactory,

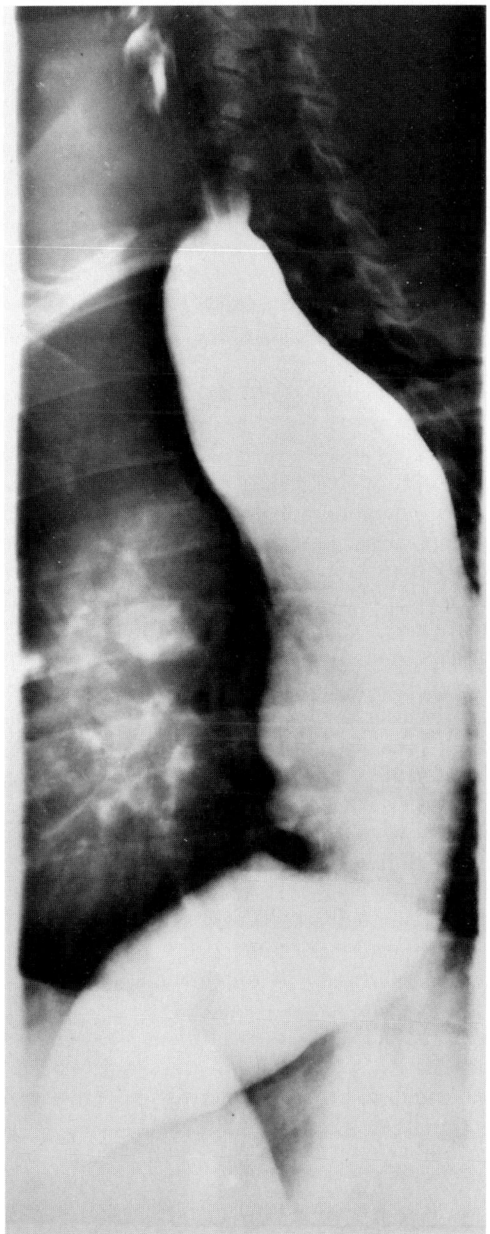

FIGURE 28–2 ■ Megaesophagus with a redundant supradiaphragmatic loop.

with rates varying from 60% to 85% as reported by Ellis and associates (1986) and by Fekete and colleagues (1982).

In selected patients with achalasia, esophagectomy with reconstruction should be considered the most appropriate treatment option. The indication for resection, as listed in Table 28–2, should be carefully established in each patient according to the type and number of previous procedures as well as on the results of radiographic, endoscopic, and esophageal function studies. Resection in patients with end-stage disease who have undergone multiple previous operations or who have experienced severe complications of GERD is well established, as suggested by Peters and co-workers (1995) and Orringer and Stirling (1989). More controversial is the issue of

TABLE 28–2 ■ **Indications for Esophagectomy in Achalasia**

Recurrent dysphagia after two or more previous myotomies
Severe esophagitis or peptic stricture after a myotomy
Dysphagia with a previous segmental esophageal resection
Dysphagia with a tortuous megaesophagus (>8 cm diameter)
Presence of esophageal carcinoma

esophagectomy for a megaesophagus without a previous attempt at an esophagus-sparing procedure, such as a myotomy or cardioplasty.

Results of esophagectomy for achalasia are summarized in Table 28–3. In Orringer and Stirling's report (1989) on 26 patients, 4 underwent resection as the primary operation for a megaesophagus whereas 22 patients had undergone one or more previous procedures. The authors argue that, in the presence of a severely distorted and tortuous esophagus, resection rather than an esophagus-sparing procedure provides better palliation for the patient.

DeMeester and coworkers presented their results with a similar group of patients (Peters et al, 1995). In their series of 19 cases, including 6 patients with a megaesophagus, all patients had had a previously failed surgical procedure before going on to esophagectomy. Resection and reconstruction was associated with a satisfactory outcome in 93% of patients, with 0% mortality. The authors concluded that although rarely necessary, resection should be considered as primary therapy for some patients with a markedly dilated and atonic megaesophagus.

The South American experience with achalasia in relation to Chagas' disease is much more extensive, as reported by Ximenes and associates (1987) and by Pinotti and colleagues (1991). In the Ximenes experience with megaesophagus, esophagectomy was not necessary. When the Thal-Hatafuku procedure, consisting of a cardioplasty and endoluminal valve, was used, results in 210 patients were satisfactory in 96% of cases, with a 0.9% mortality (Ximenes, 1991). Esophageal resection performed by this group was associated with satisfactory results in only 75% of patients, with a 7% mortality (Ximenes et al, 1987). In comparison, Pinotti and associates (1991) reported 90% satisfactory results and a low 4% mortality rate in 122 patients requiring an esophagectomy for advanced megaesophagus. Although resection is more radical, we believe that resection should be the primary operation in such patients.

Primary motor diseases of the esophagus other than achalasia include diffuse esophageal spasm (DES), supersqueeze (nutcracker) esophagus, a hypertensive LES, and nonspecific esophageal motility disorders. The list of secondary dysmotilities of the esophagus is much more extensive and varied. The most common disorders in this group include reflux esophagitis and scleroderma. Esophagectomy as primary therapy in the setting of neuromotor disease is exceedingly rare. Generally, patients requiring resection have undergone a number of previously unsuccessful esophageal procedures.

Orringer and Orringer (1982) reported their experience with 22 patients with motility disorders in whom a total of 41 prior operations had been performed before an esophagectomy. In this study, 12 patients presented with DES, 6 with achalasia, 2 with scleroderma, and 2 with a history of esophageal atresia. Orringer and Orringer believed that esophagectomy is indicated for severe, recurrent dysphagia, or for long-term complications of reflux esophagitis in patients for whom an esophagus-sparing procedure is no longer possible.

In a similar report by Waters and co-workers (1988), seven patients with DES required an esophagectomy after treatment with a myotomy and an antireflux procedure. Resection in this group of patients was indicated for continued pain, dysphagia, and weight loss directly attributable to unrelenting reflux.

Progressive systemic sclerosis, or scleroderma, is characterized by smooth muscle atrophy in the lower two thirds of the esophagus with the deposition of collagen within the esophageal wall. Manometric studies reveal low-amplitude, nonpropulsive contractions; disorganized peristalsis with impaired clearance; and a hypotonic or absent LES. Long-standing disease is associated with the development of severe erosive esophagitis, esophageal shortening with fibrous stricture, and a columnar-lined Barrett's esophagus. At times, the patients may also present with a massively dilated esophagus (Fig. 28–3).

Patients with scleroderma may be managed surgically with procedures ranging from a Nissen-type fundoplication, to a Collis-Nissen gastroplasty, to a gastric resection with Roux-en-Y reconstruction (Henderson and Pearson, 1973; Orringer et al, 1981; Poirier et al, 1994). The use of esophagectomy, however, has been reported by a limited number of authors (Akiyama et al, 1973; Fell et al, 1980; Mansour and Malone, 1988; Orringer, 1985). Surgical therapy for these patients is palliative, and thus resection and reconstruction should be considered only when all conservative measures have failed to provide relief. Esophagectomy is not indicated as primary therapy for these patients. Usually, indications for resection include the

TABLE 28–3 ■ **Results of Esophagectomy for Achalasia**

Author (Year)	*No. of Patients*	*Satisfactory Results (%)*	*Rate of Major Complications (%)*	*Mortality Rate (%)*
Orringer and Stirling (1989)	26	92	30	3.8
Peters et al (1995)	19	93	21	0
Miller et al (1995)	37	91	32	5.4
Ximenes et al (1987)	40	75	24	7.0
Pinotti et al (1991)	122	90	19	4.1

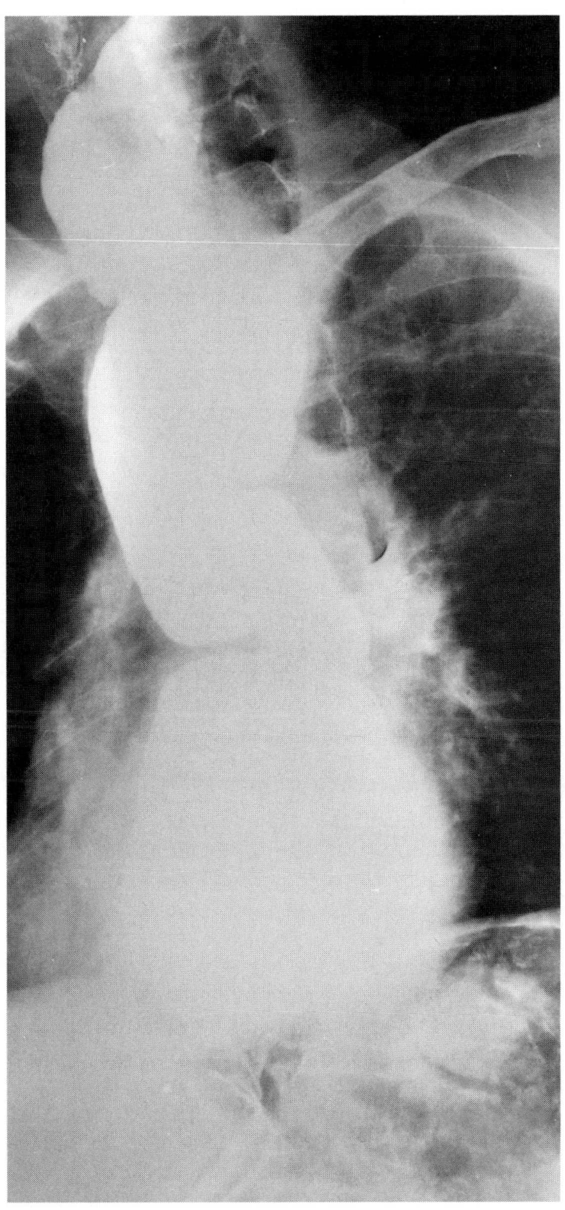

FIGURE 28–3 ■ Massively dilated esophagus with chronic reflux in a patient with scleroderma.

presence of a fixed, undilatable fibrous stricture, or severe incapacitating dysphagia after a previous operation in patients not responsive to another attempt at a reconstructive procedure (see details on surgery for scleroderma in Chapter 34).

TRAUMATIC INJURIES

Traumatic lesions of the esophagus are most often associated with perforations or corrosive injuries secondary to the ingestion of caustic substances. These injuries are serious and potentially lethal and in certain patients may call for an esophageal resection and reconstruction as definitive therapy.

The most common cause of esophageal perforation remains iatrogenic disruption. Currently, 45% to 75% of published cases of perforation are related to endoscopic manipulations or to paraesophageal surgery. Spontaneous perforations (Boerhaave's syndrome) are seen in 15% of all esophageal ruptures, whereas perforations from trauma (penetrating or blunt injuries, caustic injuries, and swallowed foreign bodies) represent approximately 20% of cases.

The clinical presentation of patients varies with the cause and location of the perforation. Main symptoms include pain, blood-tinted vomitus or hematemesis, dysphagia, odynophagia, and dyspnea. On physical examination, tachycardia and tachypnea are seen in the majority of patients. The presence of hypotension or shock suggests significant volume loss with an underlying septic process. Subcutaneous emphysema is more often palpated with a cervical perforation. Dullness or hyperresonance of the chest may suggest a pneumothorax or hydropneumothorax.

The diagnostic workup of patients with a suspected perforation must be efficient and accurate. Plain radiographs of the neck, chest, and abdomen should be performed immediately in all patients. In more than 90% of cases, the diagnosis can be suspected from these radiographs. Findings such as retroesophageal swelling on lateral neck films, air at the pharyngoesophageal level or in the upper mediastinum, lower pneumomediastinum, pleural effusion, pneumothorax, and hydropneumothorax all suggest an esophageal disruption. A water-soluble contrast esophagogram, followed if necessary by the use of liquid barium, is mandatory to confirm the diagnosis (Fig. 28–4). Occasionally, contrast medium–enhanced computed tomography may reveal extraesophageal air and thickening of the mediastinal tissue. Esophagoscopy is rarely used to diagnose a perforation for fear of spreading contamination or inducing a tension pneumothorax.

Treatment is aimed at (1) preventing further soilage from the perforation, (2) controlling and eliminating the infection produced by the disruption, (3) restoring the integrity and continuity of the gastrointestinal tract, and (4) maintaining adequate vital functions. The results of management are influenced by a number of factors, including etiology, location and size of the rupture, delay in diagnosis, extent of mediastinal and pleural contamination, and presence of an underlying esophageal disease.

Optimal therapy for patients with a perforation has remained controversial over the years because specific management guidelines did not exist and results were less than satisfactory, with high rates of morbidity and mortality. Regardless of the cause or location of a perforation, the delay between the onset of symptoms and the diagnosis remains the most influential factor in patient outcome. From the surgical literature, an early primary repair still provides the best chances of survival.

When an esophageal perforation is diagnosed in less than 24 hours, a primary repair should be the first approach to treatment. Extensive débridement of all nonviable tissue in the mediastinum and pleural cavity is undertaken. The esophagus is completely exposed, and the perforated area is identified. A myotomy is often necessary beyond the extent of the mucosal tear to expose the total length of the mucosal injury. Wide stitches in healthy tissue are used to reapproximate the edges of the perforation, without any tension and always covered with

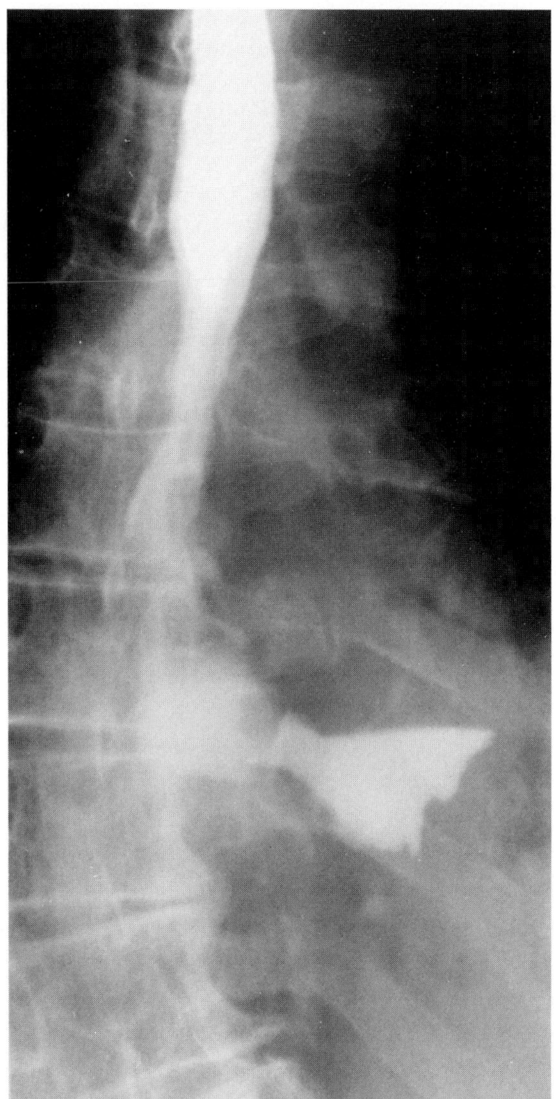

FIGURE 28–4 ■ Esophageal perforation in Boerhaave's syndrome with free-flowing contrast medium into the pleural cavity.

normal autologous tissue. Gayet and associates (1991) have proposed the use of a linear stapler to close the lacerated mucosa, also emphasizing mandatory coverage by autologous tissue after their repair. The extensively débrided mediastinum is left open for drainage after the repair.

Even early primary repairs carry a significant morbidity and mortality. Gouge and co-workers (1989) reported fistula formation in 39% of their patients, with a mortality of 25%. Both Gouge and co-workers and Gayet and colleagues (1991) suggest reinforcement or buttressing of the repair by well-vascularized autologous tissue to reduce postoperative suture line disruption. A well-mobilized gastric fundus, a Thal patch, a pleural flap, and a pedicled muscle flap taken from the diaphragm, intercostal muscle or chest wall, pericardium, or omentum may all be used to provide healthy coverage. When using this added protection, Gouge and co-workers (1989) observed a decrease of morbidity to 13% (from 39%) and a reduction of mortality to 6% (from 25%).

Esophageal perforation with late presentation or delayed diagnosis results in more contamination and further tissue necrosis and edema. An ideal repair, based on precisely identifying the esophageal wall layers, becomes more difficult, and failure often results. There is a consequent sharp rise in morbidity and mortality seen with any delay in the initiation of operative therapy. Mortality may double and even triple when the 24-hour rule for diagnosis and management cannot be respected. Radovanovic and associates (1995) reported a mortality that increased from 2.8% when patients were treated within 24 hours to 18.3% when treatment was delayed more than 24 hours. On the basis of their experience, Gouge and co-workers (1989) suggested extending this rule to 72 hours.

When a significant pathologic process exists in the esophageal wall or when extensive damage has resulted from the perforation, esophagectomy is indicated. Fear of creating an obstruction distal to the repair or the presence of failed previous attempts at repair are other indications for resection. A transhiatal or a transthoracic approach can be employed. Immediate or delayed reconstruction depends on the degree of contamination and the status of the patient. We usually delay the reconstruction unless the perforation occurs after an instrumental manipulation and is diagnosed immediately. A feeding jejunostomy and gastric decompression are mandatory after these operations. When an esophagectomy becomes necessary for an esophageal perforation, the reported mortality ranges from 25% to 30% (Boudet et al, 1996; Jones and Ginsberg, 1992).

When long-standing GERD has resulted in a stricture or when a perforated ulcer complicates a columnar-lined esophagus, esophagectomy must be considered unless a safe repair can be accomplished without any obstruction distal to the repair. If the underlying pathology is esophageal carcinoma, conservative therapy results in a high mortality. Esophagectomy and immediate reconstruction are indicated if the patient can undergo operation and has suffered an instrumental or a spontaneous perforation. If the perforation has occurred during attempts at palliative intubation, efforts at proper endoluminal positioning of the prosthesis are in order, with the hope of sealing the perforation while antibiotics and chest drainage are added. The overall mortality in this setting varies from 30% (Griffin et al, 1990) to 55% (Giudicelli et al, 1992). A perforation in association with cancer, regardless of its location, appears to be associated with higher mortality than perforations associated with benign disease or without an underlying disease (Jones and Ginsberg, 1992).

Corrosive injury to the esophagus occurs with the ingestion of a caustic substance such as alkali (lye) or a strong acid. Generally, these injuries result from accidental ingestion in young children or from suicide attempts in teenagers and adults. The entire length of the upper gastrointestinal tract may be involved, from the mouth and pharynx to the duodenum and proximal jejunum. Alkaline agents penetrate deep into the wall of the esophagus, producing liquefaction necrosis by dissolution of protein and collagen, saponification of fats, and thrombosis of blood vessels. Injury is more extensive in the esophagus than stomach and may extend by contiguity to adjacent organs. Nonalkaline agents or strong acids produce injury by coagulation necrosis, with the stomach being the preferential site of damage.

Corrosive injuries to the esophagus may be classified into three phases. The acute phase, during the first 48 to 72 hours, is associated with an intense inflammatory reaction with edema and necrosis. In the subacute or second phase, the destroyed esophageal mucosa is progressively replaced by granulation tissue. The final or chronic phase is characterized by the appearance of thick, fibrous scar tissue in the wall of the esophagus leading to the formation of stricture. In a review by Csendes and Braghetto (1992), 15% of patients during the acute phase present with severe complications from extensive necrosis, esophageal perforation, and mediastinitis. Mortality in this setting may reach 80%. In patients reaching the chronic phase, strictures develop, requiring dilatation or surgery, with a rate varying from 6% to 22% (Csendes and Braghetto, 1992; Ferguson et al, 1989).

Management options in patients presenting with caustic injuries are varied and depend on factors such as the timing of the injury, the site and extent of damage, the presence of concomitant lesions to the pharynx or stomach, and the development of complications. In the early phase, supportive measures are instituted in all patients. These include hydration with intravenous fluids, nutritional support, and antibiotic therapy. The use of corticosteroids to prevent stricture formation is no longer recommended routinely (Anderson et al, 1990; Ferguson et al, 1989; Oakes et al, 1982). Although an uncommon occurrence during the acute phase, patients with evidence of esophageal perforation or extensive gastric necrosis require urgent surgery. Esophagectomy with a cervical esophagostomy and staged reconstruction is advocated by most authors (Fig. 28–5) (Estrera et al, 1986; Ferguson et al, 1989; Gossot et al, 1987). In the chronic phase, esophageal resection is sometimes also required. Specific indications include an undilatable stricture, instrumental perforation of the esophagus, esophageal fistula with a mediastinal abscess, increased risk of malignancy in long-standing strictures, and the development of reflux with severe esophagitis. Reconstruction is carried out at the time of resection and usually consists of a gastric or colon interposition.

The detailed management of corrosive injuries may be found in Chapter 36.

ESOPHAGEAL RECONSTRUCTION AND FUNCTIONAL RESULTS

The choice of a substitute for esophageal reconstruction is still widely discussed. In regard to esophageal carcinoma, long-term survival is unlikely in most patients, and thus the choice of conduit is much less controversial. Reconstruction for benign disease, however, requires a substitute organ that is durable and associated with satis-

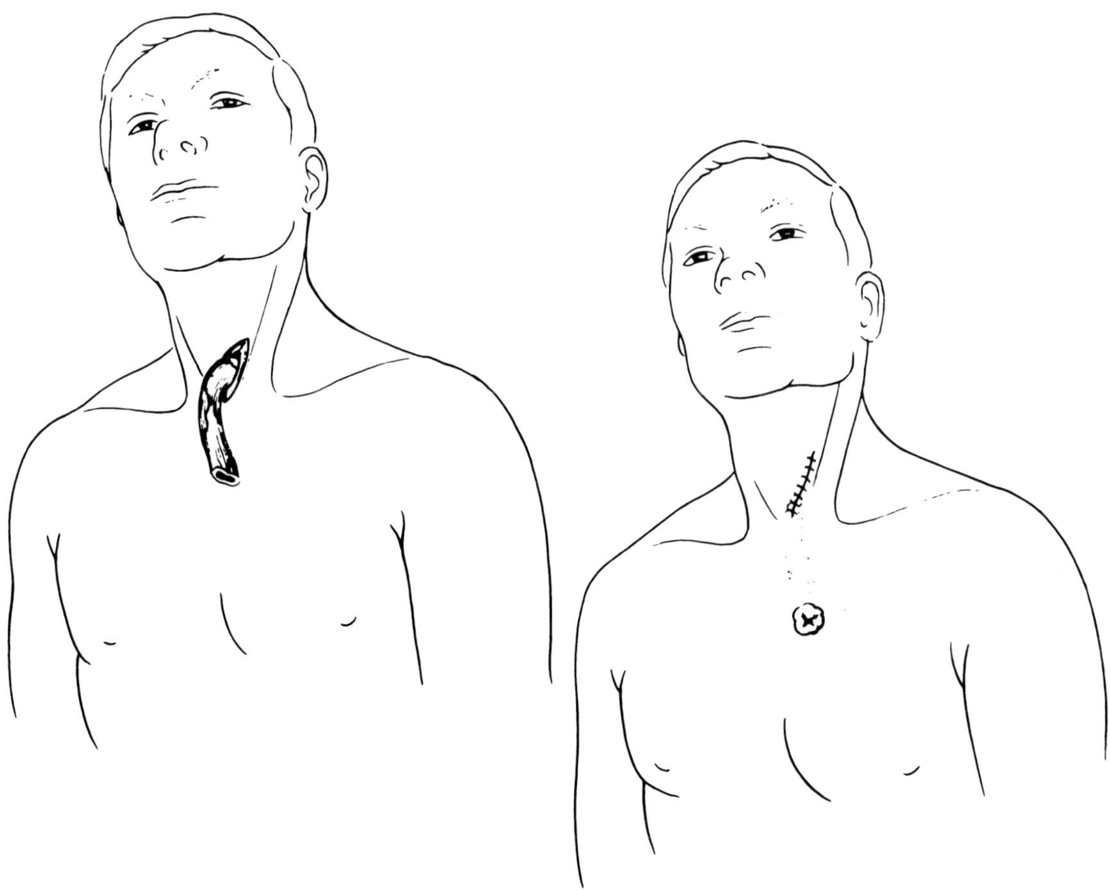

FIGURE 28–5 ■ Esophagectomy with an end-cervical esophagostomy on the anterior chest wall for delayed reconstruction.

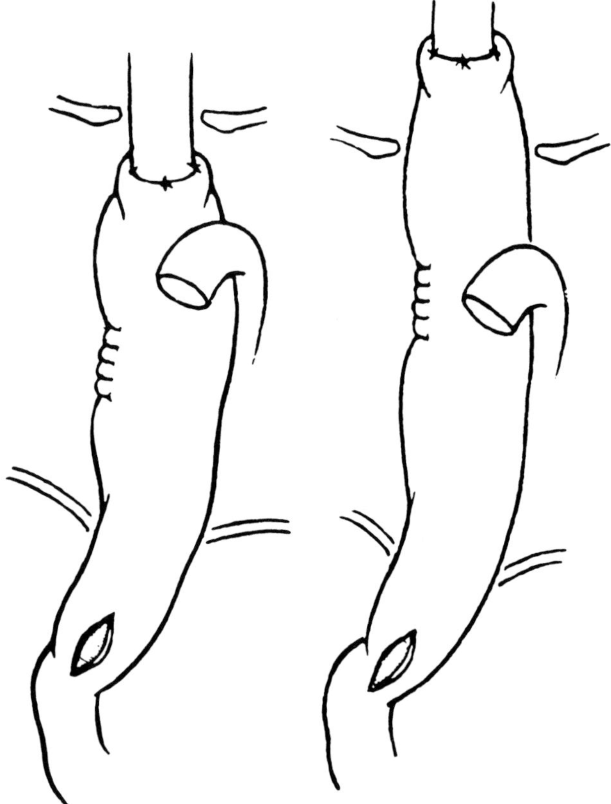

FIGURE 28–6 ■ Esophagectomy with a primary intrathoracic anastomosis *(left)* or cervical esophagogastrostomy *(right)*.

factory long-term functional results. Important factors to consider when selecting the replacement conduit include availability of organs, absence of intrinsic disease, adequacy of blood supply, patient's age, and the surgeon's own experience and proficiency.

Proponents of gastric interposition emphasize the technical ease, single anastomosis, shorter in-hospital recovery, and quicker return to normal alimentation (Fig. 28–6) (Davis and Heitmiller, 1996; Orringer et al, 1993; Saalamao et al, 1996; Waters et al, 1988). Disadvantages with the use of stomach are (1) loss of a gastric reservoir, with early satiety and dumping symptoms, and (2) the potential development of reflux disease in the remaining cervical esophagus. Authors such as DeMeester and associates (1988), Mansour and colleagues (1997), and Curet-Scott and associates (1987), however, have continued to favor the colon as an esophageal substitute. They claim that the colon retains its motor function and reservoir capacity, the stomach and duodenum remain in their normal anatomic position, GERD and duodenogastric reflux are avoided, and patients generally experience fewer symptoms after meals. The use of the colon, however, requires added technical expertise, increases the number of anastomoses from one to three, lengthens the surgical procedure, and adds to the postoperative morbidity and mortality. Experienced centers, such as those of DeMeester and associates (1988) and Cerfolio and co-workers from the Mayo Clinic (1995), reported a 9% in-hospital mortality and a rate of major complications varying from 15% to 24% with colon interposition.

Success with esophageal reconstruction for benign disease must consider long-term functional results and patient satisfaction. Orringer and Stirling (1988) reported good to excellent functional results in 91 patients who underwent esophagectomy and cervical esophagogastrostomy for benign disease. Among the 91 patients, 85% followed a regular unrestricted diet or experienced mild or intermittent dysphagia and 15% developed persistent dysphagia requiring regular dilatations. Symptoms of reflux were found in only 30% of patients, and some degree of dumping syndrome occurred in 22%. Overall, with a 3-year follow-up, all patients believed that their ability to eat with comfort had significantly improved with the surgery.

DeMeester and co-workers (1988) presented similar results, with a median follow-up of 5 years, in a group of 92 patients having undergone esophagectomy and colon interposition. Altogether, 97% of patients were satisfied with the operation, 82% believed that they were cured of their preoperative symptoms, and 18% had improved significantly. Nocturnal regurgitation or gurgling was present in 29% of patients and diarrhea or dumping in 15%.

The Mayo Clinic has presented a detailed review of functional results and patient quality of life after esophagectomy for benign disease (Young et al, 2000a, 2000b). The study group included 255 patients; in 66% the stomach was used for reconstruction, in 27% the colon, and in 7% small bowel. Generally, results seem less satisfactory than those reported by Orringer and Stirling (1988) and by DeMeester and co-workers (1988). With a median follow-up of 52 months, functional results were classified as excellent in 32% of patients, good in 10%, fair in 35%, and poor in 23%. Mild to moderate symptoms of dysphagia, heartburn, or gastric dumping were found in 51% to 72% of patients postoperatively. Although patients considered their quality of life normal in conceptual areas covering general health, as tested with a self-administered questionnaire, only 4% of patients were actually asymptomatic after their esophageal reconstruction. Factors such as age, initial diagnosis, type of reconstruction, and postoperative morbidity were not found to be predictive of long-term functional results or quality of life.

CONCLUSION

In selecting the type of reconstruction and the esophageal substitute, one finds that the available data seem conflicting as to the superiority of one organ over another. Few patients, in fact, are free of symptoms after the surgery. As such, sound preoperative decision making and careful attention to the technical aspects of the surgical procedure are essential in ensuring low postoperative morbidity and mortality rates.

■ *REFERENCES*

Akiyama H, Kogure T, Itai Y: Esophageal reconstruction for stenosis due to diffuse scleroderma: Utilizing blunt dissection of esophagus. Arch Surg 107:470–472, 1973.

Altorki NK, Skinner DB, Segalin A, et al: Indications for esophagectomy in nonmalignant Barrett's esophagus: A 10-year experience [see comments]. Ann Thorac Surg 49:724–726; discussion, 727, 1990.

Anderson KD, Rouse TM, Randolph JG: A controlled trial of corticosteroids in children with corrosive injury of the esophagus [see comments]. N Engl J Med 323:637–640, 1990.

Andersson R, Nilsson S: Perforated Barrett's ulcer with esophagopleural fistula: A case report. Acta Chir Scand 151:495–496, 1985.

Ben Rejeb M, Bouche O, Zeitoun P: Study of 47 consecutive patients with peptic esophageal stricture compared with 3880 cases of reflux esophagitis. Dig Dis Sci 37:733–736, 1992.

Bircher E: Ein Beitrag zur plastischen Bildung eines neuen Oesophagus. Zentralbl Chir 34:1479, 1907.

Bonavina L, Segalin A, Fumagalli U, et al: Surgical management of benign stricture from reflux oesophagitis. Ann Chir Gynaecol 84:175–178, 1995.

Boudet MJ, Perniceni T, Gayet B: Surgical management of esophageal perforations: A French series of 270 cases. In Perracchia A, Rosati R, Bonavina L, et al (eds): Recent Advances in Diseases of the Esophagus. Bologna, Monduzzi Editore, 1996, pp 1003–1009.

Cassella RR, Brown AL Jr, Sayre GP, et al: Achalasia of the esophagus: Pathologic and etiologic considerations. Ann Surg 160:474–486, 1964.

Cassella RR, Ellis FH Jr, Brown AL Jr: Fine structure changes in achalasia of the esophagus: Vagus nerves. Am J Pathol 46:279, 1965.

Cerfolio RJ, Allen MS, Deschamps C, et al: Esophageal replacement by colon interposition. Ann Thorac Surg 59:1382–1384, 1995.

Chen LQ, Nastos D, Hu CY, et al: Results of the Collis-Nissen gastroplasty in patients with Barrett's esophagus. Ann Thorac Surg 68:1014–1021, 1999.

Csendes A, Braghetto I: Surgical management of esophageal strictures. Hepatogastroenterology 39:502–510, 1992.

Curet-Scott MJ, Ferguson MK, Little AG, et al: Colon interposition for benign esophageal disease. Surgery 102:568–574, 1987.

Czerny V: Neue Operationen. Zentralbl Chir 4:433–434, 1877.

Dakkak M, Hoare RC, Maslin SC, et al: Oesophagitis is as important as oesophageal stricture diameter in determining dysphagia. Gut 34:152–155, 1993.

Davis EA, Heitmiller RF: Esophagectomy for benign disease: Trends in surgical results and management. Ann Thorac Surg 62:369–372, 1996.

DeMeester TR, Johansson KE, Franze I, et al: Indications, surgical technique, and long-term functional results of colon interposition or bypass. Ann Surg 208:460–474, 1988.

Denk W: Zur Radikaloperation des Oesophagus-karzinom. Zentralbl Chir 40:1065–1068, 1913.

Ellis FG: The natural history of achalasia of the cardia. Proc R Soc Med 53:633–666, 1960.

Ellis FH Jr, Olsen AM: Achalasia of the Esophagus. In Major Problems in Clinical Surgery, Vol 9. Philadelphia, WB Saunders, 1969, p 1.

Ellis FH, Crozier RE, Gibb SP: Reoperative achalasia surgery. J Thorac Cardiovasc Surg 92:859–865, 1986.

Estrera A, Taylor W, Mills LJ, et al: Corrosive burns of the esophagus and stomach: A recommendation for an aggressive surgical approach. Ann Thorac Surg 41:276–283, 1986.

Fekete F, Breil P, Tossen JC: Reoperation after Heller's operation for achalasia and other motility disorders of the esophagus: A study of eighty-one reoperations. Int Surg 67:103–110, 1982.

Fell SC, Chang P, Brenner S: Esophagectomy for scleroderma stricture of esophagus. N Y State J Med 80:942–946, 1980.

Ferguson MK, Migliore M, Staszak VM, et al: Early evaluation and therapy for caustic esophageal injury. Am J Surg 157:116–120, 1989.

Ferguson MK: Achalasia: Current evaluation and therapy. Ann Thorac Surg 52:336–342, 1991.

Ferguson MK: Medical and surgical management of peptic esophageal strictures. Chest Surg Clin North Am 4:673–695, 1994.

Gadenstätter M, Hagen JA, DeMeester TR, et al: Esophagectomy for unsuccessful antireflux operations. J Thorac Cardiovasc Surg 115:296–300, 302; discussion, 300–301, 1998.

Gayet B, Breil P, Fekete F: Mechanical sutures in perforation of the thoracic esophagus as a safe procedure in patients seen late. Surg Gynecol Obstet 172:125–128, 1991.

Giudicelli R: Esophageal perforations. Results of a national survey [French]. Ann Chir 46:183–187, 1992.

Goldblum JR, Whyte RI, Orringer MB, et al: Achalasia: A morphologic study of 42 resected specimens. Am J Surg Pathol 18:327–337, 1994.

Gossot D, Sarfati E, Celerier M: Early blunt esophagectomy in severe caustic burns of the upper digestive tract: Report of 29 cases. J Thorac Cardiovasc Surg 94:188–191, 1987.

Gouge TH, Depan HJ, Spencer FC: Experience with the Grillo pleural wrap procedure in 18 patients with perforation of the thoracic esophagus [see comments]. Ann Surg 209:612–617; discussion, 617–619, 1989.

Griffin SC, Desai J, Townsend ER, et al: Oesophageal resection after instrumental perforation. Eur J Cardiothorac Surg 4:211–213, 1990.

Hatafuku T, Maki T, Thal AP: Fundic patch operation in the treatment of advanced achalasia of the esophagus. Surg Gynecol Obstet 134:617–624, 1972.

Hedblom C: Combined transpleural and transperitoneal resection of the thoracic esophagus and cardia for carcinoma. Surg Gynecol Obstet 35:284–287, 1922.

Henderson RD, Pearson FG: Surgical management of esophageal scleroderma. J Thorac Cardiovasc Surg 66:686–692, 1973.

Henderson RD, Henderson RF, Marryatt GV: Surgical management of 100 consecutive esophageal strictures. J Thorac Cardiovasc Surg 99:1–7, 1990.

Howard PJ, Maher L, Pryde A, et al: Five year prospective study of the incidence, clinical features, and diagnosis of achalasia in Edinburgh. Gut 33:1011–1015, 1992.

Ismail-Beigi F, Horton PF, Pope CE: Histological consequences of gastroesophageal reflux in man. Gastroenterology 58:163–174, 1970.

Jones WG, Ginsberg RJ: Esophageal perforation: A continuing challenge [see comments]. Ann Thorac Surg 53:534–543, 1992.

Kadakia SC, Parker A, Carrougher JG, et al: Esophageal dilation with polyvinyl bougies, using a marked guidewire without the aid of fluoroscopy: An update. Am J Gastroenterol 88:1381–1386, 1993.

Kelling G: Oesophagoplastik mit Hilfe des Querkolon. Zentralbl Chir 38:1209–1212, 1911.

Kirschner M: Ein neues Verfahren der Oesophagoplastik. Arch Klin Chir 114:606–663, 1920.

Lilienthal H: Carcinoma of the thoracic oesophagus: Successful resection. Ann Surg 74:116–120, 1921.

Little AG, Ferguson MK, Skinner DB: Reoperation for failed antireflux operations. J Thorac Cardiovasc Surg 91:511–517, 1986.

Little AG, Naunheim KS, Ferguson MK, et al: Surgical management of esophageal strictures. Ann Thorac Surg 45:144–147, 1988.

Loof L, Gotell P, Elfberg B: The incidence of reflux oesophagitis: A study of endoscopy reports from a defined catchment area in Sweden. Scand J Gastroenterol 28:113–118, 1993.

Malthaner RA, Tood TR, Miller L, et al: Long-term results in surgically managed esophageal achalasia. Ann Thorac Surg 58:1343–1346; discussion 1346–1347, 1994.

Mansour KA, Hansen HA, Hersh T, et al: Colon interposition for advanced nonmalignant esophageal stricture: Experience with 40 patients. Ann Thorac Surg 32:584–591, 1981.

Mansour KA, Malone CE: Surgery for scleroderma of the esophagus: A 12-year experience. Ann Thorac Surg 46:513–514, 1988.

Mansour KA, Bryan FC, Carlson GW: Bowel interposition for esophageal replacement: Twenty-five-year experience. Ann Thorac Surg 64:752–756, 1997.

Meijssen MA, Tilanus HW, van Blankenstein M, et al: Achalasia complicated by oesophageal squamous cell carcinoma: A prospective study in 195 patients. Gut 33:155–158, 1992.

Meyer W: Oesophagogastrostomy after intrathoracic resection of the oesophagus. Ann Surg 50:175–189, 1909.

Miller DL, Allen MS, Trastek VF, et al: Esophageal resection for recurrent achalasia [see comments]. Ann Thorac Surg 60:922–925; discussion, 925–926, 1995.

Oakes DD, Sherck JP, Mark JB: Lye ingestion: Clinical patterns and therapeutic implications. J Thorac Cardiovasc Surg 83:194–204, 1982.

Ogilvie AL, Ferguson R, Atkinson M: Outlook with conservative treatment of peptic oesophageal stricture. Gut 21:23–25, 1980.

Orringer MB, Orringer JS, Dabich L, et al: Combined Collis gastroplasty: Fundoplication operations for scleroderma reflux esophagitis. Surgery 90:624–630, 1981.

Orringer MB, Orringer JS: Esophagectomy: Definitive treatment for esophageal neuromotor dysfunction. Ann Thorac Surg 34:237–248, 1982.

Orringer MB: Transhiatal esophagectomy for benign disease. J Thorac Cardiovasc Surg 90:649–655, 1985.

Orringer MB, Stirling MC: Cervical esophagogastric anastomosis for benign disease: Functional results. J Thorac Cardiovasc Surg 96:887–893, 1988.

Orringer MB, Stirling MC: Esophageal resection for achalasia: Indications and results. Ann Thorac Surg 47:340–345, 1989.

Orringer MB, Marshall B, Stirling MC: Transhiatal esophagectomy for benign and malignant disease. J Thorac Cardiovasc Surg 105:265–276; discussion, 276–277, 1993.

Orringer MB: Resection of the esophagus. In Shields TW (ed): General Thoracic Surgery. Philadelphia, Lippincott Williams & Wilkins, 2000, pp 1697–1722.

Patterson DJ, Graham DY, Smith JL, et al: Natural history of benign esophageal stricture treated by dilatation. Gastroenterology 85:346–350, 1983.

Pearson FG, Cooper JD, Patterson GA, et al: Gastroplasty and fundoplication for complex reflux problems: Long-term results. Ann Surg 206:473–481, 1987.

Peters JH, Kauer WK, Crookes PF, et al: Esophageal resection with colon interposition for end-stage achalasia. Arch Surg 130:632–636; discussion, 636–637, 1995.

Pinotti HW, Bettarello A: Chagasic mega-oesophagus. In Jamieson GG (ed): Surgery of the Oesophagus. New York, Churchill Livingstone, 1988, pp 471–481.

Pinotti HW, Cecconello I, Mariano du Rocha J, et al: Resection for achalasia of the esophagus. Hepatogastroenterology 38:470–473, 1991.

Poirier NC, Taillefer R, Topart P, et al: Antireflux operations in patients with scleroderma. Ann Thorac Surg 58:66–72; discussion, 72–73, 1994.

Radovanovic NS, Pesko PL, Knezevic JD, et al: Factors important for the prognosis of the esophageal perforation. In Perracchia A, Rosati R, Bonavina L, et al (eds): Recent Advances in Diseases of the Esophagus. Bologna, Monduzzi Editore, 1996, pp 1011–1015.

Rienhoff WF: Intrathoracic esophagojejunostomy for lesions of the upper third of the esophagus. South Med J 39:928–940, 1946.

Roux C: L'oesphago-jejuno-gastrostomie, nouvelle operation pour le rétrécissement infranchissable de l'oesophage. Semana Med 27:37–40, 1907.

Salamao N, Gaboury L, Duranceau A: Esophagectomy for complications of gastroesophageal reflux disease. Probl Gen Surg 13:105–111, 1996.

Sandry RJ: Pathology of reflux esophagitis. In Skinner DB, Belsey RH, Hendrix TR, et al (eds): Gastroesophageal Reflux Hiatal Hernia. Boston, Little, Brown, 1972, pp 43–58.

Singh S, Stein HJ, DeMeester TR, et al: Nonobstructive dysphagia in gastroesophageal reflux disease: A study with combined ambulatory pH and motility monitoring. Am J Gastroenterol 87:562–567, 1992.

Skinner DB, Belsey RH: Surgical management of esophageal reflux and hiatus hernia: Long-term results with 1,030 patients. J Thorac Cardiovasc Surg 53:33–54, 1967.

Skinner DB: Surgical management after failed antireflux operations. World J Surg 16:359–363, 1992.

Sonnenberg A, Massey BT, McCarty DJ, et al: Epidemiology of hospitalization for achalasia in the United States. Dig Dis Sci 38:233–244, 1993.

Stirling MC, Orringer MB: Surgical treatment after the failed antireflux operation. J Thorac Cardiovasc Surg 92:667–672, 1986.

Stirling MC, Orringer MB: Continued assessment of the combined Collis-Nissen operation. Ann Thorac Surg 47:224–230, 1989.

Stoddard CJ, Simms JM: Dilatation of benign oesophageal strictures in the outpatient department. Br J Surg 71:752–753, 1984.

Topart P, Deschamps C, Taillefer R, et al: Long-term effect of total fundoplication on the myotomized esophagus. Ann Thorac Surg 54:1046–1051; discussion, 1051–1052, 1992.

Torek F: The first successful case of resection of the thoracic portion of the oesophagus for carcinoma. Surg Gynecol Obstet 16:614–617, 1913.

Turner GG: Excision of the thoracic oesophagus for carcinoma with construction of an extra-thoracic gullet. Lancet 2:1315–1316, 1933.

Waters PF, Pearson FG, Todd TR, et al: Esophagectomy for complex benign esophageal disease. J Thorac Cardiovasc Surg 95:378–381, 1988.

Williamson WA, Ellis FHJ, Gibb SP, et al: Barrett's ulcer: A surgical disease? J Thorac Cardiovasc Surg 103:2–6; discussion, 6–7, 1992.

Wullstein L: Ueber antethorakale Oesophago-jejunostomie und Operationen nach gleichen Prinzip. Dtsch Med Wochenschr 31:734–736, 1904.

Ximenes M III, Marra O, DeBiase H, et al: Primary surgical treatment of Chagas' megaesophagus: Results of 450 cases. HFA Pub Tec Cient 2:147–161, 1987.

Ximenes M III: Chagas' megaesophagus: Current review of techniques and results. Rev Saude DF 2:207, 1991.

Yamamoto H, Hughes RWJ, Schroeder KW, et al: Treatment of benign esophageal stricture by Eder-Puestow or balloon dilators: A comparison between randomized and prospective nonrandomized trials. Mayo Clin Proc 67:228–236, 1992.

Young MM, Deschamps C, Allen MS, et al: Esophageal reconstruction for benign disease: Self-assessment of functional outcome and quality of life. Ann Thorac Surg 70:1799–1802, 2000a.

Young MM, Deschamps C, Trastek VF, et al: Esophageal reconstruction for benign disease: Early morbidity, mortality, and functional results. Ann Thorac Surg 70:1651–1655, 2000b.

CHAPTER 29

Reoperation for Failed Repairs

Reoperation for failed antireflux surgery is the most difficult operation in Thoracic Surgery.

—R. H. R. Belsey, 1959

I well remember this quote from Belsey's memorable repertoire of statements during the year that I spent as a senior house officer on his Thoracic Surgery service at Frenchay Hospital, near Bristol, England, in 1959. In the year 2001, this statement still applies. At the least, "redo surgery" for hiatal hernia and reflux remains *one* of the most challenging and technically difficult problems in our specialty. This is the only procedure for which Belsey always took primary responsibility as the operating surgeon, delegating little more than the opening and closing of the incision. Many of my colleagues, including myself, continue to manage "redo antireflux surgery" in this way. We do this for several reasons:

1. Anatomy and the usual landmarks are obscured or obliterated by adhesions.
2. During a difficult dissection, the relatively fragile walls of the esophagus, gastric cardia, and fundus are easily damaged and breached. This may impair the precise reconstruction required to obtain a good functional result. Furthermore, a postoperative leak from the esophagus or stomach is a morbid, potentially lethal complication.
3. The results after reoperation, even those obtained by the most experienced surgeons, are significantly less favorable than outcomes for "first-time" repairs: the incidence of unsatisfactory results is at least doubled after reoperation. Furthermore, the greater the number of prior failed repairs, the greater the incidence of poor results.

Since Dallemagne and colleagues' first report of a *laparoscopic* Nissen fundoplication (1991), expertise with minimally invasive, video-assisted antireflux surgery has developed in exponential fashion. Some of the most complex technical problems in this field are being successfully managed with laparoscopic methods and include reoperative surgery. Currently, significant experience reporting morbidity, mortality rates, and outcomes comparable to "open operations" is restricted to a few centers throughout the world. I have little doubt, however, that these levels of expertise will become much more widely disseminated within a few short years.

This chapter, therefore, is presented in two sections: Open Techniques and Laparoscopic Techniques.

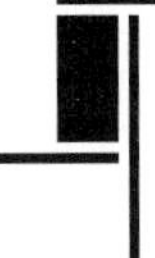

OPEN TECHNIQUES IN REOPERATION FOR FAILED REPAIRS

F. Griffith Pearson

HISTORICAL NOTE

Surgery for hiatal hernia and reflux has developed during the past 50 years and was launched by Allison's classic report, "Reflux Esophagitis, Sliding Hiatal Hernia, and the Anatomy of Repair," published in 1951.

The first formal reports of reoperation for failed prior antireflux repairs appeared about 15 years later. In 1967, Skinner reported the long-term follow-up of 1030 consecutive patients seen between 1949 and 1962 who were managed by some type of "Belsey repair" (Skinner, 1967). Ninety-one recurrent hiatal hernias were recognized, and 43 of these were managed by reoperation: Belsey repair, 28; distal esophagectomy with esophagogastrostomy, 11; and distal esophagectomy with colon replacement, 4. Orringer (1972) subsequently reported the long-term follow-up results in 892 patients managed specifically with the Belsey Mark IV repair between 1955 and 1965. Of 45 recurrences managed by reoperation, 33 underwent a second Belsey Mark IV repair and 12 were managed by resection. Hill reported his experience with reoperation in 1971 and appropriately emphasized the importance of esophageal function tests for the preoperative evaluation of these difficult patients (Hill, 1971).

HISTORICAL READINGS

Allison PR: Reflux esophagitis, sliding hiatal hernia, and the anatomy of repair. Surg Gynecol Obstet 92:419, 1951.

Hill LD: Management of recurrent hiatal hernia. Arch Surg 102:296, 1971.

Orringer MB: Long-term results of the Mark IV operation for hiatal hernia and analyses of recurrences and their treatment. J Thorac Cardiovasc Surg 63:25–33, 1972.

Skinner DB: Surgical management of esophageal reflux and hiatal hernia: Long term results with 1,030 patients. J Thorac Cardiovasc Surg 53:33–54, 1967.

CLINICAL PRESENTATION

The clinical presentation of patients undergoing reoperation for failed prior repairs is highly variable. The documentation of type and reason for failure is inconsistent and equally variable. A relatively detailed analysis is provided in reports by Little and associates (1986), Stein and co-workers (1996), Ellis and associates (1996), and Deschamps and colleagues (1997). Details of presentation and types of failure are scanty or missing in publications by Hill (1971), Polk (1980), Henderson and Marryatt (1981), Maher and associates (1985), Stirling and Orringer (1986), and Pearson and colleagues (1987). Four publications report experience with reoperation specifically for the failed Nissen fundoplication (Henderson, 1979; Hill et al, 1979; Leonardi et al, 1981; Luostarinen et al, 1993).

Recurrent Reflux

Recurrent reflux may present as symptomatic reflux, including all of the complications of reflux esophagitis and aspiration. Some patients, however, may no longer register their previous symptoms of reflux, presumably because of a reduction in sensory afferents in the distal esophagus as a result of the initial antireflux surgery. In such cases, the presenting complaint may be respiratory, caused by aspiration (e.g., sore throat, hoarseness, cough, bronchitis), or obstructive, caused by peptic esophagitis with inflammation and stricture. Such patients may not suspect that their new symptoms bear any relation to the original condition.

Recurrent Hiatal Hernia

Anatomic recurrence of a hiatal hernia may be associated with recurrent, symptomatic reflux or be totally without symptoms. If the recurrent hernia becomes incarcerated, the patient may register complaints of postprandial fullness or pain, dysphagia due to obstruction in the "crowded" diaphragmatic hiatus, or symptoms of bleeding or chronic anemia (usually seen with large, paraesophageal recurrences).

Adverse Functional Side Effects

Side effects of antireflux surgery may be disabling and warrant consideration of reoperation: "Overcorrection" of the lower esophageal sphincter (LES) valve function may result in the gas-bloat syndrome with inability to belch or vomit when necessary. Dysphagia may be due to an unduly snug closure of the hiatus or tight fundoplication. The obstructive effect of a fundoplication may be aggravated by a relative failure of peristaltic force in the body of the thoracic esophagus. Vagotomy (deliberate or inadvertent) may result in delayed gastric emptying or postprandial abdominal cramps with urgency and diarrhea. Severe impairment of gastric emptying may warrant reoperation.

Associated Primary Motor Disorder

The combination of reflux esophagitis and a primary motor disorder, such as achalasia or scleroderma, presents one of the most difficult surgical problems. In patients with achalasia (occasionally diffuse esophageal spasm), reflux esophagitis may occur at some time after an esophagomyotomy with ablation of the LES. In advanced esophageal scleroderma, the LES pressures are ablated by the disease process. In both achalasia and scleroderma, there is a complete loss of propulsive peristalsis in the body of the esophagus. When gastroesophageal reflux occurs, the failure of esophageal clearance (particularly when one is recumbent at night) frequently results in severe, erosive esophagitis and stricture. The failure rate after antireflux surgery in this group of patients is exceedingly high (Pearson et al, 1987) and results in a high incidence of reoperation.

Occasionally, symptoms of dysphagia and regurgitation from achalasia are misdiagnosed as reflux esophagitis or peptic stricture. An antireflux operation, without esophagomyotomy, inevitably fails to relieve dysphagia. The continuing dysphagia is manageable only by reoperation with dismantling of the fundoplication and performance of a myotomy.

CAUSES OF FAILURE

Failed repairs requiring reoperation may be the result of technical errors, selection of the wrong operation, or an incorrect primary diagnosis. Technical failures are undoubtedly related to the experience of the individual surgeon. There is a longer "learning curve" required for antireflux reconstructions than for most extirpative surgery of similar magnitude or complexity. Restoring a satisfactory swallowing function that prevents reflux and avoids dysphagia and functional side effects, such as the inability to belch or vomit, requires a degree of precision in the placement of sutures that has few counterparts.

Technical Errors

Technical errors are largely avoidable, yet remain the most common cause of failure resulting in reoperation. Ellis and associates (1996) attributed failure to faulty technique in 65 of 101 patients (65%) requiring reoperation. Stein and coworkers (1996) reported on 71 patients managed by reoperation and attributed the reason for failure to technical error in 40 cases (56%). Technical errors can create an unsatisfactory fundoplication, which may be unduly tight, too loose, or insecure. A Nissen fundoplication greater than 3 cm in length may produce symptoms of overcorrection of competence of the esophagogastric valvular mechanism.

Closure of the diaphragmatic hiatus may be too snug, too loose, or inadequately secured. A tight hiatus causes dysphagia. An unduly large or disrupted hiatus predisposes to recurrent herniation and reflux.

Vagal injury resulting in disabling side effects usually requires division of both vagus nerves, which occasionally results in delayed gastric emptying requiring pyloroplasty.

Damage to the esophageal wall or gastric fundus may lead to a postoperative leak into the abdomen, mediastinum, or thorax.

Wrong Operation

There is no single repair, no matter how technically well it is done, that is suitable for all of the various presentations of hiatal hernia and reflux. Selection of the optimal operation may be influenced by the presence of acquired esophageal shortening, defective esophageal motility, or significant gastric outlet obstruction. Significant acquired short esophagus is an indication for some type of esophageal lengthening procedure to reduce undue tension on the repair. Sufficient reduction in the peristaltic amplitudes of the thoracic esophagus can modify the extent of fundoplication—partial or complete. Gastric outlet obstruction may warrant the addition of pyloroplasty to the repair.

"Open" repairs may be managed more effectively through a thoracic approach in grossly obese patients and in patients with extensive abdominal adhesions resulting from previous surgery. The advent of laparoscopic repair, however, has significantly improved the facility for repair in the obese individual: The combination of gas insufflation and improved optical display has greatly improved both access and visualization.

Wrong Diagnosis

If hiatal hernia or reflux is incorrectly judged to be the cause of clinical signs and symptoms for which a repair is done, the clinical problem is not relieved. This may occur in patients with suggestive symptoms such as chest pain that is not of esophageal origin. On occasion, the adverse side effects of such a repair may warrant reoperation.

Failure to identify an underlying primary motor disorder such as achalasia or diffuse esophageal spasm results in a repair, without esophagomyotomy, which inevitably fails to relieve the clinical problem. This error most often occurs in cases of achalasia, and a repair only worsens the presenting dysphagia. Resolution requires dismantling the reconstruction and adding the myotomy. Ellis and associates (1996) attributed the need for reoperation to an incorrect diagnosis in 22 of 101 (22%) patients: achalasia, 16; diffuse spasm, 3; scleroderma, 3.

INVESTIGATION

A thorough and often extensive preoperative investigation is necessary in the evaluation of patients under consideration for reoperation. In the best of circumstances, the results of reoperation are less favorable than after the initial repair. Optimal outcomes require an appraisal of the mechanisms of failure and of the anatomy and pathophysiology of recurrence.

In all patients, the evaluation requires a detailed history of clinical presentation, contrast esophagography conducted by an informed radiologist, esophagogastroscopy by the operating surgeon, and esophageal manometry. Most surgeons consider 24-hour pH testing essential. Endoscopic examination may provide incontrovertible evidence of reflux esophagitis, but only 24-hour pH testing can provide a quantitative baseline for future reference in a group of patients in whom approximately 20% of the results after reoperation are unsatisfactory. Gastric emptying studies are often useful and are routinely advised by many practitioners. Luostarinen and colleagues observed that radionuclide transit studies were more sensitive than esophageal manometry for detecting disturbances of esophageal motility (Luostarinen et al, 1993; Russel et al, 1981). Testing for bile reflux may be useful in selected instances.

In most patients, the recurrent problem is not a significant threat to life or general health. Reoperation carries a small operative mortality risk and considerable potential morbidity. If there is any question about the need for, and possible benefit of, reoperation, it may be reasonable to delay the decision and repeat some or all of the evaluation at a subsequent time.

MANAGEMENT

The technical difficulty of this reoperative surgery is again emphasized. Prior experience with such surgery affords an enormous benefit. The usual anatomic landmarks are frequently obliterated by adhesions, the adhesions are present between fragile, easily damaged tissues, and the operative field may be further obscured if the adhesions are vascular. The learning curve to achieve expertise with this surgery is more than long—it is continuous and will continue to improve with each additional reoperation.

The selection of incision for exposure, and the choice of a specific operative procedure, are influenced by the preoperative findings; the category and presumed reason for failure; and, to some extent, the preference of the individual surgeon. Furthermore, the ultimate selection of reoperative procedure may be determined only intraoperatively in many cases.

Incision and Exposure

For open surgery, the incision and exposure may be abdominal, thoracic, or thoracoabdominal. Training and experience frequently direct the individual surgeon's choice. A few general observations may be made.

Whenever an extensive mobilization of the intrathoracic esophagus is necessary or anticipated, a thoracic exposure facilitates the dissection. By using a sixth or seventh interspace left thoracotomy incision, the surgeon can safely mobilize the esophagus circumferentially to the level of the aortic arch. If the previous repair was transthoracic and included a high level of mobilization of the mediastinal esophagus, the recommendation for a thoracic incision is even stronger.

If it is necessary to obtain access to the upper abdomen, the surgeon can simply make a curved incision in the diaphragm anteriorly, along a line that parallels its anterior costal attachment, leaving a 2- to 3-cm costal fringe for subsequent closure. Should still greater abdominal exposure be determined intraoperatively, the thoracotomy may be extended to a thoracoabdominal incision.

An open abdominal exposure is most commonly obtained with a midline, upper abdominal incision, beginning at the xiphoid to provide optimal exposure for the diaphragmatic hiatus and related structures. A good, self-retaining abdominal wall retractor and a headlight may facilitate exposure. Through the dilated diaphragmatic hiatus, it is possible to circumferentially mobilize the mediastinal esophagus under direct vision, almost to the level of the main carina. This type of mobilization is regularly achieved "transhiatally" during a transhiatal esophagectomy (see Chapter 57). Hill has used a purely transabdominal exposure in almost all of his reported cases of reoperation for failed repairs (Hill, 1971; Hill et al, 1979).

As experience has been gained with laparoscopic antireflux surgery, including reoperation, a few reports have indicated that circumferential mobilization of the mediastinal esophagus can be safely extended almost to the carinal level (Horvath et al, 2000; Swanstrom and Hansen, 1997).

Selection of Operation

The choice of reoperative procedure is determined by multiple factors:

- Presence or absence of a short esophagus
- Esophageal dysmotility
- An underlying *primary* motor disorder
- Loss of vagal nerve function
- Destruction of the anatomy of esophagogastric junction that precludes an effective antireflux reconstruction

Acquired Short Esophagus

If esophageal shortening is noted, reconstruction of an intra-abdominal antireflux barrier calls for the addition of an esophagus-lengthening procedure. For lesser degrees of shortening, extended mobilization of the intrathoracic esophagus may suffice (Gastal et al, 1999; Kauer et al, 1995; Pearson et al, 1971). Otherwise, a modification of Collis' (1957) original gastroplasty is recommended (see Chapters 15 and 24). Although an intrathoracic antireflux reconstruction can be done, adverse side effects have been reported (Maher et al, 1984).

Secondary Esophageal Dysmotility

A sufficient reduction of amplitude and frequency of peristalsis, secondary to intramural reflux damage or to prior resection of the vagus nerves, warrants a modification of the fundoplication to avoid the complication of dysphagia from a functional obstruction. This may be achieved by means of a partial, rather than complete, fundoplication or by means of a loose, short Nissen fundoplication. With either option, troublesome dysphagia may be avoided but at the expense of reduced reflux control.

Gadensstätter and colleagues (1998) reported a group of eight patients with "end-stage esophageal body dysfunction" who had undergone one earlier antireflux repair and now required reoperation.

Associated Primary Motor Disorder

As previously stated, the combination of reflux esophagitis and a primary motor disorder, such as achalasia, is a dilemma in management. These patients have had a previous esophagomyotomy for the achalasia (less commonly, diffuse esophageal spasm) and now have an ablated LES with free reflux combined with aperistalsis. Esophageal clearance depends on gravity and is absent in the recumbent position. An operation that adequately controls reflux may well result in unacceptable dysphagia, and vice versa.

Malthaner and associates (1994) reported long-term results in 35 patients managed by esophagomyotomy for achalasia, and all were observed for longer than 10 years. Severe reflux esophagitis was found in 10% of patients at 10-year follow-up and in 20% at 15-year follow-up. Ten of the 35 patients ultimately required esophagectomy for complications of achalasia, with peptic esophagitis, between 13 and 23 years after the initial esophagomyotomy.

It may be reasonable to undertake one antireflux reconstruction in selected patients, with the knowledge that long-term success is 50% at best. Orringer and Stirling (1989) favored early esophagectomy in these difficult patients.

Scleroderma can be classified as a motor disorder that is secondary to a collagen disease. The pathophysiology resembles achalasia—an ablated LES pressure and complete esophageal aperistalsis. The problem of achieving surgical control of reflux without troublesome dysphagia is identical and may be further augmented by functional obstruction in the distal stomach and bowel. Although an antireflux repair may significantly improve symptoms in selected patients (Henderson, 1987), the failure rate is high and esophagectomy may be considered in patients requiring reoperation.

Destroyed Esophagogastric Anatomy

On occasion, the distal esophagus and fundus are found to be so damaged once the previous repair is dismantled that an effective reconstruction is judged no longer possible. In this circumstance, an esophageal resection followed by reconstruction with colon, jejunum, or stomach may be indicated. If this level of difficulty is recognized before exploration, the surgeon may proceed directly to resection. If the possibility is entertained but uncertain, the patient should be prepared appropriately for this option. For example, the colon may be prepared in advance.

An alternative to resection in this difficult situation is to perform an antrectomy and Roux-en-Y gastrojejunostomy (acid suppression and bile diversion). This approach is less difficult and less dangerous than resection

TABLE 29–1 ■ **Reported Series of Reoperations with More than 30 Cases**

Author	Year	No. of Cases	> One Prior Repair	Reoperation Type	Mortality Rate (%)	Results (%) Good/Excellent	Satisfactory
Skinner	1967	43	0	Rep: 28			
				Res: 15			
Orringer	1972	45	0	Rep: 33	3	73	
				Res: 12	0	85	
Hill	1972	63	12	Rep: 63 (Hill)	3	81	
Polk	1980	36	28	Res: 28 (JEJ Interp)	4	80	
				Rep: 8	0	50	
Henderson and Marryatt	1981	121	0	Rep: 121 (Collis Nissen)	0	94	
Maher et al	1985	55	6	Rep: 55	4		80
Little et al	1986	61	27	Rep: 45			
				Res: 15	5	72	
Stirling and Orringer	1986	87	25	Rep: 73	3	67	
				Res: 23	0	76	
Pearson et al	1987	118	22	Rep: 118 (Collis Belsey)	0	80	
Low et al	1989	116		Rep: 116 (Hill)	3	86	
Siewert	1995	50	9	Rep: 42	2	70	
				Other: 5			
Stein et al	1996	71	11	Rep: 65	1		86
				Res: 6			
Ellis et al	1996	101	43	Rep: 63	1		80
				Res: 5			
				Roux Y: 18			
				Other: 15			
Deschamps	1997	185		Rep: 168 (Collis Nissen 116)	0.5		88
				Roux Y: 17			

Rep, repair, includes lesser operations such as dismantling fundoplication, removal Angelchick prostheses; Res, resection of esophagogastric junction and reconstruction with bowel or stomach; Roux Y, acid suppression and bile diversion with antrectomy ± vagotomy and Roux-en-Y jejunogastrostomy; Good/Excellent, combined total of excellent and good results; Satisfactory, combined total of excellent, good and fair results; fair results imply significant symptoms, usually; JEJ, jejunum.

and interposition. The area of previous surgery is avoided. This operation has been popularized by Ellis in America and Fekete in France (Ellis, 1994; Fekete et al, 1992).

Detailed information regarding esophageal resection and acid suppression with Roux-en-Y bile diversion for reflux disease is found in Chapters 26 and 28, respectively.

RESULTS OF REOPERATION

The reported outcomes of reoperation for failed repairs are somewhat confusing because of the lack of any accepted, standardized system of evaluation and results reporting. Nevertheless, as stated in the introductory comments for this chapter, a review of reported results clearly documents a significantly greater incidence of operative deaths, complications, and unsatisfactory outcomes. Information is summarized in Table 29–1 from publications documenting experience with groups of 35 or more cases.

Several publications focus specifically on reoperations for prior, failed Nissen repairs (Hill et al, 1979; Leonardi et al, 1981). Luostarinen and colleagues studied 15 patients who had undergone "refundoplication" for recurrent gastroesophageal reflux with a detailed, postoperative functional investigation that was done between 5 and 152 months after reoperation. The evaluation included endoscopy, manometry, 24-hour pH testing, and radionuclide transit studies. Although the symptomatic outcomes were "reasonable," results were not as good as after the primary operation. Poorer outcomes were attributed to greater impairment of esophageal motility, owing to persisting reflux, repeated surgery, or both.

The first experience with laparoscopic reoperation began in the last decade of the 20th century. At the beginning, few surgeons found these efforts other than a dangerous curiosity. Since 1999, however, it has become apparent that persistent efforts and experience combined with ever-improving instrumentation and technology have advanced laparoscopic reoperation to an increasingly prominent position in the field. The current status is well defined in the next part of Chapter 29.

■ *REFERENCES*

Allison PR: Reflux esophagitis, sliding hiatal hernia, and the anatomy of repair. Surg Gynecol Obstet 92:419, 1951.

Collis JL: An operation for hiatus hernia with short esophagus. J Thorac Cardiovasc Surg 34:768, 1957.

Dallemagne B, Weerts JM, Jehaes C, et al: Laparoscopic Nissen fundoplication: Preliminary report. Surg Laparosc Endosc 1:138–143, 1991.

Deschamps C, Trastek VF, Allen MS, et al: Long term results after reoperation for failed antireflux procedures. J Thorac Cardiovasc Surg 113:545–551, 1997.

Ellis FH, Gibb SP, Heatley GJ: Reoperation after failed antireflux surgery: Review of 101 cases. Eur J Cardiothorac Surg 10:225–233, 1996.

Ellis FH, Gibb SP: Vagotomy, antrectomy, and Roux-en-Y diversion for complex reoperative gastroesophageal reflux disease. Ann Surg 220:536–542, 1994.

Fekete F, Gayet B, Deslandes M, Dubertret M: Reintervention pour echecs de la chirurgie du reflux gastro-esophagien: A propos de cinquante reinterventions. Ann Chir 46:44–50, 1992.

Gadenstätter M, Hagen JA, DeMeester TR, et al: Esophagectomy for unsuccessful antireflux operations. J Thorac Cardiovasc Surg 115:296–302, 1998.

Gastal OL, Hagen JA, Peters JH, et al: Analysis of predictors and clinical implications. Arch Surg 134:633–638, 1999.

Henderson RD: Esophageal motor disorders. Surg Clin North Am 67:455, 1987.

Henderson RD: Nissen hiatal hernia repair: Problems of recurrence and continued symptoms. Ann Thorac Surg 28:587, 1979.

Henderson RD, Marryatt G: Recurrent hiatal hernia: Management by thoracoabdominal total fundoplication gastroplasty. Can J Surg 24:151–157, 1981.

Hill LD: Management of recurrent hiatal hernia. Arch Surg 102:296, 1971.

Hill LD, Ilves R, Stevenson JK, Pearson JM: Reoperation for disruption and recurrence after Nissen fundoplication. J Thorac Cardiovsc Surg 113:542–548, 1979.

Horvath KD, Swanstrom LL, Jobe BA: The short esophagus: Pathophysiology, incidence, presentation and treatment in the era of laparoscopic antireflux surgery. Ann Surg 232:630–640, 2000.

Kauer WKH, Peters JH, DeMeester TR, et al: A tailored approach to antireflux surgery. J Thorac Cardiovasc Surg 110:141–147, 1995.

Leonardi HK, Crozier RE, Ellis FH: Reoperation for complications of the Nissen fundoplication. J Thorac Cardiovasc Surg 81:50–56, 1981.

Little AG, Ferguson MK, Skinner DB: Reoperation for failed antireflux operations. J Thorac Cardiovasc Surg 91:511–517, 1986.

Low DE, Anderson RP, Ilves R, Hill LD: 15 to 20 year results after the Hill operation. J Thorac Cardiovasc Surg 98:444, 1989.

Luostarinen ME, Isolauri JO, Koskinen MO, et al: Refundoplication for recurrent gastroesophageal reflux. World J Surg 17:587–594, 1993.

Maher JW, Hocking MP, Woodward ER: Reoperation for esophagitis following failed antireflux procedures. Ann Surg 201:723–727, 1984.

Malthaner RA, Todd TR, Miller L, Pearson FG: Long term results in surgically managed achalasia. Ann Thorac Surg 58:1–6, 1994.

Orringer MB: Long-term results of the Mark IV operation for hiatal hernia and analyses of recurrences and their treatment. J Thorac Cardiovasc Surg 63:25–33, 1972.

Orringer MB, Stirling MC: Esophageal resection for achalasia: Indication and results. Ann Thorac Surg 47:340–345, 1989.

Pearson FG, Cooper JD, Patterson GA, et al: Gastroplasty and fundoplication for complex reflux problems. Ann Surg 206:473–481, 1987.

Pearson FG, Langer R, Henderson RD: Gastroplasty and Belsey hiatus hernia repair. J Thorac Cardiovasc Surg 61:50, 1971.

Polk HC: Jejunal interposition for reflux esophagitis and esophageal stricture unresponsive to valvuloplasty. World J Surg 4:731, 1980.

Russel COH, Hill LD, Holmes ER, et al: Radionuclide transit: A sensitive screening test for esophageal dysfunction. Gastroenterology 80:887, 1981.

Siewert JR, Stein HJ, Feussner H: Reoperations after failed antireflux procedures. Ann Chir Gynaecol 84:122, 1995.

Skinner DB: Surgical management of esophageal reflux and hiatal hernia: Long term results with 1,030 patients. J Thorac Cardiovasc Surg 53:33–54, 1967.

Stein HJ, Feussner H, Siewert JR: Failure of antireflux surgery: Causes and management strategies. Am J Surg 171:36–40, 1996.

Stirling MC, Orringer MB: Surgical treatment after the failed antireflux operation. J Thorac Cardiovasc Surg 92:667–672, 1986.

Swanstrom LL, Hansen P: Laparoscopic total esophagectomy. Arch Surg 132:943–949, 1997.

LAPAROSCOPIC TECHNIQUES IN REOPERATION FOR FAILED REPAIRS

Sean Grondin
James D. Luketich

Approximately 44% of Americans suffer from heartburn at least once a month (Isolauri et al, 1997). Lifestyle modifications and medical management with acid-suppressing medication can control symptoms in most patients, but an increasing number of patients are seeking alternative treatment options. This is particularly true in recent years owing to the application of minimally invasive techniques in the performance of antireflux procedures as well as an increasing concern regarding the cost or potential consequences of life-long medical acid suppression.

The effectiveness of laparoscopic antireflux surgery for gastroesophageal reflux disease (GERD) has been clearly demonstrated in several series reporting good to excellent patient satisfaction in approximately 90% of patients (Dallemagne et al, 1995; Trus et al, 1996). These results, in combination with a shorter hospital stay and a more rapid return to normal activities, have promoted the emergence of minimally invasive antireflux surgery, in particular, laparoscopic Nissen fundoplication, as the method of choice for the operative management of GERD (Peters and DeMeester, 1996).

The popularity of this procedure is illustrated by the increase in the number of Nissen fundoplications performed annually. The Centers for Disease Control and Prevention estimated that 12,000 fundoplications were performed by the open route in the United States in 1987 compared with 48,000 laparoscopic procedures in 1998. This increase in laparoscopic antireflux surgery has led to an increase in the number of patients presenting with recurrent symptoms after surgery. Failure of open fundoplication has been reported in 9% to 30% of cases (DeMeester et al, 1986; Hiebert and O'Mara, 1979; Shirazzi et al, 1987). Laparoscopic failure rates from published series range from 2% to 17%, and with longer follow-up higher rates may occur (Hinder, 1996; Hunter et al, 1996; Peters and DeMeester, 1996). The failure rate in nonacademic centers is largely unknown, but a well-established steep learning curve suggests that the failure rate may be even higher. Many patients with recurrent symptoms after antireflux surgery can be managed non-operatively, but from 3% to 6% require reoperation (Collard et al, 1993).

Reoperation after a failed antireflux procedure is challenging and has historically been performed using open techniques. Morbidity rates between 20% and 40% have been reported using the open technique, with a mortality rate approximating 2% (Siewert et al, 1995). Several reports have documented good results after reoperation by the laparoscopic approach. With open or laparoscopic reoperative antireflux surgery, the success of reoperation never achieves that of an initial operation in experienced hands. Despite this finding, many patients can achieve a good result after reoperation (Siewert et al, 1995). Little and colleagues (1986) reported an association between the success rate of reoperative antireflux surgery and the number of previous antireflux operations. In their series, 84% of patients with one previous antireflux operation had a good result, whereas only 42% of patients with three or more previous operations had a good outcome.

Here we present the reasons for failure after antireflux surgery, describe an approach to the evaluation of patients with recurrent symptoms, discuss management strategies, and provide an overview of laparoscopic reoperative antireflux surgery.

CAUSES OF FAILURE

The inability of antireflux surgery to relieve symptoms may include inappropriate initial patient selection because of misdiagnosis. For example, the preoperative workup may have been incomplete and the original symptoms mistaken for GERD. Laparoscopic or open approaches may result in the creation of a fundoplication that is too loose, too tight, too short, or too long or inappropriately positioned or disrupted. These technical errors may lead to recurrent GERD symptoms or a new constellation of symptoms related to dysphagia. In the era of laparoscopic antireflux surgery, the failure to adequately divide the short gastric vessels or to mobilize the esophageal fat pad may contribute to a technically poor result.

Several randomized trials of laparoscopic antireflux surgery indicate that division of the short gastric vessels may not be the critical event leading to recurrent symptoms (Blomqvist et al, 2000); nevertheless, in our experience taking down the short gastrics is more likely to result in a tension-free wrap. Other complications, such as inadvertent vagal injuries, may lead to significant bloating and even recurrent GERD.

The failure to identify acquired shortening of the esophagus, either preoperatively or intraoperatively, may lead to migration of the fundoplication into the thorax.

The failure to adequately dissect out a large hiatal hernia sac and perform a satisfactory crural repair can contribute to recurrent herniation and symptoms.

Several authors have reported on the causes of failed antireflux procedures (Low et al, 1988; O'Haranhan et al, 1990). Hinder and co-workers (1997) reported laparoscopic reoperations in 46 patients who had experienced a failed antireflux procedure; the two most common causes of failure were (1) breakdown of the fundoplication (35%) and (2) breakdown of the crural repair (22%) (Floch et al, 1999). A slipped wrap (15%) and a wrap that was too loose (8%) or too tight (8%) were less frequently observed in this series. Also in this series, nearly 70% of patients who required reoperation had recurrent symptoms within 2 years of their original surgery, suggesting that operative technique plays an important contributing role in the failure of antireflux procedures.

Failure to Recognize Esophageal Shortening

Esophageal shortening is a controversial topic for both thoracic and general surgeons. It is hypothesized by some that long-standing reflux leads to circumferential scarring and peptic strictures, and in more severe cases varying degrees of longitudinal scarring and esophageal shortening may result. In our experience, the presence of esophageal shortening should be suspected in the presence of peptic stricture, Schatzki's ring, Barrett's esophagus, and moderate to giant hiatal hernias.

The barium esophagram is helpful in recognizing patients who may have esophageal shortening. Occasionally, esophageal shortening can be detected preoperatively by the presence of an intrathoracic location of the lower esophageal sphincter (LES) on manometry or endoscopy or the presence of a shortened intersphincteric distance (i.e., the distance between the upper esophageal sphincter [UES] and the LES) on manometry (Maziak et al, 1998). A careful intraoperative evaluation is necessary to confirm clinically significant shortening. We have found dissection of the gastroesophageal fat pad to be essential to identify the true gastroesophageal junction and exclude shortening. Intraoperative endoscopy may aid recognition in borderline cases.

Laparoscopic antireflux surgery may increase the risk of missing a shortened esophagus because several intraoperative factors may mislead the surgeon. For example, the pressure of the pneumoperitoneum elevates the diaphragm and may lead to an overestimate of the tension-free intra-abdominal segment. In addition, some surgeons use a Penrose drain wrapped around the lower esophagus, and this downward traction may produce an abdominal segment of esophagus that looks adequate under tension but may subsequently retract and lead to recurrent herniation of the wrap.

Another mechanism leading to overestimation of the abdominal segment of esophagus is the placement of a rigid bougie. Although helpful in minimizing the risk of too tight a wrap, the bougie may place downward tension on the esophagus and give several centimeters of length that may again retract later when the bougie is not in place.

Laparoscopic mobilization of the mediastinal esophagus may allow the surgeon to gain enough length to allow construction of a tension-free, intra-abdominal fundoplication. If esophageal shortening is identified and adequate length with esophageal mobilization cannot be obtained, a Collis gastroplasty may minimize the incidence of subsequent diaphragmatic herniation and ultimate failure. Minimally invasive approaches to a Collis gastroplasty with good short-term results have been described by several groups (Johnson et al, 1998; Luketich et al, 2000; Swanstrom et al, 1996).

Herniation and Crural Disruption

Herniation of the antireflux wrap usually occurs secondary to disruption of the crural repair or, more commonly in our opinion, from failure to perform the initial wrap over a tension-free intra-abdominal segment of esophagus. The disruption can result from excessive tension of the primary suture repair, leading to stitches being pulled out of the crus. In our experience, careful preservation of the peritoneal layer covering the crus is helpful in maintaining the integrity of the crura before placing the closure sutures.

Occasionally, a relaxing incision of the diaphragm or a prosthetic patch (Gore-Tex; W. L. Gore and Associates, Flagstaff, Ariz.) is required to close a large esophageal hiatus. Some authors have recommended the more liberal use of mesh reconstruction of the diaphragm; however, in our report of 100 consecutive laparoscopic repairs of giant paraesophageal hernias, mesh reconstruction was required in only 3% of cases (Luketich et al, 2000).

Slipped Nissen

A "slipped Nissen" occurs when part of the stomach lies both above and below the wrap. This defect may arise as a result of slippage of the stomach through the fundoplication or incorrect positioning of the wrap around the stomach at the time of the original surgery (Hinder, 1996). Ruling out the presence of esophageal shortening and ensuring a tension-free wrap around the intra-abdominal portion of the esophagus are essential to minimize the occurrence of this complication.

Fundoplication: Too Loose or Too Tight

A wrap that is too tight or too loose remains an important cause of persistent symptoms in patients who undergo antireflux surgery. If the wrap is too floppy, the pressure created in the distal esophagus is low and may favor recurrent postoperative reflux. Conversely, if the wrap is too tight, dysphagia may occur (Leonardi et al, 1988).

Preoperative manometry findings, the patient's body habitus, and the intraoperative findings after mobilization of the stomach and distal esophagus must be carefully considered to allow the surgeon to tailor the dimensions of the wrap. At our institution, a laparoscopic Nissen fundoplication is generally performed around a Maloney bougie ranging in size from 48 to 50 French for small to average-sized (70-kg) patients. In larger patients, the fundoplication is generally wrapped around a 52 to 54 French bougie. A "shoeshine" maneuver is performed at the time of the fundoplication to allow careful assessment of any redundant wrap that may contribute to too loose of a wrap.

A recent randomized study of "bougie versus no bougie" use during laparoscopic Nissen fundoplication showed that the bougie group had a lower incidence of clinically significant dysphagia postoperatively (Patterson et al, 2000). In the patient with impaired esophageal motility, our preference is a looser Nissen wrap over a slightly larger bougie. Some reports have shown good results in patients with impaired motility using a partial fundoplication such as a Toupet or a Belsey repair. However, our experience and that of other researchers in some studies have shown this to be associated with an unacceptable rate of recurrent reflux and laparoscopic reoperation (Horvath et al, 1999).

Vagal Injury

Preservation of both vagus nerves is an important goal of antireflux repair. Injury to one or both of the vagus nerves can lead to significant sequelae. Familiarity with the anatomy and meticulous dissection in the hiatus will minimize the risk of intraoperative injury. Injury to both vagi frequently results in a marked delay in gastric emptying and dumping symptoms (Eagon et al, 1992). If an injury to both vagi is suspected or identified intraoperatively or is suspected preoperatively in a reoperative case based on an abnormal gastric emptying test, the addition of a gastric emptying procedure such as a laparoscopic pyloroplasty should be considered.

In our experience, injury to even a single vagal trunk may lead to significant exacerbations of the usually mild postoperative bloating seen in many patients after Nissen fundoplication. Careful dietary counseling and medications such as simethicone may minimize these symptoms.

EVALUATION

The evaluation of a patient with persistent or recurrent symptoms after an antireflux procedure begins with a thorough clinical evaluation. A careful review of the patient's preoperative symptoms and test results can help determine whether the fundoplication was indicated. Ruling out the presence of esophageal motility disorders (e.g., achalasia) or gastrointestinal disorders (e.g., chronic cholecystitis) is essential and may require the assistance of an experienced gastroenterologist. A careful review of the operative notes and discussion with the original surgeon may aid in the recognition of the reason for the failure.

In our experience, failure in the hands of an inexperienced surgeon may be much simpler to correct if technical errors have been made; however, a failure from a surgeon experienced in laparoscopic antireflux surgery may be more subtle and difficult to assess. Particular attention to the details of the operative notes regarding the dissection of the esophagus, short gastric vessels, and fat pad may give clues to current problems. The positioning and status of the anterior and posterior vagal fibers, nerves, bougie size, and crural repair should be noted.

Finally, a determination of the severity of the patient's symptoms, response to medical therapy, and attitude toward the initial surgical intervention can provide valuable information as to whether the initial operation was indicated. If the original diagnosis is in doubt, other diagnostic studies may be helpful.

At a minimum, our approach to the patient with a failed antireflux operation includes a barium video esophagram, chest radiograph, upper gastrointestinal endoscopy, esophageal motility, 24-hour pH testing, and a nuclear medicine gastric emptying study. The results of these tests are invaluable in determining the cause and possible solution to recurrent or new symptoms after an unsatisfactory result from antireflux surgery.

Several radiologic patterns identified on barium esophagography can assist the surgeon in determining the cause of a failed wrap (Fig. 29–1):

- A *type I* abnormality represents a near-complete or complete disruption of the wrap with recurrence of the hiatal hernia.
- A *type II* defect occurs from slippage of a portion of the stomach above the diaphragm, usually caused by incorrect positioning of the fundoplication around the upper stomach rather than esophagus. A classic "hourglass" appearance may be observed.
- A *type III* defect, commonly referred to as a "slipped Nissen," is seen when part of the stomach lies both above and below the wrap. This defect may arise as a result of slippage of the stomach through the fundoplication or incorrect positioning of the wrap around the stomach at the time of the original surgery.
- The *type IV* abnormality is seen when the entire fundoplication herniates into the chest, usually as a result of a disrupted crural repair.

Upper Gastrointestinal Endoscopy

Upper gastrointestinal endoscopy is performed to assess for esophagitis, stricture, gastritis, ulceration, or tumor and to evaluate the position and integrity of the wrap. Interpretation of the endoscopic findings requires experience and knowledge of the proposed mechanism for the failure of the antireflux procedure. For example, the presence of gastric mucosa above the wrap suggests the possibility of a "slipped Nissen." Alternatively, a widely patent gastroesophageal junction viewed on retroflexion of the endoscope positioned in the stomach suggests that the cause of recurrent symptoms may be attributed to a loose or disrupted wrap. Identifying the squamocolumnar junction and its relation to the diaphragmatic crura can make an assessment of esophageal length.

Esophageal Manometry

We recommend a repeat esophageal manometry test in the evaluation of a patient with a failed antireflux procedure. The initial manometry may have been improperly performed or interpreted, and subsequent manometry may provide valuable information regarding esophageal body motility. This can help exclude the presence of poor esophageal peristalsis or other esophageal motility

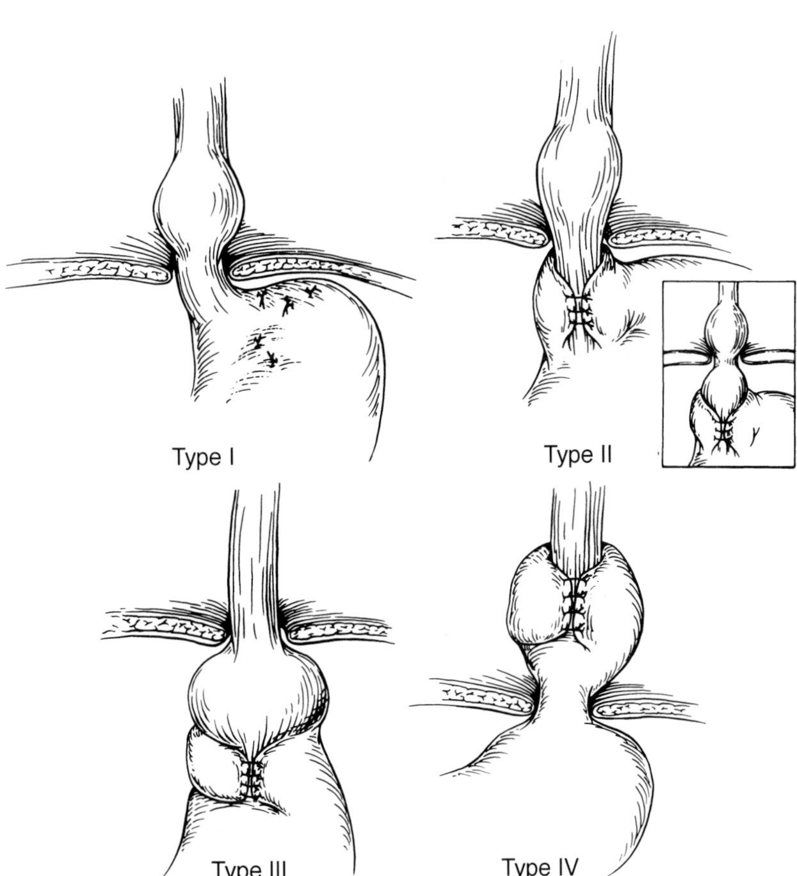

FIGURE 29–1 ■ Types of surgical failure of Nissen fundoplication. (From Hinder RA: Gastroesophageal reflux disease. In Bell RH Jr, Rikkers LF, Mulholland MW [eds]: Digestive Tract Surgery: A Text and Atlas. Philadelphia, Lippincott-Raven, 1996, p 19.)

abnormalities such as diffuse esophageal spasm or achalasia.

Assessment of LES pressures provides essential information as to whether the fundoplication has been disrupted or is too loose (i.e., low LES pressure) or whether the fundoplication is too tight, causing dysphagia (i.e., high LES pressure). The distance from the UES to LES can be measured and may suggest the presence of esophageal shortening if the distance is decreased. Pearson has reported that patients with giant paraesophageal hernia have a significant decrease in this length compared with normals (Maziak et al, 1998), and this measurement may aid in the preoperative recognition of esophageal shortening.

24-Hour pH Esophageal Studies

Twenty-four-hour esophageal pH studies are helpful in evaluating patients with recurrent symptoms after antireflux surgery (DeMeester et al, 1980). We perform this test in most patients before considering laparoscopic reoperation for failed antireflux surgery. The presence of an excessively alkaline environment suggests the possibility of duodenogastroesophageal reflux or the stasis of alkaline salivary secretions in the distal esophagus (Pelligrini et al, 1978). Some centers have begun to use biliary probes to test for bile reflux as a cause of recurrent or persistent symptoms.

MANAGEMENT STRATEGIES

Initial Evaluation

The initial workup and management of most patients with early postoperative symptomatology should be conservative. Transient symptoms of dysphagia, bloating, and dietary intolerance are common in the immediate 4 to 6 weeks postoperatively and frequently resolve. For example, mild dysphagia early in the postoperative period is often transient and secondary to edema; in contrast, extreme dysphagia with inability to tolerate a liquid diet is a warning, and early reoperation should be considered.

A particularly ominous sign is the complaint of foamy salivation or the inability to tolerate liquids immediately postoperatively. This suggests a technical error or a failure to recognize a severe esophageal motility disorder. The postoperative barium esophagram usually confirms a very tight wrap that is unlikely to improve with time and warrants consideration for early reoperation. We generally reserve dilatation for patients whose symptoms are moderate and persist beyond 2 to 3 months. In our experience, 2% to 3% of patients will require a single dilation. Persistent dysphagia despite these measures may lead to consideration for reoperation.

Some patients experience a short course of postoperative diarrhea, which is frequently related to gas bloating and often resolves with slower progression of the diet or addition of simethicone. Increased flatus and the inability to vomit or belch are other common side effects of antireflux surgery. Medications such as simethicone that help to dissipate the stomach gas bubble are occasionally helpful. If the diarrhea or gas bloating persists, injury to the vagal nerves at the time of surgery should be considered. In severe cases, diarrhea must be managed with antidiarrheal agents and gas bloating, secondary to vagal injury, may require a gastric emptying procedure such as a pyloroplasty or pyloromyotomy.

Surgical Therapy

The principles of reoperative laparoscopic surgery are similar to those of "redo" open procedures. Notably, the operation is demanding and should be undertaken only by a team of experienced laparoscopic esophageal surgeons. Operative times are frequently prolonged, with difficult cases often requiring several hours or more to complete.

After induction of anesthesia, we perform an on-the-table esophagogastroduodenoscopy. A nasogastric tube, in addition to a Foley catheter and pneumatic stockings, is positioned. An arterial line for continuous blood pressure monitoring is also placed to help guide the surgeon in adjusting the intraoperative carbon dioxide insufflation pressures and to monitor for the development of a tension pneumothorax, which can occur during the dissection of the scarred hiatus during reoperative surgery. We prefer the patient in the supine position, in the steep reverse Trendelenburg position, with the surgeon to the right of the patient (not between the legs as in lithotomy).

Initial port placement requires a direct cutdown with placement of a blunt port under direct peritoneal visualization. If dense adhesions are encountered, we generally add a more inferior and lateral port to allow better visualization and adhesiolysis. After complete adhesiolysis, we convert to our standard five access ports (Fig. 29–2). One advantage of laparoscopy over laparotomy is that this technique provides a magnified view of the operative field and the ability to easily change the angle of that view.

We prefer to use a 10-mm, 30-degree laparoscope because it provides a wider operative view. The abdomen is insufflated to an intra-abdominal pressure of 10 to 15 mm Hg. We find that lower pressures in the 8- to 10-mm Hg range are often sufficient in the dissection around the hiatus and minimize the effects of a prolonged pneumoperitoneum during a laparoscopic reoperation.

After a careful laparoscopic examination of the peritoneal cavity to exclude other intra-abdominal pathologic processes, dissection of adhesions and mobilization of the esophagogastric junction are started. The density of adhesions around the hiatus and wrap are unpredictable and can make mobilization of the stomach and distal esophagus from the liver and crus difficult, leading to injury of the stomach or esophagus. Careful and meticulous dissection with the autosonic shears (U.S. Surgical Corporation, Norwalk, Conn.) or harmonic scalpel (Ethicon, Cincinnati, Ohio) is helpful and minimizes the risk to surrounding structures and provides a relatively bloodless field. If hypotension or high ventilatory pressures are detected during the dissection of the hiatus, a pneumothorax should be suspected and treated by placement of a chest tube. At our institution, insertion of a 12 French pigtail catheter in the affected hemithorax is the preferred method to reexpand the lung.

A complete takedown of the previous repair is essential to fully evaluate the cause of failure. Full mobilization

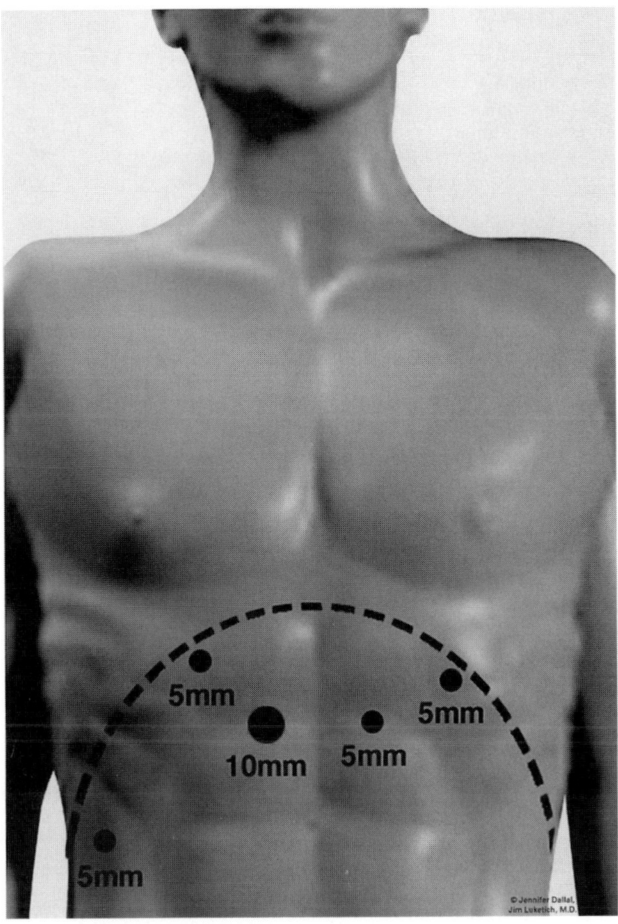

FIGURE 29–2 ■ Abdominal port sites for laparoscopic Nissen fundoplication.

of the distal esophagus, short gastric vessels, and esophageal fat pad and identification of the crus are essential to plan the repair. Early identification and removal of wrap and crural sutures will facilitate mobilization. The use of a lighted bougie can also help identify the esophagus and facilitate dissection. Once the mobilization is complete, the identification of a shortened esophagus may influence the decision to add a Collis gastroplasty to the antireflux repair. This technique is described in Chapter 24. Occasionally, a prosthetic patch (Gore-Tex) is required to perform an adequate crural reapproximation. Before performing the wrap, we insufflate the esophagus and stomach using a gastroscope to identify unrecognized enterotomies that require repair at the completion of the procedure. Once the patient is transferred to the recovery room, a baseline hematocrit is obtained and a chest radiograph is performed to rule out a pneumothorax.

In the absence of gastric ileus or abdominal distention, the nasogastric tube is removed the morning after surgery. A barium swallow is subsequently performed. If no extravasation of contrast medium is observed on the barium examination, the patient is started on a clear fluid diet. If the patient tolerates the liquid diet, discharge home usually occurs on postoperative day 2 after nutritional counseling is presented. In general, the patient remains on a soft diet for 1 to 2 weeks after surgery.

RESULTS OF LAPAROSCOPIC REOPERATIVE SURGERY

Given the increasing worldwide experience with laparoscopic antireflux surgery, reports of laparoscopic reoperative treatment of failed laparoscopic and open antireflux procedures are becoming more common. Table 29–2 lists selected studies that review the laparoscopic repair of failed antireflux surgery. Although the series are small, a few observations can be made.

First, the partial or complete breakdown or disruption of the Nissen repair is the most common cause of failure, followed by disruption of the crural repair and the "slipped Nissen" defect. In most series, a wrap that was too tight accounted for a small proportion of patients presenting with dysphagia, whereas an intact wrap that was too loose was an uncommon finding. Of note, the conversion rate from laparoscopic reoperation to open repair ranged from 0% to 55%. In this group of studies, perioperative morbidity ranged from 0% to 39%. No mortalities were reported in any of these studies. In short-term analysis, an overall patient satisfaction score above 80% was obtained in all reports.

At the University of Pittsburgh, the results of reoperative laparoscopic antireflux surgery in 28 patients have been reviewed (Ikramuddin et al, 1998). Twenty-five patients reported symptoms of recurrent GERD, such as heartburn and regurgitation. Three patients had dysphagia. At the time of surgery, seven patients experienced

TABLE 29–2 ■ **Survey of Failed Antireflux Procedures from Selected Reports (1995–1999)**

Author (Year)	*No.*	*Open Conversion*	*Morbidity*	*Mortality*	*Good Results*
Pointer et al (1999)	30	2 (7%)	39%	0	N/A
Szwerc et al (1999)	15	0%	0	0	87%
Watson et al (1999)	27	15 (55%)	0	0	93%
DePaula et al (1995)	19	1 (5%)	16%	0	84%
Curet et al (1999)	27	1 (4%)	7%	0	96%
Horgan et al (1999)	31	3 (10%)	32%	0	87%
University of Pittsburgh, Dept. of Thoracic Surgery (unpublished data) (1998)	28	3 (10%)	28%	0	85%

N/A, not available.

Data from Curet MJ, Josloff RK, Schoeb O, et al: Arch Surg 134:559, 1999; DePaula Al, Hashiba K, Bafutto M, et al: Surg Endosc 9:681, 1995; Horgan S, Pohl D, Bogetti D, et al: Arch Surg 134:809, 1999; Pointer R, Bammer T, Then P, et al: Am J Surg 178:541, 1999; Szwerc MF, Wiechmann RJ, Maley RH, et al: Reoperative laparoscopic antireflux surgery. Surgery 126:723, 1999; Watson DI, Jamieson GG, Game PA, et al: Br J Surg 86:98, 1999.

partial or complete disruption of their wraps, seven had slipped Nissens, seven had disruption of the crura, three had wraps that were too tight, and four had a shortened esophagus. There were no conversions to open procedures. Operative morbidity included one esophageal and two gastric perforations, two pneumothoraces, and two partial vagal injuries. Postoperative morbidity included three patients with urinary retention (11%), two with pleural effusions (7%), two with diarrhea (7%), one with abdominal leak (4%), one with partial small bowel obstruction (4%), and one with pulmonary embolus (4%). No operative mortalities were observed. Good to excellent short-term results were observed in 85% of patients undergoing redo operations.

CONCLUSION

Laparoscopic repair of previously failed antireflux procedures is technically challenging. Although the risk of conversion and morbidity rates are slightly higher than with first-time laparoscopic antireflux surgery, good to excellent short-term results are possible in 80% to 85% of cases using minimally invasive techniques in an experienced center, similar to results of open reoperation. A thorough evaluation by a surgeon experienced in esophageal physiology and advanced laparoscopic techniques is essential to ensure that appropriate intervention is applied.

■ *REFERENCES*

Blomqvist A, Dalenback J, Hagedorn C, et al: Impact of complete gastric fundus mobilization on outcome after laparoscopic total fundoplication. J Gastrointest Surg 4:493–500, 2000.

Collard JM, Verstraete L, Otte JB, et al: Clinical, radiological, and functional results of remedial antireflux operations. Int Surg 78:298, 1993.

Curet MJ, Josloff RK, Schoeb O, et al: Laparoscopic reoperation for failed antireflux procedures. Arch Surg 134:559, 1999.

Dallemagne B, Taziaux P, Weerts J, et al: Laparoscopic surgery for gastroesophageal reflux. Ann Chir 49:30, 1995.

Dallemagne B, Weerts JM, Markjiewicz S: Causes of laparoscopic antireflux operations. Surg Endosc 10:305, 1996.

DeMeester TR, Bonavina L, Albertucci M: Nissen fundoplication for gastroesophageal reflux disease: Evaluation of primary repair in 100 consecutive patients. Ann Surg 204:9, 1986.

DeMeester TR, Wang CI, Wernly JA, et al: Technique, indications, and clinical use of 24-hour esophageal pH monitoring. J Thorac Cardiovasc Surg 79:656, 1980.

DePaula AL, Hashiba K, Bafutto M, et al: Laparoscopic reoperations after failed and complicated antireflux operations. Surg Endosc 9:681, 1995.

Eagon JC, Miedema BW, Kelly KA: Postgastrectomy syndromes. Surg Clin North Am 72:445, 1992.

Floch NR, Hinder RA, Klingler PJ, et al: Is laparoscopic reoperation for failed antireflux surgery feasible? Arch Surg 134:733, 1999.

Hiebert CA, O'Mara CS: The Belsey operation for hiatal hernia: A twenty-year experience. Am J Surg 137:532, 1979.

Hinder RA: Gastroesophageal reflux disease. In Bell RH Jr, Rikkers LF, Mulholland MW (eds): Digestive Tract Surgery: Text and Atlas. Philadelphia, Lippincott-Raven, 1996, p 19.

Hinder RA, Klingler PJ, Perdikis G, et al: Management of the failed antireflux operation. Surg Clin North Am 77:1083, 1997.

Horgan S, Pohl D, Bogetti D, et al: Failed antireflux surgery. Arch Surg 134:809, 1999.

Horvath KD, Jobe BA, Herron DM, Swanstrom LL: Laparoscopic Toupet fundoplication is an inadequate procedure for patients with severe reflux disease. J Gastrointest Surg 3:583–591, 1999.

Hunter JG, Trus TL, Branum GD, et al: A physiologic approach to laparoscopic fundoplication for gastroesophageal reflux disease. Ann Surg 223:673–687, 1996.

Ikramuddin S, Luketich JD, Nguyen NT, Schauer PR: Reoperative laparoscopic anti-reflux surgery. Surg Endosc 12:567, 1998.

Isolauri J, Luostarinen M, Isolauri E, et al: Natural course of gastroesophageal reflux disease: 17–22 year follow-up of 60 patients. Am J Gastroenterol 92:37, 1997.

Johnson AB, Oddsdottir M, Hunter JG: Laparoscopic Collis gastroplasty and Nissen fundoplication: A new technique for the management of esophageal foreshortening. Surg Endosc 12:1055–1060, 1998.

Leonardi HK, Ellis FHS Jr: Reoperative surgery for gastroesophageal reflux. In Jamieson CG (ed): Surgery of the Oesophagus. Melbourne, Churchill Livingstone, 1988, p 291.

Little AG, Ferguson MK, Skinner DB: Reoperation for failed antireflux operations. J Thorac Cardiovasc Surg 91:511, 1986.

Low DE, Mercer CD, James EC, et al: Post Nissen syndrome. Surg Gynecol Obstet 167:1, 1988.

Luketich JD, Raja S, Fernanco HC, et al: Laparoscopic repair of giant paraesophageal hernia: 100 consecutive cases. Ann Surg 232:608–618, 2000.

Maziak DE, Todd TR, Pearson FG: Massive hiatus hernia: Evaluation and surgical management. J Thorac Cardiovasc Surg 115:53–60; discussion 61–2, 1998.

O'Hanrahan, Marples M, Bancewicz J: Recurrent reflux and wrap disruption after Nissen fundoplication: Detection, incidence and timing. Br J Surg 77:545, 1990.

Patterson EJ, Herron DM, Hansen PD, et al: Effect of an esophageal bougie on the incidence of dysphagia following Nissen fundoplication: A prospective, blinded, randomized clinical trial. Arch Surg 135:1055–1061; discussion 1061–1062, 2000.

Pelligrini CA, DeMeester TR, Wernly JA, et al: Alkaline gastroesophageal reflux. Am J Surg 135:177, 1978.

Peters JH, DeMeester TR: Indications, benefits and outcome of laparoscopic Nissen fundoplication. Dig Dis 14:169, 1996.

Pointer R, Bammer T, Then P, et al: Laparoscopic refundoplications after failed antireflux surgery. Am J Surg 178:541, 1999.

Shirazzi SS, Schulze K, Soper RT: Long-term follow-up for treatment of complicated chronic reflux oesophagitis. Arch Surg 122:548–552, 1987.

Siewert JR, Stein HJ, Feussner H: Reoperations after failed antireflux procedures. Ann Chir Gynaecol 84:122, 1995.

Skinner DB: Surgical management after failed antireflux surgery. World J Surg 16:359, 1992.

Swanstrom LL, Marcus DR, Galloway GQ: Laparoscopic Collis gastroplasty is the treatment of choice for the shortened esophagus [see comments]. Am J Surg 171:477–481, 1996.

Szwerc MF, Wiechmann RJ, Maley RH, et al: Reoperative laparoscopic antireflux surgery. Surgery 126:723, 1999.

Trus TL, Laycock WS, Branum G, et al: Intermediate follow-up of laparoscopic antireflux surgery. Am J Surg 10:32, 1996.

Watson DI, Jamieson GG, Game PA, et al: Laparoscopic reoperation following failed antireflux surgery. Br J Surg 86:98, 1999.

SECTION **V**

Neuromuscular Disorders

CHAPTER **30**

Pharyngeal and Cricopharyngeal Disorders

André Duranceau
Pasquale Ferraro

DEFINITION

Oropharyngeal dysphagia refers to difficulties in swallowing at the pharyngoesophageal level. This high, or proximal, dysphagia causes three categories of symptoms because the oropharynx is involved in the functions of swallowing, speech, and respiration:

1. Difficulty exists in propelling food or liquid from the oral cavity to the cervical esophagus. Whether the difficulty is with initiating swallows, with moving the bolus from mouth to pharynx, or with food incarceration at the cricopharyngeus level, the result is difficulty in swallowing.
2. When mechanical or functional obstruction occurs to food or liquid transit, the bolus is misdirected back toward the mouth as pharyngo-oral regurgitation or through the nasopharynx as pharyngonasal regurgitation.
3. The last category of symptoms relates to the larynx and its role in phonation and respiration. Poor coordination with hypopharyngeal stasis results in laryngeal and tracheal aspiration (Figs. 30–1 and 30–2).

Oropharyngeal dysphagia and its symptom complex is usually related to neurologic and neuromuscular diseases. Idiopathic dysfunction of the upper esophageal sphincter (UES) is a frequent cause of oropharyngeal dysphagia. Previous treatment at the oropharyngeal level, either surgery or radiation therapy, may result in proximal dysphagia. Gastroesophageal reflux or transit abnormalities at the gastroesophageal junction may result in symptoms referred to the oropharyngeal level. The causes of oropharyngeal dysphagia are summarized in Figure 30–3.

Patients with oropharyngeal dysphagia are difficult to assess. However, patients affected by these symptoms, when carefully selected, can experience great improvement after surgery on the UES.

This chapter reviews the role of surgery in managing patients with oropharyngeal symptoms.

APPROACH TO THE PATIENT

Regardless of etiology, patients with oropharyngeal dysphagia must be assessed in a systematic fashion.

TABLE 30–1 ■ **Symptom Scoring Applied to Oropharyngeal Dysphagia***

	1 Point	*2 Points*	*3 Points*	*4 Points*
I: Frequency	Occasional (less than once a month)	More often than once a month but less than once a week	More often than once a week but not as often as daily	Daily
II: Duration	Less than 6 months	More than 6 months, less than 24 months	More than 24 months, less than 60 months	More than 60 months
III: Severity	Mild, nuisance value	Moderate, spoils enjoyment of life	Marked, interferes with living normal life	Severe, terrible experience

*To calculate: add frequency to duration, multiply by severity

Mild symptoms: 1–7 Marked symptoms: 16–23
Moderate symptoms: 8–15 Severe symptoms: 24–32

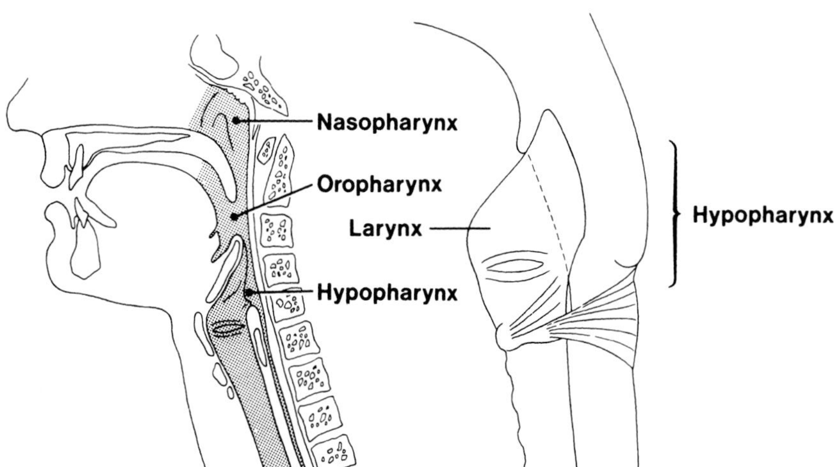

FIGURE 30–1 ■ Lateral view of pharynx and larynx. The upper esophageal sphincter (UES) and its relationship to the cricoid cartilage are shown.

Clinical assessment of symptoms remains the most important step in classifying the disorder. Although the assessment is subjective, it helps to obtain the patient's previous history. The genealogy of transmitted disease can be clarified. For more objectivity, symptoms can be quantified as has been suggested for reflux disease (De Dombal and Hall, 1979). This method is summarized in Table 30–1.

The routine use of video esophagograms to delineate anatomic and functional abnormalities of the pharyngo-esophageal junction is most important (Fig. 30–4). Conventional studies are inadequate because of the rapidity of events during the early phase of swallowing. The importance of this type of radiologic assessment is emphasized by the fact that abnormal function is sometimes confined to one or two frames projected each second (Calceterra et al, 1975). The description of specific muscle group abnormalities also requires the assistance of video technology (Curtis and Hudson, 1983; Curtis et al, 1987).

Manometric evaluation of the whole esophagus must be performed. Assessment of the esophageal body and the lower esophageal sphincter (LES) will rule out motor disorders and document the tone of the LES. Specific manometric assessment of the UES is difficult to obtain. The radial asymmetry of the sphincter requires multiple port recordings to summate the action of the sphincter (Winans, 1972) or a circumferential pressure sensing transducer (Castell and Dalton, 1992; Castell et al, 1990) (Figs. 30–5 to 30–7).

The Dent sleeve is a 6-cm perfused silicone membrane that also has the advantage of recording accurate resting pressures in the UES area (Kahrilas et al, 1988). It can record the sphincter pressure at any level along the length of the membrane even if movement displaces the sphincter. Assessment of sphincter relaxation and coordination with pharyngeal contraction is limited in its accuracy by the upward movement of the larynx during the recording (see Fig. 30–7). Castell and associates (1990, 1992) propose to position the recording sensor above the high-pressure zone of the sphincter for that purpose. Despite the sophistication of more recent manometric recordings,

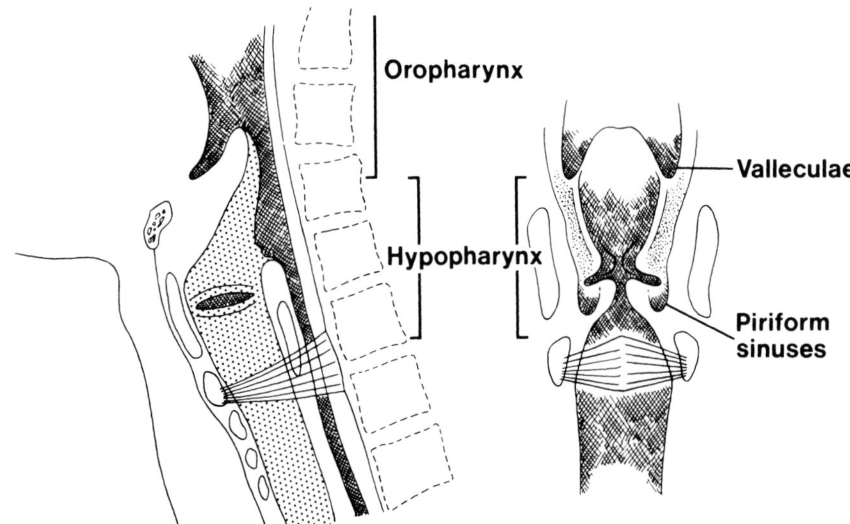

FIGURE 30–2 ■ Lateral and frontal views of the hypopharynx and larynx. The interrelation of swallowing, speech, and respiration is responsible for oropharyngeal dysphagia symptoms.

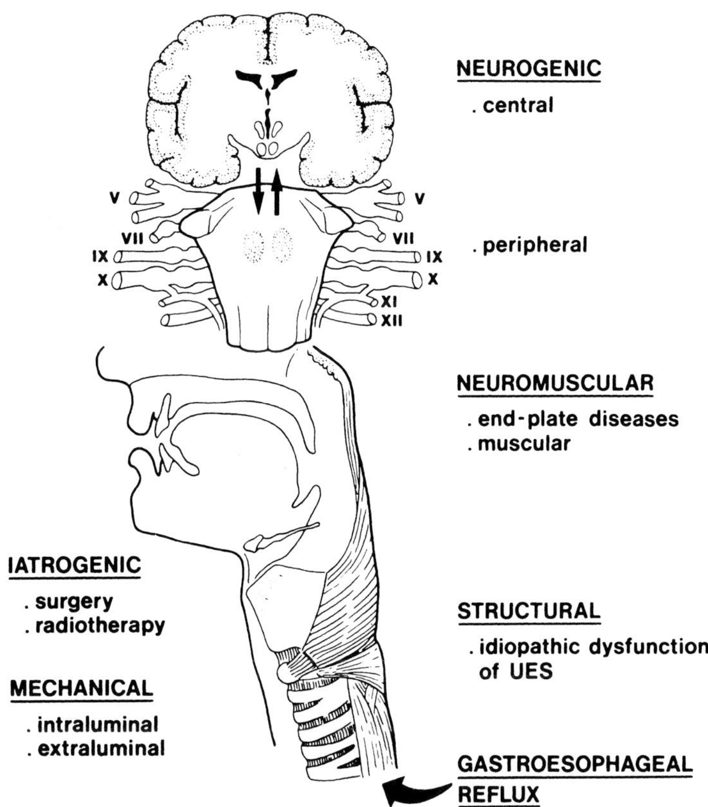

FIGURE 30–3 ■ Etiology of oropharyngeal dysphagia. (UES, upper esophageal sphincter.)

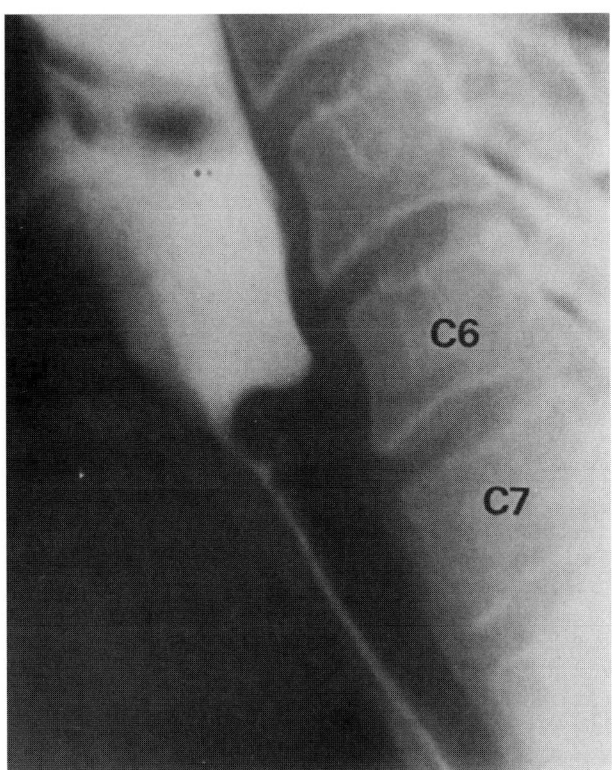

FIGURE 30–4 ■ Pharyngoesophageal junction, with the imprint of the cricopharyngeus between C6 and C7.

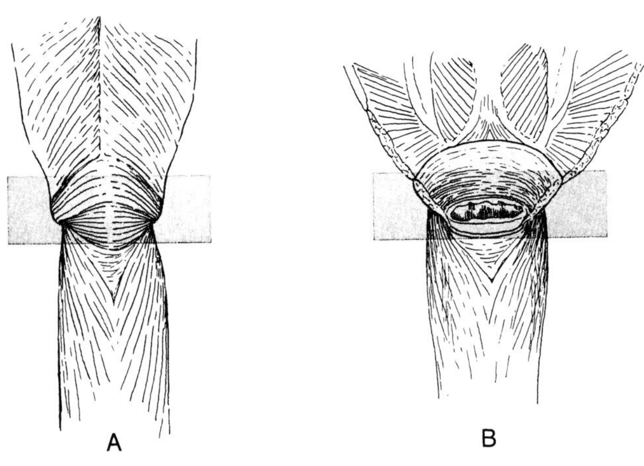

FIGURE 30–5 ■ Anatomy of the pharyngoesophageal junction with contribution of the inferior constrictor to the cricopharyngeus. *A*, Posterior closed view. *B*, Posterior open view.

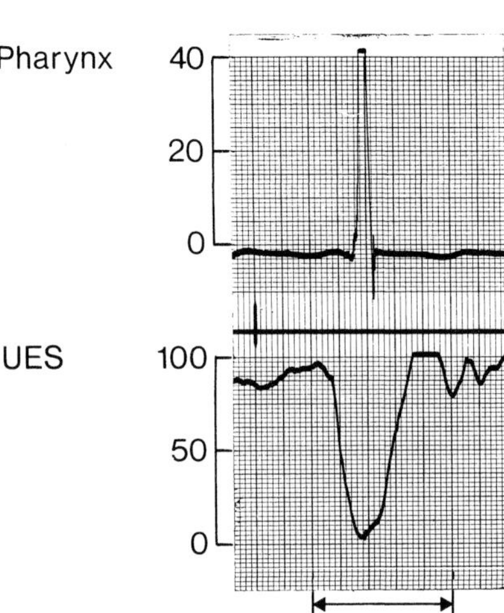

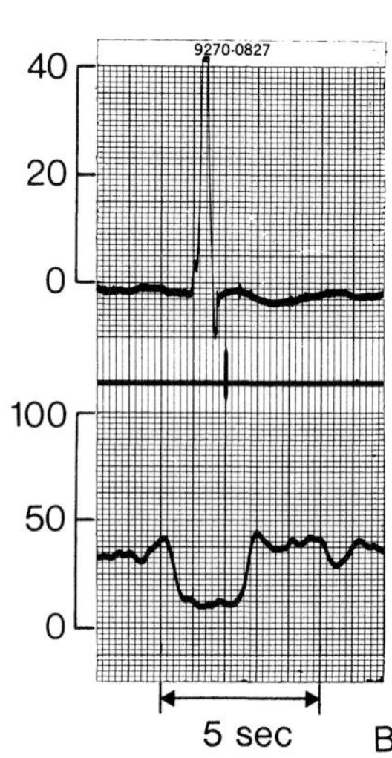

FIGURE 30–6 ■ Accurate manometric recording of the upper esophageal sphincter (UES) is difficult to obtain because of its radial asymmetry. Catheter opening in anteroposterior *(A)* and laterolateral *(B)* position.

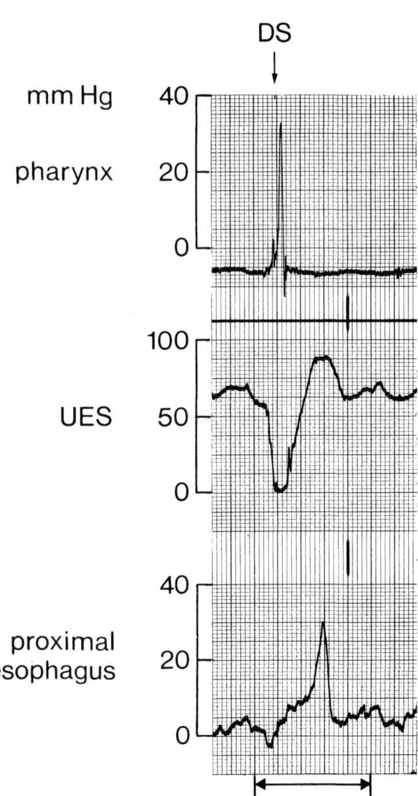

FIGURE 30–7 ■ Normal function and coordination between the pharynx, upper esophageal sphincter (UES), and cervical esophagus. The recorded UES relaxation may be partly caused by the upward excursion of the sphincter during swallowing. (DS, dry swallows.)

OROPHARYNGEAL DYSPHAGIA: ETIOLOGY AND CLASSIFICATION

Neurogenic

Central
Peripheral

Myogenic

End-plate disease
Muscular disease

Idiopathic Dysfunction of Upper Esophageal Sphincter

Isolated upper esophageal sphincter dysfunction
Upper esophageal sphincter dysfunction and pharyngoesophageal diverticulum

Iatrogenic

Surgery
Radiation therapy

Distal Esophagus Dysfunction

Gastroesophageal reflux
Motor disorder
Obstruction

Mechanical

Intrinsic
Extrinsic

Psychogenic

there is undoubtedly an underestimation of true functional abnormalities present in patients with pharyngoesophageal function disorders.

Radionuclide pharyngoesophageal transit studies are performed routinely in our assessment of patients with oropharyngeal dysphagia. These observations add quantitation to symptoms and radiologic and manometric abnormalities (Fig. 30–8). The end result of oropharyngeal dysfunction is poor emptying with solids, liquids, or both. Quantification of this end result when transit abnormalities are present should enhance objectivity, especially when any type of therapy is considered.

Endoscopic assessment of the patient with oropharyngeal dysphagia must be undertaken with great care. Anatomic abnormalities must be delineated clearly before any attempt at endoscopic evaluation. Flexible endoscopy can be used if no distortion is present. Any resistance to passage of the instrument should lead to assessment with the patient under general anesthesia.

Examination under direct vision using the laryngoscope and the short rigid esophagoscope provides detailed visualization of the larynx, pharynx, hypopharynx, and esophageal inlet. If resistance or abnormalities are present, no forceful effort should be made to pass the instrument beyond the cervical esophagus. A total assessment of the esophageal body and cardia must be obtained in patients with oropharyngeal dysphagia. If any risk is entailed in the evaluation procedures, however, therapy for the proximal condition should prevail before the investigation of the distal esophagus is completed.

Neurogenic Dysphagia

Almost any disease of the central nervous system can cause oropharyngeal dysphagia. Damage to the peripheral neurologic system may also result in significant symptoms. Tongue, soft palate, larynx and epiglottis, pharynx, and UES all must be exquisitely controlled with well-

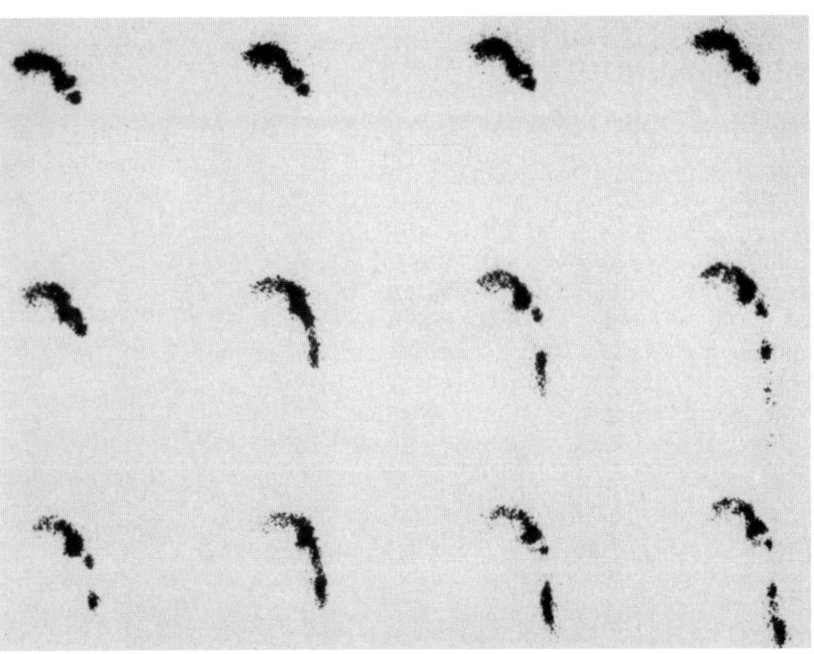

FIGURE 30–8 ■ Quantification of bolus retention above the upper esophageal sphincter using radionuclide scintiscan.

DYSPHAGIA OF NEUROGENIC ORIGIN

Central Nervous System Disease

1. Neurologic disorders
   a. Vascular disease
      (1) Cerebrovascular accident
      (2) Basilar artery thrombosis
      (3) Aneurysm and brain stem compression
   b. Amyotrophic lateral sclerosis and multiple sclerosis
   c. Bulbar disease
      (1) Poliomyelitis
      (2) Pseudobulbar palsy
      (3) Progressive bulbar palsy
      (4) Syringobulbia
   d. Degenerative disease
   e. Parkinson's disease
2. Tumors
   a. Brain stem
   b. Base of the skull
3. Trauma

Periperal Nerve Involvement

1. Neuropathy
   a. Alcohol
   b. Diabetes
2. Tumor
3. Trauma

integrated mechanisms to achieve proper phonation and deglutition. Independent of the cause, loss of control of this integrated process may result in dysfunction with resultant dysphagia symptoms.

A general classification of the etiology of neurologic dysphagia is given later. Rarer conditions are not discussed.

HISTORICAL NOTE

Reports on investigation and surgical management of neurologic dysphagia have mostly appeared since the 1960s. However, the first account of cricopharyngeal myotomy to appear in the English literature for a neurologic condition was the report of the operation of Kaplan (1951). The operation was carried out for dysphagia in a patient with bulbar poliomyelitis. Eight more cases treated by myotomy were subsequently reported by the same author. The justification for performing a myotomy in these patients came from the demonstration that even if the cricopharyngeus seemed to be functionally normal, it could "get in the way" when the patient's pharynx was unable to mount a proper pharyngeal contraction.

Further reports followed, recommending cricopharyngeal myotomy as treatment for dysphagia of neurologic origin: Bofenkamp (1958), Mills (1964), Wilkins (1964), and Lund (1968) all treated patients with cerebrovascular accidents and bulbar poliomyelitis. The low morbidity of the operation encouraged a more liberal approach, and additional reports appeared during the 1970s and the 1980s.

■ *HISTORICAL READINGS*

Bofenkamp B: The surgical correction of aphagia following bulbar poliomyelitis. Arch Otolaryngol 68:165, 1958.

Kaplan S: Paralysis of deglutition: A post-poliomyelitis complication treated by section of the cricopharyngeus muscle. Ann Surg 133:572, 1951.

Lund SW: The cricopharyngeal sphincter: Its relationship to the relief of pharyngeal paralysis and the surgical treatment of the early pharyngeal pouch. J Laryngol Otol 82:353, 1968.

Mills CP: Dysphagia in progressive bulbar palsy relieved by division of the cricopharyngeus. J Laryngol Otol 78:963, 1964.

Wilkins SA: Indications for section of the cricopharyngeus muscle. Am J Surg 108:533, 1964.

DIAGNOSIS

Clinical Features

Damage from cerebrovascular accidents may be diffuse or localized. Reduced lingual control and loss of initiation of the swallowing reflex usually cause delayed swallowing and reduced pharyngeal peristalsis (Veis and Logemann, 1985). Bilateral involvement results in more severe symptoms, whereas dysphagia from lesions confined to one cerebral hemisphere occurs more rarely. When infarcts affect the control mechanisms for the nucleus ambiguus, unilateral paralysis of the pharyngeal and laryngeal musculature occurs (Meadows, 1973). Poor closure of the larynx coupled with hypopharyngeal stasis results in aspiration (Fig. 30–9).

Pain on swallowing is rare in these patients and is usually associated with inflammatory lesions or neoplasia (Edwards, 1976). Of patients with bulbar poliomyelitis, 60% have significant oropharyngeal dysphagia for more than 1 year after the initial damage. In the condition known as amyotrophic lateral sclerosis (ALS), degeneration of motor neurons in the brain, brain stem, and spinal cord occurs. Dysphagia occurs when nerves are damaged, with resulting aspiration. Weakness, atrophy, and fasciculation of the musculature lead to poor handling of the food bolus with defective swallowing. Patients with Parkinson's disease have difficulty with the formation and preparation of the food or liquid bolus (Cotzias et al, 1969). Lack of UES opening with pulmonary aspiration may result when a delay in triggering the swallowing response occurs. Vagal lesions and selective trauma or malignant invasion of the recurrent laryngeal nerves can cause significant dysphagia. When it occurs, spontaneous improvement of dysphagia is usually observed within a few months after onset.

Radiology

During the oral phase of swallowing, cine and video radiologic studies reveal the adequacy of tongue movement and propulsion, the tone of the floor of the mouth, and the adequacy of bolus formation. Some patients with

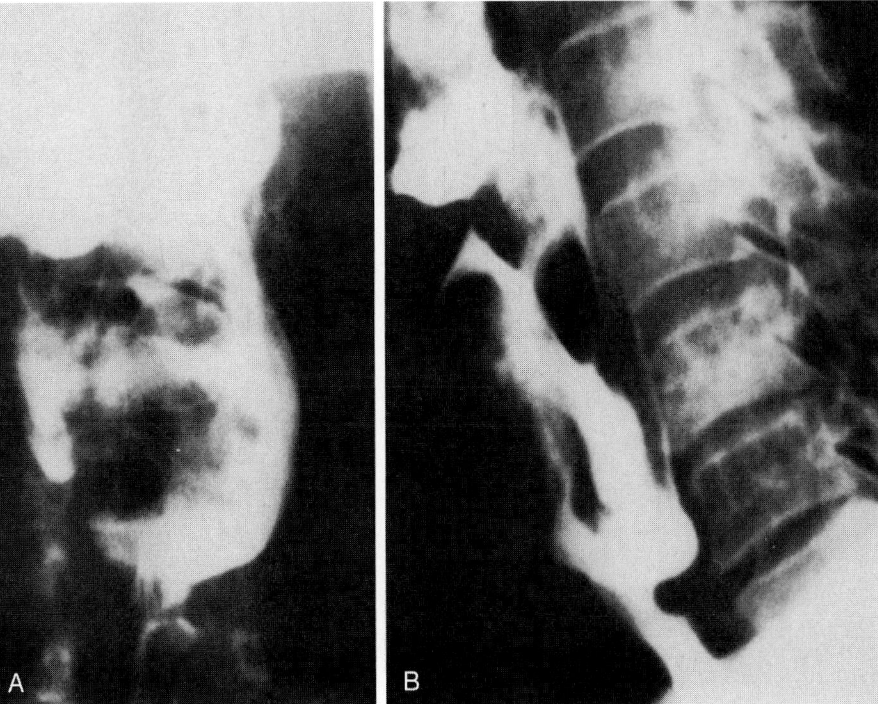

FIGURE 30–9 ■ *A*, Pseudotumor effect of the pharyngeal wall caused by paralysis of right half of the pharynx. *B*, Cricopharyngeal bar and hypopharyngeal stasis seen with paralysis of the right hemipharynx.

more diffuse neurologic damage may keep the bolus in the mouth without any attempt at initiating swallows. Hesitancy in deglutition, tremors, poor bolus formation, and back-and-forth movements of the bolus are seen in patients with Parkinson's disease and ALS.

During the pharyngeal phase of swallowing, the symmetry or asymmetry of the pharyngeal wall velopharyngeal muscles and laryngeal structures can be observed. Unilateral paralysis may be the only manifestation of a cerebrovascular accident. This condition is easily misdiagnosed as a pharyngeal tumor (see Fig. 30–9). Patients with brain stem damage exhibit reduced laryngeal closure. Pooling and stasis may be observed in valleculae and pyriform sinuses, but residual barium in the hypopharynx is considered a more reliable sign of abnormal function (Seaman, 1976).

Assessment of the third phase of swallowing, UES function, is properly assessed with video radiology. Curtis (1983) observed cricopharyngeal abnormalities in 77 patients, or 10.8% of his study group; 15% of these patients had dysphagia. Functional obstruction caused by poor opening of the UES against the contracting pharynx may cause pharyngo-oral or pharyngonasal regurgitation with laryngotracheal aspiration. Poor relaxation of the UES is a striking abnormality in patients with brain stem lesions, especially in patients with thrombosis of the posterior cerebellar artery or with bulbar paralysis. Delayed opening of the UES is seen in 30% of central degenerative disease patients (Donner and Silbiger, 1966). In our series of radiologic evaluations for neurologic dysphagia, 14 of 21 patients showed incomplete, absent, or delayed opening of the UES.

Motility Studies

Manometric tracings recorded in oropharyngeal dysphagia of neurologic origin reveal abnormalities in resting pressure, coordination, and relaxation. Bonavina and colleagues (1985) reported normal pharyngeal pressures but incomplete UES relaxation and poor opening coordination of the sphincter with the pharyngeal contraction (Fig. 30–10).

Ellis and Crozier (1981) reported UES hypertension in bulbar palsy patients after cerebrovascular accidents. Delayed relaxation and poor coordination of the UES as well as spontaneous and repetitive activity were observed in patients with amyotrophic lateral sclerosis (Carpenter et al, 1978) (Fig. 30–11). In our interpretation of motility patterns in neurologic patients, resting pressures were within normal range. Relaxation was abnormal in 7 of 20 patients (35%), 4 of whom showed abnormality in over 70% of swallows. Only 20% of all patients showed normal coordination of sphincter opening with pharyngeal contraction. Only in patients with central neurologic disease have we recorded complete absence of relaxation (achalasia) of the UES: once in a patient with basilar artery thrombosis and once in a patient who had sustained a cerebrovascular accident (Figs. 30–12 and 30–13).

Radionuclide Studies

The specific use of radionuclide studies in assessing pharyngeal and hypopharyngeal emptying in neurologic dysphagia is not implemented regularly and has not been reported frequently. Our patients were assessed with upright and supine times and activity curves, and they were

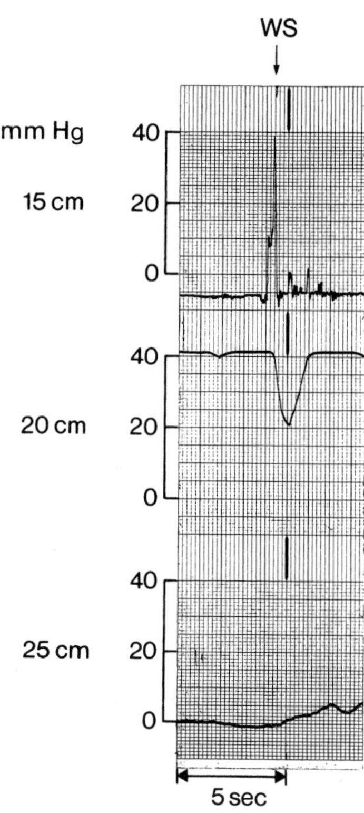

FIGURE 30–10 ■ Absent coordination between pharyngeal contraction and upper esophageal sphincter (UES) relaxation. Incomplete UES relaxation. (WS, wet swallow.)

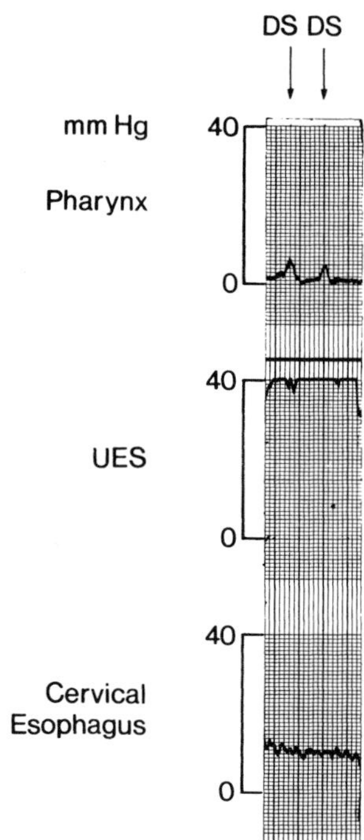

FIGURE 30–12 ■ Achalasia of the upper esophageal sphincter (UES) in a patient who suffered a basilar artery thrombosis. (DS, dry swallow.)

compared with normal subjects. When standing, 4 of 10 patients (36%) could not clear 90% of the radioactive bolus in 2 minutes. When supine, 50% of the group was unable to clear the pharynx of 90% of its content at 2 minutes. When compared with normal subjects, neurologic patients show nearly a 90% bolus retention at 20 seconds after swallowing. Preliminary results show improved emptying after cricopharyngeal myotomy when voluntary deglutition is preserved.

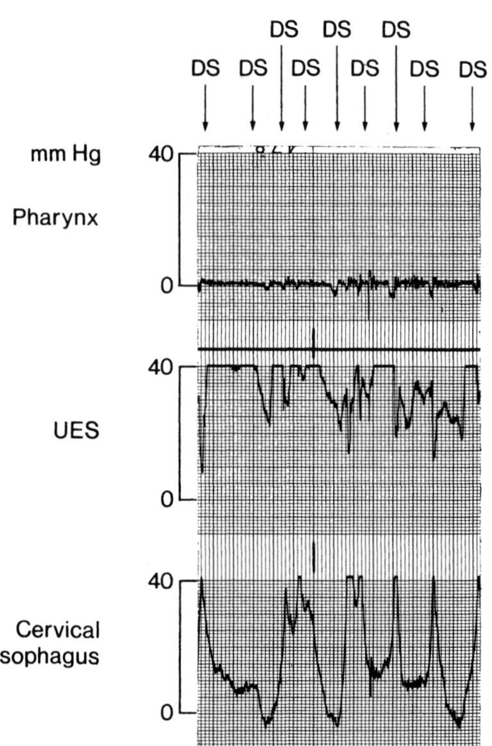

FIGURE 30–11 ■ Poor relaxation and coordination of the upper esophageal sphincter (UES) with repeated attempts at swallowing. (DS, dry swallow.)

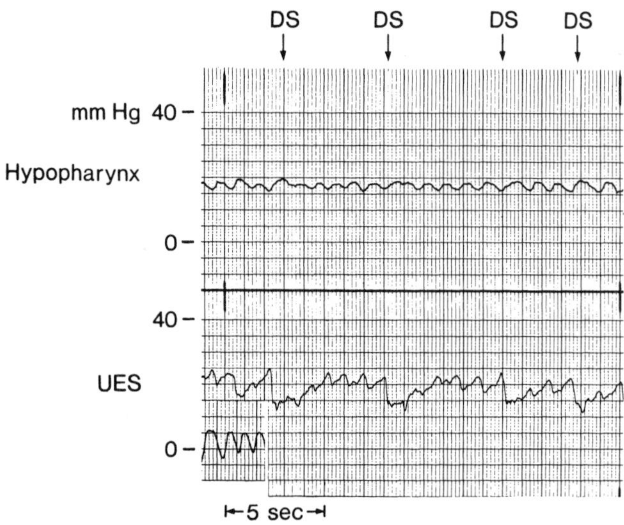

FIGURE 30–13 ■ Achalasia of the upper esophageal sphincter (UES) recorded by sleeve manometry in a patient who suffered a cerebrovascular accident. (DS, dry swallow.)

MANAGEMENT

Operation

Myotomy of the pharyngoesophageal junction is the operation of choice in patients with dysfunction of the UES after neurologic damage. Our technique is depicted in Figure 30–14 (Duranceau et al, 1983a).

The patient is placed supine with a small pillow under the shoulders. The head is in hyperextension and turned to the right. The thyroid and the cricoid cartilages are easily located, especially if the patient has a thin neck. The incision is made along the anteromedial border of the left sternomastoid muscle, covering two thirds of the distance between the ear lobe and the sternal notch (Fig. 30–14*A*).

The subcutaneous tissues and the platysma are divided. A branch of the cervical cutaneous nerve may be seen in the upper third of the field. It is protected, if feasible, because its division causes hypesthesia and dysesthesia in the submandibular skin (Fig. 30–14*B*).

The sternomastoid muscle is dissected from the underlying musculature. The omohyoid muscle and the prethyroid muscles are cut to expose the jugular vein, the carotid artery, and the thyroid gland (Fig. 30–14*C*).

The middle thyroid vein, if present, is ligated and divided. The thyroid gland, pharynx, and larynx are then retracted contralaterally, putting the deep cervical fascia under tension. The fascia is opened along the line of the incision, with care taken to identify the inferior thyroid artery immediately deep to this layer. The inferior thyroid artery is ligated as far laterally as possible where it disappears behind the carotid sheath. The recurrent laryngeal nerve, which is in the groove between the trachea and the esophagus, passes behind the branches of this inferior thyroid artery while it travels along the posterior part of the gland (Fig. 30–14*D*).

A cross-section of the neck is seen from below. The plane of access to the superior mediastinum and to the posterior pharyngoesophageal junction is depicted (Fig. 30–14*E*).

Once the inferior thyroid artery is ligated and divided, the pharynx and esophagus are dissected free from the prevertebral fascia. The recurrent laryngeal nerve is easily palpated and visualized in this groove. It is not dissected (Fig. 30–14*F*).

A 36 French mercury bougie is passed into the esophagus and used as a stent. Identification of the cricoid cartilage locates the pharyngoesophageal junction.

The assistant retracts toward the contralateral side while pushing the right side of the junction toward the left. This procedure usually affords complete exposure of the posterior pharyngoesophageal wall. Using low-intensity diathermy, the surgeon coagulates the superficial tissues over the pharynx, cricopharyngeus, and cervical esophagus, along the course of the planned myotomy. While the first assistant maintains optimal exposure, the myotomy is begun on the esophageal muscle lateral to the midline and progresses proximally. If right-handed, the surgeon holds a dissector swab in the left hand and produces lateral traction on muscle while cutting with the scalpel in the right hand. The surgeon can maintain perfect hemostasis using diathermy.

The mucosa is recognized by its bluish coloration with the submucous venous plexus that overlies it. The muscle of the cricopharyngeal area, when cut, retracts in a more pronounced fashion toward its insertion. The muscular wall of the hypopharynx is thicker. The submucous venous plexus is occasionally impressive with large tortuous veins that are easily opened, requiring a fine absorbable suture for transfixion proximally and distally. The completed myotomy extends approximately 6 cm across the posterior pharyngoesophageal junction (see Fig. 30–14*G*).

The muscularis along the myotomy line is dissected free from the mucosa along the discrete areolar plane that separates both layers. The proximal and distal limits of the myotomy are cut transversely, raising a muscle flap that is thicker on the pharyngeal side and thinner at the esophageal level. Retraction of the cricopharyngeus becomes more evident at this point. This flap of muscle is resected for histologic assessment (Fig. 30–14*H*).

The bougie is removed from the esophageal cavity, and a nasogastric tube is passed gently toward the stomach. As the gastric tube is passed in the area of the myotomized zone, 20 to 50 ml of air is injected through the tube while the myotomy is submerged under saline. This procedure ensures the integrity of the mucosa. Two small Penrose drains are left in the mediastinum for 24 hours, one at the thoracic inlet and another behind the myotomized area (Fig. 30–14*I*).

Postoperative Care

The nasogastric tube is left in place, primarily to avoid the need to insert it blindly through a freshly myotomized pharyngoesophageal junction in an emergency situation. It is usually removed the following morning after normal peristalsis is present. The patient is given a liquid diet, and the soft drains are removed after 24 hours. A hospital stay of 48 to 72 hours is considered reasonable after this operation.

Complications specific to this operation are recurrent laryngeal nerve trauma, hematoma formation, and infection with salivary fistula. Meticulous technique should prevent all of these complications. If retropharyngeal hematoma occurs, it should be evacuated because of the prolonged resorption period in patients with poor swallowing function. When aspiration persists, with absent phonation and disappearance of all protective mechanisms, pulmonary aspiration and sepsis are to be expected. In these extreme situations, we have resorted to permanent tracheostomy with laryngeal excision or exclusion (Fig. 30–15).

Results

When our own observations are added to a review of the literature, more than 201 myotomies have been reported in the treatment of pharyngeal dysphagia of exclusively neurologic origin (Table 30–2). It is difficult to extract

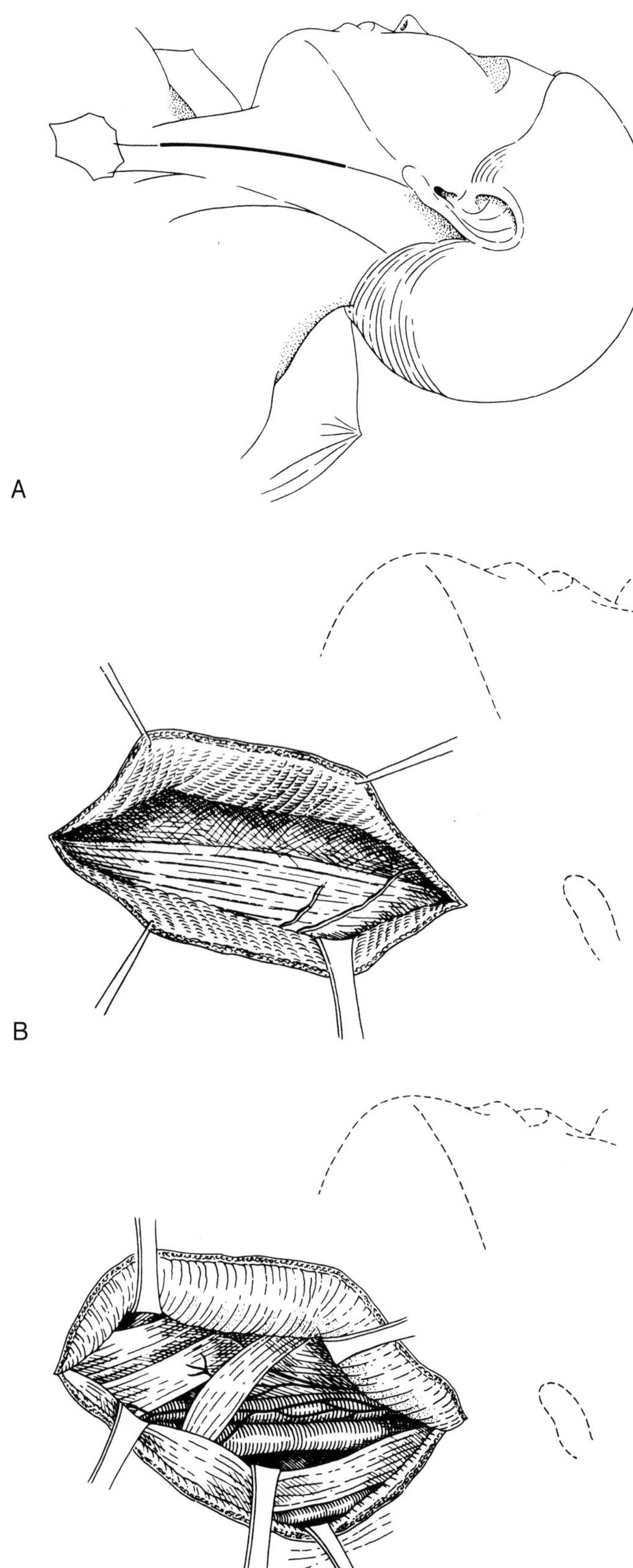

FIGURE 30–14 ■ *A–I,* Technique of pharyngoesophageal myotomy for upper esophageal sphincter dysfunction after neurologic damage. See text.

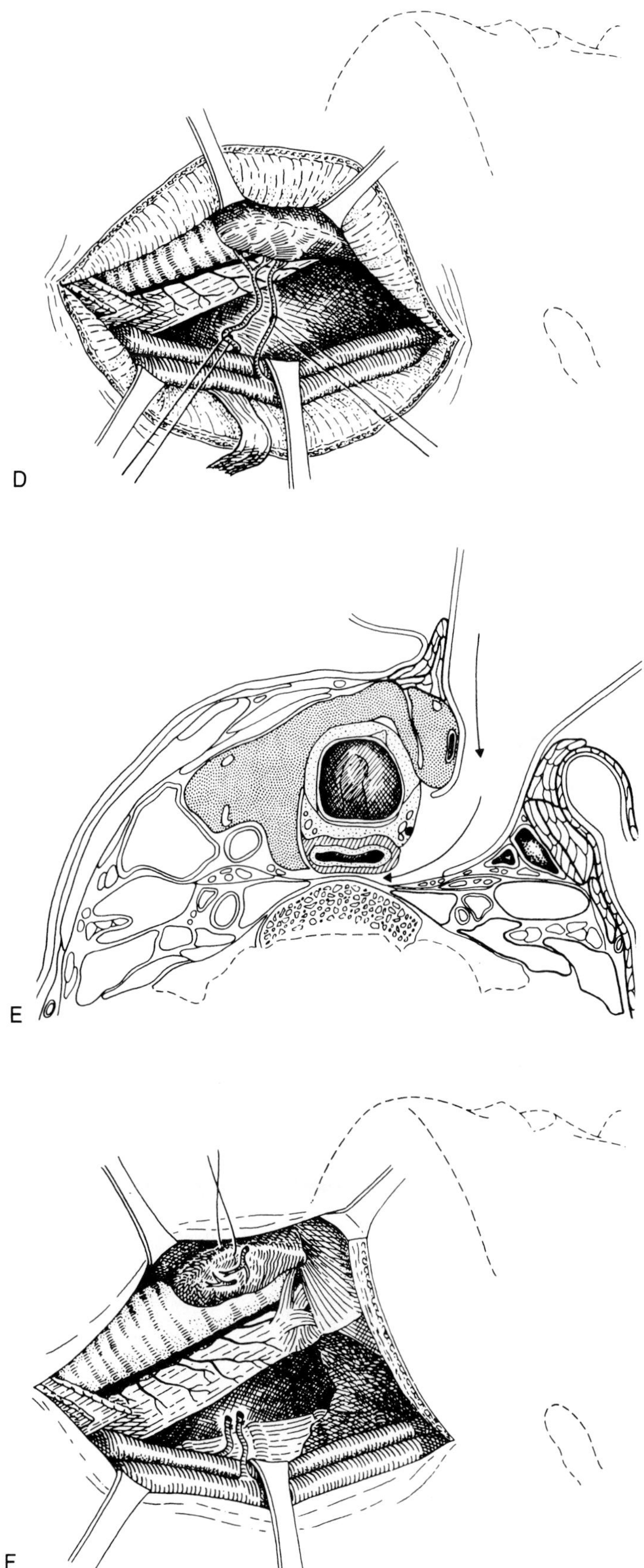

FIGURE 30–14 ■ *Continued.*

Illustration continued on following page

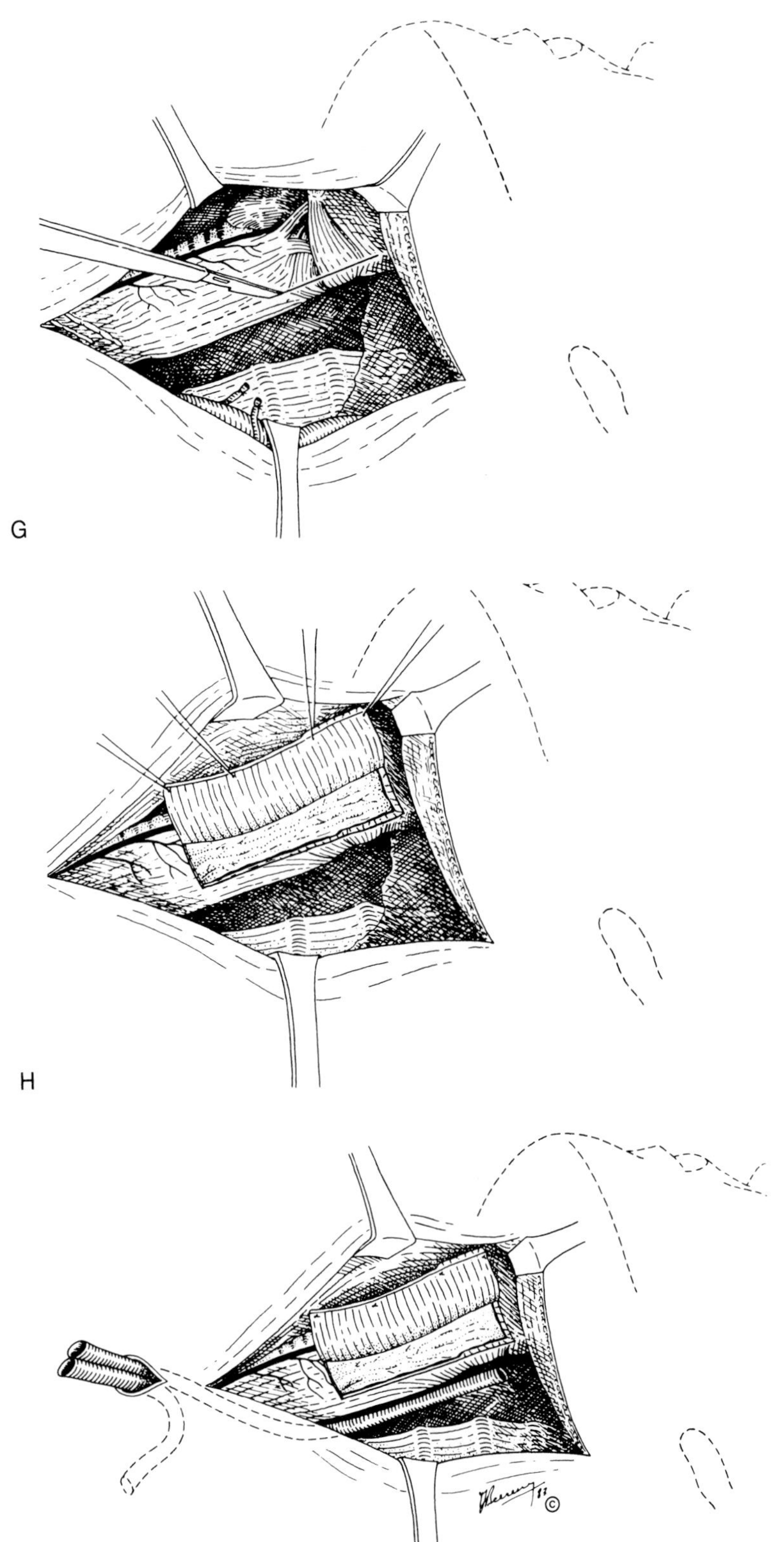

FIGURE 30–14 ■ *Continued.*

clear results from many of these reports. Consequently, numbers are incomplete and results often inconclusive.

Dysphagia caused by cerebrovascular accidents may be improved significantly by myotomy, depending on damage location; lesions in the brain stem with localized damage and basilar artery thrombosis are associated with excellent results. The same is true for dysphagia from brain stem compression by tumor or aneurysm. One third of patients in this category show excellent results, a second third show moderate improvement, and the last third remain unimproved. Mortality occurs in 12% of these victims of cerebrovascular accidents, mostly from

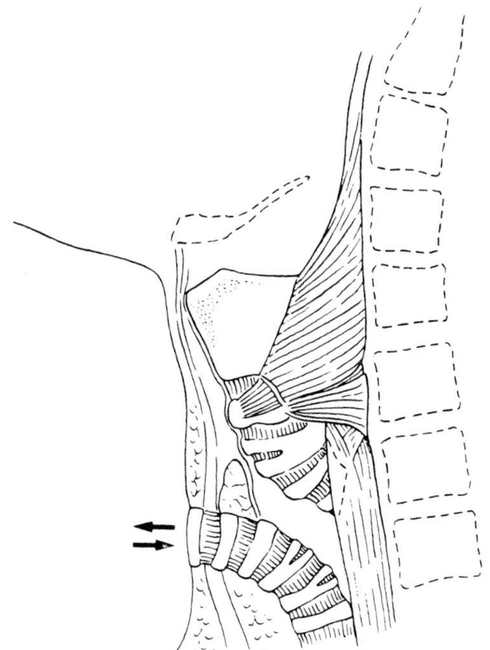

FIGURE 30–15 ■ Persistent aspiration with pulmonary soilage requires laryngeal excision or exclusion. Exclusion, as illustrated here *(arrows)*, permits eventual reconstruction if there is potential for full laryngeal activity recuperation.

pulmonary and cardiovascular causes. Morbidity results from persistent aspirations. In a summary of our results (Duranceau, 1997; Poirier et al, 1997) for cricopharyngeal myotomy in neurogenic dysphagia, we found an operative mortality of 2.5% in 40 patients. Patients were significantly improved with regard to dysphagia and aspiration in 75% of cases.

Patients with ALS or motor neuron disease may show initial improvement; however, the complete loss of voluntary deglutition results in poor improvement over time. Loizou and associates (1980) and Lebo and co-workers (1976) reported their respective experience with 25 and 35 patients. The mortality in Loizou and associates' experience was 20%, and Lebo and colleagues saw swallowing improvement in 50% of patients 6 months after the operation.

TABLE 30–2 ■ **Causes of Neurologic Dysphagia: Results with Cricopharyngeal Myotomy**

Etiology	*No. of Patients*	*Result**		
		Excellent	*Moderate*	*Poor*
Cerebrovascular disease	71	20	24	10
Amyotrophic lateral sclerosis	54	25	14	10
Bulbar and pseudobulbar palsy	21	1	7	5
Miscellaneous central causes	24	6	—	3
Trauma	10	3	—	4
Peripheral nervous system dysfunction	21	7	3	—

*As discussed in the text, results from the literature are often partial, inconclusive, and difficult to clarify.

Most of the patients with bulbar poliomyelitis and bulbar and pseudobulbar palsy showed moderate improvement after cricopharyngeal myotomy. Six of 10 patients with Parkinson's disease showed clinical improvement immediately after myotomy. The improvement in syringomyelia and in miscellaneous central lesions is comparable.

When trauma, invasion, or nerve resection resulted in oropharyngeal dysphagia, Henderson and coworkers (1974) and Mills (1973) reported excellent results with UES myotomy. All three patients treated by Akl and Blakely (1974) showed poor results.

It is an error to refuse consideration of myotomy and a potential return to comfortable swallowing in patients with central and peripheral neurologic damage. Overall, cricopharyngeal myotomy for oropharyngeal dysphagia of neurologic origin gives satisfactory to excellent results in more than 75% of treated patients. The recognized prognostic factors for improvement (Duranceau et al, 1988) in these patients are:

- Intact voluntary deglutition
- Adequate antepulsion and retropulsion of the tongue
- Normal phonation
- Absence of dysarthria

Appropriate selection of patients for cricopharyngeal myotomy in this patient category should improve those results.

Myogenic Dysphagia

Patients with muscular dystrophy are frequently affected with dysphagia at the oropharyngeal level. This is even more the case if they have the oculopharyngeal muscular variety of the disease. This disorder is hereditary and transmitted in an autosomal dominant fashion. It is characterized by late onset and in North America shows a high prevalence in families of French Canadian origin.

A study by Brais (1995) on the genetics of oculopharyngeal muscular dystrophy (OPMD) has demonstrated the locus of the OPMD gene to be on chromosome 14 of the A and B cardiac myosin heavy chain genes. This condition is now well documented in families of multiethnic origins, and it is present on five continents (Brais et al, 1995). Symptoms occur in these patients because of poor propulsive forces in the pharynx. The UES may also respond poorly, either because of a decreased stimulation response or as a result of a restrictive myopathy with diminished compliance of the pharyngoesophageal junction. This hypothesis, already well documented for the pathogenesis of pharyngoesophageal diverticulum, has not been substantiated for muscle disease dysphagia.

HISTORICAL NOTE

The initial reports on cricopharyngeal myotomy as a treatment of dysphagia in patients with muscular disease

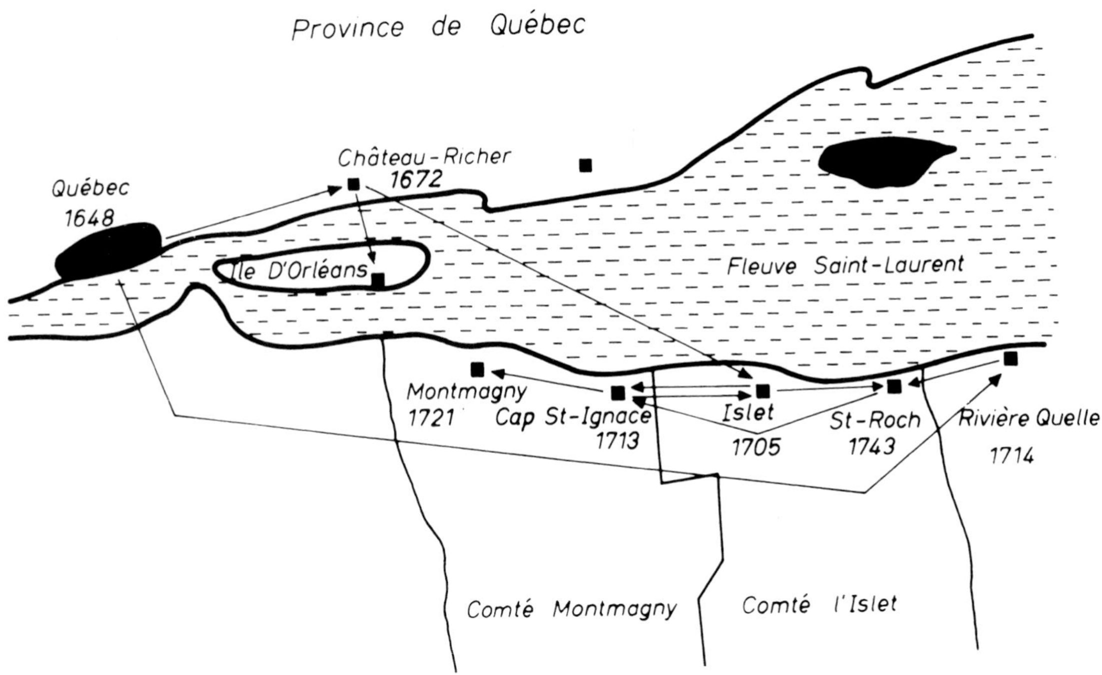

FIGURE 30–16 ■ Oculopharyngeal muscular dystrophy is traceable in French-Canadian families to the same two ancestors who emigrated from France to Canada 11 generations ago.

appeared in the early 1960s. Peterman and colleagues (1964) reported the history of a French Canadian patient living in California. He had bilateral ptosis and complained of significant dysphagia, which became markedly improved by cricopharyngeal myotomy. Previous reports on this condition had focused mostly on bilateral ptosis (Duranceau et al, 1983b).

In 1966 in Montreal, using as a starting point patients of French-Canadian origin whose cases were published in the literature, a neurologist completed a genealogical study (Barbeau, 1966, 1968) of these patients. This study concluded that the same two persons, Zacharie Cloutier and Xainte Dupont, who immigrated to Quebec from Perche, France, in 1634, were the progenitors of a form of muscular dystrophy that they transmitted in an autosomal dominant fashion to 11 generations of French Canadians (Fig. 30–16). Although well documented in families of French Canadian descent, oculopharyngeal muscular dystrophy has also been documented in families of other origin (Duranceau et al, 1983b).

These observations served as a basis to improve knowledge on clinical manifestations and evolution in these dystrophy patients. Blakeley and associates (1968) and Melgar (1968) were followed by Montgomery and Lynch (1971), who subsequently contributed their surgical experience with this disease process.

■ *HISTORICAL READINGS*

Barbeau A: The syndrome of hereditary late onset ptosis and dysphagia in French Canada. In Kuhn E: Symposium uber Progressive Musker Dystrophie. Berlin, Springer-Verlag, 1966, p 102.

Blakely WR, Gerety EJ, Smith DE: Section of the cricopharyngeus muscle for dysphagia. Arch Surg 96:745, 1968.

Montgomery WW, Lynch JP: Oculopharyngeal muscular dystrophy treated by inferior constrictor myotomy. Trans Am Acad Ophthalmol Otolaryngol 75:986, 1971.

Peterman AF, Lillington GA, Jamplis RW: Progressive muscular dystrophy with ptosis and dysphagia. Arch Neurol 10:38, 1964.

Taillefer R, Duranceau A: Manometric and radionuclide assessment of pharyngeal emptying before and after cricopharyngeal myotomy in patients with oculopharyngeal muscular dystrophy. J Thorac Cardiovasc Surg 95:868, 1988.

DIAGNOSIS

Clinical Presentation

Barbeau (1966) observed that oculopharyngeal muscular dystrophy is usually manifested by symmetric bilateral ptosis. Although dysphagia usually appears subsequently, it may on occasion become manifest simultaneously or even precede the ptosis. Both the ptosis and the dysphagia appear late and are slowly progressive.

During the evolution of the disease, two categories of symptoms have been described in patient groups assessed before surgery on the UES: (1) those that are oropharyngeal in origin and (2) those that affect the tracheobronchial tree (Duranceau et al, 1978, 1980, 1988). Dysphagia located at the oropharyngeal level is present in 65% of patients seen initially with ptosis. Frequent food incarceration followed by pharyngo-oral regurgitation is the result of a powerless pharynx that is incapable of pushing the food bolus through the UES area. Pharyngonasal regurgitation occurs frequently and is increased by the use of liquids to facilitate the swallowing of solids. Dystrophic velopharyngeal muscles account for the poor occlusion of the nasopharynx. In these patients, the time required to eat a normal meal increases significantly, such that some will eat alone, away from their families. Moreover, social embarrassment brought on by these symptoms removes the enjoyment of eating out.

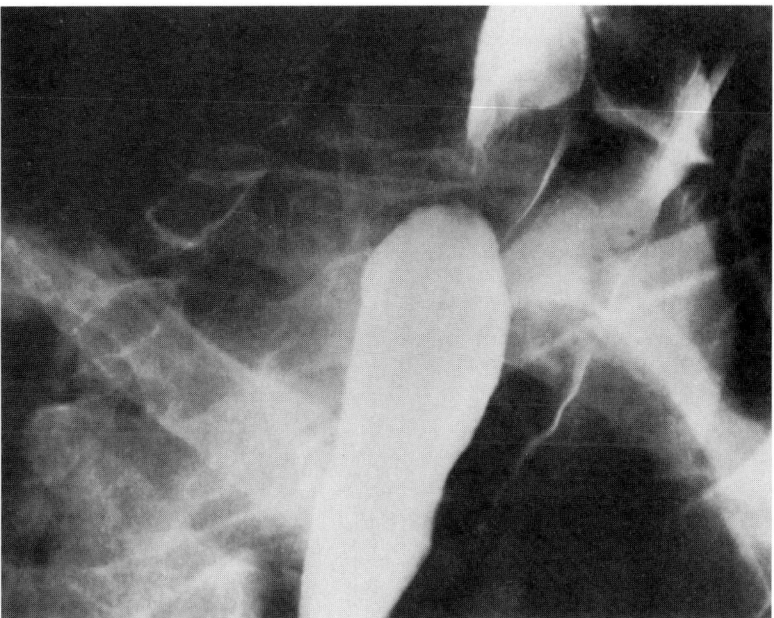

FIGURE 30–17 ■ Pseudotumor effect by a tightly closed pharyngoesophageal junction in a patient with dystrophy.

Tracheobronchial symptoms result from poor control of laryngeal muscles and parallel pharyngeal weakness and hypopharyngeal stasis. Penetration in the aditus of the larynx and tracheal aspiration may occur occasionally initially and may be present at every meal during late evolution. Repetitive aspiration leads to bronchorrhea. During daytime, these patients may frequently aspirate saliva, food, and liquids. At night, pooling and aspiration of salivary secretions create an abundant, thick, and viscous bronchorrheic mucus, which patients have to expectorate.

As long as adequate muscular strength and cough reflexes are retained, tracheobronchial toilet is maintained. Aspiration pneumonia eventually supervenes in 25% of patients during late evolution. Voice changes are present in most symptomatic patients, secondary to disease affecting tensors of the vocal cords. Dystrophy of the scapular and lower limb muscles causes weakness and gait problems in 20% of all patients affected by this condition.

Radiology

Cine radiographic findings in patients with dystrophy show impaired clearance of the radiopaque material from the pharynx. The initiation of the swallow and the voluntary phase of swallowing are usually normal. Bender (1976) reported puddling of contrast material and tracheal aspiration in 5 of 17 patients.

In a report on 16 severely symptomatic patients assessed before cricopharyngeal myotomy, Duranceau and associates (1978, 1980) reported weak or absent pharyngeal contraction in 14 of 16 patients. Pooling in the hypopharynx is seen in all patients, and pharyngonasal regurgitation was documented in 3 of the 16 patients. When assessing the UES, the radiologist suggested a smaller luminal diameter on opening, with a relaxation occurring incompletely or late in 12 of 16 patients. A cricopharyngeal bar is described in 12 patients (see Fig. 30–4). The radiologic appearance had a pseudotumor effect in two patients (Fig. 30–17). Tracheal aspiration was documented in more than 50% of the group (Fig. 30–18).

Motility Studies

Motor function of the pharynx and proximal esophageal sphincter in muscle disease patients has been reported in

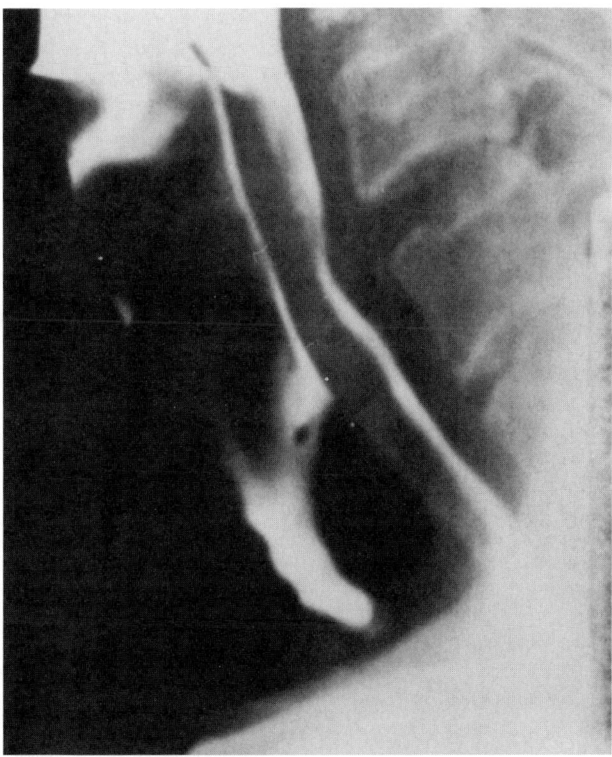

FIGURE 30–18 ■ Tracheal aspiration in a dystrophic patient. Twenty-five percent of such patients may suffer from aspiration pneumonia in the late evolution of the disease.

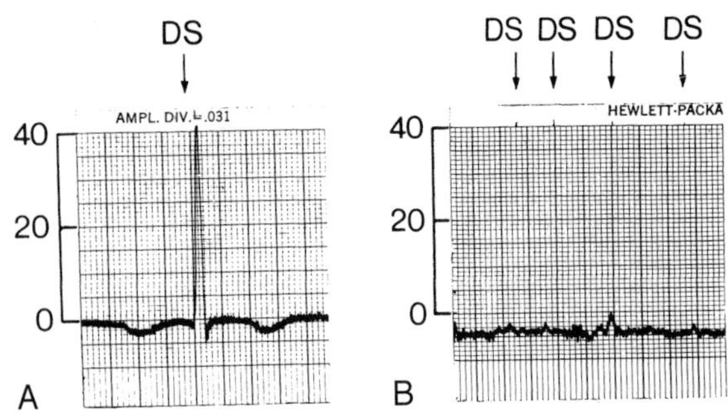

FIGURE 30–19 ■ Manometry. *A*, Normal pharynx. *B*, Repetitive efforts at swallowing in patient with dystrophy has resulted in powerless pharyngeal contractions. (DS, dry swallow.)

a number of studies. All these reports have to be analyzed with consideration of the known difficulties in recording function of the pharyngoesophageal junction.

In our initial report (Duranceau et al, 1978), pharyngoesophageal function showed a pharyngeal contraction that was significantly weaker and longer than in controls. Efforts at swallowing resulted in repetitive weak pharyngeal contractions (Figs. 30–19 and 30–20). The UES showed normal resting and contracting pressures (Fig. 30–21). Time to relaxation to a cervical esophageal resting pressure and coordination did not vary significantly from the normal. These observations are in contrast to the findings at radiology, which show significant dysfunction at the UES level.

A more definitive observation was possible when Castell and colleagues (1995) used a motility catheter with three solid-state transducers spaced at 3-cm intervals, the distal transducer being a circumferential sphincter transducer. Eleven patients with dystrophy were compared with 14 healthy controls. Abnormalities in the dystrophy group were characterized by low pharyngeal pressures and correspondingly low pharyngeal contractions. Prolonged pharyngeal contractions and associated incoordination between pharyngeal and UES relaxation were documented. Abnormal UES relaxation was found in 4 of 11 patients, with 3 showing increased residual pressures and all 4 showing an abnormal duration of relaxation. Patients with severe symptoms had a markedly abnormal manometric profile, whereas patients with mild symptoms showed a normal manometric profile.

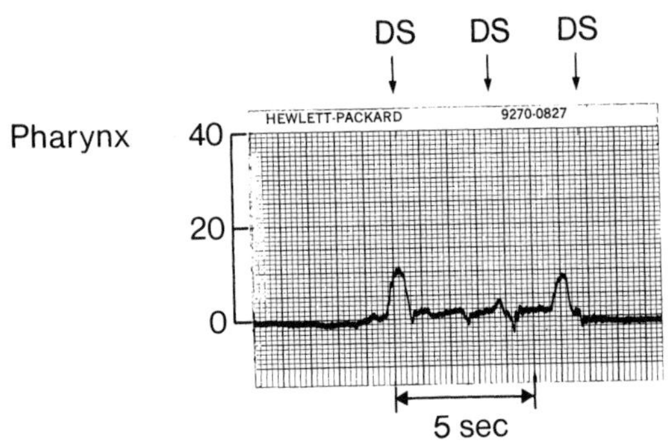

FIGURE 30–20 ■ Weak, long, and repetitive contractions seen in oculopharyngeal muscular dystrophy. (DS, dry swallow.)

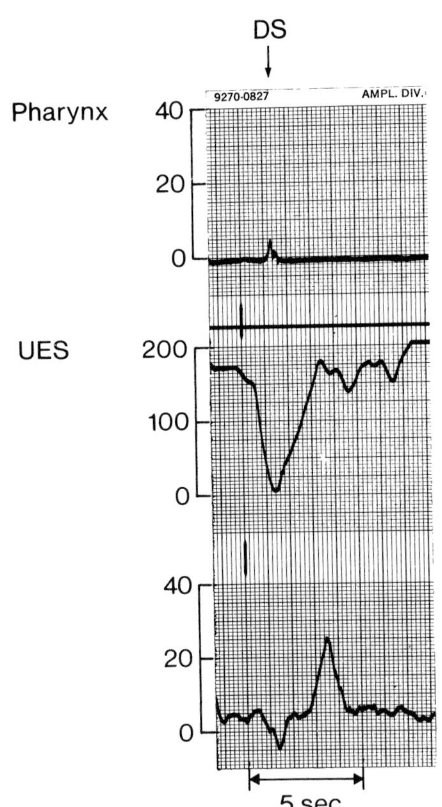

FIGURE 30–21 ■ Despite the weak pressure signal from the pharynx, the upper esophageal sphincter (UES) shows appropriate relaxation. (DS, dry swallow.)

Interestingly, esophageal body dysfunction was documented as well. Four patients showed nontransmitted contractions in the proximal esophagus, whereas nine patients of the group revealed simultaneous contractions in 20% to 100% of all swallows in the distal esophagus. The LES was considered abnormal in nine patients, showing incomplete relaxation in 33% to 100% of the swallows and being hypertensive in one case.

From these observations, abnormal transport in the esophagus may well exist even if the disease is considered to affect the striated muscle predominantly.

Radionuclide Emptying Studies

Pharyngoesophageal emptying studies have been obtained in dystrophy patients to assess pooling and emptying before and after myotomy of the pharyngoesophageal junction (Taillefer and Duranceau, 1988). The weakness of the pharynx in these patients results in poor pharyngeal transit. On average, only 20% of the liquid tracer is cleared within 1 second of voluntary swallowing. Significant retention occurs in valleculae and piriform sinuses (see Fig. 30–8). After cricopharyngeal myotomy, significant improvement in clearance at 1 second, in both the upright and the supine positions, is recorded. This finding correlates well with the substantial symptomatic improvement.

Emptying studies are noninvasive. They can be used with a bolus of variable consistency. Liquid, soft food, or solid boluses can help quantitate the capacity of the pharynx to accomplish effectively the initial phase of deglutition.

MANAGEMENT

Operation

Cricopharyngeal myotomy for muscle disorders is identical to the operation described in the section on neurogenic dysphagia (see Fig. 30–14).

Results

No medical treatment has been shown to be of any use in helping dysphagia in patients with muscular dystrophy. However, to conclude that no proven rationale exists for surgical intervention in patients with swallowing difficulties from any form of muscular dystrophy is overly pessimistic. Cricopharyngeal myotomy decreases significantly both the resting pressure and the opening time of the UES (Figs. 30–22 and 30–23) and improves pharyngoesophageal transit (Figs. 30–24 and 30–25).

Since the initial report by Peterman and associates (1964), a number of authors have reported the results of a cricopharyngeal myotomy for dysphagia in dystrophy patients. The results in 42 patients reported in a 1988 review are summarized in Table 30–3. There was one death in this series, from a gastrointestinal hemorrhage. Excellent results were reported in 75% of the group. We have reported that 8 of 11 of our initial patients have shown excellent symptomatic improvement in early follow-up (Duranceau et al, 1978). Sustained relief for 2 to 4 years has been reported by Montgomery and Lynch (1971). Peterman and associates (1964) observed a valuable improvement during the initial year after the myot-

TABLE 30–3 ■ **Myogenic Dysphagia: Results with Cricopharyngeal Myotomy**

Author (Year)	*No. of Patients*	*Result*
Peterman et al (1964)	1	Excellent for 1 year, poor after appearance of hoarseness
Melgar (1968)	1	Considerable improvement
Blakeley et al (1968)	2	Excellent
Weitzner (1969)	1	Poor, died of gastrointestinal hemorrhage
Leonard (1970)	1	Complete relief
Montgomery and Lynch (1971)	8	7 excellent, 1 poor
Nanson (1974)	2	Marked improvement
Akl (1974)	9	7 marked relief, 2 satisfactory
Desaulty (1975)	1	Spectacular improvement
Hurwitz (1975)	2	Unspecified
Mitchell (1975)	1	Excellent
Dayal (1976)	1	Excellent
Bender (1976)	1	Excellent
Duranceau et al (1978)	11	8 excellent, 3 moderate improvement

Adapted from Duranceau A, Lafontaine ER, Taillefer JR, Jamieson GG: Oropharyngeal dysphagia and operations on the upper esophageal sphincter. Surg Annu 19:317, 1987.

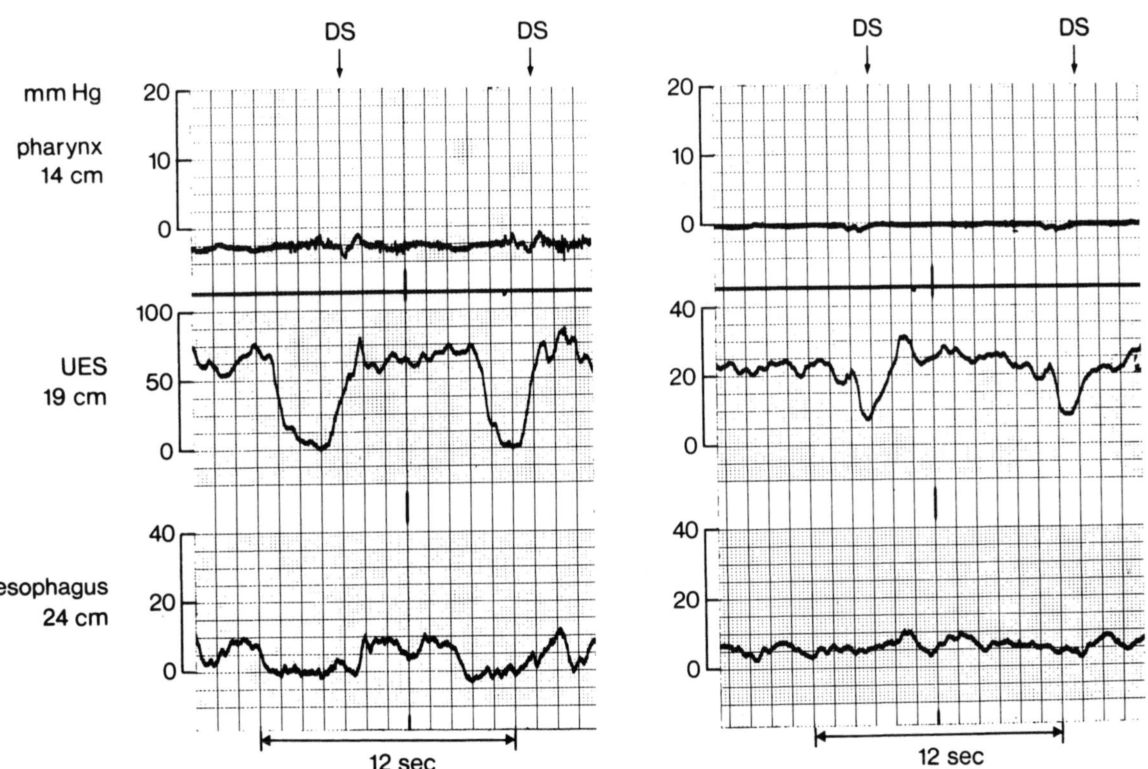

FIGURE 30–22 ■ Effects of cricopharyngeal myotomy on the upper esophageal sphincter (UES) before *(left)* and after *(right)* surgery. (DS, dry swallow.)

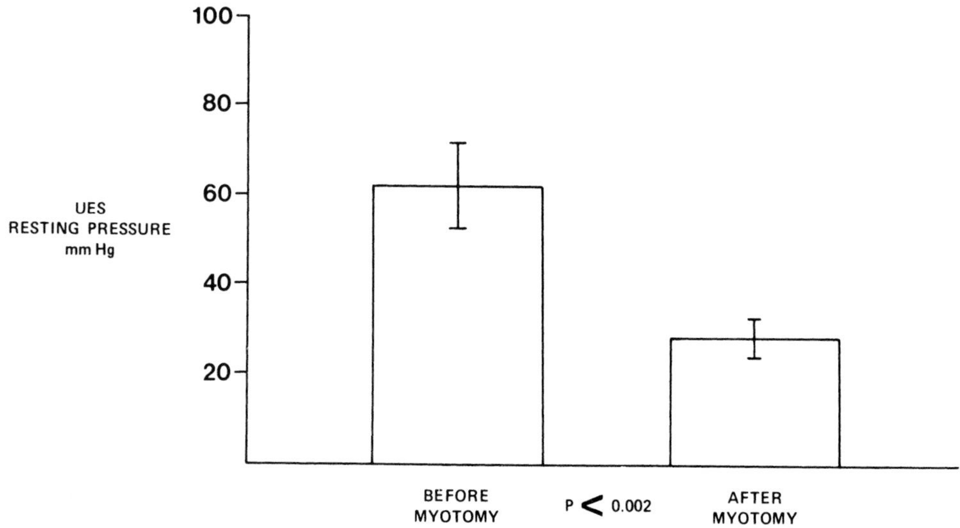

FIGURE 30–23 ■ Resting pressures of the upper esophageal sphincter (UES) are reduced significantly in oculopharyngeal muscular dystrophy. The opening phase of the UES is reduced in a similar way.

omy. However, new aspiration episodes occurred when hoarseness appeared as a symptom. A repeated myotomy at this point did not improve the aspiration episodes.

In a more recent report concentrating on the morbidity of the operation, our results were summarized for 89 operated patients (Brouillette et al, 1997). Inadvertent mucosal opening occurred in 6 patients and was repaired with fine absorbable suture without subsequent infection or fistula. One severe infection of the floor of the mouth occurred. Systemic complications were more frequent, with pulmonary infection from aspiration being the most common. Three patients went on to develop an acute respiratory distress syndrome and died of this complication. Cardiac problems, mostly arrhythmias, occurred in six patients, urinary retention occurred in three patients, and metabolic abnormalities were noted in two. The 75% excellent results reported in the literature is a constant

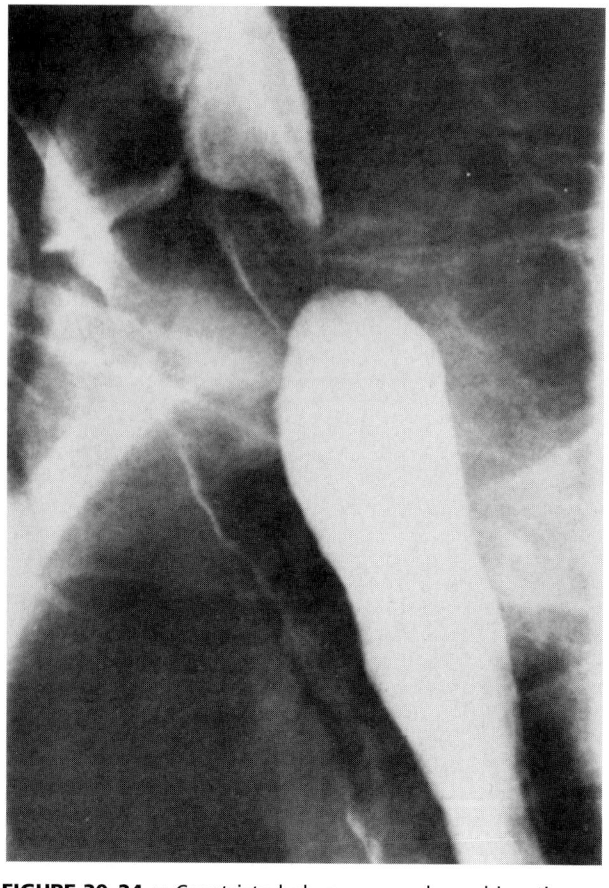

FIGURE 30–24 ■ Constricted pharyngoesophageal junction before operation.

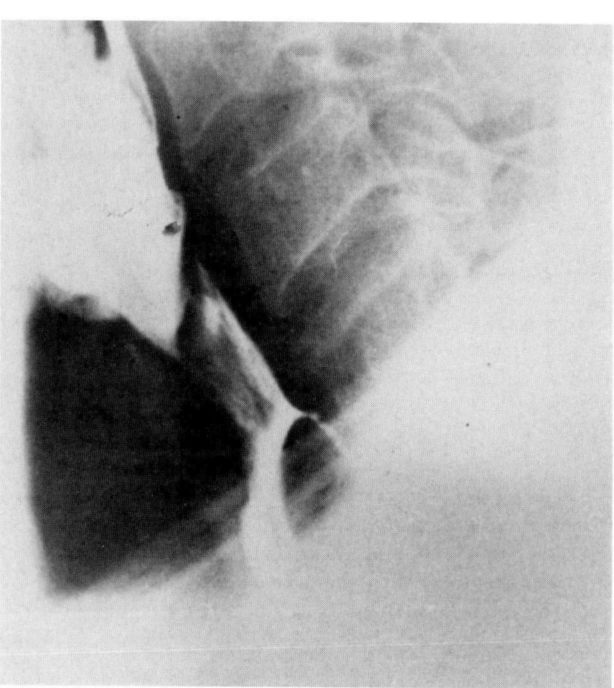

FIGURE 30–25 ■ Enlarged pharyngoesophageal opening after myotomy.

observation at early follow-up. In our long-term assessment, symptoms reappear mostly in association with new manifestations of muscular disease in other muscle groups. Voice changes and upper and lower limb muscle weakness are witness to the progression of the disease. Reappearance of oropharyngeal symptoms may also become manifest.

In our experience, hoarseness and total dysphonia are ominous prognostic signs. Absent muscular activity in the larynx encourages aspiration episodes in these patients. Four of our patients underwent permanent tracheostomy with laryngeal exclusion in two and excision in two.

Similar improvement in symptoms is reported for patients with dermatomyositis and polymyositis treated by cricopharyngeal myotomy. In these patients, the classification of their condition and the differential diagnosis from other myopathies may be difficult. Analysis of the muscle flap resected at the time of cricopharyngeal myotomy provides an objective diagnosis. In all reported cases of myositis, moderate to excellent results are obtained even after progression of the underlying disease.

Cricopharyngeal Dysfunction Without Diverticulum

Occasionally, no neurologic condition and no muscular pathology are present to explain oropharyngeal dysphagia accompanying dysfunction of the UES. The dysphagia is then classified as idiopathic or structural, suggesting primary dysfunction of the UES (Fig. 30–26). In the absence of a diverticulum, prominence of the cricopharyngeus muscle with failure of relaxation has led to the confusing term *achalasia of the upper sphincter*. This condition was seen by Belsey (1966) as an intrinsic abnormality of the cricopharyngeus manifesting itself "as recurrent attacks of obstruction aggravated by generalized nervous tension." Such suggestion of a neuropsychogenic cause for this condition has never been substantiated. However, it remains an attractive hypothesis with the observation that such patients are often high-strung individuals like those with other types of primary motor dysfunction of the esophagus.

Patients with idiopathic dysfunction of the UES present mainly with symptoms of dysphagia, pharyngo-oral regurgitation, and aspiration. Functional assessment of the pharynx and UES are anecdotal at most. Sutherland (1962) has suggested sphincteric hypertension in these patients with recognizable muscle hypertrophy at operation. A strong pharyngeal contraction should be present, and the proximal esophageal sphincter acts as a poorly relaxing functional obstruction. Whether such a hypothesis will be confirmed with true functional abnormalities of the sphincter or with abnormalities secondary to a restrictive myopathy with decreased compliance of the cricopharyngeus remains to be demonstrated. If true, development of a pharyngoesophageal diverticulum might be anticipated as a further step in the evolution of this condition.

Results after cricopharyngeal myotomy for idiopathic dysfunction of the UES, without any diverticulum present, have been reported for more than 80 patients (Table 30–4). Seven of eight treated patients have shown excellent results, and morbidity is minimal. The frequent association of a strong psychological overlay in these patients warrants the use of objective quantification of abnormalities before proceeding with cricopharyngeal myotomy. The correlation of symptoms with radiologic dysfunction, manometric abnormalities, and poor pharyngeal clearance favors good prognosis after myotomy.

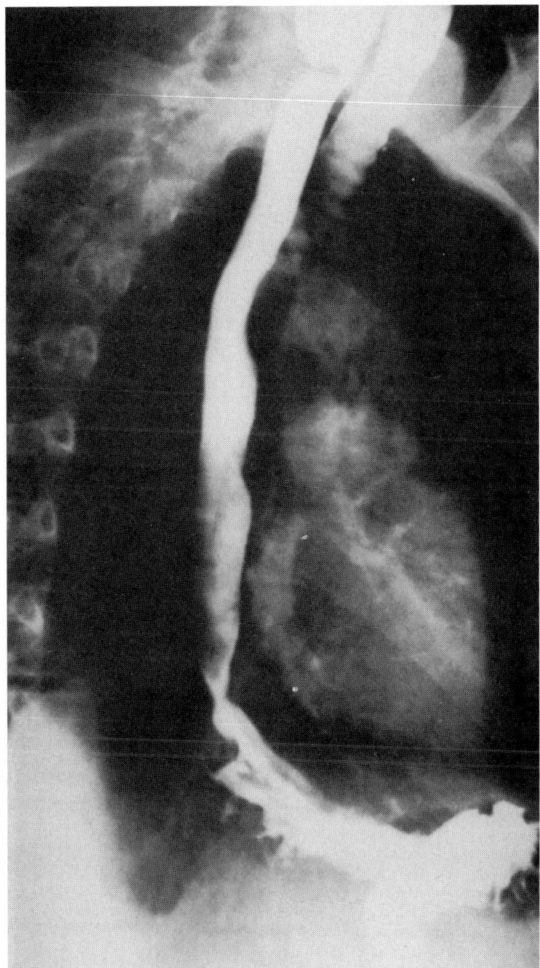

FIGURE 30–26 ■ Idiopathic dysfunction of the upper esophageal sphincter causing tracheal aspiration.

Pharyngoesophageal (Zenker's) Diverticulum

HISTORICAL NOTE

Among conditions that cause oropharyngeal dysphagia and related symptoms, a pharyngoesophageal (Zenker) diverticulum has the longest past history.

Ludlow (1769) published the first description of a pharyngoesophageal diverticulum in a patient with "obstructed deglutition." Zenker and Von Ziemssen, more than 100 years later (1878), reported 22 cases with five patients of their own. They proposed that this diverticu-

TABLE 30–4 ■ **Idiopathic Dysfunction of the Upper Esophageal Sphincter: Results with Cricopharyngeal Myotomy**

Author (Year)	*No. of Patients*	*Result*
Sutherland (1962)	8	7 excellent, 1 moderate
Bingham (1963)	1	Excellent
Belsey (1966)	32	Excellent
Parrish (1968)	1	Good
Melgar (1968)	1	Improved
Leonard (1970)	1	Excellent
Calcaterra et al (1975)	3	Excellent
Desaulty (1975)	2	Poor (fistula and stricture)
Chodosh (1975)	1	Excellent
Mitchell (1975)	1	Excellent
Hiebert (1976)	6	6 of 15 patients: 13 excellent, 2 improved
West (1977)	7	6 excellent, 1 good
Cruse (1979)	6	Unspecified
Orringer (1980)	7	6 excellent, 1 poor
Gagiz (1983)	4	3 excellent
Gay (1984)	1	Good

Adapted from Duranceau A, Lafontaine ER, Taillefer JR, Jamieson GG: Oropharyngeal dysphagia and operations on the upper esophageal sphincter. Surg Annu 19:317, 1987.

lum was the result of "pulsion" within the esophagus rather than distortion occurring by traction on the esophagus.

Early attempts at treatment failed because leakage and mediastinitis followed resection of the pouch. These problems were enough to stimulate creativity among surgeons. Wheeler (1886) described a successful excision, and Kocher (1892) subsequently performed a diverticulectomy with primary closure. With the lack of antibiotics at a time when anastomotic leakage and acute mediastinitis remained the most important problems, Schmid (1912) proposed suspension of the diverticulum to obtain better emptying while reducing morbidity and mortality.

Lahey and Warren (1954) emphasized the safety of the procedure (diverticulopexy) and the importance of freeing the diverticulum from the fibers of the cricopharyngeus muscle. They anchored the pouch mucosa to the proximal edge of the sternohyoid muscle well above the level of its junction with the esophagus. Care was taken not to transfix the diverticular wall with sutures to avoid leak and contamination. Cigarette drains were packed in the mediastinum to wall off any eventual infection from the subsequent resection. Re-exploration was carried out a week later to dissect free and resect the diverticulum. This approach significantly reduced morbidity and mortality. These authors recorded two deaths and a recurrence rate of 4.8%, with no incidence of cervical abscess or mediastinitis.

Harrington (1945) and Sweet (1956) challenged the concept of this staged approach. This led to the single-stage diverticulum resection used by Payne and Claggett (1965). The concept of adding cricopharyngeal myotomy in treating the pharyngoesophageal diverticulum appeared in 1958 with the work of Harrison. After that report, some surgeons considered the cricopharyngeus to be the number one problem and the diverticulum to be the complication of the dysfunction. Others continued to view the diverticulum itself as the main problem, maintaining diverticulectomy as the main line of treatment. An increasing number of surgeons now treat the dysfunction by myotomy and the diverticulum by either suspension or resection.

■ *HISTORICAL READINGS*

Jamieson GG, Cook IJ, Show D: The pathogenesis of Zenker's diverticulum and its normalization by cricopharyngeal myotomy (Abstract). ISDE World Congress Aug:242, 1992.

Lahey FH, Warren K: Esophageal diverticula. Surg Gynecol Obstet 98:1, 1954.

Ludlow A: A case of obstructed deglutition from a preternatural dilatation of a bag formed in the pharynx: Observations and inquiries. Soc Physicians (Lond) 3:85, 1769.

Sweet RH: Excision of diverticulum of the pharyngo-esophageal junction and lower esophagus by means of the one stage procedure. Ann Surg 143:433, 1956.

DIAGNOSIS

Clinical Presentation

Symptoms of a pharyngoesophageal diverticulum may vary with the stage of development and range from a lump sensation at the oropharyngeal level with swallowing to complete esophageal obstruction. Duranceau and Jamieson (1987) reported a series of 120 patients treated over a 32-year period, between 1950 and 1982. The mean age was 62.9 years. Forty-eight percent of the patients were symptomatic for an average of just under 2 years. Dysphagia and food regurgitation were present in all patients regardless of the size of the diverticulum. Oropharyngeal dysphagia (98%), fresh food regurgitation (85%), episodes of aspiration on swallowing (61%), cervical bruit or noise on swallowing (26%), halitosis (25%), respiratory complications (17%), and voice changes (13%) were the other symptoms recorded. Thirty-six percent of all patients reported losing weight.

In contrast, Lerut and co-workers (1987) reviewed 95 patients of their own and 390 patients from 15 different European centers. Even with the smallest form of diverticula, they observed that all patients had oropharyngeal dysphagia symptoms. Of their patients, 66% presented with severe pulmonary infections and 39 of the 95 patients had significant cachexia, suggesting a later presentation stage.

In a collected series, Postlethwait (1979) reported that 90% of the patient population was older than 40 years of age, no patient was younger than 30, and the highest incidence was seen between ages 60 and 70 years.

Radiology

On radiologic evaluation, the pharyngoesophageal diverticulum is seen as a midline protrusion at the level of the posterior hypopharyngeal wall, just above the cricopharyngeus muscle (Figs. 30–27 and 30–28). In our patient group, the diverticulum was less than 1 cm in diameter in 4% of patients, 1 to 2 cm in 20% of patients, and

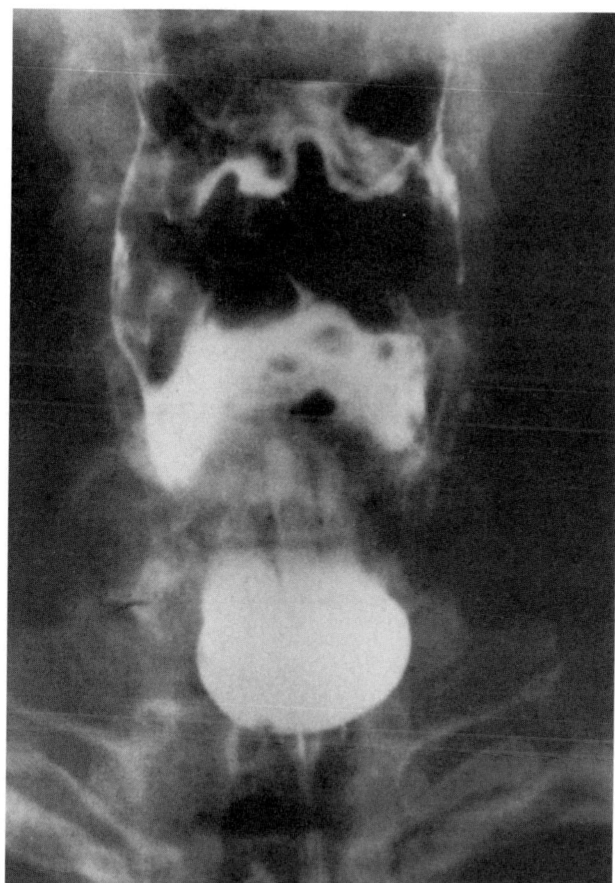

FIGURE 30–27 ■ The pharyngoesophageal diverticulum is a midline protrusion above the upper esophageal sphincter.

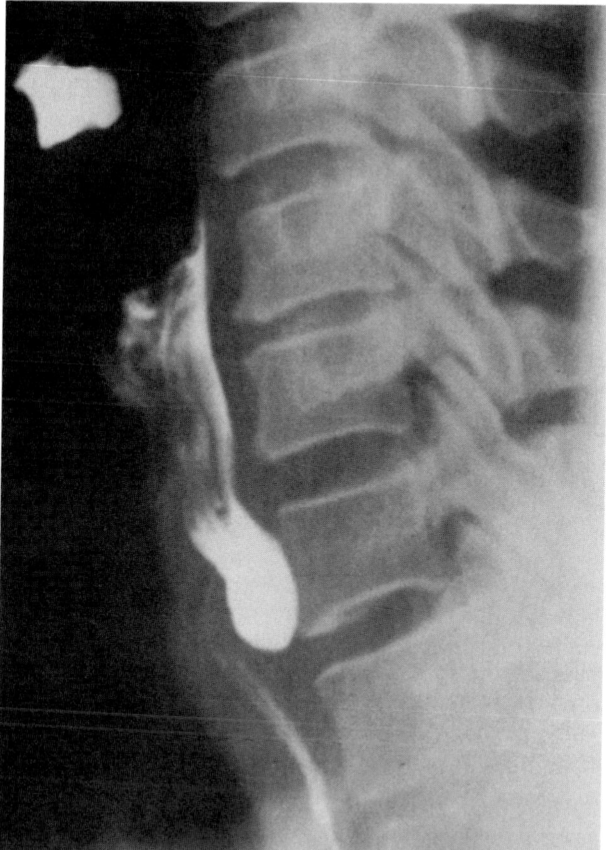

FIGURE 30–28 ■ The diverticulum descends in the mediastinum to lie between the spine and the posterior esophageal wall.

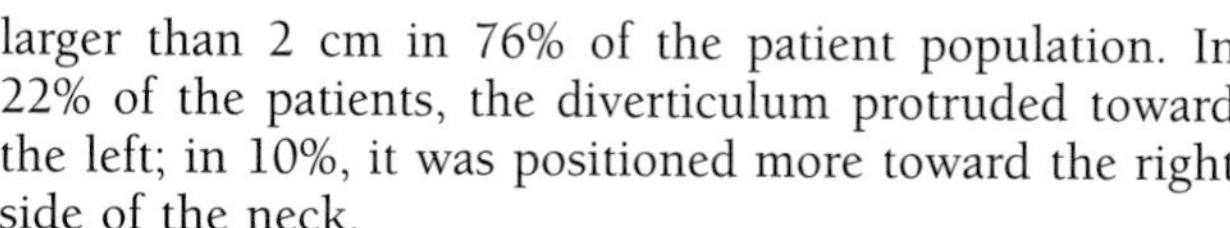

larger than 2 cm in 76% of the patient population. In 22% of the patients, the diverticulum protruded toward the left; in 10%, it was positioned more toward the right side of the neck.

The incidence of asymptomatic diverticula varies from 0.11% to 2% (Holmgren, 1946; Wheeler, 1947). Small diverticula may be transient: they have been reported in 4% to 5% of the population. It is not clear whether these transient diverticula develop into permanent pouches. Once the diverticulum is present, however, it progresses in size over time (Figs. 30–29 to 30–31).

Associated hiatal hernias have been described, with an incidence ranging from 22% (Ellis et al, 1969) to 90% (Smiley et al, 1970). No causative relationship has been established between reflux disease and the formation of a pharyngoesophageal diverticulum.

Motility Studies

It is mostly from cineradiographic studies that the presumed pathogenesis of pharyngoesophageal diverticulum formation has been proposed. Holmgren (1946) observed the appearance of small diverticula with significant impressions of the cricopharyngeus on the hypopharynx. This finding was interpreted later as a lack of relaxation of the cricopharyngeus in advance of the oncoming pharyngeal contractions.

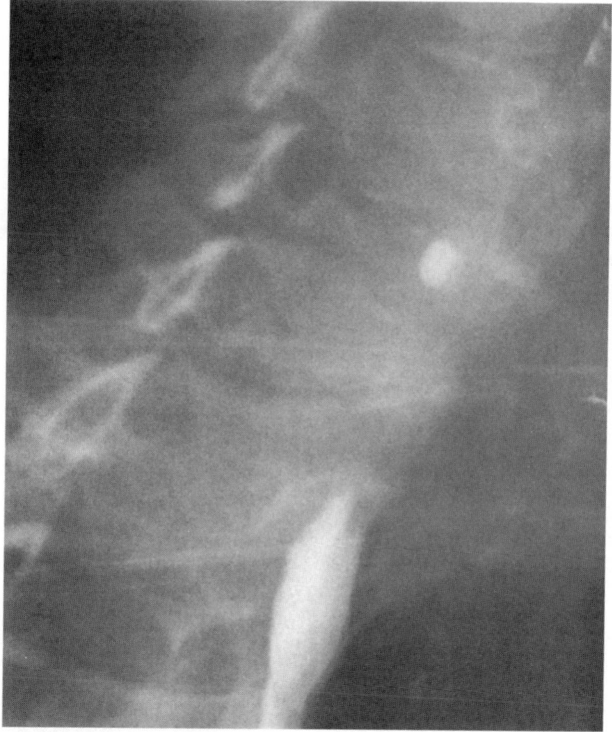

FIGURE 30–29 ■ Minute diverticulum in a patient with intermittent dysphagia.

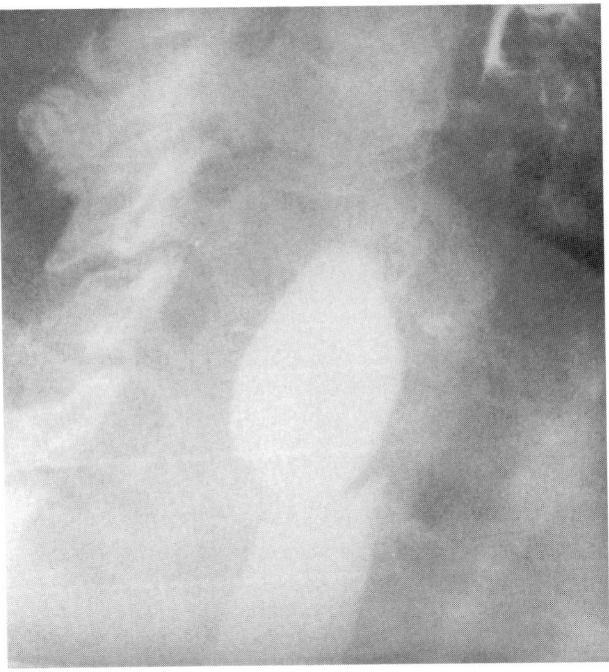

FIGURE 30–30 ■ Same patient 10 years later. The diverticulum has increased in size with progression of oropharyngeal symptoms.

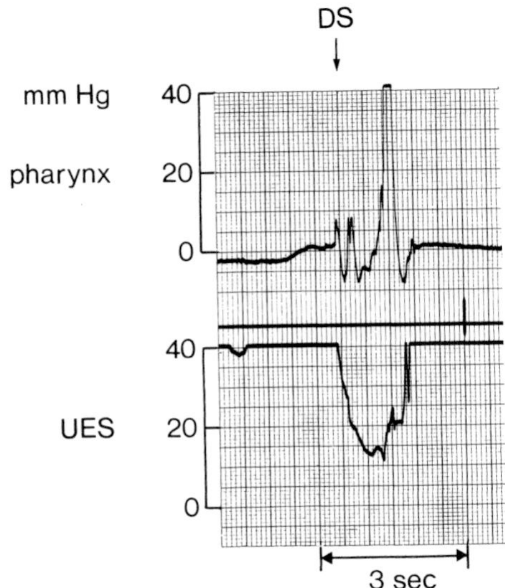

FIGURE 30–32 ■ Incoordination between pharyngeal contraction and closure of the upper esophageal sphincter (UES). (DS, dry swallow.)

These radiologic observations were never clearly recorded on motility studies. Function of the UES was reported by various authors to be either abnormal or normal. Kodicek and Creamer (1961) and Pedersen and associates (1973) reported normal function. Hunt and co-workers (1970) observed a hypertensive UES, whereas Ellis and associates (1969, 1981), Duranceau and colleagues (1983c), and Knuff and associates (1982) found low resting pressures in the sphincter. Coordination abnormalities of the sphincter with the oncoming pharyngeal contraction were suggested by Ellis and Duranceau (Fig. 30–32).

Cook and colleagues (1989) and Jamieson and associates (1992), using sophisticated manometric equipment in conjunction with video radiology of the pharyngoesophageal junction, have clarified the pathophysiology of Zenker's diverticulum formation. They computed the sphincter surface area, demonstrating that it is significantly restricted. When studied under the microscope, the excised cricopharyngeus muscle is infiltrated by fibrosis and inflammation (Cook et al, 1992a, 1992b). This constrictive pathology, causing decreased sphincter compliance, results in elevated pharyngeal and hypopharyngeal intrabolus pressures with each deglutition (Fig. 30–33*A* and *B*). Both the radiologic abnormalities and the elevated intrabolus pressures are corrected by cricopharyngeal myotomy, followed by either resection or suspension of the diverticulum (Jamieson et al, 1992).

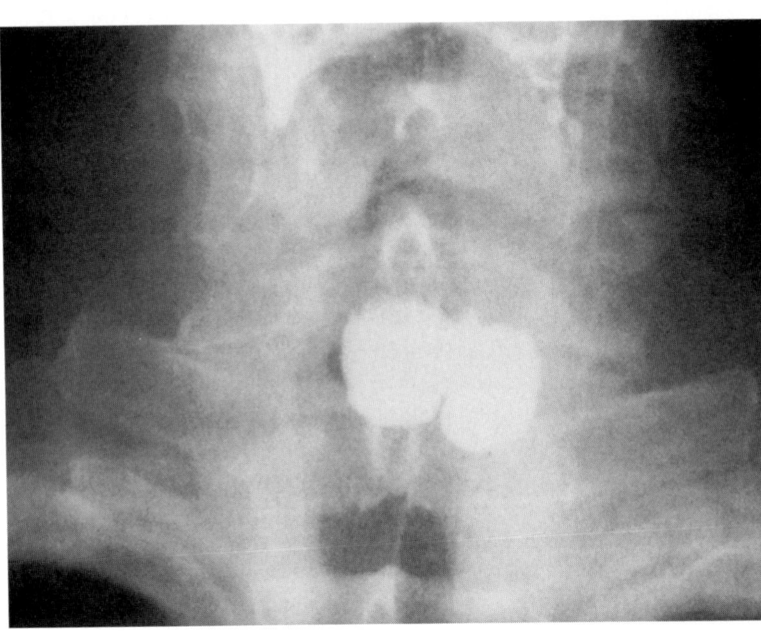

FIGURE 30–31 ■ Bilateral diverticula at the pharyngoesophageal junction.

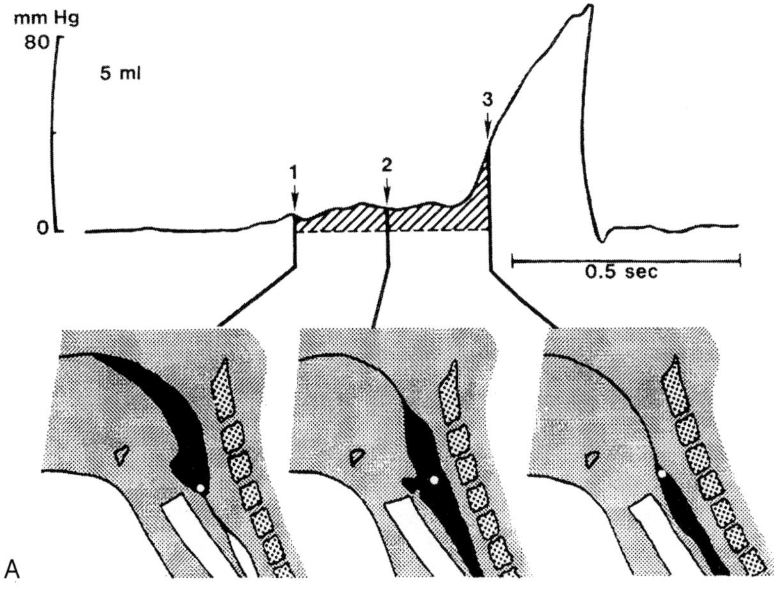

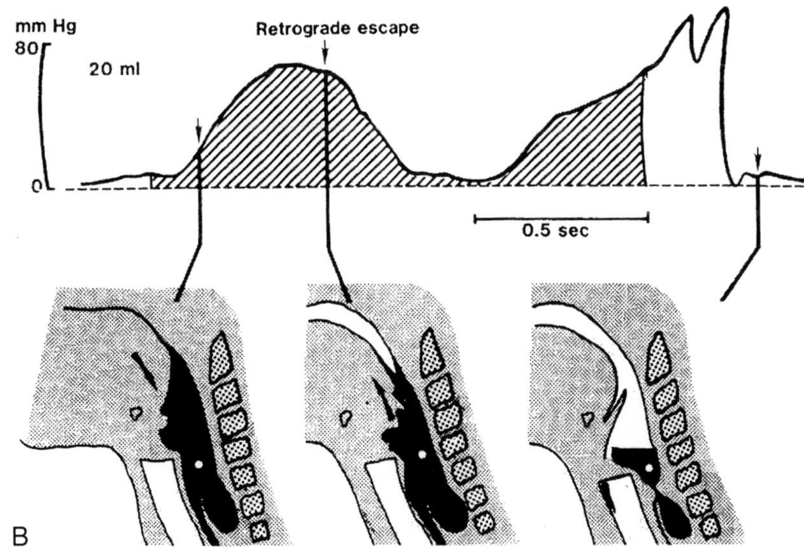

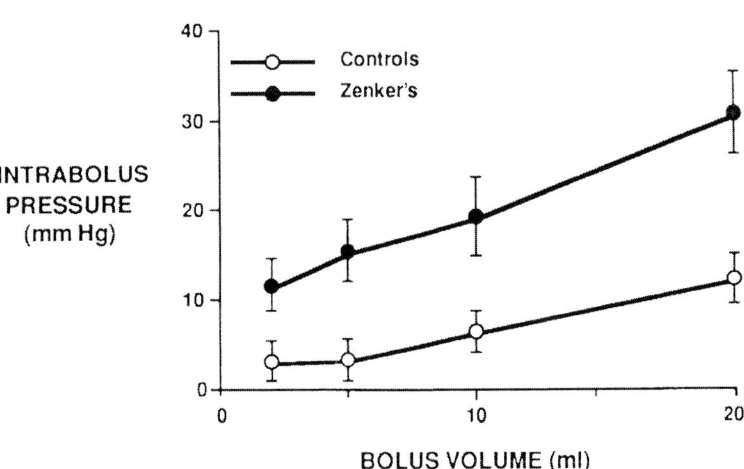

FIGURE 30–33 ■ *A*, Sleeve recording and measurement of intrabolus pressure in a normal patient. *B*, Manometric recording in a patient with Zenker's diverticulum. Hyperpressure is noted in the hypopharynx, whereas an incomplete relaxation of the sphincter is observed radiologically; this is due to restrictive disease in the sphincter. The end result over time is probably diverticulum formation. *C*, Significantly greater intrabolus pressures exist in the hypopharynx of patients with Zenker's diverticulum when compared with normal subjects. (From Cook IJ, Gabb M, Panagopoulos V, et al: Pharyngeal [Zenker's] diverticulum is a disorder of upper esophageal sphincter opening. Gastroenterology 103:1229–1235, 1992.)

Endoscopy

Although rigid esophagoscopy was used in the past in the diagnosis of a pharyngoesophageal diverticulum, rigid endoscopy today would be considered dangerous and unnecessary. One of the main arguments for using endoscopy is to rule out a carcinoma in the diverticulum, a very rare finding. Reporting on endoscopic examinations in 58 patients who eventually underwent myotomy and diverticulopexy, Lerut and associates (1987) found no lesions in any of the patients. In this setting, the risks may well outweigh the advantages. If there is reasonable suspicion of malignancy on radiologic assessment, it is ruled out by direct laryngoscopy and by using the short rigid esophagoscope.

Distal esophageal problems associated with a pharyngoesophageal diverticulum are common and may require complete endoscopic assessment. Full evaluation of the esophagus is completed only after operation on the pharyngoesophageal diverticulum, when easy transit from pharynx to esophagus has resumed.

Radionuclide Studies

The use of tracers in pharyngoesophageal diverticulum patients is not optimal for anatomic evaluation of the condition. Quantification of retention and improved clearance analysis after treatment are theoretical advantages of this technique.

THERAPEUTIC MANAGEMENT

The therapy for pharyngoesophageal diverticulum is surgical, and all patients with this condition should be considered for surgery.

Cricopharyngeal Myotomy for Small Diverticula

Lahey and Warren (1954) viewed the smallest form of pharyngoesophageal diverticulum as relatively asymptomatic. They considered that any surgical operation on these small pouches was improper. Patients were advised to await the development of a larger diverticulum.

Surgeons have used cricopharyngeal myotomy alone for this condition since the late 1950s. The number of patients undergoing myotomy has increased significantly during the past 30 years. Of all patients presenting with a diverticulum, 4% have a pouch smaller than 1 cm (Duranceau and Jamieson, 1987) that is amenable to simple cricopharyngeal myotomy. When performing a myotomy for Zenker's diverticulum, Lerut and associates (1987) left the pouch untouched when it was smaller than 2 cm. They observed no complication from this operation, and 82% of their entire group is totally asymptomatic and 95% show very good to excellent results.

Payne and King (1983) reported that cricopharyngeal myotomy alone, without attention to the diverticulum, brought permanent control of symptoms in only 78% of patients. Ellis and associates (1969, 1981) reported two failures after this operation, both in patients with small, dependent pouches.

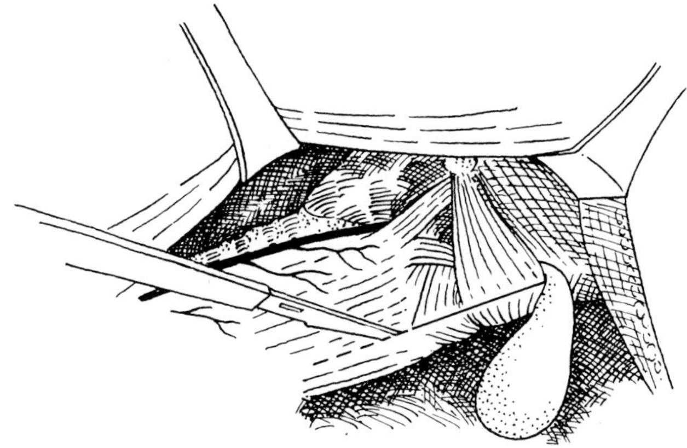

FIGURE 30–34 ■ With a 36 French mercury bougie serving as an intraesophageal stent, the myotomy is started on the cervical esophagus, progresses over the cricopharyngeus, and is extended 2 to 3 cm on the hypopharynx.

In patients with those small or minute pouches, the myotomy must extend 2 to 3 cm over the hypopharyngeal musculature and 3 to 4 cm toward the cervical esophagus. When this procedure is done, the smallest pouches simply disappear. Whenever a visible diverticulum persists after myotomy, it is important to suspend it with enough tension to eliminate any drooping of the pouch below the neck of the sac.

Cricopharyngeal Myotomy and Diverticulum Suspension

A popular option today is to treat the abnormal cricopharyngeus by myotomy and to suspend the diverticulum behind the pharynx by suturing it either to the pharyngeal musculature or to the prevertebral fascia. Initially proposed by Aubin in 1936 and first reported in the English literature by Harrison (1958), this operation has gained a wider acceptance over the past 40 years, and reported results are uniformly good to excellent. A review of these reports is summarized in a recent report (Sideris et al, 1999). The technique that we use is as follows (Figs. 30–34 through 30–36).

The approach is similar to that described for cricopha-

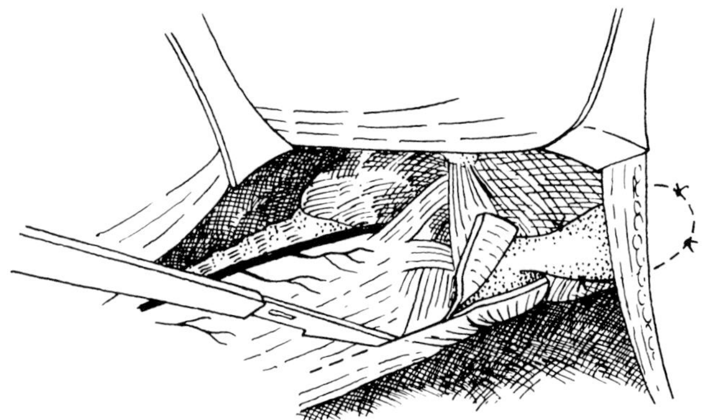

FIGURE 30–35 ■ The diverticulum is suspended and fixed by four or five stitches to the posterior pharyngeal wall.

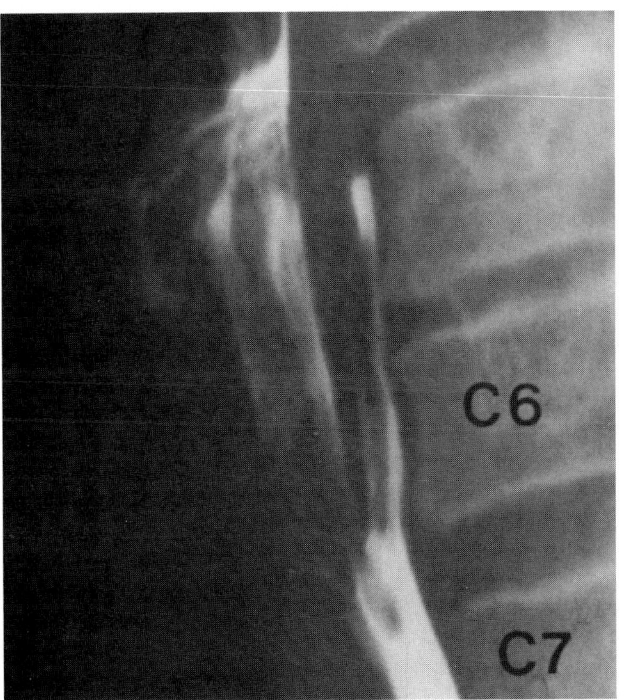

FIGURE 30–36 ■ The up-ended diverticulum should leave no prolapse of the pouch below the neck of the sac.

ryngeal myotomy for oropharyngeal dysphagia (see Fig. 30–14). After dissection and elevation of the diverticulum, a 36 French Maloney bougie is placed within the esophageal lumen. It serves as a stent, precisely locates the neck of the diverticulum, and protects the integrity of the esophageal lumen if a resection of the diverticulum is considered necessary.

The myotomy is begun on the cervical esophagus (see Fig. 30–34). The cricopharyngeus is transected, and the muscularis around the neck of the diverticulum is freed. The myotomy is then extended proximally on the hypopharynx for a distance of 2 to 3 cm. Meticulous hemostasis is maintained.

Once the myotomy is completed, the muscularis is freed from the mucosa over the posterior aspect of the pharyngoesophageal junction. The diverticulum is then suspended with four or five silk stitches, which anchor the lower end of the pouch to the posterior wall of the pharynx or, if small enough, to the muscular sides of the cleft created by the hypopharyngeal muscle transection (see Figs. 30–35 and 30–36).

We have avoided tying the diverticulum on the prevertebral fascia after treating two infections without fistula that were attributed to contamination from the sutured pouch. If a diverticulectomy is considered necessary because of the size of the diverticulum, a linear stapler is used and the mucosa transected above the neck of the diverticulum. The remaining collar is then suspended behind the pharynx as for a smaller diverticulum. Even if a diverticulectomy is performed, the myotomy is left wide open under the resection line.

Wound management is comparable to that for the simple cricopharyngeal myotomy. The rationale behind this operation is to treat the cricopharyngeal abnormality. Jamieson and colleagues (1992) have shown that the elevated intrapharyngeal pressures that occur as a result of the restrictive myopathy in the UES are normalized by cricopharyngeal myotomy.

The second argument behind the operation is to avoid opening the esophageal lumen and to prevent the complications of infections and fistula. Lerut and associates (1987) observed that the incidence of these complications was doubled when a resection of the diverticulum was performed without a myotomy, presuming an obstructive role for the cricopharyngeus. Myotomy with suspension of the diverticulum does preclude the possibility of infection and fistula formation, however. In Lerut and associates' review of 55 patients in the European community, no infection was reported but one recurrent nerve paralysis and two hematomas were noted. Orringer (1986) has reported one fistula and one vocal cord paralysis. We have now seen two fistulas after myotomy with or without diverticulum suspension.

From one review of more than 130 esophageal myotomies combined with a diverticulum suspension, good to excellent results were obtained in 95% of all patients. The exact recurrence rate for symptomatic pouches is yet to be clarified (see Fig. 30–36).

Diverticulectomy with Cricopharyngeal Myotomy

Diverticulectomy is a one-stage operation for simplified management of the pharyngoesophageal diverticulum. Sweet (1956) reported 77 patients without mortality, with a single fistula and with a 4.8% recurrence rate. Payne and King (1983) reviewed the diverticulectomy results at the Mayo Clinic in 888 patients treated between 1944 and 1978. The mortality rate was 1.2%. The most frequent complications observed were wound infection in 3% of all cases, accompanied by a fistula in 1.8% of the group. Thirty-two patients presented with a recurrence (3.6%).

Long-term follow-up of the patient after diverticulectomy, however, raises some questions. The formation of a diverticulum is a long-term process, and, as in many other esophageal problems, it is the long-term assessment of results that may clarify the underlying problems. Holinger and Schild (1969) reported on a patient presenting with a recurrent diverticulum 26 years after diverticulectomy. Nicholson (1962) followed 20 patients, and 13 showed recurrent pouches. Hansen and co-workers (1973) reported that 3 of 19 patients had a radiologic recurrence. The series by Bertelsen and Aasted (1976) showed 14 of 68 patients with a recurrence, whereas that of Einharssen (1967) revealed 17 of 20 cases with pouches. Despite these recurrences, symptoms did not seem as prominent as those recorded before operation.

It is probably for these reasons that surgeons who initially treated the pharyngoesophageal diverticulum by removal of the sac are only now adding a myotomy to the diverticulectomy (Fig. 30–37). Payne and King (1983) suggested that myotomy adds little time and morbidity to diverticulectomy. These authors were especially encouraged that no leaks occurred after their use of this

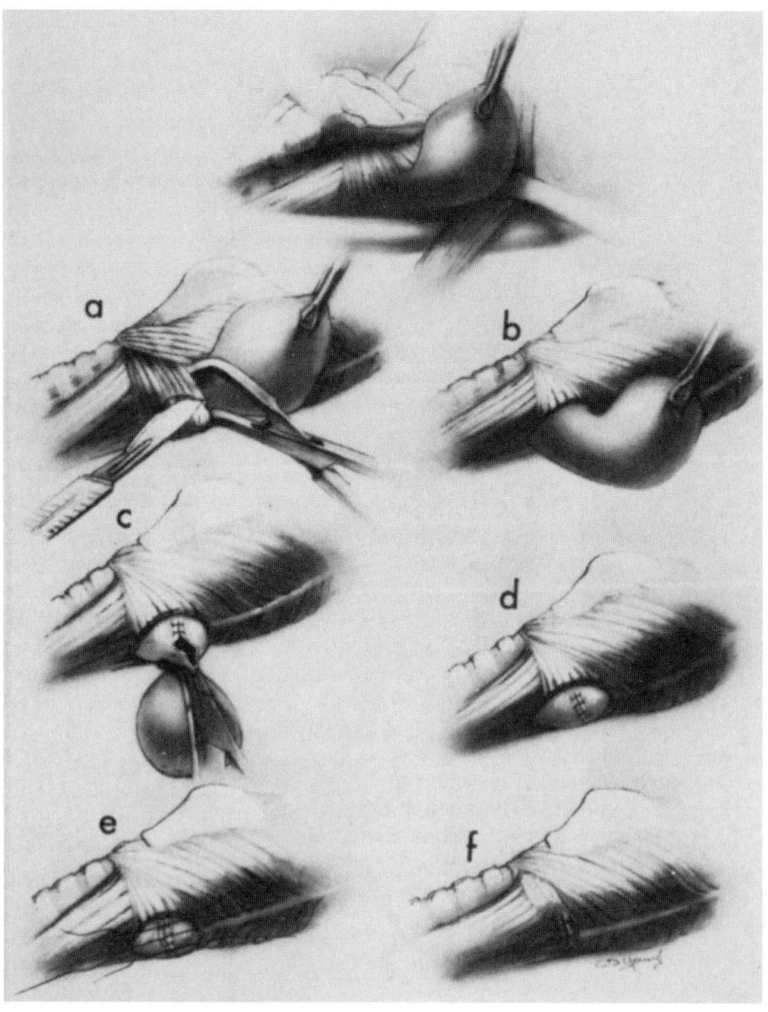

FIGURE 30–37 ■ *a–f*, Technique of myotomy and diverticulectomy proposed by the Mayo group. The muscularis is closed over the diverticulectomy site.

operation, and symptoms of anatomic recurrence were often less severe. The later documentation by Cook and colleagues (1989) and Jamieson and co-workers (1992) of the restrictive pathology in the cricopharyngeus now solidly justifies adding a myotomy whenever the pharyngoesophageal diverticulum is either removed or suspended.

The technique may vary for closure of the resection line after diverticulectomy. Payne and associates (1991) have described closure with either a hand suture technique or a linear stapler. They then re-cover the muscularis of the cervical esophagus with the hypopharyngeal wall above the mucosa at the base of the resected diverticulum, as for a two-layer anastomosis. Like Orringer (1986), we perform the diverticulectomy by leaving the myotomy wide open below the resection line. We tack the redundant mucosa posterior to the staple line to the proximal pharyngeal wall, suspending the neck of the diverticulum to avoid dependency, and add protection to the mucosal closure. This procedure has not yet resulted in fistula formation.

In summary, the results of diverticulectomy for the pharyngoesophageal diverticulum are uniformly good. Because of the known long-term recurrences and symptoms and because of the present evidence suggesting UES dysfunction, cricopharyngeal myotomy should be added to diverticulectomy.

Other Conditions Causing Oropharyngeal Dysphagia

IATROGENIC CAUSES

Any type of surgical procedure at the cervical level can result in oropharyngeal dysphagia symptoms. A good example is tracheostomy. Direct limitation to the normal laryngeal excursion is responsible for these symptoms (Bonanno, 1971). Time and rehabilitation usually alleviate the problem.

Extensive neck surgery and laryngectomy may distort innervation and muscular function at the pharyngoesophageal level (Figs. 30–38 and 30–39). A decrease in resting pressures with loss of the radial asymmetry of the sphincter has been recorded (Duranceau et al, 1976; Welch et al, 1979). Spastic contractions of the cricopharyngeus are observed in 25% of this patient category (Schobinger, 1958). Mladick and co-workers (1971) emphasized that 40% of patients after laryngectomy present with symptoms of oropharyngeal dysphagia. Cricopharyngeal myotomy may help in this setting, after objective documentation of the condition.

GASTROESOPHAGEAL REFLUX

Belsey (1966) has reported “spasmodic contraction” of the cricopharyngeus in 3.5% of 829 patients treated for

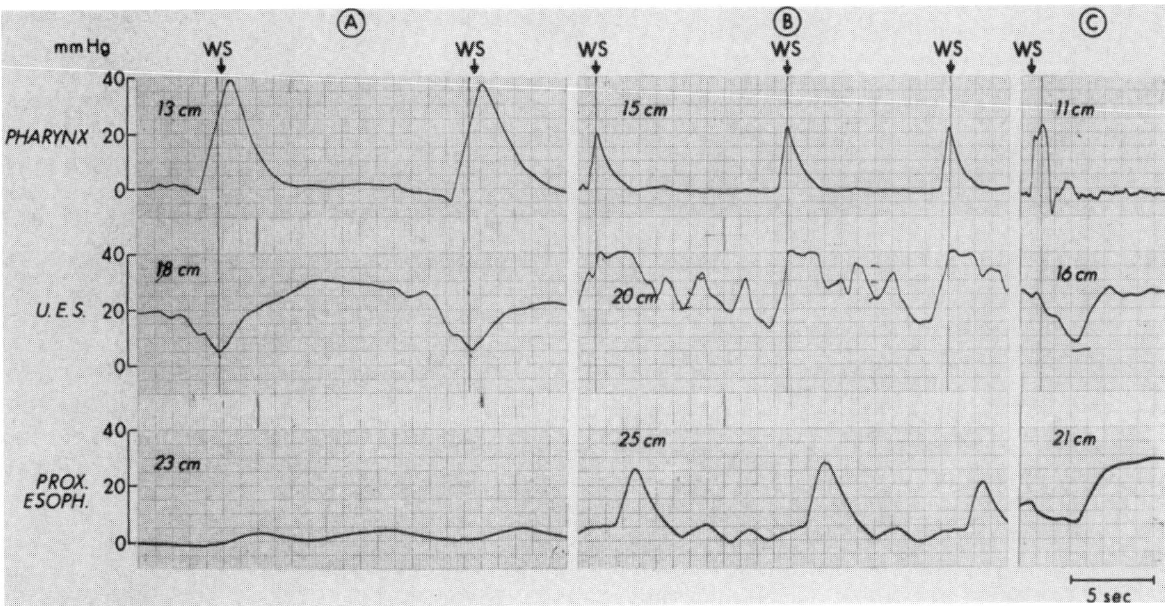

FIGURE 30–38 ■ Incoordination between pharyngeal contraction and upper esophageal sphincter (UES) closure (*A* and *B*) and opening (*C*) after laryngectomy. (WS, wet swallow.)

hiatal hernia and reflux. Henderson (1976) suggested that oropharyngeal symptoms occurred in 51% of his evaluated cases. Bonavina and associates (1985) reported that 9% of their 103 patients with well-documented gastroesophageal reflux had dysphagia referred at the cervical level.

The evidence that favors interaction between UES dysfunction and reflux disease is speculative at best.

Oropharyngeal dysphagia, asthma, and chest pain of undetermined origin represent three categories of symptoms that require, in our opinion, unequivocal proof of association with reflux episodes (by 24-hour pH monitoring), of mucosal damage (by endoscopy and biopsies), and of the physiologic dysfunction present with reflux disease (by careful motility studies), before concluding that they are related to reflux. Oropharyngeal dysphagia should be investigated and treated as such. Any association with reflux disease should also be investigated on its own. The indications for treatment in both conditions should be considered separately and independently.

Conclusion

At this writing, medication and dilatation have shown no proven benefit in managing permanent dysfunction of the cricopharyngeus. Removing the resting pressure effects of the UES in these conditions should provide significant

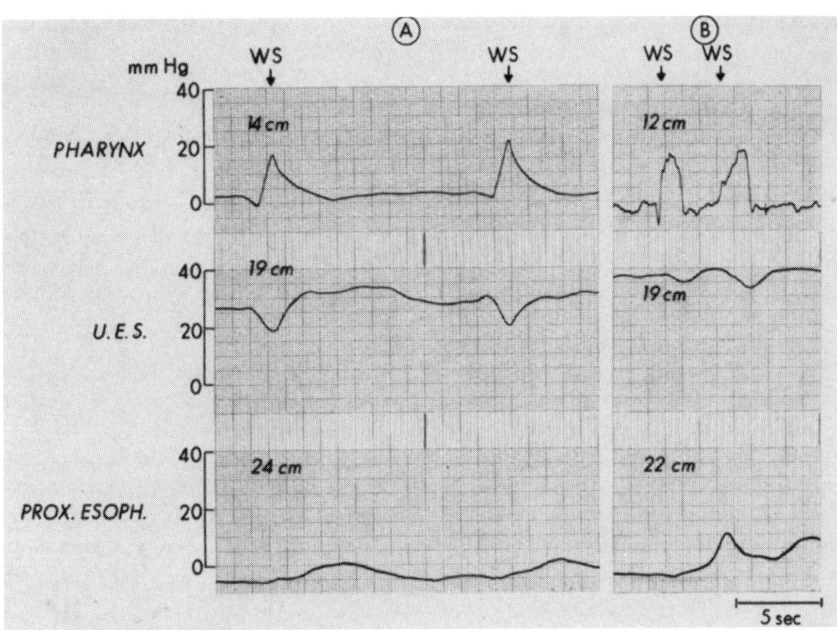

FIGURE 30–39 ■ *A* and *B*, Incomplete relaxation of the upper esophageal sphincter (UES) after laryngectomy. (WS, wet swallow.)

clinical benefit. Diminished resistance to bolus transit is probably the mechanism by which this improvement occurs (Pera et al, 1997).

Selection of patients remains the first step toward successful surgery in the surgical management of oropharyngeal dysphagia. Intact voluntary deglutition, normal movements of phonation and deglutition musculature, and correlation with radiologic and manometric abnormalities constitute the most objective prognostic criteria for improvement.

COMMENTS AND CONTROVERSIES

Drs. Duranceau and Ferraro provide a thorough and updated review of the neurogenic and myogenic causes of pharyngeal and cricopharyngeal dysphagia, the pathophysiology and management of which are not widely appreciated by many surgeons working in this field. They have offered compelling evidence, based on their extensive experience, that the swallowing disorders of neurologic origin can almost always be improved by a cricopharyngeal myotomy. The benefit may be incomplete and frequently deteriorates with time, but this surgery will provide useful palliation in a majority of carefully evaluated and selected cases. The authors present details of pathology and the investigation required for diagnosis and for the selection of surgical candidates.

The muscular dystrophies are, in general, relentlessly progressive disorders. Although the benefits of cricopharyngeal myotomy are likely to be transient, these patients may experience years of useful palliation. Similar experience has been reported in a smaller number of cases of dermatomyositis and polymyositis.

The history and subsequent reported experience with surgery for Zenker's diverticulum are concisely summarized. At present, the authors recommend cricopharyngeal myotomy alone for symptomatic but very small diverticula (<1 cm). Otherwise, it is recommended that a suspension "diverticulopexy" be combined with the myotomy. In the case of very large diverticula, the pouch may be too bulky to up-end and suspend and may warrant resection, again with the addition of myotomy.

I fully agree with these recommendations, which I learned as a resident working with Mr. Ronald Belsey in England in 1959. Although Belsey did not publish this early experience, it is clear that he developed and followed this approach beginning in the early 1950s. Belsey also taught me that very small diverticula cannot be found at surgery and will no longer be visible in a postoperative contrast esophagogram after cricopharyngeal myotomy. Furthermore, even tiny diverticula may be associated with prominent symptoms of dysphagia and aspiration. Belsey also believed that a symptomatic cricopharyngeal bar, with no associated pouch, was just an earlier stage of the same incoordinate disorder of cricopharyngeal function and could ultimately result in formation of a diverticulum. He had observed this transition in at least two patients, one of whom he had followed for 5 years before a tiny pouch was seen in the barium study.

F. G. P.

■ KEY REFERENCES

Bonavina L, Khan NA, DeMeester TR: Pharyngoesophageal dysfunctions: The role of cricopharyngeal myotomy. Arch Surg 120:541, 1985.

This article gives a careful assessment of a surgical series that includes several patients with exclusive neurologic disease.

Castell JA, Dalton CB, Castell DO: Pharyngeal and upper esophageal sphincter manometry in humans. Am J Physiol 258:G178, 1990.

Cook IJ, Gabb M, Panagopoulos V, et al: Pharyngeal (Zenker's) diverticulum is a disorder of upper esophageal sphincter opening. Gastroenterology 103:1229, 1992b.

This meticulous study documents the restrictive dysfunction of the UES as the etiologic mechanism in Zenker's diverticulum.

Curtis DJ, Cruess DF, Berg T: The cricopharyngeal muscle: A videorecording review. AJR Am J Roentgenol 142:497, 1987.

This article is a review on the radiologic assessment of the UES.

Duranceau AC, Jamieson GG, Beauchamp G: The technique of cricopharyngeal myotomy. Surg Clin North Am 63:833, 1983.

This article includes a step-by-step description of the surgical approach for a cricopharyngeal myotomy for proximal sphincter dysfunction when no diverticulum is present.

Kahrilas PJ, Dodds WJ, Dent J, et al: Upper esophageal sphincter function during deglutition. Gastroenterology 95:52, 1988.

This article describes two methods of upper esophageal motor function assessment to document physiologic abnormalities.

Taillefer R, Duranceau A: Manometric and radionuclide assessment of pharyngeal emptying before and after cricopharyngeal myotomy in patients with oculopharyngeal muscular dystrophy. J Thorac Cardiovasc Surg 95:868, 1988.

This article presents a surgical series with an effort at being objective in quantifying the results of cricopharyngeal myotomy for oropharyngeal dysphagia secondary to muscular disease.

■ REFERENCES

Akl BF, Blakeley WR: Late assessment of results of cricopharyngeal myotomy for cervical dysphagia. Am J Surg 128:818, 1974.

Aubin A: Un cas de diverticule de pulsion de l'oesophage traité par la résection de la poche associée à l'oesophagotomie extra muqueuse. Ann Otolaryngol 2:167, 1936.

Barbeau A: The syndrome of hereditary late onset ptosis and dysphagia in French Canada. In Kuhn E: Symposium uber Progressive Musker Dystrophie. Berlin, Springer-Verlag, 1966, p 102.

Barbeau A: La Myopathie Oculaire au Canada Français: Compte Rendu de Le Congrès International de Neurogénétique et de Neuro-Ophtalmologie. Basel, S Karger, 1968.

Belsey R: Functional disease of the esophagus. J Thorac Cardiovasc Surg 52:164, 1966.

Bender MD: Esophageal manometry in oculopharyngeal dystrophy. Am J Gastroenterol 62:215, 1976.

Bertelsen S, Aasted A: Results of operative treatment of hypopharyngeal diverticulum. Thorax 31:544, 1976.

Blakeley WR, Gerety EJ, Smith DE: Section of the cricopharyngeus muscle for dysphagia. Arch Surg 96:745, 1966.

Bofenkamp B: The surgical correction of aphagia following bulbar poliomyelitis. Arch Otolaryngol 68:165, 1958.

Bonanno PC: Swallowing dysfunction after tracheostomy. Ann Surg 174:29, 1971.

Bonavina L, Khan NA, DeMeester TR: Pharyngoesophageal dysfunctions: The role of cricopharyngeal myotomy. Arch Surg 120:541, 1985.

Brais B, Xie YG, Samson M, et al: The oculopharyngeal muscular dystrophy locus maps to the region of the cardiac A and B myosin heavy chain genes on chromosome 14 q 11.2–q 13. Hum Mol Genet 4:429–434, 1995.

Brouillette D, Martel E, Chen LQ, Duranceau A: Pitfalls and complications of cricopharyngeal myotomy. Chest Surg Clin North Am 7:457–475, 1997.

Calceterra TC, Kadell BM, Ward PN: Dysphagia secondary to cricopharyngeal muscle dysfunction. Arch Otolaryngol 101:726, 1975.

Carpenter RJ, McDonald TJ, Howard FM: The otolaryngologic presentation of amyotrophic lateral sclerosis. Otol AAOO 86:479, 1978.

Castell JA, Castell DO, Duranceau A, Topart P: Manometric characteristics of the pharynx, upper esophageal sphincter, esophagus, and lower esophageal sphincter in patients with oculopharyngeal muscular dystrophy. Dysphagia 10:22–26, 1995.

Castell JA, Dalton CB: Esophageal manometry. In Castell DO (ed): The Esophagus. Boston, Little, Brown, 1992, p 143.

Castell JA, Dalton CB, Castell DO: Pharyngeal and upper esophageal sphincter manometry in humans. Am J Physiol 258:G178, 1950.

Cook IJ, Blumbergs P, Cash K, et al: Structural abnormalities of the cricopharyngeus muscle in patients with pharyngeal (Zenker's) diverticulum. J Gastroenterol Hepatol 7:556–562, 1992a.

Cook IJ, Gabb M, Panagopoulos V, et al: Zenker's diverticulum: A defect in upper esophageal sphincter compliance? Gastroenterology 5(pt 2):A98, 1989.

Cook IJ, Gabb M, Panagopoulos V, et al: Pharyngeal (Zenker's) diverticulum is a disorder of upper esophageal sphincter opening. Gastroenterology 103:1229, 1992b.

Cotzias GC, Papavasiliou PS, Gellene R: Modification of Parkinsonism chronic treatment with L-dopa. N Engl J Med 280:337, 1969.

Curtis DJ, Cruess DF, Berg T: The cricopharyngeal muscle: A videorecording review. AJR Am J Roentgenol 142:497, 1987.

Curtis DJ, Hudson T: Laryngotracheal aspiration: Analysis of specific neuromuscular factors. Radiology 149:517, 1983.

De Dombal FT, Hall R: The evaluation of medical care from the clinician's point of view: What should we measure and can we trust our measurements? In Alperovitch A, De Dombal FT, Gremy F (eds): The Evaluation of the Efficacy of Medical Action. Amsterdam, North-Holland, 1979, p 13.

Donner MW, Silbiger ML: Cinefluorographic analysis of pharyngeal swallowing in neuromuscular disorders. Am J Med Sci 251:600, 1966.

Duranceau A: Cricopharyngeal myotomy in the management of neurogenic and muscular dysphagia. Neuromusc Disord 7:S85–S89, 1997.

Duranceau A, Beauchamp G, Jamieson GG, Barbeau A: Oropharyngeal dysphagia and oculopharyngeal muscular dystrophy. Surg Clin North Am 63:825, 1983b.

Duranceau A, Forand MD, Fauteux JP: Surgery in oculopharyngeal muscular dystrophy. Am J Surg 139:33, 1980.

Duranceau A, Jamieson GG: Cricopharyngeal myotomy for pharyngoesophageal diverticula. Int Trends Gen Thorac Surg 3:358, 1987.

Duranceau A, Jamieson GG, Beauchamp G: The technique of cricopharyngeal myotomy. Surg Clin North Am 63:833, 1983a.

Duranceau A, Jamieson GG, Hurwitz AL, et al: Alteration in esophageal motility after laryngectomy. Am J Surg 131:30, 1976.

Duranceau A, Lafontaine E, Taillefer R: Oropharyngeal dysphagia. In Jamieson GG (ed): Surgery of the Esophagus. London, Churchill Livingstone, 1988, p 413.

Duranceau A, LaFontaine ER, Taillefer R, Jamieson GG: Oropharyngeal dysphagia and operations on the upper esophageal sphincter. Surg Annu 19:317, 1987.

Duranceau A, Letendre J, Clermont R, et al: Oropharyngeal dysphagia in patients with oculopharyngeal muscular dystrophy. Can J Surg 21:326, 1978.

Duranceau A, Rheault MJ, Jamieson GG: Physiological response to cricopharyngeal myotomy and diverticulum suspension. Surgery 94:655, 1983c.

Edwards DAW: Discriminatory value of symptoms in the differential diagnosis of dysphagia. Clin Gastroenterol 5:49, 1976.

Einharssen S: On the treatment of esophageal diverticula. Acta Otolaryngol Stockh 64:30, 1967.

Ellis FN, Crozier RE: Cervical esophageal dysphagia: Indications for and results of cricopharyngeal myotomy. Ann Surg 194:279, 1981.

Ellis FH, Schlegel JF, Lynch VP, Payne WS: Cricopharyngeal myotomy for pharyngoesophageal diverticulum. Ann Surg 170:340, 1969.

Hansen JB, Jagt I, Gundtoft P, Sprensen HR: Pharyngoesophageal diverticula. Scand J Thorac Cardiovasc Surg 7:81, 1973.

Harrington SW: Pulsion diverticulum of the hypopharynx at the pharyngoesophageal junction: Surgical treatment in 140 cases. Surgery 18:66, 1945.

Harrison MS: The aetiology, diagnosis, and surgical treatment of pharyngeal diverticula. J Laryngol 72:523, 1958.

Henderson RD, Boszko A, Van Nostrand AWP, Pearson FG: Pharyngoesophageal dysphagia and recurrent laryngeal nerve palsy. J Thorac Cardiovascular Surg 68:507, 1974.

Henderson RD, Wool FC, Marryatt G: Pharyngoesophageal dysphagia and gastroesophageal reflux. Laryngoscope 86:1531, 1976.

Holinger H, Schild JA: The Zenker's (hypopharyngeal) diverticulum. Ann Otol 78:678, 1969.

Holmgrem BS: Inkonstante hypopharynx divertikel: Eine roentgenologische untersuchung. Acta Radiol Suppl 61:129, 1946.

Hunt PS, Connell AM, Smiley TB: Upper esophageal sphincter dysfunction in gastric reflux. Gut 11:303–306, 1970.

Jamieson GG, Cook IJ, Shaw D: The pathogenesis of Zenker's diverticulum and its normalisation by cricopharyngeal myotomy. Paper presented at Fifth World Congress of the International Society for Diseases of the Esophagus, Kyoto, 1992, p 242.

Kahrilas PJ, Dent J, Dodds WJ, et al: A method for continuous monitoring of upper esophageal sphincter pressure. Dig Dis Sci 32:121, 1987.

Kahrilas PJ, Dodds WJ, Dent J, et al: Upper esophageal sphincter function during deglutition. Gastroenterology 95:52, 1988.

Kaplan S: Paralysis of deglutition: A post-poliomyelitis complication treated by section of the cricopharyngeus muscle. Ann Surg 133:572, 1951.

Kaplan S: Paralysis of the swallowing mechanism following bulbar poliomyelitis: Surgical restoration of function. Arch Otolaryngol 65:495, 1957.

Kocher T: Das oesophagus divertikel und dessen behandlung: Coro Bl Schweiz. Aerzte Basel 22:233, 1892.

Kodicek J, Creamer B: A study of pharyngeal pouches. J Laryngol Otol 75:406, 1961.

Knuff TE, Benjamin SB, Castell DO: Pharyngoesophageal (Zenker's) diverticulum: A reappraisal. Gastroenterology 734, 1982.

Lahey FH, Warren KW: Esophageal diverticula. Surg Gynecol Obstet 98:1, 1954.

Lebo CP, Kweisang U, Norris FH: Cricopharyngeal myotomy in amyotrophic lateral sclerosis. Laryngoscope 86:862, 1976.

Lerut T, Vandekerkhof J, Leman G, et al: Cricopharyngeal myotomy for pharyngoesophageal diverticula. Int Trends Gen Thorac Surg 3:351, 1987.

Loizou LA, Small M, Dalton GA: Cricopharyngeal myotomy in motor neurone disease. J Neurol Neurosurg Psychiatry 43:42, 1980.

Ludlow A: A case of obstructed deglutition from a preternatural dilatation of and bag formed in the pharynx: Observation and inquiries. Soc Physicians (Lond) 3:85, 1769.

Lund WS: The cricopharyngeal sphincter: Its relationship to the relief of pharyngeal paralysis and the surgical treatment of the early pharyngeal pouch. J Laryngol Otol 82:353, 1968.

Meadows JC: Dysphagia in unilateral cerebral lesions. J Neurol Neurosurg Psychiatry 36:853, 1973.

Melgar A: Cricopharyngeal achalasia: An uncommon surgical syndrome. Southwestern Med 49:27, 1968.

Mills CP: Dysphagia in progressive bulbar palsy relieved by division of the cricopharyngeus. J Laryngol Otol 78:963, 1964.

Mills CP: Dysphagia in pharyngeal paralysis treated by cricopharyngeal myotomy. Lancet 1:455, 1973.

Mladick RA, Horton CE, Adamson CE: Cricopharyngeal myotomy application and technique in major oral pharyngeal resections. Arch Surg 103:1, 1971.

Montgomery WW, Lynch JP: Oculopharyngeal muscular dystrophy treated by inferior constrictor myotomy. Trans Am Acad Ophthalmol Otolaryngol 75:986, 1971.

Nicholson WF: Late results of operations for pharyngeal pouch. Br J Surg 49:548, 1962.

Orringer MB: Extended cervical esophagomyotomy for cricopharyngeal dysfunction. J Thorac Cardiovasc Surg 80:669, 1986.

Payne WS, Clagett OT: Pharyngeal and esophageal diverticula. Curr Probl Surg 1:31, 1965.

Payne WS, King RM: Pharyngoesophageal (Zenker's) diverticulum. Surg Clin North Am 63:815, 1983.

Payne WS, Pairolero PL, Trastek VF: Surgical management of esophageal diverticula. In Orringer MB (ed): Surgery of the Alimentary Tract. Philadelphia, WB Saunders, 1991, p 229.

Pedersen AS, Hansen JB, Alstrup P: Pharyngoesophageal diverticula: A manometric follow up study of ten cases treated by diverticulectomy. Scand J Thorac Cardiovasc Surg 7:87, 1973.

Pera M, Yamada A, Hiebert CA, Duranceau A: Sleeve recording of upper esophageal sphincter resting pressures during cricopharyngeal myotomy. Ann Surg 225:229–234, 1997.

Peterman AF, Lillington GA, Jamplis RW: Progressive muscular dystrophy with ptosis and dysphagia. Arch Neurol 10:38, 1964.

Poirier NC, Bonavina L, Taillefer R, et al: Cricopharyngeal myotomy for neurogenic oropharyngeal dysphagia. J Thorac Cardiovasc Surg 113:233–241, 1997.

Postlethwait RW: Diverticula of the esophagus. In Surgery of the Esophagus. New York, Appleton-Century-Crofts, 1979, p 129.

Schmid HH: Vorschlag eines einfachen Operations verfahrens zur Behandlung des Oesophages divertikels. Wien Klin Wochenschr 25:487, 1912.

Schobinger R: Spasm of the cricopharyngeal muscle as a cause of dysphagia after total laryngectomy. Arch Otolaryngol 67:271, 1958.

Seaman WB: Pharyngeal and upper esophageal dysphagia. JAMA 235:2643, 1976.

Sideris L, Chen LQ, Ferraro P, Duranceau A: The treatment of Zenker's diverticula: A review. Semin Thorac Cardiovasc Surg 11:337, 1999.

Smiley TP, Caves PK, Porter DC: Relationship between posterior pharyngeal pouch and hiatus hernia. Thorax 25:725, 1970.

Sutherland HD: Cricopharyngeal achalasia. J Thorac Cardiovasc Surg 43:114, 1962.

Sweet RH: Excision of diverticulum of the pharyngoesophageal junction and lower esophagus by means of the one stage procedure. Ann Surg 143:433, 1956.

Taillefer R, Duranceau A: Manometric and radionuclide assessment of pharyngeal emptying before and after cricopharyngeal myotomy in patients with oculopharyngeal muscular dystrophy. J Thorac Cardiovasc Surg 95:868, 1988.

Veis SL, Logemann JA: Swallowing disorders in persons with cerebrovascular accidents. Arch Phys Med Rehabil 66:372, 1985.

Welch RW, Luckmann A, Richs PM, et al: Manometry of the normal upper esophageal sphincter and its alterations in laryngectomy. J Clin Invest 63:1036, 1979.

Wheeler D: Diverticula of the fore-gut. Radiology 49:476, 1947.

Wheeler WI: Pharyngocele and dilatation of the pharynx with existing diverticulum at lower portion of the pharynx, lying posterior to the esophagus, cured by pharyngotomy being the first case of the kind recorded. Dublin J Med Sci 83:349, 1886.

Wilkins SA: Indications for section of the cricopharyngeus muscle. Am J Surg 108:533, 1964.

Winans CS: The pharyngesophageal closure mechanism: A manometric study. Gastroenterology 63:768, 1972.

Zenker FA, Von Ziemssen H: Krankheiten des oesophagus. In Handbuch der Speziellen Pathologic und Therapie. Leipzig, C Vogel, 1878.

CHAPTER **31**

Esophageal Diverticula

Toni Lerut
Clement A. Hiebert

CLASSIFICATION

Diverticula of the foregut may occur at any level, but etiology, symptoms, and surgical approach suggest a three-tiered grouping: pharyngoesophageal, parabronchial, and epiphrenic. A fourth condition—*diffuse intramural diverticulosis*—exists but is quite rare. Diverticula of the esophageal body are usefully designated as *traction* and *pulsion* types (see Figs. 31–1 and 31–3 to 31–5) and represent the result of, rather than the source of, the patient's complaint. Diverticula are associated with a motor disorder (Schima at al, 1997).

Traction Diverticula

Traction diverticula are found at the region of the tracheal bifurcation. They result from granulomatous inflammation of mediastinal lymph nodes that become anchored to the esophagus (Dukes et al, 1976). Contracting scar then tents up the adjacent esophageal wall to form a conical or tabular outpouching. Although the barium-filled diverticulum may resemble its epiphrenic cousin, it belongs to quite another family. Not only is its development different, but the uncomplicated traction diverticulum almost never causes symptoms and assumes importance only if smoldering infection at the apex eventuates in fistulous communication with a bronchus, great vessel, or pericardium (Balthazar, 1977). These complications are uncommon in the Western world; for practical purposes, a traction diverticulum is usually regarded as a sign of healed mediastinal tuberculosis or histoplasmosis (Fig. 31–1). Exceptions are rare.

Pulsion Diverticula

A pulsion diverticulum is a mucosal balloon inflated by peristaltic pulses proximal to a long-standing obstruction. The barrier is most often functional, for example, an unrelaxing sphincter as in achalasia or in chaotic surges of pseudoperistalsis reaching hypertensive levels above a spastic esophageal segment (Hurwitz et al, 1975) (see Fig. 31–1). Intraesophageal pressures as high as 250 mm Hg have been recorded (Dodds et al, 1975). Discoordinate muscle activity is the hallmark of pulsion diverticula of the esophageal body; these disorders include diffuse spasm, nutcracker esophagus, achalasia, and various unclassified anomalies (Cross et al, 1961a, 1961b; Kaye, 1974; Kramer et al, 1967; Vantrappen et al, 1979). Of 65 patients with epiphrenic diverticula reported by Debas and colleagues (1980) at the Mayo Clinic, 77% had abnormal esophageal motility, whereas 11% of the group had a distal benign stricture or hiatal hernia. Only 8 of 65 patients studied had no definable pathology. Pulsion diverticula may be single or multiple, and they can occur at any level (Figs. 31–2 to 31–4). They are sometimes called *false diverticula* because (with a nod to the nomenclature used for aneurysms) the outpocketing is less than the full thickness of esophageal wall, a quibble really. A muscle covering is present, but it is splayed out and inconsequential.

Diffuse Intramural Diverticulosis

Diffuse intramural diverticulosis is a rare condition of multiple 1- to 3-mm outpouchings associated with in-

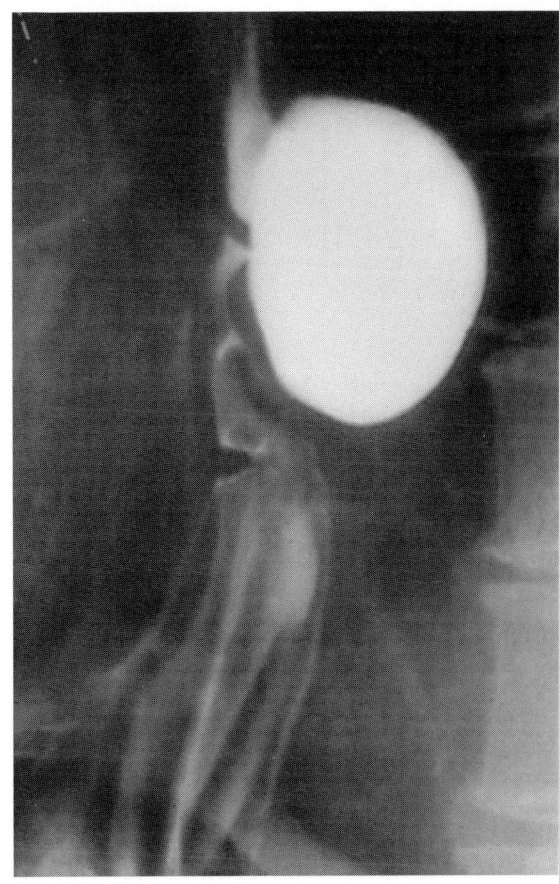

FIGURE 31–1 ■ Solitary epiphrenic diverticulum with hiatal hernia and lower esophageal ring.

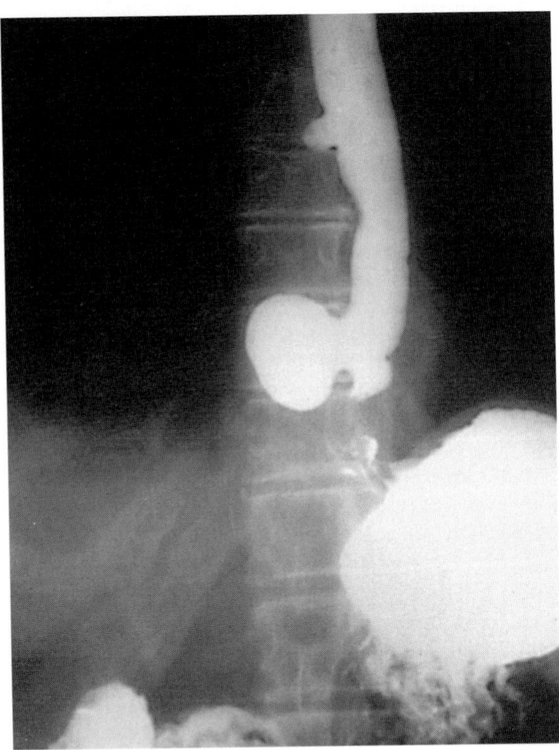

FIGURE 31–2 ■ Mid-esophageal diverticulum (plus a rather more significant epiphrenic diverticulum). The location, small size, and shape of the upper diverticulum suggest association with a healing granuloma.

flammation, fibrosis and thickening of the wall, and diffuse irregularity of the esophageal lumen on computed tomography (CT) scan (Mendl et al, 1960). The diverticulosis may be segmental or diffuse. Of the patients reported by Duranceau (1988) 91% were said to have narrowing of the esophageal lumen, half of the time in the proximal esophagus. Esophagoscopy shows esophagitis in about two thirds of patients. The tiny openings of the diverticula are not visible.

Dysphagia is the principal symptom and may be progressive. About a third of the patients have symptomatic gastroesophageal reflux. Treatment is directed toward relief of symptoms by bougienage or antireflux measures, as indicated.

HISTORICAL NOTE

The English surgeon Ludlow (1769) first described clinical and pathologic aspects of the "preternatural bag," now better known as a pharyngoesophageal or Zenker's diverticulum, after the German surgeon who painstakingly reviewed the condition more than a century ago (Zenker, 1878).

Trastek and Payne (1989) credit Deguise (1804) as being the first to describe mucosal herniation through muscle fibers in the body of the esophagus, but only recently have modern techniques for clinical investigation illuminated the probable mechanism of diverticulum production. Vinson (1934) recognized the factor of distal functional or mechanical obstruction, a point later emphasized, among others, by Goodman and Parnes (1952), Cross (1961a, 1961b), and Hurwitz and coworkers (1975). Barrett (1933) performed the first transpleural resection of an epiphrenic diverticulum.

Allen and Clagett (1965) showed the importance of relieving distal obstruction in a review of 21 patients who underwent diverticulectomy without myotomy, five of whom suffered suture line dehiscence and four others who had documented recurrence of the diverticulum. This group was compared with a subsequent series of 10 patients in whom myotomy was added and no leakage occurred.

Belsey (1966) advocated diverticulopexy for diverticula with a large orifice and stressed the importance of a long extramucosal myotomy and a loose fundoplication to prevent reflux whenever the myotomy is carried to the stomach wall.

■ *HISTORICAL READINGS*

Allen TH, Clagett OT: Changing concepts in the treatment of pulsion diverticula of the lower esophagus. J Thorac Cardiovasc Surg 50:455, 1965.

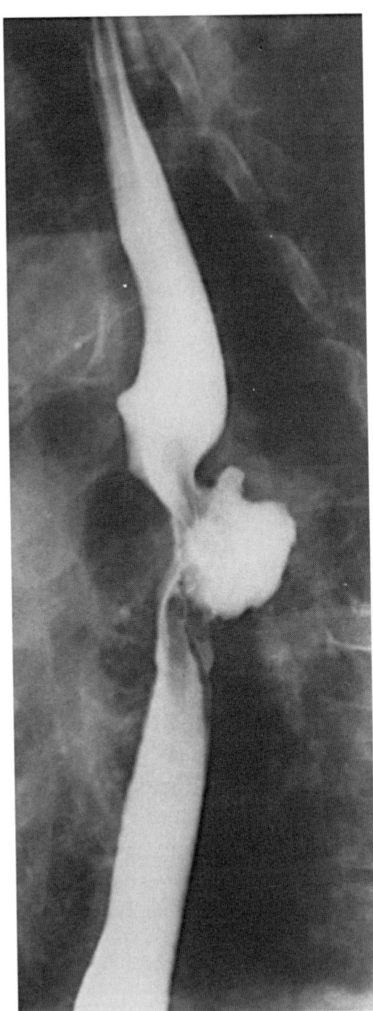

FIGURE 31–3 ■ An extremely rare midesophageal diverticulum containing an adenocarcinoma. (From Avisor E, Luketich JD: Adenocarcinoma in a mid-esophageal diverticulum: A case report. Ann Thorac Surg 69:288, 2000. Reprinted from Society of Thoracic Surgeons.)

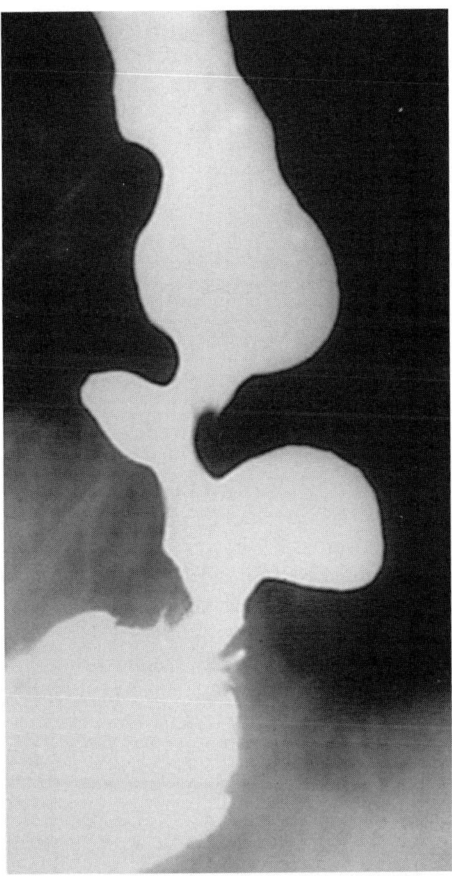

FIGURE 31–4 ■ Diffuse esophagospasm. Multiple sacs and constrictions illustrate the futility of attending to the diverticula rather than correcting the muscular obstruction.

Barrett NR: Diverticula of the thoracic oesophagus: Report of a case in which the diverticulum was successfully resected. Lancet 1:1009, 1933.

Belsey R: Functional disease of the esophagus. J Thorac Cardiovasc Surg 52:164, 1966.

Deguise F: Dissertation sur l'anérisme suivie de propositions médicales sur divers objets, et des aphorismes d'Hippocrate sur le spasme. Thesis. Paris, 1804. Cited by Trastek VF, Payne WS: Esophageal diverticula. In Shields TW (ed): General Thoracic Surgery, 3rd ed. Philadelphia, Lea & Febiger, 1989.

Vinson PP: Diverticula of the thoracic portion of the esophagus: Report of forty-two cases. Arch Otolaryngol 19:508, 1934.

Zenker FA, von Ziemssen H: Krankheiten des oesophagus. In von Ziemssen H (ed): Handbuch der speziellen Pathologic und Therapie, Vol 7, part 1 (suppl). Leipzig, FCW Vogel, 1874.

DIAGNOSIS

Clinical Features

As already noted, an uncomplicated traction diverticula by itself produces no symptoms. Pulsion diverticula of the body of the esophagus would be mostly silent, too, were it not for complaints generated by the spasm or dysfunction responsible for the diverticulum in the first place. Such symptoms include dysphagia, esophageal retention, and regurgitation occasioned by hiatal hernia, esophagitis, benign stricture, or achalasia (Cross et al, 1961b; Di Marino and Cohen, 1974; Evander et al, 1986). Perhaps as a result of the limited length of the esophageal reservoir above the higher obstructions, regurgitation and aspiration are more likely to be important symptoms with pharyngoesophageal diverticula than with epiphrenic blowouts.

In two circumstances, the sac itself may figure in the clinical picture. Both are rare. Hiebert (in an unreported operated case) found an epiphrenic diverticulum to be jammed with digitalis tablets that never arrived at the stomach. One would think that this would happen more often. A second potential hazard is the accumulation of carcinogens. Pitt (1896) reported a squamous tumor in a diverticulum, but fewer than 50 cases were found in the world literature over the next 84 years (Fujita et al, 1980). Huang and colleagues (1984) found four instances of squamous cell cancer in reviewing the records of 1249 patients treated at the Mayo Clinic for pharyngoesophageal diverticula, an incidence of 0.4%. Their data suggest that when the disease is limited, diverticulectomy alone can provide long-term survival. A single instance of *adenocarcinoma* arising in a mid-esophageal diverticulum has been reported by Avisar and Luketich (2000) (see Fig. 31–3).

Differential Diagnosis

Barium studies can usually differentiate between the small traction diverticulum with a wide mouth and lying close to the tracheal bifurcation and the globular and often huge pulsion diverticulum with abnormal esophageal contraction patterns. The pseudodiverticula seen with curling of the esophagus can be differentiated from true diverticula by the inconstancy of the barium pattern on repeated swallows. The radiologist should carry out maneuvers to identify achalasia, hiatal hernia, or another foregut pathologic process. Motility studies (Little, 1986; Vantrappen et al, 1979) may help to define the nature and extent of muscle spasm or dysfunction, as Cross argued as long ago as 1961. Combined rigid and flexible esophagoscopy is useful in clearing out residual food or fetid debris before surgery and may yield information about associated disease. Gentleness and circumspection are the watchwords for passing any esophageal instrument in any patient, especially in the presence of a blind pouch that is easily mistaken for the true lumen.

SURGICAL MANAGEMENT

Principles

The presence of a diverticulum is not by itself an indication for surgery.

Although a pulsion diverticulum of the esophagus is a tempting trophy, it can often be ignored, especially if the neck is wide and the sac is small. The pulsion diverticulum is the *result* of the problem and rarely the source of the patient's symptoms. Whether or not the surgeon elects to excise the diverticulum, the essential step is to disable the distal barrier that caused the blowout in the first place (Allen and Clagett, 1965; Skinner and Belsey, 1988). Usually, this procedure requires longitudinal division and spreading of the circular muscle from at or near the esophagogastric junction cephalad to a point above the highest diverticulum. The idea is to convert a spastic tube into a necessarily passive (but wide and open) conduit. When advanced esophagitis or stricture (rather than dysfunctional muscle) causes obstruction, esophagectomy and substitution with stomach, colon, or small bowel are in order.

Operative Technique

Points of Controversy

There are a number of controversial questions and points in regard to technique:

1. *Should the procedure include a right thoracotomy or left thoracotomy?* Arguments for a right thoracic approach include the fact that diverticula most often sprout to the right, the body of the esophagus lies mostly in the right chest, and the aortic arch is out of the way. A left thoracotomy, however, gives all important access to the esophagogastric junction that must be exposed for epiphrenic diverticula, as well as for more cephalad diverticula and for more cephalad diverticula associated with an abnormality of the lower sphincter. For exposure of the base of the diverticulum, the esophagus may be mobilized and rotated.

2. *Should the diverticulum be excised or inverted and tethered?* The factors that favor excision are a narrow neck that thwarts drainage, evidence of inflammation, malignant degeneration, and massive size of the diverticulum (Skinner and Belsey, 1988). If the diverticulum is long and has a wide mouth, the surgeon may elect to rotate the freed sac 180 degrees cephalad and tether its apex so that drainage is favored.

3. *What should be the limits of the myotomy?* The manometric features of the lower esophageal sphincter can help to settle the issue at the lower end (Fegiz et al, 1984), as do the radiographic characteristics of the barium-filled gullet. The upper limit of the myotomy may be defined by either of these studies (Little, 1986), or the surgeon may elect to extend the myotomy at least to the point where hypertrophied muscle stops.

4. *Should a concomitant antireflux operation be performed?* This issue has received considerable attention in discussions of the treatment of achalasia. Reports from the literature indicate that reflux esophagitis follows iatrogenic destruction of the lower esophageal sphincter in 3% to 48% of patients and leads to stricture and recurrence of the dysphagia in some (Black et al, 1976; Ellis et al, 1984; Ellis, 1985; Fegiz et al, 1984; Jara et al, 1979; Okike et al, 1978; Pai et al, 1984; Thompson et al, 1987). However, a timid myotomy of the lower sphincter (or none whatsoever) may leave the patient with continued obstruction and at risk for dehiscence of the esophageal suture line (Allen and Clagett, 1965).

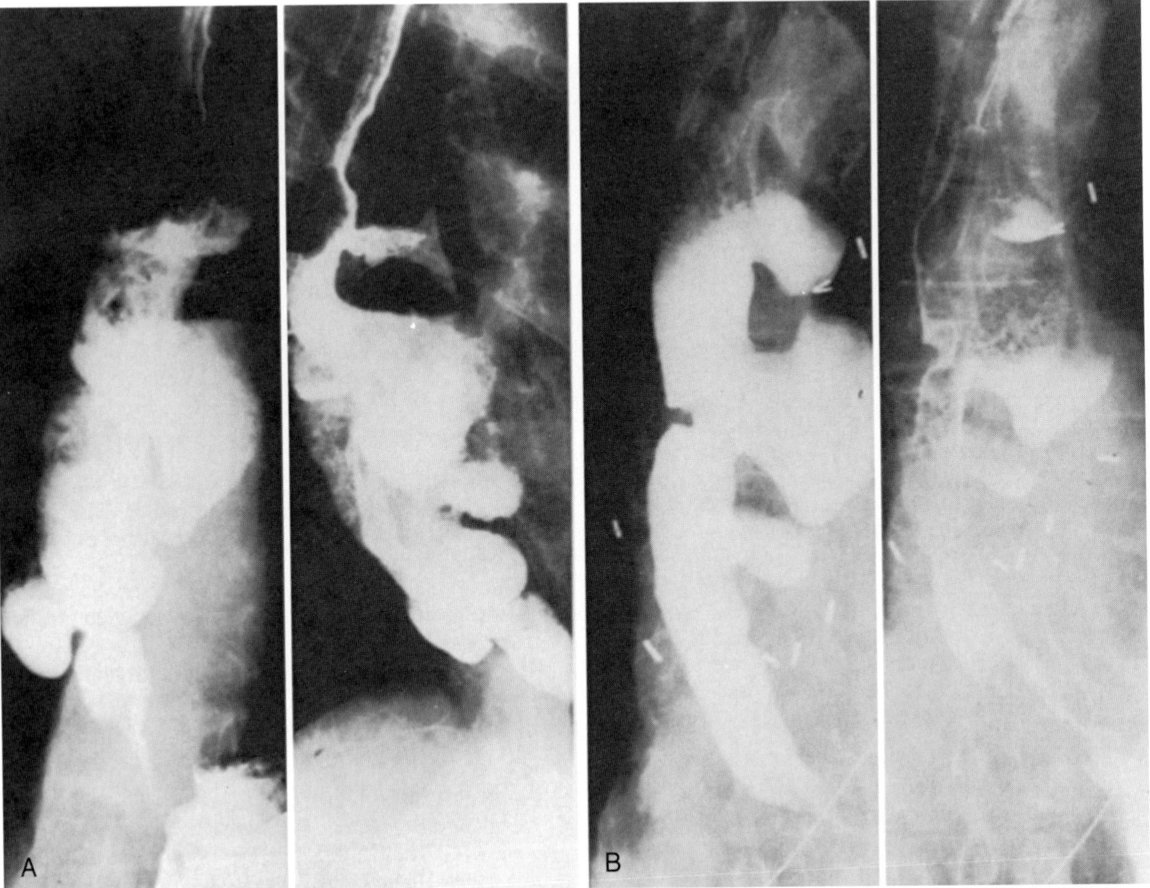

FIGURE 31–5 ■ *A*, Advanced diffuse esophagospasm and giant diverticulosis. At operation, there was intense peridiverticulitis of the entire mediastinum. A long myotomy relieved symptoms until death 12 years postoperatively. *B*, Barium study showed free passage of the contrast bolus.

Surgeons who prefer complete division of the lower esophageal sphincter usually anticipate the possibility of incompetency. A partial fundoplication of the Belsey Mark IV type prevents reflux without obstructing a patient whose peristaltic pump is feeble (Belsey, 1985; Thompson et al, 1987). The same cannot be said for the Nissen 360-degree fundoplication (Topart et al, 1992).

5. *Is there a place for minimally invasive surgery?* Such a procedure is already an acceptable approach for treatment of reflux disease and for esophageal motor disorders; trauma and pain are less, and patients can go home sooner. Moreover, advocates of minimally invasive surgery suggest that the optics afford precision otherwise unattainable. The principal drawbacks are a much longer operating time and the occasional need to convert to an open operation.

Minimally Invasive Technique

A right approach is generally selected. The patient is placed in the lateral decubitus position, and the ipsilateral lung is collapsed to obtain optimal working space. Four or five ports are required: one for the camera and up to four more for the instruments (Fig. 31–5). An endoscopic Babcock applied to the diverticulum helps with exposure (Fig. 31–6*A*). Muscle fibers are teased away from the neck of the diverticulum (Fig. 31–6*B*), and one or more cartridges of staples are applied across its base. To avoid narrowing the lumen, the surgeon passes a No. 48 Maloney bougie through the mouth before firing the stapler. The overlying muscle layer is reapproximated (Fig. 31–6*C*).

After the diverticulum has been excised, the esophagus is rotated to facilitate an extramucosal myotomy at least 90 degrees removed from the staple line. The proximal end of this cut should begin above the level of the diverticulum neck and continue caudally to the esophagogastric junction. The mucosa bulges over the length of the myotomy. Insufflation of air via a nasogastric tube helps to identify an overlooked perforation of the mucosa.

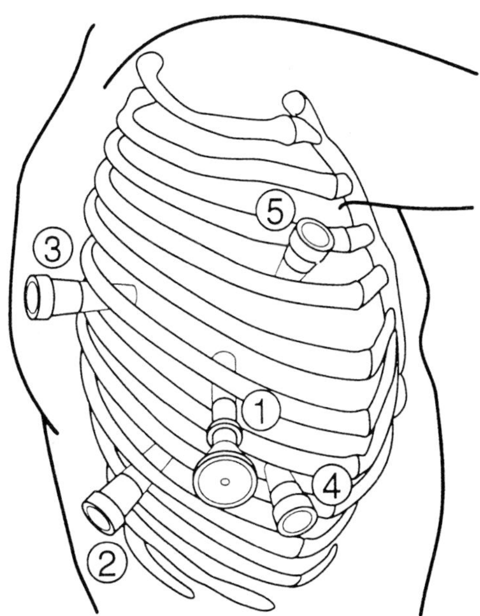

FIGURE 31–6 ■ Placement of the ports with the patient in the left lateral decubitus position. *Port 1* is used for the telescope. *Port 2* is the main operating port for the right hand of the surgeon. *Port 3* is used for the left hand. *Port 4* is used for suction probes and dissecting forceps. *Port 5* is used for the lung retractor.

The issue of whether to add an antireflux procedure after a video-assisted thoracic surgery dissection of a diverticulum is reminiscent of discussions of operations for achalasia (Rosati et al, 1998; Pellegrini, 1997; Saw et al, 1998). But the incentive to use minimally invasive surgery should not justify omission of an antireflux procedure when necessary. Rosati and colleagues (1998) successfully used minimally invasive techniques to excise the diverticulum, to perform the requisite myotomy, and to complete a partial fundoplication in four patients. This group reported satisfactory results. All the same, one must remain alert to the possibility of suture line leakage following a less than ideal closure of the stapled base of the diverticulum. It is still too early to say whether transhiatal stapling of a diverticulum, especially a large one, qualifies as acceptably safe technique.

Epiphrenic Diverticulectomy, Extended Myotomy, and Antireflux Procedure: Open Technique

The technique of epiphrenic diverticulectomy, extended myotomy, and antireflux procedure is illustrated in Figure 31–7. The chest is entered through a sixth left interspace thoracotomy. After division of the mediastinal pleura, the esophagus is identified and encircled. Generally, the diverticulum extends to the right and has to be mobilized by blunt and sharp dissection. Applying two Babcock clamps on the sac of the diverticulum, diverticulum and esophagus can be rotated laterally into the operative field. The neck of the diverticulum is now further dissected and the surrounding muscle wall identified.

At this point, a stapler device is applied on the neck of the diverticulum, with care taken to avoid extensive traction as traction might result in a narrowing of the mucosal lumen of the esophagus. In case of doubt, narrowing of the lumen can be avoided by introducing a large No. 48 Maloney bougie through the mouth.

After firing of the stapler, the diverticulum is resected. The stapler is removed, leaving a double staple line on the mucosal side. The muscular edges are approximated. The esophagus is then rotated back in its origin position and further mobilized up to the aortic arch as for a classic Belsey Mark IV antireflux procedure.

The phrenoesophageal membrane is opened, giving entrance to the greater sac of the peritoneal cavity. The upper limit of the gastrohepatic ligament is clamped and divided. After full mobilization of the cardia, two traction sutures are placed on the muscle layer of the distal esophagus, elevating the muscle layer from the underlying mucosa (Fig. 31–8*A*). The myotomy starts on the anterolateral aspect of the esophagus as the muscle layers are incised down to the submucosa, dividing all muscle fibers over the lower esophageal sphincter zone. The myotomy is extended into the stomach to ensure that the lower esophageal sphincter is completely destroyed.

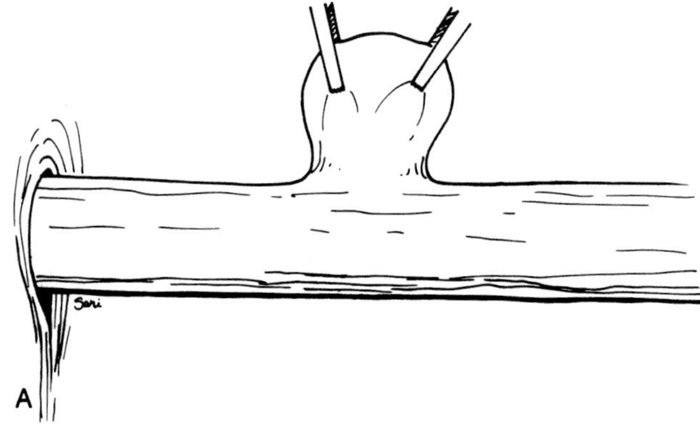

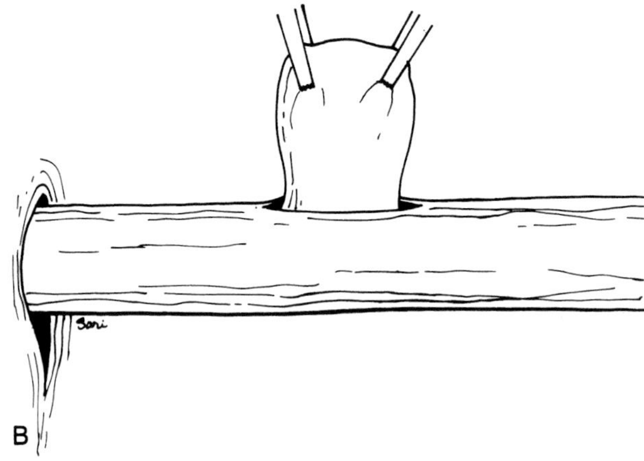

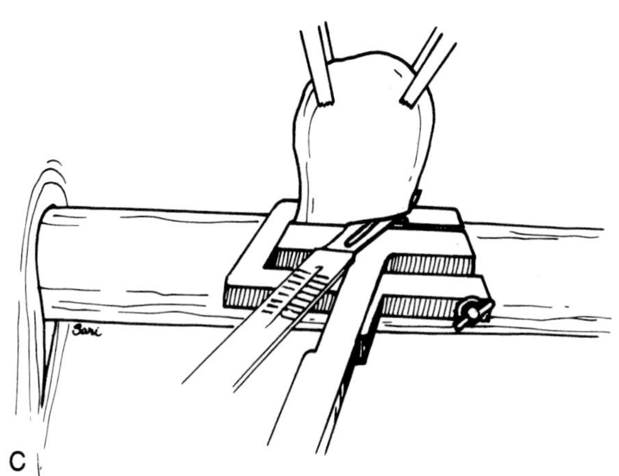

FIGURE 31–7 ■ Principles of diverticulum removal (open or video-assisted thoracoscopic surgery). *A*, The diverticulum is identified and grasped. *B*, A large Maloney bougie is passed through the mouth, and an endo stapler is used to complete the resection. Muscle closure over the resection site and contralateral myotomy (see Fig. 31–8).

When the stomach is reached, an abrupt increase in vascularity of the submucosa is noted, and the structure of the muscle layer is changing. It is important to divide all circular muscle fibers. Leaving only a few circular muscle fibers intact can prevent satisfactory relief of dysphagia.

The myotomy is extended up to the aortic arch, with care taken to preserve the vagus nerves and its branches. Usually, an oblique vagal branch connects the right and

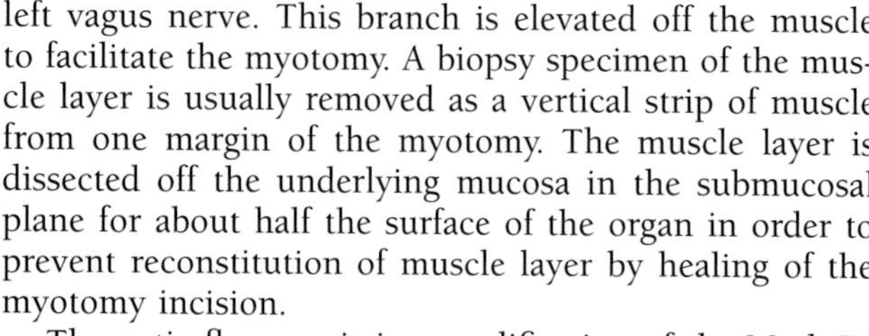

left vagus nerve. This branch is elevated off the muscle to facilitate the myotomy. A biopsy specimen of the muscle layer is usually removed as a vertical strip of muscle from one margin of the myotomy. The muscle layer is dissected off the underlying mucosa in the submucosal plane for about half the surface of the organ in order to prevent reconstitution of muscle layer by healing of the myotomy incision.

The antireflux repair is a modification of the Mark IV antireflux procedure (Belsey, 1985). Instead of two rows of three mattress sutures, only two mattress sutures are placed in each of the two rows on each side of the

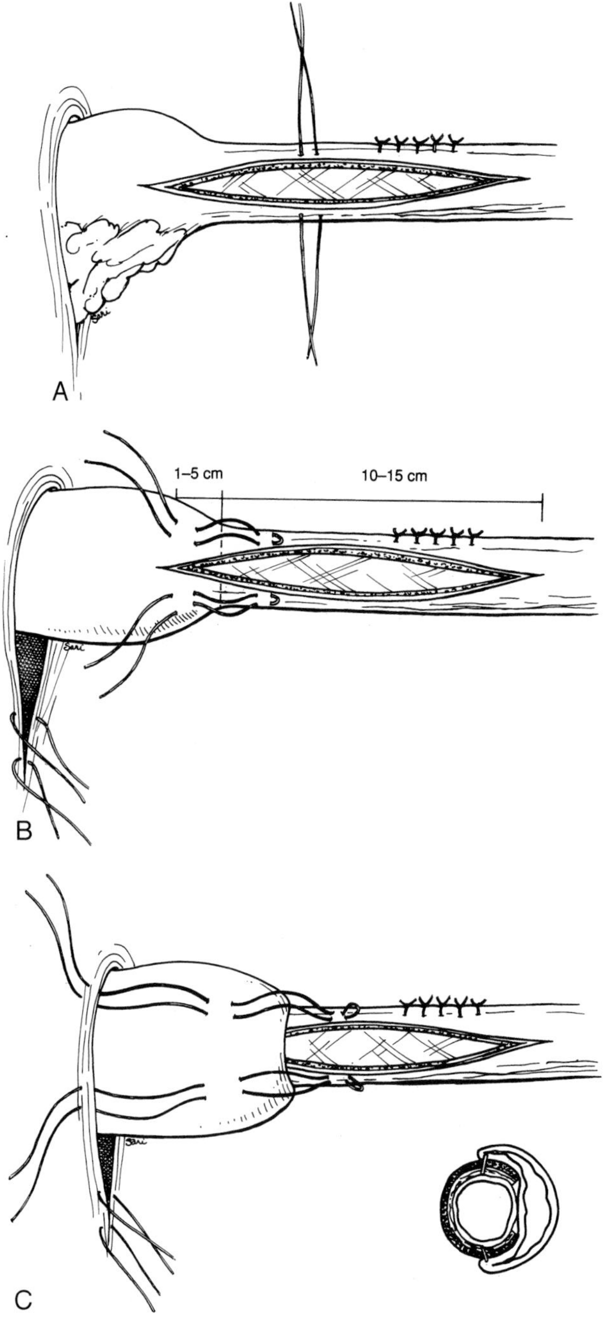

FIGURE 31–8 ■ *A–C*, Partial fundoplication. See text for details.

myotomy (Fig. 31–8*B*). The hypertrophied muscle holds sutures quite well, and a 240-degree fundoplication is readily obtained around the distal 4 to 5 cm of the esophagus (Fig. 31–8*C*).

After reduction underneath the diaphragm of the distal 4 to 5 cm of the esophagus, a posterior buttress is created through approximating the two limbs of the right crus by knotting previously placed sutures. It is important to avoid excessive narrowing of the hiatus in the absence of the esophageal body peristalsis.

Results

The experience of Lerut deals with 12 patients: Diffuse esophageal spasm was documented in six patients, achalasia in two patients, and nutcracker esophagus in one patient. Eight patients had a solitary epiphrenic diverticulum, and four patients had multiple diverticula extending to the level of the aortic arch. In one patient, strangulation was the indication for operation. A hiatal hernia was present in four patients.

Surgical treatment consisted in a simple diverticulectomy in one patient. In all other patients, a myotomy was performed. Diverticuloplexy was performed in four patients and diverticulectomy, in six patients (Table 31–1). One patient with a giant diverticulosis showed, at the time of operation, an intense peridiverticulitis in the entire mediastinum. The operation therefore consisted of a simple myotomy, resulting in a complete and definitive relief of symptoms until death from lung carcinoma 12 years later (see Fig. 31–5). In five patients, the intervention was completed with a Belsey Mark IV antireflux procedure.

No postoperative mortality, no leaks, and no major complications were found (Table 31–2). In 11 patients, follow-up continued for at least 1 year, with a maximum of 16 years. Early and transient postoperative dysphagia was seen in three patients. One patient required several dilatations for peptic stenosis at the gastroesophageal junction. Another patient was treated for an episode of food impaction, requiring endoscopic extraction. The outcome was judged excellent in six patients, very good in four patients, and good in one patient. No patient had an unsatisfactory result.

TABLE 31–1 ■ **Surgical Treatment of Esophageal Thoracic Diverticula**

Type of Operation	*No. of Patients*
Left side	11
Right side	1
Without resection (5)	
Myotomy	1
Myotomy + pexy	2
Myotomy + pexy + Belsey Mark IV	2
With resection (7)	
Diverticulectomy	1
Diverticulectomy + myotomy	3
Diverticulectomy + myotomy Belsey Mark IV	3

TABLE 31–2 ■ **Results of Surgery for Esophageal Thoracic Diverticula**

Result	*No. of Patients*
Postoperative mortality	0
Fistulas	0
Major complications	0
Long-term follow-up (*n* = 11 patients)	
Early postoperative dysphagia	3
Dilatations stenosis gastroesophageal junction (reflux?)	1
Episodes of food impaction	1
Final score	
Excellent	6
Very good	4
Good	1

■ *KEY REFERENCES*

Allen TH, Clagett OT: Changing concepts in surgical treatment of pulsion diverticula of the lower esophagus. J Thorac Cardiovasc Surg 50:455, 1965.

This landmark publication highlights the fundamental principles of surgical therapy for diverticula of the esophageal body, stressing the importance of extramucosal myotomy.

Belsey R: Functional disease of the esophagus. J Thorac Cardiovasc Surg 52:164, 1966.

This publication also stresses the association between the development of diverticula of the esophageal body and the underlying functional disorders. Besides emphasizing the importance of extramucosal myotomy, special attention is drawn to the need for an antireflux procedure in the prevention of late reflux esophagitis and stenosis.

Dukes RJ, Strimian CV, Dines DE, et al: Esophageal involvement with mediastinal granuloma. JAMA 236:2313, 1976.

This article is an overview of the causes of dysphagia, including diverticula, associated with mediastinal tuberculosis or histoplasmosis. These Mayo Clinic surgeons found it necessary to operate on fewer than 10% of such patients.

■ *REFERENCES*

Avisar E, Luketich JD: Adenocarcinoma in a mid-esophageal diverticulum: A case report. Ann Thorac Surg 69:1, 2000.

Balthazar EM: Esophagobronchial fistula secondary to ruptured traction diverticulum. Gastrointest Radiol 2:119, 1977.

Barrett NR: Diverticula of the thoracic oesophagus: Report of a case in which the diverticulum was successfully resected. Lancet 1:1009, 1933.

Belsey RH: Operative treatment of achalasia. In YK Wu, RM Peters (eds): International Practice in Cardiothoracic Surgery. Beijing, Science Press, 1985, p 530.

Black J, Vorback AN, Collis JL: Results of Heller's operation for achalasia of the esophagus: The importance of hiatal repair. Br J Surg 63:949, 1976.

Cross FS, Johnson GF, Gerein AN: Esophageal diverticula: Associated neuromuscular changes in the esophagus. Arch Surg 83:525, 1961a.

Cross FS, Johnson GF, Gerein AN: Oesophageal diverticula. Arch Surg 83:525, 1961b.

Debas HT, Payne WS, Cameron AJ, et al: Pathophysiology of lower esophageal diverticulum and its implications for treatment. Surg Gynecol Obstet 151:593, 1980.

Deguise F: Dissertation sur l'anérisme suivie de propositions médicales sur divers objets, et des aphorismes d'Hippocrate sur le spasme. Thesis, Paris, 1804. Cited by Trastek VF, Payne WS: Esophageal diverticula. In Shields TW (ed): General Thoracic Surgery, 3rd ed. Philadelphia, Lea & Febiger, 1989.

Di Marino AJ, Cohen S: Characteristics of lower esophageal sphincter function in symptomatic diffuse esophageal spasm. Gastroenterology 66:1, 1974.

Dodds WJ, Stef JJ, Hogan WI, et al: Radial distribution of esophageal peristaltic pressure in normal subjects and patients with esophageal diverticulum. Gastroenterology 69:584, 1975.

Duranceau AC: Diverticula of the oesophageal body. In Jamieson GG (ed): Surgery of the Oesophagus. New York, Churchill Livingstone, 1988.

Ellis FH Jr: Surgery for achalasia: How I do it. In YK Wu, RM Peters (eds): International Practice in Cardiothoracic Surgery. Beijing, Science Press, 1985, p 524.

Ellis FH Jr, Crozier RE, Watkins E Jr: Operation for esophageal achalasia: Results of esophagomytotomy without an antireflux operation. J Thorac Cardiovasc Surg 88:344, 1984.

Evander A, Little AG, Ferguson MK, Skinner DB: Diverticula of the mid and lower esophagus: Pathogenesis and surgical management. World J Surg 10:820, 1986.

Fegiz G, Paolini A, Di Marchi C, Torato F: Surgical management of oesophageal diverticulae. World J Surg 8:757, 1984.

Fujita H, Kakegawa T, Shima S, et al: Carcinoma within a middle esophageal (parabronchial) diverticulum: A case report and a review of the literature. Jpn Surg 10:142, 1980 (as reported by Postlewait, 1986).

Giuli R, Estienne B, Richard CA, Lortat-Jacob JL: Les diverticules de l'oesophage: À propos de 221 cas. Ann Chir 28:435, 1974.

Goodman HI, Parnes IH: Epiphrenic diverticula of the esophagus. J Thorac Cardiovasc Surg 23:145, 1952.

Huang B, Krishnan KU, Payne WS: Long-term survival following diverticulectomy for cancer in pharyngoesophageal (Zenker's) diverticulum. Ann Thorac Surg 38:207, 1984.

Hurwitz AL, Way LW, Haddad JK: Epiphrenic diverticulum in association with an unusual motility disturbance: Report of surgical correction. Gastroenterology 68:795, 1975.

Jackson C, Shallow TA: Diverticula of the oesophagus, pulsion, traction, malignant and congenital. Ann Surg 83:1, 1926.

Jara FM, Toledo-Pereyra LH, Lewis JW, Magilligan DJ Jr: Long-term results of esophagotomy for achalasia of the esophagus. Arch Surg 114:935, 1979.

Kaye MD: Oesophageal motor dysfunction in patients with diverticulae of the mid thoracic oesophagus. Thorax 29:666, 1974.

Kramer P, Harris LD, Donaldson RM Jr: Transition from symptomatic diffuse spasm to cardiospasm. Gut 8:115, 1967.

Little AG: Esophageal motility disorders. In JL Cameron (ed): Current Surgical Therapy. Toronto, BC Decker, 1986, p 3.

Mendl K, McKay JM, Tanner CH: Intramural diverticulosis of the esophagus and Rokitanski-Aschoff sinuses in the gallbladder. Br J Radiol 33:496, 1960.

Okike N, Payne WS, Neufeld DM, et al: Esophagomyotomy versus forceful dilatation for achalasia of the esophagus: Results in 899 patients. Ann Thorac Surg 28:119, 1978.

Pai GP, Ellison RG, Rubin JW, et al: Two decades of experience with modified Heller's myotomy for achalasia. Ann Thorac Surg 38:201, 1984.

Pellegrini CA: Impact and evolution of minimally invasive techniques in the treatment of achalasia. Surg Endosc 11:1–2, 1997.

Pitt GN: Epithelioma in an oesophageal pouch. Trans Pathol Soc Lond 47:44, 1896.

Postlewait RW: Surgery of the Esophagus. New York, Appleton-Century-Crofts, 1979.

Rosati R, Fumagalli U, Bona S, et al: Diverticulectomy, myotomy, and fundoplication through laparoscopy: A new option to treat epiphrenic esophageal diverticula. Ann Surg 227:174–178, 1998.

Saw EC, McDonald TP, Kam NT: Video-assisted thoracoscopic resection of an epiphrenic diverticulum with esophagomyotomy and partial fundoplication. Surg Laparosc Endosc 8:145–148, 1998.

Schima W, Schober E, Stacher G, et al: Association of midoesophageal diverticula with oesophageal motor disorders: Videofluoroscopy and manometry. Acta Radiol 38:108–114, 1997.

Skinner DB, Belsey RHR: Esophageal spasm and diverticulum. In Skinner DB, Belsey RHR (eds): Management of Esophageal Disease. Philadelphia, WB Saunders, 1988, p 431.

Thompson D, Shoenut JP, Trenholm BG, Teskey JM: Reflux patterns following limited myotomy without fundoplication of achalasia. Ann Thorac Surg 43:550, 1987.

Topart P, Deschamps C, Taillefer R, Duranceau A: Long-term effect of total fundoplication on the myotomised esophagus. Ann Thorac Surg 54:1046, 1992.

Vantrappen G, Janssens J, Hellemans J, et al: Achalasia, diffuse esophageal spasm, and related motility disorders. Gastroenterology 76:450, 1979.

Vinson PP: Diverticula of the thoracic portion of the esophagus: Report of forty-two cases. Arch Otolaryngol 19:508, 1934.

Zenker FA: Diseases of the esophagus. In von Ziemssen H (ed): Cyclopaedia of the Practice of Medicine, Vol 8. England, William Wood and Company. 1878, p 46.

CHAPTER **32**

Primary Esophageal Motor Disorders

Michael G. Wood
Jeffrey A. Hagen

The act of normal alimentation requires the movement of a bolus from the pharynx to the stomach without regurgitation or aspiration of the food contents. Conceptually, this process can be likened to two biomechanical pumps functioning in series (Bremner and DeMeester, 1997). The pharynx and tongue act as a piston pump, with the tongue functioning as a piston and the pharynx functioning as a cylinder with three valves: soft pallet, epiglottis, and cricopharyngeal sphincter. The esophagus acts as a worm drive pump, with the esophagus serving as the screw and the lower esophageal sphincter (LES) acting as the valve. Malfunction of any of these biomechanical pumps or valves leads to motility disorders resulting in dysphagia, noncardiac chest pain, or regurgitation.

Motility disorders of the esophagus can be classified as *primary* when unrelated to systemic disease and *secondary* when they occur in association with another condition. Primary motor disorders include (1) achalasia, (2) nutcracker esophagus, (3) diffuse esophageal spasm (DES), and (4) nonspecific esophageal motor disorders (NSEMDs). The common secondary motor disorders, listed in Table 32–1, are discussed elsewhere.

Achalasia

DEFINITION

Achalasia is a primary motor disorder of the esophagus characterized by absent peristalsis in the smooth muscle portion of the esophageal body and by incomplete relaxation of the LES in response to swallowing. Achalasia may be primary or secondary, depending on whether it occurs in association with other systemic diseases. A vigorous form of primary achalasia has been described with high-amplitude nonperistaltic contractions in association with the previously described findings. A number of secondary forms of achalasia have been described (Table 32–2), the most common of which include Chagas' disease in South America and cancer in the United States.

Achalasia is a relatively uncommon disorder, occurring in 0.4 to 0.6 per 100,000 population. There does not seem to be a predisposition in either gender, and it occurs most often between 20 and 50 years of age. Wong and associates (1989) described an association between achalasia and the class II antigen DQw1; 85% of their patients with achalasia had this phenotype. Familial cases of achalasia have been reported (Monnig, 1990; Senocak et al, 1990; Tryhus et al, 1989), and some estimate that these may account for as many as 1% of all cases of primary achalasia. However, a study by Mayberry and Atkinson (1985) involving 1012 first-degree relatives of 167 patients with achalasia found no documented cases of familial achalasia.

Achalasia may also occur in association with adrenal insufficiency and alacrima, in a condition termed the triple-A syndrome (Allgrove et al, 1978; Phillip et al, 1996). An association between achalasia and mental retardation has also been described (Ehrich et al, 1987; Khalifa, 1988; Tyce and Brough, 1962).

TABLE 32–1 ■ **Primary and Secondary Esophageal Motor Disorders**

Primary motor disorders
- Achalasia
- Nutcracker esophagus
- Diffuse esophageal spasm
- Nonspecific esophageal motor disorders

Secondary motor disorders
- Scleroderma
- Diabetes mellitus
- Systemic amyloidosis
- Chagas' disease
- Neuromuscular disorders of skeletal muscle
- Presbyesophagus
- Chronic idiopathic intestinal pseudo-obstruction
- Parkinson's disease

HISTORICAL NOTE

Thomas Willis described the first case of achalasia in 1679 when he wrote, "the mouth of the stomach (cardia) being always closed either by a tumor or palsie, nothing could be admitted into the ventricle (stomach) unless it were violently opened." In an attempt to manage the problem, he developed a dilator made of whalebone with a piece of sponge at the end, which the patient used each day for 15 years. Mikulicz used the term "cardiospasm" to describe the condition in 1881 and described a technique of transgastric dilatation in 1904.

Over time, open transabdominal anastomotic cardioplasty evolved as the procedure of choice for treatment of achalasia, performed in a manner similar to the pyloroplasties of the time. In 1913, Heller performed the

TABLE 32–2 ■ Forms of Achalasia

- I. Primary (idiopathic) achalasia
  - A. Classic achalasia
  - B. Vigorous achalasia
- II. Secondary achalasia
  - A. *Trypanosoma cruzi* infection (Chagas' disease)
  - B. Cancer
    - 1. Obstructing LES (pseudoachalasia)
    - 2. Remote from LES (paraneoplastic)
  - C. Infiltrating disorders of the LES
    - 1. Amyloidosis
    - 2. Fabry's disease
    - 3. Sarcoidosis
    - 4. Eosinophilic infiltration
  - D. Systemic disease
    - 1. Diabetes mellitus
    - 2. Familial adrenal insufficiency with alacrima (triple-A syndrome)
    - 3. Sicca syndrome with gastric hyposecretion
  - E. Generalized gastrointestinal dysmotility
    - 1. Intestinal pseudo-obstruction
  - F. Neuromuscular disorders
    - 1. Parkinson's disease

LES, lower esophageal sphincter.

first esophageal myotomy for achalasia, using a transabdominal double (anterior and posterior) vertical extramucosal esophagomyotomy. Zaaijer (1923) modified the technique to a single extramucosal myotomy. This procedure did not gain wide acceptance until 1949, when Barrett and Franklin published the late reflux-related complications of anastomotic cardioplasties.

■ *HISTORICAL READINGS*

Brewer LA: History of surgery of the esophagus. Am J Surg 139:730–743,1980.

Payne SW: Heller's contribution to the surgical treatment of achalasia of the esophagus. Ann Thorac Surg 48:876–881, 1989.

BASIC SCIENCE

Normal Physiology

Most of the esophagus is located in the posterior mediastinum. Only the last few centimeters, including the LES, are normally located in the positive-pressure environment of the abdomen. This relationship is essential to the competence of the LES, which depends on a normal resting pressure (>6 mm Hg), a normal overall length (>2 cm), and a normal abdominal length (>1 cm) (Zaninotto et al, 1988). Although the details of the normal physiology of the esophagus and the LES are discussed elsewhere, it is important to emphasize that the factors involved in delivery of a food bolus to the stomach include the effect of gravity, orderly peristaltic progression, the amplitude of the peristaltic wave, and adequate relaxation of the LES.

The esophagus is about 20 to 22 cm long in adults and extends from the cricopharyngeal sphincter to the LES. Two layers, an outer longitudinal layer and an inner circular layer, form this muscular tube. The upper third of the esophagus consists of skeletal muscle, the lower third and the LES consist of smooth muscle, and the middle third is a transition zone between the two. Motor innervation is derived predominately from the vagus nerve along with contributions from the glossopharyngeal and spinal accessory nerves. Sensory afferent fibers travel along the vagus nerve branches as well as with the sympathetic fibers from the upper thoracic spinal segments.

A normal "swallow-initiated contraction" is called a *primary peristaltic wave.* This wave of sequential relaxation and contraction in the esophagus travels downward at a rate of about 3 cm/sec. Interruption of the peristaltic wave, characteristic of achalasia, must be differentiated from a phenomenon called "deglutitive inhibition," described by Vantrappen and associates in 1971. In this situation, a second swallow wave, initiated while the previous swallow wave is in the striated muscle portion of the esophagus, completely inhibits the contractile activity of the first wave. When the first swallow wave has reached the smooth muscle, a second swallow wave cannot completely abolish the first wave but it decreases its amplitude and propagation. The amplitude and velocity of the primary peristaltic wave can also be affected by afferent stimuli such as bolus size (Vanek and Diamant, 1987). Luminal distention can stimulate peristalsis, even in the absence of an initial swallow (secondary peristalsis). This phenomenon is an important mechanism for clearing material not completely cleared by primary peristalsis or material that may have refluxed through the LES.

Coordination of the act of swallowing in the skeletal and smooth muscle portions of the esophagus is complex and not completely understood. In the skeletal muscle portion of the esophagus, nerve fibers from the nucleus ambiguus of the vagus nerve innervate the muscle cell directly. Orderly firing of these nerve fibers results in a sequential contraction wave. This orderly nerve stimulation of the striated portion of the esophagus is programmed by the swallowing center, located in the medulla.

Peristalsis in the smooth muscle portion of the esophagus is also predominantly under parasympathetic control. Vagal nerve fibers from the dorsal motor nucleus of the vagus, which are also under the control of the medullary swallowing center, have synapses in the ganglia of the myenteric plexus between the muscular layers of the esophageal wall. From the myenteric plexus, the postganglionic fibers directly innervate the smooth muscle cells. These postganglionic nerve fibers contain two types of effector neurons. *Excitatory* neurons cause contraction of both the circular and longitudinal muscle through a cholinergic pathway. *Inhibitory* neurons, once activated, release a noncholinergic, nonadrenergic neurotransmitter that inhibits muscle contraction in the circular muscle layer.

After swallowing occurs, it is hypothesized that the entire circular muscle of the esophagus is inhibited simultaneously through this noncholinergic, nonadrenergic pathway and that peristalsis occurs as a passive rebound contraction. The "latency period" before the postinhibition rebound contraction is shortest in the proximal smooth muscle and lengthens progressively caudally, allowing the sequential peristaltic contraction of smooth muscle (Christensen, 1987).

Sympathetic innervation originates in the thoracic spinal cord and has synapses in the cervical and thoracic ganglia. The postganglionic fibers follow blood vessels until they reach the wall of the esophagus. The afferent visceral sensory pain fibers from the esophagus travel without synapses to the first four segments of the thoracic spinal cord, following both sympathetic and vagal pathways. Interestingly, afferent pain fibers from the heart travel along the same pathway, which explains the similarity between the symptoms of cardiac and esophageal origins.

Autonomic innervation is also responsible for maintaining resting tone and proper relaxation of the LES. LES resting tone is maintained by the stimulatory neurons of the vagus. Evidence of the role of these cholinergic neurons came from the work of Holloway and associates (1986), who showed that atropine caused a substantial fall in LES pressure, whereas motilin, which acts by stimulating cholinergic nerves, caused LES contraction.

Relaxation of the LES is less completely understood. There is evidence for the involvement of a noncholinergic, nonadrenergic pathway (Torphy et al, 1986). Relaxation of the LES has been shown to be associated with increases in intracellular cyclic adenosine monophosphate (cAMP) and cyclic guanosine monophosphate (cGMP). Vasoactive intestinal polypeptide (VIP), an inhibitory neurotransmitter and stimulus for cAMP, has been found in high concentrations in the LES, suggesting an important role for this hormone (Goyal and Rattan, 1980). Because VIP does not cause an increase in intracellular cGMP, however, a second neurotransmitter must be involved. Tottrup and colleagues (1991) have suggested a physiologic role of the L-arginine/nitric oxide pathway as a possible mediator in the relaxation of the LES. This hypothesis is supported by observations of Arnold and coworkers (1977) showing increased cGMP levels in response to nitric oxide stimulation.

Pathophysiology

Achalasia is a neuromuscular disorder of the esophagus characterized by abnormal relaxation of the LES and absence of progressive peristalsis in the esophageal body. Histopathologic studies have shown inflammation in the myenteric plexus along with fibrosis and depletion of or total loss of ganglion cells (Csendes et al, 1985; Goldblum et al, 1996). Degenerative changes of the vagus nerve have also been described (Cassella et al, 1965a) along with changes of neurons in the dorsal motor nucleus of the vagus (Cassella et al, 1964; Kimura, 1929). The cause of this loss of ganglion cells is unclear. Physiologic studies have shown that patients with achalasia have impairment of the nonadrenergic, noncholinergic inhibitory nerves of the LES but intact cholinergic excitatory nerves (Holloway et al, 1986; Tottrup et al, 1990).

Aggestrup and colleagues (1983) described a reduced number of VIP-immunoreactive nerve fibers in patients with achalasia compared with control subjects, which suggests that VIP plays an important pathophysiologic role in achalasia. The question arises, however, whether the primary lesion is in the myenteric plexus or in the dorsal motor nucleus with secondary degenerative changes in vagal fibers and in the myenteric plexus. Support for the hypothesis that central vagal involvement is the primary lesion has come from the observations of Dooley and colleagues (1983) and Eckardt and associates (1989) showing impaired acid secretion and pancreatic polypeptide release with sham meals and prolonged gastrointestinal transit in patients with achalasia.

Other authors have pointed to the finding of Lewy bodies, a characteristic histopathologic feature in the brain stem of patients with Parkinson's disease, in the myenteric plexus and brain stem of patients with achalasia (Qualman et al, 1984), suggesting that both central vagal abnormalities and local myenteric plexus abnormalities may be involved.

Some authors believe that achalasia is primarily an inflammatory process, with secondary destruction of myenteric ganglion cells and nerves. Inflammation in the myenteric plexus in the region of the LES, a consistent finding in achalasia, may have an infectious and/or autoimmune etiology. Robertson and associates (1993) found increased serum antibodies to varicella-zoster virus in 58 patients with achalasia compared with control subjects. Deoxyribonucleic acid (DNA) hybridization studies showed that the virus was located in the myenteric plexus in three of nine tissue specimens analyzed. Increased serum antibody titers against the measles virus have also been reported in patients with achalasia (Jones et al, 1983), but these early studies did not check for evidence of the viral DNA in esophageal tissue. The association of achalasia with the class II human leukocyte antigen DQw1 (Wong et al, 1989) suggests that achalasia may be autoimmune-mediated in some cases, because similar associations with class II antigens have been described in such recognized autoimmune disorders as diabetes mellitus, Sjögren's syndrome, Hashimoto's thyroiditis, and celiac disease. The findings of neuronal antibodies in 7 of 18 patients with achalasia by Verne and colleagues (1997) have supported this autoimmune hypothesis.

Eosinophilic infiltrates in Auerbach's plexus have been observed in patients with achalasia (Landres et al, 1978; Tottrup et al, 1989), raising the possibility of a pathogenic role of these inflammatory cells. When Tottrup and colleagues examined tissue obtained at esophagomyotomy in patients with achalasia, they found that immunohistochemical methods for detecting eosinophil cationic protein (ECP) were positive, although eosinophils were not detected with hematoxylin-eosin staining. This ECP protein is known to be both cytotoxic and neurotoxic, a fact that might possibly explain the loss of ganglion cells in achalasia. Interestingly, eosinophils are also believed to play an important role in the clearance of the parasite *Trypanosoma cruzi* in Chagas' disease, which may explain the injury to the ganglion cells of the myenteric plexus in these patients. Additional support for the role of eosinophils comes from a case report by Fredens and associates (1989), who demonstrated eosinophilic infiltration of the LES in a patient with distal gastric cancer in whom secondary achalasia occurred as a paraneoplastic syndrome.

The effects of LES dysfunction and the resulting outflow obstruction on esophageal body motility are variable. The changes seen range from loss of peristalsis to spasm of the esophagus. Although information regarding the effect of outflow obstruction in humans is limited, animal studies (Little et al, 1986) shed some insight.

Little's group created an animal model of achalasia by placing bands measuring 110% of the resting esophageal circumference around the LES in a group of cats. The resultant interference with sphincter relaxation resulted in esophageal dilatation, development of repetitive contractions, and an increase in the number of simultaneous contractions (0% to 85% in 4 weeks) with decreased mean esophageal contraction pressures. Interestingly, when the bands were removed, there was a slow reversion of the motility to normal.

Return of peristalsis, although variable and only partial, has been reported in patients with achalasia after treatment by pneumatic dilatation or myotomy (Bielefeldt et al, 1990; Mellow, 1976). It has been proposed that with long-standing obstruction, irreversible changes in peristaltic function occur, resulting in the nonperistaltic isobaric pressure waves in patients with achalasia. These observations of apparent progression from normal motility to simultaneous contractions to aperistalsis in the animal model may explain the clinical difficulty in distinguishing between vigorous achalasia, DES, and nutcracker esophagus. It may be that all of these disorders of motility are in some cases part of a spectrum of disease, with transition of nutcracker esophagus to achalasia or DES over time (Anggiansah et al, 1990; Traube et al, 1987a; Vantrappen et al, 1988).

DIAGNOSIS

Clinical Features

Patients with achalasia often experience severe symptoms for prolonged periods of time before the correct diagnosis is established. Eckardt and associates (1997b) emphasized this point in a review of 87 cases of achalasia. They found that although most patients sought medical attention early in the course of their illness, the condition was frequently misdiagnosed. The mean time from onset of symptoms to the correct diagnosis was almost 5 years.

The most common initial symptom in most series is progressive dysphagia for both solids and liquids, which is present in nearly all patients. Regurgitation of recently ingested or undigested food, particularly at night, occurs in 85% of cases. Occasional episodes of chest pain occur in about three quarters of these patients and significant weight loss in 65%. Because the disease is slowly progressive in most cases, patients may adapt quite well for some time by greatly modifying their diet, which makes a detailed dietary history essential. The patient may experience pain, choking, or vomiting with meals and often needs additional liquids to get solid food down. The patient is often the last person to finish a meal and may avoid eating socially because of the need to regurgitate suddenly.

A history of hospitalization for food bolus obstruction may also be present. Pulmonary symptoms such as cough and wheezing may be present, and occasionally epigastric pain and heartburn may occur. True gastroesophageal reflux is rare, however, because of the nonrelaxing hypertensive LES. The sensation of heartburn in these patients may be due to dilatation of the esophagus or irritation of the esophagus by retained food. Smart and colleagues (1987) showed that the mean pH of the retained food to was 3.8, with 97% of the acidity caused by lactic acid from fermentation.

Natural History

Achalasia typically follows an indolent course, with several years of gradually progressive dysphagia. Untreated, achalasia may progress to the development of complications such as formation of lower esophageal diverticula, airway obstruction, pulmonary infection related to aspiration, and even the development of squamous cell carcinoma.

Approximately 10% of patients with achalasia have associated lower esophageal diverticula (Feldman, 1988), and their risk of cancer is estimated to be 14 to 16 times higher than that of the general population (Sandler et al, 1995; Streitz et al, 1995). Because these cancers develop in the dilated midesophagus, dysphagia is not experienced until late and the prognosis is typically poor. Long-term retention of food with inflammation and chronic esophagitis is believed to be responsible for the increased risk of cancer. Whether surveillance endoscopy is indicated, however, remains controversial. Although repeated pulmonary infections are common in these patients, upper airway obstruction secondary to a dilated esophagus is a rare complication of advanced achalasia (Berrisford et al, 1998; Morrow et al, 1982).

Differential Diagnosis

The differential diagnosis of achalasia includes anatomic obstruction caused by strictures, rings, hiatal hernias, esophageal diverticula, and benign and malignant neoplasms of the esophagus. Functional causes of dysphagia include the primary and secondary motor disorders of the esophagus listed in Table 32–1. Anatomic causes of dysphagia can usually be identified on a video esophagogram or at the time of endoscopy; correct identification of motor disorders of the esophagus requires an esophageal motility study.

Malignancies involving the gastric cardia and the distal esophagus can result in a clinical syndrome termed *pseudoachalsia*, which can be confused with *idiopathic achalasia*. Frequently, the clinical, manometric, and radiologic findings in the two disorders are indistinguishable. These tumors can cause either a functional obstruction or disturbance of LES innervation by submucosal invasion (Kahrilas et al, 1987). In such patients, a computed tomographic (CT) scan may demonstrate a mass at the cardia. Rarely, tumors remote from the LES (bronchogenic carcinoma, gastric adenoma, and pancreatic adenocarcinoma) may be associated with achalasia as a paraneoplastic syndrome similar to Eaton-Lambert syndrome (Sandler et al, 1982).

Chagas' disease is a common cause of secondary achalasia in Central America and South America. It is caused by the parasite *T. cruzi*, which is endemic in these areas. In its chronic phase, the parasite causes destruction of the parasympathetic ganglion cells throughout the body, including the heart and the gastrointestinal, urinary, and respiratory tracts. This destruction leads to cardiomyopathy, cardiac arrhythmias, and dilatation of the gastrointestinal, urinary, and respiratory tracts. The diagnosis is usually suspected on the basis of the history and physical findings in a patient from an endemic area. The diagnosis is confirmed in the acute phase by demonstration of the parasite in the blood and in the chronic phase by serologic studies. Chagas' disease of the esophagus is presented in detail in Chapter 35.

Investigative Techniques

Chest Radiography

Chest radiographic findings are usually normal, particularly in the early stages of achalasia. As the disease progresses, megaesophagus formation may lead to the appearance of a vertical shadow along the length of the mediastinum with an air-fluid level in the posterior mediastinum (Fig. 32–1). Aspiration pneumonitis may be present, and the gastric air bubble is often absent (Orlando et al, 1978).

Upper Gastrointestinal Radiography

The characteristic findings on upper gastrointestinal radiography in patients with achalasia include esophageal dilatation with a tapered narrowing distally, the so-called bird's beak deformity (Fig. 32–2). Additional information can be obtained by the use of contrast video esophagography. This technique allows one to assess esophageal clearance function as well as the degree of LES relaxation. Although the overall accuracy of video esophagography is dependent on the observer's skill, motility disorders can be correctly identified about 75% of the time (Fuller et al, 1999).

Whereas advanced achalasia with a dilated esophageal body and a nonrelaxing LES is easy to recognize, early achalasia may be difficult to differentiate from other motor disorders by upper gastrointestinal radiology alone. Pseudoachalasia may also be difficult to differentiate from idiopathic achalasia by standard radiographic studies. Dodds and associates (1986) proposed the use of amyl nitrite to distinguish between the two by video esophagography. After the administration of amyl nitrite, relaxation typically does not occur in pseudoachalasia caused by tumor infiltration of the LES but does occur in idiopathic achalasia.

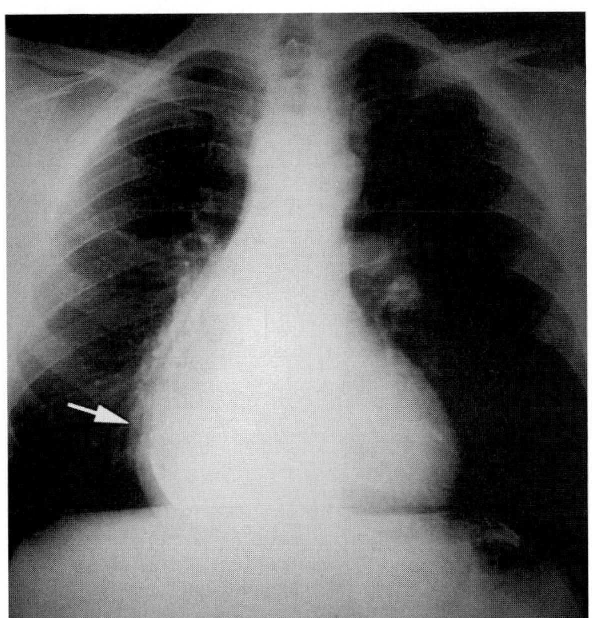

FIGURE 32–1 ■ Typical chest radiographic findings in advanced achalasia. Note the absence of a gastric air bubble with a dilated esophagus containing an air-fluid level.

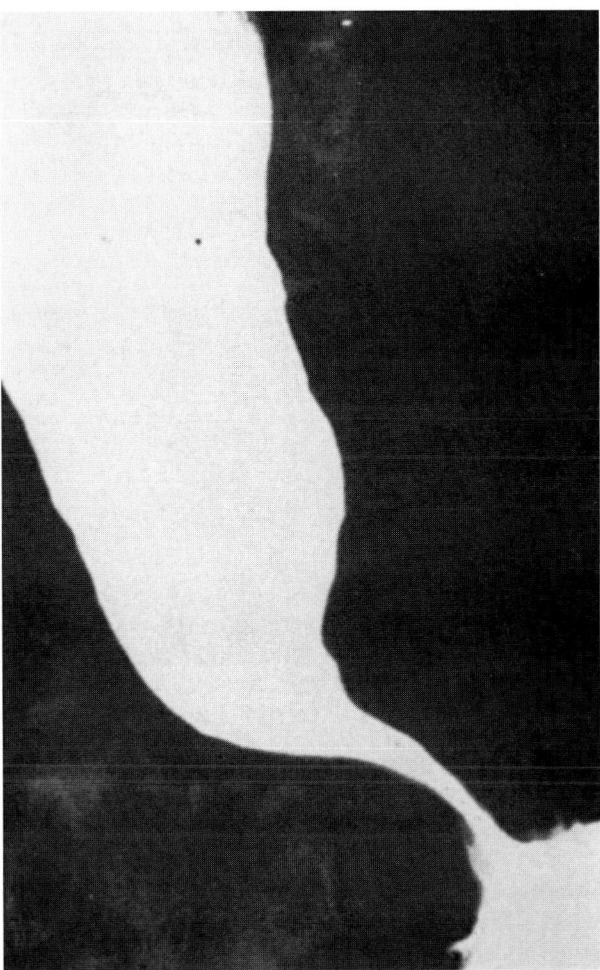

FIGURE 32–2 ■ Upper gastrointestinal radiograph showing the "bird's beak" appearance typical of achalasia. (From Dalton CB, Castell DO: Esophageal motility disorders. In Gelfand DW, Richter JE [eds]: Dysphagia Diagnosis and Treatment. New York, Igaku-Shoin, 1989, p 257.)

Endoscopy

Because a tumor in the region of the gastroesophageal junction can cause symptoms indistinguishable from those of achalasia and upper gastrointestinal radiography may not be conclusive, all patients thought to have achalasia should undergo endoscopy. In the absence of a mass, endoscopic findings are often normal, especially in early achalasia. In more advanced cases, a dilated esophagus with retained food may be seen. Esophagitis with a cobblestone appearance may be caused by stasis and fermentation of the swallowed food.

Some difficulty is often encountered in passing the endoscope through the gastroesophageal junction, but the resistance is not usually severe. When significant difficulty is encountered, pseudoachalasia related to a tumor should be suspected. Although endoscopic biopsies are too superficial to evaluate the myenteric plexus, they are useful in confirming tumor in areas of mucosal abnormalities. Finally, endoscopic ultrasonography has been reported to be useful in helping distinguish achalasia from pseudoachalasia (Deviere et al, 1989).

Manometry

Esophageal manometry is considered the "gold standard" for the diagnosis of achalasia. Characteristic findings in-

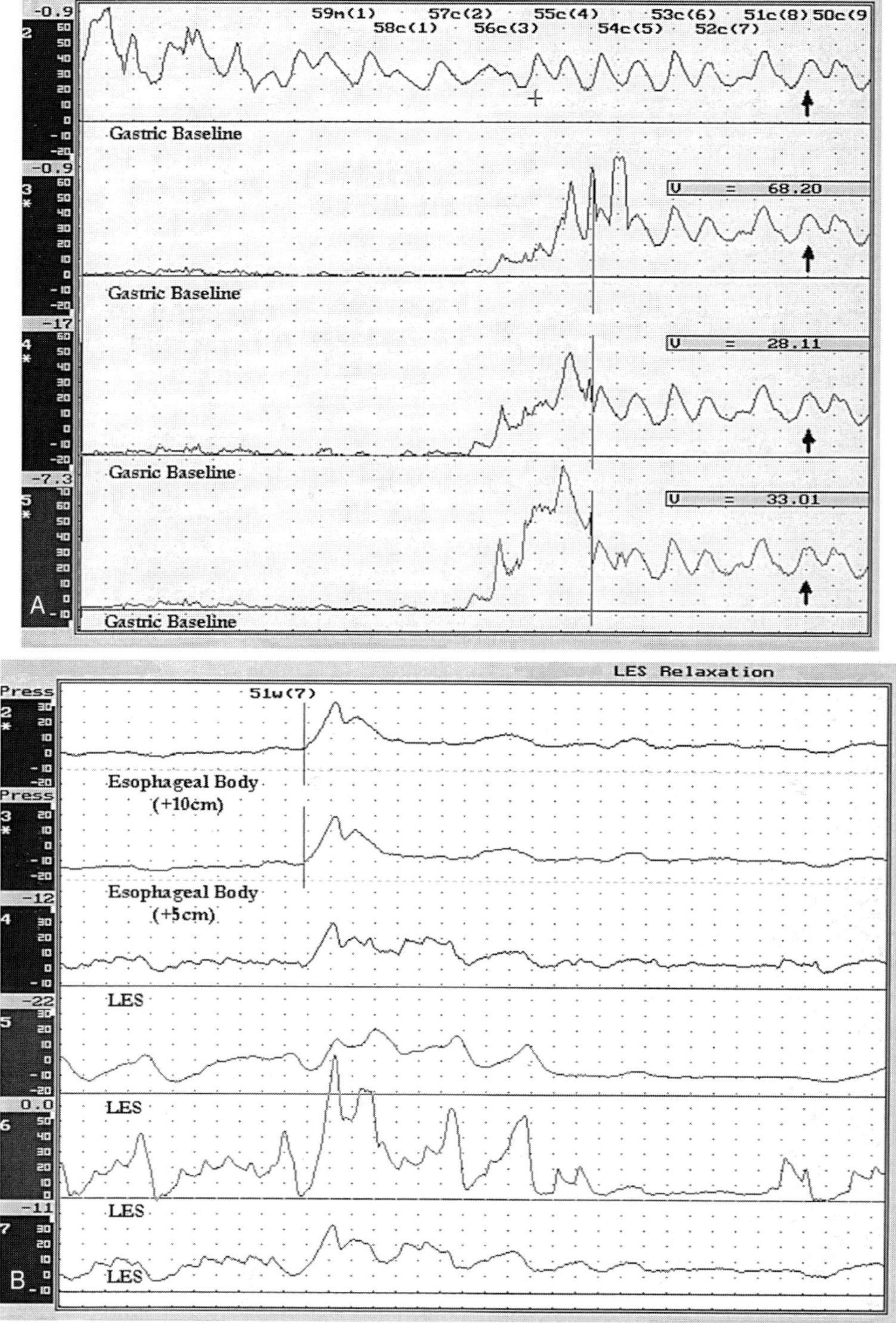

FIGURE 32–3 ■ Manometric features in achalasia. *A*, Motorized pull-through of the lower esophageal sphincter (LES) demonstrating a hypertensive LES and pressurization of the esophagus *(arrow)*. *B*, LES relaxation study using four circumferential transducers showing failure of LES relaxation. Note the simultaneous contractions in the esophageal body 5 and 10 cm above the LES.

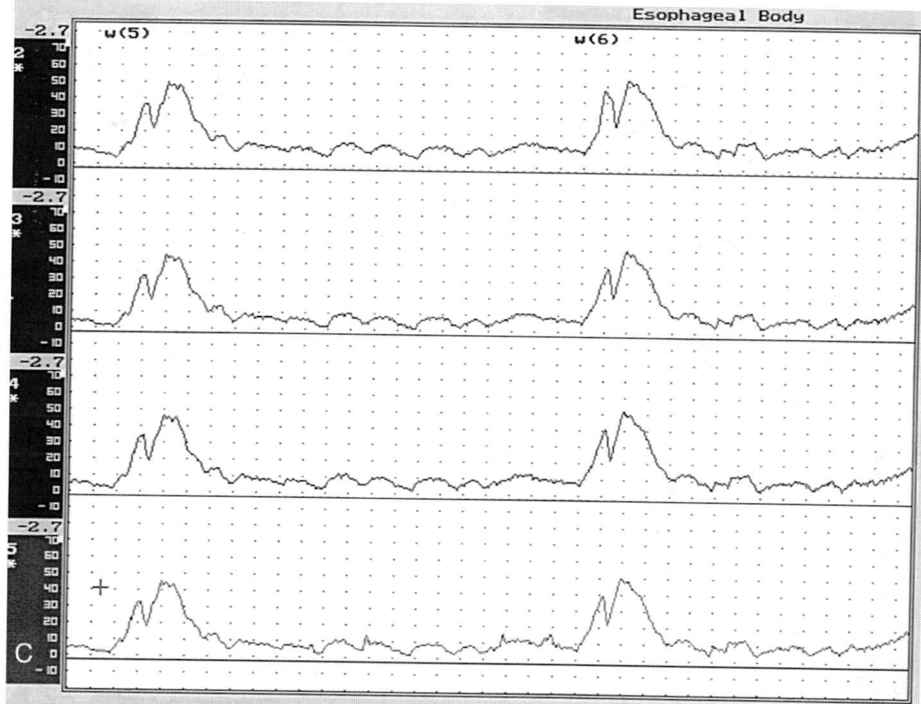

FIGURE 32–3 ■ *Continued.* *C*, Esophageal body study demonstrating absence of peristalsis, with isobaric simultaneous contractions in response to two wet swallows.

clude a high-pressure (>26 mm Hg) LES that relaxes incompletely in response to swallowing. Esophageal body peristalsis is absent, and isobaric simultaneous pressure waves are usually seen (Fig. 32–3). However, not all patients with achalasia have hypertensive sphincters, nor is incomplete relaxation a constant finding (Katz et al, 1986). Although esophageal body peristalsis is generally absent, occasional peristaltic sequences may be seen mixed with the low-amplitude isobaric pressure waves, especially in the early stages. A vigorous form of achalasia has been described (Sanderson et al, 1967), characterized by the typical LES findings of achalasia but with high-amplitude (>50 mm Hg) simultaneous pressure waves in the esophageal body.

Ambulatory manometry may be helpful when it is difficult to differentiate achalasia from other primary motor disorders (Stein and DeMeester, 1993). It may be particularly difficult to distinguish between DES (see later) and vigorous achalasia. Our experience suggests that, in addition to analyzing a much larger number of swallows, one can demonstrate pressurization of the esophagus, defined as elevation of the esophageal baseline above the gastric baseline, in nearly all cases of achalasia, particularly when the meal period is analyzed. Standard and 24-hour ambulatory manometry criteria for the diagnosis of achalasia and other primary motor disorders are shown in Table 32–3.

Radionuclide Studies

Radionuclide studies are of limited value in the diagnosis and management of achalasia. Although they lack sufficient sensitivity to be of use in diagnosis (Holloway et al, 1989; Stacher et al, 1994), these studies may be helpful in assessing clearance, particularly after treatment (Gross et al, 1979).

TREATMENT

The primary goal of therapy in achalasia is relief of outflow obstruction at the LES. All treatments for primary motor disorders, including achalasia, are merely palliative, because restoration of peristaltic function is not usually possible. As stated by DeMeester (1982), “The creation of a defect can never restore the function of an organ to normal.” Current therapeutic options include (1) medical therapy, (2) pneumatic balloon dilatation, (3) botulinum toxin (Botox) injections, and (4) surgical treatment by myotomy or resection.

Medical Therapy

Several classes of drugs, including calcium channel blockers, nitrates, β-agonists, and anticholinergics, have been effective in decreasing LES resting pressure. Each of these has been used in the treatment of achalasia.

Although calcium channel blockers clearly reduce LES resting pressure in patients with achalasia, compared with that in control subjects (Bortolotti and Labo, 1981; Traube et al, 1984), clinical improvement in patients is often limited (Short and Thomas, 1992; Triadafilopoulos et al, 1991).

Nitrates have also been shown to reduce LES pressure. Gelfond and colleagues (1981) showed that the long-acting nitrate isosorbide dinitrate improved symptoms in 19 of 23 patients with achalasia, although side effects (principally headache) frequently limited the usefulness of this drug.

The use of β-agonists also lowers LES pressures acutely (DiMarino and Cohen, 1982), but long-term clinical studies are not available. Anticholinergics have also been effective, but side effects are often severe.

As a result of the troublesome side effects demon-

TABLE 32–3 ■ **Standard and Ambulatory Motility Criteria for the Diagnosis of Primary Motor Disorders**

Disorder	*Video Esophagogram Findings*	*Stationary Manometry*	*Ambulatory Manometry*
Achalasia	Absence of peristalsis in the body of the esophagus, failure of LES to relax, occasionally dilated body with bird's beak deformity	LES: nonrelaxing Body: complete absence of peristalsis, elevation of intraluminal baseline pressure	Body: complete absence of peristalsis
Diffuse esophageal spasm	Often demonstrates simultaneous or discoordinated contractions, segmentation, or corkscrew deformity of the esophagus	LES: relaxation often inadequate or of short duration Body: must have >20% simultaneous contractions in the distal three fifths or more of the esophagus; intermittently, normal peristalsis must be present; may also have triple-peaked, prolonged duration, or high-amplitude contractions	Body: >20% simultaneous contractions with meals, >55% absence of simultaneous contractions when upright, intermittent normal peristalsis; intermittent "spastic" contractions that were multipeaked or of high amplitude
Nutcracker esophagus	Often normal or nonspecific	LES: normal Body: mean amplitude of contraction in the lower esophagus >180 mm Hg; however, normal peristaltic progression is always present	Body: mean contraction amplitude >105 mm Hg
Nonspecific esophageal motor disorder	Nonpropulsive or interrupted waves with a mild delay in transit	LES: normal or hypotensive Body: one or more abnormalities including >20% interrupted or dropped contractions, >20% multipeaked contractions, or contractions that are of prolonged duration (mean >6 sec), or low amplitude (mean <30 mm Hg)	Body: >20% multipeaked contractions, or >20% isolated contractions, or mean amplitude of contractions in the distal esophagus <25 mm Hg

LES, lower esophageal sphincter.

strated, pharmacotherapy in the management of achalasia is presently limited to use in high-risk elderly patients and patients who refuse other forms of therapy.

Pneumatic Dilatation

Forceful dilatation of the esophagus has been used to manage patients with achalasia since Thomas Willis dilated the LES with whalebone in 1679. Today, pneumatic dilatation has replaced rigid or semirigid dilatation in the treatment of achalasia. These balloon dilators are inflated in the gastroesophageal junction and forcibly rupture the LES. After dilatation, most patients are evaluated for mucosal tears or perforation with diatrizoate meglumine–diatrizoate sodium (Gastrografin) swallows and are observed for clinical signs of perforation (persistent pain, fever).

Ferguson (1991) reviewed the results of balloon dilatation in achalasia, summarizing 12 series involving a total of 1049 patients. Good to excellent results were achieved in 70% of patients after balloon dilatation, and 16.6% of the patients required repeated dilatations. Perforations occurred in 1.4%, and the overall mortality rate was 0.3%. In addition to perforation, other complications encountered include intramural hematomas and diverticula at the gastric cardia (Eckardt et al, 1997a). Reflux appears to be a common problem after pneumatic dilatation, occurring in as many as 22% of patients.

Modifications in technique, as described by Katz (1998) and Wehrmann (1995) and their associates, appear to have improved the success rate of balloon dilatation to about 85%; reflux may be less common as well. Whether these results can be generalized beyond the carefully controlled studies reported by these two groups remains to be seen.

At present, balloon dilatation remains the most common initial treatment for patients with achalasia, although it seems to be most valuable in older patients (Eckardt et al, 1992; Vantrappen and Janssens, 1983). Although myotomy has been reported to be more difficult after balloon dilatation, two long-term studies have shown that previous dilatation does not adversely affect the results of myotomy regardless of the number of previous dilatations (Ferguson et al, 1996; Little et al, 1988).

Botulinum Toxin Injection

Endoscopic injection of botulinum toxin (Botox, 80 to 100 U) in the LES has been proposed as a safe alternative to dilatation and myotomy. Examinations of series involving botulinum injections have shown initial injections to be effective in about 65%. The results, however, are usually temporary, and most patients require a second injection within 1 year (Annese et al, 1996; Cuilliere et al, 1997). Mild to moderate postprocedure pain is the only common side effect, although Eaker and associates (1997) reported a case of esophageal ulceration and hemorrhage secondary to reflux at the time of subsequent myotomy. The long-term efficacy, safety, and cost-effectiveness of repeated botulinum toxin injections need further review, but the temporary nature of the benefit is likely to limit the applicability of the procedure.

Questions have also been raised about the effects of botulinum toxin injection on the outcome of subsequent myotomy. Horgan and associates (1999) evaluated the safety of esophagomyotomy in this setting. They demonstrated an increased perforation rate and concluded that dissection in the submucosal plane was significantly more difficult.

Surgical Therapy

Choice of Operation

Although the initial treatment of choice is debated, *esophagocardiomyotomy* is considered the definitive treatment for achalasia. The goal of surgical myotomy is to relieve the functional outflow obstruction of the LES without destroying the normal mechanisms responsible for the prevention of gastroesophageal reflux. By whatever approach is used, surgical myotomy should involve limited division of the muscle in a controlled fashion, in contrast to the uncontrolled destruction of the cardia region accomplished by balloon dilatation. Since Heller performed the first myotomy via a laparotomy in 1913, several modifications in technique have been described. At present, controversy regarding the surgical approach to achalasia centers around the ideal operative approach, the extent of the myotomy, and the need for the addition of an antireflux procedure.

The operation most commonly performed for achalasia in the past several decades has been the *transthoracic modified Heller myotomy* with a partial antireflux operation. This approach allows a generous myotomy to eliminate residual outflow obstruction while avoiding the complications of reflux associated with complete disruption of the gastroesophageal junction. Some claim, however, that this additional dissection of the cardia is not necessary for adequate relief of outflow obstruction (Ellis et al, 1984; Okike et al, 1979; Pai et al, 1984). These authors emphasized that if limited dissection of the cardia is carried out, an antireflux procedure is not required. They suggest that the addition of resistance to emptying imparted by the fundoplication would lead to progressive dilatation of the esophagus and, ultimately, esophageal failure.

Proponents of the myotomy and antireflux procedure (Donahue et al, 1986; Little et al, 1988; Malthaner et al, 1994) believed that extending the myotomy precisely 5 mm onto the cardia would be difficult. An error in either direction would lead to dysphagia because of incomplete myotomy or to reflux because of an overly generous myotomy. To avoid these complications, these authors recommended a complete LES myotomy and the addition of an antireflux procedure. Although many antireflux procedures (e.g., Belsey, Dor, Toupet) have been used in conjunction with a Heller myotomy, a true Nissen fundoplication has been shown to produce dysphagia in most patients with poor esophageal motility or a myotomized esophagus and should not be used (Topart et al, 1992).

Thoracoscopic myotomy techniques have been described that allow performance of a limited esophageal myotomy, similar to that advocated by Ellis, with minimal invasiveness. Early reports of series of thoracoscopic myotomies (Maher, 1997; Pellegrini et al, 1993) show results comparable to those obtained by the open technique but with shorter hospital stays (mean, 3 days) and less postoperative pain.

Interest in the transabdominal approach has been rekindled by the proliferation of laparoscopic esophageal procedures. By definition, the abdominal approach requires full mobilization of the hiatal region in order to expose the distal esophagus and perform an adequate myotomy. As a result, an antireflux operation is always performed in combination with a *transabdominal myotomy* (Bonavina et al, 1992; Csendes et al, 1989). The advantages of a laparoscopic operation, in terms of reduced pain and shortened hospital stay, are well recognized. As with the thoracoscopic myotomy, results of the laparoscopic myotomy and partial antireflux operation have been comparable to those with the traditional techniques but with shorter hospital stays (mean, 3 days) and less postoperative pain (Graham et al, 1997; Hunter et al, 1997). Although long-term studies with detailed follow-up assessment of esophageal clearance and objective assessment of reflux are needed, the diminished pain, decreased morbidity, and shorter hospital stays associated with *minimally invasive myotomy* have resulted in this procedure becoming the preferred operative approach today in most centers around the world.

Operative Technique

The technical details of the standard transthoracic myotomy with partial antireflux procedure are described here. The minimally invasive techniques of esophageal myotomy are described elsewhere.

The operation is performed through the left chest, with the surgeon utilizing a standard thoracotomy incision. The operation begins with deflation of the left lung and division of the inferior pulmonary ligament. The left lung is then retracted superiorly. The mediastinal pleura is divided, and the lateral wall of the esophagus is exposed. The phrenoesophageal membrane is divided circumferentially, and the abdomen is entered. A nasogastric tube should be used to decompress the stomach. The fundus is then brought into the chest, and several pairs of short gastric vessels are divided to enhance mobility. The fat pad is then excised from the gastroesophageal junction.

A myotomy is performed through all muscle layers, beginning on the esophageal body. When completed, the myotomy should extend distally onto the stomach 1 to 2 cm below the gastroesophageal junction. The myotomy should extend proximally 6 to 8 cm or to approximately the level of the inferior pulmonary vein (Fig. 32–4).

To prevent rehealing of the myotomy, the surgeon separates the muscle layers from the mucosa laterally for a distance of 1 cm along the length of the myotomy (Fig. 32–5). The surgeon then reconstructs the cardia using a modified Belsey fundoplication (Fig. 32–6). Alternatively, a modified Dor partial fundoplication can be performed, as described later for the treatment of diffuse esophageal spasm (DES) (Fig. 32–7). If extensive dissection of the cardia is required, usually in the setting of a hiatal hernia, a modified Belsey antireflux repair must be done (Eypasch et al, 1992).

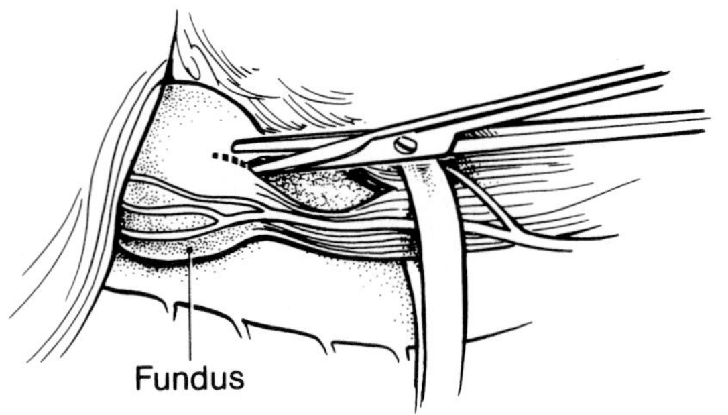

FIGURE 32–4 ■ With straight Mayo scissors, a myotomy of the circular muscle fibers is performed and carried onto the stomach for approximately 2 cm.

If an epiphrenic diverticulum is present, it should be excised before the myotomy. The neck should be carefully dissected free and stapled in the longitudinal direction. The esophageal muscles are then closed over the staple line, the esophagus is rotated 90 to 180 degrees, and a myotomy is carried out as just described.

Late Results

Even though both a randomized, prospective study by Csendes and coworkers (1989) and retrospective studies by Okike (1979) and Donahue (1986) and their associates have demonstrated superior long-term results of myotomy compared with dilatation, many gastroenterologists still argue that the low cost, short recovery time, efficacy, and safety of pneumatic dilatation are reasons to consider it as first-line therapy for achalasia. They recommend that the initial procedure of choice (and perhaps the second) in achalasia should be pneumatic dilatation and that definitive surgical therapy should be reserved for cases in which this treatment is not successful. Considering the lower success rates with balloon dilatation and the substantially diminished morbidity and mortality associated with minimally invasive operations for achalasia, the argument for dilatation before a laparoscopic myotomy is becoming more difficult for gastroenterologists to support (Spiess and Kahrilas, 1998).

The late results of myotomy in patients with achalasia follow the predictions of Barrett (1964), who wrote

> As the esophagus of a patient who has achalasia cannot be restored to physiological normality, it is probable that the late results of this disease are less satisfactory than early postoperative assessments suggest.

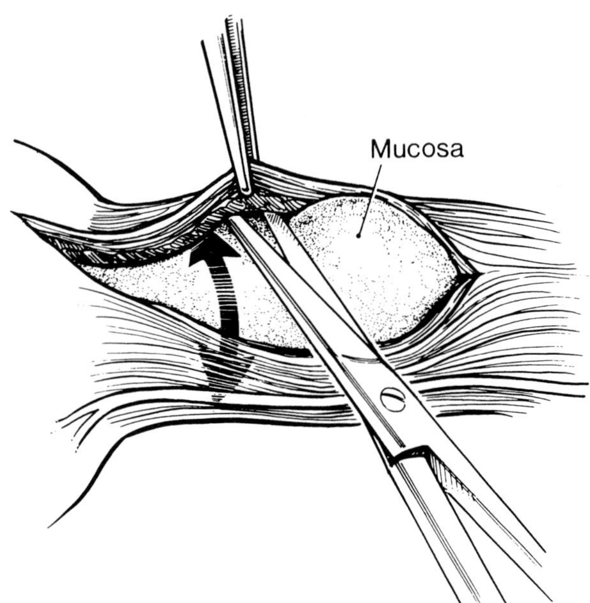

FIGURE 32–5 ■ With straight Mayo scissors, a circumferential dissection is performed in both directions of circular muscle off the mucosa to allow it to protrude.

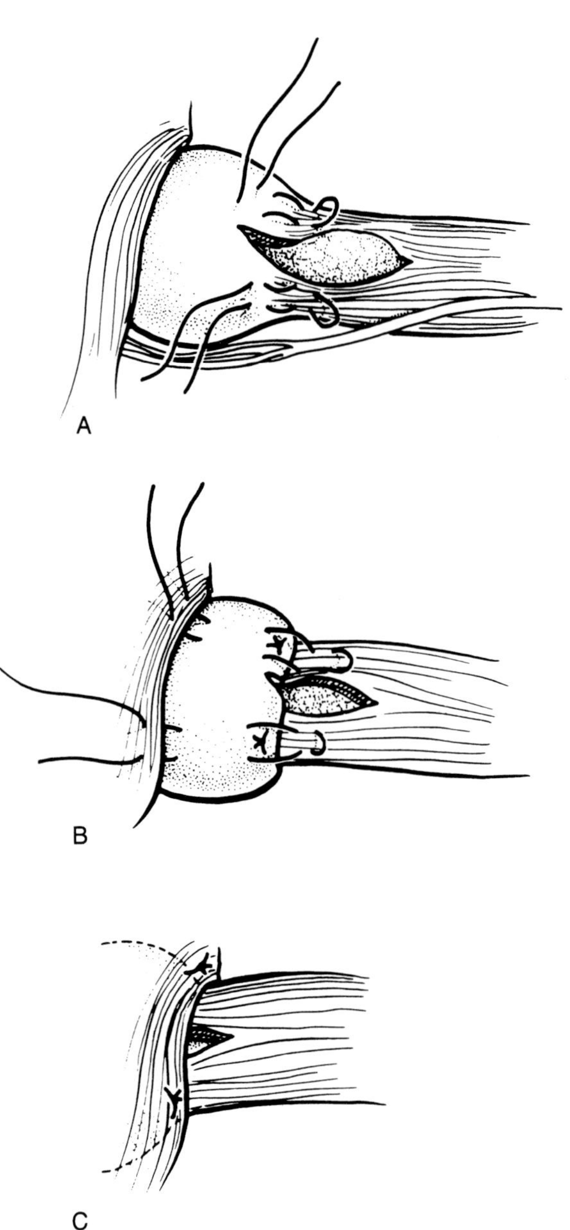

FIGURE 32–6 ■ *A,* The modified Belsey repair is carried out via vertical mattress sutures in the first layer. *B,* A second layer of sutures is placed 1 cm above the first on the esophagus, which secures the wrap to the diaphragm. *C,* The wrap is reduced into the abdomen and the second layer of sutures is secured.

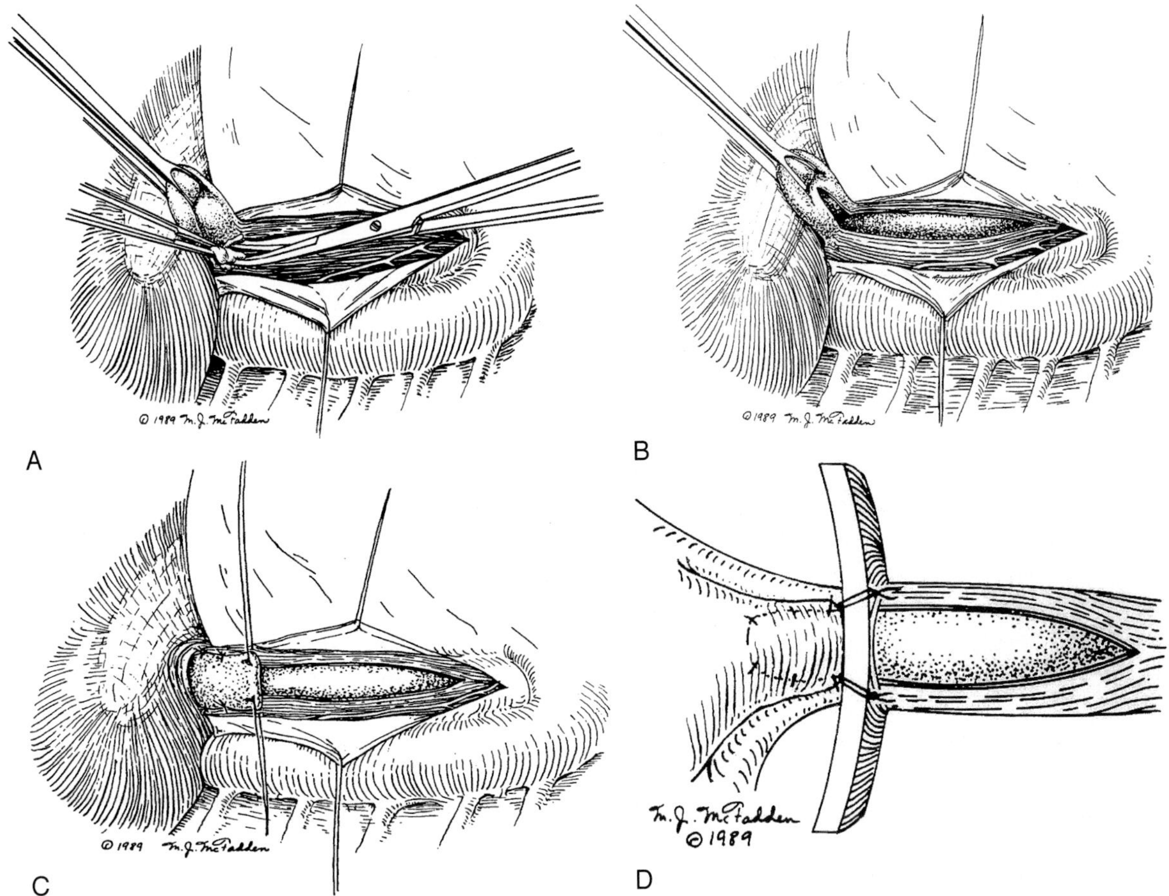

FIGURE 32–7 ■ Technical details of the long esophageal myotomy with modified Dor partial antireflux procedure. *A,* Exposure of the gastroesophageal junction with removal of the fat pad. A tongue of fundus is brought through the limited dissection of the phrenoesophageal membrane. *B,* Completed myotomy extending from below the aortic arch to 1 to 2 cm below the gastroesophageal junction onto the stomach. *C,* Reconstruction of the cardia after a myotomy with the tongue of fundus used to cover the distal 4 cm of the myotomy. *D,* Completed reconstruction of the cardia after a myotomy illustrating the subdiaphragmatic position of the gastric fundic flap. The tails of the tied apical sutures of the flap have been passed through the diaphragm and tied at the margins of the myotomy, 2 cm apart.

Although there are few series in which the long-term results of esophagomyotomy have been analyzed, 10-year follow-up in three series (Di Simone et al, 1996; Ellis, 1992; Malthaner et al, 1994) showed excellent to good results in approximately 66%, with 10% to 15% of patients requiring further surgical therapy. The major late complications of myotomy are:

- Development of gastroesophageal reflux with resulting esophagitis, Barrett's esophagus, and peptic stricture formation
- Late dysphagia
- Carcinoma

Whether these complications are due to failure of the original procedure or simply to progressive disease in the body of the esophagus with dysphagia and poor esophageal clearance is still not clear. Long-term follow-up studies after minimally invasive operations for achalasia are limited. Early reports suggest, however, that the outcome is superior with the laparoscopic approach in terms of relief of dysphagia and protection from reflux (Patti et al, 1999; Stewart et al, 1999).

In addition to myotomy, esophageal resection should be considered a surgical option for achalasia in certain circumstances; however, deciding whether to attempt another myotomy or to proceed with esophagectomy is difficult. Although the precise indicators for resection are difficult to define, a few guiding principles can be provided.

Patients with a dilated and tortuous esophagus generally do not respond well to dilatation or myotomy. The sigmoid nature of the distal esophagus in these patients (Fig. 32–8) prevents gravity clearance, resulting in esophageal stasis even in the presence of an adequate myotomy. When the patient presents late with a dilated tortuous esophagus, primary resection should be considered. Resection should also be considered when multiple prior attempts at myotomy have failed. Common causes of failure in this setting include an incomplete myotomy (usually on the gastric side), increased outflow resistance related to a fundoplication, and a stricture as the result of reflux injury.

Finally, esophagectomy should be considered for patients with significant reflux after myotomy or dilatation.

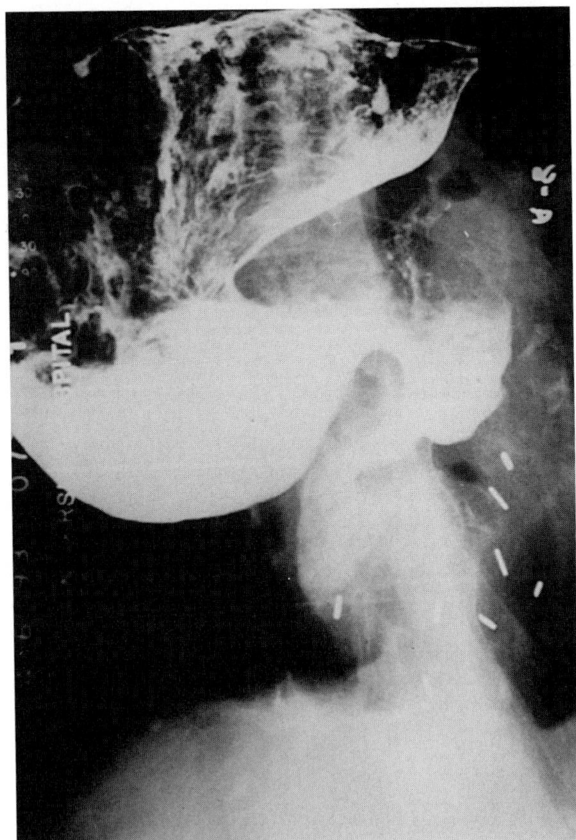

FIGURE 32–8 ■ Video esophagogram showing a massively dilated, tortuous, "sigmoid"-shaped esophagus.

In this setting, poor esophageal clearance makes medical therapy difficult, and an operation to perform an effective antireflux procedure is likely to result in dysphagia (Peters et al, 1995).

When the decision has been made to perform an esophagectomy, the type of resection and the method of reconstruction must be determined. This choice should be made on the basis of (1) the patient's age, (2) a history of previous gastric or colonic surgery, and (3) whether concurrent disease limits the choices available for reconstruction. It has been suggested that the transhiatal esophagectomy may involve an increased risk of mortality and morbidity in the setting of achalasia because of increased risk of hemorrhage. As a result, Miller and coworkers (Miller et al, 1995) have recommended a transthoracic approach, particularly when there is a history of previous myotomy.

A technique of esophageal resection has been described in which the esophagus is removed with a vein stripper (Akiyama et al, 1994). With this technique, the surgeon can remove the entire esophageal wall without entering the chest, or the esophageal stripping can be limited to the mucosal layer. The excellent upper gastrointestinal function associated with vagal nerve preservation makes this an attractive option when esophagectomy is considered for benign diseases such as achalasia. To maximize alimentary function, we prefer to use the colon for reconstruction, whenever possible, in patients with a long life expectancy.

Diffuse Esophageal Spasm

DEFINITION

DES was described by Fleshler (1967) as a

> clinical syndrome characterized by symptoms of substernal distress, dysphagia or both, the radiographic appearance of localized, non-progressive waves (tertiary contractions), and an increased incidence of non-peristaltic contractions recorded by intraluminal manometry.

By definition, patients with DES have ineffective simultaneous contractions in the distal esophagus but normal peristaltic waves intermixed with the abnormal contractions.

HISTORICAL NOTE

The first description of esophageal spasm was by Osgood (1889), who reported on the clinical features of patients with painful dysphagia. Moersch and Camp (1934) first published the radiographic features of this disorder and used the descriptive term "diffuse spasm of the lower part of the esophagus." It was not until 1958 that the manometric features of DES were described (Creamer et al, 1958).

■ *HISTORICAL READINGS*

Creamer B, Donoghue FE, Code CF: Pattern of esophageal motility in diffuse spasm. Gastroenterology 34:782, 1958.

Moersch HJ, Camp JD: Diffuse spasm of the lower part of the esophagus. Ann Otol Rhinol Laryngol 43:1165–1173, 1934.

Osgood H: A peculiar form of oesophagismus. Boston Med Surg J 120:140, 1889.

BASIC SCIENCE

The cause of DES remains unknown. Histopathologic studies of muscle biopsy specimens obtained from a long esophageal myotomy have produced conflicting results. Whereas Cassella and colleagues (1965b) described morphologic changes of the smooth muscle cells and wallerian degenerative changes of vagal nerve fibers, other authors (Eypasch et al, 1992; Friesen et al, 1983) did not show any changes in the muscle or ganglion cells.

Hypersensitivity responses to cholinergic and hormonal stimulation have been demonstrated in patients with DES. An increase in simultaneous contractions with episodes of chest pain has been shown in response to a number of pharmacologic agents, including edrophonium and bethanechol (Mellow, 1977), methacholine (Kramer, 1967), and pentagastrin (Orlando and Bozymski, 1979) in patients with DES compared with control subjects.

A study by Behar and Biancani (1993) suggested that patients with DES had a defective deglutitive inhibitory reflex that accounted for the changes seen on manometry. The investigators showed that the patients had a shorter latency in response to swallows in the distal esophagus, leading to the simultaneous contractions recorded. Administration of anticholinergic medications resulted in lengthening of the latency period, suggesting smooth muscle hypersensitivity to acetylcholine and swallow-independent discharges of acetylcholine as etiologic factors.

Other studies have shown a possible role of the nonadrenergic, noncholinergic inhibitory neurotransmitter nitric oxide. Konturek and associates (1995) demonstrated decreased duration of contractions and improvement in symptoms in five patients given glyceryl trinitrate, a nitric oxide donor. In addition, Murray and colleagues (1995) showed that systemic binding of nitric oxide by recombinant human hemoglobin induced simultaneous waves of increased duration and episodes of pain in normal subjects. Taken together, these studies suggest that DES may be caused by a hypersensitivity to cholinergic stimulation, a defect in nitric oxide neuromuscular communication, or an imbalance between the two.

Enhanced hypersensitivity to other external stimuli has been demonstrated in patients with noncardiac chest pain, including those with DES. Richter and associates (1986a) showed that balloon distention in the distal esophagus of 30 patients with noncardiac chest pain resulted in reproduction of their symptoms in 60%, compared with a 20% incidence of chest pain in the control group. The patients with chest pain also experienced pain with smaller volumes of balloon distention. These results suggest that patients with DES may have a lower visceral pain threshold similar to that reported in patients with irritable bowel syndrome.

Why these episodes of abnormal contractions cause chest pain is not fully understood. From the results of ambulatory motility studies, however, it is clear that most abnormal swallows in these patients do not cause chest pain. It may be that contractions of particularly long duration and excessive amplitude cause microvascular ischemia, resulting in episodes of chest pain (Barham et al, 1997).

DIAGNOSIS

Clinical Features

Patients with DES most commonly present with symptoms of dysphagia with or without chest pain. On the basis of symptoms alone, however, it is difficult to differentiate DES from other esophageal motility disorders with a similar presentation. In a study of 1161 patients referred for evaluation of chest pain or dysphagia, a motility disorder was present in 33% (Katz et al, 1987). Motility disorders were more common (53%) in patients with dysphagia than in those with chest pain (28%). When a motility disorder was diagnosed, DES was present in only 10% of cases. DES can occur at any age but is more common after age 50 years. There are no specific racial or gender predilections.

Chest pain in these patients may be indistinguishable from cardiac angina. Therefore, a cardiac stress test is an important part of the diagnostic evaluation. Chest pain in DES is typically described as retrosternal or epigastric and may radiate to the left arm or neck. Confusing matters further, nitrates may result in symptomatic relief. The presence of dysphagia may help in distinguishing between the two. Dysphagia in DES tends to be intermittent and can occur with both solids and liquids. Food bolus obstruction, however, is rare. Dysphagia may be precipitated by episodes of emotional stress, ingestion of cold liquids, or rapid eating. Hot-water swallows, on the other hand, have been said to decrease the amplitude and duration of contraction waves and to improve symptoms in patients with DES (Triadafilopoulos et al, 1998).

Natural History

The natural history of DES is not fully understood. There have been case reports of progression from nutcracker esophagus to DES (Dalton et al, 1988; Narducci et al, 1985; Traube et al, 1986) and from DES to achalasia (Kramer et al, 1967). The limited studies with long-term follow-up have shown that DES is a dynamic disorder and that only a minority (33%) retain manometric features of DES over time (Achem et al, 1991).

Differential Diagnosis

The differential diagnosis for patients presenting with chest pain and dysphagia involves distinguishing between anatomic and functional causes (see Achalasia earlier). As mentioned, patients with the presenting symptom of chest pain need to be evaluated for the presence of a cardiac cause. When cardiac disease has been eliminated, gastroesophageal reflux disease (GERD) must be considered because it is the most common cause of noncardiac chest pain, as shown by DeMeester and colleagues (1982). They found that as many as 46% of patients with chest pain and a normal coronary angiogram had GERD. The approach to the evaluation of dysphagia is discussed in the preceding section on achalasia.

Investigative Techniques

When anatomic causes of dysphagia have been excluded by endoscopy and upper gastrointestinal radiography, patients with dysphagia or chest pain should undergo *stationary* manometry with 24-hour pH recordings and, possibly, 24-hour *ambulatory* manometry.

Stationary Manometry

Stationary manometry is the primary tool for the diagnosis of esophageal motility disorders. Although there remains debate concerning the precise manometric definition of DES, the most commonly accepted definition includes the presence after wet swallows of more than 20% simultaneous contractions, which must be intermixed with normal peristaltic waves. When all contractions are simultaneous, a diagnosis of achalasia is usually made (see earlier). Other manometric findings that are common but not required for the diagnosis of DES include increased duration of contractions, frequent spontaneous contractions, and occasionally incomplete LES relaxation (Richter and Castell, 1984; Richter et al, 1987b).

Ambulatory Esophageal Monitoring

Twenty-four-hour pH testing is necessary to exclude GERD as a possible cause of chest pain and dysphagia (Peters et al, 1988). Using combined 24-hour motility and pH testing, Peters and colleagues showed that only 12% of chest pain episodes correlated with abnormal motor activity and that 20% of chest pain episodes were associated with acid exposure.

Radiography

Although a video esophagogram may be useful in detecting abnormal motility, its accuracy in differentiating DES from nutcracker esophagus or nonspecific esophageal motility disorders is poor (Fuller et al, 1999). Typical radiographic findings in DES include segmentation of the barium column by tertiary contractions, which has been described as "curling," "rosary beading," "pseudodiverticula," or "corkscrew" changes (Fig. 32–9). Spasm of the esophagus can compartmentalize the esophagus with development of an epiphrenic or midesophageal diverticulum. Escape of barium as a result of ineffective swallows and stasis in the body of the esophagus may also be seen. Occasionally, the diagnosis may be suggested by a CT scan with the appearance of a thickened distal esophageal wall (Nino-Murcia et al, 1997).

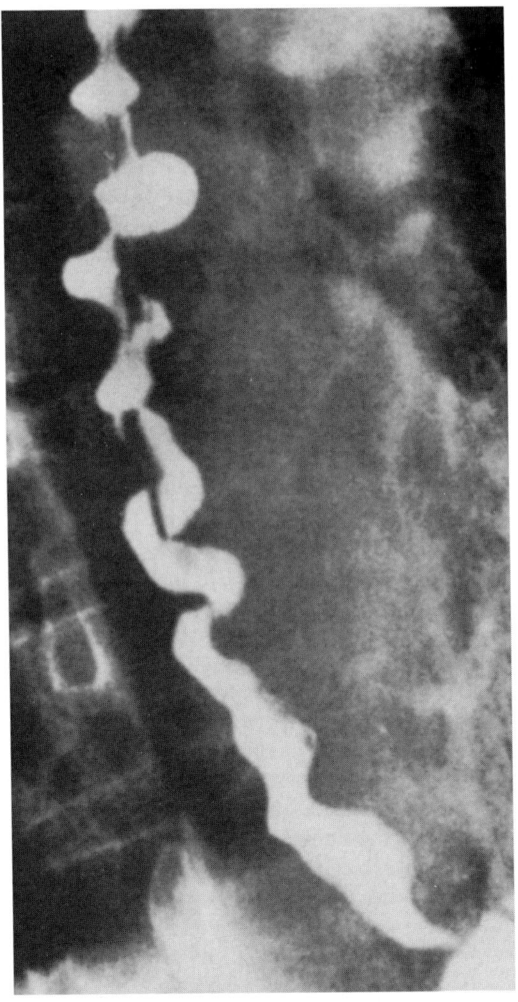

FIGURE 32–9 ■ Barium swallow in a patient with diffuse esophageal spasm. Severe segmentation is present, causing the formation of "pseudodiverticula." (From Gelfand DW: Gastrointestinal Radiology: Performing and Interpreting Fluoroscopic Examinations. New York, Churchill Livingstone, 1984, p 173.)

The availability of *24-hour ambulatory manometry* and computer-assisted analysis allows esophageal motor activity to be evaluated during normal physiologic conditions for a full circadian cycle. By use of manometry over a 24-hour period, Stein and DeMeester (1993) found that the presence of dysphagia most closely correlated with inability of the esophageal body to organize motor activity into peristaltic waves during meals (Fig. 32–10). They showed that ambulatory manometry frequently documented a more severe motor abnormality such as DES in patients thought to have normal esophageal function, NSEMD, or nutcracker esophagus on the basis of standard manometry. This discrepancy may be due to the fact that esophageal motor abnormalities are intermittent in nature and may be missed with standard manometry. Conversely, ambulatory manometry showed normal or only mildly disordered circadian motor function in patients thought to have NSEMD or nutcracker esophagus on the basis of standard manometry, suggesting that the nonphysiologic conditions of standard manometry may have acted as a trigger in patients known to have a low anxiety threshold.

The standard and 24-hour manometric criteria for diagnosis of DES and other primary motor disorders are shown in Table 32–3.

TREATMENT

Symptoms of patients with DES are often improved after the esophagus is identified as the cause of the symptoms and after reassurance and supportive intervention are provided (Richter et al, 1987b; Ward et al, 1987). Along with reassurance, medical therapy is usually instituted.

Medical Therapy

Medical therapy for DES includes (1) pharmacologic intervention, (2) dilatation, and (3) botulinum toxin injections.

Pharmacologic Therapy

The commonly used drugs used to manage DES include nitrates, calcium channel blockers, sedatives, and anticholinergics. The relative efficacy of these medications is difficult to interpret, however, because of the small number of subjects in each study and the lack of randomized, placebo-controlled investigations.

Anticholinergic medications such as pirenzepine and propantheline bromide have been shown to decrease contraction amplitude and duration in DES. Side effects associated with this class of drugs, however, limit their use. Nitrates were first used in DES by Shlemmel and coworkers (1949), who demonstrated a decrease in radiologic abnormalities and reduced chest pain. Nitrates have also been shown to correct the manometric abnormalities in DES, with reduction of contraction amplitude and duration (Orlando and Bozymski, 1973). Isosorbide dinitrate (Isordil) is the most commonly used nitrate.

Calcium channel blockers, such as nifedipine, also

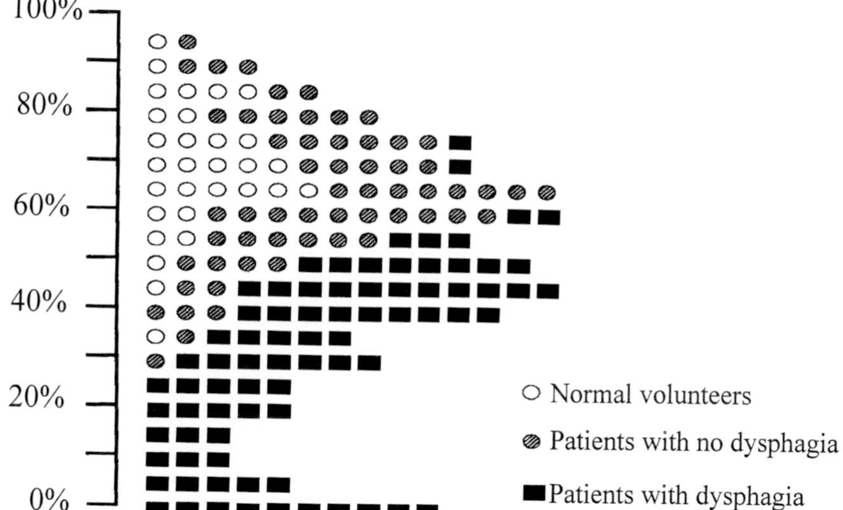

FIGURE 32–10 ■ Prevalence of effective contractions (peristaltic contractions with amplitude > 30 mm Hg) determined with 24-hour ambulatory manometry in normal volunteers and in patients with and without nonobstructive dysphagia. As the prevalence contraction fell below 50%, there was a high likelihood of having dysphagia.

decrease contraction amplitude and duration in the distal esophagus as well as LES resting tone in a dose-related fashion (Hongo et al, 1984; Richter et al, 1985). In a placebo-controlled trial, however, patients with DES who received nifedipine experienced a significant decrease in distal esophageal contraction amplitude and duration but no change in chest pain frequency or severity (Richter et al, 1987a). Nevertheless, calcium channel blockers are the most popular agents used today for DES.

The high incidence of psychiatric disturbances (affective and anxiety disorders) identified in the DES population has led to the use of psychoactive medications. Trazodone, a nontricyclic antidepressant, was shown by Clouse and associates (1987) in a placebo-controlled trial to decrease symptom scores without altering manometric results in patients with noncardiac chest pain.

Finally, it is important to remember that as many as 46% of patients with noncardiac chest pain have coexisting GERD (DeMeester et al, 1982), emphasizing the need for pH testing in these patients. The medications used to treat DES lower the LES resting pressure, resulting in increased reflux.

Dilatation

Pneumatic dilatation, a popular treatment for achalasia, has also been suggested as a possible treatment for DES. Dilatation has been helpful in the setting of DES with impaired LES function; Ebert and associates (1983) observed clinical improvement of dysphagia and regurgitation in 89% of cases. Dilatation of the esophageal body was tried by Irving and coworkers (1992), who reported a 70% success rate with one esophageal perforation.

Botulinum Toxin

Botulinum toxin has also been applied in DES as an endoscopic treatment modality. Although a response was seen in 11 of 15 patients, the results were short-lived (Miller et al, 1996).

Surgical Therapy

Surgical therapy is generally reserved for patients with recurrent, incapacitating episodes of dysphagia with or without chest pain who do not respond to medical treatment. A long esophageal myotomy in these patients abolishes (1) all contractile activity, eliminating the functional obstruction resulting from simultaneous contractions and decreased muscle compliance, and (2) any remaining propulsive contractions. Therefore, for a long esophageal myotomy to be of benefit, the degree of functional obstruction causing dysphagia must outweigh the existing propulsive activity in the esophagus.

Ambulatory manometry has been proposed as a means of identifying candidates for myotomy (Eypasch et al, 1992). These authors found that when the percentage of effective contractions fell below 50% during meals, dysphagia was common. When the percentage of effective contractions fell below 30%, surgery was beneficial.

The important technical aspects of a long esophageal myotomy include:

- Determination of the proximal and distal extent of the myotomy
- Need for an antireflux procedure
- The ideal operative approach

Esophageal manometry is a useful guide to the extent of myotomy required. The proximal extent of the myotomy should be high enough to encompass the entire length of disordered motility. Henderson and associates (1987) recommended extending the myotomy to the level of the thoracic inlet in all patients on the basis of the observation that smooth muscle can account for up to 30% of the upper thoracic esophagus. Most authors recommend the addition of an antireflux procedure when the myotomy is carried through the LES. However, there is no uniform agreement about the need to carry the myotomy onto the stomach.

The arguments regarding the distal extent of the myotomy in DES are similar to those raised in the context of achalasia. We prefer a left posterolateral thoracotomy approach in most cases. This allows easy access to the gastroesophageal junction for a complete myotomy and the addition of an antireflux procedure. We like to perform a modified Dor fundoplication (see Fig. 32–7). After completion of the myotomy, we perform the fundoplication by suturing a tongue of gastric fundus to the margins of the myotomy for a distance of 4 cm. This helps to prevent rehealing of the myotomy site and provides reflux protection. The flap of gastric fundus is allowed to retract into the abdomen and is secured in place by passing the tails of the tied apical sutures of the fundoplication through the diaphragm. Minimally invasive techniques of esophageal myotomy are described in a subsequent chapter.

LATE RESULTS

The results of long esophageal myotomy in the patient with DES have been variable. Henderson and associates (1987) reported good results in 88% of cases with a myotomy to the level of the thoracic inlet combined with a short Nissen fundoplication. A myotomy to the level of the aortic arch combined with a Dor partial fundoplication has been reported to be successful in 80% (Eypasch et al, 1992). In a retrospective review comparing medical therapy with thoracoscopic long myotomy, Patti and associates (1995) reported success in only 26% in the medical group compared with good to excellent results in 80% after surgery.

Nutcracker Esophagus

DEFINITION

The term *nutcracker esophagus* describes a syndrome characterized by high-amplitude peristaltic contractions in the distal esophagus. Patients typically present with symptoms of chest pain, which may be associated with dysphagia. For a condition to be classified as nutcracker esophagus, the average amplitude of contractions in the distal two channels must be more than 2 standard deviations above normal for the laboratory performing the motility study (>180 mm Hg).

Historical Note

Brand and associates first recognized high-amplitude peristaltic contractions as a potential cause of chest pain in 1977. Benjamin and colleagues (1979) proposed the term nutcracker esophagus in a report of patients presenting with noncardiac chest pain and peristaltic contractions with amplitudes exceeding 400 mm Hg. Other investigators have suggested terms such as *hypertensive peristalsis* or *supersqueezer esophagus*, but nutcracker esophagus has become the most widely used term to describe this syndrome.

■ *HISTORICAL READING*

Brand DL, Martin D, Pope CE: Esophageal manometrics in patients with angina-like chest pain. Am J Dig Dis 22:300–304, 1977.

BASIC SCIENCE

The etiologic mechanism of nutcracker esophagus is unknown. It is probably a part of a spectrum of esophageal motor abnormalities that includes DES and achalasia. As in DES, psychological factors may play in important role in nutcracker esophagus. On formal testing, Richter and associates (1986b) found similar psychological profiles and considerable symptom overlap between patients with irritable bowel syndrome and those with nutcracker esophagus. Both groups had high scores on scales measuring somatization, anxiety, and depression. Like patients with DES, patients with nutcracker esophagus have also had lower pain thresholds on balloon distention of the esophagus (Richter et al, 1986a).

DIAGNOSIS

Clinical Features

The most common symptom in patients with nutcracker esophagus is chest pain, present in 90%. In patients who present with noncardiac chest pain, 48% will fulfill the manometric criteria for nutcracker esophagus, making it the most common manometric abnormality in these patients (Richter et al, 1987a). Unlike patients with DES, however, these patients seldom have dysphagia. Fewer than 10% of patients referred for evaluation of dysphagia have a diagnosis of nutcracker esophagus. Although a not common occurrence, food bolus obstruction has been reported (Breumelhof et al, 1990). Other gastrointestinal symptoms (e.g., abdominal pain, flatus, constipation) may be present.

Natural History

The natural history of nutcracker esophagus is also unknown. Case reports have described progression from nutcracker esophagus to achalasia (Paterson et al, 1991) as well as from nutcracker esophagus to DES (Narducci et al, 1985). In a follow-up study by Dalton and coworkers (1988), only 9 of 17 patients with an initial diagnosis of nutcracker esophagus retained the diagnosis at follow-up manometry. Some reverted to normal, others showed findings consistent with NSEMD (see later), and the rest progressed to DES.

Differential Diagnosis

The differential diagnosis of nutcracker esophagus is similar to that of DES. The presence of chest pain, which can be indistinguishable from anginal pain, mandates a full cardiac evaluation. For the infrequent patient who presents with dysphagia, nutcracker esophagus must be differentiated from other motility disorders and mechanical causes of obstruction.

Investigative Techniques

Radiographic (Ott et al, 1986) and endoscopic examinations of patients with nutcracker esophagus are usually normal. Endoscopic ultrasonography may reveal thickening in the muscularis propria in up to 30% (Melzer et al, 1997). The diagnosis of nutcracker esophagus is made on the basis of manometry when contraction amplitudes exceed 2 standard deviations above the mean (>180 mm

Hg) in the distal esophagus. By definition, the contractions must be peristaltic. In difficult cases, ambulatory 24-hour manometry may be useful in differentiating nutcracker esophagus from other primary motility disorders (see Table 32–3).

TREATMENT

Medical Therapy

As with DES, medical therapy for patients with nutcracker esophagus most commonly includes calcium channel blockers such as diltiazem or nifedipine. Diltiazem is the only medication to date that has been shown in a placebo-controlled trial to decrease the distal esophageal contraction amplitudes and to improve symptom scores in nutcracker esophagus (Cattau et al, 1991). A similar study with nifedipine showed no significant difference compared with placebo (Richter et al, 1987a). Trazodone (Clouse et al, 1987) and imipramine (Cannon et al, 1994) have also been reported to decrease chest pain in small, uncontrolled studies.

Bougienage and pneumatic dilatation of the LES have also been used in this disorder. Winters and coworkers (1984) performed a prospective, double-blind study comparing the effectiveness of a "placebo" 24 French dilatation with that of a "therapeutic" 54 French bougie. They found that both groups had lower chest pain scores after dilatation, with no significant difference between the two groups. These studies point out the significant psychological role in the disorder and the beneficial effect that reassurance concerning an esophageal cause of the chest pain coupled with supportive follow-up has on symptoms.

Surgical Therapy

There are a few reports of the results of esophageal myotomy for nutcracker esophagus in patients refractory to medical therapy (Horton and Goff, 1986; Traube et al, 1987b). We advise caution in considering a myotomy for patients with chest pain alone, because all peristaltic contractions are abolished. It has been our experience that chest pain is not reliably alleviated in these patients, and the surgeon runs the risk of adding dysphagia to the patients' symptoms.

Nonspecific Esophageal Motility Disorders

Nonspecific esophageal motility disorders is a term used to describe a group of manometric abnormalities that, although clearly abnormal, do not fit into the definitions of named motor disorders. The common defining criteria include the presence of low-amplitude (<30 mm Hg) peristaltic contractions, nontransmitted contractions (>20% of wet swallows), spontaneous contractions, or contractions of prolonged duration (>6 seconds). In addition, isolated incomplete LES relaxation, retrograde esophageal contractions, or triple-peaked contractions may be seen. These manometric abnormalities are frequently seen in patients with chest pain, dysphagia, and gastroesophageal reflux.

When Katz and associates (1987) studied patients who presented with chest pain and dysphagia, they found that 36% of those with chest pain and 39% of those with dysphagia met manometric criteria of NSEMD. A detailed review of 61 patients classified as having NSEMD by Leite and associates (1997) showed that 98% had more than 30% ineffective contractions, which led them to propose renaming this category of manometric abnormalities as "ineffective esophageal motility" (IEM). They also found increased esophageal acid exposure, particularly in the supine position, confirming the relationship between IEM and GERD. It is still unclear, however, whether GERD leads to the development of the nonspecific motility changes seen or whether increased acid exposure is secondary to poor esophageal clearance. It is also not known whether the manometric findings revert to normal after successful medical or surgical treatment of GERD.

COMMENTS AND CONTROVERSIES

The authors provide a comprehensive but clear and concise summary of pertinent information in this chapter. Several features warrant comment:

The cause of these primary motor disorders remains obscure. Studies, however, strongly support the proposal that achalasia is an autoimmune condition. Although this observation might influence prevention or incidence in the future, it is important to realize that manifest achalasia is an incurable and inevitably progressive disease. All treatment is palliative, and long-term follow-up is critically important for the evaluation of new modalities of management.

The authors appropriately emphasize the transient benefit of botulinum toxin injection (rarely beyond 6 to 12 months in duration) in the management of achalasia. It is clearly overused by some gastroenterologists and should probably be restricted to interim management in special circumstances or to very elderly and infirm patients.

Without doubt, the most significant development since the publication of the first edition of this textbook in 1995 is the favorable and rapidly increasing experience with minimal access, video-assisted laparoscopic myotomy. There is now enough experience with this operation to state that it can be done with no more morbidity than pneumatic bag dilatation and yields a much higher percentage of good to excellent results. It is gradually and appropriately replacing pneumatic bag dilatation as the definitive, primary intervention for most patients with achalasia. As with open myotomy, the early results are good in more than 95% of patients. There is no reason to assume that these good early results will deteriorate more frequently or rapidly than the reported long-term results after open operation.

Finally, the authors highlight the still unpredictable and frequently unsatisfactory results of surgical myotomy in patients with the relatively rare conditions of diffuse spasm and nutcracker esophagus.

F. G. P.

■ KEY REFERENCES

Csendes A, Braghetto I, Henriquez A: Late results of a prospective randomized study comparing forceful dilation and oesophagomyotomy in patients with achalasia. Gut 30:299–304, 1989.

This article discusses the only prospective randomized study comparing pneumatic dilatation and surgical esophagomyotomy. The study involved 81 patients. The surgical arm of the study had significantly better late results than were obtained with dilatation.

Eypasch EP, DeMeester TR, Klingman RR, et al: Physiologic assessment and surgical management of diffuse esophageal spasm. J Thorac Cardiovasc Surg 104:859–869, 1992.

This article reviews the physiologic abnormalities in and the management of DES. It also evaluates the symptomatic and functional results of surgical therapy.

Feldman M: Esophageal achalasia syndromes. Am J Med Sci 295:60–81, 1988.

This is a comprehensive review of the pathophysiology, epidemiology, and clinical presentation of achalasia. It further discusses the different achalasia syndromes and reviews current management. It includes a comprehensive list of references that cover all aspects of achalasia.

Ferguson MK: Achalasia: Current evaluation and therapy. Ann Thorac Surg 52:336, 1991.

This article is a review of the presentation and management of achalasia. The relative efficacy and risks of pneumatic dilatation and esophagomyotomy are described. It includes a good discussion of the controversies regarding the optimal surgical technique (operative approach, proximal extent of the myotomy, need for an antireflux procedure).

Stein HJ, DeMeester TR: Indications, technique, and clinical use of ambulatory 24-hour esophageal motility monitoring in a surgical practice. Ann Surg 217:128, 1993.

This article presents ambulatory manometry values of 25 normal patients. It also compares ambulatory manometry with stationary manometry in the evaluation of patients with functional foregut disorders.

■ REFERENCES

Achem SR, Kolts BE, MacMath T, et al: Esophageal motor disorders: Patterns and understanding in a state of flux. Gastroenterology 100:A24, 1991.

Aggestrup S, Uddmman R, Sundler F, et al: Lack of vasoactive intestinal polypeptide nerves in esophageal achalasia. Gastroenterology 84:924–927, 1983.

Akiyama H, Tsurumaru M, Ono Y, et al: Esophagectomy without thoracotomy with vagal preservation. J Am Coll Surg 178:83–85, 1994.

Allgrove J, Clayden GS, Grant DB, et al: Familial glucocorticoid deficiency with achalasia of the cardia and deficient tear production. Lancet 1:1284, 1978.

Anggiansah A, Bright NF, McCullagh M: Transition from nutcracker esophagus to achalasia. Dig Dis Sci 35:1162–1166, 1990.

Annese V, Basciani M, Perri F: Controlled trial of botulinum toxin injection versus placebo and pneumatic dilation in achalasia. Gastroenterology 111:1418–1424, 1996.

Arnold WP, Mittal CK, Katsuki S: Nitric oxide activates guanylate cyclase and increases guanosine 3',5'-cyclic monophosphate levels in various tissue preparations. Proc Natl Acad Sci U S A 74:3203–3207, 1977.

Barham CP, Gotley DC, Fowler A: Diffuse oesophageal spasm: Diagnosis by ambulatory 24 hour manometry. Gut 41:151–155, 1997.

Barrett NR: Achalasia of the cardia: Reflections upon a clinical study of over 100 cases. Br Med J 1:1135–1140, 1964.

Behar J, Biancani P: Pathogenesis of simultaneous esophageal contractions in patients with motility disorders. Gastroenterology 105:111–118, 1993.

Benjamin SB, Gerhardt DC, Castell DO: High amplitude, peristaltic esophageal contractions associated with chest pain and/or dysphagia. Gastroenterology 77:478–483, 1979.

Berrisford RG, Oo A, Walshaw MJ, et al: Tracheal obstruction in achalasia: A role for airway stenting? Ann Thorac Surg 66:939–941, 1998.

Bielefeldt K, Enck P, Erckenbrect JF: Motility changes in primary achalasia following pneumatic dilatation. Dysphagia 5:152–158, 1990.

Bonavina L, Nosadini A, Bardini R: Primary treatment of esophageal achalasia: Long-term results of myotomy and Dor fundoplication. Arch Surg 127:222–227, 1992.

Bortolotti M, Labo G: Clinical and manometric effects of nifedipine in patients with esophageal achalasia. Gastroenterology 80:39–44, 1981.

Brand DL, Martin D, Pope CE: Esophageal manometrics in patients with angina-like chest pain. Am J Dig Dis 22:300–305, 1977.

Bremner RM, DeMeester TR: Current management of patients with esophageal motor abnormalities. Adv Surg 30:349–384,1997.

Breumelhof R, Van Wijk HJ, Van Es CD: Food impaction in nutcracker esophagus. Dig Dis Sci 35:1167–1171, 1990.

Cannon RO III, Quyyumi AA, Mincemoyer R, et al: Imipramine in patients with chest pain despite normal coronary angiograms. N Engl J Med 330:1411–1417, 1994.

Cassella RR, Brown AL, Sayre GP, et al: Achalasia of the esophagus, pathologic and etiologic considerations. Ann Surg 160:474–485, 1964.

Cassella RR, Ellis HF, Brown AL: Fine-structure changes in achalasia of the esophagus. I. Vagus nerves. Am J Pathol 46:279–283, 1965a.

Cassella RR, Ellis HF, Brown AL: Diffuse spasm of the lower part of the esophagus. JAMA 191:379–382, 1965b.

Cattau EL, Castell DO, Johnson DA: Diltiazem therapy for symptoms associated with nutcracker esophagus. Am J Gastroenterol 86:272–276, 1991.

Christensen J: Motor functions of the pharynx and esophagus. In Johnson LR (ed): Physiology of the Gastrointestinal Tract. New York, Raven Press, 1987, pp 595–612.

Clouse RE, Lustman PJ, Eckert TC: Low-dose trazodone for symptomatic patients with esophageal contraction abnormalities. Gastroenterology 92:1027–1036, 1987.

Creamer B, Donoghue FE, Code CF: Pattern of esophageal motility in diffuse spasm. Gastroenterology 34:782, 1958.

Csendes A, Smok G, Bragetto I, et al: Gastroesophageal sphincter pressure and histological changes in distal esophagus in patients with achalasia of the esophagus. Dig Dis Sci 30:941, 1985.

Csendes A, Braghetto I, Henriquez A: Late results of a prospective randomized study comparing forceful dilatation and oesophagomyotomy in patients with achalasia. Gut 30:299–304, 1989.

Cuilliere C, Ducrotte P, Zerbib F: Achalasia: Outcome of patients treated with intrasphincteric injection of botulinum toxin. Gut 41:87–92, 1997.

Dalton CB, Castell DO, Richter JE: The changing faces of the nutcracker esophagus. Am J Gastroenterol 83:623–628, 1988.

DeMeester TR: Surgery for esophageal motor disorders. Ann Thorac Surg 34:225–229, 1982.

DeMeester TR, O'Sullivan GC, Bermudez G, et al: Esophageal function in patients with angina-type chest pain and normal coronary angiograms. Ann Surg 196:488–498, 1982.

Deviere J, Dunham F, Rickaert F, et al..: Endoscopic ultrasonography in achalasia. Gastroenterology 96:1210–1213, 1989.

DiMarino AJ, Cohen S: Effect of an oral beta$_2$-adrenergic agonist on lower esophageal sphincter pressure in normals and in patients with achalasia. Dig Dis Sci 27:1063–1066, 1982.

Di Simone MP, Felice V, D'Errico A, et al: Onset timing of delayed complications and criteria of follow-up after operation for esophageal achalasia. Ann Thorac Surg 61:1106–1111, 1996.

Dodds WJ, Stewart ET, Kishk SM, et al: Radiologic amyl nitrite test for distinguishing pseudoachalasia from idiopathic achalasia. AJR 146:21–23, 1986.

Donahue PE, Samelson S, Schlesinger PK, Bombeck CT, Nyhus LM: Achalasia of the esophagus: Treatment controversies and the method of choice. Ann Surg 203:505–511, 1986.

Dooley CP, Taylor IL, Valenzuela JE: Impaired acid secretion and pancreatic polypeptide release in some patients with achalasia. Gastroenterology 84:809–813, 1983.

Eaker EY, Gordon JM, Vogel SB: Untoward effects of esophageal botulinum toxin injection in the treatment of achalasia. Dig Dis Sci 42:724–727, 1997.

Ebert EC, Ouyang A, Wright SH: Pneumatic dilatation in patients with symptomatic diffuse esophageal spasm and lower esophageal sphincter dysfunction. Dig Dis Sci 28:481–485, 1983.

Eckardt VF, Krause J, Bolle D: Gastrointestinal transit and gastric acid secretion in patients with achalasia. Dig Dis Sci 34:665, 1989.

Eckardt VF, Aignherr C, Bernhard G: Predictors of outcome in patients with achalasia treated by pneumatic dilation. Gastroenterology 103:1732–1738, 1992.

Eckardt VF, Kanzler G, Westermeier T: Complications and their impact after pneumatic dilation for achalasia: Prospective long-term follow-up study. Gastrointest Endosc 45:349–353, 1997a.

Eckardt VF, Kohne U, Junginger T: Risk factors for diagnostic delay in achalasia. Dig Dis Sci 42:580–585, 1997b.

Ehrich E, Aranoff G, Johnson WG: Familial achalasia associated with adrenocortical insufficiency, alacrima, and neurological abnormalities. Am J Med Genet 26:637–644, 1987.

Ellis FH Jr, Crozier RE, Watkins E: The operation for esophageal achalasia: Results of esophagomyotomy without an antireflux operation. J Thorac Cardiovasc Surg 88:344–351, 1984.

Ellis FH Jr: Esophagomyotomy for noncardiac chest pain resulting from diffuse esophageal spasm and elated disorders. Am J Med 92(Suppl 5A):129S–131S, 1992.

Ellis FH Jr, Watkins E Jr, Gibb SP: Ten- to 20-year clinical results after short esophagomyotomy without an antireflux procedure (modified Heller operation) for esophageal achalasia. Eur J Cardiothorac Surg 6:86, 1992.

Eypasch EP, DeMeester TR, Klingman RR: Physiologic assessment and surgical management of diffuse esophageal spasm. J Cardiovasc Thorac Surg 104:859–869, 1992.

Feldman M: Esophageal achalasia syndromes. Am J Med Sci 295:60–81, 1988.

Ferguson MK: Achalasia: Current evaluation and therapy. Ann Thorac Surg 52:336–342, 1991.

Ferguson MK, Reeder LB, Olak J: Results of myotomy and partial fundoplication after pneumatic dilation for achalasia. Ann Thorac Surg 62:327–330, 1996.

Fleshler B: Diffuse esophageal spasm. Gastroenterology 52:559–563, 1967.

Fredens K, Tottrup A, Kristensen IB, et al: Severe destruction of esophageal nerves in a patient with achalasia secondary to gastric cancer: A possible role of eosinophil neurotoxic proteins. Dig Dis Sci 34:297–303, 1989.

Friesen DL, Henderson RD, Hanna W: Ultrastructure of the esophageal muscle in achalasia and diffuse esophageal spasm. Am J Clin Pathol 79:319–325, 1983.

Fuller L, Huprich JE, Theisen J, et al: Abnormal esophageal body function: Radiographic-manometric correlation. Am Surg 65:911–914, 1999.

Gelfond M, Rozen P, Keren S: Effect of nitrates on LOS pressure in achalasia: A potential therapeutic aid. Gut 22:312–318, 1981.

Goldblum JR, Rice TW, Richter JE: Histopathologic features in esophagomyotomy specimens from patients with achalasia. Gastroenterology 111:648–654, 1996.

Goyal RK, Rattan S: VIP as a possible neurotransmitter of non-adrenergic inhibitory neurons. Nature 288:378–379, 1980.

Graham AJ, Finley RJ, Worsley DF: Laparoscopic esophageal myotomy and anterior partial fundoplication for the treatment of achalasia. Ann Thorac Surg 64:785–789, 1997.

Gross R, Johnson LF, Kaminski RJ: Esophageal emptying in achalasia quantified by a radioisotope technique. Dig Dis Sci 24:945–949, 1979.

Henderson RD, Ryder D, Marryatt G: Extended esophageal myotomy and short total fundoplication hernia repair in diffuse esophageal spasm: Five-year review in 34 patients. Ann Thorac Surg 43:25–31, 1987.

Holloway RH, Dodds WJ, Helm JF, et al: Integrity of cholinergic innervation to the lower esophageal sphincter in achalasia. Gastroenterology 90:924–929, 1986.

Holloway RH, Lange RC, Plankey MW, et al: Detection of esophageal motor disorders by radionuclide transit studies: A reappraisal. Dig Dis Sci 34:905–912, 1989.

Hongo M, Traube M, McAllister RG: Effects of nifedipine on esophageal motor function in humans: Correlation with plasma nifedipine concentration. Gastroenterology 86:8–12, 1984.

Horgan S, Hudda K, Eubanks T: Does botulinum toxin injection make esophagomyotomy a more difficult operation? Surg Endosc 13:576–579, 1999.

Horton ML, Goff JS: Surgical treatment of nutcracker esophagus. Dig Dis Sci 31:878–883, 1986.

Hunter JG, Trus TL, Branum GD: Laparoscopic Heller myotomy and fundoplication for achalasia. Ann Surg 225:655–665, 1997.

Irving JD, Owen WJ, Linsell J, et al: Management of diffuse esophageal spasm with balloon dilatation. Gastrointest Radiol 17:189–192, 1992.

Jones DD, Mayberry JF, Rhodes J, et al: Preliminary report of an association between measles virus and achalasia. J Clin Pathol 36:655–657, 1983.

Kahrilas PJ, Kishk SM, Helm JF, et al: Comparison of pseudoachalasia and achalasia. Am J Med 82:439–446, 1987.

Katz PO, Richter JE, Cowan R: Apparent complete lower esophageal sphincter relaxation in achalasia. Gastroenterology 90:978, 1986.

Katz PO, Dalton CB, Richter JE, et al: Esophageal testing of patients with noncardiac chest pain or dysphagia. Ann Intern Med 106:593–597, 1987.

Katz PO, Gilbert J, Castell DO: Pneumatic dilation is effective long-term treatment for achalasia. Dig Dis Sci 43:1973–1977, 1998.

Khalifa MM: Familial achalasia, microcephaly, and mental retardation. Clin Pediatr 27:509–512, 1988.

Kimura K: The nature of idiopathic esophagus dilatation. Jpn J Gastroenterol 1:199–207, 1929.

Konturek JW, Gillessen A, Domschke W: Diffuse esophageal spasm: A malfunction that involves nitric oxide? Scand J Gastroenterol 30:1041–1045, 1995.

Kramer P: Oesophageal sensitivity to Mecholyl in symptomatic diffuse spasm. Gut 8:120, 1967.

Kramer P, Harris LD, Donaldson RM: Transition from symptomatic diffuse spasm to cardiospasm. Gut 8:115–119, 1967.

Landres RT, Kuster GGR, Strum WB: Eosinophilic esophagitis in a patient with vigorous achalasia. Gastroenterology 74:1298–1301, 1978.

Leite LP, Johnston BT, Barrett J: Ineffective esophageal motility (IEM): The primary finding in patients with nonspecific esophageal motility disorder. Dig Dis Sci 42:1859–1865, 1997.

Little AG, Correnti F, Calleja IJ: Effect of incomplete obstruction on feline esophageal function with a clinical correlation. Surgery 100:430–435, 1986.

Little AG, Soriano A, Ferguson MK: Surgical treatment of achalasia: Results with esophagomyotomy and Belsey repair. Ann Thorac Surg 45:489–494, 1988.

Maher JW: Thoracoscopic esophagomyotomy for achalasia: Maximum gain, minimal pain. Surgery 122:836–841, 1997.

Malthaner RA, Todd TR, Miller L: Long-term results in surgically managed esophageal achalasia. Ann Thorac Surg 58:1343–1347, 1994.

Mayberry JF, Atkinson M: A study of swallowing difficulties in first degree relatives of patients with achalasia. Thorax 40:391–393, 1985.

Mellow MH: Return of esophageal peristalsis in idiopathic achalasia. Gastroenterology 70:1148–1151, 1976.

Mellow MH: Symptomatic diffuse esophageal spasm: Manometric follow-up and response to cholinergic stimulation and cholinesterase inhibition. Gastroenterology 73:237, 1977.

Melzer E, Ron Y, Tiomni E: Assessment of the esophageal wall by endoscopic ultrasonography in patients with nutcracker esophagus. Gastrointest Endosc 46:223–225, 1997.

Miller DL, Allen MS, Trastek VF: Esophageal resection for recurrent achalasia. Ann Thorac Surg 60:922–926, 1995.

Miller LS, Parkman HP, Schiano TD: Treatment of symptomatic nonachalasia esophageal motor disorders with botulinum toxin injection at the lower esophageal sphincter. Dig Dis Sci 41:2025–2031, 1996.

Moersch HJ, Camp JD: Diffuse spasm of the lower part of the esophagus. Ann Otol Rhinol Laryngol 43:1165–1173, 1934.

Monnig PJ: Familial achalasia in children. Ann Thorac Surg 49:1019–1022, 1990.

Morrow A, Coady TJ, Seaton D: Tracheal compression relieved by cardiomyotomy. Thorax 37:776–777, 1982.

Murray JA, Ledlow A, Launspach J: The effects of recombinant human hemoglobin on esophageal motor function in humans. Gastroenterology 109:1241–1248, 1995.

Narducci F, Bassotti G, Gaburri M, et al: Transition from nutcracker esophagus to diffuse esophageal spasm. Am J Gastroenterol 80:242–244, 1985.

Nino-Murcia M, Stark P, Triadafilopoulos G: Esophageal wall thickening: A CT finding in diffuse esophageal spasm. J Comput Assist Tomogr 21:318–321, 1997.

Okike N, Payne SW, Neufeld DM: Esophagomyotomy versus forceful dilation for achalasia of the esophagus: Results in 899 patients. Ann Thorac Surg 28:119–125, 1979.

Orlando RC, Bozymki EM: Clinical and manometric effects of nitroglycerin in diffuse esophageal spasm. N Engl J Med 289:23–25, 1973.

Orlando RC, Bozymski EM: The effects of pentagastrin in achalasia and diffuse esophageal spasm. Gastroenterology 77:472, 1979.

Orlando RC, Call DL, Bream CA: Achalasia and absent gastric air bubble (Letter). Ann Intern Med 88:60, 1978.

Osgood H: A peculiar form of oesophagismus. Boston Med Surg J 120:401, 1889.

Ott JD, Richter JE, Wu WC: Radiologic and manometric correlation in "nutcracker esophagus." AJR 147:692–695, 1986.

Pai GP, Ellison RG, Rubin JW: Two decades of experience with modified Heller's myotomy for achalasia. Ann Thorac Surg 38:201–206, 1984.

Paterson WG, Beck IT, DeCosta LR: Transition from nutcracker esophagus to achalasia. J Clin Gastroenterol 13:554–558, 1991.

Patti MG, Pellegrini CA, Arcerito M: Comparison of medical and minimally invasive surgical therapy for primary esophageal motility disorders. Arch Surg 130:609–616, 1995.

Patti MG, Pellegrini CA, Horgan S: Minimally invasive surgery for achalasia: An 8 year experience with 168 patients. Ann Surg 230:587, 1999.

Pellegrini CA, Leichter R, Patti M: Thoracoscopic esophageal myotomy in the treatment of achalasia. Ann Thorac Surg 56:680–682, 1993.

Peters JH, Werner KH, Crookes PF: Esophageal resection with colon interposition for end-stage achalasia. Arch Surg 130:632–637, 1995.

Peters L, Maas L, Petty D: Spontaneous noncardiac chest pain: Evaluation by 24-hour ambulatory motility and pH monitoring. Gastroenterology 94:878–886, 1988.

Phillip M, Hershkovitz E, Schulman H: Adrenal insufficiency after achalasia in the triple-A syndrome. Clin Pediatr 35:99, 1996.

Qualman SJ, Haupt HM, Yang P, et al: Esophageal Lewy bodies associated with ganglion cell loss in achalasia. Gastroenterology 87:848–856, 1984.

Richter JE, Castell DO: Diffuse esophageal spasm: A reappraisal. Ann Intern Med 100:242–245, 1984.

Richter JE, Castell DO: Surgical myotomy for nutcracker esophagus: To be or not to be? Dig Dis Sci 32:5–96, 1987.

Richter JE, Dalton CB, Buice RG: Nifedipine: A potent inhibitor of contractions in the body of the human esophagus. Gastroenterology 89:549–554, 1985.

Richter JE, Barish CF, Castell DO: Abnormal sensory perception in patients with esophageal chest pain. Gastroenterology 91:845–852, 1986a.

Richter JE, Obrecht WF, Bradley LA: Psychological comparison of patients with nutcracker esophagus and irritable bowel syndrome. Dig Dis Sci 31:131–138, 1986b.

Richter JE, Dalton CB, Bradley LA: Oral nifedipine in the treatment of noncardiac chest pain in patients with the nutcracker esophagus. Gastroenterology 93:21–8, 1987a.

Richter JE, Wu WC, Johns DN, et al: Esophageal manometry in 95 healthy adult volunteers: Variability of pressures with age and frequency of "abnormal" contractions. Dig Dis Sci 32:583–592, 1987b.

Robertson CS, Martin BAB, Atkinson M: Varicella-zoster virus DNA in the oesophageal myenteric plexus in achalasia. Gut 34:299–302, 1993.

Sanderson DR, Ellis FH, Schlegel JF, et al: Syndrome of vigorous achalasia: Clinical and physiologic observations. Dis Chest 52:508–517, 1967.

Sandler RS, Bozymski EM, Orlando RC: Failure of clinical criteria to distinguish between primary achalasia and achalasia secondary to tumor. Dig Dis Sci 27:209, 1982.

Sandler RS, Nyren O, Ekborn A, et al: The risk of esophageal cancer in patients with achalasia: A population based study. JAMA 274:1359–1362, 1995.

Senocak ME, Hicsonmez A, Buyukpamukcu N: Familial childhood achalasia. Z Kinderchir 45:111, 1990.

Shlemmel A, Priviter CA, Poppel MH: A study of the effects of certain drugs on curling of the esophagus. Am J Roentgenol 44:49, 1949.

Short TP, Thomas E: An overview of the role of calcium antagonists in the treatment of achalasia and diffuse oesophageal spasm. Drugs 43:177–184, 1992.

Smart HL, Foster PN, Evans DF, et al: Twenty-four hour oesophageal acidity in achalasia before and after pneumatic dilation. Gut 28:883–887, 1987.

Spiess AE, Kahrilas PJ: Treating achalasia: From whalebone to laparoscope. JAMA 280:638–642, 1998.

Stacher G, Schima W, Bergmann H, et al: Sensitivity of radionuclide bolus transport and videofluoroscopic studies compared with manometry in the detection of achalasia. Am J Gastroenterol 89:1484–1488, 1994.

Stein HJ, DeMeester TR: Indications, technique, and clinical use of ambulatory 24-hour esophageal motility monitoring in a surgical practice. Ann Thorac Surg 217:128–137, 1993.

Stewart KC, Finley RJ, Clifton JC: Thoracoscopic versus laparoscopic modified Heller myotomy for achalasia: Efficacy and safety in 87 patients. J Am Coll Surg 189:164–170, 1999.

Streitz JM, Ellis HF, Gibb PS, et al: Achalasia and squamous cell carcinoma of the esophagus: Analysis of 241 patients. Ann Thorac Surg 59:1604–1609, 1995.

Topart P, Deschamps C, Taillefer R, Duranceau A: Long-term effect of total fundoplication on the myotomized esophagus. Ann Thorac Surg 54:1046–1052, 1992.

Torphy TJ, Fine CF, Burman M, et al: Lower esophageal sphincter relaxation is associated with increased cyclic nucleotide content. Am J Physiol 251:G786–G793, 1986.

Tottrup A, Fredens K, Funch-Jensen P, et al: Eosinophil infiltration in primary esophageal achalasia: A possible pathogenic role. Dig Dis Sci 34:1894–1899, 1989.

Tottrup A, Forman A, Funch-Jensen P, et al: Effects of postganglionic nerve stimulation in oesophageal achalasia: An in vitro study. Gut 31:17–20, 1990.

Tottrup A, Knudsen MA, Gregersen H: The role of the L-arginine–nitric oxide pathway in relaxation of the opossum lower oesophageal sphincter. Br J Pharm 104:113–116, 1991.

Traube M, Hongo M, Magyar L: Effects of nifedipine in achalasia and in patients with high-amplitude peristaltic esophageal contractions. JAMA 252:1733, 1984.

Traube M, Aaronson RM, McCallum RW: Transition from peristaltic esophageal contractions to diffuse esophageal spasm. Arch Intern Med 146:1844–1846, 1986.

Traube M, Aaronson RM, McCallum RW: Transition from nutcracker esophagus to diffuse esophageal spasm. Arch Intern Med 146:1844–1847, 1987a.

Traube M, Tummala V, Baue AE: Surgical myotomy in patients with high-amplitude peristaltic esophageal contractions: Manometric and clinical effects. Dig Dis Sci 32:16–21, 1987b.

Triadafilopoulos G, Aaronson M, Sackel S: Medical treatment of esophageal achalasia: Double-blind crossover study with oral nifedipine, verapamil, and placebo. Dig Dis Sci 36:260–267, 1991.

Triadafilopoulos G, Tsang H, Segall GM: Hot water swallows improve symptoms and accelerate esophageal clearance in esophageal motility disorders. J Clin Gastroenterol 26:239–244, 1998.

Tryhus MR, Davis M, Griffith JK, et al: Familial achalasia in two siblings: Significance of a possible hereditary role. J Pediatr Surg 24:292, 1989.

Tyce FA, Brough W: The appearance of an undescribed syndrome and the inheritance of multiple diseases in three generations of a family. Psychiatr Res Rep 15:73–79, 1962.

Vanek AW, Diamant NE: Responses of the human esophagus to paired swallows. Gastroenterology 92:643–50, 1987.

Vantrappen G, Janssens J: To dilate or to operate? That is the question. Gut 24:1013–1019, 1983.

Vantrappen G, Hellemans J, Pelemans W, Janssens J: Electromyographic and manometric studies of deglutitive inhibition of the esophagus (Abstract). Gastroenterology 3:139a, 1971.

Vantrappen G, Janssens J, Hellemans J, et al: Achalasia, diffuse esophageal spasm, and related motility disorders. Gastroenterology 93:450–457, 1988.

Verne NG, Sallustio JE, Eaker EY: Anti-myenteric neuronal antibodies in patients with achalasia: A prospective study. Dig Dis Sci 42:307–313, 1997.

Ward BW, Wu WC, Richter JE, et al: Long-term follow-up of symptomatic status of patients with noncardiac chest pain: Is diagnosis of esophageal etiology helpful? Am J Gastroenterol 82:215, 1987.

Wehrmann T, Jacobi V, Jung M: Pneumatic dilation in achalasia with a low-compliance balloon: Results of a 5-year prospective evaluation. Gastrointest Endosc 42:31–36, 1995.

Winters C, Artnak EJ, Benjamin SB, et al: Esophageal bougienage in symptomatic patients with nutcracker esophagus. JAMA 252:363–366, 1984.

Wong RKH, Maydonovitch CL, Metz SJ, et al: Significant DQw1 association in achalasia. Dig Dis Sci 34:349–352, 1989.

Zaaijer JH: Cardiospasm in the aged. Ann Surg 77:615, 1923.

Zaninotto G, DeMeester TR, Schwizer W: The lower esophageal sphincter in health and disease. Am J Surg 155:104–111, 1988.

CHAPTER **33**

Chagas' Disease

Manoel Ximenes-Netto

DEFINITION

American trypanosomiasis (Chagas' disease) is a chronic disease caused by the protozoan *Trypanosoma cruzi*, discovered by Carlos Chagas in 1909. Passage to humans and animals results from contamination with feces of a blood-sucking *Triatoma* bug deposited close to the bite wound. Congenital transmission is also possible, as is transmission through blood or organs received from a contaminated donor. A nursing mother may infect her infant. Although lesions caused by the parasite may be found in any organ, the most commonly affected are the nervous, cardiovascular, and digestive systems.

More than 100 mammalian species have been contaminated with *T. cruzi*, and several patterns of parasitemia may occur with predilections for different organs. There is a wide distribution of the *Triatoma* organisms, ranging from 41°N latitude, where *Triatoma protracta* has been found in Salt Lake City, Utah, to 46°S, where *Triatoma patagonica* has been described in Patagonia in South America. There are six major triatomine vectors of Chagas' disease, namely *Triatoma dimidiata, Rhodnius prolixus, Triatoma infestans, Triatoma sordida, Panstronhylus megistus*, and *Triatoma brasiliensis*.

Of an estimated population of 360 million in the endemic countries in Latin America, 25% (90 million) are considered at risk for contracting the disease. Out of this total, 30% (5.4 million) of the infected population may manifest signs and symptoms (WHO, 1991). Among the patients with the disease, 6% to 9% have esophageal involvement (i.e., 324,000 to 486,000 patients have Chagas' megaesophagus).

Chronic cardiac disease resulting from Chagas' disease is found in 50% of patients with megaesophagus. Stomach involvement in this disease is characterized by diminished chloride-peptic secretion, delay in gastric emptying time, and pyloric hypertrophy. The duodenum is the third most frequently affected part of the digestive tract, after the esophagus and the colon. The small intestine, gallbladder, and salivary glands are less commonly involved in Chagas' disease.

HISTORICAL NOTE

Chagas' disease is perhaps the only disease in the history of medicine for which the discoverer described simultaneously the causative agent *(T. cruzi)*, the vector *(Triatoma)*, and the clinical manifestations. The patient in whom all these aspects were studied was 2 years old at the time (1909) and lived to be 82.

The first references in the Brazilian medical literature to what may have been a case of megaesophagus were by Pimenta in 1707 and by Ferreira in 1735. The term then used was *tropical dysphagia*, and the association with constipation was also noted.

With the discovery of x-rays and contrast material (bismuth salts initially) to examine the esophagus, it became possible to study the organ and verify the great dilatation, retention, and difficulty of swallowed food reaching the stomach. The association between esophageal dilatation and Chagas' disease was postulated by the scientist himself in 1916. Amorim and Correa Neto (1932) described the lesions of the myenteric parasympathetic plexus, but it remained to Koeberle (1956a, 1956b) to demonstrate the depopulation of ganglion cells not only in the esophagus but also in the entire digestive tract, heart, and bronchi.

The link between the "mega" syndromes and the chagasic etiology was clearly demonstrated by Freitas (1946) and Laranja and colleagues (1948). Both authors verified that complement fixation tests performed in patients with either megaesophagus or megacolon showed 91.2% and 97% positive serologic results, respectively. Not all accept the chagasic etiology of megaesophagus or megacolon, because in places where the disease is endemic, such as Venezuela and Central America, heart manifestations prevail instead.

In addition to possible variations in organ vulnerability, the likelihood of human infection depends on the habits of the more than 100 strains of the parasite. For example, *T. protracta, Triatoma rubida uhleri, and Triatoma gestraecheri* are found in the Midwest, Arizona, and New Mexico; however, because these organisms live in the woods and do not defecate after their blood meal, human infection is rare.

HISTORICAL READINGS

Chagas C: Tripanosomiase americana: Forma aguda da moléstia. Mem Inst Oswaldo Cruz 8:37, 1916.

Chagas C Jr: Doença de Chagas. In Cançado JR (ed): Doença de Chagas. Belo Horizonte, 1968.

Koeberle F: Chagas Krankheit: Eine Erkrankung der neurovegetative Peripherie. Wien Klin Wochenshr 68:333, 1956.

Laranja FS, Dias E, Nóbrega G: Estudo eletrocardiográfico de 81 casos de megaesôfago. Mem Inst Oswaldo Cruz 46:473, 1948.

Rezende JM, Moreira H: Chagasic megaesophagus and megacolon: Historical review and present concepts. Arq Gastroenterol 25:32, 1988.

BASIC SCIENCE

Chagas' disease was initially a *malady* of forest inhabitants. Human migration and destruction of the jungle have brought the disease to a more rural environment.

Most of the triatomines are prevalent in mud houses, in the thatched or straw roofs, and in cracks, especially at the upper level. Humans, cats, dogs, and birds are the most common source of blood for the triatomines. Rodents may play a role not only as vectors but also as predators. Once infected with the *Trypanosoma* organisms, an insect becomes a carrier for the rest of its life.

The life cycle of the *T. cruzi* begins after the triatomine takes a blood meal from a contaminated human or animal who has circulating parasites, trypomastigotes. The ingested parasites become epimastigotes and multiply in the gut of the vector insect; later, they transform once again into metacyclic trypomastigotes in the hindgut of the bug. After a subsequent blood meal, the infected insect frequently deposits the infective metacyclic form of the parasite. Once in the human organism, *Trypanosoma* organisms multiply in the cytoplasm of the blood cells, transform into motile trypomastigotes, and rupture, liberating organisms that penetrate new cells, are carried into the bloodstream to begin further cycles of multiplication, or are ingested by other vectors and initiate a new cycle (Fig. 33–1).

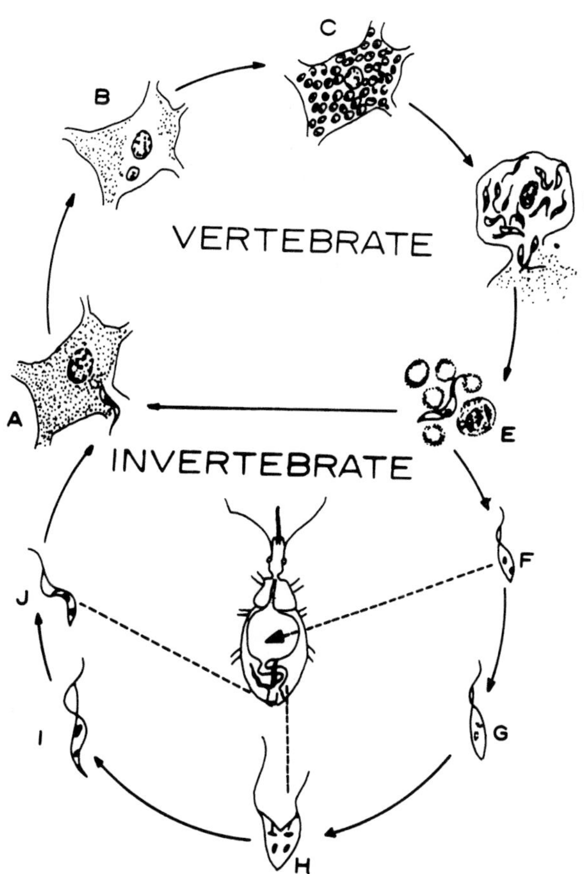

FIGURE 33–1 ■ Life cycle of *Trypanosoma cruzi*. *A*, The metacyclic *T. cruzi* penetrates into the cells. *B*, It becomes the leishmanial form. *C*, Binary multiplication fills the cytoplasm. *D*, It has transformed into metacyclic *Trypanosoma*. *E*, Rupturing into blood, *Trypanosoma* goes into other cells. *F*, It is digested by the triatomine *(arrow)*. *G* and *H*, In the duodenum of the insect, it multiplies by binary division. *I* and *J*, Difference of metacyclic tripanosoma occurs in the rectum of the triatomine. (Adapted from Chagas C Jr: Doença de Chagas. In Cancado JR: [ed]: Doença de Chagas, Belo Horizonte, 1968.)

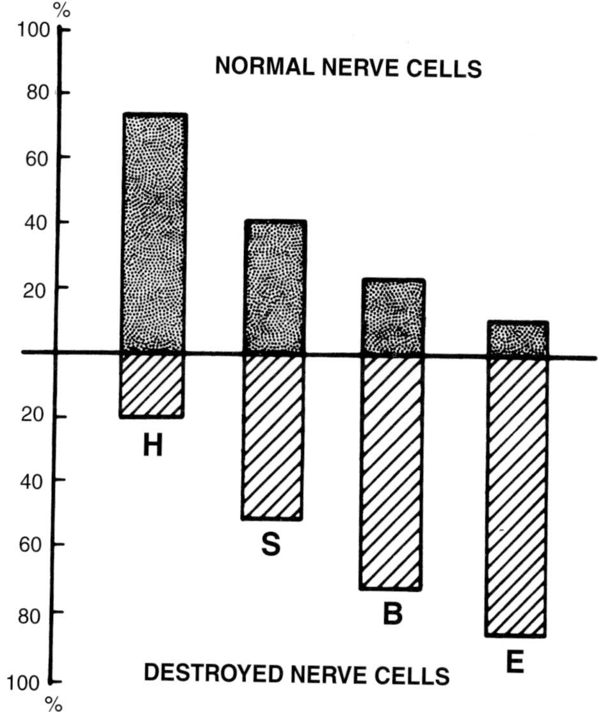

FIGURE 33–2 ■ Threshold between the number of lost ganglion cells and the appearances of symptoms in Chagas' disease. (H, heart; S, sigmoid; B, bronchi; E, esophagus.) (From Koeberle F: Chagas Krankheit: Eine erkrankun der neurovegetative peripherie. Wien Klin Wochenschr 68:333, 1956.)

Two basic pathogenic mechanisms explain the lesions caused by *T. cruzi*. The first is a local mechanism, explained by Vianna (1911), consisting of an inflammatory reaction with necrosis, tissue destruction with healing, and fibrosis. The second involves an immune reaction and is not yet completely understood.

Koeberle (1956b, 1957, 1958), Koeberle and Penha (1959), and Koeberle and Alcantara (1989) noted an acute inflammatory process followed by a chronic phase with severe symptoms related to the cardiovascular, digestive, respiratory, and nervous systems. Koeberle believed that after the disintegration of the leishmania forms of *T. cruzi* in the acute phase, there would be release of a neurolytic substance capable of destroying the nerve cells of the parasympathetic system. He postulated that lysis of the ganglion cells would occur in the acute phase and that the chronic phase was a consequence of the denervation of the affected system.

In light of these principles, Koeberle studied the ganglion cell population of the heart, colon, bronchi, and esophagus in normal and chagasic individuals and found that the threshold for the appearance of symptoms in this disease was 25% destruction of the ganglion cells in the heart, 55% in the colon, 75% in the bronchi, and 90% in the esophagus (Fig. 33–2).

Autoimmune mechanisms in the pathogenesis of the chagasic syndromes have also been investigated. Antibodies that are anti-EVI (endocardium, vessels, and interstitium), antinerves, antimuscle, and antimyocardium have been demonstrated both experimentally and in human infection. Still in the investigative phase are labeled deoxyribonucleic acid (DNA) probes and isolation of different strains by means of isoenzymes and gel electrophoresis.

DIAGNOSIS

Clinical Features

The diagnosis of Chagas' megaesophagus is quite simple on clinical grounds alone. The most common symptoms are dysphagia, regurgitation, singultus, salivation with hypertrophy of the salivary glands, cough, constipation, weight loss, and pain. A history of contact with the triatomine is almost always described by the patient.

The acute phase is found in but 1% to 2% of patients, usually in children. After an incubation period lasting approximately 1 week, induration and erythema—a so-called chagoma—can be seen at the bite site. The chagoma is frequently followed by regional adenopathy, fever, and splenomegaly. There may be periorbital swelling (Romaña's sign). One third of patients already show electrocardiographic changes, but 2% to 3% mortality in the acute phase is usually attributed to infection of the child's central nervous system.

Eight to 10 weeks after the acute stage, the patient is symptom-free but remains an important reservoir of infection. Only one third of the patients infected with Chagas' disease experience the classic cardiac, digestive, or neurologic symptoms. The time interval between infection and the symptomatic period may vary from 10 to 20 years. Any part of the digestive tract may become symptomatic, but the esophagus and colon are most commonly affected.

Dysphagia is the main symptom in megaesophagus and at the time of treatment is present in nearly all patients. It may be intermittent, depending on the type of meal ingested, and in time is present for either solid or liquid food. Sudden onset is usually associated with emotional stress and has no relation to the size of dilatation. The patient, becoming aware of this difficulty, develops characteristic maneuvers to encourage passage of food: drinking large amounts of water, taking deep breaths, deliberately swallowing air, or holding the breath. Valsalva's maneuver or arching backward is also tried in a futile attempt to empty the esophagus. Dysphagia is a result of the functional obstruction caused by loss of innervation of the body of the esophagus and consequent loss of peristalsis plus the inability of the stolid lower esophageal sphincter (LES) to open when presented with swallowed food.

Regurgitation is seen in 55% to 91% of cases of megaesophagus. It is necessary to distinguish *regurgitation* from *vomiting*, the latter being unusual. Regurgitation is the effortless flow of an undigested meal back into the pharynx. The patient at times may provoke it in order to relieve the pain or discomfort. It usually occurs at night or when lying down. Aspiration pneumonia, lung abscess, and bronchiectasis are common sequelae.

Weight loss is seen in almost 50% of patients with Chagas' esophagopathy. It is due to either inability to empty the esophagus or fear of eating because of odynophagia. When it is associated with anemia and weight loss, carcinoma should be excluded.

Retrosternal pain or discomfort is a frequent complaint. In the early stages of the disease or with vigorous achalasia, severe spontaneous substernal pain with radiation to the jaws, shoulder, and arm, lasting from a few minutes to hours, has been described. It does not seem to be related to gastroesophageal reflux or esophagitis and is frequently relieved after surgical treatment or administration of sublingual nitrates. The denervation test, which involves administration of mecholyl (Cannon's law), produces similar symptoms.

When the lower esophagus is impacted by food, pain is the predominant symptom and endoscopic removal of the food is necessary. Heartburn after inadequate surgical treatment that results in reflux is infrequent. Singultus (hiccup) may be an early sign of megaesophagus. It can be of short duration or may last for hours or days; sometimes surgical treatment is required.

Hypertrophy of the salivary glands with excessive salivation is a frequent finding in Chagas' megaesophagus. Indeed, it is characteristic of the infection (Fig. 33–3). Constipation in chagasic patients is common and results from two mechanisms: (1) the loss of ganglion cells and consequent megacolon (found in 22% of cases) and (2) swallowing of less bulky food. For these reasons, when megaesophagus and megacolon are found in the same patient, the former should be treated first.

Natural History

The long-term prognosis in patients with Chagas' megaesophagus does not seem to be influenced by the dilatation of the organ; it is associated with myocarditis, pulmonary complications, and carcinoma, which influence survival. In a review of 450 cases of Chagas' megaesophagus (Ximenes-Netto et al, 1987), we found symptomatic associated disease in the following order and frequency: megacolon, 100 cases (22%); cholelithiasis, 40 (8.8%); heart disease, 8 (5.5%); and carcinoma, 10 (2.2%).

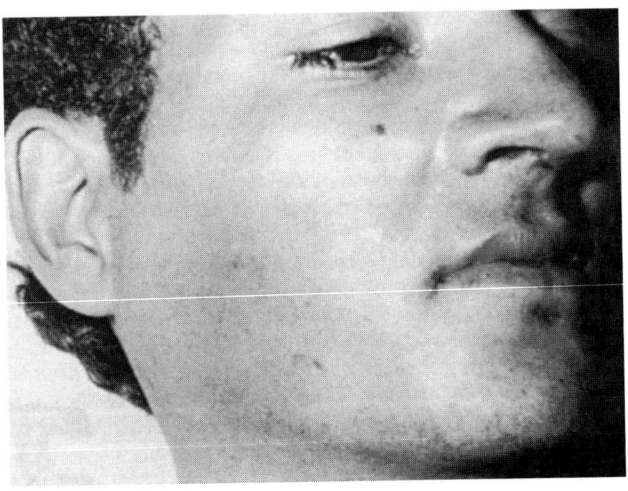

FIGURE 33–3 ■ Megaesophagus and hypertrophy of the parotid gland.

The actual incidence of megacolon and heart disease is about 50%, but many patients are asymptomatic and are not treated. Electrocardiographic changes such as arrhythmia and right bundle branch block are found in 46% of cases; heart enlargement (5.6%) and congestive heart failure (2.3%) are much less common. Biliary tract disease is found in a higher proportion of patients, probably because of the parasympathetic denervation, and because of this it justifies an abdominal approach.

Complications

In the chronic stage, 30% of infected patients manifest one of the forms of the disease, such as cardiac, pulmonary, digestive, or neurologic conditions. The pulmonary problems are caused by aspiration of regurgitated food material, which occurs particularly at night when the patient is lying down. Manifestations include cough, wheezing, and shortness of breath. Pneumonia, lung abscess, bronchiectasis, empyema, and pulmonary embolization are frequently found. Fistula between the trachea and the esophagus is a rare finding. One such case has been described (Ximenes-Netto et al, 1985).

There seems to be a difference between idiopathic achalasia and Chagas' megaesophagus regarding the incidence of carcinoma, which is less common in the latter. The incidence in carefully studied series should not exceed 3% (Ximenes-Netto et al, 1991). The diagnosis is usually delayed because of the preexisting dysphagia. One should suspect carcinoma in patients with worsening of the symptoms, weight loss, regurgitation of blood-stained material, melena, and anemia. Previous surgery does not seem to prevent the appearance of cancer.

The outlook in cases of megaesophagus and malignancy is poor. There are at least two reasons for delayed therapy: (1) the patient is rather accustomed to some degree of dysphagia and (2) because of the large caliber of the gullet, a bulkier tumor must be present before obstruction occurs.

Differential Diagnosis

Several methods are available for establishing a definite and correct diagnosis of Chagas' disease. An easy and accurate method consists of collecting blood in a capillary tube, centrifuging it, and examining the interphase between the leukocyte buffy coat and the red blood cell. The chance of confirming a diagnosis of Chagas' disease in the acute phase varies from 60% to 100%; in the chronic stage, it is below 10%.

The indirect methods are xenodiagnosis and blood culture, with 100% sensitivity in the acute stage dropping to less than 50% in the chronic stage. Several serologic tests can be used to diagnose Chagas' disease. The most commonly used are the complement fixation test (Machado-Guerreiro test), the indirect hemagglutination test, the indirect immunofluorescence test, the enzyme-linked immunosorbent assay (ELISA), and the direct agglutination test. In patients with proven parasitemia and in the chronic phase, 95% accuracy is expected.

Other conditions that may appear as megaesophagus syndrome are pseudointestinal obstruction, familial adrenal insufficiency, and postvagotomy achalasia.

Pseudointestinal obstruction affects primarily the small intestine and involves the myenteric plexus and smooth muscles. It may occasionally appear as an esophageal motility disorder with spontaneous and simultaneous contractions and abnormal function of the lower esophageal sphincter manometrically.

Familial adrenal insufficiency with achalasia was described by Allgrove and colleagues (1978). It is characterized by early recurrent hypoglycemia, increased pigmentation secondary to hypercorticism, and deficient tear production and is of unknown etiology. It is an autosomal recessive trait.

Postvagotomy achalasia is extremely rare after dissection of the cardia and is usually caused by trauma with resulting edema and hematoma. If both vagus nerves are interrupted at the cervical or thoracic level, an achalasia-like syndrome may appear, caused by the loss of the preganglionic nerves that supply the LES (Ximenes-Netto et al, 1997).

Investigative Techniques

Radiologic studies with or without contrast material are the most important tools in the diagnosis of megaesophagus. A simple chest radiograph may demonstrate several features capable of distinguishing this disorder from other organic obstructions of the esophagus. At times, the enlarged mediastinum in cases of advanced disease may be confused with a mediastinal tumor (Fig. 33–4).

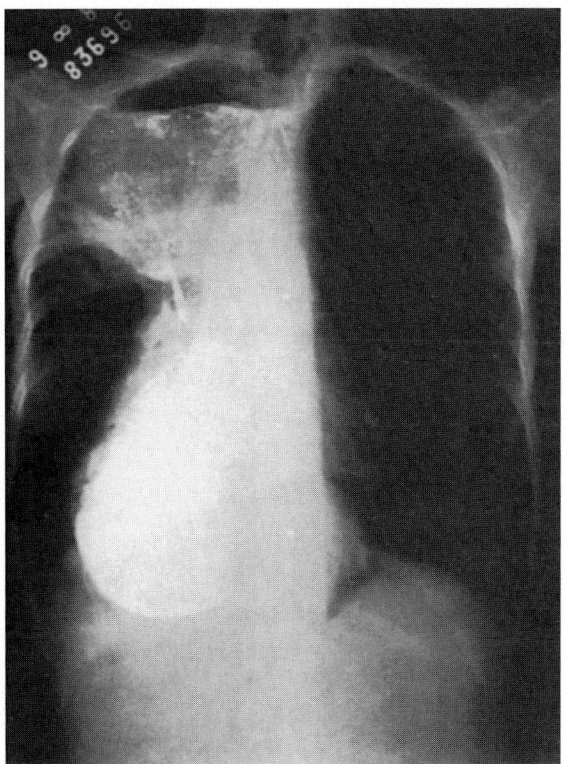

FIGURE 33–4 ■ Chest radiograph of a patient with stage IV megaesophagus. Note the air-fluid level and the absent gastric bubbles.

TABLE 33–1 ■ **Radiologic Classification of Megaesophagus**

Group	Transverse Diameter (cm)	Stasis, 10 Sec	Stasis, 5 Min	Stasis, 30 Min
I	4	Yes	No	No
II	4–7	Yes	Yes	Eventually
III	7–10	Yes	Yes	Yes
IV	Above 10	Yes	Yes	Yes

Other signs are absence of the gastric air bubble and lung alterations caused by the inflammatory changes, such as pneumonia, lung abscess, and "tumor-like shadow." On the lateral view, an air-fluid level is seen in advanced cases with displacement of the trachea.

Contrast studies of the esophagus should be preceded by lavage with a large-bore tube in order to remove residual food and facilitate examination of the patient in both lying and standing positions. With the horizontal position, the effect of gravity is eliminated, and some features of the megaesophagus may be appreciated, including the lack of esophageal emptying, discoordinated peristalsis, and lack of relaxation of the lower esophageal sphincter.

Camara-Lopes (1961), Camara-Lopes and coworkers (1958), Ferreira-Santos (1961), and Rezende (1982), on the basis of retention of contrast material, caliber of the esophagus, contractility tonicity of the lower segment, and lengthening of the organ as well as the transverse diameter, described four groups of megaesophagus (Table 33–1). A group "0" was added for cases featuring no dilatation but diminished peristalsis, and the diagnosis was established by biologic and manometric criteria. The corresponding radiologic and anatomic findings are shown in Figures 33–5 and 33–6. Treatment decisions are based on this classification; the simpler myotomy is useful in less advanced cases (group I and II), and cardioplasty or occasionally esophageal resection is required for groups III and IV.

Endoscopy

Endoscopic examination is mandatory in the patient with megaesophagus before any surgical procedure. The organ should be emptied thoroughly to facilitate complete visualization of the esophagus and stomach as well as to rule out the presence of an associated carcinoma. The flexible fiberscope has the advantage of good maneuverability and superior optics. The examination is more hazardous, and the findings of dilatation, tortuosity, and friability

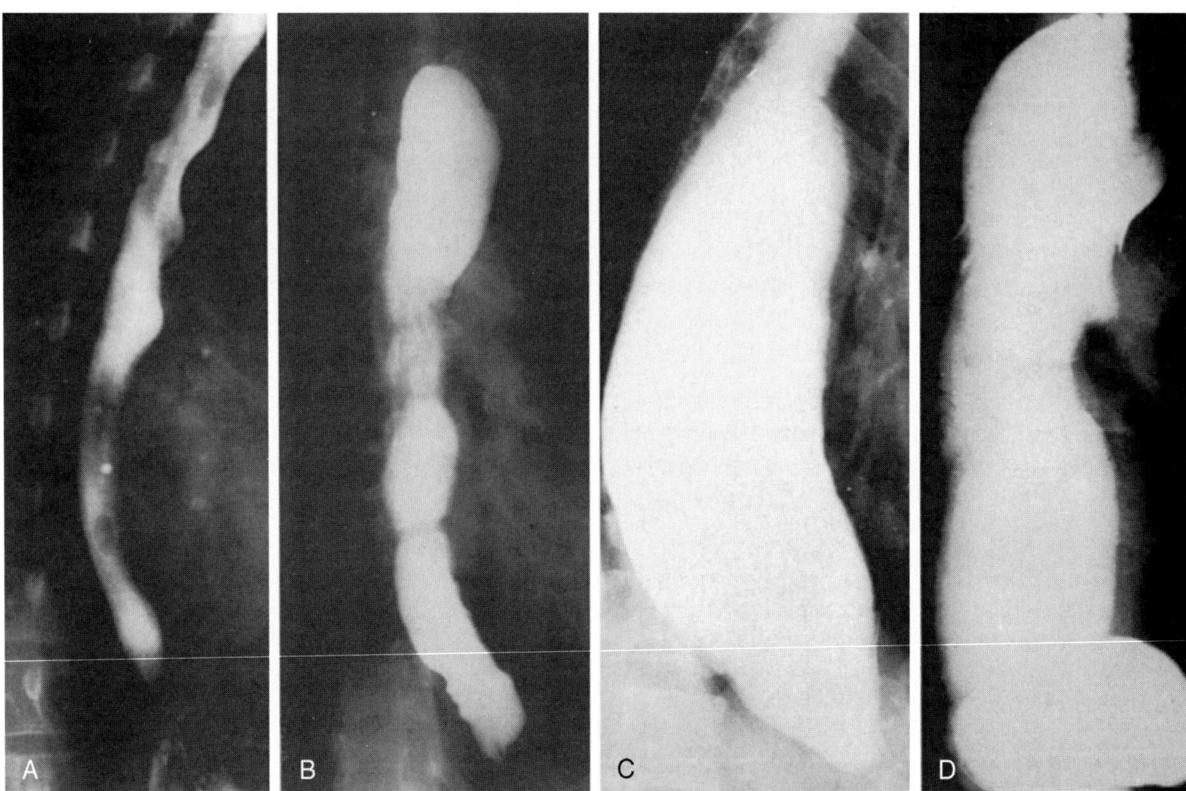

FIGURE 33–5 ■ Radiologic staging of megaesophagus in four groups based in a series of 450 surgically treated cases. *A,* Stage I, 11 patients (2.4%). *B,* Stage II, 136 patients (30.2%). *C,* Stage III, 163 patients (36.2%). *D,* Stage IV, 140 patients (31.1%).

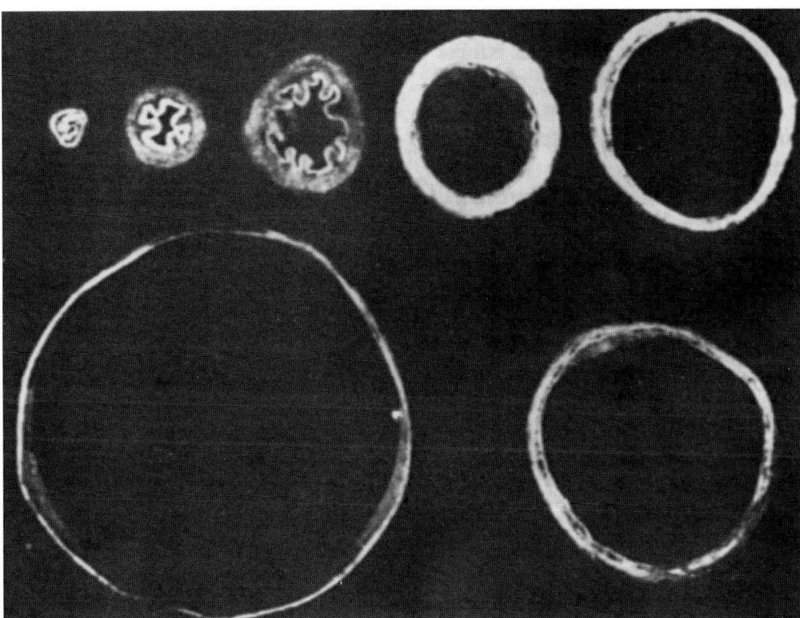

FIGURE 33–6 ■ Transverse diameter of normal esophagus *(upper left)* and the degrees of dilatation ranging from progressive hypertrophy to almost complete loss of the muscle wall and thinning. (From Koeberle F: Chagas Krankheit: Eine erkrankung der neurovegetative peripherre. Wien Klin Wochenschr 68:333, 1956.)

increase the risk of perforation. The dilatation is proportionate to the stage of the disease. Other findings described in patients include reflux esophagitis (6.4%), stasis esophagitis (3.1%), esophageal stenosis (1.3%), carcinoma (0.8%), hiatal hernia (0.7%), leukoplasia and ulcerations (0.4%), and varices (0.3%) (Rezende and Moreira, 1988).

Scintigraphy

Radioisotope scintigraphy has been used in esophageal disease to verify the transit time and dysfunction and to assess the therapeutic response to treatment. In this technique, in both the supine and sitting positions, the patient swallows a liquid or solid labeled with ^{99m}T sulfur colloid in an amount varying from 100 to 300 mCi of labeled material. Counts in the area of interest are made at fixed intervals (0.25 and 40 seconds) between the upper, middle, and lower thirds of the esophagus and stomach.

Rezende (1975) studied 13 healthy persons and 52 chagasic individuals in order to evaluate the esophageal transit time. He found an average esophageal transit time of 8.3 ± 2.2 seconds in the sitting position to be normal. When the esophageal transit time was longer than 40 seconds, he found two patterns, partial and total retention. In the cases with shuttling of material between the proximal and distal esophagus, the incoordination was classified as adynamic. Manometry confirmed the radioisotope studies in 88.5% of the author's cases. Absence of peristalsis was tantamount to retention in both sitting and supine positions, regardless of the motor status of the sphincter. However, when peristalsis was present in the upper third, partial retention was the rule.

Manometry

Pressure studies in patients with chagasic megaesophagus are particularly helpful in the initial stage of the disease and in the differential diagnosis regarding other esophageal motility disorders. Before the examination, it is important to evacuate the esophageal contents, including retained water, which may interfere with the interpretation of the results.

The basic findings in both idiopathic megaesophagus and Chagas' disease of the esophagus are lack of peristalsis, achalasia of the LES, elevation of its resting pressure, and heightened response to stimulation of the esophageal smooth muscle with cholinergic drugs. Upon deglutition in the normal individual, there are repetitive coordinated waves of contraction and opening of the LES (Fig. 33–7). In the chagasic patient, the coordinated movement of peristalsis disappears and is replaced by synchronous movement in all levels of the esophagus.

The upper esophageal sphincter (UES) is not altered in the patient with chagasic esophagus. The LES demonstrates achalasia in about 50% of patients with esophageal dilatation and in 80% of patients in whom the esophagus is dilated (Godoy, 1972; Pinotti, 1968). Total aperistalsis is seen only in advanced cases; the spontaneous motor activity of the esophagus is then caused by the stimulus produced by retained fluid, and once the esophagus is emptied, no peristalsis is seen.

The normal resting pressure of the LES varies between 7 and 17 mm Hg (average 12.7 ± 4.2); in a chagasic individual with grade II, it was 8 and 32 mm Hg (average, 19.9 ± 6.3), and in an individual with grade III, it varied between 13 and 37 mm Hg (average, 23.4 ± 6.5) (Paula-Costa and Rezende, 1978). Under normal circumstances, the LES relaxes completely with deglutition and no pressure gradient exists. In achalasic patients, a residual pressure between the stomach and esophagus effectively obstructs the cardia and contributes to stasis and dilatation. With surgery in the early stages of the disease, normal peristaltic waves may return in 10% to 30% of patients.

The denervated esophagus becomes hypertensive to cholinergic drugs such as bethanechol, pentagastrin, and cholecystokinin (Cannon's law). This motor response

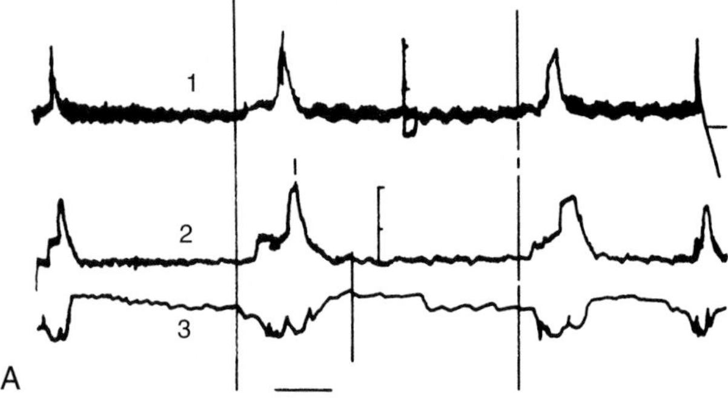

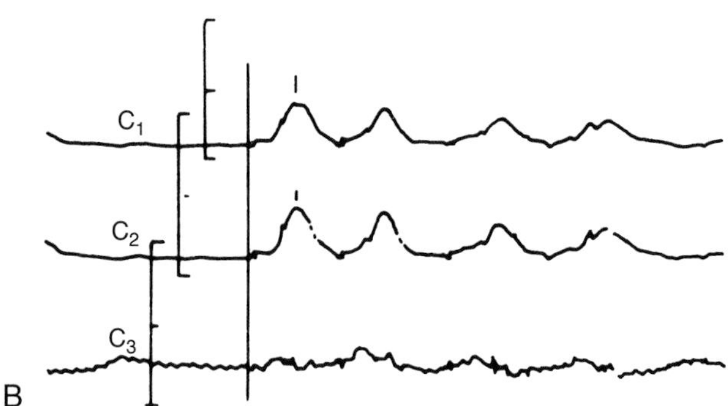

FIGURE 33–7 ■ Manometric tracings in a healthy individual *(A)* and in a chagasic patient *(B)*. The catheters were placed in the esophageal body and at the cardia. Note the peristatic waves and lower esophageal sphincter opening in the normal person and in the chagasic nonperistaltic contraction. (From Meneghelli VG: O esôfago na doneça de Chagas: Estudos fisiōlógicos, farmacológicos e clínicos. Arq Gastroenterol 24:177, 1987.)

may not be seen in the more advanced stages (groups III and IV) but is intense in earlier stages (Fig. 33–8).

MANAGEMENT

Chagas' megaesophagus is a benign disease that affects young people, and the treatment should be simple, straightforward, and capable of restoring the ability to eat as normally as possible. Morbidity and mortality rates should be close to zero.

In the acute phase of the disease, medical treatment is not only feasible but curative; in the intermediate and chronic stages, medical treatment is not advisable.

A nitrofuran derivative and a nitroimidazole are both effective drugs against trypomastigotes and amastigotes. The first is given daily in a dosage of 10 mg/kg body weight to adults and 15 mg/kg to children for 60 or 90 days, and benznidazole is used in a daily dosage of 5 to 10 mg/kg for 30 to 60 days. Allopurinol in a high dosage of 600 mg daily is being tried with promising results. For the established form of megaesophagus, pharmacologic therapy has been tried but found wanting.

Botulinum toxin injection in high-risk achalasia patients has been tried in several centers. Gordon and Eaker (1997) used 20 units of this substance in the four quadrants of the LES in 16 patients. Recurrent symptoms were noted in 32% of the patients, and within 6 months, one developed reflux, two were found to have esophageal wall inflammation. Loss of tissue planes and mediastinal adhesions were found at subsequent myotomy. Schiano and colleagues (1998) had identical results. In Chagas' megaesophagus, this drug has been used by Ferrari and coworkers (1995) but the short duration of response and untoward side effects suggesets caution.

Bougienage and Dilatation

Bougienage should not be undertaken as a primary form of treatment of megaesophagus because relief, if any, is of very short duration. Better results can be expected after pneumatic or hydrostatic balloon dilatation of the LES. Seventy-one percent of patients so treated improve, but 16% of them require more than one stretching (Table 33–2).

A good account of dilatation techniques is given by Earlam and Cunha-Mello (1981). The complications of forceful dilatation include intense pain, perforation, bleeding, aspiration, and gastroesophageal reflux leading to esophagitis and eventually stenosis as a late sequel. Table 33–3 lists the most commonly found complications.

Surgical Treatment

The question of forceful dilatation versus surgery as the initial treatment of megaesophagus has been debated for years. In many institutions, including ours, surgery is the primary form of treatment, with dilatation performed only rarely. There are few prospective randomized studies

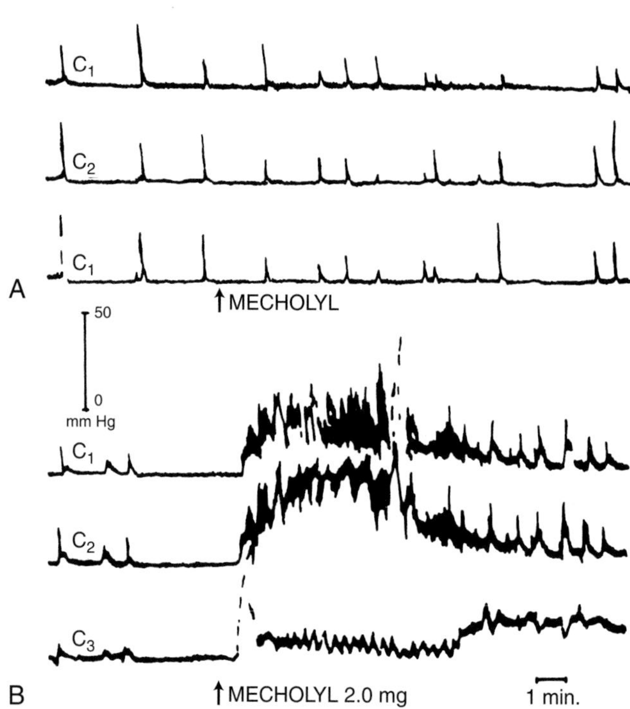

FIGURE 33–8 ■ Mecholyl test. In healthy people *(A)*, there is no response; in chagasic individuals *(B)*, there is hyperactivity. (From Meneghelli VG: O esôfago na doneça de Chagas: Estudos fisiōlógicos, farmacológicos e clinicos. Arq Gastroenterol 24:177, 1987.)

TABLE 33–2 ■ **Results of Pneumatic Dilatation for Achalasia**

Dilator	*No. of Patients*	*Improved (%)*	*Subsequent Dilatations (%)*	*Subsequent Surgery (%)*
Sippy	403	77	10	—
Browne-Moeller	50	58	38	10
Browne-McHardy	30	87	3	7
Browne-McHardy	45	86	16	2
Rider-Moeller	132	48	40	12
Mosher	37	54	11	22
Browne-McHardy	66	50	7	4
Rigiflex	24	52	8	4
Rigiflex	50	90	22	3
Witzel	45	78	11	7
Browne-McHardy	10	100	0	10
Rigiflex	10	70	20	10
Total	902	70.8	15.5	8.2

Modified from Ferguson MK: Achalasia: Current evaluation and therapy. Ann Thorac Surg 52:336, 1991. With permission from the Society of Thoracic Surgeons.

comparing both methods. Csendes and colleagues (1989) treated 39 patients by dilatation and 42 by operation. The results were considered good in 65% after dilatation compared with 95% after myotomy.

Felix and associates (1998) randomly assigned 40 patients for treatment, 20 by forceful dilation and 20 by myotomy. In their analysis, patients treated by surgery had a significantly greater reduction of the LES pressure and less reflux compared with those treated by dilatation. Anselmino and coworkers (1997) also found Heller's myotomy superior to dilatation in the treatment of achalasia in a group of 61 patients, 16 of whom had undergone surgical treatment.

As a rule, surgery should be performed in the following circumstances:

1. In advanced cases of megaesophagus associated with marked dilatation and tortuosity of the organ and difficult and hazardous positioning of the instrument.
2. In patients with associated disease, such as epiphrenic diverticulum, hiatal hernia, suspected carcinoma, cholelithiasis, or any other intra-abdominal pathologic process.
3. In patients with severe esophagitis and an esophageal wall that is friable and likely to split and perforate.
4. When previous surgery performed at the gastroesophageal junction has been unsuccessful.
5. In children and adolescents.
6. When patients prefer surgical therapy to dilatation and its implications.

Heller's Myotomy

Surgery for megaesophagus was first described by the German surgeon E. Heller, who performed the operation on April 14, 1913. The procedure was similar to a Ramstedt pyloromyotomy, with an anterior and posterior inci-

TABLE 33–3 ■ **Complications of Forceful Dilatation for Achalasia**

No. of Patients	*Perforation (%)*	*Aspiration (%)*	*Gastroesophageal Reflux Disease (%)*	*Mortality (%)*
408	3.4	—	1	0
124	1.6			
48	0	4.2	7.3	0
33	2.4	—	—	—
31	3.2	—	—	—
25	3.1	0	0	0
537	2.6	—	—	0.2
63	1.6	1.6	27	0
30	—	3.3	0	0
45	8.8	2.2	8.8	2.2
132	0.8	—	26	0
39	5.4	—	8	0
24	12.0	3	30	1.5
24	0	0	0	0
50	4	0	—	0
45	5	0	7	0
20	0	0	—	0
1678 (total)	3.4 (average)	1.4 (average)	10.5 (average)	0.27 (average)

Data from Reynolds JC, Parkman HP: Achalasia. Gastroenterol Clin North Am 18:223, 1989; and Ferguson MK: Achalasia: Current evaluation and therapy. Ann Thorac Surg 52:322, 1991.

sion, was later modified to a single incision by Groenvedeldt (1918) and Zaaijer (1923).

Several procedures were added to the myotomy, namely antireflux maneuvers with the gastric fundus, which also keep the edges of the myotomy apart and cover the esophageal mucosa as a protection in case of perforation. The most commonly used of these techniques are those described by Nissen (1951), Collis and colleagues (1954), Lortat-Jacob and coworkers (1956), Lind and associates (1965), Belsey (1966), Hill (1967), and Dor and coworkers (1967). Not all agree on the use of these added procedures, and there is even disagreement on the same procedure with different terms used, such loose, "floppy," or two-stitch fundoplication.

The critical point in all these ancillary procedures is the amount of gastric tissue that is placed around the gastroesophageal junction as a wrap. Andreollo and Earlam (1987) addressed this question, analyzing 5002 cases of achalasia, and found no difference in the incidence of postoperative reflux when an antireflux procedure was done through either a laparotomy (7.4%) or a thoracic approach (7.3%). The 360-degree plication, as described by Nissen originally, should never be applied because it creates a barrier that contradicts the basic principle of lowering LES pressure. We and others have demonstrated this (Ellis, 1997; Ellis et al, 1986; Fékété et al, 1982; Topart, 1992; Ximenes-Netto, 1987).

Laparoscopic myotomy has been used by several groups to treat esophageal achalasia. Vogt and colleagues (1997) reported 20 patients treated laparoscopically, 18 of whom also had undergone a Toupet fundoplication. Morbidity (35%) included five mucosal injuries, one bile leak, one splenic tear, and 20% reflux. The hospital stay ranged from 2 to 20 days with an average of 5 days. Maher (1997) reported that 21 patients had a conversion rate of 14% (3 patients). With increasing knowledge and technology, a laparoscopic Heller myotomy may become the method of choice (Spiess and Kahrilas, 1998).

The points that we consider important for a successful cardiomyotomy are listed in the accompanying box. The Heller myotomy and the fundoplication (Dor's) are shown in Figure 33–9. Results of the modified Heller myotomy in series with 25 cases or more and in a 20-year period are shown in Table 33–4.

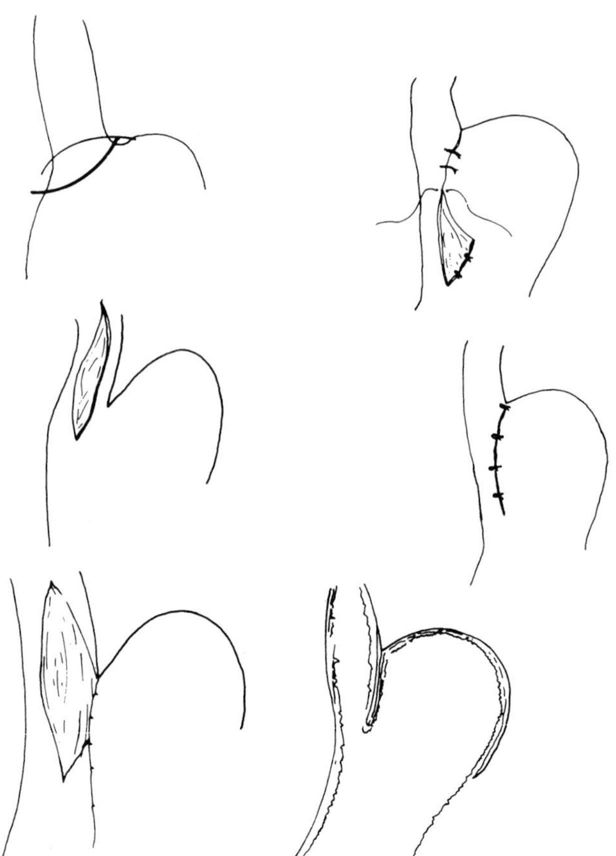

FIGURE 33–9 ■ Esophageal cardiomyotomy and anterior fundoplication.

IMPORTANT STEPS FOR A SUCCESSFUL CARDIOMYOTOMY

1. The stomach should be emptied just before surgery with a large-bore gastric tube.
2. Avoid a long incision entering the gastric wall. Stop at the first gastric vessels.
3. Avoid a short proximal incision, which may result in incomplete myotomy; up to 6 to 8 cm is sufficient.
4. Dissect the hypertrophied esophageal muscle around 50% of its circumference.
5. Never use a complete wrap around the esophagogastric junction, such as a Nissen fundoplication. It defeats the purpose of lowering the pressure in the lower esophageal.
6. A loose, 180-degree fundoplication, placed anteriorly, keeps the esophagus intra-abdominally (at least 4 cm), keeps the edges of the myotomy apart, and seals any perforation.
7. Look for an associated hiatal hernia and repair it.
8. No nasogastric tube is necessary.
9. A liquid diet may be offered on the day of surgery, and the patient may be discharged within 24 to 48 hours.

In advanced megaesophagus (stages III and IV), the Heller myotomy does not offer as good results as in less advanced cases. For this reason, we have used the principles of the onlay gastric patch as described by Thal and Hatafuku (1964), Thal and colleagues (1965), and Hatafuku and colleagues (1972).

After the original description of the cardioplasty by Wendel (1910), many modifications were made by several surgeons. The main drawback of these procedures is the reflux that follows if no other measures are taken to prevent it. After experimental work, Thal and associates (1965) demonstrated that a peptic stricture at the gastroesophageal junction could be incised and a fold of gastric fundus could be placed in such a manner that it would cover the defect. The operation was later applied to the

TABLE 33–4 ■ **Results of Esophagocardiomyotomy**

Approach	*Fundoplication*	*Results (No. of Patients) Good/Excellent (%)*	*Mortality (%)*	*Subsequent Reoperation (%)*	*Gastroesophageal Reflux Disease*
Thoracic	No	50 (78)	—	—	—
Thoracic	Yes	95 (87)	0	3	4
—	—	75 (75)	1.3	—	—
Thoracic	Yes	25 (80)	0	—	12
Thoracic	Yes	39 (79)	0	—	18
Abdominal	Both	108 (66)	0	—	19
Thoracic	No	48 (92)	5.8	4	8
Thoracic	No	102 (81)	0	—	6
Thoracic	No	25	12	—	36
Abdominal	Yes	118 (95)	0	—	5
Thoracic	No	121 (80)	0	7	52
Thoracic	No	456 (85)	0.2	—	3
Abdominal	Yes	49 (90)	2	0	0
Thoracic	Yes	32 (90)	0	0	12
Abdominal	No	103 (95)	—	—	17
Abdominal	Yes	58 (94)	0	3	6
Both	Yes	39 (64)	1.3	0	31
Thoracic	No	63 (68)	0	5	13
Abdominal	Yes	50 (76)	0	10	6
Thoracic	No	40 (95)	0	0	3
Abdominal	Yes	31 (95)	0	—	6
Abdominal	Yes	90 (88)	0	4	11
Thoracic	Yes	52 (95)	0	—	5
Thoracic	Yes	34 (95)	0	0	3
Thoracic	Yes	36 (94)	3	11	11
Thoracic	No	65 (80)	0	0	5
Both	Both	305 (96)	0.6	1.6	—
Thoracic	No	123 (92)	—	5	6
Thoracic	Yes	38 (88)	0	3	0
Abdominal	Yes	100 (92)	0	0	1
Both	Yes	43 (87)	0	0	26
Thoracic = 18 Abdominal = 9 Both = 3	Yes = 17 No = 11 Both = 2	2,613 (86)	0.93	3	12

treatment of megaesophagus electively, in case of rupture of the gastroesophageal junction, or as a remedial operation following unsuccessful treatment of megaesophagus (Ximenes-Netto, 1996; Ximenes-Netto et al, 1978, 1982). The ingenious part of this procedure is the insertion of a gusset of adjacent gastric wall in such a manner that the serosa faces into the lumen, creating an endoluminal valve.

The technique consists of full mobilization of the esophagogastric junction followed by a longitudinal full-thickness incision through the narrow segment, 6 to 8 cm in the proximal esophagus and 1 to 2 cm into the stomach (Fig. 33–10). If necessary, a few stitches are placed transversely to widen the posterior wall of the gastroesophageal junction. The next step is the formation of an antireflux valve, which is performed with three initial stitches placed parallel between the gastroesophageal junction and the gastric wall, at a point 4 cm on the angles and 2 cm in the middle. Additional suturing completes the valve.

The gastric onlay is then performed with the gastric fundus, which is sutured to the esophageal opening with interrupted nonabsorbable sutures. A few short gastric vessels may be ligated to better mobilize the gastric fundus. The completed procedure is shown in Figure 33–11.

The antireflux valve has been demonstrated both in experimental animals and in humans to be competent and capable of avoiding gastroesophageal reflux. The results of the Thal procedure have been well documented in the Brazilian literature, especially in cases of advanced megaesophagus. The results are shown in Table 33–5.

Manometric studies by Barichello and coworkers (1975) after the fundic patch operation showed the disappearance of vigorous achalasia (contractions) in more than half of the cases. One may assume an improvement of smooth muscle function because of the relief of obstruction and the absence of food stasis in the esophageal lumen after the operation. Radiologic studies performed 3 years after the Thal cardioplasty demonstrated decreases of the caliber of the esophagus to half its original size and of esophageal emptying time to less than 30 minutes in advanced disease (Fig. 33–12).

The esophageal emptying time determined with a ^{99m}Tc–diethylenetriaminepentaacetic acid (DPTA) meal also revealed a diminished curve. We were also unable to demonstrate the presence of reflux after ingestion of a 10-ml bolus of water containing 300 mCi of ^{99m}Tc sulfur colloid (Ximenes-Netto et al, 1988). This test is performed after the patient swallows substances through the mouth, pharynx, and esophagus into the stomach with

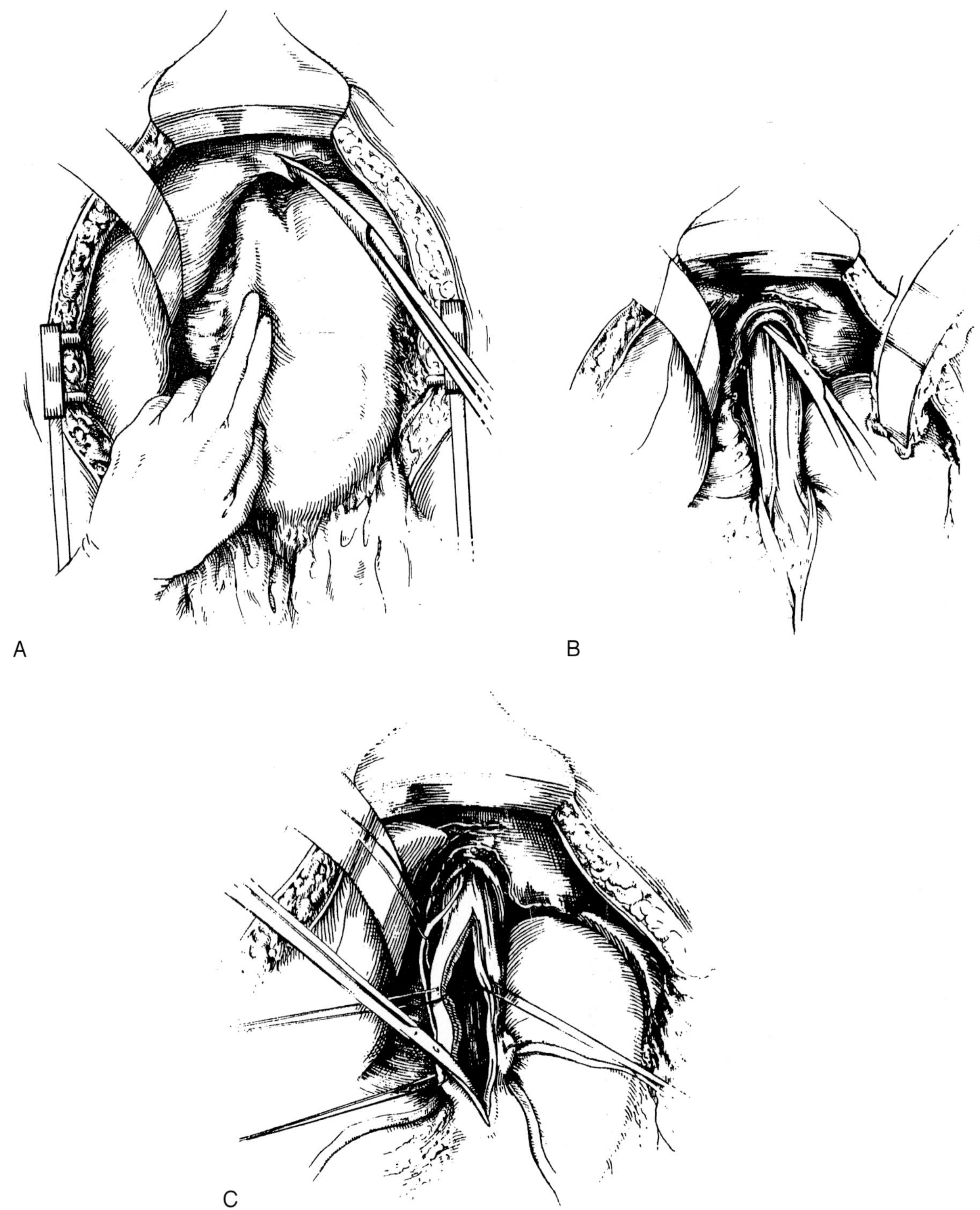

FIGURE 33–10 ■ Technique of cardioplasty with an endoluminal valve (Thal procedure). *A,* Midline laparotomy and section of the left triangular live ligament. *B,* Exposure of the gastroesophageal junction. *C,* Opening of the gastroesophageal junction 6 to 8 cm above and 2 cm below. (Courtesy H. Barreto, M.D.)

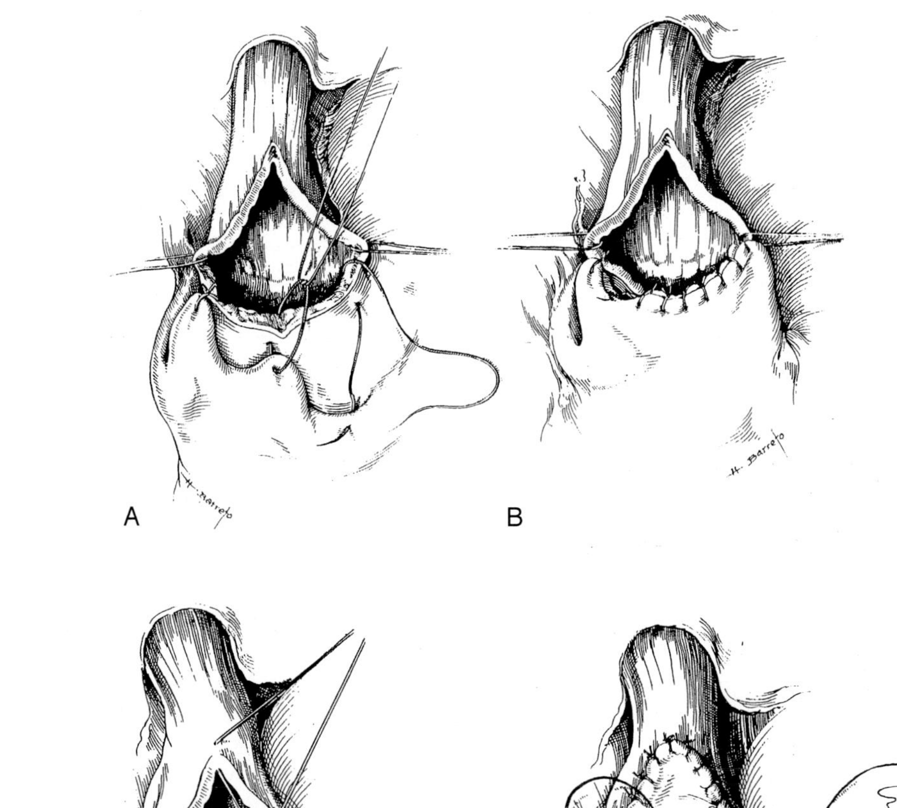

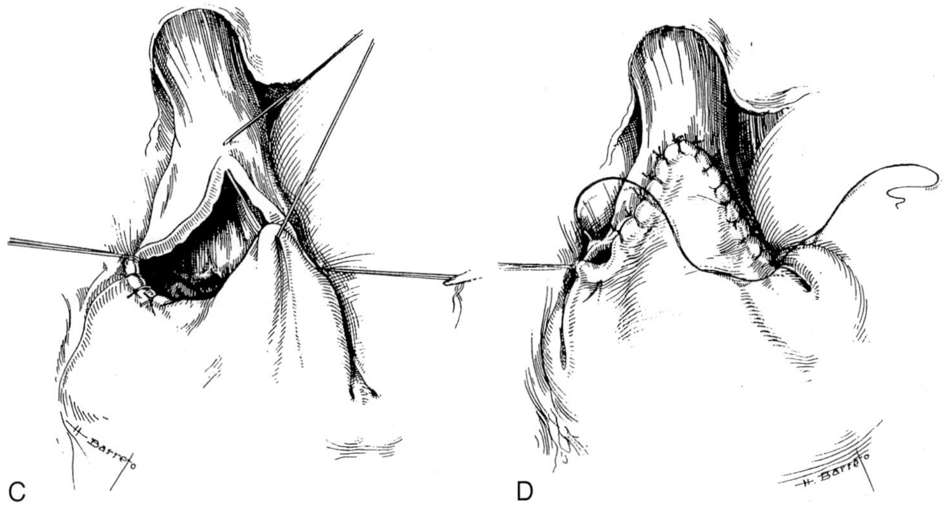

FIGURE 33–11 ■ Cardioplasty and endoluminal valve (Thal procedure). *A,* Endoluminal valve with sutures placed at the ends (4 cm) and in the middle (2 cm). *B,* Completion of the valve. *C,* Closure of the gastroesophageal junction opening with the gastric fundus and ventral surface of the stomach in a "V" shape. *D,* The procedure is completed. (Courtesy of H. Barreto, M.D.)

recording by a gamma camera. A single dry swallow is completed 30 seconds later. The procedure is repeated with another radionuclide bolus, and the radioactivity counts are averaged to obtain the final transit pattern. The data from the gamma camera are transferred to a microprocessor, where they are converted into a graphic display of radioactivity plotted against time for each area of interest.

Esophagectomy

Total removal of the thoracic esophagus in patients with Chagas' disease was first proposed in Brazil by Camara-Lopes and Ferreira-Santos (1958, 1961). The esophagectomy, with or without deliberate opening of the pleural cavities, has been performed for advanced Chagas' megaesophagus or as a remedial operation by several groups and championed by Ferreira (1973), Pinotti and col-

TABLE 33–5 ■ **Results of the Thal Operation in Chagas Megaesophagus (Brazilian Literature)**

Author	*No. of Cases*	*Mortality (%)*	*Morbidity (%)*	*Results (Good/Excellent)*
Barbosa et al (1989)	351	1.4	7.4	100
Ximenes-Netto et al (1991)	210	0.9	4.6	97
Malafaia et al (1981)	111	0	4.5	99
Sader et al (1975)	28	0	0	85.6
Guarino (1975)	20	0	10	92
Brandalise et al (1979)	20	0	0	70.3
Nakadaira et al (1977)	15	0	6.6	93.3
Total	755	0.32	4.7	91.02

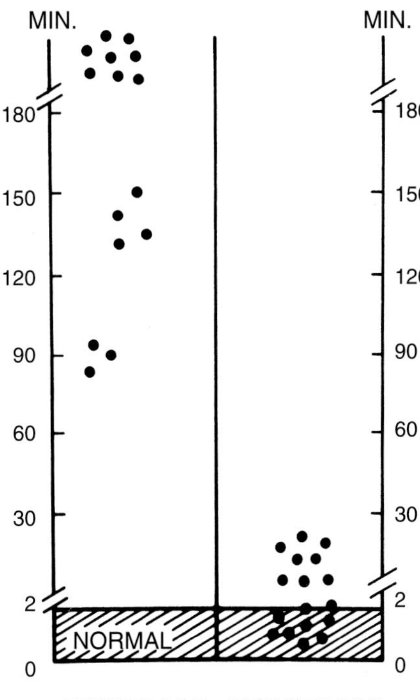

FIGURE 33–12 ■ Esophageal emptying time measured with a standard barium meal preoperatively and postoperatively, demonstrating that following surgery the time is reduced to less than 30 minutes 3 years later.

leagues (1981), Orringer and Stirling (1989), and Miller and associates (1995). These authors claim that there is a potential risk of malignancy in the dilated esophagus or that other lesser procedures are of no avail, thus justifying the removal of the organ. In our experience, the risk of malignant change is quite low, 2.2% in a series of 450 surgically treated patients (Ximenes-Netto et al, 1987).

Other experienced surgeons discount the value of esophagectomy, whether to prevent cancer, to correct stasis, or because other operations have failed. Hiebert (1989) questioned the logic of substituting one nonperistalsing bag for another. The Thal procedure or other lesser operations have been favored by Ximenes-Netto (1989, 1996), Ximenes-Netto and coworkers (1978), Mendelsohn and colleagues (1984), and Ellis (1989). The results of esophagectomy for achalasia are shown in Table 33–6.

Other Procedures

Excision of the gastroesophageal junction and replacement by a piece of jejunum or the ileocecal valve has been proposed as a form of definitive treatment of megaesophagus. Reporting on 170 patients with a jejunal interposition, DaSilva and coauthors (1987) found a mortality rate of 5.9% and complications in 31.8%. de Rezende (1973), in a series of 113 patients, reported two early deaths (1.7%) and two late ones. Complications included infection, intestinal obstruction, invagination of the transposed jejunum, fistula, duodenal obstruction, and obstruction of the transplanted bowel. Rassi (1979) reported a 14.2% death rate albeit with good results in 54% of patients.

Barbosa (1973) transplanted the ileocecal valve in 23 patients with Chagas' megaesophagus. Three of them died in the postoperative period (13%), and seven had good results (73.9%). Esophagectomy and replacement of the esophagus with the transverse colon have been used by Rassi (1979) in advanced stages of the disease in a two-stage operation. Among 48 cases that were followed, he reported three postoperative deaths (2.6%) and many complications: fistula (28%), pulmonary infection (10.9%), wound infection (23.6%), and hemothorax (9%).

Because of the large number of complications and high death rate, these procedures have not had many followers.

In cases of recurrence, antrectomy and Roux-en-Y diversion and resection of the stenotic gastroesophageal junction or esophageal gastric anastomosis has been used with much success (90%) by Ellis (1997).

COMMENTS AND CONTROVERSIES

Chagas' disease of the esophagus is a chronic, disabling affliction that affects thousands of predominantly young people. It is not malignant, and it behooves the surgeon to keep the therapy simple and safe. In Ximenes' hands, the best way to achieve these twin goals in patients with stage I and II disease is by a simple myotomy with or without a partial nonobstructing fundoplication. As with primary achalasia, the trick is to relieve the obstruction without causing reflux—a tall order, but one ordinarily achievable with morbidity and mortality close to 1%.

For patients with more advanced disease, stages III or IV, or when lesser procedures have failed, a cardioplasty

TABLE 33–6 ■ **Mortality and Complications Following Transhiatal Esophagectomy for Megaesophagus**

Author	*No. of Cases*	*Mortality (%)*	*Morbidity (%)*
Ferreira (1973)	120	2.5	22.8
Pinotti et al (1981)	108	3.7	39.9
Ferreira-Santos (1964)	54	3.0	—
Orringer and Stirling (1989)	26	3.8	21.7
Cunha (1981)	20	10	25
Pareja et al (1978)	11	0	62.7
Total	339	3.8	34.42

From Ximenes-Netto M: Megaesophagus: Current review of techniques and results. Rev Saude DF 2:209, 1991.

of the Thal type may be done. Esophageal resection is seldom indicated except for cancerous degeneration.

C. A. H.

KEY REFERENCES

Ferguson MK: Achalasia: Current evaluation and therapy. Ann Thorac Surg 52:336, 1991.

This article reviews current treatment of achalasia, with an analysis of large series, and indicates the various forms of treatment of this condition over the past 20 years.

Rezende JM: The digestive tract in Chagas disease. Mem Inst Oswaldo Cruz 79:106, 1984.

The author, who has one of the largest experiences in the world with Chagas' disease, analyzes all the aspects of this entity when it affects the digestive tract. The radiologic findings as well as the basic concepts regarding the electromanometry are described in detail.

World Health Organization (WHO): Chagas disease, Brazil: Interruption of transmission. Wkly Epidemilog Rep 75:153, 2000.

This technical report demonstrates epidemiologic and entomologic data showing a diminishing curve of vectorial transmission of Chagas disease in Brazil as a result of the national control program. This represents one insect per 10,000 houses, an infestation rate far below the minimum required for effective transmission of the parasite to new patients.

Ximenes-Netto M: Megaesophagus: Current review of techniques and results. Rev Saude DF 2:209, 1991.

All aspects of the treatment of Chagas' megaesophagus are analyzed, including the newest techniques that are available for the surgical treatment of this condition. Analysis of the results in large collected series is reported. An account of the oldest techniques is also given in a historical perspective.

REFERENCES

Allgrove J, Glayden GS, Grant DB, et al: Familial glucocorticoid deficiency with achalasia of the cardia and deficient tear production. Lancet 1:1284, 1978.

Amorim M, Correa Neto A: Histopatologia c patogênese do megaesofago e megarecto. Considerações em torno de um caso de "mal de engasgo." An Fac Med Univ Sao Paulo 8:101, 1932.

Andreollo NA, Earlam RJ: Heller's myotomy for achalasia: Is an added anti-reflux procedure necessary? Br J Surg 74:765, 1987.

Anselmino M, Perdikis G, Hinder RA, et al: Heller myotomy is superior to dilatation for the treatment of early achalasia. Arch Surg 132:233, 1997.

Barbosa H: Cardiectomia com interposição ileo-ceco-cólica no tratamento do megaesofago chagasico. Rev Goiana Med 19:137, 1973.

Barbosa H, Barichello AW, Viana AL, et al: Tratamento cirurgico do megaesôfago chagásico: Duas décadas de experiencia numa região endemica. Rev Goiana Med 35:1, 1989.

Barichello AW, Vianna AL, Souza JAG, et al: Chagas' megaesophagus: Manometric studies before and after Thal's fundic patch operation. G E N 30:25, 1975.

Belsey R: Benign strictures of the esophagus. Proc Soc Med 59:932, 1966.

Brandalise NA, Lconardi LS, Mantovani ME, Fagundes JJ: Tratamento cirúrgico do megaesôfago: Estudo comparativo entre duas técnicas de cardioplastia. Rev Col Bras Cir 6:117, 1979.

Camara-Lopes LH: Carcinoma of the esophagus as a complication of megaesophagus. Am J Dig Dis 6:742, 1961.

Camara-Lopes LH, Ferreira-Santos RE: Indicação seletiva do processo de Heller, da ressecção parcial e da ressecção subtotal do esofago no tratamento cirurgico do megaesôfago. Rev Paul Med 52:269, 1958.

Cançado JR: Doença de Chagas. Belo Horizonte, MG, 1968.

Chagas C: Tripanosomiase americana: Forma aguda da moléstia. Mem Inst Oswaldo Cruz 8:37, 1916.

Collis JL, Kelly TD, Wilwi AM: Anatomy of the crura of the diaphragm and the surgery of the hiatus hernia. Thorax 9:175, 1954.

Csendes A, Braghetto I, Mascaro J, Henriquez A: Late subjective and objective evaluation of the results of esophagomyotomy in 100 patients with achalasia of the esophagus. Surgery 104:469, 1988.

Csendes A, Braghetto I, Henriquez A, Cortes C: Late results of prospective randomised study comparing forceful dilatation and oesophagomyotomy in patients with achalasia. Gut 30:299, 1989.

Cunha EBC: Esofagectomia subtotal com anastomose esôfago-gástrica cervical transmediastinal sem toracotomia para tratamento de megaesôfago. Rev Col Bras Cir 8:159, 1981.

DaSilva AL, Conceição SA, Silva MLA: Interposição de alça jejunal no tratamento do megaesôfago chagásico. Rev Assoc Med Bras 33:94, 1987.

Dor J, Humbert P, Paoli JM, et al: Traitement du reflux par la technique ditte Heller-Nissen modifié. Press Med 75:2563, 1967.

Earlam R, Cunha-Melo JR: Benign oesophageal strictures: Historical and technical aspects of dilatation. Br J Surg 68:829, 1981.

Ellis FH Jr: Esophagectomy for achalasia: Who, when, and how much? Ann Thorac Surg 47:334, 1989.

Ellis FH Jr: Failure after esophagomyotomy for esophageal motor disorders: Causes, prevention and management. Chest Surg Clin North Am 7:477, 1997.

Ellis FH Jr, Crozie RE, Gibbs P: Reoperative achalasia surgery. J Thorac Cardiovac Surg 22:859, 1986.

Fékété F, Breil P, Tossen JC: Reoperation after Heller's operation and other motility disorders of the esophagus: A study of eighty-one reoperations. Int Surg 67:103, 1982.

Felix VN, Cecconello I, Zilberstein B, et al: Achalasia: A prospective study comparing the results of dilatation and myotomy. Hepatogastroenterology 108:97, 1998.

Ferrari AP, Siqueira ES, Brant CQ: Treatment of achalasia in Chagas' disease with botulinum toxin. N Engl J Med 23:824, 1995.

Ferreira EAB: Esofagectomia por via cérvicoabdominal combinada: Sua possivel utilização no megaesôfago. Rev Paul Med 82:133, 1973.

Ferreira-Santos R: Aperistalsis of the esophagus and colon (megaesophagus and megacolon) etiologically related to Chagas disease. Am J Dig Dis 6:700, 1961.

Ferreira-Santos R: Tratamento cirurgico do Megaesofago. In Cançado JR (ed): Doença de Chagas. Imp. Oficial, 1964, p 592.

Freitas JLP: Contribuição para o estudo do diagnóstico da moléstia de Chagas por processos de laboratório. Tese, São Paulo, S.P., Faculdade de Medicina da Universidade de São Paulo, 1946.

Godoy RA: Estudo da esofagopatia cronica por medio do método eletromamométrico e da prova de metacolina em pacientes corn e sem dilatação do esôfago. Rev Goiana Med 18:1, 1972.

Gordon JM, Eaker EY: Prospective study of esophageal botulinum toxin injection in high-risk achalasia patients. Am J Gastroenterol 92:1812, 1997.

Groenvedeldt DFR: Over cardiospassmus. Ned Tijdschr Ogeneesk 2:281, 1918.

Guarino JL: As operações de Thal no tratamento do megaesôfagor. Thesis, Universidade Federal Fluminense, Niteroi, RJ, 1975.

Hatafuku T, Maki T, Thal AP: Fundic patch operation in the treatment of advanced achalasia of the esophagus. Surg Gynecol Obstet 134:617, 1972.

Heller E: Extramukose kardioplastic beim chroniischen kardiospasmus mit dilatation des oesophagus. Mitt Grenzeg Med V Chir 45:141, 1914.

Hiebert CA: In discussion of esophageal resection for achalasia. Ann Thorac Surg 47:334, 1989.

Hill LD: An effective operation for hiatal hernia: An eight year appraisal. Ann Surg 166:681, 1967.

Koeberle F: Chagas krankheit: Eine erkrankumg der neurovegetative peripherie. Wien Klin Wochenschr 68:333, 1956a.

Koeberle F: Patogenia dos megas. Rev Goiana Med 2:105, 1956b.

Koeberle F: Uber das neurotoxin des trypanosoma cruzi. Zentribl Pathol 95:468, 1956c.

Koeberle F: Patogenia da moléstia de Chagas. Rev Goiana Med 3:55, 1957.

Koeberle F: Megaesophagus. Gastroenterology 34:460, 1958.

Koeberle F, Alcantara FG: Esôfagoneuropatias perifericas. Rev Goiana Med 35:81, 1989.

Koeberle F, Penha PD: Chagas megaesophagus. Z Tropenmed Parasitol 10:291, 1959.

Laranja FS, Dias E, Nóbrega G: Estudo cletrocardiográfico de 81 casos de megaesôfago. Mem Inst Oswaldo Cruz 46:473, 1948.

Lind JF, Bums CM, MacDouglas JJ: Physiological repair for hiatus hernia: Manometric study. Arch Surg 91:233, 1965.

Lortat-Jacob JL, Binet JP, Mailard JN: La prévention des hémorragies digestives aprés opération de Heller. Assoc Fr Chir 58:162, 1956.

Maher JW: Thoracoscopic esophagomyotomy for achalasia: Maximum gain, minimal pain. Surgery 122:836, 1997.

Malafaia O, Brenner S, Silva JT, et al: Tratamento cirúrgico do megaesôfago pela técnica de Thal. Rev Col Bras Cir 8:II1, 1981.

Mendelsohn P, Vianna AL, Barichello AW, et al: Megaesôfago chagásico recidivado: Tratamento pela cardioplastia à Thal. Rev Goiana Med 30:97, 1984.

Meneghelli VG: O esôfago na doença de Chagas: Estudos fisiológicos, farmacológicos e clinicos. Arq Gastroenterol 24:177, 1987.

Miller DL, Allen MS, Trastek VF, et al: Esophageal resection for recurrent achalasia. Ann Thorac Surg 60:922, 1995.

Nakadaira A, Benedito JM, Galetti H, et al: Tratamento do megaesôfago pela técnica de Thal. Rev Assoc Med Bras 20:371, 1977.

Nissen R: Gastropexy and fundoplication in surgical treatment of hiatal hernia. Am J Dig Dis 6:954, 1951.

Orringer MB, Stirling MC: Esophageal resection for achalasia: Indications and results. Ann Thorac Sung 47:859, 1989.

Pareja JC, Lacerda JC, Amorim JF, et al: Tratamento cirúrgico do megaesôfago grau IV pela técnica de Ferreira. Rev Assoc Med Bras 24:66, 1978.

Paula-Costa MD, Rezende JM: Pressão basal do esfincter inferior do esôfago no megaesôfago chagásico. Rev Assoc Med Bras 24:269, 1978.

Pinotti HW: Contribuição para o estudo da fisiologia do megaesôfago. Rev Goiana Med 14:137, 1968.

Pinotti HW, Zilberstein B, Pollara W, Raia A: Esophagectomy without thoracotomy. Surg Gynecol Obstet 152:345, 1981.

Rassi L: Critério seletivo na indicação da técnica cirúrgica para o megaesôfago chagásico. Rev Goiana Med 25:85, 1979.

Reynolds JC, Parknan HP: Achalasia. Gastroenterol Clin North Am 18:223, 1989.

Rezende JM: Classificação radiológica do megaesôfago. Rev Goiana Med 28:187, 1982.

Rezende JM Jr: Estudo cintilográfico do transito esofagiano na esofagopatia chagásica. Thesis, Faculty of Medicine, University of São Paulo, 1975.

Rezende JM, Moreira H: Chagasic megaesophagus: Historical review and present concepts. Arq Gastroenterol 25:32, 1988.

Rezende JS: Tratamento cirúrgico do megaesôfago chagásico: Operação de Merendino. Rev Goiana Med 19:169, 1973.

Sader AA, Carneiro JJ, Brasil JCF, et al: Gastroesofagoplastia de Thal modificada. Rev Assoc Med Bras 21:72, 1975.

Schiano TD, Parkman HP, Miller IS, et al: Use of botulinum toxin in the treatment of achalasia. Dig Dis 16:14, 1998.

Spiess AE, Kahrilas PJ: Treating achalasia: From whalebone to laparoscope. JAMA 280:638, 1998.

Thal AP, Hatafuku T: Improved operation for esophageal rupture. JAMA 188:386, 1964.

Thal AP, Hatafuku T: Improved operation for esophageal rupture. JAMA 188:826, 1965.

Thal AP, Hatafuku T, Kurtzman R: Operation for distal esophageal stricture. Arch Surg 90:464, 1965.

Topart P, Deschamps C, Taillefer R, Duranceau A: Long-term effect of total fundoplication on the myotomized esophagus. Ann Thorac Surg 45:1046, 1992.

Vianna G: Contribuição para o estudo da anatomia patológica da moléstia de Chagas. Mem Inst Oswaldo Cruz 3:276, 1911.

Vogt D, Curet M, Pitcher D, et al: Successful treatment of esophageal achalasia with laparoscopic Heller myotomy and Toupet fundoplication. Am J Surg 174:709, 1997.

Wendel W: Zur chirurgic des oesophagus. Arch Klin Chir 93:311, 1910.

Ximenes-Netto M, Andrade FOS, Cavalcanti RA, Miranda PEB: Reoperação no megaesôfago chagásico. Rev Bras Cir 66:323, 1978.

Ximenes-Netto M, Silva RO, Fleury I Jr: Thal's procedure in the management of ruptured Chagas megaesophagus. G E N 36:142, 1982.

Ximenes-Netto M, Silva RO, Fleury I Jr: Fistula traqueoesofagiana benigna: Tratamento pela exclusão bipolar c reconstrução pelo tubo gástrico invertido. Rev Bras Cir 75:151, 1985.

Ximenes-Netto M, Marra O, DeBiase H, et al: Primary surgical treatment of Chagas megaesophagus. Results of 450 cases. HFA Pub Tec Cient 2:147, 1987.

Ximenes-Netto M, Motta HJ, Piauilino MA, Ramos RN: Pesquisa de refluxo gastroesofagiano no pós operatório do megaesofago chagásico. Rev Col Bras Cir 15:75, 1988.

Ximenes-Netto M: Esophageal perforation due to pneumatic dilation for achalasia. Surg Gynecol Obstet 168:2263, 1989.

Ximenes-Netto M, Silva RO, Vicira LF, et al: Megaesôfago Chagásico. Resultados do tratamento em 537 cases. Ann XVI Meeting Brazilian Coll Surg, 1991.

Ximenes-Netto M: Esophageal resection for recurrent achalasia. Ann Thorac Surg 62:324, 1996.

Ximenes-Netto M, Gaiotto FTC: Distúrbios da motilidade esofagiana. Clin Bras Cir 2:221, 1997.

Zaaijer JH: Cardiospasmus in the aged. Ann Surg 77:615, 1923.

CHAPTER **34**

Secondary Esophageal Motor Disorders

Jocelyne Martin
Pasquale Ferraro
André Duranceau

A wide range of diseases and conditions, in addition to idiopathic motor disorders, affect normal esophageal function. The aim of this review is to identify secondary esophageal motor dysfunctions and their characteristics and to clarify the role of surgery, when indicated, in managing these conditions. A classification of secondary esophageal motor disorders is given in Table 34–1.

Collagen Diseases

SCLERODERMA

Definition

Progressive systemic sclerosis (PSS), or generalized scleroderma, is a multisystem disease of unknown cause. It is characterized by sclerosis of small arteries and arterioles associated with an abnormal amount of collagen and connective tissue deposition. This results in induration and thickening of the skin, Raynaud's phenomenon and other vascular abnormalities, musculoskeletal manifestations, and visceral involvement (LeRoy et al, 1988). It may affect many organs, especially the lungs, heart, and kidneys. The gastrointestinal (GI) tract is affected in its entire length, and collagen is found deposited in the lamina propria, the submucosa, and the serosa. It is involved in 60% of patients with symptomatic scleroderma. The esophagus is considered the most common of affected sites (Poirier and Rankin, 1972).

Scleroderma exists as a localized or a systemic disease process. Its localized form is confined to the skin and adjacent tissues and can be classified as linear or morphea. The systemic form of the disease, however, is responsible for the functional abnormalities that cause the patient to consult for lung or esophageal problems. The diagnosis of scleroderma is confirmed when:

1. Sclerodermatous changes in the skin of the hand and feet are observed.
2. Sclerodactyly, digital pitting scars, and bibasilar pulmonary fibrosis are present.

Scleroderma is rare. The annual reported incidence in the United States is 19 cases per 1 million persons, and this rate has remained stable since the 1980s. The prevalence based on hospital consultation is estimated to be 250 cases per 1 million persons (Mayes, 1997). The reported female-to-male ratio varies between 3:1 and 8:1. This ratio is higher during early adult life and becomes considerably lower in later years (Silman, 1997). The peak age of onset is around 50 years. Disease expression may be influenced by genetic, ethnic, and environmental factors (Mayes, 1996).

TABLE 34–1 ■ Secondary Esophageal Motor Disorders

1. *Collagen diseases*
   a. Scleroderma
   b. Systemic lupus erythematosus
   c. Polymyositis, dermatomyositis
2. *Peripheral neuropathy*
   a. Diabetic neuropathy
   b. Alcoholic neuropathy
3. *Infectious esophagitis*
   a. Parasitic (Chagas' disease)
   b. Viral (Behçet's syndrome)
4. *Psychiatric disorders*

Historical Note

The word *scleroderma* is derived from the Greek words *skleros* ("hard") and *derma* ("skin"). The term was first used in 1847 by Gintrac. However, different terminology had been used to describe at least three patients with scleroderma earlier in the European literature (Benedek and Rodnan, 1982).

In 1870, Day reported PSS in an American patient. Scleroderma had been considered a rarity in the United States more so than in Europe (Benedek and Rodnan, 1982). Epidemiologic studies, however, suggest that the disease occurs more commonly in the United States than anywhere else (Mayes, 1997). Ehrman (1903) reported the association of progressive dysphagia and scleroderma (Treacy et al, 1963). This was regarded as coincidental until Matsui (1924) recognized from his observations at autopsy that the visceral involvement is an inherent component of the disease. In 1945, Goetz in Capetown confirmed that scleroderma is a multiorgan disease, and he suggested the term *progressive systemic sclerosis*. He considered this to be more appropriate and descriptive than *scleroderma*, which refers to only one symptom of a systemic disease (Benedek and Rodnan, 1982).

Interestingly, art is a source of description for diseases like scleroderma. The painter Ford Madox Brown (1821–1893), who was linked stylistically and ideologically to pre-Raphaelism, probably was the first and only artist to portray systemic sclerosis in figurative art (Borroni, 1985). His 1857 portrait "Take Your Son, Sir," conserved at the Tate Gallery in London, renders a realistic portrait of a woman with an expressionless face, taut skin and loss of normal facial lines, cheeks with erythrosis, constricted opening of the mouth, tense skin on her fingers, and hardened and stiff appearance of the joints. He never finished or sold his painting, and his work was considered blasphemous, sordid, meaningless, and prosaic.

Paul Klee (1879–1940), an influential Swiss artist of the 20th century, was diagnosed with scleroderma at the age of 57. Although his productivity declined after his diagnosis, he adapted his style by using black crayon lines with his deformed hands. Klee's last themes centered around fear and death, reflecting his disfigured body, or at least how he perceived his illness. One of his drawings, entitled "Durchhalten!" ("Endure!"), shows a totally disfigured face. His work illustrated how a person with a chronic distorting disease may feel and suffer (Wolf, 1999).

Pathogenesis

In systemic sclerosis, the pathology is mostly found at the vascular and microvascular levels. There is perivascular and tissue infiltration by mononuclear inflammatory cells with increased deposition of normal matrix components in the skin and visceral organs. This deposition appears to be a response to disruption of the normal steady state of connective tissue turnover and regulated repair (Black, 1995). Theories on the etiology of systemic scleroderma have concentrated on abnormalities of the microvasculature, cytotoxic factors that may cause those anomalies, fibroblast/matrix interactions, abnormalities of the immune system, and the role of genetic and environmental factors.

The widespread vascular abnormalities have encouraged investigators to suggest that there is a vascular basis for the pathogenesis of the disease. Some evidence suggests that the capillary bed is the primary site of injury, sometimes resulting in diffuse devascularization of multiple tissues (Norton and Nardo, 1970). Scleroderma patients show a decrease in the absolute number of capillary loops in the nail folds of the fingers. The remaining capillary loops show dilatation and distortion with frank hemorrhage and reduced flow. Raynaud's phenomenon and telangiectatic lesions in patients with scleroderma are examples of these vascular abnormalities.

In contrast to large-vessel lesions, lesions of small arteries and arterioles have been observed in almost every organ. Medial hypertrophy and marked intimal proliferation are present with irregular narrowing of vascular segments. Concentric fibrosis of the intima has been found in lung and renal arterioles. Vessel-related changes also include increased platelet activity, decreased red blood cell deformability, and enhanced thrombus formation (Murrell, 1993).

The exact cause of the initial vascular injury is still not well understood. The release of oxygen free radicals secondary to noxious conditions (ischemic, autoimmune/inflammatory, or chemical) and causing necrosis of endothelial cells is one of many hypotheses (LeRoy, 1996; Murrell, 1993). Another vascular factor has been found to be the increased level of endothelin reported in the circulation of patients with scleroderma. Endothelins are the most potent vasoconstrictors known, and they have a fibrotic potential (Black, 1995). In health, the vasoconstrictive action of endothelin is balanced by the opposing action of nitric oxide. An imbalance between those two mediators may affect patients with scleroderma.

The activated immune system may play a role in causing tissue damage in these patients (White, 1996). Whether activation of the immune system is an initial or a secondary event in the disease process is unknown.

Few studies have focused on the histologic changes and the pathogenesis of esophageal involvement in scleroderma. D'Angelo and colleagues (1969) found that the esophagus was pathologically abnormal in 74% of patients with scleroderma. Smooth muscle atrophy or fibrosis, or both, is present, affecting the lower two thirds of the esophagus. These lesions affect the lower esophageal sphincter (LES) as well. None of the control subjects showed these abnormalities.

Treacy and associates (1963) reported that scleroderma involved mostly smooth muscle. They also found intimal proliferation in small arteries and collagen deposition in the adventitia, and they observed that the upper portion of the esophagus showed a relatively normal motor function that corresponded to the segment of striated muscle unaffected by the disease. Still, some segments showed decreased contraction strength despite a normal histologic appearance. These authors stated that histologic observation may not be adequate to demonstrate the first physiologic changes of scleroderma. The absence of collagen abnormalities in the stroma of the muscle or in the submucosa suggested that esophageal muscle did not undergo degeneration from the pressure or invasion of the proliferating collagen in the sclerotic tissue.

Studies of pharmacologic and hormonal agents have provided interesting insights into the pathogenesis of scleroderma-associated esophageal motility disorders. Cohen and colleagues (1972) compared the LES responses to methacholine, a parasympathomimetic agent that acts directly on muscle receptors, with LES responses to edrophonium, a cholinesterase inhibitor, and to gastrin I, acting through the release of acetylcholine. In response to direct stimulation by methacholine, the LES of scleroderma patients shows the same percent increase in pressure as in normal patients. The administration of edrophonium or gastrin, however, resulted in a significantly lower percent response in patients with scleroderma with diminished baseline peristalsis than in the normal control group.

These findings suggest that the initial lesion is a neural dysfunction and that smooth muscle atrophy is superimposed on an already existing neural problem. The mechanism responsible for this neural dysfunction has yet to be determined.

Clinical Features

Two forms of generalized scleroderma are described: (1) diffuse cutaneous systemic sclerosis and (2) limited cutaneous systemic sclerosis (LeRoy et al, 1988; Silver, 1991). Two of five cases are of the diffuse type. Differentiation between those two subsets is important in order to identify patients at risk for development of visceral complications.

Diffuse cutaneous systemic sclerosis is characterized by truncal and acral skin involvement, usually sclerodactyly, digital pitting, scarring, and bibasilar pulmonary fibrosis. The typical patient experiences an abrupt onset of fatigue and swollen hands, feet, and face associated with Raynaud's phenomenon. The widespread skin involvement may be present initially or develop over a period of a few months. It most commonly affects young or middle-aged women. These patients should be monitored closely for visceral involvement because early and significant lung disease, oliguric renal failure, and GI and myocardial disease may develop.

Limited cutaneous systemic sclerosis presents with skin involvement limited to the hands, face, and feet. The typical patient is older and describes the onset of Raynaud's phenomenon many years before presentation. Progressive slow thickening of the digits and hands associated with facial telangiectasis is usually present. Ten years or more may pass before the appearance of GI hypomotility, interstitial lung disease, or pulmonary hypertension. The limited cutaneous group includes patients with what was previously called the *CREST syndrome* (calcinosis, Raynaud's phenomenon, esophageal dysfunction, sclerodactyly, and telangiectasis).

GI disease is the most commonly recognized visceral manifestation of systemic sclerosis. In scleroderma patients who have clinical evidence of GI tract involvement, the esophagus is affected in 75% of the patients. When esophageal disease is present, the stomach, small bowel colon, and rectum are usually affected by the same process. Heartburn and dysphagia are the most frequent presenting symptoms. Heartburn is present in 50% to 80% of patients affected with scleroderma.

Sour-tasting regurgitation due to the reflux of acid and/or biliopancreatic juice into the esophagus is detected in approximately 50% of patients. This acid or mixed reflux results from an incompetent LES with the added failure of the esophageal body to clear the refluxate. However, 25% of the scleroderma patients assessed by Stentoft and colleagues (1987) and De Castro Parga and associates (1996) are asymptomatic despite significant pathology being identified in the esophagus.

In a prospective evaluation of 262 patients with scleroderma, Abu-Shakra and co-workers (1994) confirmed that heartburn or dysphagia developed in 80% of patients within 2 years of the diagnosis of scleroderma. Decreased saliva production and poor gastric emptying add to the complexity and severity of reflux disease in these patients.

The symptoms of heartburn do not differentiate the burning sensation of reflux from the infectious esophagitis appearing in stagnant secretions of the atonic esophagus. Dysphagia is present in up to 75% of patients (Weston et al, 1998), secondary to either disturbed motor function or esophagitis and stricture. When a fibrotic stricture develops, dysphagia usually increases in frequency and severity, in correlation with esophageal wall damage. If esophageal dysmotility is documented, 70% of patients report dysphagia. When ulcerative esophagitis is present, 75% of patients mention this symptom. If an esophageal stricture is identified, all patients experience dysphagia (Abu-Shakra et al, 1994). Dysphagia may also appear when a significant monilial infection is present.

Esophageal symptoms almost always indicate the presence of an abnormal esophagus (Abu-Shakra et al, 1993, 1994, 1995). However, the absence of symptoms does not exclude advanced dysfunction or mucosal disease of the esophagus; at least 25% of asymptomatic patients show abnormal results during investigation (Lock et al, 1997). Raynaud's phenomenon is considered the most important clinical finding associated with the esophageal motor dysfunction seen in patients with scleroderma (Stevens et al, 1964). These early studies suggested a direct relationship between the presence of the symptom and esophageal dysfunction.

Hurwitz and associates (1976) observed a correlation between Raynaud's phenomenon and the loss of peristalsis but without any correlation with the strength of the esophageal contraction. The presence, duration, and severity of Raynaud's phenomenon did not influence the strength of the smooth muscle contraction in the esophagus.

Patients with scleroderma, because of the nature of the disease, may present with other symptoms that suggest dysfunction of the alimentary tract. Nausea and vomiting are seen with delayed gastric emptying. Colicky abdominal pain was often associated with diarrhea (53%) or with constipation (31%). Fecal incontinence was observed in 13% of patients (Weston et al, 1998); fecal impaction must be ruled out in patients with these symptoms. Abnormal motor function may be present in the stomach, small bowel, and colon, causing discomfort related to the absence of transit. Symptoms may be similar to those of mechanical bowel obstruction. Secondary bacterial proliferation usually plays a role in altering absorption and nutrition, resulting in steatorrhea. Weight loss is common.

The prevalence of lung disease ranks second to GI tract disorders. Dyspnea and hypoxemia result from interstitial inflammation and fibrosis with secondary alveolocapillary block. These symptoms may also result from pulmonary hypertension in the absence of parenchymal lung disease. Proteinuria, urea retention, and hypertension occur in 45% of patients with systemic sclerosis. Heart disease becomes manifest with heart failure, arrhythmias, conduction disturbances, or chest pain, each of which may be the result of vascular disease and fibrosis (Silver, 1991).

Natural History

Survival is influenced by the presence and severity of internal organ involvement. Patients with diffuse systemic scleroderma are more susceptible to early and serious visceral diseases. Their prognosis from the onset of disease is significantly reduced compared with the prognosis of patients with limited cutaneous systemic sclerosis (LeRoy et al, 1988). Patients who present with the limited form of the disease die of other causes, such as cancer.

Fortunately, advances in the treatment of visceral involvement have led to a decrease in morbidity and mortality rates. Most notable are the use of angiotensin-converting enzyme (ACE) inhibitors in renal crisis and dialysis in renal failure (Mayes, 1997). Scleroderma lung disease has become the most common cause of death (Abu-Shakra and Lee, 1995; Silver, 1991). GI disease does not constitute a significant risk factor for death but contributes to the complications of systemic sclerosis (Mayes, 1996).

Using life-table analysis, a study estimated the global 3-, 6-, and 9-year survival rates at 86%, 76%, and 61%, respectively; compared with survival of the general population, there is a 4.7-fold increase in the risk of death among patients with systemic scleroderma (Abu-Shakra and Lee, 1995). The increased mortality rate seems to be linear over time (Silman, 1991).

The risk of cancer is also increased among patients with systemic sclerosis. The age-standardized incidence rate for all cancers in patients with scleroderma is approximately twice the overall rate in the general population. Lung and breast cancers and possibly non-Hodgkin's lymphoma are the most frequent. Lung carcinomas develop in the presence of pulmonary fibrosis (Abu-Shakra et al, 1993; Rosenthal et al, 1993). Esophageal adenocarcinomas develop in patients with long-standing reflux disease who have a columnar-lined esophagus. The reason cancers occur more frequently in patients with systemic sclerosis is unknown. Immunologic abnormalities may result in an altered immune response with predisposition to subsequent development of cancer.

In addition to typical reflux symptoms, scleroderma patients may complain of recurrent pulmonary infections, nocturnal cough, and morning hoarseness. Reflux disease may influence pulmonary disease resulting from occult aspiration. A significant association exists between esophageal dysmotility and reduced lung volumes (total lung capacity and forced vital capacity) and diffusion capacity (Lock et al, 1998).

Two hypotheses may explain these findings: (1) the direct effect of esophageal hypomotility on pulmonary function by repeated episodes of reflux causes microaspirations or (2) there is simultaneous involvement of esophageal and pulmonary tissues by the scleroderma process. This issue remains unresolved (Johnson et al, 1989).

The precise incidence of esophageal complications is difficult to obtain. Most observations concern patients with symptoms of varying durations.

Esophageal Investigation

Radiologic

Fraser (1966), Neschis and colleagues (1970), and Clements and associates (1979) compared their cineradiographic observations with motor function recordings in scleroderma patients. The pharynx and proximal esophagus usually show normal function. There is loss of normal activity at the junction of the proximal third and the distal two thirds of the esophageal body. Mild distention, absent or diminished peristalsis, and gravity-type emptying with a "waterfall effect" are usually observed (Figs. 34–1 to 34–3). Esophageal emptying in the recumbent position is greatly delayed. At times, marked dilatation can be observed. Intraesophageal air seen on lateral chest films can be interpreted as evidence of a common cavity between the esophagus and stomach. When seen with radiologic changes of pulmonary fibrosis, this finding suggests scleroderma (Dinsmore et al, 1966). The esophageal junction is often patulous as a result of the absence

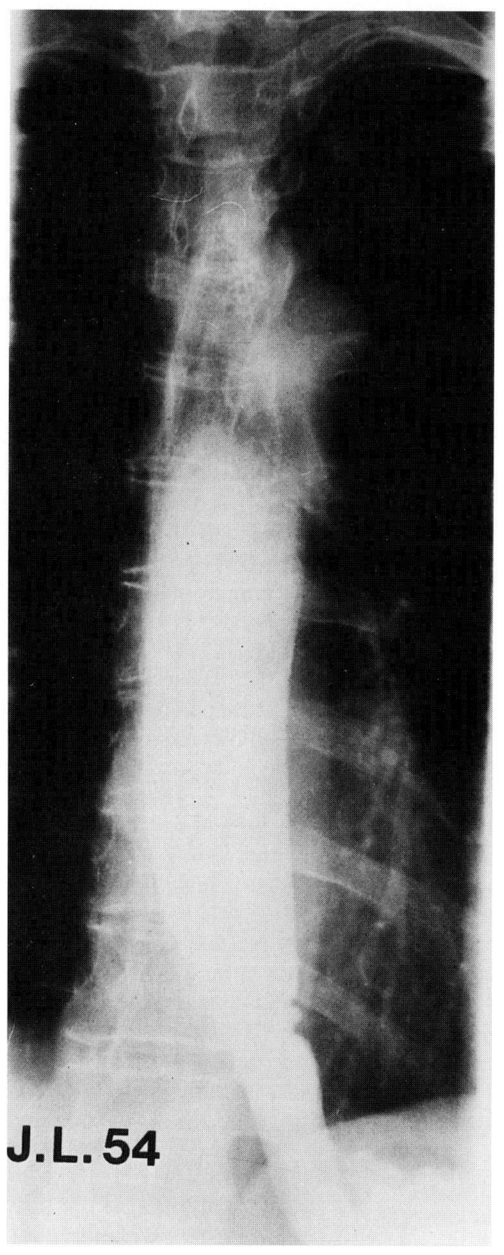

FIGURE 34–1 ■ Esophagogram of a patient with scleroderma. The esophagus is dilated, showing a loss of contractility mostly in the distal two thirds of the esophageal body.

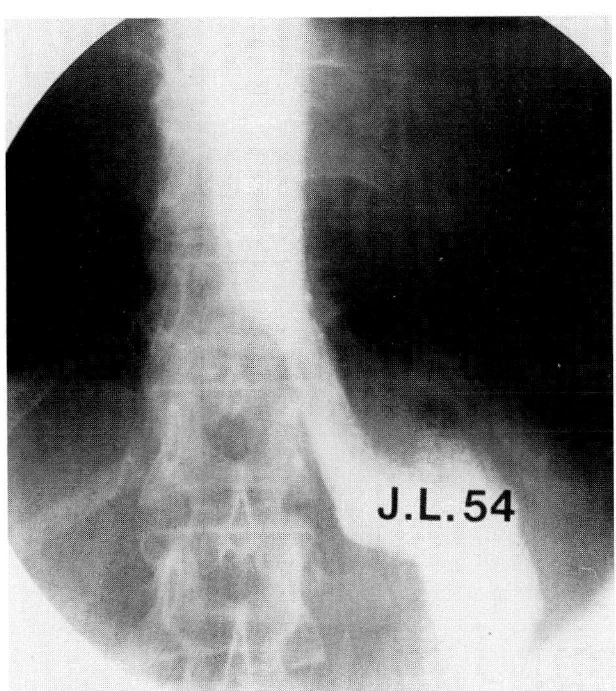

FIGURE 34–2 ■ Patulous gastroesophageal junction with free reflux observed between the stomach and the esophagus.

of LES resting tone, and free gastroesophageal reflux (GER) is commonly seen (Clements et al, 1979; Neschis et al, 1970; Yarze et al, 1993).

Although hiatal hernias are reported as frequent, this finding usually suggests a shortened esophagus with the mucosal folds of Barrett's mucosa. There is often evidence of active mucosal ulcers with a cobblestone appearance. Peptic strictures are observed more often in patients with scleroderma than in patients with idiopathic reflux (25% versus 53%), a sign of long-standing severe GER disease. Duodenal dilatation, delayed small-bowel transit, and colonic sacculation (pseudodiverticulum) are additional clues to the diagnosis when radiologic evaluation of the lower digestive tract is obtained.

Clements and associates (1979) suggested the radiologic evaluation of the esophagus as a first investigation, followed by esophageal motility studies, to document motor dysfunction.

Esophageal Emptying Scintiscan

The emptying radionuclide esophagram provides quantitative information on the functional abnormalities suggested by the radiologic evaluation. This technique was used by Drane and associates (1986) and Carette and associates (1985) as a detection test for impaired motility. In their observations, the loss of emptying capacity was proportional to the loss of distal esophageal muscle tone as recorded in motility studies.

Kaye and colleagues (1996) also used scintigraphic methods to screen patients with scleroderma for esophageal disease and to offer a new grading system for dysmotility. In their 301 patients, 246 (82%) had evidence of hypomotility. Grading patients from 0 (normal) to 4 (severe abnormality), these authors observed that 60% of patients in grades 1 and 2 had no symptoms of dysphagia. In patients with more severe (grades 3 and 4) symptoms, dysphagia correlated with the increase in severity. Radionuclide esophageal scanning characteristically shows prolongation of total transit time, often associated with delayed clearance of the esophagus for more than 60 seconds (Carette et al, 1985; Geatti et al, 1991). Compared with manometry, radionuclide transit shows a high sensitivity but lacks specificity.

The esophageal scintigram is a useful noninvasive test for detecting asymptomatic disease and providing comparative data during follow-up or after medical or surgical management.

Manometric Recording

Esophageal manometry is considered the most sensitive indicator of abnormal motility in patients with scleroderma. When patients with or without esophageal symptoms are investigated with manometry, 80% demonstrate an abnormal tracing (Bassotti et al, 1997).

Recording motor function of the esophagus in scleroderma is useful in assessing the stage of progression of the motor disturbance. These motor abnormalities may vary greatly among patients and do not depend on the duration of the disease or on the duration or severity of Raynaud's phenomenon.

Because scleroderma affects primarily smooth muscle, the striated muscle of the pharynx, upper esophageal sphincter, and cervical esophagus functions normally. The abnormal function can be identified immediately above

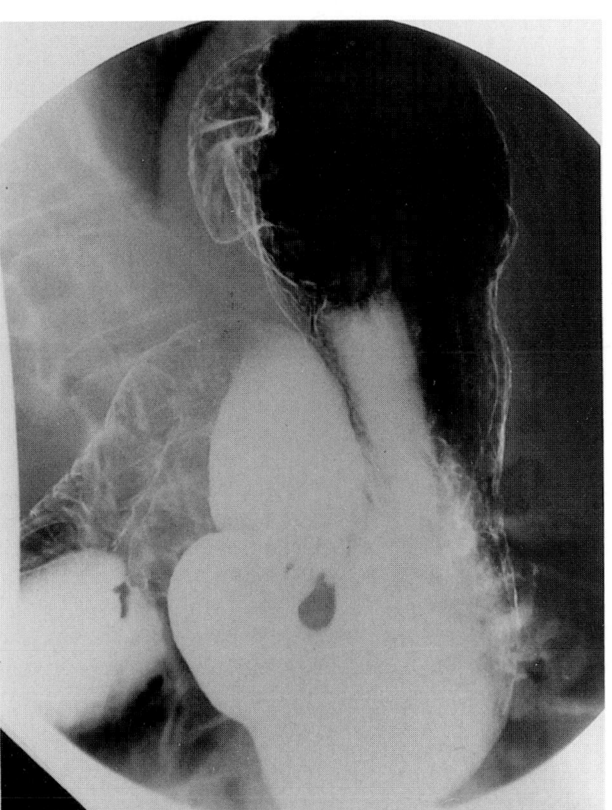

FIGURE 34–3 ■ Long atonic stomach with prolonged emptying.

the aortic arch where peak contraction pressures become weak and peristalsis is lost (Fig. 34–4*D*). This pattern of abnormal contractions is seen over the total length of the distal esophagus. The LES is frequently hypotonic and lacks adequate closing pressures. In some patients, no high-pressure zone can be identified between the esophagus and stomach. In such a situation, the stomach and esophagus form a common cavity and pressure increases in the abdominal cavity are transmitted directly into the esophagus (Fig. 34–4*E*).

Neschis and associates (1970) found LES hypotension to be an early motor abnormality in scleroderma. Treacy and colleagues (1963), however, suggested that dysfunction in the esophageal body with loss of peak contraction pressure could precede LES incompetence.

As reported by Hurwitz and colleagues (1976), four patterns of motility recordings are seen in patients with scleroderma (Fig. 34–4*A–E*):

First (and rarely), the patient reveals normal motor function in the esophageal body with the LES at the limits of hypotension. Only 1 of 12 patients reported by Hurwitz and colleagues (1976) showed this pattern. In a series of operated patients by Poirier and colleagues (1994), only one showed normal propulsion in the smooth muscle esophagus with a hypotensive LES.

In the second form, peristalsis is lost but the wave amplitude and LES resting tone may be retained.

In a third category, esophageal body contractions lose propulsion and strength, but the LES persists as a high-pressure zone.

In the final pattern, the smooth muscle esophagus is totally nonfunctional with loss of propulsion, loss of contraction force, and complete absence of LES resting pressure. As a result of the varying progression of the disease in different individuals, it is not possible to predict which motor dysfunction pattern will ensue.

The complete absence of LES resting pressure, especially in conjunction with the absence of peristaltic activity, can be used as a prognostic index for the severity of the esophagitis and the response to treatment. Zamost and associates (1987) found that no scleroderma patient with normal motility had erosive esophagitis on endoscopy; however, none of the patients with esophagitis had normal motor function. Preventive measures should be offered even if the patient is asymptomatic.

The pathologic GER that appears in scleroderma is due to the esophageal dysmotility observed in these patients. Reflux symptoms usually do not appear until LES hypotension becomes manifest. Poor distal esophageal contractions and propulsion with low or absent LES function lead to higher and longer exposure to an acid and an often mixed refluxate containing biliopancreatic secretions.

Basilisco and associates (1996) observed that the esophagus in this situation clears only with gravity, that this clearance is significantly delayed when the patient is supine, and that both the absence of propulsion and the poor contraction amplitude are responsible for these abnormalities.

Weston and associates (1998) added the observation that poor gastric emptying in most of their patients added to the complexity and severity of the reflux disease.

Documentation of Acid and Biliopancreatic Reflux

Twenty-four-hour esophageal pH monitoring and 24-hour fiberoptic monitoring of bile in the esophagus are the most objective diagnostic methods to document the exposure of the esophageal mucosa to acid and biliopancreatic refluxates (Fig. 34–5). The severity and extent of GER in patients with PSS are most closely related to the integrity of distal esophageal peristalsis (Yarze et al, 1993; Zamost et al, 1987). Regardless of esophageal symptoms, Bassotti and associates (1997) documented pathologic reflux in 78% of patients with scleroderma. Scleroderma patients with esophagitis show more and longer reflux episodes than do patients without esophagitis.

Zamost and associates (1987) documented that 11 of 32 patients had total acid exposure times exceeding 20% of the study period and that 20% of the total recording time revealed the presence of acid in the esophagus. In contrast, patients without esophagitis had less than 8% acid exposure times.

Aubert and associates (1991) reported that 20 of their 46 patients had pathologic GER (43.5%). Erosive esophagitis was common in the patients. For these authors, symptoms of reflux with poor function of the LES and abnormal acid exposure during the night were good predictors of the presence of ulcerative esophagitis.

Stentoft and associates (1987) reported on 55 patients evaluated with esophageal motility studies and 12-hour pH monitoring. Pathologic reflux was documented in 30 of 39 symptomatic patients; 33% of patients with symptoms did not have reflux damage, whereas 25% of patients without symptoms had pathologic reflux.

Johnson and colleagues (1989) suggested that, in patients with scleroderma, diffusion abnormalities, as assessed with carbon monoxide testing, correlated with proximal and distal reflux episodes. One of their conclusions was that objective documentation of acid or bile reflux is essential to ensure proper orientation of treatment.

Yarze and associates (1993) found that excessive proximal esophagus exposure to acid is documented only in patients with absent distal peristalsis. Moreover, the severity and extent of GER are closely related to the integrity of distal esophageal peristalsis.

Shoenut and coworkers (1996) tested the reproducibility of ambulatory esophageal pH monitoring in eight patients with scleroderma and demonstrated very low intrapatient variability when the tests were conducted within two consecutive 24-hour recordings. Consequently, a high level of confidence can be placed in pH monitoring as an indicator of treatment efficacy. Similarly, ambulatory 24-hour fiberoptic measurement of bilirubin is expected to be accurate and objective for the measurement of intestinoesophageal reflux.

Esophageal reflux documentation provides a precise diagnosis and an objective assessment of the adequacy of treatment.

Endoscopy

The esophageal mucosal damage in the patient with scleroderma is best assessed with endoscopy. Frequent and prolonged episodes of GER may lead to erosive esophagi-

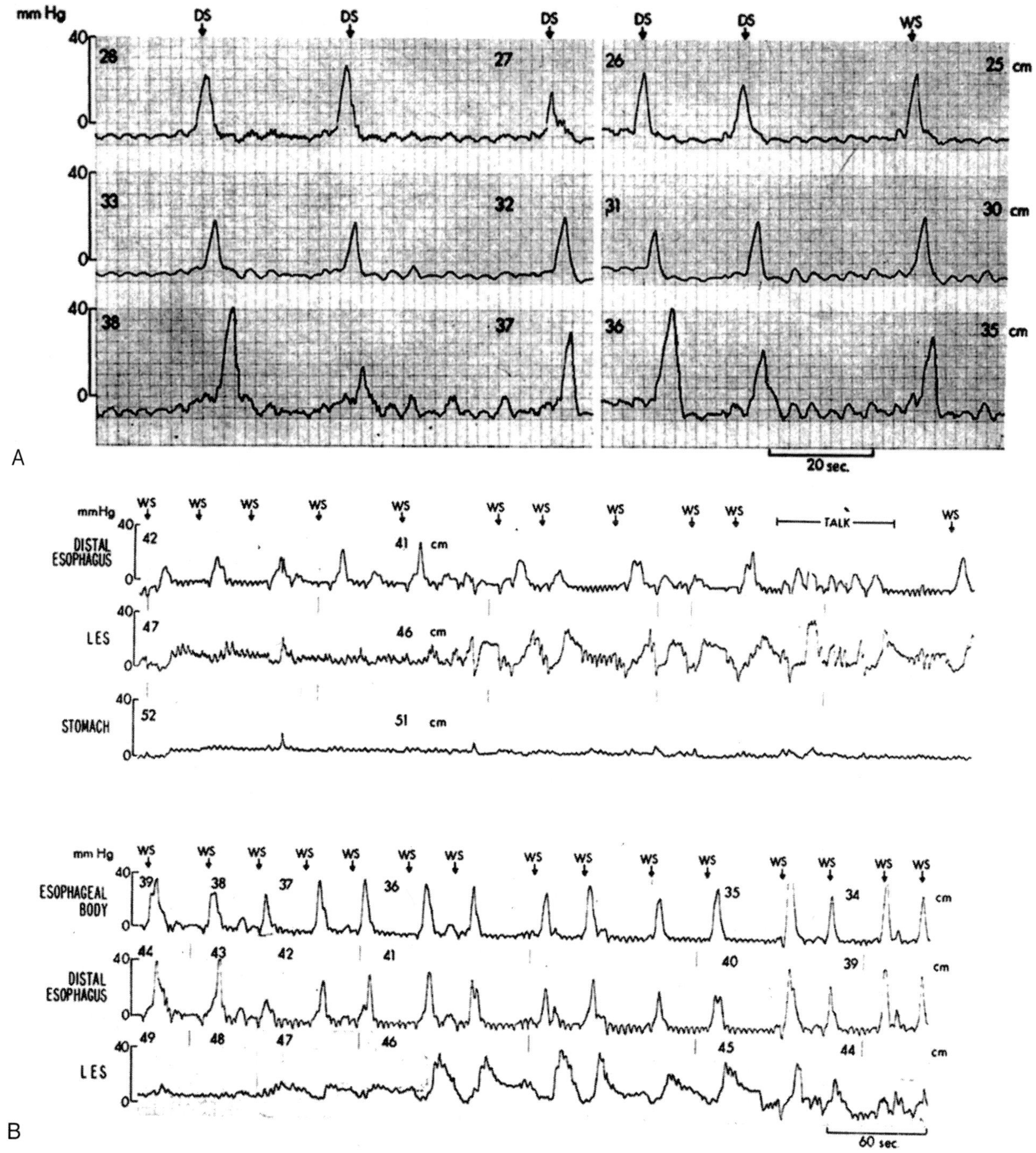

FIGURE 34–4 ■ *A,* Patterns of dysmotility in scleroderma. The contraction pattern in the esophageal body is interpreted as normal. The lower esophageal sphincter (LES) resting pressure in this situation can be normal or low. *B,* Loss of peristalsis in the esophageal body despite adequate contraction strength; the LES tone is retained.

Illustration continued on following page

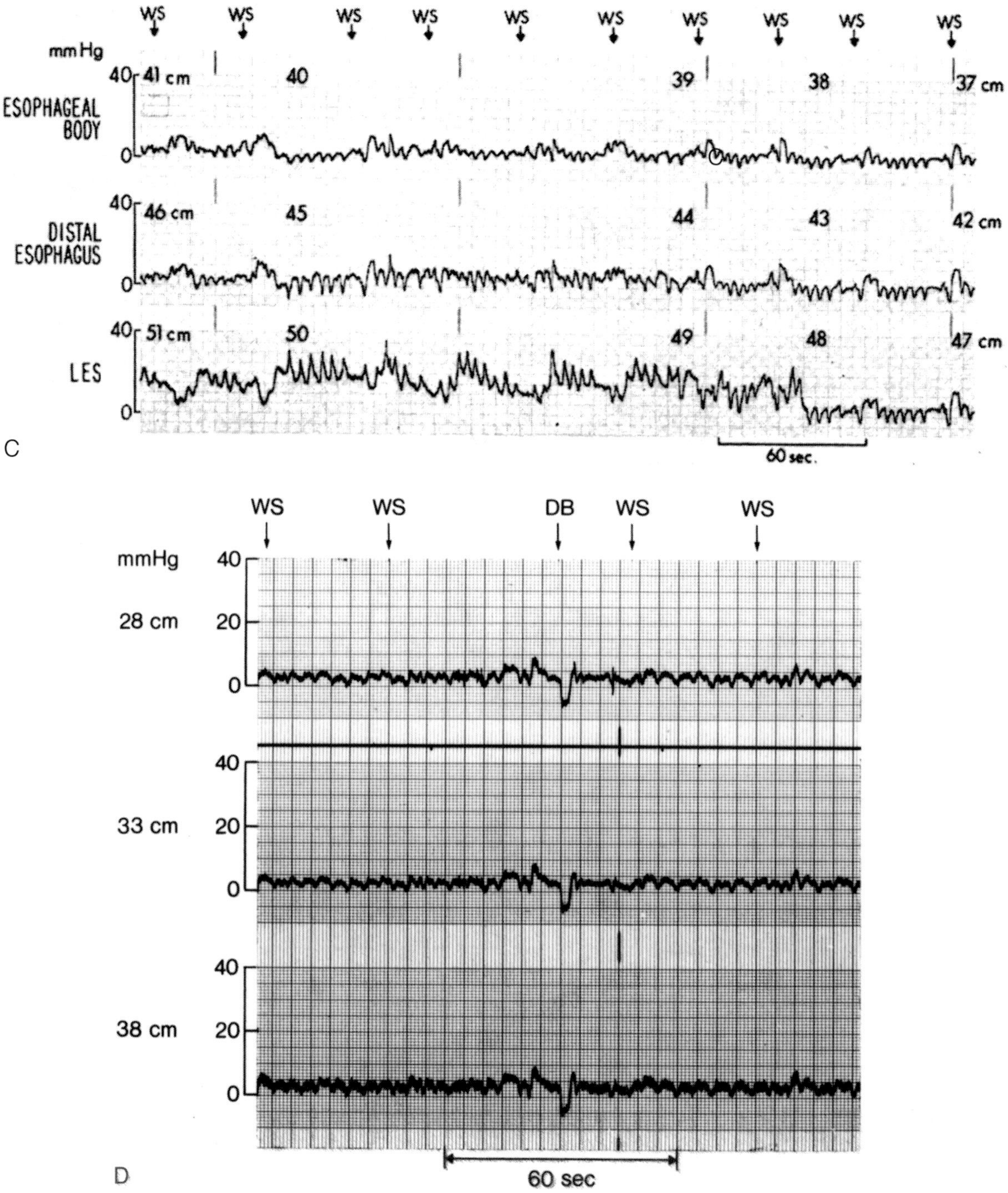

FIGURE 34–4 *(Continued)* ■ *C,* Complete loss of peristalsis with powerless contractions; the LES pressure zone is still present. *D,* Complete atony of the esophageal body.

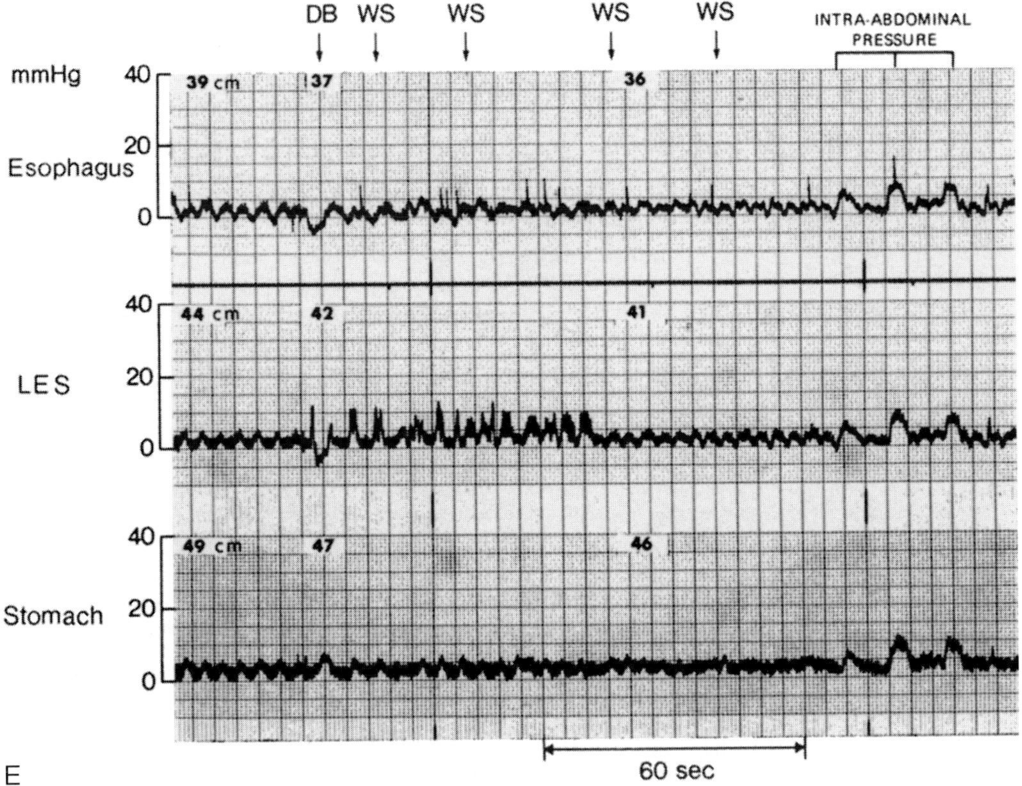

FIGURE 34–4 *(Continued)* ■ *E,* The LES pressure gradient between the stomach and the esophagus is nonexistent. The common cavity phenomenon between both organs is illustrated by the increase in recorded esophageal pressures generated by increased pressure in the abdomen.

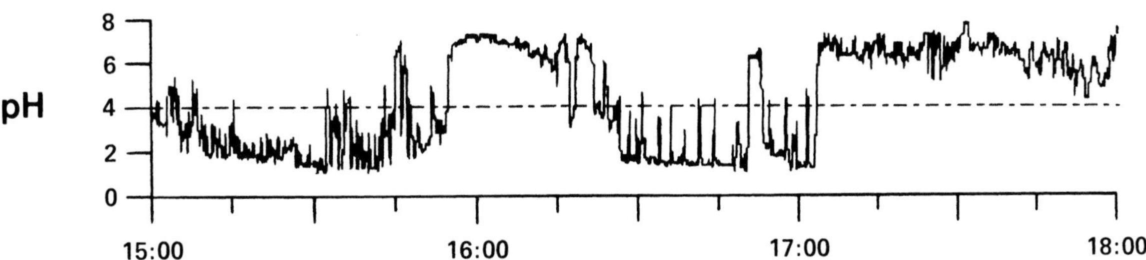

FIGURE 34–5 ■ A 24-hour pH recording is the most objective method of quantifying the presence and control of acid in the esophagus. The documentation of biliopancreatic reflux, similarly, is recorded by fiberoptic monitoring (Bilitec, Medtronic Synectics, Minneapolis).

tis, ulcerations, and stricture of the distal esophagus (Lock et al, 1997). Chronic reflux disease is also a well-known cause of Barrett's metaplasia, with its potential progression toward malignancy. Histopathology specimens obtained at endoscopy provide unequivocal documentation of the damage. Occult aspiration episodes may be anticipated when esophageal mucosal damage is documented (Lock et al, 1998).

The prevalence of erosive esophagitis varies from 50% to 60% in patients with scleroderma (Zamost et al, 1987). When Weston and colleagues (1998) assessed the esophageal mucosa of 62 patients with systemic sclerosis, they found reflux erosions in 52% and a stricture in 29%. Aubert and associates (1994) found active esophagitis in 50% of 46 patients. Esophagitis may be present in the absence of symptoms, and this is usually associated with aperistalsis. In fact, normal peristalsis was never found in any of the 31 patients with erosive esophagitis studied by Zamost and colleagues (1987), and erosive esophagitis was present in 70% of the patients.

Although uncommon, mucosal injury may be worsened by the ingestion of pills containing potassium chloride, quinidine, and particularly nonsteroidal anti-inflammatory drugs. This is explained by the increased amount of time for mucosal contact in an esophagus incapable of proper emptying.

The reported frequency of esophageal strictures in PSS ranges from 2% to 48%, with an average of 10% (Lock et al, 1997). One third of patients with dysphagia have stricture, and one third of patients with esophagitis have stricture (Lock et al, 1997; Weston et al, 1998). Strictures are more troublesome in PSS because they can cause an insurmountable barrier for a powerless esophagus. This may lead to early dysphagia and an increased risk of aspiration. Orringer (1983) found a stricture in 16 of 37 of his surgical patients. Henderson and colleagues (1987) described a stricture in 19 of 21 surgical patients. In our series (Poirier et al, 1994), 25% of the patients had a stricture.

According to Katzka and colleagues (1987), the prevalence of Barrett's metaplasia is 37% (9 of 24 of patients with esophageal symptoms referred for endoscopy). Of nine patients, two were found to have adenocarcinoma of the esophagus (8%). If, during the same period all patients seen for scleroderma at their hospital are considered, Barrett's esophagus was found in 12% (9 of 75) of scleroderma patients, and adenocarcinoma was found in 2.7% (2 of 75).

Two of 21 patients in a study by Henderson and colleagues (1987) had columnar-lined mucosa; in our series, 12 of 14 (85%) patients had documented columnar-lined mucosa. Other studies have reported a prevalence of 6% to 16% for Barrett's metaplasia in symptomatic patients (Abu-Shakra et al, 1994; Weston et al, 1998).

Without a doubt, selection and treatment group biases are present in these reports. However, because reflux disease and esophagitis are more prevalent and severe in scleroderma patients than in the general population, it is not surprising to encounter a higher number of patients with Barrett's esophagus and adenocarcinomas in this group.

Brush cytology sampling is the method of choice for the diagnosis of esophageal candidiasis. Cultures for fungi are positive in one third to one half of patients with scleroderma. When the fungal infection associated with esophagitis is treated, eradication of the fungus does not improve the esophagitis. This suggests that esophageal candidiasis itself does not play a primary role in the pathogenesis of erosive esophagitis in scleroderma (Zamost et al, 1987).

Endoluminal ultrasonography of the esophagus has been applied to the study of esophageal disease in systemic sclerosis. A hyperechoic abnormality in the normally hypoechoic muscularis propria seems to correspond to the presence of fibrosis. A strong positive correlation between the degree of hyperechoic abnormality and esophageal manometric abnormalities has been shown, but the clinical importance of this technique remains to be clarified (Miller et al, 1993).

Many authors recommend that a baseline manometry evaluation be performed in every patient in whom PSS is suspected or diagnosed whether or not symptoms of esophageal disease are present. In the case of impaired motility, endoscopy should be performed to exclude esophagitis and its complications and to orient the therapy (Lock et al, 1997; Zamost et al, 1987). If no erosive esophagitis is found, endoscopic surveillance is advisable because 80% of patients with scleroderma have abnormal motility and are at a high risk for development of erosive esophagitis.

Treatment

Medical Management

Inhibitors of collagen synthesis and corticosteroids have not affected the progression of esophageal disease (Hendel and Worning, 1989). Medical therapy in systemic sclerosis is thus directed toward palliation of the symptoms and complications of the disease.

Patients with scleroderma and esophageal reflux have a proper height-to-weight ratio. Compared with patients with idiopathic reflux, they rarely have excess weight. Esophageal reflux treatment in patients with scleroderma follows the same treatment principles as for patients with idiopathic reflux.

Despite improved pharmacologic management, the reflux seen in scleroderma is much greater than the reflux seen in the idiopathic pathologic reflux. Furthermore, even with significant symptom improvement, 50% of scleroderma patients do not experience complete healing of esophagitis because of residual, continuing GER (Hendel et al, 1992). The use of acid reflux and bile reflux monitoring, as well as endoscopic control examination, should be routine to provide quantitative information on reflux damage and its control. Repeated adjustment of maintenance doses is needed for this group of patients.

Mechanical Management. Because most exposures to reflux occur with the patient supine, elevation of the head of the bed should help to decrease episodes and the length of exposure to acid or mixed refluxates into the esophagus. The poor emptying capacity of the esophagus and stomach dictates more attention to the avoidance of meals before retiring and to active exercise in an upright position after meals.

Acid Inhibition. Inhibition of acid can decrease reflux symptoms and active esophagitis in patients with scleroderma. Histamine H_2-blockers cimetidine and ranitidine result in significant improvement of heartburn and esophagitis. If a stricture is present, however, it usually does not improve (Hendel et al, 1986; Petrobuki and Jeffries, 1979). When dysphagia results from the motor dysfunction, it will persist.

Patients who cease taking or who are not using acid-inhibiting medication show persistent or progressing esophagitis. Proton-pump inhibitors relieve heartburn and heal esophagitis (Abu-Shakra et al, 1994; Hendel et al, 1992; Shoenut et al, 1993). These authors concluded that omeprazole significantly reduces acid reflux and affords good protection against the acid component of the refluxate. Maintenance doses as high as 80 mg/day may be required to provide good control of symptoms and mucosal damage. With their deficient motor function, the patient should be receiving preventive proton-pump acid inhibition with regular surveillance of the esophageal mucosa status with endoscopy.

Prokinetic Agents. These agents act principally by facilitating acetylcholine release at the myenteric plexus level. These drugs do improve symptoms in patients with duodenogastroesophageal reflux. In patients with idiopathic reflux, they improve LES tone, esophageal emptying, and gastric emptying. In scleroderma patients, however, the response to prokinetic agents depends on the stage of the disease. The smooth muscle damage and the amount of fibrosis present in the digestive tract wall logically affect the response to the medication. Horowitz and associates (1987) and Limburg and colleagues (1991) found no significant effect of prokinetic agents in improvement of esophageal emptying in patients with PSS. Promotility drugs may have a better effect during the early stages of the disease. The prolonged use of metoclopramide may result in the appearance of neurologic symptoms.

Therapy for Esophageal Moniliasis. This disease is commonly seen because of the poor emptying capacity and consequent stasis of the esophagus. The use of nystatin (Mycostatin) improves symptoms but does not control the fungal infection. Fluconazole may be used but is contraindicated if a prokinetic agent, such as cisapride, is used in the treatment regimen. Esophageal stricture and Barrett's esophagus are seen as signs of advanced reflux disease. Bougienage, or guided dilatation, may be required to ensure proper transit. At this stage, however, when there are no compelling arguments against this approach, surgical management should be considered.

Surgical Treatment

Surgery in patients with scleroderma esophageal disease is considered when conservative treatment has failed. Thus, indications for operation are essentially the same as those for idiopathic reflux patients: ulcerative esophagitis refractory to intensive medical therapy and the development of complications (e.g., ulcers, strictures, Barrett's esophagus).

The fear of poor wound healing was expressed at first in the presence of thick abnormal skin and peripheral vascular disease. Actually, normal healing can occur in scleroderma patients even if they are receiving corticosteroid treatment (Orringer et al, 1981; Poirier et al, 1994). Patient selection is critical. In some patients, the systemic disease is too advanced to consider a major operation. Pulmonary and cardiac function assessments are essential. The early reports of surgical treatment of complications of reflux disease in scleroderma patients proposed resection and reconstruction. Significant morbidity rates were reported in these instances (Brain, 1973; Brindley and Texter, 1972; Mansour and Malone, 1988; McLaughlin et al, 1971; Murray, 1980).

Antireflux operations were first proposed by Henderson and Pearson (1973) and subsequently by Langdon and Lindberg (1973), O'Leary and associates (1975), Orringer and colleagues (1976), and Gibbon and colleagues (1982). In these reports, concern was always expressed about adding an antireflux mechanism in the presence of an atonic esophagus. The increase in resistance to bolus passage added by the repair could well result in further functional obstruction.

Surgical treatment of reflux in scleroderma is palliative. The basic systemic dysfunction persists and progresses with time. There is no ideal lasting surgical solution. Three surgical approaches may be used to palliate the complications of the disease:

1. Standard antireflux operations.
2. Acid and bile diversion.
3. Resection and reconstruction.

Antireflux Operations. Satisfied with their treatment results for dilatable peptic strictures in patients with idiopathic reflux, Henderson and Pearson (1973) offered their modification of the Collis elongation gastroplasty to 11 of 13 patients with scleroderma esophagitis. Eight of the treated patients had strictures. Follow-up for 6 to 30 months revealed no radiologic recurrence in nine patients and no or minor reflux symptoms in nine patients. Four patients had persistent dysphagia, and one patient required another postoperative dilatation (Fig. 34–6).

Orringer (1983) and associates (1976, 1981) reported on 37 patients treated with a Collis-Belsey procedure or a Collis-Nissen repair (Fig. 34–7) with a follow-up of 22 to 42 months. Reflux testing showed that acid exposure was still present in 41% of patients who underwent a gastroplasty with a partial fundoplication. In patients who underwent a gastroplasty with a total fundoplication, 25% had persistent acid reflux. Radiologic strictures were improved in 10 of 16 patients. LES manometric values were significantly higher (12 mm Hg) with a total fundoplication gastroplasty than with a partial fundoplication gastroplasty (8.6 mm Hg). In 75% of patients, the symptoms regressed and 38% complained of slow emptying.

The two patients on whom O'Leary and colleagues (1975) operated with a Thal-Nissen repair for refractory stricture showed symptom control without radiologic evidence of stricture after a follow-up of 14 and 22 months.

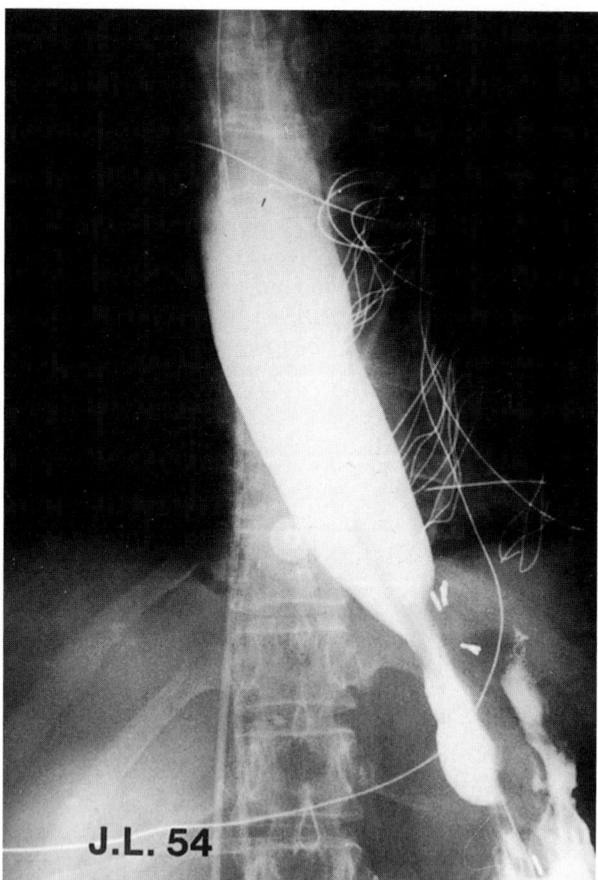

FIGURE 34–6 ■ Elongation gastroplasty with partial fundoplication in a scleroderma patient with complete atony of the esophagus. Eight years after this operation, the patient required a long limb Roux-en-Y diversion for persistent ulcerative esophagitis.

When Mansour and Malone (1988) reported their experience with 12 scleroderma patients, 8 underwent a standard partial fundoplication and 4 underwent a standard total fundoplication. All exhibited radiologic or endoscopic evidence of recurrent esophagitis, stricture, or both 1 to 8 years after the operation.

We reported our results with 14 scleroderma patients using a short total fundoplication in 10 (Fig. 34–8); 2, a gastroplasty with a short total fundoplication; 1, a gastroplasty with a partial fundoplication; and 1, a vagotomy, an antrectomy, and a Roux-en-Y diversion (Poirier et al, 1994). These patients were followed up, at the time of the report, for a mean of 65 months. Of the 14 patients, 12 (85% of the group) had a circumferential columnar-lined mucosa when treated. At manometry, these procedures increased the absolute sphincter gradient only slightly. Acid exposure in the esophagus decreased from 15% to 7.5%, although it persisted. This decrease, however, was considered sufficient to alleviate esophagitis. Strictures, ulcers, and erosions initially healed or regressed. In two patients, erosions reappeared more than 5 years after the operation. Three patients underwent another procedure of gastric resection with a Roux-en-Y reconstruction. This approach afforded complete control of reflux symptoms and the acute mucosal damage that resulted from the reflux.

Acid Suppression and Bile Diversion. None of the standard antireflux operations commonly used to treat idiopathic reflux complications appear to be as successful in treating the esophageal mucosal complications of scleroderma. Complete diversion of acid or mixed refluxate can be obtained by a partial gastrectomy, vagotomy, and a long-limb (45–60 cm) Roux-en-Y diversion or by total gastrectomy with the same Roux-en-Y reconstruction (Figs. 34–9 and 34–10).

Peix and associates (1993) and Fékété and colleagues (1996) reported subjective improvement in six scleroderma patients treated with this approach. In two patients, it was used as the initial treatment; in four, it was the operation of choice after an initial unsuccessful antireflux repair. We used partial gastrectomy with vagotomy and Roux-en-Y diversion in two patients. In an additional five patients, we resorted to total gastrectomy with a 60-cm Roux-en-Y limb.

Both operations resulted in complete control of symptoms and acute mucosal damage. Our attitude is based on the width of the scleroderma esophagus and on the type of complications present in the esophagus. If scleroderma patients present with reflux damage and a normal-sized esophagus, a standard antireflux operation is offered, identifying the temporary and palliative nature of reflux control. Total acid suppression and bile diversion are suggested for patients who have a wide, atonic esophagus in which there is no hope of creating an adequate antireflux repair without causing obstruction. It is still unclear whether a more extensive gastric resection and a longer jejunal limb are optimal to offer better control of the refluxate and better nutrition over time.

Resection. Orringer and co-workers (1993) and Mansour and Malone (1988) resorted to esophagectomy to treat advanced strictures or other complications in the scleroderma esophagus. Orringer suggested the use of transhiatal esophagectomy with a cervical esophagogastrostomy. Mansour used a short colon interposition with a distal esophagectomy.

There is very little information on the long-term functional results of these reconstructions in patients with scleroderma, who show an equally dysfunctional stomach, small bowel, and large bowel. This observation suggests that the organ used for reconstruction might well show the same atony as the resected esophagus, thus being predisposed to failure in protection of the remaining esophagus. For these reasons, we resisted the use of esophageal resections to treat reflux complications in scleroderma. Elimination and diversion of the refluxate with objective correction of the mucosal reflux damage seem to support this approach as an appropriate choice for these patients.

SYSTEMIC LUPUS ERYTHEMATOSUS

A spectrum of esophageal motor disturbances are seen in patients with systemic lupus erythematosus. Nonspecific manometric abnormalities have been reported. No rela-

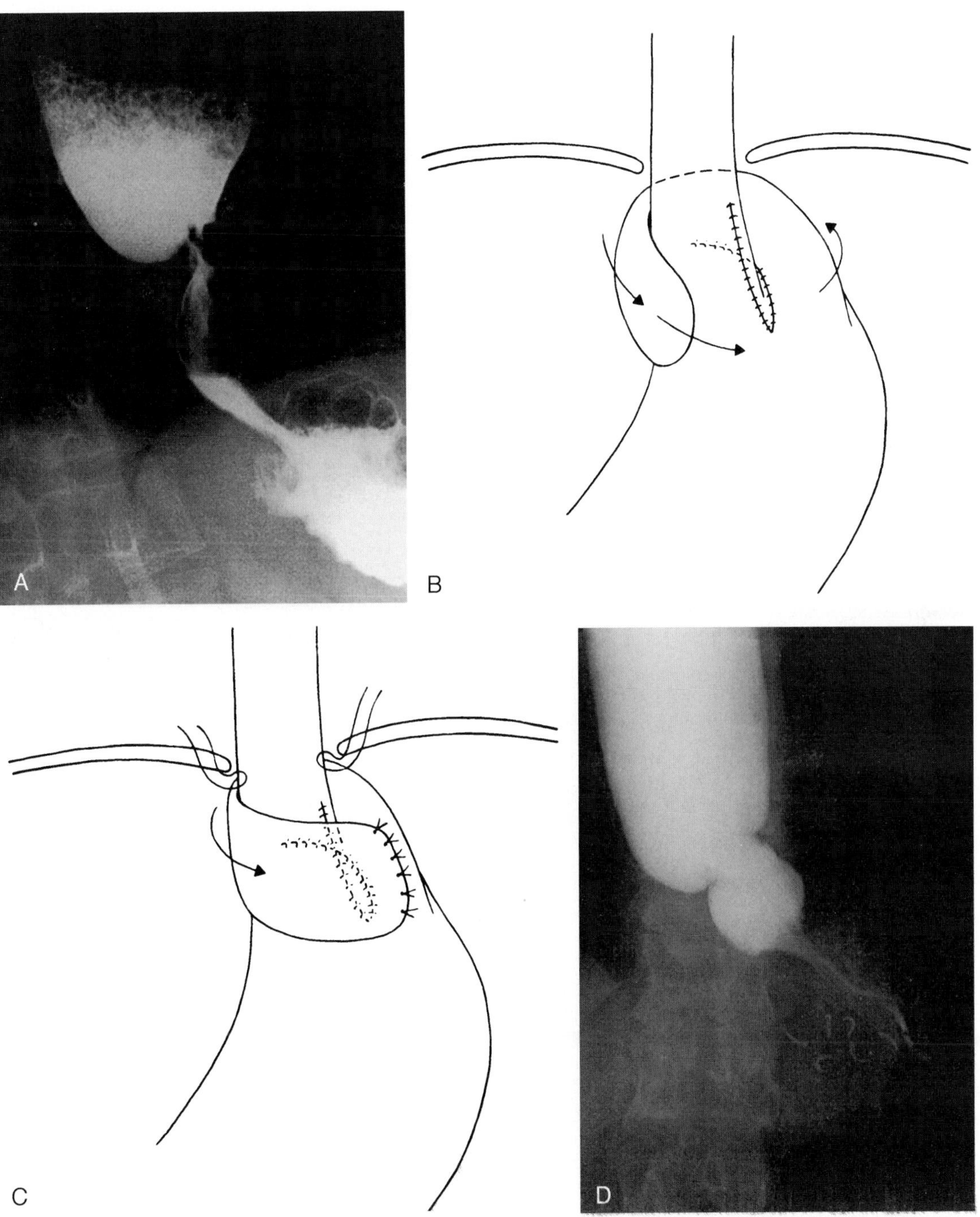

FIGURE 34–7 ■ *A,* Severe stricture in a scleroderma patient after an initial partial fundoplication. *B,* Cut elongation gastroplasty (Orringer technique). *C,* Total fundoplication around the elongation gastroplasty. The fundoplication is made shorter than in idiopathic reflux patients because of poor propulsion in these patients. *D,* Postoperative assessment shows improved stricture.

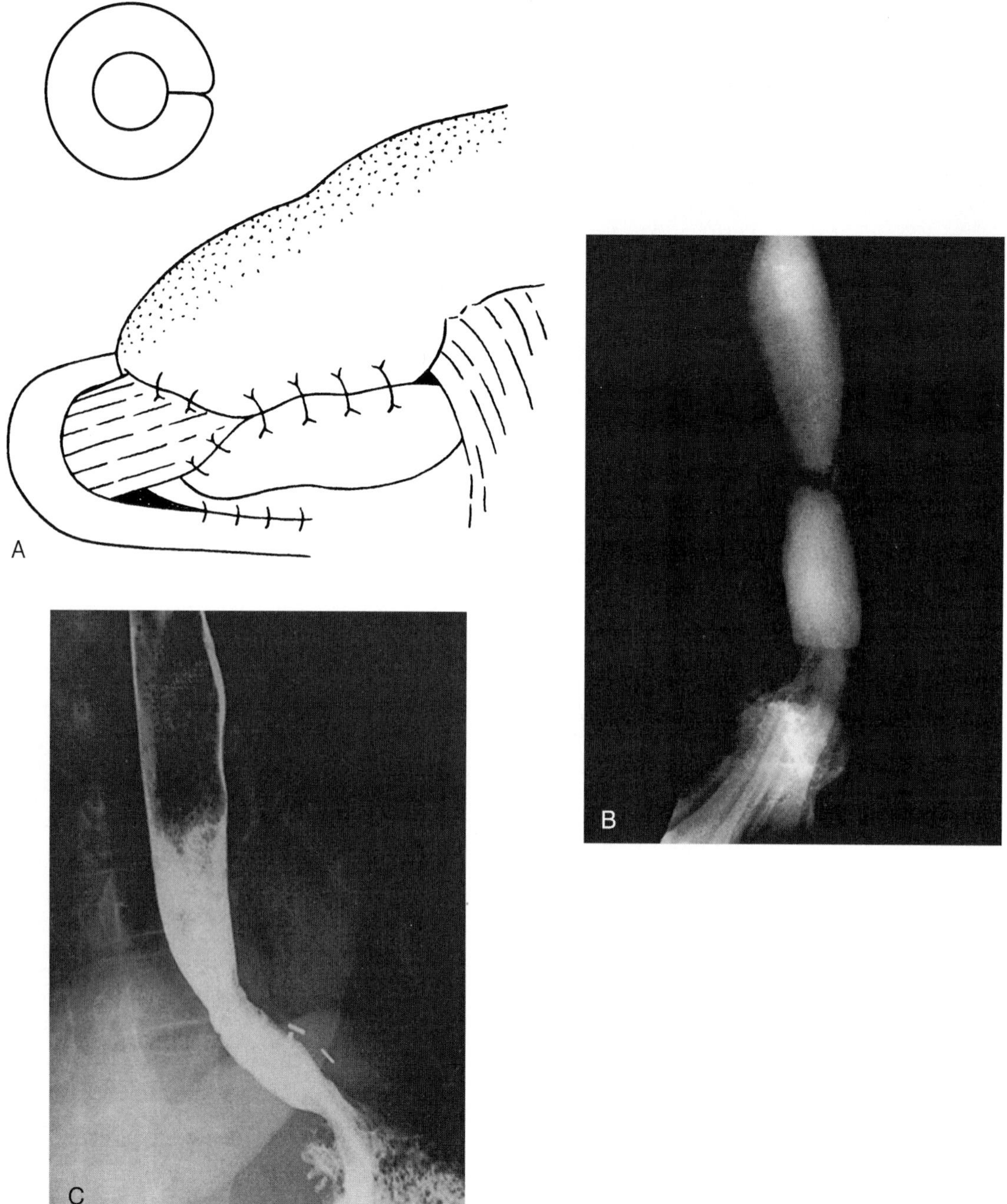

FIGURE 34–8 ■ *A,* Short (1 to 2 cm) total fundoplication created over a No. 52 to No. 56 mercury bougie alleviates esophagitis. This operation also results in slower emptying for solids. *B,* A scleroderma patient with absent peristalsis and normal esophageal diameter. The high narrowing suggests Barrett's esophagus. *C,* A total short fundoplication creates an imprint at the esophagogastric junction and palliates the effects of reflux esophagitis.

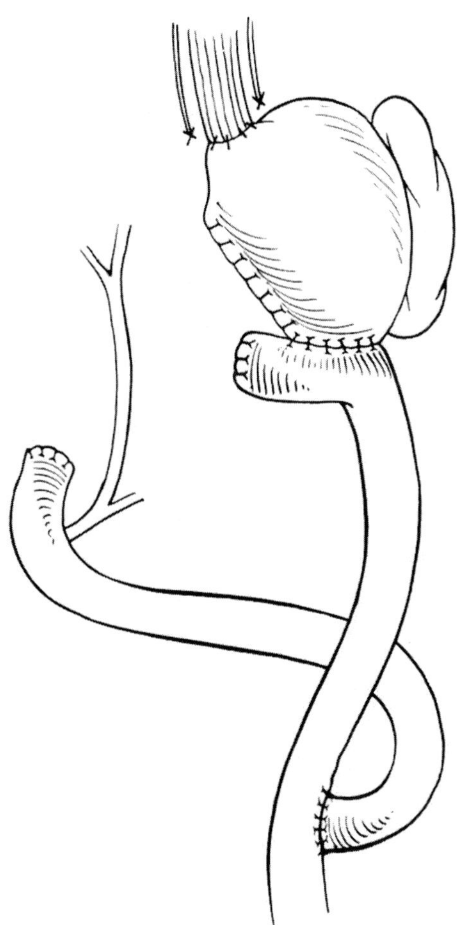

FIGURE 34–9 ■ Vagotomy antrectomy and long-limb Roux-en-Y diversion.

tionship has been established between the presence of esophageal dysfunction and activity, duration, or systemic treatment of the condition (Ramirez-Mata et al, 1974). Some have suggested a good correlation between the presence of Raynaud's phenomenon and esophageal aperistalsis (Gutierrez et al, 1982).

DERMATOMYOSITIS/POLYMYOSITIS

Polymyositis and dermatomyositis are disorders that primarily affect the skeletal musculature of the body. Abnormalities of the smooth muscle portion of the esophagus similar to those found in scleroderma have been reported. Involvement of the pharynx and of the striated-muscle portion of the esophagus is typical of polymyositis (Mukhopadhyay and Graham, 1976).

Decreased strength of the pharyngeal musculature, tongue weakness, and disordered motility of the esophagus all may interfere with normal swallowing. Cricopharyngeal achalasia has also been documented. Radiographic hypertrophy of the cricopharyngeal sphincter has been shown in barium studies and elevated proximal esophageal pressure with premature contractions and absence of relaxation has been noted in esophageal manometric studies (Kagen et al, 1985). Cricopharyngeal obstruction secondary to inflammation and/or fibrosis of the cricopharyngeus apparatus may cause dysphagia, aspiration of esophageal contents into the airways, pharyngonasal regurgitation, and secondary weight loss. These proximal symptoms do not seem to be improved by systemic medical treatment of the myositis. Although cricopharyngeal myotomy has been performed in a limited number of cases, it has provided excellent results in some chronically ill patients (Kagen et al, 1985).

Similar to abnormalities reported in scleroderma, functional abnormalities of the distal esophagus (e.g., abnormal peristalsis and esophageal dilatation) have been demonstrated in polymyositis and dermatomyositis. Unrecognized factors contribute to these distal esophageal disturbances. Distal motor function abnormalities may be present in the absence of proximal esophageal dysfunction (De Merieux et al, 1983).

Esophageal emptying has been assessed by scintigraphic techniques and has proved to be significantly delayed (Horowitz et al, 1986). Abnormal esophageal emptying as well as delayed gastric emptying correlates with the severity of peripheral skeletal muscle weakness. The esophageal dysfunction of reflux disease in patients with polymyositis and dermatomyositis is poorly documented in the literature.

Symptomatic improvement may occur with the administration of antacids and with general measures to decrease esophageal reflux symptoms, but an improvement in symptoms does not correlate with improvement in the systemic myositis. The role of surgical treatment remains limited.

Peripheral Neuropathy

DIABETIC NEUROPATHY

GI motility disorders are common in patients with diabetes mellitus. These abnormalities may be due to a combination of underlying neuropathy and metabolic derangements secondary to elevated blood glucose.

Clinical symptoms are more often seen in older patients who are insulin-dependent, in patients with poor glucose control, and in patients with evidence of peripheral neuropathy. Odynophagia in a diabetic patient should be considered a candidal esophagitis until proven otherwise.

The true pathogenesis of diabetic motility dysfunction remains unknown but appears to be related to the altered sympathetic function and cholinergic denervation (Verne and Sninsky, 1998). Typical symptoms include chest pain, heartburn, and dysphagia. However, esophageal dysfunction is often subclinical, probably because diabetes is associated with altered afferent sensory function (Russell et al, 1983).

Manometric abnormalities include spontaneous repetitive and aperistaltic contractions with decreased LES pressures (Rothstein, 1990; Stewart et al, 1976). Multipeak peristaltic contractions, usually of the two-peak variety, have also been described in the smooth muscle esophagus (Loo et al, 1985). A definitive explanation cannot be provided to account for these contractions. Scintigraphic studies may show prolonged esophageal

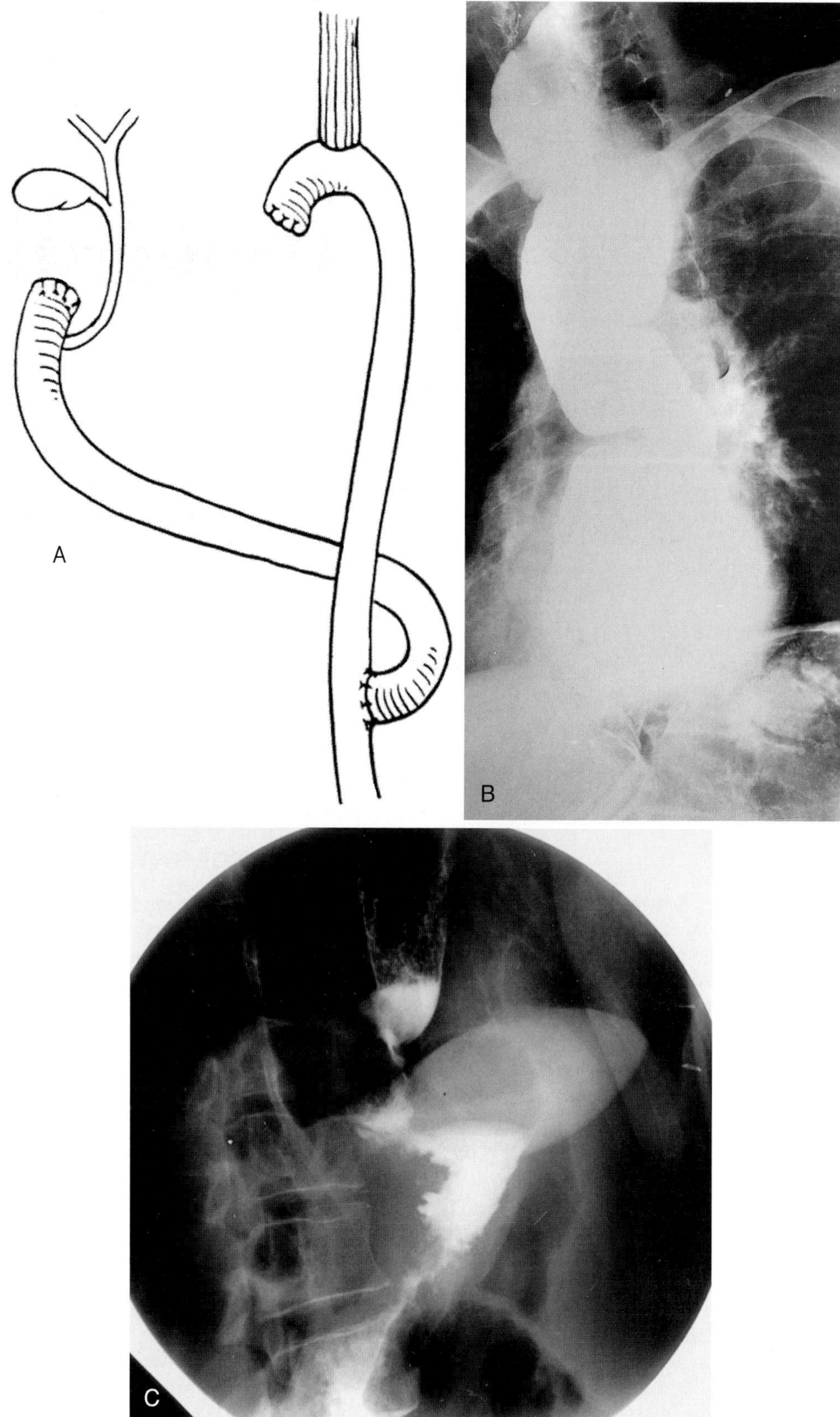

FIGURE 34–10 ■ *A,* Total gastrectomy with long-limb Roux-en-Y diversion. *B,* A patient with an 11-cm-wide scleroderma megaesophagus treated by total gastrectomy and long-limb Roux-en-Y diversion. *C,* Esophagojejunal emptying after Roux-en-Y reconstruction.

transit time (Keshaverzian et al, 1987). On concurrent esophageal manometry and radionuclide measurement of transit, it has been shown that delayed transit usually reflects either peristaltic failure or low-amplitude pressure waves (Holloway et al, 1999).

The well-documented gastroparesis observed in diabetic patients, especially if it occurs in parallel with a decreased LES pressure, predisposes to reflux disease. The treatment of reflux should follow the same therapeutic guidelines used for patients with idiopathic reflux disease.

ALCOHOLIC NEUROPATHY

The acute ingestion of alcohol results in esophageal motor dysfunction such as decreased LES pressure and decreased esophageal body peristalsis. Chronic alcohol consumption also induces esophageal dysmotility, but typical disorders are more difficult to define (Burbige et al, 1984). Esophageal studies performed on alcoholics in 1968 showed that the frequency of primary peristalsis was diminished, especially in the distal two thirds with preservation of the LES pressure. Those anomalies were believed to be associated with peripheral neuropathy (Winship et al, 1968), a fact that is not readily recognized (Grande et al, 1996; Keshaverzian et al, 1987).

Some studies, although demonstrating preservation of LES function, have shown elevated contraction amplitudes, particularly in the middle third. Grande and associates (1996) stated that these high-amplitude contractions of the middle esophagus may be a marker of excessive alcohol consumption. Surprisingly, despite high LES pressures, a significant proportion of alcoholic patients have abnormal reflux when evaluated with pH monitoring (Grande et al, 1996). Modifications of esophageal motility alone are unlikely to explain the increased risk of esophagitis in alcoholic patients. Radionuclide esophageal emptying seems slower in alcoholic patients than in control patients.

Globally, esophageal motor dysfunction is common in alcoholism, even in the absence of esophagitis and neuropathy. Abstinence is reported to favor reversal toward normal esophageal motility (Grande et al, 1996; Keshaverzian et al, 1987). It is still unclear whether esophageal motility disorders in alcoholics are due to the effects of ethanol on muscle fibers, on extrinsic neurogenic pathways, or on both.

■ *REFERENCES*

Abu-Shakra M, Guillemin F, Lee P: Cancer in systemic sclerosis. Arthritis Rheum 36:460, 1993.

Abu-Shakra M, Guillemin F, Lee P: Gastrointestinal manifestations of systemic sclerosis. Semin Arthritis Rheum 24:29, 1994.

Abu-Shakra M, Lee P: Mortality in systemic sclerosis: A comparison with the general population. J Rheumatol 22:2100, 1995.

Aubert A, Lazareth I, Vayssairat M, et al: Esophagitis in progressive systemic scleroderma: Prevalence and risk factors in forty-six patients. Gastroenterol Clin Biol 15:945–959, 1991.

Basilisco G, Carola F, Vanoli M, et al: Oesophageal acid clearance in patients with systemic sclerosis: Effect of body position. Eur J Gastroenterol Hepatol 8:205–209, 1996.

Bassotti G, Battaglia E, Debernardi V, et al: Esophageal dysfunction in scleroderma: Relationship with disease subsets. Arthritis Rheum 40:2252, 1997.

Benedek TG, Rodnan GP: The early history and nomenclature of scleroderma and of its differentiation from sclerema neonatorum and scleroedema. Semin Arthritis Rheum 12:52, 1982.

Black CM: The aetiopathogenesis of systemic sclerosis: Thick skin—thin hypotheses. J R Coll Physicians Lond 29:119, 1995.

Borroni G: Does a pre-Raphaelite painting by Ford Madox Brown depict a case of systemic sclerosis? Am J Dermatopathol 7:353, 1985.

Brain RHF: Surgical management of hiatal hernia and esophageal strictures in systemic sclerosis. Thorax 28:515–520, 1973.

Brindley GVJ, Texter ECJ: Scleroderma of the esophagus. Tex Med 68:74–80, 1972.

Burbige EJ, Lewis R, Halsted CH: Alcohol and gastrointestinal tract. Med Clin North Am 68:77–89, 1984.

Carette S, Lacoursière Y, Lavoie S et al: Radionuclide esophageal transit in progressive systemic sclerosis. J Rheumatol 12:478, 1985.

Clements PJ, Kadell B, Ippoliti A, et al: Esophageal motility in progressive systemic sclerosis: Comparison of cineradiographic and manometric evaluation. Dig Dis Sci 24:639, 1979.

Cohen S, Fisher R, Lipshutz W, et al: The pathogenesis of esophageal dysfunction in scleroderma and Raynaud's disease. J Clin Invest 51:2663, 1972.

D'Angelo WA, Fries JF, Masi AT, et al: Pathologic observations in systemic sclerosis (scleroderma): A study of fifty-eight autopsy cases and fifty-eight matched controls. Am J Med 46:428, 1969.

De Castro Parga ML, Alonso P, Garcia Porrua C, Prada JI: Lesiones mucosas esofagicas y scleroderma: Prevalencia, sintomas y factores de riesgo. Rev Espanola Enfermedades Digest 88:93–98, 1996.

De Merieux P, Verity MA, Clements PJ, et al: Esophageal abnormalities and dysphagia in polymyositis and dermatomyositis. Arthritis Rheum 26:961–968, 1983.

Dinsmore RE, Goodman D, Dreyfuss JR, et al: The air esophagram: A sign of scleroderma involving the esophagus. Radiology 87:348, 1966.

Drane WE, Karvelis K, Johnson DA, et al: Progressive systemic sclerosis: Radionuclide esophageal scintigraphy and manometry. Radiology 160:73–76, 1986.

Fékété F, Kabbej M, Sauvanet A: La diversion duodénale totale dans le traitement des oesophagites peptiques complexes. Chirurgie 121:326, 1996.

Fraser GM: The radiological manifestations of scleroderma (diffuse systemic sclerosis). Br J Dermatol 78:1–14, 1966.

Geatti O, Shapiro B, Fig LM, et al: Radiolabelled semisolid test meal clearance in the evaluation of esophageal involvement in scleroderma and Sjögren's syndrome. Am J Physiol Imaging 6:65, 1991.

Gibbon Z, Katz S, Eyal Z: Surgical aspects of multifocal involvement of the gastrointestinal tract in progressive systemic sclerosis. Int Surg 67:471–473, 1982.

Grande L, Monforte R, Ros E, et al: High amplitude contraction in the middle third of the oesophagus: A manometric marker of chronic alcoholism? Gut 38:655–662, 1996.

Gutierrez F, Valenzuela JE, Ehresmann GR, et al: Esophageal dysfunction in patients with mixed connective tissue diseases and systemic lupus erythematosus. Dig Dis Sci 27:592–597, 1982.

Hendel L, Aggestrup S, Stentoft P, et al: Long-term ranitidine in progressive systemic sclerosis (scleroderma) with gastroesophageal reflux. Scand J Gastroenterol 21:799–805, 1986.

Hendel L, Hage E, Hendel J, et al: Omeprazole in the long-term treatment of severe gastroesophageal reflux disease in patients with systemic sclerosis. Aliment Pharmacol Ther 6:565, 1992.

Hendel L, Worning H: Exocrine pancreatic function in patients with progressive systemic sclerosis. Scand J Gastroenterol 24:461–466, 1989.

Henderson RD, Marryatt G, Henderson RF: Surgical management of gastroesophageal reflux in patients with scleroderma. In Siewert JR, Hölscher AH (eds): Diseases of the Esophagus. New York, Springer-Verlag, 1987, pp 904–908.

Henderson RD, Pearson FG: Surgical management of esophageal scleroderma. J Thorac Cardiovasc Surg 66:686, 1973.

Holloway RH, Tippett MD, Horowitz M, et al: Relationship between esophageal motility and transit in patients with type 1 diabetes mellitus. Am J Gastroenterol 94:3150–3157, 1999.

Horowitz M, Maddern GJ, Maddox A, et al: Effects of cisapride on gastric and esophageal emptying in progressive systemic sclerosis. Gastroenterology 93:311, 1987.

Horowitz M, McNeil JD, Maddern GJ, et al: Abnormalities of gastric and esophageal emptying in polymyositis and dermatomyositis. Gastroenterology 90:434–439, 1986.

Hurwitz AL, Duranceau A, Postlethwait RW: Esophageal dysfunction and Raynaud's phenomenon in patients with scleroderma. Dig Dis 21:601–606, 1976.

Johnson A, Drane WE, Curran J, et al: Pulmonary disease in progressive systemic sclerosis: A complication of gastroesophageal reflux and occult aspiration? Arch Intern Med 149:589, 1989.

Kagen LJ, Hochman RB, Strong EW: Cricopharyngeal obstruction in inflammatory myopathy (polymyositis/dermatomyositis). Arthritis Rheum 28:630–636, 1985.

Katzka DA, Reynolds JC, Saul SH, et al: Barrett's metaplasia and adenocarcinoma of the esophagus in scleroderma. Am J Med 82:46, 1987.

Kaye SA, Siraj QH, Agnew J, et al: Detection of early asymptomatic esophageal dysfunction in systemic sclerosis using a new scintigraphic grading method. J Rheumatol 23:297–302, 1996.

Keshavarzian A, Iber FL, Ferguson Y: Esophageal manometry and radionuclide emptying in chronic alcoholics. Gastroenterology 92:651–657, 1987a.

Keshaverzian A, Iber FL, Nasrallah S: Radionuclide esophageal emptying and manometric studies in diabetes mellitus. Am J Gastroenterol 82:625–631, 1987b.

Langdon DE, Lindberg EF: Scleroderma and esophageal hiatal hernioplasty. Minn Med 56:643–645, 1973.

LeRoy EC: Systemic sclerosis: A vascular perspective. Rheum Dis Clin North Am 22:675, 1996.

LeRoy EC, Black C, Fleischemajer R, et al: Scleroderma (systemic sclerosis): Classification, subsets and pathogenesis. J Rheumatol 15:202, 1988.

Limburg AJ, Smit AJ, Kleibeuker JH: Effects of cisapride on the esophageal motor function of patients with progressive systemic sclerosis or mixed connective tissue disease. Digestion 49:156, 1991.

Lock G, Holstege A, Lang B, et al: Gastrointestinal manifestations of progressive systemic sclerosis. Am J Gastroenterol 92:763, 1997.

Lock G, Pfeifer M, Straub RH, et al: Association of esophageal dysfunction and pulmonary function impairment in systemic sclerosis. Am J Gastroenterol 93:341, 1998.

Loo FD, Dodds WJ, Soergel KH, et al: Multipeaked esophageal peristaltic pressure waves in patients with diabetic neuropathy. Gastroenterology 88:485–491, 1985.

Mansour KA: Surgery for scleroderma of the esophagus: A 12-year experience. Ann Thorac Surg 60:227, 1995.

Mansour KA, Malone C: Surgery for scleroderma of the esophagus: A 12-year experience. Ann Thorac Surg 46:513, 1988.

Mayes MD: Epidemiology of systemic sclerosis and related diseases. Curr Opin Rheumatol 9:557, 1997.

Mayes MD: Scleroderma epidemiology. Rheum Dis Clin North Am 22:751, 1996.

McLaughlin JS, Roig R, Woodruff MF: Surgical treatment of stricture of the esophagus in patients with scleroderma. J Thorac Cardiovasc Surg 61:641–645, 1971.

Miller LS, Liu JB, Klenn PJ, et al: Endoluminal ultrasonography of the distal esophagus in systemic sclerosis. Gastroenterology 105:31, 1993.

Mukhopadhyay AK, Graham DY: Esophageal motor dysfunction in systemic diseases. Arch Intern Med 136:583–588, 1976.

Murray GF: Operation for motor dysfunction of the esophagus. Ann Thorac Surg 29: 184–91, 1980.

Murrell DF: A radical proposal for the pathogenesis of scleroderma. J Am Acad Dermatol 28:78, 1993.

Neschis M, Siegelman SS, Rotstein J, et al: Esophagus in progressive systemic sclerosis: A manometric and radiographic correlation. Dig Dis 15:443, 1970.

Norton WL, Nardo JM: Vascular disease in progressive systemic sclerosis (scleroderma). Ann Intern Med 73:317, 1970.

O'Leary JP, Hollenbeck JI, Woodward ER: Surgical treatment of esophageal stricture in patients with scleroderma. Am Surg 41:131–135, 1975.

Orringer MB: Surgical management of scleroderma reflux esophagitis. Surg Clin North Am 63:859–867, 1983.

Orringer MB, Dabich L, Zarafonetis CJ, et al: Gastroesophageal reflux in esophageal scleroderma: Diagnosis and implications. Ann Thorac Surg 22:120, 1976.

Orringer MB, Marshall B, Stirling MC: Transhiatal esophagectomy for benign and malignant disease. J Thorac Cardiovasc Surg 105:265, 1993.

Orringer MB, Orringer JS, Dabich L, et al: Combined Collis gastroplasty-fundoplication operations for scleroderma reflux esophagitis. Surgery 90:624, 1981.

Peix JL, Maroun J, Tekinel O, et al: Traitement de l'oesophagite sclérodermique: Intérêt de la diversion duodénale. Ann Chir 47:302, 1993.

Petrobuki RJ, Jeffries GH: Cimetidine versus antacid in scleroderma with reflux esophagitis: A randomized double-blind controlled study. Gastroenterology 77(4 Pt 1):691–695, 1979.

Poirier NC, Taillefer R, Topart P, et al: Antireflux operations in patients with scleroderma. Ann Thorac Surg 58:66, 1994.

Poirier TJ, Rankin GB: Gastrointestinal manifestations of progressive systemic scleroderma based on a review of 364 cases. Am J Gastroenterol 58:30, 1972.

Ramirez-Mata M, Reyes PA, Alarcon-Segovia D, et al: Esophageal motility in systemic lupus erythematosus. Dig Dis 19:132–136, 1974.

Rosenthal AK, McLaughlin JK, Linet MS, et al: Scleroderma and malignancy: An epidemiological study. Ann Rheum Dis 52:531, 1993.

Rothstein RD: Gastrointestinal motility disorders in diabetes mellitus. Am J Gastroenterol 85:782–785, 1990.

Russell COH, Gannan R, Coatsworth J, et al: Relationship among esophageal dysfunction, diabetic gastroenteropathy, and peripheral neuropathy. Dig Dis Sci 28:289–293, 1983.

Shoenut JP, Mieflikier AB, Aldor TA, et al: Reproducibility of ambulatory esophageal pH monitoring in the aperistaltic esophagus. Dysphagia 11:248–251, 1996.

Shoenut JP, Wieler JA, Micflikier AB, et al: The extent and pattern of gastro-oesophageal reflux in patients with scleroderma oesophagus: The effect of low-dose omeprazole. Aliment Pharmacol Ther 7:509–513, 1993.

Shoenut JP, Yamashiro Y, Orr WC, et al: Effect of severe gastroesophageal reflux on sleep stage in patients with aperistaltic esophagus. Dig Dis Sci 41:372–376, 1996.

Silman AJ: Scleroderma and survival. Ann Rheum Dis 50:267, 1991.

Silman AJ: Scleroderma: Demographics and survival. J Rheumatol 24 (suppl 48):58, 1997.

Silver AM: Clinical aspect of systemic sclerosis (scleroderma). Ann Rheum Dis 50:854, 1991.

Stentoft P, Hendel L, Aggestrup S: Esophageal manometry and pH-probe monitoring in the evaluation of gastroesophageal reflux in patients with progressive systemic sclerosis. Scand J Gastroenterol 22:499–504, 1987.

Stevens MB, Siegel CI, Hookman P, et al: Aperistalsis of the esophagus in patients with connective tissue disorders and Raynaud's phenomenon. N Engl J Med 270:1218, 1964.

Stewart M, Hosking J, Preston BJ, et al: Oesophageal motor changes in diabetes mellitus. Thorax 31:278–283, 1976.

Treacy WL, Baggenstoss AH, Slocumb CH, et al: Scleroderma of the esophagus: A correlation of histology and physiologic findings. Ann Intern Med 59:351, 1963.

Verne GN, Sninsky CA: Diabetes and the gastrointestinal tract. Gastroenterol Clin North Am 27:861–874, 1998.

Weston S, Thumshirn M, Wiste J, et al: Clinical and upper gastrointestinal motility features in systemic sclerosis and related disorders. Am J Gastroenterol 93:1085, 1998.

White B: Immunopathogenesis of systemic sclerosis. Rheum Dis Clin North Am 22:695, 1996.

Winship DH, Caflisch CR, Zboralske FF, et al: Deterioration of esophageal peristalsis in patients with alcoholic neuropathy. Gastroenterology 55:173–178, 1968.

Wolf G: Endure! How Paul Klee's illness influenced his art. Lancet 353:1516, 1999.

Yarze JC, Varga J, Stampfl D, et al: Esophageal function in systemic sclerosis: A prospective evaluation of motility and acid reflux in 36 patients. Am J Gastroenterol 88:870, 1993.

Zamost BJ, Hirschberg J, Ippoliti AF, et al: Esophagitis in scleroderma: Prevalence and risk factors. Gastroenterology 92:421, 1987.

CHAPTER **35**

Achalasia: Thoracoscopic and Laparoscopic Myotomy

Richard J. Finley

DEFINITION

Achalasia is a motility disorder of the esophagus of uncertain etiology characterized manometrically by increased basal lower esophageal sphincter (LES) pressure with incomplete relaxation of the sphincter upon swallowing and aperistalsis of the body of the esophagus. Classic primary achalasia is characterized by low-amplitude, nonperistaltic, tertiary contractions of the body of the esophagus; vigorous achalasia is characterized by high-amplitude, nonperistaltic contractions.

Primary achalasia is most commonly seen in North America and Europe. The underlying pathophysiology appears to be loss of ganglion cells in the myenteric plexus of the esophagus, resulting in absence of peristalsis of the esophageal body, failure of the LES to relax with swallowing, and normal or elevated LES pressures. The estimated incidence of primary achalasia is about one case per 200,000 population (Mayberry and Atkinson, 1985). The disorder is most commonly diagnosed in patients between ages 20 and 40 years.

Achalasia secondary to ganglion cell destruction by *Trypanosoma cruzi* infection (Chagas' disease) is seen primarily in South America. In the endemic areas, Chagas' megaesophagus develops in one patient per 1000 population. (See Chapter 33 on Chagas' disease.)

HISTORICAL NOTE

Surgical therapy for achalasia has been directed at obliterating the dysfunctional LES. A myotomy of the muscles of the lower esophagus and gastroesophageal junction using both anterior and posterior incisions was first performed by the German surgeon E. Heller on April 14, 1913 (Heller, 1914). The procedure was later modified to a single incision by Groenvedeldt (1918) and Zaaijer (1923).

The surgical approach, transabdominal or transthoracic, and the need for an antireflux procedure remain controversial issues. In 1962, Professor Jacques Dor and associates at the University of Marseilles described fixing the myotomized lower esophagus in the abdomen and wrapping it using a partial anterior gastric fundoplication to compress the esophagus during elevated intragastric pressure, at which time gastroesophageal reflux usually occurs. Partial fundoplication is preferred to 360-degree fundoplication because a total fundoplication defeats the principle of lowering the high-pressure zone at the bottom of the aperistaltic esophagus. Long-term symptomatic improvement has been reported after an esophageal myotomy performed through a left thoracotomy with (Malthaner et al, 1994) and without (Ellis, 1993) a partial fundoplication.

After the popularization of minimally invasive surgery, Pellegrini and coworkers (1992) reported the first use of thoracoscopic esophagomyotomy for achalasia. Rosati and colleagues (1995) first reported excellent relief of symptoms after a laparoscopic myotomy and anterior partial fundoplication for achalasia.

■ *HISTORICAL READINGS*

Dor J, Humbert P, Dor V, et al: L'intérêt de la technique de Nissen modifiée dans la prevention de reflux après cardiomyotomie extramuqueuse de Heller. Mem Acad Chir (Paris) 88:877, 1962.

Ellis FH: Oesophagomyotomy for achalasia: A 22-year experience. Br J Surg 80:882, 1993.

Groenvedeldt DFR: Over cardiospasmus. Ned Tijdschr Ogeneeskd 2:281, 1918.

Heller E: Extra Mukose cardiaplatik beim chronisher Cardiospasmus mit Dilation Oesophagus. Mitt Grenzgeb Med Chir 27:141, 1914.

Malthaner RA, Todd TR, Miller L, et al: Long-term results in surgically managed esophageal achalasia. Ann Thorac Surg 58:1343, 1994.

Pellegrini C, Wetter LA, Leichter R, et al: Thoracoscopic esophagomyotomy: Initial experience with a new approach for the treatment of achalasia. Ann Surg 216:291, 1992.

Rosati F, Fumagalli U, Bonavina L: Laparoscopic approach to esophageal achalasia. Am J Surg 169:424, 1995.

Zaaijer JH: Cardiospasmus in the aged. Ann Surg 77:615, 1923.

DIAGNOSIS

Clinical Features

The functional obstruction at the esophagogastric junction results in symptoms of progressive dysphagia for liquids and solids. The disease usually follows an indolent course, with several years of progressive dysphagia for liquids and solids, leading eventually to regurgitation of undigested food, weight loss, wheezing, and coughing. Patients present for medical care with an average duration of symptoms of 6 years (Nelson and Castell, 1988). Over time, the esophagus slowly dilates and eventually assumes a sigmoid appearance on the barium radiograph. Burning retrosternal discomfort, secondary to acidic fermentation products of retained food, may occur at this stage.

Investigative Techniques

Early in the disease process, the chest radiograph may be normal. Later, however, manifestations of achalasia may include a widened mediastinum, an air-fluid level, absence of a gastric air bubble, and even aspiration pneumonitis. A barium swallow shows absence of peristalsis in the body of the esophagus with distal esophageal narrowing to form a "bird's beak" configuration. A sigmoid appearance of the esophagus, retention of food, and an esophageal diameter greater than 6 cm are signs of long-standing achalasia.

Upper gastrointestinal endoscopy is used to examine the esophageal mucosa for signs of esophageal cancer and the esophagogastric junction to determine whether there is any structural cause of the obstruction, such as cancer or peptic stricture, which may mimic achalasia. The endoscopist should be able to pass the tube through the esophagogastric junction with minimal pressure in classic achalasia. For biopsy of the esophagogastric junction, the instrument should be directed posteriorly, if possible, to avoid mucosal perforation in the line of the future anterior esophageal myotomy.

Radionucleotide swallows to assess esophageal transit are useful in the diagnosis and follow-up of patients with achalasia. Studies with liquid radionucleotide swallows are more reproducible than solid scintigraphic studies, which have decreased reliability because of poor mixing of the radionucleotide.

The esophageal transit time for both liquids and solids should be decreased in patients with achalasia in the supine and upright positions (Graham et al, 1997).

Esophageal manometry is the procedure of choice for the diagnosis of achalasia. Classic esophageal manometric findings include (1) an elevated LES pressure, (2) failure of the LES to relax upon swallowing, and (3) aperistalsis of the body of the esophagus. Absence of peristalsis of the body must be documented in order to confirm the diagnosis of primary achalasia (Couturier and Samama, 1991). Patients with vigorous achalasia have high-amplitude, nonperistaltic contractions in the body of the esophagus in response to swallowing and complain more often of chest pain (Cohen, 1979).

In our center, the patient's quality of life is assessed by standardized questionnaires, administered in the preoperative period and at 3, 6, and 12 months and then yearly after surgery. Postoperative dysphagia is subdivided into four classes, as described by Vantrappen and Hellemans (1980):

Class I, no dysphagia
Class II, dysphagia occurring less than once weekly
Class III, dysphagia occurring more than once weekly
Class IV, persistent dysphagia

With the same classification system, patients are questioned to determine the presence of heartburn or regurgitation; patients are also asked to state whether they are very satisfied, somewhat satisfied, or not satisfied.

MANAGEMENT

Principles of Management

The primary goal of therapy is palliation of symptoms, since the esophageal motor abnormality remains unchanged after all forms of intervention. At present, all treatment techniques are directed at relieving the functional obstruction at the level of the LES by disruption or paralysis of the esophageal muscle constituting the LES. Destruction of the LES function also places the patient at risk for pathologic gastroesophageal reflux disease (GERD). Therefore, the treatment of patients with achalasia must strike a balance between the relief of dysphagia and potential creation of pathologic gastroesophageal reflux.

Medical Therapy

Treatment approaches have involved both surgical and nonsurgical techniques. The nonsurgical techniques have consisted of passive esophageal bougienage or pneumatic dilatation of the esophagogastric junction and injection of botulinum toxin into the LES muscles.

Pneumatic dilatation forcibly disrupts the muscular fibers of the LES while preserving the esophageal mucosa. This procedure resulted in esophageal perforation in up to 4% of patients in one series (Salis Graciela et al, 1997) and other significant complications in more than 30% in another series (Eckardt et al, 1997). With experienced clinicians, long-term symptomatic relief of dysphagia and regurgitation is obtainable in 60% to 75% of patients after the first dilatation and in up to 85% after an additional procedure (Katz, 1997). In a prospective randomized trial, however, Csendes and colleagues (1989) demonstrated that esophagomyotomy of the muscles constituting the LES via laparotomy controlled dysphagia better compared with pneumatic dilatation.

Endoscopic botulinum toxin injections relaxed the smooth muscle fibers of the pathologic LES, but these effects lasted less than 6 months in most patients. Repeated injections were required for consistent long-term relief (Schiano et al, 1998). Many of these patients require other forms of treatment, and the technique is now limited to poor candidates for either pneumatic dilatation or a surgical procedure (Gordon and Eaker, 1997). Patients who have undergone botulinum injection may develop submucosal fibrosis, which may lead to a more difficult esophageal myotomy and occasional mucosal perforation (Patti et al, 1999).

Surgical Therapy

By comparison, esophagomyotomy has been the surgical procedure of choice for the treatment of achalasia since the initial description (Heller, 1914). The surgical approach—transthoracic (Ellis, 1993; Malthaner et al, 1994) or transabdominal (Bonavina et al, 1992)—and the need for concomitant fundoplication (Dor et al, 1962) remain controversial.

Long-term symptomatic improvement has been reported after an esophageal myotomy performed through a left thoracotomy with and without an antireflux procedure. Ellis (1993) reported that 74% of his patients had no or minimal dysphagia 9 years after a left thoracotomy and myotomy without an antireflux procedure. Malthaner and associates (1994) reported that 67% of their patients had minimal dysphagia 19 years after a left thoracotomy with partial fundoplication.

Pellegrini and colleagues (1992) reported the first use of thoracoscopic esophagomyotomy for achalasia. A follow-up of these thoracoscopic esophagomyotomies showed complete relief of dysphagia in 17 of 24 patients and partial relief in 4 of the 24 patients (Pellegrini et al, 1993). Five of eight patients tested in the study had experienced abnormally prolonged exposure to acid in the distal esophagus. In our center, two of the first seven patients treated with this technique had an inadequate thoracoscopic myotomy because of inability to carry the myotomy onto the stomach (Graham et al, 1997). The incidence of inadequate myotomy and gastroesophageal reflux has led us to favor laparoscopic Heller's myotomy and anterior fundoplication for the primary surgical therapy of achalasia.

Preoperative Preparation

Patients with achalasia usually present for surgical consideration with signs and symptoms of dysphagia for liquids and solids, regurgitation, weight loss, and aspiration. Severe malnutrition is treated with at least 10 days of enteral feeding before surgical intervention. Cardiopulmonary function is maximized and pulmonary sepsis is cleared before surgery. Patients who have received a previous botulinum injection are warned about the increased frequency of mucosal perforation related to submucosal fibrosis (Patti et al, 1999). However, previous botulinum injection should not be a contraindication to endoscopic Heller myotomy (Stewart et al, 1999).

Patients undergoing endoscopic esophageal myotomy should understand the risks and benefits of both laparoscopic and thoracoscopic approaches. The laparoscopic approach is preferred because of the superior long-term results (Stewart et al, 1999; Patti et al, 1999) but may not be possible if adhesions from previous upper abdominal surgery or infection prevent adequate exposure of the esophagogastric junction. In these cases, the thoracoscopic approach may be necessary. Conversely, thoracoscopic surgery may be contraindicated in patients with decreased pulmonary function that prevents the use of one-lung ventilation, which is necessary for accurate visualization of the esophagus. Thoracoscopic myotomy should be limited to patients with extensive abdominal adhesions that preclude a laparoscopic approach or to patients with diffuse esophageal spasm who do not need complete division of the LES.

All patients receive a liquid diet for 2 days before the operation and fast for 12 hours before surgery. At the time of the operation, the esophagus and the stomach are cleaned out with endoscopy before intubation and ventilation in order to avoid aspiration.

OPERATIVE TECHNIQUE

Thoracoscopic Esophagomyotomy

The objective of this operation is to perform a myotomy of the lower 6 cm of the esophagus, the esophagogastric junction, and the proximal 1 cm of the stomach using thoracoscopic techniques. With the thoracoscopic technique, the left side of the chest allows the best visualization of the lower esophagus and cardioesophageal junction.

After careful endoscopic cleansing of the esophagus and stomach before anesthesia, the trachea is intubated with a double-lumen tube, avoiding aspiration. The flexible gastroscope is then reinserted into the esophagus. Pneumatic stockings are used to avoid thromboembolic disease, and the patient is placed in the right lateral decubitus position with the head of the bed elevated 30 degrees to allow the abdominal contents and diaphragm to fall away from the operative area.

The left sixth intercostal space is marked for a posterolateral thoracotomy if this is required for an open operation (Fig. 35–1). After collapse of the left lung, the first 10-mm port (A) is introduced through a small incision in the third intercostal space in the anterior axillary line, avoiding injury to the lung. No valves are used in the ports to avoid tension pneumothorax or an air embolus. A 30-degree telescope is then introduced through the port to ensure that there are no pleural adhesions preventing the lung from collapsing and to examine the pleural space and diaphragm.

Under direct vision, a second 10-mm trocar (B) is introduced in the sixth intercostal space 5 cm posterior to the posterior axillary line, with care taken to avoid injury to the intercostal vessels or nerve. This port site is used for the 30-degree telescope for most of the operation. A third 5-mm port (C) is then placed in the sixth intercostal space in the anterior axillary line to be used for dissection or retraction of the diaphragm, and a lung retractor is then put through port A.

Once the esophagus has been well visualized, the center of the operating diamond is established and an additional two 5-mm ports (D) and (E) are placed about 15 cm apart to allow introduction of the left-hand and right-hand instruments of the operating surgeon. The left lung is retracted upward, and the inferior pulmonary ligament is divided with electrocautery up to the level of the inferior pulmonary vein. The mediastinal pleura is

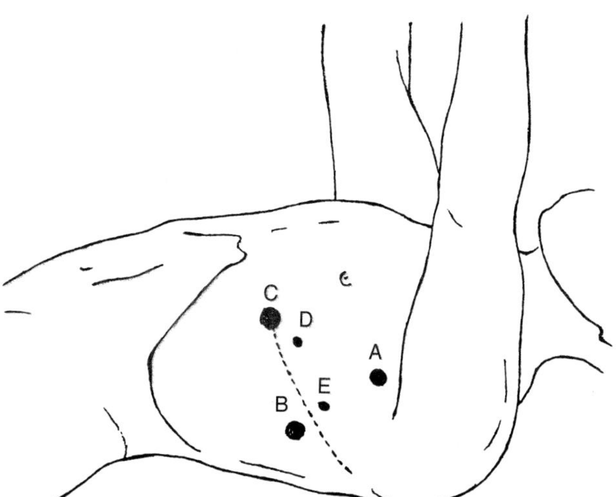

FIGURE 35–1 ■ Diagram of the left sixth intercostal space and the positions of the port sites (A through E) for thoracoscopic esophagomyotomy.

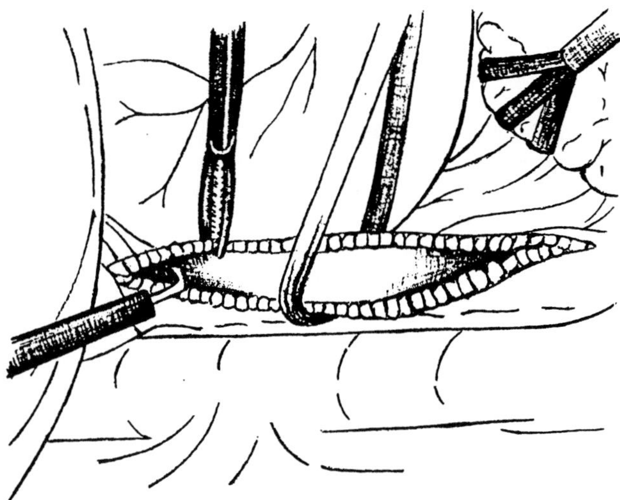

FIGURE 35–2 ■ The esophagomyotomy is started 6 to 7 cm above the diaphragmatic hiatus with a hooked cautery tip or sharp scissors dissection and brought through the phrenoesophageal ligament and on to the stomach for 1 cm.

opened, with care taken to avoid injury to the esophagus or the vagus nerve. The flexible endoscope is brought down to the lower esophagus and pointed up into the left chest to allow visualization of the esophagus. If the esophagus is not easily visualized at this time, a vascular tape is placed around the esophagus and brought out through one of the skin incisions beside the operating ports.

The esophageal myotomy is started 6 to 7 cm above the diaphragmatic hiatus and brought through the phrenoesophageal ligament and on to the stomach for 1 cm (Fig. 35–2). After the longitudinal muscle of the esophagus has been identified and marked, the incision is deepened until the circular muscle fibers are evident. The circular muscle fibers are carefully hooked away from the mucosa and divided by means of low-power electrocautery or sharp scissors dissection. The surgeon introduces the flexible endoscope into the stomach, taking care not to distend the stomach with air. The myotomy is carried distally. As the diaphragm is approached, the assistant pulls on the muscular wall of the esophagus, bringing the esophagogastric junction into the chest while the instrument through port C pushes down on the diaphragm. As the incision is carried through the esophagogastric junction, care must be taken not to injure the mucosa, which is thinner in this area and may be more difficult to separate from the muscularis than in the thoracic esophagus.

The branch of the left gastric vein running across the phrenoesophageal ligament marks the esophagogastric junction, and the myotomy should be carried on to the stomach for at least 1 cm distal to this landmark. An adequate myotomy is evident to the endoscopist as the lumen of the gastroesophageal junction suddenly becomes widely patent (open). When the lower part of the esophageal myotomy has been completed, the proximal end of the myotomy is carried toward the inferior pulmonary vein for 6 cm proximal to the esophagogastric junction. Using the endoscope as a stent, the surgeon then dissects the muscles away from the mucosa for 180 degrees.

The chest is filled with warm saline and the esophagus is distended with air to check for mucosal perforations. If the mucosa is perforated, thoracoscopic suturing may be used to close the defect. Unless the surgeon is well versed in thoracoscopic suturing, however, the esophageal defect is more safely closed with absorbable sutures through a left thoracotomy and covered, if possible, with a partial fundoplication or an intercostal muscle flap.

Port sites are then injected with 0.25% lidocaine and closed except for the anterior port, through which a No. 28 French angled chest tube is placed into the pleural cavity and attached to underwater drainage. This tube is removed 24 hours after surgery following completion of a successful esophagogram obtained by the use of water-soluble contrast material. Patients are given a "dental" soft diet for 3 weeks, after which they may resume a normal diet. Nighttime proton pump inhibitors are given to patients with symptoms of heartburn.

Laparoscopic Modified Heller Esophagogastric Myotomy with Anterior Fundoplication

The objective of the modified Heller procedure is to carry out a myotomy of the lower 6 cm of the esophagus, the esophagogastric junction, and the proximal 2 cm of the stomach, obliterating the dysfunctional LES. The antireflux barrier is augmented by fixing the lower 6 cm of myotomized esophagus below the diaphragm under the influence of positive intra-abdominal pressure and wrapping it with a partial anterior gastric fundoplication. The

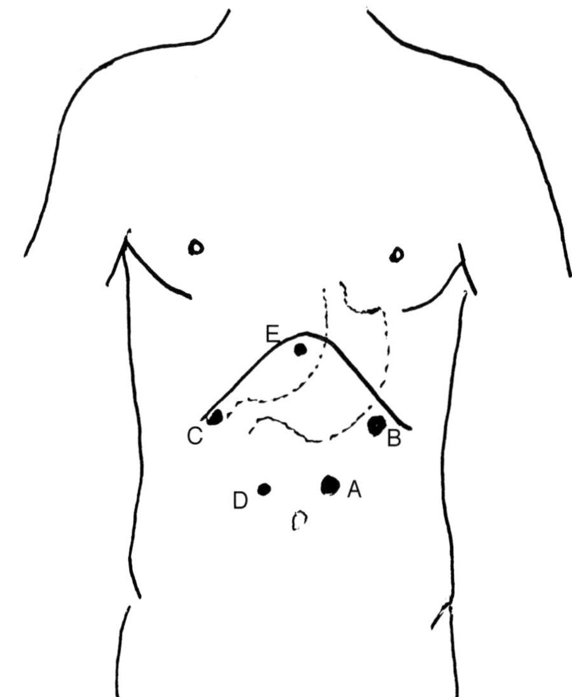

FIGURE 35–3 ■ Port placement for laparoscopic Heller myotomy and anterior fundoplication.

fundoplication results in compression of the esophagus when intragastric pressure is elevated, reducing the propensity for reflux.

All procedures are accomplished with the patient under general anesthesia after preoperative endoscopic cleaning of the esophagus and stomach in order to avoid aspiration during induction of anesthesia. Pneumatic stockings are used, and the patient is placed on the operating table in the lithotomy position with the head of the bed elevated 30 degrees.

A flexible endoscope is reinserted into the midesophagus under direct vision. After preparing and draping the abdomen, the surgeon stands between the patient's legs with the camera operator on the patient's right side. The video screen is placed at the head of the patient. The costal margin and the base of the xiphoid are marked. A pneumoperitoneum is produced using either a Veress needle in the left upper quadrant or the Hasson technique if the patient has had previous upper abdominal surgery.

Port positions are illustrated in Figure 35–3. A 10-mm port (A) is placed 15 cm below the base of the xiphoid through the left rectus sheath medial to the epigastric vessels. A 30-degree telescope is introduced through port A and a second 10-mm port (B) is placed using direct vision under the left costal margin 10 cm from the base of the xiphoid. A 5-mm trocar (C) is placed beneath the right costal margin 10 cm from the xiphoid. Through this port, the surgeon holds an atraumatic grasper with the left hand. A 5-mm trocar (D) is placed 15 cm from the base of the xiphoid through the right rectus sheath. Finally, the liver retractor is placed through a 5-mm post (E) placed in the midline just below the tip of the xiphoid. The left lobe of the liver is retracted, exposing the diaphragmatic hiatus (Fig. 35–4). A 5-mm Babcock grasper placed on the upper stomach through port D is used to retract the esophagogastric junction caudally.

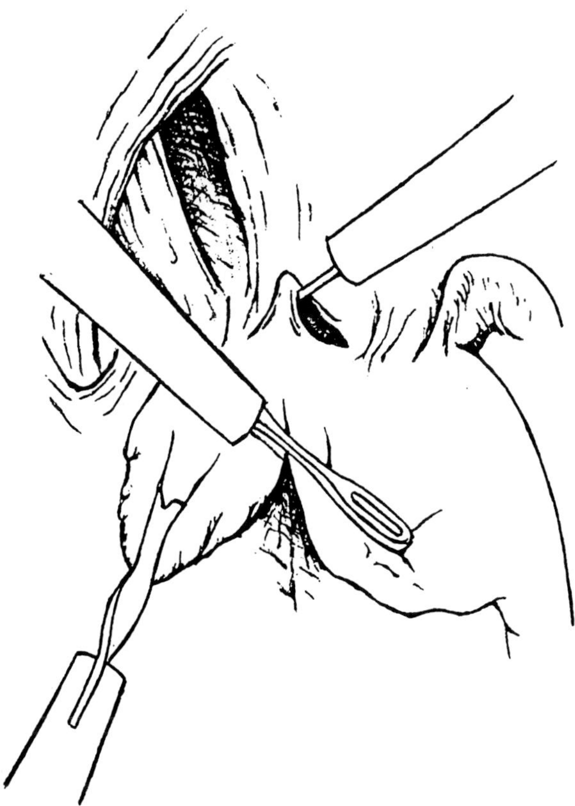

FIGURE 35–5 ■ The left crus of the diaphragm is exposed completely.

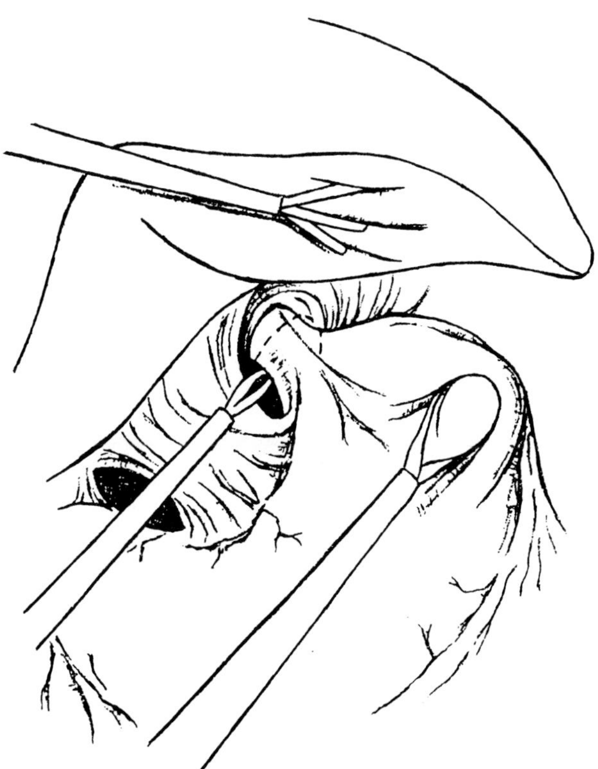

FIGURE 35–4 ■ The left lobe of the liver is retracted, exposing the diaphragmatic hiatus. The Babcock grasper is used for caudal retraction on the esophagogastric junction. Division of the gastrohepatic ligament and peritoneum overlying the abdominal esophagus begins superior to the hepatic branch of the vagus nerve and proceeds to the patient's left to the left crus of the diaphragm with care taken not to injure the anterior vagus nerve.

Division of the gastrohepatic ligament and the peritoneum overlying the abdominal esophagus begins superior to the hepatic branch of the vagus nerve and proceeds to the patient's left to the left limb of the crus of the diaphragm, with care taken not to injure the anterior vagus nerve. The left crus of the diaphragm is exposed completely (Fig. 35–5). The surgeon opens the retroesophageal space from the right side of the esophagus and encircles the esophagus with vascular tape, taking care not to injure the posterior vagus nerve or the esophagus (Fig. 35–6). With careful hemostasis maintained, 6 cm of esophagus is mobilized into the abdominal cavity.

A flexible endoscope is then placed into the stomach under direct vision. The phrenoesophageal ligament is divided between clips along the line of myotomy, with care taken to avoid injury to the anterior vagus nerve. With a hook with low-power cautery, the esophageal myotomy is started in the thickened esophagus 6 to 8 cm proximal to the phrenoesophageal ligament and carried under the anterior vagus nerve, through the esopha-

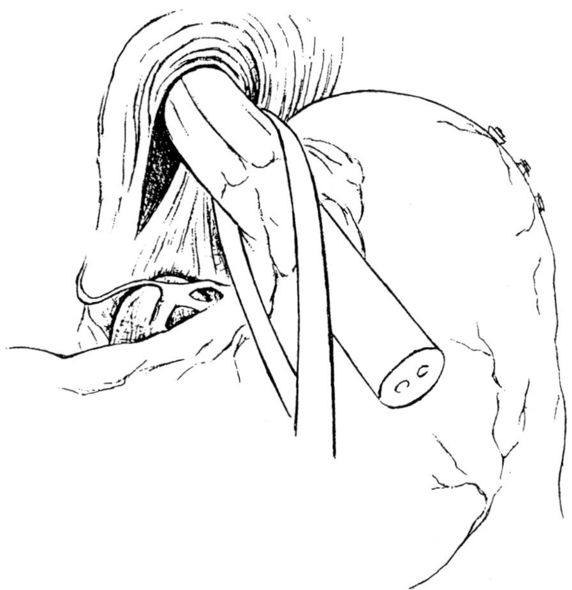

FIGURE 35–6 ■ The retroesophageal space is opened from the right side of the esophagus. The esophagus is encircled with a vascular tape. The gastroscope is placed into the stomach under direct vision.

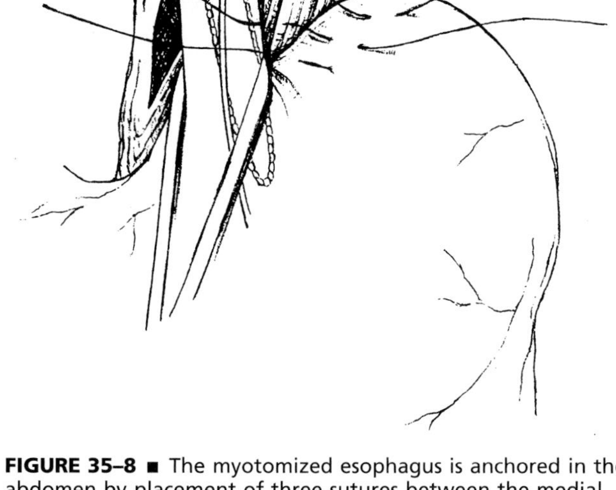

FIGURE 35–8 ■ The myotomized esophagus is anchored in the abdomen by placement of three sutures between the medial side of the fundus, the left limb of the crus of the diaphragm, and the left edge of the myotomized esophageal muscle.

gogastric junction, and on to the stomach for at least 2 cm (Fig. 35–7). This allows division of the sling fibers of the esophagogastric junction. The esophageal muscle is swept off the mucosa for 180 degrees. The surgeon removes the gastroscope, checking the esophagogastric junction for patency and the mucosa for perforations.

The myotomized esophagus is anchored in the abdomen by placement of three 2–0 silk sutures between the medial side of the fundus, the left crus of the diaphragm, and the left myotomized esophageal muscle (Fig. 35–8). The vascular tape is removed. The fundus of the stomach is anchored to the apex of the right crus. The rest of the fundus is rolled loosely over the lower esophagus and anchored in place with three sutures between the fundus, the right side of the myotomized muscle, and the right limb of the crus of the diaphragm (Fig. 35–9). The short gastric vessels are divided if the fundoplication is under tension (Fig. 35–10).

If the mucosa is perforated during the course of the procedure, the surgeon uses a laparoscopic suturing technique employing interrupted absorbable sutures to close the perforation. The perforation is then covered with the anterior fundoplication.

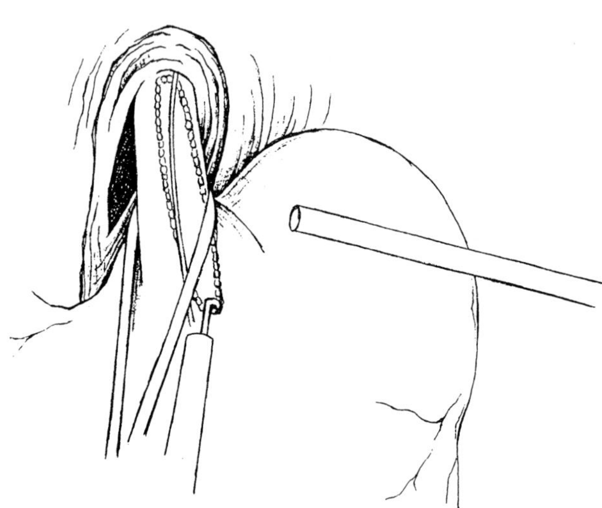

FIGURE 35–7 ■ The esophagomyotomy is started in the thickened esophagus 6 cm proximal to the phrenoesophageal ligament and carried under the anterior vagus nerve and onto the stomach for at least 2 cm via a hooked cautery.

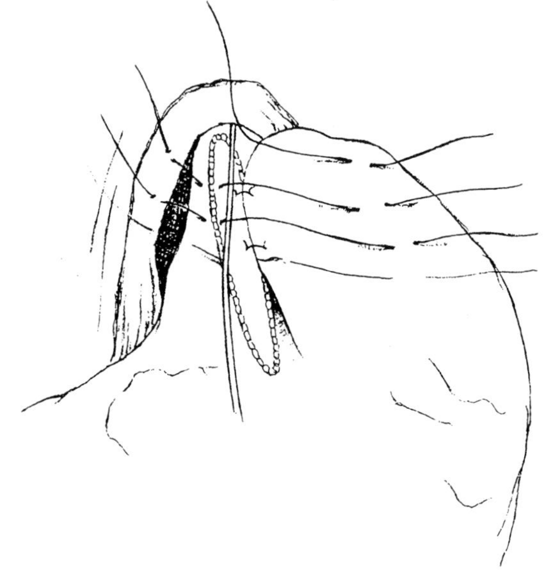

FIGURE 35–9 ■ The fundus is rolled loosely over the esophagus and anchored to the right myotomized esophagus and right crus with three or four sutures.

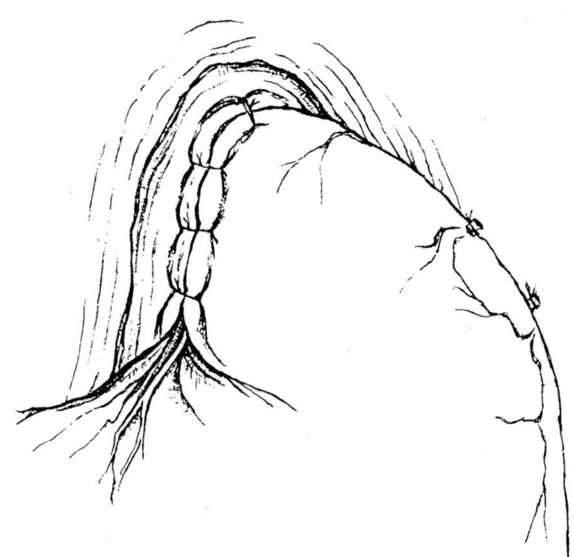

FIGURE 35–10 ■ The short gastric vessels are divided if the fundoplication is under tension.

Postoperative Care

An esophagogram with water-soluble contrast material is obtained on the first postoperative day to rule out mucosal perforations. A clear fluid diet is started, and the patient is discharged to home, usually within 36 to 48 hours. Patients are given a dental soft diet for 3 weeks postoperatively, after which a normal diet is resumed.

RESULTS

Thoracoscopic Esophageal Myotomy

In 1993, Pellegrini and colleagues reported the results for 24 patients who had undergone esophageal myotomy. Dysphagia was completely relieved in 17 of these patients and substantially, but not completely, relieved in 4 of the 24. Five of eight patients who had undergone a 24-hour pH study exhibited abnormal esophageal reflux, although they were asymptomatic. These investigators recommended that these patients be treated with nighttime proton pump inhibitors to decrease the amount of acid reflux and that they be monitored with periodic endoscopic monitoring postoperatively to make sure that mucosal damage caused by reflux was not occurring. Pellegrini's group observed that 3 of the 24 patients had residual dysphagia and concluded that the myotomy was not carried down far enough on to the stomach.

Stewart and coworkers (1999) analyzed the short-term and long-term results of thoracoscopic esophageal myotomy in 24 patients in two centers. In five patients the procedure was switched to open thoracotomy; three of the five had intraoperative esophageal perforations. These were recognized intraoperatively, and after conversion to thoracotomy, the perforations were closed and wrapped by means of a partial fundoplication using a Belsey technique. There were no postoperative leaks.

The other indication for conversion to an open procedure was poor visualization. The mean postoperative length of stay was 6 days as a result of prolonged hospitalization for the three patients with esophageal perforations. After a median follow-up of 42 months, 31% of the patients had no to minimal dysphagia, 67% had no or minimal heartburn, and 77% were satisfied with the surgical results.

Patti and colleagues (1999) reviewed the results for 35 patients who had undergone thoracoscopic esophagomyotomy in two centers. In two patients the procedure was switched to open thoracotomy. Four mucosal perforations occurred; one was repaired thoracoscopically, two were repaired by thoracotomy, and one required an esophagectomy because of end-stage disease. Excellent or good relief was observed in 73% of the patients. Symptoms of regurgitation, heartburn, and chest pain were also significantly relieved. Nine patients had persistent dysphagia secondary to an incomplete myotomy. Four of them subsequently underwent laparoscopic completion myotomies with good results.

The authors of these papers have now recommended that the laparoscopic approach to a modified Heller myotomy is the best primary surgical therapy for achalasia unless the patient has undergone previous upper abdominal surgery or has significant obesity that decreases the chance of accurate visualization of the esophagogastric junction with the laparoscopic technique.

Laparoscopic Esophageal Myotomy and Anterior Fundoplication

Using a laparoscopic myotomy and anterior fundoplication, Rosati and colleagues (1995) reported that 96% of their patients had absent or mild dysphagia postoperatively. Finley and colleagues (1999) reviewed 69 consecutive patients with achalasia who had undergone a laparoscopic Heller myotomy and anterior fundoplication by one surgeon. The median operative time was 1.9 hours, and there were no conversions to laparotomy. Operative complications included one patient with a mucosal perforation closed laparoscopically without sequelae and three patients with pneumothoraces that resolved spontaneously. Of the 64 patients available for follow-up (mean, 1 year), 96% were satisfied with their surgery. Symptoms were reported more than once a week for dysphagia in four patients, for regurgitation in three patients, and for heartburn in six patients. Liquid phase esophageal transit studies revealed significant improvement. During a 10-minute period, esophageal clearance in the supine position improved from 28% before operation to 49% after the operation and in the upright position from 55% to 81%. One patient had persistent postoperative dysphagia secondary to a tight anterior fundoplication. The dysphagia disappeared after a laparoscopic reversal of the fundoplication.

Patti and associates (1999) studied 133 patients who had undergone a laparoscopic myotomy in addition to a partial fundoplication. Mucosal perforations, which occurred in six patients, were closed laparoscopically. Eleven percent of the patients had persistent dysphagia initially, and 1% developed recurrent dysphagia after 1 year. Four of these patients had imperfectly formed Dor fundoplications, five had fibrotic transmural strictures, and two had incomplete myotomies. The incidence of preventable technical failure dropped from 23% during the early period of the study to 3% in the later experience. New gastroesophageal reflux developed in 17% of patients after laparoscopic myotomy. However, preoperative reflux was corrected in five of seven patients. The authors also reported excellent swallowing after a laparoscopic Heller myotomy, even in patients with an esophageal diameter greater than 6 cm.

The ability to mobilize and straighten a sigmoid-shaped esophagus during laparoscopic myotomy may improve esophageal emptying. For primary surgical therapy of achalasia, the laparoscopic approach to esophagomyotomy is favored over the thoracoscopic technique because the most difficult part of the dissection at the gastroesophageal junction is easiest to see laparoscopically and mucosal lacerations can be avoided. Furthermore, the laparoscopic technique avoids one-lung anesthesia and the need for chest tubes, allowing the surgeon to carry out an adequate myotomy and an antireflux procedure.

■ *REFERENCES*

Bonavina L, Nosadini A, Bardini R, et al: Primary treatment of esophageal achalasia: Long-term results of myotomy and Dor fundoplication. Arch Surg 127:222, 1992.

Cohen S. Motor disorders of the esophagus. N Engl J Med 301:184, 1979.

Couturier D, Samama J: Clinical aspects and manometric criteria in achalasia. Hepatogastroenterology 38:481, 1991.

Csendes A, Braghetto I, Henriquez A, et al: Late results of a prospective randomized study comparing forceful dilatation and oesophagomyotomy in patients with achalasia. Gut 30:299, 1989.

Dor J, Humbert P, Dor V, et al: L'intérêt de la technique de Nissen modifiée dans la prevention de reflux après cardiomyotomie extramuqueuse de Heller. Mem Acad Chir (Paris) 88:877, 1962.

Eckhardt VF, Kanzler G, Westermeien T: Complications and their impact after pneumatic dilation for achalasia: Prospective long-term follow-up study. Gastrointest Endosc 45:349, 1997.

Ellis FH: Oesophagomyotomy for achalasia: A 22-year experience. Br J Surg 80:882, 1993.

Finley RJ, Clifton JC, Stewart KC, et al: Laparoscopic Heller myotomy for achalasia: A clinical and scintigraphic swallowing follow-up. Can J Surg 42(Suppl):25, 1999.

Gordon JM, Eaker EY: Prospective study of esophageal botulinum toxin injection in high-risk achalasia patients. Am J Gastroenterol 92:1812, 1997.

Graham AJ, Finley RJ, Worsley DF: Laparoscopic esophageal myotomy and anterior partial fundoplication for the treatment of achalasia. Ann Thorac Surg 64:785, 1997.

Groenvedeldt DFR: Over cardiospasmus. Ned Tijdschr Ogeneeskd 2:281, 1918.

Heller E: Extra Mukose cardiaplatik beim chronisher Cardiospasmus mit Dilation Oesophagus. Mitt Grenzgeb Med Chir 27:141, 1914.

Katz PO, Gilbert J, Castell DO: Pneumatic dilatation for achalasia: Prospective long-term follow-up study. Gastrointest Endosc 45:349, 1997.

Malthaner RA, Todd TR, Miller L, Pearson FG: Long-term results in surgically managed esophageal achalasia. Ann Thorac Surg 58:1343, 1994.

Mayberry JF, Atkinson M: Studies of incidence and prevalence of achalasia in the Nottingham area. Q J Med 56:45, 1985.

Nelson JB, Castell DO: Esophageal motility disorders. Dis Mon 34:297, 1988.

Patti M, Pellegrini CA, Horgan S, et al: Minimally invasive surgery for achalasia: An eight year experience with 168 patients. Ann Surg 23:587, 1999.

Pellegrini CA, Leichter R, Patti M, et al: Thoracoscopic esophageal myotomy in the treatment of achalasia. Ann Thorac Surg 56:680, 1993.

Pellegrini C, Wetter LA, Leichter R, et al: Thoracoscopic esophagomyotomy: Initial experience with a new approach for the treatment of achalasia. Ann Surg 216:291, 1992.

Rosati F, Fumagalli U, Bonavina L: Laparoscopic approach to esophageal achalasia. Am J Surg 169:424, 1995.

Salis Graciela B, Garcia O, Mazzadi S, et al: Esophageal perforation after pneumatic dilatation for achalasia: Why? Acta Gastroenterol Latinoam 27:3, 1997.

Schiano TD, Parkman HP, Miller LS: Use of botulinum toxin in the treatment of achalasia. Dig Dis 16:14, 1998.

Stewart KC, Finley RJ, Clifton JC, et al: Thoracoscopic versus laparoscopic modified Heller myotomy for achalasia: Efficacy and safety in 87 patients. J Am Coll Surg 189:164–170, 1999.

Vantrappen G, Hellemans J: Treatment of achalasia and related motor disorders. Gastroenterology 79:144, 1980.

Zaaijer JH: Cardiospasmus in the aged. Ann Surg 77:615, 1923.

Trauma

CHAPTER **36**

Corrosive Injury

Kathryn D. Anderson

DEFINITION

Corrosive injury to the esophagus is usually sustained after ingestion of strong acids or strong bases. In children, almost all ingestions are accidental; in adults, a suicide gesture or a serious attempt at suicide is the cause of ingestion of corrosive substances. Children are usually in the toddler age group, and their curiosity to explore the world around them has just emerged as the driving force of their life. They can climb to apparently unscalable heights and open apparently locked doors with the greatest of ease. In addition, foolish parents may put oven cleaners, toilet bowl cleaners, and the like in attractive containers that formerly held food and drink. Because children tend to gulp things they put into their mouths, the injury is sustained on the first swallow. As a rule, the material is so noxious that the child does not ingest more than a mouthful. On the other hand, adults who are trying to commit suicide may ingest larger quantities of caustics, and the injury may extend well below the esophagus and affect the stomach and duodenum, injuries that are rare in children.

Corrosives include sulfuric and hydrochloric acids (in batteries) and sodium and potassium hydroxide (in oven cleaners, toilet bowl cleaners, drain cleaners, farm equipment cleaners). Dishwasher detergents, reagent tablets for monitoring urine glucose (Clinitest), and small batteries also contain strong alkalis. Weak bases, such as ammonia and hypochlorite solutions (household cleaners and bleach, respectively), are less caustic. Acids produce injury by coagulation necrosis and alkalis by liquefaction necrosis. Strong acids and particularly strong bases are extremely hygroscopic and penetrate deep into tissues by attaching the water of the tissue to their molecules.

In North America, the legal requirement of childproof caps has markedly decreased the incidence of corrosive esophageal injury. In countries that have no such laws, however, caustic materials are more readily accessible. In some countries, the practice persists of placing sulfuric acid crystals between double-glazed windows to absorb condensed moisture. The resulting acid solution may seep under the windows and may be ingested by the unwary toddler.

Much attention has been paid in the literature to the merits of early evaluation versus delayed evaluation of injury (Adam and Birck, 1982; Borja et al, 1969; Cardona and Daly, 1971; Viscomi et al, 1961). Those espousing the earliest examination of the esophagus for injury cite the importance of avoiding hospitalization of uninjured patients and timely treatment of those who have sustained injury (often with steroids, in an attempt to avoid stricture formation). Those who do not believe in the usefulness of steroids, and indeed some who do not advocate any esophagoscopy until a stricture is well established, believe that the risk of perforation of the injured esophagus is too great. Since the report by Spain and colleagues (1950) that corticosteroids could obviate an inflammatory response in mice and since experimental studies by and clinical impressions of several others (Haller and Bachman, 1964; Haller et al, 1971) suggested that stricture formation could be avoided by the use of steroids, steroids became part of the standard treatment regimen after ingestion of corrosive materials. The use of steroids was always controversial, and few randomized control series were available.

Stenting the esophagus by long-term placement of a nasogastric tube or silicone (Silastic) stents along the length of the esophagus has its advocates (Reyes and Hill, 1976). However, the use of these stents has never been reported in a large number of patients with a complete evaluation of the depth of the injury. It is therefore impossible to say whether stents work in the most severely injured patients. My personal opinion is that if the mucosa is destroyed circumferentially over a distance of more than a few centimeters, it is unlikely to re-epithelialize to any extent, and late strictures are inevitable. Also, because severe injuries are full thickness, stents would need to be left in place for months until the scarring had occurred to its full extent. This is not really a practical consideration because of potential complications of the stent itself.

HISTORICAL READINGS

Adam JS, Birck HG: Pediatric caustic ingestion. Ann Otol Rhinol Laryngol 91:656, 1982.

Borja AR, Ransdell HT, Thomas TV, Johnson W: Lye injuries of the esophagus. J Thorac Cardiovasc Surg 57:533, 1969.
Cardona JC, Daly JF: Current management of corrosive esophagitis. Ann Otol Rhinol Laryngol 80:521, 1971.
Haller JA, Andrews HG, White JJ, et al: Pathophysiology and management of acute corrosive burns of the esophagus: Results of treatment in 285 children. J Pediatr Surg 6:578, 1971.
Haller JA, Bachman K: The comparative effect of current therapy on experimental caustic burns of the esophagus. Pediatrics 34:236, 1964.
Reyes HM, Hill JL: Modification of the experimental stent technique for esophageal burns. J Surg Res 20:65, 1976.
Spain DM, Molomut N, Haber A: The effect of cortisone on the formation of granulation tissue in mice. Am J Pathol 26:710, 1950.
Viscomi GJ, Beekhuis GH, Whitten CF: An evaluation of early esophagoscopy and corticosteroid therapy in the management of corrosive injury of the esophagus. J Pediatr 59:356, 1961.

EARLY MANAGEMENT

Emergency Room Evaluation

If possible, the nature of the ingested material should be identified. Some predictions concerning the extent of injury can be made on the basis of this knowledge. Although household bleaches and ammonia cleansers have been reported to cause severe burns in adults (Tucker and Yarington, 1979), these materials tend to produce only mucosal injuries that do not penetrate the deeper layers of the esophagus. Such injuries usually heal without any long-term consequences. In children, who usually ingest only one mouthful of the caustic, there is rarely anything more than a superficial burn, which, in fact, has been so invariably true in my experience that I no longer perform esophagoscopy in these children. The history of actual ingestion, however, may or may not be reliable (Gaudreault et al, 1983). It has been said that unless there is a definite history of ingestion, there is no need to investigate further. One of the worst injuries that I have seen occurred in a child whose mother reported that he dipped his finger in the toilet bowl cleaner and did not ingest anything. This child eventually required a tracheostomy and esophageal replacement.

Physical examination is critically important. Oral burns are not invariably present even when esophageal injury has occurred. Although I have not personally seen esophageal injury in the absence of mouth burns in a series of 131 patients, it is reported with enough frequency that physical examination of the mouth is not considered sufficient to ascertain whether any material has been swallowed (Kirsh and Ritter 1978; Middelkamp et al, 1969; Wijburg et al, 1985). In the child particularly, intraoral and perioral burns can be extremely damaging and can result in severe cicatrix formation. Injury to the lips can produce severe narrowing of the oral cavity, requiring plastic surgery (Fig. 36–1). Scarring of the hypopharynx can result in complete closure of the esophageal inlet and extensive damage to the larynx. This condition is particularly seen with powdered lye. It is therefore extremely important to check airway patency, and if tracheal injury or laryngeal injury is suspected, laryngoscopy and bronchoscopy should be added to the diagnostic maneuvers.

Frank perforation of the esophagus and destruction of the stomach and the duodenum can occur. I have seen this condition only once in a child in more than 25 years of practice, although it is reported anecdotally (Hawkins et al, 1980; Middlekamp et al, 1969; Oakes et al, 1982). Again, with the deliberate ingestion of corrosives by adults, the stomach and duodenum are far more likely to be injured, and therefore a careful physical examination of the abdomen to rule out peritonitis and abdominal films and/or a computed tomographic (CT) scan to rule out perforation are mandatory.

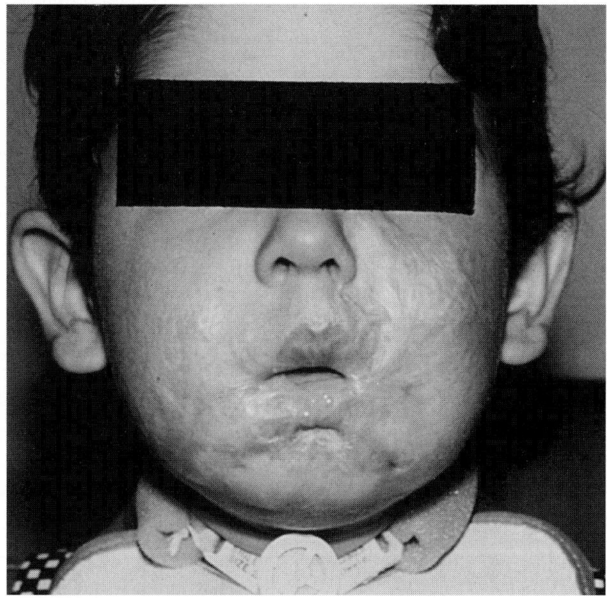

FIGURE 36–1 ■ This boy ingested lye as a toddler. He required esophageal replacement and several years later still has extensive perioral scarring, which has limited his intake of food.

All patients thought to have ingested caustic materials should be admitted to a hospital, and there are many arguments concerning which service. Gastroenterologists, otolaryngologists, and general and thoracic surgeons vie for these patients. Because I am a general pediatric surgeon, I will acquaint the reader with my own opinion.

Evaluation of injury, and indeed dilatations, can certainly be done competently by gastroenterologists and otolaryngologists. Only the general or thoracic surgeon, however, is qualified to make every single one of the management decisions, including endoscopic evaluation, handling of any complications such as perforation of the esophagus or stomach, insertion of a gastrostomy, dilatations, and, if required, eventual esophageal replacement. These management decisions are made correctly, in my opinion, only by those with experience with the entire spectrum of injury and its consequences. I strongly believe, therefore, that all such patients should be admitted to the general surgery service, which in pediatric surgery includes thoracic surgery.

Intravenous fluids are started, and the patient is given broad-spectrum antibiotics. Ampicillin or one of the cephalosporins is the antibiotic of choice. Because it was unclear whether steroids were helpful, 20 years ago a controlled randomized study was begun in my former institution after endoscopy and classification of the depth of the injury. Half of the children were treated with steroids, and half served as control subjects. The median age of the patients was 2 years. Of the 131 patients thought to have corrosive injury, 45% had significant injury and 50% of these developed strictures. Almost all of the patients who developed stricture had a third-degree burn (see later), and there was no difference between this group treated with steroids and those who served as control subjects (Anderson et al, 1990). The depth of injury, not the use of steroids, determines the development of stricture. Steroids are therefore no longer part of the management plan for our patients with caustic injury.

Endoscopic Evaluation

Because my experience with and interest in this problem began before the advent of flexible endoscopic equipment, I usually use a rigid Jesberg esophagoscope to evaluate the injury in children. I do not use magnified vision, having become adept over the years in assessing injury and stricture with an unmagnified view. With the sophistication of endoscopic equipment with magnification and good lighting, I have no argument with the advocates of flexible endoscopy (Zargar et al, 1991).

Whichever of the two methods is used, the concern must always be the vulnerability of the injured esophagus to perforation. I believe, therefore, that in the child the esophagoscope should be advanced only to the first level of the burn and no farther. If a flexible endoscope is used, it should always be the smallest size available, and air insufflation should be absolutely minimal. For adults with injury beyond the esophagus, it may be necessary to pass a flexible endoscope beyond the esophagus and into the stomach and duodenum. This procedure is safest if it is performed with a pediatric endoscope, again with minimal insufflation used (Zargar et al, 1991).

If any difficulties are encountered or if the lumen cannot be easily seen, endoscopy should be terminated. It is clear that observing only the most proximal burn may give a misleading picture of the true nature of the burn. For example, one of our patients who had severe strictures and required esophageal replacement had apparently only a relatively superficial burn as shown by esophagoscopy. It is possible that further examination, lower in the esophagus, might have shown a deeper burn.

It is also true that more than one stricture may exist, and some advocate abandoning the esophagus if this is the case (Kirsh et al, 1978; Moazam et al, 1987). Our experience has been different. Many of our patients have had successful dilatation of multiple strictures.

Burns are classified according to the depth (Kirsh and Ritter, 1976). *First-degree* injury involves only erythema and edema of the mucosa. In *second-degree* injuries, ulceration with necrotic tissue and white plaques are seen, but the injury is less than circumferential. If ulceration, white plaques, and sloughing of the mucosa are seen in a circumferential pattern, the injury is classified as *third-degree*. Other, more elaborate grading systems have been reported (Hawkins et al, 1980; Zargar et al, 1991), but this simple classification is of great value in the prediction of stricture formation.

Subsequent management depends on the depth of the burn. At the initial evaluation, if a severe injury is likely to be encountered, if large quantities of corrosive have been ingested, or if the ingestion is of an industrial-strength corrosive, such as in rural communities with dairy farms, I proceed immediately to perform a gastrostomy and place a string through the esophagus. The method of placing the gastrostomy—open or laparoscopic—is of less importance than making it large enough to pass dilators through. I recommend one or other of these methods rather than percutaneous endoscopic gastrostomy (PEG) because of the danger of esophageal perforation with the endoscope.

As discussed next, *retrograde* dilatation is much safer than *antegrade* dilatation, and because it is performed via a gastrostomy, it is useful to have the gastrostomy in place and healing for the 3 weeks or so before the stricture develops. Dilatation can then be started at that time.

In the child, the string is attached by Steri-Strips to a Phillips filiform with a small (8 French) follower and passed through the rigid scope down to the level of the stomach. It is then left in place as the esophagoscope is withdrawn.

For an adult, the filiform and follower are not long enough to reach the stomach. The string can be passed via one of the endoscopic instruments or attached to a nasogastric tube inserted under direct vision. A Stamm gastrostomy is then performed, and the string is retrieved from the stomach. One end is brought out to the gastrostomy site, the other end through the nose, and the two ends are tied together behind the patient's back. The string can be replaced with small-diameter silicone tubing between dilatations to lessen erosion of the nasolabial fold by the tense string.

In the toddler, I would place a 24 to 28 French Malecot gastrostomy catheter. Safe dilatation of the esophagus very much depends on the operator's ability to "feel" a dilator being "grabbed" by the stricture. This is not easy when the gastrostomy site is small.

The time to place a stent, if one believes in stenting, is at the initial evaluation (Mills et al, 1979; Reyes and Hill, 1976; Wijburg et al, 1989). The stents are left in place for up to 5 to 6 weeks and withdrawn after healing has taken place. I have no experience with this technique and cannot recommend it for the reasons stated earlier.

In the absence of injury, it is important to educate or counsel the individual responsible for the patient. If the patient is a child, parents must be instructed to keep all caustics away from their children. The only way to be absolutely sure of safety is to destroy the container immediately. Drain cleaners, oven cleaners, and other caustic materials should be used only once and the container washed out with gallons of water and thrown away immediately. Noxious materials should never be placed in eating or drinking vessels. Adults who have made a suicide gesture need intense psychiatric care and counseling. Follow-up of such patients can be clinical. There is no need to repeat esophagoscopy or perform any barium studies if the examiner is satisfied that no actual ingestion occurred.

Hospital Management

As stated, mouth burns can be severe. If the patient has spit out the caustic substance, injury can occur on ingestion and on egress of the material from the mouth. This problem arises particularly frequently in children, and any burn around the perimeter of the lips, especially in the corner of the mouth, can result in serious stricture formation (see Fig. 36–1). It may be necessary, therefore, to fashion stents for the mouth. These stents are left in place continuously at first and then are used only at night for several months after the injury. Pharyngeal burns can result in laryngeal injury all the way from mild hoarseness to extensive scar formation and stricture. Such patients may need a tracheostomy.

The management of the esophageal injury depends on the assessed depth of the burn. For second-degree burns, the patients are kept without food or drink and receive intravenous fluids and antibiotics until they can handle their saliva and swallow without pain. At that point, they are started on liquids, avoiding clear liquids, colas or sodas, and fruit juices, which are acidic. The diet is advanced as tolerated, and a mechanical soft diet is advised for at least 2 weeks after the injury. This diet means avoiding foods with sharp edges, such as French fries, pretzels, and potato chips.

I recommend repeated esophagoscopy in 3 weeks for patients with a second-degree injury, and at that time I examine the entire esophagus to make sure that a deeper lesion farther down in the esophagus was not missed. Flexible endoscopy gives a better view at this point. A barium swallow can be performed at this time, at the discretion of the surgeon, to examine the esophagus and the stomach and duodenum to ensure that there is no scarring.

For a third-degree injury, careful hospital follow-up of patients is required. Repeated observation to rule out intra-abdominal injury is necessary. Repeated radiographs to rule out perforation are taken as needed, and patients are kept without food or drink and receive intravenous fluids and antibiotics until they can manage saliva and until gastrointestinal function returns. When healing occurs, the patient stops drooling and can swallow without pain. Because strictures take approximately 3 weeks to become manifest, symptoms may return as a stricture becomes established.

Patients may be discharged and monitored at home when they can eat solid food, and they are re-evaluated 3 weeks after the injury. I perform an early barium swallow examination a day or two after the injury and again at 3 weeks (Kirsh and Ritter, 1976). Early evaluation by barium study may show some mucosal ulceration and may give an idea of the extent of the burn through motility disturbances in the esophagus (Fig. 36–2). In 3 weeks, the development and extent of strictures can also be evaluated by barium swallow (Stannard, 1978). Repeated endoscopy is performed, and classification of strictures, if they occur, can be made at that time.

If no stricture is present, patients are discharged with careful regular follow-up on an outpatient basis. Any symptoms such as pain on swallowing or inability to swallow solids should lead to immediate re-evaluation. If a stricture is observed at the second endoscopy, it is classified as mild, moderate, or severe, depending on the degree of compromise of the lumen. A *mild* stricture is one with minimal diminution of the size of the lumen; a *moderate* stricture, with a decrease in lumen size to one half of normal; and a *severe* stricture, with more than 50% compromise of the lumen.

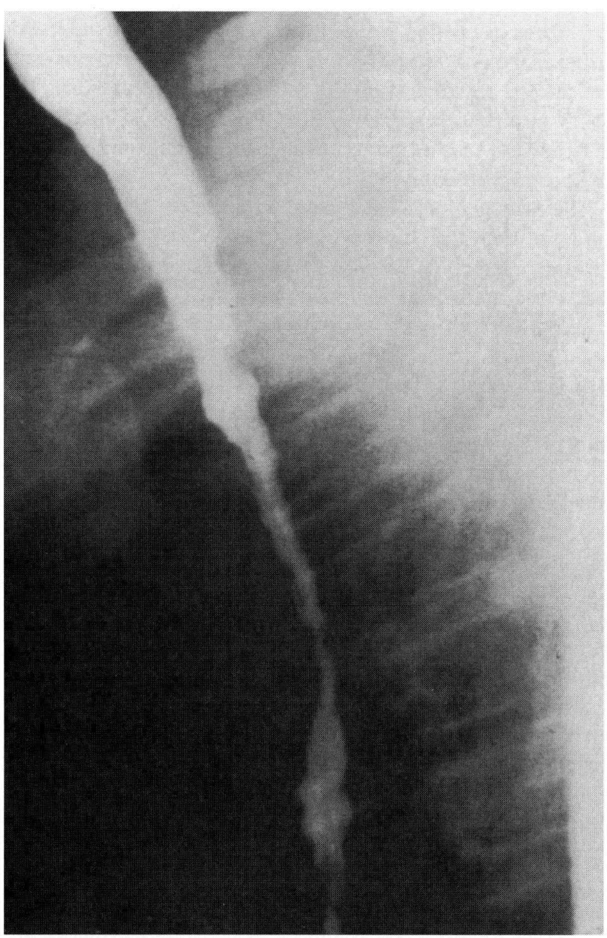

FIGURE 36–2 ■ Radiograph from barium swallow study showing ulceration of mucosa and motility abnormality of the esophagus following ingestion of a corrosive substance.

I believe that it is safest to dilate all tight strictures in retrograde fashion, and therefore a string and gastrostomy are placed at this time if this has not been done at the initial evaluation. Thus, dilatation of the stricture must be delayed for another 3 weeks until the gastrostomy is well healed. If a string has been placed or if the stricture is only moderate, gentle retrograde or antegrade dilatation can be begun at this time.

It may be important to know the length of the stricture as well as its diameter, which may be difficult to evaluate by barium swallow. If the lumen of the esophagus is severely compromised, little barium gets through the stricture and may give a false impression of a long stricture.

To define the precise length of the stricture, we have used a technique of a barium-filled Penrose drain (Tunell et al, 1971). A 1/2-inch Penrose drain is tied off at both ends. If no string is in place, a nasogastric tube is placed into the middle of the Penrose drain and tied in place. The Penrose drain is then filled with barium and advanced into the esophagus either in antegrade fashion using the nasogastric tube or tied to the string emerging

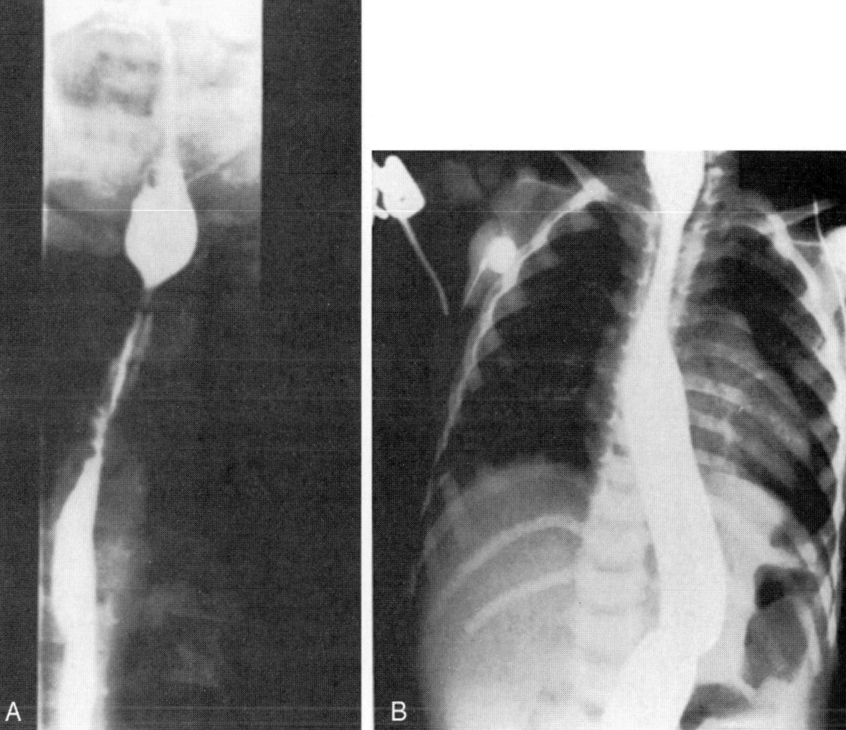

FIGURE 36–3 ■ *A*, Barium swallow with "streaming" of barium, making the extent of stricture difficult to define. *B*, Barium-filled Penrose drain in place defining precisely the severity and length of the stricture.

from the gastrostomy and gently drawn into the esophagus in a retrograde direction. A single radiograph is then taken (Fig. 36–3). This radiograph shows the extent of the stricture in terms of both diameter and length. This technique is also useful for following the extent of dilatation, films with the Penrose drain in place being taken before and after dilatation (Fig. 36–4).

The technique of dilatation is extremely important. I perform antegrade dilatation with tapered Maloney dilators. The starting size depends on an estimate of the size of the stricture. The dilator is gently advanced into the esophagus, with the operator's nondominant hand protecting the endotracheal tube and the end of the dilator being suspended by an assistant so that the dilator does

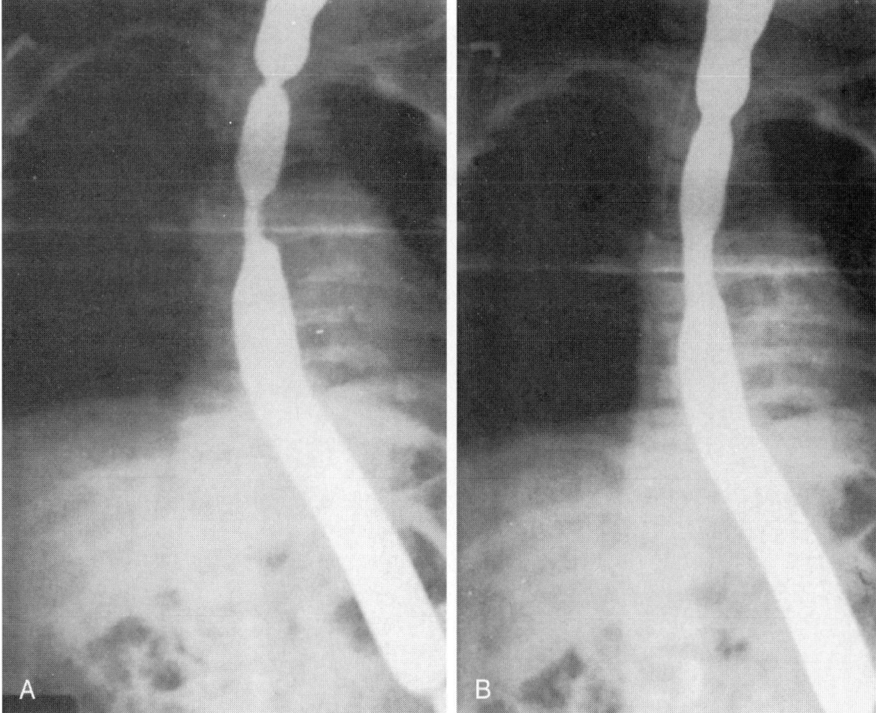

FIGURE 36–4 ■ Barium-filled Penrose drain before *(A)*, and after *(B)*, dilatation showing two strictures dilated satisfactorily.

not drag over the operator's hand. In this way, it is possible to feel the stricture "grab" the dilator. Dilators of increasing size are carefully advanced into the esophagus until they are all the way through the esophagus and can be palpated or seen through the abdominal wall. Each dilator is wiped with gauze after removal. If any blood is on the dilator, the procedure is terminated. Repeated dilatations after the appearance of blood virtually ensure that the stricture will be cracked, resulting in more severe scarring subsequently. Gentle stretching of the scar is the aim, not establishing a preconceived size of the esophagus at all cost.

The technique of retrograde dilatation is similar. Tucker graduated dilators are attached to the string emerging from the gastrostomy site (Tucker, 1974). The string is brought out through the mouth and is used to draw the dilators gradually through the esophagus. Retrograde dilatation is safest because stricture formation is often asymmetric, and the lumen of the esophagus is therefore in an eccentric position. Because the esophagus often dilates above the stricture, even if a string is used to dilate in antegrade fashion, the dilator may become impacted to one side of the lumen and perforate the esophagus.

The size to which the esophagus is dilated is again determined by the grab of the dilator by the stricture. Usually, there is a small serosanguineous stain on the dilator before the appearance of frank blood, and this sign can be used to judge a safe level of dilatation.

I have limited experience with balloon dilatation and use it only if I cannot pass a string through the stricture. A Glide Wire* can be passed through stricture followed by the balloon dilator of appropriate size. The balloon is inflated for 1 to 2 minutes, deflated fully, and withdrawn. If needed, the balloon can be filled with contrast material and radiography can be used to assess placement within the stricture, the size and length of the stricture, and the extent of dilatation accomplished. The incidence of perforation is much higher with this method.

The aim of dilatation is to keep patients at home, in school, or at work and eating a regular diet. Patients quickly learn what they can and cannot tolerate. It is interesting that foods such as potatoes and lettuce often may not go down well, possibly because of motility disturbances in the strictured esophagus. Foods such as spaghetti are often well tolerated, even by the strictured esophagus. Also, the parents and the patients are quickly able to determine when another dilatation is needed. I usually begin with a plan of dilatation electively every 2 weeks. The intervals between dilatations can then be lengthened gradually and the procedure performed on as-needed basis. In growing children, dilatations may be required from time to time when the child undergoes a growth spurt. I have noted this need particularly when the child enters puberty and begins to grow rapidly.

For strictures that totally obliterate the lumen of the esophagus, obviously the decision is made for esophageal replacement. Although some propose that esophageal replacement should be performed for an injury of extreme severity in the early days after injury (Zargar et al, 1991), I disagree because the modern treatment for replacement of the esophagus for caustic injury includes removal of the esophagus and placing the substitute through the esophageal bed rather than bypassing it and leaving it in situ. I feel it is difficult to justify this treatment in the presence of potential mediastinitis. In addition, strictures can look different in the same patient with each esophagoscopy. Unless there has been frank perforation or total sealing of the esophageal lumen, the physician simply cannot tell that the stricture is undilatable. I feel that repeated attempts at dilatation are almost always warranted.

In any case, I advocate waiting at least 6 months before deciding on esophageal replacement because seemingly intractable strictures have yielded to the dilator as the scar softens, 4 to 6 months after the burn. In addition, scar formation continues for at least 6 months, and scarring in the upper esophagus may complicate the performance of an anastomosis to the esophageal substitute.

*Glide Wire Terumo, Medi-Tech, Boston Scientific Corp., Watertown, MA.

Follow-up Evaluation

Short-term follow-up is predicated on the risk of further strictures of the esophagus in severe burns. As mentioned, the parents and/or the patient becomes adept at determining the necessity for dilatation. Long-term follow-up is essential in the growing child. As mentioned, the teenage growth spurt may produce further strictures of the esophagus, which may require further dilatations. Often, just one dilatation suffices at this time.

The risk of malignancy in the injured esophagus is considerably higher and occurs at an earlier age than in the general population (Bigelow, 1953; Ti, 1983). Esophageal carcinoma is difficult to diagnose and is often detected beyond the time when there is any hope of a cure. The parents and/or patient needs to know this risk and must always be alert to symptoms of dysphagia. For this reason also, I now perform transhiatal esophagectomy (Orringer and Sloan, 1978) when the esophagus is replaced. Even after replacement, there is still a risk of malignancy in the remaining upper esophagus. This risk may be accentuated if Barrett's esophagus develops above the anastomosis when reflux occurs in the esophageal substitute (Starnes et al, 1984).

Special Situations

Aspiration

Aspiration of corrosive material is rare and occurs most commonly in countries such as Africa, where powdered lye is the agent of injury. Lethal obstruction of the trachea and larynx may supervene, and the patient must be observed carefully for respiratory difficulties early after injury, when edema of the airway may produce obstruction, and late, when scarring narrows or obliterates the tracheal lumen.

I have had one patient who required a tracheostomy late in the course of his esophageal stricture for what was an unrecognized subglottic injury. The stricture gradually yielded to tracheal dilatations, and eventually the tracheostomy was removed. Two other patients who aspirated lye had severe laryngeal injuries. One of these injuries was repaired by a hypopharyngeal skin graft, but a later stricture necessitated a tracheostomy, which was removed during the patient's teen years. In the other patient, the tracheal lumen was entirely obliterated in the subglottic region, and he has a permanent tracheostomy.

Esophageal Perforation

Perforation of the esophagus sometimes occurs during the original injury. These perforations are usually contained and result in mediastinitis. Free perforation of the esophagus in the adult almost always requires abandoning the esophagus, and it is recommended that a cervical esophagostomy with drainage of the chest be performed on an urgent basis. Even in a child, it is doubtful whether a frank perforation can be repaired in the injured esophagus, and in most such cases the child requires esophageal replacement. Perforation during dilatation should not occur if the operator is experienced and careful. If such a mishap occurs, esophageal substitution is almost invariably required.

COMMENTS AND CONTROVERSIES

The management plan outlined in this chapter is my own, based on many years of personal experience with the entire spectrum of corrosive esophageal injuries in children. Controversies continue regarding which specialist should care for the patient, which endoscopic procedure should be performed, and the timing of the procedure. The methods of dilatation are many, and balloon dilatation has become popular, performed by gastroenterologists or even radiologists. Each method has its advantages and its drawbacks. The exquisite management of these complicated injuries is very operator-dependent, and as I have stated, my own opinion is that management by an individual experienced in the management of all aspects of the problem, rather than treatment by committee, serves the patient best.

K. D. A.

LATE MANAGEMENT

Several issues are involved in the decision to replace the injured esophagus. The first, and most obvious, one is the presence of an undilatable stricture. The second, and less obvious, one is the requirement for such frequent dilatations that the patient is unable to lead a normal life. For a child, a normal life includes the ability to eat by mouth without requiring major supplementation by gastrostomy feedings, to play normally, and to attend school without major episodes of absence. For an adult, absenteeism from work is always a problem regardless of how sympathetic supervisors are, and for both teenagers and adults, the ability to eat without embarrassment in front of family and friends is of major importance.

It is not possible to define exactly the number of dilatations that will bestow normality and how much disability is tolerable for a child or an adult. The decision to replace the esophagus is therefore a joint one made by the patient or the child's parents if the child is very young and by the physician who is responsible for the patient's care.

Preoperative Preparation

Nutrition is clearly important, and the patient may require prolonged gastrostomy feedings to ensure adequate body mass to manage the inevitable weight loss that accompanies a major operation. Close attention must be paid to the number of calories consumed by mouth and by supplemental gastrostomy.

There are a number of measures of adequate nutrition. Serum albumin and ferritin are somewhat useful, but it has always been my practice to see a steady weight gain in the child and gauge the adequacy of nutrition by direct observation. Clearly, any problems with gastrostomy stomas need to be corrected because leaking stomas make gastrostomy feedings a nightmare and, at their worst, can cause severe ulceration of the abdominal wall.

Aspiration pneumonia is relatively rare unless there is complete obliteration of the esophageal lumen. Saliva can be passed through the smallest of strictures, and in general patients with severe stricture limit oral intake so that food is rarely aspirated.

It may be necessary on rare occasions to perform a cervical esophagostomy. I recommend that the stoma be made on the left side of the neck and as low in the neck as possible to give the longest length of normal esophagus for the future anastomosis. Because the incision I make in the neck to accommodate the transposed colon or gastric tube is anterior to the sternomastoid muscle, I recommend drawing the esophagus forward of this structure to expedite the anastomosis in the major procedure. A Maloney dilator introduced into the upper portion of the esophagus allows it to be readily identified during performance of the esophagostomy.

The distal end of the esophagus is sutured or stapled closed but is left attached to the upper esophagus so that it is easily found for removal later on. The edges of the stoma are sutured to the skin; after healing of this stoma, the patient can eat by mouth wearing a colostomy bag or other device around the esophagostomy. This bag can be emptied and its contents used to supplement the nutrition by feeding the macerated diluted food or liquid into the gastrostomy. This is clearly a messy thing to do, but totally wasting the oral intake can become an expensive proposition for the patient's family.

On rare occasions, a tracheostomy has been necessary after pharyngeal or laryngeal trauma. This makes the replacement operation more difficult technically and the neck wound more susceptible to infection. Strict tracheal hygiene is necessary, and during esophageal reconstruction my practice has been to place an endotracheal tube transorally and drape the tracheostomy stoma out of the major operative field.

Surgical Options for Esophageal Replacement

There are several options for replacing the esophagus. I discuss two in some detail and mention two others.

Colon transposition has been performed for more than 40 years and has withstood the test of time well. Replacement with a reversed gastric tube has a slightly shorter history compared with colon replacement but has also held up well, particularly in children.

In the early days of esophageal replacement, particularly for malignancy, the whole stomach was transposed into the chest, and for some years this was a popular method of esophageal replacement. It has come into vogue again in children, and there are a number of good references for its use (Spitz et al, 1987). My objections to using the whole stomach are several. It functions only as a conduit, and therefore the patient essentially behaves as if he or she has had a gastrectomy, with digestive action of the stomach lost. The stomach can also be a space-occupying mass, especially in the small chest or mediastinum of the child. Acid reflux into the unprotected esophagus may well be a problem in the long term, with Barrett's esophagus and the future threat of malignancy compounding the threat of carcinoma engendered by the caustic injury itself.

The jejunum, as a pedicled viscus, has also been used in the past (Yudin, 1944) but is used to a lesser extent today. The difficulty with the jejunum is that the length of the bowel is redundant relative to the length of the mesentery, and it is difficult to obtain a straight portion of the jejunum without risking vascular compromise. The jejunum has also been transferred as a free flap using microvascular anastomoses. I leave the reader to seek technical details of these operations elsewhere, and I describe here the techniques of colon transposition and the reversed gastric tube, which is my personal preference.

Having decided on the organ to be used, the surgeon also has several choices concerning the route to the neck. Over the years, the substernal route has been the most popular and is certainly the easiest. This technique avoids dealing with the inevitable scarring in the mediastinum from the corrosive process itself, obviates a thoracotomy, and is a much less time-consuming operation. However, there are several disadvantages to the substernal route. The esophagus must take a sharp angulation forward for swallowed contents to enter the neoesophagus. This angulation sometimes causes enough functional obstruction in the adult that removal of the clavicular head is routinely recommended. This approach obviously involves some technical difficulties and also is unsightly for the patient.

The Belsey and Waterston approach via a left thoracotomy was for many years the alternative to the substernal route (Belsey, 1965; Waterston, 1964). In this approach, a thoracic incision or separate abdominal and thoracic or thoracoabdominal incisions are required. The neoesophagus is placed posterior to the root of the left lung. The esophagus is usually left in place. Alternatively, the right transthoracic route can be selected by choice or if the esophagostomy was performed on the right side of the neck.

Orringer and Sloan (1978) first described a transhiatal esophagectomy with replacement of the neoesophagus in the bed of the native esophagus. This has been my personal choice over the past decade. It has the advantage of removing the scarred esophagus with its potential for future malignancy and provides a much "straighter shot" between the neck and the stomach for the new esophagus. I always prepare the left chest, anticipating the need to do a thoracotomy as well in order to dig out the old scarred esophagus from extensive scarring in the mediastinum. This has occurred twice in my experience but never in a case of lye stricture. There is markedly decreased morbidity when a thoracotomy is avoided, and the patient has a much easier time swallowing through a tube that is essentially straight.

Preoperative Preparation

In most cases, I plan to perform a reversed gastric tube operation unless I have documented evidence of corrosive scarring of the stomach. I always perform a barium enema to make sure that the colon is normal and perform a complete bowel preparation in case the stomach is not suitable for any reason. Having decided to use a gastric tube, I have never had to resort to a colon transposition. That pitfall awaits me the first time I decide not to do the colon preparation!

Surgical Technique

Colon Transposition

Again, the surgeon must choose which portion of the colon to use. During the early days of colon transposition, the right colon with a portion of terminal ileum was placed in an isoperistaltic manner, basing the pedicle on the middle colic artery. This has worked reasonably well. The right colon tends to become redundant with time because of distensibility. Transposition of the transverse colon and left colon is my preferred method (Fig. 36–5).

As mentioned, I am always prepared to go into the left chest if a transhiatal operation is not technically feasible. Therefore, the entire abdomen, chest, neck, and left arm are prepared into the field. A sandbag is placed under the left chest, and the arm is covered with stockinette so that the arm can be placed at the patient's side or drawn forward across the chest if a thoracotomy becomes necessary. It is therefore important to request that one's anesthesia colleagues not place intravenous and intra-arterial lines or any other monitoring equipment on the left arm.

A midline incision is made, and any intra-abdominal adhesions are lysed. The gastrostomy is taken down and closed temporarily. The entire colon is inspected along with its blood supply, especially the marginal artery between the left colic and middle colic arteries. If the transverse colon and left colon are to be used in an isoperistaltic fashion, the middle colic artery is dissected down proximal to its bifurcation and a bulldog clamp placed as the artery exits from the superior mesenteric artery. This clamp is left in place for several minutes to make sure that the blood supply to the left and transverse colonic segments is preserved. The left colon is then grasped gently and advanced superiorly until it is pulled taut and a suture placed at the highest point that this portion of the colon reaches. This is the most distal portion of the neoesophagus. The distance between the midportion of the stomach and the cervical esophagus is then measured with an umbilical tape and measured off

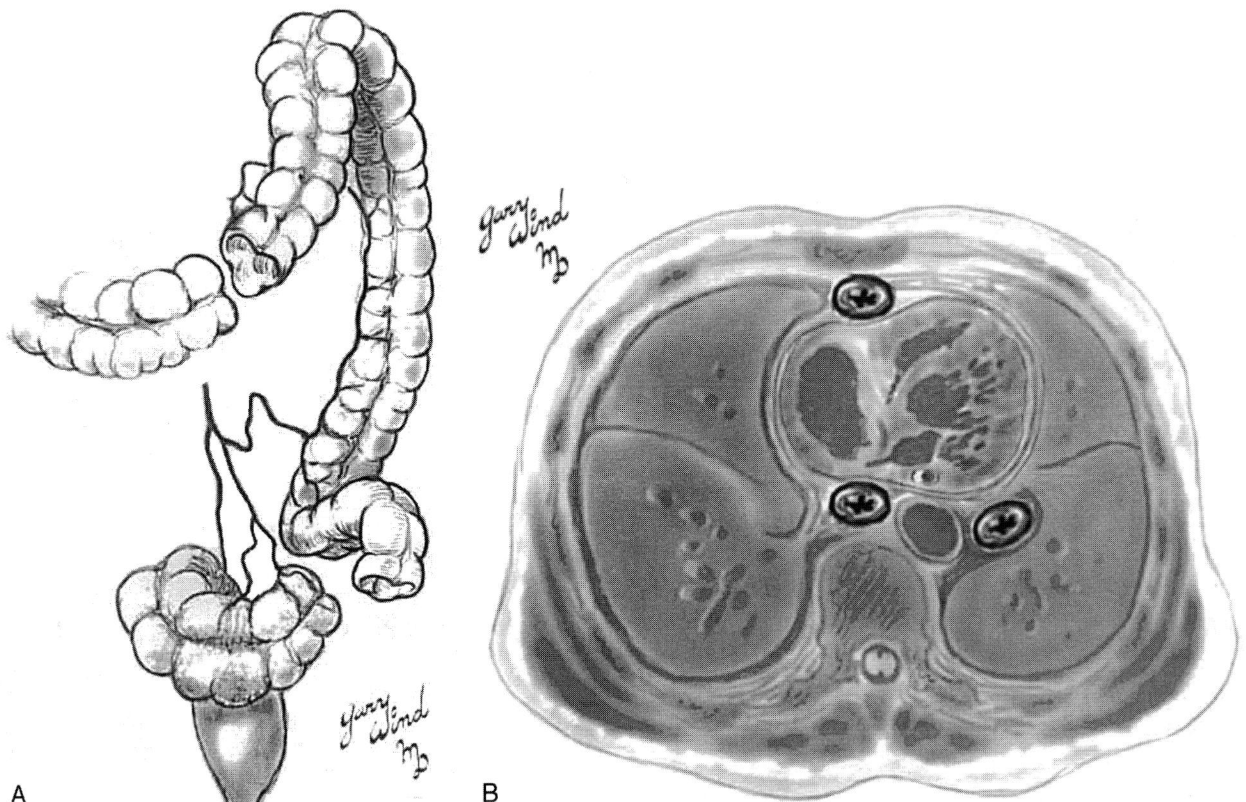

FIGURE 36–5 ■ *A* and *B*, Schema of colon used for transposition, with its blood supply, along with possible routes through the thorax.

against the colon, and a silk suture is placed proximally to indicate the length of colon needed.

The transhiatal esophagectomy is performed next. Using a combination of blunt and sharp dissection, the surgeon dissects the esophagus from below via the hiatus. As much as possible of the esophagus is separated from the mediastinal structures under direct vision as far superiorly as it is judged safe to go. A vertical cervical incision is then made along the anterior border of the sternocleidomastoid muscle. The surgeon deepens the dissection, drawing the sternocleidomastoid muscle posteriorly and the contents of the carotid sheath medially and avoiding the recurrent laryngeal nerve and the cervical sympathetic chain by staying close to the esophagus. The esophagus is surrounded with an umbilical tape.

As mentioned before, a Maloney dilator in the esophagus helps in its identification. The esophagus is then dissected distally, separating it from the mediastinal structures. Whether working from below or above or a combination, the operator must stay in the midline. This approach avoids damage to any other mediastinal structures or injury to the recurrent nerve on either side. I have performed more than 20 transhiatal esophagectomies with replacement of the esophagus via this route and have not injured the recurrent nerve in any of these.

When the esophagus is completely free in its bed, the anesthesiologist pushes the dilator into the esophagus to the level of the highest stricture. The esophagus is divided above this point. A Penrose drain is stapled to the distal cut esophagus and the esophagus drawn out into the abdominal wound, bringing the Penrose drain through to guide the neoesophagus back through this route. Alternatively, the distal esophagus can be divided at its junction with the stomach, a Penrose drain stapled at this end, and the esophagus drawn superiorly. It is important to make sure that this bed is of adequate size to carry the colon and the pedicle without any constriction and that there is also adequate room for some swelling to occur postoperatively.

Attention is then returned to the abdomen. The gastrocolic omentum is divided, with extreme care taken not to damage the inferior mesenteric vein, which can be quite short and can be seen entering the splenic vein. The middle colic artery is divided at the point where the "test" bulldog clamp was applied. The colon is then divided after the length is checked once more. Any tethering vessels from the left colic artery are divided proximal to the arcades supplying the colon itself. A portion of the colon distally may need to be trimmed if extensive division of these vessels is required. The colon is then attached to the Penrose drain and carefully brought up through the transhiatal route into the neck, being careful not to twist the vascular pedicle. The proximal end of the colon in the neck must be inspected carefully and frequently throughout the operation to ensure that its blood supply is not compromised in the transhiatal passage. For this reason, I recommend placing the transposed colon in its bed before reanastomosing the abdominal portion of colon.

Three anastomoses are then performed: (1) the colocolonic anastomosis between the transverse colon and the sigmoid colon, (2) the anastomosis between the lower

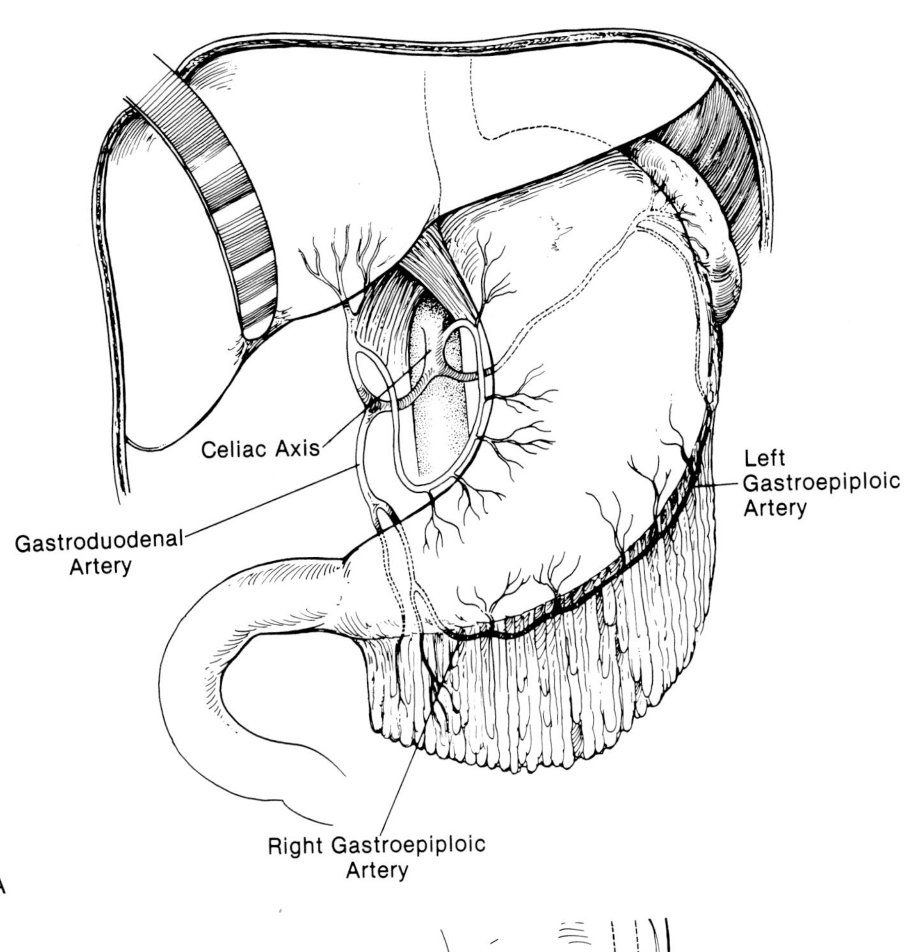

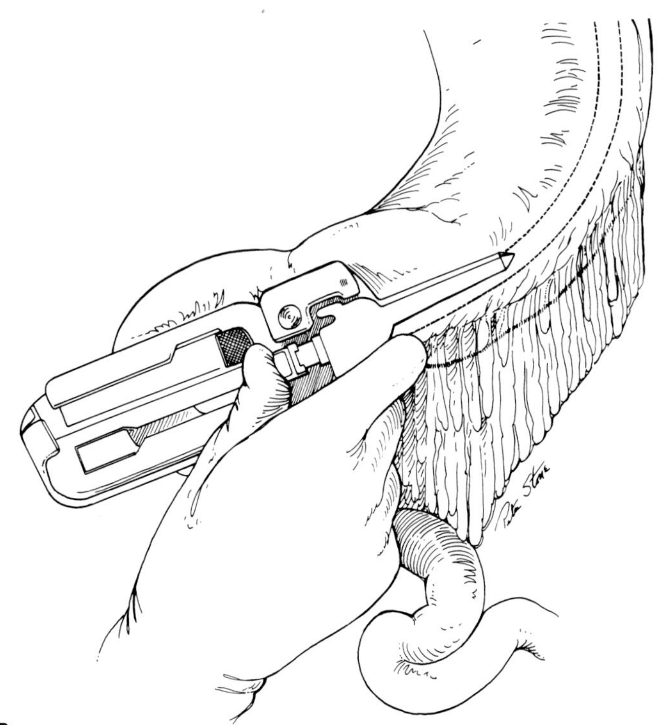

FIGURE 36–6 ■ Preparation of "reversed gastric tube." *A*, Anatomy of the area, including the blood supply of the stomach and the gastroepiploic arcade. *B*, Beginning preparation of the distal end of the gastric tube using a gastrointestinal anastomosis (GIA) stapler.

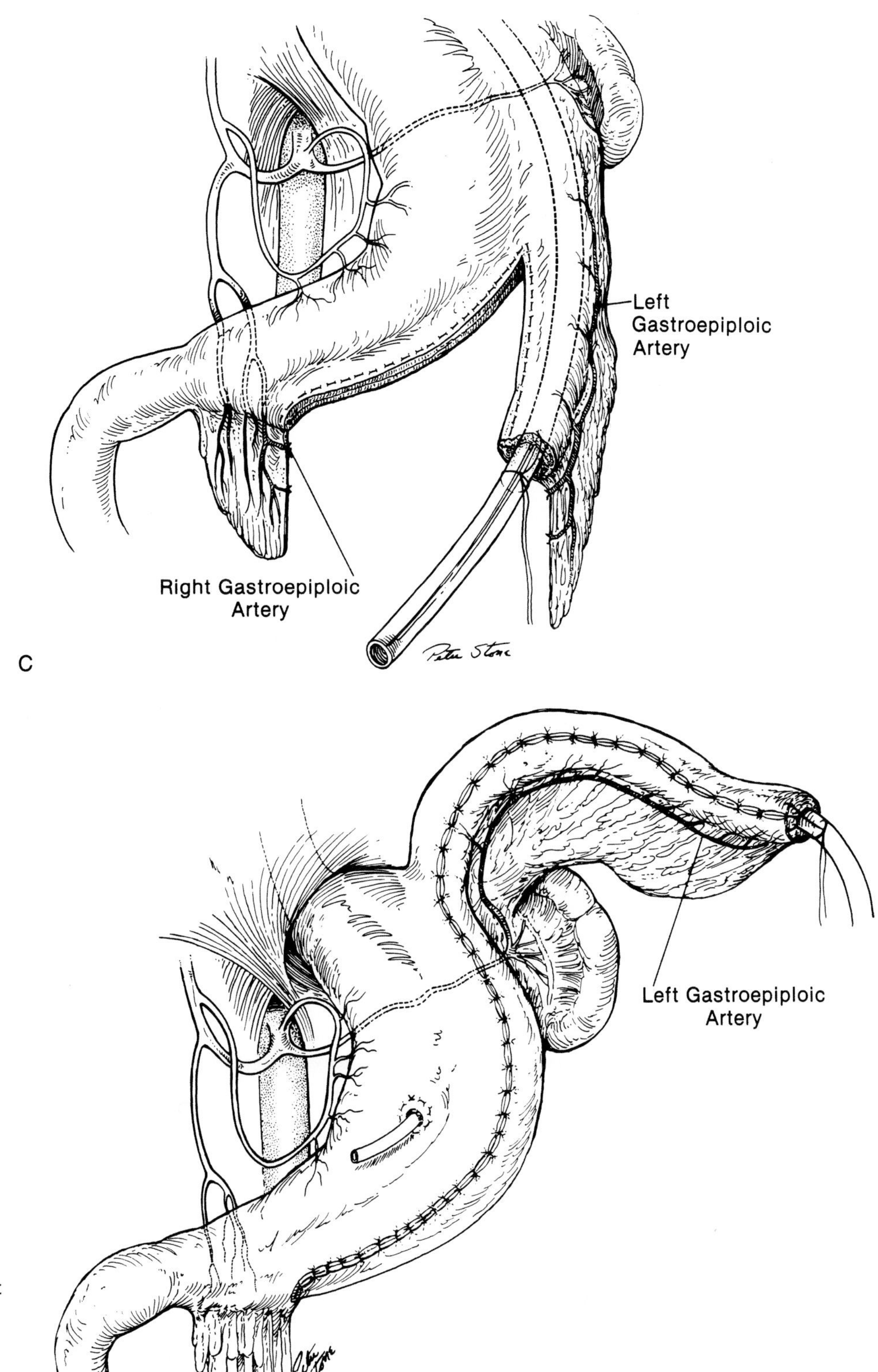

FIGURE 36–6 ■ *Continued C*, Reversed gastric tube partially formed. The right gastro-epiploic artery has been divided just proximal to the pylorus. *D*, Completed gastric tube. The spleen is preserved, and a gastrostomy is placed. The tube may be used to replace or bypass the esophagus. (From Replacement of the esophagus. In Welch KJ, Randolph JG [eds]: Pediatric Surgery, 4th ed. Chicago, Year Book Medical Publishers, 1986, p 704.)

end of the transposed colon and the stomach, and (3) the esophagocolostomy in the neck. Some advocate placing the cologastrostomy on the anterior wall, and an equal number call for placing it on the posterior abdominal wall. I do not believe that it makes much difference, and I would place it wherever it is technically easier. A cervical esophagocolostomy is then performed. The gastrostomy is re-formed and can usually be brought out through the same stab wound as before. All wounds are closed, and the neck is drained with a Penrose drain.

Gastric Tube

The incisions for the reversed gastric tube are identical to those for the colon. The gastrostomy is taken down as before, and any adhesions are lysed. With the performance of the transhiatal esophagectomy and the preparation of the cervical esophagus described in the technical details for colon transposition, I now describe only the creation of the gastric tube.

The gastroepiploic arcade running along the greater curvature of the stomach is inspected. It is not necessary for the arcade to be entirely visible outside the gastric wall. There may be an intramural anastomosis between the right and left arcades. In my experience, this is not a problem. Ideally, the gastrostomy has been placed well away from the greater curvature and the technical performance of the procedure is therefore relatively simple. If the gastrostomy has been poorly placed, however, a reversed gastric tube is still possible unless the gastrostomy has actually destroyed the arcade. I have performed several gastric tube procedures in which the closed gastrostomy became part of the tube itself. It was an interesting phenomenon but of no consequence to the child.

The surgeon can also create a large flap posteriorly and turn it anteriorly to fill in any defect created by a gastrostomy in the anterior portion of the tube. This must be done by hand suturing. I stretch the greater curvature of the stomach by having the anesthesiologist insert a nasogastric tube, and then I push it through into the duodenum. If this maneuver is precluded by the size of the stricture, the greater curvature can be stretched by hand. An umbilical tape is used to measure the length needed to reach the neck. A small series of dots is burned in the anterior serosa about 2 cm proximal to the pylorus. A point approximately 2 cm from the gastroesophageal junction is chosen at the upper end of the stomach. This point will be the distal end of the gastric tube, and the distance between these two points is measured. I have never found the length of the greater curvature to be inadequate and in one case have sutured the gastric tube into the pharynx and found it to be of a perfectly adequate length. I always make the gastric tube as long as possible (see later).

An opening is made in the anterior wall of the stomach with the electrocautery, and a chest tube of the size gauged to be correct for the size of the gastric tube is then passed along the greater curvature and held in place manually. The gastrointestinal anastomosis (GIA) stapler is placed across the anterior and posterior walls of the stomach, being guided by the intragastric chest tube, and successive portions are cut to create the tube (Fig. 36–6). The number of cuts required depends on the length of the stomach and the length of the stapler used. The gastroepiploic arcade tends to slew forward or backward as the tube is being created, and care must be taken not to allow it to be trapped in the jaws of the stapler. It is important to make sure that the upper end of the stomach at the gastroesophageal junction is not too narrow. I reinforce both staple lines by interrupted serosal sutures of silk or nylon. Theoretically, this reinforcing line of sutures is not necessary. I have never had the courage to omit it.

The gastric tube is then laid anteriorly over the chest, and it should be long enough to reach the cervical esophagus. The tube is then wrapped in warm packs as the transhiatal route is prepared. After the scarred esophagus is stapled off from the stomach and divided, I make an intussusception in the lower end of the gastric tube to create a little antireflux valve of about 270 degrees and place sutures between the serosa of the gastric tube and the stomach to hold it in place. I have found that when this is done, reflux is much less of a problem. The gastric tube is then drawn through the hiatus into the neck, and the anastomosis is completed as described for the colon. Wound closure is standard, and the neck is drained.

Postoperative Care

Prophylactic antibiotics are continued for 72 hours. The patient is given nothing by mouth and nothing by gastrostomy for 5 to 6 days. After this time, the integrity of the transposed esophagus is tested with a barium swallow. Gastrostomy feedings are begun in small volumes, especially if a gastric tube has been used, and gradually worked up to full volume. If there is no leakage at the cervical anastomosis, the patient can gradually resume oral feedings as tolerated.

Follow-up

In the case of esophageal replacement for caustic burns, it is almost inevitable that the upper anastomosis must be dilated. Dilatation is usually started approximately 3 weeks postoperatively and is done with great caution. Leaks of the anastomosis usually close spontaneously, although stricture is more likely with this problem. Dilatations are not started until the leakage has ceased.

COMMENTS AND CONTROVERSIES

Kathryn D. Anderson has accumulated a large experience with the use of a "reversed gastric tube." She reports late results that are comparable to those obtained by Belsey (1972).

Removal of the scarred esophagus is particularly important in children and young adults, who have an anticipated long life expectancy. I have seen two of my own patients (who were managed by bypass rather than resection) succumb to inoperable squamous cell carcinoma that developed in the esophageal remnant at 32 and 37 years, respectively, after the original lye ingestion.

F. G. P.

KEY REFERENCES

Anderson KD, Rouse TM, Randolph JG: A controlled trial of corticosteroids in children with corrosive injury of the esophagus. N Engl J Med 323:637, 1990.

This report describes an 18-year randomized controlled study in children with lye injury of the esophagus. The study showed that depth of injury, and not steroids, determined the outcome vis-á-vis stricture and need for replacement.

Belsey R: Reconstruction of the esophagus with left colon. J Thorac Cardiovasc Surg 49:33, 1965.

This is the "classic" reference for the technique of colon transposition in the adult.

Gaudreault P, Parent M, McGuigan M, et al: Predictability of esophageal injury from signs and symptoms: A study of caustic ingestion in 378 children. Pediatrics 71:767, 1983.

Although signs and symptoms were not absolutely predictive of esophageal injury, the children without symptoms tended to have less severe damage. Children with symptoms, especially vomiting, dysphagia, and abdominal pain, tended to have more severe injury of the esophagus.

Kirsh MM, Ritter F: Caustic ingestion and subsequent damage to the oropharyngeal and digestive passages. Ann Thorac Surg 21:74, 1976.

This article is a good review of the pathophysiology, clinical features, diagnosis, and management of caustic injuries.

Middelkamp JN, Ferguson JB, Roper CL, Hoffman LD: The management and problems of caustic burns in children. J Thorac Cardiovasc Surg 57:341, 1969.

This analysis of 95 children with caustic ingestion attempts to correlate depth of injury and steroid use with the development of stricture.

Zargar SA, Kochhar R, Mehta S, Mehta SK: The role of fiberoptic endoscopy in the management of corrosive ingestion and modified endoscopic classification of burns. Gastrointest Endosc 37:165, 1991.

This report describes a careful prospective study of the use of fiberoptic endoscopy to evaluate esophageal and upper gastrointestinal injuries for corrosive ingestion in a large group of patients, mostly adults.

REFERENCES

Adam JS, Birck HG: Pediatric caustic ingestion. Ann Otol Rhinol Laryngol 91:656, 1982.

Belsey R: The long-term clinical state after resection with colon replacement in adults. In Smith RA, Smith RE (eds): Surgery of the Esophagus. London, Butterworths, 1972.

Bigelow NH: Carcinoma of the oesophagus developing at the site of lye stricture. Cancer 6:1159, 1953.

Borja AR, Ransdell HT, Thomas TV, Johnson W: Lye injuries of the esophagus. J Thorac Cardiovasc Surg 57:533, 1969.

Cardona JC, Daly JF: Current management of corrosive esophagitis. Ann Otol Rhinol Laryngol 80:521, 1971.

Haller JA, Bachman K: The comparative effect of current therapy on experimental caustic burns of the esophagus. Pediatrics 34:236, 1964.

Haller JA, Andrews HG, White JJ, et al: Pathophysiology and management of acute corrosive burns of the esophagus: Results of treatment in 285 children. J Pediatr Surg 6:578, 1971.

Hawkins DB, Demeter MJ, Barnett TE: Caustic ingestion: Controversies in management: A review of 214 cases. Laryngoscope 90:98, 1980.

Kirsh MM, Peterson A, Brown JW, et al: Treatment of caustic injuries of the esophagus: A ten year experience. Ann Surg 88:675, 1978.

Mills LJ, Estrera AS, Platt MR: Avoidance of esophageal stricture following severe caustic burns by the use of an intraluminal stent. Ann Thorac Surg 28:60, 1979.

Moazam F, Talbert JL, Miller D, Mollitt DL: Caustic ingestion and its sequelae in children. South Med J 80:187, 1987.

Oakes DD, Sherck JP, Mark JBD: Lye ingestion: Clinical patterns and therapeutic implications. J Thorac Cardiovasc Surg 83:194, 1982.

Orringer MG, Sloan H: Esophagectomy without thoracotomy. J Thorac Cardiovasc Surg 76:643, 1978.

Reyes HM, Hill JL: Modification of the experimental stent technique for esophageal burns. J Surg Res 20:65, 1976.

Spain DM, Molomut N, Haber A: The effect of cortisone on the formation of granulation tissue in mice. Am J Pathol 26:710, 1950.

Spitz L, Kiely E, Sparnout T: Gastric transposition for esophageal replacement in children. Ann Surg 206:69, 1987.

Stannard MW: Corrosive esophagitis in children. Am J Dis Child 132:596, 1978.

Starnes VA, Adkins B, Ballinger JF, Sawyers JL: Barrett's esophagus: A surgical entity. Arch Surg 119:563, 1984.

Ti TK: Oesophageal carcinoma associated with corrosive injury: Prevention and treatment by oesophageal resection. Br J Surg 70:223, 1983.

Tucker JA: Tucker retrograde esophageal dilatations. Ann Otol 83(Suppl 16):1, 1974.

Tucker JA, Yarington CT: The treatment of caustic ingestion. Otolaryngol Clin North Am 12:343, 1979.

Tunell W, Rosser S, Anderson KD: Esophagram with a barium filled Penrose drain. J Pediatr Surg 6:667, 1971.

Viscomi GJ, Beekhuis GH, Whitten CF: An evaluation of early esophagoscopy and corticosteroid therapy in the management of corrosive injury of the esophagus. J Pediatr 59:356, 1961.

Waterston D: Colon replacement of the esophagus (intrathoracic). Surg Clin North Am 44:1441, 1964.

Wijburg FA, Beukers MM, Heymans HS, et al: Nasogastric intubation as sole treatment of caustic esophageal lesions. Ann Otol Rhinol Laryngol 94:337, 1985.

Wijburg FA, Heymans HSA, Urbanus NAM: Caustic esophageal lesions in childhood: Prevention of stricture. J Pediatr Surg 24:171, 1989.

Yudin SS: The surgical constriction of 80 cases of artificial esophagus. Surg Gynecol Obstet 78:561, 1944.

CHAPTER **37**

Foreign Bodies

ESOPHAGEAL FOREIGN BODIES IN ADULTS

Florian Lang
Philippe Pasche
Jean-Baptiste Ollyo
Philippe Monnier
Marcel Savary

DEFINITION

Foreign bodies, as well as food boluses, pills, and corrosive agents, are objects that can induce swallowing injuries to the esophagus.

HISTORICAL NOTE

Until Samuel Gross published his treatise on foreign bodies in 1854, it was common to use some form of bougie to push the offending object down into the stomach. Gross devised and advocated the use of various instruments to extract the foreign body (e.g., curved forceps, blunt metallic hooks, a piece of wire formed into a noose, a gum elastic catheter outfitted with a stylet or a piece of sponge attached to its extremity) (Clerf, 1952). The overall prognosis for patients with incarcerated esophageal foreign bodies remained poor, and according to Terracol (1951), the mortality rate was still more than 50% at the end of the 19th century. The prognosis improved with the progress in surgery but only for foreign bodies impacted in the proximal esophagus. In a series of 326 patients with external cervical esophagotomies, Balacescu and Kohn (1904) reported a mortality rate of 26.5% in the pre-antiseptic era before 1880 and of 12.6% in the aseptic era after 1900.

Real progress came with the development of rigid esophagoscopy. Bonzini was the first to visualize the upper end of the esophagus around 1795, Mackenzie used a skeleton type of esophagoscope in 1890, and Einhorn definitely improved the technique in 1902 with the introduction of the auxiliary tube in the wall of the esophagoscope as the light carrier (Clerf, 1952). With distally illuminated tubes, the overall fatality rate dropped rapidly to 12.5% in 200 cases (Lerche, 1911). In 1957, Jackson reported a 98% success rate for endoscopic removal of foreign bodies, with a 2% mortality rate. Currently, removal of esophageal foreign bodies by a rigid esophagoscope maintains a 99% success rate, and the mortality rate has continued to drop to less than 0.2% (Brossard et al, 1981; Chaikhoumi et al, 1985; Giordano et al, 1981; Roura et al, 1990). To sustain these results, precise knowledge and an adequate practical attitude must be preserved in this field.

■ *HISTORICAL READINGS*

Clerf LH: Historical aspects of foreign bodies in the air and food passages. Ann Otol Rhinol Laryngol 61:5, 1952.
Jackson CL: Foreign bodies in the esophagus. Am J Surg 93:308, 1957.
Lerche W: The esophagoscope in removing sharp foreign bodies from the esophagus. JAMA 56:634, 1911.
Terracol T: In Masson CR (ed): Les Maladies de l'Oesophage. Paris, Deuxième Edition, 1951.

EPIDEMIOLOGY

Around 1950, swallowing injuries represented the main source of esophageal trauma, being much more common than instrumental lesions. Today, they are proportionately less frequent than esophageal instrumental injuries (as a result of esophagoscopy, dilatation, malignant tumor intubation, laser application, surgery, endotracheal intubation, or tracheostomy tubes), which have increased during the last decades. However, the incidence of esophageal swallowing injuries has not decreased in absolute number (Besson and Saegesser, 1983). Foreign body ingestion remains a relatively common problem, with an estimated incidence of 120 per million population, resulting in approximately 1500 deaths each year in the United States (Smith and Peura, 1992).

The following discussion is in large part based on a clinical series of 2018 patients (age > 16 years) with a history of foreign body or food impaction who underwent esophagoscopy, which revealed a foreign body, food im-

TABLE 37–1 ■ **Outcome of Endoscopy in 2018 Adults with a History of Foreign Body or Food Impaction**

Endoscopy Outcome	*No. (%)*
Foreign body or food impaction	949 (47)
With esophageal injury	392 (19)
No foreign body but esophageal injury	447 (22)
No foreign body or esophageal injury	622 (31)

From a clinical series of patients of the ENT and Head and Neck Surgery Clinic, University of Lausanne, January 1, 1963, through December 31, 1998.

paction, or a swallowing injury in 69% of cases (Table 37–1).

AGE AND SEX DISTRIBUTION

Incarcerated esophageal foreign bodies can occur at any age, but two frequency peaks appear in most published series—one in children through the age of 10 years and one in adults older than 50 years. Both sexes are equally affected (Table 37–2). During their early learning and developmental years, children are likely to place nondigestible objects in their mouths, with subsequent accidental swallowing. Impaired vision, incomplete food mastication due to poor dentition or ill-fitting dentures, and diminished mucosal sensitivity of the palate due to dental plates account for foreign body ingestion in older adults (Röthlisberger and Savary, 1977; Smith and Peura, 1992).

RISK FACTORS

Besides those at risk just mentioned, other high-risk groups include certain professionals who tend to keep items such as pins in their mouths while working (upholsterers, dressmakers), psychotic patients, drug smugglers, prisoners, and persons with preexisting esophageal lesions (Clarkston, 1992; Jackson, 1950; Payne and Olsen, 1974; Peytral et al, 1991; Terracol, 1951; Webb, 1988) (Table 37–3).

TYPES OF FOREIGN BODIES

Most of the foreign bodies found in adults originate from food, consisting of either a soft bolus, usually a piece of meat, or a nonedible item, such as a piece of bone or a fruit pit (Table 37–4). In contrast to children, who swallow a wide variety of smooth objects (primarily toys and coins), sharp foreign bodies are predominant in adults. Bone splinters, fish bones, and dentures are among the most commonly swallowed objects. Because of the sharpness, their incarceration may produce more severe damage; injuries of the esophageal wall are common (see Table 37–1).

The nature of accidentally swallowed esophageal foreign bodies has changed. Fortunately, safety pins, hairpins, and defective dentures, which were known to produce severe esophageal injuries and to cause major mechanical difficulties during manipulation for removal, have become less common; however, objects such as disk or button-type batteries, beverage can openers, plastic pieces, and cocaine packages have become more prevalent (Clarkston, 1992; Pyman, 1974; Webb, 1988, 1995). The frequency of encountered foreign bodies also depends on geographic factors (different alimentary habits); in a series by Nandi and Ong (1978) of 2394 foreign bodies in a Chinese population, 84% of the objects were fish bones.

Finally, the type of foreign bodies reported in the literature varies according to the medical specialty of the authors. Certain treatment techniques, especially the nonendoscopic methods, imply a selection of type or localization of the foreign bodies, and the series pub-

TABLE 37–3 ■ **Risk Factors for Foreign Body Ingestion**

Childhood	
Psychiatric disease	
Altered level of consciousness	Drug use Alcohol use Dementia
Structural abnormalities	Poor vision Wearing of dentures Pathologic conditions of esophagus
Consumption of high-risk foods	Chicken bones Fish bones
Professional activities	Upholsterer Dressmaker
Illicit activities	Drug smuggling Voluntary ingestion of foreign bodies by prisoners Concealment of forbidden objects by prisoners

From a clinical series of patients of the ENT and Head and Neck Surgery Clinic, University of Lausanne, January 1, 1963, through December 31, 1998.

TABLE 37–2 ■ **Age and Sex Distribution for 949 Adults with Endoscopically Confirmed Foreign Body or Food Impaction**

	Total	*Foreign Bodies*	*Nonedible Alimentary Foreign Bodies*	*Food Impaction*
No. of patients	949	133	390	416
Male-to-female ratio (%)	52:48	60:40	38:62	62:38
Mean age (yr)	56.9	49.3	56.6	65.1

From a clinical series of patients of the ENT and Head and Neck Surgery Clinic, University of Lausanne, January 1, 1963, through December 31, 1998.

TABLE 37–4 ■ **Types of Esophageal Foreign Bodies Found in 949 Adults**

Food impaction	**426** (45%)
Meat	239
Vegetables, miscellaneous food	187
Alimentary nonedible foreign bodies	**390** (41%)
Bones (e.g., chicken, mutton)	299
Fish bones, mussel shells	64
Pits, nutshells, bay leaves	27
True foreign bodies	**133** (14%)
Dentures, teeth	34
Pills (with or without wrapping)	23
Metal objects (e.g., pins, clips, can openers)	21
Mucilages	16
Plastic objects	12
Toothpicks	6
Coins	5
Miscellaneous (e.g., disk batteries, coin bags)	16

From a clinical series of patients of the ENT and Head and Neck Surgery Clinic, University of Lausanne, January 1, 1963, through December 31, 1998.

lished by ear, nose, and throat surgeons, gastroenterologists, and radiologists differ considerably.

BASIC SCIENCE

Natural History

From 80% to 90% of swallowed foreign bodies reach the stomach without difficulty, but 10% to 20% must be removed (Webb, 1995). When the passage is difficult, damage to the esophagus can be produced in the absence of incarceration (see Table 37–1). When the foreign body is incarcerated, no mucosal damage or superficial laceration is observed on endoscopic removal in about 87% of adult patients. Deep laceration is present in 9%, whereas esophageal perforation can be diagnosed in 4% (Table 37–5). Incarcerated esophageal foreign bodies can be removed endoscopically in more than 99% of patients (Chaikhoumi et al, 1985; Giordano et al, 1981; Jackson, 1957). In 1% or 2% of patients, the extraction must be performed with surgery (Brossard et al, 1991).

Once in the stomach, most foreign bodies, even when sharp or pointed, pass the distal digestive tract without problems. However, large objects, with dimensions of greater than 2 × 5 cm, are unlikely to pass the stomach and duodenum, and endoscopic removal is recommended (Clarkston, 1992). Sometimes even small but relatively heavy metallic foreign bodies, like coins and disk batteries, do not pass the stomach. Their position should be monitored radiographically, and if they do not move uneventfully within 7 to 10 days, endoscopic extraction is mandatory (Smith and Peura, 1992). Patients with a sharp or pointed object in the stomach should be observed clinically and radiographically until natural evacuation of the foreign body has occurred; about 12% of these patients require laparotomy because of perforation (Smith and Peura, 1992).

Prognosis

In contrast to the situation in children, prolonged sojourn of an esophageal foreign body is exceptional in adults. Rare cases have been reported in which a foreign body incarcerated during childhood was discovered during adulthood (Jackson and Jackson, 1950). The prognosis for a patient with an untreated esophageal foreign body can be estimated only on the basis of the natural history to of overlooked incarcerated foreign bodies; patients with an overlooked foreign body in the esophagus do not survive longer than 5 to 6 years and usually die within 1 year (Jackson and Jackson, 1950). The prognosis thus appears catastrophic owing to perforation and its subsequent complications (see later).

Pathophysiology

Ingested foreign objects can lodge at any level of the gastrointestinal tract, but most often they become impacted in regions that are physiologically or pathologically narrowed. The normal esophagus has three anatomic sites of narrowing: the upper sphincter (cricopharyngeus muscle), the level of the aortic arch, and the lower sphincter. Indeed, 84% of true or nonedible foreign bodies lodge just above, immediately at, or just below the upper sphincter, and 42% of food impactions occur above the lower sphincter (Table 37–6). However, the presence of an anatomic narrowing cannot account for 22% of foreign bodies and 29% of food impactions in

TABLE 37–5 ■ **Esophageal Injury Due to Foreign Body Ingestion in 2018 Adults**

	Foreign Body Present (n = 949)	*No Foreign Body (n = 1069)*
Type of Injury	*No. (%)*	*No. (%)*
Superficial mucosal tear	262 (28)	384 (36)
Deep laceration with or without hematoma	88 (9)	54 (5)
Perforation	42 (4)	9 (1)
Total	392 (41)	447 (42)

From a clinical series of patients of the ENT and Head and Neck Surgery Clinic, University of Lausanne, January 1, 1963, through December 31, 1998.

TABLE 37–6 ■ **Localization of Esophageal Foreign Bodies in 949 Adults**

Location	*No. of Foreign Bodies (True and Alimentary Nonedible) (%) (n = 523)*	*No. of Food Impactions (%) (n = 426)*
Hypopharynx	116 (22)	21 (5)
Upper esophageal sphincter	209 (40)	44 (10)
Cervical esophagus	113 (22)	122 (29)
Midthoracic esophagus	46 (9)	60 (14)
Lower esophagus	39 (7)	179 (42)

From a clinical series of patients of the ENT and Head and Neck Surgery Clinic, University of Lausanne, January 1, 1963 through December 31, 1998.

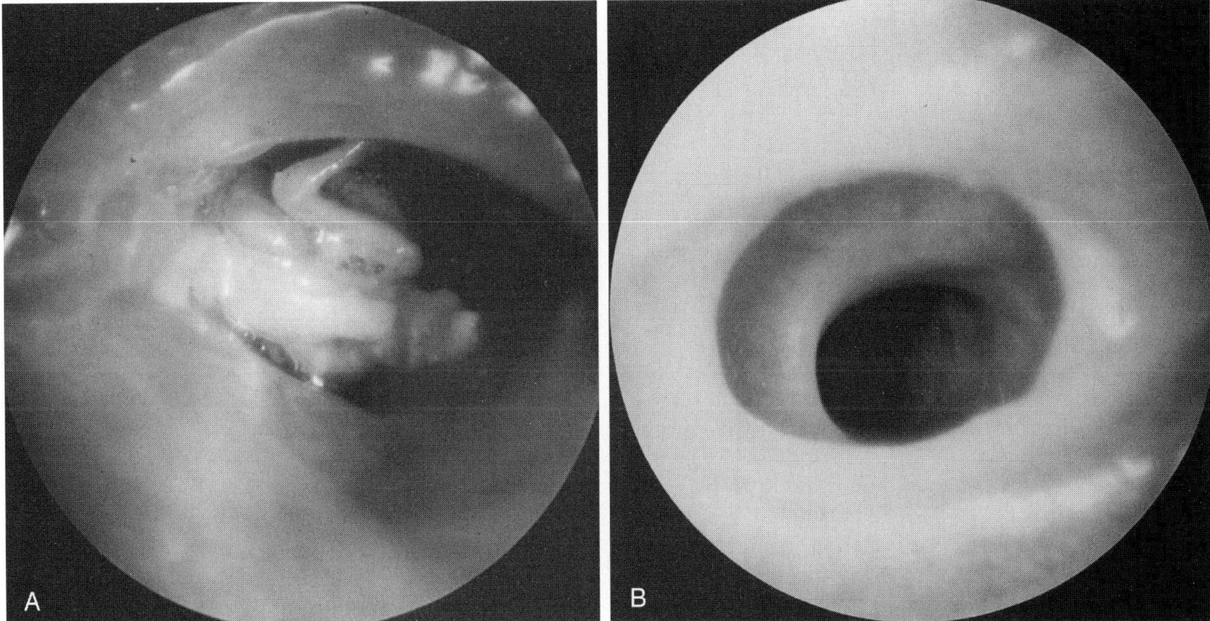

FIGURE 37–1 ■ *A,* Meat impaction in the cervical esophagus (chicken with bone). *B,* Underlying esophageal webs secondary to an epidermolysis bullosa detected during the post-extraction endoscopic follow-up evaluation.

the cervical esophagus, just below the cricopharyngeus muscle. In fact, the typical incarcerated foreign body in the cervical esophagus is located just below the posterior lip of the cricopharyngeal muscle.

The chute-like effect due to the posterior lip of the cricopharyngeal muscle, which is the chief factor in overriding a foreign body during esophagoscopy, may be of some importance. As early as 1950, Jackson suspected a weakness of the peristaltic musculature in the upper cervical esophagus, which is sufficient to carry a bolus of well-masticated and insalivated food downward but is not strong enough to carry down a physically different foreign body. Manometric studies have confirmed the presence of a segment of weak contraction amplitude in the normal proximal esophagus commonly believed to represent the area of transition from striated to smooth muscle. Particularly low in subjects with a history of foreign body, the amplitude of contraction in this area is, even in healthy volunteers, occasionally not adequate for the propulsion of an object (Mazzardi et al, 1998; Stein et al, 1992). Once the foreign body has harmlessly passed through the Killian sphincter and the cervical esophagus, it usually reaches the stomach without difficulty.

When incarceration occurs in the thoracic or lower esophagus, a much less common occurrence, an underlying esophageal disease must be suspected (see later). In contrast to the ingestion of a foreign body, esophageal food impaction occurs more frequently in the mid and lower esophagus and is related to a preexisting esophageal lesion or to a motor disorder in 65% of patients.

Underlying Esophageal Disease

Most foreign bodies that are accidentally incarcerated in the esophagus of a healthy person are found in its cervical portion. In the minority of cases in which the foreign body is located lower down, an esophageal disease must be suspected and is found in nearly 80%. In such cases, the patient's history often reveals previous or repeated episodes of foreign body incarceration (Payne and Olsen, 1974). In our series, the following pathologic esophageal conditions were found (in order of frequency): reflux esophagitis with strictures, postoperative stenoses, webs, Schatzki rings, hiatal hernia, cardioachalasia, carcinoma, diverticula, and motor disorders.

Consequently, a thorough postprocedural evaluation of the esophagus, including radiology and manometry at a minimum, should take place in the following situations:

- A foreign body incarcerated below the cervical esophagus (Fig. 37–1).
- Repeated episodes of foreign body impaction
- Meat or food impaction (see Fig. 37–1)

Complications

Esophageal injuries either are due to the sharpness of the foreign body or are secondary to pressure necrosis, as in the case of a prolonged incarceration, which is rare in adults. Regardless of whether the foreign body has spontaneously reached the stomach despite a difficult esophageal passage or has remained incarcerated, an injury is found at endoscopy in about 40% of patients with either situation (see Table 37–5). The injury is mainly a superficial mucosal tear, located in the cervical esophagus. When the foreign body has been incarcerated, severe injuries are more frequent and are detected endoscopically in 13% of the patients, with perforations occurring in 4%. Bones and fish bones cause the highest rate of injury (76%) and account for the most severe injuries (8% perforations), whereas nonalimentary foreign bodies, even sharp metallic objects (injury rate, 38%; perforation rate, 2%) and, of course, food impactions (injury rate, 11%; perforation rate, 2%) are far less dangerous.

The main complications of esophageal foreign bodies are related to esophageal perforation, either primary or secondary. The overall mortality rate coincident with perforation is substantial at 22% (Jones and Ginsberg, 1992). The more severe esophageal lesions, including perforations, are found in the upper and mid esophagus. The prognosis for patients with an esophageal perforation depends on the cause (acute perforation by sharp foreign body or slow perforation by pressure necrosis), size, location, and early recognition. Acute perforations are followed by the passage of air, saliva, or even food particles into the surrounding soft tissues with a very quick bacterial spread, resulting in the development of mediastinitis and potentially lethal septic shock (Atkins, 1985). Leaks that result from slow erosion are more likely to be contained by the subacute local inflammatory reaction, which thus limits the spread of infection, resulting more often in a local cervical or mediastinal abcess, sometimes with migration of the foreign body into the surrounding tissues or even with a complete secondary healing of the esophageal wall (Atkins et al, 1985; Nashef et al, 1992; Spitz and Hirsig, 1982; Terracol, 1951). In small puncture-like perforations, the bacterial seeding is of less importance and the reaction of the surrounding tissues is most often only local. Thoracic perforations are more feared than are cervical perforations because of the possible mediastinitis and the possible formation of fistulas between esophagus and trachea, main stem bronchi, pleura, pericardium, and major arteries (aorta, subclavian carotid), with the arterial fistulas being lethal most of the time (Hollander and Quick, 1991).

Early recognition of a perforation is vital for the prognosis (Benjamin, 1995; Segalin et al, 1996). Normally, a perforation should be diagnosed during postextraction control endoscopy (see later). If there is no initial suspicion, progressive occurrence of fever, retrosternal pain, and dysphagia during the postoperative period should alert the physician. Endoscopic recognition is easy when the laceration is large and clearly opens the mediastinum. Long, sharp, transversely incarcerated foreign bodies can also be easily recognized as transfixing the esophageal wall when they are removed. In contrast, deep, localized lacerations that extend to the muscular layer always make the endoscopist uncomfortable, arousing only a suspicion of perforation. Especially in these cases, cervical and chest radiographs should be obtained to detect cervical or mediastinal emphysema. In addition, a contrast study of the esophagus with meglumine diatrizoate (Gastrografin) should be performed.

The management of perforation should be aggressive. There are very few indications for conservative treatment: small puncture-like perforations, especially in the cervical esophagus, with no leakage of contrast medium, can be treated conservatively with intravenous fluids and antibiotics, nothing by mouth, and close monitoring; slow perforations due to pressure necrosis, when small, can also be closely monitored after the foreign body extraction (Winckler et al, 1989). If the evidence of response is not rapid, as measured by a reduction in fever, normalization of white blood cell count and radiographic appearance, and abatement of symptoms, there is a definite need for surgery. If the perforation is evident, early surgical drainage should be started within 1 to 3 hours (Atkins et al, 1985; Besson and Saegesser, 1983).

Aortoesophageal fistula is very rare (1 case in 2018 consecutive endoscopies for suspicion of foreign body in adults during a 35-year period) but is an especially serious complication, with only 9 survivors in about 500 patients reported in the literature (Ctercteko and Mok, 1980; Hollander and Quick, 1991; Quandalle et al, 1984; Wu and Wu-Wei, 1992). Clinically, aortoesophageal fistula is characterized by Chiari's triad (midthoracic pain, sentinel hemorrhage of bright red arterial blood, and exsanguination after a symptom-free interval). Most fatalities reported follow time-consuming diagnostic procedures after the sentinel hemorrhage or endoscopic extraction of the foreign body (one case in our series). Surgery at the time of exsanguination is too late. In the presence of a history of foreign body ingestion and an arterial sentinel hematemesis, *immediate* diagnostic endoscopy should be undertaken at the time of surgery, in the presence of a thoracic surgeon. As soon as the foreign body or fistula is localized, a thoracotomy for foreign body extraction and excision of the fistula with aortic and esophageal repair is necessary. Placement of a Sengstaken-Blakemore tube has demonstrated some benefit as a temporizing measure in the control of unrelenting hemorrhage (Hollander and Quick, 1991).

Esophageal strictures and tumor-like lesions are rare complications of long-standing foreign bodies in adults (Doolin, 1993; Set et al, 1992).

DIAGNOSIS

The diagnostic procedure includes the patient history, physical examination, radiology, and endoscopy.

History

The *penetration syndrome* is almost always present in adults; exceptions include some psychiatric patients and drug smugglers. This condition is described as a difficult swallowing episode with painful pharyngoesophageal passage and occasionally is associated with coughing, choking, vomiting, and, in rare instances, hematemesis. When this syndrome is absent in the adult, strong suspicion of another abnormal pharyngoesophageal condition should be aroused, but a complete diagnostic investigation nevertheless must be undertaken.

Incarceration of a foreign body results in a painful sensation that is usually felt in the lower jugular notch and is constantly exacerbated by swallowing movements, at times associated with a true dysphagia. The same symptoms may be present even if the foreign body has spontaneously reached the stomach after a difficult pharyngoesophageal passage, resulting in an esophageal injury. Total aphagia with sialorrhea may occur when the esophageal lumen is completely obstructed, such as by meat impaction. A coughing or choking attack followed by persistent dyspnea can be the result of a large foreign body, such as a piece of meat, impacted at the pharyngoesophageal junction (pseudo–café coronary). The critical

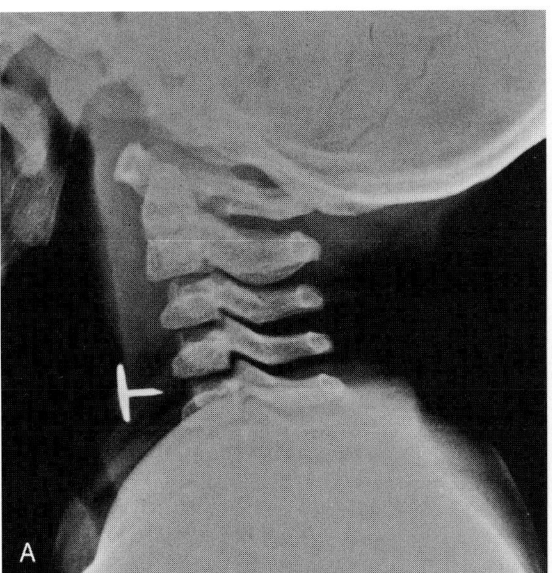

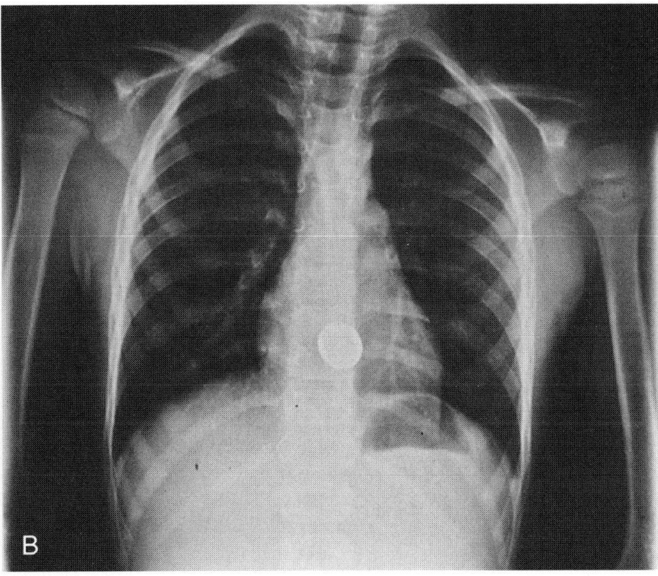

FIGURE 37–2 ■ *A,* Soft tissue lateral x-ray of the cervical region shows a drawing pin in the hypopharynx. *B,* Anteroposterior chest film shows a coin at the lower esophageal sphincter.

differentiating symptom is that in esophageal blockage, the main laryngeal functions—respiration and speech—albeit painful and impaired, always remain possible; in the true café coronary, the intralaryngeal impaction of meat induces a complete respiratory obstruction (Atkins et al, 1985).

Localization of the foreign body by the patient does not always correspond to its actual position in the esophagus. The higher the object, the better subjective localization seems to be. When the symptoms are well lateralized within the cervical region, the object is likely to be above the cricopharyngeus muscle and on the side indicated (Connolly et al, 1992). Items that are impacted below this level are poorly localized, and pain and discomfort are often felt higher up than at the effective site of incarceration. Pharyngeal innervation by the vagus and glossopharyngeal nerves seems to provide better sensation than the less-dense esophageal innervation by the vagus and cervical sympathetic nerves (Connolly et al, 1992).

In taking the patient's history, the clinician must inquire about repeated episodes of foreign body or food impaction and preexisting swallowing disorders or upper digestive diseases. The time and circumstances of the incident, the type of suspected foreign body, previous treatment trials, food and drink consumption after the time of ingestion, and the development of symptoms must be noted.

Physical Examination

The physical examination includes indirect pharyngolaryngoscopy (visible hypopharyngeal foreign body, salivary retention, edema of the arytenoid region), cervical palpation (subcutaneous emphysema, tenderness of the jugular region, painful active or passive mobilization of larynx), cardiopulmonary auscultation, abdominal palpation, and temperature determination.

Radiologic Examination

Any suspicion of an esophageal foreign body requires a lateral soft tissue radiograph of the cervical region and a chest radiograph to confirm and locate a possible radiopaque foreign body and to detect cervical or mediastinal emphysema secondary to an esophageal perforation (Fig. 37–2). An early radiologic sign of cervical emphysema is detected on the lateral cervical view, dorsal to the cricopharyngeal muscle, in the retrovisceral space in front of the sixth cervical body (sign of Minnegerode) (Fig. 37–3). In adults, it is sometimes difficult to differentiate an ingested bone splinter from calcifications of thyroid or cricoid cartilages. Contrast studies with barium are contraindicated because (1) they obscure the endoscopic view, masking the foreign body or mucosal lacerations; (2) there is a risk associated with mediastinal penetration of barium in cases of a perforation; and (3) there is a hazard of barium aspiration (Clarkston, 1992; Payne and Olsen, 1974; Peytral et al, 1991; Savary and Miller, 1978). Gastrografin contrast studies do not provide any additional useful information within the classic endoscopic management of foreign bodies.

Highly radiopaque foreign bodies such as coins, nails, and disk batteries are easily recognized. Slightly radiopaque foreign bodies are of a physical density somewhat greater than that of body tissues and form a subtler image. These substances include glass, aluminum, chicken bones, and some plastic materials. Most common commercial glass is radiopaque. Aluminum (can tops), although a metal, is of low physical density. Both glass and aluminum should be visible on a properly exposed radiograph but are difficult to visualize on radiographs with a number of superimposed structures, such as the standard chest radiograph. Foreign bodies that have the same density as that of the body (thorns, spines, some plastics, wood in situ for longer than 48 hours) are virtually impossible to detect. Radiolucent foreign bodies,

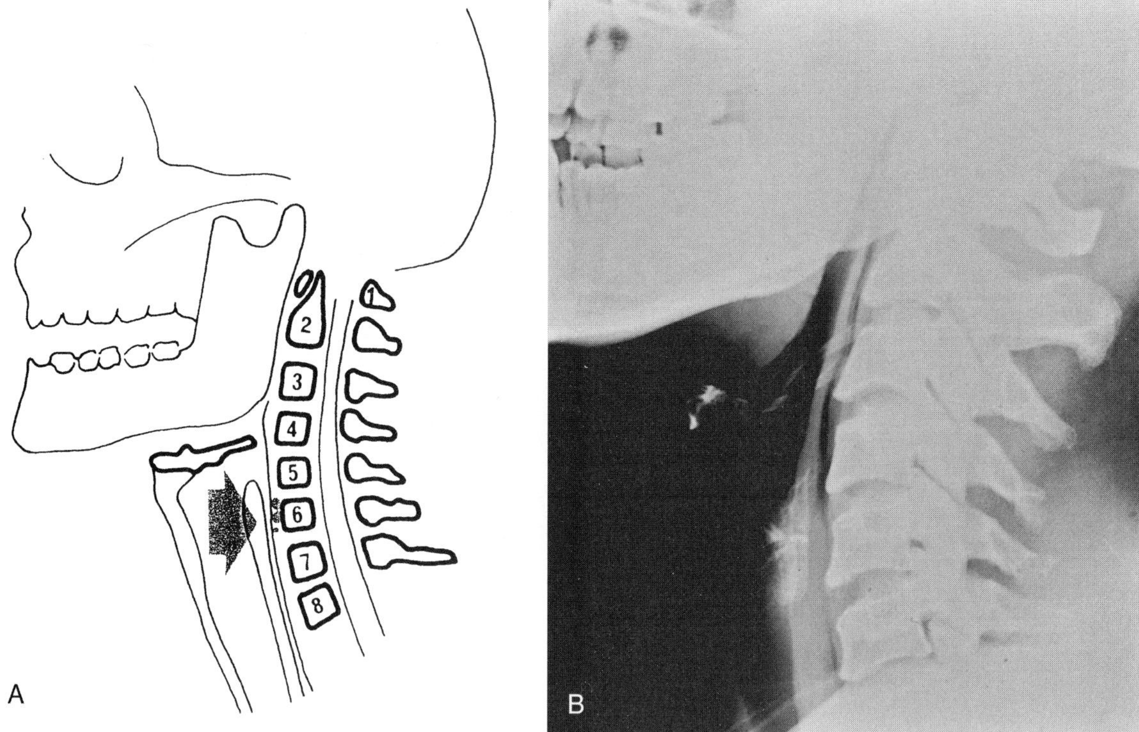

FIGURE 37–3 ■ *A,* Cervical emphysema is first detected by a soft tissue lateral x-ray of the cervical region, in the retrovisceral space in front of the sixth vertebral body (sign of Minnegerode). *B,* Cervical emphysema in the retrovisceral space.

which are of lower density than body tissues, contain mostly air (wood within a short period of injury, some plastics) and may be visualized but with difficulty. Wood (toothpicks) begins to absorb fluids immediately and within a few hours becomes equivalent in density to body tissues and thus invisible (Fodor and Malott, 1983).

Endoscopy

Any suspicion of an esophageal foreign body warrants esophagoscopy even when the results of physical and radiologic examinations have been negative (see Table 37–1). When the suspicion is based exclusively on the patient's history and no physical symptoms or radiologic signs are present, the patient is evaluated again on the next day and released if still asymptomatic. In the presence of the slightest symptom, even when physical and radiologic findings are negative, esophagoscopy is recommended. However, esophagoscopy should not be carried out with the sole purpose of making a preliminary diagnosis; it should be directly scheduled as an extraction procedure, and everything needed for removal should be at hand (Jackson and Jackson, 1950).

In patients with severe hematemesis, indicating a possible fistula with a major vessel, and in patients with cervical or mediastinal emphysema, disclosing a perforation, endoscopy should take place in the surgical unit, where surgical extraction and further treatment can be performed without delay.

ENDOSCOPIC MANAGEMENT

Indication

Endoscopic extraction is the therapy of choice for incarcerated esophageal foreign bodies (Brossard et al, 1991; Giordano et al, 1981; Jackson, 1957; Savary and Miller, 1978). An absolute contraindication to endoscopic extraction is the presence of severe hematemesis, indicating a possible fistula with a major vessel due to a perforating foreign body (Besson et al, 1981; Brossard et al, 1991).

Any evidence of perforation requires foreign body extraction as well as surgical revision for drainage and closure of the perforation. If the foreign body can be endoscopically extracted without further damage to the esophagus, the procedure may be combined (endoscopic extraction and surgical revision in the same procedure); in other cases, the entire procedure is exclusively surgical.

Timing

A foreign body that is lodged in the esophagus, regardless of its nature, must be removed under direct visualization as soon as possible; however, an emergency situation in which a complete diagnostic investigation is not possible is rare. Disk batteries should be removed without any delay because leakage of the corrosive content can rapidly perforate the esophageal wall (see later). Sharp foreign bodies can induce immediate perforations, but this event is rather unusual. We recommend extraction within the first 6 hours. Nandi and Ong (1978) report that most perforations due to sharp items occurred 24 hours after impaction; perforation occurred later in cases of smooth foreign bodies (pressure necrosis). If a perforation is evident, extraction and surgical revision procedures should take place within 1 to 3 hours.

The only true surgical emergency is a fistula with a major vessel (see earlier). If the foreign body ingestion has been followed by a sentinel hematemesis, only emergency thoracotomy can save the patient (Besson et al, 1981; Brossard et al, 1991; Grey et al, 1988; Hollander and Quick, 1991; Wilson et al, 1987; Wu and Wu-Wei, 1992).

Even the presence of a large piece of meat at the pharyngoesophageal junction (pseudo–café coronary) (see earlier) is not a critical emergency because the respiratory tract is not blocked. Nevertheless, rapid endoscopic removal is required because of the dyspnea and because of the possibility of associated compression-induced weakening or rupture of the pharyngoesophageal wall. Indeed, a number of these patients have been subjected to one or more applications of the Heimlich maneuver; in contrast to intralaryngeal meat impaction, this maneuver does not resolve the problem, because the flexibility and elasticity of the esophageal wall militate against compression-induced expulsion. Moreover, if the esophageal wall is weakened or if bits of hard material are contained in the lodged bolus, there is a chance of induced perforation with use of this maneuver (Atkins et al, 1985).

Requirements

The endoscopic procedure should be carried out in a hospital with an endoscopy suite or operating room completely equipped with facilities for general anesthesia, resuscitation, and upper aerodigestive endoscopies (laryngoscopy, bronchoscopy, esophagoscopy).

General anesthesia with tracheal intubation provides the best conditions because it prevents bronchoaspiration and provides the time and stability necessary for the extraction maneuver by ensuring respiratory function and full relaxation of the patient (Savary and Miller, 1978; Payne and Olsen, 1974; Webb, 1984). If the patient's stomach is not empty, appropriate precautions must be taken. Under no circumstances must the stomach be washed out or evacuated before examination. Usually, the extraction can be scheduled by the anesthetist within the time limits reported here.

A rigid instrument, which allows procedures with an open tube, is preferred, and either a full-lumen open tube of the Haslinger or Jackson type or a Storz Universal optical endoscope may be used (Fig. 37–4). The diameter and length of the instrument are chosen according to the location of the foreign body and the patient's age. The rigid instrument allows the various instrumental maneuvers to be carried out under conditions of perfect stability. When present above the foreign body, food particles can be properly removed. The distal lip of the rigid tube is very helpful in unfolding the mucosa and disengaging an incarcerated foreign body.

Technique

The following three steps must always be carried out: (1) endoscopic evaluation, (2) extraction, and (3) postprocedural endoscopy.

Endoscopic Evaluation

Any retained saliva or food particles are removed with a suction tube or spoon-shaped fenestrated forceps. The foreign body is brought into view, approached, and located. By shifting the instrument laterally and using the lip of the esophagoscope, the operator can identify the foreign body on the basis of its shape, size, consistency, and surface appearance. Its position is precisely determined with regard to the esophageal walls.

In cases of a large and deeply perforating foreign body or in cases of severe bleeding, we refrain from any endoscopic extraction and switch to open surgery. If there are no contraindications, the method and suitable instruments are chosen, and the endoscopic maneuvers (e.g., disengaging, detaching, turning, cutting) are determined.

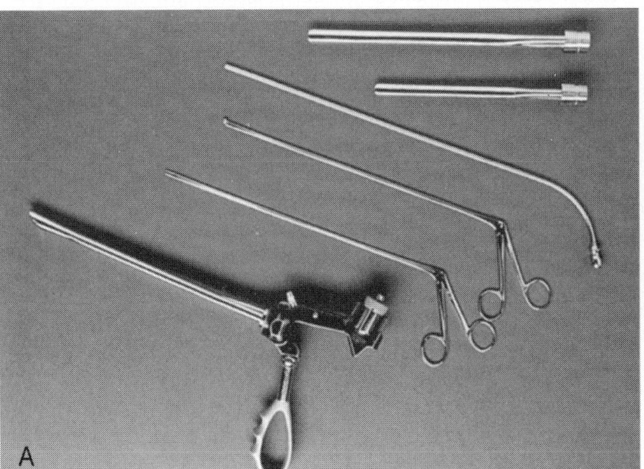

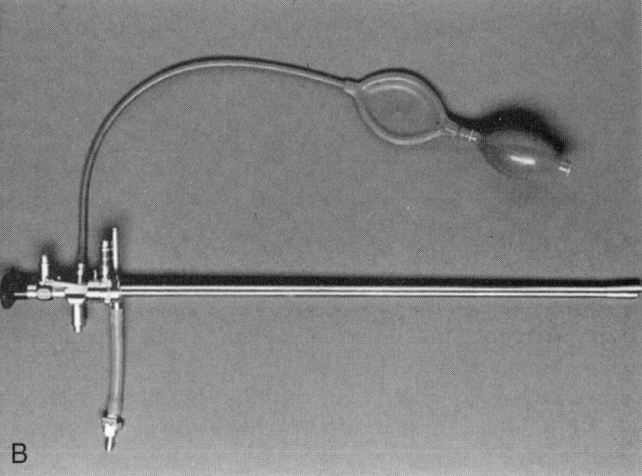

FIGURE 37–4 ■ *A,* Full-lumen open tube esophagoscope of the Haslinger type with interchangeable tubes of various diameters and lengths, foreign body forceps, and suction tube with distal opening. *B,* Storz Universal optical endoscope.

Extraction

The procedure for extraction includes the following:

1. Stabilizing the endoscope and the corresponding esophageal segment (suspension of respiratory activity).
2. Contacting the foreign body with the distal end of the instrument (the lip of the endoscope is set accordingly).
3. Gripping the chosen portion of the foreign body firmly in a single movement.
4. Drawing the foreign body into the endoscope. A foreign body is seldom retracted completely into the esophagoscope. It is not necessary to draw out that part of the foreign body that seems the most dangerous because every sharp point creates a possible hazard when being withdrawn. It is important to respect Jackson's key concept that "advancing points perforate, trailing points do not."
5. Maintaining complete stability of endoscope, forceps, and foreign body.
6. Using a slow, regular, and continuous movement for removal, ensuring that the axis of the endoscope corresponds to that of the esophagus and pharynx, with awareness of any abnormal resistance caused by friction or impaction of the foreign body.

Postextraction Endoscopy

With an optical esophagoscope, the area of entrapment is carefully explored to evaluate a possible laceration. Furthermore, the esophagus below the site of impaction is screened down to the stomach for any preexisting esophageal disease that may have caused the impaction. During removal of the endoscope, the esophagus above the site of incarceration is examined to detect any injury due to the extraction maneuver. Postoperative management depends on these findings.

Postextraction Management

When the extraction has been difficult and when deep laceration extend to the muscular layer has been detected without endoscopic and radiologic evidence of a true perforation, postoperative management is conservative, with close clinical and radiologic monitoring (see "Complications" earlier). When a puncture perforation is diagnosed endoscopically (pin or sharp bone puncture) and no mediastinal or cervical emphysema is present, management is the same, including the use of broad-spectrum antibiotics. In cases of an endoscopically or a radiologically evident perforation, surgical repair of the perforation with covering and drainage is performed within the first 3 hours, followed by the same close monitoring, which is maintained for 10 days. In all of these situations, a Gastrografin contrast study is performed before oral food intake is resumed and the patient is discharged.

SPECIAL SITUATIONS

Meat Impaction

Esophageal soft food impaction is common in adults, with large pieces of meat involved in 56% of cases (see Table 37–4). Impaction usually occurs when alcohol consumption is also involved. The patient talks while chewing food that consists of thick pieces of overcooked meat that are too hard to be effectively masticated ("backyard barbecue syndrome"; see Palmer, 1976). Food impaction may also be related to insufficient chewing by elderly, edentulous patients (Hargrove and Boyce, 1970; Payne and Olsen, 1974; Richardson, 1945; Robinson, 1962). Two preferential sites of obstruction are encountered with equal frequency—the upper portion of the esophagus and the lower esophagus (see Table 37–6). In 65% of these cases, but especially in cases that involve lower esophageal impactions, an underlying disease is revealed (see "Underlying Esophageal Disease") (Norton and King, 1963). Impactions of food other than meat are far more common in the lower esophagus.

The clinical diagnosis is evident. Swallowing of food or liquid is impossible. The patient regurgitates and may complain of retrosternal pain. There is no need for complementary radiologic investigation. The symptoms and management of food impactions at the pharyngoesophageal junction (pseudo–café coronary) have been described. The only suitable therapy is rapid endoscopic removal. Complications such as tracheobronchial aspiration or perforation are reported primarily after more than 12 hours of impaction (Clarkston, 1992).

Preoperative management should be carried out with rehydration in mind. Cautious aspiration of the fluid retained above the impacted bolus can be performed with a Levin tube (Palmer, 1976). General anesthesia with tracheal intubation is necessary to ensure safe and adequate respiratory function, the procedure often being laborious and time-consuming. Open tube endoscopes such as the Haslinger esophagoscope with interchangeable tubes of varying diameters and lengths, a large fenestrated spoon forceps, and a powerful suction tube with only one distal opening are the instruments especially suitable for this kind of procedure (see Fig. 37–4). Whenever possible, the main portion of the procedure should be performed with rigid open esophagoscopes to avoid repeated removal and reinsertion of the instrument, as is necessary with fiberscopes.

In patients with severe stiffness of the cervical spine or in kyphotic patients, a fiberscope is helpful to complete the extraction in the distal esophagus. An "overtube" can be used to avoid lesions associated with repeated reinsertion of the instrument, but it must be used with care because the mucosa can become caught between the overtube and the fiberscope, sometimes inducing perforations of the esophagus (Berkelhammer et al, 1993).

Taking into account the high percentage of underlying esophageal diseases (65%), thorough postextraction endoscopy with an optical esophagoscope is mandatory. Of a total of 21 patients with "steakhouse syndrome," Stadler and associates (1989) found 38% with malignant disease. When esophagoscopy results are negative, a swallowing disorder should be ruled out with radiology and manometry.

The endoscopic removal of a massive food impaction in an older patient in poor general condition may represent a difficult and lengthy procedure and probably is why various alternative treatments have been proposed.

Enzymatic digestion of the impacted food with papain (e.g., some meat tenderizers) has been proposed (Hargrove and Boyce, 1970; Richardson, 1945; Robinson, 1962), but it cannot be recommended. The procedure is indicated only for meat impactions. The success rate is low, and in their in vitro study, Goldner and Danley (1985) could not demonstrate any capacity of the most commonly used solutions to digest or reduce the size of an impacted meat bolus. Papain solutions have even proved to be dangerous because of underlying mucosal lesions that allow in-depth penetration of the enzymatic agent, thus significantly increasing the risk of perforation. Underlying esophageal diseases, especially esophagitis, can be worsened by the use of enzymatic solutions. Tracheobronchial aspiration of papain can cause serious pulmonary edema, and because of their high sodium content, some papain solutions have been reported to cause hyperosmolar coma when administered in large quantities (Davis, 1987; Goldner and Danley, 1985; Holsinger et al, 1968; Robinson, 1962; Stadler et al, 1989; Webb, 1988, 1995).

Glucagon, nitroglycerin, nifedipine, and diazepam have been described to induce spontaneous passage of the impacted bolus by relaxing the lower esophageal sphincter without altering the esophageal peristalsis (Bell and Eibling, 1988; DiPalma and Brady, 1987; Ferrucci and Long, 1977; Marks and Lousteau, 1979; Trenkner et al, 1983). The reported success rates, around 37%, are low (Trenkner et al, 1983). These drugs are contraindicated in a number of situations. Glucagon can cause vomiting (Webb, 1988) and serious tracheobronchial aspiration. Moreover, in a prospective placebo-controlled double-blind study, there was no significant difference in the use of glucagon, diazepam, or placebo to treat patients with impacted food boluses (Tibbling et al, 1995).

Carbonated beverages, such as cola and champagne, have also been used. The rationale is to distend the esophagus with carbon dioxide, in turn causing relaxation of the lower esophageal sphincter and free passage of the impacted bolus into the stomach (Karanjia and Rees, 1993; Rice et al, 1983; Smith et al, 1986). The success rate is mediocre, about 70% in four published series of a total of 87 patients, with a 3.4% rate of serious complications, including perforation (Levine, 1995). The method is not suitable for impactions that have been present for longer than 24 hours because of the increased risk of serious perforation (Levine, 1995). This method also may induce regurgitation, vomiting, and tracheobronchial aspiration, especially in elderly patients.

All of these treatments are very unpleasant to patients already enduring a total esophageal obstruction, because they force the patient to retain solutions that induce belching, regurgitation, and vomiting: these remedies cannot be compared with the security and comfort of endoscopic removal under general anesthesia. None of these treatments, even if successful, can spare the practitioner a mandatory postdisimpaction endoscopic examination. Finally, in consideration of the high percentage of underlying diseases, the relative inefficiency of these treatments is apparent.

Coins

Accidental coin ingestion is rare in adults (see Table 37–4) but occurs frequently during games in which a person drinks a glass containing an alcoholic beverage with a coin in the bottom and attempts to catch the coin between the teeth. Coins are the simplest and safest foreign bodies to remove endoscopically and should be removed that way.

Nevertheless, alternate blind extraction procedures with a Foley catheter under fluoroscopic control with the patient in the Trendelenburg position are still performed (Bigler, 1966; Campbell et al, 1983; Harned et al, 1997; Henry and Chamberlain, 1972; Morrow et al, 1998; Towbin et al, 1989) but only by specialists with no specific training in the care of foreign bodies in the upper aerodigestive tract (McGuirt, 1982). Success rates of around 80% (71% to 98%) have been reported, with complication rates that range between 0.4% and 1.7% (Berggreen et al, 1993; Campbell et al, 1983; Harned et al, 1997; Morrow et al, 1998; Towbin et al, 1989). However, these seemingly good results have been obtained in a group of highly selected patients (blunt foreign body in upper or midesophagus present for less than 24 hours in patients with no history of underlying disease), precisely that group of patients expected to have the lowest complication rate regardless of the method used. The method provides no control of the foreign body as it is removed. There is no airway protection. The discomfort for the patient is great; the Trendelenburg position can be associated with vomiting, especially when the stomach is not empty. The underlying pathology, if present, cannot be assessed and can give rise to complications. Cases of unrecognized (thus unextracted) foreign bodies have been described with use of this technique (Myer, 1991). If edema is evident radiologically or if the foreign body is present for longer than 24 hours, this technique should not be used. We do not use the Foley catheter technique, and we do not recommend it. It may be a treatment option only if endoscopy is not available.

Disk Batteries

Although the ingestion of disk batteries has become more frequent because of the advances in electronic miniaturization, it remains a rare event in adults (see Table 37–4). Ingestion occurs during the replacement of used cells, after the person places the new battery on the tongue to test its potency, after mistaking the battery for a tablet, or during suicide attempts (Smith and Peura, 1992). As with coins, the larger disk batteries (>21 mm in diameter) cause problems. The most common battery systems contain an alkaline electrolyte (26% to 45% potassium or sodium hydroxide) that is strong enough to cause rapid liquefaction necrosis of tissue. Zinc hearing aid and mercury oxide batteries are those most often ingested. Esophageal injury is caused through direct corrosive action, low-voltage burns, or pressure necrosis. The low-voltage current generated by the battery in gastrointestinal fluid often causes disruption of the seal and leakage of the strong alkaline content. Perforations can result, especially in the esophagus, and are rapidly complicated by esopha-

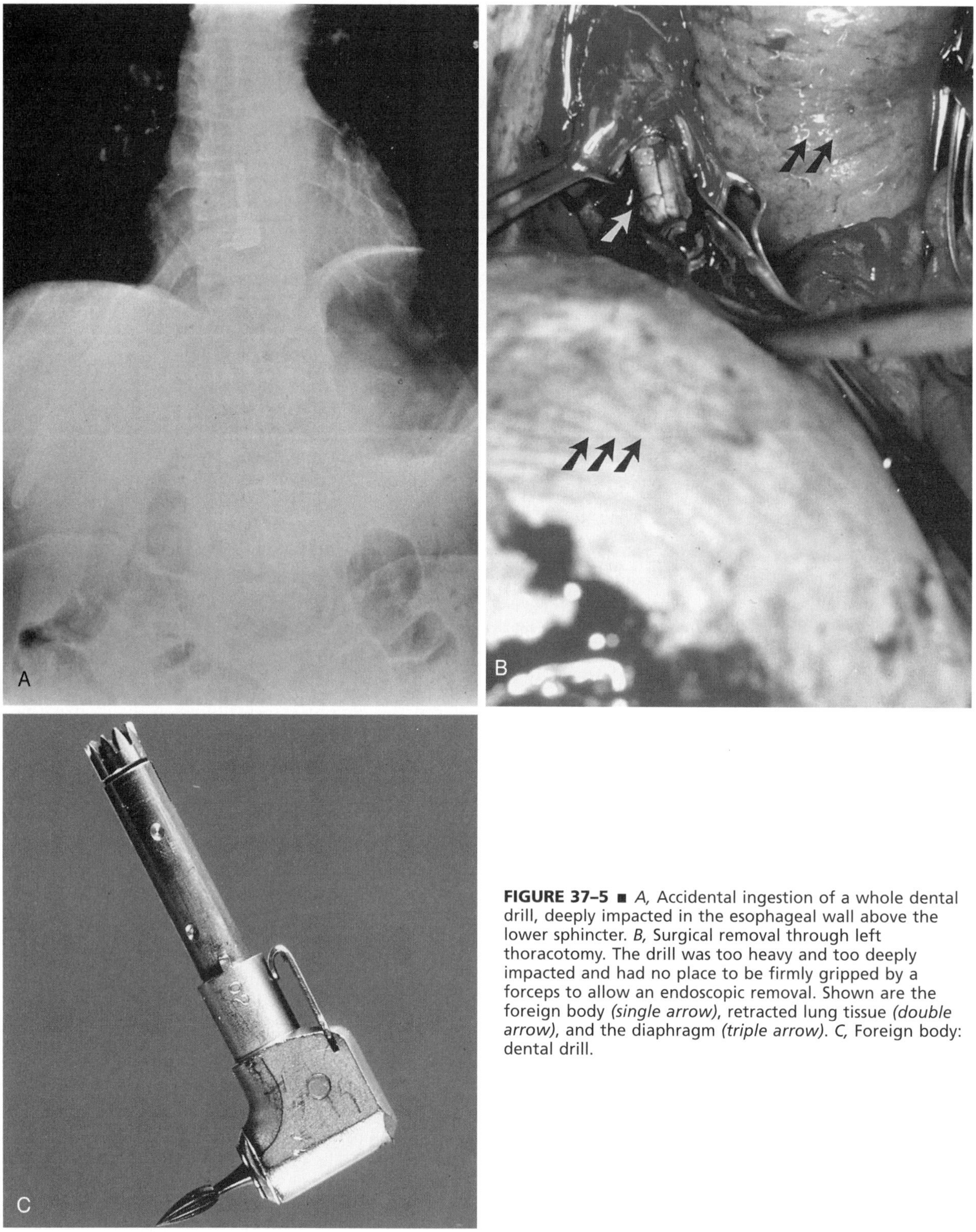

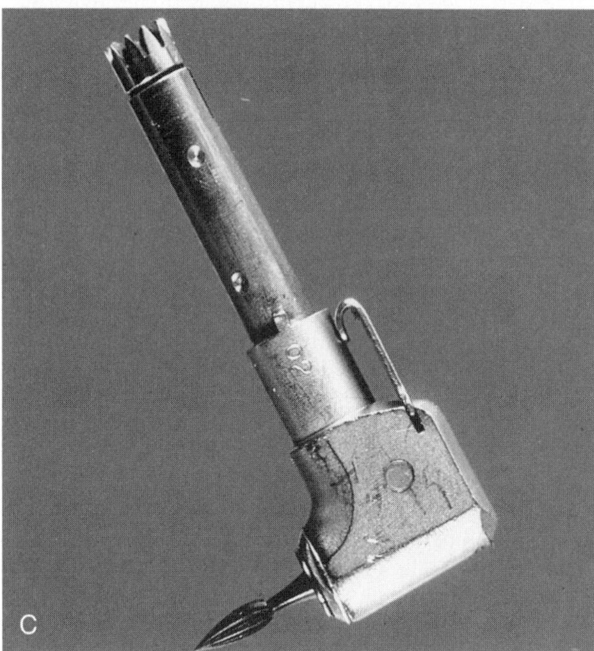

FIGURE 37–5 ■ *A,* Accidental ingestion of a whole dental drill, deeply impacted in the esophageal wall above the lower sphincter. *B,* Surgical removal through left thoracotomy. The drill was too heavy and too deeply impacted and had no place to be firmly gripped by a forceps to allow an endoscopic removal. Shown are the foreign body *(single arrow)*, retracted lung tissue *(double arrow)*, and the diaphragm *(triple arrow)*. *C,* Foreign body: dental drill.

gotracheal or esophagoaortic fistula formation (Webb, 1995).

Because of the rapid action of the alkaline substance on the esophageal wall, disk batteries should be removed without delay. Radiologically, they are easily identified by a double-density shadow in the anterior projection with rounded edges, with a step-off at the junction of the cathode and anode in the lateral projection. Endoscopic removal may be difficult because the smooth edges of the battery are difficult to grasp with a forceps (Webb, 1995); the procedure is less problematic with the use of larger forceps with rigid endoscopes. The physician can also remove the battery with a through-the-scope balloon, drawing it under direct vision, at least partially, into the rigid endoscope, and removing the balloon, battery, and endoscope as a unit. Sometimes the reaction of the adjacent tissues makes it necessary to dissect the battery free. Thorough postextraction endoscopic examination and a Gastrografin contrast study are vital for adequate further management.

If endoscopic extraction is not possible, surgical removal should be considered. Under no circumstances should the battery be left in the esophagus. Once a battery reaches the stomach, chances are excellent that it will pass distally and be evacuated. Problems in the distal digestive tract are rare. Nevertheless, clinical and radiological monitoring are required.

Drug Packages

A "body-packer" or "body-bagger" is a person who ingests packets of illicit drugs, usually cocaine, to conceal them. The condom is a favorite packet, with 3 to 5 g of cocaine usually put into a single condom. The ingestion of 1 to 3 g of cocaine in a powdered form can be fatal, and the rupture of even one package carries the risk of death (Webb, 1995). The packets can be identified on radiography in 70% to 90% of cases (Webb, 1995). Esophageal impaction is rare. In the single case in our series, the ingested package was relatively large, with a significant amount of drug being wrapped in paper inside the condom, and the symptoms were those of total esophageal obstruction. Endoscopic removal can be dangerous, and packet rupture has been described (Suarez et al, 1977). The security of the procedure must be thoroughly evaluated depending on the type of package. Even in cases of esophageal impaction in which the body-bagger is willing to cooperate, general anesthesia with airway protection is mandatory, and the use of the rigid endoscope is more secure. However, the safest means of removal remains surgery. In the management of these cases, the high probability of the presence of other packages in the lower digestive tract, with the attendant risk of toxicity, must always be considered.

SURGICAL MANAGEMENT

Surgical management is indicated:

1. When the foreign body cannot be endoscopically removed without further damage or cannot be removed at all (Fig. 37–5).
2. In the presence of an evident esophageal perforation, either for closure and drainage purposes after an endoscopic extraction or for extraction as well (Fig. 37–6).
3. As an emergency procedure in cases of associated hematemesis.

The need for primary surgical extraction of an esophageal foreign body is rare (0.8%) (Table 37–7). The earlier the intervention, the better the overall prognosis; therefore, diagnostic endoscopic or radiologic procedures to locate and evaluate the foreign body and perforation must be undertaken without delay. Immediate intravenous

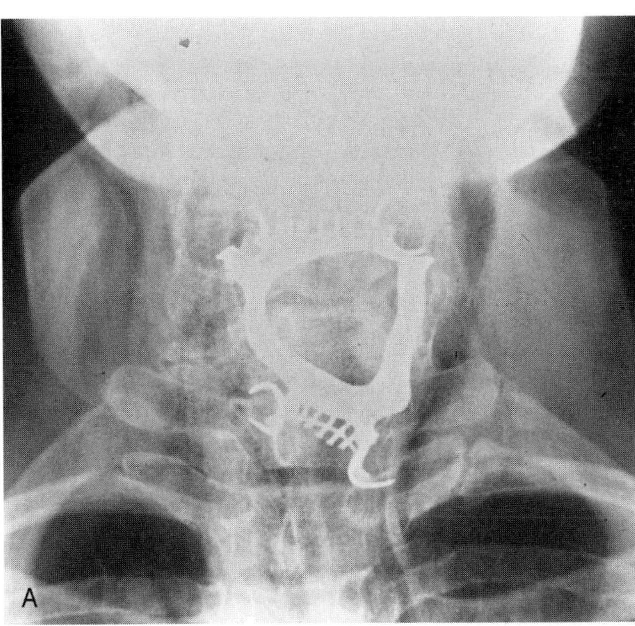

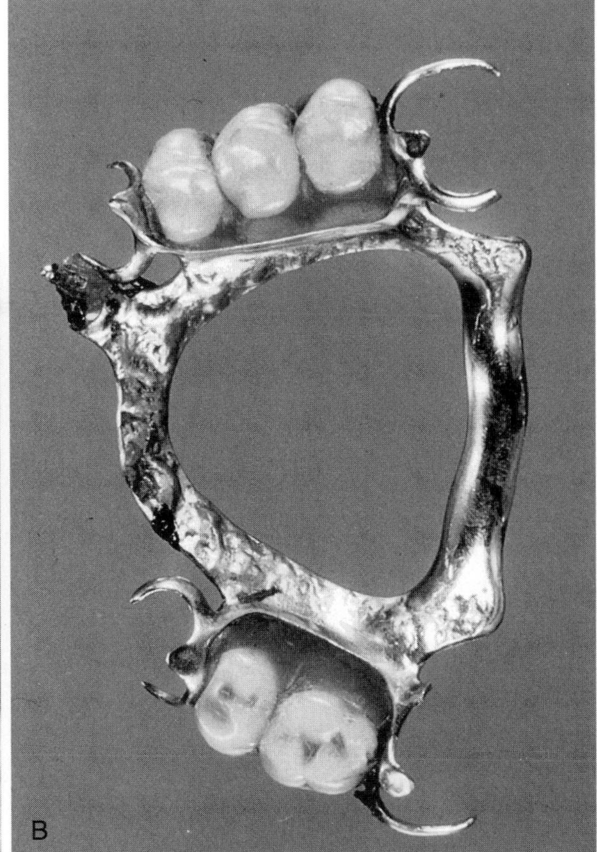

FIGURE 37–6 ■ *A,* Denture deeply impacted in the hypopharynx with evident perforation (massive cervicomediastinal emphysema). *B,* The deeply impacted, sharp-pointed hooks prevented endoscopic removal without further laceration of the esophageal wall.

TABLE 37–7 ■ **Esophageal Foreign Bodies in 949 Adults: Treatment and Final Outcome**

Outcome	Overall (n = 949) No.	(%)	Patients with Nonperforating Foreign Body (n = 907)	Patients with Perforating Foreign Body (n = 42)
Endoscopic extraction	926	(97.6)	887	39
Endoscope pushing into stomach	15	(1.6)	15	
Surgical extraction	8	(0.8)	5	3
Recovery	947	(99.8)	906	41
Death	2	(0.2)	1	1

From a clinical series of patients of the ENT and Head and Neck Surgery Clinic, University of Lausanne, January 1, 1963, through December 31, 1998.

treatment with a broad-spectrum antibiotic that covers anaerobic bacteria should be started as well. For cervical lesions, left-sided cervicotomy along the anterior border of the sternocleidomastoid is preferred, with closure of the tear in two layers and drainage of the site of perforation and the mediastinum. For upper thoracic esophageal lesions and for lesions associated with a right pleural effusion, a right posterolateral thoracotomy is required, with a large pleural drainage tube. Lesions of the distal thoracic esophagus are explored through the left side of the chest (Atkins et al, 1995) or through an upper median laparotomy (Peytral et al, 1991).

When possible, repair is made in two layers. Covering of the esophageal repair, with a strap muscle flap, pleura, or pericardium, may be helpful. If inflammatory changes in tissues or the size of the perforation makes the closure impossible, alternative methods must be considered, such as partial esophagectomy, T-tube drainage, esophageal exclusion with secondary reconstruction, or transesophageal drainage and stenting (Atkins et al, 95; Besson and Saegesser, 1983; Segalin et al, 1996).

RESULTS

In our series, 2018 patients older than 16 years underwent endoscopy, with the confirmation of an impacted foreign body in 949 cases (47%) and the presence of an esophageal injury after spontaneous passage of a foreign body in 447 cases (22%) (see Table 37–1). The endoscopic management of these esophageal foreign bodies and food impactions with rigid esophagoscopy in the patient under general anesthesia (with no exclusions as to the type or location of the foreign body and with the use of practitioners in training) was successful in 941 (99.2%) patients (see Table 37–7). In eight (0.8%) patients, the extraction was performed surgically, either because of the presence of a large perforation (three patients) or because of the danger of endoscopic removal of a very large foreign body that was already associated with deep esophageal laceration (in five patients). Two (0.2%) patients died after endoscopic extraction. One patient died from a massive hemorrhage after the endoscopic removal of a chicken bone lodged in the vicinity of the aortic arch, and the other patient, an elderly woman with massive food impaction, died after vigorous endoscopic maneuvers that caused esophageal perforation (see Table 37–7).

DISCUSSION

Endoscopic removal with rigid esophagoscopes in patients under general anesthesia appears to be efficient and safe, and the prognosis for patients with incarcerated foreign bodies of the esophagus is excellent. Nonendoscopic treatments for blunt foreign bodies of the cervical and thoracic esophagus (extraction with a balloon catheter) and for food impaction (enzymatic digestion, spasmolytic drugs, gas-forming agents) do not offer the success rate, security, innocuousness, and comfort of rigid endoscopic removal performed with general anesthesia and cannot be recommended.

Fiberoptic endoscopy has great popularity, mainly because its use does not necessitate prolonged technical training. Numerous publications have proposed the fiberoptic extraction of esophageal foreign bodies in adults and children (Classen et al, 1978; Kumagai and Makuuchi, 1987; Ricote et al, 1985; Rösch and Classen, 1972; Van Thiel and Stafan, 1974; Vizearrondo et al, 1983; Webb et al, 1984). Flexible endoscopy allows the extraction of foreign bodies from the stomach and duodenum and avoids the need for general anesthesia in the adult. The absence of protection of the respiratory tract, however, exposes patients to the risk of displacement of the foreign body with potentially severe consequences (Webb, 1988). Even with sedation, a long and difficult extraction using local anesthesia not only is unpleasant for the patient but also may create greater stress in cases of preexisting cardiorespiratory diseases than would the use of short-acting general anesthesia. The average foreign body extraction lasts approximately half as long with the rigid endoscope as with the flexible endoscope (Lim et al, 1994). This is understandable, because in the esophagus, especially in the upper sphincter and the cervical portions, despite numerous technical improvements, the efficiency of instrumental maneuvers with the fiberscope is still inferior to that of the rigid esophagoscope because of its lack of stability and the configuration of its tip (De Luca et al, 1976; Kumagai and Makuuchi, 1987). The success rate of fiberoptic esophageal foreign body removal appears to be significantly lower (76% [Vizcarrondo et al, 1983] and 85.5% [Barros et al, 1991]) than that with the use of rigid instruments (99% [Jackson, 1957], 96% (Chaikhoumi et al, 1985], and 98% [Brossard et al, 1991]). Moreover, most published reports on the fiberoptic removal of esophageal foreign bodies include patients selected according to the nature, shape, size, or location of the foreign body. Sharp and pointed foreign bodies, impacted in the upper sphincter or in the cervical or upper thoracic esophagus, which are the most frequently encountered foreign bodies in adults and the most likely to produce severe esophageal injury, are almost always managed with rigid esophagoscopes by otorhinolaryngologists or thoracic surgeons (Brossard et al, 1991; Chaikhoumi et al, 1985; Giordano et al, 1981; Peytral et al, 1991; Shamir et al, 1980). The mortality and morbidity rates for both procedures are basically the same (Webb, 1995), with this selection of foreign bodies not taken into account.

The general anesthesia required for rigid endoscopy has also been considered by many to be a significant disadvantage that reduces the cost-effectiveness of the procedure (Webb, 1988), but this is no longer true. Most of the rigid endoscopies of this series were performed on an outpatient basis, and since the introduction of the anesthetic agent propofol (Disoprivan), postprocedural discomfort is extremely low and the postoperative surveillance (3 to 4 hours) is almost the same as that after intravenous sedation. Hospitalization, which is indicated only for a suspected complication, is not dependent on the type of procedure. In our institution, there are only minor differences in charges for the two procedures. The cost of rigid endoscopic removal is about $750 ($262 endoscopist and anesthetist fees, $487 for use of the endoscopy unit), and $664 for fiberoptic removal with local anesthesia and sedation ($194 endoscopist fee, $470 for use of the endoscopy unit). These differences are not sufficient to choose fiberoptic removal—an overall less effective procedure—on the basis of cost alone.

Although the popularity of the fiberscope has led, increasingly, to the management of upper digestive foreign bodies with the flexible endoscope (Webb, 1988), one must keep in mind that in the field of esophageal foreign body removal, only rigid esophagoscopy with the patient under general anesthesia allowed a success rate of 99% with a 0.2% mortality to be reached in a comprehensive series of patients. Moreover, this occurred under conditions in which endoscopists were being trained. Novelty does not necessarily mean progress. It must first be demonstrated that basic technical innovations maintain the current level of efficiency and safety before being accepted for convenience, comfort, or economic reasons. In the future, it will still be the otorhinolaryngologist or the thoracic surgeon who is called on in difficult situations. In our experience, the need to train these specialists in rigid esophagoscopy for removal of pharyngoesophageal foreign bodies has not vanished despite the technical development of fiberoptic upper gastrointestinal panendoscopes. Optimally, the physician in charge of this field should master both rigid and fiberoptic endoscopy as well as laryngoscopy and bronchoscopy.

■ KEY REFERENCES

Atkins JP, Keane WM, Rowe LD: Foreign bodies in the esophagus: Esophageal perforation. In Berk JE (ed): Gastroenterology, 2nd ed. Philadelphia, WB Saunders, 1985.

This review article includes the clinical presentation and the treatment of "pseudo–café coronary," rules for rigid endoscopic extraction, and the diagnosis and management of esophageal perforation.

Hollander JE, Quick G: Aorto-esophageal fistula: A comprehensive review of the literature. Am J Med 91:279, 1991.

The epidemiology, etiology, clinical presentation, and management of aortoesophageal fistulas, including the place of endoscopic procedures, are provided on the basis of 106 references.

Berggreen PJ, Harrison E, Sanowski R, et al: Techniques and complications of esophageal foreign body extraction in children and adults. Gastrointest Endosc 39:626, 1993.

This discussion of rigid, fiberoptic, and alternate extraction procedures, especially with Foley catheters, is from personal experience with 76 adult and 116 pediatric cases.

Jackson C, Jackson CL: Bronchoesophagology. Philadelphia, WB Saunders, 1950.

The first and largest experience in esophageal foreign body management describes all of the basic rules of rigid endoscopic extraction.

Webb WA: Management of foreign bodies of the upper gastrointestinal tract. Gastroenterology 94:204, 1988.

Management of the different types of foreign bodies, including historical considerations, and an analysis of morbidity/mortality and cost-effectiveness, based on 118 references, are described.

■ REFERENCES

Barros JL, Caballero A Jr, Rueda JC, et al: Foreign body ingestion: Management of 167 cases. World J Surg 15:783, 1991.

Bell AF, Eibling DE: Nifedipine in the treatment of distal esophageal food impaction. Arch Otolaryngol Head Neck Surg 114:682, 1988.

Benjamin SB: Esophageal foreign bodies and perforation. In Haubrich WS, Shaffner F, Berk JE (eds): Bockus Gastroenterology, 5th ed. Philadelphia, WB Saunders, 1995.

Berkelhammer C, Madhav G, Lyon S, Roberts G: "Pinch" injury during overtube placement in upper endoscopy. Gastrointest Endosc 39:786, 1993.

Besson A, Meyer A, Savary M, et al: Etude de 58 complications intrathoraciques parmi 166 traumatismes accidentels ou iatrogènes de l'oesophage. Schweiz Med Wochenschr 111:1602, 1981.

Besson A, Saegesser F: A Color Atlas of Chest Trauma and Associated Injuries. London, Wolfe Medical Publications, 1983.

Bigler FC: The use of a Foley catheter for removal of blunt foreign bodies from the esophagus. J Thorac Cardiovasc Surg 51:759, 1966.

Brossard E, Ollyo J-B, Monnier P: Foreign bodies in the esophagus: Diagnosis and treatment. Acta Endosc 21:655, 1991.

Campbell JB, Quattromani FL, Foley LC: Foley catheter removal of blunt esophageal foreign bodies: Experience with 100 consecutive children. Pediatr Radiol 13:116, 1983.

Chaikhoumi A, Kratz JM, Crawford FA: Foreign bodies of the esophagus. Am Surg 51:173, 1985.

Clarkston WK: Gastrointestinal foreign bodies. Postgrad Med 92:46, 1992.

Classen M, Farthmann EF, Seifert E: Operative and therapeutic techniques in endoscopy. Clin Gastroenterol 7:741, 1978.

Clerf LH: Historical aspects of foreign bodies in the air and food passages. Ann Otol Rhinol Laryngol 61:5, 1952.

Connolly AAP, Birchall M, Walsh-Waring GP, et al: Ingested foreign bodies: Patient-guided localization is a useful clinical tool. Clin Otolaryngol 17:520, 1992.

Ctercteko G, Mok CK: Aorto-esophageal fistula induced by a foreign body. J Thorac Cardiovasc Surg 80:233, 1980.

Davis M: Esophagitis after papain. J Clin Gastroenterol 9:127, 1987.

De Luca RF, Ferrer JP, Wortzel EM: Polypectomy snare extraction of foreign bodies from the esophagus: Two interesting cases. Am J Gastroenterol 66:374, 1976.

DiPalma JA, Brady CE 3rd: Steakhouse spasm. J Clin Gastroenterol 9:274, 1987.

Doolin EJ: Esophageal stricture: An uncommon complication of foreign bodies. Ann Otol Rhinl Laryngol 102:863, 1993

Ferrucci JT Jr, Long JA Jr: Radiologic treatment of esophageal food impaction using intravenous glucagon. Radiology 125:25, 1977.

Fodor J III, Malott JC: The radiographic detection of foreign bodies. Radiol Technol 54:361, 1983.

Giordano A, Adams G, Boles LJ, et al: Current management of esophageal foreign bodies. Arch Otolaryngol 3:64, 1981.

Goldner F, Danley D: Enzymatic digestion of esophageal meat impaction: A study of Adolph's Meat Tenderizer. Digest Dis Sci 30:456, 1985.

Grey TC, Mittelman RE, Wetli CV, et al: Aorto-esophageal fistula and sudden death. Am J Forens Med Pathol 9:19, 1988.

Hargrove MD, Boyce HW: Meat impaction of the esophagus. Arch Intern Med 125:277, 1970.

Harned RK II, Strain JD, Hay TC, et al: Esophageal foreign bodies: Safety and efficacy of Foley catheter extraction of coins. AJR Am J Roentgenol 168:443, 1997.

Henry LN, Chamberlain JW: Removal of foreign bodies from esophagus and nose with the use of a Foley catheter. Surgery 71:918, 1972.

Holsinger JW, Fuson RL, Sealy WC: Esophageal perforation following meat impaction and papain ingestion. JAMA 204:734, 1968.

Jackson CL: Foreign bodies in the esophagus. Am J Surg 93:308, 1957.

Jones WG, Ginsberg RJ: Esophageal perforation: A continuing challenge. Ann Thorac Surg 53:534, 1992.

Karanjia ND, Rees M: The use of Coca-Cola in the management of bolus obstruction in benign esophageal stricture. Ann R Coll Surg Engl 75:94, 1993.

Kumagai Y, Makuuchi H: Practical Fiberoptic Esophagoscopy. Tokyo, Ikaku-Shoin, 1987.

Lerche W: The esophagoscope in removing sharp foreign bodies from the esophagus. JAMA 56:634, 1911.

Levine MS: Administration of gas-forming agents for the treatment of food impactions in the distal esophagus. Am J Radiol 165:480, 1995.

Lim CT, Fitch Quah R, Leong-Eam L: A prospective study of ingested foreign bodies in Singapore. Arch Otolaryngol Head Neck Surg 120:96, 1994.

Marks HW, Lousteau RJ: Glucagon and esophageal meat impaction. Arch Otolaryngol 105:367, 1979

Mazzardi S, Salis GB, Iannicillo H, et al: Foreign body impaction in the esophagus: Are they underlying motor disorders? Dis Esoph 11:51, 1998.

McGuirt WF: Use of Foley catheter for removal of esophageal foreign bodies: A survey. Ann Otol Rhinol Laryngol 91:599, 1982.

Morrow SE, Bickler SW, Kennedy AP, et al: Balloon extraction of esophageal foreign bodies in children. J Pediatr Surg 33:266, 1998.

Myer CM: Potential hazards of esophageal foreign body extraction. Pediatr Radiol 21:97, 1991.

Nandi P, Ong GB: Foreign body in the oesophagus: Review of 2394 cases. Br J Surg 65:5, 1978.

Nashef SAM, Klein C, Martigne C, et al: Foreign body perforation of the normal esophagus. Eur J Cardiothorac Surg 6:565, 1992.

Norton GW, King GD: "Steakhouse syndrome": The symptomatic lower esophageal ring. Lahey Clin Found Bull 13:55, 1963.

Palmer ED: Backyard barbecue syndrome: Steak impaction in the esophagus. JAMA 235:2637, 1976.

Payne WS, Olsen AM: The Esophagus. Philadelphia, Lea & Febiger, 1974.

Peytral C, Senechaut JP, Hazan A: Corps étrangers de l'oesophage. Encycl Med Chir Otorhinolaryngol 20835:A10, 1991.

Pyman C: The diagnostic problems of inhaled and ingested plastic foreign bodies: Is a solution possible? JFORL J Fr Otorhinolaryngol Audiophonol Chir Maxillofac 8:755, 1974.

Quandalle P, Pruvot FR, Latreille JP: Fistule aorto-oesophagienne secondaire à une perforation de l'oesophage par corps étranger. Ann Chir 38:159, 1984.

Rice BT, Spiegel PK, Dombrowski PJ: Acute esophageal impaction treated by gas-forming agents. Radiology 146:299, 1983.

Richardson JR: A new treatment of esophageal obstruction due to meat impaction. Ann Otol Rhinol Laryngol 54:328, 1945.

Ricote GC, Torre LR, De Ayala VP: Fiberendoscopic removal of foreign bodies of the upper part of the gastrointestinal tract. Surg Gynecol Obstet 160:499, 1985.

Robinson AS: Meat impaction in the esophagus treated by enzymatic digestion. JAMA 29:126, 1962.

Rösch W, Classen M: Fiberendoscopic foreign body removal from the upper gastroentestinal tract. Endoscopy 4:193, 1972.

Röthlisberger B, Savary M: Les corps étrangers de l'oesophage. Rev Fr Gastroenterol 127:41, 1977.

Roura J, Morello A, Comas J, et al: Esophageal foreign bodies in adults. ORL J Otorhinolaryngol Relat Spec 52:51, 1990.

Savary M, Miller G: The Esophagus: Handbook and Atlas of Endoscopy. Solothurn, Switzerland, Gassmann AG, 1978.

Segalin A, Bonavina L, Lazzerini M, et al: Endoscopic management of inveterate esophageal perforations and leaks. Surg Endosc 10:928, 1996.

Set PAK, Flower CDR, Stewart S: Delayed presentation of esophageal perforation simulating intrathoracic malignancy. Clin Radiol 46:331, 1992.

Shamir M, Schuman BM: Complications of the fiberoptic endoscope. Gastrointest Endosc 26:86, 1980.

Smith JC, Janower ML, Geiger AH: Use of glucagon and gas-forming agents in acute esophageal food impaction. Radiology 159:567, 1986.

Smith MT, Peura DA: Foreign bodies. In Castell DO (ed): The Esophagus. Boston, Little, Brown, 1992.

Spitz L, Hirsig J: Prolonged foreign body impaction in the esophagus. Arch Dis Child 257:551, 1982.

Stadler J, Holscher AH, Feussner H, et al: The "steakhouse syndrome": Primary and definitive diagnosis and therapy. Surg Endosc 3:195, 1989.

Stein HJ, Schwitzer W, De Meester TR, et al: Foreign body entrapment in the esophagus of healthy subjects: A manometric and scintigraphic study. Dysphagia 7:220, 1992.

Suarez CA, Arango A, Lester JL: Cocaine-condom ingestion: Surgical treatment. JAMA 238:1391, 1977.

Terracol T: In Masson CR (ed): Les Maladies de l'Oesophage. Paris, Deuxième Edition, 1951.

Tibbling L, Bjorkhoel A, Jansson E, et al: Effect of spasmolytic drugs on esophageal foreign bodies. Dysphagia 10:126, 1995.

Towbin R, Lederman HM, Dunbar JS, et al: Esophageal edema as a predictor of unsuccessful balloon extraction of esophageal foreign body. Pediatr Radiol 19:359, 1989.

Trenkner SW, Maglinte DT, Lehman GA, et al: Esophageal food impaction: Treatment with glucagon. Radiology 149:401, 1983.

Van Thiel DH, Stafan WJ: Removal of soft foreign bodies from the esophagus using a flexible instrument. Gastrointest Endosc 20:163, 1974.

Vizcarrondo FJ, Brady PG, Nord HJ: Foreign bodies of the upper gastrointestinal tract. Gastrointest Endosc 28:208, 1983.

Webb WA: Management of foreign bodies of the upper gastrointestinal tract: Update. Gastrointest Endosc 41:39, 1995.

Webb WA, McDaniel L, Jones L: Foreign bodies of the upper gastrointestinal tract: Current management. South Med J 77:1083, 1984.

Wilson RT, Dean PJ, Lewis M: Aorto-esophageal fistula due to a foreign body. Gastrointest Endosc 33:448, 1987.

Winckler AR, McClenathan DT, Borger JA, et al: Retrograde esophagoscopy for foreign body removal. J Pediatr Gastroenterol Nutr 8:536, 1989.

Wu MH, Wu-Wei L: Aortoesophageal fistula induced by foreign bodies. Ann Thorac Surg 54:155, 1992.

ESOPHAGEAL FOREIGN BODIES IN INFANTS AND CHILDREN

Blake C. Papsin
Alma Smitheringale

The ingestion of foreign bodies into the aerodigestive tract is a relatively common phenomenon at both extremes of life, namely in children younger than 3 years of age and in older adults, in whom diminished neuromuscular coordination and the presence of dental prostheses contribute to mishandling of oral contents. Foreign body ingestion occurs in children because they explore their environment through oral tactile means, have sparse dentition, and lack the cognitive ability to distinguish food from inedible objects. Of ingested foreign bodies, 70% to 80% are lodged in the esophagus, and the remainder are lodged in the laryngotracheobronchial tree (Darrow and Holinger, 1996). The resulting symptoms depend on the site and level of impaction, the size of the object, and whether the object is corrosive or sharp. Smaller, smooth objects such as coins may remain in situ for many days or weeks with minimal consequences, whereas a foreign body that can penetrate the mucosa can rapidly cause death from hemorrhage or mediastinitis.

HISTORICAL NOTE

Death by choking on foreign bodies has been known to occur for centuries, but the complex presentations of an occult indwelling foreign object were first recognized in 1838 by Ryland (Clerf, 1936), who wrote, "The diagnosis of the foreign body accident claims the most minute attention." In 1936, Jackson and Jackson described complications of esophageal foreign bodies that were not correctly diagnosed until very late.

In 1896, G. Killan first removed foreign bodies by endoscopic techniques, but it was not until the 1930s that rigid, well-illuminated endoscopy became a recognized and safe technique (Jackson and Jackson, 1936).

■ *HISTORICAL READINGS*

Clerf LH: Historical notes on foreign bodies in the air and food passages. Am Med Hist 8:547, 1936.

Jackson C, Jackson CL: Diseases of the Air and Food Passages of Foreign Body Origin. Philadelphia, WB Saunders, 1936.

DIAGNOSIS

Incidence

Children younger than 5 years account for approximately 84% of cases, and children younger than 3 years of age account for 73% (Darrow and Holinger, 1996). Several additional factors can increase the risk of foreign body impaction in children, including cerebral palsy, achalasia of the cardia, and neuromuscular disorders. Any anatomic narrowing of the esophagus (Fig. 37–7) or acquired stenotic areas (as may result from repaired tracheoesophageal fistula or repaired esophageal atresia, or strictures

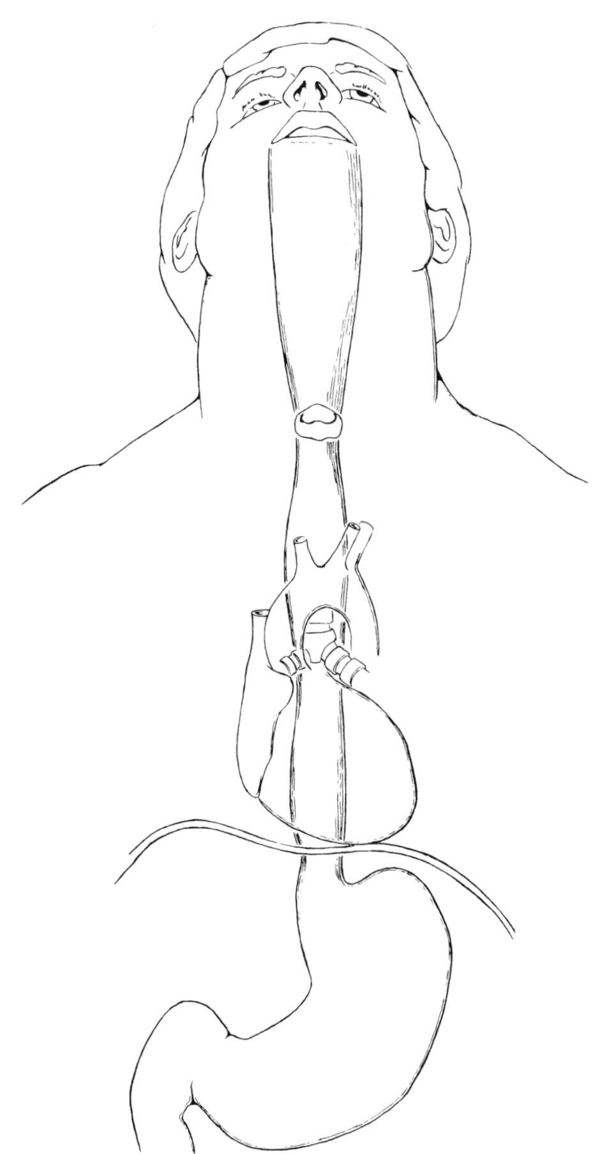

FIGURE 37–7 ■ Anatomic narrowing of the esophagus where foreign bodies are likely to become impacted.

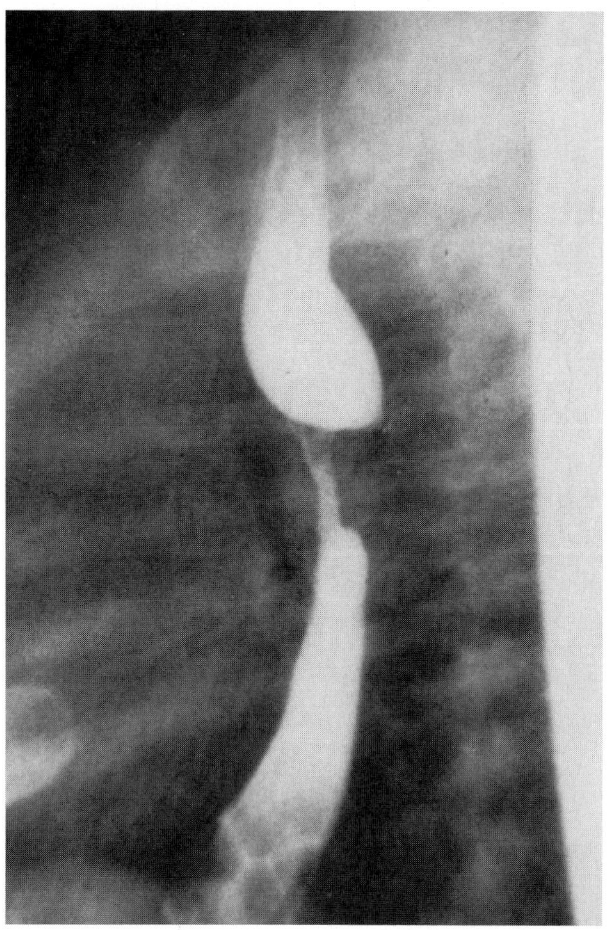

FIGURE 37–8 ■ A foreign object is likely to become impacted proximal to stenotic segment.

that form after a caustic burn or after prolonged gastroesophageal reflux) will increase the propensity for objects to lodge at the level of the narrowing (Fig. 37–8). Mental retardation, seizure disorders, and alcohol intoxication also can predispose to accidental ingestion of large objects (e.g., bottle tops) in the adolescent (Reilly and Carr, 2001).

In the older child and adolescent, fish and chicken bones often become impacted in the tonsils, vallecula, or hypopharynx. Poorly chewed meat tends to lodge lower at the gastroesophageal junction or at the site of previous surgery (tracheosophageal fistula repair). If food lodges at the cricopharyngeus or the midesophagus, bulbar palsies may be suspected.

The type of foreign body ingested has evolved over time. Metallic objects such as diaper pins are rarely seen, and plastic toy parts are seen more often. These plastic parts often are not visible on radiographs, and an effort has been made to encourage toy makers to incorporate radioopaque substances in toys for this reason (Manning and Stool, 1987). Coins remain the most common esophageal foreign body in children (Papsin and Friedberg, 1994), and unfortunately, disk or button-type batteries are increasingly found (Chiang and Chen, 2000). Esophageal foreign bodies typically lodge just below the cricopharyngeus, and if the site of impaction is lower, the possibility of an underlying stricture should be considered (Holinger, 1997).

Symptoms and Signs

The symptoms associated with esophageal foreign body vary and can be missed if not placed in context by a witness who observed the ingestion or the relatively constant brief spell of choking or gagging that occurs immediately after ingestion. Thereafter, in the absence of "classic" symptoms or signs, a high level of suspicion is helpful in the diagnosis of esophageal foreign bodies, because symptoms resemble those of general upper respiratory tract illness in children. Vomiting, dysphagia, and drooling are the most common symptoms of esophageal foreign body impaction in children (Papsin and Friedberg, 1994). There often is an asymptomatic interval after the foreign body has become lodged, which can result in a significant delay in diagnosis owing to the paucity of symptoms. An undiagnosed and unsuspected foreign body will, however, eventually cause symptoms that redirect attention to its presence; these symptoms are manifested when dysphagia, failure to thrive, or erosion into potentially dangerous structures occurs (Dahiya and Denton, 1999).

A large object that is caught in the hypopharynx or esophagus can compress the larynx and trachea, causing airway compromise and biphasic stridor. The initial event may cause coughing, choking, and cyanosis, but if the airway is completely obstructed, no sound or speech is possible, and the Heimlich maneuver (Heimlich, 1975) should be the immediate therapy. Slapping the child between the scapulae or turning a child upside down should be discouraged, because this may further lodge the foreign body (Heimlich, 1990).

When the object has passed the laryngeal inlet, choking noises cease, and the object (typically a coin) may lodge silently at the cricopharyngeus (Fig. 37–9), at the indentation of the crossing of the aortic arch at midesophagus (Fig. 37–10), or distally at the cardioesophageal sphincter. If the object totally obstructs the lumen, there is marked drooling, dysphagia, and substernal discomfort, and there may be repeated gagging (Fig. 37–11). The spillover of secretions into the larynx of the very young or debilitated patient can lead to coughing and aspiration (Fig. 37–12).

More than one object may have been ingested (Smith and Conners, 1998) (Fig. 37–13), and if a sharp object lies in the stomach, it can perforate and cause peritonitis. Perforation of the esophageal mucosa and muscular wall causes pneumomediastinum and mediastinitis with associated back pain, shortness of breath, tachycardia, and spiking fever (Fig. 37–14).

Disk or button batteries can damage the mucosa of the esophagus within 1 hour, erode into muscle in 2 to 4 hours, and perforate the esophageal wall within 8 to 12 hours. Sodium hydroxide, potassium hydroxide, and mercury leak from the battery, leading to a local caustic injury and, potentially, stricture formation, perforation, and death (Samad et al, 1999). Disk batteries can appear very much like coins on radiography, but in contradistinction, they require emergency removal and the clinical

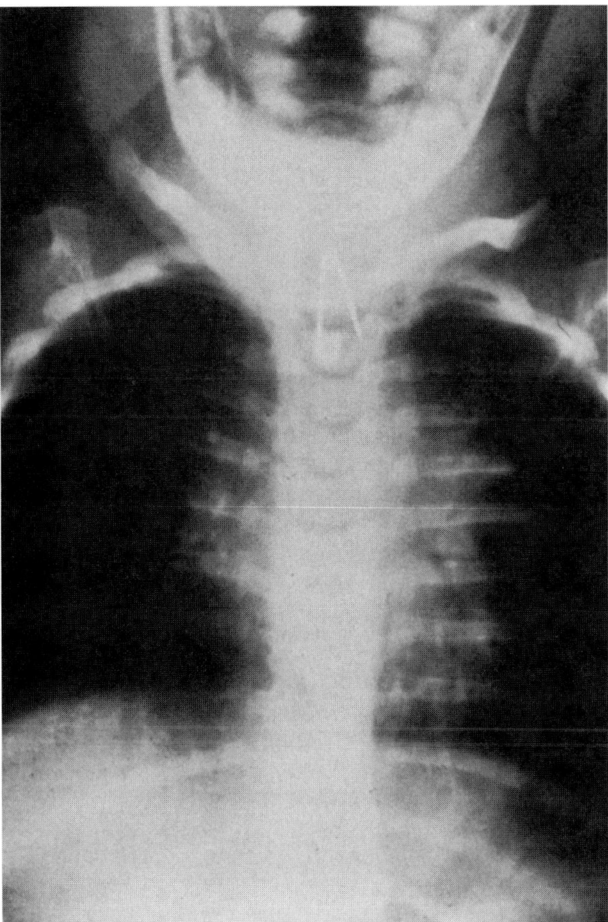

FIGURE 37–9 ■ Safety pin at the cricopharyngeus.

course taken by a child with an ingested battery is vastly different. This is the prime reason why all pediatric patients with esophageal foreign bodies should be referred to a capable endoscopist who can realize the radiographic "coin" is unusual, remove the battery on an emergency basis, and assess the esophageal damage (Fig. 37–15).

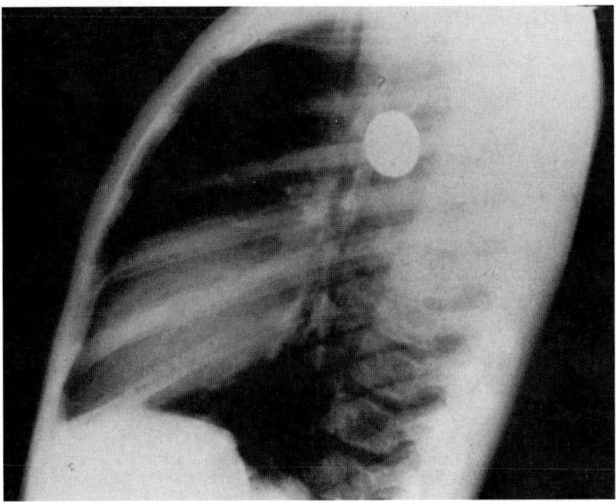

FIGURE 37–10 ■ Coin (a quarter) lodged in the esophagus at the level of the aortic arch.

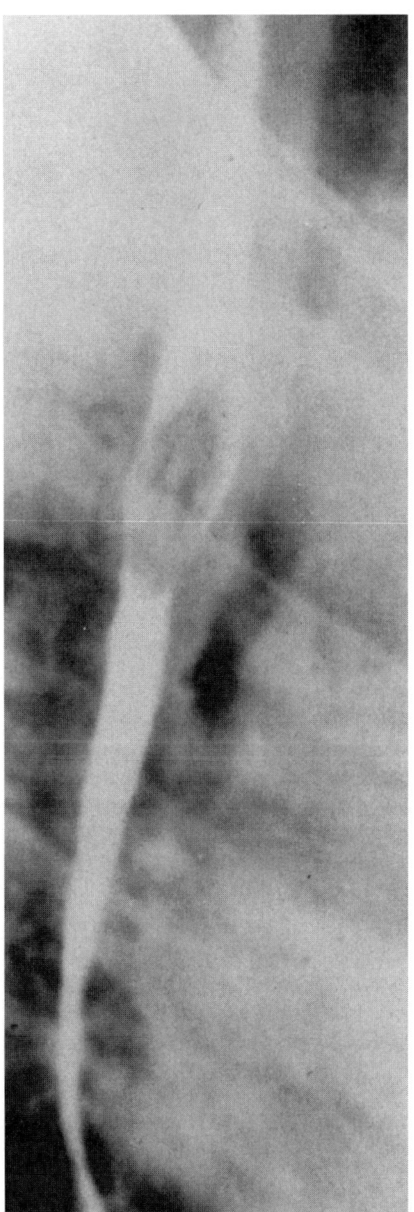

FIGURE 37–11 ■ Total obstruction, seen on barium swallow.

Chronic Complications

The presence of foreign objects that have been impacted for some time may result in progressive dysphagia, anorexia, and weight loss. This presents as failure to thrive in infants. If the object is large, it may produce progressive respiratory distress due to anterior compression of the trachea. Long-standing foreign bodies become embedded in granulation tissue, which can be friable and bleed, and occasionally the patient presents with hematemesis. Late sequelae of indwelling foreign bodies are stricture formation; fistula formation, either into the trachea (with recurrent pneumonia) or into a blood vessel, causing massive hematemesis; and perforation (Bullaboy et al, 1985).

Diagnostic Techniques

For objects that create severe airway obstruction, there is no time for investigative procedures. The patient should

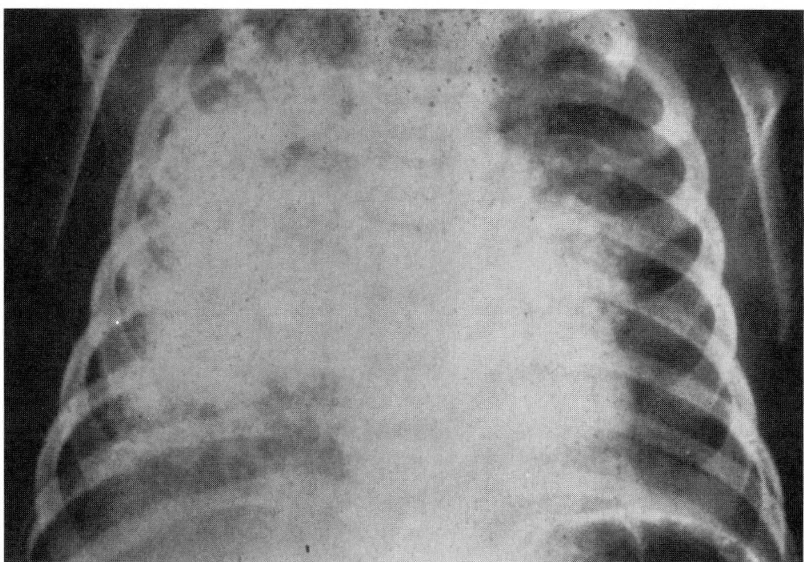

FIGURE 37–12 ■ Repeated aspiration pneumonia from spillover from an obstructed esophagus.

be taken to the operating room and anesthetized with a nonparalytic inhalation technique, and the object should be identified with use of a lit curved-blade laryngoscope and removed with Magill forceps.

In all other cases in which the airway is viable, plain neck and chest radiographs (anteroposterior and lateral views) should be obtained. The lateral view is essential to allow the identification of multiple foreign bodies. If the object is radiolucent, it can be demonstrated by means of a barium or an iohexol (Omnipaque) swallow (Manning and Stool, 1987). A small amount of the barium or iohexol suspension should be administered initially, if a complete obstruction is suspected, to prevent overflow aspiration (Fig. 37–16). If hematemesis is oc-

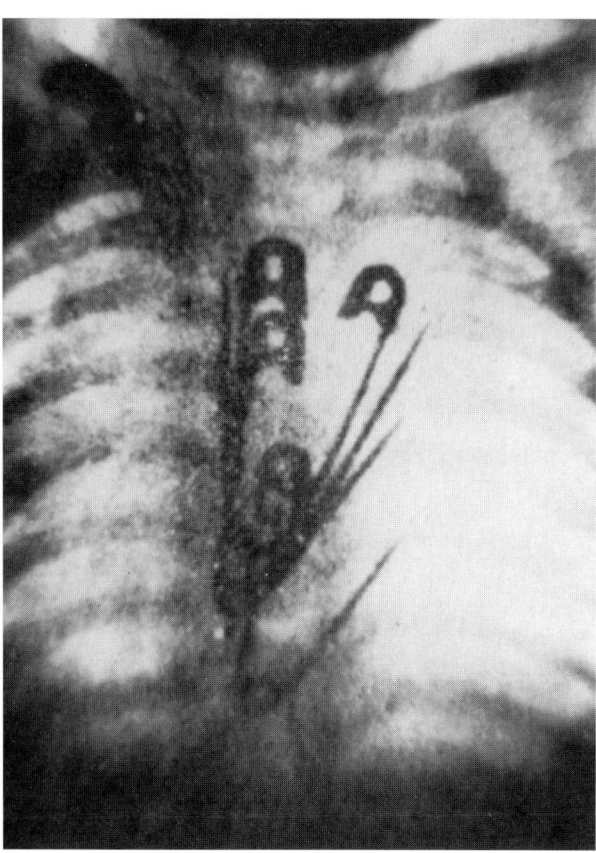

FIGURE 37–13 ■ Multiple safety pins in the esophagus (murder attempt, child abuse).

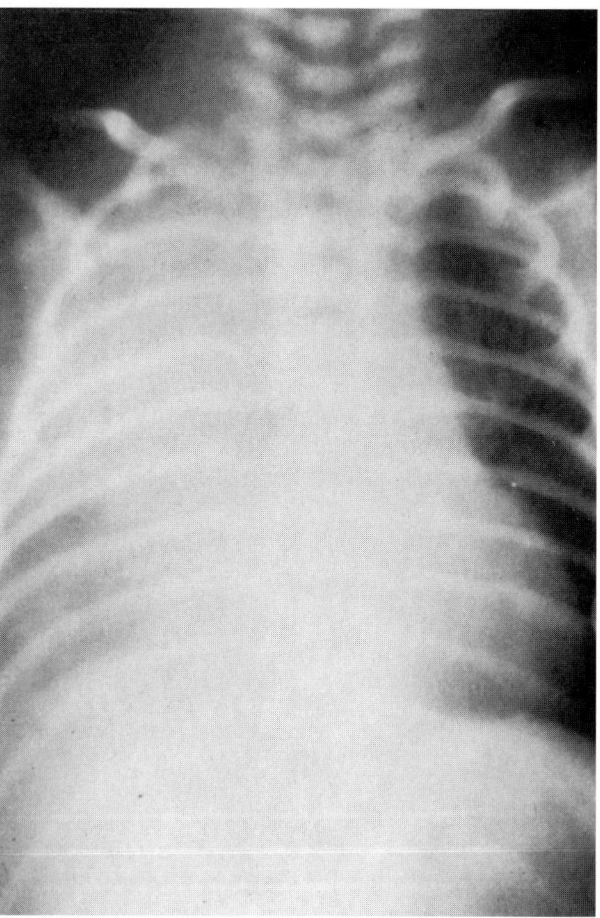

FIGURE 37–14 ■ Mediastinitis from esophageal perforation.

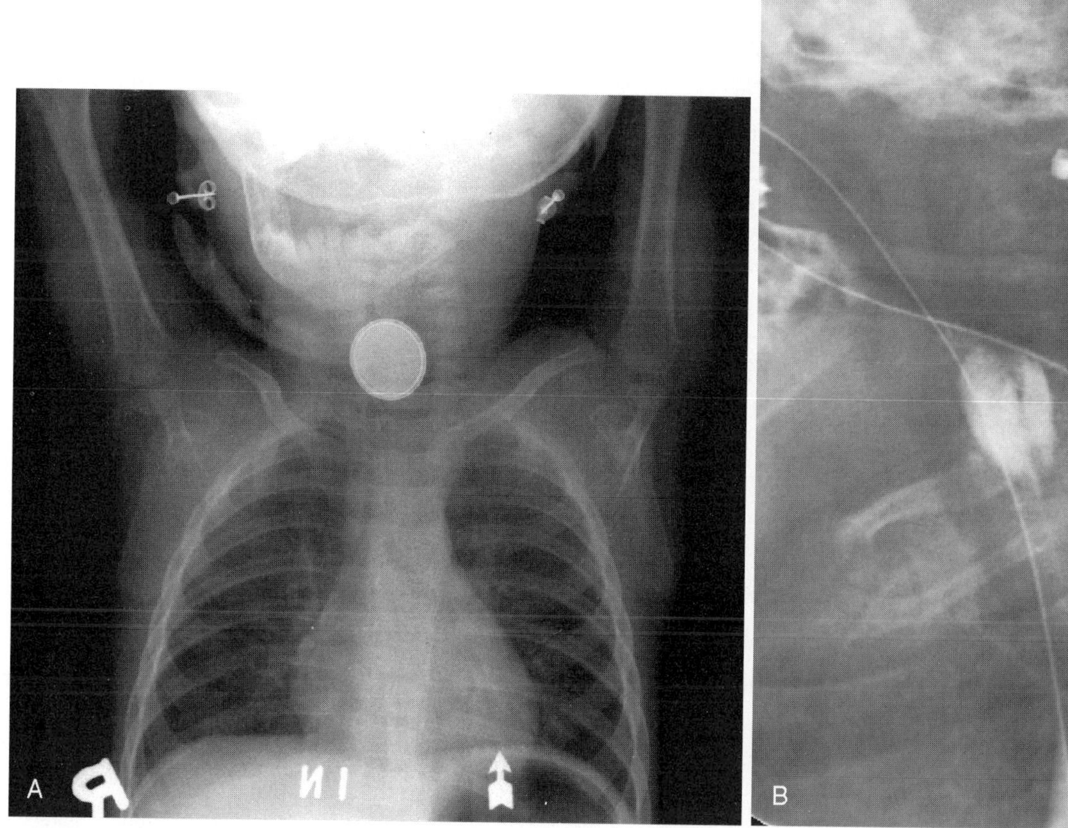

FIGURE 37–15 ■ Disk or button battery from a pocket organizer that a father thought he had thrown out the day prior to his 9-month-old's finding it. *A,* The foreign body is shown on a radiograph. Clearly not Canadian, the coin had an abnormal appearance that was explained as being Japanese money that was lying around the house. Although the battery was removed immediately when the child arrived at our institution, 5 hours had elapsed since ingestion and a considerable amount of damage had already occurred. *B,* At 1 week after ingestion, after the child was maintained on nothing-by-mouth status with a nasogastric tube, a meglumine diatrizoate (Gastrografin) swallow shows a perforation of the cervical esophagus, which was managed conservatively.

curring, it would be wise to obtain an arteriogram before any endoscopic removal is attempted in case a major artery has been eroded, in which case a thoracotomy may be required (Bullaboy et al, 1985).

If a small, sharp object such as a fish bone is suspected but not visible radiographically, a barium-dipped cotton ball or marshmallow can be used; when swallowed, it may stick onto the protruding point. If mucosal perforation by a sharp foreign object or by the presence of surgical emphysema is suspected, this may be confirmed by administering a small-volume barium swallow (Fig. 37–17).

When a metallic foreign body has been demonstrated radiographically, a commercially available metal detector can confirm its location and whether it has spontaneously passed (Gooden et al, 2000). Although this technique cannot obviate the need for initial radiographs to diagnose a foreign body (because it cannot differentiate a coin from a disk or button battery), it can eliminate the need for follow-up radiographs if some time has elapsed between initial diagnosis and arrival at the treatment facility.

MANAGEMENT

The primary objective of management should be to protect the airway from the foreign object. Hypopharyngeal large objects (dentures, plastic caps) should be removed immediately with the patient under deep inhalation anesthesia by use of a Magill forceps and a distally lit laryngoscope. When the object is at the cricopharyngeus or more distal, the patient should be intubated before manipulation of the foreign body. Use of a cuffed tube is optimal in adolescents and adults to diminish the chance of spillover of secretions into the airway. Once the airway is protected, any method of retrieval of the object is acceptable, but for the surgeon direct visualization and controlled removal with an esophagoscope are optimal.

Rigid esophagoscopes are the most versatile, because many different grasping forceps can be used through them. The Hollinger and Jesberg endoscopes were used for many years, but the Storz esophagoscope, with its far superior fiberoptic illumination, in conjunction with the internal Hopkins telescope and the telescopic forceps, have revolutionized the visibility and accessibility of most foreign bodies.

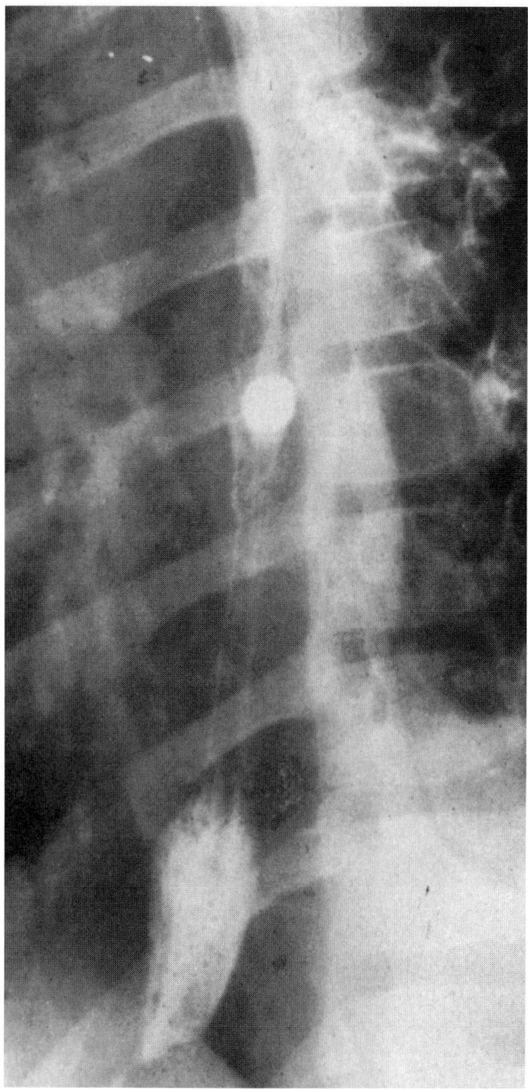

FIGURE 37–16 ■ Barium swallow can locate a radiolucent foreign body (Styrofoam ball).

When a foreign body is too large to be withdrawn through the esophagoscope, it should be withdrawn against the distal end of the esophagoscope, which is removed together with the object as a unit. Care must be taken to hold the forceps firmly at the level of the cricopharyngeus, where the object is most likely to be stripped out of the grasp of the forceps at the level of the laryngeal inlet.

Sharp foreign bodies, such as open safety pins, should be drawn into the esophagoscope as far as possible and removed with the tip trailing. If the sharp tip is pointing toward the endoscopist, it may be covered by the forceps and withdrawn using point-sheathing forceps. Alternatively, it may be closed by means of a safety pin–closing forceps or turned by means of a ring forceps, which grasps the center ring (Marsh, 1975), pushes it distally through the cardiac gastroesophageal sphincter, reverses within the stomach (endogastric version), and then pulls the ring into the esophagoscope. The Gordon bead forceps can remove oval or globular objects such as marbles.

Occasionally, an object can be seen clearly in the esophagus on radiography but not at esophagoscopy. This may occur when a small, flat object is hidden by the rugae of the esophageal mucosa. These folds can be distended by insufflation of a large volume of air to expose the contained object or by inflation of a Fogarty balloon catheter beyond the object to hold the mucosa in a distended position (Eliashar et al, 1998). This technique can be adapted to facilitate the safe removal of irregularly shaped, sharp foreign bodies such as partial dental plates or bridges.

A good technique to use to avoid missing a second foreign body is to routinely reinsert the esophagoscope down to the gastric junction and then withdraw it slowly in a repeated side-to-side sweeping motion to distend and examine every mucosal fold (Smith and Connors, 1998).

When the foreign object has been indwelling for some time, it often becomes embedded in granulation tissue. Neuropads soaked in 1:1000 epinephrine can be applied with forceps, both to shrink the tissue to afford a better view of the object and to provide hemostasis if bleeding occurs. If there is significant bleeding after the removal of such an object, the area should be tamponaded by means of a pack on a forceps or by a Foley catheter. It is very rare that bleeding is so brisk that an arteriogram with embolization is necessary for hemostasis.

Unusually shaped objects are occasionally encountered that do not conform to any available forceps. Figure 37–18 shows a circular blade from a shaving razor in midesophagus. It could not be withdrawn directly, because the upward-pointing blades would have ripped the mucosa. It was too large to be covered by an instrument or pulled into the lumen of the esophagoscope. Therefore, a small alligator-jaw forceps was used to grasp each blade tip in turn and gently roll the blade up the esophagus without causing a perforation.

If a smooth foreign body is lost into the stomach during attempts at removal, it can safely be left to pass naturally through the tract. The only exception to this is when the pylorus has been narrowed by an ulcer or a surgical procedure or when the object is caustic (e.g., an alkaline battery). In such cases, gastroscopic or surgical removal is required.

Endoscopic foreign body retrieval is a frequently performed and safe procedure. Damage to the cervical spine and trauma to the cricopharyngeus can be avoided by correct patient positioning, with a roll under the shoulders and the head extended obliquely to one side, creating a straight line from the mouth to the gastroesophageal junction (Fig. 37–19). If a deeply embedded, sharp, irregularly shaped, or excessively large foreign body cannot be removed safely with the esophagoscope, the preferred method is thoracotomy, esophagotomy, and primary closure after removal.

Finally, if a foreign body is present in an infant younger than 8 months (i.e., too young to crawl or to grasp efficiently) or if multiple foreign bodies are identified (see Fig. 37–12), child abuse should always be suspected. If multiple foreign body ingestion occurs in an adult, possible underlying causes are psychological disturbances (Jacob et al, 1990), attempts at suicide, and Munchausen syndrome.

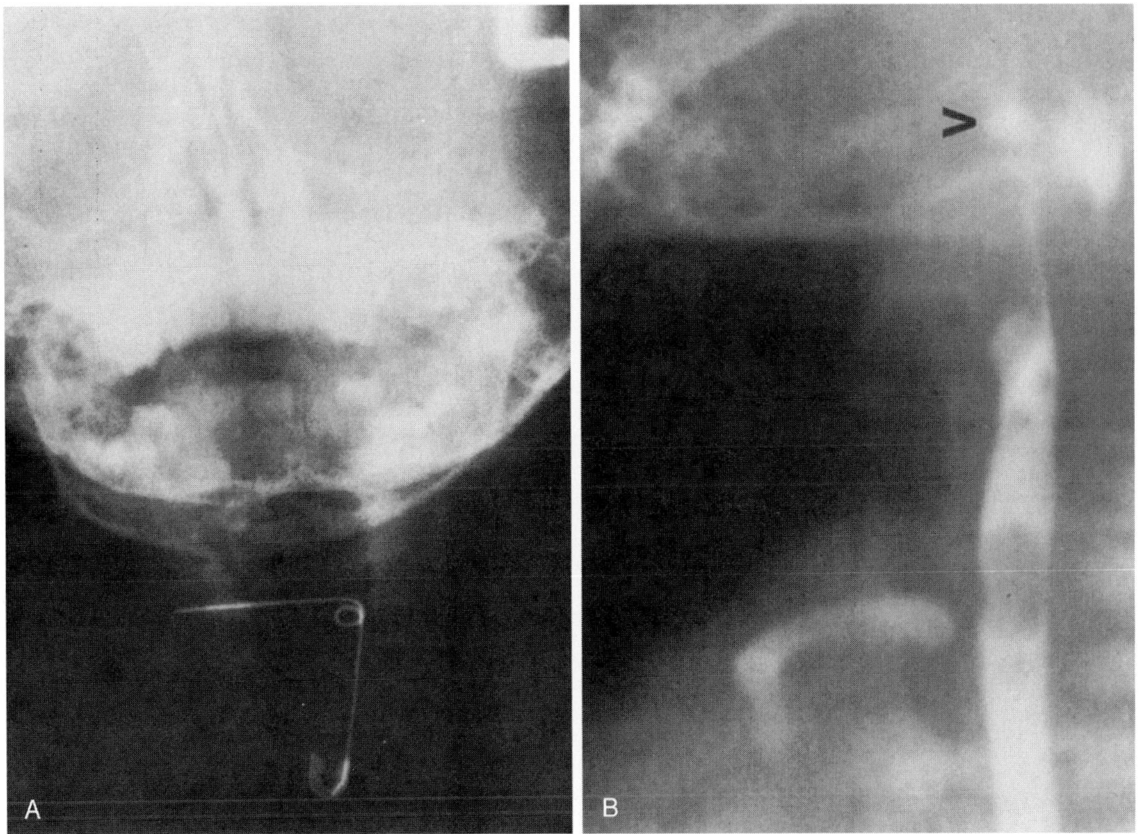

FIGURE 37–17 ■ *A,* Mucosal perforation at the right piriform fossa. *B,* Mucosal perforation at the right piriform fossa demonstrated by barium swallow (*arrowhead*).

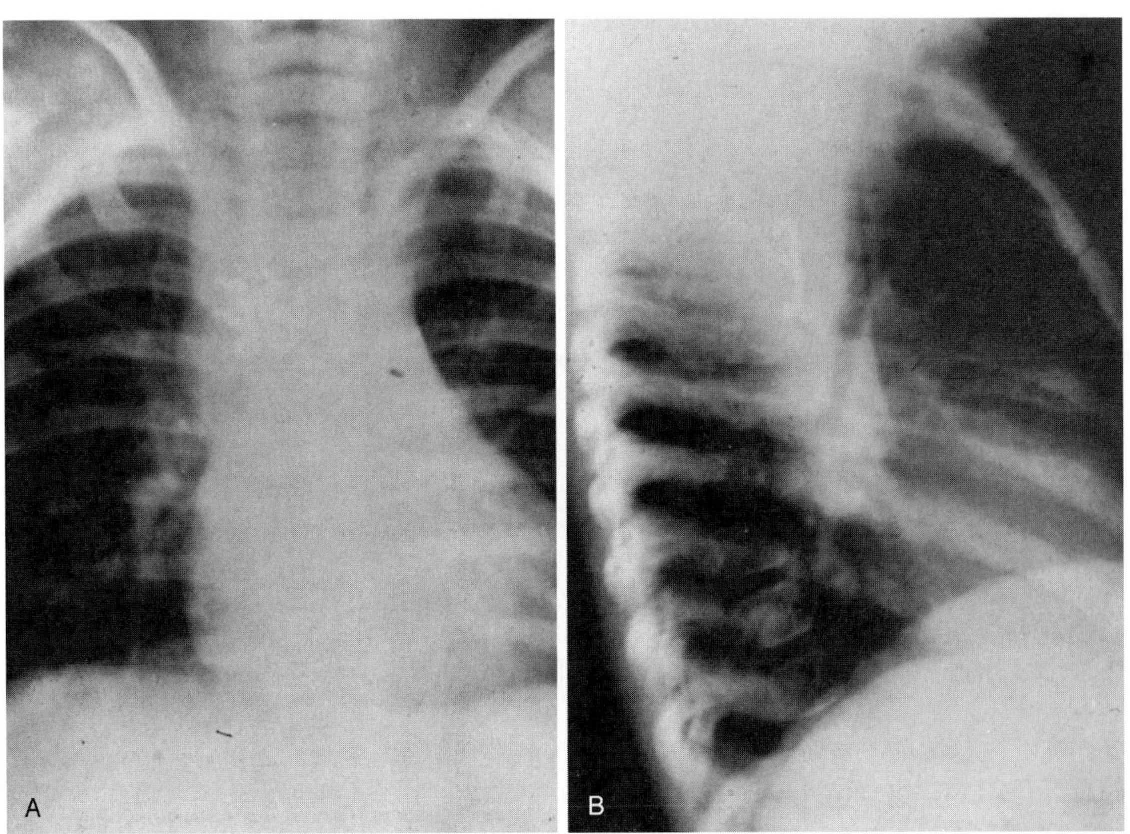

FIGURE 37–18 ■ Sharp foreign body (circular razor blade from shaver) embedded in the esophagus. *A,* Anteroposterior view. *B,* Lateral view.

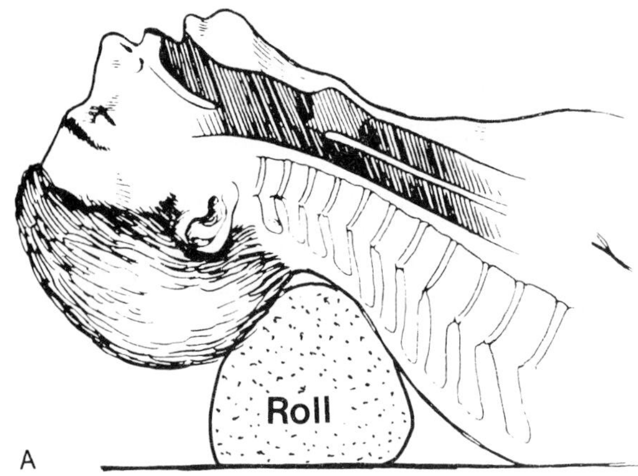

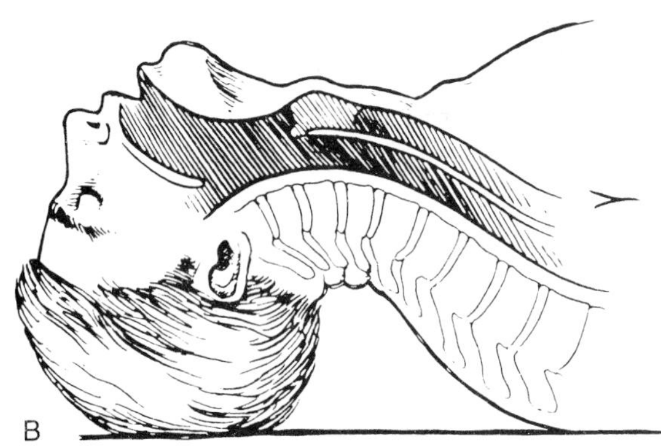

FIGURE 37–19 ■ Correct *(A)* and incorrect *(B)* positioning for rigid endoscopy.

CONTROVERSIAL METHODS OF ESOPHAGEAL FOREIGN BODY REMOVAL

Foley Catheters

There remains continued debate regarding the use of Foley catheters to remove esophageal coins from children, and these debates are predominantly fueled by economic considerations. Proponents of this method of coin removal cite the significant reduction in cost required for "safe" removal without the need for general anesthesia (Conners, 1997). This method involves passing a balloon catheter beyond the impacted foreign body under fluoroscopic guidance. Next, the balloon is inflated and withdrawn, disimpacting and removing the foreign body from the esophagus. Although there have been no serious complications reported with this method, a number of significant objections have been raised by the pediatric surgical community.

The primary objections are that the airway is not protected during removal of the foreign body and that there is an uncontrolled opportunity for the coin to become lodged in the larynx or nasopharynx (Stool and Dietch, 1973). Balloon catheter removal also is based on the presumption that the radiopaque foreign body that is visualized fluroscopically is the only one present. In addition, there is no way to assess the status of the esophageal wall during removal, which might be of concern if the object, unknowingly, has been lodged for a period of time and has caused significant esophageal ulceration. Finally, and most important, the removal procedure, which is performed with the child awake and restrained in the Trendelenburg position, can hardly be considered less traumatic than one in which the child receives a properly administered general anesthetic.

Alternative Methods

Papain

There are reports of the use of papain to "digest" impacted vegetable matter and of the use of meat tenderizer for impacted meat. This approach is inadvisable, especially in recurrent obstruction with a known stricture, because it also erodes the mucosal wall, causing florid granulations and possibly esophageal or stomach perforation (Hall and Huseby, 1988).

Drugs

Several methods have been used to relax the lower esophageal sphincter, namely the use of intramuscular diazepam, morphine, glucagon, or propantheline bromide (Pro-Banthine). These methods have had limited success but can be used under observation when a smooth object is caught at the lower esophageal sphincter.

Blind Bougienage

Finally, there have been reports of use of blind bougienage (Conners, 1999) to attempt to dilate a stricture or sphincter so as to assist the passage of a foreign body; we strongly discourage this because it may result in perforation.

These alternative methods are usually proposed by physicians unable to gain access to operating room facilities or those without surgical colleagues willing to routinely accept such cases. Esophageal foreign body removal is best undertaken by the endoscopist, who can safely and directly visualize the foreign body and gently remove it, and who is fully prepared to intervene more aggressively should the need arise.

CONCLUSION

The ingestion of foreign bodies is quite common in infants and children. Recent comprehensive reviews have been published by Holinger (1997), McGahren (1999), and Muntz (2000).

■ *KEY REFERENCES*

Holinger LD: Foreign bodies of the airway and esophagus. In Holinger LD, Lusk RP, Green CG (eds): Laryngology and Bronchoesophagology. Philadelphia, Lippincott-Raven, 1997, p 234.

McGahren ED: Esophageal foreign bodies. Pediatr Rev 20:129, 1999.

Muntz HR: Management of foreign bodies. In Wetmore RF, Muntz HR, McGill TJ (eds): Pediatric Otolaryngology. New York, Thieme Medical, 2000.

■ *REFERENCES*

Bullaboy CA, Derkal WM, Johnson DH, et al: False aneurysm of the aorta secondary to an esophageal foreign body. Ann Thorac Surg 39:275, 1985.

Chiang MC, Chen YS: Tracheoesophageal fistula secondary to disc battery ingestion. Am J Otolaryngol 21:333, 2000.

Clerf LH: Historical notes on foreign bodies in the air and food passages. Am Med Hist 8:547, 1936.

Conners GP: A literature-based comparison of three methods of pediatric esophageal coin removal. Pediatr Emerg Care 13:154, 1997.

Darrow DH, Holinger LD: Foreign bodies of the larynx, trachea and bronchi. In Bluestone CD, Stool SE, Kennam MA (eds): Pediatric Otolaryngology, 3rd ed. Philadelphia, WB Saunders, 1996, p 1390.

Dahiya M, Denton JS: Esophagoaortic perforation by foreign body (coin) causing sudden death in a 3-year-old child. Am J Forensic Med Pathol 20:184, 1999.

Eliashar R, Sichel JY, Dano I, Braverman I: Removal of a sharp esophageal foreign body using a rigid esophagoscope and a Foley catheter. J Otolaryngol 27:307, 1998.

Gooden EA, Forte V, Papsin BC: Use of a commercially available metal detector for the localization of metallic foreign body ingestion in children. J Otolaryngol 29:218, 2000.

Hall ML, Huseby JS: Hemorrhagic pulmonary edema associated with meat tenderizer treatment for esophageal meat impaction. Chest 94:640, 1988.

Heimlich HJ: The Heimlich manoeuvre: Best technique for saving any choking victim's life. Postgrad Med 87:38, 1990.

Heimlich HJ: A life saving manoeuvre to prevent food choking. JAMA 234:398, 1975.

Holinger LD: Foreign bodies of the airway and esophagus. In Holinger LD, Lusk RP, Green CG (eds): Laryngology and Bronchoesophagology. Philadelphia, Lippincott-Raven, 1997, p 234.

Jackson C, Jackson CL: Diseases of the Air and Food Passages of Foreign Body Origin. Philadelphia, WB Saunders, 1936.

Jacob B, Huckenbeck W, Barz J, Bonte W: Death, after swallowing and aspiration of a high number of foreign bodies, in a schizophrenic woman. Am J Forensic Med Pathol 11:331, 1990.

Manning S, Stool SE: Foreign body detection: Don't overlook plastic. Am J Respir Dis 8:33, 1987.

Marsh BR: The problem of the open safety pin. Ann Otol Rhinol Laryngol 84:624, 1975.

Papsin BC, Friedberg J: Aero-digestive tract foreign bodies in children: Pitfalls in management. J Otolaryngol 23:102, 1994.

Reilly S, Carr L: Foreign body ingestion in children with severe developmental disabilities: A case study. Dysphagia 16:68, 2001.

Samad L, Ali M, Ramzi H: Button battery ingestion: Hazards of esophageal impaction. J Pediatr Surg, 34:1527, 1999.

Smith SA, Conners GP: Unexpected second foreign bodies in pediatric esophageal coin ingestions. Pediatr Emerg Care 14:261, 1998.

Stool S, Dietch M: Potential danger of catheter removal of foreign body. Pediatrics 51:313, 1973.

CHAPTER **38**

*Esophageal Perforation**

Stanley C. Fell

The esophagus, strategically situated in the neck, mediastinum, and abdomen, is subject to irreparable injury; the consequences of perforation are grave and commonly result from technical misadventure.

Despite advances in diagnostic methods and supportive therapy—including ventilatory support, antibiotics, and nutrition therapy—mortality rates for esophageal perforation are 13% in patients undergoing surgery less than 24 hours after injury and 55% for those in whom therapy is delayed (Attar et al, 1990). Factors influencing mortality are (1) the age and general condition of the patient, (2) the location and cause of the perforation, and (3) the presence or absence of intrinsic esophageal disease. The common causes of esophageal perforation are discussed later. Anastomotic leaks and caustic esophageal injuries are not included in this chapter.

In a review of 511 esophageal perforations (Jones, 1992), 43% were caused by instruments, 19% were caused by trauma, 16% were spontaneous, 7% were caused by foreign bodies, 8% were caused by operative injury, and 7% were caused by tumor and miscellaneous causes. Endoscopy alone accounted for 35% of perforations by instruments, pneumatic dilatation caused 25%, and bougienage caused 20%. Faulty endotracheal intubation, Sengstaken-Blakemore tubes, nasogastric tubes, sclerotherapy, and endoesophageal prostheses caused 20% of iatrogenic perforations. In a 1974 survey of endoscopic esophageal injury, the incidence of esophageal perforation was 0.03% (Silvis, 1976). Although endoscopic procedures are performed in increasing numbers, the more frequent use of flexible endoscopy, coupled with video imaging, has probably decreased the incidence of perforations. However, the increased use of intraoperative transesophageal echocardiography for cardiac surgery has contributed another source of perforation by instruments.

Sixty percent of cervical perforations are the result of endoscopy; the remainder are caused by penetrating trauma or foreign bodies. Injury most commonly occurs during passage of the endoscope through the cricopharyngeal sphincter, the narrowest zone of the esophagus. Older people, in whom neck extension may be limited and who often have osteoarthritic spurs juxtaposed to the posterior esophageal wall, are especially at risk. The second site of esophageal narrowing, the region of the aortic arch and the left main bronchus, is more likely to be perforated by ingested foreign bodies than by instruments. The gastroesophageal junction, the third zone of esophageal narrowing, is likely to be perforated during biopsy or dilatation of both benign and malignant strictures or achalasia.

Because the clinical manifestations, radiographic findings, treatment, and prognosis of cervical perforation differ from those of thoracic and abdominal perforations, cervical perforation is best discussed as a separate entity.

Cervical Perforations

HISTORICAL NOTE

Early in the 20th century, the morbidity and mortality of cervical esophageal perforation and nasopharyngeal infections stimulated the interest of anatomists and surgeons who were studying the fascial planes of the neck and mediastinum. Pearse (1933, 1938) realized that the cervical drainage procedure described by Marschik in 1909 did not address the problem of infection that descended into the posterior superior mediastinum. He must be credited with describing the drainage procedure that is currently used and discussed in this chapter. Pearse's 1938 paper contains superb discussions by Churchill, Alexander, Lilienthal, and Wangensteen. Lilienthal (1925) described posterior inferior mediastinotomy for abscesses that occur below the level of the tracheal bifurcation, a procedure that was used by Seybold (1950). Neuhof and Jemerin (1943) and Jemerin (1948) described the pathology and compared the clinical course in patients who were treated nonoperatively with the course in patients undergoing a drainage procedure.

■ *HISTORICAL READINGS*

Jemerin EE: Results of treatment of perforation of the esophagus. Ann Surg 128:971, 1948.

Lilienthal H: Thoracic Surgery. Philadelphia, WB Saunders, 1925.

Neuhof H, Jemerin EE: Acute Infections of the Mediastinum. Baltimore, William & Wilkins, 1943.

Pearse HE: The operation for perforation of the cervical esophagus. Surg Gynecol Obstet 56:192, 1933.

Pearse HE: Mediastinitis following cervical suppuration. Ann Surg 108:538, 1938.

Seybold WD, Johnson MA, Learly WV: Perforation of the esophagus. Surg Clin North Am 30:1155, 1950.

OVERVIEW

Technical errors or omissions leading to cervical esophageal perforation include (1) inadequate sedation or anesthesia, (2) improper passage of the esophagoscope through the cricopharyngeus, (3) failure to use a rubber-tipped lumen finder and thus becoming lost in the piri-

*Supported by the Feldesman Fund for Thoracic Surgery at the Montefiore Medical Center.

CAUSES OF ESOPHAGEAL PERFORATION

Endoesophageal Instrumentation

Esophagoscopy
Transesophageal echocardiography
Bougienage
Pneumatic dilatation
Sclerosis of esophageal varices
Placement of intraesophageal tubes (nasogastric, Sengstaken-Blakemore, prostheses)
Traumatic endotracheal intubation

Periesophageal Surgery

Mediastinoscopy
Thyroid surgery
Anterior spinal surgery
Vagotomy
Pulmonary resection
Antireflux surgery
Thoracic aneurysm resection

Trauma

Penetrating
Foreign body
Caustic ingestion

Barotrauma

Postemetic
Blunt trauma—neck, thorax, abdomen
Compressed air ingestion
Miscellaneous—seizure, childbirth, defecation, brain disease

Tumor

Esophagus
Lung
Mediastinal

Infection

Tuberculosis
Histoplasmosis
Syphilis
Acquired immunodeficiency syndrome

form fossa, (4) failure to deflate the cuff of the endotracheal tube during insertion of the esophagoscope, and (5) failure to elevate the instrument anteriorly away from the cervical spine. Failure to obtain an esophagogram before endoscopy increases the risk of perforation in areas of unsuspected disease.

PATHOLOGY

A perforation occurs either as an immediate total breach of the esophageal wall or as a mucosal laceration that is followed by intraluminal abscess formation and subsequent mural rupture. Thus, there may be an interval of many hours between the endoscopy and the appearance of signs and symptoms of overt perforation. Sharp foreign bodies may perforate immediately, but blunt foreign bodies sometimes cause pressure necrosis and delayed perforation.

The thin buccopharyngeal fascia is adherent to the posterior wall of the pharynx and esophagus. Thus, the perforation can enter the retrovisceral space, allowing infection to descend into the posterior mediastinum (Fig. 38–1). The retrovisceral space becomes obliterated by fibrous tissue in the region of the tracheal bifurcation at the level of the sixth thoracic vertebra (T6). Below this point, the space continues to the diaphragm. If the pharyngoesophagus is perforated anteriorly or laterally via the piriform fossa, infection occurs in the pretracheal space and may then descend substernally.

CLINICAL FEATURES

Virtually all patients with cervical esophageal perforations complain of pain made worse by dysphagia, odynophagia, and neck flexion. The neck is tender, and crepitation may be noted on palpation or auscultation. A cervical perforation is suggested if severe pain is elicited when the examiner grasps the thyroid cartilage between the thumb and index fingers and moves it from side to side. Fever and leukocytosis develop promptly. Lateral cervical radiographs usually demonstrate loss of the normal lordosis, anterior displacement of the trachea and esophagus, and widening of the retrovisceral space. Streaks of air in the soft tissue planes are best seen in the sagittal view. Chest radiographs may demonstrate pneumomediastinum and posteriosuperior mediastinal pleural fluid collections (Fig. 38–2).

If surgery is not immediate, pleural effusion, usually right-sided, commonly develops after 24 hours. Esophagograms that are performed with water-soluble contrast material confirm perforation in approximately 80% of cases (Michel et al, 1981). The 20% incidence of false-negative results is twice that found in thoracic esophageal perforations. If findings are normal, a thin barium swallow may demonstrate the perforation. Given the clinical and radiographic findings previously described, a negative esophagogram should not deter appropriate surgical therapy. Esophagoscopy is especially valuable in cases of foreign-body perforation or penetrating trauma.

TREATMENT

Once cervical esophageal perforation is suspected, oral intake must cease, nasogastric suction should be commenced, and the patient should be given intravenous (IV) antibiotics that are effective against oral bacterial flora. Prompt surgical drainage is the basic requirement for successful management, thus reducing length of hospital stay, morbidity, and mortality. No patient is too sick for surgery. Cervical drainage may be performed with the patient under general or local anesthesia if necessary, supplemented by sedation and ventilatory support via endotracheal intubation (Neuhof and Jemerin, 1943).

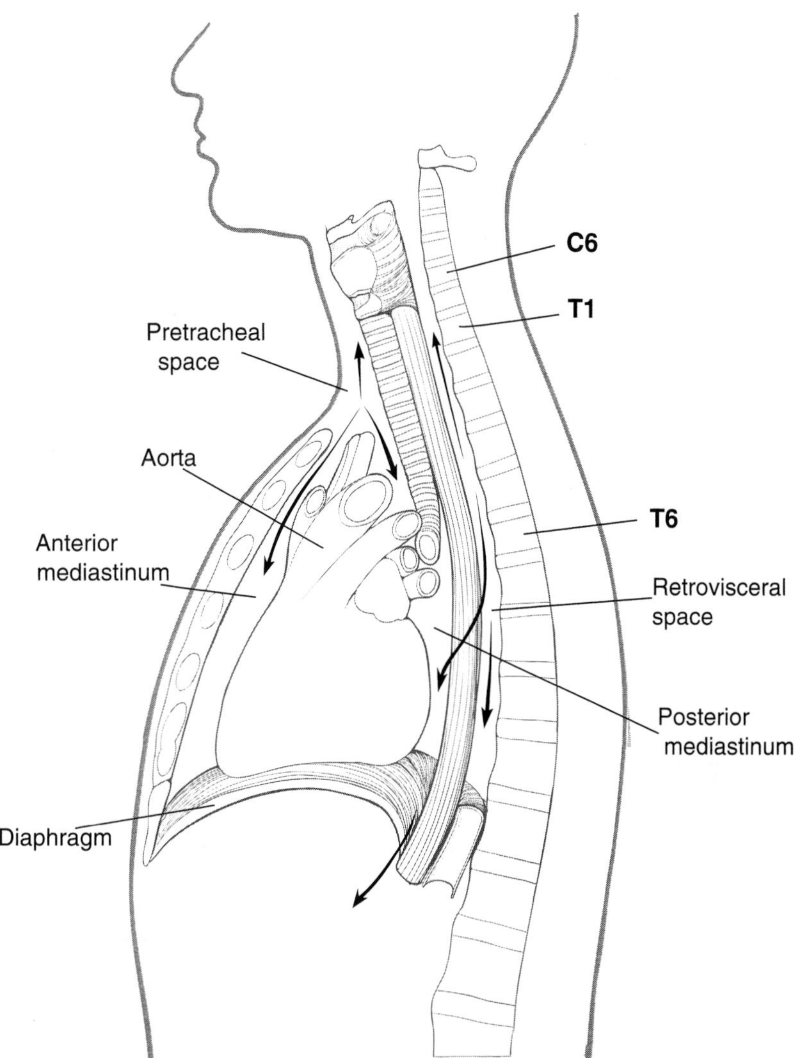

FIGURE 38–1 ■ Diagram showing pathways for spread of infection to mediastinum and pleural cavities following cervical or thoracic esophageal perforation.

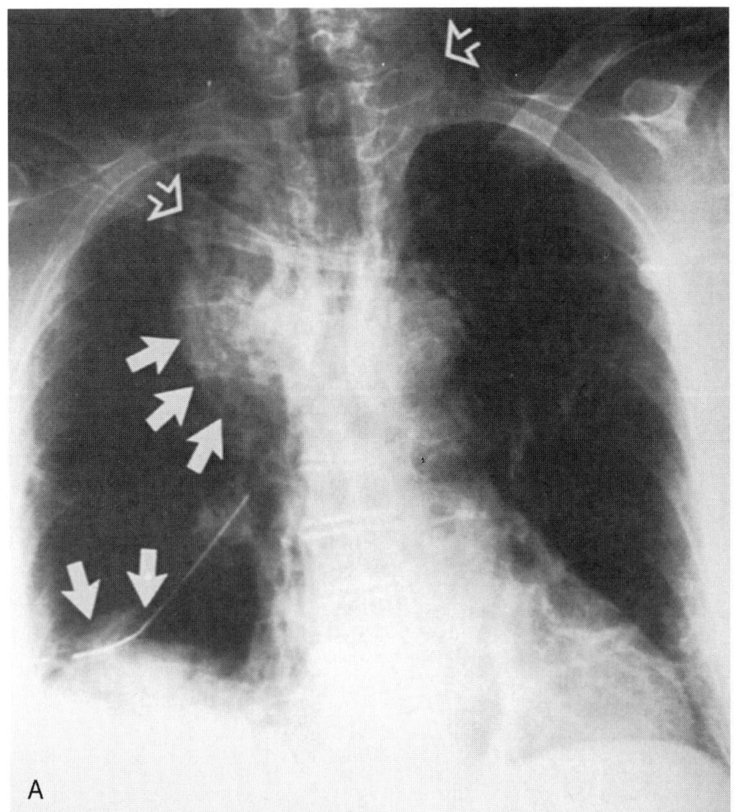

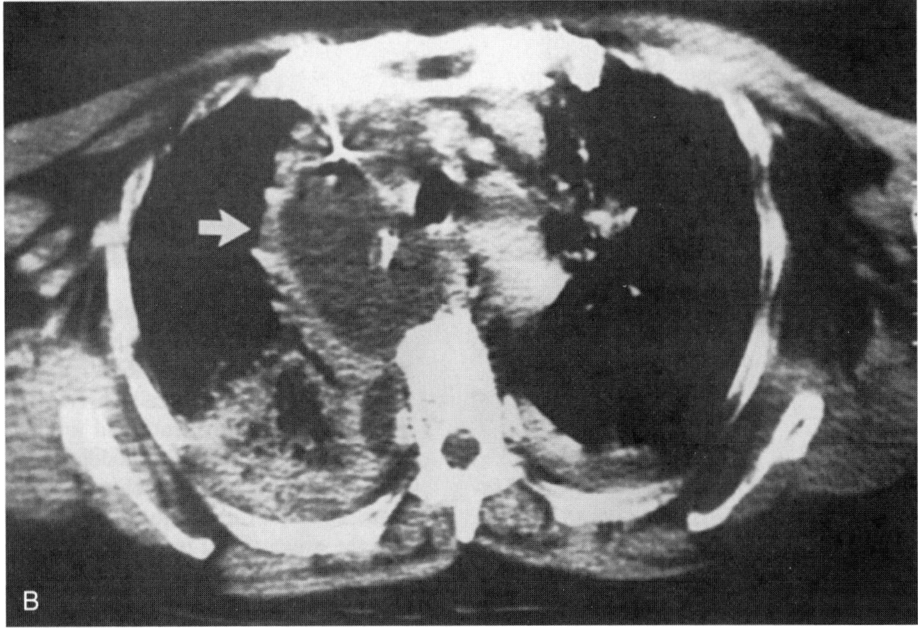

FIGURE 38–2 ■ Cervical perforation following traumatic endotracheal intubation. Treatment was delayed for 24 hours. *A*, Chest film demonstrating cervical emphysema and mediastinal *(open arrows)* and right mediastinal collection and pleural effusion *(solid arrows)*. *B*, Computed tomographic scan 24 hours following inadequate cervical drainage demonstrates right upper mediastinal fluid collection *(arrow)* and right pleural effusion. Thoracic drainage of mediastinal abscess and empyema was required.

The operative approach to cervical esophageal perforation and associated mediastinal sepsis is as follows (Fig. 38–3). An incision is made along the lower third of the anterior border of the sternocleidomastoid muscle on the side of the neck where contrast can be seen to extravasate or where significant accumulation appears in the mediastinum. Otherwise, the left-sided approach is generally preferred by right-handed surgeons. The surgeon retracts the carotid sheath and internal jugular vein laterally and divides the middle thyroid vein, if necessary, allowing the trachea and esophagus to be retracted medially. Blunt dissection leads to the retrovisceral space and the prevertebral fascia directly posterior to the esophagus. The dissection is facilitated by the edema and fluid accumulation caused by the perforation. The perforation is sought and, if found, is closed with several absorbable sutures. This step is not a requirement for successful treatment because cervical esophageal perforations heal with adequate drainage in the absence of distal obstruction.

Finger dissection is carried down into the posterior mediastinum, allowing the insertion of a suction tip. The area is copiously irrigated, and a soft suction drain is inserted into the mediastinum. Suction drainage is preferable to a Penrose drain because the drainage is uphill against gravity. The drain exits the neck through the lower angle of the incision, which is loosely closed. Perforations resulting from external trauma generally require buttressing with a pedicled flap of strap muscle or omohyoid. In cases of missile or stab wounds that cause contiguous tracheal and esophageal perforation, it is essential to interpose a pedicled muscle flap between the separate repairs.

Oral feedings are withheld, and nasogastric suction and IV antibiotics are continued until cervical drainage ceases, approximately 1 week later. An esophagogram with aqueous contrast is then obtained. After esophageal integrity is demonstrated, the drain is removed and oral feeding is gradually resumed.

Thoracic and Abdominal Perforations

OVERVIEW

In contrast to cervical perforations that are instrumental or traumatic and managed by the simple operative procedure described in the preceding section, thoracic esophageal perforations have multiple causes, including injury by instrument (Fig. 38–4), barotrauma (Fig. 38–5), caustic ingestion, carcinoma, and penetrating wounds. The management and outcome of the perforations depend on the cause, the associated esophageal disease, and the condition of the patient at the time of therapy. Risk factors for endoscopic and instrument perforation of the thoracic esophagus include:

- Poor sedation or anesthesia
- Attempts to dilate strictures using inappropriate means
- Failure to recognize a stricture that is not suitable for peroral dilatation
- Biopsy performed without proper visualization

Dilatation of strictures or pneumatic dilatation for achalasia together are responsible for 45% of esophageal perforations. Dilatation of strictures over a guidewire under fluoroscopic control should reduce the incidence of perforation. Barogenic trauma (Boerhaave's syndrome) accounts for 10% to 15% of thoracic perforations. Less commonly, perforations result from endoscopic removal of foreign bodies or gunshot wounds. Operative injuries include perforations following the performance of transthoracic or abdominal antireflux operations and unrecognized mucosal injury during esophagocardiomyotomy for achalasia. The incidence of esophageal perforation following transabdominal vagotomy is 0.54% (Postlethwait et al, 1969). The advent of laparoscopic Nissen antireflux procedures has added a new source of intraoperative esophageal injury, although with increasing experience, the rate of occurrence of this complication appears to be diminishing.

Esophagopleural fistula, an uncommon complication of pleuropneumonectomy for pulmonary tuberculosis (Takaro et al, 1960), has also occurred following radical resections for lung cancer. Mediastinal perforation of the esophagus, a rare manifestation of pulmonary tuberculosis or histoplasmosis, has been reported in association with the tuberculosis that is seen in patients with acquired immunodeficiency syndrome (AIDS) in whom the esophagus is invaded by mycobacteria from adjacent mediastinal lymph nodes (Adkins et al, 1990). Approximately 8% of middle-third esophageal carcinomas develop fistulas in the tracheobronchial tree, and occasionally esophageal carcinoma perforates into the mediastinum with abscess formation.

CLINICAL FEATURES

Perforation of the thoracic esophagus is clinically manifested by substernal or epigastric pain. Cervical subcutaneous air is noted in only 20% of cases of thoracic perforations (Sawyers et al, 1975), but mediastinal emphysema and pleural effusion are common. Because plain chest and abdominal radiographs are nondiagnostic in at least 12% of cases (Han et al, 1985), esophagograms with water-soluble agents, followed by thin barium examination if necessary, have become routine practice following the performance of pneumatic dilatation in some institutions.

Abdominal esophageal perforations that are not diagnosed and treated at the time of laparotomy cause epigastric tenderness, muscle spasm, and epigastric pain often radiating to the back or left shoulder. A history of endoscopy or periesophageal surgery makes esophageal perforation suspect. Pleural effusion, often bilateral, and subdiaphragmatic air are commonly noted radiographically. Oral contrast study confirms the diagnosis.

Boerhaave's Syndrome

HISTORICAL NOTE

Shortly before midnight, on October 29, 1723, Hermann Boerhaave, Professor of Medicine at Leyden University,

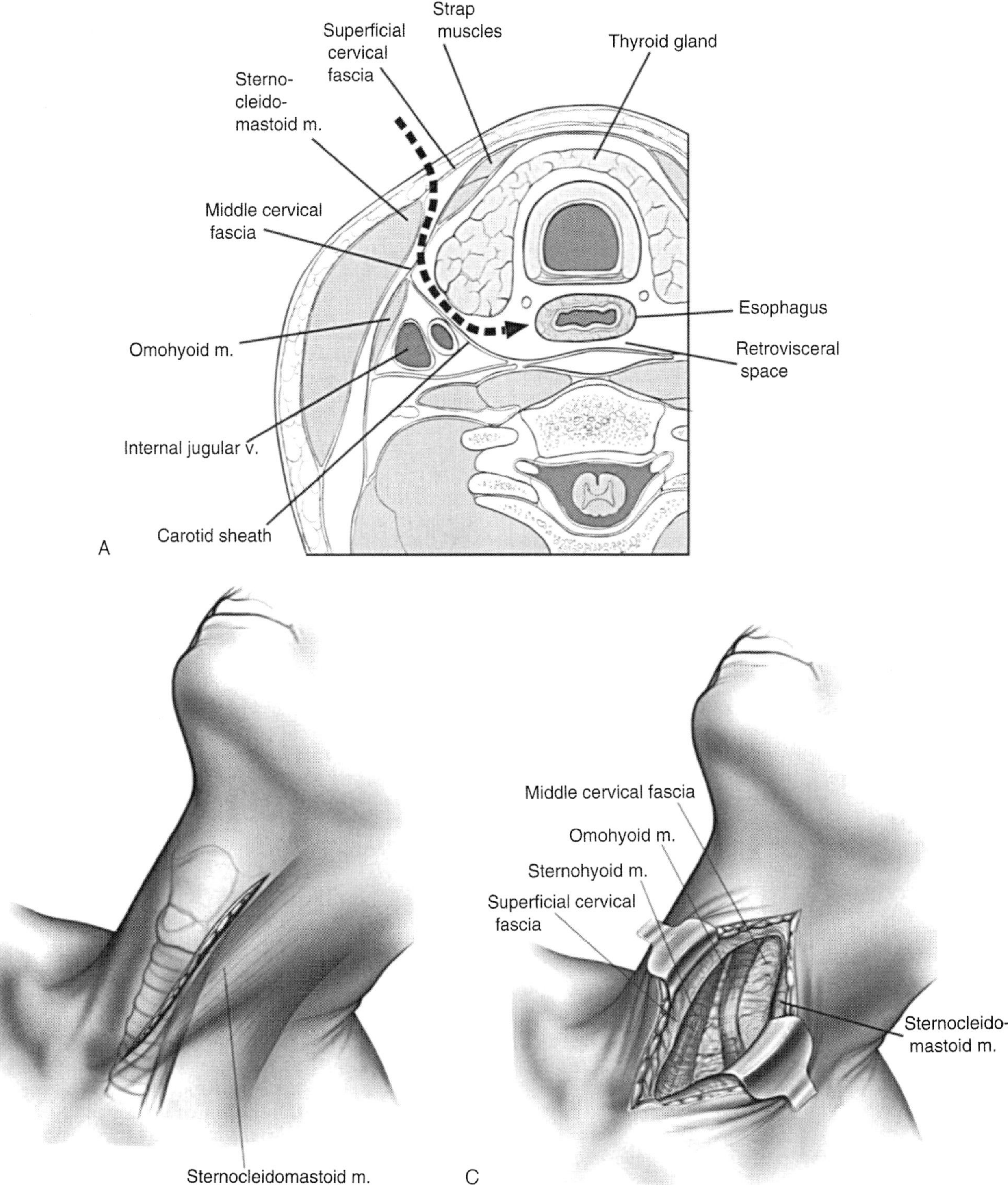

FIGURE 38–3 ■ *A–C,* Operative technique for cervical mediastinal drainage. See text for details.

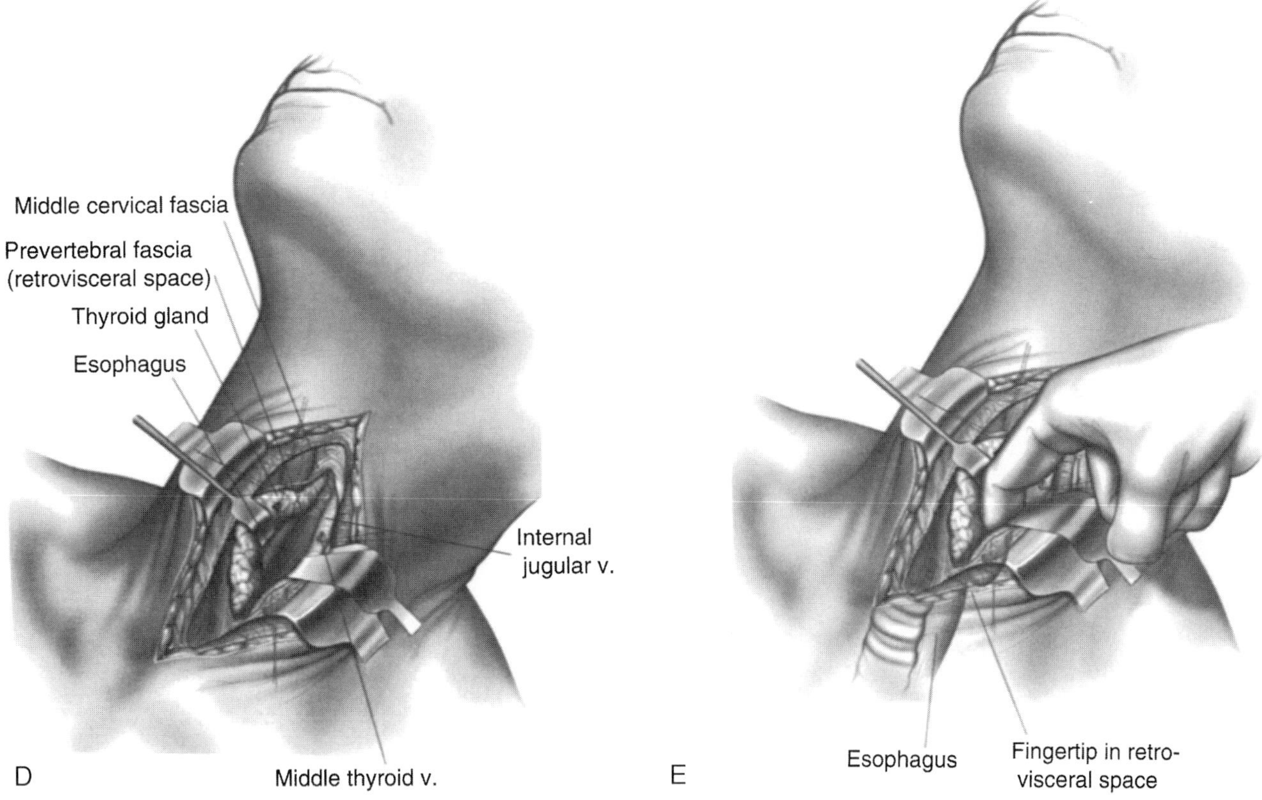

FIGURE 38–3 ■ *Continued. D* and *E, See legend on opposite page*

was summoned to attend Baron Jan van Wassenaer, grand admiral of the Holland fleet, a prodigious gourmand who often relieved his postprandial discomfort by self-induced vomiting. Having feasted richly on duck and beer early in the day, the baron vomited and gave forth a horrifying cry, complaining to his servants that something near the upper part of his stomach was torn. Thereafter, he continued to experience severe pain. Boerhaave's examination of the baron disclosed no abdominal findings. Death occurred 18 hours after onset of illness. At autopsy, Boerhaave noted emphysema of the chest wall and abdomen and a rupture of the left posterolateral wall of the esophagus, 3 inches above the diaphragm, without evidence of esophageal ulcer. He was struck by the strong odor of roasted duck and observed the olive oil, which the baron had taken as an emetic, floating in the left pleural cavity.

His 70-page autopsy protocol, "History of a Grievous Disease Not Previously Described," published in 1724, achieved wide acclaim; thus the eponym "Boerhaave's syndrome" has been applied to postemetic rupture of the normal esophagus. Using cadavers, MacKenzie (1884) reproduced the Boerhaave lesion, and Mackler (1952) confirmed these findings using intraluminal pressure of 5 pounds per square inch.

Collis and colleagues (1944) made the preoperative diagnosis of postemetic esophageal rupture and performed thoracotomy and repair, but the patient died of shock 20 hours later. Barrett (1946), having made the correct preoperative diagnosis, reported the first successful repair (performed 10 hours after the rupture). Olsen and Clagett (1947) reported a successful result in the same year.

■ HISTORICAL READINGS

Barrett NR: Spontaneous perforation of the esophagus. Thorax 1:48, 1946.

Boerhaave H: Atrocis, nec descripti prima, morbi historia. Verbatim English translation (Derbes V, Mitchell R). Bull Med Libr Assoc 43:217, 1955.

Collis JL, Humphries DR, Bond WH: Spontaneous rupture of the esophagus. Lancet 2:179, 1944.

Mackler S: Spontaneous rupture of the esophagus. Surg Gynecol Obstet 95:344, 1952.

MacKenzie M: A Manual of Diseases of the Nose and Throat. New York, William Wood, 1884.

Olsen AM, Clagett OT: Spontaneous rupture of the esophagus: Report of a case with immediate diagnosis and successful surgical repair. Postgrad Med 2:417, 1947.

PATHOPHYSIOLOGY

Similar findings are noted in cases of esophageal rupture that is unassociated with emesis, such as blunt thoracic or abdominal trauma, compressed air hose injury, epileptic seizures, defecation, and childbirth, all of which may be associated with a sudden increase in intra-abdominal pressure. All cases of barotrauma resulting in esophageal rupture may be considered to be variants of Boerhaave's syndrome, because the pathologic process and clinical course are similar. The term *spontaneous rupture of the esophagus* is inappropriate because the rupture invariably follows barotrauma. Although several reports of cases

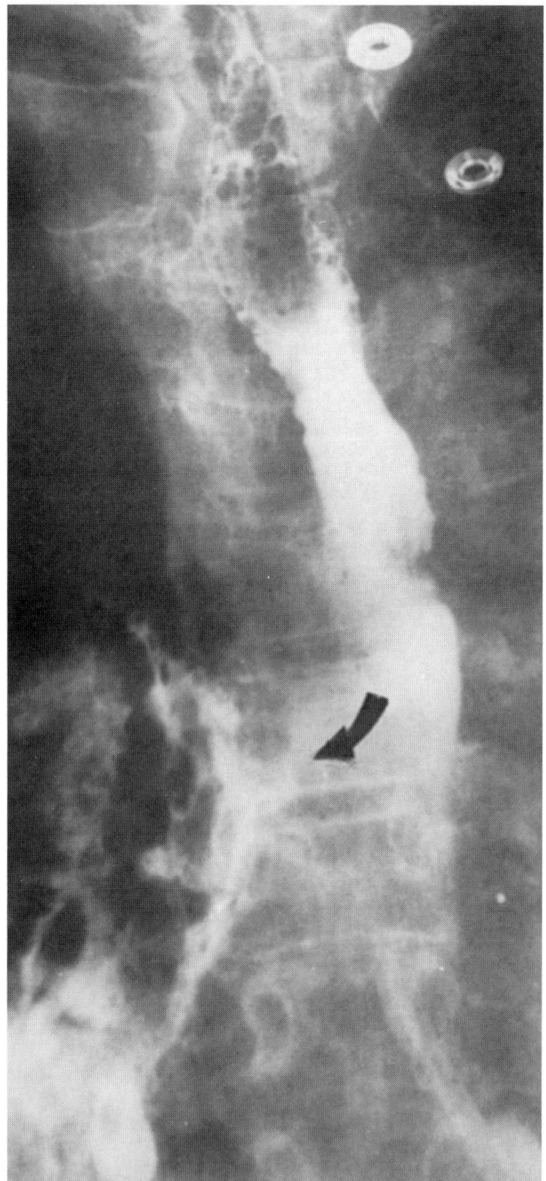

FIGURE 38–4 ■ Perforation of a normal esophagus *(arrow)* during rigid endoscopy, ineptly performed. Gastrografin esophagography had been performed because the chest radiograph revealed a right pneumothorax. Repair was performed 8 hours after injury.

have been alleged to have been truly spontaneous (Conte, 1966), these ruptures have usually been associated with motility disorders, lower esophageal ring, or food impaction.

During the normal vomiting reflex, there is coordination between the increased intra-abdominal pressure caused by rapid diaphragmatic descent and abdominal wall contraction and the relaxation of the esophagus sphincters. Alcohol ingestion, sedatives, general anesthesia, and repetitive vomiting adversely affect the reflex. Failure of the upper esophageal sphincter to relax results in an increase in intraesophageal pressure and esophageal rupture.

The *Mallory-Weiss syndrome* (massive hematemesis with or without melena) also occurs following persistent retching or vomiting but is unassociated with pain. The process consists of single or several mucosal tears at the esophagogastric junction. The pathogenesis is thought to be related to the effect of vomiting or retching when the inferior esophageal sphincter cannot relax.

The pathologic lesion in Boerhaave's syndrome is a longitudinal rent with well-defined edges, varying in length from 0.5 to 20 cm, located on the left posterolateral wall of the esophagus, 2 to 6 cm above the diaphragm in 80% of cases. The rent may involve the posterior wall or the right posterolateral wall in 8% of cases each. The anterior wall or the midesophagus is a rare site of esophageal rupture (Sealy, 1963). The predilection for the left posterolateral wall of the esophagus to be the site of rupture is thought to result from local anatomic factors, such as splaying of muscle fibers in that region or the entrance of blood vessels and nerves into the esophageal wall at that site. In rare instances, the laceration has been noted to be transverse, as it was in Boerhaave's case, or intra-abdominal.

CLINICAL FEATURES

Typically, Boerhaave's syndrome occurs in men (85% of cases) in the fourth to sixth decades, who vomit, often after overindulgence in food and drink. Eight cases have been reported in infants who were younger than 1 year of age, including three in neonates (Hohf, 1962).

Hematemesis is rare. Typically the onset of pain occurs immediately following a vomiting episode. Patients complain of a tearing substernal or epigastric pain, which may radiate to the left chest, shoulder, or back. The pain is accentuated by swallowing or bodily motion. Initially, the physical findings are minimal, perhaps only epigastric tenderness, in marked contrast to the severity of the symptoms. The differential diagnoses include perforated ulcer, acute pancreatitis, renal colic myocardial infarction, dissecting aortic aneurysm, or incarcerated paraesophageal hernia. All these diagnoses may be excluded by careful history taking, physical examination, and appropriate routine laboratory tests.

Flooding of the mediastinum with gastric content and mixed oral flora leads to a fulminant mediastinitis with hemorrhagic necrosis. The mediastinal pleura usually ruptures soon thereafter, with resultant massive pleural effusion, leading to ventilatory insufficiency, hypovolemia, and shock. In some cases, the mediastinal pleura does not rupture and the perforation is contained within the mediastinum. In such cases, the pain may be especially intense and the mediastinal phlegmon may dissect up and down the mediastinum for a considerable distance. As a result, the diagnosis may be considerably delayed because of the initial absence of a pleural effusion. Rupture into the pleural space may occur from days to weeks later.

Cervical subcutaneous emphysema is noted in 65% of cases but may not be appreciated early in the course of the disease. Plain chest radiography is the most valuable laboratory examination; mediastinal widening and cervical or mediastinal air are frequently noted, as is pleural

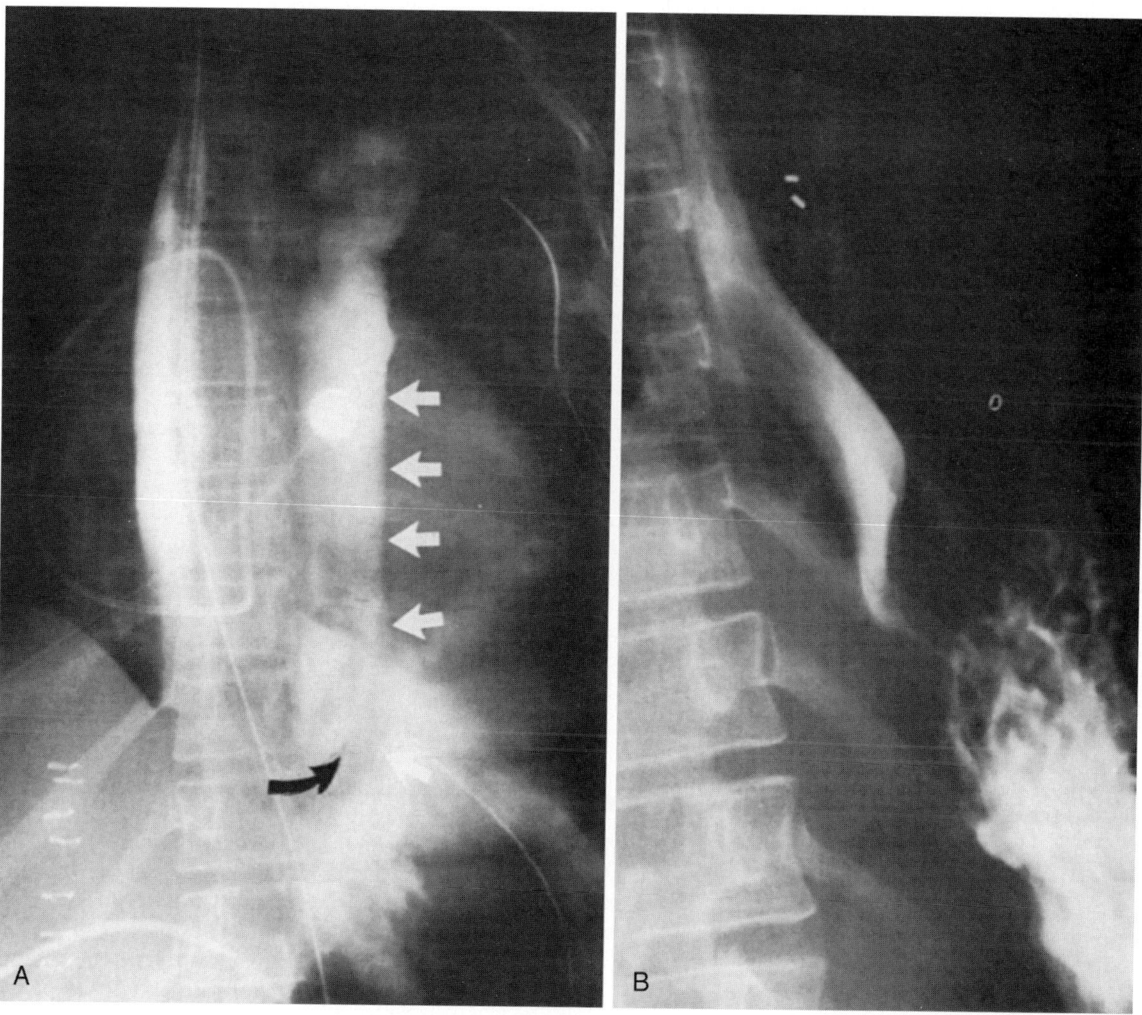

FIGURE 38–5 ■ *A*, Esophageal rupture *(curved arrow)* caused by blunt trauma (motor vehicle accident), diagnosed 3 days following laparotomy for liver laceration. Extravasation of contrast into mediastinum *(straight arrows)*. A left chest tube had been inserted for pneumothorax. *B*, Esophagogram following repair with intercostal musculopleural flap. Gastrostomy and jejunostomy were also performed.

effusion or hydropneumothorax. The effusion is most often left-sided, but may be right-sided or bilateral. Pneumothorax alone is rare. Subdiaphragmatic air has been reported in only one case (Tesler and Eisenberg, 1963).

Initially, thoracentesis yields serous fluid; following rupture of the mediastinal pleura, however, gastric content and food particles may be aspirated. These findings and a pleural fluid pH below 6 make the diagnosis indisputable. Nevertheless, an esophagogram using water-soluble contrast should be obtained (Fig. 38–6). An esophagogram may demonstrate the less common right-sided rupture. Occasionally, the water-soluble agents do not reveal the esophageal fistula, in which case thin barium swallow is recommended. In late or complicated cases, computed tomographic (CT) scans with contrast medium may be valuable in demonstrating the site of esophageal perforation or periesophageal air (Backer et al, 1990). Esophagoscopy is useful if it is not possible to obtain an esophagogram or if the study results are equivocal.

Despite the dramatic symptoms and signs of Boerhaave's syndrome, the diagnosis is frequently missed because of the rarity of the disease. Mackler (1952) stated succinctly that

> given an acutely ill patient exhibiting signs of collapse, the elicitation of a history of sudden thoracic pain occurring during or after the act of vomiting, following by the appearance of interstitial emphysema at the base of the neck, constitutes sufficient evidence to warrant a left thoracotomy.

Unfortunately, the Mackler triad is not always present in Boerhaave's syndrome; at least 40% of cases have an atypical presentation, as exemplified by the following case:

> An alcoholic man who had vomited was admitted to the medical service and treated with IV antibiotics for left lower lobe pneumonia and pleural effusion. Closed thoracostomy was performed, resulting in only partial clearing of the pleural effusion, which was considered to be empyema. Decortication was performed 1 week later, and the left lung was successfully re-expanded. Persistent copious drainage from the chest tube led to further analysis of the chest drainage. Amylase and anaerobic enterococci were detected, suggesting an esophageal

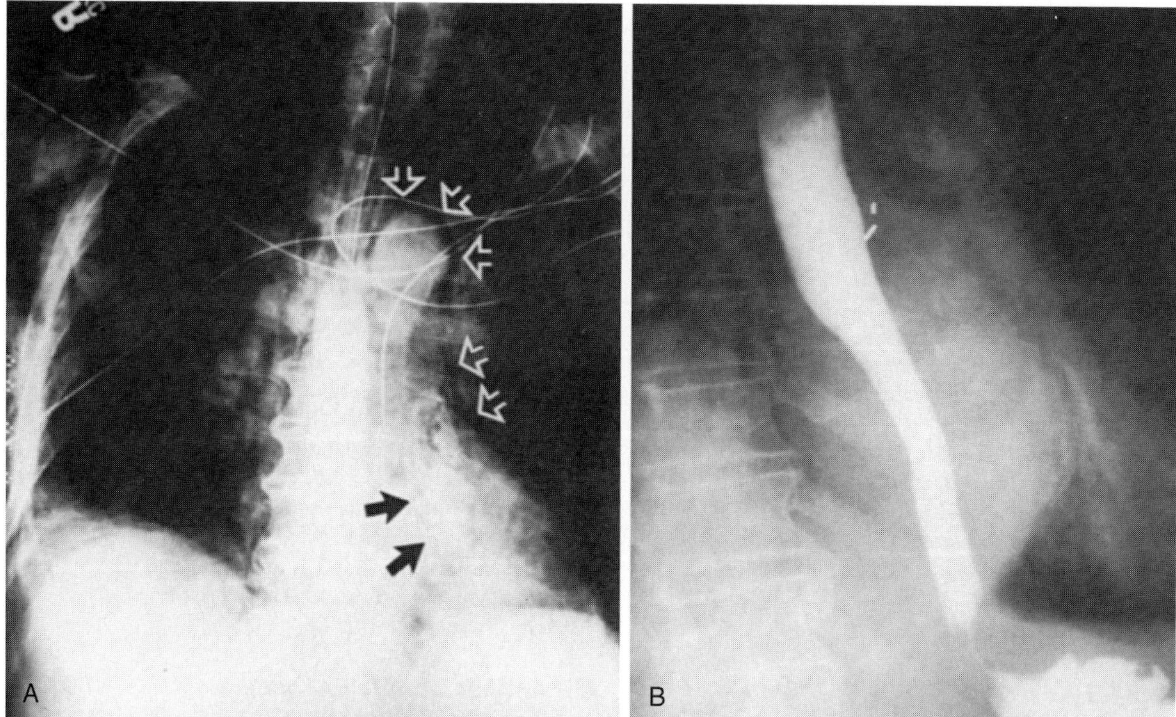

FIGURE 38–6 ■ A Boerhaave rupture of the esophagus. *A*, Mediastinal air *(hollow arrows)* and intrapleural extravasation *(solid arrows)* noted on gastrografin esophogogram. *B*, Esophagogram following primary repair and musculopleural flap.

fistula. A CT scan with oral contrast material clearly demonstrated the esophageal rupture. Healing of the esophageal rent and recovery occurred after a draining gastrostomy and feeding jejunostomy were performed.

Two lessons were learned from this case.

Lesson 1: Had the patient come to the emergency room wearing a naval admiral's uniform, voicing his complaints in Dutch, the diagnosis would still have been missed: "What one knows, one sees" (Goethe).

Lesson 2: Drainage of intrapleural sepsis, pulmonary decortication to obliterate the empyema space, gastrostomy to prevent reflux, and maintenance of nutrition by means of jejunostomy may be sufficient to allow healing of the esophageal rupture in rare cases, diagnosed late, without overwhelming sepsis.

TREATMENT OF THORACIC PERFORATION

Once the diagnosis of thoracic perforation is established, there should be no delay in bringing the patient to surgery. Preoperative measures, including hydration, IV antibiotics, and nasogastric intubation, must be expeditious. Prolonged attempts at resuscitation are not productive. The "golden" period for closure of esophageal perforations is the first 12 hours; after 24 hours the likelihood of a post-repair leak increases. Nevertheless, healing and survival may be achieved.

Upper-third and middle-third thoracic perforations are best approached by right thoracotomy through the fourth or fifth intercostal space. Lower esophageal perforations are best approached through the left sixth or seventh intercostal space.

In cases of instrument perforation that is diagnosed early, the surgeon is often afforded the luxury of operating on a fasting patient with an uncontaminated pleura. Nevertheless, the presence of pre-existing esophageal disease requires definitive management that is concomitant with esophageal repair.

Perforations resulting from pneumatic or hydrostatic dilatation for achalasia (usually longitudinal and, like postemetic rupture, situated on the left posterolateral wall of the esophagus) are managed by two-layer closure (see next section) and performance of esophagomyotomy 180 degrees away on the opposite wall of the esophagus (McKinnon and Ochsner, 1974) (Fig. 38–7). Perforation of benign strictures may often be further dilated intraoperatively and then closed and buttressed with a fundoplication such as that for an antireflux procedure. If there is esophageal shortening, a Collis gastroplasty distal to the dilated stricture may be possible. If these options are not technically feasible, esophagectomy should be considered, because healing of perforation proximal to a stricture is unlikely. In cases of carcinoma or known irreparable stricture with endoscopic perforations, either transthoracic or transhiatal esophagectomy should be considered in patients who are otherwise good surgical candidates (Blalock, 1957). Reconstruction may be either immediate or delayed, depending on the patient's condition (Orringer and Stirling, 1990).

Esophageal perforations caused by woven bougies or biopsy forceps are the easiest to repair because of their clean edges but are often difficult to find because of the

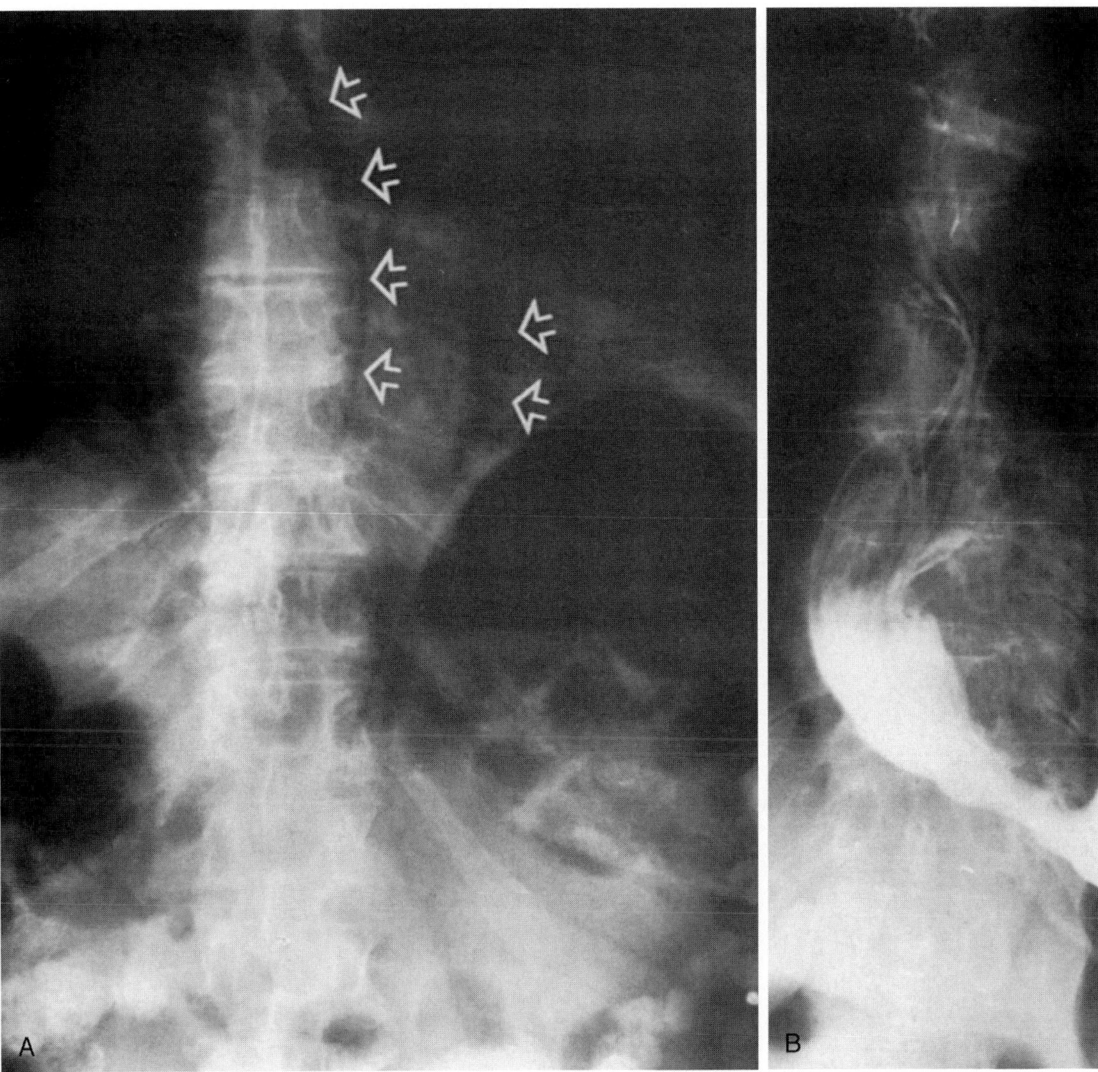

FIGURE 38–7 ■ *A*, Rupture of the terminal esophagus following pneumatic dilatation for achalasia. Note mediastinal air on the abdominal film *(arrows)*. Esophagography was not performed prior to surgery. *B*, Esophagogram following repair 3 hours after injury. Myotomy was performed on the opposite wall of the esophagus.

obliquity of their transit through the esophageal wall. Instilling methylene blue via a nasoesophageal tube to localize the site of perforation is not advised. The dye stains the tissues so intensely that it is difficult to perform an accurate repair. Milk instilled in the same way is easily visualized and does not stain the tissues. Milk taken orally is also readily visible in chest tube drainage.

Whatever the cause, once the perforation is visualized, it is essential to incise the muscular coat of the esophagus to ensure that the entire length of the mucosal defect is visualized before a two-layer closure is accomplished. Failure to do so results in inadequate repair and fistula recurrence.

The patient with a malignant esophagorespiratory fistula or perforated carcinoma with mediastinal abscess is a candidate for an endoesophageal prosthesis (Berger, 1972) (Fig. 38–8), because 80% of these patients succumb within 3 months, 9% live an additional month, and only 11% survive more than 6 months (Hill and Murray, 1989). Palliative bypass procedures carry significant morbidity and mortality and usually deprive patients of the opportunity to spend their remaining days at home with their family.

Successful management of thoracic perforations is predicated on the following:

1. Débridement and drainage of the mediastinum and pleural spaces.
2. Control of the esophageal leak.
3. Re-expansion of the lung.
4. Prevention of gastric reflux.
5. Nutrition and ventilatory support.
6. Appropriate antibiotics.
7. Postoperative localization and drainage of residual septic foci.

The methods used have been:

1. Closure with buttress or patch.
2. Exclusion and diversion.
3. T-tube fistula.

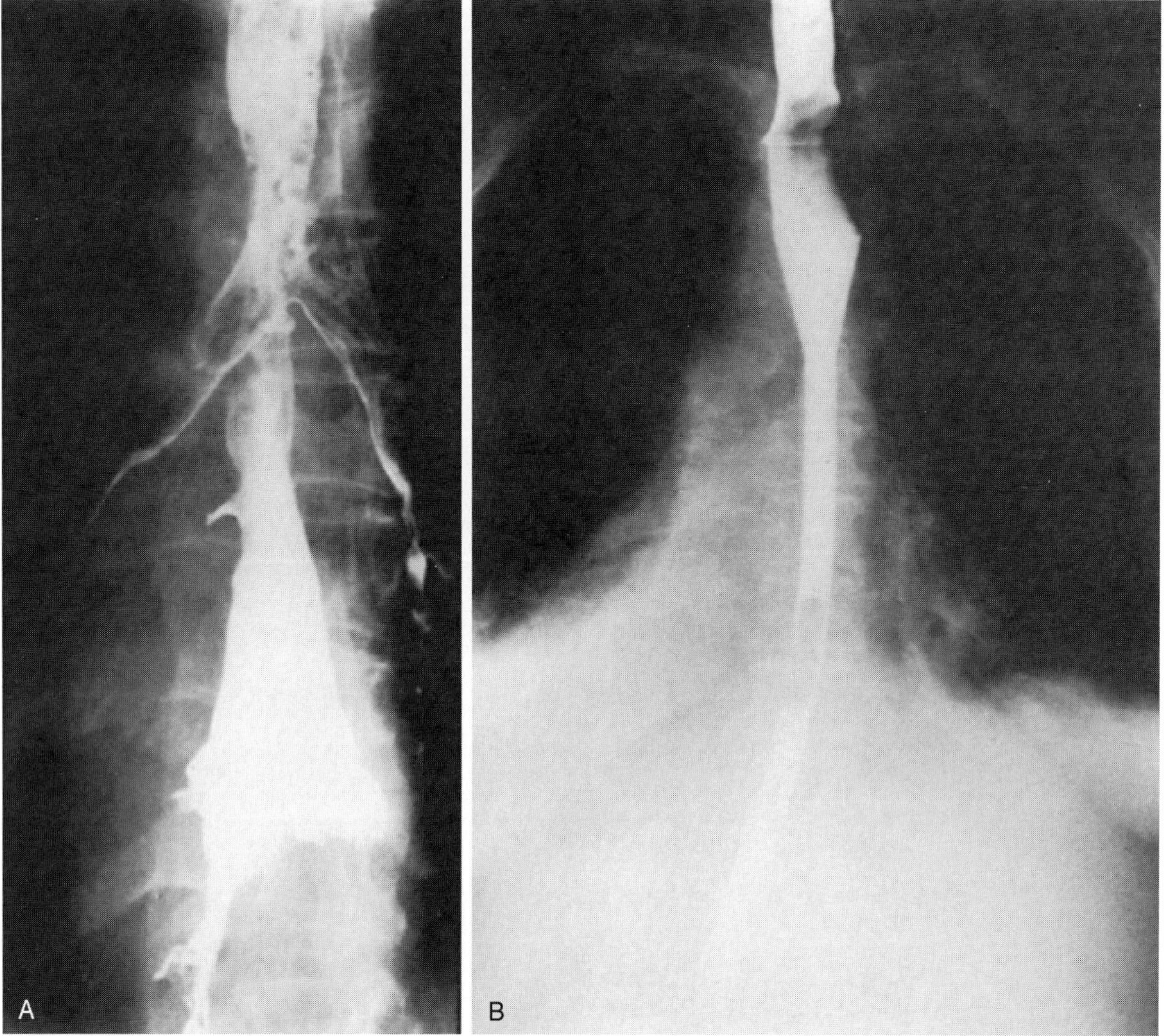

FIGURE 38–8 ■ Carcinoma of the midthoracic esophagus with tracheoesophageal fistula *(A)* treated by endoesophageal prosthesis *(B)*.

4. Thoracic drainage and irrigation.
5. Intraluminal stents.
6. Resection.

Technique of Closure

Left posterolateral thoracotomy is performed through the bed of the subperiosteally resected seventh rib. I prefer this method, rather than intercostal incision, because it facilitates the later construction of a pedicled, vascularized, intercostal musculopleural flap to buttress the esophageal suture line. Preparation and application of the flap are described in the next section.

The chest is evacuated of debris and gastric content and is copiously irrigated. The mediastinal pleura bulges and often appears as if burned by gastric secretions; it is incised from the diaphragm to the aortic arch and widely débrided of necrotic tissue (Fig. 38–9). The esophagus is then gently elevated on a silicone-like (Silastic) loop exposing the right pleural surface. This area must also be débrided to prevent the late development of a right posterior mediastinal abscess. Right pleural effusion, if present, may often be drained by passage of the suction tip into the right pleural space. Conventional closed right chest drainage is established later, after completion of the left thoracotomy if a right pleural space collection is present.

Attention is next directed to the esophageal rent. It is essential to incise the muscle layer longitudinally to ensure that the entire length of the mucosal defect is visualized. Edematous mucosal edges are trimmed, the mucosa and submucosa are closed with interrupted silk or polyglactin sutures, and the knots are placed intraluminally. The muscle coat is closed with interrupted silk. In cases diagnosed after 48 hours, the muscular closure may not be possible. Buttressed closure (see later) is then essential. A nasogastric tube is positioned above the suture line, the chest is flooded with saline, and air is gently injected into the tube. Lack of air bubbles in the chest indicates an intact suture line. The lung is then decorticated, thus ensuring full re-expansion.

At this point, consideration must be given to buttressing the repair. Despite repair within 24 hours after the injury, there is still the risk of suture line disruption and an esophagopleural fistula. Parietal pleura (Grillo

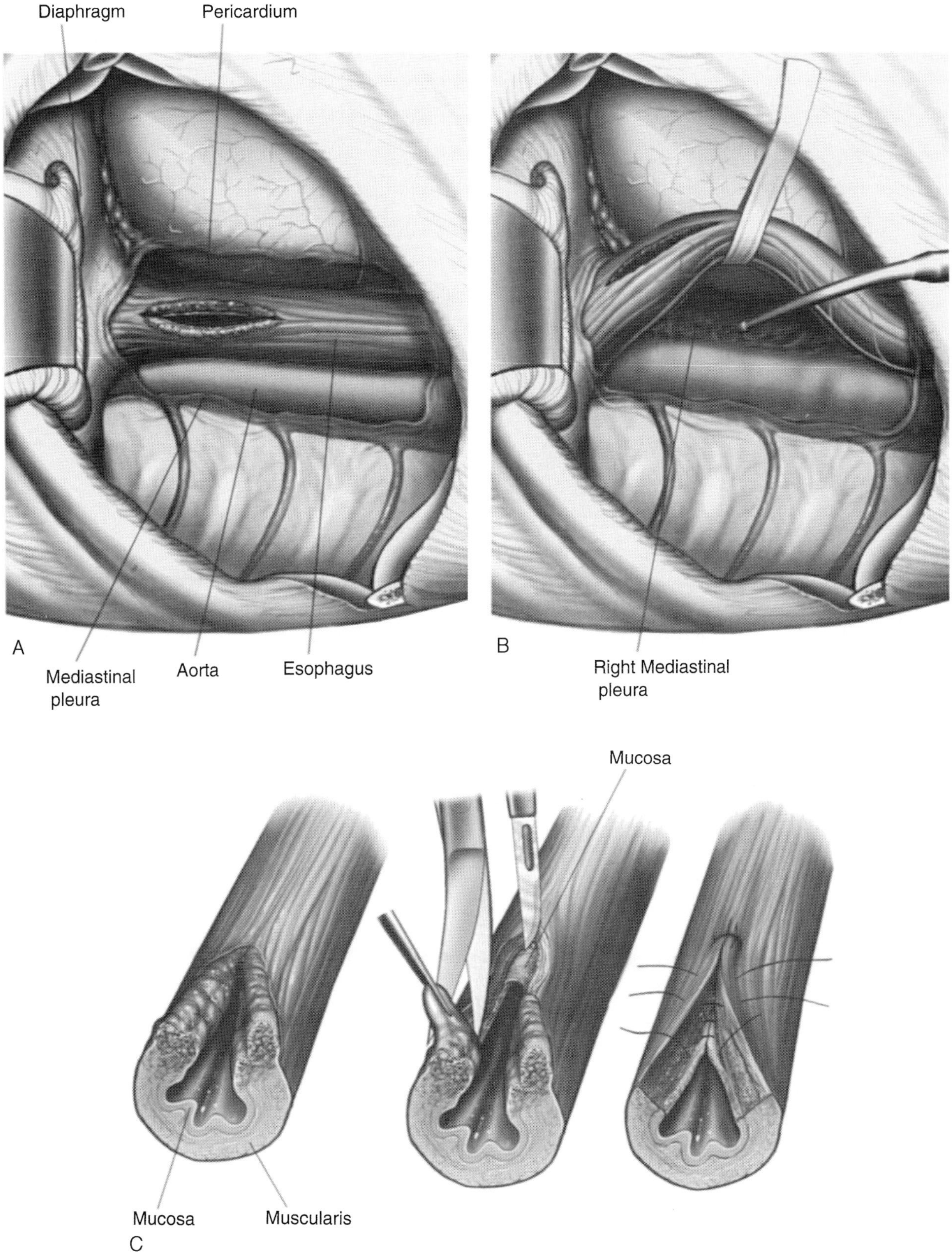

Diaphragm
Pericardium
A
Mediastinal pleura
Aorta
Esophagus
B
Right Mediastinal pleura

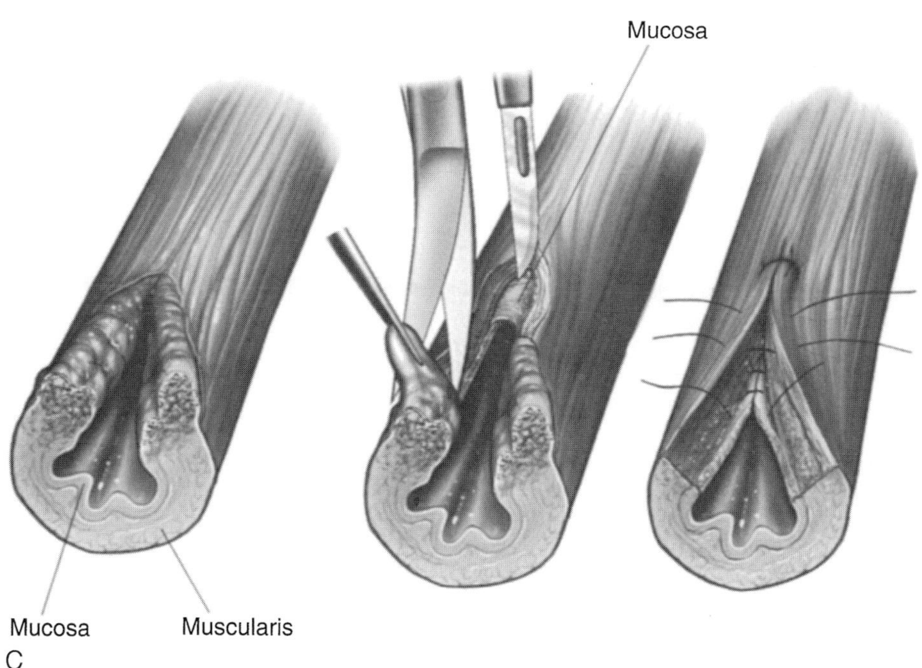

FIGURE 38–9 ■ *A*, Necrotic mediastinal pleura has been excised, and the esophageal tear has been débrided. *B*, Elevation of the esophagus on a rubber drain allows for débridement of the right mediastinal pleura if indicated. *C*, Débridement of the esophageal rupture. Muscularis is incised superiorly and inferiorly to allow visualization of the extent of mucosal defect prior to two-layer closure of the perforation if possible.

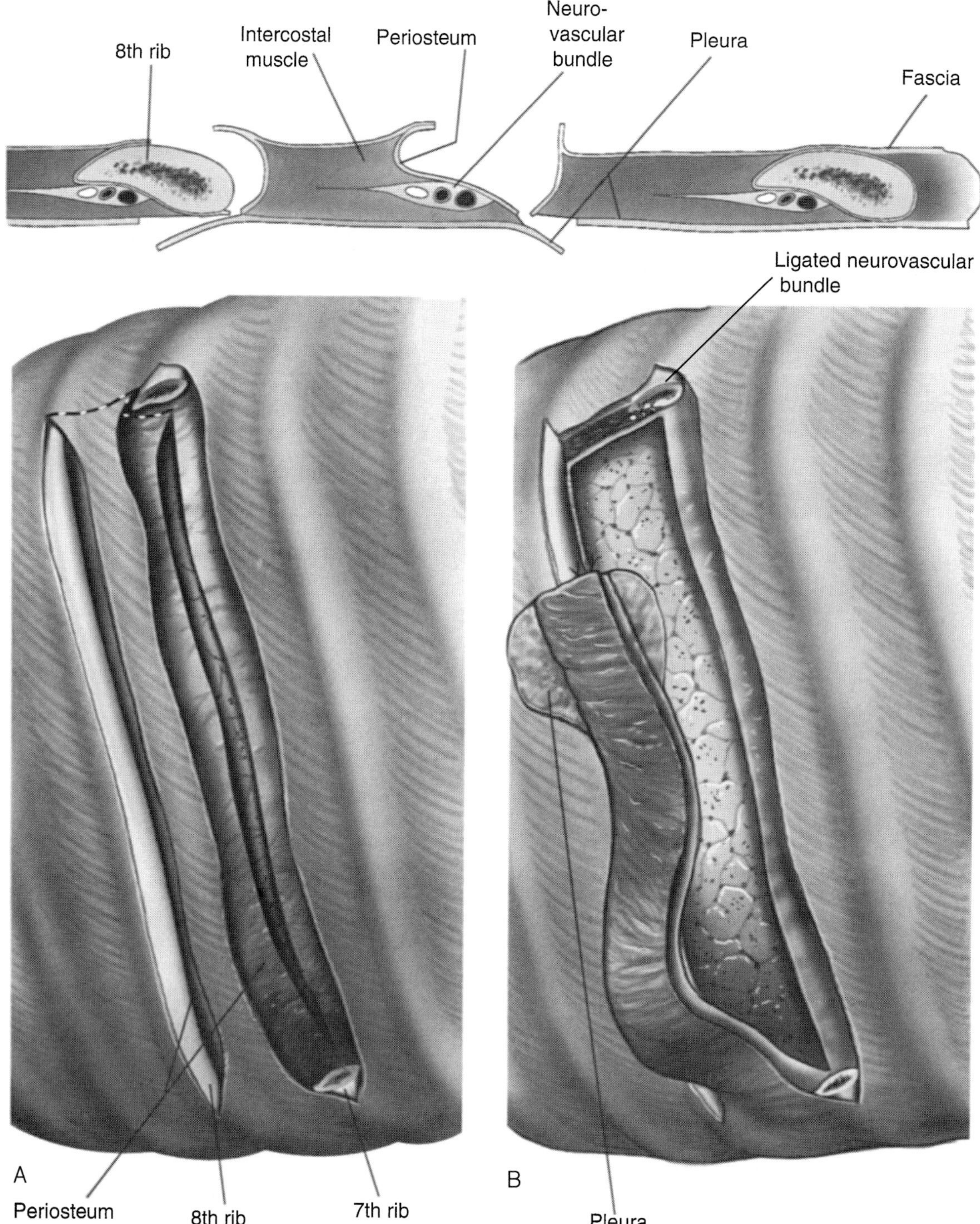

FIGURE 38–10 ■ Construction of intercostal musculopleural flap. *A*, Periosteum of the rib inferior to thoracotomy incision is incised, and the subjacent pleura is mobilized. *B*, The neurovascular bundle is divided anteriorly, and the flap is created.

and Wilkins, 1975), pedicled intercostal muscle (Dooling and Zick, 1967), diaphragm (Jara, 1979), pericardium (Millard, 1971), and omentum and gastric fundus (Thal, 1964) have all been used. Use of the latter four tissues runs the risk of infecting the peritoneal or pericardial cavities. Gastric fundus transposed to the chest may in effect create a paraesophageal hernia, with the attendant risks of late stasis ulceration and gastric mural necrosis. In early cases, the parietal pleura is thin and does not make a suitable buttress, and a pedicled intercostal musculopleural flap is preferred (Grillo and Wilkins, 1975).

A later report from the same group (Wright et al, 1995) confirmed the value of buttressing the primary repair of thoracic esophageal perforations with the pedicled intercostal muscle flap. The authors achieved primary healing in 89% of the 28 patients, 13 of whom were

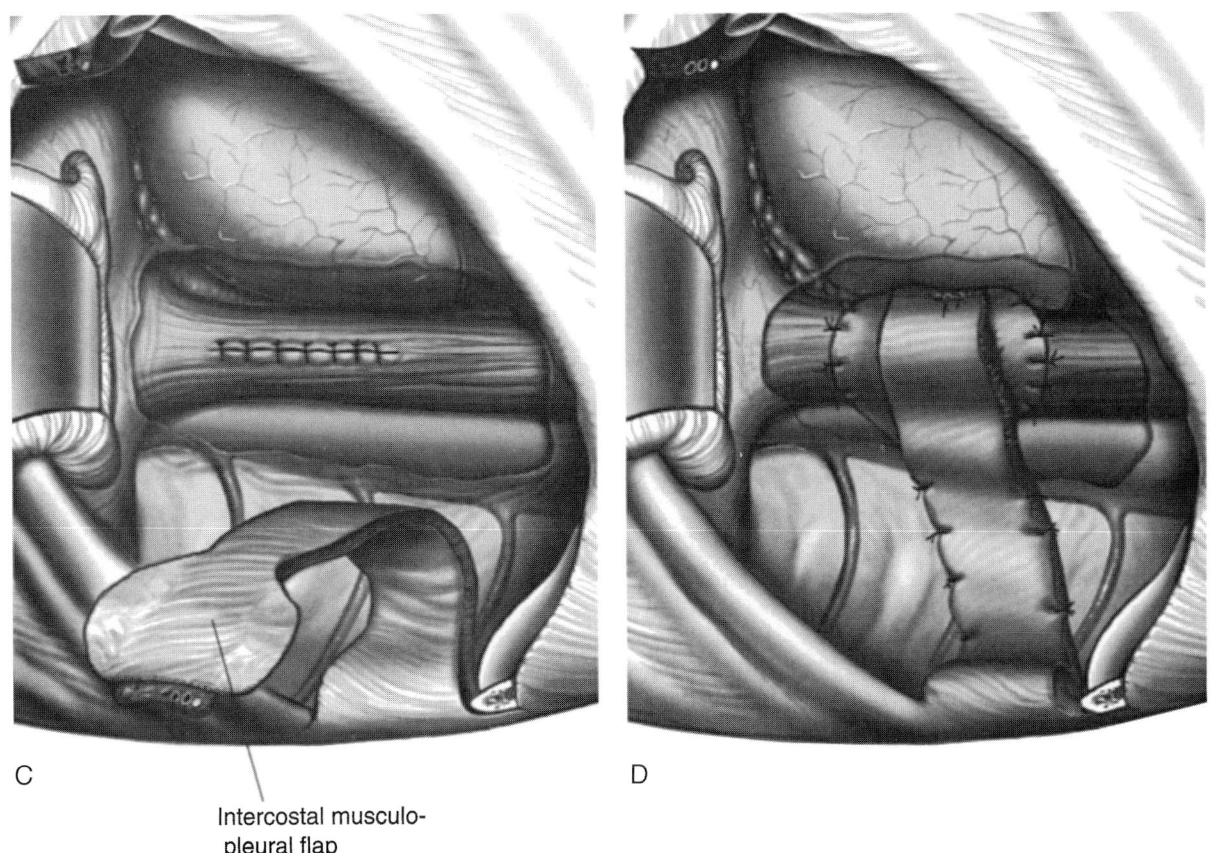

FIGURE 38–10 ■ *Continued. C,* Two-layer closure of the esophagus is performed if possible. *D,* The musculopleural flap is applied as a buttress or a patch if closure of the perforation is not possible.

treated more than 24 hours following perforation. In the seven patients with postoperative leaks, only one required reoperation. Finley reported successful management with primary closure and drainage in seven cases with delayed (>48 hrs) recognition of esophageal perforation. None of the patients required reoperation (Finley, 1980). When only mucosal repair could be accomplished, the intercostal flap was applied to the esophagus using fibrin glue; primary healing resulted (Tasdamir et al, 1996).

Preparation of the Pedicled Intercostal Musculopleural Flap

After thoracic débridement and esophageal repair, the rib spreader is removed and the ribs are partially distracted manually if necessary. The surgeon uses a length of umbilical tape to estimate the flap length required, measuring from the posterior end of the segment of rib (usually the seventh) resected at thoracotomy to the esophageal suture line.

The periosteum of the next lower rib is incised and stripped from the upper border of that rib (Fig. 38–10*A*, *B*). The periosteum, the pleura, and the intervening intercostal muscle bundle, with its associated neurovascular components, are then mobilized to the full extent of the thoracotomy incision, with a marked tape used to ensure adequate length. It is desirable to have the flap terminate in a spatulate fashion, so that a generous width of pleura is created anteriorly. The flap is transected anteriorly, and the intercostal artery and vein should bleed profusely; they are then ligated. The flap is then applied to the site of esophageal repair or defect and meticulously sutured to the muscle closure or muscle remnants (Fig. 38–10*C*, *D*).

The excess pleura is fixed to whatever mediastinal tissue is available to maintain the flap in position. The flap should not be wrapped circumferentially about the esophagus, because periosteal new bone formation may cause a "napkin-ring" constriction. Flaps constructed from the rhomboideus major (Lucas et al, 1982), pectoralis major (Siu et al, 1985), and latissimus dorsi (Richardson et al, 1985) muscles have been used to close upper thoracic esophageal perforations. The chest is drained with two large-bore catheters, one of which is juxtaposed to the esophageal repair.

Following closure of the chest, the patient is placed in the supine position, and, with a fresh surgical armamentarium, draining gastrostomy and feeding jejunostomy are performed. Gastrostomy prevents acid reflux, and jejunostomy is essential to maintain nutrition and facilitate healing.

Postoperative mechanical ventilation is mandatory for these patients with sepsis who have compromised pulmonary function. Mechanical ventilation ensures that the lung will remain fully expanded and will adhere to the esophageal repair, possibly affording additional support.

Elective use of mechanical ventilation and positive end-expiratory pressure (PEEP) may be helpful in maintaining lung expansion (Finley, 1980). Experimentally, the lung is able to seal esophageal defects (Moore et al, 1961).

If a leak develops postoperatively, a contrast esophagogram is helpful in determining the possible need for further intervention. With good drainage, nutrition support, appropriate antibiotics, and the absence of distal obstruction, the leak should eventually heal.

During early convalescence, it is not uncommon for the patient to take a turn for the worse with fever and leukocytosis associated with an unremarkable chest radiogram. A CT scan may demonstrate a residual septic focus. On occasion, this infection may be drained by catheters placed with ultrasound or CT guidance. Limited mediastinotomy may be required.

Esophageal Exclusion

The concept of esophageal exclusion for the management of thoracic perforations was advanced by Johnson and colleagues (1956), who divided and sutured the esophagogastric junction and created an end-cervical esophagostomy. Subsequently, jejunal interposition was used for reconstruction. Menguy (1971) used near-total esophageal exclusion by means of lateral cervical esophagostomy and tube gastrostomy. Urschel and associates (1974) modified the technique of total esophageal exclusion in continuity, initially tying an umbilical tape over a polytetrafluoroethylene (Teflon) band at the esophagogastric junction and performing tube gastrostomy and lateral cervical esophagostomy. Urschel modified the esophagogastric occlusion by use of a polypropylene suture snared over a Silastic band, exteriorizing the snare to obviate the need for a second laparotomy to relieve the induced esophagogastric obstruction (Urschel, 1989).

Because of difficulties in the later reconstruction of the cervical esophagus after lateral or terminal esophagostomy, proximal esophageal diversion has been accomplished by means of a mushroom catheter (Ergin et al, 1980) or T-tube with closed distal limb (Lee et al, 1991) and a Silastic occluding band applied about the esophagus and distal T-tube limb. After the esophageal perforation has healed, the band and catheter are removed. The cervical salivary fistula heals within several days.

Stapling of intestinal segments in continuity may result in restoration of the lumen (Mulholland et al, 1983). Ladin and colleagues (1989) closed a postemetic esophageal rupture and stapled the esophagus proximal and distal to the suture line, also performing cervical esophagostomy and tube gastrostomy. Six weeks later, the esophageal lumen was found to be reconstituted without stricture.

Because luminal restoration after stapling with stainless steel staples is not predictable, esophageal exclusion with absorbable staples (Lactomer) has been introduced, with esophageal recanalization reported after 2 weeks (Bardini et al, 1992). Nasoesophageal suction was used for decompression of the proximal staple line, and nutrition was maintained via jejunostomy.

T-tube Fistula and Drainage

Abbott and associates (1970) constructed a large-bore Silastic T-tube, which was inserted through the perforation. The distal portion of the short limb traversed the gastroesophageal junction, and the large limb exited from the chest. A nasogastric tube that was passed through the T-tube lumen into the stomach aided in maintaining the T-tube in position. Pleural drainage was also instituted. In a subsequent report from this group (Bufkin et al, 1996) the authors recommended that the T-tube should be brought out through a lateral incision and sutured to the diaphragm in a position that would avoid aortic erosion.

Eventual healing of the control esophageal fistula is predicated on full expansion of the lung to patch the perforation. Therefore, thorough mediastinal débridement and pulmonary decortication are required for the successful application of this technique.

Mediastinal Irrigation and Drainage

Brewer and coworkers (1986) used mediastinal antibiotic irrigation and drainage, as well as transesophageal irrigation and thoracic drainage, in selected cases. Santos and Frater (1986) used peroral, transesophageal mediastinal irrigation with drainage of the irrigant via chest tubes as a method for evacuating mediastinal sepsis. This technique requires thoracotomy for thorough débridement and well-positioned chest tubes for effective drainage.

Intraluminal Stents

The various intraluminal stents that have been used for the palliation of irresectable esophageal carcinoma have also been used to seal instrument perforations in poor-risk patients (Bergen, 1972). An expanding mesh stent placed under fluoroscopic control has been successful in the management of a Boerhaave rupture in an aging patient who could not tolerate thoracotomy (Davies, 1999). In this situation, the transabdominal route was used to drain and irrigate both the pleural cavity and the mediastinum.

As with esophageal exclusion and diversion, T-tube drainage, mediastinal irrigation, and intraluminal stents have been reserved for situations in which the condition of the patient and the size and age of the perforation indicate that optimal treatment of buttressed repair is not feasible.

Resection

Esophagectomy for the management of perforations should be considered in patients with instrument perforation, esophageal carcinoma, irremediable stricture, late diagnosed cases of Boerhaave rupture, severe traumatic disruption, and overwhelming sepsis in which successful surgical management by other means is considered unlikely to succeed or has failed. Esophagectomy may be performed via the transthoracic or transhiatal route, but mediastinal and pleural débridement are essential. The patient is left with an end-cervical esophagostomy and gastrostomy. Reconstruction by means of colon or gastric interposition via the substernal route is often best deferred for several months when mediastinitis has been controlled and the patient is in stable and satisfactory condition.

TREATMENT OF ABDOMINAL PERFORATIONS

Abdominal esophageal perforations are associated with an excellent prognosis if they are recognized at the time of injury. They are best managed by closure and partial fundic wrap as a buttress or patch. If it is not possible to use gastric fundus, an omental wrap should be performed. Complementary gastrostomy and jejunostomy are usually indicated. Berne and colleagues (1969) treated five cases of Boerhaave rupture by transabdominal repair, gastric fundoplication, and transabdominal drainage of the mediastinum. Empyemas were treated by closed thoracostomy.

RESULTS

Jones and Ginsberg (1992) analyzed the results of 13 series of esophageal perforation, totaling 598 patients, reported between 1980 and 1990. The overall mortality was 22%. Instrument and iatrogenic injuries carried a mortality rate of 19%; for Boerhaave ruptures, the rate was 39%. In their analysis of 439 patients, the mortality rate for cervical perforations was 6%; for thoracic perforations, 34%; and for abdominal perforations, 29%.

All series demonstrate that early diagnosis and surgical management favorably affected the outcome; after 24 hours, both morbidity and mortality rates increased. In Attar's series (1990), the survival in patients undergoing surgery in less than 24 hours after perforation was 87% and decreased to 55% in patients undergoing operation later. Sawyers (1990) reported no deaths in 115 patients who were managed by operation within 24 hours of perforation in the years between 1980 and 1990. Other factors that adversely influence mortality rate are pre-existing esophageal disease, perforation in a thoracic site, and anastomotic leak (Richardson et al, 1985).

Buttressing the thoracic esophageal suture line appears to decrease the incidence of recurrent esophagopleural fistula and mortality. Gouge and associates (1989) reviewed the results of 10 series of primary suture of thoracic perforations: fistulas developed in 39% of 158 patients, with a 25% mortality rate. This group included patients operated on both before and after 24 hours after perforation. In those operated on after 24 hours postperforation, the esophageal repair leaked in 50% of cases. In contrast, in 99 patients who had a buttress repair, the leakage rate was 13% and the mortality rate was 6%. These data lend credence to the concept that suture repairs of thoracic esophageal perforations should be buttressed; if suture repair is not possible, the defect should be patched, preferably with a muscle flap.

Results of Alternative Procedures

Analysis of reported series of other methods (Gouge et al, 1989) revealed mortality rates to be 36% for T-tube drainage, 35% for exclusion-diversion, and 26% for resection. Orringer and Stirling (1990) used transhiatal or transthoracic resection with either immediate or delayed reconstruction and noted a mortality rate of 13%. Pre-existing esophageal disease was present in most patients in this group.

DISCUSSION

Pearse's landmark contribution in 1933 defined the operative approach to cervical esophageal perforation and had a profound effect on survival in the pre-antibiotic era. In Jemerin's report, only 50% of patients with cervical perforations before 1936 had undergone any form of operative drainage; 70% of the entire group died. In the decade following 1936, 90% of patients underwent cervical drainage, as recommended by Pearse, and the mortality rate decreased to 17%.

The availability of potent IV antibiotics has led some physicians to advocate nonoperative treatment for small esophageal perforations. The vexing question is: How small is small? Pearse asked, "Should the esophagus be exempt from the rules, which experience has dictated, for early surgical intervention in case of perforation of other organs?"

In the absence of the radiographic findings detailed in this chapter, it is tempting to give the patient IV antibiotics and parenteral alimentation and to operate if the patient's condition deteriorates, as demonstrated by increase in fever, tachycardia, tachypnea, leukocytosis, and evidence of mediastinal and pleural fluid collections on subsequent chest films. This approach puts the patient at risk for the development of massive mediastinal sepsis; thus, the alternatives: Should one wait for mediastinal sepsis to develop and thus increase the risk of a fatal outcome, or should one operate to prevent the development of sepsis? Again, to quote Pearse, "the patient does not die of the perforated cervical esophagus per se nor does he necessarily die from the infection in the neck, but usually dies from mediastinitis, the indirect result of the perforation."

To paraphrase Groves (1966), esophageal perforation is an accepted hazard of esophageal instrumentation, yet it is difficult for endoscopists to conquer their pride and accept that perforation has occurred, and it is even more difficult to explain what happened to the patient and to the family. It is easy to succumb to the temptation to inform the patient that the esophagus has been "scratched" and to keep the patient hospitalized on an antibiotic regimen and parenteral alimentation.

The standard for management of thoracic esophageal perforations in the absence of pre-existing esophageal disease is, as detailed in this chapter, buttressed closure preceded by evacuation of mediastinal sepsis, followed by decortication of the lung, thoracic drainage tubes, gastrostomy, and jejunostomy. The reported results with gastric fundus flap for perforations at the esophagogastric junction have been excellent, provided that total fundoplication is not left above the diaphragm. The hiatus should be widened to avoid constriction of the fundus, which should be sutured circumferentially to the margins of the diaphragm. The fundus flap is ideally suited for buttressing intra-abdominal perforations. The parietal pleura, if thin, is fragile and not a satisfactory buttress. The intercostal musculopleural flap or diaphragm flap is preferred. Excellent results have been achieved with either flap without the late sequelae that occasionally occur when a portion of the stomach is transposed into the left hemithorax. The latissimus, rhomboid, and pectoralis major muscle flaps are useful in the management of middle and upper thoracic perforations.

Discussions of the merits of nonoperative management of thoracic esophageal perforation invariably refer to a report by Cameron and associates (1979). Their criteria for not performing thoracotomy are (1) contained mediastinal disruption that drains back into the esophagus and (2) minimal systemic signs and symptoms. Of the eight cases treated, five were postsurgical, including one closure of an esophageal perforation, and seven of the eight were detected from 2 to 9 days after onset and demonstrated minimal systemic findings. Although some patients with periesophageal and mediastinal fibrosis resulting from pre-existing esophageal disease do not develop fulminating mediastinitis after thoracic esophageal perforation, they are the exception rather than the rule (Fig. 38–11).

Decision-making may be difficult when esophageal perforation occurs in the presence of benign lower esophageal obstruction. Achalasia is well managed by closure of the perforation and complimentary esophagomyotomy. The management of perforation of strictures associated with reflux esophagitis requires good judgment and an experienced surgeon. If left thoracotomy is required to treat intrathoracic sepsis, intraoperative dilatation of the stricture before closure and buttress may allow healing. These strictures are frequently associated with a degree of esophageal shortening that does not allow the creation of a competent esophagogastric junction that may be repositioned beneath the diaphragm. If the esophageal stricture is considered to be irremediable, esophagectomy—either transthoracic or transhiatal—is indicated. The experience of the surgeon and anticipated technical difficulties weigh heavily in this decision. Restoration of continuity may be immediate or delayed, depending on the patient's condition.

Decision-making in cases of perforation from esophageal carcinoma is easier. If the patient is otherwise a candidate for esophagectomy, the surgeon should proceed promptly. If not, because of the extent of the disease or because of associated medical conditions, transoral insertion of an esophageal prosthesis may be a logical solution. The grave prognosis limits surgical options.

The best results in cases of Boerhaave rupture have been achieved by the operative procedure described. The necrotizing mediastinitis caused by synergistic oral bacteria and gastric content must be débrided and drained if the patient is to survive. Otherwise, the statistics are grim: Of 71 cases in the historic series of Derbes and Mitchell (1956), only 35% survived for 24 hours, 11% lived for 48 hours, and none lived longer than 1 week. Thus, closed thoracostomy, antibiotics, and ventilatory care have resulted in prolonged survival in patients with

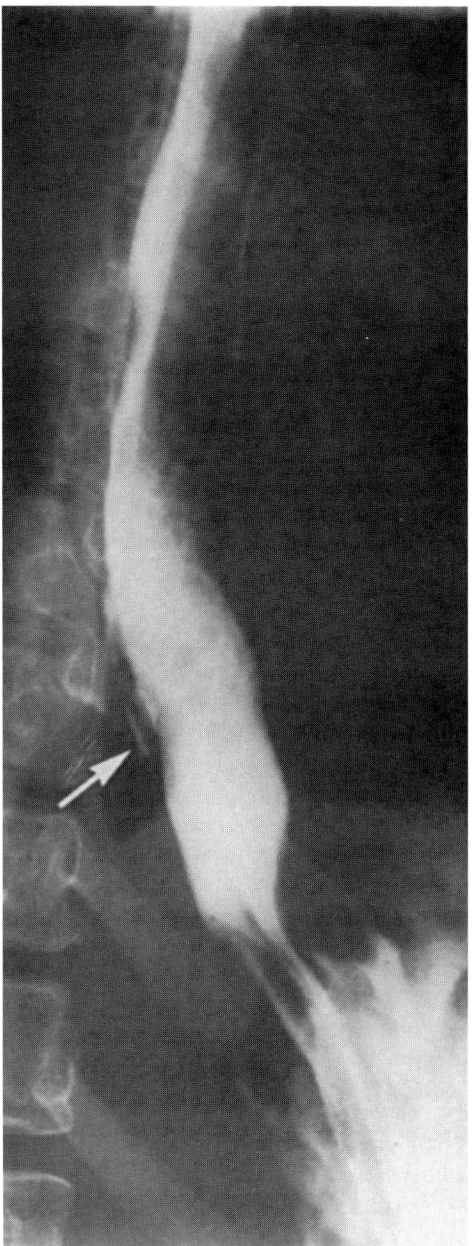

FIGURE 38–11 ■ Esophagogram following endoscopic removal of a chicken bone that perforated the thoracic esophagus *(arrow)* 2 days previously. Contained mediastinal perforation without sepsis was managed with intravenous antibiotics and parenteral alimentation.

a late diagnosis, making them candidates for repair and drainage.

The mortality rates of T-tube diversion and exclusion and diversion reflect the severity of illness in this group of patients, rather than the magnitude of the procedures. For example, a patient with cirrhosis who has hepatic failure and esophageal perforation that has been caused by a Sengstaken-Blakemore tube may not be a candidate for repair but might possibly survive following T-tube drainage or diversion and exclusion.

The objections to diversion-exclusion are that the creation of end-cervical esophagostomy presents an insurmountable problem in the restoration of esophageal continuity and that the distal cervical esophagus retracts into the mediastinum and is not retrievable. Lateral cervical esophagostomy with T-tube insertion is more acceptable; but whether it is truly more diverting than a sump nasoesophageal tube, which eliminates the need for subsequent cervical esophageal repair, is questionable. Furthermore, the sump tube allows for transesophageal instillation of antibiotic solution as an irrigant.

Is band occlusion of the esophagogastric junction significantly more efficient than a gastrostomy tube that is placed on suction? Does not the surgically created distal obstruction impede healing of the thoracic perforation, and is the band not likely to cause stricture or pressure necrosis of the esophageal wall, no matter how carefully applied? Diversion-exclusion should be used when thoracotomy is not a reasonable alternative or when attempted repair has not controlled sepsis.

Although some encouraging results have been reported for esophageal stapling in continuity, the surgeon should beware of stapling and division of the esophagus. The distal staple line is subject to dissolution, and leaving the esophagus in situ in this circumstance virtually guarantees that intrathoracic sepsis will not be controlled. If thoracotomy is being considered with this option in mind or has already been performed, esophagectomy and cervical esophagostomy are better options, with substernal gastric or colonic interposition scheduled at a later date. Advances in technology may produce more sophisticated stapling devices, lasers, or biologic adhesives for the management of perforations, but esophageal perforations will continue to pose formidable obstacles to successful management, testing the mettle of surgeons for the foreseeable future.

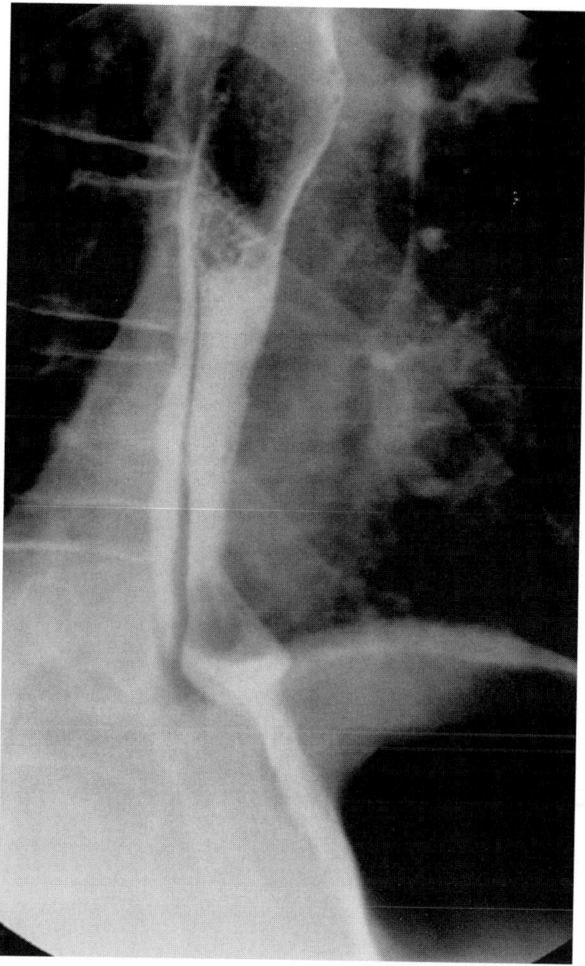

FIGURE 38–12 ■ Barium swallow obtained postoperatively in a cardiac surgical patient following intraoperative transesophageal echocardiography. The two parallel columns of contrast without extraluminal extravasation are virtually diagnostic of intramural perforation.

COMMENTS AND CONTROVERSIES

Dr. Fell's chapter is a scholarly and encyclopedic review of a complex and challenging problem. Pearson and Hiebert's comments to this chapter in the first edition of this book remain highly relevant. It should be noted that the term "perforation" has been widely used to encompass not only transmural penetration of the esophagus but also rupture of the esophagus by excessive internal distention. The latter is the mechanism usually associated with instrument disruption of the esophagus, especially endoscopy or dilatation for strictures and tumors.

I am in complete agreement with Pearson's view that careful flexible endoscopic evaluation of the esophagus should precede operative repair in virtually all cases of suspected or proven esophageal perforation. Direct visualization of the nature and extent of the injury along with presence or absence of other disease is essential in planning operative strategy. On rare occasions, endoscopy reveals an unsuspected second perforation. In the case of instrument perforation of the esophagus either by nasogastric tube or endoscope, the site of mucosal injury may be remote from the site of drainage into the mediastinum, the two sites being connected by an intramural segment of dissection. Such perforations are increasingly seen as a result of esophagoscopy and the use of transesophageal echocardiography, especially when used for intraoperative monitoring of cardiac surgical procedures.

The radiologic findings are distinct and diagnostic, as seen in Figure 38–12. The injury consists of penetration of the mucosa and dissection within the wall of the esophagus without penetration of the outer wall of the esophagus. Contrast studies demonstrate the two parallel channels of a contrast agent without mediastinal extravasation. Management in almost all cases is conservative with nasogastric tube drainage, absence of oral intake, and careful in-hospital observation for several days. Liquid oral intake can usually be safely resumed within 5 to 7 days.

Placement of a nasogastric tube in a patient receiving ventilatory assistance through an endotracheal tube may result in perforation of the piriform fossa. This is usually recognized by the aberrant location of the nasogastric tube as seen on the chest radiograph. Withdrawal of the tube, administration of antibiotics, and close observation usually result in a satisfactory outcome. Any signs of cervical sepsis should prompt immediate open drainage.

The management of esophageal perforation with delayed recognition is a particularly challenging one. At operation the mucosa is almost always viable and amenable to primary closure, whereas the muscular wall may be edematous or necrotic and not capable of closure. However, primary closure of the mucosa and buttressing, as recommended by Fell, should be the standard approach whenever possible. The notion of temporarily obliterating the esophagus distal to the site of perforation, with either an absorbable suture or staple line, has always appeared contrary to the general principles of ensuring that there is no obstruction of the gastrointestinal tract distal to a site of perforation. It is better to provide adequate drainage to the stomach and to allow esophageal contents free passage into the stomach, in addition to positioning a sump nasogastric tube in the esophagus, or to use a cervical diversion as necessary. To date, I have not encountered a situation in which occlusion of the esophageal lumen distal to a perforated site has seemed appropriate. Perhaps reversible obliteration above *the site of perforation would be rational under some circumstances.*

J. D. C.

Esophagoscopy as a Management Tool

Esophagoscopy is generally underused in the management of esophageal perforations, leaks, and injuries. Flexible esophagoscopy provides additional information from direct observation about the condition of the tissues, the extent of the injury, the presence of additional pathology, and the probability of healing. Although this information may be inferred from the esophagram and the operative findings at exploration, it is directly available from endoscopy. The risk associated with the procedure is low when it is performed carefully with a flexible instrument by a surgeon who will deal definitively with surgical or nonoperative management of the esophageal injury or leak. The hesitation to introduce an esophagoscope is related in part to infrequent use or unfamiliarity with flexible esophagoscopy on the part of the surgeon and fear of extending the injury further. My experience with using the flexible esophagoscope for evaluation of injuries or anastomatic leaks has confirmed that this policy adds useful information for management and does not complicate the problem.

Abrasions

A linear tear in the posterior cervical esophagus may be caused by a rigid esophagoscope that abrades the vertebral body or an intervertebral bony spur. When these injuries are recognized early (at the time of endoscopy), nonsurgical management by withholding feeding and administering parenteral antibiotics is justified, safe, and usually effective. The patient must be carefully monitored to ensure early recognition and drainage if a visceral space abscess develops during treatment.

Lewis Variation

An interesting variant on Urschel's exclusion technique was introduced by Lewis (1985), who recommended the use of two removable tourniquets—one around the cervical esophagus and one at the gastroesophageal junction—to provide "reversible total esophageal exclusion." The tourniquets are brought to the skin surface through catheters for later removal without a second operation. This technique, in combination with mediastinal drainage, has been effective in the management of debilitated patients who are not candidates for more extensive surgery.

F. G. P.

When it comes to woe, a hole in the esophagus is trouble in a class by itself if it is not recognized promptly or managed properly. The fact that the defect was made at all is a serious problem. The symptoms of a soiled mediastinum may be as meager as a temperature blip or as fulminant as circulatory collapse. As Fell reminds us in this chapter, delay in diagnosis is usual because (1) the condition is infrequently encountered and (2) the symptoms overlap with those of more common culprits. The crucial thing is to think about the esophagus early and hard. Diagnosis precedes treatment, *but suspicion precedes* diagnosis.

Spontaneous rupture *is a flagrant misnomer that suggests an insidious and nonviolent event. A better term is needed for this lethal explosion of acid ferment and food into the mediastinum and pleural space, classically the result of forceful or suppressed vomiting following a prodigious meal or an alcoholic debauch. The pain is sudden, unremitting, and intense. It is felt deep in the precordium and epigastric area, is worsened by movement, and is accompanied by tachypnea, cyanosis, and progressive hypotension. Suprasternal crepitus is an inconstant sign, but spasm of the upper abdomen is usual and because of it the general surgeon may be early on the scene. A second scenario is a rush to the cardiac intensive care unit to rule out the possibility of myocardial infarction, pulmonary embolism, or dissecting aneurysm. If the clinical picture remains unrecognized for 24 hours or longer, an appalling array of complications are virtually certain. Turning on the monitor is no excuse for turning off thinking.*

The essential clinical clue to Boerhaave's syndrome is chest pain following *vomiting, and the clincher is an upright chest film and esophagogram showing air and contrast medium in the mediastinum and left pleural space.*

In general, I agree with the treatment options discussed by the author. The main points are (1) control of sepsis with antibiotics, débridement, and adequate drainage of the mediastinal and pleural spaces; (2) maintenance of fluid and nutritional requirements; (3) isolation of the esophageal wound from refluxed gastric chyme (and, ideally, in my opinion, from saliva, too); and (4) construction of a dehiscence-proof suture line protected by skeletal muscle, omentum, gastric fundus, or, best of all, a pedicle of pleura, as recommended by Grillo and Wilkins. Fell's reminder to make this pedicle sufficiently long is well taken.

It remains a sobering fact that most esophageal injuries are consequent to endoscopy or intubation. Hazards of esophagoscopy include (1) the combination of a rigid scope, prominent incisor teeth, and a rigid neck; (2) cervical vertebrae with spurs; (3) mistaking the neck of a diverticulum for the main channel; (4) forceful advancement of any tube or instrument; (5) less than ideal patient cooperation, relaxation, or sedation; (6) inoculation of the mediastinum with anaerobes that originate in peridontal sepsis; (7) inexperience; and (8) lengthy examination. Even when due care and gentleness are exercised, the esophagus can be injured easily, especially at the level of the upper sphincter, near tumor, in stricture, or in the presence of a foreign body. These topics are already covered by Fell, but they are important and worthy of emphasis.

C. A. H.

■ KEY REFERENCES

Attar S, Hankins JR, Suter CM, et al: Esophageal perforation: A therapeutic challenge. Ann Thorac Surg 50:45, 1990.

In this clinical study, surgical options are reviewed and treatment plans are based on the condition of the patient. The best results were in cases treated by primary repair.

Gouge TH, Depan HJ, Spencer FC: Experience with the Grillo pleural wrap procedure in 18 patients with perforation of thoracic esophagus. Ann Surg 209:612, 1989.

This report substantiates the effectiveness of pleural flap buttress in early and late cases of thoracic esophageal perforations. It is an excellent review of earlier published reports regarding the effectiveness of various therapeutic modalities.

Grillo HC, Wilkins EW Jr: Esophageal repair following late diagnosis of intrathoracic perforation. Ann Thorac Surg 20:387, 1975.

This report establishes the principle of buttressing in the esophageal repair with a pedicled pleural flap, and it documents successful management in late cases.

Jones WG, Ginsberg R: Esophageal perforation: A continuing challenge. Ann Thorac Surg 53:534, 1992.

This comprehensive review of the etiology of esophageal perforations is based on data compiled from the literature. The treatment options are discussed, and the references are an invaluable resource.

Richardson JD, Martin LF, Borzotta AP, Polk HC: Unifying concepts in the treatment of esophageal leaks. Am J Surg 149:157, 1985.

The beneficial effects of muscle-flap buttress or patch are convincingly demonstrated. Results with exclusion-diversion were poor.

■ REFERENCES

Abbott OH, Mansour KA, Logan WD Jr, et al: A traumatic so-called "spontaneous" rupture of the esophagus: A review of 47 personal cases with comments on a new method of surgical therapy. J Thorac Cardiovasc Surg 59:67, 1970.

Adkins MS, Raccuia JS, Acinapura AJ: Esophageal perforation in a patient with acquired immunodeficiency syndrome. Ann Thorac Surg 50:299, 1990.

Backer C, Lo Cicero J, Hertz R, et al: Computed tomography in patients with esophageal perforation. Chest 98:1078, 1990.

Barrett NR: Spontaneous perforation of the esophagus. Thorax 1:48, 1946.

Barrett NR: Report of a case of spontaneous perforation of the esophagus successfully treated by operation. Br J Surg 35:216, 1947.

Bardini R, Bonavina L, Pavanello M, et al: Temporary double exclusion of the perforated esophagus using absorbable staples. Ann Thorac Surg 54:1165, 1992.

Berger RL, Donato AT: Treatment of esophageal disruption by intubation. Ann Thorac Surg 13:27, 1972.

Berne CJ, Shader AE, Doty DB: Treatment of effort rupture of the esophagus by epigastric celiotomy. Surg Gynecol Obstet 129:277, 1969.

Blalock J: Primary esophagogastrectomy for instrumental perforations of the esophagus. Am J Surg 94:393, 1957.

Boerhaave H: Atrocis, nec descripti prima, morbi historia. Verbatim English translation (Derbes V, Mitchell R) Bull Med Libr Assoc 43:217, 1955.

Brewer LA, Carter R, Mulder GA, Stiles QR: Options in the management of perforations of the esophagus. Am J Surg 152:62, 1986.

Bufkin BL, Miller JI, Mansour KA: Esophageal perforation: Emphasis on management. Ann Thorac Surg 61:1447, 1996.

Cameron JL, Kieffer RF, Hendrix TR, et al: Selective nonoperative management of contained intrathoracic esophageal disruptions. Ann Thorac Surg 27:404, 1979.

Collis JL, Humphries DR, Bond WH: Spontaneous rupture of the esophagus. Lancet 2:179, 1944.

Conte B: Esophageal rupture in absence of vomiting. J Thorac Cardiovasc Surg 51:137, 1966.

Davies AP, Vaughan R: Expanding mesh stent in the emergency treatment of Boerhaave's syndrome. Ann Thorac Surg 67:1482, 1999.

Derbes JV, Mitchell RE: Rupture of the esophagus. Surgery 39:865, 1956.

Dooling JV, Zick HR: Closure of an esophagopleural fistula using only intercostal pedicle graft. Ann Thorac Surg 3:553, 1967.

Ergin MA, Wetstein L, Griepp RB: Temporary diverting cervical esophagostomy. Surg Gynecol Obstet 151:97, 1980.

Finley RJ, Pearson FG, Weisel RD, et al: The management of nonmalignant intrathoracic esophageal perforations. Ann Thorac Surg 30:575, 1980.

Groves LK: Instrumental perforation of the esophagus: What constitutes conservative management. J Thorac Cardiovasc Surg 52:1, 1966.

Han SY, McElvein RB, Aldrete JS, Tishler JM: Perforation of the esophagus: Correlation of site and cause with plain film findings. Am J Roentgenol 145:537, 1985.

Hendren WH, Henderson BM: Immediate esophagectomy for instrumental perforation of the thoracic esophagus. Ann Surg 168:997, 1968.

Hill DC, Murray GF: Malignant tracheoesophageal fistula. In Grillo HC, Ousten WG, Wilkins EW, et al: Current Therapy in Cardiothoracic Surgery. Toronto, BC Decker, 1989.

Hohf R: Rupture of the esophagus in the neonate. JAMA 181:115, 1962.

Jara FM: Diaphragmatic pedicle flap for treatment of Boerhaave's syndrome. J Thorac Cardiovasc Surg 78:931, 1979.

Jemerin EE: Results of treatment of perforation of the esophagus. Ann Surg 128:971, 1948.

Johnson J, Schwegman CW, Kirby CK: Esophageal exclusion for persistent fistula following spontaneous rupture of the esophagus. J Thorac Surg 32:827, 1956.

Jones WG, Ginsberg R: Esophageal perforation: A continuing challenge. Ann Thorac Surg 53:534, 1992.

Ladin DA, Dunnington GL, Rappaport WD: Stapled esophageal exclusion in acute esophageal rupture: A new technique. Contemp Surg 35:45, 1989.

Lee YC, Lee ST, Chu SH: New technique of esophageal exclusion for chronic esophageal perforation. Ann Thorac Surg 51:1020, 1991.

Lewis R: Reversible total esophageal exclusion. Ann Thorac Surg 39:5, 1985.

Lilienthal H: Thoracic Surgery. Philadelphia, WB Saunders, 1925.

Loop FD, Groves LK: Esophageal perforations. Ann Thorac Surg 10:571, 1970.

Lucas A, Snow N, Tobin G, Flint L: Use of the rhomboid major muscle flap for esophageal repair. Ann Thorac Surg 33:619, 1982.

MacKenzie M: A Manual of Diseases of the Nose and Throat. New York, William Wood, 1884.

Mackler S: Spontaneous rupture of the esophagus. Surg Gynecol Obstet 95:344, 1952.

McKinnon W, Ochsner J: Immediate closure and Heller procedure after Mosher bag rupture of the esophagus. Am J Surg 127:115, 1974.

Menguy R: Near-total exclusion by cervical esophagostomy and tube gastrostomy in the management of massive esophageal perforation. Ann Surg 173:613, 1971.

Michel L, Grillo HC, Malt RA: Operative and nonoperative management of esophageal perforations. Ann Surg 194:57, 1981.

Millard AH: "Spontaneous" perforation of the oesophagus treated by utilization of a pericardial flap. Br J Surg 58:70, 1971.

Moore TC, Goldstein J, Teramoto S: Use of intact lung for closure of full-thickness esophageal defects. J Thorac Cardiovasc Surg 41:336, 1961.

Mulholland MW, Magallanes F, Quigley TM, Delaney JP: In continuity gastrointestinal stapling. Dis Colon Rectum 26:586, 1983.

Neuhof H, Jemerin EE: Acute Infections of the Mediastinum. Baltimore, William & Wilkins, 1943.

Olsen AM, Clagett OT: Spontaneous rupture of the esophagus report of a case with immediate diagnosis and successful surgical repair. Postgrad Med 2:417, 1947.

Orringer MB, Stirling MC: Esophagectomy for esophageal disruption. Ann Thorac Surg 49:35, 1990.

Pearse HE: The operation for perforation of the cervical esophagus. Surg Gynecol Obstet 56:192, 1933.

Pearse HE: Mediastinitis following cervical suppuration. Ann Surg 108:538, 1938.

Pecora DV, Brook R: Tuberculous fistula of the esophagus. J Thorac Surg 36:53, 1958.

Postlethwait R, Kim S, Dillon M: Esophageal complications of vagotomy. Surg Gynecol Obstet 128:181, 1969.

Santos GH, Frater RWM: Transesophageal irrigation for the treatment of mediastinitis produced by esophageal rupture. J Thorac Cardiovasc Surg 91:57, 1986.

Sawyers J: Discussion of Attar S, Hankins J: Esophageal perforation: A therapeutic challenge. Ann Thorac Surg 50:45, 1990.

Sawyers J, Lane C, Foster J, Daniel R: Esophageal perforation. Ann Thorac Surg 19:233, 1975.

Sealy WC: Rupture of the esophagus. Am J Surg 105:505, 1963.

Seybold WD, Johnson MA, Learly WV: Perforation of the esophagus. Surg Clin North Am 30:1155, 1950.

Silvis SE, Nebel O, Rogers G, et al: Endoscopic complications: Result of the 1974 American Society of Gastrointestinal Endoscopy survey. JAMA 235:928, 1976.

Siu K, Wei W, Lam K, Wong J: Use of the pectoralis major muscle flap for repair of a tracheoesophageal fistula. Am J Surg 150:617, 1985.

Takaro T, Walkup H, Okano T: Esophagopleural fistula as a complication of thoracic surgery. J Thorac Cardiovasc Surg 40:179, 1960.

Tasdemir O, Kucukaksu D, Karagoz H, Bayazit K: Beneficial aspects of fibrin glue on esophageal performation. Ann Thorac Surg 61:1589, 1996.

Tesler MA, Eisenberg MM: Spontaneous esophageal rupture. Int Abstr Surg 117:1, 1963.

Thal AP, Hatafuku T: Improved operation for esophageal rupture. JAMA 188:826, 1964.

Urschel HC: Discussion of Gouge TH, Depan HJ, Spencer FC: Experience with the Grillo pleural wrap procedure in 18 patients with perforation of thoracic esophagus. Ann Surg 209:612, 1989.

Urschel HC, Razzuk MA, Wood RE, et al: Improved management of esophageal perforation: Exclusion and diversion in continuity. Ann Surg 179:587, 1974.

Wright CD, Mathisen DJ, Wain JC, et al: Reinforced primary repair of thoracic esophageal performation. Ann Thorac Surg 60:245, 1995.

Neoplasms

CHAPTER 39

Benign Tumors

Farid Shamji
Thomas R. J. Todd

Benign tumors of the esophagus are rare, when compared with other esophageal disorders such as reflux esophagitis, motility disturbance, cancer, and diverticulum. They account for less than 1% of all esophageal neoplasms (Plachta, 1962; Watson et al, 1967). Among surgically resected esophageal tumors, fewer than 10% were benign. As a result, a review of accumulated experience is necessary in order to develop guidelines for therapy and to understand the variety of type and clinical effects (Arnorsson et al, 1984; Mansour et al, 1977; Plachta, 1962; Schmidt et al, 1961; Totten et al, 1953; Watson et al, 1967).

BASIC SCIENCE

Symptoms and Signs

Disorders of the esophagus present fewer difficult diagnostic problems than elsewhere in the alimentary tract for several reasons. First, the esophagus is relatively simple, a hollow muscular tube, about 23 to 25 cm long, stretching from the pharynx to the stomach with specialized sphincteric zones at either end. Second, it has a relatively simple function—to convey the bolus of food rapidly to the stomach by active peristalsis and to prevent regurgitation. Third, sensations from the esophagus readily reach consciousness. They include intense and unpleasant substernal burning sensation described as heartburn and substernal pain identical to that of coronary artery disease from distention of the lower esophagus or abnormal esophageal contractions. Fourth, the esophagus is readily accessible to investigation by contrast radiologic studies, computed tomography (CT), esophageal ultrasonography, and esophagoscopy.

Because the esophagus can accommodate the gradual growth of a benign tumor mass, most patients do not present with symptoms until late in the course of their disease. When symptoms do occur, they usually take the form of a disturbance in swallowing or substernal chest discomfort, reflecting an abnormality in the orderly peristaltic contractions; the pain can mimic cardiac pain and may be relieved with nitrates. At times, exercise testing may be necessary to differentiate esophageal pain from cardiac pain. Difficulty in swallowing is a precise symptom that must never be ignored. Because the esophagus is a transit tube in which food does not digest and usually does not stagnate, ulceration and bleeding hardly ever occur from benign tumors.

Sometimes, other conditions such as esophageal diverticulum, achalasia, hiatal hernia, and cancer may occur together with a benign tumor (Seremetis et al, 1976). In this case, the clinical picture and findings are obscure and the presence of a benign tumor may be missed. At times, a mobile pedunculated tumor on a long stalk may be regurgitated from the mouth or obstruct the larynx (Cochet et al, 1980).

Pathophysiology

Typically, a benign esophageal tumor grows very slowly and by expansion. It enlarges rather like a balloon and compresses the surrounding tissue. It neither infiltrates not metastasizes. It may calcify. If it harms the patient, it does in the following ways:

1. By an incidental complication such as obstruction of the lumen (Schmidt et al, 1961) (tumor size and shape are important—either a large annular lesion or very large eccentric growth greater than 5 cm in size).
2. By regurgitation and airway obstruction (Allen and Talbot, 1967; Cochet et al, 1980) (tumor mobility is important).
3. By pressure effects on surrounding mediastinal structures (size and location of extramural tumor are important).
4. By ulceration and bleeding (very uncommon).

Often there is spontaneous cessation of growth, and the tumor may not change in size for many years (Glanz and Grunebaum, 1977). Therefore, benign tumors of the esophagus can be present for many years and be clinically silent and sometimes are found by chance, if at all.

Several pathophysiologic features of the esophagus

will now be addressed to allow understanding of the clinical presentation of benign tumors of this portion of the alimentary tract.

Active Peristalsis

Arising within the esophageal wall, benign tumors are subjected to the forces of constant muscular contractions (Hurwitz et al, 1979). They occur in response to swallowing (primary contraction), esophageal distention or irritation (secondary contraction), or spontaneously (tertiary contraction). The striated muscle of the upper esophagus provides a rapid, short, strong contraction so that the bolus is quickly passed well into the esophagus.

In the lower esophagus, the smooth muscle provides a more leisurely peristaltic wave. Therefore, an intraluminal tumor arising in the upper esophagus is likely to become elongated on a long pedicle, a so-called pedunculated fibrovascular polyp, because of constant downward urge of food, strong esophageal contractions, and a very thin, pliable esophageal wall with loose submucosal tissue. This effect may explain the frequent origin of the fibrovascular polyps in the cervical portion of the esophagus (Avezzano et al, 1990; Van Lanschot et al, 1987). Because of its excessive mobility on a long stalk, the fibrovascular polyp may intermittently regurgitate into the mouth and obstruct the larynx; fatal asphyxiation may result (Allen and Talbot, 1967; Cochet et al, 1980). Alternatively, it may be gradually pulled down by active peristalsis into the esophagogastric junction, causing intermittent obstruction. Sometimes, these polyps grow to a great size, causing marked esophageal dilatation, resembling advanced achalasia (Barrett, 1964; Patel et al, 1984).

Anatomic Location

Most of the esophagus, except for short segments in the neck and the abdomen, occupies a position in the posterior mediastinum. An intramural tumor situated just below the cricopharyngeus muscle sphincter commonly manifests early, with the patient's difficulty in swallowing and intractable cough upon swallowing. With gradual expansion of the tumor mass within the unyielding bony thoracic inlet, the airway may become compromised, producing upper airway obstruction.

Within the mediastinum, the esophagus has important relationships to the trachea, left main bronchus, heart, aorta, and thoracic spine. As a result, a giant tumor arising from the outer surface of the esophagus encroaches upon the space available in the mediastinum and pleural cavities. Compressive effects on the mediastinal structures may produce atelectasis, "asthma," and even superior vena cava obstruction syndrome (Barrett, 1964).

Esophageal Distensibility

An intraluminal tumor, by slow progressive growth, may cause gross esophageal dilatation and may be mistaken for achalasia (Avezzano et al, 1990; Barrett, 1964; Dyke, 1927; Patel et al, 1984). Faulty diagnosis results in ineffective treatment.

Esophageal Lumen

Intramural tumors often encroach upon the lumen of the gullet eccentrically; the remainder of the circumference of the gullet becomes lengthened and stretched over the mass. Thus, the lumen is crescentic and slitlike, and it is larger than normal. Often clinically silent, obstruction of the lumen is produced only by large tumors (>5 cm in size) (Schmidt et al, 1961). Occasionally, the intramural tumor may encircle the gullet, like a collar, causing obstruction (Seremetis et al, 1976). Such annular constricting benign tumors, usually leiomyomata, are commonly located at the esophagogastric junction; they may be mistaken for benign peptic stricture or cancer, again resulting in ill-advised treatment (Fig. 39–1).

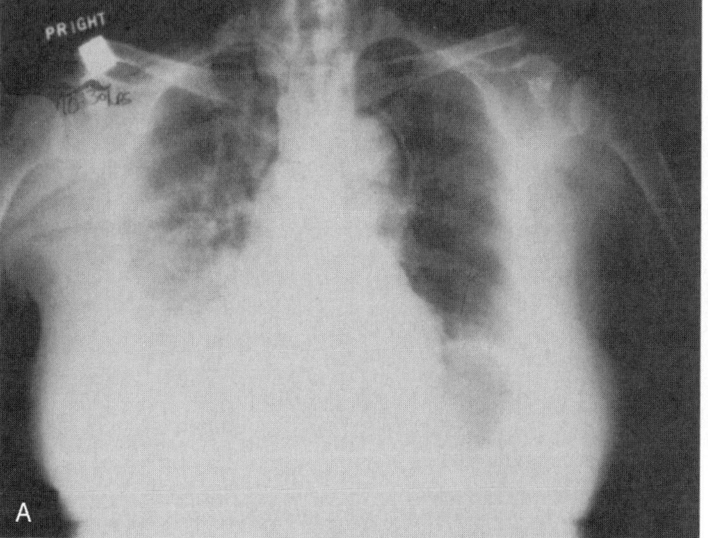

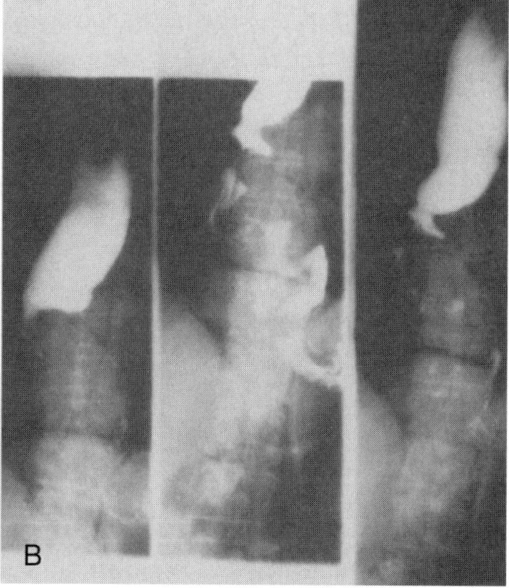

FIGURE 39–1 ■ *A*, Chest radiograph showing mediastinal emphysema following attempted esophageal dilatation of the distal esophageal stricture by the gastroenterologist. *B*, Diatrizoate meglumine (Gastrografin) swallow demonstrates perforation of the distal esophagus in the same patient.

TABLE 39–1 ■ **Human Esophagus and Histogenetic Classification of Benign Esophageal Tumors**

Esophageal Wall Tissue of Origin	*Tumor Type*	*Tissue Type*
Mucosa		
Epithelial lining		
Normal stratified squamous epithelium	Squamous cell papilloma	Epithelial
Acquired metaplastic columnar epithelium	True adenoma (rare) or adenomatous hyperplasia	Epithelial
Lamina propria		
Simple esophageal cardiac mucous gland	Mucus retention cyst	Epithelial
	True adenoma (rare)	Epithelial
Epithelial lining plus lamina propria	Inflammatory pseudotumor	Mesenchymal
	Fibrovascular polyp	Mesenchymal
Muscularis mucosae	Leiomyoma	Nonepithelial
Inflamed gastric mucosal fold at gastroesophageal junction	Inflammatory reflux polyp	Reflux polyp-fold complex
Submucosa		
Esophageal mucous gland proper	Mucus retention cyst	Epithelial
	Adenoma	Epithelial
Vascular connective tissue	Fibrovascular polyp (fibrolipoma fibromyxoma)	Mesenchymal
Blood vessel	Hemangioma	Mesenchymal
Schwann cell	Granular cell tumor	Mesenchymal
	Neurilemmoma	Mesenchymal
Muscularis propria		
Striated muscle (upper one third)	Rhabdomyoma	Mesenchymal
Smooth muscle (lower two thirds)	Leiomyoma	Mesenchymal
Nerve fiber	Neurofibroma	Mesenchymal
Schwann cell	Granular cell tumor	Mesenchymal
	Neurilemmoma	
Tunica adventitia		
Connective tissue	Fibroma	Mesenchymal
Nerve plexus	Schwannoma (neurilemmoma)	Mesenchymal
Ectopic tissues		
Sebaceous gland	Adenoma	Epithelial
Tracheobronchial rests	Choristoma	Mixed tissues

Incompetent Lower Esophageal Sphincter Mechanism

An incompetent lower esophageal sphincter (LES) leads to pathologic gastroesophageal reflux, with the harmful effects of reflux felt predominantly in the lower esophagus. Polypoid lesions may subsequently develop in the lower esophagus, such as true adenoma in the dysplastic columnar-lined esophagus (Lee, 1986; McDonald et al, 1977) and the inflammatory reflux gastroesophageal polyp (Rabin and Bremner, 1980).

Pathology

Benign tumors of the esophagus are separated into epithelial and nonepithelial types according to the tissue of origin (Table 39–1). In order to understand the variety of type and clinical effects, a knowledge of the human esophageal wall is necessary (Morson and Dawson). It consists of four layers (Fig. 39–2):

1. Inner mucosa that has three components: (a) a lining of nonkeratinizing stratified squamous epithelium, (b) a lamina propria made of loose reticular connective tissue with esophageal cardiac glands, and (c) a muscularis mucosae, a smooth muscle layer of varying thickness.
2. Submucosa, a loose connective tissue layer containing small glands, few in number and widely spaced.
3. Muscularis propria, which consists of two layers, inner circular and outer longitudinal, with the autonomic myenteric nerve plexus lying in between. Predominantly striated muscle in the upper third of the esophagus is gradually replaced by smooth muscle in the middle third, whereas the lower third is all smooth muscle.
4. Tunica adventitia, an outer layer of loose areolar tissue that is replaced by serosa in the short abdominal portion of the esophagus. The vagus nerves form a plexus on the surface.

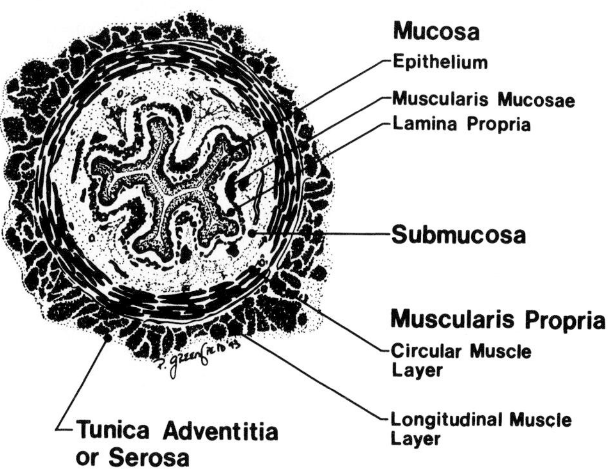

FIGURE 39–2 ■ Microanatomy of the wall of the esophagus.

Mucosa

The innermost mucosal layer may give rise to squamous cell papilloma (Weitzner and Hentel, 1968; Winkler et al, 1985), inflammatory pseudotumor (Wolf et al, 1988), mucous retention cyst, fibrovascular polyp (Van Lanschot et al, 1987), and leiomyoma (Barrett, 1964). The only examples of true adenomas have all occurred in the dysplastic, specialized columnar-lined type (Barrett's esophagus), which is believed to be secondary to gastroesophageal reflux (Lee, 1986; McDonald et al, 1977).

Submucosa

In contrast to the mucosa, the submucosa is very seldom a site of benign tumor formation. The most common benign tumors found are hemangioma and granular cell tumors (Giacobbe et al, 1988; Govoni, 1982). In theory, lipoma, fibroma, or mucous retention cysts can also arise here. It has been suggested that fibrovascular polyps may actually originate from the submucosal layer (Tasaka et al, 1982; Van Lanschot et al, 1987).

Muscularis Propria

Four types of benign tumors form in the muscularis propria: (1) leiomyoma (the most common benign intramural tumor), (2) rhabdomyoma, (3) neurofibroma, and (4) granular cell tumor. All are submucosal, and the overlying mucosa is nearly always intact, however large the tumors may be.

Tunica Adventitia (Serosa)

The outermost layer, the tunica adventitia, gives rise very rarely to a benign tumor. Schwannoma may form in the vagus nerve plexus present in this layer (Vaghei and Yost, 1991). Depending on the site of origin within the esophageal wall, the tumor may occur as an intraluminal sessile or polypoid growth or as a more deeply seated intramural submucosal tumor, or it may protrude from the outer surface of the esophagus into the mediastinum as an extramural growth.

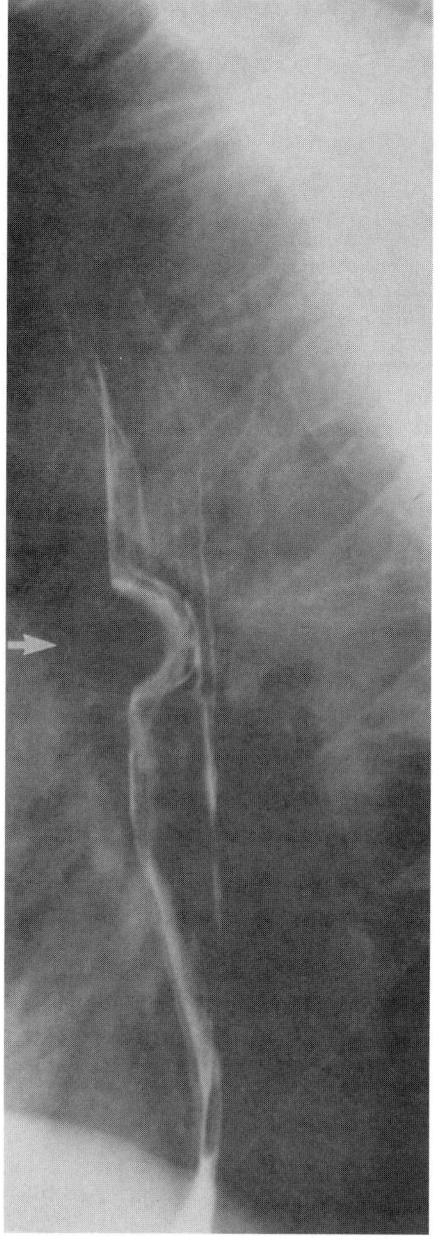

FIGURE 39–3 ■ Radiologic appearance of intramural leiomyoma *(arrow)*: smooth surface, clear-cut margins, sharp angles at upper and lower ends.

DIAGNOSIS

Clinical Presentation

Benign tumors of the esophagus can be present for many years and may be clinically silent. Many are symptomless (>85%) and found by chance, if at all, during radiologic or endoscopic examination of the esophagus. In the taking of a clinical history, a high index of suspicion should be maintained. Physical findings are negative in benign esophageal tumors. If the tumor lies just below the cricopharyngeus muscle sphincter, the presenting symptom may be "spluttering" every time the patient tries to swallow (Barrett, 1964). Rarely, the patient may have progressively increasing inspiratory stridor, upper airway obstruction caused by an enlarging tumor mass within the thoracic inlet (Pai et al, 1987). Prolonged and severe dysphagia with serious episodes of "pneumonitis" resulting from repeated spillover and aspiration should also arouse suspicion.

Sometimes, the patient may complain of a mild, intermittent difficulty with swallowing or a vague retrosternal pressure. Achalasia may be suspected. Occasionally, the history may be one of long-standing "asthma," caused by lower airway compression by the tumor. The most dramatic clinical presentation described is regurgitation of a large, fleshy soft tumor mass from the mouth. This tumor may appear and disappear suddenly and unaccountably in the mouth, and there is a serious risk of acute laryngeal obstruction (Cochet et al, 1980; Giacobbe et al, 1988). Rarely, significant hematemesis and melena may develop.

Accurate diagnosis is usually possible if taking a careful history is combined with a thorough radiographic examination and direct inspection by esophagoscopy. The endoscopic appearance is often suggestive, and biopsy is similarly often diagnostic. For example, in granular cell tumor, the tumor is immediately subepithelial and appears yellow-white. Sometimes, the pseudoepitheliomatous hyperplasia in the overlying intact epithelium may simulate squamous cell carcinoma.

Esophageal hemangioma may be diagnosed at endoscopy as a submucosal polypoid mass, blue-gray in appearance, and easily compressible (Govoni, 1982). Endoscopic biopsy should be avoided if the overlying mucosa is intact, as in intramural leiomyoma. On the other hand, biopsy proves necessary for a wartlike tumor in order to demonstrate human papilloma virus antigens and to rule out verrucous squamous carcinoma. The biopsy specimen should be analyzed by ultrastructural and immunohistologic study.

A good barium swallow examination is often diagnostic of intramural leiomyoma (Fig. 39–3). Yet a similar examination may either result in misdiagnosis or in missing the diagnosis altogether when one is dealing with pedunculated fibrovascular polyps. These tumors are known to grow to enormous size, usually larger than 10 cm (Patel et al, 1984). Progressive esophageal dilatation may occur, which may incorrectly suggest achalasia, and ill-advised esophagomyotomy has been undertaken (Barrett, 1964; Tasaka et al, 1982). Furthermore, a midesophageal tumor may be diagnosed if the tumor's pedicled attachment to the pharyngoesophageal junction is not appreciated. The diagnosis requires a combination of a full-column barium swallow examination with subsequent assessment of collapsed esophagus, cinesophagogram, double-contrast x-rays, and an index of suspicion to demonstrate a mobile pedunculated tumor with its stalk originating from the pharyngoesophageal junction (Fig. 39–4). Even at endoscopy, the tumor can be missed because it is covered with normal-appearing esophageal mucosa. Difficulty in diagnosis arises when an annular obstructing intramural leiomyoma forms at the esophagogastric junction. It may be mistaken for peptic stricture or malignant tumor. When the tumor is incorrectly diagnosed, attempts at esophageal dilatation may result in esophageal perforation (Figs. 39–1*A* and *B*).

The use of esophageal ultrasound in the diagnosis of submucosal tumors has been described (Rosch et al, 1992). By this technique, leiomyomata arise from the echo-poor layers (the second and fourth layers, i.e., the muscularis propria) and other lesions, such as cysts or fibromas, originate from the third, echo-rich layer (submucosa). Contrast CT and radionuclide angiography are two noninvasive investigative techniques that are helpful in making the diagnosis of esophageal hemangioma (Palchick et al, 1983). In the assessment of posterior mediastinal mass, whether it is calcified (which may occasionally occur in leiomyoma) or uncalcified, computed tomography is essential. The same investigation has replaced soft tissue radiographs of the neck and upper chest for further assessment of abnormal barium swallow examination (Fig. 39--5).

Description and Therapy

Squamous Cell Papilloma

By strict histologic definition, a true papilloma of the esophagus is rare. It should have a papillary architecture with a central core of vascular connective tissue stroma covered by thickened stratified squamous epithelium (Morson, 1990). The epithelium lacks atypia and shows normal differentiation. The estimated incidence in the autopsy studies is between 0.01% and 0.04% (Weitzner and Hentel, 1968). Some studies have implicated human papillomavirus as an etiologic agent (Winkler et al, 1985). The lower third of the esophagus is the most common site. Papillomas are usually small (<1.5 cm in size) and may occur multiply. At endoscopy, the papilloma appears sessile and multilobulated with a warty

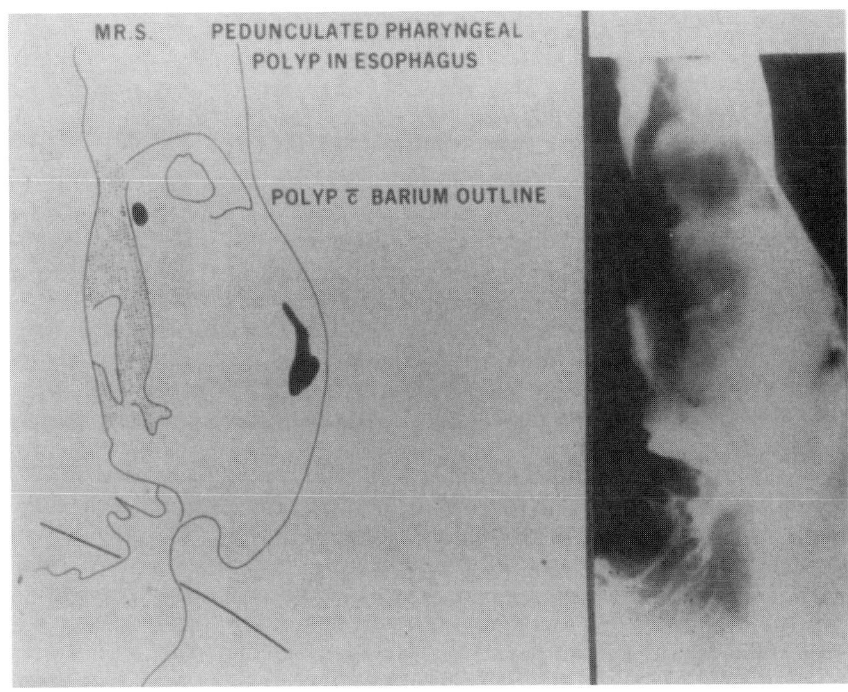

FIGURE 39–4 ■ Pedunculated intraluminal esophageal tumor. Its origin from the cervical esophagus was discovered at thoracotomy. (Courtesy of Dr. F. G. Pearson.)

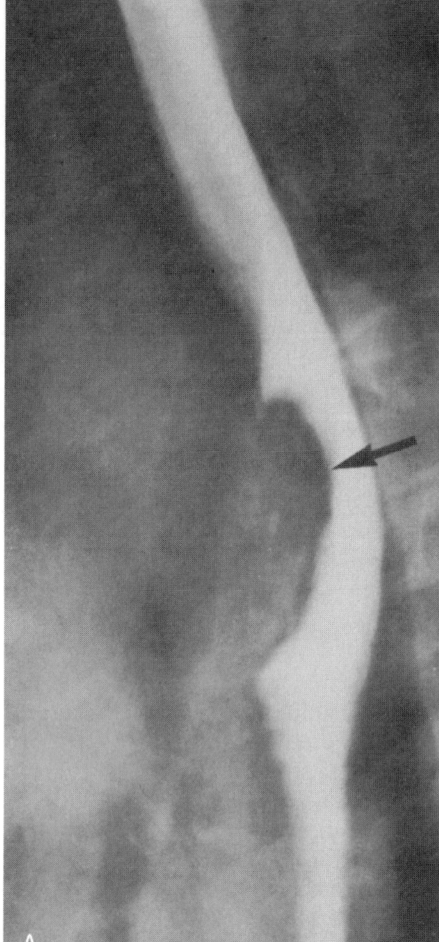

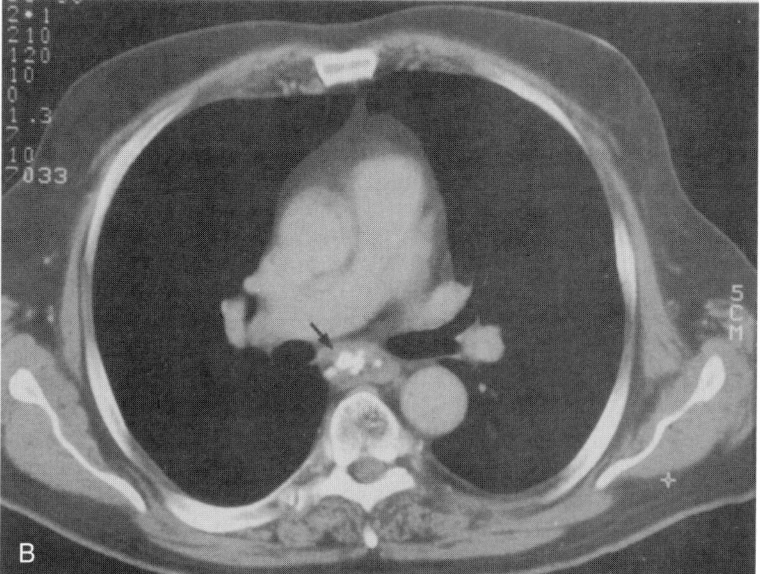

FIGURE 39–5 ■ *A,* Abnormal barium swallow in a patient complaining of mild dysphagia: well-defined, smooth filling defect with intact mucosa *(arrow)* at the level of the carina. *B,* CT examination confirms the presence of extrinsic calcified subcarinal lymph nodes *(arrow)* as the cause of abnormal barium swallow.

surface and firm consistency. It is easily confused with verrucous squamous cell carcinoma, which must be ruled out by careful biopsy (Fig. 39–6). So far, there is no evidence that squamous cell papillomas have any significant malignant potential.

The two main indications for excision of these tumors are esophageal obstruction and inability to exclude malignancy. Endoscopic removal should be attempted for an obstructing lesion. If cancer is suspected or if endoscopic removal is unsuccessful, surgical exploration of the esophagus will be necessary, with local excision, frozen-section assessment, and esophageal reconstruction to follow.

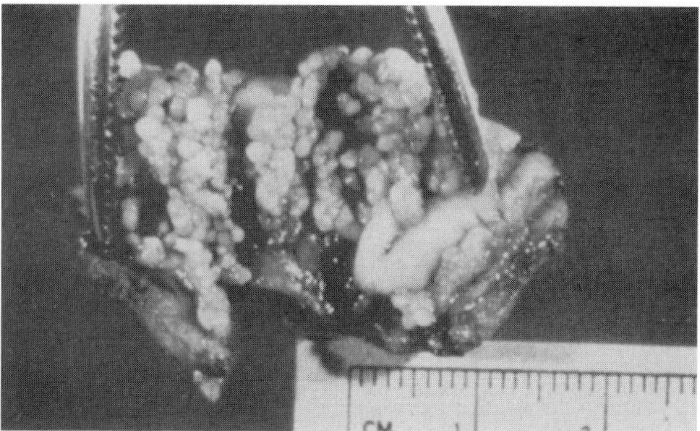

FIGURE 39–6 ■ Squamous papilloma of the esophagus. The lesion has a warty surface. (Courtesy of Dr. R. Inculet.)

Fibrovascular Polyps

Fibrovascular polyps occur frequently as solitary lesions, commonly in older men between 60 and 70 years of age. They are rare, and even large tumors often remain asymptomatic. The majority, about 85%, are located in the upper part of the esophagus (Jang et al, 1969). These polyps usually originate just below the cricopharyngeus muscle sphincter, starting as small mucosal tumors. As they grow and project into the lumen, they are gradually gripped and pulled by the constant downward urge of food and peristalsis, becoming elongated and pedunculated. Sometimes these polyps grow to a great size and have extremely long pedicles (Avezzano et al, 1990). The pedicle may be fairly thick and may contain blood vessels of considerable size; at times, the pedicle is just a thin mucosal duplication (Van Lanschot et al, 1987). The polyp itself has an appearance of a fleshy cylindrical mass (Fig. 39–7). Even when large, it may be missed on endoscopic examination because its surface appears similar to normal esophageal mucosa (Burrell and Toffler, 1973).

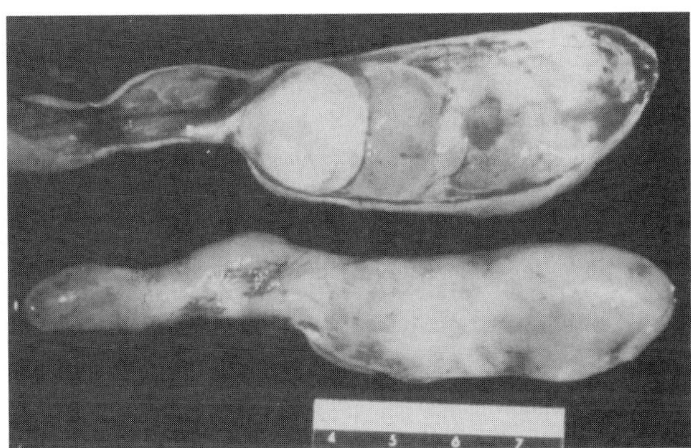

FIGURE 39–7 ■ Gross appearance of a large pedunculated fibrovascular polyp.

Fibrovascular polyps are composed of edematous connective tissue containing numerous blood vessels and a variable amount of fatty tissue, hence the histologic description of angiofibrolipomatous tissue. There is no surrounding capsule. The overlying mucosa may be ulcerated from trauma and secondary infection.

The following facts are of particular importance to the surgeon:

1. Pedunculated tumors on long stalks are mobile inside the gullet. They can range up and down over a distance of several inches.
2. To make the correct diagnosis, the physician must have the results of a proper contrast examination.
3. At endoscopy, the exact point of origin of the pedicle should be determined. The thickness of the pedicle and size of the tumor mass should be noted. Coexistent cancer in the overlying mucosa should be ruled out (Marcial-Rojas and Suan, 1959). Endoscopic ultrasound may help to assess the vessels in the pedicle, but it is not essential (Avezzano et al, 1990).
4. Esophagoscopy using topical anesthesia carries a risk of acute laryngeal obstruction if the tumor mass regurgitates during withdrawal of the scope (Tasaka et al, 1982).
5. Once the diagnosis is made, resection is indicated to prevent fatal asphyxiation from acute laryngeal obstruction (Allen and Talbot, 1967; Cochet et al, 1980).

MANAGEMENT

The surgical technique is chosen after assessment of the origin, size, and vascularity of the pedicle and the size of the tumor mass.

Small polyps (<2 cm in diameter) with a thin pedicle may be removed by endoscopic ligation and electrocoagulation of the pedicle (Tasaka et al, 1982).

Large polyps (>8 cm in length) or those with a thick, richly vascularized pedicle (when there is concern about severe bleeding) should be removed by surgical excision (Van Lanschot et al, 1987). The incision necessary to expose the esophagus depends on the site of the mucosal origin of the pedicle, since the pedicle has to be resected under direct vision.

The polyp that originates from the pharyngoesophageal junction is removed through a neck incision (Fig. 39–8). The neck incision is made on the side, right or left, opposite the origin of the tumor. This technique allows proper visualization and control of the pedicle. A 5-cm-long longitudinal incision is made in the lateral esophageal wall, starting just below the cricopharyngeus muscle. The polyp is brought out of the lumen through the esophagotomy incision. The mucosal origin of the pedicle is then either (1) securely ligated with a 3–0 vicryl and transected if thin or (2) resected and suture closed if large. The feeding vessels are first individually ligated and divided at the base of the pedicle. The base is then transected, and the resulting mucosal defect is primarily repaired with interrupted sutures of 4–0 vicryl.

The esophagotomy incision is closed in two layers using interrupted sutures of 4–0 vicryl for mucosa and interrupted sutures of 3–0 silk for muscle. Local excision is curative.

Granular Cell Tumor

In 1931, Abrikossoff described the first granular cell tumor of the esophagus. This finding was incidental at

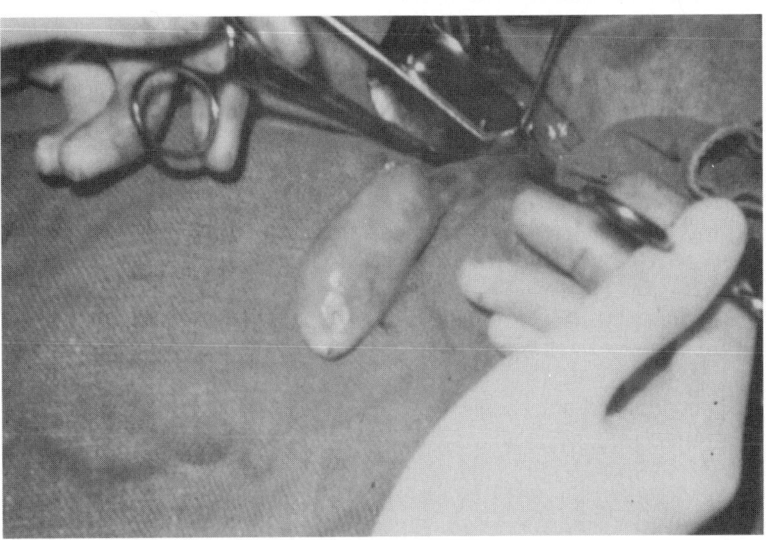

FIGURE 39–8 ■ The tumor has been taken out of the esophagus via a cervical incision.

autopsy, and the tumor was in the cervical esophagus. Since then, more than 120 examples of this uncommon tumor have been reported in the esophagus, occurring at all levels (Coutinho et al, 1985). The most common site is in the lower third of the esophagus; about 50% to 80% occur here (Andrade et al, 1987). The tumors vary in size from 8 mm to 6.5 cm.

The cell of origin is believed to be a perineural (Schwann) cell based on ultrastructural examination and immunohistologic study (Buley et al, 1988). The tumor consists of large polygonal cells containing numerous eosinophilic granules. The tumor cells show a positive reaction to specific tumor markers, namely, S-100 protein and neuron-specific enolase. The ultrastructural features include the presence of myelinoid structures in the granules and interdigitation of thin, axon-like cytoplasmic processes.

The endoscopic appearance, that of a "molar on the gingiva," frequently suggests the diagnosis. Usually, a small sessile polypoid nodule is seen, which looks yellow-white and is covered by an intact pale mucosa. The tumor feels firm to palpation with the biopsy forceps. Because it arises in the submucosa and forms immediately beneath the mucosa, which is thinned out, endoscopic biopsy is diagnostic in most cases (Andrade et al, 1987). However, one histologic feature may lead to a mistaken diagnosis of squamous cell carcinoma. This feature is the presence of pseudoepitheliomatous hyperplasia of the overlying intact squamous epithelium, which may be the only feature picked up if the biopsy sample is superficial.

Endoscopic ultrasonography should be of help in differentiating granular cell tumor from squamous cell carcinoma because the exact location and origin of the submucosal granular cell tumor can be assessed (Tada et al, 1990). Furthermore, staining the tumor surface with Lugol's solution at endoscopy, which confirms intact epithelium overlying granular cell tumor, helps to differentiate the two tumors (Tada et al, 1990). Of note, coincidental squamous cell carcinoma has been reported (Mannion et al, 1985).

Several factors influence the treatment of granular cell tumors of the esophagus:

1. They are almost always benign. Malignant change in preexisting benign tumors has not been described. However, there are reported cases of malignant forms of granular cell tumors in the esophagus, but only two; one was locally invasive, and the other had spread to regional lymph node (Brady et al, 1988).
2. Granular cell tumors have been observed to remain very stable over long duration, up to several years (Brady et al, 1988; Lack et al, 1980). During this time, the tumors have remained unchanged in size, appearance, and histology.
3. Granular cell tumors rarely cause symptoms. Asymptomatic, smaller lesions under 2 cm in size require periodic observation only. They can be safely followed with endoscopy and biopsy at 1- or 2-year intervals (Giacobbe et al, 1988), which helps to avoid the potential complications of endoscopic or surgical excision.
4. Larger, symptomatic benign tumors (>2 cm in size) and those in which malignancy cannot be excluded should be treated by local surgical excision (Coutinho et al, 1985). Benign and malignant forms of this tumor are remarkably similar on histologic examination. The appearance, which favors malignancy, is of increased cellularity and small, elongated cells. Furthermore, a tumor that grows rapidly, recurs locally after removal, or is large may be malignant.
5. Endoscopic removal of granular cell tumors is not advised because of the submucosal origin, absence of capsule, and a tendency toward local infiltration and the physician's inability to judge accurately the extent of the tumor mass preoperatively without esophageal ultrasonography. Thus, if excision is incomplete by endoscopy, not only is recurrence likely, but there is also a risk of complications such as ulceration, bleeding, and secondary infection causing perforation. The correct choice of treatment for the benign tumor type is complete local surgical excision at thoracotomy.

Inflammatory Pseudotumors

Occasional examples of an inflammatory mass have been described in the esophagus, usually in the lower third (Livolsi and Perzin, 1975). Inflammatory pseudotumors are grossly localized and commonly pedunculated masses. Their origin is uncertain, perhaps related to previous mucosal ulceration.

Inflammatory pseudotumors are important only because of their close resemblance to carcinoma; however, they are not true neoplasms. The endoscopic appearance of a polypoid mass with ulceration definitely creates a concern about malignancy. Even at histologic examination, it may be difficult to rule out squamous cell carcinoma with spindle cell features, carcinosarcoma, and Kaposi's sarcoma. The histologic examination shows fibroblast proliferation and infiltration, edematous stroma, and mixed inflammatory cell infiltrate with numerous plasma cells, eosinophils, and multinucleated giant cell (Wolf et al, 1988).

There is no specific treatment except that pseudotumors should not be confused with carcinoma; otherwise, ill-advised radical esophageal resection may be performed. Esophagectomy may be necessary if cancer of the esophagus occurs together with an inflammatory pseudotumor. This association is probably coincidental. It has not been described before and occurred in two of our patients (Figs. 39–9 and 39–10).

Inflammatory Polyp (Reflux Gastroesophageal Polyp)

Occasionally, a smooth polypoid lesion may develop near the gastroesophageal junction because of reflux esophagitis (Rabin and Bremner, 1980). The gastric folds at the squamocolumnar junction become inflamed and edematous. The resulting polyp actually represents the sessile edematous tip of a prominent gastric fold and hence is described as an inflammatory polyp fold complex. This lesion may be recognized radiologically. Biopsy of the polyp shows nonspecific inflammatory reaction in gastric mucosa. The presence of gastroesophageal reflux is confirmed by endoscopic evidence of reflux esophagitis and

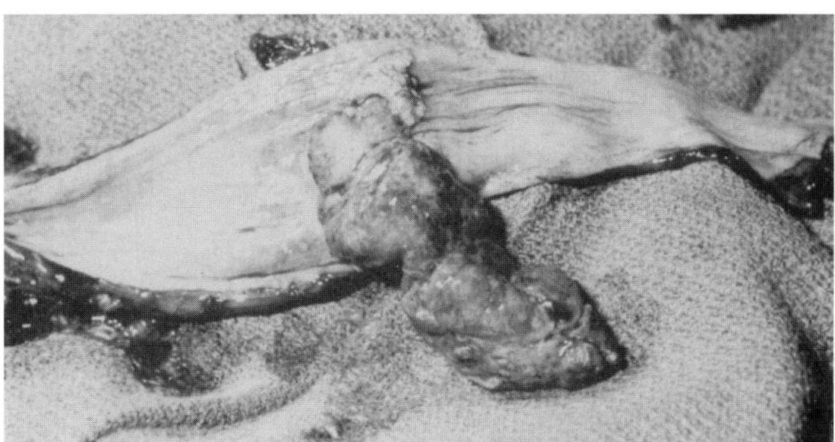

FIGURE 39–9 ■ Disabling pain on swallowing and dysphagia in an 82-year-old woman. A large polypoid mass (6 × 3 cm) is present in the thoracic esophagus. Histologic examination revealed inflammatory changes in the polypoid mass itself and the presence of a basaloid variant of squamous cell carcinoma at its base.

abnormal 24-hour esophageal pH monitoring. Treatment is necessary only for the underlying pathologic gastroesophageal reflux.

Adenomas

Polypoid masses may occasionally develop in the columnar-lined esophagus and may be classified as true adenomas (Lee, 1986; McDonald et al, 1977). In this setting, the columnar epithelium is of the specialized type, which represents a form of incomplete intestinal metaplasia, accompanied by dysplasia. Benign neoplastic proliferation occurs in the dysplastic epithelium, forming adenomatous polyps (Fig. 39–11). These adenomas have the same dysplastic histologic features as adenomas in the colon and rectum. They are composed of dysplastic glandular epithelium with a tubular or villous configuration. The adjacent flat mucosa also shows dysplasia. The appearance of high-grade dysplasia in the specialized-type columnar-lined esophagus is a worrisome finding that indicates possible subsequent malignant change. Total esophageal resection and reconstruction are indicated so that all of the abnormal dysplastic glandular epithelium is removed (Streitz et al, 1992).

There are no well-documented reports of adenomas arising from the glands in the submucosa that mimic those of the salivary glands.

Miscellaneous Uncommon Tumors

Hemangioma, neurofibroma, schwannoma, rhabdomyoma, choristoma, amyloid tumor, hamartoma, and sebaceous gland adenoma are among other uncommon tumors reported in the esophagus.

Hemangioma

Hemangiomas are tumor-like malformations that form in the submucosa, most commonly in the lower part of the esophagus (Govoni, 1982; Palchick et al, 1983). The true incidence is unknown. Dysphagia and upper gastrointestinal bleeding have been the most common symptoms reported; serious bleeding causing death has been noted as well. At endoscopy, a blue-gray polypoid tumor mass covered by normal mucosa is seen. The mass may be regular and round or irregular. The lumen may appear completely occluded but the endoscope can be advanced

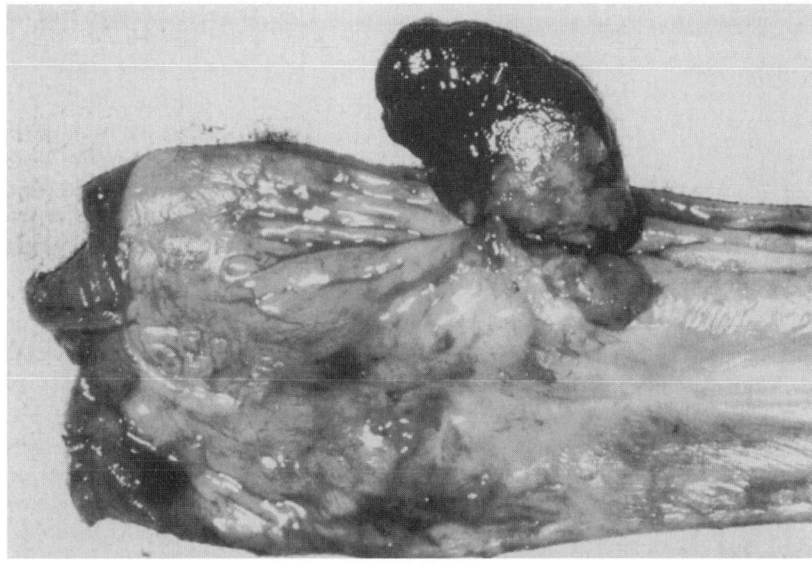

FIGURE 39–10 ■ Disabling pain on swallowing and upper gastrointestinal bleeding in an 81-year-old woman. A hemorrhagic polypoid mass (3 × 2 cm) was present in the thoracic esophagus. Histologic examination revealed vascular connective tissue with inflammatory cells and surface ulceration in the polypoid mass itself and a basal cell variant of squamous cell carcinoma at its base.

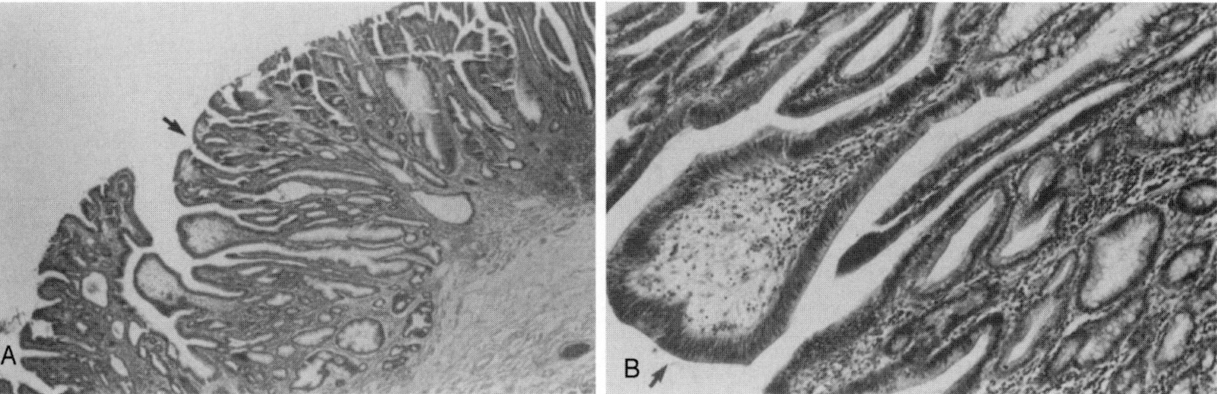

FIGURE 39–11 ■ *A*, Esophageal adenoma, a predominantly villous structure *(arrow)*. *B*, Esophageal adenoma. Hyperplasia of covering epithelium *(arrow)* with dysplasia, and glandular structures within the villous fronds. (Courtesy of Dr. M. J. Thomas, Canadian Reference Centre for Cancer Pathology.)

gently, since the mass is easily compressed. The tumor mass simply represents large dilated submucosal vessels.

The diagnosis is first suggested by the endoscopic appearance. Confirmation may be made by two noninvasive investigative techniques, contrast CT and radionuclide angiography (Palchick et al, 1983). These techniques may replace diagnostic invasive methods, which include contrast angiography, endoscopic biopsy with its attendant potential risk of serious bleeding, and surgical excisional biopsy.

Treatments described in 27 patients with esophageal hemangioma were local surgical excision in 18, some of which were probably diagnostic biopsy only; no treatment in 1; and in the remaining 7, radiotherapy or chemical fulguration (Govani, 1982).

Neurofibroma

Neurofibroma is a very rare submucosal tumor. It may be multiple as a manifestation of von Recklinghausen's disease (Morson, 1990). Endoscopically, these tumors may be suspected because of their firmness, as well as because of a brownish reticular pigmentation. Histologically, small polypoid tumors arise in the submucosa, presumably in the submucosal plexus, and larger tumors are related to the myenteric plexus.

Schwannoma

A rare case of schwannoma arising in the vagus nerve plexus on the surface of the esophagus has been reported (Vaghei and Yost, 1991). The tumor was embedded in the wall of the lower esophagus and was removed by enucleation.

Rhabdomyoma

Rhabdomyoma is a rare benign tumor arising in the striated muscle. In one case, this tumor was reported in the upper esophagus (Pai et al, 1987). The patient presented with progressive upper airway obstruction.

Lipoma

Lipoma is also a rare submucosal tumor of the esophagus. It is usually recognized endoscopically because of its yellow color, pliability, and smooth surface. The shape varies because of the squeezing effect of peristalsis. Endoscopic biopsy is difficult because the overlying mucosa tends to retract easily from the underlying fatty tumor; moreover, the biopsy incision is not deep enough to obtain diagnostic material.

Most lipomas are small, do not cause symptoms, and do not need to be removed. Occasionally, as a result of the peristaltic forces, the submucosal lipoma may become elongated, pedunculated, and mobile on a long pedicle. This condition is an indication for excision, as in fibrovascular polyps, to prevent acute laryngeal obstruction (Allen and Talbot, 1967). Rarely, lipomas become large, with central ulceration causing bleeding and pain. Again, surgical excision is curative.

Choristoma

Choristoma is an intramural tumor like mass formed from rare ectopic tracheobronchal tissue rests within the esophageal wall (Nishina et al, 1981). It is mainly cartilaginous. Approximately 10% are in the lower third of the esophagus. The majority are found in children.

Amyloid Tumor

Localized accumulation of amyloid material within the esophageal wall may produce a tumor-like mass, so-called amyloid tumor. It presents as an intramural tumor. In the case reported, it caused perforation and bleeding (Solanke et al, 1967).

Benign Pigmented Tumor

A very unusual benign pigmented tumor, probably of neural origin, has been reported in the esophagus (Morson, 1990). The patient had an asymptomatic mediastinal mass.

Hamartoma

Pedunculated hamartoma on a long stalk arising in the upper esophagus has also been described (Gupta et al, 1987).

Leiomyomata

Leiomyomata are benign tumors of smooth muscle that occur at all levels in the esophagus, more often in the lower than the upper part (Seremetis et al, 1976). Munro was the first to describe localized intramural esophageal tumor in 1797, and the histologic characteristics of esophageal leiomyoma were described by Virchow in 1863. They are the most common benign tumors of the esophagus (67%).

The usual finding, in 97% of the reported cases, is an intramural tumor mass that is solitary and grows very slowly and eccentrically in the circular muscle of the gullet (Fig. 39–12). With continued growth, the tumor bulges into the lumen eccentrically. The lumen becomes slitlike; obstruction, however, is uncommon unless the tumor is large (>5 cm in diameter) (Schmidt et al, 1961). Many leiomyomata are small and are discovered incidentally.

Furthermore, the size of the lesion may not change for many years (Glanz and Grunebaum, 1977). The overlying mucosa is nearly always intact and bleeding hardly ever occurs, except, perhaps, when the tumor extends downward across the cardia and into the stomach. Occasionally, the intramural tumor grows circumferentially to encircle the gullet, like a collar, causing disabling esophageal obstruction (Fig. 39–13). Alternatively, it may become elongated and spiral to involve a long segment of the esophagus (Fig. 39–14). The annular lesion, seen in 10% of intramural leiomyomata, may be mistaken for cancer or peptic stricture (Seremetis et al, 1976). Occasionally, in about 2%, the tumor mass protrudes from the outer surface of the esophagus into the mediastinum. Besides producing compressive symptoms, the tumors may be confused with posterior mediastinal tumors or an aneurysm of the descending thoracic aorta, especially if calcified (Barrett, 1964). Very rarely, in about 1%, leiomyomata arising from the muscularis mucosae protrude into the lumen and become elongated and pedunculated (Barrett, 1964; Seremetis et al, 1970). They are often large and mobile on long stalks and can be mistaken for fibrovascular polyps.

A typical leiomyoma is sessile, firm to the touch, rounded, and lobulated. It is gray-white on section and consists of whorls of smooth muscle surrounded by a fibrous tissue capsule. It may contain ganglion cells and fragments of nerve, which may suggest a diagnosis of neurofibroma. In practice, the difference between these two tumors is not important to the surgeon; both can be removed easily by enucleation, and, if removal is complete, neither recurs.

Leiomyomata tend to be well differentiated and composed of elongated fusiform cells with abundant eosinophilic and fibrillated cytoplasm. The tumor is not cellular. As the tumor enlarges, it accumulates more and more collagen. Calcification may occur, which may be recognized on chest radiograph and was seen in 1.8% of all cases reported (Seremetis et al, 1976).

Multiple benign smooth muscle tumors occur occasionally and must be distinguished from the rare condition of true diffuse leiomyomatosis of the esophagus (Fernandes et al, 1975; Heald et al, 1986). Multiple leiomyomata are characteristically well defined from each other, and fortunately, most of these lesions can be shelled out if necessary. In diffuse leiomyomatosis, on the other hand, the lower half of the esophagus is markedly thickened and narrowed; at times, the cardia of the stomach may be involved as well (Fig. 39–15). This condition is characterized by diffuse hyperplasia of smooth muscle in the muscularis propria and muscularis mucosae. There is also a considerable amount of intermingled fibrous tissue, hyperplasia of blood vessels and nerves, and infiltration with lymphocytes and plasma cells (Fernandes et al, 1975). Most cases occur in females in the 2nd and 3rd decades of life and occasionally are associated with vulvar leiomyomas (Wahlen and Astedt, 1965). This condition has also been described in Alport's syndrome (Guarner and Torres, 1985). The only effective treatment for true diffuse leiomyomatosis is esophagectomy and reconstruction using stomach or colon.

The histologic distinction between leiomyoma and leiomyosarcoma can be unclear. The best guides to malignancy are increased cellularity, excessive number of mitotic figures, nuclear atypia, and tumor necrosis. Leiomyoma, however, is well differentiated, not cellular, and is composed of elongated fusiform cells with abundant fibrillated cytoplasm. It is very rare for a leiomyoma to undergo malignant transformation to leiomyosarcoma (Seremetis et al, 1976).

Treatment

The recommended treatment of a clinically recognized leiomyoma has been surgical removal, whether or not

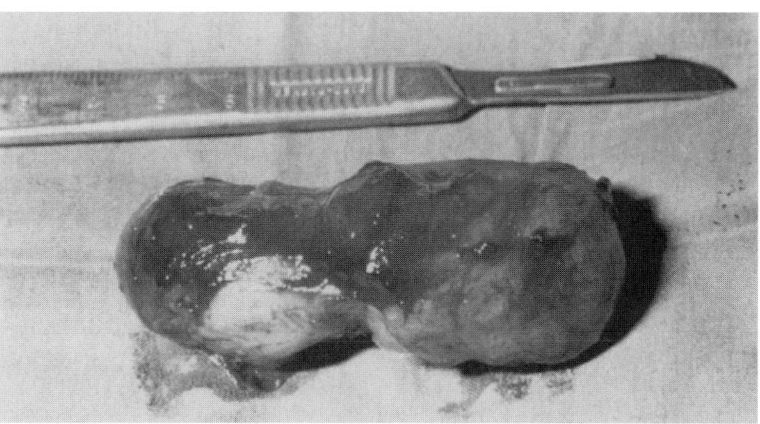

FIGURE 39–12 ■ Gross appearance of a typical solitary intramural leiomyoma after enucleation.

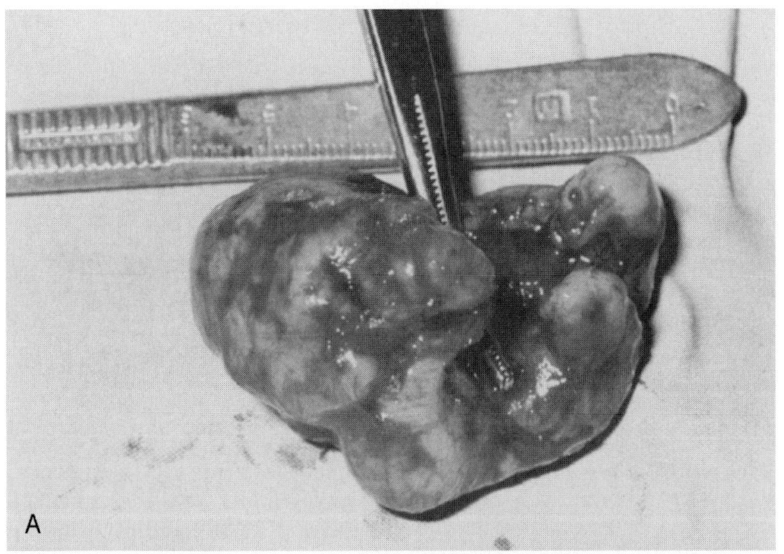

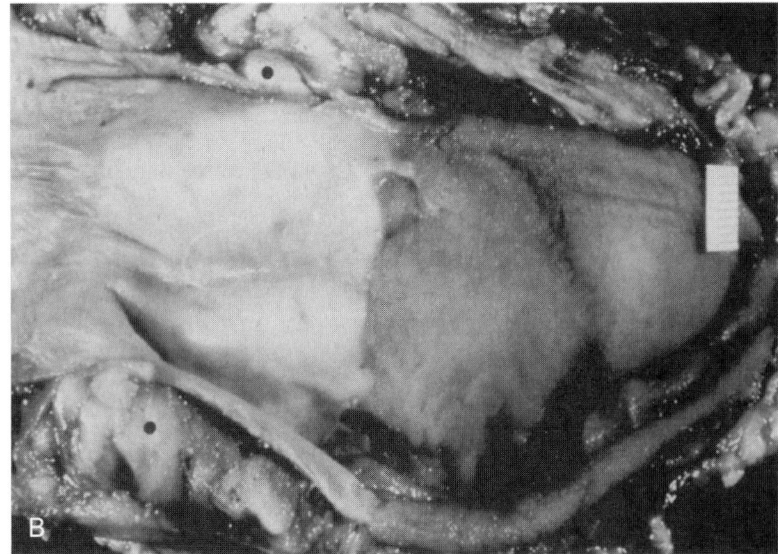

FIGURE 39–13 ■ *A*, Circumferential leiomyoma of the gastroesophageal junction removed by enucleation. *B*, The cut surface of the gastroesophageal junction was removed at operation. The tumor encircles the lumen of the lower esophagus *(circle)* and was mistaken for a peptic stricture by the gastroenterologist. The esophagus was perforated by attempted esophageal dilatation.

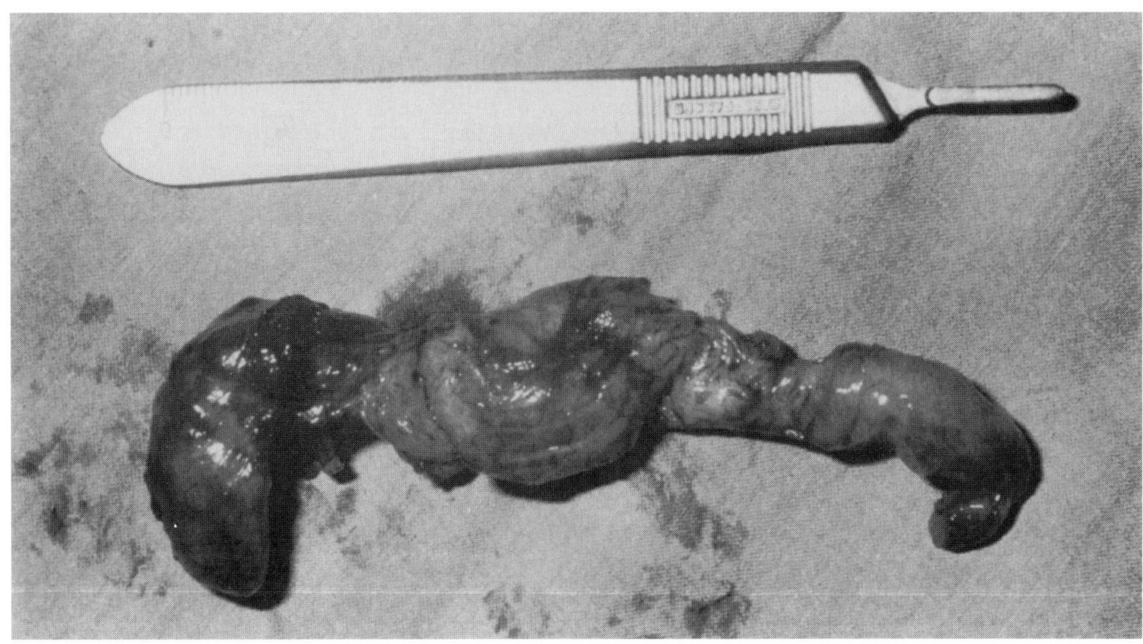

FIGURE 39–14 ■ This intramural leiomyoma, elongated and spiral, has been removed by enucleation.

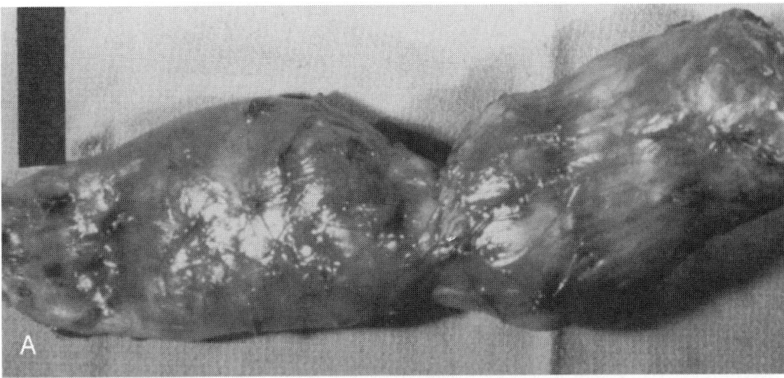

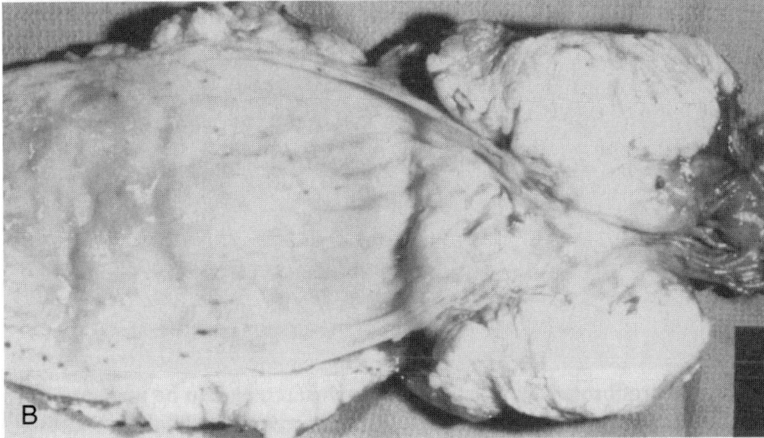

FIGURE 39–15 ■ *A*, True diffuse leiomyomatosis of the esophagus. Note the enlargement and distortion of the gullet. *B*, The specimen has been opened to show the diffuse leiomyomatous process involving the whole esophagus.

symptoms are present, despite its very slow growth, frequent absence of symptoms in the patient, and its very low risk of malignant change (Seremetis et al, 1976). On the basis of information available, several questions should be asked before proceeding to surgical intervention:

1. *Should a leiomyoma be removed because it will continue to grow?* According to Glanz and Grunebaum (1977), the tumor does maintain a stable behavior over an extended period. They monitored four patients by barium swallow examination for 3 to 15 years and found no change in the size of the tumor. Therefore, a small leiomyoma, defined as less than 5 cm in size, that is discovered incidentally and is truly asymptomatic can be watched. This tumor can be safely followed periodically at 6-month intervals with clinical assessment and esophageal ultrasound (if available) and with barium swallow examination at 1- or 2-year intervals. The patient should be advised that the tumor should be removed only if it increases in size (becoming larger than 5 cm), particularly if it grows rapidly or if symptoms develop.

2. *Is there a correlation between the tumor size and symptoms?* In the report by Seremetis and colleagues (1976), the majority of the leiomyomata that were removed were small, between 2 and 5 cm in diameter, and more than 50% of the patients were asymptomatic. Furthermore, it has been shown that these tumors seldom cause symptoms when they are less than 5 cm in diameter (Schmidt et al, 1961). According to Gray and colleagues (1961), no correlation existed between the tumor size and the duration of symptoms. Therefore, there is no reason to remove a small asymptomatic leiomyoma that has remained stable in size over an extended period of follow-up.

3. *Should a leiomyoma be removed because it may become malignant?* Leiomyosarcoma of the esophagus is rare and accounts for well under 1% of all esophageal malignancies. Most patients present with progressive dysphagia, weight loss, and pain. Only 40 reported cases were found by Seremetis and coworkers (1961) in their review. It is not even certain how many of these cases were truly leiomyosarcomas or how many of the leiomyosarcomas actually developed in previously benign leiomyomas. It seems that there were only two documented cases of such malignant transformation, an indication of the extremely low risk of malignant change. Although malignancy can be ruled out only by excision and histologic examination, it seems unreasonable to remove all small asymptomatic leiomyomata.

4. *Is there a correlation between the tumor size and malignancy?* In the study of the gastric and intestinal stromal tumors, it becomes obvious that the size of the tumor gives an indication of its aggressiveness. A stromal tumor in the stomach over 6 cm in diameter and in the intestine over 4 cm should be considered a potential sarcoma. Unfortunately, no such information is available on the size of the smooth muscle tumor of the esophagus and its potential behavior. In one study of nine such tumors of the esophagus, the size varied between 1 and 10 cm (average, 5.1 cm), and all were well-differentiated ordinary leiomyomas (Ueyama et al, 1992).

5. *Can death result from an untreated leiomyoma?* The answer is yes, but only because of misdiagnosis that

results in ineffective treatment. Death from disabling esophageal obstruction and malnutrition, due to annular constricting tumor, has been reported in a few untreated cases (Barrett, 1964). In addition, pedunculated intraluminal leiomyoma has caused fatal asphyxiation from acute laryngeal obstruction (Seremetis et al, 1976).

6. *What should be the indications for surgical removal of a leiomyoma, and how should it be removed?* Operative removal of a leiomyoma is justified, at initial diagnosis, if it is large (>5 cm in size), if the patient has symptoms, if the diagnosis is in doubt, or if the tumor is intraluminal, pedunculated, and mobile.

Surgery. Since most leiomyomas are intramural, eccentric, and well encapsulated, they can be easily shelled out (enucleated) without resorting to esophageal resection. Ohsawa of Japan was the first to perform enucleation of esophageal leiomyoma in 1933 (Seremetis et al, 1976). Enucleation is the treatment of choice for the benign smooth muscle tumor because it is curative and carries a low risk. No deaths were reported in 31 patients who underwent enucleation of the tumor (Ala-Kulju and Salo, 1987; Arnorsson et al, 1984; Mansour et al, 1977); in the immediate postoperative period, the most serious complication was esophageal leak in two patients in whom accidental opening of the mucosa was unrecognized during enucleation. Significant gastroesophageal reflux developed in seven of the nine (78%) surviving patients at 11.1 ± 6.8 (standard deviation) years follow-up (Ala-Kulju and Salo, 1987). As a result, antireflux repair should be considered under certain circumstances, as follows.

Most leiomyomas, about 89%, occur in the lower two thirds of the esophagus and must be removed through a chest incision. The right side of the chest is opened when the tumor is at or above the level of the aortic arch. A tumor present in the lower part of the esophagus is best removed through a left chest incision. Neck incision is required for the rare leiomyoma in the cervical esophagus. Either a left thoracoabdomen–left neck incision or laparotomy–left neck incision is used for the occasional annular constricting tumor at the esophagogastric junction, which requires total esophageal resection and reconstruction. The anastomosis should be placed in the neck to reduce gastroesophageal reflux.

It is important to keep in mind that leiomyoma may occasionally be intraluminal, pedunculated, and mobile on a long stalk attached to the cervical esophagus. The tumor may appear to be arising in the midesophagus, and the mucosal origin of its pedicle in the cervical esophagus may be overlooked. Failure to appreciate this possibility may result in the chest being opened unnecessarily; this tumor type should be removed through a neck incision (see Fig. 39–4) (Barrett, 1964).

Enucleation (shelling out) of the intrathoracic intramural leiomyoma is the preferred treatment and is carried out in the following manner. The chest is opened on the correct side and at the correct level, just at the tumor level. The tumor is located in the esophagus without difficulty, and the overlying mediastinal pleura is opened longitudinally, just enough for adequate exposure (Fig. 39–16). The esophagus is then mobilized at the tumor level only for manipulation. The outer longitudinal muscle layer over the tumor is often thinned out by the bulging tumor; the muscle is incised longitudinally, as in esophagomyotomy, down to the tumor level (Fig. 39–17).

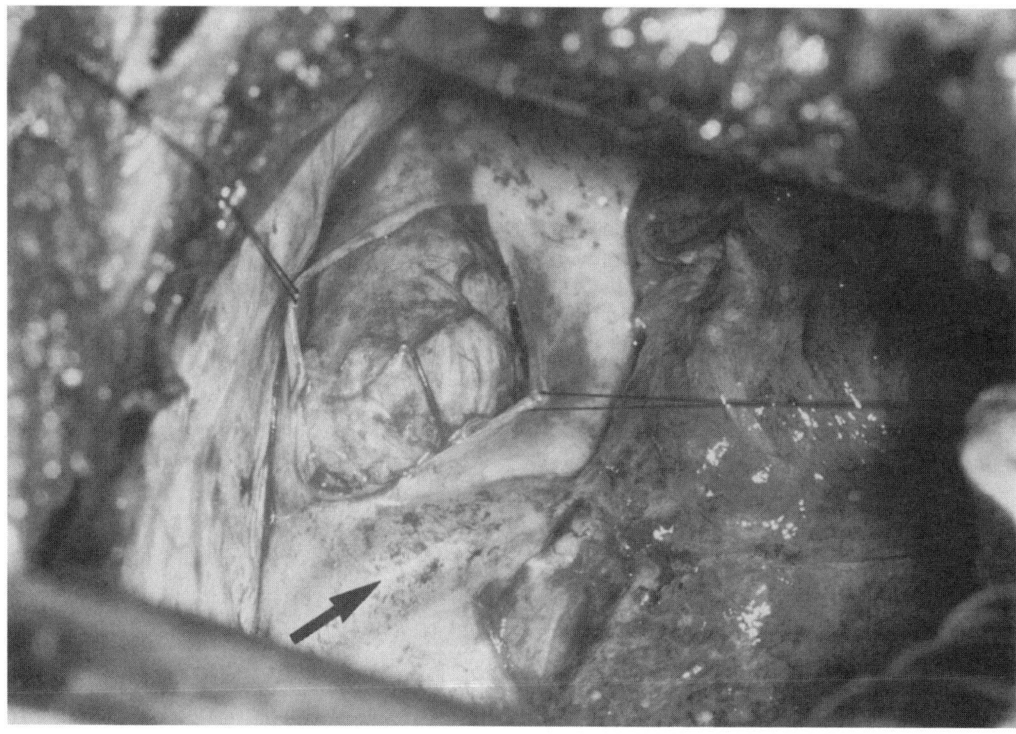

FIGURE 39–16 ■ Enucleation of a leiomyoma: the mediastinal pleural has been incised and the esophagus has been exposed. Note the bulging tumor above the azygos vein *(arrow)*.

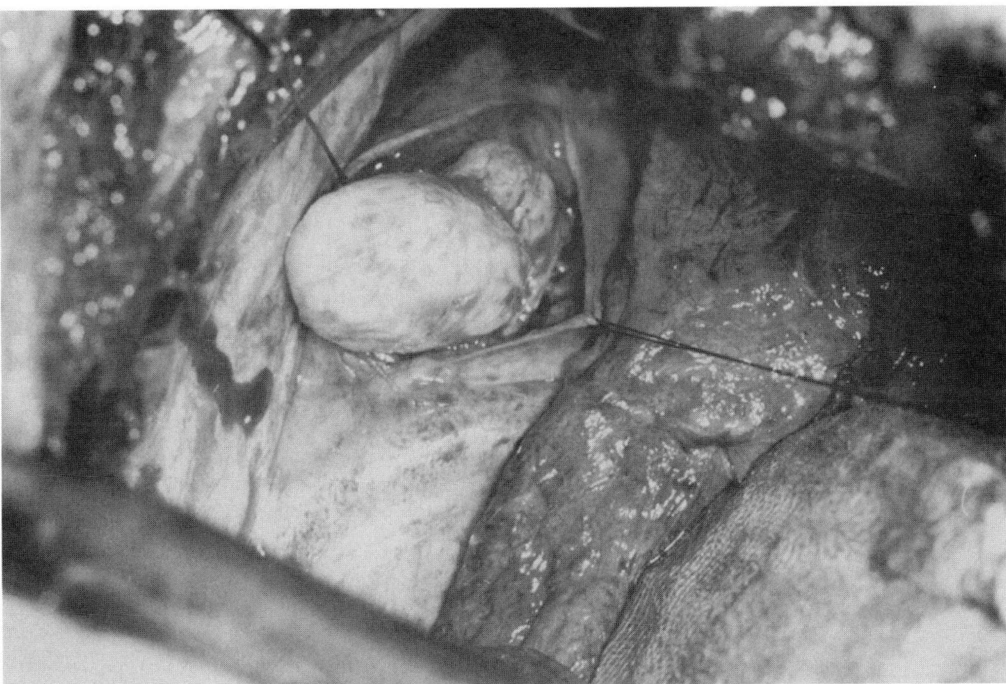

FIGURE 39–17 ■ Enucleation. Myotomy of the outer longitudinal muscle over the tumor mass and a plane of dissection developed between the tumor and the muscle layer.

The tumor often arises in the circular muscle layer. A correct plane of cleavage is found between the tumor capsule and the muscle layer of the esophagus. Careful dissection is maintained in this plane until the mucosa is reached. The tumor is then dissected off this layer, without damaging it (Fig. 39–18). The longitudinal muscle layer is reapproximated with fine nonabsorbable interrupted sutures of 4–0 silk. The mediastinal pleura is then closed over the esophagus with continuous running fine absorbable suture of 4–0 vicryl. Intramural leiomyoma in the cervical esophagus or at the gastroesophageal junction is removed in a similar manner.

If the tumor is to be removed by enucleation, the following points should be considered.

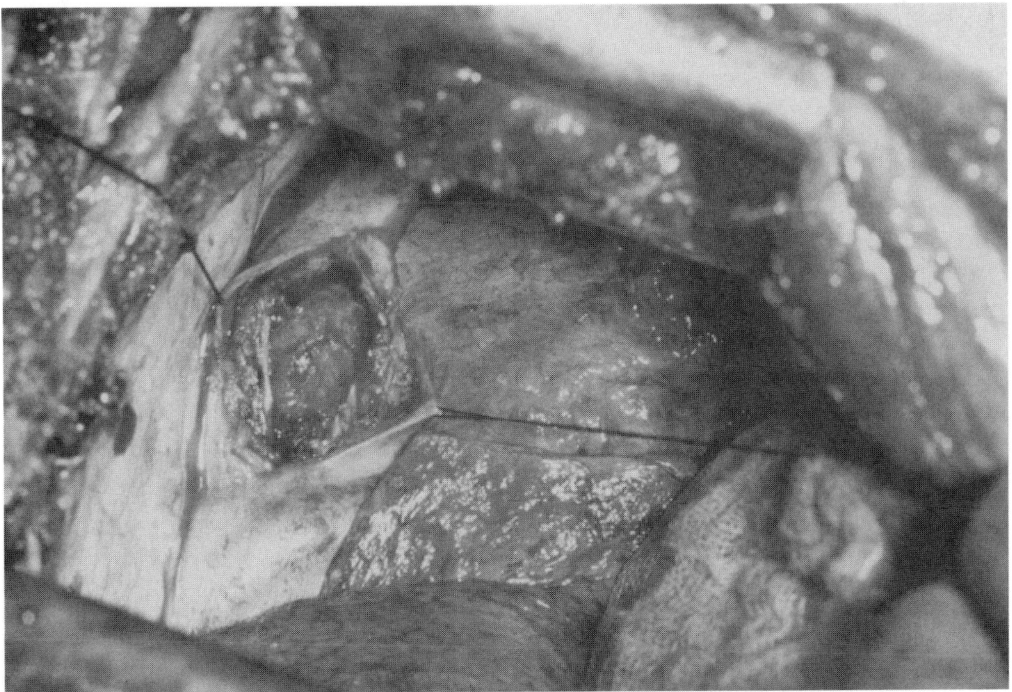

FIGURE 39–18 ■ The tumor has been enucleated without damaging the mucosa.

Postoperative Esophageal Leak. This serious complication develops because the mucosa is perforated during enucleation and is either missed or incorrectly repaired. The mucosa should always be carefully examined after the tumor has been enucleated. Any perforation that is present should be repaired with fine, absorbable, interrupted sutures of 4–0 vicryl or other absorbable suture before the muscle layer is reapproximated over the mucosa.

Postoperative Tumor Recurrence. Benign smooth muscle tumor should be removed by enucleation whenever possible. Results are excellent. The same is not true for the malignant form of this tumor because of the risk of local recurrence and progression of the tumor after enucleation; leiomyosarcoma demands excision of the tumor together with the adjacent esophagus and/or stomach, followed by reconstruction, for cure.

The clinical behavior and intraoperative appearance do not easily distinguish leiomyoma from leiomyosarcoma (Seremetis et al, 1976). The typical leiomyoma is white, lobulated, and firm to the touch and seldom undergoes necrosis. On section, gross whorling and bulging are apparent, and the tumor is surrounded by an avascular fibrous tissue capsule (Fig. 39–19). By contrast, leiomyosarcoma is yellow-brown in color and softer than leiomyoma (because of areas of hemorrhage and necrosis), and it blends imperceptibly into the surrounding muscle. Enucleation is rather tedious because there is no capsule. The main criterion by which malignancy is recognized is *immediate* intraoperative histologic examination of the tumor after removal: Malignant tumor is more cellular, with a large number of mitotic figures, nuclear atypia, and tumor necrosis.

Postoperative Gastroesophageal Reflux. Enucleation of a leiomyoma, located in the lower part of the esophagus close to the esophagogastric junction, may result in significant gastroesophageal reflux afterward (Ala-Kulju and Salo, 1987). This problem is probably related to disturbance of esophageal motility and interference with the lower esophageal sphincter mechanism.

Alternately, gastroesophageal reflux, with or without sliding hiatal hernia, may occur together with leiomyoma. Antireflux repair should be done after enucleation if gastroesophageal reflux has been documented preoperatively, if extensive mobilization of the esophagogastric junction is necessary to remove the tumor, or if sliding hiatal hernia is present.

Does Tumor Removal Require Esophageal Resection and Reconstruction Rather Than Enucleation? In 1932, Sauerbruch successfully performed an esophageal resection for a large leiomyoma (Seremetis et al, 1976). Esophageal resection and reconstruction constitute a major undertaking, with an operative risk of 5% to 10%. The specific indications are as follows:

1. An occasional giant extramural leiomyoma that not only obstructs the esophagus but also produces compression of the neighboring organs in the mediastinum and pleural cavities and cannot be enucleated.
2. A large leiomyoma that completely surrounds the esophagus and constricts it. This annular lesion usually occurs at the esophagogastric junction, and superficial ulceration may be present. Resection is necessary to rule out a malignant tumor.
3. A mucosa that is so badly damaged during enucleation of a leiomyoma that satisfactory repair is not possible. Resection is necessary to prevent postoperative esophageal leak.
4. A large leiomyoma in the distal esophagus that extends downward across the cardia and into the stomach. Superficial ulceration is common, making enucleation difficult.
5. A leiomyosarcoma that is suspected and confirmed on frozen section.

Follow-up. Careful long-term follow-up is necessary after enucleation of leiomyoma of the esophagus. Significant gastroesophageal reflux may develop years later, for which antireflux repair may be necessary.

Esophageal Cysts

The second most common tumor-like condition of the esophagus is the cyst (Arnorsson et al, 1984; Mansour et

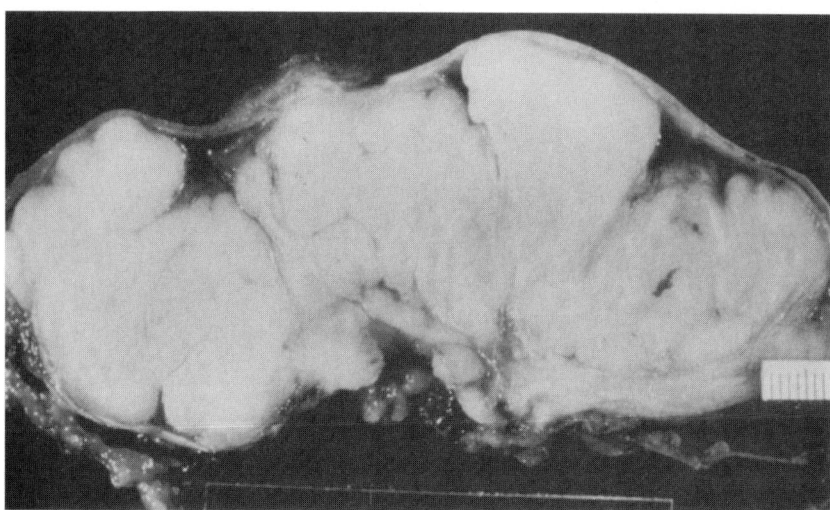

FIGURE 39–19 ■ Leiomyoma of the esophagus. Encapsulation, gross whorling, and bulging are apparent.

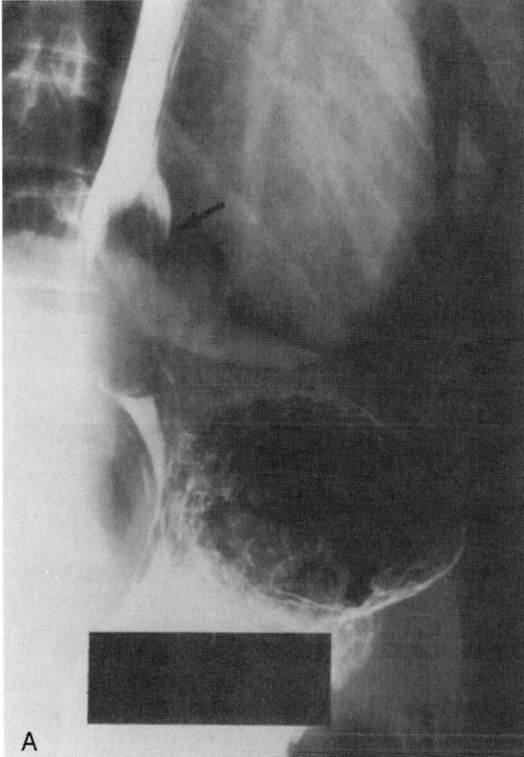

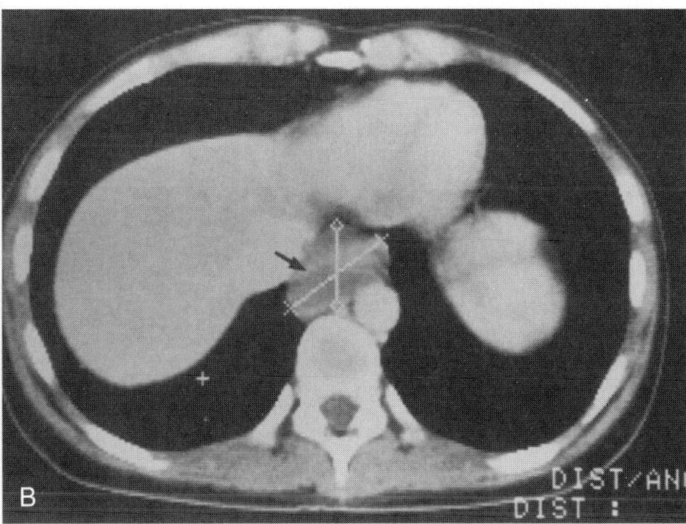

FIGURE 39–20 ■ *A*, A smooth oval mass *(arrow)* is demonstrated in the distal third of the esophagus. The mass measures 6 cm in length and appears to be intramural. *B*, CT confirms the presence of a mass intimately associated with the distal esophagus. The density readings suggest that this growth is a complicated duplication cyst.

al, 1977; Totten et al, 1953). A cyst is a pathologic fluid-filled sac bounded by an epithelium-lined wall and may be the seat of secondary infection or hemorrhage. Esophageal cysts are classified as developmental cysts arising from persistent vacuoles in the wall of the foregut during the development of the trachea and the esophagus. The cysts, therefore, are usually to be found within or close to the esophageal wall.

The esophageal cyst may increase in size, causing symptoms of esophageal obstruction and pulmonary complications. Therefore, although these cysts are not true neoplasms, they enter into the differential diagnosis of the benign esophageal tumors because of the similar clinical presentation. They can frequently be distinguished from neoplasms on CT scanning by the lower density of the fluid-filled interior (Fig. 39–20). However, because they may contain thick mucoid material, differentiation from a solid tumor may be difficult. Clinical suspicion may be confirmed by aspiration needle biopsy when feasible. If endoscopic ultrasound is available, it should be used for the assessment of benign tumors of the esophagus. By this method, cysts can be differentiated from solid benign tumors with sufficient accuracy (Rosch et al, 1992). More than 60% of esophageal cysts are present in the first year of life. Cysts of the upper third of the esophagus manifest in infancy, and those of the lower third present later in childhood. Esophageal cysts should be removed by means of an extramucosal resection whenever possible.

SUMMARY

Symptomatic benign tumors are rarely encountered in clinical practice and account for less than 1% of all esophageal neoplasms. Thus, no individual surgeon has enough experience with these tumors to be dogmatic in opinion. A review of the accumulated experience in the literature is necessary in order to understand the variety of type and clinical effects, which allows guidelines to be developed for therapy, particularly the indications for surgery.

■ *KEY REFERENCES*

Coutinho DS, Soga J, Yoshikawa T, et al: Granular cell tumours of the esophagus: A report of two cases and review of the literature. Am J Gastroenterol 80:758, 1985.

This article contains a good review of the granular cell tumors of the esophagus: 117 cases of this tumor type published through December 1984 were analyzed with respect to the clinical features, location of the tumor, malignant changes, and treatment.

Lee RG: Adenomas arising in Barrett's esophagus. Am J Clin Pathol 85:629, 1986.

Lee has clearly described three cases of the unusual esophageal adenoma, all of which arose within Barrett's esophagus. Dysplastic changes were found in the adjacent mucosa of each case.

Seremetis MG, Lyons WS, DeGuzman VC, et al: Leiomyomata of the esophagus: An analysis of 838 cases. Cancer 41:717, 1961.

The pertinent information about benign smooth muscle tumors of the esophagus can be found in the study of Seremetis and colleagues, who reviewed all reported cases through the end of 1971.

Van Lanschot JJ, Poublon RM, Zonderland HM, et al: Benign pedunculated tumor of the esophagus. Neth J Surg 39:83, 1987.

The authors describe the presentation and management of two cases of benign pedunculated tumor of the esophagus. The surgical technique has been described in detail.

Wolf BC, Khettry U, Leonardi HK: Benign lesions mimicking malignant tumors of the esophagus. Hum Pathol 19:148, 1988.

The authors describe three cases of benign lesions of the esophagus that mimicked malignant tumors. A detailed histologic description of each case has been given.

■ REFERENCES

Ala-Kulju K, Salo JA: Smooth muscle tumours of the oesophagus. Scand J Thorac Cardiovasc Surg 21:65, 1987.

Allen MS Jr, Talbot WH: Sudden death due to regurgitation of a pedunculated esophageal lipoma. J Thorac Cardiovasc Surg 54:756, 1967.

Andrade J, Bambirra EA, De Oliveira CA: Granular cell tumor of the esophagus: A study of seven cases diagnosed by histologic examination of endoscopic biopsies. S Med J 80:852, 1987.

Arnorsson T, Aberg C, Aberg T: Benign tumors of the oesophagus and esophageal cysts. Scand J Thorac Cardiovasc Surg 18:145, 1984.

Avezzano EA, Fleischer DE, Merida MA, et al: Giant fibrovascular polyps of the esophagus. Am J Gastroenterol 85:299, 1990.

Barrett NR: Benign smooth muscle tumours of the esophagus. Thorax 19:185, 1964.

Bernatz PE, Smith JL, Ellis FH Jr, et al: Benign pedunculated intraluminal tumors of the esophagus. J Thorac Surg 35:503, 1958.

Brady PG, Juergen-Nord H, Connar RG: Granular cell tumor of the esophagus: Natural history, diagnosis, and therapy. Dig Dis Sci 33:1329, 1988.

Buley ID, Gatter KC, Kelly PM, et al: Granular cell tumors revisited: An immunohistological and ultrastructural study. Histopathology 12:263, 1988.

Burrell M, Toffler R: Fibrovascular polyp of the esophagus. Am J Dig Dis 18:714, 1973.

Cochet B, Hohl P, Sans M, et al: Asphyxia caused by laryngeal impaction of an esophageal polyp. Arch Otolaryngol 106:176, 1980.

Dyke SC: Benign polyp of the oesophagus of great size. J Pathol 30:309, 1927.

Fernandes JP, Mascarenhas MJ, DaCosta JC, et al: Diffuse leiomyomatosis of the esophagus: A case report and review of the literature. Dig Dis 20:684, 1975.

Giacobbe A, Facciorusso D, Conoscitore P, et al: Granular cell tumor of the esophagus. Am J Gastroenterol 83:1398, 1988.

Glanz I, Grunebaum M: The radiological approach to leiomyoma of the oesophagus with a long-term follow-up. Clin Radiol 28:197, 1977.

Govoni AF: Hemangiomas of the esophagus. Gastrointest Radiol 7:113, 1982.

Gray SW, Skandalakis JE, Shepard D: Smooth muscle tumors of the esophagus. Int Abstr Surg 113:205, 1961.

Guarner V, Torres RG: Diffuse leiomyomatosis of the esophagus, tracheobronchial, genital, and renal Insufficiency. In DeMeester TR, Skinner DB (eds): Esophageal Disorders: Pathophysiology and Therapy. New York, Raven Press, 1985, p 447.

Gupta AK, Goyal VP, Hemani DD, et al: Pedunculated intraluminal oesophageal hamartoma. J Laryngol Otol 101:851, 1987.

Heald J, Moussalli H, Hasleton PS: Diffuse leiomyomatosis of the esophagus. Histopathology 10:755, 1986.

Heitzman EJ, Heitzman GC, Elliott CF: Primary esophageal amyloidosis. Arch Intern Med 109:595, 1962.

Hodge GB: Esophageal leiomyoma associated with an epiphrenic diverticulum and hiatus hernia. Am Surg 36:538, 1970.

Hurwitz AL, Duranceau A, Haddad JK: In Smith LE (ed): Major Problems in Internal Medicine, Vol 16: Disorders of Esophageal Motility. Philadelphia, WB Saunders, 1979, p 67.

Jang GC, Clouse ME, Fleischner FG: Fibrovascular polyp: A benign intraluminal tumor of the esophagus. Radiology 92:1196, 1969.

Lack EE, Worsham GF, Callihan MD, et al: Granular cell tumor: A clinico-pathological study of 110 patients. J Surg Oncol 13:301, 1980.

Livolsi VA, Perzin KH: Inflammatory pseudotumors (inflammatory fibrous polyps) of the esophagus: A clinico-pathology study. Am J Dig Dis 20:475, 1975.

Lu YK, Yueh-Min L, Chig-Chiang K: The coexistence of benign and malignant tumors of the esophagus. Clin Med J 82:805, 1963.

Mannion P, Honan RP, Fitzgerald MD: Contiguous granular cell myoblastoma and squamous cell carcinoma in the esophagus. Thorax 40:551, 1985.

Mansour KA, Hatcher CR, Haun CL: Benign tumors of the esophagus: experience with 20 cases. S Med J 70:461, 1977.

Marcial-Rojas RA, Suan P: Epidermoid carcinoma in mucosa overlying a pedunculated lipoma of the esophagus. J Thorac Surg 37:427, 1959.

McDonald GB, Brand DL, Thorning DR: Multiple adenomatous neoplasms arising in columnar-lined (Barrett's) esophagus. Gastroenterology 72:1317, 1977.

Morson BC: Morson and Dawson's Gastrointestinal Pathology, 3rd ed. Blackwell Science, 1990.

Nishina T, Tsuchida Y, Saito S: Congenital esophageal stenosis due to tracheobronchial remnants and its associated anomalies. J Pediatr Surg 16:190, 1981.

Pai GK, Pai PK, Kamath SM: Adult rhabdomyoma of the esophagus. J Pediatr Surg 22:991, 1987.

Palchick BA, Alpert MA, Holmes RA, et al: Esophageal hemangioma: Diagnosis with computed tomography and radionuclide angiography. S Med J 76:1582, 1983.

Patel J, Keiffer RW, Martin M: Giant fibrovascular polyp of the esophagus. Gastroenterology 87:953, 1984.

Plachta A: Benign tumors of the esophagus: Review of the literature and report of 99 cases. Am J Gastroenterol 38:639, 1962.

Rabin MS, Bremner CG: The reflux gastroesophageal polyp. Am J Gastroenterol 73:451, 1980.

Rosch T, Lorenz R, Dancygier H, et al: Endosonographic diagnosis of submucosal upper gastrointestinal tract tumors. Scand J Gastroenterol 27:1, 1992.

Schmidt HW, Clagett OT, Harrison EG Jr: Benign tumors and cysts of the esophagus. J Thorac Cardiovasc Surg 41:717, 1961.

Solanke F, Olurin EO, Nawakonobi F, et al: Primary amyloid tumor of the esophagus treated by colon transplant. Br J Surg 54:943, 1967.

Streitz JM Jr, Williamson WA, Ellis FH Jr: Current concepts concerning the nature and treatment of Barrett's esophagus and its complications. Ann Thorac Surg 54:586, 1992.

Sweet RH, Souter L, Valenzuela CT: Muscle wall tumors of the esophagus. J Thorac Surg 27:13, 1954.

Tada S, Iida M, Yao T, et al: Granular cell tumor of the esophagus: Endoscopic ultrasonographic demonstration and endoscopic removal. Am J Gastroenterol 85:1507, 1990.

Tasaka Y, Makimoto K, Yamauchi M, et al: Benign pedunculated intraluminal tumor of the esophagus. J Otolaryngol 11:111, 1982.

Totten RS, Stout AP, Humphreys GH II, et al: Benign tumors and cysts of the esophagus. J Thorac Surg 25:606, 1953.

Ueyama T, Guo K, Hashimoto H, et al: A clinicopathologic and immunohistochemical study of gastrointestinal stromal tumors. Cancer 69:947, 1992.

Vaghei R, Yost NI: Vagal schwannoma involving esophagus. Ann Thorac Surg 52:1334, 1991.

Wahlen T, Astedt B: Familial occurrence of coexisting leiomyoma of vulva and oesophagus. Acta Obstet Gynecol Scand 44:197, 1965.

Watson RR, O'Connor TM, Weisel W: Solid benign tumors of the esophagus. Ann Thorac Surg 4:80, 1967.

Weitzner S, Hentel W: Squamous papilloma of the esophagus: Case report and review of the literature. Am J Gastroenterol 50:391, 1968.

Winkler B, Capo V, Reumann W, et al: Human papillomavirus infection of the esophagus: A clinicopathologic study with demonstration of papilloma virus antigen by the immunoperoxidase technique. Cancer 55:149, 1985.

MALIGNANT NEOPLASMS

CHAPTER **40**

Biology of Esophageal Cancer

David S. Schrump
Alan G. Casson

DEFINITION

Esophageal cancers are highly lethal neoplasms; despite advances in multimodality therapy, 5-year survival generally remains less than 10% (Farrow and Vaughan, 1996). In North America and Europe, there has been a dramatic change in the epidemiology of esophageal cancer over the past 2 decades (Blot and McLaughlin, 1999; Blot et al, 1991, 1993; Parkin et al, 1993; Reed, 1991). Although the incidence of squamous cell carcinoma of the esophagus (an epithelial tumor arising from esophageal squamous mucosa) has remained stable, the incidence of primary esophageal adenocarcinomas (arising from glandular mucosa of the lower esophagus) has steadily increased, at a rate exceeding that for any other cancer.

Whereas tobacco and alcohol contribute significantly to the development of esophageal squamous cell carcinomas arising in individuals within the United States, dietary and cultural practices, nutritional deficiencies, and oncogenic human papillomaviruses have been implicated in the pathogenesis of squamous cell carcinomas arising in individuals residing in high-incidence areas of Asia, South Africa, and the Middle East (Sur and Cooper, 1998; Tao et al, 1999; Yang, 1980). These factors appear to have less impact in the pathogenesis of primary esophageal adenocarcinomas in North America and Europe (Brown et al, 1995; Francheschi et al, 1990; Gray et al, 1992; Ji et al, 1998; Levi et al, 1990; Tzonou et al, 1996), where some studies have implicated gastroesophageal reflux disease (GERD) as a significant risk factor (Chow et al, 1995; Lagergren et al, 1999). It is hypothesized that chronic acid (and bile) reflux results in acute mucosal injury (esophagitis), promotes cellular proliferation, and induces columnar metaplasia of the normal squamous epithelium lining the esophagus (Ter and Castell, 1997). The resulting columnar epithelium–lined (Barrett's) esophagus in patients with GERD appears predisposed to develop malignancy, at an estimated risk of at least 30- to 40-fold higher than in the general population (Dent et al, 1991; Ortiz-Hildago et al, 1998; Spechler, 1997; Tytgat and Hameeteman, 1992).

The etiology of esophageal cancer is unknown. As for other human solid tumors, esophageal cancers are thought to arise as a multistep process, modulated by both genetic and environmental factors. Although epidemiologic studies have implicated several environmental and life-style risk factors (see earlier), it is unlikely that a single etiologic factor could account for the marked variation in frequency of this disease worldwide. The possibility of genetic events underlying the development of esophageal cancer arose from observations of an occasional familial incidence or clustering of this disease and its association with the rare autosomal dominant disease tylosis. The tylosis–esophageal cancer gene has been mapped to a small region on chromosome 17q25 (Kelsall et al, 1996), and loss of heterozygosity (LOH) studies have further implicated this gene in sporadic esophageal tumors (Risk et al, 1999).

With the widespread application of molecular technology during the 1990s, numerous molecular genetic alterations have now been reported in esophageal tumors and premalignant lesions (for reviews, see Casson and McCart, 1995; Jankowski et al, 1999; Meltzer, 1996; Montesano et al, 1996; Roth, 1994). This chapter summarizes our current understanding of esophageal tumor biology, emphasizing the potential clinical application of molecular biology to the future practice of general thoracic surgery.

HISTORICAL NOTE

Cancer of the esophagus was apparently first described more than 2000 years ago in high-incidence regions of China (Hurt, 1991; Yang, 1980). Few accurate reports of esophageal malignancy were forthcoming, however, until the late 1800s, when improved pathologic descriptions paralleled initial attempts at surgical resection of cervical esophageal tumors (Postlethwait, 1986). Epidemiologic reports following World War II stressed the striking geographic variation in incidence of esophageal cancer. These observations stimulated laboratory studies of experimental esophageal carcinogenesis from the 1950s onward. Environmental factors and carcinogens were recognized to be essential components of esophageal tumorigenesis, leading to de-emphasis of the role of hereditary factors in cancer development.

Peptic ulceration of the lower esophagus, presumed secondary to "insufficiency of the cardia," was described in detail more than 90 years ago by Tileston (1906), who alluded to the presence of an abnormal glandular epithelium. The modern concept of a columnar epithelium–lined esophagus arose from the observations of Barrett (1950, 1957), Bosher and Taylor (1951), and Allison and Johnstone (1953), 50 years later. Morson and Belcher (1962) reported that esophageal adenocarcinomas arose from "ectopic gastric mucosa," crediting Carrie (1950) with this original observation.

Advances in molecular biology have changed our understanding of the pathogenesis of human cancer. Huebner and Todaro (1969) initially reported oncogenes in RNA tumor viruses, proposing that they were derived from proto-oncogene sequences contained in normal eukaryotic cells. Following technical advances in tumor virology, Stehlin and colleagues (1976) reported the first transforming viral gene, the *src* oncogene. Rapid progress followed, and in 1981, DNA from human tumor cells was found to transform murine fibroblasts (Krontris and Cooper, 1981; Shih et al, 1981). A year later, a transforming gene, H-*ras*, was isolated from a human bladder carcinoma cell line and sequenced (Reddy et al, 1982; Tabin et al, 1982). A point mutation in the first exon of the H-*ras* gene was found: the nucleotide guanine (G) replaced by thymidine (T) at codon 12. As a consequence of this genetic mutation, the protein product encoded by this gene was changed, and the amino acid glycine (normal) was replaced by the amino acid valine. It is thought that the normal function of cell membrane–associated p21 *ras* proteins is to modulate cellular differentiation through signal transduction, with the mutation conferring transforming potential. Mutations in the *ras* family of genes have now been reported in many human cancers and are among the most common activated oncogenes (Bos, 1989).

The 1990s saw an exponential rate of development and application of molecular biology technology in cancer research, in particular with interest in another class of cancer regulatory gene, the tumor suppressor gene (Hollingsworth and Lee, 1991; Weinberg, 1991), and gene therapy strategies (Khuri and Kurie, 2000; Melcher et al, 1997). The *p53* tumor suppressor gene appears to have a central role in human neoplasia and has been implicated in control of the cell cycle, regulation of cellular differentiation, DNA repair and synthesis, and apoptosis (Levine et al, 1991). The most frequently altered gene in human cancer (Beroud and Soussi, 1998; Greenblatt et al, 1994; Hollstein et al, 1991), the *p53* tumor suppressor gene has been proposed as a clinically relevant molecular target (Harris, 1996). However, the relative importance of individual oncogenes and tumor suppressor genes, of the sequence of gene activation and interactions, and of pathways by which genes mediate their effect or potential for modulation by gene therapy is not yet known for esophageal cancer.

■ *HISTORICAL READINGS*

Allison PR, Johnstone AS: The esophagus lined with gastric mucous membrane. Thorax 8:87, 1953.

Huebner RJ, Todaro GJ: Oncogenes of RNA tumor viruses as determinants of cancer. Proc Natl Acad Sci U S A 64:1087, 1969.

Krontris TG, Cooper GM: Transforming activity of human tumor DNAs. Proc Natl Acad Sci U S A 78:1181, 1981.

Stehlin D, Varmus HE, Bishop JM, Vogt PK: DNA related to the transforming gene(s) of avian sarcoma viruses is present in normal avian DNA. Nature 260:170, 1976.

Tileston W: Peptic ulcer of the esophagus. Am J Med Sci 132:240, 1906.

EXPERIMENTAL MODELS AND CELL LINES

Esophageal squamous cell carcinomas were induced experimentally in various species of laboratory animals through the use of chemical carcinogens, particularly the *N*-nitroso compounds. These compounds are essentially alkylating agents, acting directly or indirectly through metabolic activation (Magee and Barnes, 1967). For example, *N*-methyl-*N*-nitrosourea was used to establish an esophageal tumor model in primates (Adamson et al, 1977), *N*-nitrosodiethylamine in cats (Schmahl et al, 1978), *N*-ethyl-*N*-nitrosoguanidine in dogs (Sasajima et al, 1977), and *N*-nitrosopiperidine in hamsters (Mohr et al, 1974) and rats (Ito et al, 1971). Well-defined histologic stages of tumor development were characterized in these models, further supporting the concept of multistep tumorigenesis. Because epidemiologic observations implicated dietary nitrosamines and related compounds in high-incidence geographic regions, it was believed that such experimental systems may have relevance to the pathogenesis of human esophageal cancer.

Methyl-benzylnitrosamine (MBNA), a naturally occurring nitrosamine, was implicated as a carcinogen in human esophageal cancer in China (Yang, 1980). It induces mainly esophageal tumors in rats, regardless of route of administration (Fong et al, 1978; Hodgson et al, 1980; Yang, 1980). Defined histologic stages or pathways of esophageal tumor development in rats were characterized by Reuber (1975, 1977) as follows. After administration of MBNA, hyperplasia of the basal cells appears as an early histologic change, which progresses to invasive squamous cell carcinoma along one of two stepwise pathways, either through a dysplasia to carcinoma in situ or as a papilloma.

Wang and associates (1990b) reported activation of point mutations of the H-*ras* oncogene in DNA extracted from MBNA-induced rat esophageal papillomas. All mutations were similar in nature, constituting transitions of the normal codon 12 nucleotides guanine and cytosine to adenine and thymidine. This specificity suggested a direct mutagenic effect of MBNA and was the first report of an activated oncogene in a chemically induced esophageal tumor.

Ohgaki and colleagues (1992) reported that rat esophageal tumors induced by *N*-nitroso compounds have a high incidence of mutations in the *p53* tumor suppressor gene. These mutations comprised guanine to adenine transitions and were localized to codons 204 and 213 in exon 6 of *p53*. The importance of *p53* and *ras* mutations in chemically induced esophageal tumors was further confirmed in a study using a zinc-deficient rat model (Fong et al, 1997). Such original observations potentially link our traditional understanding of carcinogenesis with later concepts of tumor biology. It is likely, however, that esophageal tumorigenesis requires molecular alterations of several additional key genes.

Growing evidence from experimental rat models utilizing esophagojejunostomy or esophagoduodenostomy suggests that reflux of duodenal contents (especially bile) modulates esophageal tumor histology, with a resulting increase in the incidence of adenocarcinomas (Attwood et al, 1992; Goldstein et al, 1997; Miwa et al, 1996; Pera et al, 1989). In a widely quoted study by Attwood and coworkers (1992), squamous cell esophageal tumors were induced in rats exposed to 2,6-dimethyl-nitrosomorpholine (DMNM) or methyl-*N*-amyl-nitrosamine (MNAN) at a rate of 25% or 30%, respectively. The rate of malignant change in the rat esophagus was increased after esophagoduodenal anastomosis (to produce duodenoesophageal reflux) and administration of DMNM (80%) or MNAN (67%). Esophageal adenocarcinomas were found to develop with greater frequency (50%) in this experimental rat model, suggesting a role for duodenoesophageal reflux in the development of esophageal adenocarcinomas, possibly mediated by epithelial cell hyperproliferation (Pera et al, 1998).

Other laboratory models used to investigate the multiple stages of the development and progression of esophageal cancer include xenografting of primary esophageal tumors in immunodeficient laboratory animals (El-Rifai et al, 1998), transgenic animal models (Lovejoy et al, 1997), and in vitro cell culture. Experience with the establishment of cell lines from esophageal squamous cell carcinomas was reported initially from South Africa by Robinson and colleagues (1980). Few such cell lines were established as continuously growing cell lines, and it was suggested that the inherent biologic aggressiveness of the tumor (local invasion, nodal metastases, 6-month survival), rather than culture technique, correlated with successful establishment of an esophageal cell line.

Many cell lines, however, were later reported to be cross-contaminated, a finding that has hindered further development of this model (Heldin et al, 1988). Significant progress has nevertheless been made in the establishment of esophageal cancer cell lines derived from patients in North America (Banks-Schlegel et al, 1986; Washington et al, 1994), the United Kingdom (Rockett et al, 1997), China (Yang, 1980), and Japan (Nishihira et al, 1993; Shimada et al, 1992). Two reports have documented *p53* gene mutations in esophageal carcinoma cell lines (Tanaka et al, 1996; Wang et al, 1995). Techniques to increase the success rate of long-term cell culture have also been developed (Shimada et al, 1992). A novel approach to maintenance of an esophageal cell line in continuous laboratory culture by transfection of human esophageal epithelial cells with SV40 T antigen and the *hst*-1 gene was reported by Light and associates (1990) and may see increasing application in future laboratory studies.

It should be appreciated that the experimental models and studies summarized previously may not necessarily reflect the development of esophageal cancer in humans. Papillomas are rarely seen in the human esophagus. However, basal cell hyperplasia, dysplasia, and carcinoma in situ are well-recognized histologic changes of the esophageal mucosa that are frequently observed in association with invasive squamous cell carcinoma. Similar histologic findings may also be seen in Barrett's epithelium and associated primary esophageal adenocarcinomas (McArdle et al, 1992; Thurberg et al, 1999), suggesting a multistep metaplasia-dysplasia-carcinoma pathway for human esophageal adenocarcinoma.

CYTOGENETICS

Despite their relative technical difficulty, early cytogenetic studies of human solid tumors suggested regions of chromosomes that would subsequently be shown to have molecular genetic importance. Chromosome rearrangements, such as insertions and translocations, were associated with oncogene activation, whereas chromosomal deletions, causing loss or inactivation of genes, suggested the presence of tumor suppressor genes (Hollingsworth and Lee, 1991; Weinberg, 1991).

A comprehensive karyotypic analysis of human esophageal squamous cell tumor cell lines was reported by Whang-Peng and colleagues (1990). The total number of chromosomes per cell varied widely, with extensive chromosomal structural changes, the most common being nonrandom abnormalities involving deletions of chromosomes 1, 3, 9, and 11. Attempts to achieve karyotypic analysis of fresh tumors were reported to be unsuccessful.

Conventional cytogenetic techniques, applied as described previously, are limited by both the size of chromosome to be visualized (at least 5 megabases of DNA) and the requirement that cells be cultured and stimulated into mitosis for banding. More modern molecular cytogenetic techniques, such as fluorescence in situ hybridization, which can resolve smaller structural chromosomal changes (<1 kilobase of DNA), may be applied to detect multiple chromosomal changes in heterogeneous cell populations and to follow cytogenetic changes at various stages of tumor development. Since the early 1990s, comparative genomic hybridization has become the most popular molecular cytogenetic tool to analyze the entire genome (Forozan et al, 1997). These cytogenic techniques are complemented by molecular genetic techniques, such as restriction-landmark genomic scanning, differential display, serial analysis of gene expression, and microarray techniques, for genome-wide screening of copy number, structure, and expression of genes and DNA sequences.

Nonrandom chromosomal abnormalities are frequently observed in specimens of esophageal cancer as well as the precursor lesions, suggesting that these events are causally related to esophageal carcinogenesis (Aoki et al, 1994; Dolan et al, 1998; Menke-Pluymers et al, 1996; Pack et al, 1999; van Dekken et al, 1999). Cytogenetic and molecular analyses have consistently revealed evidence of allelic loss involving 2q, 3p, 5q, 9p, 11p, 12q, 13q, 17q, 17p, 18q, and Xq; interestingly, loss of Y chromosome is an extremely common and early event. Although allelic loss involving 3p, 5q, 9p, and 17p may disrupt known tumor suppressor genes, the genes specifically targeted by the remaining allelic losses have not yet been identified.

CELL CYCLE KINETICS

Tumor kinetics of esophageal squamous cell carcinomas were studied in endoscopic biopsy specimens from Chinese patients, through the use of a thymidine-labeling assay to evaluate cellular proliferation and percentage of cells in S phase (Wang et al, 1990a). An increase in the overall thymidine labeling index was seen as histologically normal esophageal epithelium progressed to hyperplasia and low-grade and high-grade dysplasia. Proliferating cells were localized to the basal layer in normal epithelium, but expansion toward the mucosal surface was seen with hyperplasia and dysplasia. This finding suggested a functional instability of the esophageal mucosa, which presumably confers greater risk for worsening dysplasia and malignant change.

Flow cytometric and molecular analyses of dysplastic squamous and Barrett's epithelia have revealed that esophageal cancers arise via widespread clonal outgrowth of cells exhibiting aberrant cell cycle regulation (Barrett et al, 1996a; Giaretti et al, 1997; Reid et al, 1993). In general, genomic instability precedes the appearance of histologic abnormalities in esophageal mucosa, and the extent of cell cycle derangements influences progression to malignancy in this setting (Fennerty et al, 1989; Galipeau et al, 1996; Jankowski et al, 1999; Krishnadath et al, 1995). Using flow cytometry techniques, Reid and colleagues (1992) prospectively evaluated 62 patients with Barrett's esophagus. Nine of 13 patients (2 with Barrett's metaplasia, 5 with low-grade dysplasia, and 2 with high-grade dysplasia) in whom these researchers found flow cytometric evidence of aberrant cell cycle regulation eventually experienced high-grade dysplasia or invasive carcinoma; none of 49 patients with normal flow cytometric findings demonstrated esophageal malignancy during the 34-month study.

In normal esophageal epithelia, proliferation is governed by complex interactions between stimulatory and inhibitory signals mediated by proto-oncogenes and tumor suppressor genes, respectively. Growth factor stimulation induces quiescent (G_0) cells to enter and progress through the G_1 phase of the cell cycle (Fig. 40–1). Progression through G_1 requires continuous external mitogenic stimulation until the restriction point is traversed, after which the cell becomes committed to divide irrespective of exogenous growth factor support. Following G_1, cells progress into S phase, in which DNA replication occurs, and then proceed through G_2 to undergo mitosis during M phase. Checkpoints at the G_1/S transition and G_2/M transition ensure genomic integrity prior to DNA replication and entry into mitosis, respectively (Hunter and Pines, 1994; Sherr, 1996).

Progression through the cell cycle occurs via the sequential formation, activation, and degradation of holoenzyme complexes consisting of specific cyclin and cyclin-dependent kinase (cdk). These complexes interact with regulatory proteins involved in cell proliferation. Cyclin D1/cdk4 (and cdk6) primarily regulates progression through early and mid-G_1, whereas cyclin E–cdk2 controls the transition from G_1 into S phase. Cyclins A and B together with cdk2 (and cdk1) govern progression through S, G_2, and M phases (Grana and Reddy, 1995; Martin-Castellanos and Moreno, 1997).

A variety of oncogene and tumor suppressor gene mutations frequently observed in esophageal cancers and their precursor lesions disrupt cell cycle regulation by perturbing the G_1 restriction point (Table 40–1). The retinoblastoma (Rb) protein governs the restriction point by sequestering E2F transcription factors (Fig. 40–2). During mid-G_1, Rb is phosphorylated by cyclin D–cdk4 or cyclin D–cdk6 complexes, thereby liberating E2F, which activates transcription of genes required for DNA synthesis in S phase. The *p16*^{INK4a} tumor suppressor gene product inhibits the association of cdk4 and cdk6 with cyclin D1. Enhanced expression of *ras*, either by mutations directly involving this proto-oncogene or by overexpression of upstream growth factor receptors, induces expression of cyclin D1 (Filmus et al, 1994; Lukas et al, 1996). Aberrant growth signals from activated oncogenes induce the expression of the *p14/ARF* gene product (see

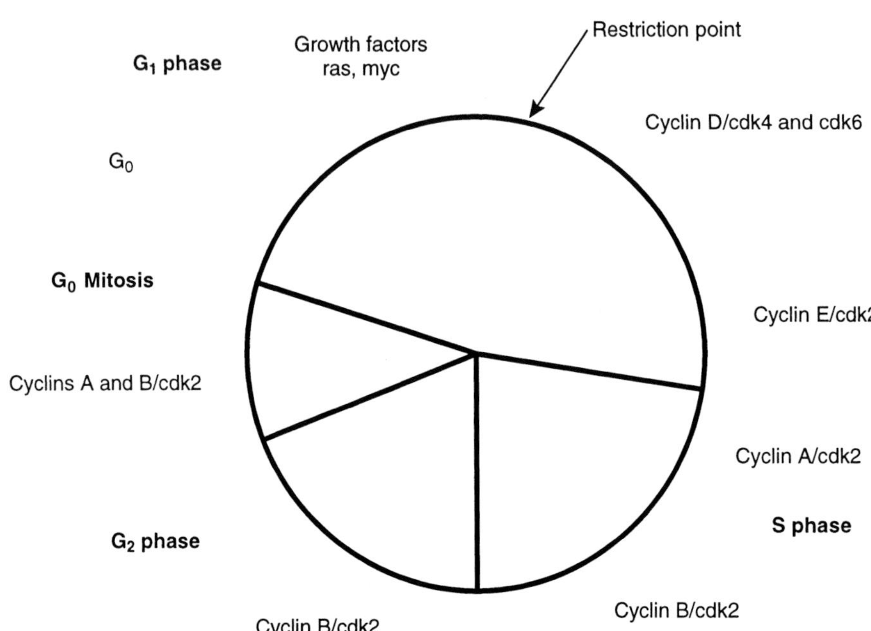

FIGURE 40–1 ■ Eukaryotic cell cycle.

TABLE 40–1 ■ Oncogene and Tumor Suppressor Gene Mutations Frequently Observed in Esophageal Cancers

Oncogenes	*Tumor Suppressors*
EGFr	3p *(FHIT)*
erbB2	Rb
Cyclin D1	*p53*
	p16
	p14/ARF
	Telomerase

EGFr, epidermal growth factor receptor; *FHIT*, fragile histidine triad.

later), which functions to stabilize the *p53* tumor suppressor gene product (Chin et al, 1998; Zhang et al, 1998). *p53* mediates apoptosis in response to activated oncogenes or genotoxic stress and induces cell cycle arrest by enhancing the expression of p21 (WAF-1), which sequesters a variety of cyclin-dependent kinases, including cdk4 and cdk6 (El-Deiry et al, 1993; Kirsch and Kastan, 1998). Hence, control of the G_1 restriction point can be circumvented by the loss of Rb, *p16*, *ARF*, or *p53* tumor suppressor gene expression or by overexpression of *ras* or *cyclin D;* all of these events result in promiscuous DNA replication and cell cycle progression.

A reciprocal relationship between Rb, cyclin D, and p16 expression has been observed in esophageal cancers. In general, esophageal cancers that lack Rb expression tend to have normal cyclin D1 and p16 expression; in contrast, cancers that retain Rb expression typically exhibit cyclin D1 overexpression, p16 inactivation, or both (Jiang et al, 1993; Schrump et al, 1996). In the majority of esophageal cancers, restriction point control is circumvented via overexpression of cyclin D1, inactivation of *p16*, or both—often in the context of *p53* mutations. Although this discussion has been highly simplified, these concepts provide a useful framework for understanding the mechanisms of esophageal carcinogenesis and for designing strategies for molecular intervention in this disease.

MOLECULAR GENETICS

Growth Factor Receptors and Proto-Oncogenes

A variety of growth factors and growth factor receptors are aberrantly expressed in esophageal cancers, some of which appear relevant to the biology and the clinical behavior of these neoplasms.

Epidermal Growth Factor Receptor

The epidermal growth factor receptor (EGFr) is a 170-kd tyrosine kinase glycoprotein that is overexpressed in approximately 80% and 30% of esophageal squamous cell cancers and adenocarcinomas, respectively (Al-Kasspooles et al, 1993; Itakura et al, 1994); nearly 40% of these tumors express transforming growth factor–α (TGF-α) which binds to EGFr to stimulate growth via autocrine mechanisms (Iihara et al, 1993). Several studies have suggested that EGFr expression may have prognostic significance in patients with esophageal cancer. Itakura and associates (1994) reported a significant correlation between EGFr immunoreactivity and poor survival after resection of esophageal squamous cell carcinomas. Iihara and colleagues (1993) observed expression of TGF-α in 35% and EGFr expression in 43% of 57 esophageal squamous cell cancers; coexpression of TGF-α and EGFr was observed in 12 tumors. Expression of either TGF-α or EGFr or coexpression of these markers correlated with diminished survival in patients with "node-positive" esophageal squamous cell carcinomas.

Kitagawa and associates (1996) evaluated the prognostic significance of EGFr expression in 107 patients with esophageal squamous cell carcinoma who had undergone curative surgery. EGFr gene amplification was detected in 13 (12%) of 107 carcinomas; multivariate analysis revealed that EGFr gene amplification was an independent prognostic factor in the predilection for lymph node metastases and diminished survival in patients with esophageal squamous cell carcinomas. In a later study, Shimada and colleagues (1999) evaluated the prognostic significance of a variety of molecular markers, including EGFr, in esophageal cancer specimens from 116 patients after potentially curative resection. Logistic regression analysis revealed that lymph node involvement, as well as overexpression of cyclin D1 and EGFr, increased the risk of hematogenous recurrence in these patients.

The erbB2 *Gene*

The *erbB2* gene encodes a 185-kd tyrosine kinase receptor molecule, p185, that is structurally related to EGFr; heregulin is the putative ligand for this receptor (Hung and Lau, 1999). p185 mediates significant mitogenic activity and appears to regulate the expression and function of a variety of other receptors, including EGFr. Data also indicate that p185 modulates interaction of cancer cells

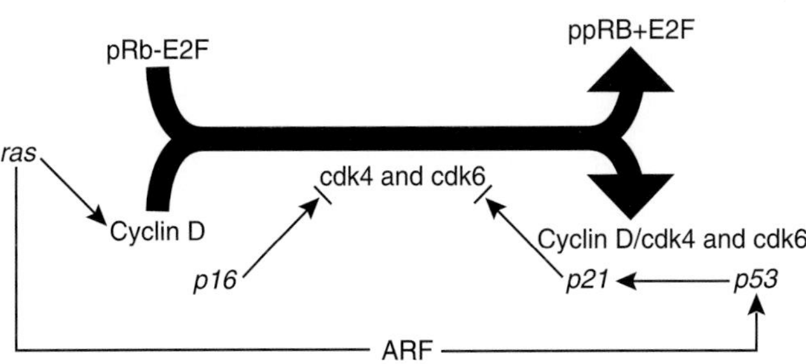

FIGURE 40–2 ■ Regulation of the G_1 restriction point.

with extracellular matrix (Roetger et al, 1998; Wiechen et al, 1999) and induces expression of vascular endothelial growth factor (VEGF), which is critical for tumor neovascularization (Petit et al, 1997). Additional studies have indicated that *erbB2* overexpression correlates with in vitro drug resistance and that abrogation of p185 expression may enhance chemosensitivity in cancer cells (Shi et al, 1992; Tsai et al, 1996).

Overexpression of *erbB2* has been observed in approximately 30% to 50% of esophageal adenocarcinomas (Al-Kasspooles et al, 1993; Moskaluk et al, 1998); however, its prognostic significance remains unclear at this time. Polkowski and associates (1999) observed overexpression of *erbB2* in 24% of adenocarcinomas of the distal esophagus and gastroesophageal junction. Interestingly, 10 of 30 stage III/IV tumors overexpressed *erbB2*, in contrast to none of 11 stage I/II cancers in this study. Cox regression analysis revealed that *erbB2* expression was not independent from clinical stage in determining patient survival. Furthermore, Wang and colleagues (1999) detected no significant correlation between *erbB2* expression and survival in 117 patients undergoing potentially curative esophagectomy. Thus, although considerable experimental data suggest that p185 overexpression is an important event during malignant transformation, the clinical significance of *erbB2* expression in esophageal cancers has yet to be defined.

ras *Mutation*

Although *ras* mutations are frequently observed in a variety of cancers, including pulmonary carcinomas, this gene is rarely mutated in esophageal malignancies (Casson et al, 1997). Thus, aberrant expression of growth factor receptors appears to be the major mechanism by which ras signaling is enhanced during esophageal carcinogenesis.

Cyclin D1

Overexpression of cyclin D1 has been observed in nearly 40% to 60% of esophageal adenocarcinomas and squamous cell carcinomas and in nearly 30% of biopsy specimens from patients with precancerous Barrett's epithelium (Adelaide et al, 1995; Arber et al, 1996; Jiang et al, 1992; Yoshida et al, 1993). Gene amplification as well as overexpression due to mutations involving upstream growth factor receptors such as EGFr and p185 may contribute to aberrant cyclin D1 expression in esophageal cancers (Roncalli et al, 1998). Abrogation of cyclin D1 overexpression via antisense techniques inhibits the proliferation and tumorigenicity of esophageal cancer cells (Zhou et al, 1995), suggesting that cyclin D1 overexpression is an important molecular event during esophageal carcinogenesis.

Several studies have indicated that overexpression of cyclin D1 may also have prognostic significance in patients with esophageal cancer. Shimada and colleagues (1999) observed a correlation among cyclin D1 overexpression, hematogenous recurrence, and diminished survival in 116 patients undergoing potentially curative resection. Takeuchi and associates (Takeuchi et al, 1997) noted a correlation between cyclin D1 overexpression and distant metastases as well as diminished survival in 111 patients after esophagectomy. Roncalli and coworkers (1998) evaluated the expression of a variety of molecular markers, including cyclin D1, in a series of 74 esophageal carcinomas. Amplification of cyclin D1 was observed in 17 (31%) of 55 cases and was particularly frequent in squamous cell carcinomas. Overexpression of cyclin D1 correlated in a statistically significant manner with lymph node metastases, advanced tumor stage, and reduced overall survival. Irrespective of the mechanisms by which it occurs, overexpression of cyclin D1 appears to be a significant factor in modulation of the malignant phenotype of esophageal carcinoma cells.

Tumor Suppressor Genes

Fragile Histidine Triad Gene

Deletions involving 3p have been detected in 60% to 100% of esophageal cancers as well as a significant percentage of specimens derived from Barrett's esophagus; 3p allelic loss appears to be a very early molecular event associated with Barrett's adenocarcinogenesis (Jankowski et al, 1999; Krishnadath et al, 1995). Although the tumor suppressors that are silenced by 3p mutations have not been identified conclusively, one major target appears to be the fragile histidine triad (*FHIT*) gene, which is involved in hydrolyzing dinucleotide triphosphates and modulates cell cycle progression and apoptosis (Brenner et al, 1999; Sard et al, 1999).

Restoration of *FHIT* expression inhibits in vitro proliferation and tumorigenicity of cancer cells, suggesting that *FHIT* functions as a tumor suppressor gene (Ji et al, 1999). Point mutations or deletions in this gene result in the loss of FHIT protein expression; promoter methylation is an additional mechanism of *FHIT* inactivation (Ohata et al, 1996; Tanaka et al, 1998). Aberrant expression of *FHIT* has been observed in 50% to 90% of esophageal cancers and 85% of specimens derived from Barrett's esophagus examined to date (Chen et al, 1997; Michael et al, 1997). Although the prognostic significance of *FHIT* mutations in esophageal cancers has not been defined, these mutations correlate with greater tobacco exposure and diminished survival in patients with lung cancer (Nelson et al, 1998; Tomizawa et al, 1998).

Retinoblastoma (Rb) Gene

The retinoblastoma (*Rb*) gene, located on 13q14, encodes a 105-kd nuclear phosphoprotein that governs the G_1 restriction point (Chen et al, 1995). A variety of regulatory proteins, including cyclin-dependent kinases, transcription factors, and viral oncoproteins, interact with Rb and related proteins (p107 and p130) to regulate cell cycle progression (Ewen, 1994). Rb is a critical mediator of cell cycle arrest after DNA damage (Harrington et al, 1998). Restoration of Rb expression by gene transfer techniques induces cell cycle arrest in cancer cells (Demers et al, 1998).

Mutations involving the retinoblastoma gene frequently disrupt RNA splicing, resulting in the loss of Rb protein expression (Dolan et al, 1998; Harbour et al, 1988; Jiang et al, 1993; Reid et al, 1993). *Rb* mutations have been observed in approximately 20% to 40% of esophageal cancers as well as Barrett's esophagus; *Rb* mutations occur more frequently in tumors that also exhibit mutations involving *p53* (Xing et al, 1999c). Studies suggest that loss of Rb expression correlates with advanced stage of disease, nodal metastases, and diminished survival in patients with esophageal cancer (Roncalli et al, 1998).

The *p16* Gene

The *p16* tumor suppressor gene product encoded on 9p21 inhibits the activity of cdk4 and cdk6, thus preventing cyclin D–dependent phosphorylation of the Rb protein at the restriction point (Grana et al, 1995). Inactivation of *p16* by allelic deletion or point mutation has been detected in approximately 20% of esophageal squamous cell cancers (Esteve et al, 1996; Xing et al, 1999b). Barrett and colleagues (1996b) observed LOH involving 9p21 in 24 of 32 (75%) aneuploid cell populations derived from esophageal adenocarcinomas as well as 7 of 7 samples of premalignant Barrett's epithelia from patients whose tumors had *p16* mutations. Allelic loss involving *p16* preceded the onset of aneuploidy in 13 of 15 specimens. Somatic mutation silenced the remaining *p16* allele in 23% of the aneuploid cell samples. Promoter silencing by methylation mechanisms contributes to *p16* inactivation in an additional 50% of squamous cell or adenocarcinomas of the esophagus (Wong et al, 1997; Xing et al, 1999b). Data also suggest that *p16* inactivation correlates with cyclin D1 overexpression and diminished survival in patients with esophageal cancer (Takeuchi et al, 1997). Restoration of *p16* expression by gene therapy techniques profoundly inhibits the proliferation and tumorigenicity of esophageal cancer cells (Schrump et al, 1996), attesting to the significance of *p16* inactivation during esophageal carcinogenesis.

The *p14* Gene

The *p14/ARF* gene product is encoded by an alternate reading frame in the *p16* locus; studies indicate that *ARF* prevents interaction of p53 with MDM2, a protein that facilitates p53 degradation (Zhang et al, 1998). *ARF* mediates *p53*-dependent apoptosis in response to activated proto-oncogenes such as *myc* and *ras* (Palmero et al, 1998); however, *ARF* does not appear to be involved in regulating p53 response to genotoxic stress, a fact that may explain the simultaneous loss of *ARF* and *p53* expression in many cancers (Gazzeri et al, 1998).

The *p16/ARF* gene locus is unique, in that it encodes two separate protein products that link the *Rb* and *p53* tumor suppressor pathways (Bates et al, 1998); thus, it is not surprising that mutations involving 9p21 have significant ramifications for cell cycle regulation. Inactivation of *ARF* occurs by allelic deletion as well as methylation mechanisms that simultaneously inactivate *p16* (Robertson and Jones, 1998). Expression of *ARF* in esophageal cancers and their precursor lesions has not been systematically analyzed; however, Xing and associates (1999a) performed a comprehensive analysis of the mechanisms responsible for silencing expression of *p14/ARF* and *p16* in 40 esophageal cancers. Aberrant promoter methylation involving *ARF* or *p16* was observed in 15% and 40% of specimens, respectively. Whereas most of the *p16* methylations were exclusive, nearly all of the methylations involving *ARF* also involved *p16*. Homozygous deletions involving *ARF* and *p16* were seen in 33% and 18% of specimens, respectively. Collectively, these data indicate that in esophageal squamous cell cancers, *p14/ARF* is a primary target for homozygous deletion, whereas *p16* appears to be more frequently silenced by hypermethylation.

The different mechanisms responsible for silencing these tumor suppressor genes in esophageal cancers highlight the complexities inherent in esophageal carcinogenesis and indicate the level of sophistication necessary to target specific genetic alterations in esophageal cancers. Conceivably, inactivation of *p14/ARF* is a major mechanism by which *p53* pathways are circumvented in esophageal cancers that retain *p53* expression.

The *p53* Gene

The *p53* gene encodes a 53-kd polypeptide that regulates cell cycle progression, DNA repair, apoptosis, and neovascularization in normal and malignant cells via highly complex DNA as well as protein interactions (Kastan et al, 1995). As previously discussed, oncogene activation is mediated to *p53* via *ARF*; however, genotoxic stress resulting from DNA damage or telomeric shortening (see later) directly induces *p53* expression (Saretzki et al, 1999; Sherr, 1998). A nonspecific DNA binding domain in the carboxy-terminal region of *p53* interacts with single-stranded (mutated) DNA; depending on the extent of DNA damage, a sequence-specific DNA binding site in the central region of the *p53* molecule induces either cell cycle arrest and DNA repair or apoptosis (Kastan et al, 1991). *p53* mediates cell cycle arrest in part by inducing the expression of p21 (*WAF-1*), which sequesters a variety of cyclin-dependent kinases facilitating G_1 as well as G_2/M arrest (El-Deiry et al, 1994). *p53* mediates apoptosis by a variety of mechanisms, including caspase activation, upregulation of FAS and FAS ligand, as well as the proapoptotic protein BAX; *p53* may also induce apoptosis via transcription-independent mechanisms (Kastan et al, 1995). *p53* may influence the metastatic potential of tumor cells by inhibiting expression of VEGF (Fontanini et al, 1998). Restoration of *p53* expression by gene therapy techniques induces apoptosis and confers sensitivity to radiation and chemotherapeutic agents in esophageal cancer cells (Matsubara et al, 1999; Schrump and Nguyen, 1999).

p53 gene mutations were reported first in esophageal squamous cell carcinomas (Hollstein et al, 1990) and subsequently in primary esophageal adenocarcinomas and associated Barrett's epithelium (Casson et al, 1991). Examples of a *p53* gene mutation and *p53* protein distribution in Barrett's epithelium are shown in Figures 40–3 and 40–4, respectively. *p53* gene alterations in esophageal carcinomas have now been confirmed by several other investigators (Bennett et al, 1992; Campomenosi et al, 1996; Casson et al, 1998; Gao et al, 1994; Gleeson et al, 1995; Huang et al, 1993; Jankowski et al, 1992; Moskaluk et al, 1996; Neshat et al, 1994; Schneider et al, 1996).

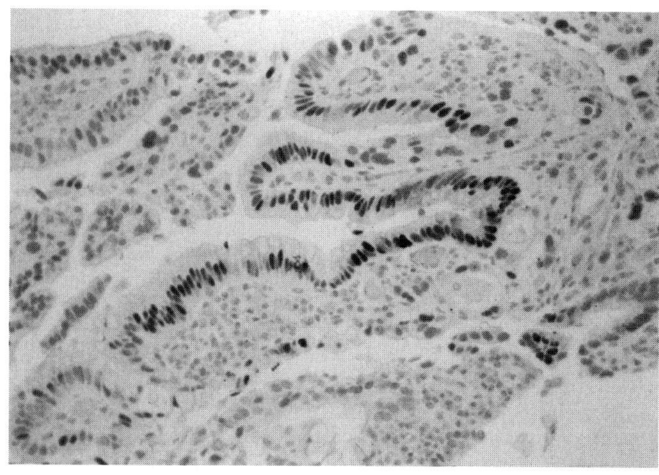

FIGURE 40–3 ■ Photomicrograph showing distribution of *p53* protein (dark nuclear staining) in Barrett's epithelium (DO7 monoclonal anti-*p53* antibody; ×300.)

The majority of *p53* mutations occur in evolutionarily conserved residues within the sequence-specific DNA binding domain (Hainaut et al, 1998).

Because p53 regulates the expression or function of multiple genes involved in cell cycle control (Robert et al, 2000), mutations involving this tumor suppressor gene might be expected to enhance the malignant phenotype of esophageal cancers. In the most comprehensive study of primary esophageal adenocarcinomas (defined by strict clinicopathologic criteria) reported to date, *p53* mutations were associated with poorly differentiated tumors and reduced disease-free and overall survival (Casson et al, 1998).

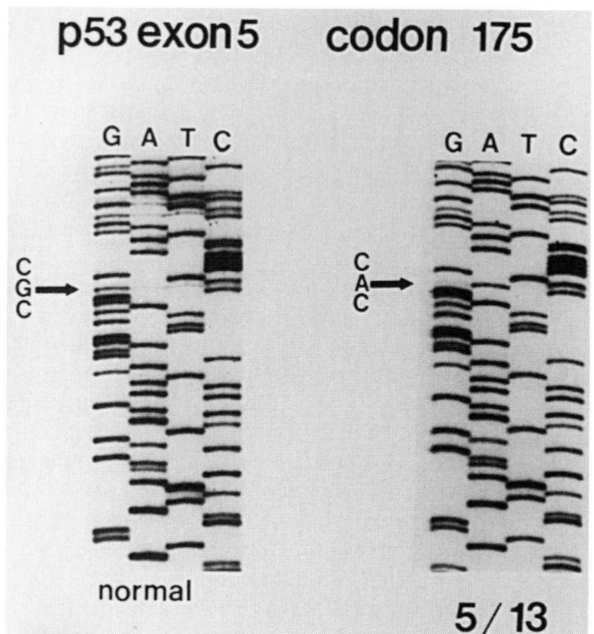

FIGURE 40–4 ■ Sequence analysis of Barrett's epithelium (5/13) and corresponding histologically normal esophageal mucosa (*left panel*). A point mutation (CAC) is found at codon 175 (exon 5) of *p53* in the Barrett's specimen. The normal sequence at codon 175 is CGC. Nucleotides: G, guanine; A, adenine; T, thymidine; C, cytosine.

Telomerase

Following a finite number of divisions, normal cells undergo senescence—a state of irreversible cell cycle arrest due to activation of *Rb* and *p53* in response to genotoxic stress and shortening of chromosomal ends (telomeres) during DNA synthesis (Vaziri and Benchimol, 1999). Mutations involving *Rb* or *p53* relieve the senescent state, allowing cells to undergo additional divisions with progressive loss of telomere length until *crisis* occurs, escape from which is possible only by overexpression of telomerase, a ribonucleoprotein that adds hexameric DNA repeats to chromosomal ends to prevent further loss of telomere length (Cerni, 2000). Telomerase has two components, telomerase RNA (TR) and telomerase reverse transcriptase protein (TERT). TR appears to be present in most normal cells, whereas TERT is expressed only in transformed cells. Overexpression of TR has been observed frequently in esophageal cancers as well as Barrett's esophagus (Hiyama et al, 1999).

Koyanagi and associates (1999) detected telomerase expression in 100% of 57 esophageal squamous cell cancers, compared with 5 of 50 (10%) normal tissue samples, 4 of which had tumor cells infiltrating vessels in the mucosa or submucosa. Morales and associates (1998) evaluated TR levels in a variety of formalin-fixed, paraffin-embedded tissues obtained from specimens of esophageal adenocarcinoma and Barrett's esophagus. One hundred percent of adenocarcinomas and high-grade dysplasias exhibited high-level expression of telomerase; in contrast, weak to moderate expression was detected in 70% of Barrett's metaplasias, and moderate expression was seen in the vast majority of low-grade dysplasias.

Asai and colleagues (1998) observed no correlation between tumor doubling time and telomerase activity in a panel of cultured esophageal cancer lines; however, cell lines with short telomeres—but not those with relatively long telomers—appeared to be resistant to cisplatin. Although the clinical relevance of telomerase activity in esophageal cancers has not been defined (Takubo et al, 1997), the fact that abrogation of telomerase activity is sufficient to induce death in cultured cancer cells (Hahn et al, 1999) strongly suggests that telomerase may significantly influence the malignant behavior of these neoplasms.

Implications for Therapy

Although the prognostic significance of each of these molecular alterations remains unclear, abundant data confirm that mutations involving growth factor receptors, *cyclin D1, Rb, p16, p53,* and *telomerase* are appropriate targets for intervention in esophageal cancers and their precursor lesions. A variety of pharmacologic agents and antibodies antagonize signal transduction from cell surface growth factor receptors implicated in carcinogenesis and chemoresistance. These include novel compounds that specifically inhibit the tyrosine kinase activity of EGFr, or erbB2, and enhance the efficacy of conventional cytotoxic agents. Nguyen and associates (manuscript in preparation) evaluated the effects of 17-allylamino geldanamycin (17-AAG, a pharmacologic inhibitor of p185 expression) in cultured esophageal cancer cells. Dose-dependent depletion of p185 protein expression and diminished in vitro proliferation were observed with an inhibitory concentration 50% (IC 50) of 116 nanomolar for esophageal adenocarcinomas, and of 320 nanomolar for epidermoid cancer cells that overexpressed cyclin D1. Reduced doses of 17-AAG (20 to 40 nanomolar) that by themselves exhibited minimal inhibitory activity synergistically potentiated the effects of paclitaxel in esophageal cancer cells irrespective of histology. Enhanced paclitaxel sensitivity following 17-AAG treatment correlated with cell cycle arrest and apoptosis in these cells. Chemotherapeutic regimens that exploit these observations are currently under evaluation at the National Cancer Institute.

Present delivery systems for gene transfer are not practical for treatment of local or disseminated disease; however, novel pharmacologic agents have been identified that specifically target the *Rb* tumor suppressor pathway, which is disrupted in virtually all esophageal cancers. Flavopiridol, is a synthetic flavone that inhibits several cyclin-dependent kinases (including cdk4 and cdk6), reduces *cyclin D1* and *BCL-2* expression, and induces cell cycle arrest and apoptosis in a variety of cancer cells (Carlson et al, 1996; Konig et al, 1997). Schrump and colleagues (1998) reported that flavopiridol mediates profound cell cycle arrest and apoptosis in esophageal cancer cells irrespective of both histology and *Rb, p53, cyclin D1*, or *p16* expression. In their study, flavopiridol inhibited cyclin *D1* mRNA expression and diminished Rb and p107 protein levels, effects that preceded the onset of apoptosis in these cells. Additional studies have revealed that pretreatment of esophageal cancer cells with flavopiridol markedly enhances their sensitivity to paclitaxel by synchronizing them at the G_2-M interface, where sensitivity to paclitaxel is maximal (Schrump and Nguyen, 1999).

In addition to being a novel agent for the treatment of esophageal cancers, flavopiridol may be a potential chemoprevention agent because it effectively targets three mutational events (i.e., cyclin D1 overexpression as well as *Rb* and *p16* inactivation) that are known to occur early during multistep esophageal carcinogenesis. These data have provided the preclinical rationale for a phase 2 study involving sequential flavopiridol-paclitaxel administration in patients with esophageal cancer.

Approximately 50% of esophageal cancers exhibit loss of *p16* expression due to promoter hypermethylation. Studies by Weiser and colleagues (2000a) at the National Cancer Institute have revealed that the demethylating agent 5-Aza-2′-deoxycytidine (DAC) markedly enhances *p16* expression in esophageal cancer cells; furthermore, these investigators have observed that the histone deacetylase inhibitor depsipeptide (DP) FR901228 synergistically enhances apoptosis in these cells. Interestingly, growth arrest and apoptosis following sequential DAC/DP treatment do not appear to correlate with *p16, Rb*, or *p53* expression in these cells. Additional studies have revealed that sequential DAC/DP treatment enhances expression of the tumor antigens MAGE-3 and NY-ESO-1 in esophageal cancer cells and enables their recognition by HLA-restricted cytolytic T cells specific for NY-ESO-1 (Weiser et al, 2000b). Clinical trials designed to evaluate the ability of DAC and DP to mediate target gene induction and apoptosis in patients with esophageal cancer are currently under way in the Thoracic Oncology Section, Surgery Branch of the National Cancer Institute.

Data from other studies provide the rationale for molecular interventions specifically targeting mutations involving growth factor receptors as well as the *Rb* tumor suppressor pathway in esophageal cancers and their precursor lesions. These agents, together with compounds that have been discovered to target *p53* mutations and telomerase expression in cancer cells (Hahn et al, 1999; Foster et al, 1999), may ultimately facilitate the development of more precise and efficacious treatment for highly lethal esophageal neoplasms.

COMMENTS AND CONTROVERSIES

Advances in molecular biology have influenced our current understanding of the pathogenesis of human cancer. Molecular genetic changes have been described in esophageal cancers, although their biologic significance is currently unknown. It is likely that many more genes will be associated with various stages of the development and progression of esophageal cancer, providing further insight into esophageal tumor biology. This insight is currently of importance, as the incidence of primary esophageal adenocarcinomas is rising in North America.

Study of such molecular markers may have potential clinical application in the early diagnosis of esophageal cancer in high-risk patients. Patients with Barrett's epithelium who are enrolled in endoscopic surveillance programs would appear to represent a particularly promising population providing relatively easy endoscopic access to a relevant human model tumor system. In the future, molecular markers may be incorporated into conventional clinicopathologic staging systems, either as stratification factors in future clinical trials of adjuvant therapies for esophageal cancer or as targets for novel anticancer therapies.

D. S. S.
A. G. C

KEY REFERENCES

Jankowski JA, Wright NA, Meltzer SJ, et al: Molecular evolution of the metaplasia-dysplasia-adenocarcinoma sequence in the esophagus. Am J Pathol 154:965, 1999.

This article reviews the molecular biology of esophageal cancer.

Schrump DS, Nguyen DM: Strategies for molecular intervention in esophageal cancers and their precursor lesions. Dis Esophagus 12:181, 1999.

Part of a symposium on the molecular biology of esophageal cancer (VIIth World Congress, International Society for Diseases of the Esophagus, Montreal, September 1998), this manuscript summarizes evolving strategies for the molecular therapy of esophageal cancer.

■ REFERENCES

Adamson RK, Krolikowski FL, Correa P, et al: Carcinogenicity of N-methyl-N-nitrosurea in chickens and domestic cats. J Natl Cancer Inst 59:415, 1977.

Adelaide, J, Monges, G, Derderian C, et al: Oesophageal cancer and amplification of the human cyclin D gene CCND1/PRAD1. Br J Cancer 71:64, 1995.

Al-Kasspooles, M, Moore, JH, Orringer, MB, Beer, DG: Amplification and over-expression of the EGFR and erbB-2 genes in human esophageal adenocarcinomas. Int J Cancer 54:213, 1993.

Allison PR, Johnstone AS: The esophagus lined with gastric mucous membrane. Thorax 8:87, 1953.

Aoki T, Mori T, Xiqun D, et al: Allelotype study of esophageal carcinoma. Genes Chromosomes Cancer 10:177, 1994.

Arber N, Lightdale C, Rotterdam H, et al: Increased expression of the cyclin D1 gene in Barrett's esophagus. Cancer Epidemiol Biomarkers Prev 5:457, 1996.

Asai A, Kiyozuka Y, Yoshida R, et al: Telomere length, telomerase activity and telomerase RNA expression in human esophageal cancer cells: Correlation with cell proliferation, differentiation and chemosensitivity to anticancer drugs. Anticancer Res 18:1465, 1998.

Attwood SEA, Smyrk TC, DeMeester TR, et al: Duodenoesophageal reflux and the development of esophageal adenocarcinoma in rats. Surgery 111:503, 1992.

Banks-Schlegel SP, Quintero J: Growth and differentiation of human esophageal squamous carcinoma cell lines. Cancer Res 46:250, 1986.

Barrett MT, Galipeau PC, Sanchez CA, et al: Determination of the frequency of loss of heterozygosity in esophageal adenocarcinoma by cell sorting, whole genome amplification and microsatellite polymorphisms. Oncogene 12:1873, 1996a.

Barrett MT, Sanchez CA, Galipeau PC, et al: Allelic loss of 9p21 and mutation of the CDKN2/p16 gene develop as early lesions during neoplastic progression in Barrett's esophagus. Oncogene 13:1867, 1996b.

Barrett NR: Chronic peptic ulcer of the esophagus and esophagitis. Br J Surg 38:175, 1950.

Barrett NR: The lower esophagus lined by columnar epithelium. Surgery 41:881, 1957.

Bates S, Phillips AC, Clark PA, et al: p14ARF links the tumour suppressors RB and p53. Nature 395:124, 1998.

Bennett WP, Hollstein MC, Metcalf RA, et al: p53 mutation and protein accumulation during multistage human esophageal carcinogenesis. Cancer Res 52:6092, 1992.

Beroud C, Soussi T: p53 gene mutation: Software and database. Nucleic Acids Res 26:200, 1998.

Blot WJ, Devesa SS, Fraumeni JF: Continuing climb in rates of esophageal adenocarcinoma: An update. JAMA 270:1320, 1993.

Blot WJ, Devesa SS, Kneller RW, Fraumeni JF: Rising incidence of adenocarcinoma of the esophagus and gastric cardia. JAMA 265:1287, 1991.

Blot WJ, McLaughlin JK: The changing epidemiology of esophageal cancer. Semin Oncol 26:2, 1999.

Bos JL: *ras* oncogenes in human cancer: A review. Cancer Res 49:4682, 1989.

Bosher LH, Taylor FH: Heterotrophic gastric mucosa in the esophagus with ulceration and stricture formation. J Thorac Surg 21:306, 1951.

Brenner C, Bieganowski P, Pace HC, Huebner K: The histidine triad superfamily of nucleotide-binding proteins. J Cell Physiol 181:179, 1999.

Brown LM, Swanson CA, Gridley G, et al: Adenocarcinoma of the esophagus: Role of obesity and diet. J Natl Cancer Inst 87:104, 1995.

Campomenosi P, Conio M, Bogliolo M, et al: p53 is frequently mutated in Barrett's metaplasia of the intestinal type. Cancer Epidemiol Biomarkers Prev 5:559, 1996.

Carlson BA, Dubay MM, Sausville EA, et al: Flavopiridol induces G_1 arrest with inhibition of cyclin-dependent kinase (CDK) 2 and CDK4 in human breast carcinoma cells. Cancer Res 56:2973, 1996.

Carrie A: Adenocarcinoma of upper end of esophagus arising from ectopic gastric epithelium. Br J Surg 37:474, 1950.

Casson AG, McCart JA: Genetic modulation in the pathogenesis and treatment of cancer. Chest Surg Clin North Am 5:17, 1995.

Casson AG, Mukhopadhyay T, Cleary KR, et al: p53 gene mutations in Barrett's epithelium and esophageal cancer. Cancer Res 51:4495, 1991.

Casson AG, Tammemagi M, Eskandarian S, et al: p53 alterations in esophageal cancer: Association with clinicopathologic features, risk factors and survival. Mol Pathol 51:71, 1998.

Casson AG, Wilson SE, McCart JA, et al: ras mutation and expression of the ras regulated genes osteopontin and cathepsin L, in human esophageal cancer. Int J Cancer 72:739, 1997.

Cerni C: Telomeres, telomerase, and myc: An update. Mutat Res 462:31, 2000.

Chen PL, Riley DJ, Lee WH: The retinoblastoma protein as a fundamental mediator of growth and differentiation signals. Crit Rev Eukaryot Gene Expr 1:79, 1995.

Chen YJ, Chen PH, Lee MD, Chang JG: Aberrant FHIT transcripts in cancerous and corresponding non-cancerous lesions of the digestive tract. Int J Cancer 72:955, 1997.

Chin L, Pomerantz J, Depinho RA: The INK4a/ARF tumor suppressor: One gene—two products—two pathways. Trends Biochem Sci 23:291, 1998.

Chow WH, Finkle WD, McLaughlin JK, et al: The relation of gastroesophageal reflux disease and its treatment to adenocarcinomas of the esophagus and gastric cardia. JAMA 274:474, 1995.

Demers GW, Harris MP, Wen S-F, et al: A recombinant adenoviral vector expressing full-length human retinoblastoma susceptibility gene inhibits human tumor cell growth. Cancer Gene Ther 5:207, 1998.

Dent J, Bremner CG, Collen MJ, et al: Barrett's esophagus. J Gastroenterol Hepatol 6:1, 1991.

Dolan K, Garde J, Gosney J, et al: Allelotype analysis of oesophageal adenocarcinoma: Loss of heterozygosity occurs at multiple sites. Br J Cancer 78:950, 1998.

El-Deiry WS, Harper JW, O'Connor PM, et al: WAF1/CIP1 is induced in p53-mediated G1 arrest and apoptosis. Cancer Res 54:1169, 1994.

El-Deiry WS, Tokino T, Velculescu VE, et al: WAF1, a potential mediator of p53 tumor suppression. Cell 75:817, 1993.

El-Rifai W, Harper JC, Cummings OW, et al: Consistent genetic alterations in xenografts of proximal stomach and gastroesophageal junction adenocarcinomas. Cancer Res 58:34, 1998.

Esteve A, Martel-Planche G, Sylla BS, et al: Low frequency of p16/CDKN2 gene mutations in esophageal carcinomas. Int J Cancer 66:301, 1996.

Ewen ME: The cell cycle and the retinoblastoma protein family. Cancer Metastasis Rev 13:45, 1994.

Farrow DC, Vaughan TL: Determinants of survival following the diagnosis of esophageal adenocarcinoma (United States). Cancer Causes Control 7:322, 1996.

Fennerty MB, Sampliner RE, Way D, et al: Discordance between flow cytometric abnormalities and dysplasia in Barrett's esophagus [see comments]. Gastroenterology 97:815, 1989.

Filmus J, Robles AI, Shi W, et al: Induction of cyclin D_1 overexpression by activated *ras*. Oncogene, 9:3627, 1994.

Fong LYY, Lau KM, Huebner K, Magee PN: Induction of esophageal tumors in zinc-deficient rats by single low doses of N-nitrosomethylbenzylamine (NMBA): Analysis of cell proliferation, and mutations in H-ras and p53 genes. Carcinogenesis 18:1477, 1997.

Fong LY, Sivak A, Newberne PM: Zinc deficiency and methylbenzylnitrosamine-induced esophageal cancer in rats. J Natl Cancer Inst 61:145, 1978.

Fontanini G, Boldrini L, Vignati S, et al: Bc12 and p53 regulate vascular endothelial growth factor (VEGF)–mediated angiogenesis in non-small cell lung carcinoma. Int J Cancer 34:718, 1998.

Forozan F, Karhu R, Kononen J, et al: Genome screening by comparative genomic hybridization. Trends Cell Biol 13:405, 1997.

Foster BA, Coffey HA, Morin MJ, Rastinejad F: Pharmacological rescue of mutant p53 conformation and function. Science 286:2507, 1999.

Francheschi S, Talamini R, Barra S, et al: Smoking and drinking in relation to cancers of the oral cavity, pharynx, larynx and esophagus in Northern Italy. Cancer Res 50:6502, 1990.

Galipeau PC, Cowan DS, Sanchez CA, et al: 17 p (p53 allelic losses, 4N (G2/tetraploid) populations, and progression to aneuploidy in Barrett's esophagus. Proc Natl Acad Sci U S A 93:7081, 1996.

Gao H, Wang LD, Zhou Q, et al: p53 tumor suppressor gene mutation in early esophageal precancerous lesions and carcinoma among high-risk populations in Henan, China. Cancer Res 54:4342, 1994.

Gazzeri S, Valle VD, Chaussade L, et al: The human p19ARF protein encoded by the beta transcript of the p16INK4a gene is frequently lost in small cell lung cancer. Cancer Res 58:3926, 1998.

Giaretti W: Aneuploidy mechanisms in human colorectal preneoplastic lesions and Barrett's esophagus: Is there a role for K-ras and p53 mutations? Anal Cell Pathol 15:99, 1997.

Gleeson CM, Sloan JM, McGuigan JA, et al: Base transitions at CpG dinucleotides in the p53 gene are common in esophageal adenocarcinoma. Cancer Res 55:3406, 1995.

Goldstein SR, Yang GY, Curtis SK, et al: Development of esophageal metaplasia and adenocarcinoma in a rat surgical model without the use of a carcinogen. Carcinogenesis 18:2265, 1997.

Grana X, Reddy EP: Cell cycle control in mammalian cells: Role of cyclins, cyclin dependent kinases (CDKs), growth suppressor genes and cyclin-dependent kinase inhibitors (CKIs). Oncogene 11:211, 1995.

Gray JR, Coldman AJ, MacDonald WC: Cigarette and alcohol use in patients with adenocarcinoma of the gastric cardia or lower esophagus. Cancer 69:2227, 1992.

Greenblatt MS, Bennett WP, Hollstein M, Harris CC: Mutations in the p53 tumor suppressor gene: Clues to cancer etiology and molecular pathogenesis. Cancer Res 54:4855, 1994.

Hahn WC, Stewart SA, Brooks MW, et al: Inhibition of telomerase limits the growth of human cancer cells [see comments]. Nat Med 5:1164, 1999.

Hainaut P, Hernandez T, Robinson A, et al: IARC database of p53 gene mutations in human tumors and cell lines: Updated compilation, revised formats and new visualization tools. Nucleic Acids Res 26:205, 1998.

Harbour JW, Lai S-L, Whang-Peng J, et al: Abnormalities in structure and expression of the human retinoblastoma gene in SCLC. Science 241:353, 1988.

Harrington EA, Bruce JL, Harlow E, Dyson N: pRB plays an essential role in cell cycle arrest induced by DNA damage. Proc Natl Acad Sci U S A 95:11945, 1998.

Harris CC: Structure and function of the p53 tumor suppressor gene: Clues for rational cancer therapeutic strategies. J Natl Cancer Inst 88:1442, 1996.

Heldin PD, Wild IJF, Albrecht CF, et al: Cross-contamination of human esophageal squamous carcinoma cell lines detected by DNA fingerprint analysis. Cancer Res 48:5660, 1988.

Hiyama T, Yokozaki H, Kitadai Y, et al: Overexpression of human telomerase RNA is an early event in oesophageal carcinogenesis. Virchows Arch 434:483, 1999.

Hodgson RM, Wiessler M, Kleihues P: Preferential methylation of target organ DNA by the esophageal carcinogen *N*-nitrosomethylbenzylamine. Carcinogenesis 1:861, 1980.

Hollingsworth RE, Lee WH: Tumor suppressor genes: New prospects for cancer research. J Natl Cancer Inst 83:91, 1991.

Hollstein MC, Metcalf RA, Walsh JA, et al: Frequent mutation of the p53 gene in human esophageal cancer. Proc Natl Acad Sci U S A 87:9958, 1990.

Hollstein M, Sidransky D, Vogelstein B, Harris CC: *p53* mutations in human cancers. Science 253:49, 1991.

Huang Y, Meltzer SJ, Yin J, et al: Altered messenger RNA and unique mutational profiles of p53 and Rb in human esophageal carcinomas. Cancer Res 53:1889, 1993.

Huebner RJ, Todaro GJ: Oncogenes of RNA tumor viruses as determinants of cancer. Proc Natl Acad Sci U S A 64:1087, 1969.

Hung MC, Lau YK: Basic science of HER-2/neu: A review. Semin Oncol 26:51, 1999.

Hunter T, Pines J: Cyclins and cancer II: Cyclin D and CDK inhibitors come of age. Cell 79:573, 1994.

Hurt R: Surgical treatment of carcinoma of the esophagus. Thorax 46:528, 1991.

Iihara K, Shiozaki H, Tahara H, et al: Prognostic significance of transforming growth factor-alpha in human esophageal carcinoma: Implication for the autocrine proliferation. Cancer 71:2902, 1993.

Itakura Y, Sasano H, Shiga C, et al: Epidermal growth factor receptor overexpression in esophageal carcinoma: An immunohistochemical study correlated with clinicopathologic findings and DNA amplification. Cancer 74:795, 1994.

Ito N, Kamamoto Y, Hiasa Y, et al: Histopathological ultrastructural studies of esophageal tumors in rats treated with *N*-nitrosopiperidine. Gann 62:445, 1971.

Jankowski J, Coghill G, Hopwood D, et al: Oncogenes and oncosuppressor genes in adenocarcinoma of the esophagus. Gut 33:1033, 1992.

Jankowski JA, Wright NA, Meltzer SJ, et al: Molecular evolution of the metaplasia-dysplasia-adenocarcinoma sequence in the esophagus. Am J Pathol 154:965, 1999.

Ji BT, Chow WH, Yang G, et al: Dietary habits and stomach cancer in Shanghai, China. Int J Cancer 76:659, 1998.

Ji L, Fang B, Yen N, et al: Induction of apoptosis and inhibition of tumorigenicity and tumor growth by adenovirus vector-mediated fragile histidine triad (FHIT) gene overexpression. Cancer Res 59:3333, 1999.

Jiang W, Kahn SM, Tomita N, et al: Amplification and expression of the human cyclin D gene in esophageal cancer. Cancer Res 52:2980, 1992.

Jiang W, Zhang Y-J, Kahn SM, et al: Altered expression of the cyclin D1 and retinoblastoma genes in human esophageal cancer. Proc Natl Acad Sci U S A 90:9026, 1993.

Kastan MB, Canman CE, Leonard CJ: p53, cell cycle control and apoptosis: Implications for cancer. Cancer Metastasis Rev 14:3, 1995.

Kastan MB, Onyekwere O, Sidransky D, et al: Participation of p53 protein in the cellular response to DNA damage. Cancer Res 51:6304, 1991.

Kelsall DP, Risk JM, Leigh IM, et al: Close mapping of the focal non-epidermolytic palmoplantar keratoderma (PPK) locus associated with esophageal cancer (TOC). Hum Molec Genet 5:857, 1996.

Khuri FR, Kurie JM: Antisense approaches enter the clinic. Clin Cancer Res 6:1607, 2000.

Kirsch DG, Kastan MB: Tumor-suppressor p53: Implications for tumor development and prognosis. J Clin Oncol 16:3158, 1998.

Kitagawa Y, Ueda M, Ando N, et al: Further evidence for prognostic significance of epidermal growth factor receptor gene amplification in patients with esophageal squamous cell carcinoma. Clin Cancer Res 2:909, 1996.

Konig A, Schwartz GK, Mohammad RM, et al: The novel cyclin-dependent kinase inhibitor flavopiridol downregulates Bcl-2 and induces growth arrest and apoptosis in chronic B-cell leukemia lines. Blood 90:4307, 1997.

Koyanagi K, Ozawa S, Ando N, et al: Clinical significance of telomerase activity in the non-cancerous epithelial region of oesophageal squamous cell carcinoma [see comments]. Br J Surg 86:674, 1999.

Krishnadath KK, Tilanus HW, van Blankenstein M, et al: Accumulation of genetic abnormalities during neoplastic progression in Barrett's esophagus. Cancer Res 55:1971, 1995.

Krontris TG, Cooper GM: Transforming activity of human tumor DNAs. Proc Natl Acad Sci U S A 78:1181, 1981.

Lagergren J, Bergstrom R, Lindgren A, Nyren O: Symptomatic gastroesophageal reflux as a risk factor for esophageal adenocarcinoma. N Engl J Med 340:825, 1999.

Levi F, Ollyo JB, La Vecchia C, et al: The consumption of tobacco, alcohol and the risk of adenocarcinoma in Barrett's oesophagus. Int J Cancer 45:852, 1990.

Levine AJ, Momand J, Finlay CA: The p53 tumor suppressor gene. Nature 351:453, 1991.

Light B, Stoner GD, Gerwin B, et al: *hst-1* induced tumorigenicity in SV40 T antigen immortalized, non-tumorigenic human esophageal epithelial cells. Proc Am Assoc Cancer Res 31:136, 1990.

Lovejoy EA, Clarke AR, Harrison DJ: Animal models and the molecular pathology of cancer. J Pathol 181:130, 1997.

Lukas J, Bartkova J, Bartek J: Convergence of mitogenic signalling cascades from diverse classes of receptors at the cyclin D-cyclin-dependent kinase-pRb-controlled G_1 checkpoint. Mol Cell Biol 16:17, 1996.

Magee PN, Barnes JM: Carcinogenic nitroso compounds. Adv Cancer Res 10:163, 1967.

Martín-Castellanos C, Moreno S: Recent advances on cyclins, CDKs and CDK inhibitors. Trends Cell Biol 7:95, 1997.

Matsubara H, Kimura M, Sugaya M, et al: Expression of wild-type p53 gene confers increased sensitivity to radiation and chemotherapeutic agents in human esophageal carcinoma cells. Int J Oncol 14:1081, 1999.

McArdle JE, Lewin KJ, Randall G, Weinstein W: Distribution of dysplasias and early invasive carcinoma in Barrett's esophagus. Hum Pathol 23:479, 1992.

Melcher AA, Garcia-Ribas I, Vile RG: Gene therapy for cancer—managing expectations. BMJ 315:1604, 1997.

Meltzer SJ: The molecular biology of esophageal carcinoma. Recent Rev Cancer Res 142:1, 1996.

Menke-Pluymers MBE, van Drunen E, Vissers KJ, et al: Cytogenetic analysis of Barrett's mucosa and adenocarcinoma of the distal esophagus and cardia. Cancer Genet Cytogenet 90:109, 1996.

Michael D, Beer DG, Wilke CW, et al: Frequent deletions of FHIT and FRA3B in Barrett's metaplasia and esophageal adenocarcinomas. Oncogene 15:1653, 1997.

Miwa K, Sahara H, Segawa M, et al: Reflux of duodenal or gastro-duodenal contents induces esophageal carcinoma in rats. Int J Cancer 67:269, 1996.

Mohr U, Reznick G, Schuller HR: Carcinogenic effects of N-nitrosomorpholine and N-nitrosopiperidine on hamsters. J Natl Cancer Inst 53: 231, 1974.

Montesano R, Hollstein M, Hainaut P: Genetic alterations in esophageal cancer and their relevance to etiology and pathogenesis: A review. Int[ED1] J Cancer (Pred Oncol) 69:225, 1996.

Morales CP, Lee EL, Shay JW: In situ hybridization for the detection of telomerase RNA in the progression from Barrett's esophagus to esophageal adenocarcinoma. Cancer 83:652, 1998.

Morson BC, Belcher JR: Adenocarcinoma of the esophagus arising from ectopic gastric mucosa. Br J Cancer 6:127, 1962.

Moskaluk CA, Heitmiller R, Zahurak M, et al: p53 and p21 gene products in Barrett's esophagus and adenocarcinoma of the esophagus and esophagogastric junction. Hum Pathol 27:1211, 1996.

Moskaluk CA, Hu J, Perlman EJ: Comparative genomic hybridization of esophageal and gastroesophageal adenocarcinomas shows consensus areas of DNA gain and loss. Genes Chromosomes Cancer 22:305, 1998.

Nelson HH, Wiencke JK, Gunn L, et al: Chromosome 3p14 alterations in lung cancer: Evidence that FHIT exon deletion is a target of tobacco carcinogens and asbestos. Cancer Res 58:1804, 1998.

Neshat K, Sanchez CA, Galipeau PC, et al: p53 mutations in Barrett's adenocarcinoma and high-grade dysplasia. Gastroenterology 106:1589, 1994.

Nguyen DM, Stewart JH, Chen GA, Schrump DS: In vitro enhancement of paclitaxel sensitivity in thoracic malignancies by 17-allylamino 17-demethoxy-geldanamycin: Targeting ErbB2. Submitted.

Nishihira T, Hashimoto Y, Katayama M, et al: Molecular and cellular features of esophageal cancer cells. J Cancer Res Clin Oncol 119:441, 1993.

Ohata M, Inoue H, Cotticelli MG, et al: The FHIT gene, spanning the chromosome 3p14.2 fragile site and renal carcinoma-associated t(3;8) breakpoint, is abnormal in digestive tract cancers. Cell 84:587, 1996.

Ohgaki H, Hard GC, Hirota N, et al: Selective mutation of codon 204 and 213 of the p53 gene in rat tumors induced by alkylating *N*-nitroso compounds. Cancer Res 52:2995, 1992.

Ortiz-Hildago C, De La Vega G, Aguirre-Garcia J: The histopathology and biologic prognostic factors of Barrett's esophagus. J Clin Gastroenterol 26:342, 1998.

Pack SD, Karkera JD, Zhuang Z, et al: Molecular cytogenetic fingerprinting of esophageal squamous cell carcinoma by comparative genomic hybridization reveals a consistent pattern of chromosomal alterations. Genes Chromosomes Cancer 25:160, 1999.

Palmero I, Pantoja C, Serrano M: p19ARF links the tumour suppressor p53 to Ras. Nature 395:125, 1998.

Parkin DM, Pisani P, Ferlay J: Estimates of the worldwide incidence of eighteen major cancers in 1985. Int J Cancer 54:594, 1993.

Pera M, Cardesa A, Bombi JA, et al: Influence of esophagojejunostomy on the induction of adenocarcinoma of the distal esophagus in Sprague-Dawley rats by subcutaneous injection of 2,6-dimethylnitrosomorpholine. Cancer Res 49:6803, 1989.

Pera M, Grande L, Gelabert M, et al: Epithelial cell hyperproliferation after biliopancreatic reflux into the esophagus of rats. Ann Thoracic Surg 65:779, 1998.

Petit AM, Rak J, Hung MC, et al: Neutralizing antibodies against epidermal growth factor and ErbB-2/neu receptor tyrosine kinases down-regulate vascular endothelial growth factor production by tumor cells in vitro and in vivo: Angiogenic implications for signal transduction therapy of solid tumors. Am J Pathol 151:1523, 1997.

Polkowski W, van Sandick JW, Offerhaus GJ, et al: Prognostic value of Lauren classification and c-erbB-2 oncogene overexpression in adenocarcinoma of the esophagus and gastroesophageal junction. Ann Surg Oncol 6:290, 1999.

Postlethwait RW: Surgery of the Esophagus, 2nd ed. East Norwalk, CT, Appleton & Lange, 1986.

Reddy EP, Reynolds RK, Santos E, Barbacid M: A point mutation is responsible for the acquisition of transforming properties by the T24 human bladder carcinoma oncogene. Nature 300:149, 1982.

Reed PI: Changing pattern of oesophageal cancer. Lancet 338:178, 1991.

Reid BJ, Blount PL, Rubin CE, et al: Flow-cytometric and histological progression to malignancy in Barrett's esophagus: Prospective endoscopic surveillance of a cohort. Gastroenterology 102:1212, 1992.

Reid BJ, Sanchez CA, Blount PL, Levine DS: Barrett's esophagus: Cell cycle abnormalities in advancing stages of neoplastic progression. Gastroenterology 105:119, 1993.

Reuber MD: Carcinomas of the esophagus in rats ingesting diethylnitrosamine. Eur J Cancer 11:97, 1975.

Reuber MD: Histopathology of preneoplastic and neoplastic lesions of the esophagus in BFU rats ingesting diethylnitrosamine. J Natl Cancer Inst 58:313, 1977.

Risk JM, Mills HS, Garde J, et al: The tylosis esophageal (TOC) locus: More than just a familial cancer gene. Dis Esophagus 12:173, 1999.

Robert V, Michel P, Flaman JM, et al: High frequency in esophageal cancers of p53 alterations inactivating the regulation of genes involved in cell cycle and apoptosis. Carcinogenesis 21:563, 2000.

Robertson KD, Jones PA: The human ARF cell cycle regulatory gene promoter is a CpG island which can be silenced by DNA methylation and down-regulated by wild-type p53. Mol Cell Biol 18:6457, 1998.

Robinson KM, Haffejee AA, Anghorn IB: Tissue culture and prognosis in carcinoma of the esophagus. Clin Oncol 6:125, 1980.

Rockett JC, Larkin K, Darnton SJ, et al: Five newly established esophageal carcinoma cell lines: Phenotypic and immunological characterization. Br J Cancer 75:258, 1997.

Roetger A, Merschjann A, Dittmar T, et al: Selection of potentially metastatic subpopulations expressing c-erbB-2 from breast cancer tissue by use of an extravasation model. Am J Pathol 153:1797, 1998.

Roncalli M, Bosari S, Marchetti A, et al: Cell cycle-related gene abnormalities and product expression in esophageal carcinoma. Lab Invest 78:1049, 1998.

Roth JA: The cell and molecular biology of esophageal cancer. Chest Surg Clin North Am 4:205, 1994.

Sard L, Accornero P, Tornielli S, et al: The tumor-suppressor gene FHIT is involved in the regulation of apoptosis and in cell cycle control. Proc Natl Acad Sci U S A 96:8489, 1999.

Saretzki G, Sitte N, Merkel U, et al: Telomere shortening triggers a p53-dependent cell cycle arrest via accumulation of G-rich single stranded DNA fragments. Oncogene 18:5148, 1999.

Sasajima K, Kawachi T, San T, et al: Esophageal and gastric cancers in metastases induced in dogs by *N*-ethyl-*N*-nitrosoguanidine. J Natl Cancer Inst 58:1789, 1977.

Schmahl D, Habs M, Ivankovic S: Carcinogenesis of *N*-nitrosodiethylamine in chickens and domestic cats. Int J Cancer 22:552, 1978.

Schneider PM, Casson AG, Levin B, et al: Mutations of p53 in Barrett's esophagus and Barrett's cancer: A prospective study of 98 cases. J Thorac Cardiovasc Surg 111:323, 1996.

Schrump DS, Chen A, Consuli U, et al: Inhibition of esophageal cancer proliferation by adenoviral-mediated delivery of $p16^{INK4}$. Cancer Gene Ther 3:357, 1996.

Schrump DS, Matthews W, Chen GA, et al: Flavopiridol mediates cell cycle arrest and apoptosis in esophageal cancer cells. Clin Cancer Res 4:2885, 1998.

Schrump DS, Nguyen DM: Strategies for molecular intervention in esophageal cancers and their precursor lesions. Dis Esophagus 12:181, 1999.

Sherr CJ: Cancer cell cycles. Science 274:1672, 1996.

Sherr CJ: Tumor surveillance via the ARF-p53 pathway. Genes Dev 12:2984, 1998.

Shi D, He G, Cao S, et al: Overexpression of the c-erbB-2/neu-encoded p185 protein in primary lung cancer. Carcinogenesis 5:213, 1992.

Shih C, Padhy LC, Murray M, Weinberg RA: Transforming genes of carcinomas and neuroblastomas introduced into mouse fibroblasts. Nature 290:261, 1981.

Shimada Y, Imamura M, Watanabe G, et al: Prognostic factors of oesophageal squamous cell carcinoma from the perspective of molecular biology. Br J Cancer 80:1281, 1999.

Shimada Y, Imamura M, Wagata T, et al: Characterization of 21 newly established esophageal cancer cell lines. Cancer 69:277, 1992.

Spechler SJ: The columnar-lined esophagus: History, terminology and clinical issues. Gastroenterol Clin North Am 26:455, 1997.

Stehlin D, Varmus HE, Bishop JM, Vogt PK: DNA related to the transforming genes of avian sarcoma viruses is present in normal avian DNA. Nature 260:170, 1976.

Sur M, Cooper K: The role of the human papillomavirus in esophageal cancer. Pathology 30:348, 1998.

Tabin CJ, Bradley SM, Borgmann CI, et al: Mechanism of activation of a human oncogene. Nature 300:143, 1982.

Takeuchi H, Ozawa S, Ando N, et al: Altered p16/MTS1/CDKN2 and cyclin D1/PRAD-1 gene expression is associated with the prognosis of squamous cell carcinoma of the esophagus. Clin Cancer Res 3:2229, 1997.

Takubo K, Nakamura K, Izumiyama N, et al: Telomerase activity in esophageal carcinoma. J Surg Oncol 66:88, 1997.

Tanaka H, Shibagaki I, Shimada Y, et al: Characterization of p53 gene mutations in esophageal squamous cell carcinoma cell lines: Increased frequency and different spectrum of mutations from primary tumors. Int J Cancer 65:372, 1996.

Tanaka H, Shimada Y, Harada H, et al: Methylation of the 5′ CpG island of the FHIT gene is closely associated with transcriptional inactivation in esophageal squamous cell carcinomas. Cancer Res 58:3429, 1998.

Tao X, Zhu H, Matanoski GM: Mutagenic drinking water and risk of male esophageal cancer: A population-based case-control study. Am J Epidemiol 150:443, 1999.

Ter RB, Castell DO: Gastroesophageal reflux disease in patients with columnar-lined esophagus. Gastroenterol Clin North Am 26:549, 1997.

Thurberg BL, Duray PH, Odze RD: Polypoid dysplasia in Barrett's esophagus: A clinicopathologic, immunohistochemical, and molecular study of five cases. Hum Pathol 30:745, 1999.

Tileston W: Peptic ulcer of the esophagus. Am J Med Sci 132:240, 1906.

Tomizawa Y, Nakajima T, Kohno T, et al: Clinicopathological significance of FHIT protein expression in stage I non-small cell lung carcinoma. Cancer Res 58:5478, 1998.

Tsai CM, Levitzki A, Wu, LH, et al: Enhancement of chemosensitivity by tyrphostin AG825 in high-p185(neu) expressing non-small cell lung cancer cells. Cancer Res 56:1068, 1996.

Tytgat GNJ, Hameeteman W: The neoplastic potential of columnar-lined (Barrett's) esophagus. World J Surg 16:308, 1992.

Tzonou A, Lipworth L, Garidou A, et al: Diet and risk of esophageal cancer by histologic type in a low risk population. Int J Cancer 68:300, 1996.

van Dekken H, Geelen E, Dinjens WN, et al: Comparative genomic hybridization of cancer of the gastroesophageal junction: Deletion of 14Q31-32.1 discriminates between esophageal (Barrett's) and gastric cardia adenocarcinomas. Cancer Res 59:748, 1999.

Vaziri H, Benchimol S: Alternative pathways for the extension of cellular life span: Inactivation of p53/pRb and expression of telomerase. Oncogene 18:7676, 1999.

Wang D, You L, Sneddon J, et al: Frameshift mutation in codon 176 of the p53 gene in rat esophageal epithelial cells transformed by benzo[a]pyrine dihydrodiol. Molec Carcinog 14:84, 1995.

Wang L, Chow K, Chi K, et al: Prognosis of esophageal squamous cell carcinoma: Analysis of clinicopathological and biological factors. Am J Gastroenterol 94:1933, 1999.

Wang LD, Lipkin M, Qui SL, et al: Labelling index and labelling distribution of cells in esophageal epithelium of individuals at increased risk for esophageal cancer in Huixian, China. Cancer Res 50:1591, 1990a.

Wang Y, You M, Reynolds SH, et al: Mutational activation of the cellular Harvey *ras* oncogene in rat esophageal papillomas induced by methylbenzylnitrosamine. Cancer Res 50:1591, 1990b.

Washington K, Gottfried MR, Telen MJ: Tissue culture of epithelium derived from Barrett's esophagus. Gut 35:879, 1994.

Weinberg RA: Tumor suppressor genes. Science 254:1138, 1991.

Weiser TS, Ohnmacht GA, Guo ZS, . . . Schrump DS: Induction of MAGE-3 expression in lung and esophageal cancer cells. Ann Thorac Surg 71:295, 2001.

Weiser TS, Guo ZS, Ohnmacht GA, . . . Schrump DS: Sequential 5-Aza-2′-deoxycytidine-depsipeptide FR901228 treatment induces apoptosis preferentially in cancer cells and facilitates their recognition by cytolytic T lymphocytes specific for Ny-Eso-1. J Immunother 24:151, 2001.

Whang-Peng J, Banks-Schlegel SP, Lee EC: Cytogenetic studies of esophageal carcinoma cell lines. Cancer Genet Cytogenet 45:101, 1990.

Wiechen K, Karaaslan S, Dietel M: Involvement of the c-erbB-2 oncogene product in the EGF-induced cell motility of SK-OV-3 ovarian cancer cells. Int J Cancer 83:409, 1999.

Wong DJ, Barrett MT, Stoger R, et al: p16INK4a promoter is hypermethylated at a high frequency in esophageal adenocarcinomas. Cancer Res 57:2619, 1997.

Xing EP, Nie Y, Song Y, et al: Mechanisms of inactivation of p14ARF, p15INK4b, and p16INK4a genes in human esophageal squamous cell carcinoma. Clin Cancer Res 5:2704, 1999a.

Xing EP, Nie Y, Wang LD, et al: Aberrant methylation of p16INK4a and deletion of p15INK4b are frequent events in human esophageal cancer in Linxian, China. Carcinogenesis 20:77, 1999b.

Xing EP, Yang GY, Wang LD, et al: Loss of heterozygosity of the Rb gene correlates with pRb protein expression and associates with p53 alteration in human esophageal cancer. Clin Cancer Res 5:1231, 1999c.

Yang CS: Research on esophageal cancer in China: A review. Cancer Res 40:2633, 1980.

Yoshida T, Sakamoto H, Terada M: Amplified genes in cancer in upper digestive tract. Semin Cancer Biol 4:33, 1993.

Zhang Y, Xiong Y, Yarbrough WG: ARF promotes MDM2 degradation and stabilizes p53: ARF-INK4a locus deletion impairs both the Rb and p53 tumor suppression pathways. Cell 92:725, 1998.

Zhou P, Jiang W, Zhang YJ, et al: Antisense to cyclin D1 inhibits growth and reverses the transformed phenotype of human esophageal cancer cells. Oncogene 11:571, 1995.

CHAPTER **41**

Epidemiology of Malignant Neoplasms

Harry Henteleff
Alan G. Casson

Carcinoma of the esophagus is one of the most common malignancies wordwide (Parkin et al, 1988). The epidemiology of this disease is characterized by a striking geographic variation in incidence, not only between countries but also within distinct geographic regions and among ethnic groups. These observations distinguish esophageal cancer from many other solid tumors in humans.

Although squamous cell carcinoma remains the most common histologic subtype of esophageal cancer globally, early reports from North America (Blot et al, 1991) and Europe (Reed, 1991) confirmed clinical suspicions that primary esophageal adenocarcinomas were being seen more frequently. Throughout the 1990s, the incidence of adenocarcinoma surpassed that of squamous cell carcinoma in white males in North America (Devesa et al, 1998).

The cause of esophageal cancer is not known. Epidemiologic studies from high-incidence geographic areas suggest an association between various environmental factors and the development of esophageal tumors. Alcohol and tobacco, diet, and nutritional deficiencies have consistently been implicated, but the relative influence of each factor appears unique to the region studied. Further epidemiologic observations, together with advances in molecular biology, may offer further insight into the development and progression of esophageal cancer, including the changing biology of esophageal adenocarcinomas.

The following discussion summarizes the salient epidemiologic features of this disease and emphasizes the contribution of such observations to our current understanding of the biology of esophageal cancer.

HISTORICAL NOTE

The remarkable variability of incidence of esophageal cancer worldwide led to numerous epidemiologic studies attempting to delineate risk factors for the disease. Both genetic and environmental factors were implicated in the causation of esophageal cancer. Careful analysis of patients with esophageal cancers suggested that tobacco carcinogens and alcohol might play an important role in the development of these cancers (Wynder and Bross, 1961).

Early detection became an ideal of cancer control programs when cytologic screening of exfoliated cells for the diagnosis of cancer was developed and validated. More than 40 years ago, ingenious balloons covered with a mesh were devised for brushing the esophagus. This technique did not achieve wide application because of the relatively low prevalence of the targeted tumor in the general population; surgeons continued to deal with advanced disease at presentation, with discouraging results. When a localized geographic area of high prevalence of esophageal cancer was identified in northern China, esophageal balloons were introduced in an early screening program. Early detection was effective and economical, yielding an encouraging improvement in surgical results.

In the United States, the widespread use of flexible upper gastrointestinal endoscopy for the diagnosis of gastric complaints has led to the incidental detection of early-stage esophageal cancers in a small number of patients, facilitating surgical treatment with an improved prospect for cure. Although the appropriate target population is not yet clearly defined, the identification of geographic areas of high prevalence and the first steps toward genetic identification of people at increased risk bring us to the threshold of a new era in which physicians may detect and treat esophageal cancer more effectively.

■ *HISTORICAL READING*

Wynder EL, Bross IJ: A study of etiologic factors in cancer of the esophagus. Cancer 14:389, 1961.

STATISTICS

Geography

Estimates of the incidence of common human cancers have documented squamous cell carcinoma of the esophagus to be one of the ten most common malignancies worldwide, preceded by carcinomas of the prostate, stomach, lung, breast, colon, uterine cervix, and oropharynx (Parkin et al, 1988). Cancers of the esophagus exhibit a marked geographic variation in incidence, perhaps greater than that for any other tumor. High-incidence areas (expressed as crude incidence per 100,000 for males) are China (21 per 100,000); temperate South America, especially Uruguay and northern Argentina (13 per 100,000); western Europe, notably France (11 per 100,000); southern Africa (10 per 100,000); Japan (9 per 100,000); and northern Europe and the former Soviet

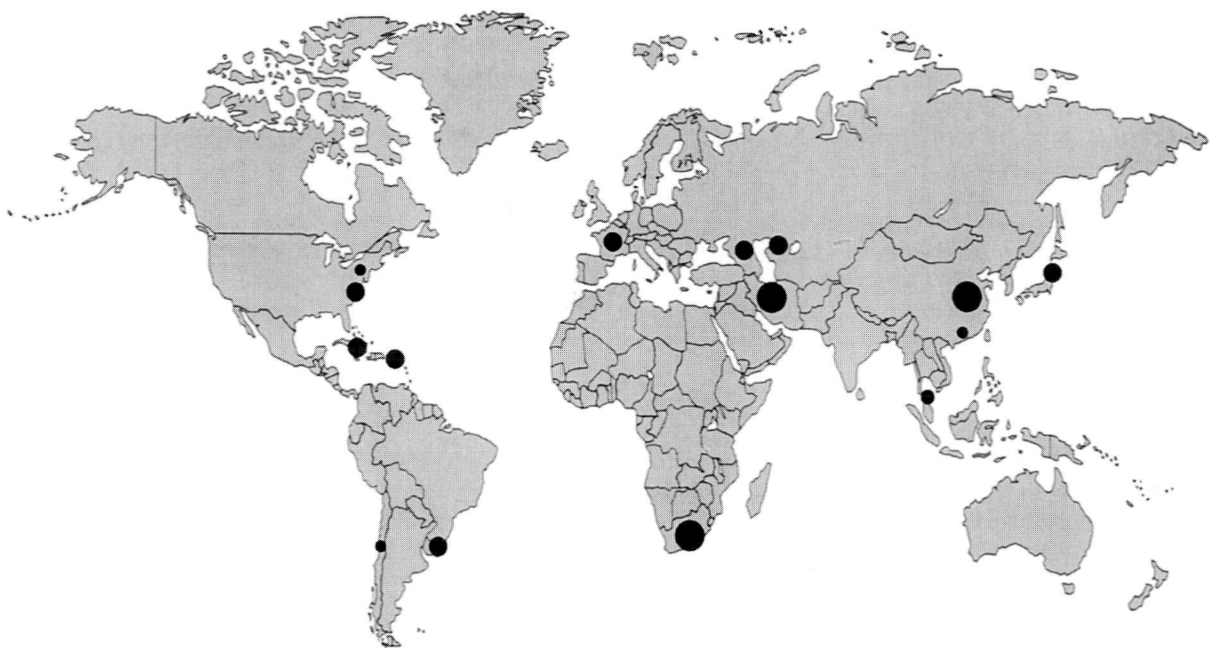

FIGURE 41–1 ■ World map showing geographic regions of high incidence of esophageal cancer.

Union (8 per 100,000 each) (Fig. 41–1). Low-incidence areas (<1.5 per 100,000 for males) include middle, western, and northern Africa, Central America, western Asia, and Polynesia.

Within each of these broad geographic areas are identifiable smaller regions in which the incidence of esophageal cancer may be 10 to 50 times as high. In three central and northern Chinese provinces (Henan, Hebei, and Shanxi), for example, the crude age-adjusted mortality rates for esophageal cancer are higher than those for for the country overall, approaching 37 per 100,000. Within these provinces, rates vary from 140 per 100,000 in Hebei County to 1.5 per 100,000 in Hunyuan County. In Linxian (Henan Province), where a registry was started in 1959, average incidence and prevalence rates for esophageal squamous cell carcinoma were reported as 109 per 100,000 and 379 per 100,000, respectively (Li et al, 1989; Yang, 1980). Squamous cell carcinoma of the esophagus is the second most common cause of cancer death among men in this region (Huang, 1988).

Similar regional trends are found in other high-incidence geographic areas. In other countries of the Far East in which accurate registries are kept, esophageal cancer is most frequent in southern Thailand (Chanvitan, 1990), mountainous regions of Japan (Hirayama, 1979), and along the southern coast of China (DeJong et al, 1974; Li, 1982). In certain regions of Iran bordering the Caspian Sea, the incidence is reported to be greater than 100 per 100,000 (Mahboudi and Aramesh, 1980). In southern Africa, esophageal cancer is now the most common cancer among black males in the southern Transkei (Rose, 1978), central Kenya, and southern Zimbabwe (Day and Munoz, 1982). In contrast to areas in which esophageal cancer has been endemic for centuries, the increasing incidence of this tumor in southern Africa appears to be relatively recent (Cook-Mozaffari et al, 1979). A marked regional variation in incidence is also seen within the so-called developed countries of Europe and North America. High-incidence clusters of the disease are reported in the French provinces of Brittany, Normandy, and Pays de Loire (Day and Munoz, 1982), northeastern Italy (Franceschi et al, 1990), and certain industrial cities of central England (Reed, 1991). In the United States, further regional variation is seen, with high-incidence areas reported around the District of Columbia and along coastal regions of the southeastern states (Fraumeni and Blot, 1977).

The real importance of the epidemiologic observations just presented relates to their potential contribution to our understanding of the etiology and pathogenesis of esophageal cancer. Human solid tumors are thought to arise as a multistep process modulated by both genetic and environmental factors. Such geographic variations in incidence suggest a predominant role for environmental factors in esophageal tumorigenesis, although it seems unlikely that a single etiologic factor accounts for such a dramatic variation in the worldwide frequency of the disease. The contribution of environmental factors to the pathogenesis of esophageal cancer are reviewed in the following discussion. The molecular genetic aspects of the disease have been covered in the previous discussion of its biology.

Histology

Although squamous cell carcinoma is still the most common histologic subtype of primary esophageal cancer worldwide, epidemiologic observations from North America (Blot et al, 1991; Kirby et al, 1994; Yang and Davis, 1988) and Europe (Powell and McConkey, 1990; Reed, 1991) indicate a rising incidence for adenocarcinomas of the esophagus. Although controversial, it has been suggested that adenocarcinomas may be considered to have a primary esophageal origin on the basis of the following criteria, determined by radiologic, endoscopic, operative, or pathologic studies (Casson et al, 1991, 1998):(1) the finding of an associated columnar epithelium–lined esophagus (Barrett's epithelium), (2) more than 75% of the tumor mass involving the tubular esophagus, (3) minimal gastric involvement, (4) direct invasion of periesophageal tissues, and (5) clinical symptoms of esophageal obstruction (dysphagia).

Reporting more than 9000 esophageal cancers registered in nine National Cancer Institute Surveillance, Epidemiology, and End Results program areas, Blot and associates (1991) found that adenocarcinomas of the lower esophagus accounted for 17% of primary esophageal tumors overall. Between 1976 and 1987, the average annual rate of increase for primary esophageal adenocarcinomas exceeded that for any other cancer (Fig. 41–2). By the end of the study (1984 to 1987), adenocarcinomas accounted for 34% of all esophageal tumors in white males. A 1998 update of this study found that the rise in the rates of incidence of adenocarcinoma of the esophagus and esophagogastric junction in white North American males exceeded 350% from 1976 to 1994 (Devesa et al, 1998). In the United States, by 1993, 48.1% of all cancers in the lower-third esophagus were adenocarcinomas (Daly et al, 1996).

The reasons for this indicated increase in incidence are unclear, and to date no single environmental factor has been implicated. Many adenocarcinomas appear to arise in association with Barrett's epithelium (Barrett's esophagus), which is thought to be an acquired metaplasia resulting from chronic gastroesophageal reflux. Prevalence rates for Barrett's esophagus of 10% for symptomatic patients and less than 1% for the asymptomatic general population have been reported (Cameron and Lomboy, 1992; Dent et al, 1991). Prospective studies estimated that patients with Barrett's epithelium are at higher (at least 30- to 40-fold) risk for development of invasive esophageal adenocarcinoma and that Barrett's epithelium should be considered premalignant (Cameron et al, 1985; Spechler et al, 1984). Mutations of the p53 tumor suppressor gene have been found in Barrett's epithelium and primary esophageal adenocarcinomas (Casson et al, 1991), implicating this gene in tumor progression to invasive cancer (Casson et al, 1998). In the future, molecular epidemiologic studies of esophageal cancer, correlating patterns of genetic mutations with carcinogen exposure, may provide further insight into the changing biology of this disease (Jones et al, 1991).

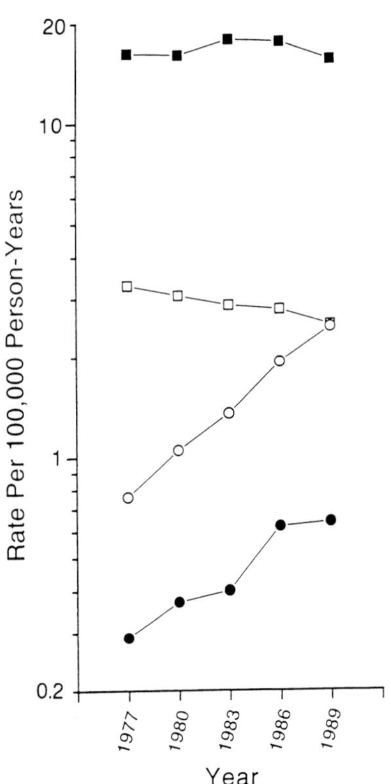

FIGURE 41–2 ■ Trends in age-adjusted incidence rates of squamous cell carcinomas and adenocarcinomas of the esophagus among American men by race: ■, squamous cell carcinoma, black men; □, squamous cell carcinoma, white men; ●, adenocarcinoma, black men; ○, adenocarcinoma, white men. (Courtesy of Dr. W. J. Blot.)

RISK FACTORS

Age, Sex, and Race

In general, esophageal cancers are seen infrequently in early adulthood, and growing incidence parallels increasing age. In high-incidence regions of northern China, the occurrence of squamous cell esophageal cancer increases gradually after age 25 years, with the highest mortality rates for men seen between ages 60 and 70 years (Yang, 1980). In nearby regions of lower incidence, however, the average age for development of esophageal cancer is generally higher. In the United States, both squamous cell carcinoma and adenocarcinoma of the esophagus have been reported infrequently before age 40 years, beyond which the incidence of each subtype continues to rise with each decade of life (Yang and Davis, 1988).

Worldwide, males of all ages are more commonly affected than females, although as a general rule, the sex ratio narrows in high-incidence regions. In France, the male-to-female ratio approximates 9:1, with higher ratios (17:1) seen in the high-incidence province of Brittany (Sons, 1987). The male-to-female ratio for squamous cell carcinoma in the United States ranges from 2.1:1 to 3.7:1 for all age groups; in contrast, that for primary esophageal adenocarcinomas varies among age groups, peaking at 13:1 in the fifth decade of life (Yang and Davis, 1988). In northern China, the male-to-female ratio ranges from 2.6:1 in low-incidence regions to 1.4:1 in high-incidence regions (Yang, 1980). In high-incidence regions of the Caspian littoral of Iran, the sex ratio is reversed, and esophageal cancers are reported more frequently in females (Mahboudi and Aramesh, 1980). Despite these striking observations, however, there is no evidence that sex hormones play a role in the etiology of esophageal carcinoma (Lagergren and Nyren, 1998).

Racial or ethnic differences have been reported from high-incidence areas of the world, although the significance of these observations is unclear. In western China, higher incidence of esophageal cancer is seen in peoples of the Kazak ethnic group but not in the neighboring Uygurs (Li, 1982). The black populations of South Africa (Rose, 1978) and North America (Yang and Davis, 1988) appear to be at increased risk for development of esophageal squamous cell tumors, especially before age 55 years; such a high black-to-white ratio is seen for no other cancer in this region (Blot and Fraumeni, 1987). In contrast, the rising incidence of primary esophageal adenocarcinomas predominates among white males (Blot et al, 1991; Yang and Davis, 1988).

Alcohol and Tobacco

Heavy alcohol intake has been implicated as an etiologic factor in esophageal cancer, both by clinical observations and by epidemiologic studies (Bradshaw and Schonland, 1974; Dean et al, 1979; Franceschi et al, 1990; Hakulinen et al, 1974; Jensen, 1979; Schmidt and Popham, 1981). This factor has also been tested by cohort studies, which demonstrated a progressively higher risk of squamous cell esophageal cancer among heavy drinkers of hard liquor (Hakulinen et al, 1974; Schmidt and Popham, 1981). Two cohort studies of beer drinkers reported an increased risk of esophageal cancer among brewery workers in Denmark (Jensen, 1979) but not in Ireland (Dean et al, 1979). Most studies in which accurate data were obtained, however, originated in developed countries. Later studies of esophageal adenocarcinomas suggest that heavy alcohol intake may not be a significant risk factor for the development of this histologic subtype (Gray et al, 1992; Levi et al, 1990). In certain high-incidence regions of the world, such as Iran, where alcohol is forbidden for religious reasons, other environmental factors probably assume greater importance in the pathogenesis of esophageal cancer.

In high-incidence regions of China, the smoking of locally grown tobacco is common but has not been clearly correlated with the development of esophageal cancer (Yang, 1980). Several retrospective and prospective studies, however, have consistently demonstrated a 5-fold to 6-fold higher risk of esophageal squamous cell carcinoma among cigarette smokers (Bradshaw and Schonland, 1974; Doll and Peto, 1976; Hammond, 1966; Rogot and Murray, 1980; Schmidt and Popham, 1981). Furthermore, smokers of cigars and pipes appear to be at increased risk (Doll and Peto, 1976; Franceschi et al, 1990; Hammond, 1966). The relationship between smoking and development of esophageal adenocarcinoma is less clear, with two later reports suggesting no clear association (Gray et al, 1992; Levi et al, 1990).

Perhaps the most interesting observation is the higher relative risk (>100-fold) for development of esophageal cancer when cigarette smoking is combined with heavy alcohol consumption (Bradshaw and Schonland, 1974; Franceschi et al, 1990; Tuyns, 1983; Warwick, 1973; Wynder and Bross, 1961). Although this observation suggests synergy between chemical mutagens that frequently contaminate tobacco and alcoholic drinks, the contribution of each agent to human esophageal carcinogenesis is still undefined. Alcohol, particularly when consumed hot (Launoy et al, 1997) may serve as a promoter by (1) increasing the rate of proliferation of the epithelium, exacerbating its vulnerability to tobacco carcinogens, or (2) increasing the permeation of carcinogens to the premitotic cells below the surface epithelium.

In high-incidence areas of the world where tobacco smoking is uncommon, other local habits are associated with the development of esophageal cancers. These habits include the chewing of opium residue in Iran (Cook-Mozaffari et al, 1979), of betel in India (Gupta et al, 1982; Jussawalla and Desphande, 1971) and southern Thailand (Chanvitan, 1990), and of pipe tobacco residue in southern Africa (Hewer and Rose, 1978).

Diet and Nutrition

Perhaps more than any other risk factor, dietary and nutritional factors have been consistently implicated in the pathogenesis of esophageal cancer (VanRensburg et al, 1985). In general, populations living in high-incidence areas of the world have been shown to have poor diets, often with specific nutritional deficiencies, or to be exposed to common dietary carcinogens. Epidemiologic observations have been reproduced in subsequent laboratory studies using animal models, providing additional compelling evidence for diet in the pathogenesis of esophageal cancer. In the future, dietary supplementation and improved nutritional status may reduce the frequency of esophageal cancer in high-risk populations.

Several nutritional surveys of high-incidence regions worldwide have suggested that diets rich in carbohydrate and low in animal protein, green vegetables, and fruit were associated with the development of esophageal cancer (Schottenfeld, 1984; Silber, 1985; Yang, 1980; Ziegler et al, 1981). Consumption of cholesterol in the form of butter may contribute to a large proportion of the excess incidence of esophageal cancer in high-risk areas in France (Launoy et al, 1998). Although overt clinical malnutrition was uncommon in the populations studied in these surveys, most diets were also deficient in vitamins, trace elements, or minerals. For example, deficiency of vitamin A has been associated with esophageal tumorigenesis in humans (Decarli et al, 1987; Yang, 1980) and laboratory animals (Gabrial et al, 1982). Dietary supplementation with vitamin A was found to prevent carcinogen-induced esophageal tumors in animals (Sporn and Newton, 1979). Prospective dietary intervention studies (Blot and Li, 1985; Li et al, 1985), in which high-risk populations in China are receiving supplements of multiple vitamins and minerals, are ongoing to assess the efficacy of this approach to cancer prevention.

Epidemiologic studies also supported a role for direct ingestion of dietary carcinogens in esophageal cancer, because the esophagus is frequently the first mucosal site to contact potentially harmful dietary components. Specifically, exposure to nitrosamines and their precursors (nitrates and nitrites) has been shown to be common in high-incidence regions of northern China for both humans and domestic animals having common water and food sources (Lu et al, 1986; Singer et al, 1986; Yang, 1980). Similarly, greater exposure to nitrosamines has been reported in Iran (Mahboudi and Aramesh, 1980), southern Africa (Rose, 1978; Silber, 1985), India (Siddiqi and Preussmann, 1989), and southern Thailand (Chanvitan, 1990). Nitrosamines have to induced esophageal tumors experimentally in laboratory animals (Terzaghi et al, 1981; Yang, 1980). Carcinogenic *N*-nitroso compounds are formed endogenously by reaction of nitrates with secondary or tertiary amines. Major sources of ingested nitrates are pickled vegetables, cured meats and fish, and alcoholic drinks. Fungal contamination of such foods may further raise levels of dietary amines and promote increased nitrosamine formation (Chang et al, 1992; Garner, 1980; Yang, 1980). High levels of carcinogenic polycyclic aromatic hydrocarbons in food has been suggested as a cause of the high incidence of esophageal cancer in the Linxian province of China (Roth et al, 1998).

Intrinsic Esophageal Disease

Various intrinsic diseases of the esophagus have been reported to be associated with the development of esophageal cancer, although patient numbers are inevitably small and statistical correlation is difficult. Many of the conditions discussed here, however, are now considered premalignant.

Plummer-Vinson (Paterson-Kelly) Syndrome

Larrson and co-workers (1975) found atrophy of the oropharyngeal and esophageal mucosa secondary to iron and vitamin (nicotinamide and lactoflavin) deficiency, also known as Plummer-Vinson (Paterson-Kelly) syndrome, to be associated with increased risk for development of upper aerodigestive tract cancers, especially cancers of the cervical esophagus and hypopharynx. This Scandinavian study also reported that correction of iron deficiency anemia reduced the incidence of these tumors.

Columnar Epithelium–Lined (Barrett's) Esophagus (Barrett's Epithelium)

The diagnosis of Barrett's epithelium is confirmed when metaplastic columnar epithelium is found to extend at least 3 cm proximal to the esophagogastric junction or by the presence of specialized "intestinal-type" epithelium. Although this disorder is a controversial entity (DeMeester, 1993; Dent et al, 1991), it is now thought to represent an acquired change related to prolonged gastroesophageal reflux, but Barrett's epithelium may also be seen in association with other intrinsic esophageal diseases, including scleroderma (McKinley and Sherlock, 1984), achalasia (Kortan et al, 1981), and lye stricture (Spechler et al, 1981). Barrett's esophagus has also been reported to develop following anticancer chemotherapy (Sartori et al, 1991).

The importance of Barrett's epithelium is its association with malignancy, particularly primary esophageal adenocarcinoma. The increase in incidence noted for this tumor underlies the importance of the putative premalignant condition. Patients with Barrett's epithelium are estimated to be at least 30 to 40 times as likely to experience esophageal cancer as the general population (Cameron et al, 1985; Spechler et al, 1984). Unfortunately, retrospective studies suggest that most patients with esophageal adenocarcinoma do not have a previous diagnosis of Barrett's esophagus (Bytzer et al, 1999). Although Barrett's epithelium appears to link benign gastroesophageal reflux disease and esophageal malignancy, no clear biologic mechanism has been established to explain this association.

Stricture

Occasional case reports suggest that esophageal tumors may develop as a late complication of acid-induced or lye-induced esophageal strictures (Applequist and Salma, 1980; Hopkins and Postlethwait, 1981; Kiviranta, 1952). Experimental studies in rats with surgically induced esophageal strictures demonstrated increased numbers of carcinogen-induced esophageal tumors at the site of esophageal narrowing compared with control rats without stenosis (Sons et al, 1985).

Achalasia

Squamous cell carcinoma has been reported as a late complication of achalasia (Just-Viera and Haight, 1969). Wychulis and colleagues (1971) reported the development of 13 tumors in more than 1300 patients with achalasia, a rate suggesting this complication to be an infrequent occurrence. A population-based study from Sweden documented a 16-fold higher risk of esophageal cancer from 1 to 24 years after the diagnosis of achalasia (Sandler et al, 1995). Although the precise etiologic mechanism of this functional esophageal disorder is unknown, prolonged mucosal exposure to ingested carcinogens secondary to stasis is proposed as a possible factor predisposing to malignancy.

Diverticula

Esophageal diverticula are rare and are commonly associated with functional esophageal disorders. A few case reports have documented an association between esophageal cancer and pharyngoesophageal diverticula (Nanson, 1976; Sarks, 1933; Wychulis et al, 1969), midesophageal diverticula (Kuwano et al, 1982), and epiphrenic diverticula (Gwande et al, 1972).

Miscellaneous Conditions

Esophageal mucosal injury from long-term ingestion of hot liquids or foods has been associated with development of cancer in high-risk regions of France (Launoy et al, 1997), China (DeJong et al, 1974; Yang, 1980), Iran (Ghadirian, 1987), Japan (Nakachi et al, 1988), Thailand (Chanvitan, 1990), Brazil (Munoz et al, 1987), Paraguay (Rolon et al, 1995), and Uruguay (Vassallo et al, 1985). Casson and associates (1998) reported the percentage of esophageal tumors with p53 mutations to rise significantly with increasing consumption of hot beverages. Reports of higher risk secondary to occupational exposure to asbestos (Selikoff et al, 1979) and rubber (Norell et al, 1983) are infrequent.

Multiple Primary Tumors of the Upper Aerodigestive Tract

Patients with cancers of the upper aerodigestive tract are increasingly recognized to be at greater risk for development of second, or multiple, primary tumors (Choy et al, 1992; Cooper et al, 1989; Licciardello et al, 1989). Chung and associates (1993) reported discordant p53 gene mutations in multiple primary cancers of the upper aerodigestive tract, suggesting that such tumors may arise as independent events.

Infectious Causes

Evidence pointing to infectious agents in the pathogenesis of aerodigestive cancer is derived from the close association between human papillomavirus and herpes simplex virus and oral cancer (Scully, 1989; Scully et al, 1988); Epstein-Barr virus and nasopharyngeal cancer (Graffey and Weiss, 1990); *Helicobacter pylori* infection and gastric cancer (Parssonet et al, 1991); and *H. pylori* infection and Barrett's epithelium (Graham, 1988). Using molecular techniques, Furihata and colleagues (1993) demonstrated human papillomavirus DNA in 24 of 71 Japanese squamous cell cancers. However, epidemiologic studies have not conclusively linked esophageal cancer with seropositivity for human papillomavirus (Lagergren et al, 1999b).

H. pylori infection plays a controversial role in the pathogenesis of esophageal cancer, with several studies suggesting a protective effect of the infection (el-Serag and Sonnenberg, 1998; Richter et al, 1998). If eradication of *H. pylori* proves to be a risk factor for development of esophageal cancer, a radical change in the management of peptic ulcer disease may result.

Familial and Genetic Factors

The possibility that genetic factors might predispose to the development of esophageal cancer arose initially from two unrelated observations: an association with tylosis, a rare autosomal dominant disorder, and the occasional familial incidence or clustering of this disease.

Observations of familial clusterings of esophageal cancer raise the question of whether the affected individuals were at higher risk because of underlying genetic factors or because of exposure to a common environmental factor, such as a dietary carcinogen. Earlier reports of esophageal cancer in families from Iran (Pour and Ghadirian, 1974) and China (Wu and Ran, 1979) initially suggested no apparent genetic predisposition. Slight associations were reported of esophageal cancers with blood group A, HLA-A2, and HLA-B40 (Zhu et al, 1982) and with cytogenetic aneuploidy (Wu and Ran, 1979) in high-risk families in Linxian, China. The first formal genetic segregation analysis of 221 high-risk families in Linxian suggested an autosomal recessive mendelian inheritance, however, with the putative gene present at a frequency of 19% in this subpopulation (Carter et al, 1992).

Tylosis is an uncommon familial syndrome characterized by thickening, or hyperkeratosis, of the skin of the soles of the feet and the palms of the hands. In the largest series, consisting of four families with tylosis, almost 40% of family members had squamous cell carcinoma of the esophagus by their mid-40s (Harper et al, 1970). It was estimated that members of these four families would have a 95% risk of development of esophageal cancer by age 65 years. Similarly, members of the first American family described with this condition were estimated to have at least a 90% percent risk of having esophageal malignancy by age 65 years (Marger and Marger, 1993). Through the use of linkage analysis of United Kingdom and American family members, the tylosis esophageal cancer gene has been localized to a small region on chromosome 17q25 (Kelsell et al, 1996).

COMMENTS AND CONTROVERSIES

Technologic advances such as flexible endoscopy and cytologic examination of desquamated cells from the esophagus, lung, colon, and uterine cervix suggest the possibility of early detection of esophageal cancer, with the implication that curative therapy can be achieved in a larger fraction of patients. This goal has been accomplished when screening studies have been conducted successfully in regions of high prevalence (Huang et al, 1982; Japanese Committee for Registration of Esophageal Carcinoma, 1985).

The low prevalence of esophageal cancer in nonendemic areas of the world makes screening programs impractical, but the strategy is effective in endemic areas. The use of esophageal balloon cytologic examination in the Linxian district resulted in early detection and encouraging results of surgical treatment. The cost-to-benefit ratio of such screening becomes unacceptably high in nonendemic areas.

It is encouraging to record that genetic markers, such as p53, have been discovered that may identify patients at higher risk for esophageal cancer. If costs can be brought to a reasonable level, more specific screening of a subpopulation at higher risk through the use of endoscopy might be rationally applied at reasonable cost. At present, routine endoscopic screening is prohibitively expensive and inconvenient. If an inexpensive and reliable screening probe can be developed to identify appropriate patients for endoscopic or balloon cytologic surveillance, the current results of all modalities of therapy for esophageal cancer will be dramatically improved. There seems to be little question that the proliferation of flexible upper gastrointestinal endoscopy has led to detection of more early carcinomas of the esophagus and stomach.

Many surgeons and physicians are concerned that the rising incidence of esophageal cancer may be linked to gastroesophageal reflux disease. A history of reflux symptoms has been strongly linked to the later development of esophageal adenocarcinoma (Lagergren, et al, 1999a). The development of effective agents to suppress gastric acid has led to an interest in bile reflux as a possible contributor to esophageal carcinogenesis (Fein et al, 1998). The rise in the incidence of esophageal adenocarcinoma is not nearly as marked in countries where acid suppression therapy has not been widely available (Bollschweiler et al, 1998). However, the use of histamine

(H_2) receptor blockers has not been shown to be a risk factor for esophageal cancer in a case-control study (Fioretti et al, 1997). The eventual clarification of this relationship will be an interesting chapter in the history of cancer epidemiology.

H. H.
A. G. C.

■ KEY REFERENCES

Devesa SS, Blot WJ, Fraumeni JF: Changing patterns in the incidence of esophageal and gastric carcinoma in the United States. Cancer 83:2049, 1998.

This study updates a brief report from 1991 that documented the recent increase in incidence of primary esophageal adenocarcinomas in the United States.

Yang CS: Research on esophageal cancer in China: A review. Cancer Res 40:2633, 1980.

Although dating back to 1980, this frequently cited review documents extensive epidemiologic and experimental studies from a high-incidence area of the world, China.

■ REFERENCES

Applequist P, Salmo M: Lye corrosion carcinoma of the esophagus. Cancer 45:2655, 1980.

Blot WJ, Devesa SS, Kneller RW, Fraumeni JF: Rising incidence of adenocarcinoma of the esophagus and gastric cardia. JAMA 265:1287, 1991.

Blot WJ, Fraumeni JF: Trends in esophageal cancer mortality among U.S. blacks and whites. Am J Public Health 77:296, 1987.

Blot WJ, Li JY: Some considerations in the design of a nutrition intervention trial in Linxian. Natl Cancer Inst Monogr 69:29, 1985.

Bollschweiler E, Gutschow C, Holscher AF: Rising incidence of adenocarcinoma in the gastroesophageal junction: Differences between USA and Europe? Can J Gastroenterol 12:152B, 1998.

Bradshaw E, Schonland M: Smoking, drinking, and oesophageal cancer in African males in Johannesburg, South Africa. Br J Cancer 30:157, 1974.

Bytzer P, Christensen PB, Damkier P, et al: Adenocarcinoma of the esophagus and Barrett's esophagus: A population-based study. Am J Gastroenterol 94:86, 1999.

Cameron AJ, Lomboy CT: Barrett's esophagus: Age, prevalence, and extent of columnar epithelium. Gastroenterology 103:1241, 1992.

Cameron AJ, Ott BJ, Payne WS: The incidence of adenocarcinoma in columnar-lined (Barrett's) esophagus. N Engl J Med 313:857, 1985.

Carter CL, Hu N, Wu M, et al: Segregation analysis of esophageal cancer in 221 high-risk Chinese families. J Natl Cancer Inst 84:771, 1992.

Casson AG, Mukhopadhyay T, Cleary KR, et al: p53 gene mutations in Barrett's epithelium and esophageal cancer. Cancer Res 51:4495, 1991.

Casson AG, Tammemagi M, Eskandarian S, et al: p53 alterations in oesophageal cancer: Association with clinicopathologic features, risk factors, and survival. J Clin Pathol Mol Pathol 51:71, 1998.

Chang F, Syrjanen S, Wang L, Syrjanen K: Infectious agents in the etiology of esophageal cancer. Gastroenterology 103:1336, 1992.

Chanvitan A: Oesophageal Cancer Studies in Southern Thailand. Bangkok, Medical Media Publisher, 1990.

Choy ATK, van Hasselt CA, Chrisholm EM, et al: Multiple primary cancers in Hong Kong Chinese patients with squamous cell cancer of the head or neck. Cancer 70:815, 1992.

Chung KY, Mukhopadhyay T, Kim J, et al: Discordant p53 gene mutations in primary head and neck cancers and corresponding secondary primary cancers of the upper aerodigestive tract. Cancer Res 53:1676, 1993.

Cook-Mozaffari PJ, Azordkegan F, Day NE, et al: Oesophageal cancer studies in the Caspian littoral of Iran: Results of a case-control study. Br J Cancer 39:293, 1979.

Cooper JS, Pajak TF, Rubin P, et al: Second malignancies in patients who have head and neck cancer: Incidence, effect on survival, and implications based on the RTOG experience. Int J Radiat Oncol Biol Phys 17:449, 1989.

Daly JM, Karnell LH, Menck HR: National Cancer Data Base Report on Esophageal Carcinoma. Cancer 78:1820, 1996.

Day NE, Munoz N: Esophagus. In Schottenfeld D, Fraumeni J (eds): Cancer Epidemiology and Prevention. Philadelphia, WB Saunders, 1982.

Dean G, MacLennan R, McLoughlin H, et al: Causes of death of blue-collar workers at a Dublin brewery. Br J Cancer 40:581, 1979.

Decarli A, Liati P, Negri E, et al: Vitamin A and other dietary factors in the etiology of esophageal cancer. Nutr Cancer 10:29, 1987.

DeJong UW, Breslow N, Hong JG, et al: Aetiological factors in oesophageal cancer in Singapore Chinese. Int J Cancer 13:291, 1974.

DeMeester T: Barrett's esophagus. Surgery 113:239, 1993.

Dent J, Bremner CG, Collen MJ, et al: Barrett's esophagus. J Gastroenterol Hepatol 6:1, 1991.

Devesa SS, Blot WJ, Fraumeni JF: Changing pattens in the incidence of esophageal and gastric carcinoma in the United States. Cancer 83:2049, 1998.

Doll R, Peto R: Mortality in relation to smoking: 20 years observation on male British doctors. Br Med J 2:1525, 1976.

El-Serag HB, Sonnenberg A: Opposing time trends of peptic ulcer and reflux disease. Gut 43:327, 1998.

Fein M, Peters JH, Ritter MP, et al: Induction of esophageal cancer by reflux of duodenal juice. Can J Gastroenterol 12:153B, 1998.

Fioretti F, Tavani A, La Vecchia C, Franceschi S: Histamine$_2$-receptor antagonists and oesophageal cancer. Eur J Cancer Prev 6:143, 1997.

Franceschi S, Talamini R, Barra S, et al: Smoking and drinking in relation to cancers of the oral cavity, pharynx, larynx, and esophagus in northern Italy. Cancer Res 50:6502, 1990.

Fraumeni JF, Blot WJ: Geographic variation in esophageal cancer mortality in the United States. J Chron Dis 30:759, 1977.

Furihata M, Ohtsuki Y, Ogoshi S, et al: Prognostic significance of human papillomavirus genomes (type-16, -18) and aberrant expression of p53 protein in human esophageal cancer. Int J Cancer 54:226, 1993.

Gabrial GN, Schrazer TF, Newberne PM: Zinc deficiency, alcohol, and a retinoid: Association with esophageal cancer in rats. J Natl Cancer Inst 68:785, 1982.

Garner RC: Carcinogenesis by fungal products. Br Med Bull 36:47, 1980.

Ghadirian P: Thermal irritation and oesophageal cancer in northern Iran. Cancer 60:1909, 1987.

Graffey MJ, Weiss LM: Viral oncogenesis: Epstein-Barr virus. Am J Otolaryngol 11:375, 1990.

Graham DY: *Campylobacter pylori* and Barrett's esophagus. Mayo Clin Proc 63:1258, 1988.

Gray JR, Coldman AJ, MacDonald WC: Cigarette and alcohol use in patients with adenocarcinoma of the gastric cardia or lower esophagus. Cancer 69:2227, 1992.

Gupta P, Pindborg J, Mehta FS: Comparison of carcinogenicity of betel quid with and without tobacco: An epidemiologic review. Ecol Dis 4:213, 1982.

Gwande AS, Batiuchock WB, Barman AA, Mule JE: Carcinoma within a lower esophageal (epiphrenic) diverticulum. N Y State J Surg 10:1749, 1972.

Hakulinen T, Lehtimaki L, Lehtonen M, et al: Cancer morbidity among two male cohorts with increased alcohol consumption. J Natl Cancer Inst 52:1711, 1974.

Hammond EC: Smoking in relation to death rates of one million men and women. Natl Cancer Inst Monogr 19:127, 1966.

Harper PS, Harper RMJ, Howel-Evans AW: Carcinoma of the esophagus with tylosis. Q J Med 34:317, 1970.

Hewer T, Rose E, Ghadririan P, et al: Ingested mutagens from opium and tobacco pyrolysis products and cancer of the oesophagus. Lancet 2:494, 1978.

Hirayama T: Diet and cancer. Nutr Cancer 1:67, 1979.

Hopkins RA, Postlethwait RW: Caustic burns and carcinoma of the esophagus. Ann Surg 194:146, 1981.

Huang GJ: Epidemiology of esophageal cancer in China. In Siewert JR, Holscher AH (eds): Diseases of the Esophagus. Berlin, Springer-Verlag, 1988.

Huang KD, et al: Diagnosis and surgical treatment of early esophageal carcinoma. In Stipa S, Belsey RHR, Moraldi A (eds): Medical and Surgical Problems of the Esophagus: Serona Symposia, vol 43. New York, Academic Press, 1982, p 296.

Japanese Committee for Registration of Esophageal Carcinoma: A proposal for a new TNM classification of esophageal carcinoma. Jpn J Clin Oncol 14:625, 1985.

Jensen OM: Cancer morbidity and causes of death among Danish brewery workers. Int J Cancer 23:454, 1979.

Jones PA, Buckley JD, Henderson BE, et al: From gene to carcinogen: A rapidly evolving field in molecular epidemiology. Cancer Res 51:3617, 1991.

Jussawalla DJ, Desphande VA: Evaluation of cancer risk in tobacco chewers and smokers: An epidemiologic assessment. Cancer 28:244, 1971.

Just-Viera JO, Haight C: Achalasia and carcinoma of the esophagus. Surg Gynecol Obstet 128:1081, 1969.

Kelsell DP, Risk JM, Leigh IM, et al: Close mapping of the focal non-epidermolytic palmoplantar keratoderma (PPK) locus associated with esophageal cancer (TOC). Hum Mol Genet 5:857, 1996.

Kirby TJ, Rice TW: The epidemiology of esophageal carcinoma. Chest Surg Clin North Am 4:217, 1994.

Kiviranta UK: Corrosion carcinoma of the esophagus. Acta Otol Laryngol 42:89, 1952.

Kortan P, Warren RE, Gardner J, et al: Barrett's esophagus in a patient with surgically treated achalasia. J Clin Gastroenterol 3:357, 1981.

Kuwano H, Sugimachi K, Inokuchi K, et al: Squamous cell carcinoma in a middle esophageal (parabronchial) diverticulum: Report of a case. Jpn J Surg 12:266, 1982.

Lagergren J, Bergstrom R, Lindgren A, Nyren O: Symptomatic gastroesophageal reflux as a risk factor for esophageal adenocarcinoma. N Engl J Med 340:825, 1999a.

Lagergren J, Nyren O: Do sex hormones play a role in the etiology of esophageal adenocarcinoma? Cancer Epidemiol Biomarkers Prev 7:913, 1998.

Lagergren J, Wang Z, Bergstrom R, et al: Human papillomavirus infection and esophageal cancer: A nationwide seroepidemiologic case-control study in Sweden. J Natl Cancer Inst 91:156, 1999b.

Larrson LG, Sandstrom A, Westling P: Relationship of Plummer-Vinson disease to cancer of the upper alimentary tract in Sweden. Cancer Res 35:3308, 1975.

Launoy G, Milan C, Day NE, et al: Diet and squamous cell cancer of the oesophagus: A French multicentre case-control study. Int J Cancer 76:7, 1998.

Launoy G, Milan C, Day NE, et al: Esophageal cancer in France: Potential importance of hot alcoholic drinks. Int J Cancer 71:917, 1997.

Levi F, Ollyo JB, La Vecchia C, et al: The consumption of tobacco, alcohol, and the risk of adenocarcinoma in Barrett's oesophagus. Int J Cancer 45:852, 1990.

Li JY: Epidemiology of esophageal cancer in China. Natl Cancer Inst Monogr 62:113, 1982.

Li JY, Ershow AG, Chen ZJ, et al: A case-control study of cancer of the esophagus and gastric cardia in Linxian. Int J Cancer 43:755, 1989.

Li JY, Li GY, Zheng SF, et al: A pilot nutrition intervention trial in Linxian. Natl Cancer Inst Monogr 69:29, 1985.

Licciardello JTW, Spitz MR, Hong WK: Multiple primary cancer in patients with cancer of the head and neck: Second cancer of the head and neck, esophagus, and lung. Int J Radiat Oncol Biol Phys 17:467, 1989.

Lu SH, Ruggero M, Zhang MS, et al: Relevance of *N*-nitrosamines to esophageal cancer in China. J Cell Physiol 4:51, 1986.

Mahboudi EO, Aramesh B: Epidemiology of esophageal cancer in Iran, with special reference to nutritional and cultural aspects. Prev Med 9:613, 1980.

Marger RS, Marger D: Carcinoma of the esophagus and tylosis: A lethal genetic combination. Cancer 72:17, 1993.

McKinley M, Sherlock P: Barrett's esophagus with adenocarcinoma in scleroderma. Am J Gastroenterol 79:438, 1984.

Munoz N, Victora CG, Crespi M, et al: Hot maté drinking and precancerous lesions of the esophagus: An endoscopic survey in southern Brazil. Int J Cancer 39:708, 1987.

Nakachi K, Imai K, Hoshivama Y, Sasaba T: The joint effects of two factors in the aetiology of oesophageal cancer in Japan. Epidemiol Commun Health 42:355, 1988.

Nanson EM: Carcinoma in a long-standing pharyngeal diverticulum. Br J Surg 63:417, 1976.

Norell S, Ahblom A, Lipping H, et al: Oesophageal cancer and vulcanization work. Lancet 1:462, 1983.

Parkin DM, Laara E, Muir CS: Estimates of worldwide frequency of sixteen major cancers in 1980. Int J Cancer 41:184, 1988.

Parssonet J, Friedman GD, Vandersteen DP, et al: *Helicobacter pylori* infection and the risk of gastric carcinoma. N Engl J Med 325:1127, 1991.

Pour P, Ghadirian P: Familial cancer of the esophagus in Iran. Cancer 33:1649, 1974.

Powell J, McConkey CE: Increasing incidence of adenocarcinoma of the gastric cardia and adjacent sites. Br J Cancer 62:440, 1990.

Reed PI: Changing patterns of esophageal cancer. Lancet 338:178, 1991.

Richter JE, Falk GW, Vaesi MF: *Helicobacter pylori* and gastroesophageal reflux disease: The bug may not be all bad. Am J Gastroenterol 93:1800, 1998.

Rogot E, Murray JL: Smoking and causes of death among U.S. veterans: 16 years of observation. Public Health Rep 95:127, 1980.

Rolon PA, Castellsague X, Benz M, et al: Hot and cold maté drinking and esophageal cancer in Paraguay. Cancer Epidemiol Biomarkers Prev 4:595, 1995.

Rose EF: Cancer of the oesophagus. S Afr J Hosp Med 4:110, 1978.

Roth MJ, Strickland KL, Wang GQ, et al: High levels of carcinogenic polycyclic aromatic hydrocarbons present within food from Linxian, China, may contribute to that region's high incidence of oesophageal cancer. Eur J Cancer 34:757, 1998.

Sandler RS, Nyren O, Ekbom A, et al: The risk of esophageal cancer in patients with achalasia: A population based study. JAMA 274:1359, 1995.

Sarks JV: Report of a case of pharyngeal diverticulum containing a neoplasm in its wall. Br J Radiol 6:233, 1933.

Sartori S, Nielsen I, Indelli M, et al: Barrett's esophagus after chemotherapy with cyclophosphamide, methotrexate, and 5-fluorouracil (CMF): An iatrogenic injury? Ann Intern Med 114:210, 1991.

Schmidt W, Popham RE: The role of drinking and smoking in mortality from cancer and other causes in male alcoholics. Cancer 47:1031, 1981.

Schottenfeld D: Epidemiology of cancer of the oesophagus. Semin Oncol 11:92, 1984.

Scully C: Orofacial herpes simplex virus infections: Current concepts in the epidemiology, pathogenesis, and treatment, and disorders in which the virus may be implicated. Oral Surg Oral Med Oral Pathol 68:701, 1989.

Scully C, Cox MF, Prime SS, Maitland N: Papillomavirus: The current status in relation to oral disease. Oral Surg Oral Med Oral Pathol 65:526, 1988.

Selikoff IJ, Hammond EC, Seidman H: Mortality experience of insulation workers in the United States and Canada. Ann N Y Acad Sci 330:91, 1979.

Siddiqui M, Preussmann R: Esophageal cancer in Kashmir—an assessment. J Cancer Res Clin Oncol 115:111, 1989.

Silber W: Carcinoma of the oesophagus: Aspects of epidemiology and aetiology. Proc Nutr Soc 44:101, 1985.

Singer GM, Chuan J, Roman J, et al: Nitrosamines and nitrosamine precursors in foods from Linxian, China, a high incidence area for esophageal cancer. Carcinogenesis 7:733, 1986.

Sons HU: Etiologic and epidemiologic factors of carcinoma of the esophagus. Surg Gynecol Obstet 165:183, 1987.

Sons HU, Borchard F, Muller-Jah K, Sandmann H: Accelerated tumor induction by distal esophageal constriction in the rat under the influence of *N*-ethyl-*N*-butyl-nitrosamine. Cancer 56:2617, 1985.

Spechler SJ, Robbins AH, Rubins HB, et al: Adenocarcinoma and Barrett's esophagus: An overrated risk? Gastroenterology 87:927, 1984.

Spechler SJ, Schimmel EM, Dalton JW: Barrett's epithelium complicating lye ingestion with sparing of the distal esophagus. Gastroenterology 81:580, 1981.

Sporn MB, Newton DL: Chemoprevention of cancer with retinoids. FASEB J 38:2528, 1979.

Terzaghi M, Nellesheim P, Yarita T, et al: Epithelial focus assay for early detection of carcinogen-altered cells in various organs of rats exposed in situ to *N*-nitrosoheptamethyleneimine. J Natl Cancer Inst 67:1057, 1981.

Tuyns AJ: Oesophageal cancer in non-smoking drinkers and nondrinking smokers. Int J Cancer 32:443, 1983.

VanRensburg SJ, Bradshaw ES, Bradshaw D, et al: Oesophageal cancer in Zulu men, South Africa: A case-control study. Br J Cancer 51:399, 1985.

Vassallo A, Correa P, DeStefani E, et al: Esophageal cancer in Uruguay: A case control study. J Natl Cancer Inst 75:1005, 1985.

Warwick GP: Some aspects of the epidemiology and aetiology of oesophageal cancer with particular emphasis on the Transkei, South Africa. Adv Cancer Res 17:81, 1973.

Wu YC, Ran SZ: Genetic etiology of oesophageal cancer: Cytogenetic study of individuals in five cancer families in Linxian. Acta Genet Sin 6:277, 1979.

Wychulis AR, Cunnulangsson GH, Lagett OT: Carcinoma occurring in pharyngeal-oesophageal diverticulum. Surgery 66:976, 1969.

Wychulis AR, Woolam GL, Anderson HA, Ellis FH: Achalasia and carcinoma of the esophagus. JAMA 215:1638, 1971.

Wynder EL, Bross IJ: A study of etiological factors in cancer of the esophagus. Cancer 14:389, 1961.

Yang CS: Research on esophageal cancer in China: A review. Cancer Res 40:2633, 1980.

Yang PC, Davis S: Incidence of cancer of the esophagus in the U.S. by histologic type. Cancer 61:612, 1988.

Zhu XK, Li GS, He QQ, et al: A preliminary report on the possible association of esophageal cancer and HLA. Clin J Oncol 4:257, 1982.

Ziegler RG, Morris LE, Blot WJ, et al: Esophageal cancer among black men in Washington DC: I. Role of nutrition. J Natl Cancer Inst 67:1199, 1981.

CHAPTER **42**

Pathology of Malignant Esophageal Neoplasms

Victoria A. Marcus
Mark Redston
James B. Cullen

DEFINITION

An estimated 80% of primary esophageal neoplasms are malignant. Squamous cell carcinoma has traditionally accounted for more than 90% of these cancers. Although only 6% have been estimated to be adenocarcinoma, the incidence of the latter has been rising over the past two decades and more than half of esophageal carcinomas seen at most centers are now adenocarcinomas. In addition, there is a host of rare malignant primary esophageal neoplasms (Table 42–1). Because the thoracic surgeon deals predominantly with squamous cell carcinoma and adenocarcinoma of the esophagus, the discussion focuses mainly on these two diagnoses. The frozen-section analysis as well as prognostic indicators within a pathology report are also presented.

BASIC SCIENCE

Squamous Cell Carcinoma

Until 1990, squamous cell carcinoma was the most prevalent type of esophageal cancer in the United States. Patients are usually male and between 50 and 70 years of age. In the United States, squamous cell carcinoma occurs more commonly in African Americans than in the rest of the population. Approximately 55% of these neoplasms are located between the level of the tracheal carina and the inferior pulmonary veins (in the middle third of the esophagus); 15% and 30% are located in the upper third and lower third of the esophagus, respectively (Lewin et al, 1992).

Histogenesis

Squamous cell carcinoma is associated with risk factors (particularly the use of alcohol and tobacco) and predisposing conditions (e.g., celiac disease, achalasia) (see Chapter 41). Like other tumors of the gastrointestinal tract, squamous cell carcinoma appears to follow the dysplasia-carcinoma sequence. *Squamous dysplasia* and *carcinoma in situ* are premalignant lesions, defined as neoplastic squamous cells replacing part and all of the epithelial thickness, respectively, with an intact basement membrane. Detection of these premalignant lesions before the development of invasive carcinoma may be accomplished by mass screening in high-risk populations. In China, for example, exfoliative cytologic examination using an inflatable balloon covered with an abrasive nylon mesh has more than 90% sensitivity and specificity. More than 80% of lesions detected by screening cytologic examination are in early stage and may be cured by resection (Lewin et al, 1992). Although the interval between carcinoma in situ and invasive carcinoma is not known, it has been estimated to be 3 to 4 years (Guanrei et al, 1982).

Pathology

Superficial squamous cell carcinoma is characterized by invasion confined to the lamina propria or submucosa,

TABLE 42–1 ■ **Classification of Malignant Neoplasms of the Esophagus**

EPITHELIAL
Squamous cell carcinoma
Typical
Verrucous carcinoma
Spindle cell carcinoma
Small cell carcinoma
Basaloid carcinoma
Adenocarcinoma
Other
Adenosquamous carcinoma
Adenoacanthoma
Adenoid cystic carcinoma
Mucoepidermoid carcinoma
Neuroendocrine/small cell carcinoma
Choriocarcinoma
MESENCHYMAL
Leiomyosarcoma
Rhabdomyosarcoma
Synovial sarcoma
LYMPHOPROLIFERATIVE
Malignant non-Hodgkin's lymphoma
Hodgkin's lymphoma
OTHER
Malignant melanoma
NEOPLASMS METASTATIC TO THE ESOPHAGUS

regardless of lymph node involvement (Lewin and Appelman, 1996). At endoscopy, the lesion may be difficult to identify, sometimes appearing as only a subtle mucosal irregularity. The use of Lugol's iodine dye may help to differentiate normal glycogenated squamous mucosa from neoplastic epithelium, which does not stain (Dawsey et al, 1998). In addition to these occult lesions, the gross appearance of early squamous cell carcinoma may also be erosive or ulcerated, papillary, or, more commonly, plaque-like (Fig. 42–1). Although most superficial squamous cell carcinomas are small, some may involve the entire circumference of the esophagus.

In contrast to superficial carcinoma, most esophageal squamous cell carcinomas are at an advanced stage at presentation. Grossly, they may appear as primarily exophytic or endophytic lesions. Exophytic tumors are more common and include fungating, polypoid, and plaque-like tumors, which may contain deep ulceration with raised everted edges (Fig. 42–2). Endophytic or infiltrating neoplasms, accounting for 15% of tumors, show extensive intramural spread and are located at or below the level of adjacent mucosa. These tumors may elicit a desmoplastic response, which results in stricture formation. Multiple neoplasms may be present in 15% of cases, either as separate primary neoplasms reflecting field carcinogenesis or as proximal submucosal metastases (Kuwano et al, 1988).

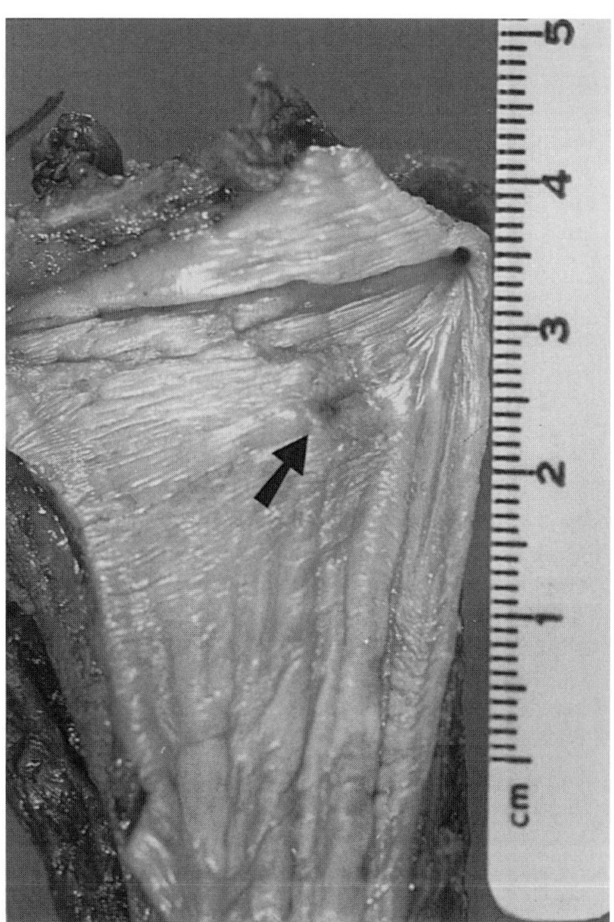

FIGURE 42–1 ■ Nearly occult superficial squamous cell carcinoma (*arrow*) with central ulceration.

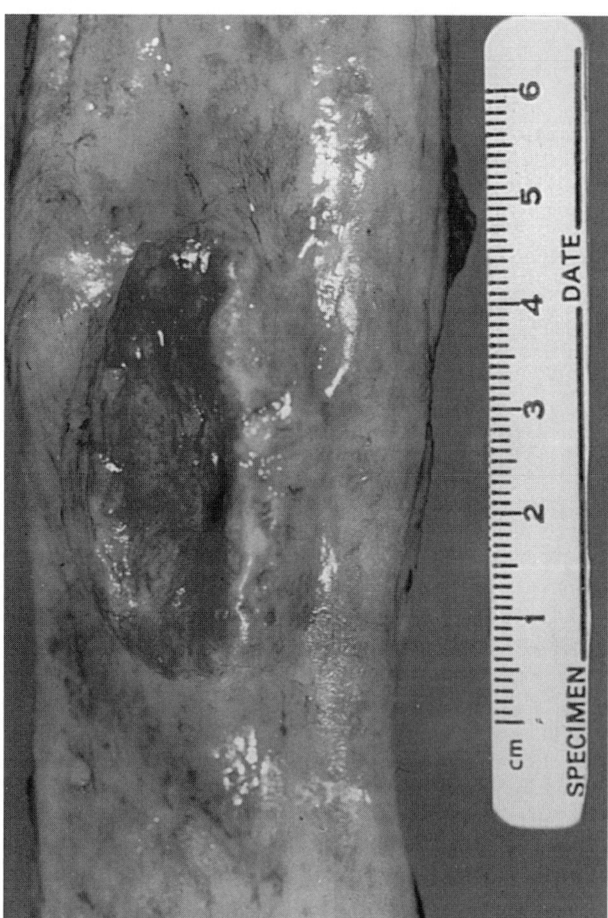

FIGURE 42–2 ■ Advanced squamous cell carcinoma with raised edges and deep ulceration.

At microscopy, the appearance of squamous cell carcinoma ranges from the well-differentiated type, with keratin pearls and intercellular bridging, to the poorly differentiated type, with nests of pleomorphic cells and few squamous features (Fig. 42–3).

Unlike the rest of the gastrointestinal tract, the esophagus has no serosal layer. Advanced carcinomas penetrating the adventitia may therefore easily infiltrate adjacent organs. Invasion of the tracheobronchial tree is most common (40%) and may lead to fistula formation (10% to 15%) (Mandard et al, 1981). In addition to tracheobronchial or pulmonary involvement, malignant neoplasms involving the upper third of the esophagus may invade the thoracic duct and the left recurrent nerve; those of the middle third may involve and rupture the aorta; and malignancies of the lower third may invade the diaphgram, stomach, and liver. Metastases to regional and distant lymph nodes may also be present. The site of lymph node involvement, however, does not necessarily reflect the site of the primary malignancy because 40% of upper-third tumors metastasize to abdominal lymph nodes, and an equal percentage of lower-third neoplasms involve cervical lymph nodes (Mandard et al, 1981). Hematogenous metastases to distant organs are present in approximately one third of cases, specifically to the lung, liver, pleura, bone, and kidney, in decreasing order of frequency (Anderson and Lad, 1982; Chan et al, 1986).

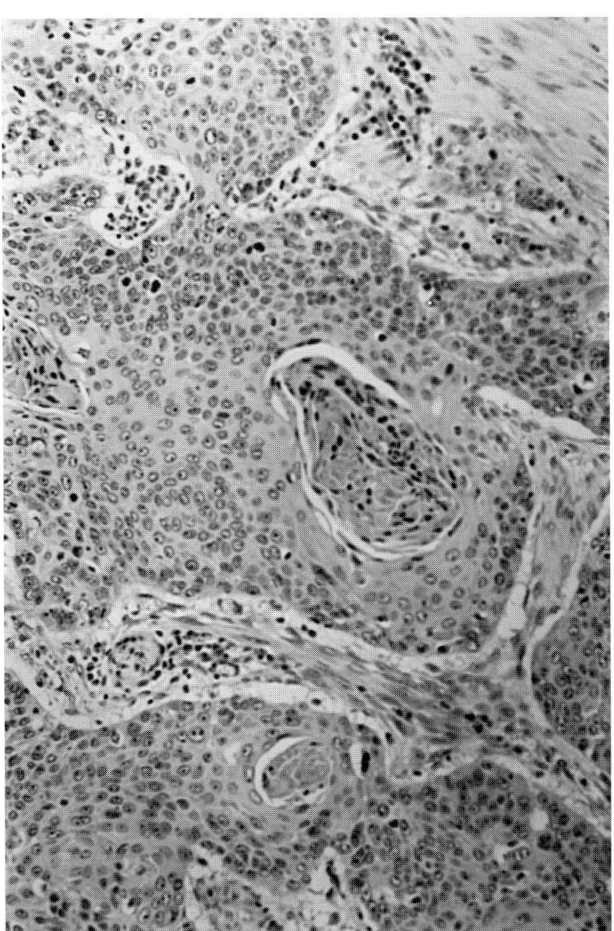

FIGURE 42–3 ■ Moderately differentiated squamous cell carcinoma with keratin formation.

Adenocarcinoma

The incidence of esophageal adenocarcinoma has been rising, and these tumors account for more than half of malignant esophageal neoplasms in many centers (Blot et al, 1991; Gore, 1997; Kirby and Rice, 1994; Mayer, 1993). The typical patient is a 60-year-old white man with a lower esophageal tumor. Differentiating esophageal adenocarcinoma at the gastroesophageal junction from gastric adenocarcinoma is difficult, if not impossible. There is evidence, however, that these tumors may have a similar biology (Mandard et al, 1995). Indeed, differentiating between esophageal and gastric origins currently has no effect on treatment.

Histogenesis

Esophageal adenocarcinoma may arise in various settings (Table 42–2). Most, however, arise in the background of *Barrett's metaplasia. Barrett's esophagus* typically occurs in white men aged 40 to 60 years. It is located in the lower esophagus and is usually secondary to prolonged gastroesophageal reflux, often in a setting of hiatus hernia. About 12% of patients with chronic gastroesophageal reflux experience Barrett's esophagus (Winters et al, 1987).

At endoscopy, the squamocolumnar junction (Z line) is proximally displaced. The mucosa in Barrett's esophagus is pink and stains blue if sprayed with acetic acid followed by toluidine blue, like gastric mucosa. It is vital to supply the pathologist with information regarding the location of the biopsy site in relation to the true gastroesophageal junction. On histologic examination, Barrett's esophagus is characterized by the replacement of squamous epithelium with columnar epithelium.

Traditionally, three forms of Barrett's metaplasia have been described: (1) *cardiac type* (resembling gastric cardia), (2) *fundic type* (resembling gastric fundus), and (3) *specialized type* epithelium (Ming and Goldman, 1998). The latter, also known as the *distinctive type* of Barrett's epithelium, is characterized by goblet cells (intestinal metaplasia) and is particularly susceptible to neoplastic transformation. Most pathologists now require the identification of specialized type of epithelium for the diagnosis of Barrett's metaplasia (Lewin et al, 1992; Riddell, 1996).

Although the time course is unknown, Barrett's metaplasia may progress to dysplasia and carcinoma (Streitz, 1994). Approximately 5% to 10% of patients with Barrett's metaplasia eventually demonstrate esophageal adenocarcinoma, representing a 30- to 40-fold higher risk over that for the general population (Cameron et al, 1985; Spechler et al, 1984). A history of smoking or alcoholism may increase the risk. On the other hand, neither the duration of existence nor the physical length of Barrett's metaplasia affects risk for malignant transformation. In fact, most Barrett's adenocarcinomas occur in relatively short segments of Barrett's metaplasia (Lewin et al, 1992).

Finally, antireflux therapy may lead to pseudoregression of Barrett's epithelium by allowing squamous mucosa to cover metaplastic glands. There is no evidence, however, that either medical or surgical antireflux therapy can prevent the development of carcinoma.

Surveillance for early detection of neoplastic transformation in Barrett's esophagus is usually performed every 1 to 2 years (Mandard et al, 1995). The pathologist must distinguish reactive atypia (due to inflammation) from dysplasia (low grade or high grade), a task that is often difficult. High-grade dysplasia is an ominous finding because up to half of affected patients actually have invasive adenocarcinoma in resected esophagectomy specimens.

TABLE 42–2 ■ **Origins of Esophageal Adenocarcinoma**

Sources of Adenocarcinoma	*Comments*
Barrett's esophagus	Most common
Esophageal mucosal glands	Cardiac-type; in lamina propria; upper and lower thirds of esophagus
Esophageal submucosal glands	Mucus-secreting (rarely serous); in submucosa; upper to lower esophagus
Ectopic gastric mucosa	Upper third; cardiac- or fundic-type glands
Nonesophageal sources	Direct extension (e.g., stomach) or metastasis

For this reason, a diagnosis of high-grade dysplasia, confirmed by a second experienced pathologist, is considered an indication for surgery in suitable surgical candidates (Clark et al, 1996; Edwards et al, 1996; Heitmiller et al, 1996; Wright, 1997). Interestingly, however, in approximately 40% of patients with adenocarcinoma, Barrett's esophagus is diagnosed only at the time of resection (Haggitt and Dean, 1985; Mandard et al, 1995). These patients have had no prior symptoms of gastroesophageal reflux and would not have been involved in surveillance.

Pathology

The gross appearances of adenocarcinoma are comparable to those of squamous cell carcinoma, varying from the occult lesion to the deeply infiltrating endophytic tumor to the large exophytic mass (Fig. 42–4). Most adenocarcinomas are flat and ulcerated. Occlusion of the lumen may occur. The adjacent background mucosa is often red, reflecting the associated Barrett's metaplasia (Fig. 42–5). Some large malignancies, however, may obliterate the preexisting Barrett's epithelium.

The histologic appearance of esophageal adenocarcinoma is similar to that of its gastric counterpart. Well-differentiated to moderately differentiated adenocarcinoma forming tubular or acinar structures (Fig. 42–6) is most commonly present (Paraf et al, 1995). Some neoplasms are mucinous, and rare signet ring–type adenocarcinoma may occur.

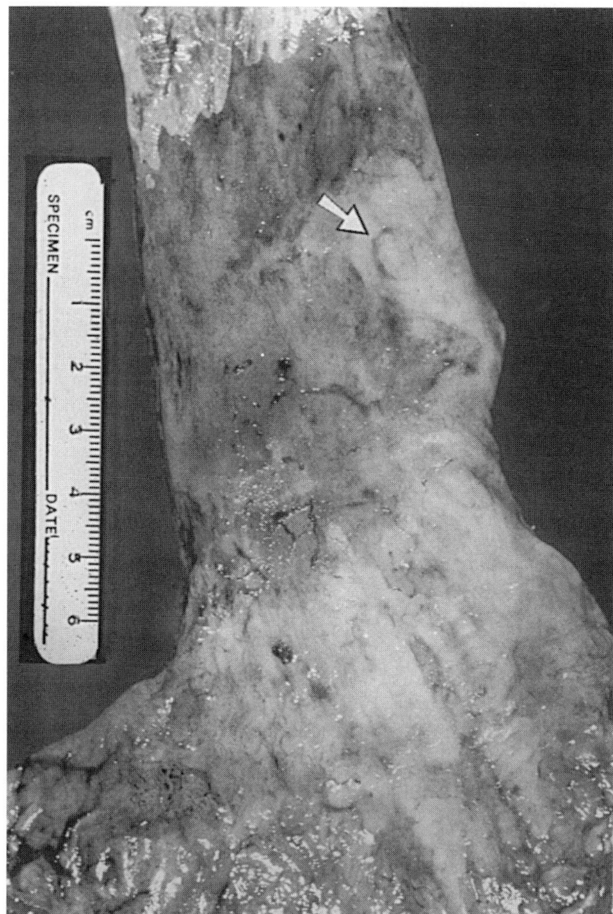

FIGURE 42–5 ■ Barrett's metaplasia with occult adenocarcinoma (*arrow*).

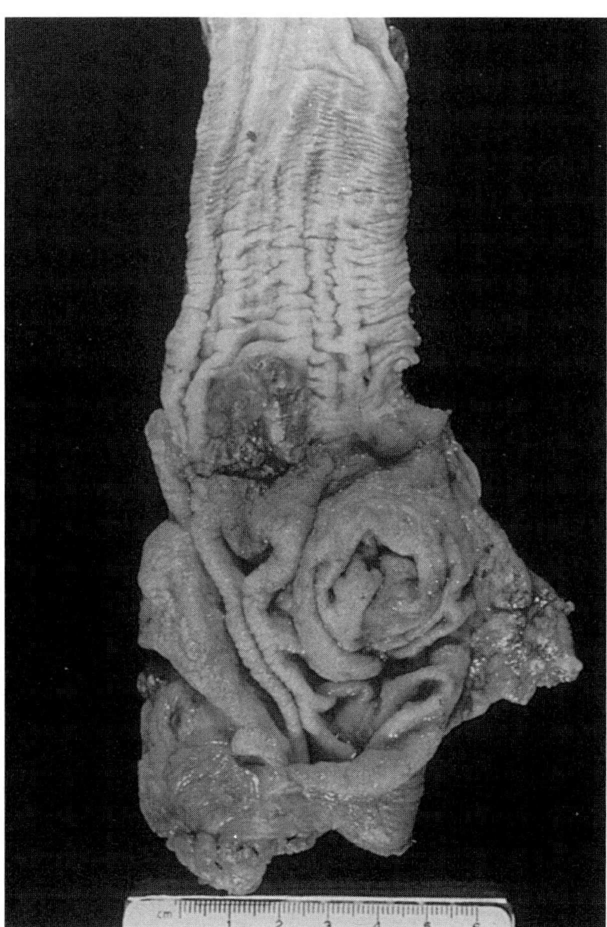

FIGURE 42–4 ■ Exophytic adenocarcinoma at the gastroesophageal junction.

As with squamous cell carcinoma, most adenocarcinomas are advanced at the time of diagnosis. Direct extension to adjacent organs, particularly diaphragm, stomach, and liver, is more common than tracheobronchial involvement, as would be expected by its usual distal

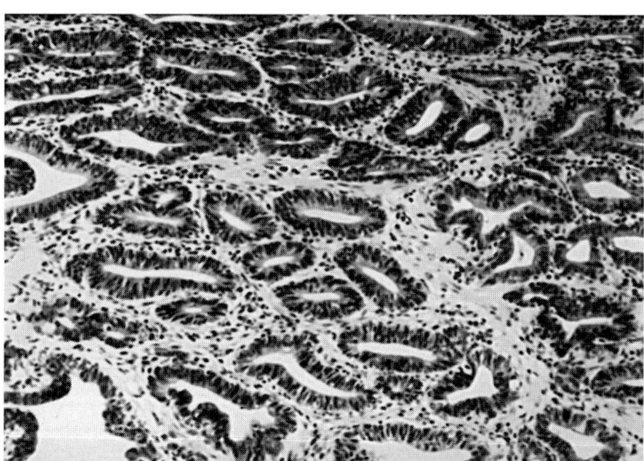

FIGURE 42–6 ■ Moderately differentiated esophageal adenocarcinoma with formation of tubules.

location. Lymph node or distant metastases or both occur in nearly 75% of cases (Ming and Goldman, 1998). Survival rates for adenocarcinoma are comparable to those for squamous cell carcinoma.

Other Malignant Neoplasms of the Esophagus

Aside from squamous cell carcinoma and adenocarcinoma, there are numerous other types of primary esophageal malignancies. Although they are rare, brief mention is made of the more important ones. Detailed descriptions are available in other publications (Lewin and Appelman, 1996). Some of the malignancies listed in Table 42–1, such as choriocarcinoma and malignant lymphoma of the esophagus, are too rare to justify further discussion.

Verrucous carcinoma is a slow-growing variant of squamous cell carcinoma. Although gradually invasive, it usually remains superficial and rarely metastasizes. It is an exophytic, cauliflower-like tumor. Histologic diagnosis is difficult because only minimal dysplasia is noted at microscopy. Indeed, a superficial biopsy specimen may be reported as a benign squamous papilloma. Correct diagnosis often requires close clinicopathologic correlation.

Spindle cell carcinoma, another variant of squamous cell carcinoma, occurs in men aged 50 to 60 years. Usually found in the middle to lower esophagus, it is an exophytic, polypoid tumor often with superficial ulceration and a pedicle. Although they may measure up to 15 cm, spindle cell carcinomas tend not to infiltrate deeply into the esophageal wall. Typically, at microscopy, there is a malignant squamous component admixed with a more predominant malignant spindle cell component, which may be indistinguishable from a sarcoma. The latter may even contain smooth muscle, cartilage, bone, or other types of mesenchymal differentiation.

Small cell carcinoma of the esophagus may either represent a variant of squamous cell carcinoma or may be a primary neuroendocrine carcinoma. Metastatic small cell carcinoma from the lung must first be ruled out. Usually occurring in the middle to lower third, primary small cell carcinoma of the esophagus is more common in males in the fifth to seventh decades. Grossly, these tumors are large exophytic lesions, often with ulceration and necrosis. They are composed of anaplastic cells in solid sheets or ribbons. Approximately 30% of small cell carcinomas have focal evidence of squamous differentiation. Although they may have immunohistochemical evidence of adrenocorticotropic hormone (ACTH), Cushing's syndrome has not been documented in association with such findings. Hypercalcemia and syndrome of inappropriate antidiuretic hormone, however, have been reported. Primary small cell carcinoma of the esophagus is an aggressive neoplasm that manifests in a late stage; most patients with this tumor die within 6 months of diagnosis.

Adenoid cystic carcinoma occurs equally in the two genders, usually in the seventh decade, and is located in the middle to lower third of the esophagus. Its origin, although debated, may be either the squamous epithelium or the submucosal ducts or glands. Grossly, adenoid cystic carcinomas are large exophytic masses. They have a cribriform pattern with abundant basement membrane material. Although histologically similar to their salivary gland counterparts, these neoplasms are more aggressive in the esophagus because they usually manifest with widespread distant metastases.

Mucoepidermoid carcinoma, which also occurs in older adults, is located in the middle to lower third of the esophagus. Its proposed origins are similar to those of adenoid cystic carcinoma. These tumors are characterized by islands of neoplastic cells, often with well-differentiated squamous cell carcinoma at the periphery, closely admixed with glandular elements within the center. Mucoepidermoid carcinomas are aggressive; lymph node metastases are common at presentation.

Primary malignant melanoma of the esophagus occurs more commonly in males in their sixth to seventh decades. Located in the middle to lower third of the esophagus, these tumors are large, exophytic, polypoid lesions usually with a smooth surface. Approximately 10% are amelanotic. Before a primary esophageal malignant melanoma is diagnosed, metastatic spread from the more common origins must be ruled out, particularly the skin, the eyes, and the mucosa of the anus or vagina. Although present in only 40% of cases, junctional melanocytic activity in adjacent esophageal mucosa is considered diagnostic of primary esophageal melanoma (Kreuser, 1979). Esophageal malignant melanoma usually is an advanced tumor, often with distant metastases at presentation; most patients die within 1 year of diagnosis.

Metastatic tumors to the esophagus may arise from lymphatic or hematogenous spread, but more commonly, secondary involvement of the esophagus by tumor occurs by direct extension (Lewin and Appelman, 1996). Extension may occur, for example, from the larynx, thyroid, lung, or stomach. In addition, metastatic tumor to periesophageal lymph nodes, usually from primary tumors in the lung or breast, may subsequently invade the esophagus. Metastatic lesions are usually asymptomatic and small. Because most are submucosal, histologic examination of a superficial biopsy specimen may be nondiagnostic, revealing only normal squamous epithelium. These lesions, however, have higher risk for perforation, and caution must be taken with collection of deep biopsy specimens. Lastly, although not metastatic in origin, synchronous or metachronous carcinoma of the esophagus occurs at high incidence in patients with squamous carcinoma of the head and neck, likely because of exposure to identical carcinogens, most notably tobacco.

MANAGEMENT

Role of the Frozen-Section Analysis

Esophageal carcinomas tend to spread in submucosal lymphatics. Although such spread may form satellite nodules, the extension usually is grossly imperceptible, being detectable only on microscopy. Typically, the lymphatic spread is proximal and may extend for several centimeters. It is very difficult for a surgeon to determine the adequacy of the proximal resection margin without analysis of a frozen section of tissue. An intraoperative frozen-section analysis from the proximal margin is indicated

TABLE 42–3 ■ **TNM Staging of Esophageal Carcinoma**

Stage	*Primary Tumor (T)*	*Regional Lymph Nodes (N)*	*Distant Metastasis (M)*
	Tx: Cannot be assessed	Nx: Cannot be assessed	Mx: Cannot be assessed
	T0: No primary tumor	N0: no metastases to regional lymph nodes	M0: No distant metastases
0	Tis: Carcinoma in situ	N0	M0
I	T1: Invasion of lamina propria or submucosa	N0	M0
IIA	T2: Invasion into muscularis propria	N0	M0
	T3: Invasion into adventitia	N0	M0
IIB	T1 or T2	N1: Metastases to regional lymph nodes	M0
III	T3	N1	M0
	T4: Invasion into adjacent structures	Any N	M0
IV	Any T	Any N	M1: Distant metastases

only if further proximal resection can be performed should carcinoma be detected at the margin. Optimally, a ring of the entire esophageal resection line should be examined. Frozen-section analysis may therefore avert the performance of direct anastomosis through malignancy, thereby reducing the likelihood of anastomotic recurrence and improving the chances for cure.

Some surgeons request a frozen-section analysis of celiac lymph nodes at the beginning of the thoracoabdominal approach. If tumor is detected, the surgeon is aware that cure is unlikely. Indeed, celiac node metastases are present in 40% of patients without clinical evidence of metastatic disease (Lewin et al, 1992). The presence of metastatic disease does not necessarily negate surgery, however, because resection is often an effective form of palliation.

Pathologic Prognostic Indicators

The most important prognostic indicators are included in the tumor-node-metastasis (TNM) staging system as proposed by the American Joint Commission on Cancer (Table 42–3) (Fleming et al, 1997). First, the depth of infiltration correlates independently with prognosis. A patient with a neoplasm limited to the lamina propria or submucosa (i.e., T1), has a 5-year survival rate greater than 60%, whereas a patient with an advanced malignancy invading adjacent structures (T4) has a 5-year survival rate less than 10%. Second, although related to depth of infiltration, the presence of lymph node metastases is an independent prognostic indicator. The number of involved lymph nodes, not their location, may also affect prognosis, and some groups define N1 as one to four affected lymph nodes and N2 as five or more positive regional lymph nodes (Ming and Goldman, 1998). The presence of distant metastases is an ominous sign, and in affected patients, 5-year survival rate is negligible.

Gross morphology, histologic grade, and tumor type are not independent prognostic factors. Some tumor types, such as verrucous carcinoma and spindle cell carcinoma, carry a better outcome, but this effect is related to tumor stage. Size of tumor less than 5 cm was previously thought to convey a better prognosis. Although tumor size may affect resectability, as shown by multivariate analysis, this variable is not an independent prognosticator and is no longer included in the staging system. In addition, vascular invasion, perineural invasion, and fistula formation have no definite prognostic significance (Lewin et al, 1992).

Techniques other than pathologic staging may also have prognostic importance. DNA aneuploidy, detected through flow cytometry, may correlate with increased postoperative recurrence. In addition, immunohistochemical analysis of p53, as well as elevation of epidermal growth factor, epidermal growth factor receptor, and transforming growth factor-α, may prove to correlate with worse outcome (Ming and Goldman, 1998).

■ KEY REFERENCES

Lewin KJ, Appelman HD: Atlas of Tumor Pathology: Tumors of the Esophagus and Stomach. Washington, DC, Armed Forces Institute of Pathology, 1996.

Like all AFIP fascicles, this monograph remains the standard for tumor pathology.

Lewin KJ, Riddell RH, Weinstein WM: Gastrointestinal Pathology and its Clinical Implications. New York, Igaku-Shoin, 1992.

This two-volume book is a classic text combining pathology with clinical practice. A new edition may be available soon.

■ REFERENCES

Anderson LL, Lad TE: Autopsy findings in squamous-cell carcinoma of the esophagus. Cancer 50:1587, 1982.

Blot WJ, Devesa S, Kneller RW, et al: Rising incidence of adenocarcinoma of the esophagus and gastric cardia. JAMA 265:1287, 1991.

Cameron AJ, Ott BJ, Payne WS: The incidence of adenocarcinoma in columnar-lined (Barrett's) esophagus. N Engl J Med 313:857, 1985.

Chan KW, Chan EY, Chan CW: Carcinoma of the esophagus: An autopsy study of 231 cases. Pathology 18:400, 1986.

Clark GW, Ireland AP, DeMeester TR: Dysplasia in Barrett's esophagus: Diagnosis, surveillance and treatment. Dig Dis 14:213, 1996.

Dawsey SM, Fleischer DE, Wang GQ, et al: Mucosal iodine staining improves endoscopic visualization of squamous dysplasia and squamous cell carcinoma of the esophagus in Linxian, China. Cancer 83:220, 1998.

Edwards MJ, Gable DR, Lentsch AB, Richardson JD: The rationale for esophagectomy as the optimal therapy for Barrett's esophagus with high-grade dysplasia. Ann Surg 223:585, 1996.

Fleming ID, Cooper JS, Henson DE, et al: AJCC Cancer Staging Manual, 5th ed. Philadelphia, Lippincott-Raven, 1997.

Gore RM: Esophageal cancer: Clinical and pathologic features. Radiol Clin North Am 35:243, 1997.

Guanrei Y, He H, Sungliang Q, et al: Endoscopic diagnosis of 115 cases of early esophageal carcinoma. Endoscopy 14:157, 1982.

Haggitt RC, Dean PJ: Adenocarcinoma in Barrett's epithelium. In Spechler SJ, Goyal RK (eds): Barrett's Esophagus: Pathophysiology, Diagnosis, and Management. New York, Elsevier, 1985, pp 153–166.

Heitmiller RF, Redmond M, Hamilton SR: Barrett's esophagus with high-grade dysplasia: An indication for prophylactic esophagectomy. Ann Surg 224:66, 1996.

Kirby TJ, Rice TW: The epidemiology of esophageal carcinoma: The changing face of a disease. Chest Surg Clin North Am 4:217, 1994.

Kreuser ED: Primary malignant melanoma of the esophagus. Virchows Arch (A) 385:49, 1979.

Kuwano H, Ohno S, Matsuda H, et al: Serial histologic evaluation of multiple primary squamous cell carcinomas of the esophagus. Cancer 61:1635, 1988.

Lewin KJ, Appelman HD: Atlas of Tumor Pathology: Tumors of the Esophagus and Stomach. Washington, DC, Armed Forces Institute of Pathology, 1996.

Lewin KJ, Riddell RH, Weinstein WM: Gastrointestinal Pathology and its Clinical Implications. New York, Ikagu-Shoin, 1992.

Mandard AM, Chasle J, Marnay J, et al: Autopsy findings in 111 cases of esophageal cancer. Cancer 48:329, 1981.

Mandard AM, Whitehead R, Li L, et al: Other tumours of the oesophagus. In Whitehead R (ed): Gastrointestinal and Oesophageal Pathology, 2nd ed. New York, Churchill Livingstone, 1995, pp 777–822.

Mayer RJ: Overview: The changing nature of esophageal cancer. Chest 103:404S, 1993.

Ming SC, Goldman H: Pathology of the Gastrointestinal Tract, 2nd ed. Baltimore, Williams & Wilkins, 1998.

Paraf F, Flejou JF, Pignon JP, et al: Surgical pathology of adenocarcinoma arising in Barrett's esophagus: Analysis of 67 cases. Am J Surg Pathol 19:183, 1995.

Riddell RH: Early detection of neoplasia of the esophagus and gastroesophageal junction. Am J Gastroenterol 91:853, 1996.

Spechler SJ, Robbins AH, Rubins HB, et al: Adenocarcinoma and Barrett's esophagus: An overrated risk? Gastroenterology 87:927, 1984.

Streitz JM Jr: Barrett's esophagus and esophageal cancer. Chest Surg Clin North Am 4:227, 1994.

Winters C Jr, Spurling TJ, Chobanian SJ, et al: Barrett's esophagus: A prevalent, occult complication of gastroesophageal reflux disease. Gastroenterology 92:118, 1987.

Wright TA: High-grade dysplasia in Barrett's oesophagus. Br J Surg 84:760, 1997.

MANAGEMENT

CHAPTER **43**

Esophageal Carcinoma

DIAGNOSIS AND STAGING OF ESOPHAGEAL CARCINOMA

Thomas W. Rice

DIAGNOSIS

The clinical diagnosis of esophageal carcinoma is obtained from a history, physical examination, and barium esophagogram. In the Western world, the classic presentation is solid dysphagia in a middle-aged to elderly white man with a long-standing history of reflux and a known hiatal hernia. This is treated as an esophageal adenocarcinoma until proven otherwise. Physical examination typically reveals a robust man without weight loss, with potential comorbidities, and without clinically detectable metastases to nonregional lymph nodes (supraclavicular) or to distant sites (liver, pleura).

In contradistinction, a patient with squamous cell carcinoma is usually from an endemic area and a lower socioeconomic class, with a history of dysphagia, weight loss, heavy smoking and drinking, and an advanced stage of carcinoma. Barium esophagogram, the first investigation in the evaluation of dysphagia and the clinical diagnosis of esophageal carcinoma (Fig. 43–1), has been replaced by flexible fiberoptic videoesophagoscopy in many centers (Fig. 43–2) (see Color Plate). In patients with esophageal carcinoma, however, barium esophagogram has been reported to detect a lesion in 98% of barium studies, was suggestive or diagnostic of esophageal carcinoma in 96% of studies, and had an estimated positive predictive value of 42% (Levine et al, 1997). For many physicians, barium esophagogram remains the principal test for the clinical diagnosis of esophageal carcinoma.

The clinical diagnosis of esophageal carcinoma requires tissue confirmation. Flexible esophagoscopy is the procedure of choice for the pathologic diagnosis of esophageal carcinoma (see Chapter 6, Esophagoscopy). Cytology brushings and multiple biopsies are diagnostic in most patients (Figs. 43–3 and 43–4) (see Color Plate). In the exceptional case of a patient for whom the results of esophagoscopy and biopsy fail to confirm the clinical diagnosis, endoscopic esophageal ultrasound (EUS) and fine-needle aspiration (FNA) of the abnormal esophageal wall are useful in the diagnosis of malignant strictures that are not endoscopically accessible (Faigel et al, 1998). FNA or open biopsy of suspected distant metastases provides a pathologic diagnosis and crucial staging.

Surveillance of high-risk groups allows the diagnosis of early-stage disease in asymptomatic patients. This process is cost-effective compared with other cancer surveillance programs (Provenzale et al, 1999; Streitz et al, 1998). In North America, patients with a columnar-lined esophagus should undergo esophagoscopy and biopsy (four quadrant biopsy samples every 2 cm) every 1 to 2 years.

STAGING

TNM staging of esophageal carcinoma is obtained through the evaluation of primary *tumor* invasion (T)

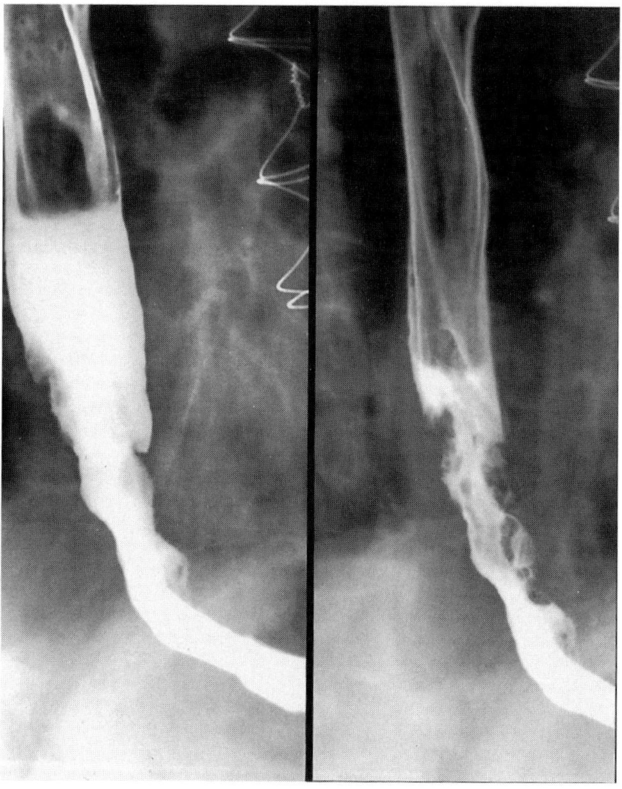

FIGURE 43–1 ■ Barium esophagogram of a malignant esophageal stricture. This long irregular stricture has mucosal destruction and irregular filling defects obstructing the esophageal lumen.

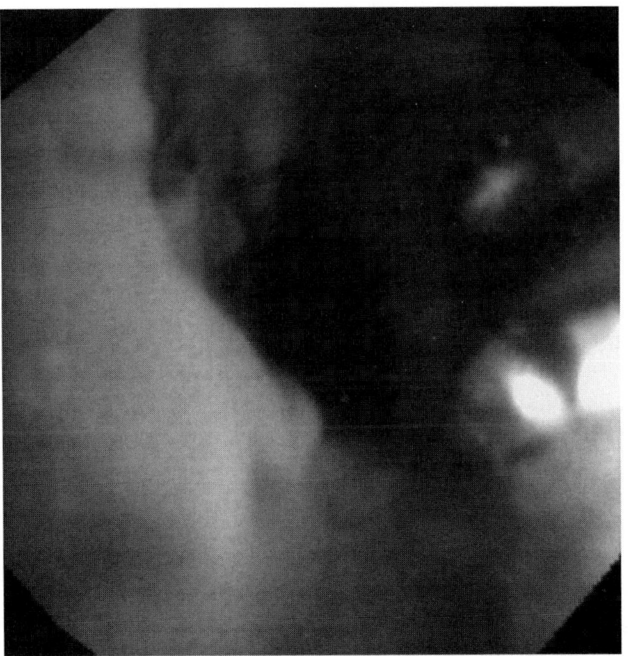

FIGURE 43–2 ■ Esophagoscopy and biopsy, following brush cytology, of a malignant esophageal stricture. (See Color Plate.)

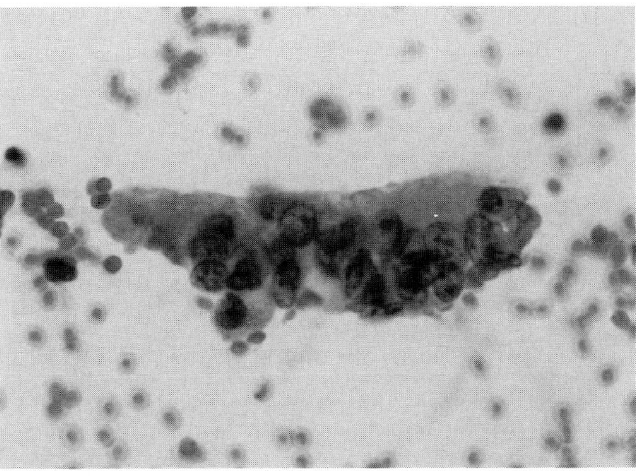

FIGURE 43–3 ■ Adenocarcinoma cells obtained from brushing of Barrett's esophagus. Shown are clusters of neoplastic cells with hyperchromatic, pleomorphic nuclei and loss of polarity but retained columnar configuration and cytoplasmic mucin. (See Color Plate.)

and the status of regional lymph *nodes* (N) and distant sites *(metastases)* (M) (Table 43–1) (Fleming et al, 1997).

Classification

Primary Tumor

Primary tumor (T) is defined only by the depth of invasion (Fig. 43–5).

Tis tumors are intraepithelial malignancies, which are confined to the epithelium without invasion of the basement membrane (high-grade dysplasia).

T1 tumors breach the basement membrane to invade the lamina propria, muscularis mucosa, or submucosa but do not invade beyond the submucosa. The broad definition of T1 carcinomas has prompted the clinically accepted practical subdivision of this subset into T1 intramucosal carcinomas (T1a), which invade the lamina propria or muscularis mucosa, and T1 submucosal carcinomas (T1b).

T2 tumors invade into but not beyond the muscularis propria.

T3 tumors invade beyond the esophageal wall into the paraesophageal tissue but do not invade adjacent structures.

T4 tumors directly invade structures in the vicinity of the esophagus.

Regional Lymph Nodes

Regional lymph nodes (N) are characterized only by the absence (N0) or presence (N1) of metastases to lymph nodes in the area of the primary tumor (see Table 43–1 and Fig. 43–5). Distinction of a regional lymph node from a nonregional lymph node may be problematic de-

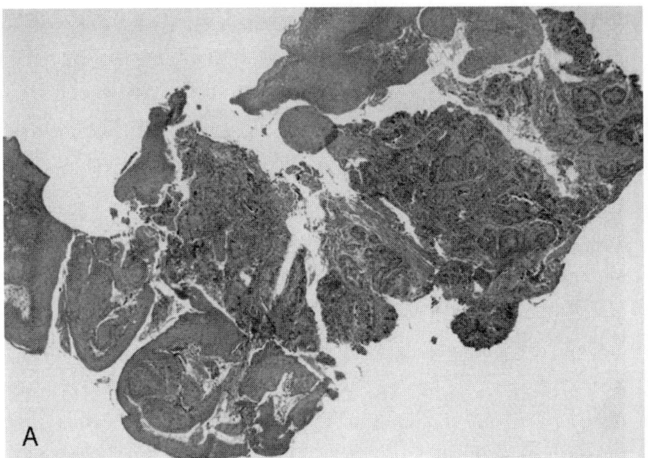

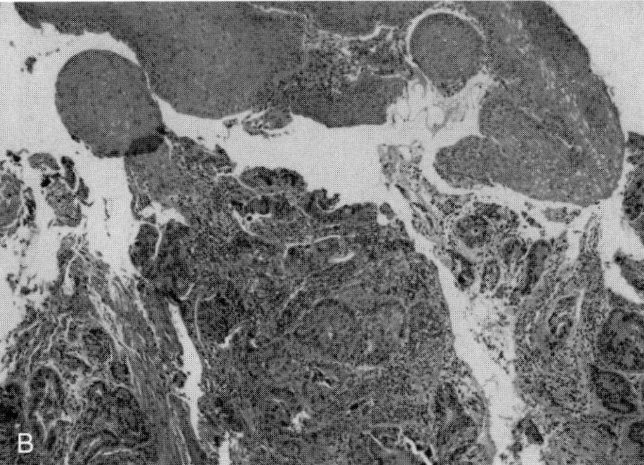

FIGURE 43–4 ■ *A*, Superficial mucosal biopsy demonstrates malignant glands undermining intact squamous mucosa. This is at least intramucosal cancer. No goblet cells are seen. *B*, Higher magnification demonstrates malignant glands infiltrating the lamina propria below the squamous epithelium. (See Color Plate.)

TABLE 43–1 ■ **Tumor-Node-Metastasis (TNM) Staging of Esophageal Carcinoma**

T:	PRIMARY TUMOR	
	TX	Tumor cannot be assessed
	T0	No evidence of tumor
	Tis	High-grade dysplasia
	T1	Tumor invades the lamina propria, muscularis mucosa or submucosa; does not breach the submucosa
	T2	Tumor invades into but not beyond the muscularis propria
	T3	Tumor invades the paraesophageal tissue but does not invade adjacent structures
	T4	Tumor invades adjacent structures
N:	REGIONAL LYMPH NODES	
	NX	Regional lymph nodes cannot be assessed
	N0	No regional lymph node metastases
	N1	Regional lymph node metastases
M:	DISTANT METASTASES	
	MX	Distant metastases cannot be assessed
	M1a	Upper thoracic esophagus metastatic to cervical lymph nodes
		Lower thoracic esophagus metastatic to celiac lymph nodes
	M1b	Upper thoracic esophagus metastatic to other nonregional lymph nodes or other distant sites
		Midthoracic esophagus metastatic to either nonregional lymph nodes or other distant sites
		Lower thoracic esophagus metastatic to other nonregional lymph nodes or other distant sites

STAGE GROUPINGS	T	N	M
Stage 0	Tis	N0	M0
Stage I	T1	N0	M0
Stage IIA	T2	N0	M0
	T3	N0	M0
Stage IIB	T1	N1	M0
	T2	N1	M0
Stage III	T3	N1	M0
	T4	Any N	M0
Stage IVA	Any T	Any N	M1a
Stage IVB	Any T	Any N	M1b

spite the broad definition in the staging manual (Fleming et al, 1997). The regional lymph node map is crucial for clinical staging and lymph node sampling (Fig. 43–6).

The lack of subclassification of N1 is a shortcoming of the present staging system. N1 lymph node burden is a prognosticator, and many physicians substage N1, depending on the total number of N1 nodes (less than four) and the percentage of resected lymph nodes that are N1.

Distant Metastases

Similarly, distant sites (M) are characterized by the presence (M1) or absence (M0) of metastases (see Table 43–1). Revision of the staging system for esophageal carcinoma subdivides distant metastatic carcinomas (M1) into M1a (distant, nonregional lymph node metastases) and M1b (other distant metastases) (Fleming et al, 1997). M1a disease is classified further by tumor location. M1a tumors of the upper thoracic esophagus have metastasized to cervical nodes and M1a tumors of the lower thoracic esophagus have metastasized to celiac lymph nodes. No M1a subdivision for midthoracic esophageal carcinomas exists because these tumors metastatic to nonregional lymph nodes have a prognosis equivalent to that of tumors metastatic to other distant sites. Although this subclassification has anatomic and statistical significance, the clinical relevance is questionable (Christie et al, 1999).

Summary

TNM descriptors are grouped into stages to assemble subgroups with similar behavior and prognosis (see Table 43–1). Despite shortcomings, the present staging system is an essential tool in the evaluation and treatment of esophageal carcinoma.

Clinical Staging

All information obtained before definitive treatment is used to establish clinical stage (cTNM). Evidence is derived from physical examination, imaging, esophagoscopy, laparoscopy, thoracoscopy, biopsy, and needle aspiration. Clinical stage provides the baseline for treatment evaluation and is the basis for rational treatment decisions.

Determination of Clinical Tumor (cT) Stage

EUS is the only clinical tool that provides a detailed examination of the esophageal wall. It is the procedure of choice for determining cT (see part 3 of Chapter 5). The muscularis propria (fourth ultrasound layer) is critical in differentiating T1, T2, and T3 tumors also. EUS is used to evaluate the interface between the primary tumor and adjacent structures.

Tumors are defined as follows:

- cT by EUS
- cT1 if there is no invasion of the muscularis propria (fourth ultrasound layer)
- cT2 if invasion is into the muscularis propria
- cT3 if invasion is beyond the muscularis propria
- cT4 if there is invasion of adjacent structures

In a review of 21 series, the accuracy of EUS for T determination was 84% (Rösch, 1995). Accuracy is not constant; it varies with T. In this meta-analysis, for T1 carcinomas accuracy was 83.5% with 16.5% of tumors overstaged; for T2, it was 73% with 10% understaged and 17% overstaged; for T3, it was 89% with 5% understaged and 6% overstaged; and for T4 it was 89% with 11% understaged. A review of the literature shows variation in accuracy with T: 75% to 82% for T1, 64% to 85% for T2, 89% to 94% for T3, and 88% to 100% for T4 (Saunders et al, 1997). The most unreliable of cT EUS determinations is that for cT2 (Heidemann et al, 2000).

Exclusion of cT4 carcinomas, demonstrated by the preservation of fat planes between an esophageal cancer and adjacent structures, is the only role of computed

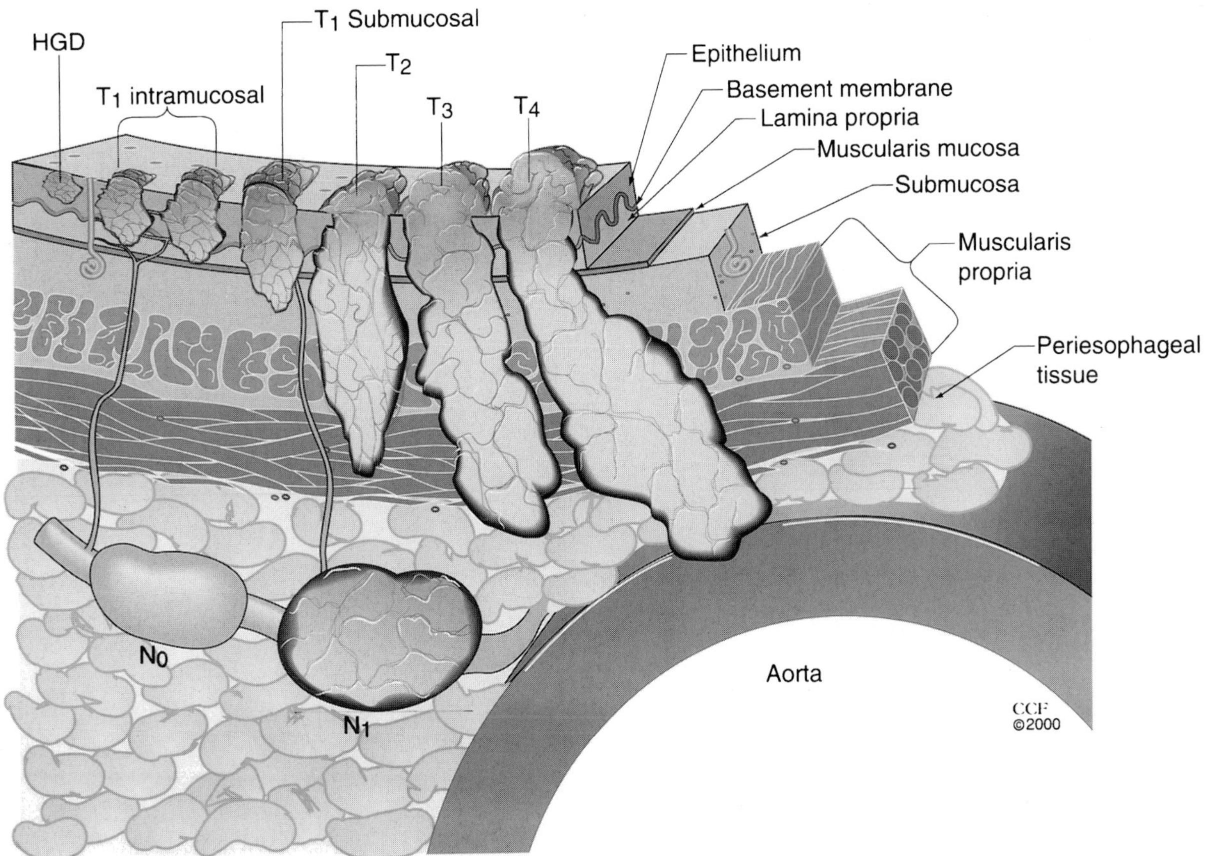

FIGURE 43–5 ■ Primary tumor status (T) is defined by depth of tumor invasion. Regional lymph node (N) status is defined by the absence (N0) or presence (N1) of regional nodal metastases. (HGD, high-grade dysplasia). (Courtesy of Cleveland Clinic Foundation.)

tomography (CT) in determining cT (Fig. 43–7). Contiguous soft tissues provide radiographic contrast necessary to define the esophagus; however, these planes may be absent in cachectic patients. In normal patients, fat may be absent between an esophageal carcinoma and aorta, trachea, left main bronchus, or pericardium. Physiologic absence of fat planes complicates the assessment of the invasion of adjacent structures. Alternate CT findings have been devised to predict T4 status. Aortic invasion is suggested by an arc of contact between the tumor and the aorta that is more than 90 degrees, although this is not an absolute confirmation of a T4 tumor. Thickening or indentation of the normally flat or slightly convex posterior membranous wall of the intrathoracic trachea or left main bronchus suggests airway invasion but may be produced by the mass effect of the adjacent tumor without actual airway involvement. On occasion, a tumor in the airway lumen or a fistula between the esophagus and airway may be visualized, but bronchoscopic confirmation with biopsy is necessary. Pericardial invasion is suspected if pericardial thickening, pericardial effusion, or indentation of the heart with loss of the pericardial fat plane at the level of the tumor is demonstrated. Magnetic resonance imaging (MRI) offers no significant advantage over CT.

Theoretically, thoracoscopy can exclude a cT4 tumor but requires dissection of the primary tumor from the adjacent structure presumed to be invaded. Although mentioned as a possible staging tool for cT4 detection (Buenaventura and Luketich, 2000; Krasna, 1997), the only documentation of T staging has been the detection of cT4 disease in 14% of patients undergoing thoracoscopy and laparoscopy for regional lymph node staging (Krasna et al, 1999).

Positron emission tomography (PET) using 2-[^{18}F]fluoro-2-deoxy-D-glucose (FDG) has been reported to accumulate in 92% to 100% of esophageal cancers (Flanagan et al, 1997; Rankin et al, 1998). However, FDG-PET and other imaging modalities do not provide definition of the esophageal wall or paraesophageal tissue and therefore have no value in the determination of cT.

Determination of cN (Regional) and cM1 (Nonregional) Lymph Node Status

EUS is used to evaluate nodal size, shape, border, and internal echo characteristics in regional lymph node assessment (see part 3 of Chapter 5). In a retrospective review of 100 EUS examinations, the EUS determination of N was 89% sensitive, 75% specific, and 84% accurate (Catalano et al, 1994). The positive predictive value of EUS for N1 disease was 86%; the negative predictive value was 79%. In a meta-analyses of 21 series, the accuracy of EUS determination was 77% for N, 69% for N0, and 89% for N1 (Rösch, 1995). Endosonography-directed FNA (EUS-FNA) further refines clinical staging by adding tissue sampling to endosonographic findings.

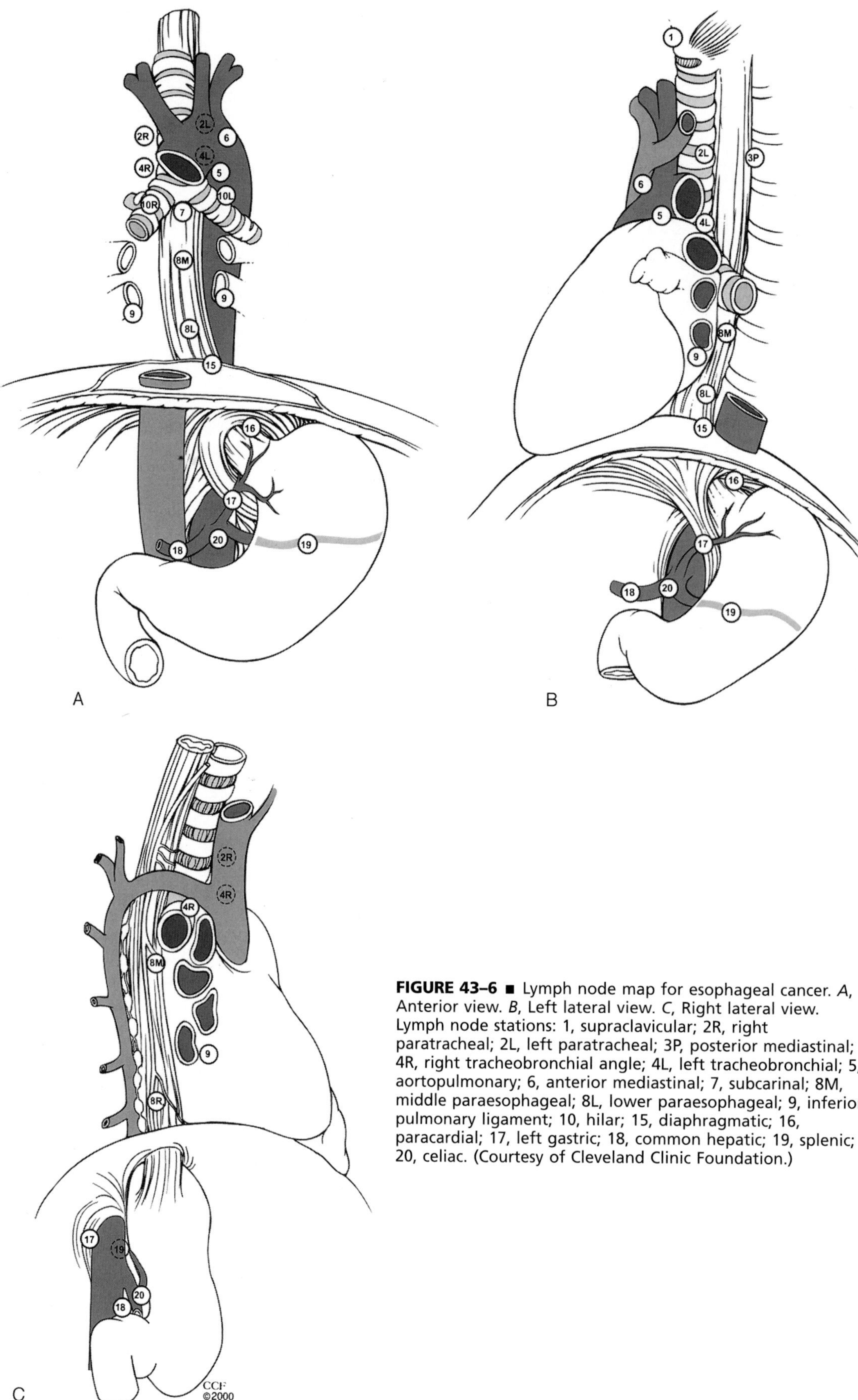

FIGURE 43–6 ■ Lymph node map for esophageal cancer. *A*, Anterior view. *B*, Left lateral view. *C*, Right lateral view. Lymph node stations: 1, supraclavicular; 2R, right paratracheal; 2L, left paratracheal; 3P, posterior mediastinal; 4R, right tracheobronchial angle; 4L, left tracheobronchial; 5, aortopulmonary; 6, anterior mediastinal; 7, subcarinal; 8M, middle paraesophageal; 8L, lower paraesophageal; 9, inferior pulmonary ligament; 10, hilar; 15, diaphragmatic; 16, paracardial; 17, left gastric; 18, common hepatic; 19, splenic; 20, celiac. (Courtesy of Cleveland Clinic Foundation.)

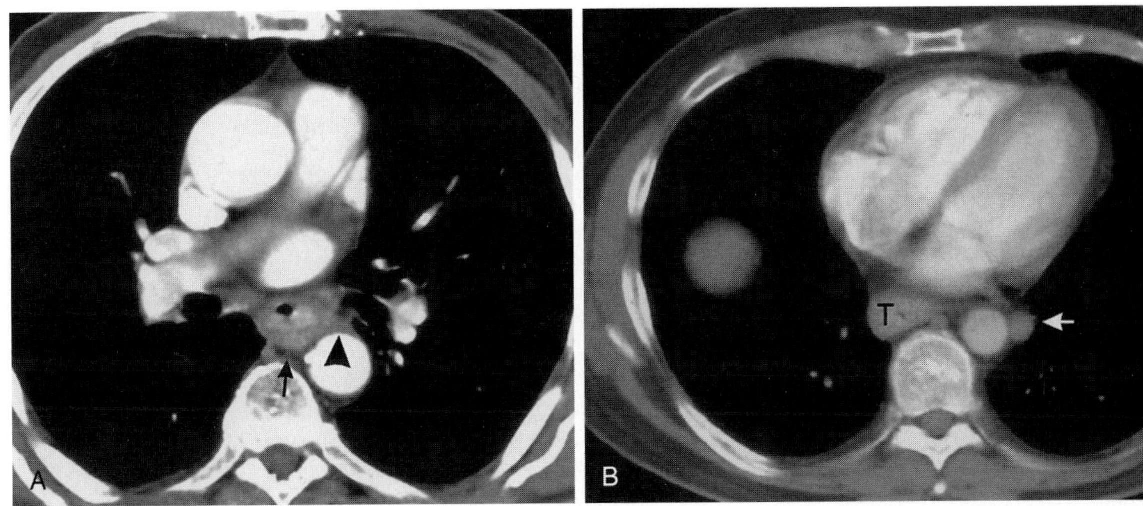

FIGURE 43–7 ■ *A*, Nonspecific CT finding of esophageal cancer is thickening of the esophageal wall. CT does not discriminate between cTis, cT1, cT2, and cT3 tumors. Preservation of periesophageal fat excludes cT4 cancer. In this study, preservation of the posterior fat plane (*arrow*) excludes invasion of the prevertebral fascia. Though suggestive of aortic invasion, the absence of a fat plane between the tumor and aorta (*arrowhead*) is not diagnostic. *B*, Esophageal cancer (T) is surrounded by fat. An enlarged thoracic lymph node (*arrow*) is seen.

In a multicenter study, 171 patients had EUS-FNA of 192 lymph nodes (Wiersema et al, 1997). In the determination of lymph node status EUS-FNA had a sensitivity of 92%, specificity of 93%, positive predictive value of 100%, and negative predictive value of 86%. The combination of EUS and endosonography-directed FNA of celiac lymph nodes deemed positive by EUS had a sensitivity of 72%, a specificity of 97%, a positive predictive value of 95%, and a negative predictive value of 82% (Reed et al, 1999). FNA confirmed positive EUS M1a disease in 88% of patients.

Surface ultrasound examination of cervical lymph nodes has been reported to detect nonpalpable metastasis in patients with squamous cell carcinoma (Doldi et al, 1998; Natsugoe et al, 1999).

Thoracoscopic and laparoscopic staging has been used to evaluate cN and cM1 lymph node status. A combination of thoracoscopic and laparoscopic staging was reported to be 94% accurate in detecting lymph node metastases (Krasna et al, 1999). For thoracic lymph nodes, sensitivity, specificity, and positive predictive value were 63%, 100%, and 100%, respectively. For abdominal lymph nodes, sensitivity, specificity, and positive predictive value were 85%, 100%, and 100%, respectively. Of 88 patients entered into the study, thoracoscopy was performed in 82 (93%), laparoscopy in 55 (63%), and both in 49 (57%). Induction chemoradiotherapy was administered to 34 (39%) patients. Only 47 (53%) patients underwent resection, making comparative pathologic stage available in only 13 (15%) patients. The best operative time and hospital stay reported are 3.6 hours and 1.8 days, respectively (Luketich et al, 1997a). These procedures are not without serious morbidity (Gilbert et al, 1999).

An enlarged lymph node on CT suggests nodal metastasis (see Fig. 43–7). The short axis of these nodes is easily measured; intrathoracic and abdominal lymph nodes larger than 1 cm are considered enlarged. Supraclavicular lymph nodes with a short axis larger than 0.5 cm and retrocrural lymph nodes larger than 0.6 cm are pathologic (van Overhagen and Becker, 1998). However, the probability that cN status can be determined by lymph node size alone is small (Doi et al, 1999). Normal-sized nodes may contain metastatic deposits, and metastatic nodes in direct contact with the tumor may be indistinguishable from the primary tumor. These situations result in false-negative examinations and influence the sensitivity and negative predictive value. Not all enlarged lymph nodes are malignant. Inflammatory nodes are the most common cause of a false-positive examination and lower specificity and positive predictive value. CT assessment of lymph nodes varies with anatomic site; accuracies of 61% to 96%, sensitivities of 8% to 75%, and specificities of 60% to 98% were reported for cervical, mediastinal, and abdominal nodes (Chandawarkar et al, 1996). Again, MRI offers no important advantage over CT.

The physiologic evaluation of esophageal carcinoma provided by FDG-PET relies not only on the size of the metastatic deposit but also on the intensity of FDG uptake and decay. Theoretically, it is possible to identify microscopic metastases if glucose metabolism is sufficient to concentrate large quantities of FDG. FDG-PET cannot differentiate adjacent N1 from the primary tumor (Flanagan et al, 1997) (Fig. 43–8). The accuracy of FDG-PET in detecting lymph node metastases from esophageal carcinomas is highly variable, ranging from 37% to 90% (Block et al, 1997; Kole et al, 1998; Luketich et al, 1997b, Rankin et al, 1998). Compared with the detection of lymph node metastases in lung carcinoma, FDG-PET is much less accurate in esophageal carcinoma (Luketich et al, 1999).

Because of its high sensitivity, the main role of FDG-PET is to confirm cN0 status (Flamen et al, 2000). The addition of [methyl-^{11}C]choline PET to FDG PET has been reported to increase the accuracy of PET cN1 staging (Kobori et al, 1999).

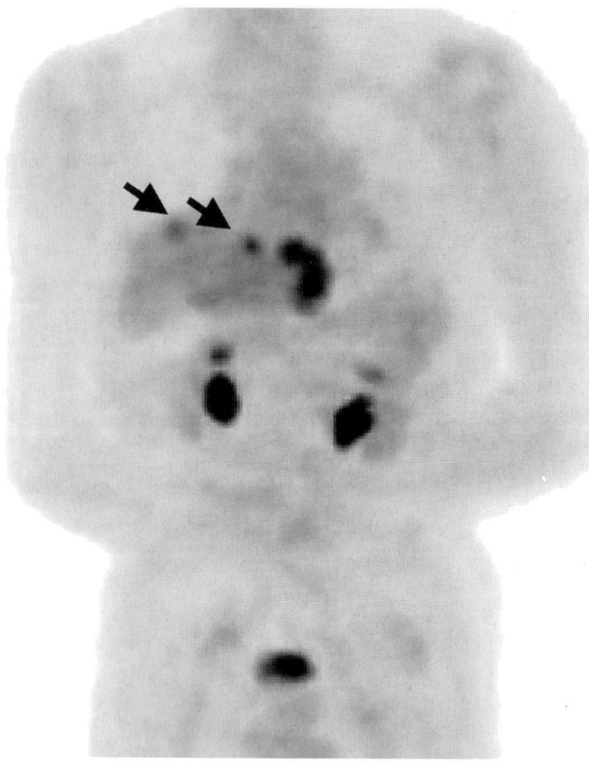

FIGURE 43–8 ■ PET scan of a T3 N1 M1B esophageal cancer. Primary tumor and regional lymph nodes cannot be differentiated and appear as one large mass. There are two hepatic metastases (*arrows*). The kidneys excrete and the bladder stores fluorodeoxyglucose.

Determination of Non-nodal M1b Status

In patients with recently diagnosed esophageal carcinoma, metastases are found in the liver (35% of patients), lungs (20%), bone (9%), adrenal gland (2%), brain (2%), and the pericardium, pleura, soft tissues, stomach, pancreas, and spleen (1% each) (Quint et al, 1995). Except for the brain, CT scans of the esophagus include all or a portion of all other sites. Contrast-enhanced CT scanning, with imaging during the portal venous phases of contrast distribution, provides both screening for and diagnosis of masses in these areas.

Hepatic metastases appear as ill-defined, low-density lesions of varying sizes (Fig. 43–9). Conventional CT imaging (dynamic incremental scanning with intravenous bolus contrast enhancement) is excellent in detecting hepatic metastases larger than 2 cm (Wernecke et al, 1991). Sensitivity is 70% to 80% (van Overhagen and Becker, 1998). Although no study is available for esophageal cancer, spiral CT produced similar results as conventional CT in the detection of colorectal liver metastases; a sensitivity of 76% and a positive predictive value of 90% have been reported (Valls et al, 1998). Subcentimeter metastases are frequently not recognized by CT; they are the main cause of false-negative examinations and the low sensitivity of CT in the detection of liver metastases.

To distinguish benign from malignant nodules, ultrasound is used for the diagnosis of benign cysts and MRI is used for the diagnosis of hemangiomas. Adrenal metastases cause heterogeneous, focal enlargement of the adrenal gland. Contrast-enhanced CT is a sensitive but nonspecific screening tool for adrenal masses. Non–contrast-enhanced CT, MRI, percutaneous FNA, or laparoscopy may be required to confirm the nature of these nodules.

In a cohort of patients with predominant squamous cell carcinoma of the esophagus, solitary lung metastases were rare at diagnosis of the primary cancer and most lung lesions were either a benign nodule or synchronous primary lung cancer (Margolis et al, 1998). Although multiple lung metastases were uncommon at diagnosis, they became increasingly common during the late stages of the disease. Many were not visualized on chest radiography. CT is very sensitive in the detection of pulmonary nodules; however, histologic confirmation of these abnormalities is required if their nature alone is to determine therapy.

The presence of ascites, pleural effusion, or nodules in the omentum or pleura is strongly suggestive of metastases to these mesothelium-lined surfaces. Laparoscopy or thoracoscopy can confirm these findings.

Brain metastases are reported in 2% to 4% of patients who present with esophageal carcinoma (Gabrielsen et al, 1995; Quint et al, 1995). They tend to occur in patients with large adenocarcinoma of the esophagogastric junction that have invaded locally or metastasized to lymph nodes. A pretreatment CT scan of the brain may be reasonable in these patients.

Despite improved technology, CT has a sensitivity of 37% to 66% in screening for distant metastases in patients with esophageal cancer (Block et al, 1997; Kole et al, 1998; Luketich et al, 1999; O'Brien et al, 1995). FDG-PET is superior to CT in detecting M1b disease. In 91 patients undergoing 100 FDG-PET studies, distant metastatic disease was detected in 39 scans at 51 sites (Luketich et al, 1999); 70 distant metastases were confirmed by biopsy or at resection. For FDG-PET, sensitivity was 69%, specificity was 93%, and overall accuracy was 84%. In this series, sensitivity of CT was 46%, specificity was 74%, and accuracy was 63%. FDG-PET did not detect distant metastases in the liver (10 patients), pleura (4), lungs (2), and peritoneum (1). All metastases were

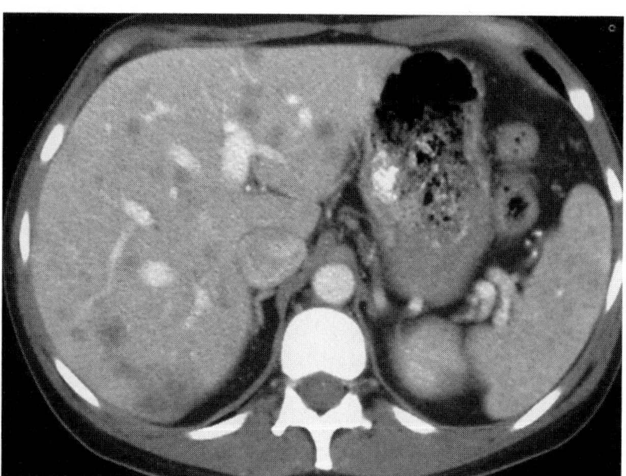

FIGURE 43–9 ■ In this CT scan, hepatic metastases appear as ill-defined, low-density lesions of variable size.

less than 1 cm in diameter. Of 21 false-negative CT scans, FDG-PET identified distant metastases in 11 (62%); of 12 false-negative FDG-PET scans, CT was accurate in 4 (33%). These mature results are less favorable than those from an earlier report by the same group, in which the sensitivity of FDG-PET in the detection of distant metastases was 88%, the specificity was 93%, and the accuracy was 91% (Luketich et al, 1997b).

FDG-PET identified five (71%) of seven patients with distant metastatic disease (Flanagan et al, 1997). A liver metastasis that was less than 1 cm in diameter was not visualized, and a pancreatic metastasis was misinterpreted as a left gastric lymph node metastasis. There were no false-positive findings in 36 patients. During a similar time period, the same group reported 17 distant metastases in 59 patients with FDG-PET. There were no false-negative results, but transhiatal esophagectomy was commonly used to obtain pathologic stage (Block et al, 1997).

FDG-PET detects radiographically occult distant metastatic disease in 10% to 20% of patients with esophageal cancer (Block et al, 1997; Kole et al, 1998; Luketich et al, 1997b, 1999). The combination of FDG-PET and CT has a diagnostic accuracy of 80% to 92% (Block et al, 1997; Kole et al, 1998) and prevents unnecessary surgery in 90% of patients (Kole et al, 1998). FDG-PET provided additional staging information in 22% of patients, upstaging 15% and downstaging 7% (Flamen et al, 2000).

Laparoscopy has been reported to change therapy in 10% of patients, allowing resection in 2% who were overstaged and avoiding resection in 8% with undetected M1b disease (Bonavina et al, 1997). The sensitivities of laparoscopy in detecting peritoneal and liver metastases were 71% and 86%, respectively. Laparoscopic ultrasonography does not improve accuracy of staging by laparoscopy alone (Bemelman et al, 1995; Romijn et al, 1998).

EUS has limited value in screening for distant metastases (M1b). The distant organ must be in direct contact with the upper gastrointestinal tract (e.g., the left lateral segment of the liver and retroperitoneum) for EUS to be useful.

Pathologic Staging

The pathologic stage is the clinical stage modified by additional information acquired from surgery and from pathologic examination of the resection specimen and biopsies of distant sites. Pathologic assessment of the primary tumor, pT, requires resection (primary tumor mobilization and biopsy in the case of pT4 tumors) sufficient in extent to evaluate the highest pT category (Fleming et al, 1997). Pathologic assessment of regional lymph nodes pN also entails the removal of a sufficient number of lymph nodes to evaluate the highest pN category (Fleming et al, 1997). Biopsy of distant metastasis without removal of the primary tumor is necessary to confirm pM1b.

Although recommendations are available for the handling of esophageal resection specimens, no uniform criteria exist for examination of the resection specimen (Haggitt et al, 2000; Ibrahim, 2000; Lee and Compton, 1997). An acceptable method of sectioning requires only

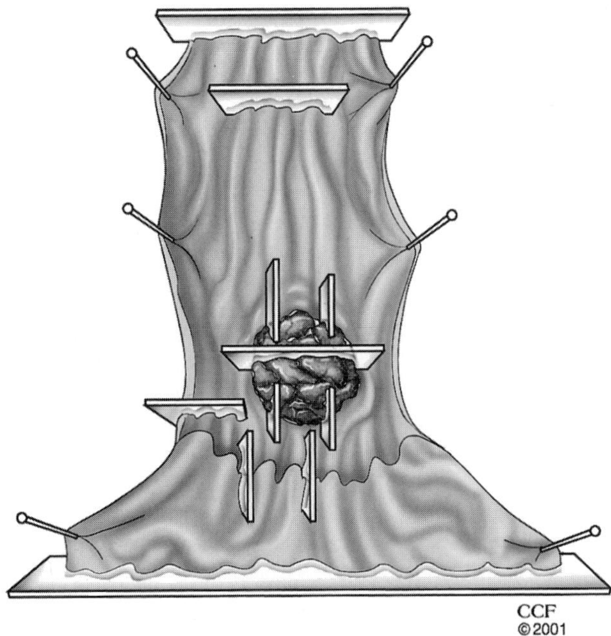

FIGURE 43–10 ■ Pathologic evaluation of an esophagectomy specimen. Sections are taken at the proximal resection margin, the distal resection margin, the esophagus proximal to the tumor, the esophagus distal to the tumor, and the esophagogastric junction. The specimen soft tissue margin should be inked, and the tumor should be sectioned at its largest point. The superior and inferior boundaries of the tumor should be sectioned. All lymph nodes should be dissected from the resection specimen and be evaluated with the lymphadenectomy specimen. (Courtesy of Cleveland Clinic Foundation.)

8 to 11 sections to be evaluated (Fig. 43–10). Lymphadenectomy specimens and lymph nodes removed from the resection specimen are evaluated on the basis of single representative sections of each individual lymph node. The histologic determination of pT and pN is subject to sampling error.

Re-treatment Staging

After primary treatment and a disease-free interval, the stage of recurrent cancer is called the *re-treatment stage*. Biopsy or FNA cytology is used to determine this stage. Local recurrence of tumor, rT, can usually be established by endoscopy and biopsy. The determination of rN and rM may require mediastinoscopy, thoracoscopy, or laparoscopy. Open biopsy may be necessary. Imaging, although less accurate in the re-treatment staging, directs these biopsy procedures.

EUS is not accurate in determination of rT and rN after effective chemoradiotherapy. It cannot distinguish tumor from inflammation and fibrosis produced by chemoradiotherapy, and it cannot detect microscopic residual disease. From the experience of restaging after induction chemoradiotherapy, EUS was reported to be accurate in determining rT for only 27% to 59% of patients (Beseth et al, 2000; Bowrey et al, 1999; Isenberg et al, 1998; Laterza et al, 1999; Zuccaro et al, 1999).

The most common mistake made in determining rT

was overstaging. Similar difficulties in distinguishing tumor from postchemoradiotherapy inflammation and fibrosis have also been reported with EUS staging of rectal cancers (Fleshman et al, 1992). EUS accuracy for rN after chemoradiotherapy has been reported to be 58% to 71% (Beseth et al, 2000; Bowrey et al, 1999; Laterza et al, 1999; Zuccaro et al, 1999). The accuracy of rN determination after chemoradiotherapy is less than that of cN due to alteration in the ultrasonographic appearance of nodes after chemoradiotherapy, to the extent that established EUS criteria do not apply and residual foci of cancer within the nodes are too small for detection by any modality other than pathologic analysis.

EUS has been useful in restaging patients with anastomotic recurrences that are not endoscopically visible (Catalano et al, 1995; Lightdale et al, 1989).

The role of FDG-PET in restaging is still being defined. Although it may not differentiate anastomosis recurrence from stricture it is valuable in detecting regional and distant recurrences (Paulus et al, 1997; Skehan et al, 2000).

CT is inaccurate in determining rT and rN after chemoradiotherapy (Jones et al, 1999). CT detection of a mass in the field of resection or a distant metastasis is helpful in determining the re-treatment stage.

Autopsy Staging

Every effort should be made to obtain a postmortem examination to determine autopsy stage (aTNM). Therapeutic assessment in treated patients and a natural history in untreated patients constitute valuable information (Anderson and Lad, 1982; Attah and Hajdu, 1968; Cilley et al, 1989; Soares et al, 1991).

CONCLUSION

Stage, as defined by anatomic extent (TNM), is invaluable in the treatment and study of esophageal carcinoma. Stage is determined at four intervals:

- Before treatment, or the clinical stage (cTNM)
- After resection, or the pathologic stage (pTNM)
- At the time of recurrence, or the re-treatment stage (rTNM)
- At death, or the autopsy stage (aTNM)

The clinical stage of an esophageal carcinoma has prognostic and therapeutic importance. CT is readily available to all patients. It is relatively inexpensive and usually reimbursed. It provides exquisite anatomic detail of the chest and abdomen in patients with esophageal cancer. The only reliable use of CT in the determination of T is to exclude T4 tumors, suggested by the preservation of fat planes. Enlarged lymph nodes suggest metastatic disease but call for further study or tissue sampling if nodal metastases are to determine treatment. The major use of CT is in detection of distant metastatic disease, but 30% to 60% of distant metastases may be radiographically occult.

Because there is a significant learning curve for EUS clinical staging of esophageal cancer, this study should be performed at an institution where there is a dedicated, experienced endoscopic ultrasonographer with adequate instrumentation to allow specialty imaging and endosonography-directed FNA. EUS is the best means of clinically determining T. The addition of endosonography-directed FNA to routine EUS evaluation of lymph nodes allows an accuracy similar to that of EUS determination of T. EUS has no significant role in the assessment of non-nodal distant metastatic disease. However, the serendipitous finding of a distant metastasis in adjacent structures visualized during the evaluation of the primary tumor and lymph nodes has, on occasion, detected M1b disease.

FDG-PET represents an advancement over CT in screening for distant metastases. Major problems with FDG-PET staging of esophageal cancer are the failure to detect metastatic deposits smaller than 1 cm in diameter and a lack of anatomic definition. FDG-PET cannot determine T and has been inaccurate in the detection of adjacent lymph node metastases. Because this test is not readily available, is expensive, and is not routinely reimbursible, its use in staging esophageal cancer, unfortunately, continues to be limited.

Today, CT and EUS are the mainstays in the clinical staging of esophageal carcinoma. When possible, FDG-PET should be added to CT to improve the evaluation of non-nodal M1b disease. Results of these studies should determine the necessity of invasive staging techniques, such as thoracoscopy and laparoscopy, and should direct their use.

Meticulous handling and analysis of the resection specimen are necessary for accurate pathologic staging. Because pathologic stage is built on clinical stage, a precise pathologic stage requires a precise clinical stage. The tools of clinical staging are all that are available to determine retreatment stage. However, imaging in treated patients is less accurate. Results of these studies should determine the necessity of invasive staging and should direct its use. Responsibility to patients with esophageal carcinoma extends beyond death. The autopsy stage is invaluable to the study of the disease, its treatment, and the mode and extent of treatment failure. A postmortem examination should be requested in every patient.

COMMENTS AND CONTROVERSIES

This chapter by Dr. Rice is authoritative, comprehensive, and well illustrated. It reflects the meticulous application and evaluation of EUS undertaken by Dr. Rice and his colleagues. In our experience, preoperative EUS seldom alters the decision regarding resectability but frequently determines the treatment protocol to be followed, especially concerning the use of neoadjuvant therapy.

Dr. Rice notes the inaccuracy of PET scanning in detecting lymph node metastases. This is certainly true for lymph nodes adjacent to the primary tumor, which, because of the limits of spatial resolution of PET scanning, cannot be distinguished from the primary tumor. Nonetheless, the value of PET scanning in the detection of distant nodal metastases or other known nodal metastases is far better than any other noninvasive method of staging esophageal carcinoma.

In our experience, PET scanning has detected distant metastases in 20% of patients thought on the basis of CT scan analysis to show no distant metastases. Pathologic confirmation of such PET-detected metastasis must be made by needle biopsy or open biopsy. In the case of suspected cervical or supraclavicular lymph nodes not palpable on physical examination, ultrasonography-guided, fine-needle aspiration may be very useful. It is our practice to use both PET and CT scanning for the evaluation of all patients with esophageal carcinoma before treatment planning, with the exception of patients found to have high-grade dysplasia at the time of surveillance endoscopy and biopsy, for the presence of columnar-lined esophagus.

J. D. C.

REFERENCES

Anderson LL, Lad TE: Autopsy findings in squamous cell carcinoma of the esophagus. Cancer 50:1587, 1982.

Attah EB, Hajdu SI: Benign and malignant tumors of the esophagus at autopsy. J Thorac Cardiovasc Surg 55:396, 1968.

Bemelman WA, van Delden OM, van Lanschot JJ, et al: Laparoscopy and laparoscopic ultrasonography in staging of carcinoma of the esophagus and gastric cardia. J Am Coll Surg 181:421, 1995.

Beseth BD, Bedford R, Isacoff WH, et al: Endoscopic ultrasound does not accurately assess pathologic stage of esophageal cancer after neoadjuvant chemoradiotherapy. Am Surg 66:827, 2000.

Block MI, Patterson GA, Sundaresan RS, et al: Improvement in staging of esophageal cancer with the addition of positron emission tomography. Ann Thorac Surg 64:770, 1997.

Bonavina L, Incarbone R, Lattuada E, et al: Preoperative laparoscopy in management of patients with carcinoma of the esophagus and of the esophagogastric junction. J Surg Oncol 65:171, 1997.

Bowrey DJ, Clark GW, Roberts SA, et al: Serial endoscopic ultrasound in the assessment of response to chemoradiotherapy for carcinoma of the esophagus. J Gastrointest Surg 3:462, 1999.

Buenaventura P, Luketich JD: Surgical staging of esophageal cancer. Chest Surg Clin North Am 10:487, 2000.

Catalano MF, Sivak MV Jr, Rice TW, et al: Endosonographic features predictive of lymph node metastases. Gastrointest Endosc 40:442, 1994.

Catalano MF, Sivak MV Jr, Rice TW, et al: Postoperative screening for anastomotic recurrence of esophageal carcinoma by endoscopic ultrasonography. Gastrointest Endosc 42:540, 1995.

Chandawarkar RY, Kakegawa T, Fujita H, et al: Comparative analysis of imaging modalities in the preoperative assessment of nodal metastasis in esophageal cancer. J Surg Oncol 61:214, 1996.

Christie NA, Rice TW, DeCamp MM, et al: M1a/M1b esophageal carcinoma: Clinical relevance. J Thorac Cardiovasc Surg 118:900, 1999.

Cilley RE, Strodel WE, Peterson RO: Cause of death in carcinoma of the esophagus. Am J Gastroenterol 84;147, 1989.

Doi N, Aoyama N, Tokunaga M, et al: Possibility of pre-operative diagnosis of lymph node metastasis based on morphology. Hepatogastroenterology 46:977, 1999.

Doldi SB, Lattuada E, Zappa MA, et al: Ultrasonographic evaluation of the cervical lymph nodes in preoperative staging of esophageal neoplasms. Abdom Imaging 23:275, 1998.

Faigel DO, Deveney C, Phillips D, et al: Biopsy-negative malignant esophageal stricture: Diagnosis by endoscopic ultrasound. Am J Gastroenterol 93:2257, 1998.

Flamen P, Lerut A, Van Cutsem E, et al: Utility of positron emission tomography for the staging of patients with potentially operable esophageal carcinoma. J Clin Oncol 15:3202, 2000.

Flanagan FL, Dehdashti F, Siegel BA, et al: Staging of esophageal cancer with ^{18}F-fluorodeoxyglucose positron emission tomography. AJR Am J Roentgenol 168:417, 1997.

Fleming ID, Cooper JS, Henson DE, et al: Digestive system: Esophagus. In Fleming ID (ed): AJCC Cancer Staging Manual, 5th ed. Philadelphia, Lippincott Williams & Wilkins, 1997, pp 65–69.

Fleshman JW, Myerson RJ, Fry RD, et al: Accuracy of transrectal ultrasound in predicting stage of rectal cancer before and after preoperative radiation therapy. Dis Colon Rectum 35:823, 1992.

Gabrielsen TO, Eldevik OP, Orringer MB, et al: Esophageal carcinoma metastatic to the brain: Clinical value and cost-effectiveness of routine enhanced head CT before esophagectomy. Am J Neuroradiol 16:1915, 1995.

Gilbert TB, Goodsell CW, Krasna MJ: Bronchial rupture by a double-lumen endobronchial tube during staging thoracoscopy. Anesth Analg 88:1252, 1999.

Haggitt RC, Appelman HD, Lewin KJ, et al: Recommendations for the reporting of resected esophageal carcinomas. Associations of Directors of Anatomic Surgical Pathology. Hum Pathol 31:1188, 2000.

Heidemann J, Schilling MK, Schmassmann A, et al: Accuracy of endoscopic ultrasonography in preoperative staging of esophageal carcinoma. Dig Dis Sci 17:219, 2000.

Ibrahim NB: ACP. Best practice No 1. Guidelines for handling oesophageal biopsies and resection specimens and their reporting. J Clin Pathol 53:89, 2000.

Isenberg G, Chak A, Canto MI, et al: Endoscopic ultrasound in restaging of esophageal cancer after neoadjuvant chemoradiation. Gastrointest Endosc 48:158, 1998.

Jones DR, Parker LA Jr, Detterbeck FC, et al: Inadequacy of computed tomography in assessing patients with esophageal carcinoma after induction chemoradiotherapy. Cancer 85:1026, 1999.

Krasna MJ: Minimally invasive staging for esophageal cancer. Chest 112:191S, 1997.

Krasna MJ, Mao YS, Sonnett J, et al: The role of thoracoscopic staging of esophageal cancer patients. Eur J Cardiothorac Surg 16 (Suppl):S31, 1999.

Kobori O, Kirihara Y, Kosaka N, et al: Positron emission tomography of esophageal carcinoma using (11)C-choline and (18)F-fluorodeoxyglucose: A novel method of preoperative lymph node staging. Cancer 86:1638, 1999.

Kole AC, Plukker JT, Nieweg OE, et al: Positron emission tomography for staging of oesophageal and gastroesophageal malignancy. Br J Cancer 78:521, 1998.

Laterza E, deManzoni G, Guglielmi A, et al: Endoscopic ultrasonography in the staging of esophageal carcinoma after preoperative radiotherapy and chemotherapy. Ann Thorac Surg 67:1466, 1999.

Lee RG, Compton CC: Protocol for the examination of specimens removed from patients with esophageal carcinoma: A basis for checklists. The Cancer Committee, College of American Pathologists, and the Task Force on the Examination of Specimens from Patients with Esophageal Cancer. Arch Pathol Lab Med 121:925, 1997.

Levine MS, Chu P, Furth EE, et al: Carcinoma of the esophagus and esophagogastric junction: Sensitivity of radiographic diagnosis. AJR Am J Roentgenol 168:1423, 1997.

Lightdale CJ, Botet JF, Kelson DP, et al: Diagnosis of recurrent upper gastrointestinal cancer at the surgical anastomosis by endoscopic ultrasound. Gastrointest Endosc 35:407, 1989.

Luketich JD, Friedman DM, Weigel TL, et al: Evaluation of distant metastases in esophageal cancer: 100 Consecutive positron emission tomography scans. Ann Thorac Surg 68:1133, 1999.

Luketich JD, Schauer P, Landreneau R, et al: Minimally invasive surgical staging is superior to endoscopic ultrasound in detecting lymph node metastases in esophageal cancer. J Thorac Cardiovasc Surg 114:817, 1997a.

Luketich JD, Schauer PR, Meltzer CC, et al: Role of positron emission tomography in staging esophageal cancer. Ann Thorac Surg 64:765, 1997b.

Margolis ML, Howlett P, Bubanj R: Pulmonary nodules in patients with esophageal carcinoma. J Clin Gastroenterol 26:245, 1998.

Natsugoe S, Yoshinaka H, Shimada M, et al: Assessment of cervical lymph node metastasis in esophageal carcinoma using ultrasonography. Ann Surg 229:62, 1999.

O'Brien MG, Fitzgerald EF, Lee G, et al: A prospective comparison of laparoscopy and imaging in the staging of esophagogastric cancer before surgery. Am J Gastroenterol 90:2191, 1995.

Paulus P, Hustinx R, Daenen F, et al: Usefulness of ^{18}FDG positron emission tomography in detection and follow-up of digestive cancers. Acta Gastroenterol Belg 60:278, 1997.

Provenzale D, Schmitt C, Wong JB: Barrett's esophagus: A new look at surveillance based on emerging estimates of cancer risk. Am J Gastroenterol 94:2043, 1999.

Quint LE, Hepburn LM, Francis IR, et al: Incidence and distribution of distant metastases in newly diagnosed esophageal carcinoma. Cancer 76:1120, 1995.
Rankin SC, Taylor H, Cook GJ, et al: Computed tomography and positron emission tomography in the pre-operative staging of oesophageal carcinoma. Clin Radiol 53:659, 1998.
Reed CE, Mishra G, Sahai AV, et al: Esophageal cancer staging: Improved accuracy by endoscopic ultrasound of celiac lymph nodes. Ann Thorac Surg 67:319, 1999.
Romijn MG, van Overhagen H, Spillenaar Bilgen EJ, et al: Laparoscopy and laparoscopic ultrasonography in staging of oesophageal and cardial carcinoma. Br J Surg 85:1010, 1998.
Rösch T: Endosonographic staging of esophageal cancer: A review of literature results. Gastrointest Endosc Clin North Am 5:537, 1995.
Saunders HS, Wolfman NT, Ott DJ: Esophageal cancer: Radiologic staging. Radiol Clin North Am 35:281, 1997.
Skehan SJ, Brown AL, Thompson M, et al: Imaging features of primary and recurrent esophageal cancer at FDG PET. Radiographics 20:713, 2000.
Soares FA, Landell GA, de Olivera JA: Pulmonary tumor embolism from squamous cell carcinoma of the oesophagus. Eur J Cancer 27:495, 1991.
Streitz JM Jr, Ellis FH Jr, Tilden RL, et al: Endoscopic surveillance of Barrett's esophagus: A cost effectiveness comparison with mammographic surveillance of breast cancer. Am J Gastroenterol 93:911, 1998.
Valls C, Lopez E, Guma A, et al: Helical CT versus CT arterial portography in the detection of hepatic metastases of colorectal carcinoma. AJR Am J Roentgenol 170:1341, 1998.
van Overhagen H, Becker CD: Diagnosis and staging of carcinoma of the esophagus and gastroesophageal junction, and detection of postoperative recurrence, by computed tomography. In Meyers MA (ed): Neoplasms of the Digestive Tract: Imaging, Staging and Management. Philadelphia, Lippincott-Raven, 1998, pp 31–48.
Wernecke K, Rummeny E, Bongartz G, et al: Detection of hepatic masses in patients with carcinoma: Comparative sensitivities of sonography, CT and MR imaging. AJR Am J Roentgenol 157:731, 1991.
Wiersema MJ, Vilmann P, Giovannini M, et al: Endosonography-guided fine-needle aspiration biopsy: Diagnostic accuracy and complication assessment. Gastroenterology 112:1087, 1997.
Zuccaro G Jr, Rice TW, Goldblum JR, et al: Endoscopic ultrasound cannot determine suitability for esophagectomy after aggressive chemoradiotherapy for esophageal cancer. Am J Gastroenterol 94:906, 1999.

VIDEO-ASSISTED APPROACHES TO STAGING OF ESOPHAGEAL CARCINOMA

Mark J. Krasna
Joshua R. Sonett
Ziv Gamliel

In the United States, esophageal cancer accounts for 1% to 3% of all cancers and 10% of all gastrointestinal cancers (Kirby and Rice, 1994). Approximately 13,000 new cases of esophageal cancer were diagnosed in 1998; of these, almost 12,000 patients died within 1 year. Although some progress has been made in the treatment of this devastating disease, morbidity and mortality rates remain exceptionally high (Ellis, 1979). Early diagnosis has been shown to improve survival. Appropriate staging and, if indicated, preoperative combined modality treatment followed by surgery may offer the patient with esophageal cancer a chance for improved survival but may well increase overall morbidity and treatment time. Accurate staging of esophageal cancer is of paramount importance both clinically and academically.

The incidence of adenocarcinoma now exceeds 50% of all patients with esophageal cancer, with fewer patients having a history of tobacco and alcohol abuse. These lesions occur most frequently in the distal third of the thoracic esophagus, with a male-to-female ratio of 3:1. Like its gastric counterpart, early lymphatic spread and local tissue invasion characterize adenocarcinoma of the esophagus (Blot et al, 1991).

Only a minority of esophageal carcinomas are diagnosed at an early stage. These lesions have aggressive biologic behavior that results in widespread early lymphatic involvement, local infiltration, and metastatic hematogenous spread. The site of the primary tumor does not necessarily indicate which nodal groups will be involved at the site of initial spread. The tumors tend to locally invade adjacent tissues. Middle-third and upper-third tumors may extend to invade the aorta, tracheobronchial tree, and left recurrent laryngeal nerve. Lower-third lesions may invade the diaphragm, pericardium, and stomach. Local invasion of periesophageal tissues has been described in 70% of individuals at the time of diagnosis (Bardini et al, 1990).

The lack of an esophageal serosa may explain the propensity for locoregional spread of esophageal cancer. The lymphatic drainage of the esophagus consists of two interconnecting longitudinal networks. A mucosal network is connected to a submucosal network through transverse interconnections. It is estimated that the longitudinal flow via lymphatics is at least six times that of the transverse flow, and this is thought to explain the tendency of this tumor to spread longitudinally to distant lymph nodes. Flow may occur freely in either direction and can be influenced by intrathoracic pressure differences and/or obstruction of lymphatic channels (Rice et al, 1998). Typically, the cervical esophagus drains into the internal jugular and supraclavicular nodes, the mid-esophagus drains into the paraesophageal and periesophageal nodes, and the inferior esophagus drains below the diaphragm to the region of the cardia, left gastric vessels, lesser curve of the stomach, and celiac axis (Shields, 1989).

The *AJCC Cancer Staging Manual** (Fleming, 1997) incorporates revisions that allow better discrimination between stages of esophageal carcinoma. Like the previous system, the new system is applicable to clinical as well as pathologic criteria and should improve the ability to provide meaningful prognostication. This new system takes into account the extent of tumor invasion (T stage), the presence and level of nodal involvement (N stage), and the presence of distant metastatic disease (M stage).

Evidence of distant spread or extensive local direct invasion into surrounding structures by an esophageal carcinoma precludes curative resection (Rankin and Manson, 1993). Precise preoperative evaluation of the extent of disease that includes the presence of distant disease, lymph node invasion, and invasion of local structures may avoid unnecessary surgical procedures and may identify individuals who may be favorable candidates for aggressive chemotherapy and radiation therapy regimens. The optimal preoperative staging modality should provide an accurate assessment of the extent of tumor invasion, including the precise depth of the mural lesion, the extent of extraesophageal spread of disease, and the presence or absence of both lymphatic and hematogenous metastatic disease (Takemoto et al, 1986).

The importance of staging esophageal carcinoma is demonstrated by evaluating surgical series of esophageal cancer treatment that report survival by stage (Huang, 1988). Accurate pretreatment staging of these tumors would allow stage-specific treatment. This may involve curative resection for low-stage tumors, whereas higher-stage tumors may be targeted for palliative surgical treatments and/or chemotherapy and radiation. Several diagnostic modalities are used in the workup and staging of esophageal carcinoma; the most common are computed tomography (CT) and endoscopic ultrasound (EUS). Innovations include the application of positron emission tomography (PET) scanning and EUS-guided fine-needle aspiration to stage esophageal cancer.

NONINVASIVE STAGING

Although several early studies reported favorable results with preoperative staging of esophageal carcinoma using CT, investigations have discovered several limitations in its use (Halvorsen and Thompson, 1989). The efficacy of CT in the preoperative staging of esophageal carcinoma varies according to the location of the primary lesion. Whereas it is highly effective in the assessment of mediastinal esophageal carcinomas, it is less helpful in the staging of cervical or gastroesophageal junction carcinomas.

CT also has limitations in terms of staging lymph node involvement. CT is unable to differentiate among small nodes, normal-sized nodes, and nodes that are small but invaded by tumor. Likewise, it cannot differentiate between hyperplastic and neoplastic nodes. It has been suggested that mediastinal nodes of more than 1 cm in diameter in the short axis be classified as pathologic and that subdiaphragmatic nodes of more than 8 mm in diameter be considered abnormal. With these criteria, CT has a sensitivity that approaches 100% but a specificity of only 43%, because many involved lymph nodes are of a normal size (Inculet et al, 1985). CT is very accurate (94% to 100%) in determining the presence of liver metastases if intravenous contrast medium is administered.

One of the newer modalities used in the staging of esophageal carcinoma is EUS. Extensive information can be obtained with minimal patient risk. Ultrasonic imaging of the gastrointestinal tract shows distinct layers of alternating echogenicity. It has been demonstrated that EUS is accurate in assessing the depth of tumor invasion in 89% of cases by determining alterations in the orderly alignment of the layers of the esophageal wall as well as in clearly demonstrating the transition between normal and pathologic esophagus (Tio et al, 1989). This modality is not applicable in about 25% of cases, which are stenotic and obstructive to the probe (Tio et al, 1990). EUS is able to diagnose lymph node metastasis but may fail to differentiate enlarged nonmetastatic nodes from those with metastasis (accuracy of 81%, sensitivity of 95%, specificity of 50%). It is not accurate in the assessment of distant metastatic disease such as liver metastasis. Although lymph nodes less than 5 mm on EUS are not likely to be malignant, lymph nodes of more than 10 mm in the region of the primary are malignant 48% of the time (Botet et al, 1991).

In studies that used EUS for the preoperative staging of esophageal carcinoma, high sensitivity has been reported. Rice and associates (1991) used EUS to document response to preoperative chemotherapy and found that EUS predicted the pathologic T stage with an accuracy of 82% and the N stage with an accuracy of 73%. They have shown that obstruction to the scope, and therefore advanced T stage, is the single most important predictor of lymph node spread (Rice et al, 1998).

A new development is the use of EUS-guided biopsy to stage the mediastinal nodes. This technique, akin to transbronchial biopsy of mediastinal lymph nodes, holds much promise. Preliminary data of its use in lung cancer and reports in staging celiac lymph nodes in esophageal cancer are promising (Reed et al, 1999; Silvestri et al, 1996). Tachimori and colleagues (1994) described the use of transcervical ultrasound to screen cervical lymph nodes. The use of ultrasound detected lymph nodes in 18 of 143 patients. When combined with manual palpation, a diagnostic accuracy of 91.7% was achieved (Tachimori et al, 1994).

The utility of PET in staging thoracic malignancies is still being investigated. PET, with the glucose analog 2-[^{18}F]fluoro-2-deoxy-D-glucose (FDG), takes advantage of the metabolic differences between tumor and benign cells. Studies have shown PET to be useful in identifying malignant pulmonary nodules and in staging mediastinal disease in non–small cell lung cancer (Abe et al, 1990).

*AJCC, American Joint Committee on Cancer.

Its limitations stem from the fact that some infectious processes also contain macrophages, which have a high FDG uptake. In addition, the resolution limits of PET may prevent detection of lesions less than 1 cm or nodal involvement adjacent to the primary tumor site. There are preliminary data from one report of the use of PET in conjunction with lymph node thoracoscopy/laparoscopy (TSLN/LSLN) to stage esophageal cancer (Luketich et al, 1999). A new Intergroup study of PET staging in esophageal cancer will begin through the American College of Surgery Oncology group (ACS 000210).

SURGICAL STAGING

Surgical treatment of esophageal cancer remains the gold standard for both palliation and curative treatment. Reports have shown excellent survival in patients with stage I and stage II tumors (Ellis et al, 1997; Steup et al, 1996). Long-term cures with advanced lesions are infrequent despite protocols that combine the use of surgery, radiation therapy, and chemotherapy. Because lesions are typically advanced before symptoms occur and are frequently associated with submucosal spread, lymph node involvement (75%), and extension to surrounding structures, this is hardly surprising (Shields, 1989). The lack of a satisfactory routinely applicable method to preoperatively stage esophageal carcinoma has resulted in a disparity between pathologic stage and clinical stage in two thirds of cases.

Akiyama and associates (1981) studied lymph node spread in esophageal cancer and found that lymph node metastases commonly occur along the lesser curvature and celiac axis. Tumors frequently spread to distant lymph nodes at all levels, with most patients having spread to at least one thoracic lymph node station regardless of the level of tumor. Abe and colleagues (1991) described the pattern of lymph node metastasis in patients with resectable esophageal cancer, showing the incidence of spread to mediastinal and celiac nodes from all levels of esophageal cancer. Skinner and colleagues (1986) described the importance of lymph node staging in selection of the type of procedure for patients with esophageal cancer, using extensive resections for patients with spread to periesophageal lymph nodes. Reports on the role of three-field lymphadenectomy for esophageal cancer demonstrate that despite questions regarding the impact of lymph node resection on survival, careful lymph node staging is possible with appropriate prognostication. These series point out the importance of lymph node stage as a prognosticator independent of the surgical procedure or treatment option chosen.

The major handicap in allocating and comparing treatment modalities for esophageal cancer is the lack of precise preoperative staging. Mediastinoscopy has been used successfully in preoperative staging for lung cancer and for allocation of therapy according to disease stage. Preoperative surgical staging in esophageal cancer may separate advanced disease from early local disease. Prognostication of patients with esophageal cancer might allocate chemotherapy/radiation therapy more appropriately, thus reducing the morbidity and mortality of the treatment of esophageal cancer. This is especially important in comparing results from different protocols and different centers.

Murray and associates (1977) used mediastinoscopy and minilaparotomy prospectively in 30 patients with esophageal cancer. Dagnini and colleagues (1986) performed routine laparoscopy for esophageal cancer in 369 patients; intra-abdominal metastases were noted in 14% and celiac lymph node metastases were noted in 9.7%, so unnecessary resection was avoided in these patients. The use of intra-abdominal ultrasound, laparoscopy, and peritoneal lavage identified unsuspected intra-abdominal metastases in 18% to 30% of patients (Jiao et al, 2000). With the advances in video technology, thoracoscopy has been developed as a useful tool in thoracic surgery (Krasna and McLaughlin, 1994). These techniques have been used as a complement to mediastinoscopy, replacing the Chamberlain procedure as a preoperative lymph node staging technique (Fiocco and Krasna, 1992).

Krasna and McLaughlin (1993) first described the efficacy of thoracoscopic lymph node staging in esophageal cancer in 19 patients. Although the thoracic lymph node staging was correct in 14 patients, 2 of the 14 had celiac lymph nodes found at the time of esophageal resection. In a follow-up series from three institutions of Cancer and Leukemia Group B, thoracoscopy and laparoscopy were used to stage the chest and abdomen, with a success rate of greater than 90% (Krasna et al, 1995). A report from 1996 (Krasna, 1996) of 65 patients demonstrated a 94% accuracy with laparoscopy and a 91% accuracy with thoracoscopy for esophageal cancer staging. Similar results confirmed the efficacy of thoracoscopic and laparoscopic staging (Luketich et al, 1999).

TECHNIQUE

The operating room is set up similarly for both right and left thoracoscopic procedures, with the first assistant and instrument table usually opposite the surgeon (Fig. 43–11). Placement of video monitors at the head and foot of the operating table eliminates mirror-image awkwardness when changing views from the apex to the base of the chest. The light source, irrigation and suction, and video cable are usually placed behind the first assistant. A thoracotomy instrument set should always be available in the room. Carbon dioxide insufflation is not usually required but can greatly facilitate the procedure if deflation of the lung cannot be achieved quickly. When used, the pleural pressure should be set at 10 to 15 mm Hg maximum with flow rates of less than 2.5 L/min (Wolfer et al, 1994).

The patient is initially placed supine on the operating room table. If the lesion abuts the airway, bronchoscopy is performed via an endotracheal tube after the induction of general endotracheal anesthesia. A double-lumen tube is then placed, and the patient is turned onto the appropriate side for thoracoscopy. The hips should be placed below the break in the bed such that flexion of the bed will not interfere with the thoracoscope, especially when looking at the apex. An axillary roll and rolls for each side of the patient should be placed for support. Flexible bronchoscopy should be performed now to confirm placement of the double-lumen endotracheal tube. A ster-

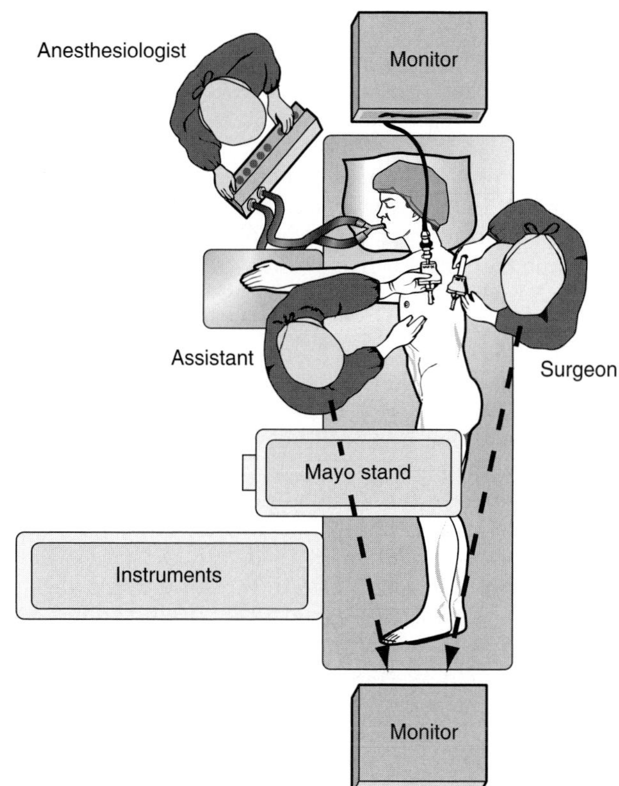

FIGURE 43–11 ■ Room setup for thoracoscopy/laparoscopy staging. (From Krasna MJ, Mach M: Atlas of Thoracoscopic Surgery. St. Louis, Quality Medical Publishing, 1993, p 19.)

ile preparation and drape should provide wide exposure of the chest to the spine posteriorly, the sternum anteriorly, the shoulder superiorly, and the iliac crest inferiorly. A right thoracoscopic approach is preferred because this allows greater exposure of the esophagus and periesophagus lymph nodes without interference from the aorta.

Right Thoracoscopy

As with all video-assisted surgery, proper port placement is critical. Lymph node dissection on the right requires adequate exposure of the right paratracheal area, which requires mobilization of the azygos vein. This provides access to the level 2 and level 4 nodes superior to the azygos vein and to the level 10 nodes, which are inferior to the azygos vein. In addition, the subcarinal (level 7), paraesophageal (level 8), and inferior pulmonary ligament (level 9) nodes should be sampled for complete staging. An "inverted pyramid" arrangement of three ports provides the access to all of these nodes (Fig. 43–12).

The first port should be placed two fingerbreadths below the tip of the scapula, at approximately the sixth intercostal space near the posterior axillary line. A 1.5-cm transverse skin incision should be made directly over the intercostal space. The surgeon must be sure that the right lung has been deflated while single-lung ventilation of the left lung is performed. This can be done while draping the patient. A Crile clamp is best suited to enter the pleural space perpendicular to the chest wall. Finger exploration should verify collapse of the lung and absence of adhesions. An 11.5-mm blunt-tip port is then

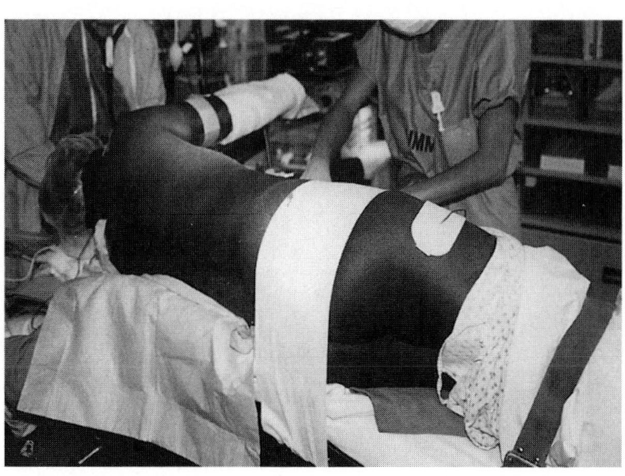

FIGURE 43–12 ■ Patient positioning for right thoracoscopic lymphatic node staging.

placed into the right pleural cavity, followed by the thoracoscope, preferably an operating scope. The surgeon now performs asystematic exploration of the right chest, specifically searching for metastatic nodules on the parietal pleura, pericardium, or diaphragm. The lung should be examined for synchronous lesions and for iatrogenic injury from the trocar insertion. The presence of effusion should be noted, and fluid samples should be sent for cytologic examination. The primary lesion should be fully assessed to determine whether there is T3 or T4 involvement.

Two additional 5- to 11.5-mm ports should now be inserted under videoscopic vision. The second port should be at the anterior axillary line at the same approximate level as the first (fifth or sixth intercostal space). The third port should be inferior to the other two, in the midaxillary line at the seventh or eighth intercostal space.

The dissection is begun by retracting the right upper lobe inferiorly and anteriorly to identify the azygos vein. A large blunt instrument placed through the second port is used to manipulate the lung, with grasping of the lung avoided if possible. The mediastinal pleura superior to the azygos vein is grasped at the border between the trachea and esophagus. With the use of cautery attached to endoshears, the pleura is incised up to the level of the subclavian vessels. Level 3p (posterior paraesophageal) lymph nodes are teased away, with any attachments clipped to reduce bleeding, and are labeled and sent for pathologic examination.

This dissection should extend inferiorly to the azygos vein (Fig. 43–13). The azygos vein should then be mobilized carefully using blunt dissection above and below. This allows retraction of the vein and exposure of level 10 nodes behind and inferior to the vein (Fig. 43–14). Rarely does division of vein become necessary to improve exposure, but an endovascular stapler can be used to perform this step easily. The level 10 nodes are sampled, again with liberal use of the clip applicator for any vascular attachments.

Level 7 (subcarinal) and level 8 (paraesophageal) node dissection requires repositioning of the lung to improve exposure. The right lower lobe should be retracted anteriorly and superiorly, again with the lung grasped only if necessary with an atraumatic grasper. Placing the patient in Trendelenburg position also improves exposure. The mediastinal pleura is lifted and incised along a line running between the trachea and the esophagus. At the level of the carina, posterior subcarinal nodes (level 7) can be bluntly removed with the application of hemaclips (Fig. 43–15) (see Color Plate). Dissection inferiorly along the esophagus will allow biopsy of level 8 nodes.

The inferior pulmonary ligament lymph nodes are the final nodes to undergo biopsy on the right. The first and second ports are initially used to retract the lung superiorly. Grasping of the right lower lobe and retraction toward the apex help to expose the inferior pulmonary ligament. A grasping instrument can then be placed with cautery to manipulate the inferior pulmonary ligament. Endoshears placed through the operating scope inferiorly can then be used to incise the pleura. Careful blunt dissection will expose the level 9 nodes, which are just inferior to the pulmonary vein (Fig. 43–16) (see Color Plate). Hemaclips should be placed on any adherent tissue. All surgical sites should be inspected for bleeding. A single No. 28 French chest tube is then placed into the chest through the most inferior trocar site (the third port). The thoracoscope confirms that the chest tube is placed posteriorly for optimal drainage. Two-lung ventilation should be resumed, and the ipsilateral lung should be inspected for full reexpansion.

Left Thoracoscopy

When preoperative noninvasive staging shows suspicious lymph nodes on the left, a left thoracoscopy can be done.

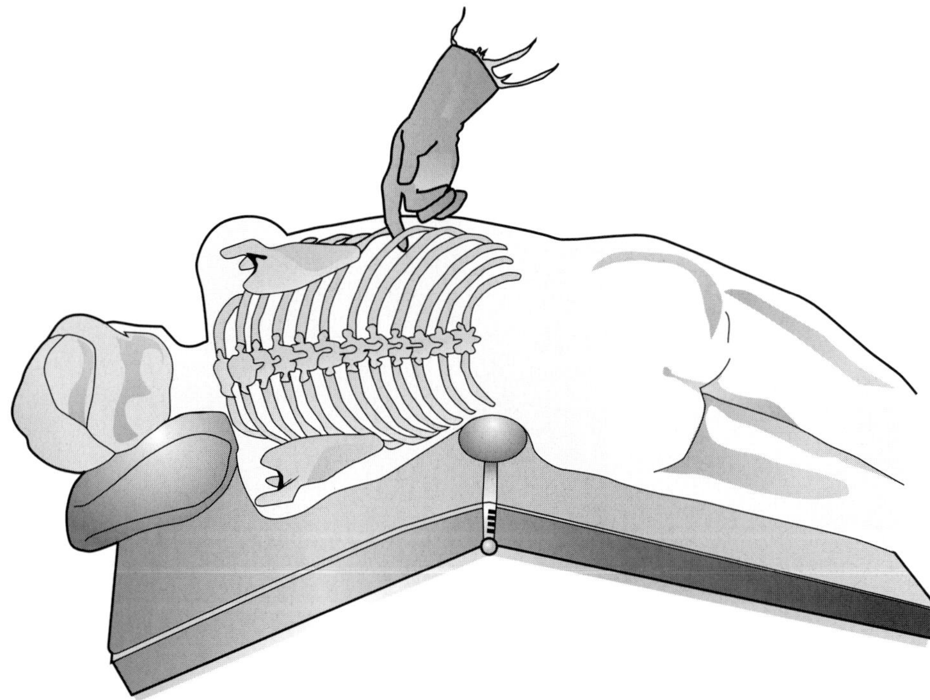

FIGURE 43–13 ■ Finger exploration of the chest. (From Krasna MJ, Mach M: Atlas of Thoracoscopic Surgery. St. Louis, Quality Medical Publishing, 1993.)

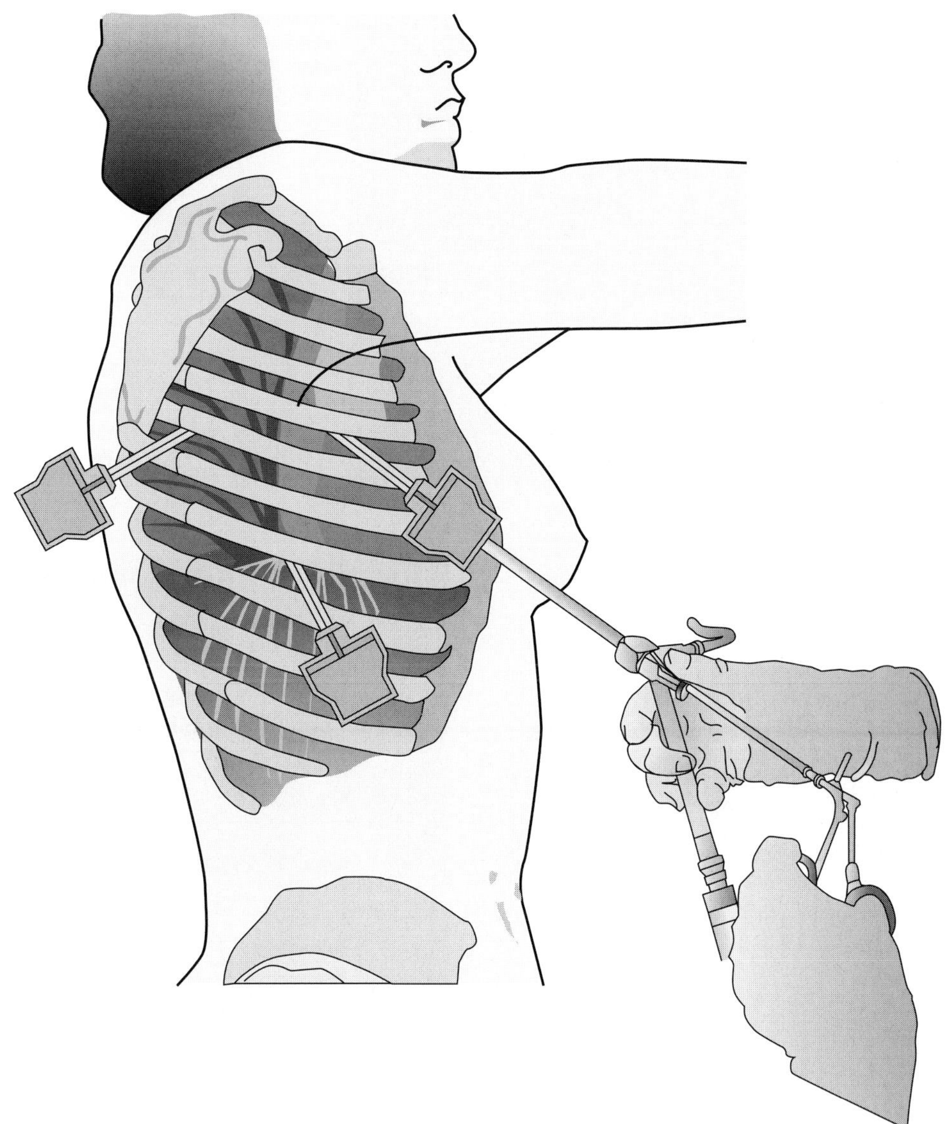

FIGURE 43–14 ■ Port placement for right thoracoscopic lymph node staging.

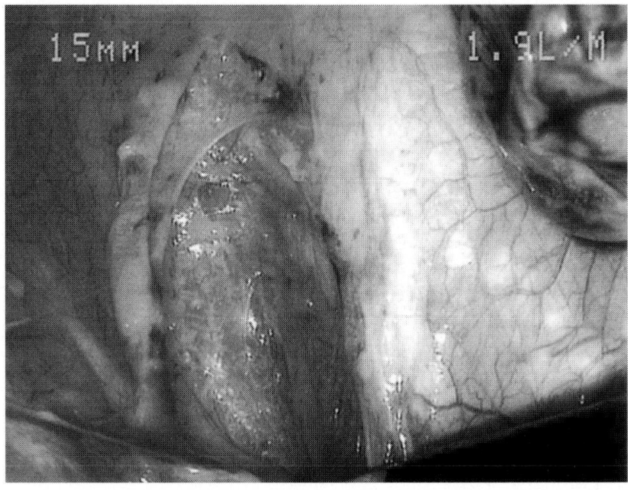

FIGURE 43–15 ■ Upper paraesophageal lymph node dissection. (See also Color Plate.)

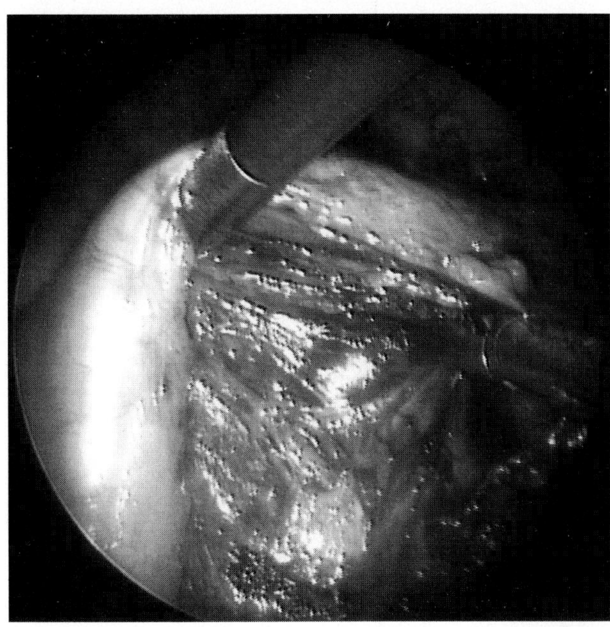

FIGURE 43–16 ■ Subazygous region during lymph node dissection. (See also Color Plate.)

FIGURE 43–17 ■ *A* and *B*, Subcarinal lymph node dissection. (From Krasna MJ, Mach M: Atlas of Thoracoscopic Surgery. St. Louis, Quality Medical Publishing, 1993.) (See also Color Plate for *A*.)

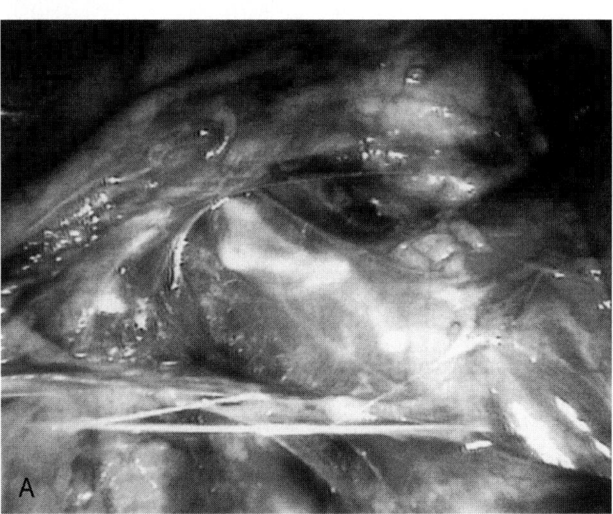

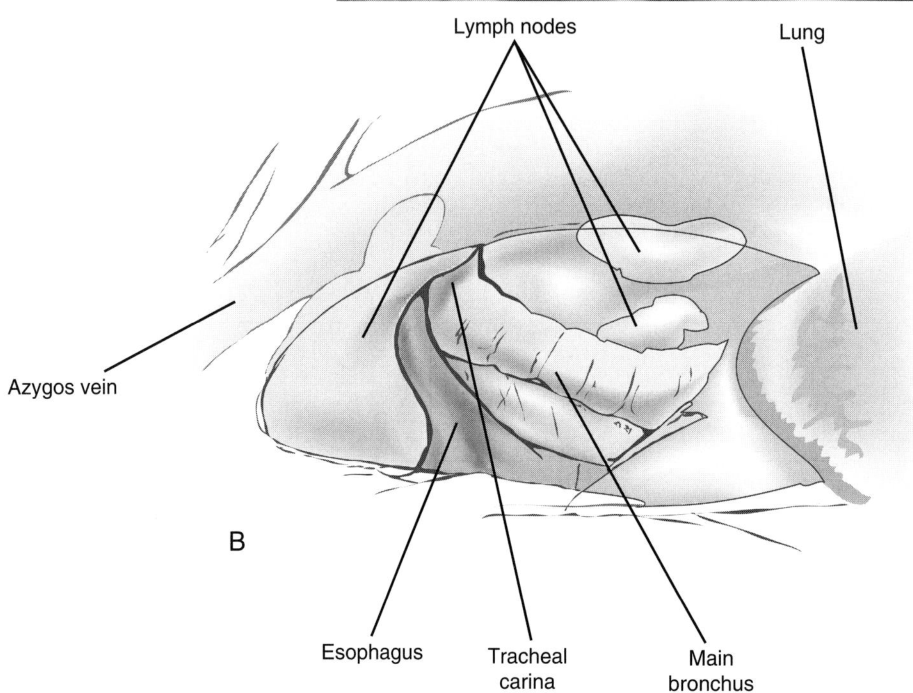

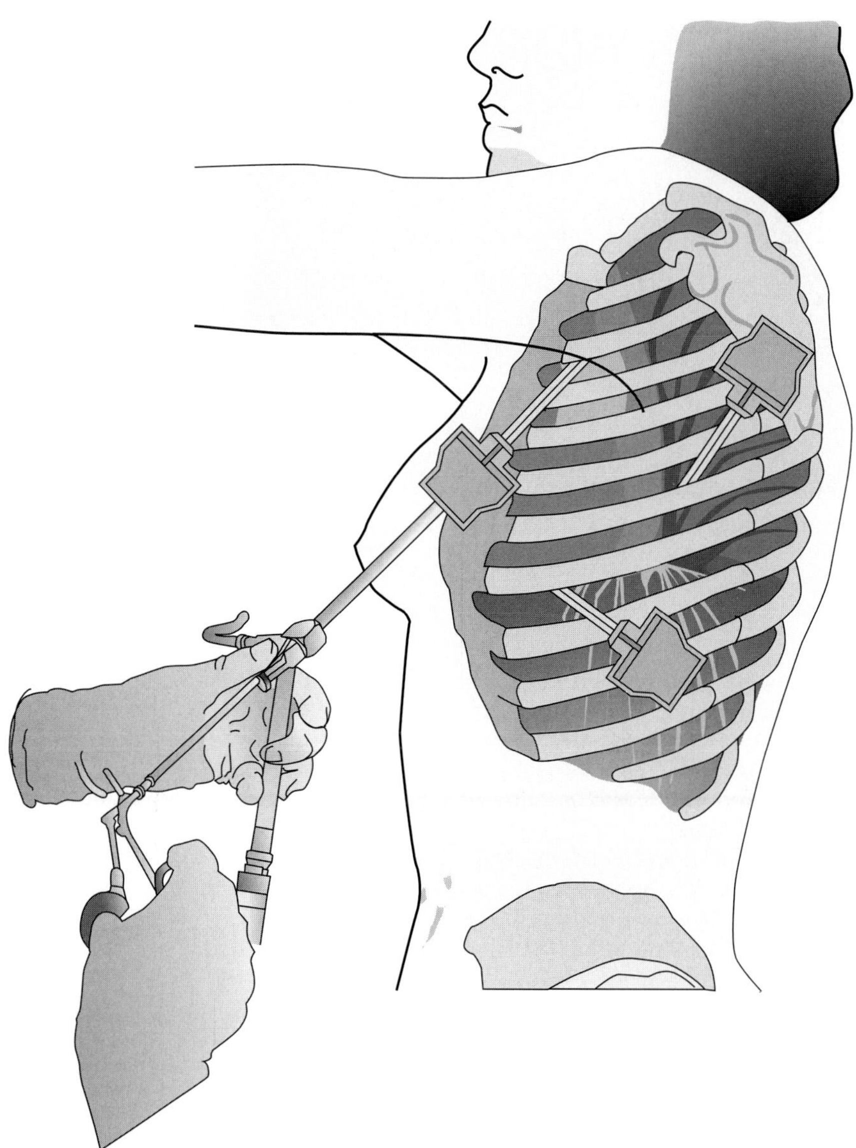

FIGURE 43–18 ■ Port placement for left thoracoscopic lymph node staging. (From Yim A, Hazelrigg S, Izzat M, et al [eds]: Minimal Access Cardiothoracic Surgery. Philadelphia, WB Saunders, 2000, p 190.)

If enlarged anteroposterior lymph nodes are present, the left chest is explored via the sixth intercostal space. Two additional incisions are then made in the anterior axillary line, one in the third intercostal space and the other in the seventh interspace (Fig. 43–17) (see Color Plate).

The mediastinal pleura overlying the lymph nodes is incised with an electrocautery scissors from the phrenic and vagus nerves superiorly to the left main pulmonary artery inferiorly (Fig. 43–18). Lymph nodes are grasped using a Babcock/Allis-type grasper. The vascular pedicle is ligated with an endoscopic clip applicator. Additional lymph node biopsies are performed from the inferior pulmonary ligament as described earlier.

LAPAROSCOPIC LYMPH NODE STAGING

The patient is placed in the supine position and prepared for a standard laparotomy. The first incision is made above the umbilicus in the midline, and a Veress needle used to insufflate the abdomen. Two additional ports are then placed in the right upper quadrant and left upper quadrant, as is done for laparoscopic fundoplication. A liver retractor is used on the right side and an atraumatic grasper is used on the left. We generally start with an operating scope and use an additional 5-mm incision if necessary. The lesser curvature is identified, and the stomach is grasped and retracted to the left. This allows visualization of the lesser omentum, which is incised with a cautery scissors. The lesser sac is now entered, and the stomach is retracted superiorly and to the left. The right crus is identified and dissected laterally, thus allowing biopsy of lesser curvature and parahiatal lymph nodes (levels 15 and 16). The left gastric vessels are noted and are traced to their origin as the stomach is retracted up to the abdominal wall. This exposes the celiac axis and allows biopsy of levels 17 to 20 (Fig. 43–19) (see Color Plate). If needed, a feeding jejunostomy, mediport, or both can be placed at this time as well.

RESULTS AT UNIVERSITY OF MARYLAND

After the initial 14 patients were staged through the left chest, thoracoscopy was routinely approached via the

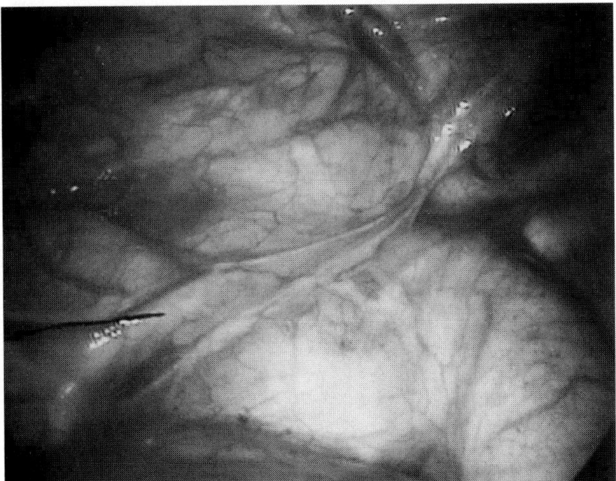

FIGURE 43–19 ■ Exposure of anteroposterior window and lymph nodes at the thoracoscopic lymph node. (See also Color Plate.)

right chest. This allowed maximal dissection of paraesophageal lymph nodes while avoiding the aortic arch. One patient with lymph node enlargement predominantly in the aortopulmonary window (level 5) had a left-side exploration. After TSLN is completed, laparoscopic staging is performed.

CT and EUS examinations, followed by thoracoscopy and laparoscopy, were used to stage 88 patients with esophageal cancer (Krasna and Mao, 1999). The pathology of the patients included squamous cell carcinoma (49 patients), adenocarcinoma (35), small cell carcinoma (2), and poorly differentiated carcinoma (2). There were 72 men and 16 women with a mean age of 60.7 years (age range, 38 to 78 years). Chest and abdominal CT was performed in 82 patients, and chest and abdominal magnetic resonance imaging (MRI) was performed in 52 patients. We have since abandoned the use of MRI because it adds little to CT and EUS except to rule out liver metastases in patients with lesions seen on CT. Sixty-two patients underwent EUS.

Thoracoscopic staging was successfully performed in 82 patients and was aborted in 3 patients because of adhesions. Three patients had laparoscopy alone to confirm suspected peritoneal metastases. Fifty-five patients had laparoscopic staging. Of these patients, 49 underwent both thoracoscopic and laparoscopic staging. Thirty-nine patients did not undergo resection after staging because of an advanced lesion (T4 in 12 patients, M1 in 3 patients), refusal (4 patients), poor health status (9 patients), or failure to complete chemoradiation (1 patient).

Thoracoscopic/laparoscopic staging detected 13 patients with T4 lesions; 3 patients with M1 lesions (2 with pulmonary M1 and 1 with liver M1) were also identified. Thoracic lymph node staging demonstrated N0 status in 71 patients and N1 status in 11 patients. Celiac lymph nodes were negative in 34 patients and positive in 21 patients. Esophagectomy was performed in 47 patients after thoracoscopic staging (33 after laparoscopic staging). Of these 47 patients who underwent resection, thoracoscopic staging showed N0 lymph node status in 42 patients and N1 in 5 patients. Three of the 42 (6.3%) patients with N0 disease on thoracoscopy were found at resection to have paraesophageal lymph node involvement (N1). Thoracoscopic staging was accurate in detecting the presence of diseased thoracic lymph nodes in 44 of 47 (93.6%) patients. Laparoscopic staging correctly detected normal celiac lymph nodes in 20 patients and diseased lymph nodes in 11 patients. Two patients who were deemed to have N0 disease by laparoscopic staging actually had N1 lymph nodes at esophagectomy. Thus, laparoscopic staging was accurate in 31 of 33 (93.9%) patients.

Thirty-four patients were treated with neoadjuvant chemoradiation followed by surgery. Of 17 patients found to have positive lymph nodes on thoracoscopy/laparoscopy, 12 (70.6%) were downstaged to N0 after chemoradiation. Twenty-five (71.4%) patients were downstaged by T and/or N stage and 15 (44.8%) patients had a complete pathologic response after chemoradiation.

Compared with the resection specimen pathology (Table 43–2), the sensitivity, specificity, and positive predictive value of thoracoscopic staging for N1 disease in chest were 62.5%, 100%, and 100%, respectively, for CT. The sensitivity, specificity, and positive predictive value for the detection of thoracic N1 disease were 27.3%, 74.2%, and 15.0%, and values were 62.5%, 60.8%, and 20.0%, respectively, for EUS. For the detection of N1 disease in the abdomen, the results for laparoscopy were 84.6%, 100%, and 100%, compared with 23.8%, 94.3%, and 71.4% for CT and 47.1%, 95.2%, and 88.8% for EUS, respectively.

DISCUSSION

It has been suggested that preoperative chemotherapy with radiotherapy may improve the survival of patients with esophageal cancer who demonstrate a complete pathologic response (Krasna and Mao, 1999; Orringer et al, 1990; Urba et al, 2001; Walsh et al, 1996). To evaluate the results of preoperative neoadjuvant chemotherapy with radiotherapy, accurate TNM staging and definition

TABLE 43–2 ■ **Sensitivity, Specificity, and Positive Predictive Value of Thoracoscopy/Laparoscopy, Computed Tomography, and Endoscopic Ultrasound Compared with Resection**

	Sensitivity (%)	*Specificity (%)*	*Positive Predictive Value (%)*
Chest N1			
Thoracoscopy	62.5	100.0	100.0
Computed tomography	27.3	74.2	15
Endoscopic ultrasound	62.5	60.8	20
Abdominal N1			
Laparoscopy	84.6	100.0	100.0
Computed tomography	23.8	94.3	71.6
Endoscopic ultrasound	47.1	95.2	88.8

of standard staging methods for esophageal cancer are very important. If accurate TNM staging for patients with esophageal cancer could be obtained, surgeons would know which group of patients might benefit from preoperative chemotherapy with radiotherapy. CT, MRI, and endoscopic esophageal ultrasonography are the nonoperative staging methods generally used for esophageal cancer.

CT is sensitive in the detection of the presence of lymphadenopathy in the chest but is not sensitive in T staging. EUS has a higher sensitivity in detection of the depth of the lesion invading the esophageal wall (T staging) but is limited when the lesion is advanced and occludes the esophageal lumen or when lymph nodes are distant from the esophagus. The reported accuracy of these noninvasive methods is sometimes suspect because pathologic comparison was not included. Preoperative staging by thoracoscopy and laparoscopy has been shown to be effective, safe, and accurate in patients with esophageal cancer. The positive predictive value of thoracoscopy and laparoscopy staging for N1 in the chest and abdomen was 100.0% because it allows direct visualization, biopsy, and pathologic examination. The greater accuracy afforded by thoracoscopy and laparoscopy staging is essential for patients who will undergo preoperative chemoradiation. It might be most useful to combine nonoperative staging tools such as CT and EUS with minimally invasive staging tools like thoracoscopy and laparoscopy.

Another advantage of thoracoscopy/laparoscopy staging is that it can provide pretreatment specimens that document the presence of lymph node metastasis and the changes in lymph nodes before and after chemoradiation in different stages of esophageal cancer (Izbicki et al, 1997; Krasna et al, 2001). Biomarkers detectable by immunohistochemical staining, such as Ber-Ep4 (Izbicki et al, 1997; Krasna et al, 2000), may improve the specificity and accuracy of the detection of occult lymph node metastasis. Even though concurrent chemoradiotherapy has a higher pathologic complete response (PCR) than other regimens, about 50% of patients have only a partial response or have no response (Krasna et al, 1999b). Thoracoscopy/laparoscopy staging may help select early-stage patients without any lymph node metastasis who can directly undergo resection, avoiding the unnecessary morbidity produced by chemoradiation (Krasna et al, 1999b; Krasna et al, 2000).

Patients with esophageal cancer who undergo trimodality therapy need a clearly dedicated regimen of preoperative chemotherapy and radiotherapy to decrease the morbidity and mortality during the perioperative period. The use of thoracoscopy/laparoscopy can provide preoperative pathologic documentation of lymph node metastasis in the chest and abdomen, allowing individualized preoperative radiation field design for every patient to avoid unnecessary morbidity due to extended radiation field (Suntharalingam et al, 1996).

A prospective trial as a Thoracic Intergroup study has been completed using thoracoscopic and laparoscopic lymph node staging for esophageal cancer (Cancer and Leukemia Group B 9380) The results of this study are expected to define the efficacy of this technique and its role in the management of esophageal cancer (Krasna et al, 2001).

COMMENTS AND CONTROVERSIES

The importance of accurate staging has been well demonstrated in lung cancer. Unfortunately, there is far less stage-specific information available for esophageal cancer. With continuing refinements in radiotherapy, chemotherapy, and perioperative care, the need for large trials of multimodality treatment regimens in esophageal cancer has never been greater. Such trials can be of only limited value, however, in the absence of accurate staging information. As with lung cancer, both prognosis and choice of treatment regimen are dependent on disease stage in esophageal cancer.

Despite impressive advances in various imaging techniques for lung cancer staging, including spiral CT scanning and PET scanning, there often is no substitute for thorough evaluation of the mediastinal lymph nodes by mediastinoscopy. Similarly, there often is no substitute for detailed thoracoscopic and laparoscopic assessment of the primary tumor and regional lymph nodes in esophageal cancer. Lymph nodes enlarged on CT scans may simply be hyperplastic. Unenlarged lymph nodes containing metastatic tumor may escape detection by PET scans due to insufficient uptake of FDG. EUS may be unable to identify lymph node metastases and may be unreliable for discriminating between T3 and T4 primary tumor stages.

With the widespread and ever-increasing use of thoracoscopy and laparoscopy, a versatile array of sophisticated instrumentation is available. The morbidity associated with these techniques is exceedingly low. Because there is only minimal discomfort and no need for lengthy hospitalization, patient acceptance of these minimally invasive staging methods is high. The time has come to refine the quest for effective treatment regimens for esophageal cancer through aggressive and accurate staging.

M. J. K.
J. R. S.
Z. G.

This chapter outlines a method for detailed pathologic staging of esophageal carcinoma that is expensive, time consuming, and invasive. Features include the need for general anesthesia, a double-lumen endotracheal tube, video-assisted thoracoscopy with multistation nodal sampling, and laparoscopy.

As the authors note, esophageal carcinoma, unlike lung carcinoma, is not as predictable in its pattern of nodal spread, and hence there is a need to stage the chest, the abdomen, and the cervical region regardless of the level of the primary tumor. One of the main benefits of accurate staging is the ability to compare series from different institutions and to conduct multicenter trials with a uniform staging protocol. It is unlikely that the video-assisted staging technique will gain sufficient acceptance or consistency to provide this benefit. In addition, the favorable experience with use of PET scanning for staging esophageal carcinoma will further limit the need for invasive staging. Its major value may be to confirm suspected sites of metastases identified on PET scans when the sites are not accessible to fine-needle aspiration biopsy. Confirmation of such suspected metastases may well reduce the incidence of exploratory procedures that lead to nonresection.

J. D. C.

REFERENCES

Abe S, Tachibana M, Shiraishi M, et al: Lymph node metastasis in resectable esophageal cancer. J Thorac Cardiovasc Surg 100:287–291, 1991.

Abe Y, Matsauzawa J, Fijiwaar T, et al: Clinical assessment of therapeutic effects on cancer using ^{18}F-2-fluoro-2-deoxy-D-glucose and positron emission tomography: Preliminary study of lung cancer. Int J Radiat Oncol Biol Phys 19:1005–1010, 1990.

Akiyama H, Tsurumaru M, Kawamura T, et al: Principles of surgical treatment for carcinoma of the esophagus. Ann Thorac Surg 194:438–446, 1981.

Bardini R, Castoro C, Sorrentino P, et al: Prognostic factors for squamous cell carcinoma of the thoracic esophagus after curative resection. In Ferguson MK, Little AG, Skinner DB (eds): Diseases of the Esophagus, vol I: Malignant Diseases. Armonk, NY, Futura Publishing Company, 1990, pp 219–228.

Blot WJ, Devesa SS, Kneller RW, et al: Rising incidence of adenocarcinoma of the esophagus and gastric cardia. JAMA 265:1287–1289, 1991.

Botet JF, Lightdale CJ, Zauber AAG, et al: Preoperative staging of esophageal cancer: Comparison of endoscopic ultrasound and dynamic CT. Radiology 181:419–425, 1991.

Dagnini G, Caldironi MW, Marin G, et al: Laparoscopy in abdominal staging of esophageal carcinoma. Gastrointest Endosc 32:400–402, 1986.

Ellis FH Jr: Carcinoma of the distal esophagus and esophagogastric junction. Mod Tech Cardiothorac Surg 13:1–10, 1979.

Ellis F, Heatley G, Balogh K: Proposal for improved staging criteria for carcinoma on the esophagus and cardia. Eur J Cardiothorac Surg 12:361–364, 1997.

Fiocco M, Krasna MJ: Thoracoscopic lymph node dissection. J Laparoendosc Surg 2:111–115, 1992.

Fleming ID (ed): AJCC Cancer Staging Manual, 5th ed. Philadelphia, Lippincott Williams & Wilkins, 1997.

Halvorsen RA Jr, Thompson WM: CT of oesophageal neoplasms. Radiatr Clin North Am 136:1051–1056, 1989.

Huang GJ: Natural progression in esophageal carcinoma. Int Trends Gen Thorac Surg 87–89, 1988.

Inculet RI, Keller SM, Swyer A: Evaluation of noninvasive tests for the preoperative staging of carcinoma of the esophagus. Ann Thorac Surg 40:561–565, 1985.

Izbicki J, Hosch S, Pichlmeier U, et al: Prognostic value of immunohistochemically identifiable tumor cells in lymph nodes of patients with completely resected esophageal cancer. N Engl J Med 337:1188–1194, 1997.

Jiao X, Zhang M, Wen Z, et al: Pleural lavage cytology in esophageal cancer without pleural effusions: Clinicopathologic analysis. Eur Cardiovasc Thorac Surg 17:575–579, 2000.

Kirby TJ, Rice TW: The epidemiology of esophageal carcinoma: The changing face of a disease. Chest 4:217–225, 1994.

Krasna MJ, Flowers JL, Attar S, McLaughlin J: Combined thoracoscopic/laparoscopic staging of esophageal cancer. J Thorac Cardiovasc Surg 111:800–807, 1996.

Krasna MJ, Mao YS: Making sense of multimodality therapy for esophageal cancer. In Locicero J (ed): Surgical Oncology Clinics of North America. Philadelphia, WB Saunders, 1999, pp 259–278.

Krasna MJ, Mao YS, Jiao X, et al: Correlation of clinicopathology, biological markers (p53, TS) and occult lymphatic metastasis with response, recurrence and survival in esophageal carcinoma treated with trimodality treatment. Paper presented at Proceedings of the 91st Annual Meeting of The American Association for Cancer Research, San Francisco, April 1–5, 2000.

Krasna MJ, Mao YS, Sonett JR, et al: P53 gene protein overexpression predicts results of trimodality therapy in esophageal cancer patients. Ann Thorac Surg 68:2021–2024, 1999a.

Krasna MJ, Mao YS, Sonett JR, et al: The role of thoracoscopic staging of esophageal cancer patients. Eur J Cardiothorac Surg 16 (Suppl 1):S31–S33, 1999b.

Krasna MJ, McLaughlin JS: Thoracoscopic lymph node staging for esophageal cancer. Ann Thorac Surg 56:671–674, 1993.

Krasna MJ, Reed C, Hollis D, et al: A prospective trial of the feasibility of thoracoscopy/laparoscopy in the staging of esophageal cancer: Preliminary results of Cancer and Leukemia Group B (CALGB) 93. Ann Thorac Surg 71:1073–1079, 2001.

Krasna MJ, Reed C, Jaklitsch MT, et al: Thoracoscopic staging of esophageal cancer: A prospective multi-institutional trial. Ann Thorac Surg 60:1337–1340, 1995.

Luketich JD, Friedman D, Weigel T, et al: Evaluation of distant metastases in esophageal cancer: 100 Consecutive positron emission tomography scans. Ann Thorac Surg 68:1133–1136, 1999.

Murray GF, Wilcox BR, Stared PIK: The assessment of operability of esophageal carcinoma. Ann Thorac Surg 23:393, 1977.

Orringer MB, Forastiere AA, Perez-Tamayo C, et al: Chemotherapy and radiation therapy before transhiatal esophagectomy for esophageal carcinoma. Ann Thorac Surg 119:348–355, 1990.

Rankin S, Manson R: Staging of esophageal carcinoma. Clin Radiatr 46:373–377, 1993.

Reed CE, Mishra G, Sahai AV, et al: Esophageal cancer staging: Improved accuracy by endoscopic ultrasound of celiac lymph nodes. Ann Thorac Surg 67:319–322, 1999.

Rice TW, Boyce GA, Sivak MV, et al: Esophageal ultrasound and the preoperative staging of carcinoma of the esophagus. J Thorac Cardiovasc Surg 101:536–544, 1991.

Rice TW, Zuccaro G, Adelstein DJ, et al: Esophageal carcinoma: Depth of tumor invasion is predictive of regional lymph node status. Ann Thorac Surg 65:787–792, 1998.

Shields TW: Lymphatic drainage of the esophagus. In Shields TW (ed): General Thoracic Surgery. Philadelphia, Lea & Febiger, 1989, pp 76–86.

Silvestri G, Hoffman B, Bhutani M, et al: Endoscopic ultrasound with fine-needle aspiration in the diagnosis and staging of lung cancer. Ann Thorac Surg 61:1441–1446, 1996.

Skinner DB, Ferguson MK, Little AG, et al: Selection of operation for esophageal cancer based on staging. Ann Surg 204:391–401, 1986.

Steup WH, Leyn PD, Deneffe G, et al: Tumors of the esophagogastric junction: Long-term survival in relation to the lymph node metastasis and a critical analysis of the accuracy or inaccuracy of pTMN classification. J Thorac Cardiovasc Surg 111:85–95, 1996.

Suntharalingam M, Vines E, Krasna MJ: Surgical staging prior to chemoradiation followed by esophagectomy: A preliminary analysis of a single institutional experience with esophageal cancer. ASCO Proc 15:215, 1996.

Tachimori Y, Kato H, Watanabe H, et al: Neck ultrasonography for thoracic esophageal carcinoma. Ann Thorac Surg 57:1180–1183, 1994.

Takemoto T, Ito T, Aibe T, et al: Endoscopic ultrasonography in the diagnosis of esophageal carcinoma with particular regard to staging it for operability. Endoscopy 18 (Suppl 3):22–25, 1986.

Tio TL, Cohen P, Coene P, et al: Endosonography and computed tomography of esophageal carcinoma. Gastroenterology 96:1478–1486, 1989.

Tio TL, Cohen P, den Hartog Jager FC, et al: Preoperative TNM classification of esophageal carcinoma by endosonography. Hepatogastrology 37:376–381, 1990.

Urba S, Orringer MB, Turrisi A, et al: Randomized trial of preoperative chemoradiation versus surgery alone in patients with locoregional esophageal carcinoma. J Clin Oncol 19:305–313, 2001.

Walsh TN, Noonan N, Hollywood D, et al: A comparison of multimodal therapy and surgery for esophageal adenocarcinoma. N Engl J Med 335:462–467, 1996.

Wolfer RS, Krasna MJ, Hasnain JU, et al: Hemodynamic effects of carbon dioxide insufflation during thoracoscopy. Ann Thorac Surg 58:404–408, 1994.

CHAPTER **44**

Management of Squamous Cell Carcinoma of the Esophagus

Simon Y. K. Law
John Wong

HISTORICAL NOTE

One of the earliest descriptions of esophageal cancer was in the second century AD, when Galen described a fleshy obstructing growth in the esophagus that was responsible for the inability to swallow and that led to emaciation and death. In the 10th century, Avicenna described various conditions leading to dysphagia, of which tumors were a common cause. Since then, numerous descriptions of cancer of the esophagus have appeared in the literature. Surgery of the esophagus began with the first recorded procedure by the Egyptians in 2500 BC, when "repair of the gullet" after perforation was reported. The history of esophagectomy for cancer was well narrated by Brewer. In 1877, Czerny performed the first successful resection of a cervical esophageal cancer, and the patient lived for 15 months. Rehn carried out the first, although unsuccessful, attempt at resection of thoracic esophageal cancer in 1898.

It was Torek who, in 1913, performed the first successful transthoracic resection. A 67-year-old woman had a squamous cell cancer of the midesophagus. Through a left thoracotomy, the esophagus was resected. The proximal cervical esophagus was brought out through an incision anterior to the sternocleidomastoid muscle and tunneled subcutaneously along the anterior chest wall, where a cutaneous esophagostomy was fashioned. The patient was fed via a rubber tube connecting the esophagostomy with a gastrostomy. The patient lived for 13 years.

The high mortality rates associated with transthoracic resection led to attempts using different techniques of esophagectomy. The transhiatal approach to esophageal resection was introduced by Denk in 1913 and refined by Turner in 1931. The technique became more popular after LeQuesne and Rauger in 1966 and Ong in 1970 described its use for cancer of the hypopharynx and cervical esophagus.

During the 1920s and 1930s, feeding was re-established by gastrostomy, with or without esophageal resection, with interposition of a plastic tube, skin tubes, or flaps. Later, various new approaches to esophageal reconstruction were described. In 1920, Kirschner described the use of the stomach, which was brought up subcutaneously to anastomose to the cervical esophagus, in experimental animals. The method was adapted to humans, and the first successful resection of a thoracic esophageal cancer with reconstruction using the stomach was performed by Ohsawa, a Japanese surgeon in Kyoto, who reported use of the technique in 18 patients. In 1946, Ivor Lewis described esophageal resection using a two-phase approach via a right thoracotomy and laparotomy. Tanner independently also described the procedure in 1947. Since then, other methods of reconstruction, including use of the colon and small bowel, have been described. The first surgeon to use a free jejunal graft for reconstruction was Seidenberg, who reported his experience in 1959. Free jejunal graft transfers to replace the cervical esophagus have gained popularity with advances in microvascular surgery.

HISTORICAL READINGS

Akiyama H: History, epidemiology, and related factors. In Gardner N (ed): Surgery for Cancer of the Esophagus. Baltimore, Williams & Wilkins, 1990, p 1.

Breasted JH: The Edwin Smith Surgical Papyrus. Chicago, University of Chicago Press, 1930, p 312.

Brewer LA: History of surgery of the esophagus. Am J Surg 139:730, 1980.

Kirschner M: Ein neues Verfahren der Oesophagoplastik. Arch Klin Chir 114:606, 1920.

LeQuesne LP, Rauger D: Pharyngolaryngectomy, with immediate pharyngogastric anastomosis. Br J Surg 53:105, 1966.

Lewis I: The surgical treatment of carcinoma of the esophagus with special reference to a new operation for growths of the middle third. Br J Surg 34:18, 1946.

Ohsawa T: Esophageal surgery. J Jpn Surg Soc 34:1518, 1933.

Ong GB: Cancer of the oral and pharyngeal cavities. J R Coll Surg Edinb 15:250, 1970.

Seidenberg B, Rosenak SS, Hurwitt ES, Som LM: Immediate reconstruction of the cervical esophagus by a revascularized isolated jejunal segment. Ann Surg 149:162, 1959.

Tanner NC: The present position of carcinoma of the esophagus. Postgrad Med J 23:109, 1947.

BASIC SCIENCE

Epidemiology and Etiology

There is marked geographic variation in the incidence of cancer of the esophagus. The disease is especially common in certain areas of Asia, the so-called Asian esophageal cancer belt, which stretches from eastern Turkey and east of the Caspian Sea through northern Iran, northern Afghanistan, and southern areas of the former Soviet Union, such as Turkmenistan, Uzbekistan, and Tajikistan, to northern China and India. High incidences are also found in the Transkei province of South Africa and in

Kenya. In high-incidence areas, the occurrence of esophageal cancer is 50- to 100-fold higher than in the rest of the world. In Henan province of China, esophageal cancer is the second most common cause of cancer death in adult men following lung cancer. In contrast, squamous cell esophageal cancer is relatively uncommon in the United States, Canada, and most areas of Europe, with notable exceptions in France and Italy. In low-incidence areas, the occurrence of esophageal cancer is 2 to 3 per 100,000 population and accounts for less than 2% of all malignant diseases. Esophageal cancer most commonly occurs in the sixth and seventh decades of life, and the male-to-female ratio ranges from 1.5:1 to 8:1.

Certain lesions have been described in the malignant transformation of the esophageal epithelium, including chronic esophagitis, papilloma, atrophy, dysplasia, and carcinoma in situ. Endoscopic surveys in high-risk groups have demonstrated the presence of chronic esophagitis in 84%, atrophy in 10%, and dysplasia in 8%. This distribution suggests that esophageal cancer may start with esophagitis, which in predisposed individuals progresses to atrophy, dysplasia, and cancer (Munoz et al, 1982).

Alcohol and tobacco are well-established risk factors. From case-control studies, alcohol is associated with a relative risk of 2.3 to 15.5 and smoking with a relative risk of 2.5 to 19 (Ribeiro et al, 1996). Pipe and cigar smokers have a greater risk for development of cancer than cigarette smokers. Smoking and drinking are independent contributing factors, as shown by prospective studies of patients who drink but do not smoke and, conversely, of patients who smoke but do not drink (Cheng et al, 1995; Tuyns, 1983). In addition to drinking and smoking, dietary and environmental factors are important, especially in Asian countries.

Nitrosamines and their precursors (nitrate, nitrite, and secondary amines) are incriminated in high-risk areas. In Linxian province in China, these substances are detected in various common foods and drinking water. Urinary levels of excreted nitrosamine-related compounds are also high. A positive correlation between the mortality rate for esophageal cancer and the consumption of these foods was demonstrated. Pickled vegetables are known to contain high levels of *N*-nitroso compounds, which strengthens the evidence that such chemicals are carcinogenic (Cheng et al, 1992).

Nutritional depletion of certain micronutrients together with an inadequate protein intake predisposes the esophageal epithelium to neoplastic transformation. Diets deficient in vitamin A, vitamin C, vitamin E, niacin, riboflavin, and fresh fruits and vegetables have been suggested. There is an inverse correlation between the mortality rate for esophageal cancer and the soil content of trace elements such as molybdenum, manganese, zinc, magnesium, and silicon. Molybdenum is a cofactor of the enzyme nitrate reductase, which affects the nitrite and nitrate contents of plants, and thus may be protective (Yang, 1980). Other dietary risk factors include consumption of hot beverages, opium smoking, betel nut chewing, and maté drinking in South American countries.

Concerning an infective etiologic mechanism, human papillomavirus (HPV) involvement was first suggested in 1992. HPV DNA sequences have been detected in esophageal cancer. In high-risk populations of China, HPV was found in up to 67% of patients with invasive cancer (Chang et al, 1992; He et al, 1997), although in other localities this was not universally reported (Lam et al, 1997). Other infectious agents implicated include certain fungi belonging to the genera *Fusarium, Alternaria, Geotrichum, Aspergillus, Cladosporium,* and *Penicillium.* The fungi may interact with foodstuffs in the production of nitroso- compounds.

Diseases that are known to predispose to esophageal cancer are few. The risk associated with achalasia is estimated to be 7-fold to 33-fold, but symptoms of achalasia are present for an average of 15 to 20 years before the emergence of cancer (Ribeiro et al, 1996). Chronic stasis of partially degraded foodstuffs in the esophagus produces chronic esophagitis, which may predispose to cancer. The incidence of lye corrosive strictures in esophageal cancer is about 0.8% to 5%. The time from a caustic burn to the emergence of carcinoma is about 40 years (Csikos et al, 1985). Other less common diseases associated with esophageal cancer include Plummer-Vinson syndrome, tylosis, and celiac disease.

Patients with other aerodigestive malignancies are at increased risk for squamous cell carcinoma of the esophagus, presumably because both malignancies involve exposure to similar environmental carcinogens. In the authors' unit, with esophageal cancer used as the index tumor, multiple primary cancers were found in 9.5% of patients; 70% of the tumors were in the aerodigestive tract (Poon et al, 1998b). The overall incidence of synchronous or metachronous esophageal cancer in patients with primary head and neck cancer is estimated to be 3% (Atabek et al, 1990; Shaha et al, 1988).

Clinical Pathology

In Asian countries, more than 80% of esophageal cancer is of squamous origin, whereas in Western countries there has been a dramatic rise in adenocarcinoma (Blot et al, 1991; 1993). In the United States, among white males, the incidence of adenocarcinoma of the esophagus rose by more than 350% from the mid-1970s, and surpassed that of squamous cell cancer around 1990 (Devesa et al, 1998). In many reports, adenocarcinoma now accounts for more than 50% of cancers seen. Gastroesophageal reflux disease and Barrett's intestinal metaplasia are implicated. Other less common tumors found in the esophagus (Lam and Ma, 1997) include mucoepidermoid cancer, adenosquamous cancer (Fegelman et al, 1994; Lam et al, 1994), small cell cancer (Law et al, 1994a), basaloid squamous tumor (Lam et al, 1998), sarcomatoid carcinoma, lymphoma, melanoma (Lam et al, 1999), and various subtypes of stromal tumors (Lam et al, 1996a, 1996b). The following discussion focuses on squamous cell cancers.

From a clinical standpoint, the pathologic information that is most important in management decision making is (1) the relationship between depth of tumor infiltration and lymphatic spread and (2) the propensity for intramural and longitudinal lymphatic spread of esophageal cancer. Patients who have early-stage cancers have a much better prognosis than patients with more advanced cancers.

Superficial cancer is usually defined as tumors limited to the mucosa or submucosa. *Mucosal* lesions can be further divided into m1 to m3. *Intraepithelial* cancer or cancer that barely breaks the basement membrane is defined as m1; cancer that is close to or that infiltrates the lamina muscularis mucosae, m3; and lesions between these two, m2. In a national survey in Japan, the incidences of lymph node involvement in m1, m2, and m3 tumors were 0%, 3.3%, and 12.2%, respectively. Similarly, *submucosal* lesions can be divided into Sm1, Sm2, and Sm3 categories. The incidences of lymph node involvement were 26.5%, 35.8%, and 45.9%, respectively (Kodama and Kakegawa, 1998). When the tumor has penetrated into the submucosa, the incidence of metastases increases and the prognosis is correspondingly poorer. For mucosal cancers, 5-year survival rates are mostly 80% to 100%; for submucosal cancers, the rates are 50% to 65% (Holscher and Siewert, 1997).

The Japanese Society for Esophageal Diseases (JSED) has classified the morphologic appearance at endoscopy of superficial cancer into different types:

- 0-I, superficial protruding type
- 0-IIa, superficial flat-elevated type
- 0-IIb, superficial flat-flat type
- 0-IIc, superficial flat-depressed type
- 0-III, superficial and depressed type

More advanced lesions (Dittler et al, 1992) are divided into:

- I, protruding type
- II, ulcerative and localized type
- III, ulcerative and infiltrative type
- IV, diffusely infiltrative type

There is some correlation between endoscopic appearance and pathologic depth of infiltration, but the accuracy is suboptimal and its use in guiding treatment is limited. In Japan, the reported occurrence of early esophageal cancer is around 10% (Holscher and Siewert, 1997). Outside Japan, the more commonly encountered squamous cell cancers are more advanced ones in which tumor has already extended to the muscularis propria and the adventitia and not uncommonly has infiltrated adjacent organs and metastasized to regional lymph nodes.

Spread of squamous cell carcinoma is by direct infiltration, intramural extension, and lymphatic and bloodborne metastasis. The esophageal wall has a rich network of submucosal lymphatics and thus is susceptible to longitudinal spread of tumor. Intramural metastases may be seen microscopically as subepithelial spread, skip lesions, or satellite nodules, all of which may be found some distance away from the main tumor. The incidence of intramural metastasis and multiple tumors is up to 30% (Lam et al, 1996c). Subepithelial spread is not uncommon, and this must be taken into consideration in decisions concerning surgical resection, especially the extent of axial resection margin required.

Another important pathologic aspect of esophageal cancer is the potential for widespread lymph node metastases, not uncommonly involving the thorax, abdomen, and cervical regions. When preoperative endoscopic injection of technetium-labeled rhenium colloid into the esophageal wall has been performed, radioactivity can be detected in lymph nodes. Lymphatic flow of the upper and middle thirds of the esophagus drains mainly to the neck and upper mediastinum, and the flow from the lower third drains mainly into the abdomen. Lymphatics of the thoracic esophagus can therefore drain to all three fields, but there is usually one predominant area of drainage, depending on the location of the tumor (Tanabe et al, 1986). From a therapeutic viewpoint, the most important group of lymph nodes lies along the recurrent laryngeal nerves, which traverses the thoracic inlet. This widespread lymphatic spread forms the basis of three-field lymphadenectomy, in which lymphatic dissection of all three fields is carried out, although its value remains unproven.

DIAGNOSIS

Symptoms and Signs

The spectrum of symptoms varies, depending on the extent of disease. The duration of symptoms does not necessarily correlate with tumor stage, curability, or resectability. Most patients with early cancers are asymptomatic or have only mild symptoms; the tumors are usually detected on routine medical examination or during investigation of other, unrelated conditions. The common complaints of these patients are mild pain, discomfort, and a mild hold-up sensation while eating, which are unrelated to tumor obstruction. It is thus important that in localities where the disease is not rare, even minor complaints be thoroughly investigated.

In advanced cases, the most common presenting symptom is dysphagia (80% to 95%), initially for solids and later for liquids as the obstruction becomes complete. Dysphagia may not be apparent until two thirds of the esophageal lumen has been obliterated, however, and many patients may delay seeking medical attention until severe dysphagia and weight loss have occurred. Many patients take water with their meals to help "force" the food down the gullet. Regurgitation is common. With high-grade obstruction, this symptom may be worse at night when the patient lies supine. Fluid regurgitation can lead to bouts of coughing, aspiration, and even chest infection. Odynophagia (retrosternal pain associated with swallowing) is not uncommon. It may be due to an ulcerated area of the tumor or to esophageal peristalsis attempting to overcome the obstruction. Persistent back pain between the scapulae is more ominous and may indicate extraesophageal invasion. Hoarseness is the result of recurrent laryngeal nerve compression; and the left nerve is more commonly affected because of its longer intrathoracic course and the fact that most tumors are located in the middle third of the esophagus. Right recurrent laryngeal nerve palsy indicates a proximal tumor or metastatic lymph node to the apex of the right chest or in the neck.

General examination may reveal evidence of weight

loss, muscle wasting, and dehydration. Examination of the chest may show the presence of pneumonia, which is due to aspiration or the development of a tracheo-esophageal fistula. Patients are often heavy smokers, and thus signs of chronic obstructive airway disease may be present. Lymph nodes should be searched for in the supraclavicular regions.

Investigation

Diagnosis of Early Disease

Advanced disease, which is present in most patients, is easily diagnosed. Suggestive symptoms prompting a contrast study or endoscopy can lead to a confident diagnosis, especially in areas of high prevalence. Early disease, however, is mostly asymptomatic. Because the prognosis is superior with early cancer, there has been interest in mass screening of high-risk populations.

The most common primary screening technique for the early detection for esophageal cancer is abrasive cytology. Two principal types of samplers have been used: an inflatable balloon developed in China (Shen, 1984; Shu, 1983) and an encapsulated sponge sampler developed in Japan (Nabeya et al, 1990). The balloon is made of rubber covered with a cotton tube and is swallowed by the patient. Once inside the stomach, it is inflated with 20 to 30 ml of air and then gradually pulled back. After removal, the balloon is smeared onto glass slides for examination. The sponge sampler is made of a sphere of polyurethane mesh compressed inside a gelatin capsule and attached to a thin solid plastic stylet. The sponge is swallowed and is left in the stomach for 5 minutes to allow the gelatin capsule to dissolve and the sponge to expand, after which it is pulled back into the esophagus. The sponge is shaken in fluid, which is centrifuged, and the "cell pellet" is then resuspended to make slides for examination.

The largest experience in the use of cytologic screening is in Linxian province in China, where the incidence of esophageal cancer is extremely high. In symptomatic individuals, these samplers were reported to have high sensitivities (73% to 99%) for detecting cancer. For asymptomatic individuals, however, the accuracy is lower. In one study, the sensitivity and specificity of the balloon for detecting biopsy-proven squamous cell cancer were 44% and 99%, respectively, and the corresponding figures for the sponge sampler were 10% and 100% (Roth et al, 1997). These values are not far below the sensitivity of current cytologic screening for uterine cervical cancer. Long-term follow-up studies showed a consistent progression of risk for development of esophageal cancer with increasing severity of the initial cytologic diagnosis of hyperplasia, dysplasia, and "near-cancer" (Liu et al, 1994).

Primary endoscopic screening has also been reported in alcoholic individuals and smokers in Japan and France, with the prevalence of esophageal cancer reported to be 3.3% to 8.2% of individuals screened (Ban et al, 1998; Meyer et al, 1997; Yokoyama et al, 1995). Widespread use of this method is limited by the cost and expertise required.

Chromoendosopy is an useful adjunct in the diagnosis of early esophageal cancer. The most commonly used stain is Lugol's iodine solution. This solution stains non-keratinized squamous cell epithelium dark brown to black because of its glycogen content. Inflammatory, dysplastic, and malignant tissues remain unstained. Another stain used in the esophagus is toluidine blue, which is absorbed by nucleic acid material of malignant epithelium (Acosta and Boyce, 1998). The use of such stains probably only moderately improves the diagnostic accuracy of video endoscopy. It does aid in the targeted biopsy of dysplastic areas and defines unexpected extension of the primary cancerous lesion for planning of the radiotherapy field and surgical resection. Intraoperative use to ensure an adequate resection margin has also been advocated (Mori et al, 1993; Sugimachi et al, 1992).

Staging Investigations

Refinement in surgical techniques and their appropriate selection (e.g., transhiatal esophagectomy) and employment of neoadjuvant therapies have made precise local staging more important. Staging information is also essential in the context of clinical trials; accurate staging enhances the value of the trials and helps to avoid bias. The tumor-node-metastasis (TNM) staging system has been modified. Cervical or celiac lymph nodes were previously classified as distant nodes but are now subdivided according to the level of the primary tumor. Cervical lymph node involvement for *upper third tumors* and celiac lymph node involvement for lower third tumors are assigned as M1a. Cervical lymph node for *lower third tumors* and celiac lymph node for upper third tumors are assigned as M1b. Lymph nodes in both regions are grouped as M1b for *middle third tumors.*

A chest radiograph should be obtained; with an advanced tumor, a widened mediastinum, tracheal compression, or a deviation may be seen. There may be evidence of aspiration pneumonia, lung metastases, or concomitant pulmonary parenchymal disease. Typical features in a contrast barium study include mucosal irregularity and shouldering, narrowing by the lumen, and proximal dilatation of the esophageal lumen. The study gives a longitudinal graphic view of the tumor in relation to other mediastinal structures, especially the trachea and main bronchi. It is a useful guide to the endoscopist, and it is sensitive in depicting a trachea-airway fistula. Tortuosity, angulation, axis deviation from the midline, sinus formation, and fistulation to the bronchial tree are signs indicative of advanced tumor that has traversed the adventitia and involved the neighboring fixed organs (Akiyama et al, 1972).

Use of the fiberoptic endoscope allows histologic confirmation of the cancer by biopsy or brush cytology. Flexible bronchoscopy is performed to assess tumor involvement of the tracheobronchial tree. Signs of involvement include a widened carina, external compression, tumor infiltration, and fistulization. The last two signs contraindicate resection (Cheung et al, 1988). Unless obvious tumor is seen on bronchoscopy, diagnosis of tumor infiltration can be difficult and can be helped by biopsy and brush cytologic examination of suspected areas. In one detailed prospective study, macroscopic abnormalities were detected in the trachea and main bronchi in 32% of patients with esophageal cancer located above the tracheal bifurcation. Proof of cancer could be obtained in only 3.6% of these abnormalities. Macroscopic appearance, therefore, is not sufficiently accurate to exclude patients from curative resection unless there is histologic evidence. The overall accuracy of bronchoscopy with multiple brush cytology and biopsy sampling in otherwise operable patients was 95.8%. Bronchoscopy was the sole decisive staging procedure, resulting in exclusion from surgery of 9.7% of patients because of airway invasion (Riedel et al, 1998).

The main value of a computed tomographic (CT) scan in staging of esophageal cancer is in its ability to detect distant disease. For the detection of metastases to liver, lungs, bone, and kidney, the accuracy of CT was reported to be 95% (Thompson et al, 1983). In defining the T and N stages, the accuracy is much lower at 59% to 64% for T stage and 48% to 74% for N stage (Holscher et al, 1994). Obliteration of the fat plane between the esophagus and aorta by more than 90 degrees of the circumference was suggested to predict aortic involvement with 80% accuracy (Picus et al, 1983). The frequent absence of mediastinal fat in nutritionally depleted patients makes this criterion unreliable. The sensitivity for detecting mediastinal and abdominal nodal involvement was poor because normal-sized lymph nodes may contain metastatic deposits and enlargement of lymph nodes may be due to reactive hyperplasia. Overall, agreement between CT scan and operative staging was seen in about 50% of patients, and preoperative underestimation of tumor growth by CT was noted in almost 40% (Lanfermann et al, 1990). Experience with magnetic resonance imaging (MRI) has shown limitations similar to those of CT, especially with respect to the low detection rate of mediastinal lymph nodes (Lehr et al, 1988). Positron emission tomographic (PET) scans for staging esophageal cancer have demonstrated greater sensitivity for detecting metastatic disease than CT scans (Orringer et al, 2000). The use of PET scans for staging esophageal cancer is discussed in Chapter 5.

Endoscopic ultrasound (EUS), or endosonography, allows definition of the esophageal wall as five discrete layers. A conventional 7.5-MHz EUS system distinguishes T1 from T2 lesions but is inadequate for finer discrimination. Use of a higher frequency (up to 20 MHz) allows distinction of mucosal and submucosal cancers. Intraepithelial cancer (m1), tumor involving the lamina propria (m2), and tumor penetrating the lamina muscularis mucosae (m3) can be distinguished. The diagnostic accuracy was 80% when the muscularis mucosae was seen (Yanai et al, 1996). Such information is of particular importance when endoscopic mucosal resection is a treatment option. Echo features of lymph nodes that suggest malignant involvement include size greater than 1 cm, hypoechoic pattern, sharp border, and round shape (Catalano et al, 1994). Each of these features when present alone was found to be inaccurate in detecting metastatic lymph node; when all four features were present, the accuracy was 80%. All features were present in only 25% of malignant nodes, however (Bhutani et al, 1997). Some authors have found different rates of accuracy for different lymph node locations. Accuracy is highest for paraesophageal nodes and varies inversely with the axial distance of the nodes from the esophageal axis (Chandawarkar et al, 1996). The value of EUS was demonstrated by a multicenter study of the American Endosonography Club. For 24% of patients who underwent EUS staging, the information led to a change in management plan (Nickl et al, 1996). Only those who performed the EUS study were surveyed, however, and depending on local treatment policy bias and preference, the extra information provided by EUS may not result in a change in management. This is especially true if surgery is the preferred treatment even when the intent is palliative (Fok et al, 1992).

The accuracy of EUS in local regional staging is not questioned. Comparative studies of EUS and CT proved the superiority of the former. The accuracy of EUS for T and N staging averaged 85% and 75% compared with 58% and 54% for CT (Rosch, 1995). One main limitation of EUS is inability to pass the endoscope through the tumor stricture, which occurs in about one third of patients (Bumm, 1996; Fok et al, 1992). High-grade nontraversible tumors, however, usually indicate T3 or T4 disease with lymph node metastases (Van Dam et al, 1993; Vickers and Alderson, 1998). Miniaturized ultrasound catheter probes passed through the working channel of a conventional endoscope showed accuracy comparable to that of conventional EUS. With a 6 French, 12.5-MHz miniprobe, the overall accuracy in the assessment of tumor infiltration depth was 90%. Lymph node involvement was accurately diagnosed in 78% of the patients (Hunerbein et al, 1998). The value of miniprobe scanning in the assessment of advanced tumors may be limited by the imaging depth of the probe (~3 cm). EUS-guided, fine-needle aspiration allows direct puncture of lymph nodes and aspiration of cells for cytologic examination and thus increases the diagnostic accuracy of EUS (Hunerbein et al, 1996).

Thoracoscopy and laparoscopy with laparoscopic ultrasonography have also been advocated to provide accurate staging information. Thoracoscopic staging usually involves a right-sided approach, with opening of the mediastinal pleura from below the subclavian vessels to the inferior pulmonary vein with lymph node sampling. Laparoscopic staging involves celiac lymph node biopsy and the use of laparoscopic ultrasonography for detecting liver metastases. Thoracoscopic lymph node staging has been 93% accurate in detecting thoracic lymph nodes, and a corresponding figure of 94% has been reported for laparoscopic staging of abdominal lymph nodes (Krasna, 1998; Krasna et al, 1995). Staging was claimed to be superior to EUS (Luketich et al, 1997a). The examination, is invasive, however, and general anesthesia and one-lung anesthesia are required. It is not widely practiced, and its true value remains to be seen. Another novel staging technique is the use of intra-aortic ultrasonography for determining tumor involvement of the thoracic aorta (Akiyama et al, 1997).

MANAGEMENT

Most patients presenting with esophageal cancer are old, frail, and malnourished. Late presentation, locally advanced disease, or even distant metastases are not uncommon when patients are first seen. Traditionally, after exclusion of moribund patients or patients with distant widespread metastases, who were to receive palliative care only, the choice of treatment has usually been between radiotherapy and surgical resection. The latter was often associated with a high mortality rate. Alternative endoscopic methods for palliation include intubation with a plastic prosthesis and laser therapy. With refinements in surgical technique and perioperative care and the emergence of new chemotherapeutic drugs, ways to deliver radiotherapy, and new endoscopic procedures, optimal therapy for the individual patient has become more difficult to define. Quality of life issues are also assuming more importance.

Surgical Treatment of Esophageal Cancer

Surgery has been the mainstay of treatment of esophageal cancer against which other modalities should be compared. Surgery is justified only when acceptably low morbidity and mortality rates can be achieved even for advanced disease; otherwise, the benefits gained by those who survive the operation are offset by the deaths of others (Wong, 1987).

Results of surgical resection have improved. In a review of 83,783 patients in 122 publications over a 20-year period from 1969 to 1979, the operability rate was 58%, the resectability rate was 39%, mortality associated with resection was 29%, and overall 5-year survival was only 4% (Earlam and Cunha-Melo, 1980a). Ten years later, in a review of 76,911 patients in 130 publications from 1980 to 1988, the resectability rate was 56%, the mortality rate 13%, and the 5-year survival 10% (Muller et al, 1990). In subsequent publications, mortality rates of less than 10% and even 2% were reported (Akiyama et al, 1994; DeMeester et al, 1988b; Law et al, 1992; Orringer et al, 1993; Zhang et al, 1994). There is no doubt that a significant learning curve exists for esophagectomy, but in specialized centers with experience, it is now an operation of acceptable risk (Matthews et al, 1986; Patti et al, 1998; Sutton et al, 1998). Improvements in surgical outcome can be achieved by (1) identifying patients with prohibitively high risk and excluding them from surgery, (2) optimizing the patients' physiologic status before surgery, and (3) refinements of surgical technique and perioperative care.

Most patients with esophageal cancer are heavy smokers and drinkers and have concomitant chronic disease. Risk factors often implicated include advanced age, presence of chronic lung and cardiovascular diseases, diabetes, cirrhosis, weight loss and malnutrition secondary to decreased food intake and malignancy, and disease stage (Law and Wong, 1999) Esophagectomy in older adults has been shown to be as safe as in their younger counterparts. Disease-specific long-term survival was also not inferior when compared with that of younger patients. Thus, selection on the basis of age alone is not adequate, and more objective evaluation is warranted (Ellis et al, 1998; Poon et al, 1998a).

Although poor nutritional status is often cited as a cause of a poor outcome, definite evidence that preoperative hyperalimentation can improve surgical outcome is lacking (Law and Wong, 1999). Various risk models have been generated to predict the outcome after esophagectomy. Risk stratification to different degrees is possible (Ferguson et al, 1996; Indahl et al, 1993; Law et al, 1994b; Lund et al, 1990; Muehrcke et al, 1989; Nagawa et al, 1994; Saito et al, 1993). With models so generated, the accuracy is about 75% to 80%. The value of these models is often questioned, however, because they are usually generated using retrospective data and rarely validated by prospective evaluation. Furthermore, preoperative risk analysis could not take into account intraoperative events and mishaps, which have a significant bearing on the development of postoperative complications. In one well-conducted study, the patient's general status and poor cardiac, hepatic, and respiratory functions were identified as independent predictors of a fatal postoperative course. On the basis of these impaired organ functions, a composite score was generated and prospectively validated. Including the score in the process of selection of patients and choice of surgical procedure resulted in a decrease of postoperative mortality rate from 9.1% to 1.6% (Bartels et al, 1998). When patients are judged fit to undergo surgical resection, existing diseases should be treated to optimize their physiologic status. Simple measures of cessation of smoking, active chest physiotherapy, and hyperalimentation are often adequate as preoperative preparations.

Resectability rates differ among reports. These rates depend on many factors, including (1) the referral patterns of individual centers, (2) the prevailing treatment philosophy, (3) the availability of alternative therapies, and (4) the possible mortality that the surgeon is prepared to accept even when resection is palliative for advanced tumors. In the authors' practice, most patients who are seen are not preselected for surgery and are representative of the general population. In 1097 patients, the resectability rate was 66% (Fig. 44–1). In the West, in patients not preselected by the referring physicians, the resectability rate is about 40% (Watson, 1994).

Surgery for esophageal cancer is fraught with difficulties. Two or three body cavities are traversed (neck, thorax, and abdomen), resulting in great surgical stress. Techniques in both resection and reconstruction are complex. The margin of error is also small. Versatility is required, since no single operation can address cancers at all levels of the esophagus. Surgeons therefore must possess a repertoire of procedures that can be employed for tumors at various locations and of different stages (Table 44–1).

Surgical Approach to Resection

Cervical Esophageal Cancer

About 6% of esophageal cancers arise in the cervical portion of the esophagus. Traditionally, treatment was radiotherapy because tumor extirpation requires a laryngectomy. Ong and Lee (1960) first described the procedure of pharyngo-laryngo-esophagectomy (PLE) as an one-stage, three-phase operation that involved cervical, abdominal incisions and a thoracotomy. Tumors involving the hypopharyngeal and upper cervical esophageal region

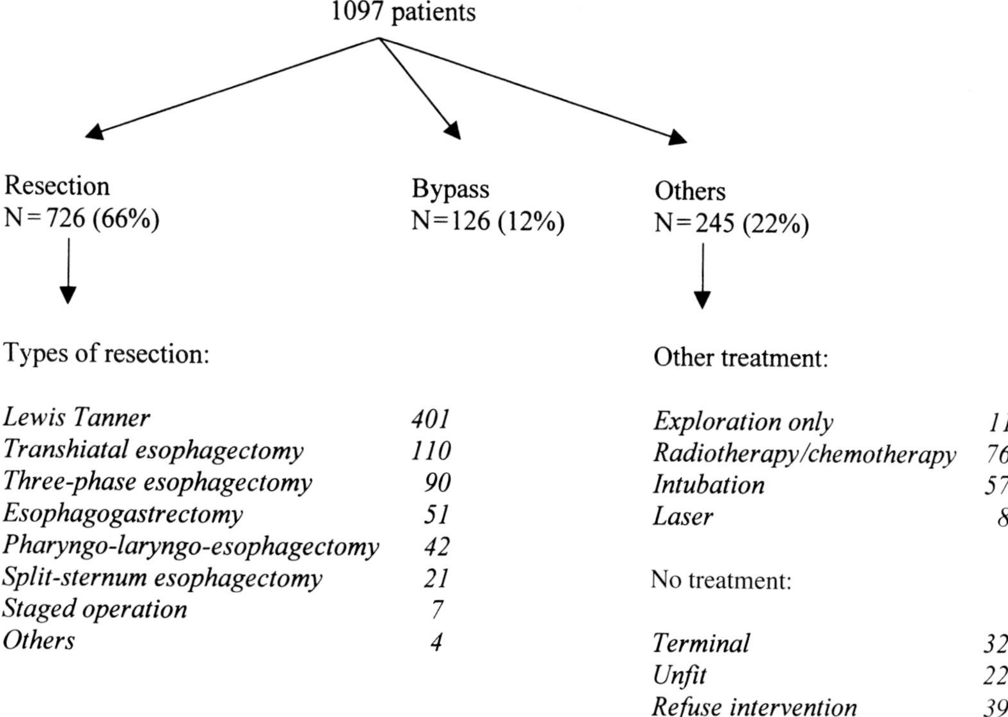

FIGURE 44–1 ■ Summary of primary treatment given to 1097 patients with squamous cell cancer of the esophagus managed at the University of Hong Kong Medical Center, Queen Mary Hospital, between 1982 and 1998.

were resected together with the whole esophagus, and the stomach was delivered via the posterior mediastinum to the neck for pharyngogastric anastomosis. A terminal tracheostomy was constructed. The thoracotomy was later replaced by transhiatal esophageal mobilization. This operation was associated with significant morbidity and mortality. Improvements in surgical results have made PLE an operation with a risk similar to that associated with resection of esophageal tumors from other locations. In the authors' experience, in 317 PLEs performed from 1966 to 1995, the mortality rate has decreased from 31% to 9% (Wei et al, 1998b). Thoracoscopic esophageal mobilization is also carried out now in lieu of the transhiatal technique.

TABLE 44–1 ■ **Common Surgical Approaches to Resection and Bypass for Squamous Cell Cancer of the Esophagus**

Tumor Location	*Resection (Thoracotomy)*	*Resection (No Thoracotomy)*	*Bypass*
Cervical	Pharyngo-laryngo-esophagectomy (transthoracic approach)	Pharyngo-laryngo-esophagectomy (transhiatal, minimal access approach) Free jejunal graft	None
Superior mediastinal segment	Three-phase esophagectomy (McKeown's approach)	Split-sternum esophagectomy	Kirschner bypass
		Transhiatal esophagectomy Minimal access approach	Colonic bypass
Middle third	Lewis Tanner esophagectomy Three-phase esophagectomy	Transhiatal esophagectomy Minimal access approach	Kirschner bypass Colonic bypass
Lower third	Lewis Tanner esophagectomy Three-phase esophagectomy Left thoracotomy or thoracoabdominal approach	Transhiatal esophagectomy Minimal access approach	Kirschner bypass Colonic bypass
Tumors involving the cardia	Esophagogastrectomy (abdominal–right chest or left thoracoabdominal approach)	Esophagogastrectomy (transhiatal approach)	Jejunal bypass

For tumors confined to the proximal portion of the cervical esophagus, with sufficient distal margin, a free jejunal interposition graft or deltopectoral or pectoralis major myocutaneous flaps are options for reconstruction after resection. The use of a free jejunal graft is advantageous because it avoids mediastinal dissection, although expertise in performing microvascular anastomosis must be acquired. Graft necrosis, fistula formation, and later graft strictures are specific problems (Takooda et al, 1991). When it is compared with gastric pull-up, graft survival and leakage rates are similar. Stricture was the most common late complication for free jejunal transfers, whereas reflux was more common in gastric pull-ups, as reported by Schusterman and colleagues (1990). Functional study showed a satisfactory swallowing mechanism in all patients (Reece et al, 1995). The jejunal graft has been shown to be tolerant to postoperative radiotherapy (Reece et al, 1995; Wei et al, 1998a).

Upper Thoracic Esophageal Cancer

About 7% of squamous esophageal tumors are located in the transitional cervicothoracic region, which is relatively inaccessible by conventional thoracotomy or cervical approaches. Blind mobilization carries significant risk because of the close proximity of the tumor to the membranous trachea and great vessels, together with the fact that many of the cancers are advanced at presentation. The split-sternum approach to cancer of the superior mediastinum allows direct visualization and dissection of important structures and also avoids position change of the patient during operation. A thoracotomy is also avoided. Our experience as well as that of others with this approach has been favorable (Moorehead et al, 1989; Ong et al. 1978; Orringer, 1984).

For tumors in the upper thoracic esophagus at and above the level of the aortic arch, obtaining a sufficient proximal resection margin demands an anastomosis placed in the neck. For this reason, resection is best carried out by a three-phase esophagectomy, or the McKeown approach (McKeown, 1976). During this procedure, a right thoracotomy is first carried out to mobilize the thoracic esophagus together with lymphadenectomy; this is followed by abdominal and neck incisions for the mobilization of the esophageal substitute, with the anastomosis placed in the neck.

Middle and Lower Third Esophageal Cancer

Most squamous esophageal cancers are located in the intrathoracic portion. About 61% of these occur in the middle and 26% in the lower thoracic segment. The most widely used approach was that described independently by Lewis (1946) and Tanner (1947). The operation begins with an abdominal phase, in which the stomach is prepared; a right thoracotomy and resection of the tumor together with lymphadenectomy follow. The stomach is then brought up into the chest for anastomosis, with the proximal esophagus at the apex of the pleural cavity. A commonly employed alternative approach involves a single left thoracotomy incision as described by Adams and Phemister (1938) and popularized by Ellis and colleagues (1983). Through a left thoracotomy and incision in the diaphragm, both the esophagus and stomach would be mobilized and resection carried out. This approach is also widely employed in China. The disadvantage is that the heart and proximally the aortic arch preclude adequate access to the esophageal bed, the latter in particular causing mobilization of the proximal esophagus and subsequent anastomosis to be difficult. The approach is therefore more suitable for cancer of the cardia or the distal esophagus, where an adequate resection margin is obtained below the aortic arch.

Transhiatal versus Transthoracic Resections

For patients with limited cardiopulmonary reserve who are not candidates for thoracotomy, a transhiatal resection may be performed. In this procedure, the thoracic part of the esophagus is mobilized by blunt, and often blind, dissection through the enlarged esophageal hiatus. The mobilized stomach is then delivered to the neck and anastomosed to the cervical esophagus. There is continuing controversy over whether a transthoracic esophagectomy (TTE) or a transhiatal esophagectomy (THE) approach is optimal for intrathoracic esophageal cancer. THE appears to result in less pulmonary complications and mortality compared with TTE (Muller et al, 1990). There are added advantages of a shorter operating time and placing the upper esophageal anastomosis in the cervical region where a longer resection margin is obtained. Anastomotic leakage in the neck is often cited as being less lethal. Long-term survival is not inferior to that with TTE. Proponents of TTE criticize THE for providing inadequate oncologic clearance because an adequate thoracic lymphadenectomy cannot be performed and state that the claimed advantage of a lower pulmonary complication rate is unproved. A review of the literature in the 1980s showed an overall mortality rate of 7% in 1353 patients who had THE (Katariya et al, 1994). In experienced centers, mortality is as low as 5% (Orringer et al, 1993). Almost all comparative studies of the two approaches have been retrospective (Bolton et al, 1992; Hankins et al, 1989; Mathisen et al, 1988; Shahian et al, 1986; Tilanus et al, 1993), making them less than adequate for proper and unbiased evaluation. A retrospective analysis in the authors' institute showed that pulmonary-related deaths were associated less frequently with THE than TTE in patients with high pulmonary risks for surgery (Fok et al, 1993a). Others have obtained similar results (Bolton et al, 1992).

Randomized controlled trials comparing the two procedures are few, partly because both procedures are not practiced at the same institutions with equal skill and preference. One such trial compared the clinical outcomes of 67 patients with squamous cell cancer randomly assigned to THE or TTE. There were no difference in morbidity rates (THE 56% versus TTE 46%) and especially in the incidence of pulmonary complications (THE 19% versus TTE 20%). Mortality rates were also similar (THE 6.2% versus TTE 8.5%) (Goldminc et al, 1993). In our trial with 39 patients randomly assigned, intraoperative hypotension was more common in the THE group. This was probably the result of the operator's hand and forearm in the posterior mediastinum reducing venous return as well as compressing the heart. THE took less time to perform. Perioperative morbidity, mortality, and long-term survival did not differ. In this study, however, only patients with lower-third tumors were included and both groups of patients were judged to have sufficient pulmonary reserve to undergo TTE before randomization (Chu et al, 1997).

Specific complications of THE include bleeding, tumor rupture and contamination, chylothorax, tracheobronchial injury, Horner's syndrome, and recurrent nerve paresis. A worse outcome with middle third tumors has been reported (Fok et al, 1993a; Hurley and Keeling, 1990). This is not surprising, since this is a "blind" area of blunt dissection. Advances in staging technique, especially with EUS, make prediction of extraesophageal spread more accurate and the application of THE in cancer of this location less hazardous. In our experience, we reserve THE for patients with lower or upper third tumors, where the dissection of the esophagus can be carried out under vision, and for patients with reduced pulmonary reserve or patients with an obliterated pleural cavity. More recently, we have used the thoracoscopic approach in lieu of THE for patients with similar indications and have largely abandoned THE except where the pleural cavity cannot be entered because of adhesions.

Minimal Access Surgery

Minimal access surgery, as applied to esophageal resection, has taken many forms, including thoracoscopic esophageal mobilization (Peracchia et al, 1997), video-assisted transmediastinal esophageal mobilization using a laparoscope inserted through the diaphragmatic hiatus (Sadanaga et al, 1994), laparoscopic gastric mobilization followed by thoracotomy (Perniceni et al, 1996), laparoscopic gastric and esophageal mobilization (DePaula et al, 1995), and mediastinoscopic dissection (Bumm et al, 1993). The thoracoscopic approach with open laparotomy for preparation of the esophageal substitute and a cervical anastomosis is most common. In the authors' institute, thoracoscopic esophageal mobilization took a median time of 110 minutes. When it was compared with open thoracotomy resections, no significant difference in morbidity and mortality rates was found. However, patients selected for thoracoscopy had an increased surgical risk (significantly worse Eastern Cooperative Oncology Group [ECOG] scores compared with those who underwent open thoracotomy resections) (Law et al, 1997d).

The lack of clear advantages of minimal access techniques over conventional approaches may be related to the learning curve, selection of patients, and the multifactorial nature of the genesis of cardiopulmonary complications. The benefit of smaller port sites compared with open thoracotomy may be offset by the reported lengthened time of single-lung anesthesia. The surgical trauma of mediastinal dissection is also independent of the incision size. Improvements in pain relief and perioperative care also lessen the deleterious effects of thoracotomy and laparotomy (Tsui et al, 1997). Port site recurrence is another concern. Review of the literature showed similar results (Peracchia et al, 1997). All except one report have demonstrated no obvious advantage in postoperative morbidity. One report showed that pulmonary morbidity was reduced from 33% to 20% compared with open thoracotomy. Incidence of hoarseness was also reduced. Extensive animal experimentation was carried out before clinical use, and this may have eliminated the learning curve that was present in other series (Akaishi et al, 1996).

Reconstruction and Surgical Complications

After resection, selection of a suitable substitute organ and selection of the appropriate anastomotic technique are important operative decisions. The organ most commonly used for reconstruction after esophagectomy is the stomach. The stomach can rely on the right gastroepiploic artery alone, with the best blood supply to a 4-cm-wide gastric tube on the greater curvature (Liebermann-Meffert et al, 1992). It is of sufficient length to be brought up for anastomosis without tension to the chest or neck.

When the stomach is not used for reconstruction, the colon or small bowel may be selected. The colon's blood supply is more variable, but preoperative arteriography may help in identifying reliable vasculature and lessen the risk of graft failure. Arterial anatomic features are favorable in at least 80% of patients with arteriographic examination, and the incidence of anastomotic leakage and graft failure can be less than 2% (Peters et al, 1995). An isoperistaltic loop can be constructed from either the left-sided or right-sided colon. The jejunal loop is less reliable, and in about 25% of cases the arrangement of the arcade precludes its use.

Anastomotic leakage is a feared complication because of its high morbidity and mortality. A review of reports in the 1980s revealed an average leakage rate of 12% (Muller et al, 1990), and even after that leakage rates of up to 30% were still reported (Hsu et al, 1992). Technical errors probably account for most leaks. In our study, a detailed analysis of the causes of leaks showed that 53% were associated with an identifiable technical error and were thus protentially avoidable (Law et al, 1994b). The use of stapling devices was shown to decrease leakage rates (Wong et al, 1987). Stapling devices are perhaps less operator dependent. Pooled data from randomized trials comparing stapled with hand-sewn esophagogastric anastomoses showed no significant difference for leaks (stapled 9%, hand-sewn 8%) but a higher incidence of strictures in stapled anastomoses (stapled 27%, hand-sewn 16%) (Beitler and Urschel, 1998). In a randomized trial performed in the authors' unit, leakage rates were not significantly different at 4.9% and 1.6% for stapled and hand-sewn anastomoses, but stricture was more frequent in the group receiving staples (40% versus 9.1%) (Law et al, 1997c).

Pyloric drainage is necessary to prevent gastric stasis, especially in the early postoperative period. In 13% of patients without drainage, symptomatic outlet obstruction developed in the early postoperative period, with more patients having persistent problems with eating compared with those who had had a pyloroplasty (Fok et al, 1991). A pyloromyotomy is an equally effective alternative (Law et al, 1997a).

Other less commonly encountered surgical complications include gangrene of the esophageal substitute and chylothorax (Lam et al, 1979; Moorehead and Wong, 1990). Routine ligation of the thoracic duct is recommended to prevent chylothorax. Should it occur, early reexploration with thoracic duct ligation is recommended. Guidelines for surgery may include (1) chyle leak of 1 L/day for more than 5 days, (2) persistent leak for more than 2 weeks despite conservative treatment, and (3) nutritional or metabolic complications (Merrigan et al, 1997).

With careful selection of patients for surgery, meticulous surgical technique, and anesthetic and perioperative care, esophagectomy has been made a safe operation in specialized centers (Table 44–2). Improvement in long-term prognosis remains a more difficult goal to achieve.

Extent of Resection for Esophageal Cancer

One of the most controversial aspects of treating gastrointestinal malignancies is the appropriate extent of resection to achieve the best outcome, and this debate is best exemplified by esophageal cancer (Wong, 1993). Some surgeons have a minimalist attitude toward cancer of the esophagus and believe that surgical resection is mostly palliative and a cure is a chance phenomenon attained only in those with very early tumors. Transhiatal resection is partly based on this reasoning (Orringer et al, 1993). Conventional transthoracic resection usually involves a "standard" lymphadenectomy, which entails removing the nodes and periesophageal tissue below the level of the carina (Bumm and Wong, 1994). More aggressive surgeons practice extended radical resection of the primary tumor as well as lymphadenectomy, extending the field of dissection to the neck and abdomen even for intrathoracic cancers. Although improvement in survival is the ultimate test for different philosophies of resection, locoregional recurrence after apparently successful surgical resection remains an important cause of death and produces symptoms difficult to palliate. Ways to achieve local control, if not cure, should be sought, hence the importance of defining the appropriate extent of resection.

An R0 resection is consistently identified as the most important prognostic factor for long-term survival. An R0 resection results in total removal of the tumor mass (primary and lymph nodes) with a clear proximal, distal, and lateral margin (Hermanek, 1995). The need for an adequate longitudinal margin in the prevention of anastomotic recurrence is well recognized. The incidence of intramural metastasis and multiple tumors is up to 30% (Lam et al, 1996c). An adequate margin is required to guard against the development of anastomotic recurrence, the risk for which was shown to be related to the length of resection margin attained at operation (Law et al, 1992, 1998). A negative histologic margin indicated by frozen section at the time of surgery is no guarantee against subsequent anastomotic recurrence because skip lesions can be present. Taking into account shrinkage of the specimen after resection (Siu et al, 1986), an in situ margin of 10 cm provides a less than 5% chance of anastomotic recurrence.

The issue of lateral margin and lymphadenectomy is more difficult to define. Microscopic involvement of the lateral margin (macroscopically clear) results in a poorer prognosis with an increased chance of local recurrence (Sagar et al, 1993). The site of the tumor has some bearing on the ability to widen this margin. For supracarinal tumors, the close proximity of the trachea makes widening the margin difficult except in T1 or T2 cancers. For tumor of any location, most agree that for T4 tumors with infiltration to adjacent mediastinal organs, aggressive resection together with involved organs is not justified.

The optimal extent of lymphadenectomy is perhaps most controversial. The lack of appropriate randomized controlled trials is a main reason. Lymph node involvement occurs early in esophageal cancer and is closely related to depth of invasion in the esophageal wall. For tumors reaching the muscularis mucosae, between 8% and 30% of patients had pathologic lymph nodes; a corresponding figure of up to 58% has been reported for tumors reaching the submucosa (Akiyama et al, 1994; Isono et al, 1991; Kato et al, 1993; Kodama and Kakegawa, 1998). For truly intraepithelial cancer (m1) and cancer that has not reached the lamina muscularis mucosae (m2), lymphatic spread is infrequent and therefore simple esophagectomy without radical lymphadenectomy is justified. In Japan, endoscopic mucosal resection is commonly employed for the treatment of these tumors with gratifying results (Kodama and Kakegawa, 1998). It has been claimed that high-frequency EUS can reliably distinguish these tumors from those with deeper infiltration (Yanai et al, 1996). For more advanced lesions, more extensive lymphadenectomy seems indicated.

In a multicenter survey conducted by the Groupe Européen pour l'Étude des Maladies de l'Oesophage (GEEMO) for early squamous cell cancers (Tis–T1 N0 M0), the 5-year survival rate in patients with submucosal tumor was higher after TTE than after THE (54.2% versus 25.5%). For mucosal cancers, this survival advantage was not seen (Bonavina, 1995). However, advocates of THE without systematic lymphadenectomy claim long-term survival rates similar to those for open thoracotomy resections, and this issue remains unsettled without well-conducted randomized trials (Orringer et al, 1993).

TABLE 44–2 ■ **Mortality Rates of 726 Patients with Squamous Cell Cancer of the Esophagus After Esophageal Resection in Three Different Time Periods**

	1982–1987	*1988–1993*	*1994–1998*
No.	272	277	177
30-day mortality	11 (4%)	14 (5%)	0 (0%)
>30-day mortality	40 (14%)	23 (8%)	5 (2.8%)
*Hospital mortality**	51 (18%)	37 (13%)	5 (2.8%)

*Hospital mortality includes all deaths occurring in the hospital after resection.

Three-Field Lymphadenectomy

The detailed locations of lymph node metastases painstakingly delineated by Japanese surgeons, showing that lymph node involvement frequently occurs in the neck and the upper abdomen, were the theoretical justification for three-field lymphadenectomy (3-FL) with dissection of the neck, mediastinum, and upper abdomen. In addition, recurrence patterns in patients after conventional esophagectomy have shown a 46% to 49% incidence of lymphogenic recurrences, most located in the upper mediastinal and cervical region (Fujita et al, 1994). There is less controversy regarding removing abdominal lymph nodes in the paracardiac region and left gastric and celiac trifurcation because of its relative ease and lack of significant morbidity. Extending lymphadenectomy to the cervical and upper thoracic region is debated because of technical difficulty and associated morbidity. The nodes along the recurrent laryngeal nerves are most commonly involved. This "cervicothoracic" group can be considered as one entity, and when assessed together, lymph nodes are involved in up to 63.4% of proximal-third, 45.2% of middle-third, and 42.0% of lower-third cancers in patients undergoing 3-FL (Akiyama et al, 1994).

A nationwide survey from Japan reported significant differences in 5-year survival rates for 3-FL and two-field lymphadenectomy (2-FL) of the mediastinum and abdomen, both for N0 and N1 diseases (57% versus 45% and 33% versus 29%, respectively) in favor of the more extensive approach (Isono et al, 1991). Two randomized trials have been published comparing 3-FL with 2-FL. One showed a higher postoperative mortality for 2-FL and a survival advantage for 3-FL. Patients who had 2-FL, however, were older and had more proximal tumors. 3-FL and 2-FL were performed by two different groups of surgeons, although patients were apparently randomly allocated. Patients were also not stratified for postoperative adjuvant therapies (Kato et al, 1991). In the other trial, 5-year survival rates were not statistically different at 66.2% and 48% for 3-FL and 2-FL, respectively. The small number of patients (n = 73) were highly selected. Only 64 of 264 patients who had undergone surgery during the recruiting period were eventually analyzed. Most patients had T1 or T2 disease only, the rate of cervical metastases in the 3-FL group was low, and patients were also randomly assigned to postoperative adjuvant therapy (Nishihira et al, 1998).

Although these randomized trials were insufficient to prove an advantage with 3-FL, results from nonrandomized studies indicate that significant subgroups of patients may benefit from 3-FL. Early superficial cancers confined to the mucosa show low incidence of pathologic lymph nodes, and for these 3-FL is not recommended (Nishimaki et al, 1993). In a study of 51 patients with submucosal tumors who underwent 3-FL, the incidence of positive lymph nodes was 57% with 20% having cervical lymph node spread. The overall 5-year survival rate was 68%; the corresponding figure in the GEEMO study was only 44.3%. This suggests a benefit with 3-FL for submucosal tumors (Bonavina, 1995; Nishimaki et al, 1999).

Overall, for all tumor stages except for mucosal tumors, a 5-year survival rate of 52.2% was reported for 3-FL (Akiyama et al, 1994). This result is better than that in reports on conventional lymphadenectomy, which has a corresponding figure of only 35% to 40%. A survival advantage was demonstrable only for upper-third and middle-third cancers by various investigators, probably because of the preferential lymphatic spread of tumors from these sites to the neck and the fact that cervical node involvement is a late event for lower-third cancer (Akiyama et al, 1994; Baba et al, 1994; Fujita et al, 1995; Nishimaki et al, 1997). Other poor prognostic factors included (1) metastatic nodes in all three fields, (2) a lower-third tumor having positive cervical nodes, and (3) involvement of five or more lymph nodes. These situations indicate advanced metastatic disease and are associated with such a poor prognosis that 3-FL may not be justified (Nishimaki et al, 1998).

Whether patients with or without pathologic cervical nodes benefit from neck dissection is controversial. Patients with negative neck nodes had a 5-year survival rate of 56.6% after 3-FL. Even when cervical nodes were involved, a surprising 5-year survival rate of 25.3% was achieved, suggesting that cervical lymph nodes could be regarded as "regional" nodes and that 3-FL had the potential of eliminating neck disease with long-term survival (Akiyama et al, 1994). The national survey in Japan demonstrated better survival with 3-FL in N0 or N1 disease (Isono et al, 1991).

3-FL is carried out with minimal mortality in Japan, mostly below 5%; however, there is no doubt that such extensive surgery is associated with increased operating time and significant morbidity (Nishimaki et al, 1999). Recurrent laryngeal nerve palsy, related to extensive dissection of the recurrent laryngeal nerve chain, can reach 70% (Fujita et al, 1995). Recurrent nerve palsy influences not only immediate postoperative recovery but also long-term quality of life, in particular speech and swallowing ability (Baba et al, 1998). In two Western studies reporting on 3-FL, however, recurrent laryngeal nerve palsy was seen in only 5% and 6% of patients (Altorki and Skinner, 1997; Lerut et al, 1994). It is not certain whether the consistently higher rates of hoarseness reported in Japan are due to more thorough dissection of the recurrent laryngeal nerve chain. In any case, with its attendant potential morbidity, 3-FL should be carried out only in experienced centers.

The optimal extent of lymphadenectomy thus remains controversial. A summary at the Consensus Conference for the International Society for Diseases of the Esophagus in Milan in 1995 concluded that data from the literature were in favor of a transthoracic approach for lymphadenectomy in a fit patient with curative intent. For supracarinal cancers, a total mediastinal lymphadenectomy with cervical dissection should be carried out. No clear conclusions could be drawn about infracarinal cancers (Fumagalli, 1996).

Multimodality Treatment

Radiotherapy alone used to be the only effective alternative to surgery. The best results of radiotherapy as the primary therapeutic modality for esophageal cancer were reported by Pearson (1966). A 1-year survival of 44% and a 5-year survival of 22% were achieved. However, this series included mainly tumors of the cervical esophagus, and similar results have not been confirmed by others. In a large review, the 1-, 2-, and 5-year survival rates for more than 8000 patients with radiotherapy as the primary treatment of esophageal carcinoma were 18%, 8%, and 6%, respectively (Earlam and Cunha-Melo, 1980b). The treatment dose is usually 55 to 65 Gy. Mostly because of treatment preference, radiotherapy tends to be given either because of high surgical risk or to patients with advanced or metastatic disease that is not amenable to curative surgery. An attempt by the Medical Research Council (MRC) in the United Kingdom to conduct a randomized controlled trial comparing surgery with radiotherapy alone resulted in premature study termination after 18 months because of lack of sufficient recruitment. Only 31 patients entered from 16 centers (Earlam, 1991). Although many still advocate radiotherapy as first-line treatment, the emphasis has been shifted to multimodality treatment, in which chemotherapy is given in addition to radiotherapy. The role of surgery in such treatment programs has to be redefined.

In theory, multimodality treatments can down-stage the tumor and improve local control and, in this regard, may replace radical lymphadenectomy. More limited surgery might then be justified. In addition, chemotherapy may help control systemic micrometastases. However, no randomized controlled trial so far has provided convincing evidence that multimodality treatment is superior (Thomas, 1997).

Trials of neoadjuvant radiotherapy have failed to show increased resection rate or improved survival compared with surgery alone (Arnott et al, 1992; Gignoux et al, 1987; Launois et al, 1981; Nygaard et al, 1992; Wang et al, 1989). Postoperative radiotherapy can reduce local recurrence, especially tracheobronchial recurrence in a subgroup of patients with residual mediastinal disease after palliative resection, but there was no demonstrable survival benefit (Fok et al, 1993b; Ténière et al, 1991; Zieren et al, 1995). Neoadjuvant chemotherapy resulted in significant down-staging of disease in approximately 50% of patients, but a pathologic complete response (p-CR) rate was achieved in less than 10%. Subgroup analysis showed that a survival benefit, if any, appeared to exist only in objective responders (Law et al, 1997b; Roth et al, 1988; Schlag, 1992). Only in one trial reported, in abstract form, was a significant survival advantage shown (Kok et al, 1998), and this was not supported by other studies. The latest multicenter study of neoadjuvant chemotherapy versus surgery alone recruited 440 patients (of whom about half had squamous cell cancers). No survival benefit was demonstrated; 2-year survival rates were 35% and 37% for patients who did and did not receive chemotherapy, respectively (Kelsen et al, 1998). The results of similar large multi-institutional trial, the MRC protocol OE02, are awaited.

Currently, the most intensive investigations center on chemoradiation. The Radiation Therapy Oncology Group (RTOG 85-01) randomized trial is widely believed to provide convincing evidence of the superiority of chemoradiation over radiation alone (Al-Sarraf et al, 1997; Herskovic et al, 1992). The 2- and 5-year survival rates were 36% and 27% in the chemoradiation group and 10% and 0% in the radiotherapy-alone group. Reduction in both local and distant failures was reported. Toxicities, however, were substantial. The combination of chemoradiation with surgery has resulted in significant disease down-staging, has increased the p-CR rate to 25%, and has increased the proportion of R0 resections. A consistent survival advantage, however, has not been in evidence. A survival advantage with neoadjuvant chemoradiation over surgery alone was shown in one trial, which included patients with adenocarcinoma only (Walsh et al, 1996). Three-year survival rates were 32% for the preoperative treatment group and 6% for surgery alone. This trial has been criticized on the grounds of inadequate preoperative staging, unclear surgical procedure, a large number of protocol violations, and exceptionally poor survival in the surgery group.

Another report on 100 patients who underwent THE (75% of whom had adenocarcinoma) showed a p-CR rate of 28%. A 3-year survival advantage was seen (32% versus 15%), with reduction of locoregional recurrence (39% versus 19%) (Urba et al, 1997). Similar results were not shown in trials that included squamous cell cancers only (Apinop et al, 1994; Bosset et al, 1997; Le Prise et al, 1994). The results of these trials are conflicting and inconclusive.

From the limited data available, it seems that chemoradiation may help local disease control when applied in addition to surgical resection. However, no randomized trial has directly compared chemoradiation with surgery alone as monotherapy (whether with standard lymphadenectomy or extensive lymphadenectomy).

It has been suggested that chemoradiation alone can be adequate without surgical resection. Four considerations argue against the omission of surgery:

1. Chemoradiation alone provides inferior local disease eradication when surgical resection is omitted. In approximately 50% of patients who had chemoradiation alone, persistent local or locally recurrent tumors were found. The addition of surgery reduces local disease recurrence (Fink et al, 1995).
2. False complete responses are commonly seen, and a true p-CR can be ascertained only after resection.
3. Persistent nodal disease despite sterilization of the primary tumor requires surgical clearance.
4. The ability to relieve dysphagia also differs. The restoration of normal eating ability with radiotherapy was far inferior to that with surgery. In one report, only 45% of the patients could eat satisfactorily after radiotherapy and the remaining 55% could tolerate fluids or had complete obstruction, whereas all patients who underwent resection could eat solids (Chakkaphak et al, 1989). In another prospective study, the incidence of stricture (benign and malignant) was 16% after surgery and 50% after radical radiotherapy (O'Rourke et al, 1992). Malignant strictures responded to dilatation poorly, and most patients required a further endoscopic procedure, such as intubation, to relieve dysphagia. The need for a further procedure is uncommon after resection. Surgical treatment thus provides palliation of dysphagia with much greater certainty.

Further clinical studies are needed to identify the best multimodality regimens, their dose levels, and the methods and schedules of administration. Meanwhile, surgery remains the standard treatment for resectable esophageal cancer. For those judged unfit for surgery or those with locally advanced disease, chemoradiation seems a reasonable first alternative.

Surgical Palliative Treatment

In the presence of locally advanced or metastatic disease, palliation is the goal of treatment. "Quality of life" issues assume more importance than long-term prognosis. Major symptoms of dysphagia, pain, and tumor bleeding should clearly be eliminated, but the patient's attitude, anxiety, and other aspects of quality of life should be taken into account when treatment is planned. Surgery plays a significant part in palliation. Tumor resection can readily alleviate dysphagia, pain related to the tumor, and bleeding. It also prevents the local complications of tumor perforation, fistula formation, and airway obstruction. In esophageal cancer, dysphagia is a major component of quality of life. In a study of laser therapy and intubation, the degree of dysphagia was found to correlate well with a Linear Analogue Self-Assessment (LASA) test, which assessed the patient's physical and psychological well-being and symptom control. LASA also correlated strongly with a Quality of Life Index (Loizou et al, 1992).

Esophagectomy offers excellent palliation for diet-related symptoms. Our study showed that both curative esophagectomy and palliative esophagectomy resulted in significant improvement in the type and quantity of food intake and other diet-related symptoms for at least 1 year after surgery. More important, these symptomatic improvements were equally well maintained in the curative and palliative groups. After 3 months, more than 90% of patients were asymptomatic with regard to swallowing or had only occasional difficulty with solid food. However at 9 months after resection, pain status and global QOL score were worse for the palliative group than for the curative group (Branicki et al, 1998).

Resection is therefore valuable even if the intent is only palliative. When surgery is offered, it must be done with minimal morbidity and mortality and a short hospital stay. Second, a reasonably long life expectancy should be anticipated. O'Rourke and co-workers (1992) evaluated palliation in patients who had surgery, radiotherapy, intubation, or no treatment. The quality of palliation was quantified graphically using Karnofsky scores, pain severity, and swallowing ability. Surgery provided poorer palliation in the first 3 months but no differences in pain or performance were detectable for the second 3 months at which time superior swallowing efficiency scores were evident in the surgical group. Thus, distant organ metastases, a malignant fistula into the airway, and spread to multiple nonregional lymph nodes, which all suggest a short life expectancy, should discourage palliative resections and other palliative options should be explored instead.

Surgical bypass using stomach, colon, and jejunal loops, if successful, offers rapid and durable palliation in terms of dysphagia (DeMeester et al, 1988a; Lam et al, 1982; Ong et al, 1982). The procedure most commonly employed is the Kirschner operation, in which the stomach is brought up to the neck by the retrosternal or subcutaneous route to anastomose with the cervical esophagus. The thoracic esophagus is drained by a Roux-en-Y jejunal loop to the distal esophagus (Kirschner, 1920; Ong, 1973; Wong et al, 1981). Operative morbidity and mortality rates are, however, substantial in patients with very advanced disease, who often have a poor surgical risk. Mortality of near 40% has been reported (Orringer and Sloan, 1975; Wong et al, 1981). There is no doubt that successful bypass provides excellent relief of dysphagia, but the operative magnitude, short life expectancy, and the availability of low-risk alternatives make bypass a less practical procedure. When unresectable disease is encountered intraoperatively at the time of a planned resection, a bypass procedure is justified. In this situation, a lesser procedure is performed for a patient judged fit to undergo tumor extirpation and in whom surgical exploration is already being performed.

Nonsurgical Palliative Treatment

Radiotherapy and Chemotherapy

External beam radiation (external radiation therapy, ERT) is an important method of palliation. The need for 4 to 6 weeks of treatment and 30% to 50% incidence of severe mucositis, radiation stricture, and fistula formation are significant problems reducing its efficacy (Albertsson et al, 1989).

Brachytherapy has been used in the treatment of esophageal cancer. It has the potential for improving the therapeutic ratio, that is, delivery of a relatively high dose of radiation to the tumor with relative sparing of the surrounding tissues, particularly the lungs and adjacent spinal cord. It has been advocated as the sole primary treatment for early cancers, as a boost therapy to follow external ERT, or as a palliative treatment option. In some studies comparing ERT with and without a brachytherapy boost, improvements in survival, local control, and swallowing ability were claimed with addition of a boost. Guidelines have been published by the American Brachytherapy Society on its indications and recommended regimen. The use of radiotherapy and chemotherapy for palliation is discussed in greater detail in Chapter 50.

Endoscopic Palliation

The simplest form of endoscopic procedure is dilatation. It is simple and inexpensive, but relief is short-lived. Risks of bleeding and perforation are present. It remains an option for those with a short life expectancy, especially when local economic factors do not allow a more expensive modality.

The two most common forms of endoscopic palliative treatment employed are esophageal stenting and laser therapy. These modalities are discussed in Chapters 65 and 66.

Comparisons of intubation and laser therapy have been addressed in clinical trials. Earlier studies comparing conventional plastic prostheses with laser therapy suggested slightly higher complication rates with intubation and found that the quality of food eaten may also be better with laser therapy (Bown, 1991; Carter et al, 1992). In subsequent reports comparing laser therapy and plastic and metallic stents, relief of dysphagia was similar, although complications may still be more frequent with stents (Gevers et al, 1998). The disadvantage of restenosis after laser therapy makes stenting the preferred method in patients with a reasonably long life expectancy. The two modalities should be viewed as complementary. The argon beam coagulator has been used in a similar fashion to laser therapy. A jet of argon is ionized to conduct high-frequency electrical energy of uniform intensity to the target area. It clears blood from the area being cauterized and allows a no-touch technique, which provides effective hemostasis, dessication, and thermal coagulation. Experience with this method is limited. It has also been used in conjunction with intubation to ablate overgrowth tumor (Robertson et al, 1996).

Photodynamic therapy (PDT) is unique, in that it is selective in the destruction of tumor tissue. A photosensitizing agent, a hematoporphyrin derivative, is injected into the bloodstream. The compound is selectively taken up by tumor and is activated by a laser with a wavelength of 630 mm. Local cytotoxic effects are mediated by singlet oxygen. A multicenter trial of 218 patients comparing PDT with laser therapy showed that relief of dysphagia was similar. Fewer sessions were required for PDT, but more side effects occurred, including sunburn (19%), nausea (8%), fever (16%), and pleural effusion (10%). Perforation was more common with the laser (7% versus 1%) (Lightdale et al, 1995). PDT is not widely available, given its cost of installation.

Intralesional injection of various substances has been tried. Alcohol injection causes necrosis of tumor tissue. Several uncontrolled series (about 150 patients) showed its effectiveness in restoring swallowing; the duration of response was similar to that with laser therapy. Major complications included mediastinitis and an esophagus-airway fistula, which occurred in less than 2% of patients. Transient low-grade fever and pain may also occur (Saidi and Marcon, 1998). Other less commonly used substances include the sclerosant polidocanol, cytotoxic agents such as 5-fluorouracil or peplomycin, bleomycin, mitomycin, methotrexate, and cisplatin. Immunomodulators such as tumor necrosis factor and OK432, combined with radiotherapy or given preoperatively, were found in small studies to improve dysphagia and outcome (Mukai et al, 1995).

The BICAP heater probe delivers bipolar electrocoagulation energy to the tumor. It consists of an "olive" with a circumferential heating unit in the center. The treatment results, palliative efficacy, and safety of the BICAP probe were similar to those of the laser (Jensen et al, 1988). The advantage of the BICAP is its portability, low equipment cost, and ability to treat long or high cancer strictures in a single session.

The use of hyperthermia is based on the selective heat sensitivity of neoplastic cells compared with normal cells. This method was shown to enhance the anticancer effect of radiation and chemotherapy, and the improvement varied with the cytotoxics selected (Saeki et al, 1998). An uncontrolled study showed that response and survival rates were higher for the 136 patients receiving preoperative hyperthermia-chemoradiation therapy than for the 107 patients undergoing preoperative chemoradiation only (Kuwano et al, 1995).

Various methods have been described, some well tested and some novel, and the method should be selected according to individual needs. Tumor characteristics and availability are important considerations. No one method is superior and applicable in all situations.

PROGNOSIS

The ability to achieve an R0 resection, the depth of tumor invasion, and the presence and number of lymph node metastases have consistently been shown to reflect the long-term prognosis after surgical resection. Lymph node ratio, the number of lymph nodes found positive on histopathologic examination divided by the number of lymph nodes sampled, may also indicate the prognosis (Fumagalli, 1996; Roder et al, 1994). In the authors' institute, the median survival calculated from presentation for all patients with squamous cell cancer regardless of treatment is 8.8 months, with a 5-year survival rate of 14%. All resections are associated with a 5-year survival rate of 19%. Curative resections yield a median survival of 32 months and a 5-year survival rate of 34%, compared with respective figures of 7.5 months and 8% for palliative resections. Five-year survival rates for patients with stage I, IIa, IIb, III, and IV disease are 60%, 30%, 40%, 13%, and 3% (Figs. 44–2 and 44–3).

THE FUTURE

Great steps have been made in improving surgical results. Once an operation with the highest mortality, esophagectomy has become a relatively safe procedure through improved selection of patients, well-conducted operations, and better perioperative care. The long-term prognosis in this disease, however, remains suboptimal. In

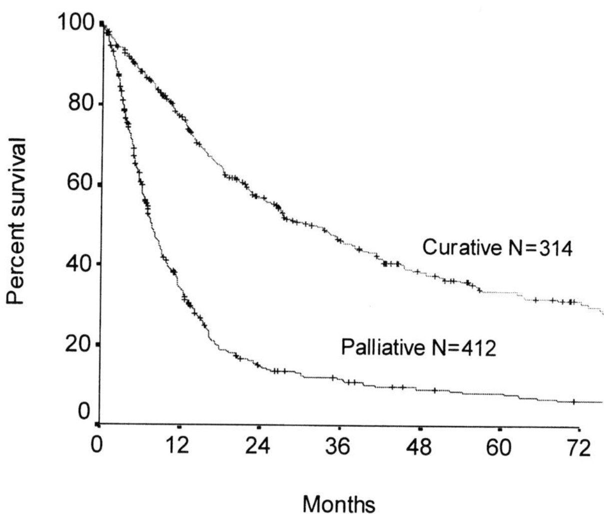

FIGURE 44–2 ■ Cumulative survival curves for patients who underwent curative and palliative resections for squamous cell cancer of the esophagus. The 5-year survival rates were 34% and 8%, respectively, for curative and palliative resections.

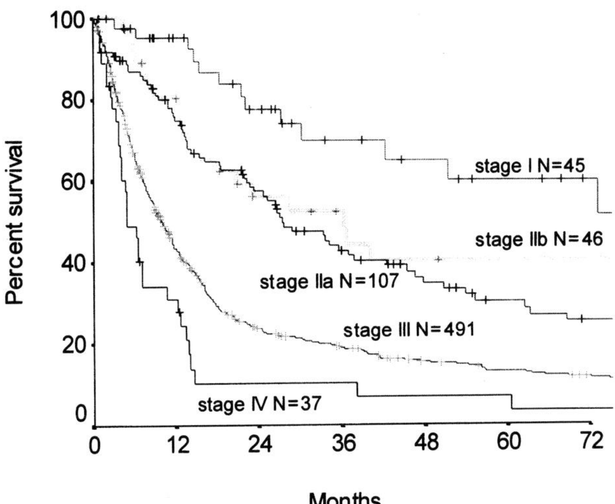

FIGURE 44–3 ■ Cumulative survival curves, according to the American Joint Committee on Cancer classification of tumor stage, for patients who underwent resection. Five-year survival rates for stages I, IIa, IIb, III, and IV were 60%, 30%, 40%, 13%, and 3%, respectively.

terms of improving the prognosis, the greatest controversies concern the optimal extent of lymphadenectomy and combined multimodality treatment. Subgroups of patients who may benefit from extended surgery should be better defined. Advances in technology will contribute to more accurate preoperative staging, guide proper selection of therapeutic modalities, and help in monitoring the response to adjuvant therapies. In particular, it is most important that responders to chemotherapy and radiotherapy can be predicted so that potentially harmful treatments are not given to those who are unlikely to respond while good-quality survival is provided to those who can benefit. The prevalence of systemic spread prompts discovery of newer and more effective chemotherapeutic agents to treat this deadly disease.

COMMENTS AND CONTROVERSIES

This chapter by Professors John Wong and Simon Y. K. Law clearly reflects extensive experience in dealing with squamous cell carcinoma of the esophagus and thoughtfulness in addressing the many difficult and often vexing issues related to the choice of appropriate therapy for patients who often have a poor prognosis.

As noted, most squamous cell carcinomas occur in the middle portion of the esophagus with the concomitant possibility of direct involvement of the trachea or main bronchi. I personally favor the use of both rigid and flexible bronchoscopic examination when evaluating possible airway involvement. The tip of the rigid bronchoscope is used to "palpate" the membranous wall of the trachea and main bronchi, looking for loss of mobility, or fixation, which may be the only sign of tumor extension to the membranous wall. Even if the airway mucosa is intact, biopsy of such sites may reveal infiltrating tumor. Obvious displacement of the posterior tracheal wall alone does not necessarily indicate tumor infiltration.

Slow-growing, constricting carcinomas in the region of the cervical esophagus may be difficult to diagnose at esophagoscopy in spite of repeated attempts. Rigid bronchoscopy, with biopsy of the posterior subglottic airway, may yield the diagnosis. On rare occasions, open biopsy of the esophageal wall may be the only means of obtaining tissue confirmation.

We have found the use of PET extremely valuable for the staging of esophageal carcinoma and now use it routinely to complement CT scan evaluation for esophageal carcinoma. The PET scan is particularly useful for detecting previously unsuspected nodal or other distant metastases, but it is inferior to the CT scan in determining the size and the depth of penetration (T status). On the other hand, the T status alone influences the patient's candidacy for resection much less frequently than does the presence of nodal or distant metastases. In this regard, a more accurate determination of tumor depth by endoscopic ultrasonography plays little role in choosing patients for resection but may be important in recommending neoadjuvant therapy or in accurately staging patients for clinical trials.

When comparing surgical resection with chemoradiation therapy, the authors correctly emphasize that surgical treatment provides a much greater certainty of palliation of dysphagia for the lifetime of the patient. Thus, a resection that turns out to be palliative rather than curative in nature may still be of considerable benefit to the patient. This may be especially true in cases of esophageal carcinoma adjacent to the tracheal bronchial tree. The incidence of the dreaded complication of tracheal esophageal fistula in such cases is significantly reduced by surgical resection compared with chemoradiation therapy.

Of the various conduits utilized for reconstruction after esophagectomy, none, in my opinion, has the safety and efficacy of the stomach. An esophagogastric anastomosis high in the chest or in the neck is associated with excellent swallowing ability and minimal reflux, regurgitation, or esophagitis in the remaining esophagus. Drs. Wong and Law note the increased incidence of esophagogastric anastomotic leak when the transhiatal approach is used compared with the transthoracic approach. This experience has been almost uniform.

Several reasons have been given for the increase leak rate associated with a transhiatal procedure, including greater tension on the anastomosis because of its more proximal location or compromise of the arterial or venous circulation by compression of the stomach at the thoracic inlet. In addition, the use of a cervical anastomosis, in the case of a transhiatal resection, is often associated with a very short proximal esophageal length. In this situation, extension of the neck or elevation of the larynx with swallowing can increase the tension on the anastomosis. If several extra centimeters of cervical esophagus are retained, the completed esophagogastric anastomosis can be repositioned to lie just below the thoracic inlet, which may reduce the incidence of anastomotic complications. Orringer has reported a significant reduction in the anastomotic leak rate with use of a linear stapler to create a side-to-side esophagogastric anastomosis. This technique is associated with a longer proximal esophageal stump than usual for hand-sewn anastomoses and does create a very strong, tension-resistant connection between the esophagus and stomach.

After esophagectomy and reconstruction by means of a gastric conduit, Drs. Wong and Law advocate routine use of a pyloromyotomy or pyloroplasty. It has been my practice not to incorporate either procedure unless there has been preexisting duodenal ulcer disease. Gastric stasis is rare after transhiatal esophagectomy with the stomach suspended vertically within the mediastinum. After esophagectomy with the aid of a right thoracotomy, however, postoperative gastric stasis is more common. In such cases, gastric stasis is usually due to angulation of the stomach as it passes from the right chest through the hiatus and not to a tight pylorus. Repositioning the stomach in the mediastinum at the end of a transthoracic esophageal resection helps reduce this complication. On rare occasions after esophagectomy with gastric replacement, a tight pylorus may be associated with gastric retention. This can usually be dealt with effectively by means of endoscopic balloon dilatation.

J. D. C.

■ KEY REFERENCES

Akiyama H, Tsurumaru M, Udagawa H, et al: Radical lymph node dissection for cancer of the thoracic esophagus. Ann Surg 220:364, 1994.

The results of three-field lymphadenectomy for esophageal cancer emanated from a single author's experience. A landmark paper discussing the topic from a surgeon with extensive experience with esophageal cancer.

Law S, Wong J: Complications: prevention and management. In Daly JM, Hennessy TPJ, Reynolds JV (eds): Management of Upper Gastrointestinal Cancer. London, WB Saunders, 1999, pp 240–262.

A comprehensive review of complications after esophagectomy. The etiology, means of prevention, and treatment are discussed.

Lewis I: The surgical treatment of carcinoma of the esophagus with special reference to a new operation for growths of the middle third. Br J Surg 34:18, 1946.

Lewis first described the two-phase right-sided thoracotomy approach for esophageal cancer in 1946. In 1947, Norman Tanner independently performed a similar procedure. Commonly referred to as the Lewis-Tanner operation, the procedure has become the most commonly performed operation for carcinoma of the middle third of the esophagus.

Muller JM, Erasmi H, Stelzner M, et al: Surgical therapy of oesophageal carcinoma. Br J Surg 77:845, 1990.

A comprehensive literature review of surgical results in the treatment of esophageal cancer in the 1980s. This is particularly interesting when compared with a similar review published by Earlam and Cunha-Melo 10 years earlier of results in the 1960s and 1970s. Morbidity and mortality associated with resections had improved, but long-term survival remained suboptimal.

■ REFERENCES

Acosta MM, Boyce HW Jr: Chromoendoscopy: Where is it useful? J Clin Gastroenterol 27:13, 1998.

Adams WE, Phemister DB: Carcinoma of the lower thoracic esophagus: Report of a successful resection and esophagogastrectomy. J Thorac Surg 7:62, 1938.

Akaishi T, Kaneda I, Higuchi N, et al: Thoracoscopic en bloc total esophagectomy with radical mediastinal lymphadenectomy. J Thorac Cardiovasc Surg 112:1533, 1996.

Akiyama H: History, epidemiology, and related factors. In Gardner N (ed): Surgery for Cancer of the Esophagus. Baltimore, Williams & Wilkins, 1990, p 1.

Akiyama H, Kogure T, Itai Y: The esophageal axis and its relationship to the resectability of carcinoma of the esophagus. Ann Surg 176:30, 1972.

Akiyama H, Tsurumaru M, Udagawa H, et al: Radical lymph node dissection for cancer of the thoracic esophagus. Ann Surg 220:364, 1994.

Akiyama S, Sekiguchi H, Fujiwara M, et al: Intra-aortic ultrasonography in advanced esophageal cancer. Semin Surg Oncol 13:234, 1997.

Albertsson M, Ewers SB, Widmark H, et al: Evaluation of the palliative effect of radiotherapy for esophageal carcinoma. Acta Oncol 28:267, 1989.

Al-Sarraf M, Martz K, Herskovic A, et al: Progress report of combined chemoradiotherapy versus radiotherapy alone in patients with esophageal cancer: An intergroup study [published erratum appears in J Clin Oncol 15:866, 1997]. J Clin Oncol 15:277, 1997.

Altorki NK, Skinner DB: Occult cervical nodal metastasis in esophageal cancer: Preliminary results of three-field lymphadenectomy. J Thorac Cardiovasc Surg 113:540, 1997.

Apinop C, Puttisak P, Preecha N: A prospective study of combined therapy in esophageal cancer. Hepatogastroenterology 41:391, 1994.

Arnott SJ, Duncan W, Kerr GR, et al: Low dose preoperative radiotherapy for carcinoma of the oesophagus: Results of a randomized clinical trial. Radiother Oncol 24:108, 1992.

Atabek U, Mohit TM, Rush BF, et al: Impact of esophageal screening in patients with head and neck cancer. Am Surg 56:289, 1990.

Baba M, Aikou T, Natsugoe S, et al: Quality of life following esophagectomy with three-field lymphadenectomy for carcinoma, focusing on its relationship to vocal cord palsy. Dis Esophagus 11:28, 1998.

Baba M, Aikou T, Yoshinaka H, et al: Long term results of subtotal esophagectomy with three-field lymphadenectomy for carcinoma of the thoracic esophagus. Ann Thorac Surg 219:310, 1994.

Ban S, Toyonaga A, Harada H, et al: Iodine staining for early endoscopic detection of esophageal cancer in alcoholics. Endoscopy 30:253, 1998.

Bartels H, Stein HJ, Siewert JR: Preoperative risk analysis and postoperative mortality of oesophagectomy for resectable oesophageal cancer. Br J Surg 85:840, 1998.

Beitler AL, Urschel JD: Comparison of stapled and hand-sewn esophagogastric anastomoses. Am J Surg 175:337, 1998.

Bhutani MS, Hawes RH, Hoffman BJ: A comparison of the accuracy of echo features during endoscopic ultrasound (EUS) and EUS-guided fine-needle aspiration for diagnosis of malignant lymph node invasion. Gastrointest Endosc 45:474, 1997.

Blot WJ, Devesa SS, Fraumeni JF Jr: Continuing climb in rates of esophageal adenocarcinoma: An update (Letter). JAMA 270:1320, 1993.

Blot WJ, Devesa SS, Kneller RW, et al: Rising incidence of adenocarcinoma of the esophagus and gastric cardia. JAMA 265:1287, 1991.

Bolton JS, Sardi A, Bowen JC, et al: Transhiatal and transthoracic esophagectomy: A comparative study. J Surg Oncol 51:249, 1992.

Bonavina L: Early oesophageal cancer: Results of a European multicentre survey. Br J Surg 82:98, 1995.

Bosset JF, Gignoux M, Triboulet JP, et al: Chemoradiotherapy followed by surgery compared with surgery alone in squamous-cell cancer of the esophagus. N Engl J Med 337:161, 1997.

Bown SG: Palliation of malignant dysphagia: Surgery, radiotherapy, laser, intubation alone or in combination? Gut 32:841, 1991.

Branicki FJ, Law SY, Fok M, et al: Quality of life in patients with cancer of the esophagus and gastric cardia: A case for palliative resection. Arch Surg 133:316, 1998.

Breasted JH: The Edwin Smith Surgical Papyrus. Chicago, University of Chicago Press, 1930, p 312.

Brewer LA: History of surgery of the esophagus. Am J Surg 139:730, 1980.

Bumm R: Staging and risk-analysis in esophageal carcinoma. Dis Esophagus 9:20, 1996.

Bumm R, Wong J: Extent of lymphadenectomy in esophagectomy for squamous cell esophageal carcinoma: How much is necessary? Dis Esophagus 7:151, 1994.

Bumm R, Holscher AH, Feussner H, et al: Endodissection of the thoracic esophagus: Technique and clinical results in transhiatal esophagectomy. Ann Surg 218:97, 1993.

Carter R, Smith JS, Anderson JR: Laser recanalization versus endoscopic intubation in the palliation of malignant dysphagia: A randomized prospective study. Br J Surg 79:1167, 1992.

Catalano MF, Sivak MV Jr, Rice T, et al: Endosonographic features predictive of lymph node metastasis. Gastrointest Endosc 40:442, 1994.

Chakkaphak S, Krishnasamy S, Walker SJ, et al: Treatment of carcinoma of the proximal esophagus. Surg Gynecol Obstet 168:307, 1989.

Chandawarkar RY, Kakegawa T, Fujita H, et al: Endosonography for preoperative staging of specific nodal groups associated with esophageal cancer. World J Surg 20:700, 1996.

Chang F, Syrjanen S, Wang L, et al: Infectious agents in the etiology of esophageal cancer. Gastroenterology 103:1336, 1992.

Cheng KK, Day NE, Duffy SW, et al: Pickled vegetables in the aetiology of oesophageal cancer in Hong Kong Chinese. Lancet 339:1314, 1992.

Cheng KK, Duffy SW, Day NE, et al: Oesophageal cancer in never-smokers and never-drinkers. Int J Cancer 60:820, 1995.

Cheung HC, Siu KF, Wong J: A comparison of flexible and rigid endoscopy in evaluating esophageal cancer patients for surgery. World J Surg 12:117, 1988.

Chu KM, Law SY, Fok M, et al: A prospective randomized comparison of transhiatal and transthoracic resection for lower-third esophageal carcinoma. Am J Surg 174:320, 1997.

Csikos M, Horvath O, Petri A, et al: Late malignant transformation of chronic corrosive oesophageal strictures. Langenbecks Arch Chir 365:231, 1985.

DeMeester TR, Johansson KE, Franze I, et al: Indications, surgical technique, and long-term functional results of colon interposition or bypass. Ann Surg 208:460, 1988a.

DeMeester TR, Zaninotto G, Johansson KE: Selective therapeutic approach to cancer of the lower esophagus and cardia. J Thorac Cardiovasc Surg 95:42, 1988b.

DePaula AL, Hashiba K, Ferreira EA, et al: Laparoscopic transhiatal esophagectomy with esophagogastroplasty. Surg Laparosc Endosc 5:1, 1995.

Devesa SS, Blot WJ, Fraumeni JF Jr: Changing patterns in the incidence of esophageal and gastric carcinoma in the United States. Cancer 83:2049, 1998.

Dittler HJ, Pesarini AC, Siewert JR: Endoscopic classification of esophageal cancer: Correlation with the T stage. Gastrointest Endosc 38:662, 1992.

Earlam R: An MRC prospective randomised trial of radiotherapy versus surgery for operable squamous cell carcinoma of the oesophagus. Ann R Coll Surg Engl 73:8, 1991.

Earlam R, Cunha-Melo JR: Oesophageal squamous cell carcinoma: I. A critical review of surgery. Br J Surg 67:381, 1980a.

Earlam R, Cunha-Melo JR: Oesophageal squamous cell carcinoma: II. A critical review of radiotherapy. Br J Surg 67:457, 1980b.

Ellis FH Jr, Gibb SP, Watkins E: Esophagogastrectomy: A safe, widely applicable, and expeditious form of palliation for patients with carcinoma of the esophagus and cardia. Ann Surg 198:531, 1983.

Ellis FH Jr, Williamson WA, Heatley GJ: Cancer of the esophagus and cardia: Does age influence treatment selection and surgical outcomes? J Am Coll Surg 187:345, 1998.

Fegelman E, Law SY, Fok M, et al: Squamous cell carcinoma of the esophagus with mucin-secreting component: Mucoepidermoid carcinoma. J Thorac Cardiovasc Surg 107:62, 1994.

Ferguson MK, Martin TR, Reeder LB, et al: Determinants of pulmonary complications following esophagectomy. In Peracchia A, Rosati R, Bonavina L, et al (eds): Disease of the Esophagus. Bologna, Monduzzi Editore, 1996, pp 527–532.

Fink U, Stein HJ, Wilke H, et al: Multimodal treatment for squamous cell esophageal cancer. World J Surg 19:198, 1995.

Fok M, Cheng SW, Wong J: Pyloroplasty versus no drainage in gastric replacement of the esophagus. Am J Surg 162:447, 1991.

Fok M, Cheng SW, Wong J: Endosonography in patient selection for surgical treatment of esophageal carcinoma. World J Surg 16:1098; discussion 103, 1992.

Fok M, Law S, Stipa F, et al: A comparison of transhiatal and transthoracic resection for oesophageal carcinoma. Endoscopy 25:660, 1993a.

Fok M, Sham JS, Choy D, et al: Postoperative radiotherapy for carcinoma of the esophagus: A prospective, randomized controlled study. Surgery 113:138, 1993b.

Fujita H, Kakegawa T, Yamana H, et al: Lymph node metastasis and recurrence in patients with a carcinoma of the thoracic esophagus who underwent three-field dissection. World J Surg 18:266, 1994.

Fujita H, Kakegawa T, Yamana H, et al: Mortality and morbidity rates, postoperative course, quality of life, and prognosis after extended radical lymphadenectomy for esophageal cancer: Comparison of three-field lymphadenectomy with two-field lymphadenectomy. Ann Surg 222:654, 1995.

Fumagalli U: Resective surgery for cancer of the thoracic esophagus: Results of a Consensus Conference held at the VIth World Congress of the International Society for Diseases of the Esophagus. Dis Esophagus 9:30, 1996.

Gevers AM, Macken E, Hiele M, et al: A comparison of laser therapy, plastic stents, and expandable metal stents for palliation of malignant dysphagia in patients without a fistula. Gastrointest Endosc 48:383, 1998.

Gignoux M, Roussel A, Paillot B, et al: The value of preoperative radiotherapy in esophageal cancer: Results of a study of the E.O.R.T.C. World J Surg 11:426, 1987.

Goldminc M, Maddern G, Le Prise E, et al: Oesophagectomy by a transhiatal approach or thoracotomy: A prospective randomized trial. Br J Surg 80:367, 1993.

Hankins JR, Attar S, Coughlin TR Jr, et al: Carcinoma of the esophagus: A comparison of the results of transhiatal versus transthoracic resection. Ann Thorac Surg 47:700, 1989.

He D, Zhang DK, Lam KY, et al: Prevalence of HPV infection in esophageal squamous cell carcinoma in Chinese patients and its relationship to the *p53* gene mutation. Int J Cancer 72:959, 1997.

Hermanek P: pTNM and residual tumor classifications: Problems of assessment and prognostic significance. World J Surg 19:184, 1995.

Herskovic A, Martz K, al Sarraf M, et al: Combined chemotherapy and radiotherapy compared with radiotherapy alone in patients with cancer of the esophagus. N Engl J Med 326:1593, 1992.

Holscher AH, Dittler HJ, Siewert JR: Staging of squamous esophageal cancer: Accuracy and value. World J Surg 18:312, 1994.

Holscher AH, Siewert JR: Surgical treatment of early esophageal cancer. Dig Surg 14:70, 1997.

Hsu HK, Hsu WH, Huang MH: Prospective study of using fibrin glue to prevent leak from esophagogastric anastomosis. J Surg Assoc ROC 25:1248, 1992.

Hunerbein M, Dohmoto M, Rau B, et al: Endosonography and endosonography-guided biopsy of upper-GI-tract tumors using a curved-array echoendoscope. Surg Endosc 10:1205, 1996.

Hunerbein M, Ghadimi BM, Haensch W, et al: Transendoscopic ultrasound of esophageal and gastric cancer using miniaturized ultrasound catheter probes. Gastrointest Endosc 48:371, 1998.

Hurley JP, Keeling P: Transhiatal oesophagectomy: Its role for tumours of the middle third of the intrathoracic oesophagus. Ir Med J 83:23, 1990.

Imdahl A, Munzar T, Schulte-Monting J, et al: Perioperative risk factors in esophageal cancer: A prospective study of independent variables. Zentralbl Chir 118:190, 1993.

Isono K, Sato H, Nakayama K: Results of a nationwide study on the three fields of lymph node dissection in esophageal cancer. Oncology 48:411, 1991.

Jensen DM, Machicado G, Randall G, et al: Comparison of low-power YAG laser and BICAP tumor probe for palliation of esophageal cancer strictures. Gastroenterology 94:1263, 1988.

Katariya K, Harvey JC, Pina E, et al: Complications of transhiatal esophagectomy. J Surg Oncol 57:157, 1994.

Kato H, Tachimori Y, Mizobuchi S, et al: Cervical, mediastinal, and abdominal lymph node dissection (three-field dissection) for superficial carcinoma of the thoracic esophagus. Cancer 72:2879, 1993.

Kato H, Watanabe H, Tachmimori Y, et al: Evaluation of neck lymph node dissection for thoracic esophageal carcinoma. Ann Thorac Surg 51:931, 1991.

Kelsen DP, Ginsberg R, Pajak TF, et al: Chemotherapy followed by surgery compared with surgery alone for localized esophageal cancer. N Engl J Med 339:1979, 1998.

Kirschner MB: Ein neues Verfahren der Oesophagoplastik. Arch Klin Chir 114:606, 1920.

Kodama M, Kakegawa T: Treatment of superficial cancer of the esophagus: A summary of responses to a questionnaire on superficial cancer of the esophagus in Japan. Surgery 123:432, 1998.

Kok TC, van Lanschot JJ, Siersema PD, et al: Neoadjuvant chemotherapy compared with surgery in esophageal squamous cell cancer. Can J Gastroenterol 12:297, 1998.

Krasna MJ: Advances in staging of esophageal carcinoma. Chest 113:107S, 1998.

Krasna MJ, Reed CE, Jaklitsch MT, et al: Thoracoscopic staging of esophageal cancer: A prospective, multiinstitutional trial: Cancer and Leukemia Group B Thoracic Surgeons. Ann Thorac Surg 60:1337, 1995.

Kuwano H, Sumiyoshi K, Watanabe M, et al: Preoperative hyperthermia combined with chemotherapy and irradiation for the treatment of patients with esophageal carcinoma. Tumori 81:18, 1995.

Lam KH, Lim STK, Wong J, et al: Chylothorax following resection of the oesophagus. Br J Surg 66:105, 1979.

Lam KH, Wong J, Lim ST, et al: Intrathoracic gastric bypass for carcinoma of oesophagus found unresectable at exploration. Br J Surg 69:71, 1982.

Lam KY, Dickens P, Loke SL, et al: Squamous cell carcinoma of the oesophagus with mucin-secreting component (muco-epidermoid carcinoma and adenosquamous carcinoma): A clinicopathologic study and a review of literature. Eur J Surg Oncol 20:25, 1994.

Lam KY, He D, Ma L, et al: Presence of human papillomavirus in esophageal squamous cell carcinomas of Hong Kong Chinese and its relationship with p53 gene mutation. Hum Pathol 28:657, 1997.

Lam KY, Law S, Wong J: Malignant melanoma of the esophagus: Clinicopathologic features, p53 over-expression, steroid receptors analysis and a review of the literature. Eur J Surg Oncol 25:168, 1999.

Lam KY, Law SY, Chan KW, et al: Glomerulonephritis associated with basaloid squamous cell carcinoma of the oesophagus: A possible unusual paraneoplastic syndrome. Scand J Urol Nephrol 32:61, 1998.

Lam KY, Law SY, Chu KM, et al: Gastrointestinal autonomic nerve tumor of the esophagus: A clinicopathologic, immunohistochemical, ultrastructural study of a case and review of the literature. Cancer 78:1651, 1996a.

Lam KY, Law SY, Loke SL, et al: Double sarcomatoid carcinomas of the oesophagus. Pathol Res Pract 192:604, 1996b.

Lam KY, Ma L: Pathology of esophageal cancers: Local experience and current insights. Chin Med J Engl 110:459, 1997.

Lam KY, Ma LT, Wong J: Measurement of extent of spread of oesophageal squamous carcinoma by serial sectioning. J Clin Pathol 49:124, 1996c.

Lanfermann H, Krestin GP, Muller JM, et al: [The value of computed tomography for the staging of esophageal carcinoma]. Rontgenblatter 43:241, 1990.

Launois B, Delarue D, Campion JP, et al: Preoperative radiotherapy for carcinoma of the esophagus. Surg Gynecol Obstet 153:690, 1981.

Law S, Arcilla C, Chu KM, et al: The significance of histologically infiltrated resection margin after esophagectomy for esophageal cancer. Am J Surg 176:286, 1998.

Law S, Cheung MC, Fok M, et al: Pyloroplasty and pyloromyotomy in gastric replacement of the esophagus after esophagectomy: A randomized controlled trial. J Am Coll Surg 184:630, 1997a.

Law S, Fok M, Chow S, et al: Preoperative chemotherapy versus surgical therapy alone for squamous cell carcinoma of the esophagus: A prospective randomized trial. J Thorac Cardiovasc Surg 114:210, 1997b.

Law S, Fok M, Chu KM, et al: Comparison of hand-sewn and stapled esophagogastric anastomosis after esophageal resection for cancer: A prospective randomized controlled trial. Ann Surg 226:169, 1997c.

Law S, Fok M, Chu KM, et al: Thoracoscopic esophagectomy for esophageal cancer. Surgery 122:8, 1997d.

Law SY, Fok M, Cheng SW, et al: A comparison of outcome after resection for squamous cell carcinomas and adenocarcinomas of the esophagus and cardia. Surg Gynecol Obstet 175:107, 1992.

Law SY, Fok M, Lam KY, et al: Small cell carcinoma of the esophagus. Cancer 73:2894, 1994a.

Law SY, Fok M, Wong J: Risk analysis in resection of squamous cell carcinoma of the esophagus. World J Surg 18:339, 1994b.

Law SYK, Wong J: Complications: Prevention and management. In Daly JM, Hennessy TPJ, Reynolds JV (eds): Management of Upper Gastrointestinal Cancer, 1st ed. London, WB Saunders, 1999, pp 240–262.

Lehr L, Rupp N, Siewert JR: Assessment of resectability of esophageal cancer by computed tomography and magnetic resonance imaging. Surgery 103:344, 1988.

Le Prise E, Etienne PL, Meunier B, et al: A randomized study of chemotherapy, radiation therapy, and surgery versus surgery for localized squamous cell carcinoma of the esophagus. Cancer 73:1779, 1994.

LeQuesne LP, Rauger D: Pharyngolaryngectomy, with immediate pharyngogastric anastomosis. Br J Surg 53:105, 1966.

Lerut TE, de Leyn P, Coosemans W, et al: Advanced esophageal carcinoma. World J Surg 18:379, 1994.

Lewis I: The surgical treatment of carcinoma of the esophagus with special reference to a new operation for growths of the middle third. Br J Surg 34:18, 1946.

Liebermann-Meffert DMI, Meier R, Siewart JR: Vascular anatomy of the gastric tube used for esophageal reconstruction. Ann Thorac Surg 54:1110, 1992.

Lightdale CJ, Heier SK, Marcon NE, et al: Photodynamic therapy with porfimer sodium versus thermal ablation therapy with Nd:YAG laser for palliation of esophageal cancer: A multicenter randomized trial. Gastrointest Endosc 42:507, 1995.

Liu SF, Shen Q, Dawsey SM, et al: Esophageal balloon cytology and subsequent risk of esophageal and gastric-cardia cancer in a high-risk Chinese population. Int J Cancer 57:775, 1994.

Loizou LA, Rampton D, Atkinson M, et al: A prospective assessment of quality of life after endoscopic intubation and laser therapy for malignant dysphagia. Cancer 70:386, 1992.

Luketich JD, Schauer P, Landreneau R, et al: Minimally invasive surgical staging is superior to endoscopic ultrasound in detecting lymph node metastases in esophageal cancer. J Thorac Cardiovasc Surg 114:817, 1997a.

Luketich JD, Schauer PR, Meltzer CC, et al: Role of positron emission tomography in staging esophageal cancer. Ann Thorac Surg 64:765, 1997b.

Lund O, Kimose HH, Aagaard MT, et al: Risk stratification and long-term results after surgical treatment of carcinomas of the thoracic esophagus and cardia: A 25-year retrospective study. J Thorac Cardiovas Surg 99:200, 1990.

Mathisen DJ, Grillo HC, Wilkins E Jr, et al: Transthoracic esophagectomy: A safe approach to carcinoma of the esophagus. Ann Thorac Surg 45:137, 1988.

Matthews HR, Powell DJ, McConkey CC: Effect of surgical experience on the results of resection for oesophageal carcinoma. Br J Surg 73:621, 1986.

McKeown KC: Total three-stage oesophagectomy for cancer of the oesophagus. Br J Surg 63:259, 1976.

Merrigan BA, Winter DC, O'Sullivan GC: Chylothorax. Br J Surg 84:15, 1997.

Meyer V, Burtin P, Bour B, et al: Endoscopic detection of early esophageal cancer in a high-risk population: Does Lugol staining improve videoendoscopy? Gastrointest Endosc 45:480, 1997.

Moorehead RJ, Paterson I, Wong J: The split-sternum approach to carcinoma of the superior mediastinal esophagus. Dig Surg 6:114, 1989.

Moorehead RJ, Wong J: Gangrene in esophageal substitutes after resection and bypass procedures for carcinoma of the esophagus. Hepatogastroenterology 37:364, 1990.

Mori M, Adachi Y, Matsushima T, et al: Lugol staining pattern and histology of esophageal lesions. Am J Gastroenterol 88:701, 1993.

Muehrcke DD, Kaplan D, Donnelly RJ: Oesophagogastrectomy in patients over 70. Thorax 44:141, 1989.

Mukai M, Kubota S, Morita S, et al: A pilot study of combination therapy of radiation and local administration of OK-432 for esophageal cancer: Five-year survival and local control rate. Cancer 75:2276, 1995.

Muller JM, Erasmi H, Stelzner M, et al: Surgical therapy of oesophageal carcinoma. Br J Surg 77:845, 1990.

Munoz N, Crespi M, Grassi A, et al: Precursor lesions of oesophageal cancer in high-risk populations in Iran and China. Lancet 1:876, 1982.

Nabeya K, Hanaoka T, Onozawa K, et al: Early diagnosis of esophageal cancer. Hepatogastroenterology 37:368, 1990.

Nagawa H, Kobori O, Muto T: Prediction of pulmonary complications after transthoracic oesophagectomy. Can J Surg 81:860, 1994.

Nickl NJ, Bhutani MS, Catalano M, et al: Clinical implications of endoscopic ultrasound: The American Endosonography Club Study. Gastrointest Endosc 44:371, 1996.

Nishihira T, Hirayama K, Mori S: A prospective randomized trial of extended cervical and superior mediastinal lymphadenectomy for carcinoma of the thoracic esophagus. Am J Surg 175:47, 1998.

Nishimaki T, Suzuki T, Kanda T, et al: Extended radical esophagectomy for superficially invasive carcinoma of the esophagus. Surgery 125:142, 1999.

Nishimaki T, Suzuki T, Suzuki S, et al: Outcomes of extended radical esophagectomy for thoracic esophageal cancer. J Am Coll Surg 186:306, 1998.

Nishimaki T, Suzuki T, Tanaka Y, et al: Evaluating the rational extent of dissection in radical esophagectomy for invasive carcinoma of the thoracic esophagus. Surg Today 27:3, 1997.

Nishimaki T, Tanaka O, Suzuki T, et al: Tumor spread in superficial esophageal cancer: Histopathologic basis for rational surgical treatment. World J Surg 17:766, 1993.

Nygaard K, Hagen S, Hansen HS, et al: Pre-operative radiotherapy prolongs survival in operable esophageal carcinoma: A randomized, multicenter study of pre-operative radiotherapy and chemotherapy: The second Scandinavian trial in esophageal cancer. World J Surg 16:1104; discussion, 1110, 1992.

Ohsawa T: Esophageal surgery. J Jpn Surg Soc 34:1518, 1933.

Ong GB: Cancer of the oral and pharyngeal cavities. J R Coll Surg Edinb 15:250, 1970.

Ong GB: The Kirschner operation: A forgotten procedure. Br J Surg 60:221, 1973.

Ong GB, Lam KH, Lam PH, et al: Resection for carcinoma of the superior mediastinal segment of the esophagus. World J Surg 2:497, 1978.

Ong GB, Lee Y: Pharyngogastric anastomosis after oesophago-pharyngectomy for carcinoma of the hypopharynx and cervical oesophagus. Br J Surg 48:193, 1960.

Ong GB, Lam KH, Lim ST, et al: Jejunal loop bypass and fundoplication for malignant esophagobronchial fistula. Surg Gynecol Obstet 154:165, 1982.

O'Rourke IC, McNeil RJ, Walker PJ, et al: Objective evaluation of the quality of palliation in patients with oesophageal cancer comparing surgery, radiotherapy and intubation. Aust N Z J Surg 62:922, 1992.

Orringer MB: Partial median sternotomy: Anterior approach to the upper thoracic esophagus. J Thorac Cardiovasc Surg 87:124, 1984.

Orringer MB, Marshall B, Iannettoni MD: Eliminating the cervical esophagogastric anastomotic leak with a side-to-side stapled anastomosis. J Thorac Cardiovasc Surg 119:277, 2000.

Orringer MB, Marshall B, Stirling MC: Transhiatal esophagectomy for benign and malignant disease. J Thorac Cardiovasc Surg 105:265, 1993.

Orringer MB, Sloan H: Substernal bypass of the excluded thoracic esophagus for palliation of esophageal carcinoma. J Thorac Cardiovasc Surg 70:836, 1975.

Patti MG, Costantini M, Godwin DH, et al: A hospital's annual rate of esophagectomy influences the operative mortality rates. J Gastrointest Surg 2:186, 1998.

Pearson JG: The radiotherapy of carcinoma of the oesophagus and post cricoid region in South East Scotland. Clin Radiol 17:242, 1966.

Peracchia A, Rosati R, Fumagalli U, et al: Thoracoscopic esophagectomy: Are there benefits? Semin Surg Oncol 13:259, 1997.

Perniceni T, Boudet MJ, Le Guillou JL, et al: Laparoscopic gastrolysis and esogastric resection for esophageal cancer: A prospective study in 27 patients. O.E.S.O. Fifth World Polydisciplinary Congress, The Esophagogastric Junction, Paris, Abstract book: V30, 1996.

Peters JH, Kronson JW, Katz M, et al: Arterial anatomic considerations in colon interposition for esophageal replacement. Arch Surg 130:858, 1995.

Picus D, Balfe DM, Koehler RE, et al: Computed tomography in the staging of esophageal carcinoma. Radiology 146:433, 1983.

Poon RT, Law SY, Chu KM, et al: Esophagectomy for carcinoma of the esophagus in the elderly: Results of current surgical management. Ann Surg 227:357, 1998a.

Poon RT, Law SY, Chu KM, et al: Multiple primary cancers in esophageal squamous cell carcinoma: Incidence and implications. Ann Thorac Surg 65:1529, 1998b.

Reece GP, Schusterman MA, Miller MJ, et al: Morbidity and functional outcome of free jejunal transfer reconstruction for circumferential defects of the pharynx and cervical esophagus. Plast Reconstr Surg 96:1307, 1995.

Ribeiro U, Posner MC, Safatle RA, et al: Risk factors for squamous cell carcinoma of the oesophagus. Br J Surg 83:1174, 1996.

Riedel M, Hauck RW, Stein HJ, et al: Preoperative bronchoscopic assessment of airway invasion by esophageal cancer: A prospective study. Chest 113:687, 1998.

Robertson GS, Thomas M, Jamieson J, et al: Palliation of oesophageal carcinoma using the argon beam coagulator. Br J Surg 83:1769, 1996.

Roder JD, Busch R, Stein HJ, et al: Ratio of invaded to removed lymph nodes as a predictor of survival in squamous cell carcinoma of the oesophagus. Br J Surg 81:410, 1994.

Rosch T: Endosonographic staging of esophageal cancer: A review of literature results. Gastrointest Endosc Clin North Am 5:537, 1995.

Roth JA, Pass HI, Flanagan MM, et al: Randomized clinical trial of preoperative and postoperative adjuvant chemotherapy with cisplatin, vindesine, and bleomycin for carcinoma of the esophagus. J Thorac Cardiovasc Surg 96:242, 1988.

Roth MJ, Liu SF, Dawsey SM, et al: Cytologic detection of esophageal squamous cell carcinoma and precursor lesions using balloon and sponge samplers in asymptomatic adults in Linxian, China. Cancer 80:2047, 1997.

Sadanaga N, Kuwano, H, Watanabe M, et al: Laparoscopy-assisted surgery: A new technique for transhiatal esophageal dissection. Am J Surg 168:355, 1994.

Saeki H, Kawaguchi H, Kitamura K, et al: Recent advances in preoperative hyperthermochemoradiotherapy for patients with esophageal cancer. J Surg Oncol 69:224, 1998.

Sagar PM, Johnston D, McMahon MJ, et al: Significance of circumferential resection margin involvement after oesophagectomy for cancer. Br J Surg 80:1386, 1993.

Saidi RF, Marcon NE: Nonthermal ablation of malignant esophageal strictures: Photodynamic therapy, endoscopic intratumoral injections, and novel modalities. Gastrointest Endosc Clin North Am 8:465, 1998.

Saito T, Shimoda K, Kinoshita T, et al: Prediction of operative mortality based on impairment of host defense systems in patients with esophageal cancer. J Surg Oncol 52:1, 1993.

Schlag PM: Randomized trial of preoperative chemotherapy for squamous cell cancer of the esophagus: The Chirurgische Arbeitsgemeinschaft Fuer Onkologie der Deutschen Gesellschaft Fuer Chirurgie Study Group. Arch Surg 127:1446, 1992.

Schusterman MA, Shestak K, de Vries EJ, et al: Reconstruction of the cervical esophagus: Free jejunal transfer versus gastric pull-up. Plast Reconstr Surg 85:16, 1990.

Seidenberg B, Rosenak SS, Hurwitt ES, Som LM: Immediate reconstruction of the cervical esophagus by a revascularized isolated jejunal segment. Ann Surg 149:162, 1959.

Shaha AR, Hoover EL, Mitrani M, et al: Synchronicity, multicentricity, and metachronicity of head and neck cancer. Head Neck Surg 10:225, 1988.

Shahian DM, Neptune WB, Ellis FH Jr, et al: Transthoracic versus extrathoracic esophagectomy: Mortality, morbidity, and long term survival. Ann Thorac Surg 41:237, 1986.

Shen Q: Diagnostic cytology and early detection. In Huang GJ, Kai W (eds): Carcinoma of the Esophagus and Gastric Cardia. Berlin, Springer-Verlag, 1984, pp 155–190.

Shu YJ: Cytopathology of the esophagus: An overview of esophageal cytopathology in China. Acta Cytol 27:7, 1983.

Siu KF, Cheung HC, Wong J: Shrinkage of the esophagus after resection for carcinoma. Ann Surg 173, 1986.

Sugimachi K, Kitamura K, Baba K, et al: Endoscopic diagnosis of early carcinoma of the esophagus using Lugol's solution. Gastrointest Endosc 38:657, 1992.

Sutton DN, Wayman J, Griffin SM: Learning curve for oesophageal cancer surgery. Br J Surg 85:1399, 1998.

Takooda S, Nishijima W, Usui H, et al: [Reconstruction of hypopharynx and cervical esophagus using a free jejunal graft.] Nippon Jibiinkoka Gakkai Kaiho 94:41, 1991.

Tanabe G, Baba M, Kuroshima K, et al: [Clinical evaluation of the esophageal lymph flow system based on RI uptake of dissected regional lymph nodes following lymphoscintigraphy.] Nippon Geka Gakkai Zasshi 87:315, 1986.

Tanner NC: The present position of carcinoma of the esophagus. Postgrad Med J 23:109, 1947.

Téniére P, Hay J-M, Fingerhut A, et al: Postoperative radiation therapy does not increase survival after curative resection for squamous cell carcinoma of the middle and lower esophagus as shown by a multicenter controlled trial. Surg Gynecol Obstet 173:123, 1991.

Thomas CR Jr: Biology of esophageal cancer and the role of combined modality therapy. Surg Clin North Am 77:1139, 1997.

Thompson WM, Halvorsen RA, Foster WL Jr, et al: Computed tomography for staging esophageal and gastroesophageal cancer: Reevaluation. Am J Roentgenol 141:951, 1983.

Tilanus HW, Hop WC, Langenhorst BL, et al: Esophagectomy with or without thoracotomy: Is there any difference? J Thorac Cardiovasc Surg 105:898, 1993.

Tsui SL, Law S, Fok M, et al: Postoperative analgesia reduces mortality and morbidity after esophagectomy. Am J Surg 173:472, 1997.

Tuyns AJ: Oesophageal cancer in non-smoking drinkers and in non-drinking smokers. Int J Cancer 32:443, 1983.

Urba S, Orringer MB, Turrisi A, et al: A randomized trial comparing surgery (S) to preoperative concomitant chemoradiation plus surgery in patients (pts) with resectable esophageal cancer (CA): Updated analysis. Proc Annu Meet Am Soc Clin Oncol 16:A983, 1997.

Van Dam J, Rice TW, Catalano MF, et al: High-grade malignant stricture is predictive of esophageal tumor stage: Risks of endosonographic evaluation. Cancer 71:2910, 1993.

Vickers J, Alderson D: Influence of luminal obstruction on oesophageal cancer staging using endoscopic ultrasonography. Br J Surg 85:999, 1998.

Walsh TN, Noonan N, Hollywood D, et al: A comparison of multimodal therapy and surgery for esophageal adenocarcinoma. N Engl J Med 335:462, 1996.

Wang M, Gu XZ, Yin WB, et al: Randomized clinical trial on the combination of preoperative irradiation and surgery in the treatment of esophageal carcinoma: Report on 206 patients. Int J Radiat Oncol Biol Phys 16:325, 1989.

Watson A: Operable esophageal cancer: Current results from the West. World J Surg 18:361, 1994.

Wei WI, Lam LK, Yuen PW, et al: Mucosal changes of the free jejunal graft in response to radiotherapy. Am J Surg 175:44, 1998a.

Wei WI, Lam LK, Yuen PW, et al: Current status of pharyngolaryngo-esophagectomy and pharyngogastric anastomosis. Head Neck 20:240, 1998b.

Wong J: Esophageal resection for cancer: The rationale of current practice. Am J Surg 153:18, 1987.

Wong J: Surgery in esophageal cancer: How radical should it be? Dig Surg 10:164, 1993.

Wong J, Cheung HC, Lui R, et al: Esophagogastric anastomosis performed with a stapler: The occurence of leakage and stricture. Surgery 101:408, 1987.

Wong J, Lam KH, Wei WI, et al: Results of the Kirschner operation. World J Surg 5:547, 1981.

Yanai H, Yoshida T, Harada T, et al: Endoscopic ultrasonography of superficial esophageal cancers using a thin ultrasound probe system equipped with switchable radial and linear scanning modes. Gastrointest Endosc 44:578, 1996.

Yang CS: Research on esophageal cancer in China: A review. Cancer Res 40:2633, 1980.

Yokoyama A, Ohmori T, Makuuchi H, et al: Successful screening for early esophageal cancer in alcoholics using endoscopy and mucosa iodine staining. Cancer 76:928, 1995.

Zhang DW, Cheng GY, Huang GJ, et al: Operable squamous esophageal cancer: Current results from the East. World J Surg 18:347, 1994.

Zieren HU, Muller JM, Jacobi CA, et al: Adjuvant postoperative radiation therapy after curative resection of squamous cell carcinoma of the thoracic esophagus: A prospective randomized study. World J Surg 19:444, 1995.

CHAPTER **45**

Adenocarcinoma of the Esophagus and Esophagogastric Junction

Richard J. Finley

DEFINITION

The incidence of adenocarcinomas of the esophagus and esophagogastric junction has risen rapidly in the United States and Western Europe (Blot et al, 1991; Powell and McConkey, 1992). Adenocarcinomas of the tubular esophagus are well delineated. In the past, however, there was confusion about the classification and optimal management of cancers of the esophagogastric junction. At a Consensus Conference of the International Gastric Association and the International Society for Diseases of the Esophagus, adenocarcinomas of the esophagogastric junction were defined as tumors whose centers are within 5 cm proximal and distal to the anatomic cardia (Siewert and Stein, 1998).

Three distinct tumor entities within this area were identified.

- *Type I* tumors are adenocarcinomas of the distal esophagus located at least 1 cm above the esophagogastric junction and usually arising from an area of specialized intestinal metaplasia (Barrett's esophagus).
- *Type II* tumors are true carcinomas of the cardia arising from the cardiac epithelium or short segments of intestinal metaplasia at the esophagogastric junction.
- *Type III* tumors are subcardial gastric carcinomas that infiltrate the esophagogastric junction or distal esophagus or both.

The assignment of a lesion to one of these types is morphologic, based on (1) the anatomic location of the tumor center or, (2) in patients with an advanced tumor, the location of the tumor mass. Although carcinomas arising in the vicinity of the esophagogastric junction have several common features, distinct epidemiologic and morphologic characteristics are seen in all three types of tumors.

Patients with type I tumors are more likely to have a hiatus hernia and a long history of gastroesophageal reflux disease (GERD). Specialized intestinal epithelial metaplasia is found in 80% of type I, 40% of type II, and 10% of type III tumors. There is an increased prevalence of poor differentiation and nonintestinal growth pattern in subcardial gastric cancers. Lymphographic studies show that the main lymphatic pathways for cancers originating in the lower esophagus advance both cephalad into the mediastinum and caudad along the celiac axis, whereas cancers of the gastric cardia and subcardial region preferentially make their way to the celiac axis, the splenic hilum, and the periaortic lymph nodes (Aikou and Shimazu, 1989).

This chapter concentrates on the management of adenocarcinomas of the esophagus (type I esophagogastric tumors) and adenocarcinomas confined to the cardia (type II esophagogastric tumors).

HISTORICAL NOTE

Adenocarcinoma in an esophagus lined with columnar epithelium (columnar-lined esophagus) was first recognized by Ortmann (1901). Barrett (1950) published a well-researched review of the literature, asserting that the columnar-lined segment was intrathoracic stomach abnormally situated by congenital esophageal shortening and rejecting the concept of columnar metaplasia of the esophageal mucosa. He retracted this view after Allison and Johnstone (1953) carefully documented the relative positions of the true anatomic gastroesophageal junction and the squamocolumnar mucosal junction and thus confirmed the existence of columnar-lined esophagus.

Adler (1963) first suggested that patients with Barrett's esophagus were at increased risk for esophageal adenocarcinoma. Naef and colleagues (1975) stressed the importance of dysplasia in the development of 12 adenocarcinomas in 140 patients with Barrett's esophagus.

Surgical therapy for carcinomas of the esophagus and esophagogastric junction has evolved along the principles of complete resection of the tumor, the abnormal esophagus, and draining lymph nodes. Swallowing is restored by the interposition of the stomach, small bowel, or colon (Ellis et al, 1959). Tumors of the esophagogastric junction can be resected by (1) total gastrectomy with Roux-en-Y intestinal reconstruction (Akiyama et al, 1979), (2) partial esophagogastrectomy through a left thoracotomy incision of the diaphragm (Phemister, 1943), (3) left thoracoabdominal incision (Garlock, 1967), or (4) transhiatal esophagogastrectomy with gastric interposition to the neck (Orringer and Sloan, 1978).

Cancers of both the upper and middle thoracic esophagus can be resected by laparotomy and right thoracotomy with interposition of the stomach to the esophagus in the upper chest (Lewis, 1946) or laparotomy, right thoracotomy, and cervical incision with esophagogastric anastomosis in the neck (McKeown, 1972). Radical esophagogastrectomy may improve survival for patients with advanced disease (Skinner, 1983).

■ *HISTORICAL READINGS*

Adler RH: The lower esophagus lined by columnar epithelium: Its association with hiatal hernia, ulcer stricture and tumor. J Thorac Cardiovasc Surg 45:13, 1963.

Akiyama H, Miyazono H, Tsurumaru M, Hashimoto C: Thoraco-abdominal approach for carcinoma of the cardia of the stomach. Am J Surg 137:345, 1979.

Allison PR, Johnstone AS: The oesophagus lined with gastric mucous membrane. Thorax 8:87, 1953.

Barrett NR: Chronic peptic ulcer of the oesophagus and 'oesophagitis'. Br J Surg 38:175, 1950.

Ellis FH, Jackson RC, Kkrueger JT, et al: Carcinoma of the esophagus and cardia: Results of treatment, 1946 to 1956. N Engl J Med 260:351, 1959.

Garlock JH: Garlock's Surgery of the Alimentary Tract. East Norwalk, CT, Appleton & Lange, 1967, p 77.

Lewis I: The surgical treatment of carcinoma of the oesophagus with special references to a new operation for growths of the middle third. Br J Surg 34:18, 1946.

McKeown KC: Trends in oesophageal resection for carcinoma with special reference to total oesophagectomy. Ann R Coll Surg Engl 51:213, 1972.

Naef AP, Savary M, Ozzello L: Columnar-lined lower esophagus: An acquired lesion with malignant predisposition. J Thorac Cardiovasc Surg 70:826, 1975.

Orringer MB, Sloan H: Esophagectomy without thoracotomy. J Thorac Cardiovasc Surg 76:643, 1978.

Ortmann K: Klinische Beitrage zur Erkrankung des Äsophagus durch Ulcus e digestione. Munch Med Wochenschr 48:387, 1901.

Phemister DB: Transthoracic resection for cancer of the cardiac end of the stomach. Arch Surg 46:915, 1943.

Skinner DB: En bloc resection for neoplasm of the esophagus and cardia. J Thorac Cardiovasc Surg 85:58, 1983.

BASIC SCIENCE

Epidemiology and Etiology

Barrett's esophagus is an eponym for the syndrome characterized by metaplastic replacement of the usual stratified squamous epithelium of the esophagus with columnar epithelium. The diagnosis is confirmed when the squamocolumnar junction is 3 cm above the endoscopically determined gastroesophageal junction or when biopsies within 3 cm of this junction demonstrate specialized intestinal columnar epithelium. Barrett's esophagus would be of only passing interest were it not for the associated 30- to 100-fold increased risk for development of primary adenocarcinoma (Spechler and Goyal, 1986). Gauging the importance of this association requires an estimate of both the frequency of Barrett's esophagus and the risk of development of adenocarcinoma in patients with the syndrome.

The prevalence of columnar-lined esophagus in patients undergoing endoscopy for symptoms of esophageal reflux varies from 5% to 15% and increases to 44% in patients with esophageal strictures. Cameron and coworkers (1990) observed the prevalence of Barrett's esophagus at postmortem examination (376 per 100,000) to be approximately 20 times higher than that observed in clinical practice (18 per 100,000). This finding suggests that Barrett's esophagus may occur much more frequently than previously estimated. The incidence of adenocarcinoma that develops in a columnar-lined esophagus gives a more accurate picture of the actual risk. Prospective screening of patients with a columnar-lined esophagus showed rates of one case of adenocarcinoma per 52 to 150 patient-years. Excluding three studies with possibly anomalous and high cancer incidence rates, the consensus incidence is approximately one per 200 patient-years (Kim et al, 1997).

The annual age-adjusted incidence of adenocarcinoma in a columnar-lined esophagus tripled from 0.8 per 100,000 to 2.5 per 100,000 among white men between 1976 and 1996 in the United States, surpassing the incidence of squamous cell carcinoma in 1990 (Devesa et al, 1998). Rates also rose among black males but remain at much lower levels (white-to-black ratio of 3:1). To a lesser extent, there was a continuing increase in adenocarcinoma of the gastric cardia among males to 4.2 cases per 100,000 people, which nearly equaled the rates for noncardia tumors of the stomach. The upward trend for both tumors was much greater among older than younger men. The mean age at diagnosis was 58 years, with a range of 15 to 88 years. Although the incidence also rose among females, rates remained much lower than among males (male-to-female ratio 7:1). Similar increases in the incidence of adenocarcinoma of the esophagus and cardia have also been observed in Western Europe (Powell and McConkey, 1992).

The reasons for the rising incidence are unknown, and only a few moderately strong risk factors have been identified. Gastroesophageal reflux (GER) appears to play an important role in the development of adenocarcinomas of the esophagus and cardia (Lagergren et al, 1999). Among people with recurrent symptoms of gastroesophageal reflux, compared with those without such symptoms, the odds ratios for development of cancer were 7 for esophageal adenocarcinoma and 2 for adenocarcinoma of the cardia. The more frequent, the more severe, and the longer-lasting the symptoms of reflux, the greater the risk. Among people with long-standing and severe symptoms of reflux, the odds ratios were 43 for esophageal adenocarcinoma and 4 for adenocarcinoma of the cardia.

The risks of esophageal squamous cell carcinoma were not associated with reflux. There is no evidence that the incidence of gastroesophageal reflux disease, estimated to be present in 4% to 9% of adults, has increased. It is ironic that the incidence of adenocarcinoma of the esophagus has increased dramatically in the period in which highly effective therapeutic agents, such as proton pump inhibitors, have provided symptomatic relief and mucosal healing.

Case-control studies have implicated cigarette smoking in esophageal adenocarcinoma, with an odds ratio of 2.0 for smokers of more than one pack/day. Cessation of smoking did not confer a protective effect (Gammon et al, 1997). The rising incidence of esophageal adenocarcinoma, especially among white men of high socioeconomic class, runs counter to the parallel decline in smoking in this group, arguing against tobacco as a major factor.

The risk of esophageal adenocarcinoma increases significantly with obesity, with an odds ratio of 3 to 1 for the heaviest compared with the lightest quartile of body mass (Chow et al, 1998). The rising incidence of esophageal adenocarcinoma also parallels the increase in body cell mass index over a similar period. Diets high in fat and low in vitamins A, E, and C are associated with an increased risk of adenocarcinoma. Agents that relax the lower esophageal sphincter (LES), such as calcium channel blockers and bronchodilators, are not associated with an increased risk of cancer.

Pathogenesis

The lining of the fetal esophagus is ciliated columnar epithelium until about the 17th week of development. Subsequently, it is replaced by squamous epithelium, starting in the middle of the esophagus and extending in both directions to cover the entire organ by birth. Remnants of ciliated columnar epithelial may be found, most commonly in the cervical region, which is the last area to develop squamous epithelium. Occasional foci of heterotopic or ectopic gastric epithelium and superficial cardiac glands also persist in the lamina propria of the distal esophagus.

Although these areas of columnar epithelium have no histopathologic resemblance to Barrett's epithelium, they may undergo malignant degeneration. Histologically, Barrett's esophagus can be categorized into three types of columnar epithelium:

1. Junctional epithelium resembles the normal lining of the gastric cardia.
2. Epithelium of the gastric fundus type resembles that of the body and fundus of the stomach.
3. Specialized columnar epithelium, the most common type, resembles intestinal epithelium and is most likely to undergo malignant degeneration.

Another important aspect of histology is dysplasia. Current thinking, as summarized by Kim and colleagues (1997), is that adenocarcinoma results from a progression of dysplastic changes from low-grade to high-grade dysplasia to in situ and, finally, to invasive adenocarcinoma.

The pathophysiology of Barrett's esophagus has not been fully elucidated. Barrett (1950) initially considered the lesion to be congenital, but the frequent association of Barrett's esophagus with gastroesophageal reflux and its usual occurrence in patients in the middle and older age groups support an acquired origin. A study of pediatric patients by Dahms and Rothstein (1984) indicated that Barrett's esophagus in children, as in adults, is usually due to gastroesophageal reflux.

Dent and coworkers (1991) summarized the role of gastroesophageal reflux with particular emphasis on two factors: (1) the intense exposure of the esophagus to gastric contents and (2) the unusually aggressive nature of this reflux material. Compared with other patients with reflux esophagitis, patients with Barrett's esophagus have a significantly longer duration of esophageal exposure to gastric contents. This exposure appears to be related to incompetence of the LES and poor clearance of the refluxed material by the esophagus. In addition, refluxed materials are particularly damaging because of their high acid content and the presence of increased amounts of duodenal contents, such as bile acids (Marshall et al, 1997).

Barrett's esophagus is an excellent model for the progression of a premalignant lesion to frank neoplasia. Dysplasia is currently the only risk factor identified for the development of adenocarcinoma in patients with columnar-lined esophagus. The presence of low-grade dysplasia may be helpful in identifying patients who progress to high-grade dysplasia and adenocarcinoma. Dent and coauthors (1991) reviewed 50 patients with high-grade dysplasia who were monitored with regular endoscopy for up to 5 years; adenocarcinoma developed in 32%. In five patients observed by Hameeteman and associates (1989), carcinoma developed 1 to 10 years after the initial diagnosis of dysplasia. In all cases, high-grade dysplasia or adenocarcinoma originated in specialized columnar-lined esophagus resembling intestinal epithelium.

In addition to dysplasia, the length of the columnar-lined esophagus, the severity of peptic esophagitis, and genetic factors have been implicated in the development of adenocarcinoma in the columnar-lined esophagus. Robertson and colleagues (1988) suggested that the incidence of adenocarcinoma is greater when the length of columnar-lined esophagus exceeds 8 cm. Weston and coworkers (1997) showed that the prevalence of dysplasia in short-segment (<3 cm) Barrett's esophagus was 8% versus 24% in long-segment Barrett's esophagus. Neither high-grade dysplasia nor cancer developed in short-segment Barrett's esophagus. There is insufficient evidence to suggest that persistent peptic esophagitis has any independent effect on risk of adenocarcinoma.

Cancer develops in Barrett's esophagus through the stepwise accumulation of genetic events that lead to progressive loss of growth regulation. Reid (1991) observed that adenocarcinoma developed in 70% of patients with deoxyribonucleic acid (DNA) aneuploidy and high-grade dysplasia, whereas none of the 49 patients without aneuploidy had tumors. Familial aggregation of GERD has been documented in patients with Barrett's esophagus and esophageal adenocarcinoma (Romero and Cameron, 1997). The high prevalence of 17p allelic deletions in esophageal adenocarcinoma suggests that inactivation of the *p53* tumor suppressor gene may be an early event in the neoplastic transformation of the metaplasia (Blount et al, 1991; Casson et al, 1991). Inactivation of *p53* leads to loss of cell cycle arrest and apoptosis. The autocrine growth factors epidermal growth factor receptor (EGF-R) and transforming growth factor type 2 (TGF-2) increase in concentration from the gastric fundus type of mucosa to junctional type to specialized intestinal type and finally to adenocarcinoma, suggesting an increased autocrine growth loop in adenocarcinoma of the esophagus (Jankowski et al, 1992).

Gastroesophageal reflux of acid and bile has been linked to the development of dysplasia and adenocarcinoma. Intestinal metaplasia developed in animals subjected to acid and pancreatic juice reflux (Miwa et al, 1994). Intermittent acidification rather than steady-state acidification appeared to cause proliferation of columnar cells (Fitzgerald, 1998).

Pathology

Adenocarcinoma of the esophagus may arise in ectopic islands of columnar-lined epithelium, in subepithelial gastric glands, or in an acquired columnar-lined epithelium. Adenocarcinoma of the esophagus is thought to progress through the stages of metaplasia, low-grade dysplasia, high-grade dysplasia, carcinoma in situ, and finally invasive carcinoma. Carcinoma of the esophagogastric junction probably goes through a similar progression, although it is not as clearly defined.

Patients with early-stage cancers, in which tumors are confined to the epithelium and lamina mucosa, have a low incidence of lymph node metastasis and a much better prognosis than patients with more advanced tumors that invade the rich lymphatic pathways of the submucosa and beyond. In 350 cases in which resection was performed, Ruol and coworkers (1997) observed that the prevalence of early adenocarcinoma was 4% for cardia and 27% for Barrett's esophagus. Among early cancers, 16% were mucosal and 54% submucosal tumors. Approximately 30% of the latter had metastases. Overall, the survival rate was 100% in the absence of lymph node metastases and 43% in the presence of node metastases.

Despite the increase in surveillance for Barrett's esophagus, the adenocarcinoma most commonly encountered in most centers is an advanced cancer in which tumor has already extended to the muscularis propria and the adventitia and, not uncommonly, has infiltrated the adjacent organs and metastasized to regional lymph nodes. Approximately 20% of the patients have nonresectable tumors because of distant metastases or their medical condition at the time of diagnosis. Of 122 patients undergoing primary resection for adenocarcinoma of the cardia, 74% had lymph node metastases (Graham et al, 1998). Those patients with no evidence of lymph involvement had a 5-year survival rate of 45%, and those with malignant nodes had a 5-year survival of 9%. Tumor stage was classified as T1 in 2%, T2 in 31%, T3 in 61%, and T4 in 6%. Advanced tumor stage was also found to be associated with decreased survival. Histologic differentiation was classified as poorly differentiated in 46%, moderately differentiated in 38%, and well differentiated in 16%. Aneuploid DNA was found in 78% of the resected specimens and was associated with decreased survival.

In 165 patients who underwent esophagogastrectomy for adenocarcinoma of the esophagus (Hölscher et al, 1995), the T stage classification was T1 in 23%, T2 in 26%, T3 in 35%, and T4 in 15%. Lymph node metastases were not detected in mucosal cancers (T1A) but were observed in 18% of submucosal cancers (T1B), 77% of T2, 83% of T3, and 96% of T4. The 5-year survival rate for patients with less than 30% invaded nodes was 45% compared with 0% for more than 30% invaded nodes. Patients with no lymph node metastases had a 5-year survival rate of 63%. Patients with lymph node metastases had a 5-year survival rate of 27%. In all studies, lymph node metastasis appeared to be the most significant prognostic indicator for survival.

DIAGNOSIS

Symptoms

The spectrum of symptoms varies according to the extent of disease (Table 45–1). Symptom severity or duration does not necessarily correlate with tumor stage, operability, or resectability. Most patients with early-stage cancer are asymptomatic, and the diagnosis is usually established by screening for a columnar-lined esophagus or by endoscopy for symptoms of GERD.

TABLE 45–1 ■ **Symptoms Experienced by 290 Patients with Adenocarcinoma of the Esophagus or Cardia on Presentation**

	% of Patients	
Symptom	*Esophagus* (*n* = 110)	*Cardia* (*n* = 180)
Dysphagia	84	93
Weight loss	62	66
Heartburn	39	24
Regurgitation	23	20
Odynophagia	14	14
Chest pain	17	9
Hoarseness	7	3
Cough	4	2
Bone pain	4	3
Melena	4	3
Hematemesis	2	2

The symptoms experienced by 110 patients with esophageal adenocarcinoma and 180 patients with adenocarcinoma of the cardia seen in our center are outlined in Table 45–1. Dysphagia and weight loss are the most common symptoms. Dysphagia is less common in patients with esophageal adenocarcinoma because of the increased number of early-stage cancers picked up by screening for columnar-lined esophagus. Dysphagia for solids may not be apparent until two thirds of the esophageal lumen has been obliterated. Therefore, by the time of diagnosis many patients have advanced-stage disease. In our series of 290 patients, 9% presented with symptoms of distant metastatic disease, 7% were found to have had asymptomatic distant metastatic disease on preoperative investigations, and 4% were found to have nonresectable cancer at the time of surgery. Symptoms that suggest local invasion of the cancer into vital structures include (1) back pain, secondary to celiac lymph node involvement or malignant invasion of the spine; (2) shortness of breath, secondary to pleural effusions or tracheoesophageal fistula; and (3) hoarseness caused by recurrent laryngeal nerve involvement.

Physical examination may reveal evidence of unilateral neurologic abnormalities suggesting brain metastasis, bone pain or tenderness suggesting bone metastasis, or hepatomegaly suggestive of liver metastasis. Cervical lymphadenopathy was found in 2% of our patients. Tracheal esophageal fistula is an uncommon complication of adenocarcinoma of the esophagus.

Investigation

After a thorough history and physical examination, the physician carries out investigations to determine the diagnosis and resectability of the tumor. The diagnosis is usually confirmed by a contrast barium swallow and flexible esophagogastroscopy. The barium findings may be normal in patients with early carcinomas but usually show mucosal irregularities or constrictions that must be distinguished from benign peptic strictures or achalasia. Tortuosity, angulation, axis deviation from the midline, and a fistula to the tracheobronchial tree are signs of an advanced tumor that has traversed the esophageal wall and involved the neighboring organs. A barium swallow also shows the extent of tumor infiltration of the stomach as well as tumor level and length.

Fiberoptic esophagogastroscopy allows the identification of a columnar-lined esophagus and histologic confirmation of the cancer by biopsy or brush cytology. Biopsy specimens may be examined histologically for cell type and differentiation and by flow cytometric DNA analysis for aneuploidy. For patients with nodularity and ulceration of the columnar-lined esophagus, biopsy specimens should be obtained with large forceps. Patients with a columnar-lined segment should undergo biopsies of each quadrant at 2-cm intervals for metaplasia and 1-cm intervals for high-grade dysplasia. Identification of abnormal areas or early carcinoma in situ may be facilitated by the use of vital staining with Lugol's iodine or by autofluorescence. The length and circumference of the tumor should be recorded. Gastric involvement can be documented by retroflexion of the flexible scope in the stomach.

When the diagnosis of cancer has been established, patients with symptoms suggestive of distant metastatic disease should undergo a computed tomographic (CT) scan of the chest and upper abdomen as well as a bone scan. Ultrasonography of the liver may show small metastases not seen on a CT scan. Chest radiography may show a hilar mass, tracheal compression or deviation, aspiration pneumonia, or pulmonary metastasis.

Therapeutic strategies for adenocarcinoma of the esophagus and esophagogastric junction depend on the tumor stage at diagnosis. CT scans are accurate in detecting extraesophageal tumor spread and metastasis, but a comparison of CT and surgical staging of the primary tumor has established that the accuracy of CT scans is poor, with sensitivity ranging from 0 to 67% and specificity from 71% to 100%. Preoperative underestimation of the stages of tumor growth in almost 40% of patients has been noted (Lanferman et al, 1990). Accuracy decreases for cancers around the esophagogastric junction compared with cancers of the esophagus. In our center, sensitivity and specificity have been improved by placing the patient in the prone position during CT scans, allowing the esophagogastric junction tumors to fall away from the aorta and celiac axis.

Experience with magnetic resonance imaging (MRI) shows limitations similar to those with CT, especially with respect to the low detection rate of cancer in the mediastinal lymph nodes. The questionable value of CT scans and MRI as staging modalities has led to the search for other methods that may increase the accuracy of preoperative assessment of the esophageal cancer. Endoscopic ultrasonography is more accurate than CT in staging intrathoracic esophageal tumors, provided that the ultrasound probe can be passed through the tumor. Endoscopic ultrasonography allows direct visualization of the five discrete layers of the esophageal wall, and paraesophageal lymph nodes are identified by their size, shape, margin, internal echoes, and structures. Nodes that exceed 10 mm in diameter have a high incidence of tumor involvement.

Compared with surgical staging, endoscopic ultrasonography determines T stages accurately in more than 80% of cases and lymph node metastasis in more than 70% of cases. Inability to pass the endoscopic ultrasound probe occurred in fewer than 20% of the cases, which usually involve at least T3 or T4 disease. CT scanning is superior to endoscopic ultrasonography in advanced-stage disease (Krasna, 1999).

When compared with surgical staging, positron emission tomography (PET) (69% sensitivity, 93% specificity, 84% accuracy) was more accurate than CT scanning (46% sensitivity, 73% specificity, and 63% accuracy) in detecting distant metastasis (Luketich et al, 1999). Preoperative thoracoscopy and laparoscopy in conjunction with endoscopic ultrasonography and CT scanning of the chest and abdomen are emerging as safe, effective, and accurate methods for staging carcinoma of the esophagus and esophagogastric junction (Krasna, 1999).

Flexible bronchoscopy is performed to assess involvement of the tracheobronchial tree in adenocarcinoma of the esophagus above the inferior pulmonary view. Signs of involvement include a widened carina, external compression, tumor infiltration, and fistulization.

Differential Diagnosis

Blot and colleagues (1991) observed that 80% of adenocarcinomas associated with Barrett's esophagus arose in the distal esophagus. Thus, such adenocarcinomas must be distinguished from benign ulcers of the esophagus as well as from all histologic types of carcinomas involving the distal esophagus and proximal stomach. Benign esophageal ulcers must be observed closely with multiple esophageal biopsies and cytologic brushings. If the carcinoma is definitely within the esophagus, Barrett's carcinoma must be differentiated from other esophageal carcinomas.

A well-differentiated squamous cell carcinoma with keratin formation and intercellular bridges is easy to distinguish from a well-differentiated adenocarcinoma. Distinguishing a poorly differentiated squamous cell carcinoma growing in cords and nests or solid sheets from a poorly differentiated Barrett's adenocarcinoma is much more difficult. In these cases, the presence of carcinoma in situ in the squamous or columnar surface component may identify the epithelium of origin. Use of special stains and electron microscopy may be necessary to identify distinguishing features of the tumor. Endocrine carcinoma arising from the esophagus usually resembles oat cell or small cell undifferentiated carcinoma of the lung but may at times contain cell clusters similar to those in adenocarcinoma. Diagnosis of this unusual tumor depends on the demonstration of typical endocrine-type secretory granules by special stains. Rarely, an adenocarcinoma appears to arise intramurally with no detectable surface component; these tumors probably originate from esophageal submucosal glands or ducts.

The major diagnostic problem, however, arises in distinguishing adenocarcinomas associated with Barrett's esophagus from usual adenocarcinomas of the cardia. Adenocarcinoma located in the tubular esophagus and in the presence of the columnar-lined esophagus is classified as *Barrett's adenocarcinoma*. Carcinomas of the cardia are usually associated with in situ adenocarcinoma or dysplasia in the surrounding mucosa of the cardia.

NATURAL HISTORY

Robertson and coworkers (1988) observed the progression of columnar-lined esophagus during relatively ineffective medical therapy. In a follow-up of 1 to 5 years, 11 of 56 patients showed a 2- to 6-cm extension of their columnar lining. Conversely, 45 patients in this study experienced no detectable progression.

Hameeteman and colleagues (1989) noted that it took 1 to 8 years for low-grade dysplasia to develop from metaplasia but only 1 to 2 years for severe dysplasia to develop in five patients with Barrett's esophagus who had carcinoma. Furthermore, in three patients with established microscopic carcinoma but with very high surgical risk, no evidence of invasive tumor was found in follow-up periods of 12, 45, and 54 months.

Although rates of early carcinoma appear to have been increasing because of the availability of screening, early adenocarcinoma still represents fewer than 20% of diagnosed Barrett's carcinomas. Most patients present with tumors with locoregional spread and no previous history of a columnar-lined esophagus.

MANAGEMENT

Overview

Initial management of adenocarcinoma of the esophagus and esophagogastric junction is directed toward determining the resectability of the tumor and operability of the patient. Because the median survival of these patients is 9 months, investigation and treatment should be as timely and effective as possible. Patients with distant metastatic disease should receive palliative treatment for their symptoms. If the patient suffers from dysphagia, the esophageal lumen may be re-established by esophageal dilatation, laser fulguration, brachytherapy and/or external beam radiotherapy, chemoradiotherapy, or intubation, preferably with an expansile stent. In rare circumstances, patients with a tracheoesophageal fistula may benefit from an esophageal bypass or covered esophageal or tracheal stent. Improving the quality of life is paramount for these patients.

Locally invasive tumors may be resectable after preoperative radiotherapy or chemotherapy. Failure to reduce the stage of the tumor with preoperative therapy may result in esophageal bypass or stenting in order to relieve symptoms. During therapy, adequate nutrition is maintained by oral liquid supplementation, nasogastric feedings, percutaneous endoscopic gastrostomy feeding, jejunostomy feeding, or parenteral nutrition in rare circumstances. Placing a percutaneous endoscopic gastrostomy in the lesser curve of the stomach allows the use of a gastric tube with a greater curve for esophageal replacement at a later date.

It may not be possible to operate if severe dysfunction of the cardiovascular, respiratory, cerebrovascular, or hepatorenal system is present. Patients with severe cardiopulmonary dysfunction appear to tolerate a transhiatal esophagectomy better than a transthoracic esophagectomy.

The primary objectives of therapy are to relieve dysphagia and, if possible, to cure the patient. In our series of 290 patients, 16% had tumors considered to be nonresectable because of distant metastatic disease. At the time of operation, 4% had tumors found to be nonresectable because of undiagnosed liver metastasis or direct invasion of the tumor into vital structures. The median survival of these patients was less than 6 months. If the tumor appears to be resectable and the patient can tolerate the operation, surgical therapy is directed toward complete resection of the cancer, the draining lymph nodes, and the diseased esophagus and restoration of swallowing with either a gastric interposition, a small bowel transposition, or, if necessary, a left colon interposition.

Despite the operative risks, surgery remains the primary mode of therapy for adenocarcinoma of the esophagus and the esophagogastric junction because of the poor cure rate and persistence of symptoms after therapy with other modalities. The follow-up of our surgical patients showed that 90% have been able to take solid meals and to enjoy normal living.

Barrett's Esophagus

Although no data from well-controlled studies indicate whether persistent peptic esophagitis influences the risk of adenocarcinoma, Dent and coworkers (1991) recommended that esophagitis be healed by either medical or surgical means in patients with columnar-lined esophagus. Medical therapy with a continued high level of suppression of gastric acid should be undertaken preferentially when other medical problems or advanced age makes antireflux surgery unusually hazardous. Fit young patients with uncomplicated esophagitis should undergo antireflux surgery with closure of the crura and a Nissen fundoplication, preferably with the laparoscopic approach. Patients with an esophageal stricture may require esophageal lengthening with a Collis gastroplasty at the time of the hiatus hernia repair. When severe alkaline reflux follows gastric surgery, a Roux-en-Y procedure is indicated. The presence of high-grade dysplasia or microscopic carcinoma is an absolute contraindication to antireflux surgery.

Dysplasia is the only factor that identifies patients at especially high risk for development of adenocarcinoma. When Barrett's esophagus is diagnosed initially, an energetic search for adenocarcinoma or dysplasia by means of closely spaced biopsy sampling is essential. Diligent surveillance is the only method of reducing mortality in this disease. If dysplasia is observed in biopsy specimens, the slides should be reviewed by a pathologist with expertise in the field. If the diagnosis of high-grade dysplasia or adenocarcinoma is uncertain, endoscopic examination must be repeated without delay to obtain further biopsy specimens.

For patients with no evidence of dysplasia in a columnar-lined esophagus, Dent and colleagues (1991) recommended that closely spaced biopsy sampling be undertaken at 18-month intervals. If low-grade dysplasia is reported, it may be due to the inflammatory changes of esophagitis, and the situation should be clarified by repeated biopsy after vigorous acid suppression therapy for 12 weeks. Patients found to have low-grade dysplasia are not considered to be at sufficiently high risk for adenocarcinoma to justify resectional surgery. However, closely spaced biopsies every 6 months are recommended in view of the evidence that high-grade dysplasia develops in sequence from low-grade dysplasia.

Using flow cytometric analysis of the DNA content of columnar epithelium, Reid (1991) observed that aneuploidy with or without elevated G2-tetraploid fractions are the strongest predictors of progression of low-grade dysplasia to high-grade dysplasia or cancer. In addition, he suggested that the combination of high-grade dysplasia and multiple aneuploid cell populations may identify patients at especially high risk for adenocarcinoma.

Endoscopic ultrasonography in patients with high-grade dysplasia without endoscopic evidence of carcinoma failed to define two of three intramucosal carcinomas and had a false-positive rate of 33% for predicting invasive carcinoma (Falk et al, 1994). The current generation of endoscopic ultrasound devices does not reliably differentiate malignant from benign wall thickening.

For surgically fit patients with confirmed high-grade dysplasia, resection should be the treatment of choice. At the Mayo Clinic, 19 patients with high-grade dysplasia and no preoperative evidence of invasive carcinoma underwent esophagectomy (Pera et al, 1992). Nine patients had no cancer, six patients had stage I disease, and three patients had stage II disease. The 5-year survival rate for the patients with high-grade dysplasia was 100% and for those with stage I and stage II disease was 36%.

Thirty consecutive patients with high-grade dysplasia underwent esophagectomy, with one operative death (Heitmiller et al, 1996). Invasive adenocarcinoma was found in 43% of the patients, and no cancer-related deaths occurred in the 57% of patients with no adenocarcinoma.

In our series of 21 patients undergoing esophagectomy for high-grade dysplasia, there was one postoperative death. Fourteen patients had evidence of adenocarcinoma (six with stage I, seven with stage II, and one with stage III). No patient with high-grade dysplasia alone died of cancer. The 5-year survival rate of patients with cancer was 42%.

Streitz and colleagues (1993) observed that patients who had surveillance of a columnar-lined esophagus had earlier stage disease and better survival than patients with Barrett's adenocarcinoma who did not undergo surveillance.

If a patient with high-grade dysplasia is unable to have an operation, the patient should receive ongoing antireflux therapy and have repeated biopsies every 3 months. Ablation of high-grade dysplasia and intramucosal esophageal adenocarcinoma has been reported with a neodymium:yttrium-aluminum-garnet (Nd:YAG) laser (Ertan et al, 1995) or photodynamic therapy (Overholt and Panjehpour, 1995). For these patients, the incidence of esophageal stricture after circumferential mucosal ablation is high.

Surgical Resection

The goals of operative treatment of adenocarcinomas of the esophagus and cardia are (1) to resect completely the primary tumor, the adjacent lymph nodes, and the premalignant columnar-lined esophagus and (2) to restore swallowing with gastric or intestinal interposition. Because adenocarcinoma of the esophagus tends to demonstrate both cephalad and caudal spread, total esophagectomy is usually indicated. The esophagectomy can be carried out by either a transhiatal or a transthoracic technique. Gastrointestinal continuity can be established with anastomosis high in the right chest or in the left neck.

Adenocarcinoma of the esophagogastric junction tends to infiltrate up the esophagus and down into the stomach. Resection margins of at least 5 cm on both the stomach and esophageal margins are required. This resection can be done as either a total gastrectomy, a partial esophagogastrectomy, or a transhiatal esophagogastrectomy. Anastomosis can be carried out transabdominally, in the left chest, high in the right chest, or in the left neck.

The primary therapeutic modality for adenocarcinoma of esophagus is surgery. Resection is indicated for patients with high-grade dysplasia or adenocarcinoma in the columnar-lined esophagus, provided that neither a major associated disease that imposes prohibitive operative mortality nor obvious distant metastases are present. This recommendation concurs with that of Skinner and colleagues (1985) that the entire columnar segment be resected to remove the risk of further adenocarcinomas in the residual columnar-lined esophagus.

How radical the resection should be, however, remains controversial. Skinner (1985) and DeMeester (1988) and their coworkers advocated a radical en bloc resection in patients without transmural tumor extension, lymph node involvement, or systemic metastasis. Hagen and colleagues (1993) showed that survival was significantly better for patients with early lesions after en bloc resection than for patients with transhiatal resection (75% versus 20%) and patients with advanced lesions (27% versus 9%).

Collard and associates (1997) carried out en bloc resection of the esophagus and local regional lymph nodes in 55 patients with adenocarcinoma of the esophagus. The 5-year survival rate after complete resection for invasive carcinoma was 59%. The 5-year survival rate was 73% for patients without lymph node involvement, 61% for patients with less than five lymph nodes involved, and 0% for patients with more than five nodes involved.

Lerut and associates (1994) carried out radical en bloc resection in 66 patients with Barrett's carcinoma. Pathologic staging showed the following:

- Stages 0 and I, 38%
- Stage II, 21%
- Stage III, 22%
- Stage IV, 19%

Survival of patients was as follows:

- Stage I, 100%
- Stage II, 87%
- Stage III, 22%
- Stage IV, 0%

Hölscher and coworkers (1995) performed a radical transhiatal esophagectomy in 134 patients and reported an overall 5-year survival rate of 35%. The 5-year survival for patients without postoperative residual tumor was 41% and for those without lymph node metastasis was 63%. Five-year survival for patients with less than 30% invaded nodes was 40%, compared with 0% for patients with more than 30% invaded nodes.

Finley and Inculet (1989) reported a 3% operative mortality rate and a 50% 2-year survival rate (stages I and II) for patients with adenocarcinomas of the esophagus treated with transhiatal esophagectomy. Neither Goldfaden and colleagues (1986) nor Shahian and associates (1986) found an advantage for transthoracic over transhiatal esophagectomy in the management of adenocarcinoma of the distal esophagus. Establishment of gastrointestinal continuity in the neck and that in the chest appear to involve comparable morbidity and mortality. Colon interposition is associated with more complications and perioperative deaths than gastric interposition.

Patients with adenocarcinoma of the cardia usually present with late-stage disease. At the time of surgical resection, Graham and colleagues (1998) found stage I, 14%; stage II, 23%; stage III, 52%; and stage IV, 11%. Cancers with stages T3 and T4 were observed in 67%, and lymph node metastases were present in 74%.

The advanced-stage presentation is consistent with the reports by Launois and coauthors (1993), who found lymph node metastasis in 70% and a stage of T3 or higher in 86%, and Jakl and colleagues (1995), who reported that 70% of patients had cancer of stage T3 or greater. Consequently, 5-year survival rates for the disease remain below 20% in most centers.

Radiation Therapy

In our institution, 32 patients with adenocarcinoma of the esophagus and cardia refused surgical therapy and underwent primary radiation therapy. The 5-year survival rate was 6% with a median survival of 9 months. Of the patients, 40% experienced significant dysphagia related to radiation strictures. Herskovic and colleagues (1992) showed that addition of chemotherapy to radiation therapy improved short-term survival in patients with squamous cell carcinoma. Kelsen and Ilson (1995) have shown the efficacy of primary chemotherapy, particularly *cis*-platinum–based multimodality therapy, for the treatment of esophageal cancer.

Adjuvant Chemoradiotherapy

Surgery and radiotherapy directed at local control, although important, are not sufficient. Up to 25% of patients with adenocarcinoma of the esophagus or cardia develop distant metastatic disease after radiotherapy or surgical treatment. Herskovic and colleagues (1992) have shown the efficacy of adding chemotherapy to radiation therapy in treating squamous cell cancer of the esophagus. Kelsen and Ilson (1998), however, were unable to show a significant improvement in survival with the addition of preoperative chemotherapy to esophagectomy for patients with esophageal cancer, 55% of whom had an adenocarcinoma. They reported a 24% complete response rate in 213 patients undergoing high-dose chemotherapy before esophagectomy. The 2-year survival rate of both groups was 27%, and the median survival was 16 months.

Walsh and co-workers (1996) reported results of a randomized clinical trial of preoperative chemotherapy and radiotherapy, followed by surgery compared with surgery alone for adenocarcinoma of the esophagus and cardia. Of the patients enrolled in this study, 34% had adenocarcinoma of the cardia. The Walsh trial showed a median survival of 16 months for the preoperative chemoradiotherapy and surgery group and 11 months for the group treated with surgery alone. The study was weakened by poor preoperative staging and a low 5-year survival rate for the control group.

Forastiere and associates (1993) used preoperative 5-fluorouracil, *cis*-platinum, and radiotherapy for 42 patients who underwent resection and showed a median survival of 32 months and a 5-year survival rate of 34%. Patients with complete response of the tumor had a survival of 70 months and 60% were alive at 5 years.

For the controlled trials of preoperative chemoradiotherapy with positive outcomes (Forastiere et al, 1993; Walsh et al, 1996) concurrent preoperative chemotherapy and radiation therapy were primarily used; in the negative trials, chemotherapy and radiation therapy were given sequentially. Keller and colleagues (1998) showed that increasing the dose in preoperative radiotherapy to 60 Gy did not improve survival but did not increase operative morbidity and mortality.

COMMENTS AND CONTROVERSIES

Adenocarcinoma of the esophagus and cardia remains one of the most difficult solid tumors to cure. A better understanding of the etiology and molecular biology of the disease is needed to reduce the incidence of this disease. The molecular events that occur during the progression of Barrett's esophagus from metaplasia to adenocarcinoma are being defined. The importance of stopping reflux and ablating the premalignant columnar-lined esophagus is still unknown. Biologic markers and improved staging techniques are required in order to identify patients with adenocarcinoma who would benefit from adjuvant therapies.

Using prospective randomized trials, surgeons should determine the influence of the surgical approach or the use of radical resections on the outcomes of this disease. New agents, such as matrix metalloproteinase inhibitors, are required to combat the detrimental effects of metastases and angiogenesis. Effective and safe therapies need to be developed that are not only curative but improve the quality of life of patients with adenocarcinoma of the esophagus and cardia.

R. J. F.

KEY REFERENCES

Dent J, Bremner CG, Collen MJ, et al: Barrett's esophagus. J Gastroenterol Hepatol 6:1, 1991.

This report of the Working Party on Barrett's Esophagus to the World Congress of Gastroenterology in 1990 examines controversy related to the diagnosis and pathogenesis of adenocarcinoma in the columnar-lined esophagus. The report makes recommendations on screening for cancer risk, as well as for the surgical management of adenocarcinoma, in patients with Barrett's esophagus.

Devesa SS, Blot WJ, Fraumeraf F: Changing patterns in the incidence of esophageal and gastric carcinoma in the United States. Cancer 80:249, 1998.

Data from nine areas of the United States revealed steadily rising rates of adenocarcinoma of the esophagus and gastric cardia between 1976 and 1996. In contrast, rates for squamous cell carcinoma of the esophagus were relatively stable and those for adenocarcinoma of the more distal portions of the stomach declined slightly.

Lerut T, Coosemans W, Van Raemdonck D, et al: Surgical treatment of Barrett's carcinoma: Correlations between morphologic findings and prognosis. J Thorac Cardiovasc Surg 107:1059, 1994.

The incidence, etiology, and pathogenesis of malignant degeneration in Barrett's esophagus are reviewed. Surveillance of patients with nonmalignant Barrett's esophagus permits detection of early cancers, resection of which results in excellent long-term survival. The role of surgical resection of adenocarcinoma in a columnar lined esophagus is reviewed.

REFERENCES

Adler RH: The lower esophagus lined by columnar epithelium: Its association with hiatal hernia, ulcer stricture and tumor. J Thorac Cardiovasc Surg 45:13, 1963.

Aikou T, Shimazu H: Difference in main lymphatic pathways from the lower esophagus and gastric cardia. Jpn J Surg 19:290, 1989.

Allison PR, Johnstone AS: The oesophagus lined with gastric mucous membrane. Thorax 8:87, 1953.

Barrett NR: Chronic peptic ulcer of the oesophagus and oesophagitis. Br J Surg 38:175, 1950.

Blot WJ, Devesa SS, Kneller RW, et al: Rising incidence of adenocarcinoma of the esophagus and gastric cardia. JAMA 265:1287, 1991.

Blount PL, Ramel S, Raskind WH, et al: 17p allelic deletions and p53 protein overexpression in Barrett's adenocarcinoma. Cancer Res 51:5482, 1991.

Cameron AJ, Zinmeister AR, Ballard DJ, et al: A prevalence of columnar-lined (Barrett's) esophagus: Comparison of population based clinical and autopsy findings. Gastroenterology 99:918, 1990.

Casson AG, Mukopadhyay T, Cleary KR, et al: p53 gene mutations in Barrett's epithelium and esophageal cancer. Cancer Res 51:4495, 1991.

Chow WH, Blot WJ, Vaughan TL, et al: Body mass index and risk of adenocarcinoma of the esophagus and gastric cardia. J Natl Cancer Inst 90:150, 1998.

Collard JM, Romagnoli R, Hermans BP, et al: Radical esophageal resection for adenocarcinoma arising in the Barrett's esophagus. Am J Surg 174:307, 1997.

Dahms BB, Rothstein FC: Barrett's esophagus in children: A consequence of gastroesophageal reflux. Gastroenterology 86:318, 1984.

DeMeester TR, Zaninotto G, Johnnsson K: Selective therapeutic approach to cancer of the lower esophagus and cardia. J Thorac Cardiovasc Surg 95:42, 1988.

Dent J, Bremner CG, Collen MJ, et al: Barrett's esophagus. J Gastroenterol Hepatol 6:1, 1991.

Devesa SS, Blot WJ, Fraumeraf F: Changing patterns in the incidence of esophageal and gastric carcinoma in the United States. Cancer 80:249, 1998.

Ertan A, Zimmerman M, Younes M: Esophageal adenocarcinoma associated with Barrett's esophagus: Long-term management with laser ablation. Am J Gastroenterol 90:2201, 1995.

Falk GW, Catalano MF, Sivak MV Jr, et al: Endosonography in the evaluation of patients with Barrett's esophagus and high-grade dysplasia. Gastrointest Endosc 40:207, 1994.

Finley RJ, Inculet RI: The results of esophagogastrectomy without thoracotomy for adenocarcinoma of the esophagogastric junction. Ann Surg 310:535, 1989.

Fitzgerald R: Sodium hydrogen exchange activity as a mechanism for acid induced hyperproliferation with Barrett's esophagus. Am J Physiol 275:47, 1998.

Forastiere AA, Orringer M, Perez-Tanoyo C, et al: Preoperative chemoradiation followed by transhiatal esophagectomy for carcinoma of the esophagus: Final report. J Clin Oncol 11:1118, 1993.

Gammon MD, Schoenberg JB, Ahsan H, et al: Tobacco, alcohol and socioeconomic status and adenocarcinoma of the esophagus and gastric cardia. J Natl Cancer Inst 89:1277, 1997.

Goldfaden D, Orringer MB, Appelman HD, et al: Adenocarcinoma of the distal esophagus and gastric cardia: Comparison of results of transhiatal esophagectomy and thoracoabdominal esophagogastrectomy. J Thorac Cardiovasc Surg 91:242, 1986.

Graham AJ, Finley RJ, Clifton J, et al: Surgical management of adenocarcinoma of the cardia. Am J Surg 175:481, 1998.

Hagen JA, Peters JH, DeMeester TR: Superiority of extended en bloc esophagogastrectomy for carcinoma of the lower esophagus and cardia. J Thorac Cardiovasc Surg 106:850, 1993.

Hameeteman W, Tytgat GNJ, Houthoff HJ, et al: Barrett's esophagus: Development of dysplasia and adenocarcinoma. Gastroenterology 96:1249, 1989.

Heitmiller RF, Redmond M, Hamilton SR: Barrett's esophagus with high-grade dysplasia: An indication for prophylactic esophagectomy. Ann Surg 224:66, 1996.

Herskovic A, Martz K, Al-Sarraf M, et al: Combined chemotherapy and radiotherapy compared with radiotherapy alone in patients with cancer of the esophagus. N Engl J Med 326:1593, 1992.

Hölscher AH, Bollschweiler E, Siewart RJ, et al: Prognostic factors of resected adenocarcinoma of esophagus. Surgery 118:845, 1995.

Jakl R, Miholic J, Koller R, et al: Prognostic factors in adenocarcinoma of the cardia. Am J Surg 69:316, 1995.

Jankowski J, McMenemin R, Yu C, et al: Proliferative cell nuclear antigen in oesophageal disease: Correlation with transforming growth factor expression. Gut 33:587, 1992.

Keller SM, Ryan LM, Coia LR, et al: High dose chemoradiotherapy followed by esophagectomy for adenocarcinoma of the esophagus and gastroesophageal junction: Results of a phase II study of the Eastern Cooperative Oncology Group. Cancer 83:1908, 1998.

Kelsen DP, Ginsberg R, Pajak TF, et al: Chemotherapy followed by surgery compared with surgery alone for localized esophageal cancer [see comments]. N Engl J Med 339:1979, 1998.

Kim R, Weissfeld J, Reynolds J, et al: Etiology of Barrett's metaplasia and esophageal adenocarcinoma. Cancer Epidemiol Biomarkers Prev 6:369, 1997.

Krasna MJ: Surgical staging and surgical treatment in esophageal cancer. Semin Oncol 26:9, 1999.

Lagergren, J, Bergström R, Lingren A, et al: Symptomatic gastroesophageal reflux as a risk factor for esophageal adenocarcinoma. N Engl J Med 340:825, 1999.

Lanferman H, Krestin GP, Muller JM, et al: The value of computed tomography for the staging of esophageal carcinoma. Roentgenblatter 43:241, 1990.

Launois B, Bourdonnec P, Bardaxoglou E, et al: The influence of the extent of the gastrectomy on survival in adenocarcinoma of the cardia. Dis Esoph 6:41, 1993.

Lerut T, Coosemans W, Van Raemdonck D, et al: Surgical treatment of Barrett's carcinoma: Correlations between morphologic findings and prognosis. J Thorac Cardiovasc Surg 107:1059, 1994.

Luketich JD, Friedman DM, Weigel TL, et al: Evaluation of distant metastases in esophageal cancer: 100 consecutive positron emission tomography scans. Ann Thorac Surg 68:1133, 1999.

Marshall RE, Anggiansah A, Owen WJ: Bile in the oesophagus: Clinical relevance and ambulatory detection. Br J Surg 84:21, 1997.

Miwa K, Segawa M, Takano Y, et al: Induction of the oesophageal and forestomach carcinomas in rats by reflux of duodenal contents. Br J Cancer 70:185, 1994.

Overholt BF, Panjehpour M: Photodynamic therapy in Barrett's esophagus: Reduction of specialized mucosa, ablation of dysplasia, and treatment of superficial esophageal cancer. Semin Surg Oncol 11:372, 1995.

Pera M, Trastek VF, Carpenter HA, et al: Barrett's esophagus with high-grade dysplasia: An indication for esophagectomy? Ann Thorac Surg 54:199, 1992.

Powell J, McConkey CC: The rising trend in oesophageal adenocarcinoma and gastric cardia. Eur J Cancer Prev 1:265, 1992.

Reid BJ: Barrett's esophagus and esophageal adenocarcinoma. Gastroenterol Clin North Am 20:817, 1991.

Robertson CS, Mayberry JF, Nicholson DA, et al: Value of endoscopic surveillance in the detection of neoplastic change in Barrett's esophagus. Br J Surg 75:760, 1988.

Romero Y, Cameron AJ: Familial aggregation of gastroesophageal reflux in patients with Barrett's esophagus and esophageal adenocarcinoma. Gastroenterology 113:1449, 1997.

Ruol A, Merigliano S, Baldan N, et al: Prevalence, management and outcome of early adenocarcinoma (pT1) of the esophagogastric junction: Comparison between early cancer in Barrett's esophagus (type I) and early cancer of the cardia (type II). Dis Esoph 10:190, 1997.

Shahian DM, Neptune WB, Ellis FH Jr, et al: Transthoracic versus extrathoracic esophagectomy: Mortality, morbidity and long-term survival. Ann Thorac Surg 41:237, 1986.

Siewert JR, Stein HJ: Classification of adenocarcinoma of the esophagogastric junction. Br J Surg 85:1457, 1998.

Skinner DB, Walther BC, Little AG: Surgical treatment of Barrett's esophagus. In Spechler SK, Goyal RK (eds): Barrett's Esophagus: Pathophysiology, Diagnosis and Management. New York, Elsevier, 1985, p 211.

Spechler SJ, Goyal RK: Barrett's esophagus. N Engl J Med 315:362, 1986.

Streitz JM Jr, Andrews CW Jr, Ellis FH Jr: Endoscopic surveillance of Barrett's esophagus. Does it help? J Thorac Cardiovasc Surg 105:383, 1993.

Walsh TN, Noonan N, Hollywood D, et al: Comparison of multimodal therapy and surgery for esophageal adenocarcinoma. N Engl J Med 225:462, 1996.

Weston AP, Krmpotich PT, Cherian R, et al: Prospective long-term endoscopic and histological follow-up of short segment Barrett's esophagus: Comparison with traditional long segment Barrett's esophagus. Am J Gastroenterol 92:407, 1997.

CHAPTER **46**

Management of Dysplasia and Superficial Carcinoma

Manuel Pera

Victor F. Trastek

In 1906, Tileston first reported on peptic-like ulcerations arising in the lower esophagus lined by columnar epithelium. In 1950, Norman Barrett described a condition characterized by a columnar epithelium–lined tube extending below the squamocolumnar junction in patients with hiatal hernia and reflux. Barrett postulated that the tube was an attenuated part of the stomach pulled up into the chest by a shortened esophagus. Subsequently, Allison and Johnstone (1953) suggested the condition described was indeed a columnar epithelium–lined lower esophagus with upper displacement of the squamocolumnar junction above the anatomic esophagogastric junction.

Soon after this description by Barrett (1950), Morson and Belcher (1952) reported an association of adenocarcinoma with columnar cell lining of the distal esophagus. They observed an adenocarcinoma arising in a segment of a "glandular mucous membrane" lining the distal esophagus with chronic inflammation and atrophic changes and containing intestinal-type epithelium with goblet cells.

At the 1962 Annual Meeting of the American Association for Thoracic Surgery, Adler (1963) first suggested that patients with *Barrett's esophagus* (BE) were at increased risk for development of esophageal adenocarcinoma. Naef and colleagues (1975) subsequently found a 10% incidence of adenocarcinoma in a series of 140 patients with BE.

Over time, a clearer picture of the developmental morphology, complications, and implications of BE has evolved. Today, Barrett's ulcer, Barrett's stricture, and Barrett's carcinoma have all been well described, and it has been suggested that the process and the associated complications should be described as *Barrett's disease.* The ability to define the carcinogenic process from squamous epithelium through columnar-lined esophagus to dysplasia and, ultimately, adenocarcinoma is of key importance in treatment of adenocarcinoma of the esophagus. Early diagnosis and intervention, either at or just before the development of dysplasia, might allow interruption of the process before it becomes invasive adenocarcinoma and eventually spreads throughout the lymph nodes and body.

BARRETT'S ESOPHAGUS

Definition

Columnar-lined esophagus, or BE, is an acquired condition in which the normal stratified squamous epithelium lining the distal esophagus is replaced to a variable extent by metaplastic columnar epithelium containing goblet cells, also known as specialized intestinal metaplasia (Weinstein and Ippoliti, 1996). This is the epithelial phenotype in which adenocarcinoma of the esophagus usually arises. Investigators recommend maintaining the distinction between endoscopically apparent long segments (>3 cm) and short segments (<3 cm) of specialized intestinal metaplasia because most of our current knowledge of the pathophysiology, incidence, prevalence, and risk of malignant transformation of BE has come from studies of patients with long-segment BE (Spechler, 1997).

Pathophysiology

BE is commonly associated with gastroesophageal reflux, as many patients with reflux have had the distal esophagus exposed to the injurious effects of secretions of acid and duodenal contents (Kauer et al, 1995). Components present in the reflux material damage the squamous epithelium, promoting a metaplastic process by changing the phenotype of the exposed squamous multipotential stem cells into a mucus-secreting phenotype (Jankowski, 1993).

Prospective endoscopic studies have shown that 10% to 13% of patients with frequent reflux symptoms have *long segments* of BE (LSBE) (Mann et al, 1989; Winters et al, 1987). In subsequent endoscopic studies, however, about 3% of patients (male and female) with reflux symptoms were found to have LSBE (Abo et al, 1995; Cameron et al, 1995; Cameron and Carpenter, 1997). The inclusion of some patients with columnar-lined epithelium but without specialized intestinal metaplasia in earlier series may explain their higher prevalence rates of LSBE because later series included only cases with specialized intestinal metaplasia. The observed prevalence of *short segments* of BE (SSBE) in this group of patients is 9% to 13% (Cameron et al, 1995; Cameron and Carpenter, 1997; Spechler et al, 1994). The overall prevalences of LSBE and SSBE in patients having endoscopy for any clinical reason are about 1% and 6%, respectively (Hirota et al, 1999).

Current data suggest that a "silent majority" of patients with BE remain unrecognized in the general population and that BE may not be diagnosed unless complications such as adenocarcinoma develop. Studies of patients with esophageal adenocarcinomas showed that fewer than 10% of them were known to have BE before seeking medical attention because of symptoms of esophageal cancer (Bytzer et al, 1999; Menke-Pluymers et al, 1992). The major clinical significance of BE is that it is a premalignant condition; patients with BE are at increased risk for development of an esophageal adenocarcinoma through a multistep sequence of events that leads to dysplasia and, finally, to adenocarcinoma.

Assessment of the presence and degree of dysplasia in esophageal biopsy specimens after endoscopic surveillance is the present method of choice in assessing the risk for development of invasive cancer in patients with BE. This chapter reviews current aspects of the diagnosis, natural history, and management of dysplasia in patients with BE.

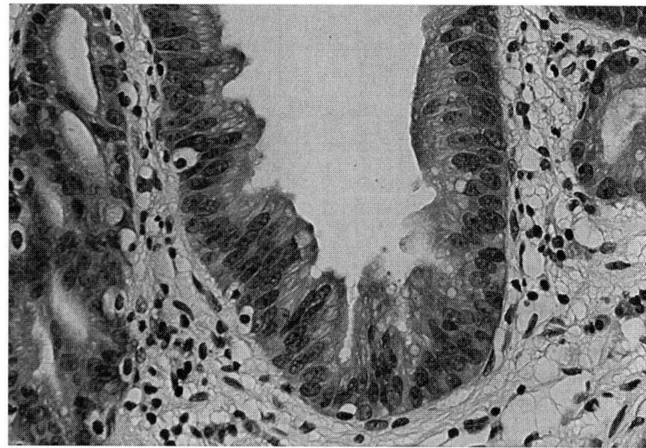

FIGURE 46–1 ■ Microscopic view of Barrett's epithelium with low-grade dysplasia. (Courtesy of Dr. H. A. Carpenter.)

DYSPLASIA IN BARRETT'S ESOPHAGUS

Definition

Histologically, *dysplasia* is defined as an unequivocal neoplastic change in the epithelium characterized by architectural and cytologic abnormalities (Antonioli and Wang, 1997; Haggitt, 1994). Architectural criteria of dysplasia vary and include such features as glandular irregularity and budding, an exaggerated villous conformation, and a crowded or cribriform growth pattern in the specialized epithelium.

Nuclear dysplasia comprises a spectrum of progressive abnormalities characterized by nuclear and cytoplasmic variability in size and shape, increased density of nuclear staining (hyperchromatism), presence of large nucleoli, and increased number of mitoses, usually associated with crowding of cells, loss of nuclear polarity, cellular dedifferentiation (loss of mucin production), and stratification of nuclei within the cell cytoplasm. Epithelial abnormalities in Barrett's dysplasia form a continuous spectrum from relatively mild changes to extreme changes that pathologists must subdivide by morphologic criteria in order to classify dysplasia.

Grading of Dysplasia

Dysplasia in BE can be classified as *low grade* or *high grade* according to the same system used for dysplasia in inflammatory bowel disease (Riddell et al, 1983) (Table 46–1).

In *low-grade dysplasia*, the crypt architecture tends to be preserved; distortion, if present, is mild. Nuclear stratification is confined to the lower part of the cells without reaching the luminal surface, and goblet and columnar cell mucin production is markedly diminished. The cellular abnormalities extend to the surface of the mucosa (Fig. 46–1).

In contrast, the criteria for *high-grade dysplasia* include marked architectural changes with branching and lateral budding of crypts, a villiform configuration of the mucosal surface, or formation of intraluminal cellular bridges leading to a cribriform pattern of "back-to-back" glands (Fig. 46–2). Nuclear stratification extends through the entire thickness of the epithelium, and goblet and columnar cell mucus is usually absent.

Finally, early invasive adenocarcinoma is recognized by the presence of groups of carcinoma cells or single cells infiltrating beyond the basement membrane into the lamina propria or muscularis mucosae (Fig. 46–3).

The task of determining the existence and the degree of dysplasia is not as simple as merely applying the

TABLE 46–1 ■ **Dysplasia Grading for Barrett's Esophagus**

Negative
Indefinite
Positive
Low-grade
High-grade
Carcinoma

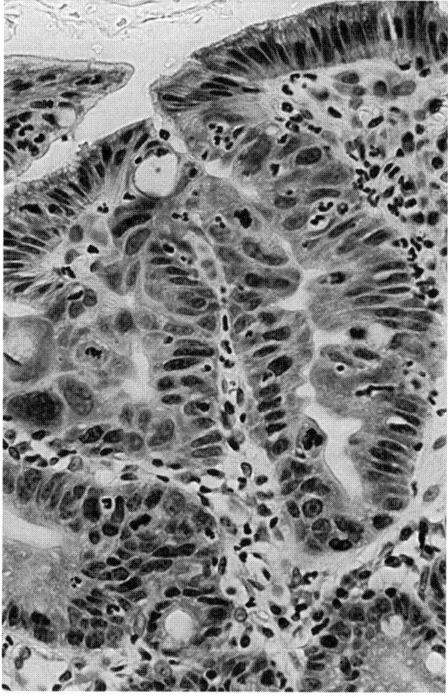

FIGURE 46–2 ■ Microscopic view of Barrett's epithelium with high-grade dysplasia. (Courtesy of Dr. H. A. Carpenter.)

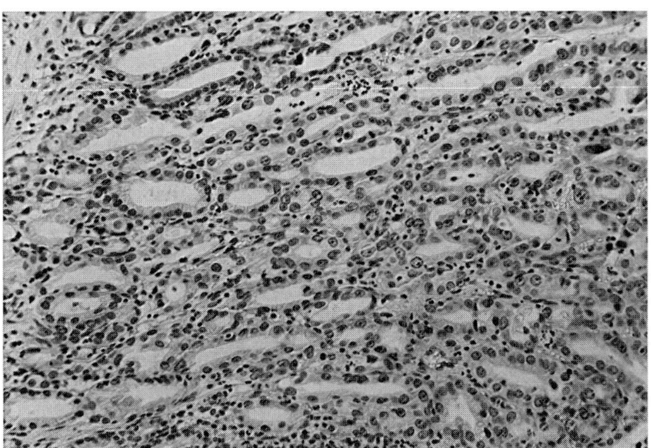

FIGURE 46-3 ■ Microscopic view of Barrett's epithelium with intramucosal carcinoma. (Courtesy of Dr. H. A. Carpenter.)

criteria mentioned earlier. In particular, differentiating reactive/regenerative epithelial changes caused by active inflammation or ulceration from mild true epithelial dysplasia is difficult. When there is doubt about the significance of epithelial abnormalities in a biopsy specimen, the diagnosis of "indefinite for dysplasia" is usually made.

Significant intraobserver and interobserver variation in the diagnosis and grading of dysplasia exists, particularly at the indefinite/low-grade interface (Antonioli and Wang, 1997; Reid et al, 1988a). For this reason, pathologists combine the indefinite and low-grade categories for practical purposes; however, there is greater interobserver and intraobserver agreement in differentiating high-grade dysplasia or intramucosal carcinoma from lesser degrees of dysplasia. The interobserver variability in grading dysplasia has led investigators to explore less subjective markers of cancer risk that might be able to supplement the current grading system, as discussed later.

Prevalence, Distribution, and Natural History of Dysplasia

For patients with no apparent tumor in BE, the prevalence of dysplasia in previous series after standard random biopsies was 5% to 10% (Spechler and Goyal, 1986). A later study prospectively examined a large cohort of patients to determine the prevalence of LSBE and SSBE in addition to dysplasia and cancer (Hirota et al, 1999). The overall dysplasia rate was 15.4% for LSBE and 8.0% for SSBE. Of the two patients with LSBE with dysplasia, one had high-grade dysplasia, confirmed histologically after esophagectomy. All four patients with SSBE and dysplasia had low-grade dysplasia. Two patients with cancer were noted in the LSBE group and one with cancer in the SSBE group.

Other authors have noted a similar prevalence of dysplasia in patients with SSBE (Sharma et al, 1997; Weston et al, 1997). The evidence suggests that patients with LSBE may have a slightly greater cancer risk (Iftikhar et al, 1992); however, patients with even very short segments are at risk and cannot be ignored (Schnell et al, 1992). The distribution of dysplasia and early adenocarcinoma in Barrett's specialized epithelium is usually patchy and irregular.

Most of this information is derived from histologic maps of esophagectomy specimens of patients who have undergone surgery for high-grade dysplasia or early invasive adenocarcinoma with no endoscopic evidence of cancer (Cameron and Carpenter, 1997; McArdle et al, 1992). Cameron and Carpenter (1997) mapped 30 esophagectomy specimens and found that the median surface area of total BE was 32 cm^2, of low-grade dyplasia 13 cm^2, of high-grade dysplasia 1.3 cm^2, and of adenocarcinoma 1.1 cm^2. The surface areas of the three smallest carcinomas were 0.02, 0.3, and 0.4 cm^2. They observed that invasive carcinoma was associated with either focal or extensive areas of high-grade dysplasia. Of interest, they also found that microscopic areas of different grades of dysplasia were commonly intermingled. All of these findings clearly explain the difficulties inherent in biopsy diagnosis of adenocarcinoma in BE with high-grade dysplasia.

Relatively little information exists regarding the temporal course of development of dysplastic lesions in patients with uncomplicated BE. During endoscopic surveillance, biopsy sampling error related to the multifocal distribution of dysplasia in BE makes the assessment of the natural history of dysplasia difficult. Despite these limitations, data from some prospective endoscopic studies provide some insights into the time course of development of dysplasia and cancer in BE.

Katz and associates (1998) assessed 97 patients with BE without any dysplasia or adenocarcinoma at baseline; by 3 years of follow-up, dysplasia (low grade or higher) had developed in approximately 8% of these patients. A significant fraction (7%) of patients with nondysplastic BE had low-grade dysplasia within the first 2 years of follow-up. In contrast, high-grade dysplasia or adenocarcinoma did not develop in patients with nondysplastic BE until more than 2 years had elapsed after the initial diagnosis. A similar pattern has been observed in other follow-up studies (Drewitz et al, 1997; Hameeteman et al, 1989; Reid et al, 1992).

Levine and colleagues (1996) examined the natural history of high-grade dysplasia in 70 patients. They found early carcinoma on prompt follow-up endoscopy within 2 months in 12 (17%) patients, and early-stage carcinoma developed in 15 of the 58 (26%) other patients during a median follow-up of 24 months. The remaining patients either continued to have high-grade dysplasia (47%) or were found to have lesser lesions on follow-up (27%).

Basic Science

Cancer develops in BE by a multistep process in which specialized columnar epithelium progresses to dysplasia and, eventually, to adenocarcinoma (Jankowski et al, 1999). Dysplastic epithelial alterations of varying degrees represent the histomorphologic features of this sequential process normally preceding the appearance of adenocarcinoma, making these dysplastic lesions the target of current surveillance strategies. An improved understanding of the molecular mechanisms directing the metaplasia-dysplasia-carcinoma sequence is essential to identify reliable biomarkers of risk of malignant transformation in BE (Souza and Meltzer, 1997). This will make it possible to develop strategies for the optimal management of patients with BE.

The progression to cancer in patients with BE is characterized by loss of cell cycle regulation, accumulation of multiple genetic abnormalities, and the appearance of aneuploid cell populations, one of which acquires the capability for invasion and becomes an early carcinoma (Neshat et al, 1994). Genetic lesions lead to hyperproliferation, genomic instability, and clonal expansion. Elevated proliferative activity characterizes the specialized intestinal metaplasia, with expansion of the normal proliferative compartment from the glands and the lower part of the crypt toward the upper part of the crypt and the surface of the epithelium.

By utilizing monoclonal antibodies against a proliferation-associated antigen (Ki-67), Hong and colleagues (1995) demonstrated a good correlation between the pattern of Ki-67 expression and the degree of dysplasia. Areas with low-grade dysplasia demonstrated a greater percentage of positive nuclei in the lower crypt zone and, in some cases, extended upward to involve both the upper crypt and the surface epithelium. The pattern of Ki-67 staining was significantly different in high-grade dysplasia, in which the percentage of positive nuclei was much higher in the upper crypt and surface epithelial zones (Table 46–2). These changes may reflect disturbance of the normal cell cycle control mechanism leading to continued deoxyribonucleic acid (DNA) synthesis and replacement of differentiated cells by immature proliferating cells near the surface of the epithelium. These cells, which have lost the ability to exit the cell cycle, may be more susceptible to genetic alterations, allowing clonal expansion of cells associated with dysplasia.

A number of molecular genetic abnormalities are involved in the pathogenesis or progression of Barrett's adenocarcinomas, including nonrandom loss of heterozygosity (LOH) involving multiple chromosome arms (4q, 5q, 9p, 13q, 17p, and 18q) (Gleeson et al, 1998). These regions of LOH include specific tumor-suppressor genes that are involved in neoplastic progression. In particular, 17p LOH and 9p21 LOH occur as early events during progression to cancer in BE and are associated with inactivation of the cell cycle–regulatory protein p53 and the cyclin-dependent kinase inhibitor CDKN2/p16. Inactivation of p53 and CDKN2/p16 occurs in premalignant diploid cells before aneuploidy and cancer during neoplastic progression in BE (Barrett et al, 1996; Blount et al, 1994) (Fig. 46–4).

Inactivation of p53 by 17p LOH and mutation is linked with the development of increased 4N (G2/tetraploid) populations that are strongly predictive of the subsequent development of aneuploidy (Galipeau et al, 1996). In a number of cases, the same p53 and CDKN2/p16 mutation has been detected both in premalignant BE and in adjacent esophageal adenocarcinoma and has been detected in both diploid and aneuploid cell populations (Barrett et al, 1996; Blount et al, 1994). These observations of shared molecular abnormalities in premalignant BE and adjacent adenocarcinoma suggest a process of clonal expansion underlying the proposed histologic pathway of tumor development.

Subsequently, p16 promoter hypermethylation was assessed as an alternative mechanism for p16 gene inactivation during neoplastic progression in BE (Klump et al, 1998). In that study, p16 promoter hypermethylation was detected in 3% (2 of 67) of the samples without dysplasia, 60% (3 of 5) of the samples with lesions indefinite for dysplasia, 55.6% (10 of 18) of the specimens with low-grade dysplasia, and 75% (3 of 4) of the specimens with high-grade dysplasia.

Loss of expression and function of the E-cadherin/catenin membrane complex can result in loss of cell adhesion and contribute to invasive or metastatic potential in carcinomas. Two studies found that abnormal expression of β-catenin, α-catenin, and E-cadherin was significantly associated with higher degrees of dysplasia in BE (Bailey et al, 1998; Washington et al, 1998). Fourteen of 16 cases of high-grade dysplasia and 7 of 7 cases of intramucosal adenocarcinoma showed abnormal expression of β-catenin, compared with 3 of 6 cases indefinite for dysplasia and 11 of 17 cases with low-grade dysplasia. These findings demonstrate that inappropriate expression of cadherins and catenins occurs early in the dysplasia-carcinoma sequence in BE, suggesting their role in the process of tumorigenesis.

Diagnostic Techniques

Normal-appearing BE may harbor focal areas of dysplasia and carcinoma. Currently, the combination of annual or biannual esophageal endoscopy and multiple biopsies is the standard method of screening patients with BE for dysplasia. However, even a careful endoscopy and biopsy protocol cannot eliminate the chance of missing a small area of dysplasia or carcinoma. Therefore, new techniques are being assessed in order to reveal and target hidden foci of dysplasia in the extensive landscape of BE.

TABLE 46–2 ■ **Correlation of Expansion of Ki-67 Proliferative Compartment with Degree of Dysplasia***

	Normal Gastric Mucosa	*Intestinal Epithelium without Dysplasia*	*Low-Grade Dysplasia*	*High-Grade Dysplasia*
Surface	0	0	7.8 ± 13	33.3 ± 15.2
Upper crypt	0	0.3	5.1 ± 10.4	25.3 ± 14.7
Lower crypt	7.9 ± 4.6	24.3 ± 12	31.3 ± 19.6	12.2 ± 6.2
Glands	12.8 ± 5.9	33.5 ± 18	40.5 ± 23.3	10.4 ± 10

*Ki-67 scores for each histologic subtype and for each tissue zone. Values are mean ± SD.
Modified with permission from Hong MK, Laskin WB, Herman BE, et al: Expansion of the Ki-67 proliferative compartment correlates with degree of dysplasia in Barrett's esophagus. Cancer 75:423, 1995.

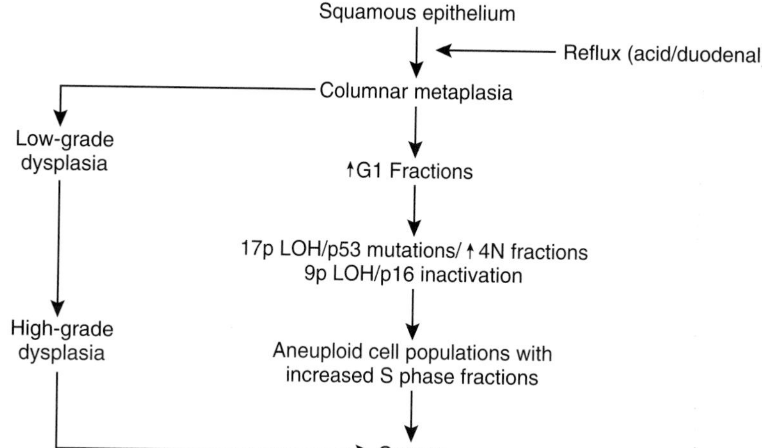

FIGURE 46–4 ■ Current hypotheses suggest that clinical progression from normal Barrett's, through dysplastic Barrett's, and finally to adenocarcinoma appears to parallel a progressive acquisition of multiple genetic abnormalities. Inactivation of tumor-suppressor genes (p53, p16) together with other genetic abnormalities might be responsible for the sequence of cell cycle abnormalities which lead to the development of cancer. (LOH, loss of heterozygosity.)

Endoscopy

Experts recommend a rigorous endoscopic surveillance program utilizing a systematic biopsy protocol characterized by four-quadrant biopsies with a large-particle (jumbo) forceps at intervals of 2 cm or less, accompanied by biopsies of any suggestive lesion, such as ulceration, erosion, plaque, nodule, or stricture in the Barrett's segment (Levine et al, 1993; Reid et al, 1988b). Prospective studies have shown a smaller risk of missing carcinoma, provided that endoscopy shows no suspicious lesion and that this systematic endoscopic protocol is applied to the entire BE.

When multiple, large biopsy specimens were taken with a large-channel endoscope, no carcinoma was missed in seven patients who underwent operations for high-grade dyplasia (Levine et al, 1993). Using the same endoscopic protocol but taking biopsy specimens with standard forceps, Cameron and Carpenter (1997) found that 2 of 19 (10.5%) patients who had undergone resection for high-grade dysplasia had very small areas of submucosal cancer in the resected esophagus. In general, the endoscopic appearance of BE, although suggestive of coexisting adenocarcinoma in cases with nodularity or ulcer, does not permit a distinction between high-grade dysplasia and early adenocarcinoma (Cameron and Carpenter, 1997).

A later study evaluated the prevalence of unsuspected carcinoma at esophagectomy in patients with BE with high-grade dysplasia after endoscopic surveillance with a large-particle (jumbo) forceps compared with standard biopsy forceps (Falk et al, 1999). No patients had endoscopic evidence of carcinoma. Standard biopsy forceps have a sample volume that ranges from 4 to 7 mm^3, whereas jumbo forceps have a sample volume that ranges from 14 to 18 mm^3. Unsuspected cancer was found in 4 of 12 (33%) patients in the jumbo biopsy group compared with 6 of 16 (38%) in the standard biopsy group. All six cancers in the standard biopsy group were intramucosal, whereas two were intramucosal and two were submucosal in the jumbo biopsy group. The authors concluded that unsuspected cancer is commonly found in patients with BE who are undergoing esophagectomy for high-grade dysplasia whether or not a rigorous jumbo biopsy protocol is used. Despite these results, and waiting for more accurate methods to target areas of dysplasia or cancer, most investigators support the use of the jumbo biopsy technique for every 2 cm of BE and the addition of brush cytology in order to reduce the chance of missing areas of dysplasia and carcinoma.

Chromoendoscopy

Vital staining, or chromoendoscopy, refers to staining of endoscopic tissue or topical application of chemical stains or pigments to alter tissue appearances and thereby improve localization, characterization, or diagnosis (Canto, 1999). In theory, vital staining should aid in diagnosis of BE and areas of high-grade dysplasia and early carcinoma and, therefore, aid in selection of patients for different surveillance and therapeutic options.

Four vital stains have been used in patients with BE: (1) Lugol's solution, (2) methylene blue, (3) toluidine blue, and (4) indigo carmine. Unlike methylene blue, Lugol's solution and toluidine blue do not improve the diagnosis of dysplasia and cancer. Methylene blue is a vital stain taken up by actively absorbing tissues, such as small intestine and colonic epithelium. Methylene blue does not stain nonabsorptive epithelium, such as squamous or gastric mucosa. Methylene blue appears to be highly accurate for selective staining of specialized columnar epithelium, which defines BE and is the histologic subtype most associated with risk of carcinoma.

Canto and associates (1996a) studied 43 patients with biopsy-proven BE and specialized columnar epithelium. These patients underwent both four-quadrant jumbo random biopsy and methylene blue–directed jumbo biopsy in a randomized order. Compared with random biopsy, methylene blue–directed biopsy led to identification of a much larger proportion of specialized intestinal metaplasia in endoscopic biopsy samples. Despite fewer biopsies per patient, methylene blue–directed biopsy led to the diagnosis of dysplasia or cancer in significantly more biopsy samples (12% versus 6%) and more patients (44% versus 28%) than random biopsy. It resulted in the diagnosis in five more patients with low-grade dysplasia, one more with high-grade dysplasia, and one more with cancer.

Subsequently, the methylene blue staining characteristics of dysplastic and malignant BE were studied prospectively in parallel in vivo and ex vivo experiments by Canto and associates (1996b). They noted that increased heterogeneity and decreased methylene blue stain intensity were significant independent predictors of high-grade dysplasia or cancer and may help direct biopsies. However, the sensitivity and specificity of vital staining are known to be significantly affected by the presence of ulcers and esophagitis. Therefore, this technique is best performed after aggressively treating esophagitis with proton pump inhibitors and noting the presence and location of erosions and ulcers (Canto, 1999).

Canto (1999) suggested a possible explanation for the differential staining of dysplastic and nondysplastic BE—the decreases in cytoplasm (increased nuclear-to-cytoplasmic ratio) and in the number of goblet cells that are characteristic of dysplastic epithelium. Future prospective studies have been proposed in order to verify the potential of methylene blue–directed biopsy in combination with magnification endoscopy to decrease the number of biopsies performed and increase the diagnostic yield of dysplasia and early adenocarcinoma (Canto, 1999).

Cytology

Cytologic studies have potential advantages over endoscopic biopsy for diagnosing BE and monitoring for dysplasia. Because foci of dysplasia may be difficult to identify endoscopically, they may be missed by the relatively limited sampling inherent in random mucosal biopsy. Theoretically, esophageal brushing samples a much greater area of the mucosal surface and may allow detection of lesions that are invisible to the endoscopist. Because dysplastic cells are generally less cohesive and tend to exfoliate from mucosal surfaces, brushing should selectively sample these dyshesive elements (Hughes and Cohen, 1998). In addition, because esophageal cytology is less expensive than biopsy, it has potential as a cost-effective alternative or adjunct to biopsy.

In an earlier study, Geisinger and associates (1992) reviewed 65 consecutive, paired esophageal brushing and biopsy specimens from 42 patients with BE. Agreement between the diagnoses on the basis of the two techniques was 72% (47 of 65). In 13 of the 18 discrepancies, the cytologic diagnosis indicated a higher level of abnormality than the concurrent biopsy diagnosis. Furthermore, 10 esophagectomy specimens were available for review; two showed high-grade dysplasia, and eight showed invasive adenocarcinoma. Preoperative cytologic specimens contained cells interpreted as adenocarcinoma in all 10, whereas endoscopic biopsy specimens were predictive of cancer in only 6 instances. A later study confirmed the excellent yield of brush cytology performed at the time of endoscopy (Falk et al, 1997). Brush cytology missed no cases of cancer or high-grade dysplasia, although it was disappointing for detecting low-grade or indefinite dysplasia.

In summary, brush cytology has the potential to be a useful technique for detecting most high-grade glandular lesions and adenocarcinomas of the esophagus. However, the detection of low-grade lesions remains extremely difficult.

Laser-Induced Fluorescence Spectroscopy

Experience with laser-induced tissue fluorescence spectroscopy, using either autofluorescence of endogenous fluorophores or exogenously induced porphyrin fluorescence after sensitization with porphyrins, has shown promising results in the detection of dysplasia and carcinoma in normal-appearing BE on the basis of its spectral pattern. Fluorescence can guide the physician during endoscopy in selecting biopsy sites in suspicious areas indicated by high fluorescence ratios. In theory, the probability of finding early malignant tumors might be higher than with the random biopsy approach.

During this procedure, optical fibers are used to excite tissue with laser light at different wavelengths. The fluorescent light emitted by the tissue can then be collected and analyzed mathematically.

Panjehpour and colleagues (1996), applying laser-induced autofluorescence to 36 patients with BE, found that 70% of patients (16 of 23) without dysplasia were correctly classified as having benign disease and all seven patients with high-grade dysplasia were correctly classified as having premalignant disease. However, all six cases of low-grade dysplasia were classified as benign.

Other investigators have encountered considerable overlap between normal mucosa, Barrett's epithelium, and all grades of dysplasia, limiting the current use of this technique (Staël von Holstein et al, 1996). In addition, this technique does not permit simultaneous optical and tissue biopsies because the optical fiber and biopsy forceps must be introduced, one after the other, into the biopsy channel of the instrument.

Aminolevulinic acid (ALA)–induced endogenous photosensitization is a novel approach to tumor detection that utilizes the heme biosynthetic pathway to produce endogenous porphyrins, particularly protoporphyrin IX (PPIX), an effective photosensitizer (Dougherty et al, 1998). Preferential accumulation of ALA-induced porphyrins in rapidly proliferating neoplastic cells provides the possibility of photodetection of the porphyrin fluorescence in tumor cells.

Messmann and colleagues (1999) performed fluorescence-guided biopsies of two patients with BE after sensitization with 20 mg/kg 5-ALA orally enabled them to detect areas of high-grade and low-grade dysplasia. The endoscope was adapted to a camera with an image-processing module that delivered real-time fluorescence pictures. The dysplastic areas containing high PPIX concentrations had a characteristic red fluorescence after illumination with blue light. These preliminary results are promising because this technique has the potential to allow more selective sampling in patients with a large surface area of BE.

Aids in the Surveillance of Dysplasia

Measurement of DNA Content of Epithelial Nuclei by Flow Cytometry

Flow cytometric analysis of DNA content in esophageal biopsies may play a role in the management of patients with BE. The presence of DNA aneuploidy and an elevated G2/tetraploid fraction of cells correlates well with the diagnosis of dysplasia and predicts which patients are at greatest risk for progressing to development of high-grade dysplasia or cancer (Reid et al, 1992). This technique may be of potential value in stratifying patients under surveillance into high-risk and low-risk groups to be observed at different intervals. For instance, patients whose results are negative for dysplasia and whose results for flow cytometry are normal appear to have little risk and can be monitored at longer intervals. Patients with aneuploidy or increased G2/tetraploidy having indefinite or low-grade dysplasia should be followed up at shorter intervals (Reid et al, 1992).

p53 Immunostaining

Overexpression of p53 has been detected in all stages of the dysplasia spectrum, from negative for dysplasia to invasive carcinoma, although it tends to be increasingly found with increasing degrees of dysplasia (Ramel et al, 1992). Although all these changes presumably play a role in the pathogenesis of dysplasia and cancers in BE, their potential as a marker in dysplasia remains uncertain (Kubba et al, 1999).

Younes and associates (1997) examined the utility of p53 immunostaining as a marker of malignant potential in 61 patients with BE. Nine of 25 patients with low-grade dysplasia had a p53-positive biopsy specimen, and 5 of these 9 patients went on to develop high-grade dysplasia. None of the 16 patients with low-grade dysplasia whose p53-negative biopsy was negative went on to have high-grade dysplasia (Fig. 46–5). This study suggests that p53 immunostaining may be a better marker of cancer risk in patients with low-grade dysplasia than the histologic diagnosis of dysplasia. Since p53 immunostaining is practical and relatively inexpensive, this study shows that tailoring of surveillance programs to cancer risk may be practical in the future.

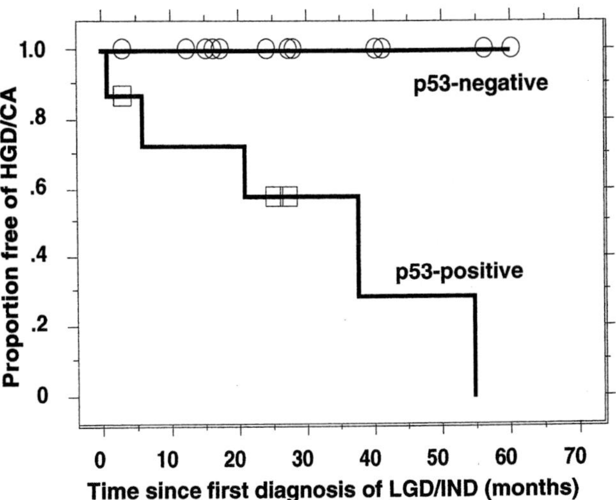

FIGURE 46–5 ■ Kaplan-Meier curves for the development of high-grade dysplasia/carcinoma (HGD/CA) in 25 patients with low-grade dysplasia/indefinite (LGD/IND) according to p53 protein accumulation. While none of the patients with LGD/IND and p53-negative biopsies progressed to development of HGD/CA, 40% of those with LGD/IND and p53-positive biopsies progressed to development of HGD/CA 24 months after first diagnosis of LGD/IND and 65% after 42 months. (From Younes M, Ertan A, Lechago LV, et al: p53 Protein accumulation is a specific marker of malignant potential in Barrett's metaplasia. Dig Dis Sci 42:697, 1997.)

MANAGEMENT OF DYSPLASIA IN BARRETT'S ESOPHAGUS

Low-Grade Dysplasia

Patients with BE and low-grade dysplasia should undergo extensive examination of Barrett's epithelium and standard four-quadrant biopsies every 2 cm through the length of Barrett's segment. In patients not receiving medical treatment, there is potential for confusion between inflammatory reactive changes and true low-grade dysplasia, and surveillance biopsies should be repeated after approximately 8 to 12 weeks of intensive acid suppression therapy with proton pump inhibitors.

Immunohistochemical analysis of p53 expression and the Ki-67 staining pattern in biopsies can be a valuable tool for discriminating between various grades of dysplasia in cases in which the diagnosis is difficult (Gimenez et al, 1998; Hong et al, 1995; Polkowski et al, 1998). Subsequently, one possible management scheme would be to perform further surveillance endoscopies with multiple biopsies at 6 and 12 months after the first diagnosis of low-grade dysplasia and then yearly (Sampliner, 1998).

For young patients with a long history of severe gastroesophageal reflux disease (GERD), antireflux surgery should be indicated. This is the subgroup of patients who are at high risk for esophageal adenocarcinoma (Lagergren et al, 1999). An additional argument favoring early antireflux surgery is that patients with BE generally need high doses of proton-pump inhibitor to suppress acid reflux completely, and even with this intensive antisecretory therapy, the esophagus may be exposed to acid during some part of the nocturnal period (Anderson et al, 1998). The existence of GERD during this period of acid breakthrough may be especially injurious because of delayed clearance at night.

Although there is no clear evidence that either acid suppression therapy or antireflux surgery prevents malignant transformation in BE, studies have suggested the role of an effective antireflux operation in protecting against neoplastic transformation of BE (Katz et al, 1998; Ortiz et al, 1996). Patients who are unfit for surgery should receive intensive medical therapy. If low-grade dysplasia regresses, surveillance can then be performed on a 1- to 2-year basis. This time interval seems reasonable on the basis of data showing that high-grade dysplasia or adenocarcinoma did not develop in patients with nondysplastic BE until more than 2 years had elapsed after the first diagnosis of BE (Katz et al, 1998). Patients with persistent low-grade dysplasia after an effective antireflux procedure or medical treatment might be considered in the future for some kind of endoscopic ablative therapy (Fig. 46–6).

High-Grade Dysplasia

The optimal management of patients with high-grade dysplasia but no evidence of invasive adenocarcinoma on

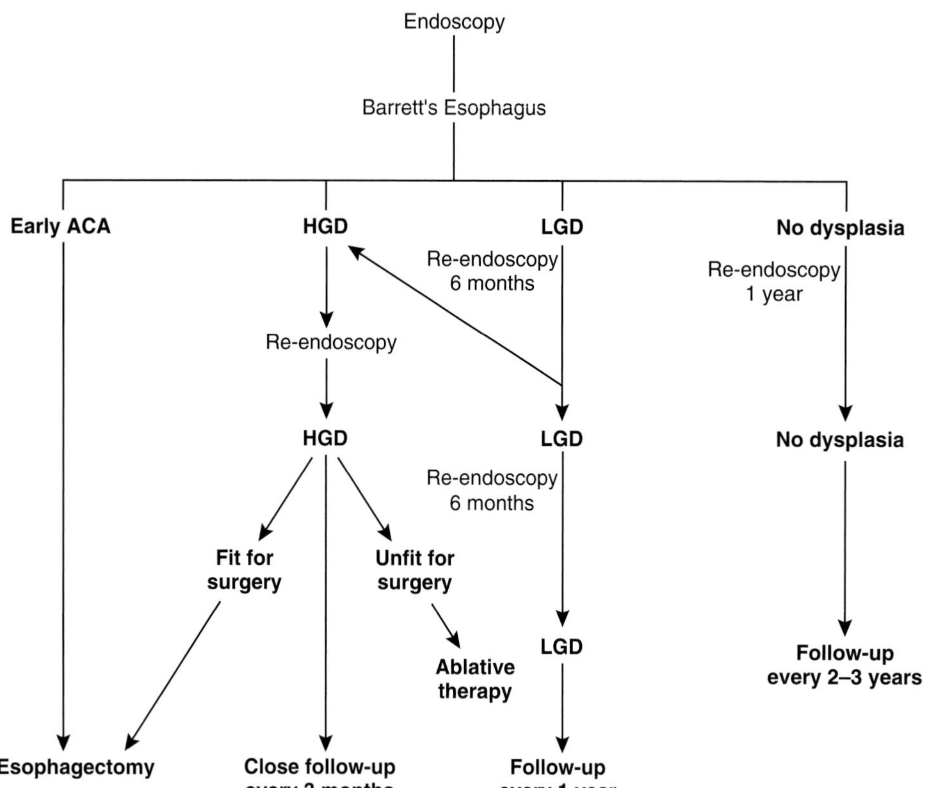

FIGURE 46–6 ■ Barrett's esophagus: grade of dysplasia and proposed follow-up. ACA, adenocarcinoma; HGD, high-grade dysplasia; LGD, low-grade dysplasia.

endoscopy and biopsy remains controversial. Patients with an endoscopic diagnosis of high-grade dysplasia may already have an adenocarcinoma. The prevalence of invasive carcinoma among patients who undergo resection for high-grade dysplasia approaches 50% (Ferguson and Naunheim, 1997; Pera et al, 1992). In addition, two studies have reported progression from high-grade dysplasia to adenocarcinoma in 15 of 58 (26%) and in 8 of 42 (19%) patients, whereas adenocarcinoma did not develop in the remaining patients (Levine et al, 1996; Schnell et al, 1996).

The observed high prevalence of invasive carcinoma in esophagectomy specimens in early series may have been due to the fact that endoscopic biopsy protocols were not rigorous enough to rule out the presence of adenocarcinoma before surgery (Levine, 1997). Despite the use of a systematic biopsy protocol, however, a lower but still worrisome prevalence of unsuspected cancer (33%) was found in patients with high-grade dysplasia undergoing esophagectomy (Falk et al, 1999).

The proponents of esophagectomy have used these data to justify resection (Ferguson and Naunheim, 1997). Others, however, recommend endoscopic follow-up with extensive biopsies until early adenocarcinoma is detected (Levine, 1997; Schnell et al, 1996). They propose that high-grade dysplasia can be accurately distinguished from early esophageal adenocarcinoma and that patients with high-grade dysplasia can be safely monitored using their systematic and rigorous endoscopic biopsy protocol. They also suggest that surgical therapy involves high mortality and morbidity and that, with this conservative alternative, unnecessary esophagectomy in patients with high-grade dysplasia without associated cancer can be reduced.

Diagnosis of small associated invasive carcinomas in LSBE with high-grade dysplasia can be difficult. It is more demanding to follow up with multiple biopsies for patients who have LSBE than for patients who have SSBE. The detection of malignant cells beyond the basement membrane in the lamina propria confirms the presence of an adenocarcinoma, but distinction between high-grade dysplasia and early adenocarcinoma with endoscopic pinch biopsies is not easy and interobserver variation may occur.

A missed unsuspected adenocarcinoma may already have lymph node metastases if the tumor has invaded through the lamina propria and muscularis mucosae into the mucosa and submucosa. The prevalence of regional lymph node metastases in patients with intramucosal and submucosal adenocarcinomas is about 3% and 25%, respectively, because of the rich lymphatic supply of the esophagus that extends into the lamina propria (Rice et al, 1998; Siewert and Stein, 1997). The goal of surveillance is to decrease mortality resulting from adenocarcinoma, and intervention before frank adenocarcinoma is reasonable. To date, no clear answer can be given to the problem of high-grade dysplasia in BE, but a selective approach assessing all endoscopic results and characteristics of the patient should be followed, with esophageal resection favored for young patients who have a low surgical risk.

One possible management scheme for a patient with high-grade dysplasia would be as follows. The patient would undergo repeated endoscopy with multiple biopsies, according to the protocol previously described, in order to rule out the presence of an invasive adenocarcinoma. Biopsy specimens would also be taken from any abnormal area (shallow ulcer, small nodule) in the Barrett's surface. If an invasive adenocarcinoma is detected, the patient would be evaluated for esophageal resection. For all other patients, serial histologic sections would be reviewed by a second expert pathologist. If high-grade dysplasia is not confirmed by the second pathologist, the patient would be reassessed at 3-month intervals.

If two experienced pathologists unequivocally confirm the diagnosis of high-grade dysplasia, the patient would be offered the choice of esophageal resection if he or she were young, had long segments of Barrett's metaplasia, had mucosal abnormalities (stricture, ulcer, nodule), and had a low surgical risk. Treatment would be given at an institution with large experience in esophageal surgery and where the mortality is below 5%. The opportunity for early intervention and cure in an otherwise lethal disease might outweigh the risks of the operation in this situation.

In certain patients, such as those with normal-appearing SSBE in whom the whole BE segment can easily be sampled, endoscopic reassessment every 3 to 6 months would be an alternative.

Finally, patients with high-grade dysplasia on repeated endoscopic examinations who are not good candidates for surgery because of age or associated disease might undergo endoscopic ablative therapy in combination with intensive acid suppressive therapy (see Fig. 46–6).

The goals of resection are complete removal of all areas of Barrett's metaplasia and thorough histologic examination of lymph nodes. Complete removal must be emphasized because high-grade dysplasia and adenocarcinoma have been reported to arise in residual BE after esophagectomy. Use of both an Ivor Lewis and a transhiatal esophagectomy with associated lymphadenectomy can attain these goals. The prevalence of unsuspected cancer and the mortality after esophagectomy in patients with BE and high-grade dysplasia are shown in Table 46–3.

Superficial Adenocarcinoma

Because early adenocarcinoma in BE rarely causes symptoms, detection of cancer at an early, curable stage can be achieved only by surveillance. Several studies have found that patients with BE who develop cancer while in a surveillance program have earlier-stage disease, fewer lymph node metastases, and improved survival (Streitz et al, 1993; van Sandick et al, 1998).

Surgical resection is the mainstay of therapy for patients with superficial or early adenocarcinoma who are fit for surgery. Complete removal of the primary tumor and its lymphatic drainage must be the primary goal of any surgical approach to early adenocarcinoma of the esophagus. Because lymph node metastases may already be present in patients with cancer limited to the mucosa and submucosa, a lymph node dissection is required, both prognostically and therapeutically, in patients with early adenocarcinoma. Subtotal esophagectomy has the best potential for long-term survival (Collard et al, 1997; Holscher et al, 1997). A transhiatal or transthoracic approach can be used. Lymphatic metastases of adenocarcinoma usually involve the lower thoracic, paraesophageal, and paracardial nodes (Clark et al, 1994; Holscher et al, 1995).

Holscher and colleagues (1997) reported their results with transhiatal subtotal esophagectomy in 41 patients with early adenocarcinoma; 31 patients had infiltration of the submucosa, and 10 had carcinoma limited to the mucosa. No patient with mucosal adenocarcinoma had lymph node involvement. The operative mortality was 4.8%, and the 5-year survival rate of the total group of 41 patients, including postoperative mortality, was 83%. All 10 patients with adenocarcinoma limited to the mucosa were alive at 5 years; of the 31 patients with submucosal infiltration, 79% survived to 5 years. Patients without lymph node metastases had a 5-year survival rate of 81%, compared with 50% for those in the positive lymph node (pN1) category.

These results emphasize the need to detect esophageal adenocarcinoma in the T1 (tumor) stage because the prognosis is significantly correlated with the pT category. The most significant variation in long-term survival is found between pT1 and pT2 tumors caused by an increase in lymph node metastases.

Endoscopic Ablative Therapy for High-Grade Dysplasia and Early Adenocarcinoma

Destruction of Barrett's epithelium is followed by squamous re-epithelialization in an antacid environment (Ber-

TABLE 46–3 ■ **Esophagectomy for High-Grade Dysplasia in Barrett's Esophagus**

Author	*No. of Patients*	*No. of Patients with Carcinoma No. (%)*	*Mortality (No.)*
Altorki et al, 1991	8	4 (50)	0
Pera et al, 1992	18	9 (50)	0
Rice et al, 1993	16	6 (38)	1
Levine et al, 1993	7	0	1
Peters et al, 1994	9	5 (55)	0
Edwards et al, 1996	11	8 (73)	0
Heitmiller et al, 1996	30	13 (43)	1
Collard et al, 1997	12	4 (33)	0
Ferguson and Naunheim, 1997	15	8 (53)	0
Cameron and Carpenter, 1997	19	2 (10.5)	0

enson et al, 1993). On the basis of this observation, enthusiasm has developed for eradication of Barrett's epithelium with dysplasia and early adenocarcinoma by means of *photodynamic therapy* (PDT) or thermal coagulation combined with intense acid suppression accomplished by fundoplication or pharmacologic means.

The outcome of these therapeutic modalities clearly depends on complete destruction of the specialized epithelium with subsequent persistent squamous re-epithelialization without leaving any focus of intestinal metaplasia beneath the new squamous epithelium. The end point of these therapies has been either to "downgrade" the degree of dysplasia (i.e., from high-grade to low-grade) or to eliminate the Barrett segment (Wang, 1999). The possibility of eliminating Barrett's epithelium harboring areas of dysplasia and early adenocarcinoma with minimal morbidity and preserving the native esophagus is an attractive proposition that needs to be confirmed on a long-term basis.

This alternative has been questioned for two reasons:

1. Intramucosal carcinomas, although in a small percentage, may already have lymph node metastases.
2. Differentiation of intramucosal tumors from submucosal carcinomas, which are associated with poorer survival, by endoscopic ultrasonography is extremely difficult.

Therefore, such an approach would have the potential to leave lymph nodes untreated or residual tumor in the esophageal wall.

Photodynamic Therapy

A tumor-localizing photosensitizing agent, which may require metabolic synthesis (i.e., a prodrug), is administered, followed by activation of the agent by light of a specific wavelength. This therapy causes a sequence of photochemical and photobiologic processes that cause irreversible photodamage to tumor tissues.

The largest PDT study was carried out by Overholt and associates (1999) and involved 100 patients with dysplasia or superficial carcinoma. Porfimer sodium (Photofrin) 2.0 mg/kg was injected, with light delivery of 630 nm 48 hours later by means of a 1.5- to 2.5-cm cylindrical diffuser or a windowed centering esophageal balloon. After PDT and a mean follow-up of 19 months, Barrett's mucosa completely disappeared in 43 patients. Neodymium:yttrium-aluminum-garnet (Nd:YAG) laser ablation was also used in 35 of these patients to destroy small areas of residual BE. Dysplasia was eliminated in 69 of the 87 (79%) patients without cancer. Of the 73 patients with high-grade dysplasia, 7 continued to have high-grade dysplasia, 8 experienced a switch to low-grade dysplasia, and 2 had a diagnosis of cancer. Surgery revealed high-grade dysplasia without cancer in the latter two patients. High-grade dysplasia was eliminated in the remaining 56 patients. Low-grade dysplasia was cleared in 13 of 14 patients, but high-grade dysplasia developed in 1 patient in areas both treated and not treated with PDT. Of the 13 patients with superficial cancers, the malignancy persisted in three after PDT. Complications included stricture in 34 patients, and 11 patients required multiple dilations.

Gossner and associates (1998) reported on their experience with ALA and PDT in 10 patients with high-grade dysplasia and 22 patients with superficial cancer followed for a mean of 9 months after therapy. Dysplasia was eliminated in all 10 patients and cancer in 17 of 22 patients. Partial re-epithelialization with squamous mucosa was noted in all, and subsquamous intestinal metaplasia was found in two patients.

Using the same technique, Barr and colleagues (1996) treated five patients with high-grade dysplasia in BE. In each of the five patients, PDT with 5-ALA resulted in re-epithelialization with squamous epithelium. No patients had persistence of high-grade dysplasia. Mucosal biopsy specimens of two patients showed columnar mucosa without dysplasia beneath the regenerated squamous mucosa. One concern in using ALA and PDT is that the superficial destruction of BE may leave untreated foci of intramucosal and submucosal carcinoma.

Further investigation is needed before PDT becomes an accepted modality in the management of high-grade dysplasia. Current technology for PDT, including the laser wavelength, the photosensitizer, and the laser diffusion system, is not perfect, and underpenetration is a problem in some areas. The result is incomplete and irregular destruction of BE, with a potential for persistence of Barrett's mucosa or the occurrence of dysplasia or cancer in mucosa that remains beneath the new squamous epithelium.

In the Overholt series, a small island of metaplastic mucosa with high-grade dysplasia under areas completely covered with squamous epithelium developed in two patients 18 and 22 months after treatment (Overholt et al, 1999). In another patient, a subsquamous 2 × 4 mm adenocarcinoma occurred 6 months after PDT.

Another important aspect of the Overholt study was the high recurrence rate of high-grade dysplasia in patients with intractable GERD. At present, optimal candidates for PDT might be those who are not good candidates for surgical resection in whom the risk of malignant degeneration might be reduced with this technique.

Thermal Ablation

Thermal ablation using a laser, multipolar electrocoagulation (MPEC), or argon plasma coagulation in combination with aggressive acid suppression has been used to eradicate BE with and without dysplasia (Sampliner, 1999). Barham and associates (1997) reported the short-term results of laser photothermal ablation with adjunctive acid suppression for the management of BE in 16 patients. An average of three treatments resulted in elimination of the endoscopically visible BE with squamous regeneration in 13 patients who completed the study. However, for 11 of the 13 patients, some biopsy specimens revealed persisting Barrett's glands under areas of squamous epithelium.

Gossner and colleagues (1999) treated 10 patients with SSBE or traditional BE and histologically proven low-grade dysplasia, high-grade dysplasia, or early adenocarcinoma with potassium titanyl phosphate (KTP) laser superficial vaporization in combination with acid suppression therapy. An average of 2.4 sessions per patient was required for ablation of BE. After a mean follow-up of 10.6 months, a complete response was obtained for all 10 patients. Biopsy specimens of two patients showed specialized mucosa beneath the restored squamous cell epithelial layer.

It has been suggested that the technique of thermal destruction of BE may be used mainly to manage focal or short dysplastic Barrett's segments. For tubular, circumferential segments (>2 cm) or longer Barrett's segments (>3 cm), especially in those with multifocal high-grade dysplasia, PDT appears to offer greater advantage (Gossner et al, 1999).

CONCLUSION

Little did Norman Barrett and all of those who contributed along the way realize the importance of their observations concerning columnar-lined esophagus. The treatment of Barrett's disease, in particular the diagnosis and management of dysplasia and superficial carcinoma, is one of the most exciting areas of general thoracic surgery. The ability to intervene in the carcinogenic process that results in adenocarcinoma of the esophagus provides an opportunity to improve survival and quality of life for those afflicted by this dreadful disease.

COMMENTS AND CONTROVERSIES

Although the incidence of Barrett's-associated carcinoma of the esophagus is rising rapidly, the cause remains unclear. It seems unlikely that an increasing incidence of gastroesophageal reflux in the general population is the cause, although the pattern of increasing obesity in the United States population has probably resulted in an increase in reflux-related problems. Some suggest that the increasing use of histamine$_2$ blockers or proton pump inhibitors in the treatment of reflux might be implicated, but this remains conjectural. Whatever the reason, the increased awareness of the malignant potential of Barrett's epithelium and the need for surveillance programs has significantly transformed the spectrum of esophageal adenocarcinoma referred to the thoracic surgeon. More patients are seen in the asymptomatic state; as a result, esophagectomy for adenocarcinoma of the esophagus now results in a significant cure rate—a happy occurrence for both patient and thoracic surgeon.

Whether or not the presence of Barrett's esophagus in itself is an indication for an antireflux operation is unanswered, but to date there is no evidence that an antireflux procedure reduces the subsequent incidence of adenocarcinoma in Barrett's esophagus. A conservative approach to antireflux surgery in the asymptomatic patient with Barrett's esophagus seems warranted, and continued endoscopic surveillance is essential if an antireflux operation is performed for relief of reflux symptoms. On the other hand, an aggressive approach toward esophagectomy in the presence of severe dysplasia seems warranted unless there are significant contraindications to surgical resection.

The presence of coexistent early carcinoma or subsequent development of carcinoma in the setting of severe dysplasia poses a significant threat. Operative mortality associated with esophagectomy at major centers is less than 5%, and the risk-benefit ratio is tipped in favor of resection. I completely agree with the author's suggestion that ablation of severely dysplastic epithelium, by means of PDT or laser, should be reserved for patients with prohibitive operative risks.

M. P.
V. F. T.

REFERENCES

Abo SR, Stevens PD, Abedi M, et al: Prevalence of short-segment Barrett's epithelium in patients with gastroesophageal reflux disease. Gastroenterology 108:A43, 1995.

Adler R: The lower esophagus lined by columnar epithelium: Its association with hiatal hernia, ulcer, stricture and tumor. J Thorac Cardiovasc Surg 13:45, 1963.

Allison PR, Johnstone AS: The oesophagus lined with gastric mucous membrane. Thorax 8:87, 1953.

Altorki NK, Sunagawa M, Little AG, Skinner DB: High-grade dysplasia in the columnar-lined esophagus. Am J Surg 161:97, 1991.

Anderson C, Katz P, Khoury D, Castell D: Distal esophageal reflux accompanies nocturnal gastric acid breakthrough in patients with gastroesophageal reflux disease (GERD) on proton pump inhibitors (PPI) BID (Abstract). Gastroenterology 114:A56, 1998.

Antonioli DA, Wang HH: Morphology of Barrett's esophagus and Barrett's-associated dysplasia and adenocarcinoma. Gastroenterol Clin North Am 26:495, 1997.

Bailey T, Biddlestone L, Shepherd N, et al: Altered cadherin complexes in Barrett's esophagus-dysplasia-adenocarcinoma sequence. Am J Pathol 152:135, 1998.

Barham CP, Jones RL, Biddlestone LR, et al: Photothermal laser ablation of Barrett's oesophagus: Endoscopic and histologic evidence of squamous re-epithelization. Gut 41:281, 1997.

Barr H, Shepherd NA, Dix A, et al: Eradication of high-grade dysplasia using 5-ALA and acid suppression: A (photo)dynamic duo. Lancet 348:584, 1996.

Barrett MT, Sanchez CA, Galipeau PC, et al: Allelic loss of 9p21 and mutation of the *CDKN2/p16* gene develop as early lesions during neoplastic progression in Barrett's esophagus. Oncogene 13:1867, 1996.

Barrett NR: Chronic peptic ulcer of the esophagus and esophagitis. Br J Surg 38:175, 1950.

Berenson MM, Johnson TD, Markowitz NR, et al: Restoration of squamous mucosa after ablation of Barrett's esophageal epithelium. Gastroenterology 104:1686, 1993.

Blount PL, Galipeau PC, Sanchez CA, et al: 17p Allelic losses in diploid cells of patients with Barrett's esophagus who develop aneuploidy. Cancer Res 54:2292, 1994.

Bytzer P, Christensen PB, Damkier P, et al: Adenocarcinoma of the esophagus and Barrett's esophagus: A population-based study. Am J Gastroenterol 94:86, 1999.

Cameron AJ, Carpenter HA: Barrett's esophagus, high-grade dysplasia and early adenocarcinoma: A pathological study. Am J Gastroenterol 92:586, 1997.

Cameron AJ, Kamath PS, Carpenter HA: Barrett's esophagus: The prevalence of short and long segments in reflux patients (Abstract). Gastroenterology 108:A65, 1995.

Cameron AJ, Kamath PS, Carpenter HA: Prevalence of Barrett's esophagus and intestinal metaplasia at the esophagogastric junction (Abstract). Gastroenterology 112:A82, 1997.

Canto MI: Vital staining and Barrett's esophagus. Gastrointest Endosc 49:S9, 1999.

Canto MI, Setrakian S, Petras RE, et al: Methylene blue staining of dysplastic and nondysplastic Barrett's esophagus: An in vivo and ex vivo study (Abstract). Gastrointest Endosc 43:164, 1996a.

Canto MI, Setrakian S, Willis J, et al: Methylene blue–directed biopsy for improved detection of intestinal metaplasia and dysplasia in Barrett's esophagus: A controlled sequential trial (Abstract). Gastrointest Endosc 43:165, 1996b.

Clark GWB, Peters JH, Ireland AP, et al: Nodal metastases and sites of recurrence after en bloc esophagectomy for adenocarcinoma. Ann Thorac Surg 58:646, 1994.

Collard JM, Romagnoli R, Hermans BP, Malaise J: Radical esophageal resection for adenocarcinoma arising in Barrett's esophagus. Am J Surg 174:307, 1997.

Dougherty TJ, Gomer CJ, Henderson BW, et al: Photodynamic therapy. J Natl Cancer Inst 90:889, 1998.

Drewitz DJ, Sampliner RE, Garewal HS: The incidence of adenocarcinoma in Barrett's esophagus: A prospective study of 170 patients followed 4.8 years. Am J Gastroenterol 92:212, 1997.

Edwards MJ, Gable DR, Lentsch AB, Richardson JD: The rationale for esophagectomy as the optimal therapy for Barrett's esophagus with high-grade dysplasia. Ann Surg 223:585, 1996.

Falk GW, Chittajallu R, Goldblum JR, et al: Surveillance of Barrett's esophagus for dysplasia and cancer with balloon cytology. Gastroenterology 112:1787, 1997.

Falk GW, Rice TW, Goldblum JR, Richter JE: Jumbo biopsy forceps protocol still misses unsuspected cancer in Barrett's esophagus with high-grade dysplasia. Gastrointest Endosc 49:170, 1999.

Ferguson MK, Naunheim KS: Resection for Barrett's mucosa with high-grade dysplasia: Implications for prophylactic photodynamic therapy. J Thorac Cardiovasc Surg 114:824, 1997.

Galipeau PC, Cowan DS, Sanchez CA, et al: 17p (p53) allelic losses, 4N (G2/tetraploid) populations, and progression to aneuploidy in Barrett's esophagus. Proc Natl Acad Sci U S A 93:7081, 1996.

Geisinger KR, Teot LA, Richter JE: A comparative cytopathologic and histologic study of atypia, dysplasia, and adenocarcinoma in Barrett's esophagus. Cancer 69:8, 1992.

Gimenez A, Minguela A, Parrilla P, et al: Flow cytometric DNA analysis and p53 protein expression show a good correlation with histologic findings in patients with Barrett's esophagus. Cancer 83:641, 1998.

Gleeson CM, Sloan JM, McGuigan JA, et al: Barrett's oesophagus microsatellite analysis provides evidence to support the proposed metaplasia-dysplasia-carcinoma sequence. Genes Chromosomes Cancer 21:49, 1998.

Gossner L, May A, Stolte M, et al: KTP laser destruction of dysplasia and early cancer in columnar-lined Barrett's esophagus. Gastrointest Endosc 49:8, 1999.

Gossner L, Stolte M, Sroka R, et al: Photodynamic ablation of high-grade dysplasia and early cancer in Barrett's esophagus by means of 5-aminolevulinic acid. Gastroenterology 114:448, 1998.

Haggitt RC: Barrett's esophagus, dysplasia, and adenocarcinoma. Hum Pathol 25:982, 1994.

Hameeteman W, Tygat GNJ, Houthoff HJ, et al: Barrett's esophagus: Development of dysplasia and adenocarcinoma. Gastroenterology 96:1249, 1989.

Heitmiller RF, Redmon M, Hamilton SR: Barrett's esophagus with high-grade dysplasia. Ann Surg 224:66, 1996.

Hirota WK, Loughney TM, Lazas DJ, et al: Specialized intestinal metaplasia, dysplasia, and cancer of the esophagus and esophagogastric junction: Prevalence and clinical data. Gastroenterology 116:277, 1999.

Holscher AH, Bollschweiler E, Bumm R, et al: Prognostic factors of resected adenocarcinoma of the esophagus. Surgery 118:845, 1995.

Holscher AH, Bollschweiler E, Schneider PM, Siewert JR: Early adenocarcinoma in Barrett's oesophagus. Br J Surg 84:1470, 1997.

Hong MK, Laskin WB, Herman BE, et al: Expansion of the Ki-67 proliferative compartment correlates with degree of dysplasia in Barrett's esophagus. Cancer 75:423, 1995.

Hughes JH, Cohen MB: Is the cytologic diagnosis of esophageal glandular dysplasia feasible? Diagn Cytopathol 18:312, 1998.

Iftikhar SY, James PD, Steele RJC, et al: Length of Barrett's oesophagus: An important factor in the development of dysplasia and adenocarcinoma. Gut 33:1155, 1992.

Jankowski JA: Gene expression in Barrett's mucosa: Acute and chronic adaptive responses in the oesophagus. Gut 34:1649, 1993.

Jankowski JA, Wright NA, Meltzer SJ, et al: Molecular evolution of the metaplasia-dysplasia-adenocarcinoma sequence in the esophagus. Am J Pathol 154:965, 1999.

Katz D, Rothstein R, Schned A, et al: The development of dysplasia and adenocarcinoma during endoscopic surveillance of Barrett's esophagus. Am J Gastroenterol 93:536, 1998.

Kauer W, Peters J, DeMeester TR, et al: Mixed reflux of gastric and duodenal juices is more harmful to the esophagus than gastric juice alone. Ann Surg 222:525, 1995.

Klump B, Hsieh CJ, Holzmann K, et al: Hypermethylation of the CDKN2/p16 promoter during neoplastic progression in Barrett's esophagus. Gastroenterology 115:1381, 1998.

Kubba AK, Poole NA, Watson A: Role of p53 in management of Barrett's esophagus. Dig Dis Sci 44:659, 1999.

Lagergren J, Bergströn R, Lindgren A, Nyrén O: Symptomatic gastroesophageal reflux as a risk factor for esophageal adenocarcinoma. N Engl J Med 340:825, 1999.

Levine DS: Management of dysplasia in the columnar-lined esophagus. Gastroenterol Clin North Am 26:613, 1997.

Levine DS, Haggit RC, Irvine S, Reid BJ: Natural history of high-grade dysplasia in Barrett's esophagus (Abstract). Gastroenterology 110:A550, 1996.

Levine DS, Haggitt RC, Blount PL, et al: An endoscopy biopsy protocol can differentiate high-grade dysplasia from early adenocarcinoma in Barrett's esophagus. Gastroenterology 105:40, 1993.

Mann NS, Tsai MF, Nair PK: Barrett's esophagus in patients with symptomatic reflux esophagitis. Am J Gastroenterol 84:1494, 1989.

McArdle JE, Lewin KJ, Randall G, Weinstein W: Distribution of dysplasias and early invasive carcinoma in Barrett's esophagus. Hum Pathol 23:479, 1992.

Menke-Pluymers MB, Schoute NW, Mulder AH, et al: Outcome of surgical treatment of adenocarcinoma in Barrett's esophagus. Gut 33:1454, 1992.

Messmann H, Knüchel R, Bäumler W, et al: Endoscopic fluorescence detection of dysplasia in patients with Barrett's esophagus, ulcerative colitis, or adenomatous polyps after 5-aminolevulinic acid–induced protoporphyrin IX sensitization. Gastrointest Endosc 49:97, 1999.

Morson BC, Belcher JR: Adenocarcinoma of the esophagus and ectopic gastric mucosa. Br J Cancer 6:127, 1952.

Naef AP, Savary M, Ozello L: Columnar-lined lower esophagus: An acquired lesion with malignant predisposition. J Thorac Cardiovasc Surg 71:826, 1975.

Neshat K, Sanchez CA, Galipeau PC, et al: Barrett's esophagus: The biology of neoplastic progression. Gastroenterol Clin Biol 18:D71, 1994.

Ortiz A, Martinez de Haro LF, Parrilla P, et al: Conservative treatment versus antireflux surgery in Barrett's oesophagus: Long-term results of a prospective study. Br J Surg 83:274, 1996.

Overholt BF, Panjehpour M, Haydek JM: Photodynamic therapy for Barrett's esophagus: Follow-up in 100 patients. Gastrointest Endosc 49:1, 1999.

Panjehpour M, Overholt BF, Vo-Dinh T, et al: Endoscopic fluorescence detection of high-grade dysplasia in Barrett's esophagus. Gastroenterology 111:93, 1996.

Pera M, Trastek VF, Carpenter HA, et al: Barrett's esophagus with high-grade dysplasia: An indication for esophagectomy? Ann Thorac Surg 54:199, 1992.

Peters JH, Clark GWB, Ireland AP, et al: Outcome of adenocarcinoma arising in Barrett's esophagus in endoscopically surveyed and nonsurveyed patients. J Thorac Cardiovasc Surg 108:813, 1994.

Polkowski W, Baak JPA, van Lanschot JJ, et al: Clinical decision making in Barrett's oesophagus can be supported by computerized immunoquantification and morphometry of features associated with proliferation and differentiation. J Pathol 184:161, 1998.

Ramel S, Reid BJ, Sanchez CA, et al: Evaluation of p53 protein expression in Barrett's esophagus by two-parameter flow cytometry. Gastroenterology 102:1220, 1992.

Reid B, Haggitt R, Rubin C, et al: Observer variation in the diagnosis of dysplasia in Barrett's esophagus. Hum Pathol 19:166, 1988a.

Reid BJ, Weinstein WM, Lewin KJ, et al: Endoscopic biopsy can detect high-grade dysplasia or early adenocarcinoma in Barrett's esophagus without grossly recognizable neoplastic lesions. Gastroenterology 94:81, 1988b.

Reid BJ, Blount PL, Rubin CE, et al: Flow-cytometric and histological progression to malignancy in Barrett's esophagus: Prospective endoscopic surveillance of a cohort. Gastroenterology 102:1212, 1992.

Rice TW, Falk GW, Achkar E, Petras RE: Surgical management of high-grade dysplasia in Barrett's esophagus. Am J Gastroenterol 88:1832, 1993.

Rice TW, Zuccaro G, Adelstein DJ, et al: Esophageal carcinoma: Depth of tumor invasion is predictive of regional lymph node status. Ann Thorac Surg 65:787, 1998.

Riddell RH, Goldman H, Ransohoff DF: Dysplasia in inflammatory bowel disease: A standardized classification with provisional clinical applications. Hum Pathol 14:931, 1983.
Sampliner RE: Practice guidelines on the diagnosis, surveillance, and therapy of Barrett's esophagus. Am J Gastroenterol 93:1028, 1998.
Sampliner RE: Barrett's esophagus: Electrocoagulation. Gastrointest Endosc 49:S17, 1999.
Schnell T, Sontag S, Chejfec G: Adenocarcinomas arising in tongues or short segments of Barrett's esophagus. Dig Dis Sci 37:137, 1992.
Schnell T, Sontag SJ, Chejfec G, et al: High grade dysplasia (HGD) is not an indication for surgery in patients with Barrett's esophagus (BE) (Abstract). Gastroenterology 110:A590, 1996.
Sharma P, Morales TG, Bhattacharyya A, et al: Dysplasia in short-segment Barrett's esophagus: A prospective 3-year follow-up. Am J Gastroenterol 92:2012, 1997.
Siewert JR, Stein HJ: Barrett's cancer: Indications, extent, and results of surgical resection. Semin Surg Oncol 13:245, 1997.
Souza RF, Meltzer SJ: The molecular basis for carcinogenesis in metaplastic columnar-lined esophagus. Gastroenterol Clin North Am 26:583, 1997.
Spechler SJ: Short and ultrashort Barrett's esophagus: What does it mean? Semin Gastrointest Dis 8:59, 1997.
Spechler SJ, Goyal RK: Barrett's esophagus. N Engl J Med 315:362, 1986.
Spechler SJ, Zeroogian JM, Antonioli DA, et al: Prevalence of metaplasia at the gastro-oesophageal junction. Lancet 344:1533, 1994.
Staël von Holstein C, Nilsson AMK, Anderson-Engels S, et al: Detection of adenocarcinoma in Barrett's esophagus by means of laser induced fluorescence. Gut 39:711, 1996.
Streitz JM, Andrews CW, Ellis FH: Endoscopic surveillance of Barrett's esophagus: Does it help? J Thorac Cardiovasc Surg 105:383, 1993.
Tileston, W: Peptic ulcer of the esophagus. Am J Med Sci 132:240, 1906.
van Sandick JW, van Lanschot JJB, Kuiken BW,et al: Impact of endoscopic biopsy surveillance of Barett's oesophagus on pathological stage and clinical outcome of Barrett's carcinoma. Gut 43:216, 1998.
Wang KK: Current status of photodynamic therapy of Barrett's esophagus. Gastrointest Endosc 49:S20, 1999.
Washington K, Chiappori A, Hamilton K, et al: Expression of β-catenin, α-catenin, and E-cadherin in Barrett's esophagus and esophageal adenocarcinoma. Mod Pathol 11:805, 1998.
Weinstein WM, Ippoliti AF: The diagnosis of Barrett's esophagus: Goblets, goblets, goblets. Gastrointest Endosc 44:91, 1996.
Weston AP, Krmpotich PT, Cherian R, et al: Prospective long-term endoscopic and histological follow-up of short segment Barrett's esophagus: Comparison with traditional long segment Barrett's esophagus. Am J Gastroenterol 92:407, 1997.
Winters C, Spurling TJ, Chobanian SJ, et al: Barrett's esophagus: A prevalent, occult complication of gastroesophageal reflux disease. Gastroenterology 92:118, 1987.
Younes M, Ertan A, Lechago LV, et al: p53 Protein accumulation is a specific marker of malignant potential in Barrett's metaplasia. Dig Dis Sci 42:697, 1997.

CHAPTER **47**

Adjuvant and Neoadjuvant Therapy for Cancer of the Esophagus

Patrick Yau
Glyn G. Jamieson

The mainstay of treatment for cancer of the esophagus is surgical resection; however, the cure rate from resection is poor, even though at operation all macroscopic disease can usually be removed. Patterns of recurrence indicate that about 50% of patients undergo local recurrence of the cancer before any more widespread disease becomes evident, and about half of the remainder experience local recurrence and systemic recurrence at about the same time (Daly et al, 1996). Therefore it has seemed rational to suggest that treatments should be added to surgery to prevent such recurrences.

The Latin verb *adjuvare* means to help. As treatments were added in order to complement surgery, the adjective *adjuvant* became appended to treatments such as "adjuvant" radiotherapy, "adjuvant" chemotherapy, or "adjuvant" immunotherapy. These therapies were given preoperatively, postoperatively, or indeed sometimes both.

Adjuvant radiotherapy has been studied the most, its primary aim being to eradicate the high rate of local recurrence seen with surgery alone. Adjuvant chemotherapy was developed later because chemotherapeutic agents were discovered later than radiotherapy. Chemotherapeutic agents have the potential to prevent local recurrence as well as systemic recurrence.

When both radiotherapy and chemotherapy were combined as adjuvant therapy, as this was a new way of using the modalities, the term *neoadjuvant therapy* was coined. The term has been used somewhat loosely since then, and some authors consider the term synonymous with *preoperative*. This makes no sense, because "preoperative" is a much more exact term, whose meaning is clear.

Which patients with esophageal cancer are candidates for adjuvant or neoadjuvant therapy? Some say that patients with early or locally confined cancer (e.g., stages 0, I, and IIA) should have surgery alone. Since most patients present with stage IIB disease or higher, most patients are still regarded as candidates for some form of therapy adjunctive to surgery. However, perhaps with the exception of stage 0 (Tis) disease, it has not been established that surgery alone is the optimal treatment for stage I and IIA disease.

ADJUVANT THERAPY

Adjuvant Radiotherapy

The potential benefits of giving radiotherapy preoperatively include sterilization of the surgical field of viable cancer cells and shrinkage of the tumor to improve the possibility of complete resection.

Five randomized trials in which radiotherapy and surgery were compared to surgery alone revealed no significant survival advantage for the adjuvant treatment arm. One of the trials (Nygaard et al, 1992) also included a neoadjuvant therapy arm; when their radiotherapy groups were combined, a significant improvement in survival over surgery without radiotherapy was noted. However, chemotherapy as adjuvant therapy was used in another group; thus, there were confounding variables in this study to the use of radiotherapy. Combining the results from the randomized studies (Table 47–1) indicates that radiotherapy has not improved 5-year survival compared to surgery alone. A meta-analysis of 1147 patients did not demonstrate a significant survival benefit with preoperative radiation (Arnott et al, 1998).

Two randomized controlled trials of postoperative radiotherapy have been published, one of 221 patients (Fok et al, 1993) and the other of 60 patients (Teniere et al, 1991). Radiotherapy in the larger study was associated with a lower rate of local recurrence (30% versus 15%) but no difference in 5-year survival (19% in both groups). The smaller study similarly showed no difference in 5-year survival. Almost all of these studies have been of squamous cell carcinoma; since this tumor is usually regarded as more radiosensitive than adenocarcinoma of the esophagus, radiotherapy alone, as adjuvant therapy for esophageal cancer appears to have little to recommend it.

Adjuvant Chemotherapy

As mentioned earlier, antitumor drug therapy not only has the potential to affect the primary tumor, but also can kill micrometastases in lymph nodes and in the systemic circulation. Many agents have been used in both preoperative and postoperative settings and as single agents and in combination. Agents studied have included 5-fluorouracil, mitomycin, cisplatinum, bleomycin, methotrexate, and the newer agents paclitaxel and vinorelbine.

Generally, the results of chemotherapy as adjuvant therapy alone have been disappointing (Ruol et al, 1996); so far, only results of phase II studies have been pub-

TABLE 47–1 ■ **Compilation of Randomized Controlled Trials of Preoperative Adjuvant Radiotherapy (RT) with Surgery Versus Surgery Alone**

	No. of Patients		*No. of Patients (Operative Mortality)*		*No. of Patients (Five-Year Survival)*	
Author	*Surgery*	*Surgery + Preoperative RT*	*Surgery*	*Surgery + Preoperative RT*	*Surgery*	*Surgery + Preoperative RT*
Arnott et al (1998)	86	90	7	9	14	8
Nygaard et al (1992)	50	58	6	7	5	12
Wang et al (1989)	102	104	5	5	38	34
Launois et al (1981)	57	67	6	9	6	7
Gignoux et al (1987)	106	102	19	24	11	9
TOTAL	401	421	43 (10.7%)	54 (12.8%)	74 (18.5%)	70 (16.6%)

lished. One study (in abstract form) of a randomized controlled trial from the Netherlands has compared surgery alone with preoperative chemotherapy in the form of cisplatinum and etoposide (Kok et al, 1998). In this trial, the 3-year survival rate in 67 patients having chemotherapy followed by surgery was 41%, compared with 21% of patients having surgery alone. The complete pathologic response rate in the chemotherapy-treated patients was 6%, which is considerably lower than rates achieved with chemoradiotherapy (see later). Other larger randomized controlled trials are in progress, but this form of adjuvant therapy seems less likely than neoadjuvant therapy to influence outcome.

In some ways, the use of postoperative chemotherapy has more appeal, as at least patients can be staged; all patients with stage N1 disease, for instance, might be singled out for a course of chemotherapy. The only randomized study of the use of chemotherapy in this way comes from Japan (Ando et al, 1997). Two courses of cisplatinum and vindesine were given postoperatively to one group of patients. The other patients had surgery alone. No difference in 5-year survival was found between the two groups. Thus, unless and until more studies appear, such as the one from the Netherlands reported in abstract form, there is unlikely to be much enthusiasm for this form of therapy.

NEOADJUVANT THERAPY

There are several theoretical reasons why combining chemotherapy with radiotherapy might be better than using either modality alone. First, there is independent activity of each treatment mode (i.e., radiotherapy for the primary site and chemotherapy for both primary site and micrometastatic disease). Because the toxicity of each mode tends to be different, there is a summation of antitumor activity without summation of toxic effects. Second, there may be a synergistic effect, with the total effect on the tumor being greater than expected from a simple addition of individual effects. This may be related to chemotherapy's making the tumor more sensitive to radiotherapy, or vice versa, or perhaps both (Vokes, 1993; Steel and Peckham, 1979). Many phase II studies have now been published with regard to neoadjuvant therapy for esophageal cancer, and approximately two thirds of them suggest a survival advantage compared with historical controls. However, the problem of comparing a new treatment to historical or nonrandomized controls is well known (Law and Wong, 1997), and it is thus important for an assessment of this treatment in the context of randomized controlled trials (Table 47–2). So far, three randomized controlled trials have been published in this field, and at least one other major North American trial is nearing completion.

In all three published trials, the postoperative mortality rate was higher in the patients undergoing neoadjuvant therapy. This was for surgery alone versus chemoradiotherapy and surgery, respectively (13% versus 24%, 2% versus 7%, 4% versus 13%). Despite this increased postoperative mortality, there was also a higher 3-year survival in each of the groups undergoing neoadjuvant therapy; rates were, respectively, 11% versus 18%, 6%

TABLE 47–2 ■ **Compilation of Randomized Controlled Trials of Preoperative Neoadjuvant Therapy with Surgery Versus Surgery Alone**

	No. of Patients		*No. of Patients (Operative Mortality)*		*No. of Patients (Three-Year Survival)*	
Author	*Surgery*	*Surgery + CRT*	*Surgery*	*Surgery + CRT*	*Surgery*	*Surgery + CRT*
Nygaard et al (1992)	38	34	5	8	4	6
Walsh et al (1996)	55	58	1	4	4	19
Bosset et al (1997)	139	143	6	18	57	61
TOTAL	232	235	12 (5.2%)	30 (12.8%)	65 (28%)	86 (37%)

CRT, chemoradiotherapy.

versus 32%, and 41% versus 43%. If we include the trial of Urba and colleagues (1997), published only in abstract form, the statistical significance of the meta-analysis findings is further strengthened.

These results clearly suggest that neoadjuvant therapy in the form of synchronous chemotherapy and radiotherapy before surgery is increasing survival rate in patients with cancer of the esophagus.

Nevertheless, there are clear differences between treatment protocols used in these trials, and it is equally clear that if the increased postoperative mortality associated with neoadjuvant therapy could be made comparable to the operative mortality of surgery alone, the survival advantage of neoadjuvant therapy over surgery alone is likely to be even greater. The task remains to find the most effective anticancer dosages associated with the fewest side effects for chemotherapeutic agents and for radiotherapy.

Even if other current randomized controlled trials find similar results, we still do not know whether all patients with esophageal cancer or only subgroups should be treated in this way. In other words, if it can be established that the cancer is only at stage 0 or stage I, it seems unlikely that neoadjuvant therapy has much to offer in treatment above resection alone. But what of stage IIA disease? Or stage IV? Many questions in this field remain to be answered.

COMMENTS AND CONTROVERSIES

This chapter succinctly outlines the attempts to improve results of surgical resection for esophageal carcinoma with the use of adjuvant therapies. The need for randomized clinical trials in this area is obvious but has been hampered in the past by the inability to accurately stage cancer of the esophagus preoperatively—an essential requirement for evaluating the effect of preoperative (neoadjuvant) therapies. However, with the use of endoscopic ultrasound to evaluate the "T" status of the tumor in combination with positron emission tomography to detect metastatic tumor, the ability to accurately stage esophageal carcinoma has greatly improved. This in turn should facilitate randomized clinical trials to evaluate the role of neoadjuvant chemotherapy and radiotherapy in the overall management of esophageal carcinoma.

J. D. C.

REFERENCES

Ando N, Iizuka T, Kakegawa T, et al: A randomized trial of surgery with and without chemotherapy for localized squamous carcinoma of the thoracic esophagus: The Japan Clinical Oncology Group Study. J Thorac Cardiovasc Surg 114:205–209, 1997.

Arnott SJ, Duncan W, Gignoux M, et al: Preoperative radiotherapy in esophageal carcinoma: A meta-analysis using individual patient data (Oesophageal Cancer Collaborative Group). Int J Radiat Oncol Biol Phys 41:579–583, 1998.

Arnott SJ, Duncan W, Kerr GD, et al: Low-dose preoperative radiotherapy in esophageal cancer: Results of a randomized clinical trial. Radiother Oncol 24:108–113, 1992.

Bossett J-F, Gignoux M, Triboulet J-P, et al: Chemoradiotherapy followed by surgery compared with surgery alone in squamous cell cancer of the esophagus. N Engl J Med 337:161–167, 1997.

Daly JM, Karnell L, Menck H: National cancer database report on esophageal cancer. Cancer 78:1820–1828, 1996.

Fok M, Sham JST, Choy D, et al: Postoperative radiotherapy for carcinoma of the esophagus: A prospective randomized controlled study. Surgery 113:138–147, 1993.

Gignoux M, Roussel A, Paillot B, et al: The value of preoperative radiotherapy in esophageal cancer: Results of a study of the EORTC. World J Surg 11:426–432, 1987.

Kok T, van Lanschot J, Siesema PD, et al: Neoadjuvant chemotherapy compared with surgery in esophageal squamous cell cancer (Abstr 297). Can J Gastroenterol 12(Suppl B):99B, 1998.

Launois B, Delarue D, Campion JP, Kerbaol M: Preoperative radiotherapy for carcinoma of the esophagus. Surg Gynecol Obstet. 153:690–692, 1981.

Law S, Wong J: Esophageal cancer surgery: The value of controlled clinical trials. Semin Surg Oncol 13:281–287, 1997.

Nygaard K, Hagen S, Hansen HS, et al: Preoperative radiotherapy prolongs survival in operable esophageal carcinoma: A randomized, multicenter study of preoperative radiotherapy and chemotherapy. The second Scandinavian trial in esophageal cancer. World J Surg 16:1104–1109, 1992.

Ruol A, Bonadonna G, Chanvitan A, et al: Multimodality treatment for non-metastatic cancer of the thoracic esophagus. Dis Esophagus 9(Suppl I):39–35, 1996.

Steel GG, Peckham MJ: Exploitable mechanisms in combined radiotherapy chemotherapy: The concept of additivity. Int J Radiat Oncol Biol Phys 5:85–91, 1979.

Teniere P, Hay J-M, Fingerhut A, Fagniez P: Postoperative radiation therapy does not increase survival after curative resection for squamous cell carcinoma of the middle and lower esophagus as shown by a multicenter controlled trial. Surg Gynecol Obstet 173:123–130, 1991.

Urba S, Orringer M, Turrisi A, et al: A randomized trial comparing surgery to preoperative concomitant chemoradiation plus surgery in patients with resectable esophageal cancer: Updated analysis (Abstract 983). Proc Am Soc Clin Oncol 16:277a, 1997.

Vokes EE: Interactions of chemotherapy and radiation. Semin Oncol 20:70–79, 1993.

Walsh TN, Noonan N, Hollywood D, et al: A comparison of multimodal therapy and surgery for esophageal adenocarcinoma. N Engl J Med 335:462–467, 1996.

Wang M, Gu XZ, Yin WB, et al: Randomized clinical trial on the combination of preoperative irradiation and surgery in the treatment of esophageal carcinoma: Report on 206 patients. Int J Radiat Oncol Biol Phys 16:325–327, 1989.

CHAPTER **48**

Chemotherapy and Radiotherapy as Primary Treatment of Esophageal Cancer

David H. Ilson

Bruce D. Minsky

Esophageal cancer, an uncommon but highly virulent malignancy in the United States, will have been responsible for 12,200 deaths in 1999 (Landis et al, 1999). The majority of patients who have esophageal cancer die of the disease, which represents the seventh leading cause of cancer death in American men. Although esophageal cancer remains relatively uncommon in the United States, it is a major cause of cancer worldwide. Particularly high incidences are observed in northern China, the Caspian littoral, and the Transkei province of South Africa (Kmet and Mahoubi, 1972; McGlashan, 1969; Wu et al, 1982). The epidemiologic factors responsible for the geographic variability in incidence of esophageal cancer, including potential dietary and environmental carcinogens, are under active investigation. In Western countries, an association with abuse of tobacco and alcohol and the development of squamous cell carcinoma of the esophagus is generally accepted (Rosenberg et al, 1989).

Although the incidence of squamous cell carcinoma of the esophagus has remained relatively constant in the United States, adenocarcinoma of the esophagus is increasing at an epidemic proportion in this and other Western countries. Esophageal adenocarcinoma now exceeds squamous cell carcinoma in incidence in white men, and esophageal adenocarcinoma has shown the most rapid rate of increase of any solid tumor malignancy in the past 20 years (Devesa et al, 1998).

Epidemiologic studies have implicated tobacco use and obesity as potential risk factors (Chow et al, 1998; Gammon et al, 1997). One prospective study identified chronic symptoms of esophageal reflux as substantially raising the risk of esophageal adenocarcinoma independently of other factors (Lagergren et al, 1999).

The prognosis for patients with esophageal cancer treated with the standard approaches of surgery or radiation therapy is suboptimal. The largest retrospective series of patients treated with either surgery alone or radiotherapy alone, reviewed by Earlam and Cunha-Melo (1980a, 1980b), reported equally poor 2-year survivals of 6% to 8% and 5-year survivals of 4% to 6%. The operative mortality for surgically treated patients in this review was 29%. However, this 1980 report is out of date and at variance with current results. Later surgical series from single institutions have reported operative mortality rates of 5% to 15%. Muller and associates (1990) reported an overall operative mortality rate of 12.5% in a review of the surgical literature, with 10% of patients achieving a 5-year survival. Ultimately, most patients treated with either surgery or radiation therapy alone are destined to die of their disease.

The failure of standard surgery or radiation therapy in patients with disease clinically limited to the local-regional area prior to treatment is due both to a high incidence of local-regional failure of treatment and to early systemic dissemination of disease. Autopsy series bear out the frequent systemic nature of squamous cell carcinoma, even at the time of or shortly after initial presentation (Anderson and Ladd, 1982; Bosch et al, 1980; Chan et al, 1986; Mandard et al, 1981). Despite the brief duration of illness in these patients, most were found to have evidence of distant metastatic disease at autopsy whether or not residual local disease was present.

Adenocarcinoma of the distal esophagus or gastroesophageal junction appears to have a natural history of disease similar to that of esophageal squamous cell carcinoma, with equally poor survival after surgical therapy due to a combination of local and systemic recurrence of disease (Nanus et al, 1989). The clear need to address the early systemic spread of esophageal carcinoma with systemic treatment has led to the development of combined-modality therapy with the incorporation of chemotherapy. Concurrent use of chemotherapy and radiotherapy is now a standard of care in the nonsurgical management of locally advanced esophageal cancer. The study of preoperative chemoradiotherapy is the subject of ongoing investigation.

Approximately 50% of patients with a diagnosis of esophageal cancer present with overt metastatic disease, and chemotherapy is the mainstay of palliation in this setting. With the high likelihood of the development of metastatic disease in patients with initial local-regional cancer, systemic chemotherapy is ultimately required in the majority of patients. This review focuses on the use of systemic chemotherapy in the treatment of esophageal cancer and of radiation-based therapy in the primary management of locally advanced esophageal cancer.

SINGLE-AGENT CHEMOTHERAPY

The antitumor activity for single-agent chemotherapy in esophageal carcinoma is summarized in Table 48–1. Early

TABLE 48–1 ■ **Activity of Single-Agent Chemotherapy**

Agent	Cell Type	No. of Patients	No. of Responses	Response Rate (%)	95% Confidence Intervals (%)	Author
ANTIBIOTICS						
Bleomycin	S	80	12	15	7–23	Bonadonna et al (1972), Clinical Screening Group (1970), Kolaric et al (1976), Ravry et al (1973), Stephens (1973), Tancini et al (1974), Yagoda et al (1972)
Mitomycin	S	58	15	26	15–37	Desai et al (1969), Engstrom et al (1983), Whittington & Close (1970)
Doxorubicin	S	38	7	18	5–31	Ezdinli et al (1980), Kolaric et al (1977)
ANTIMETABOLITES						
5-Fluorouracil	S	26	4	15	1–29	Ezdinli et al (1980)
	A + S	13	11	85	60–100	Lokich et al (1987)
Methotrexate	S	65	23	35	24–47	Advani et al (1985), Ezdinli et al (1980)
PLANT ALKALOIDS						
Vindesine	S	86	19	22	14–32	Bedikian et al (1979), Bezwoda et al (1984), Kelsen et al (1979), Popkin et al (1983)
Navelbine (vinorelbine)	S	30	6	20	4–36	Conroy et al (1996)
HEAVY METALS						
Cisplatin	S	152	42	28	20–35	Davis et al (1980), Murthy et al (1990), Panettiere et al (1981), Ravry et al (1985)
	A	12	1	8	0–26	Ajani et al (1984)
Carboplatin	S	59	3	5	0–11	Mannell & Winters (1989), Queisser et al (1990), Sternberg et al (1985)
	A	11	1	9	0–26	Einzig et al (1985)
TAXANES						
Paclitaxel	S	18	5	28	8–48	Ajani et al (1994)
	A	32	11	34	15–51	Ajani et al (1994)
Paclitaxel (96-hour)	A + S	14	0	—	—	Xiao et al (1998)
Docetaxel	A	8	2	25	0–55	Einzig et al (1996)
TOPOISOMERASE INHIBITORS						
Etoposide	A + S	27	0	—	—	Coonley et al (1983), Kelsen et al (1983)
	S	26	5	19	4–34	Harstrick et al (1992)
OTHER DRUGS						
Ifosfamide	S	22	2	8	1–23	Ansell et al (1989)
Lomustine	S	19	3	16	0–32	Moertel et al (1976)
Mitoguazone	S	45	9	20	8–31	Falkson (1971), Kelsen et al (1982)

S, squamous cell carcinoma; A, adenocarcinoma.

studies evaluated only squamous cell carcinoma. Modest antitumor activity for a broad range of chemotherapy drugs is seen in esophageal carcinoma, but the duration of response to single-agent chemotherapy is generally brief and on the order of 4 to 6 months. Early chemotherapy trials, such as the studies of bleomycin, were performed on small numbers of patients often in the context of broad phase 1 or 2 trials in diverse solid tumors. Such trials also included patients with prior, often extensive chemotherapy treatment. More modern trials, however, have been larger phase 2 trials and have generally limited new drug evaluation to patients without prior chemotherapy exposure. Later studies have also employed a population size large enough to quantify a major antitumor response with some degree of statistical significance. These trials have included patients with adenocarcinoma, reflecting the rising incidence of this disease.

For some single agents, variable response proportions

in different trials have been reported. In general, higher response rates for single agents have been observed in patients treated with local-regional disease (often prior to definitive local surgery or radiotherapy) than in patients with distant metastatic disease. Greater response rates have also been seen in trials treating chemotherapy-naive patients rather than pretreated patients. In trials employing higher drug doses, higher response rates have also been observed. Despite the disparate response rates for some single agents, the confidence limits of response overlap among different trials in most cases.

Antibiotics, Antimetabolites, and Plant Alkaloids

Antitumor antibiotics have been evaluated only in squamous cell carcinoma. Bleomycin has demonstrated a pooled response rate of 15%. The largest of these trials, conducted by Tancini and colleagues (1974), achieved a 14% response rate in 29 patients. However, 41% of patients (12) suffered severe pulmonary toxicity, two of whom died. High-dose mitomycin C (20 mg/m^2) every 4 weeks and then every 6 weeks was used in an Eastern Cooperative Oncology Group (ECOG) trial evaluating this agent (Engstrom et al, 1983). Of 24 previously untreated patients, 42% had a major response. Cumulative grade III/IV hematologic toxicity was, however, noted in 42% of patients. Lower doses of mitomycin C have shown lower response rates but more acceptable levels. The anthracycline doxorubicin has also been evaluated in phase 2 trials, with an overall response rate in only 18% in 38 patients treated in two phase 2 trials (Ezdinli et al, 1980; Kolaric et al, 1977).

The ECOG has also evaluated single-agent methotrexate and bolus single-agent 5-fluorouracil (5-FU) in patients with previously untreated, metastatic or unresectable squamous cell carcinoma (Ezdinli et al, 1980). Major responses were noted in 12% of patients treated with methotrexate and in 15% of patients treated with 5-FU. In a small study by Lokich and coworkers (1987), continuous infusion 5-FU had a higher response rate. Patients in this study had localized disease only, however, and this higher response rate has not been confirmed in other, similar studies.

The vinca alkaloid vindesine has shown consistent antitumor activity in squamous cell carcinoma (Bezwoda et al, 1984; Kelsen et al, 1979). One study by Kelsen and associates (1979) showed a 17% response rate in 23 mostly pretreated patients. Toxicity, however, was significant, with peripheral neuropathy in 50% of patients and one treatment-related death.

A newer plant alkaloid, vinorelbine, has shown less toxicity with a similar response rate. In a trial by the European Organization for Research and Treatment of Cancer (EORTC), vinorelbine 25 mg/m^2 was given weekly to 46 patients with measurable squamous cell carcinoma (Conroy et al, 1996). Six of 30 previously untreated patients (20%) and 1 of 16 previously treated patients (6%) showed a major response. The median duration of response in the untreated group was 21 weeks. The entire group had a median survival of 6 months. Grade III/IV granulocytopenia was seen in 59% of patients, yet there was no significant peripheral neuropathy and no treatment-related deaths occurred.

Platinum Analogs

Since its introduction in 1980, cisplatin has become the cornerstone of combination chemotherapy in esophageal cancer. As a single agent, cisplatin has a pooled response rate of 20%. The largest trial, conducted by the Southwest Oncology Group, treated squamous cell carcinoma patients with cisplatin, 50 mg/m^2, on days 1 and 8 every 28 days (Panettiere et al, 1984). Nine of 35 evaluable patients (26%) had a major response. A second study by ECOG gave a relatively low dose of cisplatin (50 mg/m^2) once every 3 weeks (Engstrom et al, 1983). This group reported a 25% response rate in 24 previously untreated patients. Treatment was well tolerated in both trials, with no treatment-related deaths.

Carboplatin, by contrast, has shown a disappointingly low 0 to 9% response rate in both squamous cell carcinoma (Mannell and Winters, 1989; Queisser et al, 1990; Steinberg et al, 1985) and adenocarcinoma (Einzig et al, 1985). Oxaliplatin is a promising new platinum analog that, in combination with 5-FU, can salvage patients with colorectal cancer refractory to 5-FU (Bleiberg and de Gramont, 1998). The efficacy of oxaliplatin in esophageal cancer has as yet not been determined.

Taxanes

Paclitaxel is one of the most active single agents in esophageal cancer and has also been evaluated in combination chemotherapy trials. Initial results were reported by Ajani and colleagues (1994) in a joint Memorial Sloan-Kettering Cancer Center (MSKCC) and M.D. Anderson Cancer Center trial. In this study, paclitaxel was given as a 250 mg/m^2 infusion over 24 hours with G-CSF (granulocyte colony-stimulating factor) support every 21 days. Of 32 patients with adenocarcinoma, 11 patients (34%) showed a complete or partial response. Similarly, 5 of 18 patients with squamous cell carcinoma (28%) had a major response. The median duration of response was 17 weeks, and the median survival was 13.2 months. Therapy was generally well tolerated. Although 86% of patients had grade III and IV neutropenia, only 18% were hospitalized for neutropenic fever.

After earlier work in breast and ovarian cancer, other infusion schedules for paclitaxel have been developed. Three-hour paclitaxel is the most commonly used schedule, but it has not been tested as a single agent in esophageal cancer. On the basis of a successful salvage regimen for metastatic breast cancer, esophageal cancer patients who experienced progression of disease while receiving a shorter infusion schedule of paclitaxel were treated with 96-hour paclitaxel at a dose of 35 mg/m^2 per day every 21 days at MSKCC (Xiao et al, 1998). Of the 8 patients evaluated initially, none had an objective response. This study has now been completed, and there were no responses in 14 patients.

In breast and ovarian cancer, 1-hour weekly paclitaxel has shown significant antitumor activity with greater total dose and lower neutropenia than with the original, more protracted infusions. Weekly paclitaxel is currently undergoing phase 2 evaluation at MSKCC and other centers.

Docetaxel has been evaluated in an ECOG study of 33 patients with gastric cancer and 8 patients with esophageal adenocarcinoma (Einzig et al, 1996). Previously untreated patients received 1-hour docetaxel, 100 mg/m^2, every 3 weeks. Two of the eight patients with esophageal adenocarcinoma (25%) had a major response. Overall, grade IV neutropenia occurred in 88% of patients and neutropenic fever in 46%. There are no comparative studies of docetaxel and paclitaxel. In vitro, however, docetaxel has been more active than paclitaxel in 10 esophageal cancer cell lines (histology not given by the authors) (Kawamura et al, 1997).

Topoisomerase Inhibitors

The topoisomerase I inhibitor etoposide (VP-16) has been studied in both adenocarcinoma and squamous cell carcinoma (Coonley et al, 1983; Kelsen et al, 1983b). In mostly pretreated patients, Kelsen and associates (1983b) reported no activity in 7 patients with adenocarcinoma and no major responses in 20 patients with squamous cell carcinoma. In a later study of previously untreated patients with squamous cell carcinoma, however, Harstrick and colleagues (1992) observed 5 partial responses in 26 patients (19%) treated with a higher dose of etoposide.

The topoisomerase II inhibitor irinotecan has shown promising activity in gastric cancer, and reports of the use of irinotecan in combination with cisplatin in both esophageal and gastric cancer also indicate significant activity. As a single agent, irinotecan is currently in a phase 2 trial at the Dana-Farber Cancer Institute.

COMBINATION CHEMOTHERAPY

With modest activity demonstrated for several single chemotherapy agents, combination chemotherapy has also been extensively studied (Table 48–2). In earlier trials,

TABLE 48–2 ■ **Activity of Combination Chemotherapy**

Agent	*Cell Type*	*No. of Patients*	*No. of Responses*	*Response Rate (%)*	*95% Confidence Intervals (%)*	*Author*
BLEOMYCIN						
Cisplatin-bleomycin	S	110	28	26	14–37	Bosset et al (1983), Bromer et al (1984), Coonley et al (1984), Izquierdo et al (1993)
Cisplatin-vindesine-bleomycin	S	191	91	47	40–54	Dinwoodie et al (1986), Kelsen et al (1983), Kelsen et al (1990), Roth et al (1988), Schlag et al (1988)
Cisplatin-vindesine/vinblastine-mitoguazone	S	90	29	32	24–40	Chapman et al (1987), Forastiere et al (1987), Kelsen et al (1986)
	A	16	5	33	8–54	Forastiere et al (1983)
Cisplatin-bleomycin-vincristine–5-FU	S	10	6	60	30–90	El Akkad et al (1983)
Cisplatin-bleomycin-etoposide	S	16	5	31	8–54	Forastiere et al (1983)
CISPLATIN/METHOTREXATE						
Cisplatin-methotrexate	S	43	32	76	63–89	Advani et al (1985)
Cisplatin-methotrexate-bleomycin	S	41	13	32	18–46	De Besi et al (1984), Vogl et al (1981)
Cisplatin-methotrexate-vincristine	S	28	17	61	43–79	Resbeut et al (1985)
Cisplatin-methotrexate-bleomycin-mitoguazone	S	14	9	64	39–89	Vogl et al (1985)
CISPLATIN/ETOPOSIDE						
Cisplatin-etoposide	S	15	3	20	0–40	Burton et al (1986)
	S	65	31	48	36–60	Kok et al (1996)
	A	27	13	48	29–67	Spiridonidis et al (1996)
Cisplatin-etoposide-doxorubicin	A	25	13	52	32–72	Ajani et al (1991)
CISPLATIN/5-FU						
Cisplatin vs. Cisplatin–5-FU	S	89	NS	11	—	Bleiberg et al (1991)
			NS	36		Bleiberg et al (1991), Hilgenberg et al (1988), Kies et al (1984), Vignoud et al (1990)
Cisplatin–5-FU	S	238	116	49	43–55	Ajani et al (1995), Charlois et al (1992), De Besi et al (1986)

patients with both local-regional and with metastatic disease were treated with the same protocols, although patients with local-regional disease usually underwent subsequent definitive surgery or radiation therapy. Virtually all studies used cisplatin. Cisplatin-based combination chemotherapy has yielded antitumor activity in metastatic squamous cell carcinoma of the esophagus in the range of 25% to 35% of patients. The response rate observed in local-regional disease has been consistently higher, on the order of 45% to 75%. Despite higher response rates seen with combination therapy than with single-agent chemotherapy, the duration of response to combination therapy has also been relatively brief, on the order of 4 to 6 months. Unfortunately, the higher response rates achieved with cisplatin combinations have not translated into significantly longer response duration or improved survival. In this primarily palliative setting, the potentially greater response rate for combination chemotherapy must be balanced with a frequently higher toxicity and an increasingly complex and time-consuming schedule.

Early trials combined bleomycin with cisplatin and other agents. Coonley and associates (1984) reported activity of bleomycin and cisplatin in 61 patients with squamous cell carcinoma, only 15% of whom showed a major response.[39] Comparable response proportions were seen in patients with local-regional disease treated preoperatively (given only one cycle of preoperative chemotherapy) and in patients with advanced or metastatic disease. Duration of response in metastatic disease ranged from 5 to 9.5 months. Three other smaller trials showed similar antitumor activity for the combination of bleomycin and cisplatin (Bosset et al, 1983; Bromer et al, 1984; Izquierdo et al, 1993). Overall, a response proportion of 25.5% has been observed.

Cisplatin in combination with vindesine and bleomycin has been studied in three phase 2 trials and two phase 3 trials. In the largest phase 2 trial, reported by Kelsen and coworkers (1983a), major responses were seen in 28 of 44 patients with local-regional disease (63%) after 1 or 2 cycles of preoperative therapy, and in 8 of 24 patients (33%) with advanced or metastatic disease.

TABLE 48–2 ■ **Activity of Combination Chemotherapy** *Continued*

Agent	*Cell Type*	*No. of Patients*	*No. of Responses*	*Response Rate (%)*	*95% Confidence Intervals (%)*	*Author*
Cisplatin–5-FU-mitomycin	S	33	20	61	47–78	Iop et al (1996)
Cisplatin–5-FU–doxorubicin	S	21	7	33	13–53	Gisselbrecht et al (1983)
Cisplatin–5-FU–doxorubicin-etoposide	S	24	17	71	61–81	Bedikian et al (1987)
Cisplatin–5-FU–etoposide	S	20	13	65	47–83	Preusser et al (1988)
	A	35	17	49	32–66	Ajani et al (1990)
Cisplatin–5-FU–bleomycin	S	43	23	53	38–68	Spielmann et al (1989)
Cisplatin–5-FU–vindesine	S	32	16	53	36–70	Spielmann et al (1987)
BIOMODULATION						
5-FU–leucovorin	S	35	6	17	5–29	Alberts et al (1992)
Cisplatin–5-FU–leucovorin	S	56	27	48.2	37–59	Hayashi et al (1992), Zaniboni et al (1987)
Cisplatin–5-FU–leucovorin-etoposide	S	38	22	58	42–73	Wilke et al (1992)
5-FU–interferon	A + S	57	15	26	15–37	Kelsen et al (1992), Wadler et al (1993)
5-FU–interferon-cisplatin	A + S	26	13	50	31–69	Ilson et al (1995)
5-FU–interferon-cisplatin	S	45	34	76	63–89	Pai et al (1998), Wadler et al (1996)
13-*cis*-retinoic acid–interferon	A + S	41	0	—	—	Enzinger et al (1999), Kok et al (1997), Slabber et al (1996)
CISPLATIN/PACLITAXEL						
Cisplatin-paclitaxel–5-FU	A + S	60	29	48	35–61	Ilson et al (1998)
Cisplatin-paclitaxel–5-FU	S	17	12	71	49–93	Garcia-Alfonso et al (1998)
Cisplatin-paclitaxel	A + S	32	15	46	26–66	Costa et al (1997)
Cisplatin-paclitaxel	A + S	20	11	55	34–76	Petrasch et al (1998)
Cisplatin-paclitaxel	A + S	59	31	52	39–65	Kok et al (1997)
OTHER COMBINATIONS						
Carboplatin-paclitaxel	A	9	4	44	12–76	Philip et al (1998)
Cisplatin-irinotecan	A + S	35	20	57	41–73	Ilson et al (1999)
Bleomycin-Adriamycin	S	16	3	19	1–37	Kolaric et al (1980)
Mitomycin-etoposide	A	15	2	13	0–30	Braybrooke et al (1997)

A, adenocarcinoma; S, squamous cell carcinoma; 5-FU, 5-fluorouracil.

Schlag and associates (1988) reported major responses in 45% of patients with squamous cell carcinoma treated preoperatively, two of whom had pathologically confirmed complete responses (5%). Dinwoodie and colleagues (1986) reported major responses in 7 of 27 patients (29%) with advanced or metastatic disease (Dinwoodie et al, 1986). In phase 3 trials, preoperative cisplatin, vindesine, and bleomycin were compared with either surgery alone (Roth et al, 1988) or preoperative radiotherapy (Kelsen et al, 1990), with major responses seen in 47% to 55% of patients and pathologically confirmed complete responses in 6% to 8%. Of a total of 192 patients treated with cisplatin, vindesine, and bleomycin, 91 (47%), responded, with consistently different response proportions seen in patients with local-regional disease (54%) and metastatic disease (29%). Bleomycin-induced pulmonary toxicity was substantial in many of these trials.

Cisplatin in combination with mitoguazone and vindesine or vinblastine was studied in three separate phase 2 trials, with one trial treating both adenocarcinoma and squamous cell carcinoma (Chapman et al, 1987; Forastiere et al, 1987; Kelsen et al, 1988). Overall, 15 of 30 patients with local regional squamous cell carcinoma had a major response (50%) with two pathologically confirmed complete responses (7%), and 14 of 60 patients with advanced or metastatic disease had a major response (23%). Duration of response in metastatic disease was brief, lasting a median of 3 to 4 months. Other cisplatin-based combinations have been reported, including combinations with methotrexate and other agents, with response proportions of 20% to 76% in pooled series of patients with metastatic or local-regional disease (see Table 48–2). One reported preoperative trial of etoposide, adriamycin, and cisplatin in esophageal adenocarcinoma reported a response in 52% of patients (Ajani et al, 1991). The combination of cisplatin and etoposide achieved a 48% response rate in 27 patients with advanced adenocarcinoma (Spiridonidis et al, 1996) and in 65 patients with advanced squamous cell carcinoma (Kok et al, 1996). Toxicity was primarily neutropenia.

Cisplatin and 5-Fluorouracil

The combination of cisplatin and 5-FU given by continuous infusion for 4 to 5 days has been studied extensively, primarily on the basis of the activity of this regimen in squamous cell carcinoma of the head and neck, and with interest waning in the use of bleomycin-containing regimens because of the pulmonary toxicity observed in surgical and radiation therapy protocols. Toxicity observed for the combination of cisplatin and 5-FU, mainly mucositis and myelosuppression, has been substantial but tolerable. Kies and associates (1987) reported the first use of 5-FU and cisplatin in local-regional squamous cell carcinoma of the esophagus, with 11 major responses observed in 26 patients treated preoperatively with three cycles (42%). The duration of response was indeterminate because most of the patients underwent surgical resection or later received radiotherapy.

Subsequent reports have noted similar response proportions in patients predominantly with local-regional disease (Ajani et al, 1992; Charlois et al, 1992; De Besi et al, 1986; Hilgenberg et al, 1988; Vignoud et al, 1990). Of a total of 238 patients treated with squamous carcinoma, the majority of whom had local-regional disease and were treated preoperatively or prior to local radiotherapy, 116 (48.7%) showed a major response. Occasionally pathologically confirmed complete responses have been observed in patients treated preoperatively (14 patients, 7.0%).

In the trials of patients with metastatic or unresectable disease, the response to cisplatin and 5-FU has been lower, ranging from 35% to 40% (Bleiberg et al, 1991; De Besi et al, 1986). Efforts have been made to improve upon this regimen by adding other agents. In one study, mitomycin C (6 mg/m^2) was added to the cisplatin–5-FU regimen in 33 mostly untreated patients with unresectable or metastatic squamous cell carcinoma and yielded a 61% major response rate (Iop et al, 1996). Toxicity was reported as mild, yet 46% of patients required a treatment delay. The additions of doxorubicin (Gisselbrecht et al, 1983), doxorubicin and etoposide (Bedikian et al, 1987), or allopurinol (De Besi et al, 1986) to 5-FU and cisplatin in squamous cell carcinoma have shown no significant improvement over cisplatin and 5-FU alone. Similarly, in adenocarcinoma, the addition of etoposide alone (Ajani et al, 1990) or leucovorin with etoposide (van der Gaast et al, 1997) has shown no advantage.

Despite the increasingly common use in the community of the combination of 5-FU and cisplatin for the treatment of esophageal carcinoma, only one trial has directly addressed the issue of the comparative efficacy of single-agent cisplatin and the combination of 5-FU and cisplatin (Bleiberg et al, 1997). This phase 2 study in locally advanced or metastatic squamous cell carcinoma randomly assigned patients to receive either cisplatin (100 mg/m^2) plus continuous infusion 5-FU (1000 mg/m^2/day, days 1–5) or to cisplatin (100 mg/m^2) alone, both regimens repeated every 3 weeks. The cisplatin–5-FU arm had a higher response rate (35%) and better median survival (33 weeks) than the cisplatin arm (19% and 28 weeks, respectively), but these findings were not statistically significant. Cisplatin–5-FU was also more toxic, with 16% treatment-related deaths for the combination, compared with no such deaths for cisplatin alone.

Overall, cisplatin-based combination chemotherapy has significant antitumor activity in esophageal cancer. Most studies have evaluated patients with locally advanced disease with squamous cell carcinoma, with response proportions for metastatic disease consistently lower than for local-regional disease. Activity for cisplatin-based chemotherapy is also noted for adenocarcinoma; however, the trials conducted in this disease have mainly been of preoperative chemotherapy for local-regional, resectable disease.

Biomodulation Combination Chemotherapy

On the basis of results first reported in colorectal cancer, efforts were made to improve response rates in esophageal cancer with biomodulation therapy. Leucovorin, which enhances the cytotoxic activity of 5-FU by potentiating the inhibition of the enzyme thymidylate synthase, enhances the clinical antitumor response of 5-FU in patients with colorectal carcinoma (Schmoll et al, 1992). Alberts and colleagues (1992) studied leucovorin as a potential biomodulator of 5-FU antitumor activity in patients with esophageal squamous cell carcinoma who received the Mayo Clinic regimen. Of 35 patients with metastatic or locally advanced squamous cell carcinoma, 6 showed a major response (17%), with a median duration of response of 32 weeks. No improvement was seen in antitumor response compared with the reported experience with single-agent 5-FU. Cisplatin in combination with infusional 5-FU and leucovorin was studied in 56 patients with locally advanced disease who were treated preoperatively or had metastatic disease (Hayashi et al, 1992; Hoffman et al, 1992; Ilson and Kelsen, 1993); Zaniboni et al, 1987). Twenty-seven (48.2%) patients experienced a major response, no different from the results achieved without leucovorin (48.7%).

Interferon, another potential biomodulator of 5-FU, has also been evaluated in the metastatic disease setting. Kelsen and associates (1992) first tested the combination of interferon and 5-FU in patients with locally advanced or metastatic disease. Ten of 37 evaluable patients (27%) had a major response. The response rate was somewhat better in adenocarcinoma (38%) than in squamous cell carcinoma (21%); however, the patient numbers were small. A confirmatory study by Wadler and colleagues (1993) showed similar results. To improve the response rate, Ilson and coworkers (1995) added cisplatin to the interferon–5-FU combination in patients with previously untreated metastatic or unresectable esophageal carcinoma. Thirteen of 26 evaluable patients (50%) had a major response. A higher response rate was noted in squamous cell carcinoma (73%) than in adenocarcinoma (33%), although only a small number of patients in this trial (12) has squamous cell carcinoma. Toxicity was significant, and two treatment-related deaths occurred. Similar response rates, toxicities, and deaths with this combination were reported by Wadler and associates (1996) and Pai and colleagues (1998) in patients with previously untreated squamous cell carcinoma of the esophagus.

Others have investigated biomodulation therapy in esophageal cancer with 13-*cis*-retinoic acid and interferon alfa. Unfortunately, no major responses were seen in a total of 28 patients in three phase 2 studies of squamous cell carcinoma or in a separate trial of 13 patients with adenocarcinoma. (Enzinger et al, 1999; Kok et al, 1997b; Slabber et al, 1996).

Taxane-Platinum Combination Therapy

Paclitaxel, which had shown significant promise as a single agent, was added to the cisplatin–5-FU regimen in a phase 2 multicenter study (Ilson et al, 1998a). Paclitaxel (175 mg/m²/3 hr, day 1), cisplatin (20 mg/m², days 1–5), and continuous-infusion 5-FU (750 mg/m², days 1–5) were given to patients with metastatic or recurrent esophageal cancer on a 28-day treatment cycle without G-CSF support. A 3-hour schedule of paclitaxel was selected on the basis of results of a prior phase 1 trial reported by Bhalla and associates (1994), who had used the regimen in an attempt to reduce myelosuppression and permit the delivery of full doses of 5-FU and cisplatin. Of 60 patients evaluable for response in the multicenter study, 29 patients (48%) had major responses. Similar response rates were seen in patients with adenocarcinoma (46%) and patients with squamous cell carcinoma (50%). The median duration of response was 5.7 months, and the median survival was 10.8 months. Toxicity was severe, with 48% of patients requiring a dose attenuation. Half the patients were hospitalized for toxicity, yet there were no treatment-related deaths. An impressive 20% clinical complete response rate was observed in patients with squamous cell carcinoma.

An alternative schedule of cisplatin, 5-FU, and paclitaxel has been given to patients with unresectable or metastatic squamous cell carcinoma (Garcia-Alfonso et al, 1998). In this phase 1 study reported from Spain, paclitaxel was given on day 14 instead of day 1. Paclitaxel dosage was escalated from 135 mg/m² to 225 mg/m², at which point one toxicity-related death occurred. The maximum tolerated dose for paclitaxel was 200 mg/m². Complete responses were noted in 24% of patients, and partial responses in 47%.

Because of the severe toxicity seen with the cisplatin, 5-FU, and paclitaxel combination, a United States multicenter group initiated a trial of paclitaxel, 200 mg/m² over 24 hours, and cisplatin, 75 mg/m², without 5-FU but with G-CSF support (Costa et al, 1997). Patients with predominantly metastatic disease were treated. The trial has now been completed, and in 32 patients, an overall response rate of 46% was seen. Gastrointestinal toxicity was less severe with the elimination of 5-FU from the regimen, but myelosuppression remained significant, with grade III to IV neutropenia in 55% of patients and treatment-related deaths in 11%.

Two European groups have evaluated a biweekly schedule of paclitaxel and cisplatin. Petrasch and coworkers (1998) gave 3-hour paclitaxel (90 mg/m²) with cisplatin (50 mg/m²) every 14 days in a phase 2 trial to patients with unresectable or metastatic disease. Of 20 patients with either adenocarcinoma or squamous cell carcinoma, 40% had a major response, and the complete response rate was 15%. Grade III to IV toxicity was limited to neutropenia (10%) and neurotoxicity (5%). Kok and associates (1997) reported a phase 1 trial of cisplatin, 60 mg/m², and escalating doses of 3-hour paclitaxel without G-CSF support in 31 patients with adenocarcinoma and 28 patients with squamous cell carcinoma. Paclitaxel was increased from 100 mg/m² to 200 mg/m². Grade III to IV granulocytopenia was the predominant toxicity, yet sensory neuropathy was dose-limiting, with a maximum tolerated paclitaxel dose of 180 mg/m². Of 58 evaluable patients, 30 (52%) had an objective response, the rates being 53% in those with adenocarcinoma and 50% in those with squamous cell carcinoma. No treatment-related deaths were reported in either trial.

Carboplatin has also been combined with 3-hour paclitaxel (200 mg/m²) every 3 weeks in 23 patients with upper gastrointestinal malignancies (Philip et al, 1998). In this study, nine patients with unresectable local-regional esophageal cancer had a 44% response rate. Severe neutropenia was reported in 55% of patients, yet other toxicity was mild.

Irinotecan-Cisplatin Combination Therapy

On the basis of the promising results observed in lung, colon, and gastric cancer by Japanese investigators, Saltz and colleagues (1998) developed a regimen of irinotecan, 65 mg/m^2, and cisplatin, 30 mg/m^2, given weekly for 4 weeks followed by a 2-week rest period. A phase 2 trial of this regimen was then initiated in patients with previously untreated, metastatic esophageal cancer (Ilson et al, 1999). A 57% response rate in 35 evaluable patients has been observed. Response rates for patients with adenocarcinoma (52%) and with squamous cell carcinoma (66%) were similar. Toxicity was relatively mild, with tolerable myelosuppression and rare grade III diarrhea.

Non–Cisplatin-Based Combination Chemotherapy

There are very few combination chemotherapy regimens in esophageal cancer that do not incorporate cisplatin. An early trial of bleomycin in combination with doxorubicin showed relatively modest activity (Kolaric et al, 1980). Braybrooke and associates (1997) investigated the combination of mitomycin C and oral etoposide in patients with advanced adenocarcinoma of the upper gastrointestinal tract. Of 28 evaluable patients, 15 had esophageal or gastroesophageal junction cancers. In this group, only 2 patients (13%) had a major response.

Response Rates in Adenocarcinoma and Squamous Cell Carcinoma

Generally, it appears that adenocarcinoma and squamous cell carcinoma have overlapping response rates to combination chemotherapy, similar to the experience with non–small cell lung cancer. Few single agents have been tested in both cell types, and the number of patients treated in such studies has been small.

Combination chemotherapy trials, incorporating such agents as cisplatin, 5-FU, and paclitaxel, have mostly shown overlapping response rates, that are slightly higher in squamous cell carcinoma. An interesting exception is the combination of cisplatin, 5-FU, and interferon. Three trials have shown a remarkably high pooled response rate of 70% (42 of 60 patients) for use of this combination in squamous cell carcinoma but only a modest 33% response rate (5 of 15 patients) in one trial of its use in adenocarcinoma.

CURRENT AND FUTURE CHEMOTHERAPY TRIALS

On the basis of our favorable experience with the combination of weekly irinotecan and cisplatin at MSKCC, we are currently adding to this regimen escalating doses of 1-hour weekly paclitaxel in a phase 1 trial. Similarly, a trial of combination weekly cisplatin, irinotecan, and 5-FU is to be initiated soon. The group at Villejuif in France is investigating the combination of oxaliplatin and irinotecan in gastrointestinal malignancies (Wasserman et al, 1997). Other groups in Europe are testing the combination of cisplatin and vinorelbine. New agents, including paclitaxel, docetaxel, irinotecan, and vinorelbine, are also under active investigation in combination with concurrent radiotherapy in locally advanced disease. Of great interest is the identification of biochemical markers in tumors that may be predictive of chemotherapy response and resistance. Thymidylate synthase, the enzyme targeted by 5-FU, appears to be a potential marker of chemotherapy response: An increase in expression of thymidylate synthase may lead to resistance to 5-FU in gastroesophageal cancers (Lenz et al, 1996).

The search for effective antitumor agents in the treatment of esophageal cancer continues, given the modest activity of currently available agents and brief duration of antitumor responses observed. Future strategies in the treatment of esophageal carcinoma will undoubtedly be based on advances in the understanding of the molecular biology of the disease. Ongoing studies indicate a role for numerous oncogenes and tumor suppressor genes in the mechanism of tumorigenesis, and these factors may be important biologic prognostic factors as well as potential targets for the development of new antitumor drugs.

Laboratory studies have revealed evidence of enhanced expression and amplification of the epidermal growth factor (EGF) receptor gene (Hollstein et al, 1988; Lu et al, 1988) and amplification of the *c-myc* oncogene (Lu et al, 1988) in esophageal squamous cell carcinoma. Immunohistochemical studies of EGF and EGF receptor protein expression in resected esophageal squamous cancers have shown that higher degree of expression of EGF or EGF receptor protein correlates with a worse outcome with poorer survival. (Mukaida et al, 1991). A high degree of expression of the HER-2 receptor has also been demonstrated in esophageal adenocarcinoma and Barrett's esophagus, and like the EGF receptor, HER-2 is a tyrosine kinase growth factor receptor (Jankowski et al, 1992). Antibodies to both the EGF receptor and HER-2 are under active clinical investigation because these agents may lead to tumor growth inhibition and may act synergistically with chemotherapy and possibly with radiotherapy to increase antitumor response (Baselga et al, 1998; Mendelsohn, 1997). An antibody to HER-2 is now available commercially as the drug herceptin; its delivery along with paclitaxel, leads to an enhanced tumor response and longer median survival in patients with metastatic breast cancer, whose tumors overexpress HER-2 (Slamon et al, 1998).

Inhibitors of protein kinase C and cyclin-dependent kinases are also the subject of investigation, including the agents flavopiridol (Schwartz et al, 1998) and bryostatin (Kaubisch et al, 1999), as these agents appear to act synergistically to trigger cellular apoptotic death when coadministered with chemotherapy agents, including paclitaxel (Kaubisch et al, 1999; Schwartz et al, 1999). Cell cycle regulatory proteins that also appear to be affected in squamous cell and adenocarcinomas include mutation of the tumor suppressor gene p53 (Casson et al, 1991; Hollstein et al, 1990; Jiang et al, 1992), loss of heterozygosity of the retinoblastoma tumor suppressor gene (Boynton et al, 1991), and gene amplification of cyclin D (Jiang et al, 1992). All are potential targets for new drug therapy intervention.

PALLIATION

Most chemotherapy trials in metastatic esophageal cancer report on the response rate of single-agent or combination therapy. Secondary end points in these trials include median patient survival and toxicity of therapy. Few trials reported on either the symptom palliation or the quality of life achieved on these trials. Later studies, however, have included symptomatic relief in response assessment, and increasingly, quality of life measures are being included in patient assessment of palliative chemotherapy programs.

Three chemotherapy trials showed significant palliation of patient dysphagia with chemotherapy alone (Costa et al, 1997; Ilson et al, 1999; Spiridonidis et al, 1996). Spiridonidis and colleagues (1996) treated patients who had unresectable or metastatic esophageal cancer with cisplatin and etoposide. Of 18 evaluable patients with dysphagia, 89% experienced relief of dysphagia within 3 weeks of initiating chemotherapy. The results of dysphagia relief with chemotherapy have been reported in two serial chemotherapy trials in metastatic disease (Costa et al, 1997; Ilson et al, 1999). Of 25 patients with dysphagia prior to therapy with cisplatin and paclitaxel, 18 showed complete resolution (72%) and 2 had partial resolution of dysphagia (8%) with chemotherapy.

In a subsequent trial using a combination of weekly irinotecan and cisplatin, 20 patients had evaluable dysphagia; 14 patients (70%) had complete resolution and 4 patients (20%) experienced improvement of dysphagia, with improvement occurring after a median of one treatment cycle. Quality of life was assessed in this trial as well, with responding patients showing a statistically significant improvement in quality of life as measured by two quality-of-life scales (Ilson et al, 1999). The rate of dysphagia relief reported in these trials correlated with antitumor response rates, ranging from 40% to 50%. Given the often substantial toxicity of combination chemotherapy used to palliate metastatic disease, symptom relief and quality of life assessment of patients will play an increasing role in the future assessment of the clinical benefit of systemic chemotherapy programs.

NEOADJUVANT CHEMOTHERAPY

The use of preoperative chemotherapy in locally advanced esophageal carcinoma has been the subject of numerous trials. Most of these trials were single-arm phase 2 studies evaluating preoperative chemotherapy given from one to six cycles, followed by a definitive surgical procedure. Later trials, however, have given chemotherapy both preoperatively and postoperatively. Virtually all preoperative chemotherapy trials in esophageal cancer have employed cisplatin-based combination chemotherapy. Earlier trials involved predominantly squamous cell carcinoma, but with the higher incidence of adenocarcinoma, both cell types have been treated with the same preoperative protocols.

Early trials combined bleomycin with cisplatin and other agents. Because of the marginal antitumor activity observed for cisplatin and bleomycin, vindesine was added to cisplatin and bleomycin in subsequent trials in squamous cell carcinoma. (Kelsen et al, 1983a, 1990; Roth et al, 1988; Schlag et al, 1988). Given the pulmonary toxicity associated with bleomycin, and the limited antitumor activity observed for the combination of bleomycin and cisplatin in preoperative therapy and in metastatic disease, other cisplatin-based combinations were studied in phase 2 preoperative chemotherapy trials. Cisplatin in combination with mitoguazone and vindesine or vinblastine was studied in two phase 2 trials (Forastiere et al, 1987; Kelsen et al, 1986). The combination of cisplatin and 5-FU given by continuous infusion for 4 to 5 days has also been extensively studied in preoperative chemotherapy trials (Ajani et al, 1992; Hilgenberg et al, 1988; Kies et al, 1987; Vignoud et al, 1990). Subsequent trials combined etoposide with cisplatin and 5-FU (Ajani et al, 1990) or cisplatin, doxorubicin (Adriamycin), and etoposide (Ajani et al, 1991) in adenocarcinoma of the gastroesophageal junction or of the distal esophagus. Other reported series of patients have been treated with preoperative 5-FU and cisplatin in combination with doxorubicin (Gisselbrecht et al, 1983) doxorubicin and etoposide (Bedikian et al, 1987), etoposide (Preusser et al, 1988), leucovorin (Hoffman et al, 1992), leucovorin and etoposide (Wilke et al, 1992), and carboplatin (Cure et al, 1993). Toxicity observed for these trials, mainly mucositis, myelosuppression, and nephrotoxicity, has been substantial but tolerable.

Overall, preoperative chemotherapy with cisplatin-based combination chemotherapy has achieved a major response in 17% to 66% of patients, with pathologically confirmed complete responses in 3% to 10% of patients. Rate of operability after chemotherapy has ranged from 50% to 100%, and the rate of resectability of operated tumors has ranged from 40% to 90%, with the operative mortality after preoperative chemotherapy comparable to that of surgical series alone. These results indicate that the administration of preoperative chemotherapy is safe and without a demonstrably adverse effect on surgical outcome. The overall survival of patients treated with preoperative chemotherapy has been disappointing, however, with a median survival ranging from 10 to 26 months in larger series. An improvement in the percentage of patients achieving long-term survival has been suggested in preoperative chemotherapy trials, with a trend toward better survival in patients manifesting a major objective response to chemotherapy. Whether response to chemotherapy is independent of other favorable prognostic factors is unclear.

The duration of chemotherapy delivered in preoperative chemotherapy trials has also undergone evolution. Whereas earlier trials administered only one or two cycles of chemotherapy preoperatively without subsequent postoperative therapy, more recent trials have given up to three or more cycles of preoperative therapy and two or three cycles of postoperative chemotherapy. The treatment outcomes of the earlier and late trials may not be

TABLE 48–3 ■ Esophageal Cancer Preoperative Chemotherapy Phase 3 Trials

Author	*Regimen*	*Cell Type*	*No. of Patients*	*Resectable Tumors (%)*	*Operative Mortality (%)*	*Median Survival (Months)*	*Survival (%)*
Roth et al (1988)	Cisplatin-bleomycin-vindesine	S	17	35	12	9	25 (3-year)*
	Surgery		19	21	0	9	5 (3-year)
Schlag (1991)	Cisplatin–5-FU	S	29	71	21	8	—
	Surgery		40	77	12	9	—
Nygaard et al (1992)	Cisplatin-bleomycin	S	50	58	15	NS	3 (3-year)
	Surgery		41	69	13	NS	9 (3-year)
	RT 3500 cGy		48	54	11	NS	21 (3-year)*
	RT/Cisplatin-bleomycin		47	66	24	NS	17 (3-year)*
Kelsen et al (1990)	Cisplatin-bleomycin-vindesine	S	48	58	11	10	20†
	RT		48	65	14	12	
Kelsen et al (1998)	Cisplatin–5-FU	A + S	213	62	7	14.9	20%
	Surgery		227	59	6	16.1	20%
Kok et al (1996)	Cisplatin-etoposide	S	74	63	NS	18.5‡	—
	Surgery		74	63	NS	11	—

*Not statistically significant.
†Survival of all patients.
‡P = .002.
A, adenocarcinoma; RT, radiation therapy; S, squamous cell carcinoma; 5-FU, 5-fluorouracil.

directly comparable, particularly in regard to the impact of additional cycles of systemic therapy on systemic recurrence of disease. Postoperative radiation therapy was also delivered in some trials, but later trials have not routinely included postoperative radiotherapy.

The role of preoperative chemotherapy in the treatment of local-regional esophageal carcinoma can be clearly defined only in the context of random assignment trials with a surgery-only control arm (Table 48–3). Four small randomized trials have compared surgery alone with preoperative chemotherapy and surgery, and a fifth trial compared preoperative chemotherapy with preoperative radiotherapy.

Roth and colleagues (1988) randomly assigned patients to receive preoperative chemotherapy with cisplatin, bleomycin, and vindesine or to undergo surgery alone. Schlag and associates (1991) randomly assigned patients to undergo surgery alone or to receive three cycles of preoperative chemotherapy with 5-FU and cisplatin. Nygaard and coworkers (1992) randomly assigned patients to receive either surgery alone, preoperative chemotherapy with cisplatin and bleomycin, preoperative radiotherapy, or preoperative treatment with sequential chemotherapy and radiotherapy. Kok and associates (1996) randomly assigned patients to two cycles of preoperative etoposide plus cisplatin, with responding patients receiving a total of four cycles. Kelsen and colleagues (1990) randomly assigned patients to treatment either with preoperative high-dose radiotherapy, 5500 cGy delivered over 5.5 to 6 weeks by a multified technique, or with preoperative chemotherapy consisting of cisplatin, vindesine, and bleomycin.

Of these four small randomized trials, only one trial demonstrated a survival advantage for preoperative chemotherapy, with the Kok and associates (1996) reporting a median survival advantage for chemotherapy (18.5 months) over surgery alone (11 months). Schlag and associates (1991) reported no difference in survival between patients receiving 5-FU and cisplatin and those undergoing surgery alone. No survival benefit was conveyed by preoperative chemotherapy in the study reported by Nygaard and coworkers (1992), and the patients with the poorest survival at 3 years (5%) had received preoperative chemotherapy. The use of a probably suboptimal chemotherapy regimen may have diminished the effect of chemotherapy in this study. In the trial reported by Kelsen and colleagues (1990), a survival comparison between the two treatment groups could not be made because the trial design permitted a postoperative crossover to the other treatment modality, and most patients received both chemotherapy and radiation therapy. The actuarial survival rate observed for all patients was 20% at 5 years, superior to that for historical controls, with the subgroup of patients with responses to either chemotherapy or radiotherapy showing a trend toward improved survival.

The large American Intergroup Trial (INT) 0113, reported by Kelsen and associates (1998), is the most definitive trial to date of preoperative chemotherapy in esophageal cancer. In this landmark trial, 227 patients were randomly assigned to undergo immediate surgery, and 213 patients to receive three preoperative cycles of cisplatin and 5-FU, surgery, and two postoperative cycles of cisplatin and 5-FU. The trial showed no benefit for neoadjuvant chemotherapy over surgery alone. Median survival for patients undergoing surgery alone was 16.1 months compared with 14.9 months for patients receiving chemotherapy, not a significant difference. Overall survival at 2 years (37% for surgery alone versus 35% for chemotherapy) and 5 years (20% for both treatment groups) was also not significantly different for the two patient groups, and there was also no difference in 2-year disease-free survival for either group (20%). Curative resections with negative surgical margins (R-0 resection) were equivalent in the two groups (59% for surgery alone and 62% for preoperative chemotherapy), and surgical mortality was also comparable (6% operative mortality for surgery alone and a 7% operative mortality for preoperative chemotherapy). Two percent of patients died of chemotherapy-related complications.

At the present, time, for surgically treated patients, surgery alone remains the standard of care and the value of preoperative chemotherapy outside an investigational setting is unproven. The combined use of concurrent radiotherapy and chemotherapy as preoperative treatment remains the subject of intense and ongoing investigation.

PRIMARY RADIATION THERAPY

Primary treatment of esophageal cancer is either surgical therapy or nonsurgical, usually radiation-based, therapy. Although the overall results of these approaches are similar, it must be emphasized that the patient population selected for treatment with each modality is usually different, resulting in a selection bias against nonsurgical therapy.

First, patients with poor prognostic features are more commonly selected for treatment with nonsurgical therapy. These features include patients who are not surgical candidates because of medical contraindications or who have primary unresectable or metastatic disease. Second, surgical series report results on the basis of pathologic staging of tumors, whereas nonsurgical series report results on the basis of clinical staging. Pathologic staging has the advantage of excluding some patients with metastatic disease. Third, because some patients treated without surgery are approached in a palliative rather than a curative fashion, the intensity of chemotherapy and the doses and techniques of radiation therapy can be suboptimal.

Radiation Therapy Alone

Many series have reported results of external-beam radiation therapy alone. Most include patients with unfavorable features such as clinical T4 disease and positive lymph nodes. For example, in the series reported by De-Ren (1989), 184 of the 678 patients had stage IV disease. Overall, the 5-year survival rate for patients treated with radiation therapy alone is 0 to 10% (De-Ren, 1989; Newaishy et al, 1982; Okawa et al, 1989). The use of radiation therapy as a potentially curative modality requires doses of at least 5000 cGy at 180 to 200 cGy per fraction. Furthermore, given the large size of many unresectable esophageal cancers, doses of 6000 cGy or greater are probably required. However, even in the radiation therapy alone arm of the Radiation Therapy Oncology Group (RTOG) 85-01 trial, in which patients received 6400 cGy with modern techniques, all patients were dead of disease by 3 years (Al-Sarraf et al, 1996; Herskovic et al, 1992).

There is one report of radiation therapy alone for patients with clinically early-stage disease. The trial reported by Sykes and colleagues (1998) was limited to 101 patients (90% squamous cell carcinoma) with tumors smaller than 5 cm, who received 4500 to 5250 cGy in 15 or 16 fractions. The 5-year survival was 20%.

In summary, radiation therapy alone should be reserved for palliation or for patients who are medically unable to receive chemotherapy. As discussed later, the results of combined-modality therapy are more favorable and this approach represents the standard of care.

COMBINED-MODALITY THERAPY

Conventional Approaches

There are a number of single-arm, nonrandomized trials of combined-modality therapy alone (Coia et al, 1991; Izquierdo et al, 1993; John et al, 1989; Seitz et al, 1990; Valerdi et al, 1994). Selected series are summarized in Table 48–4. The series reported by Coia and associates (1991) is the only one in which patients with early-stage disease (clinical stages I and II) were analyzed separately from those with more advanced disease. These patients received 5-FU and mitomycin C concurrently with 6000 cGy. Combining results for patients with clinical stages I and II diseases, the local failure rate was 25%, the 5-year actuarial local relapse–free survival was 70%, and the 5-year actuarial survival was 30%.

The Southwest Oncology Group (SWOG) 9060 trial reported by Poplin and associates (1996) included 32 patients who received 5-FU–cisplatin concurrently with

TABLE 48–4 ■ **Combined-Modality Therapy Alone for Esophageal Cancer: Selected Nonrandomized Series**

Series	*Clinical Stage*	*No. of Patients*	*Cell Type*	*Local Failure (%)*	*Actuarial Overall Survival (%)*	*Local Relapse Free Survival (%)*
Coia et al (1991)	I	13	S + A	26	73 (5-year)	100 (5-year)
	II	44	S + A	45	20	59
	All	16	A	—	38	71
	All	39	S	—	27	58
	Total	57	S + A	25	30	70
John et al (1989)	I–III	30	S + A	27	29 (2-year)	—
Seitz et al (1990)	I–III	35	S	—	21 (2-year)	—
Izquierdo et al (1993)	"Unresectable"	25	S	—	8 (4-year) 8 months (median)	—

A, adenocarcinoma; S, squamous cell carcinoma.

TABLE 48–5 ■ **Radiation Therapy versus Combined-Modality Therapy for Esophageal Cancer: Randomized Trials**

Series	*No. of Patients*	*Overall Survival (%)*	*Median Survival (Months)*	*Local Failure (%)*	*Author*
RTOG					
Radiation alone	62	0 (5-year)*	9	68†	Herskovic et al (1992)
Combined-modality	61	27	14	45‡	
Combined-modality*	69	N/A	17	54	
NCI Brazil					
Radiation alone	31	6 (5-year)		84	Araujo et al (1991)
Combined-modality	28	16		61	
EORTC (Roussel)					
Radiation alone	69	6 (3-year)			Roussel et al (1988)
Combined-modality	75	12			
Scandinavia					
Radiation alone	51	6 (3-year)			Nygaard (1992)
Combined-modality	46	0			
Pretoria§					
Radiation alone	36		5		Slabber et al (1998)
Combined modality	34		6		
ECOG EST-1282‖					
Radiation alone	60	7 (5-year)	9‡		
Combined-modality	59	9	15		

*Nonrandomized group treated following early closure of the randomization.
†RTOG reported local failure as local persistence + local failure.
‡Statistically significant.
§Limited to patients with squamous cell cancer with T3 disease.
‖Approximately 50% in each arm underwent surgery.
ECOG, Eastern Cooperative Oncology Group; EORTC, European Organization for Research and Treatment of Cancer; NCI, National Cancer Institute; RTOG, Radiation Therapy Oncology Group.

5000 cGy followed by two cycles of 5-FU–cisplatin. Because the choice of further management (observation, radiation, chemotherapy, surgery) was based on the tumor response, this trial cannot be considered a pure combined-modality therapy series. Although the median survival was 20 months, Poplin and associates (1996) concluded that the complexity and toxicity precluded further use of this approach.

Six randomized trials have been reported comparing radiation therapy alone with combined modality therapy (Table 48–5) (Al-Sarraf et al, 1997; Araujo et al, 1991; Herskovic et al, 1992; Nygaard et al, 1992; Roussel et al, 1988; Slabber et al, 1998; Smith et al, 1998). Of the six trials, five used suboptimal doses of radiation, and three used inadequate doses of systemic chemotherapy. For example, in the series reported by Araujo and colleagues (1991), patients received only 1 cycle of 5-FU, mitomycin C, and bleomycin. The EORTC trial used subcutaneous methotrexate (Roussel et al, 1988). In the Scandinavian trial reported by Hatlevoll and associates, patients received low doses of chemotherapy (cisplatin, 20 mg/m^2, and bleomycin, 10 mg/m^2, for a maximum of two cycles) (Nygaard et al, 1992).

In the Eastern Cooperative Oncology Group (ECOG) EST-1282 trial, patients who received combined-modality therapy had a significantly increased median survival than those receiving radiation alone (15 months vs. 9 months; $P = .04$) but had no improvement in 5-year survival (9% versus 7%). However, this trial was not a purely nonsurgical trial because approximately 50% of patients in each arm underwent surgery after receiving 4000 cGy. Furthermore, the decision to perform surgery depended on the individual investigator's preference. The operative mortality was 17%.

Finally, the Pretoria trial reported by Slabber and coworkers (1998), which was limited to a total of 70 patients with T3 squamous cell cancers, used a low-dose (4000 cGy), split-course radiation schedule.

The only trial that was designed to deliver adequate doses of systemic chemotherapy with concurrent radiation therapy was the RTOG 85-01 trial reported by Herskovic and colleagues (1992) and Al-Sarraf and coworkers (1997). This Intergroup trial primarily included patients with squamous cell carcinoma. Patients received 4 cycles of 5-FU (1000 mg/m^2/24 hr for 4 days) and cisplatin (75 mg/m^2, day 1). Radiation therapy (5000 cGy at 200 cGy/day) was given concurrently with day 1 of chemotherapy. Curiously, cycles 3 and 4 of chemotherapy were delivered every 3 weeks (weeks 8 and 11) rather than every 4 weeks (weeks 9 and 13). This intensification may explain, in part, why only 50% of the patients finished all four cycles of the chemotherapy. The control arm consisted of radiation therapy alone, albeit a higher dose (6400 cGy) than that given in the combined-modality therapy arm.

Patients who received combined-modality therapy had a significant improvement in median survival (14 months versus 9 months), and 5-year survival (27% versus 0%; $P < .0001$) (Al-Sarraf et al, 1997). The 2-year actuarial incidence of local failure as the first site of failure was also significantly lower in the combined-modality arm (45% versus 66%; $P = .0123$). The study was closed early because of the positive results. Following this early closure, an additional 69 patients were treated with the same combined-modality therapy regimen and similar results were seen (30% 3-year survival).

Combined-modality therapy not only yields better results than radiation alone but also is associated with a higher incidence of acute toxicity. In the RTOG 85-01 trial, patients who received combined-modality therapy had a higher incidence of acute grade III toxicity (44% versus 25%) and acute grade IV toxicity (20% versus 3%) than those undergoing radiation therapy alone. Including the one treatment-related death (2%), the incidence of total acute grade III or higher toxicity was 66%. Although the incidence of this complication was higher with combined-modality therapy than with radiation therapy alone (35% versus 12%), there was little difference in the incidence of late toxicity (29% versus 23%).

The positive results of the RTOG 85-01 trial, demonstrate that the conventional nonsurgical treatment for esophageal carcinoma is combined-modality therapy. Notwithstanding, the local failure rate in the study's combined-modality therapy arm is 45% and there is room for improvement. Therefore, new approaches, such as intensification of combined-modality therapy and escalation of the radiation dose, have been developed in an attempt to improve the results.

Intensification of Combined-Modality Therapy

The phase 2 Intergroup Trial (INT) 0122 (ECOG PE-289, RTOG 90-12) was designed to intensify the RTOG 85-01 combined-modality arm (Minsky et al, 1999). The development of the neoadjuvant chemotherapy approach used in INT 0122 was based, in part, on the results of a randomized trial of preoperative radiation therapy (5500 cGy) versus preoperative chemotherapy (5-FU/cisplatin-vindesine) reported from Memorial Sloan-Kettering Cancer Center (MSKCC) (Kelsen et al, 1990). This trial revealed that the rates of resectability (65% versus 58%), objective response (64% versus 55%), and local failure (15% versus 6%) for preoperative radiation therapy and preoperative chemotherapy were similar. Both the chemotherapy and radiation therapy in INT 0122 were intensified as follows:

1. The 5-FU continuous infusion (1000 mg/m^2/24 hours) was increased from 4 days to 5 days.
2. The total number of cycles of chemotherapy was increased from four to five.
3. Three cycles of full-dose neoadjuvant 5-FU–cisplatin were delivered prior to the start of combined-modality therapy.
4. The radiation dose was increased from 5000 cGy to 6480 cGy.

Eligibility was limited to patients with squamous cell carcinoma, and 45 patients were entered in the trial, of whom 38 were ultimately eligible to participate.

The final results of INT 0122 have been reported. (Minsky et al, 1999). For the 38 eligible patients, the primary tumor response rate was 47% complete and 8% partial; 3% had stable disease. The first site of clinical failure was local in 39% of patients and distant in 24%. For the total patient group, there were six deaths during treatment, of which 9% (4/45) were treatment-related. The median survival was 20 months, and the 5-year actuarial survival was 20%. Therefore, this intensive neoadjuvant approach did not appear to offer a benefit over conventional doses and techniques of combined-modality therapy. The higher radiation dose (6480 cGy) was tolerable, however, and is being further tested in trial INT 0123, which replaced trial RTOG 85-01.

A limited number of phase 2 trials have tested the use of neoadjuvant chemotherapy prior to radiation therapy or combined-modality therapy. Valerdi and colleagues (1994) reported results for 40 patients with clinical stage 2 or 3 squamous cell carcinoma who received two cycles of neoadjuvant cisplatin-vindesine-bleomycin (days 1 and 29) followed by 6000 cGy.[125] In contrast with INT 0122, no chemotherapy was delivered with the radiation therapy in this trial. The complete response rate was 53%. With a median follow-up of 78 months, the local failure rate was 62%, the median survival was 11 months, and the 5-year actuarial survival was 15%. These results are similar to those obtained with the combined-modality arm of RTOG 85-01, with the exception of the higher treatment-related death rate of 5%.

Using a five-drug neoadjuvant regimen, Roca and colleagues (1996) treated 55 patients (54 with squamous cell carcinoma) with bolus cisplatin–5-FU/leucovorin/bleomycin/mitomycin C for 15 days followed by 6000 cGy plus concurrent 5-FU/leucovorin-cisplatin. No maintenance chemotherapy was delivered. Patients with disease at all anatomic sites within the esophagus were eligible for participation, and 53% had clinical stage III disease. Although the treatment-related mortality was only 4% and the 3-year survival was 35%, the local failure rate (as a component of failure) was 42%, similar to the 45% reported for the combined-modality therapy arm of RTOG 85-01.

In summary, neoadjuvant chemotherapy, as delivered in the trials described, does not appear to improve the results of combined-modality therapy. New trials using taxol-based neoadjuvant chemotherapy are in progress (Kelsen et al, 1999).

Intensification of the Radiation Dose

Another approach to the dose intensification of combined-modality therapy is to increase the radiation dose to more than 6000 cGy. There are two methods by which the radiation dose to the esophagus can be increased: brachytherapy and external-beam therapy.

Brachytherapy

Intraluminal brachytherapy allows the escalation of the dose to the primary tumor while protecting the surrounding dose-limiting structures, such as the lung, heart, and spinal cord (Armstrong, 1993). A radioactive source is placed intraluminally via bronchoscopy or a nasogastric tube. Brachytherapy has been used both as primary therapy (Jager et al, 1995) and boost following external-beam radiation therapy (Calais et al, 1997; Moni et al, 1996). It can be delivered by high or low dose rate (Caspers et al, 1993). Although there are technical and radiobiologic differences between the two dose rates, there are no clear therapeutic advantages.

As a primary therapy, brachytherapy results in a local control rate of 25% to 35% (Moni et al, 1996; Sur et al, 1992). In the randomized trial reported by Sur and colleagues (1992), there was no significant difference in local control or survival between high-dose-rate brachytherapy and external-beam irradiation.

A major limitation of brachytherapy is the effective treatment distance. The primary isotope is ^{192}Ir, which is usually prescribed to treat to a distance of 1 cm from the source. Therefore, any portion of the tumor that is farther from the source receives a suboptimal radiation dose.

Encouraging results were reported in a phase 2 trial by Calais and associates (1997). A total of 53 patients with clinically unresectable adenocarcinoma or squamous cell carcinoma of the esophagus received 6000 cGy plus three cycles of concurrent 5-FU/cisplatin–mitomycin C followed by high-dose-rate intraluminal brachytherapy (500 cGy/week for 2 weeks) prescribed to 0.5 cm. With a median follow-up of 39 months, the 3-year and 5-year actuarial survivals were 27% and 18%, respectively. Severe late toxicity occurred in 11% of patients. One patient died of treatment-related toxicity. Although fistulas developed in two patients (4%), both were due to tumor progression. Swallowing function was "good" in 75%. The local failure rate was 43% (23/53). The results are comparable with those of other trials of combined-modality therapy; therefore, the benefit of adding intraluminal brachytherapy is unclear.

In the RTOG 92-07 trial, reported by Gaspar and associates (1997b), 75 patients with squamous cell cancers (92%) or adenocarcinomas (8%) of the thoracic esophagus received the RTOG 85-01 combined-modality regimen (5-FU/cisplatin ×4 with concurrent 5000 cGy) followed by a boost during cycle 3 of chemotherapy with either low-dose-rate (19 patients) or high-dose-rate (56 patients) intraluminal brachytherapy. The choice of the dose rate was at the discretion of the investigator. Owing to low accrual of patients, the low-dose-rate option was discontinued and the analysis was limited to patients who received the high-dose-rate treatment. High-dose-rate brachytherapy was delivered in weekly fractions of 500 cGy during weeks 8, 9, and 10. After the development of several fistulas, the fraction delivered at week 10 was discontinued.

The rate of complete response was 73%, but with a median follow-up of only 11 months, the rate of local failure as the first site of failure was 27%. Rates and levels of acute toxicity were 58% for grade III, 26% for grade IV, and 8% for grade V (treatment-related death). The cumulative incidence of fistula was 18% per year, and the crude incidence was 14%. Of the six treatment-related fistulas, three were fatal. Given the significant toxicity, this treatment approach should be used with caution.

The American Brachytherapy Society has developed guidelines for esophageal brachytherapy (Gaspar et al, 1997). For patients treated in the curative setting, brachytherapy should be limited to tumors 10 cm or smaller with no evidence of distant metastasis. Contraindications include tracheal or bronchial involvement, cervical esophagus location, and stenosis that cannot be bypassed. The applicator should have an external diameter of 6 to 10 cm. If combined-modality therapy is used (defined as 5-FU–based chemotherapy plus 4500–5000 cGy), the recommended doses of brachytherapy are (1) high dose rate, 1000 cGy in 2 weekly fractions of 500 cGy each or (2) low dose rate, 2000 cGy in a single fraction at 40 to 100 cGy/hr. The doses should be prescribed to 1 cm from the midsource. Lastly, brachytherapy should be delivered after the completion of external-beam irratiation and not concurrently with chemotherapy.

External-Beam Irradiation

Data examining the tolerance of external-beam irradiation doses of 6000 cGy or higher when delivered concurrently with chemotherapy are limited. In a toxicity analysis, Coia and associates (1991) reported results of combined chemotherapy and radiation therapy in 90 patients with clinical stages I to IV squamous cell carcinomas and adenocarcinomas of the esophagus. The incidence of grade III toxicity was 22% and of grade IV toxicity, 6%. There were no treatment-related deaths.

Calais and associates (1994) reported the results in 53 patients with clinically unresectable disease who received 5-FU–cisplatin–mitomycin C plus 6500 cGy. The full dose of radiation could be delivered in 96% of patients. The incidence of World Health Organization (WHO) grade III or higher toxicity was 30%, and the overall 2-year survival was 42%. The chemotherapy in this trial was not delivered at doses adequate to treat systemic disease.

On the encouraging side, almost all the patients in both INT 0122 and the Calais trials (96% and 94%, respectively) who started radiation therapy completed the full dose (6480–6500 cGy). Therefore, this higher dose of radiation was considered tolerable and is used in the experimental arm of the INT 0123 (RTOG 94-05). In this trial, patients with either squamous cell carcinomas or adenocarcinomas who are selected for a nonsurgical approach are randomly assigned to receive either a slightly modified RTOG 85-01 combined-modality regimen, with 5040 cGy or the same chemotherapy with 6480 cGy.

The modifications to the original RTOG 85-01 combined modality therapy arm include the following:

1. Use of 180 cGy fractions to 5040 cGy rather than 200 cGy fractions to 5000 cGy.
2. Treatment with 5 cm proximal and distal margins for 5040 cGy rather than treating the whole esophagus for the first 300 cGy followed by a "cone down" with 5 cm margins to 5000 cGy.
3. Cycle 3 of 5-FU/cisplatin, beginning only after 4 weeks after the completion of radiation therapy rather than 3 weeks.
4. Cycles 3 and 4 of chemotherapy delivered every 4 weeks rather than every 3 weeks.

INT 0123 opened in late 1994, and accrual is complete. A preliminary analysis suggests no improvement in local control with the increased 6480-cGy dose of radiotherapy.

TABLE 48–6 ■ **High-Dose Accelerated Fractionation or Hyperfractionated Combined-Modality Therapy: Selected Series**

Series	*No. of Patients*	*Treatment*	*Survival (%)*	*Toxicity*
Villejuif	88	6500 cGy ± 5-FU/CDDP before radiation	12 (3-year)	13% Gr 3 +
Kyoto	28	5400 cGy 5-FU/CDDP × 4	29 (5-year)	50% Gr 3 +

CDDP, *cis*-diaminedichloroplatinum; 5-FU, 5-fluorouracil.

In addition to increasing the total dose, radiation can be intensified by accelerated fractionation or hyperfractionation. Selected series using this approach are summarized in Table 48–6 (Girinsky et al, 1997; Jeremic et al, 1998; Powell et al, 1997). Although these approaches are reasonable, most series report an increase in acute toxicity without any clear therapeutic benefit. Therefore, these regimens remain investigational.

Palliation of Dysphagia with Nonsurgical Therapy

Dysphagia is a common problem in patients with esophageal cancer. It not only is the most common presenting symptom but also can remain a problem up to the time of the patient's death.

Major weaknesses of the series examining palliation are that they are retrospective and most do not use objective criteria to define and assess dysphagia. Some do not report the number of patients presenting with dysphagia or the percentage who experience palliation until the time of death. Furthermore, few series carefully examine other variables that may influence the results, such as histology, stage, and the location of the primary tumor.

As seen in Table 48–7, a limited number of series have examined the palliative benefits with either radiation alone (Caspers et al, 1988; Petrovich et al, 1991; Roussel et al, 1988; Wara et al, 1976; Whittington et al, 1990) or combined-modality therapy (Algan et al, 1995; Gill et al, 1992; Izquierdo et al, 1993; Seitz et al, 1990; Urba and Tumsi, 1995; Whittington et al, 1990). Overall, external-beam radiation therapy alone offers palliation of dysphagia in approximately 70% to 80% of patients.

The most comprehensive and carefully performed analysis of swallowing function in patients receiving combined-modality therapy is has reported by Coia and associates (1993). Using a swallowing score modified from that developed by O'Rourke and colleagues (1988), these researchers analyzed 102 patients treated with three 5-FU–based combined modality regimens. Prior to the start of therapy, 95% of patients had some degree of dysphagia. Within 2 weeks after the start of treatment, 45% experienced an improvement in dysphagia; by the completion of the 6-week therapy, 83% showed improvement; overall, 88% experienced an improvement. The median time to maximum improvement was 4 weeks (range, 1–21 weeks), and all but two patients could swallow at least soft or solid foods at the time of maximum symptomatic improvement.

TABLE 48–7 ■ **Palliation of Dysphagia with Radiation Therapy with or without Chemotherapy**

		*Palliation of Dysphagia**	
Series	*No. of Patients*	*At End of Treatment (%)*	*Duration of Palliation*
Radiation therapy alone			
Wara et al (1976)	103	89	6 months average
Petrovich et al (1991)	133	87	34% ≥ 6 months 18% ≥ 3 months 35% ≤ 3 months
Roussel et al (1988)	69	70	—
Caspers et al (1988)	127	71	54% until death
Whittington et al (1990)	25	—	5% at 9 months
Combined-modality therapy			
Coia et al (1993)	102	88	67–100% until death
Seitz et al (1990)	35	100†	—
Whittington et al (1990)	26	—	87% 3-year actuarial
Algan et al (1995)	8	100	—
Gill et al (1992)	71	60	—
Urba et al (1995)	27	—	59% until death
Izquierdo et al (1993)	25	64	Median 5 months

*See text for definition and number of patients presenting with dysphagia.
†Patients underwent dilation or laser therapy at the start of treatment.

Variables such as intent of treatment, histology, and tumor location were examined. All of the 25 patients treated with a curative intent who survived more than 1 year were able to eat soft or solid foods after treatment. The rate of *benign stricture* (a stricture in the absence of recurrent disease) was 12%. Of patients treated in the noncurative setting, 91% experienced an initial improvement in swallowing and 67% enjoyed palliation of dysphagia until the time of death.

Histology and stage had no impact of the rate of palliation. However, patients with lesions in the distal third of the esophagus had a significantly higher rate of improvement in dysphagia than those with tumors of the upper two thirds (95% versus 79%; $P < .05$).

Intraluminal brachytherapy is also an effective, albeit more limited, method of palliation. It achieves palliation of dysphagia in 40% to 90% of patients. (Moni et al, 1996; Sur et al, 1992). As previously discussed, because this therapy is usually prescribed to 1 cm from the source, it may undertreat gross disease. There is a selection bias against brachytherapy because it is commonly used either for patients in whom external-beam irradiation has failed or who cannot to travel for daily outpatient treatment. Even accounting for these selection biases, however, given its limited effective range, this modality is usually not as successful as external-beam irradiation in treating the entire tumor volume.

In summary, external-beam radiation therapy, either alone or in combination with chemotherapy, offers palliation of dysphagia in approximately 80% of patients, with half enjoying palliation until the time of death. If a patient requires rapid palliation (within a few days), alternative approaches, such as laser therapy or the use of a stent, are recommended. Although external-beam radiation with or without chemotherapy requires at least 2 weeks to obtain palliation, the palliation once achieved is more durable than that achieved with other palliative modalities because radiotherapy treats the problem (the gross tumor mass), not just the symptom. If external-beam radiation is not possible, brachytherapy should be considered.

Acute and Long-Term Toxicity of Nonsurgical Therapy

The toxicity of radiation therapy is a function of total dose, technique, and whether the patient has received chemotherapy. Toxicity data in patients who received conventional doses of radiation therapy are limited.

The most carefully documented data for acute radiation-related toxicity are from the control arm of RTOG 85-01, in which patients received radiation therapy alone to a dose of 6400 cGy (Al-Sarraf et al, 1997; Herskovic et al, 1992). The incidence of acute grade III toxicity was 25% and of grade IV toxicity, 3%. There were no treatment-related deaths.

As with surgery, radiation therapy can produce esophageal strictures. The total incidence of stricture (benign plus malignant) in patients receiving radiation therapy alone or combined with chemotherapy is 20% to 40% in modern series and up to 60% in historical series (Minsky, 1994). Almost half of these strictures are malignant because they are associated with a local recurrence of tumor. Furthermore, the incidence of stricture is lower when careful radiation techniques have been used. For example, Coia and associates (1993) examined a subset of 25 patients whose tumors were locally controlled and who survived at least 1 year. The incidence of benign stricture in this group was 12%.

One series examined the functional results in patients who experienced benign or malignant strictures (O'Rourke et al, 1988). Eighty patients received 4500 to 5600 cGy, and 53% received some form of chemotherapy. Of the 24 patients in whom a benign stricture developed (30%), 71% were able to tolerate a full or soft diet and required dilation, with a median interval between dilations of 5 months. Therefore, even in the subset of patients who experience a benign stricture, dilation is effective in most cases. In contrast, in the 28% of patients who had a malignant stricture, dilation was unsuccessful and esophageal intubation was required.

The high incidence of fistulas reported in the RTOG 92-07 trial of combined-modality therapy plus intraluminal brachytherapy (18% actuarial, 14% crude) has not been reported in series using radiation therapy or combined-modality therapy without intraluminal brachytherapy. The incidence of other long-term grade III or higher toxicities, such as pneumonitis or pericarditis, is 5%. If appropriate radiation doses and techniques are used, spinal cord myelitis should not occur.

Treatment-Related Deaths

The issue of treatment-related deaths in patients receiving combined-modality therapy in Intergroup Trials is complex. Although the incidence was only 2% in RTOG 85-01, subsequent trials have reported a higher treatment-related mortality rate (i.e., 9% in INT 0122, and 8% in RTOG 92-07). These mortality rates are lower than the 10% to 15% reported in the historical surgical series, although only slightly higher than the 6% reported in the surgical control arm of INT 0113. It is interesting to note that as the mortality rate for surgery has decreased, there has been a corresponding increase in the treatment-related mortality rate reported in the nonoperative trials. As previously discussed, this trend may be related, in part, to selection bias against patients treated with the nonoperative approach. Only a randomized trial of surgical versus nonsurgical therapy can address this issue.

SURGICAL THERAPY

Like results of radiation therapy alone, most of the results reported for surgery alone are from historical series. Surgical trials report 5-year survivals of 5% to 20%. The results of the surgical control arms from two randomized trials of preoperative chemotherapy in patients with clinically resectable disease offer a more accurate assessment of results. In these trials, patients underwent an Ivor Lewis or transhiatal esophagectomy.

In the Dutch trial of preoperative chemotherapy reported by Kok and associates (1996), the 160 patients in the surgical control arm had a median survival of 11 months. Similar results were reported in the 234 patients

(110 with squamous cell carcinoma and 124 with adenocarcinoma) in the surgical control arm of INT 0113 (RTOG 89-11) (Kelsen et al, 1998). The operative mortality rate was 6%. With a median follow-up of 55 months, the median survival was 16 months, the 5-year survival was 20%, and the incidence of local failure as the first site of failure in the 59% of patients who underwent a complete resection with negative margins (R-O resection) was 31%.

Some surgeons, primarily based in Japan, advocate a three-field dissection rather than a more conventional Ivor Lewis or transhiatal esophagectomy. With this unusually aggressive surgical approach, regardless of the location of the primary tumor, patients undergo dissection of the lymph nodes in the neck, mediastinum, and celiac axis. In a report by Bhansali and colleagues (1997), of 90 patients with squamous cell cancers (57% of whom received preoperative chemotherapy or radiation therapy), the 5-year survival was 39%. However, the local failure rate was still 72%, and there was high incidence of postoperative complications (i.e., 74% for recurrent laryngeal nerve paralysis, 32% for anastomotic leak, 26% for aspiration pneumonia). Nishimaki and associates (1998) reported a 58% morbidity rate in 190 patients treated with this technique. In summary, most investigators outside Japan do not advocate for this more aggressive surgical approach.

COMPARISON OF NONSURGICAL THERAPY AND SURGICAL THERAPY

Because of the selection bias favoring surgery, by which patients have clinically resectable disease and are medically fit for an operation, it is difficult to compare the results of nonsurgical and surgical approaches in the absence of a randomized trial. Despite the adverse selection factors, a comparison of the results of these respective treatment approaches from the national Intergroup Trials reveals that the nonsurgical approaches offer a survival rate the same as, if not better than, that for surgery as well as an improvement in palliation of dysphagia.

For example, the median and 5-year survivals were 14 months and 27%, respectively, in the combined-modality therapy arm of RTOG 85-01 and 20 months and 20%, respectively, in INT 0122. In comparison, the median survival in the surgical control arm of the Dutch trial reported by Kok and associates (1996) was 11 months, and the median and 5-year survivals in the surgical control arm of INT 0113 were 16 months and 20%, respectively; likewise, local failure rates were similar. The incidence of local failure (local failure plus local persistence of disease) as the first site of failure was 45% in RTOG 85-01 and 39% in INT 0122. Although local failure as the first site of failure in INT 0113 was 31%, this analysis was limited to patients who underwent a complete resection with negative margins (R-O resection). An additional 30% of patients had residual local disease; therefore, if one were to score these patients as having local persistent disease (as in the RTOG 85-01 analysis), the comparable local failure rate with surgery alone would be 30% plus 31%, or 61%. The treatment-related mortality rates were also similar (2% in RTOG 85-01, 9% in INT 0122, and 6% in INT 0113).

In summary, the rates of local failure, survival, and treatment-related mortality are similar for nonsurgical and surgical therapies. Although the results are comparable, it is clear that both nonsurgical and surgical approaches have limited success. Therefore, trials that have combined the two approaches (surgery plus preoperative or postoperative adjuvant therapy) have been developed.

SMALL CELL CARCINOMA

Small cell carcinoma of the esophagus is an uncommon histologic subtype of esophageal carcinoma, with fewer than 100 cases reported in the literature. The incidence ranges from less than 1% to 3% of cases of esophageal cancer diagnosed (Nichols and Kelsen, 1989; Saito et al, 1992; Tateishi et al, 1976). Staging of small cell carcinoma of the esophagus is similar to that of small cell carcinoma of the lung, with *limited-stage disease* defined as local-regional disease with or without local regional lymph node involvement. *Extensive-stage disease* is defined as distant metastatic disease outside the local-regional area. As in small cell carcinoma in the lung, there is a clear association between development of the disease in the esophagus with tobacco use, and distant metastatic disease is frequently present at diagnosis. Also, like small cell cancer of the lung, esophageal small cell carcinoma appears to be highly responsive to radiotherapy and to a broad spectrum of chemotherapeutic agents (Nichols and Kelsen, 1989; Remick and Ruckdeschel, 1992).

The almost universal development of metastatic disease in small cell carcinoma of the esophagus has led to the general acceptance of chemotherapy as part of combined-modality therapy in the treatment of small cell carcinoma of the esophagus. However, despite treatment of limited-stage disease with a combination of chemotherapy and surgery and or radiotherapy, reports of long-term survivors with small cell carcinoma of the esophagus are anecdotal. Median survival of patients with small cell carcinoma of the esophagus ranges from 3 months to 7.5 months. For local control of disease, it seems more logical to use radiotherapy rather than to subject the patient to the risks associated with esophagectomy. However, the appropriate role of surgery or radiotherapy for control of the primary tumor remains to be established.

COMMENTS AND CONTROVERSIES

To the surgeon, a recitation of the numerous chemotherapy and radiotherapy protocols for treating a particular type of cancer can be mind-numbing, leaving the surgeon with little appreciation for the subtle nuances of differences between various protocols. However, the preceding exhaustive almost encyclopedic catalog of the various clinical trials and treatments for esophageal cancer is well organized and gives insight into the difficulties of conducting and evaluating clinical trials. The chapter conveys the step-by-step approach required for making and recognizing progress, and the specifics of the various protocols are perhaps less important than an understanding of the process. The chapter also illustrates the difficulties in interpreting trial results and the importance of randomized clinical trials in defining what is real from what is apparent. One of the main difficulties in conducting clinical trials relates to the task of accurately staging esophageal cancer from a clinical standpoint. The availability of small-diameter endoscopic ultrasound probes, combined with the use of computed tomography and positron emission tomography, now permits much more accurate staging.

The authors of the chapter note that in terms of local failure rate, survival rate, and treatment-related mortality, there is little difference between surgical and nonsurgical treatment modalities for esophageal cancer—probably because most cases of esophageal cancer are discovered at a late stage. However, with improved detection of early-stage esophageal cancer and the declining mortality rate for esophagectomy, surgical resection coupled with adjuvant therapy will continue to be the mainstay of treatment. With improved staging techniques, many patients who formerly would have been selected for surgical therapy may now be considered candidates for nonsurgical treatment on the basis of an identification of more advanced tumor stage.

J. D. C.

■ REFERENCES

Advani SH, Saikia TK, Swaroop S, et al: Anterior chemotherapy in esophageal cancer. Cancer 56:1502–1506, 1985.

Ajani J, Ilson D, Daugherty K, et al: Activity of taxol in patients with squamous cell carcinoma and adenocarcinoma of the esophagus. J Natl Cancer Inst 86:1086–1091, 1994.

Ajani J, Kantarjian H, Kanojia M, et al: Phase II trial of *cis*-platinum in advanced upper gastrointestinal cancer (abstract). Proc Am Soc Clin Oncol 2:147, 1984.

Ajani JA, Roth JA, Ryan B, et al: Evaluation of pre- and postoperative chemotherapy for resectable adenocarcinoma of the esophagus or gastroesophageal junction. J Clin Oncol 8:1231–1238, 1990.

Ajani J, Roth J, Ryan B, et al: High-dose chemotherapy with GM-CSF for resectable adenocarcinoma of the esophagus (ACE) (Meeting Abstract). Proceedings of the American Society of Clinical Oncology, Vol 10, 1991, p A472.

Ajani JA, Ryan B, Rich TA, et al: Prolonged chemotherapy for localised squamous carcinoma of the oesophagus. Eur J Cancer 28A:880–884, 1992.

Alberts AS, Schoeman L, Burger W, et al: A phase II study of 5-fluorouracil and leucovorin in advanced carcinoma of the esophagus. Am J Clin Oncol 15:35–36, 1992.

Algan O, Coia LR, Keller SM, et al: Management of adenocarcinoma of the esophagus with chemoradiation alone or chemoradiation followed by esophagectomy: Results of sequential nonrandomized phase II studies. Int J Radiat Oncol Biol Phys 32:753–761, 1995.

Al-Sarraf M, Martz K, Herskovic A, et al: Superiority of chemoradiotherapy (CT-RT) vs radiotherapy (RT) in patients with esophageal cancer. Final report of an Intergroup Randomized and Confirmed Study (Abstract). Proceedings of the American Society of Clinical Oncology, Vol 15, 1996, p 206.

Al-Sarraf M, Martz K, Herskovic A, et al: Progress report of combined chemoradiotherapy versus radiotherapy alone in patients with esophageal cancer: An intergroup study. J Clin Oncol 15:277–284, 1997.

Anderson I, Ladd T: Autopsy findings in squamous cell carcinoma of the esophagus. Cancer 50:1587–1590, 1982.

Ansell SM, Alberts AS, Falkson G: Ifosfamide in advanced carcinoma of the esophagus: A phase II trial with severe toxicity. Am J Clin Oncol 12:205–207, 1989.

Araujo CMM, Souhami L, Gil RA, et al: A randomized trial comparing radiation therapy versus concomitant radiation therapy and chemotherapy in carcinoma of the thoracic esophagus. Cancer 67:2258–2261, 1991.

Armstrong JG: High dose rate remote afterloading brachytherapy for lung and esophageal cancer. Semin Radiat Oncol 4:270–277, 1993.

Baselga J, Norton L, Albanell J, et al: Recombinant humanized anti-HER2 antibody (Herceptin) enhances the antitumor activity of paclitaxel and doxorubicin against HER2/neu overexpressing human breast cancer xenografts. Cancer Res 58:2825–2831, 1998.

Bedikian A, Valdivieso M, Bodey G, et al: Phae II evaluation of vindesine in the treatment of colorectal and esophageal tumors. Cancer Chemother Pharmacol 2:263, 1979.

Bedikian AY, Deniord R, El-Akkak S: Value of pre-op chemotherapy for esophageal carcinoma (Meeting Abstract). Proceedings of the American Society of Clinical Oncology, Vol 6, 1987, p A375.

Bezwoda WR, Derman DP, Weaving A, et al: Treatment of esophageal cancer with vindesine: An open trial. Cancer Treat Rep 68:783–785, 1984.

Bhalla KN, Kumar GN, Walle T, et al: Phase I and pharmacokinetic trial of a 3 hour infusion of taxol, cisplatin plus 5-fluorouracil in advanced solid tumors (Abstract). Proceedings of the American Society of Clinical Oncology, Vol 13, 1994, p 165.

Bhansali MS, Fujita H, Kakegawa T, et al: Pattern of recurrence after extended radical esophagectomy with three-field lymph node dissection for squamous cell carcinoma in the thoracic esophagus. World J Surg 21:275–281, 1997.

Bleiberg H, Conroy T, Paillot B, et al: Randomized phase II study of cisplatin and 5-FU versus cisplatin alone in advanced squamous cell oesophageal cancer. Eur J Cancer 33:1216–1220, 1997.

Bleiberg H, de Gramont A: Oxaliplatin plus 5-fluorouracil: Clinical experience in patients with advanced colorectal cancer. Semin Oncol 25:32–39, 1998.

Bleiberg H, Jacob JH, Bedenne L, et al: Randomized phase II trial of 5-fluorouracil (5FU) and cisplatin (DDP) vs DDP alone in advanced esophageal cancer (Meeting Abstract). Proceedings of the American Society of Clinical Oncology, Vol 10, 1991, p A447.

Bonadonna G, De Lena M, Monfardini S, et al: Clinical trials with bleomycin in lymphomas and in solid tumors. Eur J Cancer 8:205–215, 1972.

Bosch A, Frias Z, Pellett JR: Carcinoma of the esophagus: Twenty-five years' experience at the University of Wisconsin Hospitals. Wisconsin Med J 79:23–26, 1980.

Bosset J, Hurteloup P, Bontemas P, et al: A phase II trial of bleomycin and cisplatin in advanced esophagus carcinoma (Abstract). Proceedings of the 13th International Cancer Congress, Vol 41, 1983.

Boynton RF, Huang Y, Blount PL, et al: Frequent loss of heterozygosity at the retinoblastoma locus in human esophageal cancers. Cancer Res 51:5766–5769, 1991.

Braybrooke JP, O'Byrne KJ, Saunders MP, et al: A phase II study of mitomycin C and oral etoposide for advanced adenocarcinoma of the upper gastrointestinal tract. Ann Oncol 8:294–296, 1997.

Bromer R, Abbruzzese J, Karp D, et al: Ineffectiveness of cisplatin-bleomycin induction chemotherapy for esophageal cancer (Abstract). Proceedings of the American Society of Clinical Oncology, Vol. 3, 1984, p 143.

Burton GV, Wolfe WG, Crocker IR, et al: Esophageal carcinoma: Response to cisplatin and etoposide chemotherapy (Meeting Abstract). Proceedings of the American Society of Clinical Oncology, Vol 5, 1986, p 86.

Calais G, Dorval E, Louisot P, et al: Radiotherapy with high dose rate brachytherapy boost and concomitant chemotherapy for stages IIB and III esophageal carcinoma: Results of a pilot study. Int J Radiat Oncol Biol Phys 38:769–775, 1997.

Calais G, Jadaud E, Chapet S, et al: High dose radiotherapy (RT) and concomitant chemotherapy for nonresectable esophageal cancer: Results of a phase II study (Abstract). Proceedings of the American Society of Clinical Oncology, Vol 13, 1994, p 197.

Caspers RJL, Welvaart K, Verkes RJ, et al: The effect of radiotherapy on dysphagia and survival in patients with esophageal cancer. Radiother Oncol 12:15–23, 1988.

Caspers RJL, Zwinderman AH, Griffioen G, et al: Combined external beam and low dose rate intraluminal radiotherapy in oesophageal cancer. Radiother Oncol 27:7–12, 1993.

Casson AG, Mukhopadhyay T, Clear KR, et al: p53 gene mutations in Barrett's epithelium and esophageal cancer. Cancer Res 51:4495–4499, 1991.

Chan KW, Chan EY, Chan CW: Carcinoma of the esophagus: An autopsy study of 231 cases. Pathology 18:400–405, 1986.

Chapman R, Fleming TR, Van Damme J, et al: Cisplatin, vinblastine, and mitoguazone in squamous cell carcinoma of the esophagus: A Southwest Oncology Group Study. Cancer Treat Rep 71:1185–1187, 1987.

Charlois T, Burtin P, Ben-Bouali AK, et al: Predictive factors of response to chemotherapy for esophageal squamous cell carcinoma: Study of 60 patients and proposal of a response score. Gastroenterol Clin Biol 16:134–140, 1992.

Chow WH, Blot WJ, Vaughan TL, et al: Body mass index and risk of adenocarcinomas of the esophagus and gastric cardia. J Natl Cancer Inst 90:150–155, 1998.

Clinical Screening Group: Study of the clinical efficiency of bleomycin in human cancer. Br Med J 2:643–645, 1970.

Coia LR, Engstrom PF, Paul AR, et al: Long-term results of infusional 5-FU, mitomycin-C, and radiation as primary management of esophageal cancer. Int J Radiat Oncol Biol Phys 20:29–36, 1991.

Coia LR, Soffen EM, Schultheiss TE, et al: Swallowing function in patients with esophageal cancer treated with concurrent radiation and chemotherapy. Cancer 71:281–286, 1993.

Conroy T, Etienne PL, Adenis A, et al: Phase II trial of vinorelbine in metastatic squamous cell esophageal carcinoma. J Clin Oncol 14:164–170, 1996.

Coonley CJ, Bains M, Heelan R, et al: Phase II study of etoposide in the treatment of esophageal carcinoma. Cancer Treat Rep 67:397–398, 1983.

Coonley CJ, Bains M, Hilaris B, et al: Cisplatin and bleomycin in the treatment of esophageal carcinoma: A final report. Cancer 54:2351–2355, 1984.

Costa F, Ilson D, Forastiere A, et al: Phase II study of paclitaxel and cisplatin in patients with advanced adenocarcinoma (A) and squamous cell (S) carcinoma of the esophagus (Abstract). Proceedings of the American Society of Clinical Oncology, Vol 16, 1997, p 262a.

Cure H, Pezet D, Slim K, et al: High response rate in non-operable esophageal cancer with a neoadjuvant chemotherapy using carboplatin, cisplatin and 5-fluorouracil. Proceedings of the American Society of Clinical Oncology, Vol 12, 1993, p A574.

Davis S, Shanmugathasa M, Kessler W: *cis*-Dichlorodiammineplatinum (II) in the treatment of esophageal carcinoma. Cancer Treat Rep 64:709–711, 1980.

De Besi P, Salvagno L, Endrizzi L, et al: Cisplatin, bleomycin and methotrexate in the treatment of advanced oesophageal cancer. Eur J Cancer Clin Oncol 20:743–747, 1984.

De Besi P, Sileni VC, Salvagno L, et al: Phase II study of cisplatin, 5-FU, and allopurinol in advanced esophageal cancer. Cancer Treat Rep 70:909–910, 1986.

De-Ren S: Ten-year follow-up of esophageal cancer treated by radical radiation therapy: Analysis of 869 patients. Int J Radiat Oncol Biol Phys 16:329–334, 1989.

Desai P, Borges E, Vohrs V, et al: Carcinoma of the esophagus in India. Cancer 23:979–989, 1969.

Devesa SS, Blot WJ, Fraumeni JF Jr. Changing patterns in the incidence of esophageal and gastric carcinoma in the United States. Cancer 83:2049–2053, 1998.

Dinwoodie WR, Bartolucci AA, Lyman GH, et al: Phase II evaluation of cisplatin, bleomycin, and vindesine in advanced squamous cell carcinoma of the esophagus: A Southeastern Cancer Study Group Trial. Cancer Treat Rep 70:267–270, 1986.

Earlam R, Cunha-Melo JR: Oesophageal squamous cell carcinoma: I. A critical review of surgery. Br J Surg 67:381–390, 1980a.

Earlam R, Cunha-Melo JR: Oesophageal squamous cell carcinoma: II. A critical view of radiotherapy. Br J Surg 67:457–461, 1980b.

Einzig A, Kelsen DP, Cheng E, et al: Phase II trial of carboplatin in patients with adenocarcinomas of the upper gastrointestinal tract. Cancer Treat Rep 69:1453–1454, 1985.

Einzig AI, Neuberg D, Remick SC, et al: Phase II trial of docetaxel (Taxotere) in patients with adenocarcinoma of the upper gastrointestinal tract previously untreated with cytotoxic chemotherapy: The Eastern Cooperative Oncology Group (ECOG) results of protocol E1293. Med Oncol 13:87–93, 1996.

El Akkad S, Amer M, Kerth W: Combination chemotherapy, surgery, and radiotherapy for esophageal cancer. Proceedings of the 13th International Cancer Congress, Vol 40, 1983.

Engstrom PF, Lavin PT, Klaassen DJ: Phase II evaluation of mitomycin and cisplatin in advanced esophageal carcinoma. Cancer Treat Rep 67:713–715, 1983.

Enzinger PC, Ilson DH, Saltz LB: Phase II clinical trial of 13-*cis*-retinoic acid and interferon alpha-2a for patients with advanced esophageal carcinoma. Cancer 85:1213–1217, 1999.

Ezdinli EZ, Gelber R, Desai DV, et al: Chemotherapy of advanced esophageal carcinoma: Eastern Cooperative Oncology Group experience. Cancer 46:2149–2153, 1980.

Falkson G: Methyl-GAG (NSC 32946) in the treatment of esophageal cancer. Cancer Chemother Rep 55:209–212, 1971.

Forastiere AA, Gennis M, Orringer MB, et al: Cisplatin, vinblastine, and mitoguazone chemotherapy for epidermoid and adenocarcinoma of the esophagus. J Clin Oncol 5:1143–1149, 1987.

Forastiere A, Patel H, Hankins J, et al: Cisplatin, bleomycin and VP-16-213 in combination for epidermoid carcinoma of the esophagus. Proceedings of the American Society of Clinical Oncology, Vol 2, 1983, p A127.

Gammon MD, Schoenberg JB, Ahsan H, et al: Tobacco, alcohol, and socioeconomic status and adenocarcinomas of the esophagus and gastric cardia. J Natl Cancer Inst 89:1277, 1997.

Garcia-Alfonso P, Guevara S, Lopez P, et al: Taxol and cisplatin + 5-fluorouracil sequential in advanced esophageal cancer (Abstract). Proceedings of the American Society of Clinical Oncology, Vol 17, 1988, p 998.

Gaspar LE, Nag S, Herskovic A, et al: American Brachytherapy Society (ABS) consensus guidelines for brachytherapy of esophageal cancer. Int J Radiat Oncol Biol Phys 38:127–132, 1997.

Gaspar LE, Qian C, Kocha WI, et al: A phase I/II study of external beam radiation, brachytherapy and concurrent chemotherapy in localized cancer of the esophagus (RTOG 92-07): Preliminary toxicity report. Int J Radiat Oncol Biol Phys 37:593–599, 1997.

Gill PG, Denham JW, Jamieson GG, et al: Patterns of treatment failure and prognostic factors associated with the treatment of esophageal carcinoma with chemotherapy and radiotherapy either as sole treatment of followed by surgery. J Clin Oncol 10:1037–1043, 1992.

Girinsky T, Auperin A, Marsiglia H, et al: Accelerated fractionation in esophageal cancers: A multivariate analysis on 88 patients. Int J Radiat Oncol Biol Phys 38:1013–1018, 1997.

Gisselbrecht C, Calvo F, Mignot L, et al: Fluorouracil (F), Adriamycin (A), and cisplatin (P) (FAP): Combination chemotherapy of advanced esophageal carcinoma. Cancer 52:974–977, 1983.

Harstrick A, Bokemeyer C, Preusser P, et al: Phase II study of single-agent etoposide in patients with metastatic squamous-cell carcinoma of the esophagus. Cancer Chemother Pharmacol 29:321–322, 1992.

Hayashi K, Ide H, Shinoda M, et al: Phase II study of cisplatin (CDDP) plus 5-fluorouracil (5-FU) and leucovorin (LCV) for squamous cell carcinoma (SCC) of the esophagus (Meeting Abstract). Proceedings of the American Society of Clinical Oncology, Vol 11, 1992, p A526.

Herskovic A, Martz LK, Al-Sarraf M, et al: Combined chemotherapy and radiotherapy compared with radiotherapy alone in patients with cancer of the esophagus. N Engl J Med 326:1593–1598, 1992.

Hilgenberg AD, Carey RW, Wilkins EW Jr, et al: Preoperative chemotherapy, surgical resection, and selective postoperative therapy for squamous cell carcinoma of the esophagus. Ann Thorac Surg 45:357–363, 1988.

Hoffman P, Vokes E, Ferguson M, et al: Induction chemotherapy, surgery and concomitant chemoradiotherapy for carcinoma of the esophagus (Meeting Abstract). Proceedings of the American Society of Clinical Oncology, Vol II, 1992, p A588.

Hollstein MC, Mewtcalf RA, Welsh JA, et al: Frequent mutation of the p53 gene in human esophageal cancer. Proc Natl Acad Sci U S A 87:9958–9961, 1990.

Hollstein MC, Smits AM, Galiana C, et al: Amplification of epidermal growth factor receptor gene but no evidence of *ras* mutations in primary human esophageal cancers. Cancer Res 48:5119–5123, 1988.

Ilson DH, Ajani J, Bhalla K, et al: Phase II trial of paclitaxel, fluorouracil, and cisplatin in patients with advanced carcinoma of the esophagus. J Clin Oncol 16:1826–1834, 1998.

Ilson D, Kelsen D: Chemotherapy in esophageal cancer. Anticancer Drugs 4:287–299, 1993.

Ilson DH, Saltz L, Enzinger P, et al: A Phase II trial of weekly irinotecan plus cisplatin in advanced esophageal cancer. J Clin Oncol 17:3270–3275, 1999.

Ilson DH, Sirott M, Saltz L, et al: A Phase II trial of interferon alpha-2A, 5-fluorouracil, and cisplatin in patients with advanced esophageal carcinoma. Cancer 75:2197–2202, 1995.

Iop A, Cartei E, Vigevani E, et al: Combination chemotherapy (mitomycin C, cisplatin, 5-fluorouracil) in poor prognosis squamous cell carcinomas. Proceedings of the American Society of Clinical Oncology, Vol 15, 1996, p 900.

Izquierdo MA, Marcuello E, Gomez de Segura G, et al: Unresectable nonmetastatic squamous cell carcinoma of the esophagus managed by sequential chemotherapy (cisplatin and bleomycin) and radiation therapy. Cancer 71:287–292, 1993.

Jager J, Langendijk H, Pannebakker M, et al: A single session of intraluminal brachytherapy in palliation of esophageal cancer. Radiother Oncol 37:237–240, 1995.

Jankowski J, Coghill G, Hopwood D, et al: Oncogenes and oncosuppressor gene in adenocarcinoma of the oesophagus. Gut 33:1033–1038, 1992.

Jeremic B, Shibamoto Y, Acimovic L, et al: Accelerated hyperfractionated radiation therapy and concurrent 5-fluorouracil/cisplatin chemotherapy for locoregional squamous cell carcinoma of the thoracic esophagus: A phase II study. Int J Radiat Oncol Biol Phys 40:1061–1066, 1998.

Jiang W, Kahn SM, Tomita N, et al: Amplification and expression of the human cyclin D gene in esophageal cancer. Cancer Res 52:2980–2983, 1992.

John MJ, Flam M, Ager Mowry PA, et al: Radiotherapy alone and chemoradiation for nonmetastatic esophageal carcinoma. Cancer 63:2397–2403, 1989.

Kaubisch A, Kelsen DP, Saltz L, et al: A phase I trial of weekly sequential bryostatin-1 (BRYO) and paclitaxel in patients with advanced solid tumors (Abstract). Proceedings of the American Society of Clinical Oncology, Vol 18, 1999, p 166a.

Kawamura H, Terashima M, Ikeda K, et al: Antitumor activities of Taxotere and Taxol against human esophageal cancer (Abstract). Proceedings of the Annual Meeting of the American Association for Cancer Research, Vol 38, 1997, p A1540.

Kelsen DP, Bains MS, Cvitkovic E, et al: Vindesine in the treatment of esophageal carcinoma. A phase II study. Cancer Treat Rep 63:2019–2021, 1979.

Kelsen D, Chapman R, Bains M, et al: Phase II study of methyl-GAG in the treatment of esophageal carcinoma. Cancer Treat Rep 66:1427–1429, 1982.

Kelsen DP, Fein R, Coonley C, et al: Cisplatin, vindesine, and mitoguazone in the treatment of esophageal cancer. Cancer Treat Rep 70:255–259, 1986.

Kelsen DP, Ginsberg R, Pajak TF, et al: Chemotherapy followed by surgery compared with surgery alone for localized esophageal cancer. New Engl J Med 339:1979–1984, 1998.

Kelsen D, Hilaris B, Coonley C, et al: Cisplatin, vindesine, and bleomycin chemotherapy of local-regional and advanced esophageal carcinoma. Am J Med 75:645–652, 1983a.

Kelsen D, Ilson D, Lipton R, et al: A phase I trial of radiation therapy (RT) plus concurrent fixed dose cisplatin (C) with escalating doses of paclitaxel (P) as a 96-hour continuous infusion in patients (PTS) with localized esophageal cancer (EC) (Abstract 1039). Proceedings of the American Society of Clinical Oncology, Vol 18, 1999.

Kelsen D, Lovett D, Wong J, et al: Interferon alfa-2a and fluorouracil in the treatment of patients with advanced esophageal cancer. J Clin Oncol 10:269–274, 1992.

Kelsen DP, Magill GB, Cheng E, et al: Phase II trial of etoposide in adenocarcinomas of the upper gastrointestinal tract. Cancer Treat Rep 67:509–510, 1983b.

Kelsen DP, Minsky B, Smith M, et al: Preoperative therapy for esophageal cancer: A randomized comparison of chemotherapy versus radiation therapy. J Clin Oncol 8:1352–1361, 1990.

Kies MS, Rosen ST, Tsang TK, et al: Cisplatin and 5-fluorouracil in the primary management of squamous esophageal cancer. Cancer 60:2156–2160, 1987.

Kmet J, Mahoubi E: Esophageal cancer in the Caspian littoral of Iran: Initial studies. Science 175:846–853, 1972.

Kok TC, Janschot JV, Siersema PD: Neoadjuvant chemotherapy in operable esophageal squamous cell cancer: Final report of a randomized controlled trial. Rotterdam Esophageal Tumor Study Group. European Organization for Research and Treatment of Cancer (EORTC) Gastrointestinal Symposium, 1996.

Kok TC, van der Gaast A, Dees J, et al: Cisplatin and etoposide in oesophageal cancer: A phase II study. Br J Cancer 76:980–984, 1996.

Kok TC, van der Gaast A, Kerfhofs L, et al: Biweekly administration of cisplatin and increasing doses of paclitaxel in patients with advanced esophageal cancer (Abstract). Proceedings of the American Society of Clinical Oncology, Vol 17, 1997a, p 997.

Kok TC, van der Gaast A, Splinter TAW: 13-*cis*-Retinoic acid and alpha-interferon in advanced squamous cell cancer of the oesophagus (Letter). Eur J Cancer 33:165–166, 1997.

Kolaric K, Maricic Z, Dujmovic I, et al: Therapy of advanced esophageal cancer with bleomycin, irradiation and combination bleomycin and irradiation. Tumori 62:255–262, 1976.

Kolaric K, Maricic Z, Roth A, et al: Adriamycin alone and in combination with radiotherapy in the treatment of inoperable esophageal cancer. Tumori 63:485–491, 1977.

Kolaric K, Maricic Z, Roth A, et al: Combination of bleomycin and Adriamycin with and without radiation in the treatment of inoperable esophageal cancer: A randomized study. Cancer 45:2265–2273, 1980.

Lagergren J, Bergstrom R, Lindgren A, et al: Symptomatic gastroesophageal reflux as a risk factor for esophageal adenocarcinoma. Engl J Med 340:825–831, 1999.

Landis SH, Murray T, Bolden S, et al: Cancer Statistics, 1999. CA Cancer J Clin 49:8–31, 1999.

Lenz HJ, Leichman CG, Danenberg KD, et al: Thymidylate synthase mRNA level in adenocarcinoma of the stomach: A predictor for primary tumor response and overall survival. J Clin Oncol 14:176–182, 1996.

Lokich JJ, Shea M, Chaffey J: Sequential infusional 5-fluorouracil followed by concomitant radiation for tumors of the esophagus and gastroesophageal junction. Cancer 60:275–279, 1987.

Lu SH, Hsieh LL, Luo FC, et al: Amplification of the EGF receptor and *c-myc* genes in human esophageal cancers. Int J Cancer 42:502–505, 1988.

Mandard AM, Chasle J, Marnay J, et al: Autopsy findings in 111 cases of esophageal cancer. Cancer 48:329–335, 1981.

Mannell A, Winters Z: Carboplatin in the treatment of oesophageal cancer. S Afr Med J 76:213–214, 1989.

McGlashan ND: Esophageal cancer and alcoholic spirits in central Africa. Gut 10:643, 1969.

Mendelsohn J: Epidermal growth factor receptor inhibition by a monoclonal antibody as anticancer therapy. Clin Cancer Res 3 (12 Pt 2):2703–2707, 1997.

Minsky BD: Radiation therapy in the treatment of esophagus cancer. Chest Surg Clin North Am 4:285–297, 1994.

Minsky BD, Neuberg D, Kelsen DP, et al: Final report of Intergroup Trial 0122 (ECOG PE-289, RTOG 90-12): Phase II trial of neoadjuvant chemotherapy plus concurrent chemotherapy and high-dose radiation for squamous cell carcinoma of the esophagus. Int J Radiat Oncol Biol Phys 43:517–523, 1999.

Moertel C, Schutt A, Reitemeier R, et al: Therapy for gastrointestinal cancer with the nitrosoureas alone in drug combination. Cancer Treat Rep 60:729, 1976.

Moni J, Armstrong JG, Minsky BD, et al: High dose rate intraluminal brachytherapy for carcinoma of the esophagus. Dis Esophagus 9:123–127, 1996.

Mukaida H, Toi M, Hirai T, et al: Clinical significance of the expression of epidermal growth factor and its receptor in esophageal cancer. Cancer 68:142–148, 1991.

Muller JM, Erasmi H, Stelzner M, et al: Surgical therapy of oesophageal carcinoma. Br J Surg 77:845–857, 1990.

Murthy SK, Prabhakaran PS, Chandrashekar M, et al: Neoadjuvant *cis*-DDP in esophageal cancers: An experience at a regional cancer centre, India. J Surg Oncol 45:173–176, 1990.

Nanus DM, Kelsen DP, Niedzwiecki D, et al: Flow cytometry as a predictive indicator in patients with operable gastric cancer. J Clin Oncol 7:1105–1112, 1989.

Newaishy GA, Read GA, Duncan W, et al: Results of radical radiotherapy of squamous cell carcinoma of the esophagus. Clin Radiol 33:347–352, 1982.

Nichols GL, Kelsen DP: Small cell carcinoma of the esophagus: The Memorial Hospital experience 1970 to 1987. Cancer 64:1531–1533, 1989.

Nishimaki T, Suzuki T, Suzuki S, et al: Outcomes of extended radical esophagectomy for thoracic esophageal cancer. J Am Coll Surg 186:306–312, 1998.

Nygaard K, Hagen S, Hansen HS, et al: Pre-operative radiotherapy prolongs survival in operable esophageal carcinoma: A randomized, multicenter study of pre-operative radiotherapy and chemotherapy. The second Scandinavian trial in esophageal cancer. World J Surg 16:1104–1110, 1992.

Okawa T, Kita M, Tanaka M, et al: Results of radiotherapy for inoperable locally advanced esophageal cancer. Int J Radiat Oncol Biol Phys 17:49–54, 1989.

O'Rourke IC, Tiver K, Bull C, et al: Swallowing performance after radiation therapy for carcinoma of the esophagus. Cancer 61:2022–2026, 1988.

Pai C, Bazarbashi S, Rahal M, et al: Phase II study of cisplatin, 5-fluorouracil and interferon alpha-2b in advanced metastatic epidermoid esophageal carcinoma (Abstract). Proceedings of the American Society of Clinical Oncology, Vol 17, 1998, p 1158.

Panettiere FJ, Leichman L, O'Bryan R, et al: *Cis*-diamminedichloride platinum(II), an effective agent in the treatment of epidermoid carcinoma of the esophagus: A preliminary report of an ongoing Southwest Oncology Group study. Cancer Clin Trials 4:29–31, 1981.

Panettiere FJ, Leichman LP, Tilchen EJ, et al: Chemotherapy for advanced epidermoid carcinoma of the esophagus with single-agent cisplatin: Final report on a Southwest Oncology Group study. Cancer Treat Rep 68:1023–1024, 1984.

Petrasch S, Welt A, Reinacher A, et al: Chemotherapy with cisplatin and paclitaxel in patients with locally advanced, recurrent or metastatic oesophageal cancer. Br J Cancer 78:511–514, 1998.

Petrovich Z, Langholz B, Formenti S, et al: Management of carcinoma of the esophagus: The role of radiotherapy. Am J Clin Oncol 14:80–86, 1991.

Philip PA, Gadgeel S, Hussain M, et al: Phase II study of paclitaxel and carboplatin in patients with advanced gastric and esophageal cancers (Abstract). Proceedings of the American Society of Clinical Oncology, Vol 17, 1998, p 1001.

Popkin J, Bromer R, Bryne R, et al: Continuous 48-hour infusion of vindesine in squamous cell carcinoma of the upper aero-digestive tract. (Abstract). Proceedings of the 13th International Cancer Congress, Vol 40, 1983.

Poplin EA, Jacobson J, Herskovic A, et al: Evaluation of multimodality treatment of locoregional esophageal carcinoma by Southwest Oncology Group 9060. Cancer 78:1851–1866, 1996.

Powell MEB, Hoskin PJ, Saunders MT, et al: Continuous hyperfractionated accelerated radiotherapy (CHART) in localized cancer of the esophagus. Int J Radiat Oncol Biol Phys 38:133–136, 1997.

Preusser P, Wilke H, Achterrath W, et al: Disease oriented phase II study with cisplatin (P), etoposide (E), and 5FU (F) (PEF) in advanced squamous cell carcinoma of the esophagus (Meeting Abstract). Proceedings of the American Society of Clinical Oncology, Vol 7, 1988, p A388.

Queisser W, Preusser P, Mross KB, et al: Phase II evaluation of carboplatin in advanced esophageal carcinoma: A trial of the Phase I/II Study Group of the Association for Medical Oncology of the German Cancer Society. Onkologie 13:190–193, 1990.

Ravry M, Moertel CG, Schutt AJ, et al: Treatment of advanced squamous cell carcinoma of the gastrointestinal tract with bleomycin (NSC 125066). Cancer Chemother Rep 57:493–495, 1973.

Ravry MJ, Moore MR, Omura GA, et al: Phase II evaluation of cisplatin in squamous carcinoma of the esophagus: A Southeastern Cancer Study Group trial. Cancer Treat Rep 69:1457–1458, 1985.

Remick SC, Ruckdeschel JC: Extrapulmonary and pulmonary small-cell carcinoma: Tumor biology, therapy, and outcome. Med Pediatr Oncol 20:89–99, 1992.

Resbeut M, Le Prise-Fleury E, Ben-Hassel M, et al: Squamous cell carcinoma of the esophagus: Treatment by combined vincristine-methotrexate plus folinic acid rescue and cisplatin before radiotherapy. Cancer 56:1246–1250, 1985.

Roca E, Pennella E, Sardi M, et al: Combined intensive chemoradiotherapy for organ preservation in patients with resectable and non-resectable oesophageal cancer. Eur J Cancer 32A:429–432, 1996.

Rosenberg JC, Lichter AS, Leichman LP: Cancer of the esophagus. In DeVita VT, Hellman S, Rosenberg SA (eds): Cancer: Principles & Practice of Oncology, Philadelphia, JB Lippincott, 1989, pp 725–764.

Roth JA, Pass HI, Flanagan MM, et al: Randomized clinical trial of preoperative and postoperative adjuvant chemotherapy with cisplatin, vindesine, and bleomycin for carcinoma of the esophagus. J Thorac Cardiovasc Surg 96:242–248, 1988.

Roussel A, Jacob JH, Jung GM, et al: Controlled clinical trial for the treatment of patients with inoperable esophageal carcinoma: A study of the EORTC gastrointestinal tract cancer Cooperative Group. In Schlag P, Hoheberger P, Metger G (eds): Results in Cancer Research. Berlin, Springer-Verlag, 1988, pp 21–30.

Saito T, Hikita M, Kohno K, et al: Different sensitivities of human esophageal cancer cells to multiple anti-cancer agents and related mechanisms. Cancer 70:2402–2409, 1992.

Saltz LB, Spriggs D, Schaaf LJ, et al: Phase I clinical and pharmacologic study of weekly cisplatin combined with weekly irinotecan in patients with advanced solid tumors. J Clin Oncol 16:3858–3865, 1998.

Schlag P: Preoperative chemotherapy in localized squamous cell carcinoma of the esophagus: Results of a prospective randomized trial. Eur J Cancer 27:S76, 1991.

Schlag P, Herrmann R, Raeth V, et al: Preoperative chemotherapy in esophageal cancer: A phase II study. Acta Oncologica 27:811–814, 1988.

Schmoll HJ, Hiddemann W, Rustum Y, et al: Recent developments in biomodulation: Second International Workshop on Gastrointestinal Cancer. Semin Oncol 19:1992.

Schwartz GK, Kaubisch A, Saltz L, et al: Phase I trial of sequential pacitaxel and the cyclin dependent kinase inhibitor flavopiridol (Abstract). Proceedings of the American Society of Clinical Oncology, Vol 18, 1999, p 160a.

Schwartz GK, Werner JL, Maslak P: Flavopiridol enhances the biologic effects of paclitaxel: A phase I trial in patients with advanced solid tumors (Abstract). Proceedings of the American Society of Clinical Oncology, Vol 17, 1998, p A725.

Seitz JF, Giovannini M, Padaut-Cesana J, et al: Inoperable nonmetastatic squamous cell carcinoma of the esophagus managed by concomitant chemotherapy (5-fluorouracil and cisplatin) and radiation therapy. Cancer 66:214–219, 1990.

Slabber CF, Falkson G, Burger W, et al: 13-*cis*-Retinoic acid and interferon alpha-2a in patients with advanced esophageal cancer: A phase II trial. Invest New Drugs 14:391–394, 1996.

Slabber CF, Nel JS, Schoeman L, et al: A randomized study of radiotherapy alone versus radiotherapy plus 5-fluorouracil and platinum in patients with inoperable, locally advanced squamous cell cancer of the esophagus. Am J Clin Oncol 21:462–465, 1998.

Slamon D, Leyland-Jones B, Shak S, et al: Addition of Herceptin (Humanized Anti-HER Antibody) to first line chemotherapy for HER2 overexpressing metastatic breast cancer HER2 + /MBC) markedly increases anticancer activity: A randomized, multinational controlled phase III trial (Abstract). Proceedings of the American Society of Clinical Oncology, Vol 17, 1998, p 98a.

Smith TJ, Ryan LM, Douglass HO, et al: Combined chemoradiotherapy vs. radiotherapy alone for early stage squamous cell carcinoma of the esophagus: A study of the Eastern Cooperative Oncology Group. Int J Radiat Oncol Biol Phys 42:269–276, 1998.

Spielmann M, Guillot T, Kac J, et al: Phase II trial of cisplatin (P) and continous infusion (CI) of bleomycin (B) and 5-fluorouracil (F) in advanced esophageal cancer (ESO CA) (Meeting Abstract). Proceedings of the American Society of Clinical Oncology, Vol 8, 1989, p A393.

Spielmann M, Kac J, Rougier P, et al: Phase II study of 5-fluorouracil (FU) infusion, *cis*-platin (DDP) and vindesine (VDS) in squamous carcinoma of the esophageal (Meeting Abstract). Proceedings of the American Society of Clinical Oncology, Vol 6, 1987, p 94.

Spiridonidis CH, Laufman LR, Jones JJ, et al: A phase II evaluation of high dose cisplatin and etoposide in patients with advanced esophageal adenocarcinoma. Cancer 77:2070–2077, 1996.

Stephens FO: Bleomycin—a new approach in cancer chemotherapy. Med J Aust 1:1277–1283, 1973.

Sternberg C, Kelsen D, Dukeman M, et al: Carboplatin: A new platinum analog in the treatment of epidermoid carcinoma of the esophagus. Cancer Treat Rep 69:1305–1307, 1985.

Sur RK, Singh DP, Sharma SC: Radiation therapy of esophageal cancer: Role of high dose rate brachytherapy. Int J Radiat Oncol Biol Phys 22:1043–1046, 1992.

Sykes AJ, Burt PA, Slevin NJ, et al: Radical radiotherapy for carcinoma of the oesophagus: An effective alternative to surgery. Radiother Oncol 48:15–21, 1998.

Tancini G, Bajetta E, Bonadonna G: Terapia con bleomycin da sola o in associazione con methotrexate nel carcinoma epidermoide dell'esofago. Tumori 60:65–71, 1974.

Tateishi R, Taniguchi K, Horai T, et al: Argyrophil cell carcinoma (APUDoma) of the esophagus: A histopathological entity. Virchows Arch (A) 371:283–294, 1976.

Urba SG, Turrisi AT: Split-course accelerated radiation therapy combined with carboplatin and 5-fluorouracil for palliation of metastatic or unresectable carcinoma of the esophagus. Cancer 75:435–439, 1995.

Valerdi JJ, Tejedor M, Illarramendi JJ, et al: Neoadjuvant chemotherapy and radiotherapy in locally advanced esophagus carcinoma: Long term results. Int J Radiat Oncol Biol Phys 27:843–847, 1994.

van der Gaast A, Kok TC, Splinter TA, et al: Phase II study of cisplatin etoposide, 5-FU and leucovorin in patients with adenocarcinoma of the esophagus (Abstract). Proceedings of the American Society of Clinical Oncology, Vol 16, 1997, p 1087.

Vignoud J, Visset J, Paineau J, et al: Preoperative chemotherapy in squamous cell carcinoma of the esophagus: Clinical and pathological analysis, 48 cases (Abstract). Ann Oncol 1:45, 1990.

Vogl SE, Camacho F, Berenzweig M, et al: Chemotherapy for esophageal cancer with mitoguazone, methotrexate, bleomycin, and cisplatin. Cancer Treat Rep 69:21–23, 1985.

Vogl SE, Greenwald E, Kaplan BH: Effective chemotherapy for esophageal cancer with methotrexate, bleomycin, and *cis*-diamminedichloroplatinum: II. Cancer 48:2555–2558, 1981.

Wadler S, Fell S, Haynes H, et al: Treatment of carcinoma of the esophagus with 5-fluorouracil and recombinant alfa-2a-interferon. Cancer 71:1726–1730, 1993.

Wadler S, Haynes H, Beitler JJ, et al: Phase II clinical trial with 5-FU, recombinant interferon-alpha-2b, and cisplatin for patients with metastatic or regionally advanced carcinoma of the esophagus. Cancer 78:30–34, 1996.

Wara WM, Mauch PM, Thomas AN, et al: Palliation for carcinoma of the esophagus. Radiology 121:717–720, 1976.

Wasserman E, Cvitkovic E, Goldwasser F, et al: Oxaliplatin/CPT-11 combination: Preliminary results of a phase I study of an active combination in gastrointestinal malignancies (Abstract). Proceedings of the American Association for Cancer Research, Vol 38, 1997, p A1508.

Whittington R, Close H: Clinical experience with mitomycin-C. Cancer Chemother Rep 54:195–198, 1970.

Whittington R, Coia LR, Haller DG, et al: Adenocarcinoma of the esophagus and esophago-gastric junction: The effects of single and combined modalities on the survival and patterns of failure following treatment. Int J Radiat Oncol Biol Phys 19:593–603, 1990.

Wilke H, Stahl M, Preusser P, et al: Phase II trial with 5-FU (F), folinic acid (L), etoposide (E), and cisplatin (P; FLEP) ± surgery in advanced esophageal cancer (Meeting Abstract). Proceedings of the American Society of Clinical Oncology, Vol 11, 1992, p A494.

Wu YK, Huang GJ, Shao LF, et al: Honored Guest's Address: Progress in the study and surgical treatment of cancer of the esophagus in China, 1940–1980. J Thorac Cardiovasc Surg 84:325–333, 1982.

Xiao H, O'Reilly E, Ilson D, et al: A phase II trial of 96 hour paclitaxel in patients with previously treated esophageal carcinoma (Abstract). Proceedings of the American Society of Clinical Oncology, Vol 17, 1998, p 1179.

Yagoda A, Mukherji B, Young C, et al: Bleomycin, an antitumor antibiotic: Clinical experience in 274 patients. Ann Intern Med 77:861–870, 1972.

Zaniboni A, Simoncini E, Tonini G, et al: Cisplatin, high dose folinic acid and 5-fluorouracil in squamous cell carcinoma of the esophagus: A pilot study. Chemioterapia 6:387–389, 1987.

CHAPTER **49**

Surgical Palliation of Esophageal Cancer

Robert J. Korst
Steven R. DeMeester

Carcinoma of the esophagus is a deadly disease, with cure to be expected in only 5% to 10% of patients. The mainstay of curative therapy is surgical resection; however, fewer than 50% of patients present with disease confined to the esophagus or regional lymph nodes, and the remainder have evidence of distant spread (Postlethwait, 1986). These patients with distant metastases need a mechanism to control symptoms attributable to the primary tumor because they are not candidates for esophagectomy.

Systemic palliative chemotherapy, used primarily for symptom relief, has been poorly studied. Given the debilitated condition and poor performance status of many of these patients, it is not surprising that chemotherapy-related toxicity can be significant in this setting (Alberts et al, 1992). External beam radiotherapy relieves symptoms of esophageal obstruction with success rates of more than 50% in patients with squamous cell carcinoma, but the treatment course is prolonged and complications occur in approximately one third of cases (Caspers et al, 1988).

The addition of chemotherapy to external beam radiotherapy has sometimes prolonged survival in patients with unresectable or metastatic esophageal cancer (Herskovic et al, 1992), although other authors have disputed these findings (Slabber et al, 1998). There was no significant difference in the improvement of swallowing between patients receiving only radiotherapy and those receiving chemoradiotherapy in the trial reported by Herskovic and coworkers (1992). They did note that the side effects of chemoradiotherapy were severe in 44% and life-threatening in 20% of patients. Furthermore, Leichman and colleagues (1987) noted that 20% of the patients receiving chemoradiotherapy had persistent, intractable dysphagia. For patients with a malignant esophagorespiratory tract fistula, chemoradiotherapy has a limited role and may exacerbate rather than improve the problem.

UNRESECTABLE ESOPHAGEAL CANCER

Patients who present with systemic metastases from esophageal carcinoma are not candidates for curative resection, yet they require palliation for their symptoms. The median survival for these patients is less than 6 months (Postlethwait, 1979). Consequently, it is important that palliative procedures have a low morbidity and mortality rate and work well in the short term. The symptoms requiring palliation result mainly from esophageal obstruction or fistulization.

Clinical Features

Dysphagia

Esophageal obstruction in patients with carcinoma usually manifests as dysphagia. Typically, the difficulty begins with solid foods; as the tumor progresses, many patients become unable to swallow liquids and even saliva. Of concern, saliva may spill over into the airway and cause repetitive aspiration episodes. Historically, patients with unresectable or metastatic esophageal cancer were offered palliative surgical bypass. Given the poor prognosis of these weakened patients, many of whom have lost a large amount of weight, bypass procedures are associated with high morbidity and mortality rates (Table 49–1). Currently, safe and effective palliation for esophageal obstruction can be accomplished with endoscopic stent placement in most patients. Consequently, with rare exception, bypass procedures have been abandoned for esophageal obstruction.

Fistulization

Fistulization between the lumen of the esophagus and the tracheobronchial tree is not uncommon in patients with unresectable carcinoma of the esophagus (Little et al, 1984). Typically, the fistulous tract opens into either the trachea or the main bronchus, but it may also communicate with the segmental airways. Many of these patients present with refractory pneumonia, and the fistula is evident with a contrast esophagram. Historically, esophageal exclusion and bypass or insertion of plastic "funnel-shaped" tubes has been used. As with palliation

TABLE 49–1 ■ **Operative Mortality and Anastomotic Leaks After Esophageal Bypass Using a Substernal Gastric Pull-up**

Reference	*No. of Patients*	*Operative Mortality (%)*	*Anastomotic Leaks (%)*
Robinson et al, 1982	16	36	38
Conlan et al, 1983	71	21	24
Orringer, 1984	37	24	20
Mannell et al, 1988	116	11	20

for the patient with dysphagia, the development of expandable coated metal stents represents a significant advance in the treatment of this difficult problem and has nearly eliminated the need for surgical intervention.

Current Techniques and Devices

Tumor Dilatation

Tumor dilatation, one of the oldest palliative measures for patients with esophageal cancer, can be accomplished by the use of Maloney or Savary bougies or a "through the scope" (TTS) balloon. Care must be taken to dilate the tumor gently to avoid a perforation. Relief from dysphagia after bougienage alone is so short-lived that this technique is rarely applicable as a solitary procedure (Lundell et al, 1989). Dilatation is often necessary, however, in preparation for other palliative measures, such as stent placement. The stricture must be dilated up to about 14 mm before traditional plastic tube placement but only to about 10 mm before insertion of a self-expanding metal stent.

A feared complication of dilatation for tumors located in the upper and middle esophagus is creation of a tracheoesophageal fistula. For any patient thought to have a fistula, dilatation should not be attempted.

Esophageal Endoprostheses

Plastic Tubes. Intubation of the obstructed esophagus with prosthetic tubes was first performed more than 100 years ago (Symonds, 1887). Since then, many different designs and materials have been used. The most commonly employed tubes in recent years have been made of silicone with the Atkinson design. Polyethylene Celestin tubes have also been popular (Fig. 49–1).

Important features of these tubes include a distal flange to help prevent migration and a proximal funnel to help guide ingested food through the lumen of the prosthesis (Fig. 49–2). Some tubes may also have a detachable distal "introducer" to facilitate placement via the traction technique.

The use of these plastic tubes has diminished tremendously since the introduction of endoscopically placed

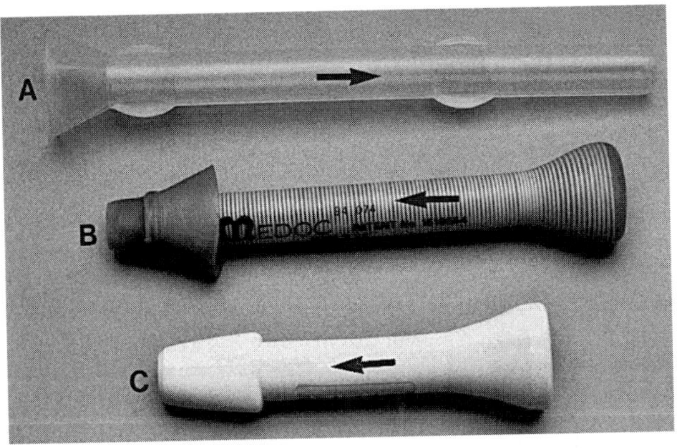

FIGURE 49–1 ■ Traditional "plastic" endoesophageal tubes. *A*, Soft, thin, salivary tube. *B*, Celestin tube. *C*, Atkinson tube. *Arrows* indicate direction of flow.

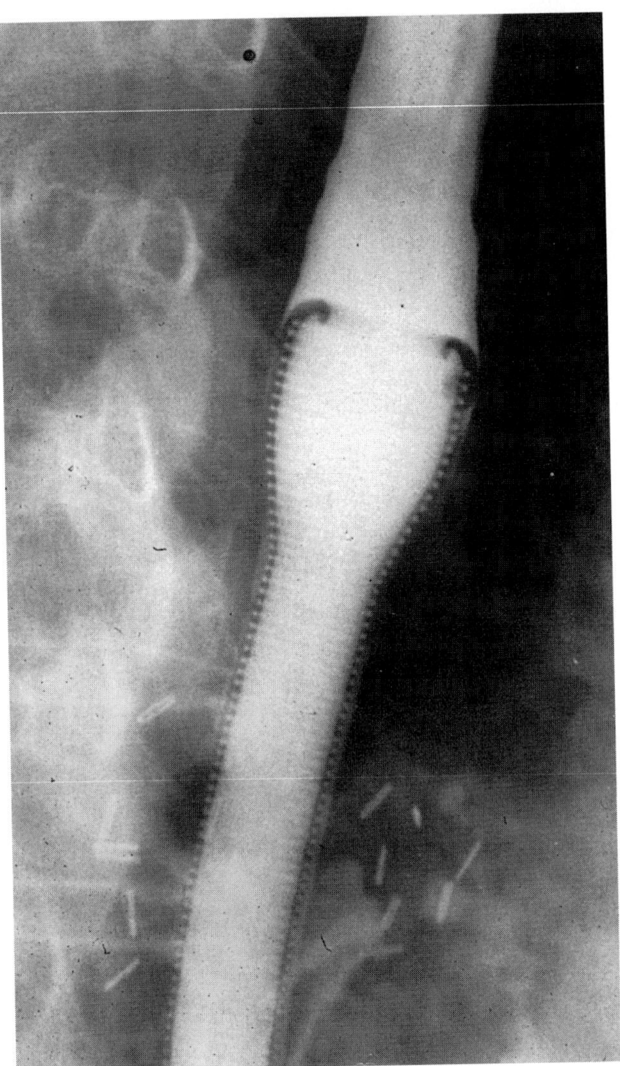

FIGURE 49–2 ■ Contrast radiograph of a Celestin tube placed for the palliation of malignant dysphagia.

self-expanding metal stents. Occasionally, these tubes are still used when there is a possibility that the tube would be needed for only a short time and then would be removed or when the obstruction is just below the cricopharyngeus.

An important consideration in placement of esophageal tubes is the location of the obstruction. For mid-esophageal lesions, approximately 4 cm of the prosthesis should protrude beyond the tumor in either direction. Gastroesophageal junction lesions present a particular problem because passage of the tube into the stomach invites gastroesophageal reflux and makes the tube more likely to migrate. If a tube is placed in this location, it may be sutured to the stomach wall to prevent migration (Celestin, 1959). If unrelenting gastroesophageal reflux occurs, the tube may have to be removed. For high, cervical obstructions, the foreign body sensation may be unbearable for the patient, especially if the proximal funnel is above the cricopharyngeus. The softer, thinner salivary tube may work better in this situation (see Fig. 49–1).

One must bear in mind the debilitated state of these patients and the simplistic tube design when interpreting results of tube placement. Most patients are unable to eat normally, although the majority can handle soft solid food. Approximately one third of patients, however, are restricted to a diet consisting only of liquids (Watson, 1982). Complications of tube placement include (1) perforation in 5% to 10%, (2) pressure necrosis with or without fistulization, (3) obstruction, (4) tube migration, and (5) reflux (Liakakos et al, 1992).

Mortality after tube placement reflects the devastating nature of advanced esophageal cancer and ranges from approximately 3% to nearly 40%, depending on technique of insertion (Cusumano et al, 1992; Liakakos et al, 1992; Proctor, 1980). In general, the "pull," or traction, technique is associated with a higher operative mortality than the "push" technique (Girardet et al, 1974).

Self-Expanding Metal Stents. Endoluminal metallic stents have revolutionized the management of unresectable esophageal carcinoma. They have virtually eliminated the need for palliative resection or bypass and have severely narrowed the indications for the placement of rubber tubes or laser therapy.

There are many advantages of the expandable stents over traditional tubes:

1. Metal stents are simpler to place, with most patients requiring only intravenous sedation and flexible esophagoscopy with fluoroscopic guidance. In contrast, general anesthesia and rigid esophagoscopy are often necessary when a plastic tube is placed.
2. The delivery system is more compact (8 to 12 mm), eliminating the requirement for dilatation in many patients.
3. Expandable metal stents are more flexible, and their internal diameters (18 to 22 mm) far exceed those of traditional tubes.
4. If the stent migrates or tumor ingrowth occurs, a second stent can be placed and "telescoped" into the first stent to restore patency (Fig. 49–3).

Complications of stent insertion are few. Many studies confirm the ease of insertion and low early complication rates in patients with esophageal cancer (Table 49–2). When used for malignant esophagorespiratory fistulas, coated self-expanding stents adequately occlude the fistula in more than 90% of patients (Low and Kozarek, 1998; May and Ell, 1998). Three randomized trials comparing expandable metal stents with traditional tubes all confirmed the greater ease and safety associated with use

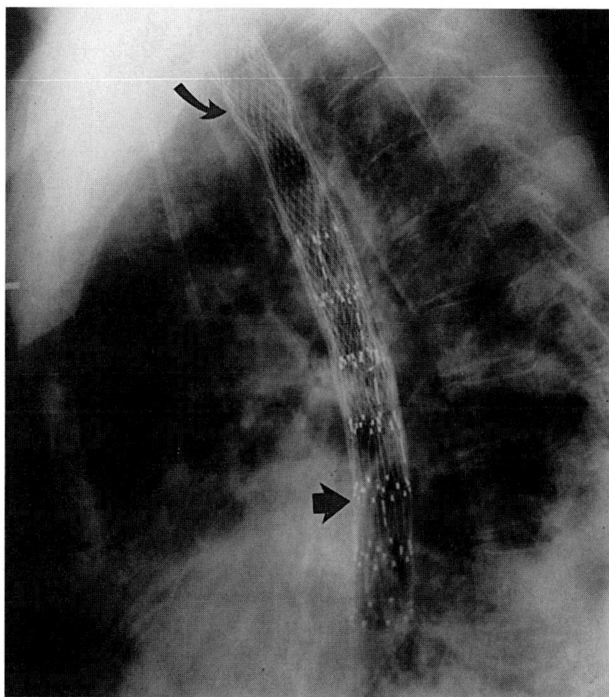

FIGURE 49–3 ■ Lateral chest radiograph displaying a Schneider Wallstent (*curved arrow*) "telescoped" into a Wilson-Cook Z-stent (*straight arrow*) for the palliation of malignant dysphagia. Following placement of the Z-stent, the tumor grew over the upper aspect, requiring insertion of another stent.

of self-expanding stents (Table 49–3). Longer-term failure rates were similar in both groups, however. More specifically, rates of recurrent dysphagia were comparable regardless of the choice of prosthesis.

Despite their clear advantages over plastic tubes, self-expanding metal stents do have drawbacks:

1. Once metal stents are placed, it can be difficult to remove them.
2. Tumor ingrowth may occur through the mesh, although this problem has largely been eliminated by the use of a coated stent.
3. Placement of these stents across the gastroesophageal junction can lead to wide-open reflux, but new designs are available that may help limit this problem.

Four models of self-expanding stents are available for use.

Wallstent. The Wallstent (Schneider, Boston Scientific) consists of a woven steel mesh and is available in several

TABLE 49–2 ■ **Technical Success, Early Complications, and Late Failures After Insertion of Self-Expanding Metal Stents for Malignant Dysphagia**

Reference	*No. of Patients*	*Stent*	*Technical Success (%)*	*Early Complications (%)*	*Late Failures (%)*
Pescatore and Manegold, 1995	29	Z-stent	100	14	28
Jiminez et al, 1996	35	Wallstent	100	0	17
Wengrower et al, 1998	81	Esophacoil	100	14	22
May et al, 1996	35	Ultraflex	100	37	35

TABLE 49–3 ■ Randomized Trials of Traditional Plastic Tubes Versus Expandable Metal Stents for Inoperable Carcinoma of the Esophagus

Reference	*Prosthesis*	*No. of Patients*	*Complications (%)*	*Recurrent Dysphagia (%)*
Siersema et al, 1998	Gianturco-Rosch	37	16	24
	Celestin	38	47	26
DePalma et al, 1996	Ultraflex	19	0	38
	Wilson-Cook	20	22	54
Knyrim et al, 1993	Wallstent	21	0	33
	Wilson-Cook	21	43	33

different lengths. The proximal and distal ends are flared to allow easier passage of food and to anchor the stent in place (see Fig. 49–3). This prosthesis comes in both covered and uncovered versions, with the polyurethane layer covering only the central portion. The uncoated ends allow tissue ingrowth and discourage migration. An added feature of the deployment system is that the stent can be partially deployed, and if the position is not satisfactory it can be re-employed and repositioned appropriately.

Esophacoil. The Esophacoil model (Instent, Medtronics) is a coiled spring made of a nickel-titanium alloy. It is tightly wound onto the deployment catheter and shortens when placed (Fig. 49–4). Although it is available only in an uncovered version, tumor ingrowth has not been more of a problem than with coated stents. The ends of the stent are flared to discourage migration and to allow easy passage of food. In addition, the Esophacoil expands with more force than the other models, which may be advantageous when it is placed through a constricting tumor. Whether this expansile force contributes to a higher incidence of pressure necrosis is unclear.

Two additional features of the Esophacoil are worth mentioning. First, this prosthesis can be deployed in one of three fashions: proximal to distal, distal to proximal, or from the center outward. Second, with the use of flexible endoscopy, it is possible to remove the Esophacoil completely after it has been placed: An overtube is inserted into the esophagus just proximal to the stent, the end of the coil is grasped with biopsy forceps, and the stent is withdrawn through the overtube to prevent trauma to the esophagus.

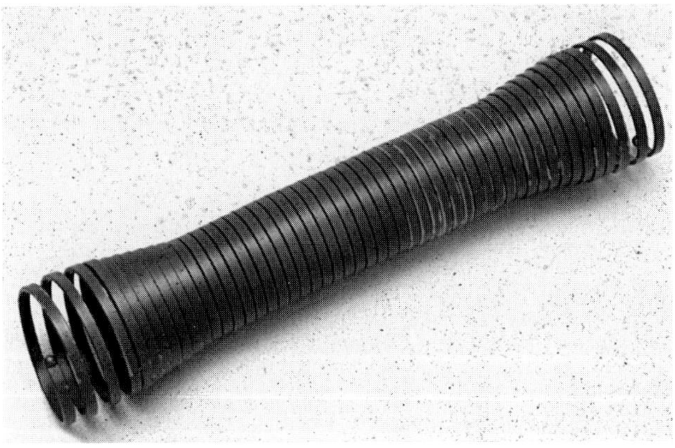

FIGURE 49–4 ■ Esophacoil (Instent) stent in its fully expanded form.

Ultraflex. The Ultraflex esophageal stent (Microvasive) is made from nitinol and is available in both a polyurethane-coated and an uncoated version (Fig. 49–5). The stents self-expand to 18 mm and flare at each end to 23 mm. An easy-to-use catheter delivery system allows deployment to proceed from either proximal to distal or distal to proximal (Fig. 49–6). As with most stents, the flared ends are uncoated to facilitate anchoring of the stent. The compressed stent shortens as it is deployed. Radiopaque markers on the catheter delivery device demonstrate where the ends of the fully deployed stent are located.

One can gradually deploy the stent by pulling on a string that binds the stent to the catheter delivery device. Consequently, the stent can easily be manipulated into precise position prior to complete deployment. The op-

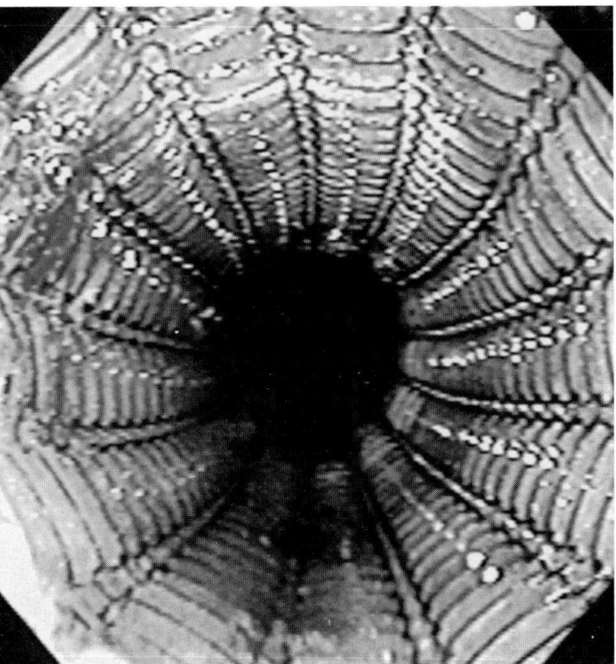

FIGURE 49–5 ■ Endoscopic view of an Ultraflex (Microvasive) expandable metal stent deployed across a malignant esophageal obstruction.

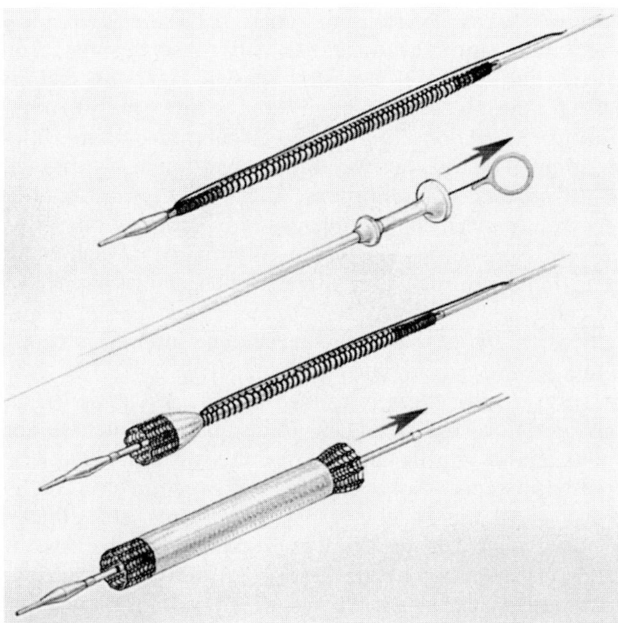

FIGURE 49–6 ■ Deployment system for the Ultraflex (Microvasive) expandable metal stent. Retraction of the string causes deployment of the stent.

tion to deploy the stent initially, either proximally or distally, is useful for tumors located at one or the other end of the esophagus. For cervical esophageal tumors, it is best to deploy the stent from proximal to distal, starting just below the cricopharyngeus. For tumors near the gastroesophageal junction, the distal release stent may be the best option.

Z-Stent. Two types of esophageal stents (Wilson-Cook) are coated with nitinol and constructed according to the Gianturco "Z" design. Consequently, they do not shorten with deployment. Both stents are flared at each end, and one of the stents is fitted with a "Dua" antireflux valve (Fig. 49–7). The Dua valve, which consists of a windsock-type appendage off the distal end of the stent, is designed to reduce the possibility of reflux when the stent is positioned across the gastroesophageal junction.

Both stents are deployed by means of an overtube-type assembly, and at the appropriate location the stent is pushed out from within the tube and allowed to expand. The deployment system allows release only from distal to proximal.

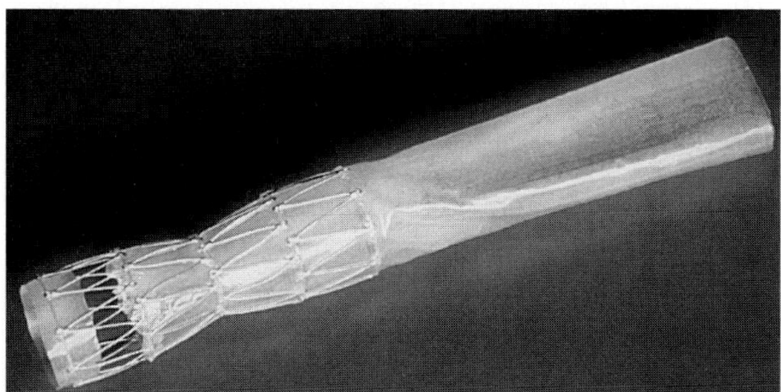

FIGURE 49–7 ■ Fully deployed Wilson-Cook Z-stent with accompanying "Dua" antireflux valve for use across the gastroesophageal junction.

Laser Ablation

For nearly 20 years, the neodymium:yttrium-aluminum-garnet (Nd:YAG) laser has been used to restore luminal patency in patients with esophageal cancer. As with palliative resection and bypass, the development of expandable metal stents has restricted the indications for laser palliation for patients with this disease. Tumor characteristics ideally suited for laser ablation include the following:

- An exophytic or fungating morphology
- A noncircumferential short stricture with no angulation
- A location in the middle or distal esophagus.

Advantages of the Nd:YAG laser include its ease of use with a flexible endoscope and its excellent coagulating and tissue penetration properties. Technical success is achieved in most patients, with luminal patency restored in over 90% of cases in most series; however, more than half of these patients required repeated treatment prior to death (Reed, 1994). Furthermore, technical success does not always translate into functional success, since only 70% to 80% of patients actually experience restored ability to eat. The main complications are bleeding and perforation, but in most series these manifestations occur in only 4% to 10% of patients.

Photodynamic Therapy

Photodynamic therapy (PDT) has also been used to restore luminal patency in patients with obstruction secondary to esophageal carcinoma (Marcon, 1994). With this modality, a systemically administered photosensitizing agent is taken up preferentially by malignant cells. The agent is then activated by a specific wavelength of light, which is administered via a low-energy laser with or without a diffusing mechanism. Oxygen free radicals are liberated, and cell death ensues. Patients with less advanced disease tend to have a better palliative result. Tumor ingrowth through expandable metal stents has also been treated with some success with PDT (Scheider et al, 1997). Like laser therapy, PDT has no role in the palliation of malignant esophagorespiratory fistulas.

PDT has been compared with Nd:YAG thermal ablation for the palliation of malignant dysphagia in a randomized, prospective, multicenter trial (Lightdale et al, 1995). Twenty-four institutions participated, and 236 patients were randomly assigned to the treatments. Dysphagia was palliated equally in both groups; however, patients receiving PDT had a better objective tumor response at 1 month, as measured by luminal diameters. Although there were more complications after PDT, these were usually minor, with sunburn being the most common (19%). Esophageal perforation occurred more frequently after laser therapy than after PDT (1% versus 7%, respectively).

Other Palliative Measures

In patients with end-stage disease in whom attempts at functional palliation have failed, the placement of either a gastrostomy or jejunostomy tube may be beneficial to allow nutrition and hydration. In addition, feeding tubes have been useful for augmenting nutritional intake in patients who have successfully undergone other palliative procedures, such as a tube or stent insertion. Obviously, feeding tube placement does nothing to address problems associated with esophageal obstruction or fistulization, and in these patients aspiration continues to be a significant concern.

Other strategies, such as direct injection of the tumor with chemicals that cause necrosis or direct electrocautery of the lesion, have been used intermittently for palliation, but these methods seem to be less versatile than laser ablation or stent placement and often require repeated treatments. As a result, these techniques are rarely utilized.

LOCALLY RECURRENT ESOPHAGEAL CANCER

Recurrence After Definitive Radiation Therapy

Locally recurrent or persistent tumor following treatment with radiation therapy is common, documented in 65% of patients in the series of Leichman and colleagues (1987). Despite previous high-dose radiation, some patients are candidates for esophagectomy. In others, the presence of systemic metastases makes an endoprosthesis a better choice. Frequently, in order to place a stent in these patients, the strictured area must be dilated. Particular care needs to be taken during dilatation because of the risk of perforation. Again, self-expanding metal stents are superior to traditional tubes because the stricture does not need to be dilated as widely before stent placement. Furthermore, the metal stents continue to expand slowly after insertion, an attractive quality when dealing with these "fragile" strictures.

As with plastic tubes, studies have suggested that metal stent placement is associated with higher risk of perforation after radiation therapy (Tytgat, 1990; Vermeijden et al, 1995). However, when placement is performed carefully in experienced centers, the perforation rate should be quite low. For patients who are not deemed candidates for stents, either laser or PDT may be an option. In rare circumstances, surgical bypass may be appropriate.

Recurrence Following Esophagectomy

Surgery for esophageal cancer has two goals: (1) to attempt cure of the patient's cancer and (2) to provide successful palliation of the patient's symptoms. Local recurrence after esophagectomy represents a failure to achieve the first goal and may compromise the goal of palliation as well.

Dysphagia associated with local recurrence can be produced by obstruction at a number of levels. Anastomotic recurrence or recurrence within mediastinal, celiac, or hepatoduodenal nodes can impair the passage of food and liquids into the intestines and cause dysphagia or obstruction. A close or positive gastric resection margin at the time of esophagectomy and gastric pull-up may lead to recurrence along the lesser curvature suture line. In some patients, this produces obstructive symptoms. Unfortunately, obstruction or fistulization from locally recurrent cancer after esophagectomy can be difficult to palliate. This underscores the importance of achieving good local control when surgery is used for esophageal cancer.

Most patients with local recurrence after esophagectomy are not candidates for any type of re-resection or surgical procedure, although in selected patients re-resection for cure has been accomplished. Increasingly, stents are being utilized; however, the success rate associated with stenting for recurrences after esophagectomy is worse than the success rate when stents are utilized primarily in esophageal cancer. In part, this is because of the altered anatomy after esophagectomy. In addition, recurrences at the esophagogastric anastomosis are often quite proximal, and it can be difficult to position a stent and remain below the cricopharyngeus. Unless the stricture or recurrent tumor holds the stent snugly in place, the stents often migrate distally into the gastric conduit. Another option for these patients is to insert a soft rubber salivary tube (see Fig. 49–1) across the lesion, with the funnel positioned above the cricopharyngeus. Most patients tolerate this quite well with little associated foreign body sensation.

Esophagorespiratory fistulas after esophagectomy are a particularly vexing problem. A coated, self-expanding stent positioned in the esophagus so that the fistula is covered by the coated portion of the stent often works well to occlude the fistulous tract and to prevent soiling of the airway. In some circumstances, there may be an advantage to "double stenting," whereby stents are placed to occlude both the esophageal and the tracheal end of the fistula (Colt et al, 1992). However, one must use caution when placing self-expanding stents adjacent to each other in both the esophagus and the trachea because compression of the esophagus and membranous wall of the trachea between the two stents may lead to ischemia and extension of the fistula. One consideration is to use a salivary tube in the esophagus and a coated self-expanding tracheal stent if necessary.

If the recurrent disease is truly well localized, resection with both palliative and curative intent may be attempted. Kurtzman and colleagues (1990) reported a small series of five patients with locally recurrent esophageal adenocarcinoma following esophagectomy who underwent re-resection. One patient was alive without disease 15 months after re-resection, and another died 18 months after the operation of an unrelated cause. In the remaining three patients, recurrent disease developed 8, 11, and 24 months after re-resection.

CONCLUSION

Local symptoms associated with inoperable carcinoma of the esophagus are caused primarily by obstruction or airway fistulization. The development of self-expanding metal stents has revolutionized the care of patients with these problems. Morbidity associated with insertion is low, and palliation for obstruction is effective. Long-term durability, however, is no better than that seen with traditional rubber tubes. Palliative surgical resection or bypass is now rarely performed, but in unusual, selected circumstances an operative approach may be indicated. Laser therapy and PDT are other options, but neither seems to offer significant advantages over stent placement alone.

Symptomatic locally recurrent disease after esophagectomy remains a difficult problem because of the limited effectiveness of esophageal endoprostheses. In these circumstances, palliative procedures need to be individually tailored to each patient's situation. Some patients may benefit from re-resection, although these complex procedures should be undertaken only in centers experienced with esophageal surgery.

COMMENTS AND CONTROVERSIES

This chapter, although entitled "Surgical Palliation of Esophageal Cancer," deals almost entirely with endoscopic procedures for palliation. This reflects the authors' appreciation for the fact that the major, risky, and often fruitless procedures used to bypass or resect persistent esophageal cancer have little place today. The technical aspects of such procedures are presented in Chapter 62.

In the rare circumstance in which nonsurgical treatment of esophageal cancer has resulted in a refractory stricture, persistent or recurrent cancer, or a tracheal esophageal fistula, yet the patient is apparently free of metastatic tumor, a bypass procedure may be warranted. Various conduits have been used, usually via the substernal route. The cervical esophagus is divided with the proximal end used for the anastomosis and the distal end turned in. Conduits include the reversed and nonreversed gastric tubes, whole stomach, colon, and rarely isolated jejunal grafts. In the case of whole stomach or intestinal bypass techniques, drainage of the distal esophagus is advisable, adding further to the complexity of the undertaking.

J. D. C.

■ KEY REFERENCES

Liakakos TK, Ohri SK, Townsend ER, Fountain SW: Palliative intubation for dysphagia in patients with carcinoma of the esophagus. Ann Thorac Surg 53:460, 1992.

This article describes a large series of Atkinson tube placement using the "push" technique.

Lightdale CJ, Heier SK, Marcon NE, et al: Photodynamic therapy with porfimer sodium versus thermal ablation therapy with Nd:YAG laser for palliation of esophageal cancer: A multicenter randomized trial. Gastrointest Endosc 42:507, 1995.

A randomized trial of PDT versus laser for palliation of dysphagia is presented.

Mannell A, Becker PJ, Nissenbaum M: Bypass surgery for unresectable oesophageal cancer: Early and late results in 124 cases. Br J Surg 75:283, 1988.

A large series of esophageal bypass with one of the lowest operative mortality rates is described.

Siersema PD, Hop WCJ, Dees J, et al: Coated self-expanding metal stents for esophagogastric cancer with special reference to prior radiation and chemotherapy: A controlled, prospective study. Gastrointest Endosc 47:113, 1998.

This is the largest randomized trial of self-expanding metal stents versus traditional tubes for palliation of dysphagia.

■ REFERENCES

Alberts AS, Burger W, Greeff F, et al: Severe complications of 5-fluorouracil and cisplatin with concomitant radiotherapy in inoperable non-metastatic squamous cell oesophageal cancer after intubation: Early termination of a prospective, randomized trial. Eur J Cancer 28A:1005, 1992.

Caspers RJ, Welvaart K, Verkes RJ, et al: The effect of radiotherapy on dysphagia and survival in patients with esophageal cancer. Radiother Oncol 12:15, 1988.

Celestin LR: Permanent intubation in inoperable cancer of the oesophagus and cardia. Ann R Coll Surg Engl 25:165, 1959.

Colt HG, Meric B, Dumon JF: Double stents for carcinoma of the esophagus invading the tracheobronchial tree. Gastrointest Endosc 38:485, 1992.

Conlan AA, Nicolaou N, Hammond CA, et al: Retrosternal gastric bypass for inoperable esophageal cancer: A report of 71 patients. Ann Thorac Surg 36:396, 1983.

Cusumano A, Ruol A, Segalin A: Push-through intubation: Effective palliation in 409 patients with cancer of the esophagus and cardia. Ann Thorac Surg 53:1010, 1992.

DePalma DG, Di Matteo E, Romano G, et al: Plastic prosthesis versus expandable metal stents for palliation of inoperable esophageal thoracic carcinoma: A controlled, prospective study. Gastrointest Endosc 43:478, 1996.

Girardet RE, Ransdell HT Jr, Wheat MW Jr: Palliative intubation in the management of esophageal carcinoma (collective review). Ann Thorac Surg 18:417, 1974.

Herskovic A, Martz K, Al-Sarraf M, et al: Combined chemotherapy and radiotherapy compared with radiotherapy alone in patients with cancer of the esophagus. N Engl J Med 326:1593–1598, 1992.

Jiminez FJ, Urtosun F, Barborena J, et al: "Wallstent" self expanding prostheses for palliation of malignant dysphagia. Endoscopy 28:S3, 1996.

Knyrim K, Wagner HJ, Bethge N, et al: A controlled trial of an expansile metal stent for palliation of esophageal obstruction due to inoperable cancer. N Engl J Med 329:1302, 1993.

Kurtzman SH, Turnbull AD, Bains MS: Recurrence of resected esophagogastric adenocarcinoma: Results of re-resection. J Surg Oncol 45:224, 1990.

Leichman L, Herskovic A, Leichman CG, et al: Nonoperative therapy for squamous-cell cancer of the esophagus. J Clin Oncol 5:365–370, 1987.

Liakakos TK, Ohri SK, Townsend ER, Fountain SW: Palliative intubation for dysphagia in patients with carcinoma of the esophagus. Ann Thorac Surg 53:460, 1992.

Lightdale CJ, Heier SK, Marcon NE, et al: Photodynamic therapy with porfimer sodium versus thermal ablation therapy with Nd:YAG laser for palliation of esophageal cancer: A multicenter randomized trial. Gastrointest Endosc 42:507, 1995.

Little AG, Ferguson MK, DeMeester TR, et al: Esophageal carcinoma with respiratory tract fistula. Cancer 53:1322, 1984.

Low DE, Kozarek RA: Comparison of conventional and wire mesh expandable prostheses and surgical bypass in patients with malignant esophagorespiratory fistulas. Ann Thorac Surg 65:919, 1998.

Lundell L, Leth R, Lind T, et al: Palliative dilatation in carcinoma of the esophagus and esophagogastric junction. Acta Chir Scand 155:179, 1989.

Mannell A, Becker PJ, Nissenbaum M: Bypass surgery for unresectable oesophageal cancer: Early and late results in 124 cases. Br J Surg 75:283, 1988.

Marcon NE: Photodynamic therapy and cancer of the esophagus. Semin Oncol 21(6 Suppl 15):20, 1994.

May A, Ell C: Palliative treatment of malignant esophagorespiratory fistulas with Gianturco Z stents: A prospective clinical trial and review of the literature on covered metal stents. Am J Gastroenterol 93:532, 1998.

May A, Hahn EG, Ell C: Self-expanding metal stents for palliation of malignant obstruction in the upper gastrointestinal tract: Comparative assessment of three stent types implemented in 96 implantations. J Clin Gastroenterol 22:261, 1996.

Orringer M: Substernal gastric bypass of the excluded esophagus: Results of an ill-advised operation. Surgery 96:467, 1984.

Pescatore P, Manegold BC: Results of coated Gianturco Z-stents in the palliative management of esophageal stricture. Gastrointest Endosc 43:343, 1995.

Postlethwait RW: Surgery of the Esophagus. New York, Appleton-Century Crofts, 1979, pp 393–394.

Postlethwait RW: Surgery of the Esophagus, 2nd ed. East Norwalk, CT, Appleton-Century Crofts, 1986.

Proctor DS: Esophageal intubation for carcinoma of the esophagus. World J Surg 4:451, 1980.

Reed CE: Endoscopic palliation of esophageal carcinoma. Chest Surg Clin North Am 4:155, 1994.

Robinson JC, Isa SS, Spees EK, et al: Substernal gastric bypass for palliation of esophageal carcinoma: Rationale and technique. Surgery 91:305, 1982.

Scheider DM, Siemans M, Cirocco M, et al: Photodynamic therapy for the treatment of tumor ingrowth in expandable esophageal stents. Endoscopy 29:271, 1997.

Siersema PD, Hop WCJ, Dees J, et al: Coated self-expanding metal stents for esophagogastric cancer with special reference to prior radiation and chemotherapy: A controlled, prospective study. Gastrointest Endosc 47:113, 1998.

Slabber C, Johan N, Schoeman L, et al: A randomized study of radiotherapy alone versus radiotherapy plus 5-fluorouracil and platinum in patients with inoperable, locally advanced squamous cancer of the esophagus. Am J Clin Oncol 21:462–465, 1998.

Symonds CJ: The treatment of malignant stricture of the oesophagus by tubage or permanent catheters. Br Med J 1:870, 1887.

Tytgat GN: Oesphageal perforation: Diagnosis, prevention and therapy. Eur J Gastroenterol Hepatol 2:198, 1990.

Vermeijden JR, Bartelsman JRWM, Fockens P, et al: Self expanding metal stents for palliation of esophagocardial malignancies. Gastrointest Endosc 41:58, 1995.

Watson A: A study of the quality and duration of survival following resection, endoscopic intubation, and surgical intubation in oesophageal carcinoma. Br J Surg 69:585, 1982.

Wengrower D, Fiorini A, Valero J, et al: Esophacoil: Long-term results in 81 patients. Gastrointest Endosc 48:376, 1998.

CHAPTER **50**

Unusual Malignancies

Robert J. Korst

The majority of esophageal malignancies are either squamous cell carcinoma or adenocarcinoma, many of which arise in a metaplastic (Barrett's) esophagus. In most parts of the world, squamous cell carcinoma is the predominant histologic type, with the incidence in some specific regions of China and Iran reaching endemic levels (Huang, 1988). In Western Europe and North America, however, adenocarcinoma has become more common than squamous cell carcinoma, a change occurring over the past 20 years (Devesa et al, 1998).

In rare instances, a malignant tumor arising in the esophagus does not resemble one of these two common cell types. During the 53-year period 1946 through 1999, 3081 patients with primary malignant lesions of the esophagus were seen and their cases entered into the tumor registry at Memorial Sloan-Kettering Cancer Center. Of these, 71 (2.3%) had tumors that were not typical squamous cell carcinoma or adenocarcinoma (Fig. 50–1). Similarly, malignant tumors other than squamous cell carcinoma were found in 2.1% of esophagectomy specimens in a study encompassing 68 institutions in Japan (Suzuki and Nagayo, 1980). It is important to note that in this earlier Japanese report, adenocarcinoma was a rare finding as well.

Given the wide range of cell types found in these unusual tumors, it is not surprising that the associated clinical features and biologic behavior as well as the histogenesis differ significantly from lesion to lesion.

HISTOGENESIS OF RARE TUMORS

The esophagus is a tubular organ whose wall is composed of four distinct layers: mucosa, submucosa, muscularis propria, and adventitia. The mucosa consists of three layers: (1) an inner lining of nonkeratinized, stratified squamous epithelium; (2) the immediately subjacent layer of thin connective tissue called the lamina propria; and (3) the muscularis mucosa. Unusual esophageal tumors may be classified according to their respective layer of origin and cell or tissue of origin (Table 50–1).

Small cell carcinoma and carcinoid tumors of the esophagus are thought to arise from cells of the amine precursor uptake and decarboxylation (APUD) system (Bensch et al, 1968). These cells are classified as either argyrophilic or argentaffinic, a distinction based on their response to defined silver stains. The cells of origin of small cell carcinoma are the argyrophilic cells, a cell type shown to be present in the epithelial layer of approximately 28% of esophagi (Tateishi et al, 1974). In addition, melanocytes have been found in the basilar aspect of the normal esophageal epithelium, an observation that may explain the occurrence of primary malignant melanoma of the esophagus (De la Pava et al, 1963; Tateishi et al, 1974).

The cell of origin of carcinosarcoma (pseudosarcoma) of the esophagus has been the subject of debate, but these mixed tumors probably result from the sarcomatous dedifferentiation of an established carcinoma (Battifora, 1976; Gal et al, 1987). Similarly, although primary choriocarcinoma of the esophagus may arise from displaced nests of germ cells, a more likely explanation is that these rare tumors result from dedifferentiation of an adenocarcinoma because most gastrointestinal tract choriocarcinomas contain adenocarcinomatous elements (Kikuchi et al, 1988). Verrucous carcinoma is a morphologic variant of squamous cell carcinoma of the esophagus, arising from squamous epithelium. This lesion, however, should be regarded as an entity distinct from typical squamous cell carcinoma because of its unusual morphology and vastly different biologic behavior (Malik et al, 1996).

The normal lamina propria contains connective tissue as well as small blood vessels, scanty diffuse lymphatic tissue, and occasional small lymphatic nodules. Tumors arising from these elements include the malignant lymphoproliferative disorders (non-Hodgkin's lymphoma, Hodgkin's disease, and plasmacytoma) and primary sarcomas of the esophagus. The muscularis mucosa is formed by longitudinal smooth muscle fibers, a possible site of origin of leiomyosarcoma of the esophagus.

The submucosa is a wide layer composed of loose connective and adipose tissue. In addition, it contains networks of lymphatics, small blood vessels, and nerves. The esophageal glands, or tubuloalveolar mucous glands, arise in the submucosa. The epithelium of these glands, which resemble minor salivary glands, is in direct continuity with the stratified squamous epithelium of the mucosa. Given the highly mesenchymal nature of the submucosa, sarcomatous tumors may arise from this layer. The glandular epithelium may also give rise to epithelial tumors, including mucoepidermoid carcinoma, adenoid cystic carcinoma, and adenocarcinoma (not associated with Barrett's metaplasia, or the "true" esophageal adenocarcinoma) (Ming, 1982). Nerves in the submucosa may give rise to granular cell tumors of the esophagus, a lesion with questionable malignant potential (Goldblum et al, 1996).

The muscularis propria contains mainly skeletal muscle in the upper third of the esophagus, smooth muscle in the lower third, and a mixture of these two types of muscle in the middle third. The adventitia, or outermost layer, is a connective tissue layer that exists in continuity with surrounding structures, such as the trachea. These

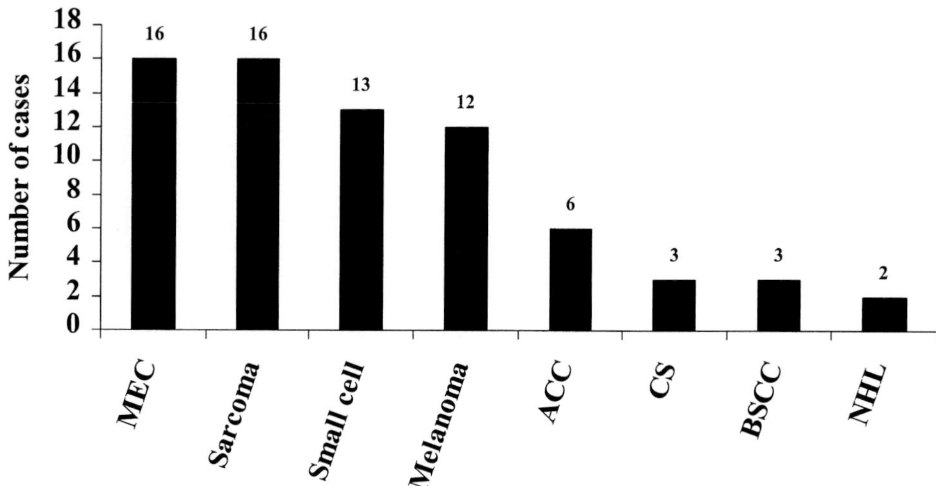

FIGURE 50–1 ■ Histologic distribution of 71 unusual esophageal malignancies seen at Memorial Sloan-Kettering Cancer Center from 1946 to 1999. (MEC, mucoepidermoid carcinoma; ACC, adenoid cystic carcinoma; CS, carcinosarcoma; BSCC, basaloid–squamous cell carcinoma; NHL, non-Hodgkin's lymphoma.)

two layers may also be responsible for the generation of malignant mesenchymal tumors of the esophagus.

TUMOR CHARACTERISTICS AND BIOLOGY

Gross Morphology

The gross, macroscopic appearance of squamous cell carcinoma and adenocarcinoma of the esophagus ranges from polypoid, exophytic, and protuberant lesions to ulcerative and stricture-forming lesions (Akiyama, 1990). Similarly, unusual tumors that arise in the esophageal epithelium may also assume any of these morphologic features. Several epithelial tumors, however, possess characteristic macroscopic features worth further discussion.

TABLE 50–1 ■ **Histologic Origin of Unusual Esophageal Malignancies**

Layer of Origin	*Cell or Tissue of Origin*	*Tumor*
Mucosa		
Epithelium	Argyrophilic cells	Small cell carcinoma
	Argyrophilic, argentaffinic cells	Carcinoid
	Melanocytes	Malignant melanoma
	Epithelial squamous cells	Verrucous carcinoma Carcinosarcoma Basaloid–squamous cell carcinoma
Lamina propria	Lymphocytes	Malignant lymphoproliferative disorders
	Connective tissue	Sarcomas
Muscularis mucosa	Smooth muscle	Leiomyosarcoma
Submucosa	Tubuloalveolar mucous glands	Adenoid cystic carcinoma Mucoepidermoid carcinoma
	Lymphocytes	Malignant lymphoproliferative disorders
	Connective tissue	Sarcomas
	Nerves	Granular cell tumor
Muscularis propria	Smooth and striated muscle	Sarcomas
Adventitia	Connective tissue	Sarcomas

Carcinosarcomas (pseudosarcomas) are polypoid in the majority of cases. In one review of more than 150 such lesions, more than 90% were found to be polypoid (Iascone and Barreca, 1999). In fact, these tumors have been referred to as "polypoid carcinomas" in some reports (Murray and Vasilakis, 1994). Verrucous carcinoma is also a protuberant lesion but has a characteristic warty or cauliflower-like appearance.

Primary malignant melanoma of the esophagus also usually manifests as a polypoid mass with ulceration, but the lesion is pigmented in 75% to 90% of cases (Taniyama et al, 1990). Other gross findings associated with melanoma are the presence of satellite nodules and melanosis of the surrounding mucosa in 12% and 25% of cases, respectively (Di Constanzo and Urmacher, 1987). Choriocarcinomas are characteristically very friable tumors, and they bleed easily at endoscopy.

Tumors that originate from deeper in the esophageal wall are frequently protuberant masses with a smooth surface, indicating normal overlying mucosa. Morisaki and colleagues (1996), in a review of adenoid cystic carcinoma, found that 16 of 35 tumors had this appearance and were covered with squamous mucosa. Mucoepidermoid carcinoma, lymphoma, and sarcomas of the esophagus also commonly manifest in a similar fashion. Endoscopic biopsy of a nonulcerated portion of a deeper tumor may reveal only normal mucosa (Morisaki et al, 1996). In this regard, such tumors must be distinguished from benign submucosal tumors, such as leiomyomas (see Chapter 41).

Tumor Location

Most squamous cell carcinomas arise in the middle third of the esophagus (Akiyama et al, 1981). Adenocarcinoma has a predilection for the lower esophagus, a tendency that is not surprising when one considers its common

TABLE 50–2 ■ **Distribution of Unusual Malignancies in the Esophagus**

	Distribution (%)		
Tumor	*Cervical/Upper Thoracic*	*Middle Thoracic*	*Lower Thoracic*
Small cell carcinoma	6	46	49
Carcinoid	14	29	57
Carcinosarcoma	10	60	30
Malignant melanoma	10	37	53
Adenoid cystic carcinoma	7	62	31
Mucoepidermoid carcinoma	20	55	25
Verrucous carcinoma	45	18	36
Basaloid–squamous cell carcinoma	N/A	N/A	N/A
Choriocarcinoma	0	20	80
Non-Hodgkin's lymphoma	28	39	33
Hodgkin's disease	40	40	20
Solitary plasmacytoma	0	0	100
Sarcoma	26	32	42

N/A, data not available.

association with Barrett's esophagus and gastroesophageal reflux. Table 50–2 summarizes the distribution of the uncommon esophageal malignancies as reported in the literature. Although any tumor can arise in any location, two general trends can be appreciated:

1. Epithelial tumors tend to be located farther down the esophagus, usually in the middle or lower third.
2. Tumors arising from deeper layers of the esophageal wall (sarcoma, lymphoma) seem to be more evenly distributed throughout the body of the esophagus.

Patterns of Spread

Malignant tumors of the esophagus, regardless of cell type, have the potential to spread via the following four mechanisms (Table 50–3):

- Intraesophageal spread
- Wall penetration with invasion of neighboring structures
- Spread to regional and distant lymph nodes
- Systemic hematogenous dissemination

Typical squamous cell carcinoma and adenocarcinoma as well as some unusual lesions (small cell carcinoma, carcinoid, adenoid cystic carcinoma, mucoepidermoid carcinoma) spread readily via all four mechanisms (Casas et al, 1997; Fegelman et al, 1994; Lindberg et al, 1997; Morisaki et al, 1996). Interestingly, some lesions associated with a relatively good prognosis in other organs (pulmonary carcinoid, adenoid cystic carcinoma of the major salivary glands) carry a very high mortality rate when they arise in the esophagus because of their significant metastatic potential.

Other rare esophageal tumors tend to spread by one mechanism, but not others, reflecting the varying biology of these lesions. An example is verrucous carcinoma. Although a variant of squamous cell carcinoma, it is a slow-growing tumor. In a review of existing cases, Garrard and colleagues (1994) found that only 1 of 14 reported cases involved metastasis to lymph nodes, whereas distant metastases have not been reported. Death from esophageal verrucous carcinoma usually results from the consequences of local invasion. Carcinosarcoma and malignant melanoma, in contrast, tend not to penetrate the esophageal wall but spread via lymphatic and hematogenous routes (Iascone and Barreca, 1999; Joob et al, 1995). In all five reported cases of choriocarcinoma, widespread metastases were present at autopsy (Burt, 1995; Wasan et al, 1994).

CLINICAL FEATURES

Patient Demographics

Squamous cell carcinoma and adenocarcinoma of the esophagus are diseases of older adults, with men typically affected at a higher rate than women. Similarly, unusual esophageal tumors are most likely to present in men in their seventh decade of life (Table 50–4) (Burt, 1995; Casas et al, 1997; Fegelman et al, Garrard et al, 1994; Iascone and Barreca, 1999; Joob et al, 1995; Lindberg et al, 1997; Morisaki et al, 1996). Primary sarcomas of the

TABLE 50–3 ■ **Patterns of Spread Seen with Unusual Esophageal Malignancies**

Tumor	***Transmural***	***Submucosal***	***Lymph***	***Blood***
Small cell carcinoma	+	+	+	+
Carcinoid	+	+	+	+
Carcinosarcoma	−	−	+	+
Malignant melanoma	−	+	+	+
Adenoid cystic carcinoma	+	+	+	+
Mucoepidermoid carcinoma	+	+	+	+
Verrucous carcinoma	+	−	−	−
Basaloid–squamous cell carcinoma	+	+	+	+
Choriocarcinoma	±	+	+	+
Non-Hodgkin's lymphoma	N/A	N/A	N/A	N/A
Hodgkin's disease	N/A	N/A	N/A	N/A
Solitary plasmacytoma	N/A	N/A	N/A	N/A
Sarcoma				
Polypoid	−	−	±	−
Infiltrative	+	+	+	+

+, frequent occurrence; ±, moderate occurrence; −, infrequent occurrence; N/A, not applicable.

TABLE 50–4 ■ **Median Age and Male-to-Female Ratio of Patients with Unusual Esophageal Malignancies**

Tumor	*Median Age*	*Male/Female Ratio*
Small cell carcinoma	64*	1.6:1
Carcinoid	57	6:1
Carcinosarcoma	62	4.5:1
Malignant melanoma	60	2:1
Adenoid cystic carcinoma	65†	5:1
Mucoepidermoid carcinoma	66‡	9:1
Verrucous carcinoma	58	1.4:1
Basaloid–squamous cell carcinoma	— §	3.3:1
Choriocarcinoma	44	1.5:1
Non-Hodgkin's lymphoma	61	1.6:1
Hodgkin's disease	42	5:1
Solitary plasmacytoma	— ‖	1:1
Sarcoma	55	1.3:1

*Mean age; range 38–89 years.
†Mean age; range 49–79 years.
‡Mean age; ± 9.4 years.
§Data not available.
‖Only two patients, ages 59 and 67 years.

esophagus as well as choriocarcinomas have a predilection for slightly younger men (in the sixth and fifth decades of life, respectively) (Burt, 1995; Kikuchi et al, 1988; McKechnie and Fechner, 1971; Sasano et al, 1969; Trillo et al, 1979; Wasan et al, 1994).

Presenting Symptoms

Dysphagia and weight loss remain the most common presenting symptoms in patients with any malignant lesion of the esophagus, regardless of cell type, with one exception: All five reported patients with esophageal choriocarcinoma presented with gastrointestinal bleeding (Kikuchi et al, 1988; McKechnie and Fechner, 1971; Sasano et al, 1969; Trillo et al, 1979; Wasan et al, 1994). In fact, all but one of these patients died as a result of hemorrhagic complications, either from the primary tumor or from a metastatic lesion.

Diagnosis

Although the histologic diagnoses of squamous cell carcinoma and adenocarcinoma of the esophagus are routinely made via endoscopic biopsy in the preoperative setting, the diagnoses of many rare tumors of this organ are frequently not confirmed until the esophagectomy specimen is examined. Examples are carcinosarcoma, adenoid cystic carcinoma, mucoepidermoid carcinoma, verrucous carcinoma, and choriocarcinoma. In a review of 127 carcinosarcomas and 56 pseudosarcomas of the esophagus reported in the literature, Iascone and Barreca (1999) found that the correct diagnosis was obtained by means of endoscopic biopsy in less than one third of cases. Similarly, in a series of 32 cases of adenoid cystic carcinoma compiled from the Japanese literature, diagnosis was made through preoperative biopsy in only eight cases (Morisaki et al, 1996).

There are three reasons for the poor diagnostic yield of endoscopic biopsy:

1. The index of suspicion is low because these tumors are very uncommon.
2. A small biopsy specimen may not reveal the characteristic cell type and tissue architecture because many of these rare tumors contain components that resemble typical squamous cell carcinoma or adenocarcinoma.
3. Adequate endoscopic biopsy specimens of submucosal lesions are difficult to obtain unless ulceration is present.

Treatment

Because many of these uncommon esophageal malignancies are misdiagnosed as ordinary squamous cell carcinoma or adenocarcinoma prior to therapy, treatment usually consists of esophagectomy if the disease is thought to be localized to the chest. When an unusual cell type is confirmed before treatment, however, many different therapeutic modalities have been employed, either alone or in combination. Unfortunately, no consensus exists concerning the most appropriate treatment for some of these lesions, and the numbers are so small that no significant conclusions can be drawn regarding treatment-specific survival. Despite these inadequacies, some general trends can be appreciated that may help direct therapy for these unusual tumors (see following discussion).

SPECIFIC UNUSUAL TUMOR TYPES

Figure 50–2 displays the distribution of unusual esophageal malignancies as reported in the English literature. An accurate count of each tumor type is difficult and sometimes impossible to determine because a significant number of cases are reported more than once. Therefore, the figures quoted are approximations.

Epithelial Tumors

Neuroendocrine Tumors: Small Cell Carcinoma, Carcinoid

The unusual esophageal malignancy that has been reported most frequently is small cell, or oat cell, carcinoma. It was first described in 1952 in an autopsy series by McKeown (1952). The esophagus is actually the most common extrapulmonary site of small cell carcinoma (Ibrahim et al, 1984). At Memorial Sloan-Kettering Cancer Center, my colleagues and I have seen 13 cases of primary small cell carcinoma of the esophagus between 1946 and 1999, representing 18% of the 71 rare esophageal malignancies observed at this institution.

The tumor is usually present in the lower two thirds of the esophagus, and the diagnosis is suggested by the small, lymphocyte-like appearance of the cells at histologic examination. Immunohistochemical analysis may demonstrate the presence of neuron-specific enolase, whereas a Grimelius stain may reveal cytoplasmic argyrophilia in approximately half the cases (Casas et al, 1997). A mixed histologic appearance, in which squamous dif-

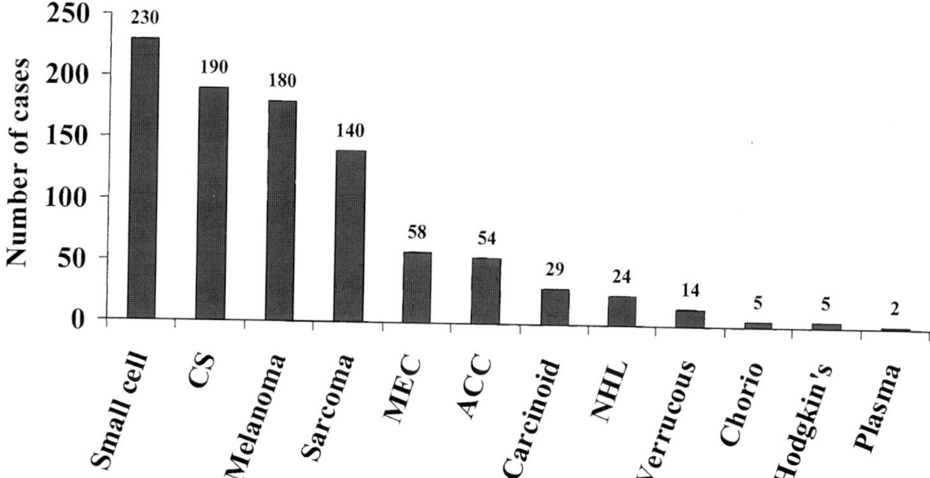

FIGURE 50–2 ■ Histologic distribution of unusual esophageal malignancies reported in the English literature. (CS, carcinosarcoma; MEC, mucoepidermoid carcinoma; ACC, adenoid cystic carcinoma; NHL non-Hodgkin's lymphoma; chorio, choriocarcinoma; plasma, plasmacytoma.)

ferentiation occurs, is present in up to a third of tumors; the majority are pure small cell carcinoma (Casas et al, 1997).

In a comprehensive review of 199 cases of esophageal small cell carcinoma collected from the literature, Casas and associates (1997) found that 93 patients presented with disease confined to the chest, and 95 with metastatic disease; in 11 cases, no stage was reported. Of the patients with metastatic disease, 65 received systemic chemotherapy and 30 underwent no treatment. Systemic therapy prolonged the median survival in this group of patients from 1 month to 6 months, but only one patient survived to 2 years.

When distant metastases have not been detected, patients have been treated with local therapy (surgical resection or radiotherapy) with or without the addition of chemotherapy. Of the 93 patients in the Casas review who had local disease, 50 were treated with either surgery or radiotherapy alone and systemic chemotherapy was added to the treatment regimen for 43 patients. Figure 50–3 shows the actuarial survival curves for these two groups of patients. These data suggest that patients with small cell carcinoma of the esophagus benefit from multimodal treatment strategies when no distant metastases are present. No significant differences in survival were found with regard to different types of local treatment (surgery versus radiotherapy) when they were carried out along with systemic treatment.

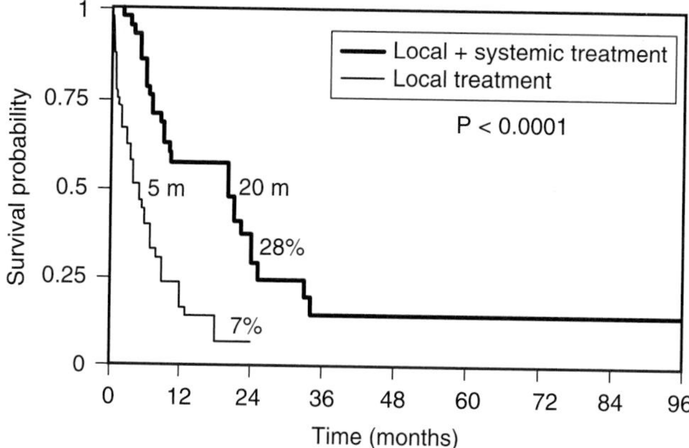

FIGURE 50–3 ■ Survival probability for patients with localized small cell carcinoma of the esophagus according to treatment strategy. (Modified from Casas F, Ferrer F, Farrus B, et al: Primary small cell carcinoma of the esophagus: A review of the literature with emphasis on therapy and prognosis. Cancer 80:1366, 1997.)

Primary carcinoid tumor of the esophagus represents another malignancy arising from cells of APUD system. This tumor was first described in 1969 by Brenner and associates. Since then, 29 reported cases of esophageal carcinoid have been published (Soga, 1998; Tanida et al, 1998). We have never documented a case of this unusual neoplasm at Memorial Sloan-Kettering Cancer Center.

In the 29 described cases, two patients presented with symptoms that could be attributed to the carcinoid syndrome. Preoperative endoscopic biopsy was not accurate in more than 75% of cases. This diagnostic inaccuracy may explain why the majority of reported patients presented without evidence of distant metastases and underwent resection consisting of esophagectomy or local excision. It is likely that more cases of esophageal carcinoid exist but are misdiagnosed on endoscopic biopsy as typical squamous cell carcinoma or adenocarcinoma. If distant metastases are present, the diagnosis is not confirmed by esophagectomy.

After resection, the development of distant metastases is common. In the review reported by Soga (1998), the 5-year actuarial survival for 21 patients who underwent resection for primary carcinoid tumor of the esophagus was 32%.

In summary, primary small cell carcinoma of the esophagus is an aggressive disease with a grave prognosis, and it behaves similarly in the lung. The mainstay of treatment seems to be systemic chemotherapy, but for patients with no detectable distant metastases, radiation should be added as a means of local therapy. Surgical resection probably does not offer a survival advantage for these patients. Primary esophageal carcinoid is a very rare tumor, also with an aggressive phenotype. When carcinoid is properly diagnosed and there is no evidence of distant spread, the best choice of therapy remains resection.

Carcinosarcoma

Carcinosarcoma is a malignant neoplasm that histologically contains both carcinomatous and sarcomatous elements. It was first described in the esophagus in 1903 by Hansemann, but not until 1949 was an operation carried out for this disease (Stout et al, 1949). Several decades ago, it had been suggested that carcinosarcoma and pseudosarcoma were different disease entities, but later reports comparing clinicopathologic data have confirmed that these two lesions probably represent the same type of tumor (Table 50–5) (Iascone and Barreca, 1999). Since the initial reports, nearly 190 cases of carcinosarcoma or pseudosarcoma have been described in the literature (Iascone and Barreca, 1999). At Memorial Sloan-Kettering Cancer Center, we have seen only three cases of carcinosarcoma of the esophagus between 1946 and 1999, or 4% of the 71 rare esophageal malignancies observed at this institution.

Several theories have arisen to explain the origin of carcinosarcoma:

1. The lesions may result from the coincidental "collision" of two separate tumors, one epidermal and one mesenchymal, arising in close proximity to each other.
2. The mesenchymal portion may represent stromal reactive hyperplasia, and not malignancy.
3. Both types of cells may originate from one "stem" cell, with the sarcomatous cells representing "dedifferentiation" of the carcinomatous elements.

Electron microscopy as well as immunohistochemical evidence supports the theory that both histologic elements of carcinosarcoma result from a common, epithelial cell–type carcinoma (Battifora, 1976; Gal et al, 1987; Wang et al, 1992).

Carcinosarcoma typically manifests as a polypoid mass in the lower two thirds of the thoracic esophagus. In contrast to patients with small cell carcinoma, most patients with carcinosarcoma do not have evidence of distant metastases at the time of presentation, allowing surgical resection to be performed in most reported cases.

TABLE 50–5 ■ **Clinicopathologic Similarities Between Carcinosarcoma and Pseudosarcoma of the Esophagus**

	Carcinosarcoma	*Pseudosarcoma*
Age (range in years)	49–86	44–84
Sex (male/female ratio)	4.1:1	4.7:1
Morphology (polypoid) (%)	83	96
Wall Penetration (%)		
Submucosa	40	46
Muscularis propria	27	23
Adventitia	17	4
Location in middle third (%)	89	94
Survival (%)		
Dead of disease within 3 years	34	40
No evidence of disease *or* dead from other causes after 5 years	16	9

In an extensive review of the literature, Iascone and Barreca (1999) found that 86% of patients with this tumor type underwent surgical resection. Esophagectomy was the most common procedure performed (95%), and a small number of patients underwent polypectomy with or without adjuvant radiation or chemotherapy. Lymph node metastases were found in approximately 50% of patients.

Excluding operative deaths (15.7%), follow-up data were available for 77 patients who underwent resectional therapy for carcinosarcoma or pseudosarcoma. Of these patients, 60% were either alive without disease or dead from an unrelated cause at a mean of 2.5 years after surgery (range, 3 months to 7 years) (Iascone and Barreca, 1999). In an earlier survival analysis, a 5-year actuarial survival rate of 54% was found for patients who underwent esophagectomy for carcinosarcoma of the esophagus (Fig. 50–4). In this report, survival data were considered adequate for 34 cases available from the literature at that time (Burt, 1995).

Recurrence following resection may be local-regional, distant, or both. In addition, both the carcinomatous and mesenchymal portions of the tumor have been reported to metastasize to distant sites, which include liver, brain, bone, and lung (Iyomasa et al, 1990; Osamura et al, 1978).

In summary, carcinosarcoma and pseudosarcoma of the esophagus most likely represent the same lesion. Despite its polypoid appearance, this tumor has significant metastatic potential. Treatment should consist of esophagectomy with an adequate lymph node dissection. Local or endoscopic resection (polypectomy) should be avoided because of the high incidence of lymph node metastases seen with this tumor. Although the number of reported cases is small, available evidence suggests that survival after resection of this lesion may be better than that obtained for patients with typical squamous cell carcinoma or adenocarcinoma of the esophagus.

Malignant Melanoma

Although malignant melanoma is most commonly a primary tumor of the skin, extracutaneous sites have been described. The most frequent location of extracutaneous melanoma is the eye, although this tumor has also been reported to arise in the esophagus (Scotto et al, 1976). Primary esophageal melanoma was first described in 1906, and for many years it was unclear whether the lesion represented primary or metastatic disease (Baur, 1906). In 1963, De la Pava and colleagues found melanocytes in the epithelium of 4 of 100 normal esophagi at autopsy, suggesting that primary melanoma could indeed arise in this organ. A Japanese study later confirmed these results with the finding of melanocytes in 8% of normal esophagi studied (Tateishi, 1974).

Since the initial report, more than 180 cases of primary malignant melanoma of the esophagus have been described (Dematos et al, 1997; Joob et al, 1995; Sabanathan et al, 1989). At Memorial Sloan-Kettering Cancer Center, my associates and I have documented 12 patients with this tumor between 1946 and 1999, accounting for 17% of all unusual esophageal malignancies seen. Typi-

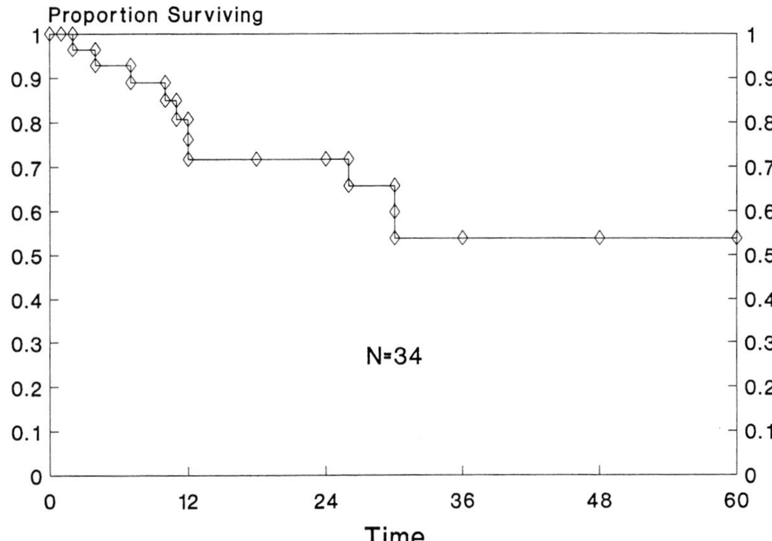

FIGURE 50–4 ■ Overall actuarial survival of 34 patients surviving resection for primary carcinosarcoma of the esophagus (5-year survival, 54%).

cally, the lesion manifests as a polypoid, ulcerated, pigmented mass in the lower two thirds of the thoracic esophagus. Satellite lesions and more diffuse melanosis may also be present. Approximately 50% of patients have some form of metastatic disease at the time of presentation (Sabanathan et al, 1989). The most common sites of distant metastases are liver, lung, brain, and pleura, although spread to any organ may occur.

Surgical resection represents the most commonly utilized therapeutic option for patients with esophageal melanoma, provided that the disease appears to be localized to the chest. An evaluation of the outcome for 46 patients with local-regional disease who survived esophagectomy found a 5-year actuarial survival of only 19%, with most patients experiencing distant recurrences (Burt, 1995). The number of absolute 5-year survivors was only four, underlining the need for effective systemic therapy for this disease (De Mik et al, 1992; Hamdy et al, 1991; Suehs, 1961; Suzuki and Nagayo, 1980).

In summary, primary malignant melanoma of the esophagus is an aggressive tumor that is usually disseminated at the time of diagnosis. Esophagectomy is the only viable option for patients without evidence of metastases. Despite complete resection, however, long-term survival is rare.

Adenoid Cystic Carcinoma, Mucoepidermoid Carcinoma

Although distinct entities, the epithelial tumors adenoid cystic carcinoma and mucoepidermoid carcinoma share many clinical and biologic characteristics (Table 50–6). The first case report of esophageal adenoid cystic carcinoma, also known as cylindroma, was from Bergmann and Charnas in 1958; since that time, approximately 54 cases have been described in the English literature (Kitada et al, 1997; Lieberman et al, 1994; Morisaki et al, 1996). Primary mucoepidermoid carcinoma (adenosquamous carcinoma, adenoacanthoma) of the esophagus is similarly rare, with approximately 58 cases having been reported (Fegelman et al, 1994; Lieberman et al, 1994; Mafune et al, 1995; Sakata et al, 1998). At Memorial Sloan-Kettering Cancer Center, we have seen 6 cases of adenoid cystic carcinoma and 16 cases of mucoepidermoid carcinoma between 1946 and 1999; they account for 8.5% and 22.5%, respectively, of the 71 unusual esophageal malignancies observed at our institution.

Both of these rare tumors are thought to arise from cells that compose the tubuloalveolar mucous glands of the esophagus: adenoid cystic carcinoma from the ductal cells, and mucoepidermoid carcinoma from the mucus-secreting glandular cells (Bell-Thompson et al, 1980; Nelms and Luna, 1972; Pourzand et al, 1975). Histologically, these tumors resemble their counterparts in the salivary glands; however, they tend to have a higher number of mitotic figures and more necrosis. These pathologic findings are consistent with the aggressive nature of both lesions when found in the esophagus; when the tumors are diagnosed in the salivary glands, the 5-year survival is much more favorable, ranging from 60% to 70% (Spiro et al, 1978, 1979).

Typically, both adenoid cystic carcinoma and mucoepidermoid carcinoma of the esophagus manifest as submucosal protuberant masses in the middle third of the thoracic esophagus. These tumors spread readily via both

TABLE 50–6 ■ **Clinical Features of Esophageal Adenoid Cystic and Mucoepidermoid Carcinomas**

	Adenoid Cystic Carcinoma	*Mucoepidermoid Carcinoma*
No. of reported cases	54	58
Age (mean in years)	65	66
Sex (male/female ratio)	5:1	9:1
Location in middle third (%)	62	55
Operability (%)	89	95
Median survival (months)	12	9.5

lymphatic and hematogenous routes (see Table 50–3); most tumors in the esophagus, however, are considered resectable at the time of presentation. In a review of 37 patients with adenoid cystic carcinoma of the esophagus in Japan, 33 (89%) underwent esophagectomy with curative intent (Morisaki et al, 1996). Similarly, in the largest reported series of esophageal mucoepidermoid carcinoma, 19 of 20 (95%) patients were deemed to have resectable tumors (Fegelman et al, 1994). These figures are appreciably higher than those for typical squamous cell carcinoma and adenocarcinoma in this organ. Because adenoid cystic carcinoma and mucoepidermoid carcinoma are aggressive tumors, a likely explanation for the high rate at which they are deemed resectable preoperatively is the common misinterpretation of endoscopic biopsy specimens of such tumors as poorly differentiated squamous carcinoma. Only after esophagectomy is the correct diagnosis secured. Therefore, many cases of inoperable adenoid cystic carcinoma or mucoepidermoid carcinoma are probably misdiagnosed because they never undergo resection.

Survival after resection of these two unusual epithelial tumors, unfortunately, is dismal. In a Kaplan-Meier survival analysis of data from 22 patients who survived esophagectomy for adenoid cystic carcinoma, there were no 5-year survivors (Lieberman et al, 1994). The 1-year survival was 70%; the 3-year survival, 35%; and the median survival, 24 months. Most recurrences are in the form of systemic metastases after resection. Similarly, in the largest reported series of esophageal mucoepidermoid carcinoma, there were no 5-year survivors and the 2-year survival was 39% (Fegelman et al, 1994).

In summary, adenoid cystic carcinoma and mucoepidermoid carcinoma have many clinical and biological similarities. Unfortunately, they are both aggressive tumors that are not usually diagnosed until after resection is performed. Unlike survival of their counterparts in the salivary glands, survival of patients with these esophageal tumors is dismal despite resection.

Unusual Variants of Squamous Cell Carcinoma: Verrucous Carcinoma and Basaloid–Squamous Cell Carcinoma

Verrucous carcinoma is a rare squamous cell variant characterized by its slow, local growth and warty, cauliflower-like appearance. We have seen no examples of this variant at Memorial Sloan-Kettering Cancer Center, and only 14 cases have been reported in the literature (Garrard et al, 1994; Malik et al, 1996). Interestingly, 6 of the 14 patients reported had preexisting esophageal disorders; 3 had a history of achalasia, and 3 had previous lye injury. In 9 of the 14 patients, tumor had invaded through the esophageal wall into neighboring structures, and only 7 patients underwent esophageal resection.

The biology of verrucous carcinoma is unique among esophageal malignancies, in that no patients had evidence of distant metastatic disease and only one had lymphatic disease. In fact, the most common cause of death (in both operated and unoperated patients) was some complication of esophagorespiratory fistula. The etiology of this lesion is unclear but may be related to esophageal injury, given the aforementioned preexisting disorders. No consistent association with human papillomavirus (HPV) has been demonstrated for verrucous carcinoma of the esophagus, in contrast to verrucous carcinomas arising in other sites (Malik et al, 1996). Because this unusual tumor is mainly a local problem, esophagectomy remains the best choice for treatment if it is technically feasible.

Basaloid–squamous cell carcinoma (BSCC) is an unusual esophageal malignancy that had not been recognized in the literature until approximately a decade ago. Histologic criteria for light microscopy examination have since been published (Wain et al, 1986). In one report, 17 of 150 squamous cell carcinomas of the esophagus were reclassified as BSCC after pathologic reanalysis using the published criteria (Sarbia et al, 1997). This tumor can be very difficult to distinguish histologically and immunohistochemically from adenoid cystic carcinoma and is often misdiagnosed as typical squamous cell carcinoma because it commonly has squamous components.

We have documented three cases of BSCC at Memorial Sloan-Kettering Cancer Center (4.2% of 71 unusual esophageal malignancies seen). Only scattered case reports and three small series of patients with esophageal BSCC exist in the literature, but this tumor is probably more common than indicated because of the ease with which it is misdiagnosed (Abe et al, 1996; Sarbia et al, 1997; Tsang et al, 1991). Treatment is with esophagectomy, and survival is similar to that of typical squamous cell carcinoma of the esophagus.

Choriocarcinoma

Immunohistochemically, as many as 10% and 21% of gastrointestinal adenocarcinomas stain positive for alpha-fetoprotein (AFP) and human chorionic gonadotropin (HCG), respectively (Abelov, 1971; Brownstein et al, 1973). Significantly elevated serum levels of these hormones are present in far fewer instances, however, and germ cell tumor morphology is usually absent. Primary germ cell tumors of the esophagus are extremely rare, with only five reported cases in existence (Kikuchi et al, 1988; McKechnie and Fechner, 1971; Sasano et al, 1969; Trillo et al, 1979; Wasan et al, 1994). In all cases, the patients had choriocarcinoma, with one patient also having areas of yolk sac differentiation (Wasan et al, 1994).

Primary extragonadal choriocarcinoma of the gastrointestinal tract usually occurs in the stomach (85%), the five reported esophageal cases constituting only 7% of the total (Kikuchi et al, 1988). We have seen no patients with this disease at Memorial Sloan-Kettering Cancer Center. The histogenesis of primary choriocarcinoma of the esophagus is debated, but the fact that 67% of choriocarcinomas arising in the stomach also contained elements of adenocarcinoma or undifferentiated carcinoma implies that these tumors probably result from adenocarcinomas through a process of dedifferentiation or metaplasia (Kikuchi et al, 1988).

All five patients with choriocarcinoma of the esophagus presented with gastrointestinal hemorrhage, and endoscopy showed very friable tumors in the lower two thirds of the thoracic esophagus. All patients died with diffuse metastases, and none was treated with resection, although two received systemic chemotherapy. This lesion, although rare, must be considered in the younger patient who presents with gastrointestinal bleeding and a friable esophageal tumor.

Malignant Lymphoproliferative Disorders

Non-Hodgkin's Lymphoma

The gastrointestinal tract is the most common site of extranodal non-Hodgkin's lymphoma (NHL), and up to 50% of all patients with NHL are found at autopsy to have alimentary tract involvement (Hermann et al, 1980). The esophagus, however, represents the least common of these sites. The unusual instance in which the esophagus is involved with NHL usually results from invasion by mediastinal disease or upward extension from the stomach (Rosenberg et al, 1961).

Primary, extranodal NHL is not an unusual event. In the collected series from the End Results Section of the National Cancer Institute, 12,357 patients had NHL, of whom 1497 (12%) had extranodal NHL of all sites (Freeman et al, 1972). Only three patients had primary esophageal NHL. In fact, only 24 cases of primary esophageal NHL have been reported in the English literature (Field et al, 1984; Gupta et al, 1996; Kirsch et al, 1983; Nissan et al, 1974; Orvidas et al, 1994; Pearson and Borg-Grech, 1991; Worgan and Baldock, 1976). At Memorial Sloan-Kettering Cancer Center, we have seen only two patients with this entity in the 53-year period 1946 through 1999, representing 2.8% of all unusual esophageal malignancies seen. Similarly, in a series of patients with NHL involving the esophagus reported from the Mayo Clinic, only three cases of primary esophageal NHL were seen over a 47-year period (Orvidas et al, 1994).

The usual presentation of primary esophageal NHL is one of dysphagia caused by a submucosal mass that is present with equal frequency throughout the length of the esophagus. Men are affected more than women (see Table 50–4), at a median age of 61 years. Pathologically, these lesions are usually of the B cell immunophenotype, with nearly two thirds being large cell, B cell lymphomas. Lymph node involvement has been documented in 17% of patients, but an accurate assessment of nodal status cannot be made because not all patients underwent resection. When nodes are not involved, the disease is staged as IE, whereas nodal involvement classifies the disease as stage IIE.

A survival analysis performed for 18 of the 24 patients with primary NHL of the esophagus revealed an actuarial survival rate of 49% (Burt, 1995). The data are difficult to interpret both because of the small numbers and the fact that treatment strategies for this disease have varied widely (Table 50–7). All but one of the long-term survivors, however, received systemic chemotherapy with or without local therapy (resection or radiation therapy), suggesting that perhaps chemotherapy with radiation therapy should be the first choice for treatment.

TABLE 50–7 ■ **Therapeutic Strategies Used to Treat Primary Non-Hodgkin's Lymphoma of the Esophagus in 17 Patients**

Strategy	*No. of Patients*
Chemotherapy alone	4
Chemotherapy and radiotherapy	4
Esophagectomy alone	3
Local resection alone	2
Esophagectomy and chemotherapy	1
Radiotherapy alone	1
Esophagectomy, radiotherapy, and chemotherapy	1
None	1

Hodgkin's Disease

In contrast to non-Hodgkin's lymphoma, primary extranodal Hodgkin's disease is a rare entity. A review of the Armed Forces Medical Registry determined that approximately 0.3% of patients with this disease present in this fashion, for a total of 354 known cases (Wood and Coltman, 1973). To date, only five cases of primary esophageal Hodgkin's disease have been reported (Chiolero, 1935; Leroux-Robert et al, 1951; Meriel et al, 1953; Stein et al, 1981). We have seen no cases at Memorial Sloan-Kettering Cancer Center.

An obvious problem in the diagnosis of primary esophageal Hodgkin's disease is the ability to distinguish it from secondary esophageal involvement resulting from mediastinal nodal disease. To qualify as primary esophageal disease, the tumor must contain histologic features of Hodgkin's disease and must involve only the esophagus or limited contiguous nodes. In addition, distant disease must be excluded. Patients with these findings would be classified as having either stage IE disease (involvement of a single extranodal site) or stage IIE disease (involvement of a single extranodal site plus its contiguous lymph node chain) (Carbone et al, 1971).

Like non-Hodgkin's lymphoma, primary esophageal Hodgkin's disease presents as a submucosal mass. If biopsy reveals the correct diagnosis, an extensive search for other sites of disease should be undertaken. If no other sites of tumor are found, treatment should probably consist of primary radiotherapy because long-term survival has been achieved with this modality.

Solitary Plasmacytoma

Solitary extramedullary plasmacytoma constitutes the presentation of approximately 4% of patients with multiple myeloma. Most extramedullary plasmacytomas manifest in the nasopharynx, oropharynx, and upper respiratory tract (Meis et al, 1987). Only two cases of esophageal plasmacytoma have been described in the English literature (Ahmed et al, 1976; Morris and Pead, 1974).

For the diagnosis of primary extramedullary plasmacytoma of the esophagus, the following criteria must be met:

- Absence of Bence Jones proteinuria
- Normal serum electrophoresis values
- Normal result of bone marrow biopsy
- Normal bone and liver scans
- Histologic appearance of esophageal tumor consistent with plasmacytoma

The two patients reported in the literature were both treated with resection. Follow-up is important because approximately one fourth to one third of patients with extramedullary plasmacytoma of all sites go on to experience multiple myeloma, usually within 2 years (Holland et al, 1992; Meis et al, 1987).

Malignant Mesenchymal Tumors

Malignant mesenchymal tumors, or sarcomas, can arise nearly anywhere in the body, including the esophagus. Primary esophageal sarcomas are uncommon, however, with approximately 140 reported cases existing in the English literature as of 1995 (Burt, 1995). At Memorial Sloan-Kettering Cancer Center, we have seen 16 cases of primary esophageal sarcoma in the 53-year period 1946 through 1999, accounting for 22.5% of all unusual esophageal malignancies seen. The most common histologic type of esophageal sarcoma encountered is leiomyosarcoma, which constitutes nearly two thirds of these unusual neoplasms (Perch et al, 1991). All other subtypes are mainly curiosities, with fewer than 20 cases of each being reported.

Leiomyosarcoma

Leiomyosarcoma of the esophagus was first reported in 1902 by Howard, and more than 80 cases have been described since then (Perch et al, 1991). The lesions in these cases are distributed equally throughout the esophagus, and the gross appearance can be either polypoid or infiltrative (Rocco et al, 1998). Distinguishing between leiomyoma and leiomyosarcoma can be difficult both clinically and histologically. Typically, the more microscopic evidence of cellular proliferation, the more aggressive the tumor. In most cases, however, therapeutic decisions must be based on clinical behavior and gross appearance of the tumor.

Resection with curative intent should be the standard of care for patients with this disease because of the significant long-term survival observed for this approach. In the largest series (17 patients), the 5-year survival was 80% after curative resection (Rocco et al, 1998). Long-term survival has also been achieved with enucleation or polypectomy alone for some well-differentiated, polypoid leiomyosarcomas of the esophagus (Choh et al, 1986). Despite these results, both local and distant recurrences are seen after local resection techniques, leaving esophagectomy as the best hope for cure if the patient can tolerate the procedure.

Factors enhancing survival with esophagectomy are (1) the performance of a complete resection, (2) early tumor stage, (3) low tumor grade, (4) polypoid growth pattern, and (5) a thoracic, rather than cervical, tumor location (Rocco et al, 1998). Unlike patients with other esophageal tumors, patients with esophageal leiomyosarcoma who have distant metastatic disease can experience long-term survival after resection (Matsumori et al, 1992; Takayama et al, 1996).

In summary, leiomyosarcoma is the most common esophageal sarcoma described in the literature. Cure can be achieved in a significant percentage of cases with a complete resection, especially for well-differentiated, polypoid tumors. The presence of limited metastatic disease should not preclude resection.

Other Sarcomas

Sarcomas other than leiomyosarcoma that have been reported in the esophagus are listed in Table 50–8. Because of the rarity of these tumors and the incompleteness of available information regarding treatment and survival, it is difficult to draw conclusions that will dictate therapy. However, esophagectomy can currently be performed with minimal operative mortality and it is the only modality that has consistently achieved long-term survival in patients with these tumors. Unless other treatment strategies can demonstrate an advantage, resection will remain the best choice for esophageal sarcomas.

One lesion deserving special mention is *Kaposi's sarcoma* of the esophagus. This tumor may be associated with immunodeficient states (Beral et al, 1990) or may occur endemically in certain regions of Africa and southern Europe (Kaloterakis et al, 1984; Templeton and Bhana, 1975). In one series of 87 patients with cutaneous Mediterranean Kaposi's sarcoma, 22% had esophageal lesions consistent with the disease (Kolios et al, 1995). Kaposi' sarcoma has also been described in the esophagus in the absence of disease at any other sites (Pass et al, 1984). Treatment of isolated Kaposi's sarcoma of the esophagus must be individualized for each patient and depends on the overall clinical condition.

Granular cell tumors of the esophagus have also been described (Goldblum et al, 1996). Usually asymptomatic and occurring more commonly in black women, these lesions have been diagnosed more frequently over the last two decades as a result of increased detection by means of flexible endoscopy. Malignant granular cell tumors originating elsewhere in the body have been described, but it is unclear whether this entity exists in the esophagus. There are three questionable reports of the malignancy in the literature, but in all three instances either histologic details or follow-up were not reported (Crawford and DeBakey, 1953; Obiditsh-Mayer et al, 1961; Ohmori et al, 1987). Given their typically benign nature, these lesions can usually be observed, with resection reserved for symptomatic tumors that either are large (>2 cm) or show infiltration into the esophageal wall, as demonstrated with endoscopic ultrasonography (Goldblum et al, 1996).

TABLE 50–8 ■ **Histology of Esophageal Sarcomas Other Than Leiomyosarcoma**

Fibrosarcoma
Rhabdomyosarcoma
Liposarcoma
Synovial cell sarcoma
Malignant hemangiopericytoma
Desmoid
Malignant peripheral nerve tumor
Chondrosarcoma
Osteogenic sarcoma
Malignant fibrous histiocytoma
Kaposi's sarcoma

SUMMARY

Unusual malignancies arising in the esophagus represent a wide spectrum of diseases. Similar to typical squamous cell carcinoma and adenocarcinoma, most patients with unusual tumors present with dysphagia and weight loss. Evaluation of these lesions resembles that for the common esophageal carcinomas, although preoperative endoscopic biopsy is much less reliable for diagnosis of these rare tumors.

Because of their infrequency and the use of multiple therapeutic approaches, survival data are confusing to interpret, making it difficult to draw conclusions regarding the best therapeutic strategy. As a result, treatment usually consists of esophageal resection; however, some histologic types may be best approached with nonoperative strategies.

■ *KEY REFERENCES*

Burt M: Unusual malignancies. In Pearson FG, Deslauriers J, Ginsberg RJ, et al (eds): Esophageal Surgery. New York, Churchill Livingstone, 1995, pp 629–647.

This chapter from the first edition contains a fairly comprehensive reference list for unusual esophageal tumors.

Casas F, Ferrer F, Farrus B, et al: Primary small cell carcinoma of the esophagus: A review of the literature with emphasis on therapy and prognosis. Cancer 80:1366, 1997.

This article is a comprehensive review of small cell carcinoma of the esophagus resulting from an intensive literature search.

Garrard CL, Sheih WJ, Cohn RA, et al: Verrucous carcinoma of the esophagus: Surgical treatment for an often fatal disease. Am Surg 60:613, 1994.

Details on most of the existing cases of verrucous carcinoma are summarized.

Iascone C, Barreca M: Carcinosarcoma and pseudosarcoma of the esophagus: Two names, one disease—comprehensive review of the literature. World J Surg 23:153, 1999.

This exhaustive review summarizes all important data concerning this entity.

Ming SC: Tumors of the Esophagus and Stomach. Atlas of Tumor Pathology, Fascicle 7. Washington, DC, Armed Forces Institute of Pathology, 1982.

This classic work describes the pathologic and clinical findings of esophageal tumors, both benign and malignant. It is highly recommended reading.

Morisaki Y, Yoshizumi Y, Hiroyasu S, et al: Adenoid cystic carcinoma of the esophagus: Report of a case and review of the Japanese literature. Surg Today 26:1006, 1996.

This article gives a clear, concise review of adenoid cystic carcinoma of the esophagus.

Rocco G, Trastek VF, Deschamps C, et al: Leiomyosarcoma of the esophagus: Results of surgical treatment. Ann Thorac Surg 66:894, 1998.

The largest single-institution series of leiomyosarcoma of the esophagus is presented.

Sabanathan S, Eng J, Pradham GN: Primary malignant melanoma of the esophagus. Am J Gastroenterol 84:1475, 1989.

The authors review 139 cases of primary esophageal melanoma in the literature. This review is by far the best for this entity.

■ *REFERENCES*

Abe K, Sasano H, Itakura Y, et al: Basaloid-squamous carcinoma of the esophagus: A clinicopathologic, DNA ploidy, and immunohistochemical study of seven cases. Am J Surg Pathol 20:453, 1996.

Abelov GI: Alpha-fetoprotein in oncogenesis and its association with malignant tumors. Adv Cancer Res 14:295, 1971.

Ahmed N, Ramos S, Sika J, et al: Primary extramedullary esophageal plasmacytoma. Cancer 38:943, 1976.

Akiyama H: Surgery for Cancer of the Esophagus, Baltimore, Williams & Wilkins, 1990.

Akiyama H, Tsurumaru M, Kawamura T, et al: Principles of surgical treatment for carcinoma of the esophagus: Analysis of lymph node involvement. Ann Surg 194:438, 1981.

Battifora H: Spindle cell carcinoma: Ultrastructural evidence of squamous origin and collagen production by tumor cells. Cancer 37:2275, 1976.

Baur E: Ein fall von primarem melanom des oesophagus. Arb Geb Pathol Anat Inst Tuebingen 5:343, 1906.

Bell-Thompson J, Haggitt RC, Ellis HR: Mucoepidermoid and adenoid cystic carcinomas of the esophagus. J Thorac Cardiovasc Surg 79:438, 1980.

Bensch KG, Corrin B, Pariente R, Spencer H: Oat-cell carcinoma of the lung: Its origin and relationship to bronchial carcinoid. Cancer 22:1163, 1968.

Beral V, Peterman TA, Berkelman RL, et al: Kaposi's sarcoma among persons with AIDS: A sexually transmitted infection? Lancet 335:123, 1990.

Bergmann M, Charnas RM: Tracheobronchial rests in the esophagus: Their relation to some benign strictures and certain types of cancer of the esophagus. J Thorac Surg 35:97, 1958.

Brenner S, Heimlich H, Widman M: Carcinoid of esophagus. N Y State J Med 69:1337, 1969.

Brownstein GD, Vaitukaitis JL, Carbone PP, Ross GT: Ectopic production of human chorionic gonadotropin by neoplasms. Ann Intern Med 78:39, 1973.

Carbone PP, Kaplan HS, Musshoff K, et al: Report of the Committee on Hodgkin's Disease Staging Classification. Cancer Res 31:1860, 1971.

Chiolero J: Un cas de lymphogranulomatos primitive de l'oesophage. Policlinico (Med) 12:305, 1935.

Choh JH, Khazei AH, Ihm HJ: Leiomyosarcoma of the esophagus: Report of a case and review of the literature. J Surg Oncol 32:223, 1986.

Crawford ES, Debakey ME: Granular cell myoblastoma: Two unusual cases. Cancer 6:786, 1953.

De la Pava S, Nigogosyan G, Pickren JW, et al: Melanosis of the esophagus. Cancer 16:48, 1963.

Dematos P, Wolfe WG, Shea CR, et al: Primary malignant melanoma of the esophagus. J Surg Oncol 66:201, 1997.

De Mik JI, Kooijman CD, Hoekstra JBL, et al: Primary malignant melanoma of the esophagus. Histopathology 20:77, 1992.

Devesa SS, Blot WJ, Fraumeni JF Jr: Changing patterns in the incidence of esophageal and gastric carcinoma in the United States. Cancer 83:2049, 1998.

Di Constanzo DP, Urmacher C: Primary malignant melanoma of the esophagus. Am J Surg Pathol 11:46, 1987.

Fegelman E, Law SYK, Fok M, et al: Squamous cell carcinoma of the esophagus with mucin-secreting component: Mucoepidermoid carcinoma. J Thorac Cardiovasc Surg 107:62, 1994.

Field SP, Sachar DB, Childs CC, Rubin KP: Steroid-responsive dysphagia: A clue to the diagnosis of esophageal lymphoma. Mt Sinai J Med 51:451, 1984.

Freeman C, Berg JW, Cutler SJ: Occurrence and prognosis of extranodal non-Hodgkins lymphomas. Cancer 29:252, 1972.

Gal AA, Martin SE, Kernen JA, Patterson MJ: Esophageal carcinoma with prominent spindle cells. Cancer 60:2244, 1987.

Goldblum JR, Rice TW, Zuccaro G, et al: Granular cell tumors of the esophagus: A clinical and pathologic study of 13 cases. Ann Thorac Surg 62:860, 1996.

Gupta NM, Goenka MK, Jindal A, et al: Primary lymphoma of the esophagus. J Clin Gastroenterol 23:203, 1996.

Hamdy FC, Smith JHF, Kennedy A, Thorpe JAC: Long survival after excision of a primary malignant melanoma of the oesophagus. Thorax 46:397, 1991.

Hansemann D: Das gleichzeitige vorkommen verschiedenartiger geschwulste bei derselben person. Z Krebsforschung 1:183, 1903.

Hermann R, Panahon A, Barcos MP, et al: Gastrointestinal involvement in non-Hodgkin's lymphoma. Cancer 46:215, 1980.

Holland J, Trenkner DA, Wasserman TH, Fineberg B: Plasmacytoma:

Treatment results and conversion to myeloma. Cancer 69:1513, 1992.
Howard WT: Primary sarcoma of the esophagus and stomach. JAMA 38:392, 1902.
Huang GJ: Epidemiology of esophageal cancer in China. In Siewert JR, Holscher AH (eds): Diseases of the Esophagus. Berlin, Springer-Verlag, 1988, p 3.
Ibrahim NBN, Briggs JC, Corbishley CM: Extrapulmonary oat cell carcinoma. Cancer 54:1645, 1984.
Iyomasa S, Kato H, Tachimori Y, et al: Carcinosarcoma of the esophagus: A twenty-case study. Jpn J Clin Oncol 20:99, 1990.
Joob AW, Haines GK III, Kies MS, et al: Primary malignant melanoma of the esophagus. Ann Thorac Surg 60:217, 1995.
Kaloterakis A, Stratigos J, Trichopolous D, et al: Mediterranean Kaposi's sarcoma. Bull Soc Pathol Exot 77:570, 1984.
Kikuchi Y, Tsuneta Y, Kawai T, Aizawa M: Choriocarcinoma of the esophagus producing chorionic gonadotropin. Acta Pathol Jpn 38:489, 1988.
Kirsch HL, Cronin DW, Stein GN, et al: Esophageal perforation: An unusual presentation of esophageal lymphoma. Dig Dis 28:371, 1983.
Kitada H, Yamaguchi K, Takashima M, et al: Adenoid cystic carcinoma of the esophagus: Report of a case. Surg Today 27:238, 1997.
Kolios G, Kaloterakis A, Filiotou A, et al: Gastroscopic findings in Mediterranean Kaposi's sarcoma (non-AIDS). Gastrointest Endosc 42:336, 1995.
Leroux-Robert S, Ennuyer A, Calle R, Rousseay S: Les localisations ésophagiennes de la maladie Hodgkin's. Chir Cervicofac 68:573, 1951.
Lieberman MD, Franceschi D, Marsan B, et al: Esophageal carcinoma: The unusual variants. J Thorac Cardiovasc Surg 108:1138, 1994.
Lindberg GM, Molberg KH, Vuitch MF, et al: Atypical carcinoid of the esophagus: A case report and review of the literature. Cancer 79:476, 1997.
Mafune K-I, Takubo K, Tanaka Y, et al: Sclerosing mucoepidermoid carcinoma of the esophagus with intraepithelial carcinoma or dysplastic epithelium. J Surg Oncol 58:184, 1995.
Malik AB, Bidani JA, Rich HG, et al: Long-term survival in a patient with verrucous carcinoma of the esophagus. Am J Gastroenterol 91:1031, 1996.
Matsumori M, Mukai T, Tsukube T, et al: A two-stage operation successfully performed for giant leiomyosarcoma of the esophagus with hepatic metastasis. Jpn J Surg 22:543, 1992.
McKechnie JC, Fechner RE: Choriocarcinoma and adenocarcinoma of the esophagus with gonadotropin secretion. Cancer 27:694, 1971.
McKeown F: Oat-cell carcinoma of the oesophagus. J Pathol Bact 64:889, 1952.
Meis JM, Butler JJ, Osborne BM, Ordonez NG: Solitary plasmacytomas of bone and extramedullary plasmacytomas: A clinicopathologic and immunohistochemical study. Cancer 59:1475, 1987.
Meriel PC, Darnaud C, Denard Y, et al: Malignant lymphogranulomatosis with esophageal localization. Sangre 24:627, 1953.
Morris WT, Pead JL: Myeloma of the oesophagus. J Clin Pathol 25:537, 1972.
Murray GF, Vasilakis A: Less common malignant tumors of the esophagus. In Shields TW (ed): General Thoracic Surgery, 4th ed. Baltimore, Williams & Wilkins, 1994, pp 1681–1693.
Nelms DC, Luna MA: Primary adenocystic carcinoma (cylindromatous carcinoma) of the esophagus. Cancer 29:440, 1972.
Nissan S, Bar-Moar JA, Levy E: Lymphosarcoma of the esophagus: A case report. Cancer 34:1321, 1974.
Obiditsh-Mayer I, Salzer-Kuntschik M: Malignes, "gekirntzelliges Neurom" soganntes Myoblastemmoym des Oesophagus. Beitr Pathol Anat 125:357, 1961.
Ohmori T, Arita N, Uraga N, et al: Malignant granular cell tumor of the esophagus: A case report with light and electron microscopic, histochemical and immunohistochemical study. Acta Pathol Jpn 37:775, 1987.
Orvidas LJ, McCaffrey TV, Lewis JE, et al: Lymphoma involving the esophagus. Ann Otol Rhinol Laryngol 103:843, 1994.
Osamura RY, Watanabe K, Shimamura K, et al: Polypoid carcinoma of the esophagus: A unifying team for "carcinosarcoma" and "pseudosarcoma." Am J Surg Pathol 2:201, 1978.
Pass HT, Potter DA, Macher AM, et al: Thoracic manifestations of the acquired immune deficiency syndrome. J Thorac Cardiovasc Surg 88:654, 1984.
Pearson JM, Borg-Grech A: Primary Ki-1(CD 30)–positive, large cell, anaplastic lymphoma of the esophagus. Cancer 68:418, 1991.
Perch SJ, Soften EM, Whittington R, Brooks JJ: Esophageal sarcomas. J Surg Oncol 48:194, 1991.
Pourzand A, Freant L, Levin R, et al: Primary adenoid cystic carcinoma of the esophagus. J Thorac Cardiovasc Surg 69:785, 1975.
Rosenberg SA, Diamond HD, Jaslowitz B, et al: Lymphosarcoma: A review of 1269 cases. Medicine 40:31, 1961.
Sakata K, Ishida M, Hiraishi H, et al: Adenosquamous carcinoma of the esophagus after endoscopic variceal sclerotherapy: A case report and review of the literature. Gastrointest Endosc 47:294, 1998.
Sarbia M, Verreet P, Bittinger F, et al: Basaloid–squamous cell carcinoma of the esophagus: Diagnosis and prognosis. Cancer 79:1871, 1997.
Sasano N, Abe S, Satake O, et al: Choriocarcinoma mimicry of an esophageal carcinoma with urinary gonadotropic activities. Tohoku J Exp Med 100:153, 1969.
Scotto J, Fraumeni JF, Lee JAH: Melanomas of the eye and other noncutaneous sites: Epidemiologic aspects. J Natl Cancer Inst 56:489, 1976.
Soga J: Esophageal endocrinomas—an extremely rare tumor: A statistical comparative evaluation of 28 ordinary carcinoids and 72 atypical variants. J Exp Clin Cancer Res 17:47, 1998.
Spiro RH, Huvos AG, Berk R, Strong EW: Mucoepidermoid carcinoma of salivary gland origin: A clinicopathologic study of 367 cases. Am J Surg 136:461, 1978.
Spiro RH, Huvos AG, Strong EW: Adenoid cystic carcinoma: Factors influencing survival Am J Surg 138:579, 1979.
Stein HA, Murray D, Warner HA: Primary Hodgkin's disease of the esophagus. Dig Dis Sci 26:457, 1981.
Stout AP, Humphreys GH, Rottenberg LA: A case of carcinosarcoma of the esophagus. Am J Roentgenol 61:461, 1949.
Suehs OW: Malignant melanoma of the esophagus. Ann Otol Rhinol Laryngol 70:1140, 1961.
Suzuki H, Nagayo T: Primary tumors of the esophagus other than squamous cell carcinoma: Histologic classification and statistics in the surgical and autopsied material in Japan. Int Adv Surg Oncol 3:73, 1980.
Takayama T, Kato H, Tachimori Y, et al: Treatment of rupture of a liver metastasis from esophageal leiomyosarcoma. Jpn J Clin Oncol 26:248, 1996.
Tanida S, Miyamoto T, Katagiri K, et al: Carcinoid of the esophagus located in lamina propria. J Gastroenterol 33:541, 1998.
Taniyama K, Suzuki H, Sakuramachi S, et al: Amelanotic malignant melanoma of the esophagus: Case report and review of the literature. Jpn J Clin Oncol 20:286, 1990.
Tateishi R, Taniguchi H, Wada A, et al: Argyrophil cells and melanocytes in esophageal mucosa. Arch Pathol 98:87, 1974.
Templeton AC, Bhana D: Prognosis in Kaposi's sarcoma. J Natl Cancer Inst 55:1301, 1975.
Trillo AA, Accettullo LM, Yeiter TL: Choriocarcinoma of the esophagus: histologic and cytologic findings—a case report. Acta Cytol 23:69, 1979.
Tsang WYW, Chan JKC, Lee KC, et al: Basaloid-squamous carcinoma of the upper aerodigestive tract and so-called adenoid cystic carcinoma of the oesophagus: The same tumour type? Histopathology 19:35, 1991.
Wain SL, Kier R, Vollmer RT, et al: Basaloid-squamous carcinoma of the tongue, hypopharynx and larynx: Report of 10 cases. Hum Pathol 17:1158, 1986.
Wasan HS, Schofield JB, Krausz T, et al: Combined choriocarcinoma and yolk sac tumor arising in Barrett's esophagus. Cancer 73:514, 1994.
Wood NL, Coltman CA: Localized primary extranodal Hodgkin's disease. Ann Intern Med 78:113, 1973.
Worgan D, Baldock CR: Lymphosarcoma of the oesophagus. J Laryngol Otol 90:207, 1976.

SECTION **VIII**

Operative Techniques

CHAPTER **51**

Overview of Operative Techniques

Joel D. Cooper

No area of thoracic surgery is more challenging or more daunting than that of esophageal resection and reconstruction. The extirpative portion of the procedures are often technically demanding, but reconstruction is by far the most challenging aspect. The quality of life for the remainder of the patient's existence depends on the functional outcome produced.

The succeeding chapters summarize a wide variety of approaches and techniques and are not intended to replace an atlas but, rather, to depict and illustrate the breadth of available options, any one of which might, on occasion, be the ideal approach for a specific patient. Many of the procedures are mainly of a stark interest but nonetheless may be summoned up as needed to solve a difficult problem.

Most of us who have spent the majority of our career in the 20th century have at one time or another used almost every technique depicted. To date, however, most cases of esophageal resection and reconstruction can be well handled by choosing from a relatively small number of surgical options, thus potentially limiting the armamentarium available to the next generation of esophageal surgeons. However, surgeons who do not familiarize themselves with the indications and techniques of a wide variety of surgical options do so to their own limitation and to the potential detriment of patients referred for management of complicated esophageal problems.

The following chapters represent a distillation of a vast amount of experience on the part of the distinguished authors who prepared them. I recommend their periodic review by thoracic surgeons who wish to maintain familiarity with the broadest possible surgical armamentarium.

CHAPTER **52**

Selection and Placement of Conduits

Clement A. Hiebert

Carl E. Bredenberg

Except for excision of the second portion of the duodenum, there is no greater surgical challenge in the digestive tract than resection and replacement of the esophagus. Owing to the inelastic character of the esophagus, the beguilingly simple option of resection and end-to-end anastomosis is ordinarily denied the esophageal surgeon, who must match elaborate replacement strategy with the best approach to removal of the afflicted organ. This chapter looks at what is available in the abdominal "closet" of spare parts, takes the measure of likely conduits, and scouts spaces and tunnels through which the new gullet might be routed.

CRITERIA FOR ORGAN SELECTION

Ideally, the transposed organ should preserve as many functions of the normal esophagus as possible: agreeable transport, a barrier to reflux and aspiration, and provision for vomiting and belching. One may have to settle for less, for when all is said and done, enabling the patient to swallow without aspirating is the ultimate goal. A modest amount of reflux may be acceptable when the operation is performed for cancer, but the ideal for a young person with a benign condition ought to include not only restoration of agreeable swallowing but also long-term freedom from heartburn, esophagitis, and stricture.

A second criterion for selecting an esophageal substitute relates to the morbidity and mortality of the procedure itself. Esophageal resections are among the most difficult operations in the surgeon's repertoire. Tradeoffs are the rule. A cancerous cervical esophagus *can* be replaced with a revascularized jejunal graft that spares normal esophagus, but such an operation usually requires two teams, five anastomoses, and as many hours of operating. The functional result may be excellent, but are the risks justified when there may be a simpler option, such as pedicled graft of stomach or colon (Fig. 52–1)? One may favorably influence morbidity and mortality by choosing not merely what is easier but what is familiar.

STOMACH

Mobilized and released from its short gastric and left gastric vascular tethers, the fundus of the intact stomach can be detached from the esophagus and advanced to the cervical esophagus and, usually, the pharynx (Akiyama et al, 1978; Moores et al, 1983). Relocating the stomach requires but one anastomosis. It travels, moreover, with its own omental "security blanket" with which to wrap the suture line. The stomach is not the least bit shy and springs to the fore, whether uncovered through a left chest, left thoracoabdominal, or abdominal approach. The stomach is a clean and convenient substitute for the esophagus. It can even be mobilized through the undivided diaphragmatic hiatus, as reported by Belsey and Hiebert (1974) in 191 patients who underwent surgery via an exclusive right thoracic approach. The stomach, tubed or intact, remains the overwhelming choice for an esophageal substitute. Huang (2000) used the stomach in 98.2% of 1874 patients who required esophagectomy for either benign or malignant disease.

Transposing the stomach has both short- and long-term risks. The bête noire of every resection is vascular insufficiency at the anastomosis or, even worse, necrosis of the explant. This is something of a paradox, considering that for years it has been taken as common knowledge that the stomach has a robust blood supply fully capable of tolerating minor abuse from clamps, forceps, or fingers. Liebermann-Meffert and colleagues (1992) showed with corrosion cast studies that robustness of the blood supply peters out at the upper end of the gastroepiploic arcade. After the left and short gastric vessels are divided and ligated, survival of the fundus depends on submucosal microvascular channels. It is obvious that bruising this vascular network can set the stage for devastating tissue breakdown. Petechial hemorrhages, mottled serosa, pale mucosa, and dark oozing are familiar signs that augur poorly for optimal healing. A bruised stomach needs to be warmed, straightened out, or trimmed back or to have its tunnel widened. It should be kept in mind that a mauled organ "remembers," and one should treat the stomach with consideration.

Using the stomach as an esophageal substitute has a second, major long-term risk occasioned by the valveless joining of esophagus and stomach. Almost a third of patients so treated experience esophagitis, stricture, and aspiration (Bender and Walbaum, 1987; Skinner and Belsey, 1988). Orringer and colleagues (1999), using a cervical anastomosis, noted occasional regurgitation of gastric contents after overeating in 32% of his patients. Seven percent required postural elevation to prevent nocturnal reflux. Efforts to curb reflux by encircling the anastomosis with a collar of fundus (Pearson et al, 1969) or

Organ	Technique	No. of Anastomoses	Inherent Morbidity Difficulty	Upper Level of Usefulness	Disadvantages
Stomach	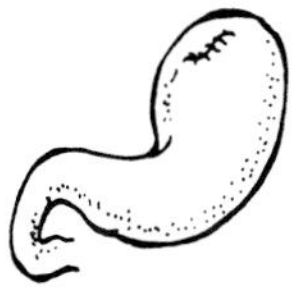	1	+	Cervical Esophagus and Pharynx	Bulky Reflux Risk
Greater Curvature Tube	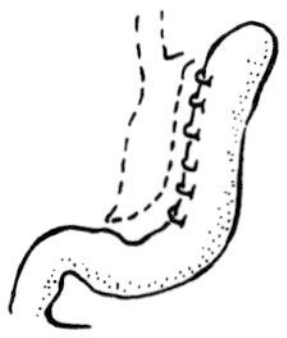	1	+	Cervical Esophagus and Pharynx	Reflux Risk
Reversed Gastric Tube	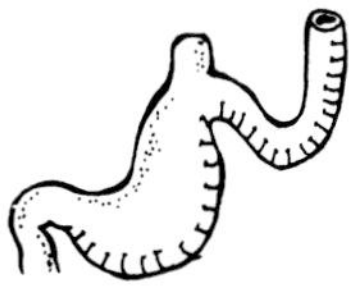	1	+++	Cervical Esophagus and Pharynx	Long Suture Line Limited Blood Supply
Non-reversed Gastric Tube	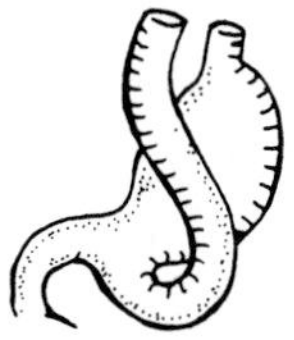	1	++	Lower Cervical Esophagus	Long Suture Line
Right Colon	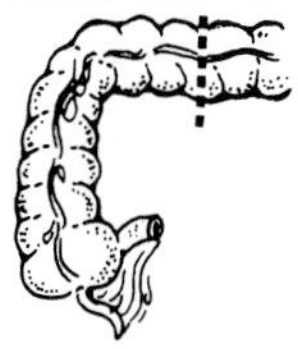	3	+++	Lower Cervical Esophagus	Thin-walled Bulky Short Pedicle
Left Colon	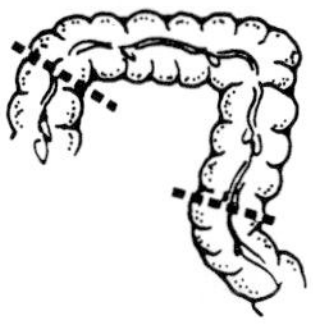	3	++++	Most versatile organ for use at any level Lower third to Pharynx	Extensive operation Redundancy over time
Jejunum	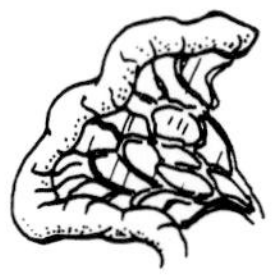	2 (Roux Loop) 3 (Interposition)	++	Lower Third	Limited graft length without revision of pedicle or bowel
Free Graft	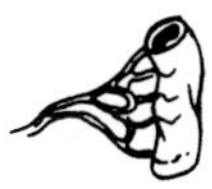	5 (2 micro-vascular)	+++++	Pharynx and Cervical Esophagus	Microvascular anastomoses required

FIGURE 52–1 ■ Comparative usefulness of various esophageal substitutes.

intercostal muscle (Demos and Biele, 1980) have been advocated, but most surgeons agree with Sweet's observation (1945) that the higher the anastomosis, the less the reflux.

Greater Curvature Tube

The most commonly employed gastric tube is created by excision of the upper two thirds of the lesser curvature in continuity with the celiac nodes and esophagus. Lateral release of the duodenum (Kocher's maneuver) and ligation and division of the left and short gastric vessels allow the tube to be advanced to the neck. The vascular main, on which the transplant depends, is that most serviceable of vessels, the right gastroepiploic artery. The right gastric artery, according to Liebermann-Meffert and colleagues (1992), makes an insignificant contribution.

Specific disadvantages to a greater curvature tube are few. Stapling or careful sewing has reduced, but not eliminated, the possibility of dehiscence of the long suture line, and positioning the anastomosis in the neck has lessened the gravity of any leak. Provided that reflux esophagitis has not supervened, long-term functional results are generally satisfactory (Orringer et al, 1999; Skinner and Belsey, 1988).

Reversed Gastric Tube

Replacement of the entire esophagus with a reversed greater curvature tube was invented by Beck and Carrell (1905), first used successfully in a patient by Ropke (1912), rediscovered by Gavriliu (1965, 1975, 1988), and championed by a variety of surgeons, including Heimlich (1972), Ximenes-Netto (1986), and Lortat-Jacob and Giuli (1973). Anderson and Randolph (1978) showed its usefulness in children. Gavriliu (1988) reported using the reversed tube technique in 93.5% of 768 patients of all ages undergoing esophagectomy for both benign and malignant conditions. The ostensible advantages of the technique include the ability to reach the pharynx via one of several routes, the absence of kinking, and the satisfactory restoration of swallowing.

Blood supply of the reversed gastric tube depends on the microcirculation plus the variable communication of a mediocre left gastroepiploic artery with the right gastroepiploic artery, a connection described by Liebermann-Meffert and colleagues (1992) as "of minor vascular diameter." Most surgeons find the prospect of a long suture line and the tenuous blood supply to be daunting. The spleen is easily injured, and Skinner (1991) cautions against continuing the operation if splenectomy is necessary. Fistula formation was a problem in 7.5% and anastomotic strictures occurred in 12.5% of Gavriliu's (1965, 1975) patients. Theoretical concern about retrograde peristalsis has not been borne out by manometric studies (Postlethwait, 1986).

Nonreversed Gastric Tube

Postlethwait (1986) described creation of an isoperistaltic greater curvature tube to bypass or replace the thoracic esophagus. Like its reversed cousin, this tube allows the esophagus to drain into the stomach. Postlethwait has found the technique to be especially useful in bypass performed in patients with carcinoma invading the airway. Substernal interposition was used in 31 such patients; half of the members of this very sick group experienced anastomotic leaks, and 22.6% of the total group died (Postlethwait, 1979). We have used this operation successfully in the case of a child with a severe caustic burn in whom the presence of mediastinitis militated against esophagectomy.

As with the creation of a reversed gastric tube, a rather long suture line is required, but the right gastroepiploic artery is a reliable blood supply. Because vagal nerves are undisturbed, the need for a pyloroplasty is obviated.

JEJUNUM

Jejunum may replace the lower esophagus as (1) an intact loop, (2) a Roux-en-Y reconstruction, (3) an interposition between intrathoracic esophagus and stomach, or (4) a free tissue graft transposed to the neck, where its artery and vein are anastomosed with microvascular techniques to suitable vessels in the cervical area.

Jejunum is readily available and, being an isoperistaltic segment, is a reliable transporter of food. It does not require a bowel preparation, and its diameter is a convenient match for that of the esophagus. The jejunal wall, moreover, is just the right thickness for comfortable placement of sutures. As an interposed isoperistaltic conduit, the jejunum becomes an effective barrier against gastroesophageal reflux, especially if its overall length is at least 15 cm and if the intra-abdominal portion is sufficient to allow anastomosis well down on the posterior wall of the stomach (Skinner and Belsey, 1988).

The limiting factor with jejunum is the tight radius of the looping branches of the superior mesenteric artery, which resemble parachute shrouds pulling down from the edge of the canopy. The limiting factor is not the length of the viscus, but the configuration of the vascular arcades (Wong, 1988). For jejunum to reach above the level of the pulmonary hilum, redundant bowel in the middle of the loop must be excised (Kasai et al, 1965). In North America, the popularity of interposed small bowel has waned but jejunum remains an excellent replacement organ for resections of the lower third of the esophagus.

Roux-en-Y reconstruction using jejunum can substitute for the excised lower esophagus and stomach (Roux, 1907). It provides an excellent barrier to reflux and is useful when other operations have failed (Mannell, 1988). The details of the Roux-en-Y acid suppression–alkaline diversion procedure can be found in Chapter 26.

LEFT COLON

A pedicled segment of left colon is a versatile substitute for excised esophagus in the treatment of a wide variety of maladies, from benign to malignant in patients from infancy to old age. Colon is the organ to which the surgeon likely turns when the stomach has been truncated by caustic burn, scar, ulceration, or previous operation. Proponents of isoperistaltic colon substitution have used the organ for a wide variety of conditions, including long-segment esophageal atresia, malignant tracheo-esophageal fistula, benign stricture, lye burns, perforation, and failed gastric pull-up as well as after unsuccessful operations for achalasia (Belsey, 1989; DeMeester et al, 1988; Hiebert, 1991).

The most popular technique uses the left and transverse colon based on the ascending branch of the left colic artery. Transposed left colon ordinarily reaches to the neck; if necessary, however, the surgeon may gain additional length by dividing the transverse colon near the hepatic flexure. Before doing so, the surgeon must ascertain the adequacy of communications between the left and midcolic vessels. In contrast to the exasperating limitations imposed by vascular arcades of the small bowel, the marginal vessels of the colon lie straight and close to the viscus, making early redundancy and kinking of large intestine less of a problem. The wall of the left colon is agreeably thick for suturing, and the caliber of its lumen matches that of the esophagus.

Other advantages of the left colon as an isoperistaltic substitute include its memory, albeit variable, for propelling a solid bolus (Belsey, 2000). Colon has a mucous shield to protect it from reflux. Any acid that manages to sneak in is greeted with a peristaltic rush, a worthy trait for an organ recruited to serve both as a conduit and as a barrier to reflux (Jones et al, 1973).

Disadvantages of using an isoperistaltic segment of left colon are few. A bowel preparation begun the day before is desirable to lessen the chances of empyema or wound sepsis. Repositioning of the colon, therefore, is hardly an ad hoc maneuver to be used in the event of intraoperative disappointment with another organ. Extensive mobilization and three anastomoses make for a long operation, even with two teams working synchronously. Over the years, the colon, like other transposed viscera—indeed, like the rest of the body—has a tendency to sag, broaden, and lose tone.

Contraindications to the use of large intestine as an esophageal substitute include severe mesenteric arteriosclerosis, anatomic discontinuity of the marginal artery, and the presence of intrinsic colonic disease. Belsey (2000) states that mild diverticulosis does not seem to matter, but diverticulitis prohibits its use. Hirschsprung's disease in the infant or an atonic colon in the adult also disqualifies use of this organ. Wilkins (1991) recommends preoperative evaluation of the colon with colonoscopy, mesenteric arteriography, and barium enema.

RIGHT COLON

Compared with the left colon, the right colon is thin-walled, bulky, and sluggish. When used as an esophageal substitute, it barely reaches to the neck. Retaining the terminal ileum and using it for the upper anastomosis may occasionally be advantageous, but angulation and uncertainty about the blood supply of the ileal segment cast shadows over the technique. The main problem with the right colon consists of the lack of a marginal artery in two thirds of cases and the taut sheath of right colic and ileocolic vessels that sets the upper limit of the organ's usefulness. The right colon, like the small bowel, is best regarded as an option when the stomach or the left colon is unavailable.

REVASCULARIZED FREE TRANSPLANTS

Before the mid-20th century, cancer or caustic burns of the pharynx, hypopharynx, and upper cervical esophagus were usually managed with local excision or radiation. If the lesion was circumferential, a sleeve resection might be performed, followed by two-stage reconstruction using a pedicled tube of skin and subcutaneous tissue (Wookey, 1942). Seidenberg and associates (1959) reported the free transfer of jejunum; two years later, Hiebert and Cummings (1961) reported the free transfer of revascularized gastric antrum. Another decade passed, however, before free tissue transfer emerged from sporadic reporting of feats to the realm of clinical acceptability (Jurkiewicz, 1984; Paletta and Jurkiewicz, 1991; Perrachia, 1985; Trastek et al, 1994). Where are we now?

Esophageal surgeons have generally shied away from using revascularized grafts, in large part because of the development of alternatives simpler than a 6- to 10-hour operation involving a couple of teams committed to the construction of five anastomoses, including two lilliputian "tedio-meticulostomies" (Richardson, personal communication, 1961). All the same, free grafting has the following three benefits not found in other approaches:

1. The normal esophagus is retained.
2. The surgeon may resect the tumor, completely confident that proximal and distal anastomoses will be tension-free.
3. It is the best hope for rescuing a conventionally transposed viscus that has been spoiled by necrosis at the anastomosis.

If less than the full circumference of the original organ is affected, the jejunal transplant may be opened longitudinally and applied as a gusset (Trastek et al, 1994). Except for rescue missions, however, most surgeons who operate for cancer of the cervical esophagus have stayed with familiar, if less dazzling, operations (see Fig. 52–1).

Having used both jejunum and stomach as esophageal substitutes, a surgeon can see clearly that the right gastroepiploic vessels are stouter and easier to sew than the vessels supplying the small bowel. Transposed stomach has the further advantage of "forgetting" its peristaltic past and being able to settle comfortably into service as a funnel. In the jejunum, peristalsis continues after transfer but is not synchronized with swallowing (Paletta and Jurkiewicz, 1991). Any surgeon wishing to revisit the subject of which is the better organ for this use is likely to be daunted by the knowledge that there is but one stomach in the abdominal "stockroom," whereas there is jejunum galore.

SKIN OR MYOCUTANEOUS FLAPS

Flaps of skin, subcutaneous tissue, and muscle represent yet another fallback option for repair of secondary leaks or fistulas. Alternatively, the flap may be rolled up into a bulky tube to bridge a short circumferential gap. Pectoralis major myocutaneous flap is popular with plastic surgeons, but free revascularized flaps from the forearm or leg are sometimes used (Chen et al, 1991; Lam et al, 1988). The forearm cutaneous flap based on the radial artery has become especially popular among otorhinolaryngology surgeons and is quite reliable and versatile.

EXTERNAL BYPASS WITH A PROSTHESIS

External prosthetic replacement of the esophagus may be considered in those exceptional circumstances in which disease or previous surgery has ablated the stomach and colon and in which disease or previous surgery has ablated the stomach and colon and in which small bowel is unavailable because of adhesions or inadequate vascular architecture. Akiyama and Hatano (1968) devised a mushroom-tipped silicone catheter prosthesis, one end of which is inserted into an esophagostomy and the other into a gastrostomy, echoing the replacement procedure used by Thorek (1913) in the first successful esophagectomy. Thorek's patient was enabled to swallow and maintain nutrition for more than 13 years. Skinner and colleagues (1988) reported favorably on the subject.

RESECTION AND END-TO-END ANASTOMOSIS

At the opposite end of the continuum of surgical complexity is the very short or partial esophageal resection that allows reapproximation. Three examples are (1) for congenital atresia of the esophagus, (2) in the repair of a fistula resulting from an operation to divert saliva, and (3) after removal of a small tumor (Billroth, 1871; Davidson, 1967; Little, et al, 1985; Orringer, 1984).

POSITIONING OF THE CONDUIT

Ideally, the substituted organ should lie in a straight line. There should be neither encroachment on the lumen of the viscus nor embarrassment of its blood supply. Advantages and disadvantages of the five available routes are depicted in Figure 52–2. The eventual choice, however, is most often determined by the position of the patient and the incisions required to resect the gullet and mobilize the intended substitute. In a word, the planned limits of resection determine the operation and organ; these, in turn, define the incisions, which in turn dictate the logical tunnel or space through which the transposed organ should be routed.

Presternal Subcutaneous Route

The presternal subcutaneous route has such an obvious cosmetic disadvantage that, at least in the Western world, it is a tunnel of last resort. Nonetheless, this route obviates encroachment of transposed viscus on the heart or lungs and seems to modify the catastrophic consequences of an infarcted graft.

Retrosternal Route

The retrosternal route is created by blunt separation of inconsequential connections between the sternum in front and the pericardium, thymus gland, and innominate vein behind. This channel may prove a godsend when the posterior mediastinum is frozen or when vascular adhesions block safe crossing of the pleural space. At other times, the retrosternal route may be chosen as a matter of convenience.

Disadvantages of the retrosternal route include possible interference with operations, either past or contemplated, on the heart, aortic arch, or great vessels. Because the transposed organ above the manubrium must spiral around the trachea, the swallowing route is not direct. At the lower end, the graft must angle posteriorly from the xiphoid to the stomach. These curves assume importance if bougienage is needed for an anastomotic stricture.

Transpleural Route

The transpleural route may be elected as part of Sweet's transthoracic technique for performing a high esophagogastrostomy lateral to the aortic arch (Sweet, 1945). The transpleural route is the obvious one to use if an unresectable tumor at the cardia is to be bypassed, but it makes little sense for a tumor requiring a cervical anastomosis.

Posterior Mediastinal Route

The posterior mediastinal route is in the bed of the resected esophagus, allowing both upper and lower anastomoses to be in line with the axis of the transplant. The posterior mediastinal channel can be used from the abdomen or via a thoracotomy on either side. According to Maillard and Hay (1988), this corridor is up to 25% (5 to 10 cm) shorter than the retrosternal route.

Endoesophageal Route

The endoesophageal route is the brainchild of Saidi and associates (1990), who discovered that the normal esophagus is easily stripped of its mucosa, leaving a distensible muscle sleeve through which colon or stomach may be passed to the neck. The technique ostensibly avoids vascular hazards of conventional transhiatal esophagectomy in which the plane of dissection is outside the esophagus. The best use of the endoesophageal route appears to be in situations in which full-thickness excision of the thoracic esophagus adds little to the likelihood of cure, for example, for lesions limited to the cardia or situated in the cervical esophagus. In addition to ease and safety of dissection, the technique ensures (at least for the short term) a straight lie of transposed stomach or colon.

CONCLUSION

Before we conclude this discussion of conduit selection and placement, it is appropriate to remember that most esophagectomies are performed for cancer. In such cases, success is ordinarily defined in months, not years. Stoller and coworkers (1977) defined *palliation* as the number of days at home with the ability to swallow—to which I might add "and the desire to do so." Choosing the proper

Route	Procedure	Advantages	Disadvantages
Sub-cutaneous	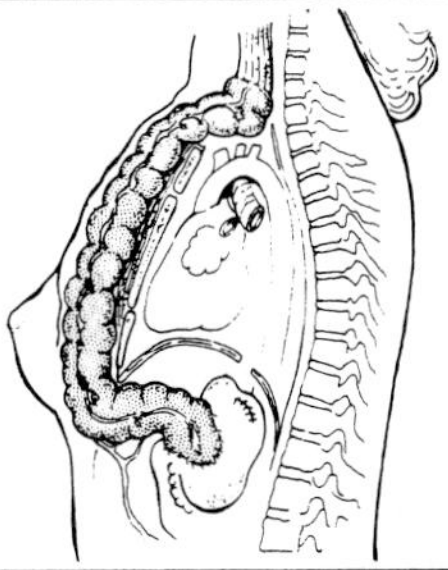	Ease of construction. Avoids encroachment on heart or lungs. Facilitates early detection of graft failure.	Cosmetically far from ideal. Longest course of any route.
Substernal	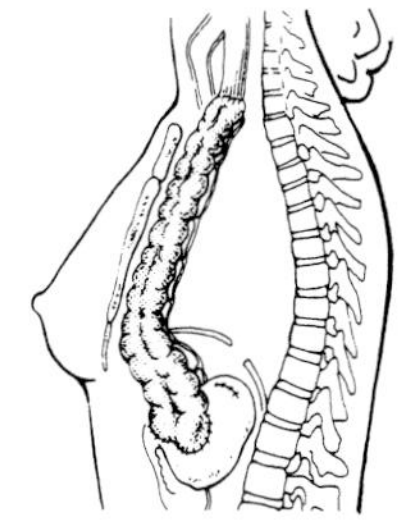	Ease of construction. Useful when mediastinum is unavailable.	Long route. Graft angulation. Cardiac surgery concerns (past or proposed).
Transpleural	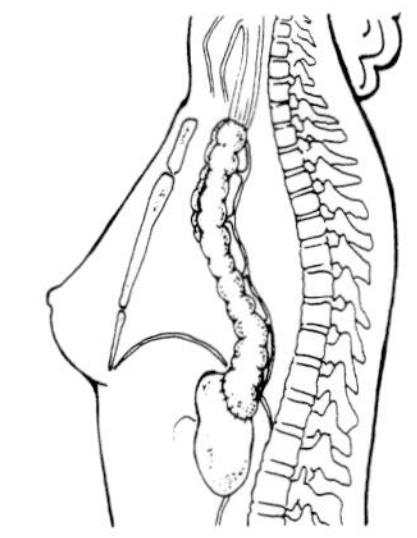	Convenient from left thoracic approach.	Displaces lung.
Posterior Mediastinal	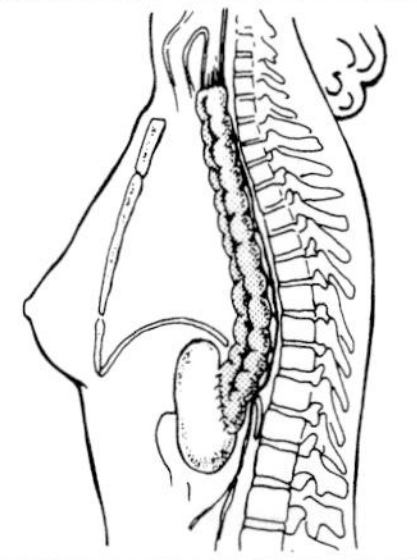	Short and direct.	Mediastinum may be unavailable if inflamed, scarred, or involved with cancer.
Endo-esophageal	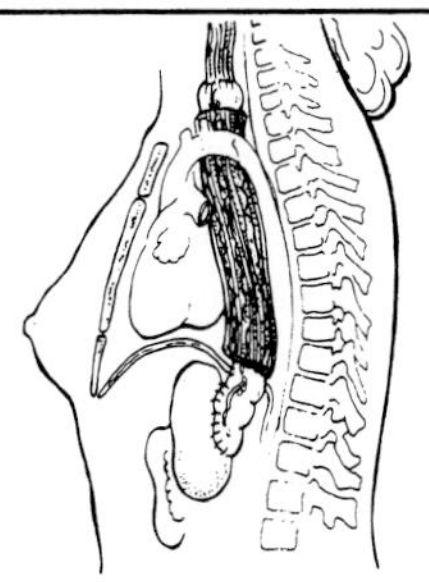	Lessened risk of bleeding. Short and direct. Promotes a straight lie of the viscus.	? Compromise of cancer operation. ? Possibility for constriction.

FIGURE 52–2 ■ Advantages and disadvantages of available routes for positioning the esophageal substitute. (Adapted from Hiebert CA: Surgical options for esophageal replacement: Colon interposition. In Baue AE, Geha AS, Hammond GL, et al: [eds]: Glenn's Thoracic and Cardiovascular Surgery, Vol II, 5th ed., East Norwalk, CT, Appleton & Lange, 1991, p 811).

replacement organ and skillfully suturing it where it will work best is the "right stuff" of our specialty, but equally important is to do no harm to those doomed patients for whom the best replacement organ may be no organ at all.

COMMENTS AND CONTROVERSIES

The preceding chapter by Drs. Hiebert and Bredenberg is an entertaining and informative mixture of philosophy, prose, and pragmatism. Reconstruction or bypass of the esophagus is a demanding, often daunting task, and the quality of the patient's remaining life will be greatly affected by the functional result. Probably no area of reconstructive surgery demands more versatility of approach and technique.

It has become clear that the stomach is by far the most suitable conduit for esophageal replacement with generally excellent long-term functional results. As the authors point out, however, the blood supply to the apex of the gastric tube can be somewhat tenuous. It is for this reason that postoperative hypotension or low cardiac output must be avoided, as these factors can jeopardize the viability of the gastric side of the esophagogastric anastomosis. The authors refer to Sweet's observation, in 1945, that the higher the anastomosis, the less the reflux. Certainly, this dictum has stood the test of time. It is one of the principal reasons why subtotal esophagectomy with a high anastomosis has virtually replaced the left thoracoabdominal approach with its resulting midthoracic esophagogastric anastomosis and its frequent consequence of disabling symptoms of reflux esophagitis.

During preparation of the gastric conduit, excision of the lesser curvature not only permits en bloc resection of the left gastric and celiac axis lymph nodes but also adds significant length to the remaining gastric conduit. In fact, if a gastric conduit is too short to easily reach the cervical esophagus, re-excision of an additional portion of the lesser curvature frequently results in marked lengthening of the conduit.

The authors advocate pyloroplasty or pyloromyotomy when using the stomach as an esophageal replacement. Although this step is common practice, it has been my own preference not to incorporate either procedure unless there is obvious scarring of the duodenum from previous peptic ulcer disease. My concern is that enlarging the pylorus may increase the incidence of bile reflux. Rarely has postoperative gastric emptying been a problem in my experience, and on such occasions simple endoscopic balloon dilatation of the pylorus has solved the problem. When poor gastric emptying does occur, it usually follows an Ivor Lewis approach using the right thoracotomy. In this situation, the stomach tends to fall into the right pleural space posteriorly. Angulation of the distal stomach as it rests on the diaphragm and takes a 90-degree turn to descend through the hiatus is usually the cause of delayed emptying and gastric distention. One benefit of the transhiatal route is the containment of the stomach within the mediastinum, which predisposes to improved gastric emptying.

Both reversed and nonreversed gastric tubes are associated with a high rate of anastomotic leakage. The nonreversed gastric tube, however, has a much more secure blood supply and is by far the preferred method of the two.

The authors refer to the endoesophageal route proposed by Saidi and colleagues (1990), namely, the stripping of the esophageal mucosa and the use of the remaining muscular tube as a route to bring either stomach or colon to the neck. In the normal esophagus, the resulting muscular tube is of insufficient diameter in most cases, although the proposal may have merit in the patient with achalasia. Another possible use of this route is in the patient with a previously irradiated carcinoma of the hypopharynx or cervical esophagus who needs esophageal reconstruction because of complications or recurrence of tumor. The stomach is the ideal conduit for such cases, but resection of the irradiated cervical esophagus is commonly associated with subsequent necrosis of the membranous wall of the adjacent trachea, leading to a fatal outcome. In such a situation, I have stripped the esophageal mucosa, as proposed by Saidi and colleagues, and then split the resulting muscular tube longitudinally along its posterior aspect to allow the gastric conduit to be brought to the neck without the need for dissecting the back wall of the trachea. This approach has resulted in a very satisfactory outcome.

R. J. G.

KEY REFERENCES

Bender EM, Walbaum PR: Esophagastrectomy for benign esophageal stricture. Ann Surg 205:385, 1987.

The authors report on a series of 89 patients with an intrathoracic anastomosis. Although heartburn was present only 8% of the time, variable degrees of dysphagia were experienced by 30% to 40% of the group who required esophageal dilatation over a prolonged period. The authors conclude that an intrathoracic esophagogastric anastomosis is inappropriate for benign disease.

DeMeester TR, Johansson KE, Franze I, et al: Indications, surgical technique, and long-term functional results of colon interposition or bypass. Ann Surg 208:460, 1988.

This detailed review of 92 patients undergoing colon interposition or bypass performed by an experienced esophageal surgeon has an excellent description of operative details, including drawings and follow-up.

Liebermann-Meffert DMI, Meier R, Siewert JR: Vascular anatomy of the gastric tube used for esophageal reconstruction. Ann Thorac Surg 54:1110, 1992.

In this elegant study of the anatomy of gastric blood and the intragastric collaterals, emphasis is placed on the blood supply to the greater curvature used for construction of a gastric tube. The study demonstrates that the critical part of the greater curve aspect of the fundus on which the reversed gastric tube is based has the poorest collateral supply, depending entirely on the submucosal and mucosal microvascular network.

Orringer MB, Marshall B, Iannettoni MD: Transhiatal esophagectomy: Clinical experience and refinements. Ann Surg 230:392, 1999.

This article contains the most recent summary of Orringer's experience with transhiatal esophagectomy. With benign disease, good or excellent functional results were achieved in nearly 70% of patients after a cervical esophagogastric anastomosis. Seventy-seven percent required one or more anastomotic dilatations, but only 4% had persistent anastomotic strictures. Clinically troublesome "nocturnal reflux" occurred in 7% usually managed successfully with elevation of the torso. The authors conclude that transhiatal esophagectomy is feasible in most patients requiring esophageal resection for either benign or malignant disease. The total series consisted of 1085 patients: 285 treated for benign disease and 800 for malignant disease.

Payne WS, Trastek VF, Fisher J: Free intestinal transfer and microvascular techniques in reconstruction of the esophagus. In Shields TW (ed): General Thoracic Surgery, 4th ed. Baltimore, Williams & Wilkins, 1994, p 1500.

This succinct chapter is well written, well illustrated, and well referenced on the use of free jejunal grafts as cervical microvascular anastomoses in either primary or secondary reconstruction of the cervical and upper mediastinal esophagus.

■ REFERENCES

Akiyama H, Hatano S: Esophageal cancer: Palliative treatment. Jpn J Surg 21:391, 1968.

Akiyama H, Miyazono H, Tsurumaru M, et al: Use of the stomach as an esophageal substitute. Ann Surg 188:606, 1978.

Anderson K, Randolph J: Reversed gastric tube for esophageal replacement in children. Ann Thorac Surg 25:521, 1978.

Beck C, Carrell A: Demonstration of specimens illustrating a method of formation of a prethoracic esophagus. Ill Med J 7:463, 1905.

Belsey RHR: Replacement of the esophagus with colon. In Shields TW, Lo Cicero J III, Ponn RB (eds): General Thoracic Surgery, 5th ed. Philadelphia, Lippincott Williams & Wilkins, 2000, p 1733.

Belsey R, Hiebert CA: An exclusive right thoracic approach for cancer of the middle third of the esophagus. Ann Thorac Surg 18:1, 1974.

Bender EM, Walbaum PR: Esophagogastrectomy for benign esophageal stricture. Ann Surg 205:385, 1987.

Billroth T: General Surgical Pathology and Therapeutics, 1871 (translated from the German by Hackley CE, Special Ed, Classics of Surgery Library). New York, Appleton, 1984.

Chen H, Tang Y, Noordhoff MS: Posterior tibial artery flap for reconstruction of the esophagus. Plastic Reconstr Surg 88:980, 1991.

Davidson JS: Resection of squamous cell carcinoma of the oesophagus with end-to-end oesophageal anastomosis. Br J Surg 54:63, 1967.

DeMeester TR, Johansson KE, Franze I, et al: Indications, surgical technique, and long-term functional results of colon interposition or bypass. Ann Surg 208:460, 1988.

Demos N, Biele R: Intercostal pedicle method for control of postresection esophagitis. J Thorac Cardiovasc Surg 80:17, 1980.

Gavriliu D: Aspects of esophageal surgery. Curr Probl Surg 12:1, 1975.

Gavriliu D: The replacement of the esophagus by a gastric tube. In Jamieson GG (ed): Surgery of the Oesophagus. New York, Churchill Livingstone, 1988.

Gavriliu D: Report on the procedure of reconstruction of the esophagus by gastric tube. Int Abstr Surg 121:655, 1965.

Heimlich HJ: Esophagoplasty with reversed gastric tube: Review of 53 cases. Am J Surg 123:80, 1972.

Hiebert CA: Surgical options for esophageal replacement: Colon interposition. In Baue AE, Geha AS, Hammond GL, et al (eds): Glenn's Thoracic and Cardiovascular Surgery, Vol I, 5th ed., East Norwalk, CT, Appleton & Lange, 1991, p 811.

Hiebert CA, Cummings GO Jr: Successful replacement of the cervical esophagus by transplantation and revascularization of a free graft of gastric antrum. Ann Surg 154:103, 1961.

Huang GJ: Replacement of the esophagus with the stomach. In Shields TW, Lo Cicero J III, Ponn RB (eds): General Thoracic Surgery, 5th ed. Philadelphia, Lippincott Williams & Wilkins, 2000, p 1723.

Jones EL, Skinner DB, DeMeester TR, et al: Response of the interposed human colonic segment to an acid challenge. Ann Surg 177:75, 1973.

Jurkiewicz MJ: Reconstructive surgery of the cervical esophagus. J Thorac Cardiovasc Surg 88:893, 1984.

Kasai M, Abols SI, Makino K, et al: Reconstruction of the cervical esophagus by a pedicled jejunal graft. Surg Gynecol Obstet 121:102, 1965.

Lam K, Ho C, Lau W, et al: Immediate reconstruction of pharyngoesophageal defects. Arch Otolaryngol 115:608, 1988.

Liebermann-Meffert DMI, Meier R, Siewert JR: Vascular anatomy of the gastric tube used for esophageal reconstruction. Ann Thorac Surg 54:1110, 1992.

Little AG, DeMeester TR, Skinner DB: Strictures of the proximal esophagus. In DeMeester TR, Skinner DB (eds): Esophageal Disorders: Pathophysiology and Therapy. Raven Press, New York, 1985, p 227.

Lortat-Jacob JL, Giuli R: Esophageal replacement. Prog Surg 12:77, 1973.

Maillard JN, Hay M: Surgical anatomy of available routes for oesophageal bypass. In Jamieson GG (ed): Surgery of the Oesophagus, New York, Churchill Livingstone, 1988, p 723.

Mannell A: Distal oesophagectomy: Left-sided thoracoabdominal approach. In Jamieson GG (ed): Surgery of the Oesophagus. New York, Churchill Livingstone, 1988, p 647.

Moores D, Ilves R, Cooper J, et al: One stage reconstruction for pharyngolaryngectomy. J Thorac Cardiovasc Surg 85:330, 1983.

Orringer MB: Partial median sternotomy: Anterior approach to the upper thoracic esophagus. J Thorac Cardiovasc Surg 87:124, 1984.

Orringer MB, Marshall B, Iannettoni MD: Transhiatal esophagectomy: Clinical experience and refinements. Ann Surg 230:392, 1999.

Paletta CE, Jurkiewicz MJ: Esophageal replacement: Microvascular jejunal transplantation. In Baue AE, Geha AS, Hammond GL (eds): Glenn's Thoracic and Cardiovascular Surgery, Vol I, 5th ed., East Norwalk, CT, Appleton & Lange, 1991.

Peracchia A, Ancona E, Tremolada C, et al: Comparison between different techniques for the reconstruction of the cervical esophagus resected for cancer. In DeMeester TR, Skinner DB (eds): Esophageal Disorders: Pathophysiology and Therapy. New York, Raven Press, 1985.

Pearson FG, Henderson RD, Parrish RM: An operative technique for control of reflux following esophagogastrectomy. J Thorac Cardiovasc Surg 58:688, 1969.

Postlethwait RW: Technique for isoperistaltic gastric tube for esophageal bypass. Ann Surg 189:673, 1979.

Postlethwait RW: Surgery of the Esophagus, 2nd ed. Norwalk, CT, Appleton-Century-Crofts, 1986.

Ropke W: Ein neuses Verfahren fur die Gastrostomie und Oesophagoplasti, Zntralbl Chir 39:1569, 1912 (cited by Bernatz and Hopkins: Replacement of the cervical esophagus. Surg Clin North Am 43:1171, 1963).

Roux C: L'oesophago-jejuno-gastrome: Nouvelle operation pour retrécissement infranchissable de l'oesophage. Semaine Medica (Paris) 27:37, 1907.

Saidi F, Abbassi A, Shadmehr M, et al: Endothoracic endoesophageal pull-through operation. J Thorac Cardiovasc Surg 102:43, 1990.

Seidenberg B, Rosenak SS, Hurwitt ES, et al: Immediate reconstruction of the cervical esophagus by a revascularized isolated jejunal segment. Ann Surg 149:162, 1959.

Skinner DB: Atlas of Esophageal Surgery. New York, Churchill Livingstone, 1991.

Skinner DB, Belsey RHR: Management of Esophageal Disease. Philadelphia, WB Saunders, 1988.

Stoller JL, Samer KJ, Toppin DI, et al: Carcinoma of the oesophagus: A new proposal for the evaluation of treatment. Can J Surg 20:454, 1977.

Sweet RH: Transthoracic resection of esophagus and stomach for carcinoma: Analysis of postoperative complications, causes of death, and late results of operations. Ann Surg 121:272, 1945.

Thorek F: The first successful case of resection of the thoracic portion of the oesophagus for carcinoma. Surg Gynecol Obstet 16:614, 1913.

Trastek VF, Payne WS, Fisher J: Free intestinal transfer techniques in reconstruction of the esophagus. In Shields TW (ed): General Thoracic Surgery, 4th ed. Baltimore, Williams & Wilkins, 1994, p 1500.

Wilkins EW: Techniques of esophageal reconstruction. In Zuidema GD (ed): Shackelford's Surgery of the Alimentary Tract, Vol I, 3rd ed. Philadelphia, WB Saunders, 1991.

Wong J: The use of small bowel for oesophageal replacement following oesophageal resection. In Jamieson GG (ed): Surgery of the Oesophagus. New York, Churchill Livingstone, 1988.

Wookey H: The surgical treatment of carcinoma of the pharynx and upper esophagus. Surg Gynecol Obstet 75:499, 1942.

Ximenes-Netto M: Esophageal reconstruction for benign disease. G E N 40:173, 1986.

CHAPTER **53**

Left Thoracoabdominal Approaches

CLASSIC LEFT THORACOABDOMINAL APPROACHES

Earle W. Wilkins, Jr.

The left thoracic approach was the first, and remains the standard, approach for resection of a carcinoma of the lower esophagus and cardia. Sweet (1954), in his early textbook *Thoracic Surgery*, called this posterolateral approach the standard thoracotomy incision. It may be extended anteriorly across the costal margin to provide the true thoracoabdominal incision for the exposure of upper abdominal viscera or upward in a parascapular fashion to provide access to the entire length of the intrathoracic esophagus.

HISTORICAL NOTE

Meade (1961), in his comprehensive *A History of Thoracic Surgery*, describes the evolution of surgical operations on the esophagus, beginning with Billroth in 1877.

Success with transthoracic approaches to the intrathoracic esophagus begins, however, with Voelcker (1908), who was described by Meade as reporting "the first case of successful resection of the cardia." This was one success of the three attempted. He used a left paramedian abdominal incision. If the tumor was deemed resectable, a second incision was added to resect ribs seven, eight, or nine, as necessary for exposure. (This principle may still be applied today; the thoracoabdominal incision may be used when the resectability of extensive carcinoma of the cardia of the stomach or distal esophagus remains in question despite the findings of diagnostic imaging techniques or laparoscopy.)

Kirschner (1920) described the technique of gastric mobilization for replacement of the esophagus. This has become the standard today. By dividing the left gastric, left gastroepiploic, and short gastric arteries in dogs and human cadavers, "he then could bring the stomach up over the costal margin and up to the clavicle without trouble." He apparently was not successful in attempting the technique in patients with carcinoma but, in principle, preferred its use to small or large intestine for replacement of the esophagus. Roux (1907) had described the use of jejunum, and Kelling (1911) reviewed the transverse colon. Kirschner's operation perpetuated the then-prevalent concept of avoiding intrathoracic placement of the stomach.

Eggers (1931) described the left transthoracic route for access to the esophagus in his successful partial esophagectomy for carcinoma. (He had administered the anesthesia during Torek's first successful esophagectomy in 1913.) The details of Egger's esophageal resection were not unlike the standard mediastinal dissection of today. Replacement of the esophagus was not included, however. The proximal esophagus was brought out through a cervical incision subcutaneously down to the level of the anterior third rib, and the distal end was closed and placed below the diaphragm.

Transpleural dissection of an esophageal carcinoma and replacement with a mobilized stomach were finally combined by Adams and Phemister (1938) in their successful resection and esophagogastrostomy for carcinoma of the lower esophagus. The details of their pioneering technique of anastomosis merit quotation.

> An inner layer of through-and-through interrupted linen sutures was then introduced, and the anastomosis completed by burying this anteriorly with a row of external interrupted linen sutures. . . . Great care was taken that no tension was placed on the gastroesophageal suture line.

Their principles of a two-layer interrupted suture anastomosis and avoidance of tension remain basic.

The technique of anastomosis was perfected by Churchill and Sweet (1942), who emphasized the essential residual blood supply of the stomach through the right gastric and right gastroepiploic arteries and the interrupted-suture two-layer anastomosis (in their hands, with fine silk). Churchill commented that "the mucous membrane sutures are placed with the exactitude and with the degree of tension that we would use in the fine plastic procedure on the lip." Sweet added, "We have had no strictures in our cases. Perhaps we have paid unusual attention to the detail of the anastomosis." This anastomosis always requires "unusual attention" and "exactitude."

After struggling with the troubling techniques of antethoracic plastic procedures to connect the cervical esophagostomy and the Beck-Jianu gastrostomy after middle-third esophagectomy, Sweet (1945) reported on the intrathoracic supra-aortic resection and anastomosis, which brings the stomach to the apex of the left hemithorax. His original exposure with this operation was an eighth rib resection with "shingling," or posterior division, of ribs four to seven. This rather ruthless bit of rib carpentry was later replaced by the double-rib resection (ribs eight and four) through the elongated parascapular skin incision.

Thus, the historical evolution of the left transthoracic esophageal resection with intrathoracic esophagogastrostomy was complete—in a span of 37 years. The principles contained therein remain absolute as follows: (1) determination of resectability, (2) use of the stomach with retention of its right-sided blood supply, (3) the left transpleural route for controlled complete resection of the esophagus and lymph node dissection, (4) carefully exact anastomosis, and (5) extension of the technique to any intrathoracic level of the esophageal carcinoma.

■ *HISTORICAL READINGS*

Adams WE, Phemister DB: Carcinoma of the lower thoracic esophagus: Report of a successful resection and esophagogastrostomy. J Thorac Surg 7:621, 1938.

Churchill ED, Sweet RH: Transthoracic resection of tumors of the stomach and esophagus. Ann Surg 115:897, 1942.

Eggers C: Resection of the thoracic portion of the esophagus for carcinoma. Surg Gynecol Obstet 52:739, 1931.

Kirschner M: Eines neues Verfahren der Ösophagoplastik. Arch Klin Chir 114:606, 1920.

Sweet RH: Surgical management of carcinoma of the midthoracic esophagus: Preliminary report. N Engl J Med 233:1, 1945.

Voelcker F: Über Exstirpation der Cardia wegen Carcinoms. Verh Dtsch Ges Chir 37:126, 1908.

MANAGEMENT

Operative Technique

Preparation

Preoperative considerations involve (1) an assessment of the nutritional and general medical conditions of the patient, (2) the use of prophylactic broad-spectrum antibiotics, and (3) a determination of the type of anesthesia.

A positive nitrogen balance is important in the patient's safe passage through the rigors of this major operation and its postprocedural stress. Hyperalimentation may be necessary. In extreme situations, a feeding gastrostomy in the obstructed patient may convert a physiologically inoperable individual to one able to tolerate the operation. In this type of surgery, in which the mediastinum is extensively dissected and the bacteriologically contaminated esophagus is opened, the use of prophylactic antibiotics is mandatory. One dose is administered intramuscularly on call to the operating room, and the drug is continued intravenously throughout the procedure. One of the cephalosporins is the drug of choice. General anesthesia is used, and the placement of a double-lumen endotracheal tube or a left main bronchial blocker simplifies the left transpleural dissection in every way.

One other preoperative consideration, not within the scope of this discussion, is the use of neoadjuvant therapy—multiagent chemotherapy, mediastinal irradiation, or both.

The Incision

The right decubitus position and the placement of the left thoracic approach to the esophagus are illustrated in Figure 53–1. The basic incision is made from the level of the costal cartilage in front to the paravertebral region at the angle of the scapula behind, resecting the seventh rib or using the seventh intercostal space. Through the fundamental thoracotomy, the stomach may be approached, often adequately, in a technique described (Page et al, 1990) as "esophagogastrectomy via left thoracophrenotomy." In this description, the diaphragm is "opened in line with the wound." Division of the diaphragm circumferentially preserves more of the phrenic innervation, which is desirable for its help in postoperative lung ventilation.

As illustrated, the incision may be extended anteriorly across the costal margin (the true thoracoabdominal technique), with the left rectus muscle divided transversely. This particular technique is especially useful for the dissection of tumors of the cardia that necessitate splenectomy and/or distal partial pancreatectomy. Should there be an unsettled concern about resectability, the limited abdominal portion of the incision may be made first to permit exploration and determine resectability. Sweet (1954) termed this an *abdominothoracic* (not thoracoabdominal) incision to reflect semantically the orderly making of the incision.

The basic incision may be extended upward between the scapula and the vertebral column to the base of the neck. This allows the resection of a higher rib, usually the fourth, to gain access to the supra-aortic dissection of the esophagus and to permit an easier high intrathoracic anastomosis.

Mediastinal Dissection

The principles of mediastinal dissection are (1) wide dissection of the esophagus to bare its mediastinal visceral margins, such as the aorta; (2) complete lymph node dissection; and (3) adequate length of the margins on either end of the esophageal neoplasm.

The esophagus is freed from the hiatus to a level at least 5 cm above the tumor. To avoid dissection too close to the tumor, the descending aorta is completely bared; its esophageal branches on the adventitia of the aorta are divided. The pulmonary ligament or, if necessary, a wedge of the lung itself is taken with the tumor. The pericardium is dissected free, the right mediastinal pleura is entered, if necessary, and the right lung parenchyma is resected. The excision of the parenchyma of either lung is facilitated by the use of the mechanical stapler. All mediastinal lymph nodes are removed in continuity with the esophagus. The vagus nerves are divided at the level of esophageal transection. The thoracic duct is usually protected beyond the descending aorta in the left transthoracic approach, but chylothorax can ensue if the dissection is carried widely in this direction. It would then be wise to check for possible damage to the duct.

In many patients who have undergone an operation for curative resection, it is necessary to extend mobilization of the esophagus to the right of and above the aortic arch. Division of the intercostal aortic branches may be

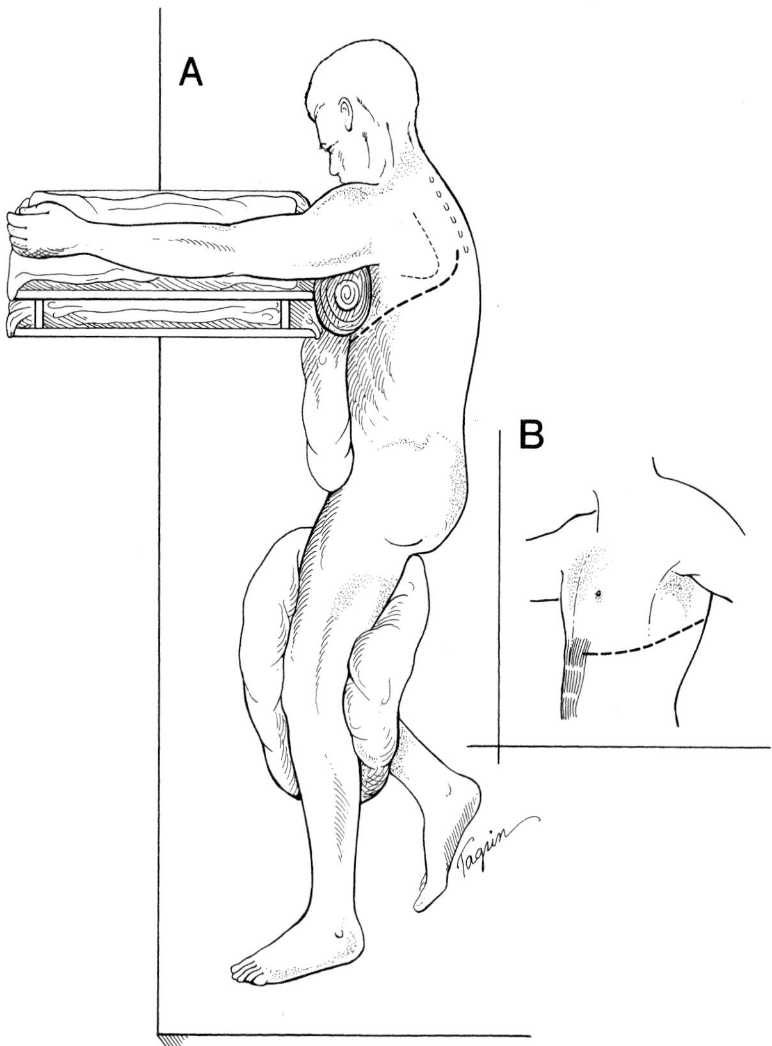

FIGURE 53–1 ■ Placement of the standard left thoracotomy incision for esophageal resection, including anterior and posterior extensions when necessary. *A*, The right decubitus position, left side uppermost, with the usual posterolateral skin incision. *B*, The thoracoabdominal incision.

necessary to help in the mobilization of the arch itself. In general, such mobilization is required only if the tumor lies behind the arch. The left recurrent nerve is carefully preserved. It is in the exposure of the esophagus above the arch that the thoracic duct is most vulnerable to injury (Fig. 53–2). If the thoracic duct is injured, it must be ligated both above and below the point of injury. The azygos arch can be injured from the left side, and this must be carefully avoided. The left main bronchus is examined for possible injury to its membranous portion.

Gastric Mobilization

The Wilkins (1996) description of gastric mobilization is used here. It is a refinement of the Sweet (1954) technique. The essential principles are (1) preservation of the blood supply by preserving the right gastric and right gastroepiploic vessels and arcades and (2) obtaining the maximal length by using the longer greater curvature for positioning the anastomosis.

The initial step in the detachment of the stomach is the division of the greater omentum outside the gastroepiploic arcade with preservation of the right gastroepiploic artery (Fig. 53–3). The surgeon facilitates this division, grasping the transverse colon, lifting it out of the incision caudally, and entering the lesser omental sac at a point where the omentum is thinnest and most transparent. The dissection is carried to the level of the pylorus; the rather small omental branches of the epiploic arcade are divided. These vessels may be coagulated, clipped, or ligated. Fine ligatures are preferred to avoid any retrograde clotting, which might compromise the integrity of the gastroepiploic arcade, and to avoid metal clips, which might compromise the clarity of detail of subsequent computed tomography (CT) scans.

The dissection is then directed toward the spleen, where the left gastroepiploic artery is ligated at the upper end of the arcade above the last segmental artery to the stomach wall. The short gastric (gastrolienal) arteries are divided carefully between hemostatic forceps and are ligated securely. The more proximal of these vessels may be very short and require the application of suture ligatures. Ligatures on the stomach end must be tied securely; sometimes these ties have slipped off the stomach, which later became distended within the thorax.

Finally, there is a posterior branch from the splenic artery to the back of the cardia of the stomach that is

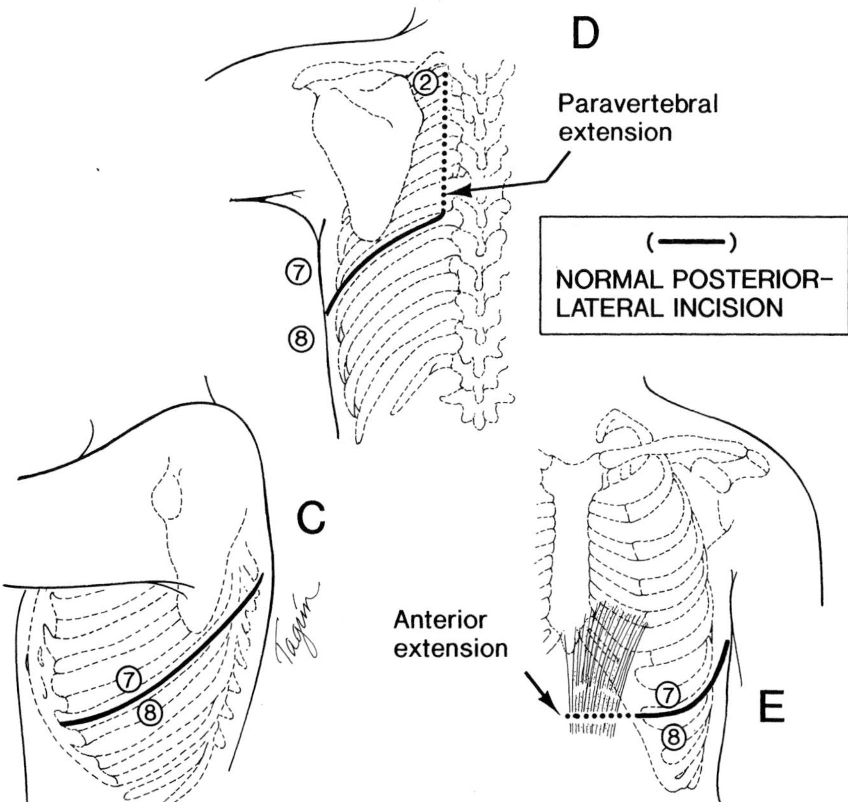

FIGURE 53–1 ■ *Continued. C,* At the costal level, the *solid line* shows the positioning of a seventh interspace incision. *D,* The cephalad paravertebral extension is shown by the *dotted line.* Carrying this to the second rib permits a fourth rib resection for better access to the supra-aortic esophagus. Scapular retraction is facilitated by the surgeon placing the patient's left arm, rotated internally at the shoulder, at the patient's side in front of the abdomen. *E,* The thoracoabdominal anterior extension is shown; the *dotted line* crosses the left rectus muscle to the midline. The operating table is rotated laterally to the left to permit this abdominal exposure.

constant; its division completes the liberation of the greater curvature of the stomach.

Attention is directed toward exposure of the origin of the left gastric artery at the trifurcation of the celiac axis. This structure is approached most easily from behind the stomach, which is elevated to the right by the assistant who applies traction on the Penrose tape (see Fig. 53–3).

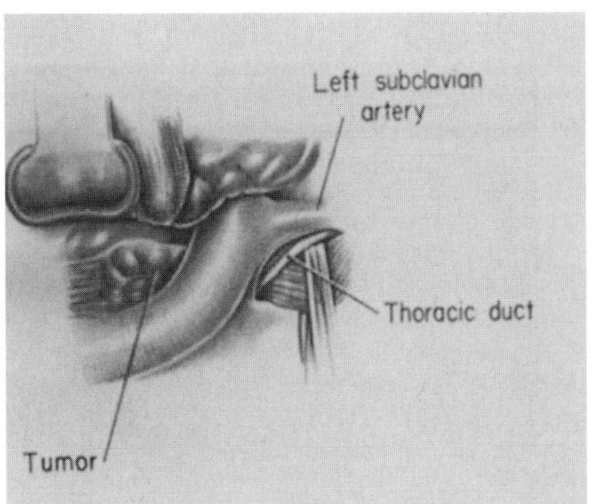

FIGURE 53–2 ■ Course of the thoracic duct as it crosses the esophagus in the superior mediastinum above the arch of the aorta. The duct is easily injured. Particular attention should be directed to this possibility. If continuity has been impaired, ligature should be carried out both above and below the point of injury. (From Sweet RH: Thoracic Surgery, 2nd ed. Philadelphia, WB Saunders, 1954.)

It is necessary to divide the filmy, avascular adhesions between the back of the stomach and the retroperitoneum, which extend from the pylorus to the superior edge of the pancreas. The left gastric artery is exposed by palpation as the surgeon's thumb and forefinger encircle what is left of the lesser curvature attachments. It is doubly ligated at its origin from the celiac axis with a heavy nonabsorbable suture. The first ligature is placed and firmly tied before the artery is actually divided so that should the ligature break during tying, a freely spurting major artery is avoided. Two hemostatic clamps are applied distal to this ligature, and the artery is divided between them. A second tie or transfixion stitch is placed on the left gastric artery distal to the first tie. The artery on the gastric side is best managed with a secure stitch ligature. The left gastric vein is usually identifiable separately from the artery and is handled in a similar fashion.

Lymph nodes along the left gastric artery and celiac axis are thus dissected carefully so that they remain in continuity with the stomach. The stomach itself is transsected from a greater curvature point opposite the level of emergence of the left gastroepiploic artery to a point on the lesser curvature below the lowest branch of the left gastric artery with the gastrointestinal anastomosis (GIA) stapler. This lesser curvature point of transection may actually be carried distally to a point below the incisura. The stapled gastric margin is then turned in with interrupted Lembert 3–0 silk sutures.

Gastric Drainage

It has never been conclusively settled whether a special maneuver is necessary to promote gastric drainage after

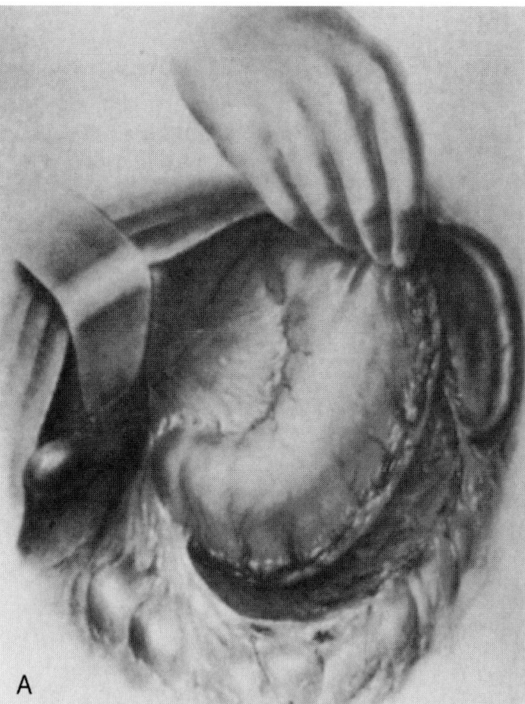

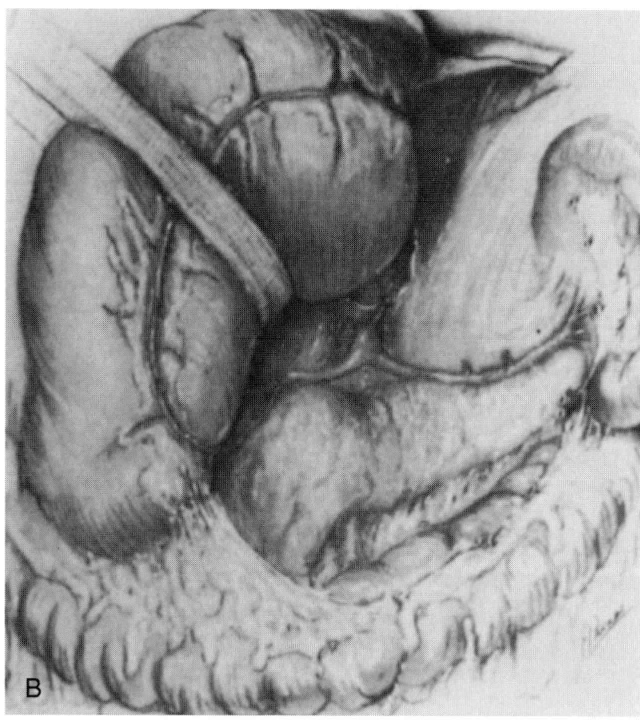

FIGURE 53–3 ■ Two steps in the mobilization of the stomach. *A*, Separation of the greater omentum and the spleen from the stomach with preservation of the gastroepiploic arcade. (From Postlethwait RW: Substernal isoperistaltic gastric tube for esophageal bypass. Surg Rounds 7:20, 1984.) *B*, Upward pull on the tape for retraction of the stomach, which permits exposure of the left gastric artery and the celiac lymph node dissection from behind the stomach. (From Postlethwait RW: Surgery of the Esophagus, 2nd ed. Norwalk, CT, Appleton-Century-Crofts, 1986, p 496.)

esophagectomy with its accompanying bilateral vagectomy. From a physiologic standpoint, gastric drainage seems to make particularly good sense. Because gastroesophageal reflux is fairly common after an intrathoracic anastomosis of the esophagus and stomach and the threat of a peptic stricture is always a possibility, most experienced general thoracic surgeons use a drainage procedure. Pyloromyotomy is preferred because it does not detract from the length of stomach when it must be brought high into the thorax, and the pyloric muscle retains some of its capacity to prevent the reflux of bile and pancreatic juice into the stomach with the threat of alkaline gastritis. Should the mucosa be entered during the completion of the pyloromyotomy, the opening may be sutured and covered with omentum, or the pyloromyotomy may then be converted into a limited pyloroplasty of the Heineke-Mikulicz type.

The Anastomosis

The anastomosis discussed here is the Sweet (1954) or Massachusetts General Hospital technique, a manual layered technique that evolved from the Churchill and Sweet (1942) method. It has been described by Mathisen and associates (1988) and Wilkins (1996).

With completion of the mediastinal dissection and gastric mobilization, the stomach can be brought to any level within the thorax by gentle traction on the upper end of the greater curvature. This is where the maximal length of the viscus can be obtained. Traction on the gastroesophageal specimen upward as a sort of handle permits an end (esophagus)-to-side (stomach) esophagogastric anastomosis. A small circle is then scored through the gastric serosa at least 2 cm from the gastric turn in and nearer the gastroepiploic arcade on the greater curvature. The intramural plexus of vessels is suture-ligated around the circumference of this circle; this minimizes ooze and preserves an unobscured view for suture placement (Fig. 53–4).

A first row of 4–0 silk sutures is placed in a horizontal mattress fashion between the muscularis of the esophagus and the musculoserosa of the stomach. This forms the outer posterior row. Approximately four of these are placed first and then tied carefully by the surgeon, who always draws the stomach upward to the esophagus by positioning the tying forefinger above the point of the actual approximation of tissue. The esophagus is a fixed structure that cannot be brought down distally; its serosaless muscular coats are more fragile and do not hold sutures as well as the stomach. The outer posterior row of sutures covers only about one third of the circumference; this limitation permits more accessible exposure for the placement of the next layer of sutures. The corner ties are left long and marked with hemostats.

Only now is the esophagus opened, always with the sharp scalpel and not cautery, about 4 to 5 mm distal to the outer row of stitches. The incision is extended around each corner. The mucosal layer of the stomach is opened, and the scored button of gastric wall is excised. The pinkish gray esophageal mucosa is exposed carefully (it tends to retract) by the surgeon, who spreads (does not grasp) the opening in the esophagus. The inner posterior sutures, also of 4–0 silk, are placed and tied as the

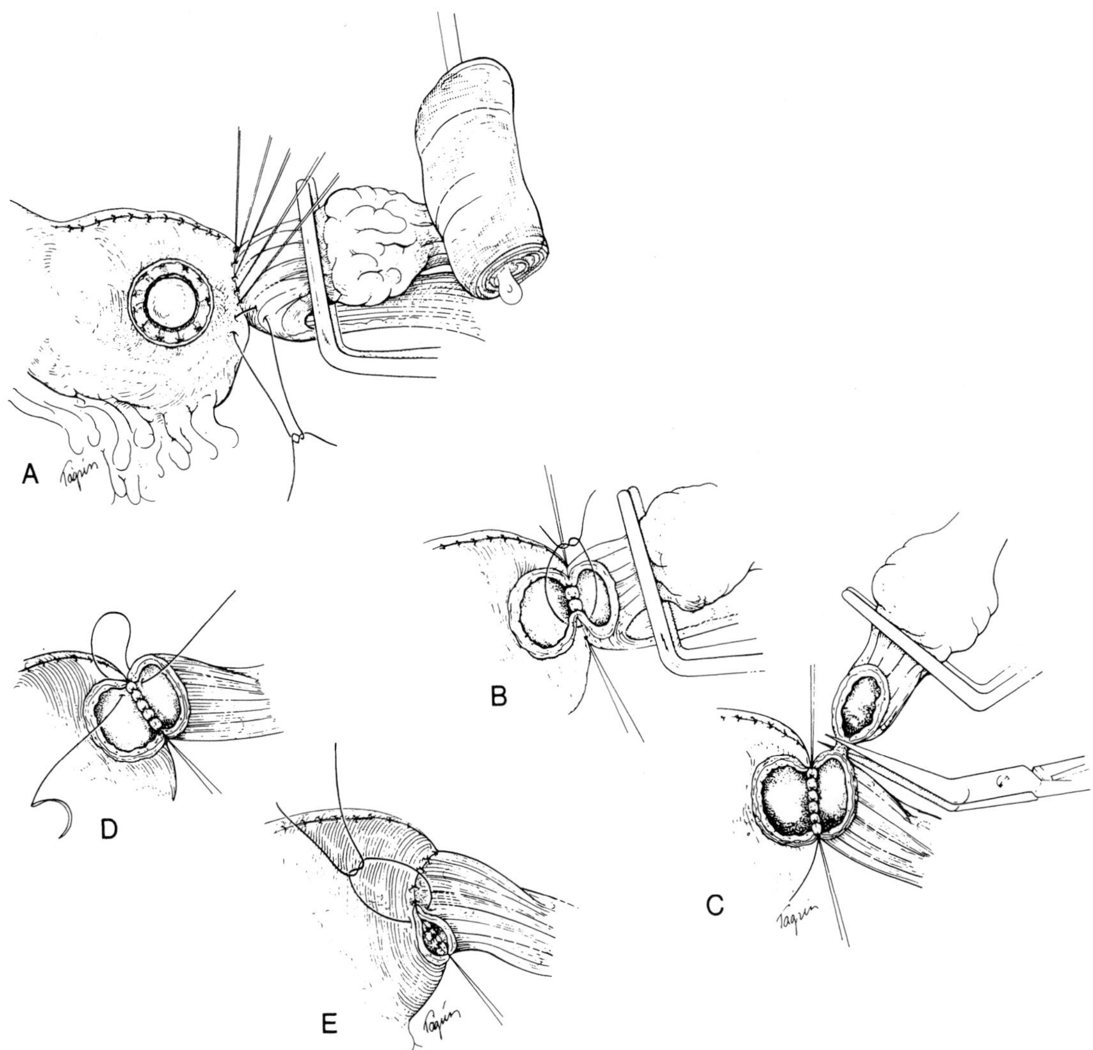

FIGURE 53–4 ■ The Sweet esophagogastric anastomosis, developed at the Massachusetts General Hospital, 1942 to 1988.

A, An end-to-side anastomosis is initiated with excision of a button of gastric wall. This button is actually placed closer to the greater curvature than illustrated; care is taken not to be close to the gastric turn-in, which would compromise the blood supply to that corner of the anastomosis. The outer posterior row of the anastomosis is carried out with interrupted mattress sutures of fine silk placed across the longitudinal muscle fibers of the esophagus. Each suture approximates the muscle of esophagus to the musculoserosa of the stomach. These sutures are placed in horizontal mattress fashion (not as actually demonstrated) so that there is less risk of cutting through.

B, The gastric button has been excised. The gastroesophageal specimen is still attached and, with a right-angle clamp placed to avoid spillage, acts as a handle for exposure of the suture line. The mucosa of the esophagus and stomach are approximated with interrupted fine silk sutures.

C, Completion of the posterior inner row and excision of the specimen.

D, The corner of the anastomosis is being turned to begin the anterior row of sutures. These are placed, again in interrupted fashion, with the knots tied on the inside.

E, Completion of the anastomosis with mattress sutures of interrupted silk in the outer anterior row.

(From Mathisen DJ, Wilkins EW Jr: Techniques of esophageal reconstruction. In Zuidema GD [ed]: Shackelford's Surgery of the Alimentary Tract, 4th ed, Vol 1. Philadelphia, WB Saunders, 1996, p 402.)

surgeon proceeds. Each stitch is placed about 5 mm back from the cut margin. The gastric mucosa is picked up with a similar bite of tissue. The needle must be pulled through each edge separately; an attempt to include both mucosal edges in one application of the needle causes tearing of the tissue. The use of atraumatic grasping forceps is necessary to place this first stitch. Subsequent grasping by the surgeon of the mucosa is unnecessary. Elevation of the prior stitch guides the placement of the next. The full posterior mucosal row is completed; the corner sutures are left uncut. Transection of the esophagus and removal of the specimen are now completed. A nasogastric tube is directed downward through the anastomosis to the level of the gastric antrum and is fixed by the anesthetist to the patient's nose to prevent later inadvertent withdrawal.

The anterior inner row is continued in an interrupted fashion; the stitches are placed so that the knots are always tied within the lumen. The assistant holds the previous tie down and away as the surgeon secures each subsequent stitch. This method allows complete inversion of the mucosal layer. The prior suture is then cut after each subsequent stitch is tied. This row of sutures is tied from either end toward the middle so that a final horizontal mattress suture can be placed anteriorly to complete the anterior mucosal row.

The outer anterior row is placed in a horizontal mattress fashion over the remaining two thirds of the circumference of the esophagus. The serosa of the stomach is brought as much as 1 cm above the inner mucosal layer. Because the anastomosis has been placed 2 cm or more down from the apex of the stomach posteriorly and the stomach has been folded upward anteriorly, a valve-like luminal orifice has been created that helps to minimize the possibility of gastroesophageal reflux.

The anterior aspect of the anastomosis may further be buttressed by a flap of omentum, which remains at the upper end of the gastroepiploic arcade. The stomach is suspended by a series of nonabsorbable sutures to the fascia that overlies the thoracic spine. This helps to avoid downward traction on the anastomosis suture line.

Closure

The diaphragm is closed circumferentially where it has been divided and is also sutured to the wall of the stomach to prevent prolapse of intra-abdominal contents into the thorax. Two No. 28 Argyle chest catheters are used for drainage. One is placed low in the gutter posteriorly and one toward the apex of the chest but not adjacent to the anastomosis, where it might incur foreign body trauma. The chest wall is closed in layers with pericostal sutures of catgut about the ribs and careful approximation of the muscles of the chest wall to avoid interference with postoperative shoulder function.

Postoperative Care

Early management is best conducted in an intensive care unit where tracheal extubation and expert respiratory therapy can be executed. The management of the upper digestive system is solely the surgeon's responsibility. The nasogastric tube is left in situ until peristalsis has returned or gastric drainage has become minimal. There is no rush to begin oral feeding. Clear liquids in small hourly amounts may be begun after the tube is removed. Fluids are then increased as tolerated, and a checkup barium swallow is obtained between day 7 and day 10. Only when an intact anastomosis is verified are soft solids permitted. Feedings then should be frequent and in small portions. If the patient's preoperative nutritional status were precarious, a feeding jejunostomy would have been advisable at the time of the surgical procedure.

Results

The results have been best expressed in the reported Massachusetts General Hospital (Mathisen et al, 1988) and Broadgreen Hospital, Liverpool (Page et al, 1990) experiences. These results, from the teaching hospital units of Dr. Hermes Grillo and Mr. Raymund Donnelly, compared the techniques of manual layered and stapled anastomoses (Table 53–1). The Massachusetts General Hospital experience may be unique. We performed 104 consecutive esophageal resections and anastomoses; 90% were performed by residents under supervision, with a 2.9% hospital mortality rate and no anastomotic leaks (verified by barium esophagography in all 101 survivors).

TABLE 53–1 ■ **Comparison of Manual Layered and Stapled Anastomoses***

Aspect	*Massachusetts General Hospital*	*Broadgreen Hospital*
Time interval	1980–1986	1983–1989
No. of resections	104	115
Gender ratio (M/F)	78/26	80/35
Mean age (yr)	62	63
Operative mortality (rate)	3 (2.9%)	10 (8.7%)
Anastomotic leakage	0	2 (1.7%)
Anastomoses requiring dilatation	5 (4.8%)	16 (13.9%)
Hospital stay (days)	13.7	13
Survival (3 yr)	18%	22%

*Comparable series from the United States and England compared hand-sewn and stapled anastomoses. Note is made that all the Broadgreen Hospital (Liverpool, England) series patients were resected by left thoracophrenotomy; the Massachusetts General Hospital series consisted of 64 patients treated by the thoracoabdominal and 40 by the Ivor Lewis approach.

CONCLUSION

Our preference is for thoracic residents in training to become experienced in the manual-layered anastomosis as their basic technique.

COMMENTS AND CONTROVERSIES

This chapter discusses an approach that is mainly of historic interest and seldom used today. However, the principles of esophagogastric anastomosis, including meticulous attention to detail, as are so well conveyed by Dr. Wilkins' lucid text remain highly relevant today. His description, based on the techniques developed by his mentors Drs. Churchill and Sweet, and the results achieved with this technique remain the "gold standard" for esophagogastric anastomoses.

Currently, most esophagectomies are carried out either through the transhiatal approach or through the abdomen, the right thoracotomy (Ivor Lewis) approach. The main advantage of the left thoracoabdominal approach is the excellent exposure of the distal esophagus and proximal stomach. This is of particular value when there has been previous surgery in this region or when a tumor involves both the proximal stomach and distal esophagus. The liabilities of the thoracoabdominal approach include the extensive nature of the incision, including the partial division of the diaphragm, the painful consequences of interruption of the costal arch, and the high incidence of poor functional outcome due to severe gastroesophageal reflux when the anastomosis is positioned in the mid to lower chest. If the thoracoabdominal approach is deemed necessary, the esophagogastric anastomosis can still be performed high in the chest, as described by Sweet, or in the neck. With the use of fixed retraction devices to improve exposure, the transhiatal dissection of the distal esophagus can be every bit as radical as that achieved through the left thoracotomy approach.

If the thoracic duct is injured in the course of the dissection, ligation both above and below the injury should be performed. In my own experience, ligation inferior to the site of injury is sufficient. When there is any doubt as to possible injury to the thoracic duct, ligation just above the hiatus can easily be performed.

It is my preference not to add a pyloromyotomy or pyloroplasty to avoid bile reflux. Postoperative delayed gastric emptying is rare and can usually be well managed by prokinetic agents or by the use of endoscopic balloon dilatation of the pylorus on rare occasions.

J. D. C.

■ *KEY REFERENCES*

Mathisen DJ, Grillo HC, Wilkins EW Jr, et al: Transthoracic esophagectomy: A safe approach to carcinoma of the esophagus. Ann Thorac Surg 45:137, 1988.

This report from the Massachusetts General Hospital summarizes 104 consecutive esophageal resections; 2.9% mortality and 0% leak rates were found. It demonstrates that transthoracic esophagectomy is indeed a safe approach to carcinoma of the esophagus.

Mathisen DJ, Wilkins EW Jr: Techniques of esophageal reconstruction. In Zuidema GD (ed): Shackelford's Surgery of the Alimentary Tract, 4th ed, Vol 1. Philadelphia, WB Saunders, 1996.

This is an up-to-date summary not only of the standard left thoracotomy for dissection of the esophagus with gastric replacement but also of all avenues of approach to the esophagus at any level and the various visceral replacements of the esophagus.

Sweet RH: Thoracic Surgery, 2nd ed. WB Saunders, Philadelphia, 1954.

In this, the first thoracic surgical textbook devoted to the personal experience of one individual, an early master reports his preference for the approach to carcinoma of the esophagus at all levels from the left thorax. His technique of anastomosis derived directly from the two-layer interrupted linen suture anastomosis of Adams and Phemister and led to the reliable manual anastomosis required of all general thoracic surgical residents in training.

■ *REFERENCES*

Adams WE, Phemister DB: Carcinoma of the lower thoracic esophagus: Report of a successful resection and esophagogastrostomy. J Thorac Surg 7:621, 1938.

Churchill ED, Sweet RH: Transthoracic resection of tumors of the stomach and esophagus. Ann Surg 115:897, 1942.

Eggers C: Resection of the thoracic portion of the esophagus for carcinoma. Surg Gynecol Obstet 52:739, 1931.

Kelling G: Ösophagoplastik mit Hilfe des Querkolon. Zentralbl Chir 38:1209, 1911.

Kirschner MB: Eines neues Verfahren der Ösophagoplastik. Arch Klin Chir 114:606, 1920.

Meade RH: A History of Thoracic Surgery. Springfield, IL, Charles C Thomas, 1961.

Page RD, Khalil JF, Whyte RI, et al: Esophagogastrectomy via left thoracophrenotomy. Ann Thorac Surg 49:763, 1990.

Postlethwait RW: Surgery of the Esophagus, 2nd ed. Norwalk, CT, Appleton-Century-Crofts, 1986.

Postlethwait RW: Substernal isoperistaltic gastric tube for esophageal bypass. Surg Rounds 7:20, 1984.

Roux C: L'esophago-jejuno-gastronome, nouvelle operation pour rétrécissement infranchisable de l'oesophage. Semaine Med 27:37, 1907.

Sweet RH: Surgical management of carcinoma of the mid-thoracic esophagus: Preliminary report. N Engl J Med 223:1, 1945.

Torek F: The first successful case of resection of the thoracic portion of the esophagus for carcinoma. Surg Gynecol Obstet 16:614, 1913.

Voelcker F: Über Exstirpation der Cardia wegen Carcinoms. Verh Dtsch Ges Chir 37:126, 1908.

LEFT THORACOABDOMINAL CERVICAL APPROACH

Robert J. Ginsberg

Anastomoses below the arch of the aorta do not allow for the near-total esophagectomy required for many tumors (especially those with Barrett changes). Because of the level of the anastomosis, bile acid reflux, esophagitis, and strictures are more frequently encountered.

For this reason, when a left thoracic approach is required, I have used a modification of the standard left thoracoabdominal approach, as described by Dr. Wilkins in the previous subchapter, for a variety of lower esophageal lesions to permit a near-total esophagectomy to be performed. This approach has the distinct advantage of excellent exposure of the lower half of the esophagus and proximal stomach and allows for a high thoracic or cervical anastomosis. It is not valuable in lesions that extend above the carina, when a right thoracotomy is more appropriate.

TECHNIQUE

The patient is placed in the full right lateral position with the left side uppermost and is draped as shown in Figure 53–5. The patient's neck is exposed for the anastomosis, and the left arm is draped free so it can be moved out of the way for the cervical portion of the procedure. Rather

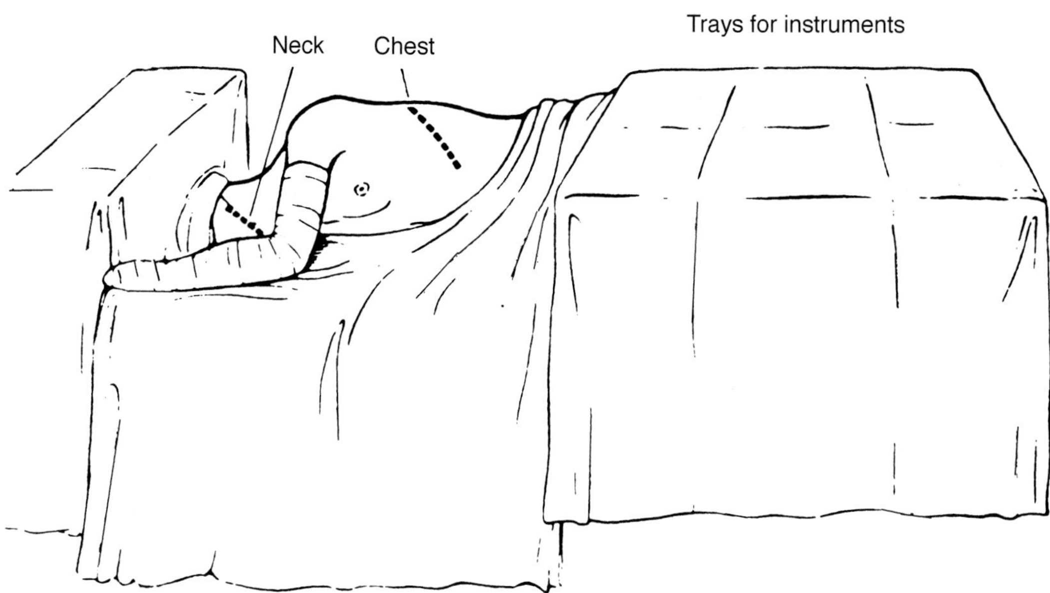

FIGURE 53–5 ■ The patient is placed in the full right lateral decubitus position with the abdomen, chest, and left neck exposed.

than use the seventh intercostal space incision, as described earlier by Dr. Wilkins, I prefer to use a sixth or fifth intercostal space incision, although I realize that two cartilages of the costal margin may have to be divided. There is no disadvantage to the patient. With the higher interspace incision, a full thoracotomy can be performed with access to the apex of the chest and abdomen (Fig. 53–6). I do not excise a rib, preferring a simple division of intercostal muscle to open the interspace.

Unlike the approach of Dr. Wilkins, the abdominal portion of the incision is extremely short and extends only to the lateral border of the rectus. I rarely, if ever, divide the rectus because the approach to the abdomen is through the diaphragm. Once the costal arch is divided, the diaphragm is opened circumferentially 2 cm from its attachments to the anterior and lateral chest wall until a significant exposure of the upper abdomen is available. (See Dr. Wilkins' section for techniques of dividing the diaphragm circumferentially.) Similarly, the initial gastric and esophageal mobilization is identical to that of Dr. Wilkins.

With the higher fifth or sixth intercostal space incision, a more direct access to the aortic arch is available if a full posterolateral incision is used. To mobilize the esophagus above the arch, I open the mediastinum just behind the subclavian artery (Fig. 53–7). If necessary, one or two of the highest intercostal branches can be divided, although care must be taken to avoid the fourth intercostal branch, which may give off the anterior spinal artery. Mobilization of the esophagus medial to the arch is accomplished with sharp and blunt dissection, which is facilitated by the placement of tapes around the esoph-

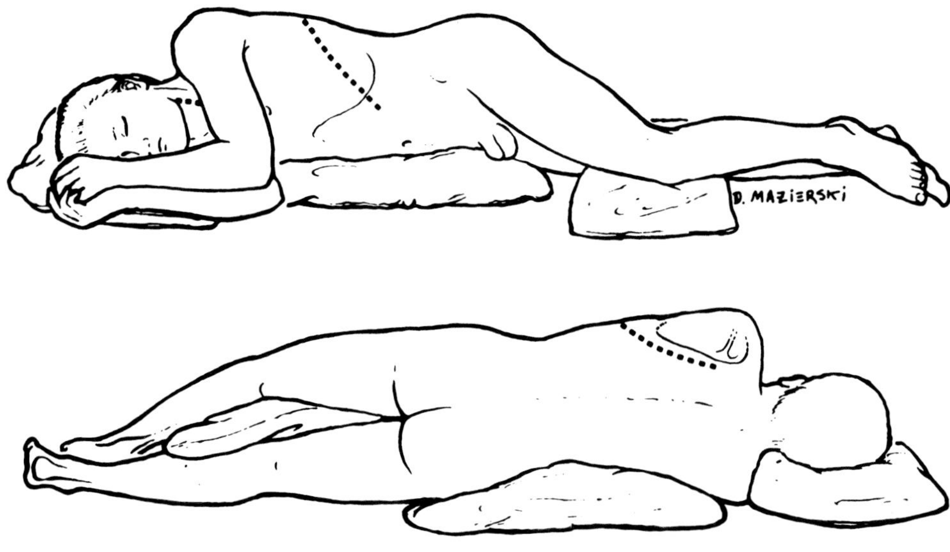

FIGURE 53–6 ■ A full thoracotomy is made with a minor extension over the costal arch. The approach to the abdomen is through the divided diaphragm.

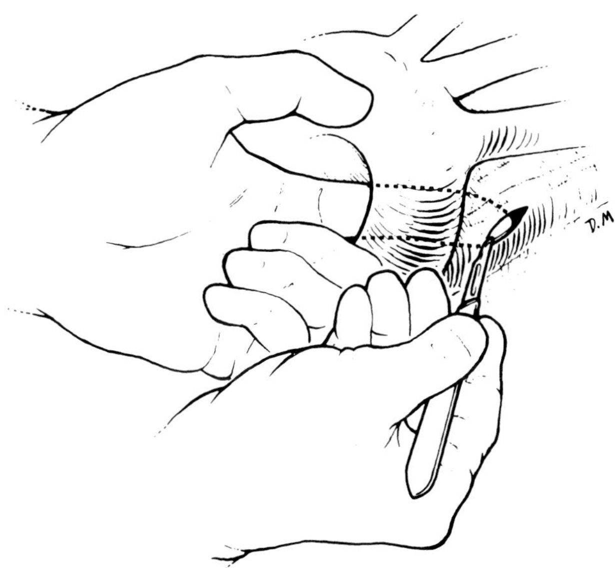

FIGURE 53–7 ■ The superaortic esophagus is mobilized with care to avoid the vagus and recurrent nerves and the thoracic duct.

agus above and below the arch (Fig. 53–8). Care must be taken to avoid injury to the thoracic duct, which is found just beside the subclavian artery in the area of dissection. If possible, this should be identified, divided, and removed en bloc with the esophagus. Similar care must be taken to avoid injury to the left vagus nerve and recurrent nerve in its course around the arch and up the tracheoesophageal groove. It is preferable to include a complete upper abdominal and lower mediastinal lymph node dissection together with an en bloc resection of the lower esophagus and stomach.

Further dissection of the proximal esophagus is now carried out. This approach is most appropriate when no disease is present in the upper esophagus. I perform a simple sharp and blunt dissection of the upper esophagus, separating it from the back wall of the trachea to preserve the recurrent nerve. Finger dissection of the esophagus into the neck, with the surgeon gently freeing all structures and avoiding the two recurrent nerves, completes the esophageal mobilization.

Once the esophagus is totally freed, standard preparation of the gastric tube can be made within the chest. The esophagus, surrounding tissue, and lymph nodes can then be removed through division of the esophagus in the distal cervical or high thoracic region.

The cervical anastomosis can be accomplished with the patient still in the full lateral decubitus position. Alternatively, if preferred, after the thoracoabdominal incision is closed, the patient is turned to a supine position reprepared and redraped. (With this approach, the gastric tube is tacked to the divided esophagus and then brought up to the neck after the neck exposure is complete.) When the anastomosis is to be made in the neck, a standard incision is made following the anterior border of the sternomastoid, and further dissection to mobilize the esophagus is carried out before its division.

The stomach is positioned medial to the aorta in an orthotopic position, and care is taken to position it correctly, without torsion. The lesser curvature faces right and the greater curvature, left.

I prefer a hand-sewn anastomosis in the neck in two layers, utilizing absorbable polyglycolic acid sutures for both layers (Fig. 53–9). The gastric tube is secured in both the neck and thorax with tacking sutures.

If desired, a high intrathoracic anastomosis can be achieved with a hand-suturing (see previous subchapter) or a circular stapling technique. The gastric tube is placed

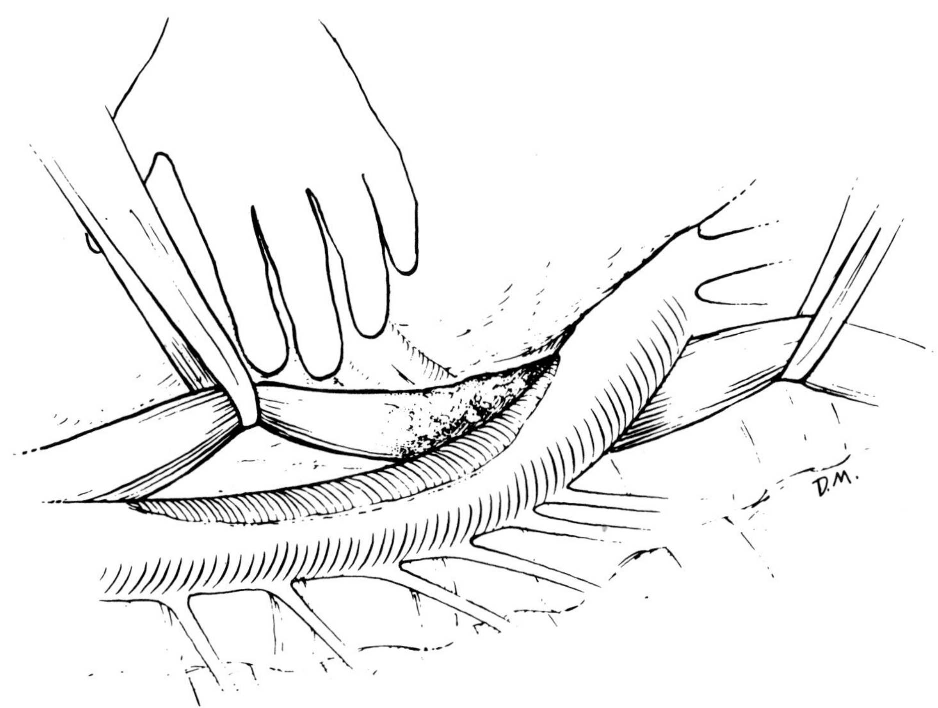

FIGURE 53–8 ■ After complete mobilization of the esophagus, tapes are placed around the esophagus to complete a wide dissection.

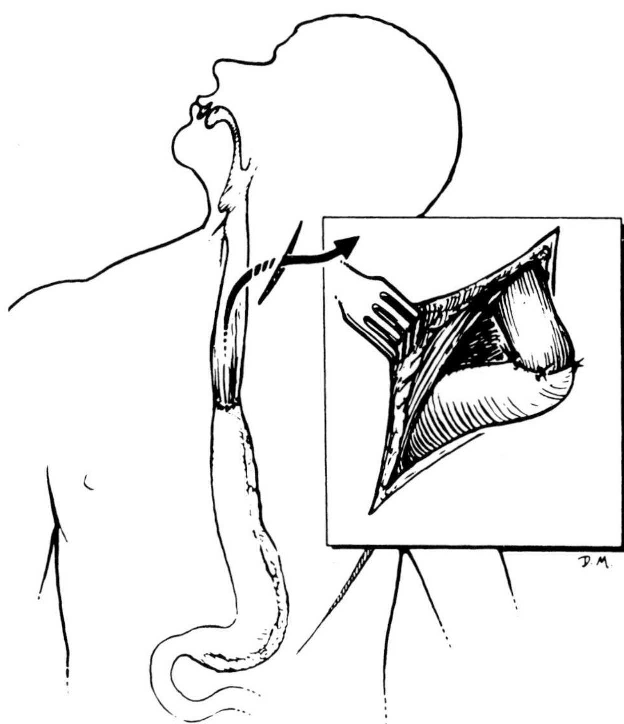

FIGURE 53–9 ■ The hand-sewn anastomosis in the neck has been completed. This can be accomplished either with the patient remaining in the full lateral decubitus position or, after closure of the thoracoabdominal wound, by placing the patient in a supine position.

either orthotopically or lateral to the aorta to avoid the esophageal bed (Fig. 53–10).

When an intrathoracic anastomosis is preferred, it can be performed with the stomach either in the orthotopic position or placed lateral to the aortic arch. If it is performed with the stomach in the orthotopic position, the apex of the gastric tube and the esophagus are brought out posterior to the great vessels for anastomosis and then replaced orthotopically once the anastomosis is completed. If the stomach is placed lateral to the aortic arch, the proximal esophagus is brought out posterior to the great vessels high in the chest, and either a hand-sewn or stapled anastomosis can be accomplished.

The thoracoabdominal incision is closed, as described by Dr. Wilkins. A short segment of costal cartilage can be excised to avoid overriding or, if the cartilage is malleable, one or two monofilament nonabsorbable sutures can be placed to approximate the cartilage and then fix it. The soft tissues of the diaphragm and internal oblique muscles are used to firmly buttress the reconstructed costal arch.

CONCLUSION

With either a fifth or sixth interspace full posterolateral incision for the thoracoabdominal approach, the esophagus can be totally mobilized. A near-total esophagectomy can be easily performed with the esophagogastric anastomosis in the neck or, if preferred, at the apex of the chest. If a high intrathoracic anastomosis is desired, the gastric tube can be placed orthotopically (medial to the aortic arch) or, if preferred, lateral to the aortic arch, which avoids problems if disease recurs within the bed of the original esophagus. I have found that this approach allows superb exposure to the upper abdomen and a full length of the esophagus and is well tolerated by patients.

COMMENTS AND CONTROVERSIES

The left thoracoabdominal cervical approach described by Dr. Ginsberg, like the left thoracoabdominal approach

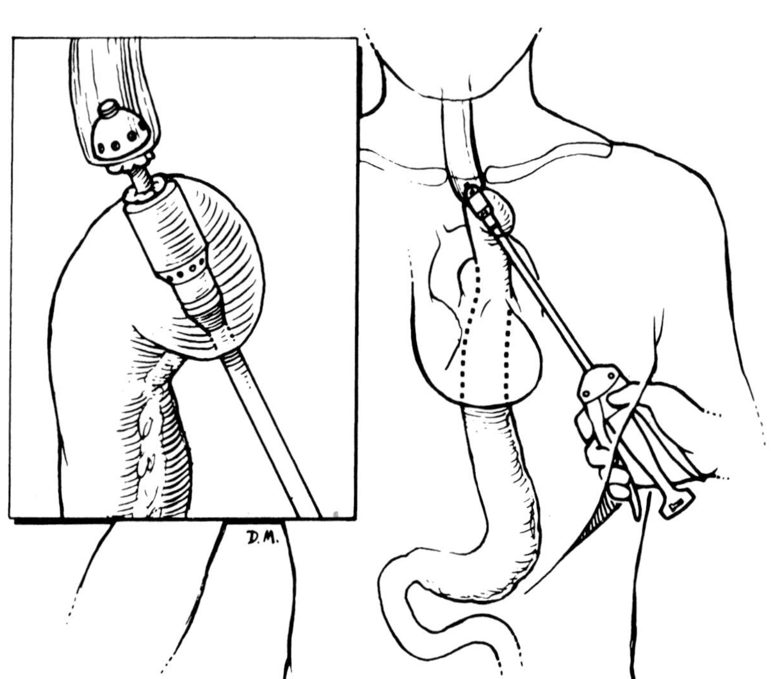

FIGURE 53–10 ■ A high intrathoracic anastomosis is being completed with a circular stapler placed through the fundus of the stomach. In this illustration, the gastric tube has been placed lateral to the aorta to avoid the esophageal bed.

described by Dr. Wilkins, is mainly of historical interest with few present indications. However, familiarity with this technique adds an important option to the armamentarium of the esophageal surgeon. It provides the excellent exposure of the distal esophagus afforded by left thoracotomy plus the functional advantage of a high esophagogastric anastomosis. Thus, for a patient who has had previous surgery on the lower esophagus or esophagogastric region or for a patient who has a contraindication to right thoracotomy for an Ivor Lewis approach, the procedure described by Dr. Ginsberg may be of value.

The use of the fifth or sixth intercostal incision, as described by Dr. Ginsberg, does provide better exposure to the upper esophagus but may negate some of the advantages of the traditional thoracoabdominal approach. This higher approach may be of disadvantage if there has been previous surgery in the upper abdomen or if mobilization of the duodenum or creation of a pyloromyotomy or pyloroplasty is desired. The division of one or more costal cartilages to facilitate the upper abdominal exposure does, in my opinion, create additional morbidity risk in terms of postoperative pain. If this approach is used, resection of a portion of the cartilage together with reattachment of the ends with heavy monofilaments suture is desirable to prevent both overriding and movement of the ends of the cartilage.

I emphasize the importance of mobilizing the cervical esophagus through the chest, which is easily accomplished, before closure of the thoracotomy. This is especially important if the cervical portion of the operation is performed without repositioning the patient. Finally, the free draping of the left arm, as demonstrated in Figure 53–5, is essential if the cervical portion of the procedure is to be accomplished without repositioning the patient.

J. D. C.

LEFT TRANSTHORACIC ESOPHAGECTOMY

Bernard J. Park
Robert J. Ginsberg

Since the first successful resection of the thoracic esophagus for carcinoma by Torek (1913), a variety of one-stage operative approaches for resection of the esophagus and cardia have been developed and advocated. Among the first published series was that of Ohsawa (1933), who reported on 18 patients who underwent transpleural esophagogastrectomy with end-to-side esophagogastrostomy via left thoracotomy. Eight patients survived the procedure. In the United States, Marshall (1938) of the Lahey Clinic and Adams and Phemister (1938) are credited with the first case reports of successful esophagogastrectomy through a left thoracotomy for patients with distal esophageal carcinoma. Churchill and Sweet (1942) subsequently described a series of 11 patients who underwent resection of lower esophageal and cardia carcinomas via the left thoracophrenotomy approach. They emphasized the importance of meticulous anastomotic technique and lack of tension on the suture line, achieving a perioperative mortality rate of 9.1%. After these initial successes, esophageal surgery evolved to include a variety of surgical approaches for esophagectomy to provide optimal therapy while minimizing morbidity and mortality. In most centers, the thoracoabdominal approach has replaced the left thoracotomy.

Although the left thoracotomy method has not received as much attention, it remains a viable alternative and appears to be used by an increasing number of surgeons, including Ellis and colleagues (1981, 1997), Krasna (1995), Lu and associates (1987), Sabanathan (1992), and Page and coworkers (1990). Advocates of this approach point to its excellent access to the thoracic esophagus, especially the distal third and cardioesophageal junction; the ease of gastric mobilization through the diaphragm; the shorter operative time required; and the comparable results, including morbidity and mortality rates. One weakness of the left thoracotomy approach is the failure of an initial abdominal exploration to rule out intra-abdominal metastases or other reasons for inoperability. Other drawbacks during the abdominal portion of the dissection include difficulty in executing a Kocher maneuver, performance of a pyloroplasty or pyloromyotomy for gastric drainage, and placement of a feeding jejunostomy.

TECHNIQUE

The technique of esophagectomy through a transthoracic approach is well described in the two previous subchapters by Drs. Wilkins and Ginsberg, respectively. The major difference between a thoracoabdominal approach and a pure thoracic approach is the choice of the incision level and the exposure of the abdomen through the diaphragm. These are discussed in detail here. (See the previous subchapters for steps in esophageal and gastric mobilization, choices of anastomotic sites, and similar issues. Where these differ, a more detailed explanation is provided.)

Incision and Exposure

After the administration of general anesthesia and endotracheal intubation with a double-lumen tube, the patient is placed in the right lateral decubitus position with the arm flexed 45 degrees at the elbow and shoulder. The table is flexed to widen the intercostal spaces. The sixth and seventh ribs are identified and marked. Preparation and draping of the patient include the upper abdomen in the event that a laparotomy or thoracoabdominal incision is required. The incision extends from the costal margin to at least the posterior axillary line. The chest is entered through the sixth or seventh intercostal space or by resection of the sixth or seventh rib. The anterior costal margin is left intact.

After a thorough, systematic exploration of the pleural cavity, the inferior pulmonary ligament is mobilized to the level of the inferior pulmonary vein, and the lymph nodes within it are removed. The mediastinal pleura overlying the esophagus is incised medial to the aorta and lateral to the pleural reflection at the pericardium, and the tumor is identified and assessed for resectability. Further mobilization of the esophagus is deferred until an exploration of the abdomen is performed once the diaphragm is opened.

Incision of the Diaphragm

There are four approaches to opening the diaphragm for the abdominal phase: (1) a circumferential incision, (2) an incision through the central tendon (septum transversum incision), (3) enlargement of the hiatus, and (4) a radial incision. Before the seminal work of Merendino and associates (1956), who reported the anatomic distribution of the phrenic nerve within the diaphragm, radial incisions were customarily used. However, it is well established that these incisions result in near-complete diaphragmatic paralysis. To understand where to place incisions that preserve phrenic innervation, the anatomy, as characterized by Merendino and associates (1956) and reviewed by Fell (1998), must be appreciated.

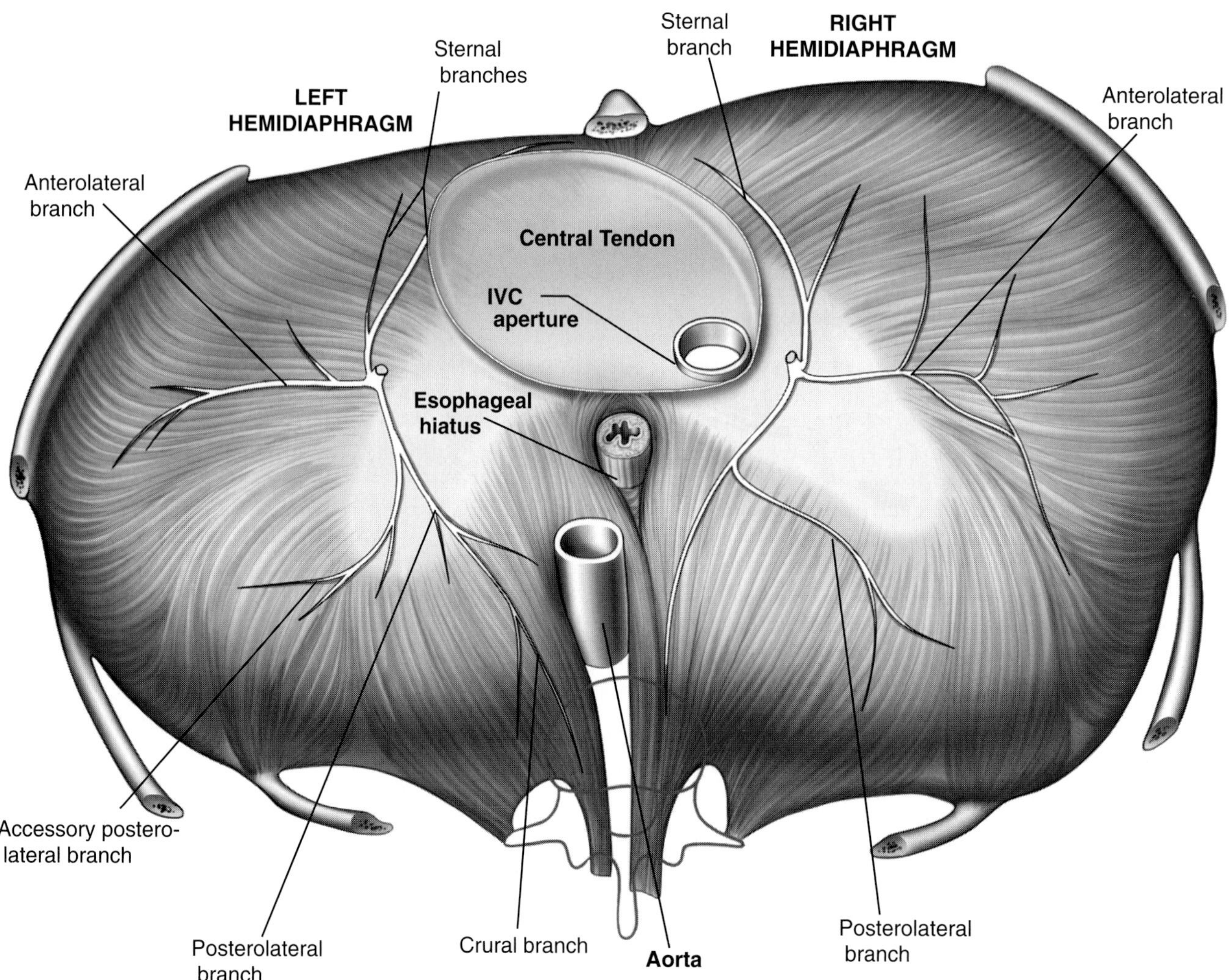

FIGURE 53–11 ■ Anatomy of the diaphragm with special reference to phrenic innervation. IVC, inferior vena cava.

The phrenic nerve, both right and left, divides into several terminal branches at the level of the diaphragm or 1 to 2 cm above it. With the exception of two or three fine branches to the pleural and peritoneal surfaces of the diaphragm, the phrenic nerve continues through the diaphragm as muscular rami. These rami pierce the diaphragm and supply four major areas of distribution with some, but generally little, overlap. The number of rami may vary from two to four, but most commonly there are three rami. The first courses anteromedially toward the sternum and is termed the *sternal*, or *anterior, branch*. The second, the *anterolateral branch*, runs laterally anterior to the lateral leaf of the central tendon. The third branch is directed posteriorly and quickly divides into one that runs laterally posterior to the lateral leaf of the central tendon (*posterolateral branch*) and one that runs posteriorly and medially to the region of the crus (*crural branch*) (Fig. 53–11). Based on the anatomy, Merendino and associates (1956) designated "safe" areas in the diaphragm where incisions would preserve the branches of the phrenic nerve in the diaphragm (Fig. 53–12).

The circumferential incision is made along the periphery of the diaphragm. We recommend making the incision with cautery 2 to 5 cm from the costal margin, beginning anteriorly (see Fig. 53–12). The left inferior phrenic vessels on the undersurface of the diaphragm will be encountered and should be suture-ligated. This circumferential incision can end posteriorly at a distance from the hiatus once adequate exposure of the abdominal contents has been obtained. With this approach, when the esophagus is mobilized at the hiatus, a cuff of hiatal musculature is usually removed en bloc with the attached phrenoesophageal ligaments. Alternatively, the incision may be carried to the esophageal hiatus. The incision may be carried to the esophageal hiatus with resection of the diaphragm with the tumor if it is adherent. Traction sutures are placed through the cut edges of the diaphragm for exposure (Fig. 53–13).

Another approach to the diaphragmatic incision is the septum transversum incision reported by Sicular (1992). This incision is placed through the central tendon medial to the main left phrenic nerve and has the advantages of ease of application and rapid reconstruction (see Fig. 53–12). Merendino and associates (1956) originally described a variant of this incision for use with a thoracoabdominal incision. The latter incision extends medially and inferiorly between the entrance of the phrenic nerve into the diaphragm and the attachment of the pericardium. As in the septum transversum incision, the anterior or sternal branch of the phrenic nerve is severed, but the majority of phrenic innervation is preserved (see Fig. 53–13).

Adams and Phemister (1938), in one of the first reports of successful esophagogastrectomy via left thoracotomy, used an incision beginning 2 inches from the hiatus and extending to it with subsequent mobilization of the

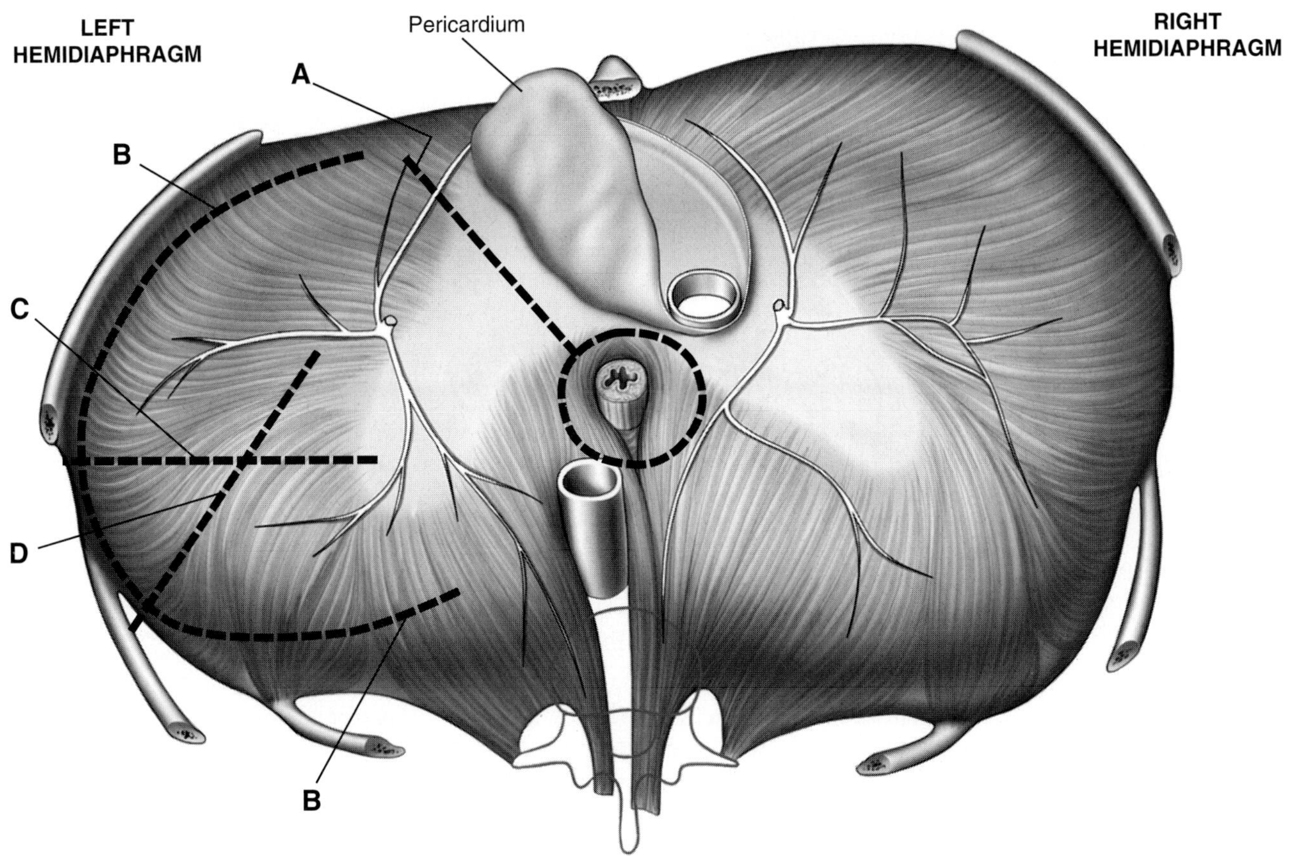

FIGURE 53–12 ■ The various incisions available to expose the abdomen include septum transversus (*A*), circumferential (*B*), radial (*C* and *D*), and hiatal enlargement (*E*) (not labeled).

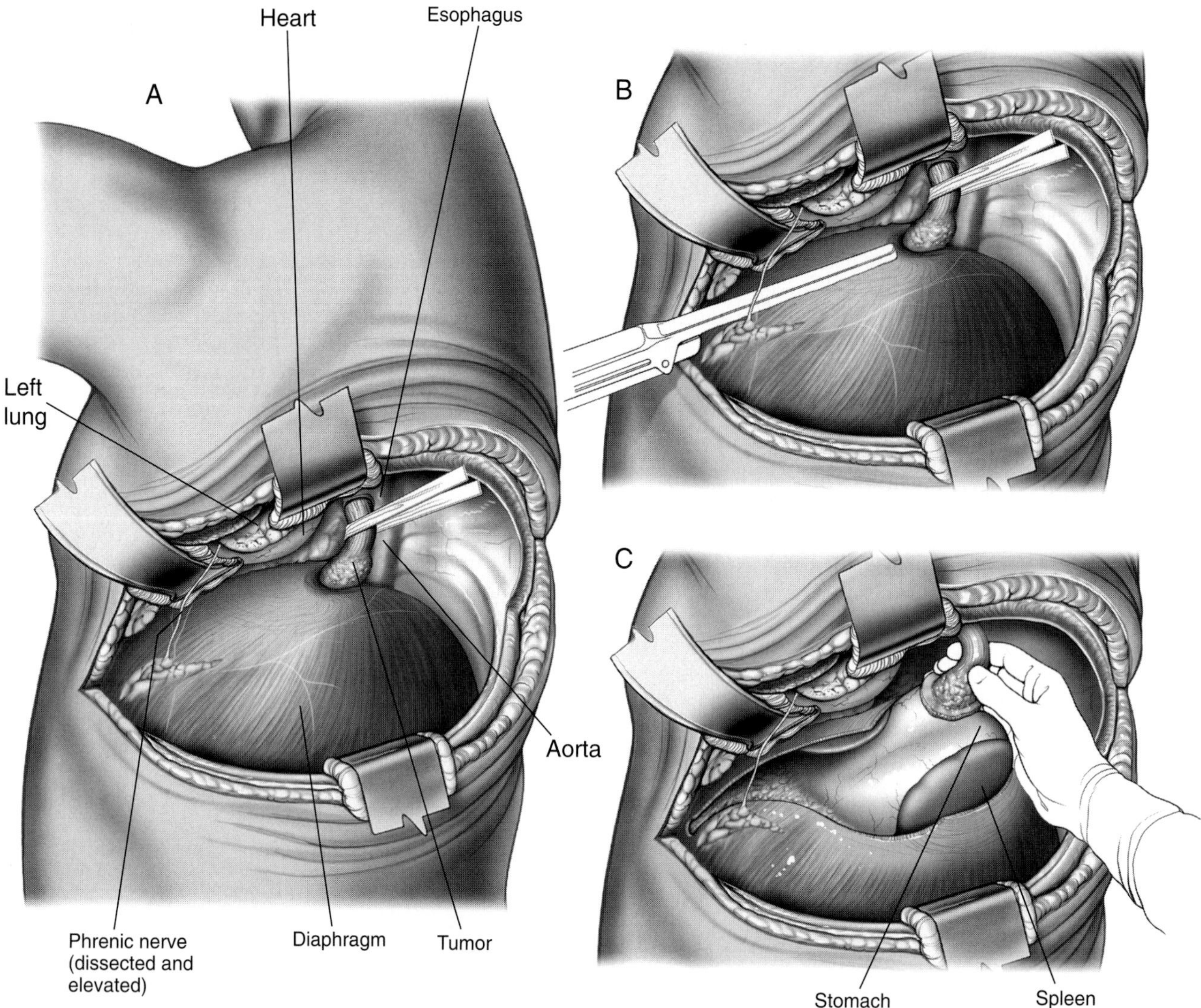

FIGURE 53–13 ■ *A,* A full thoracotomy incision has been made. The esophagus has been mobilized. The pericardium has been elevated off the anterior portion of the diaphragm, and the phrenic nerve insertion onto the diaphragm is isolated to protect it. *B,* A stapler is used to divide the diaphragm, thus preserving most of the phrenic nerve innervation other than a medial twig. *C,* Through this incision, the surgeon can easily mobilize the stomach to prepare it for transposition into the chest.

esophagus and cardia (see Fig. 53–13). After completion of the resection, the cut edges of the diaphragm are sutured to the stomach below the site of anastomosis.

The radial diaphragmatic incision was commonly used before the work by Merendino and associates (1956) and is still used by some surgeons. Extending more laterally from the costal margin to the esophageal hiatus, it results in near-complete denervation of the diaphragm and may be a major factor in postoperative morbidity and mortality from ineffective cough, lower lobe atelectasis, and resultant pneumonia (see Fig. 53–12). As reviewed by Zhao and associates (1985), unilateral diaphragmatic paralysis results in a 20% to 30% decrease in vital capacity, a 20% decrease in oxygen uptake on the affected side, and decreased residual volume and total lung capacity. For these reasons, radial incisions in the diaphragm should be avoided.

Exploration of the Abdomen

No matter the diaphragmatic incision, once it has been accomplished the upper abdomen is explored to assess complete resectability. To assess the area of the celiac axis, the lesser sac should be entered by dividing the gastrohepatic omentum as well as the short gastric vessels. From this approach, as with the thoracoabdominal approach, the right lobe of the liver can be palpated but not directly visualized. The greater omentum, transverse colon mesentery, and small bowel mesentery should be inspected for sites of peritoneal metastases.

Esophagogastric Mobilization

With this exposure, esophagogastric mobilization is carried out, as with a thoracoabdominal incision (see previous subchapters by Drs. Wilkins and Ginsberg).

After completion of the esophagogastric resection, the site of anastomosis is chosen according to oncologic principles. If the lesion approaches the middle third of the esophagus, it may be necessary to mobilize the portion of the esophagus behind and above the aortic arch. In such cases, it is important to choose entry into the chest as high as possible (through the sixth interspace or by resection of the sixth rib). Although a pyloromyotomy or pyloroplasty is somewhat difficult, it can be accomplished, as can a feeding jejunostomy. Once the anastomosis has been completed, the surgeon secures the stomach using interrupted sutures to the mediastinum and the enlarged hiatus.

Closure of the Diaphragm

We prefer to close the diaphragm with interrupted horizontal mattress sutures of nonabsorbable heavy polypropylene. This may be reinforced with a second, continuous layer of the same material. Usually, no drainage is required in the abdomen, and one or two chest tubes are inserted in the chest, with at least one of the tubes being placed and secured near the anastomosis.

COMMENTS AND CONTROVERSIES

Although many authors use this approach for all lower third esophageal carcinomas, I reserve it for small tumors at the hiatus, believing that a thoracoabdominal incision (if a left thoracotomy is to be used) provides a somewhat better exposure below the diaphragm without a significant increase in pain or morbidity. The significant advantage of a left thoracotomy–only approach is the speed of closure. Therefore, in somewhat debilitated individuals who require a small resection, I use this as the approach of choice.

R. J. G.

REFERENCES

Adams WE, Phemister DB: Carcinoma of the lower thoracic esophagus: Report of a successful resection and esophagogastrostomy. J Thorac Cardiovasc Surg 7:621, 1938.

Churchill ED, Sweet RH: Transthoracic resection of tumors of the stomach and esophagus. Ann Surg 115:897, 1942.

Ellis FH, Jr, Heatley GJ, Krasna MJ, et al: Esophagogastrectomy for carcinoma of the esophagus and cardia: A comparison of findings and results after standard resection in three consecutive eight-year intervals with improved staging criteria. J Thorac Cardiovasc Surg 113:836, 1997.

Ellis FH, Jr, Maggs PR: Surgery for carcinoma of the lower esophagus and cardia. World J Surg 5:527, 1981.

Fell SC: Surgical anatomy of the diaphragm and phrenic nerve. Chest Surg Clin North Am 8:281, 1998.

Krasna MJ: Left transthoracic esophagectomy. Chest Surg Clin North Am 5:543, 1995.

Lu YK, Li YM, Gu YZ: Cancer of the esophagus and esophagogastric junction: Analysis of results of 1,025 resections after 5 to 20 years. Ann Thorac Surg 43:176, 1987.

Marshall SF: Carcinoma of the esophagus: Successful resection of lower end of esophagus with re-establishment of esophageal gastric continuity. Surg Clin North Am 18:643, 1938.

Merendino KA, Johnson RJ, Skinner HH, Maguire RX: The intradiaphragmatic distribution of the phrenic nerve with particular reference to the placement of diaphragmatic incisions and controlled segmental paralysis. Surgery 39:189, 1956.

Ohsawa T: Surgery of the oesophagus. Arch Jpn Chir 10:665, 1933.

Page RD, Khalil JF, Whyte RI, et al: Esophagogastrectomy via left thoracophrenotomy. Ann Thorac Surg 49:763, 1990.

Sabanathan S: Left thoracotomy approach for resection of carcinoma of the oesophagus and cardia. Ann Ital Chir 63:25, 1992.

Sicular A: Direct septum transversum incision to replace circumferential diaphragmatic incision in operations on the cardia. Am J Surg 164:167, 1992.

Torek F: The first successful case of resection of the thoracic portion of the oesophagus for carcinoma. Surg Gynecol Obstet 16:614, 1913.

Zhao H, D'Agostino R, Pitlick P, et al: Phrenic nerve injury complicating closed cardiovascular surgical procedures for congenital heart disease. Ann Thorac Surg 39:445, 1985.

CHAPTER **54**

Right Thoracoabdominal Approaches

IVOR LEWIS–McKEOWN PROCEDURES

Douglas J. Mathisen

The primary goal of treatment of esophageal carcinoma remains cure of the neoplasm, with relief of dysphagia as an important secondary concern. Until proven otherwise, the best chance for cure includes an operation that encompasses the entire tumor and draining of lymph nodes with adequate proximal and distal margins. Some studies suggest adjuvant therapy may improve survival for patients with squamous carcinoma of the esophagus and possibly adenocarcinoma of the esophagus as well (Carey and Mathisen, 1993; Forastiere et al, 1997; Naunheim et al, 1995; Orringer et al, 1990; Walsh et al, 1994; Wright et al, 1997). The more widespread use of preoperative adjuvant therapy for carcinoma of the esophagus argues for operative approaches that provide as much biologic and staging information as possible to allow better evaluation of the results of such treatment.

Choice of operation for carcinoma of the esophagus depends on a number of factors: preference of the surgeon, location of the tumor, body habitus, prior operations, condition of the patient, choice of esophageal substitute, and prior irradiation. Remote irradiation for other diseases, although an uncommon occurrence, is an important consideration. If the dose of irradiation exceeded 50 Gy and was given more than 1 year before the contemplated surgery, the risk of complications after esophagectomy is greatly increased. In this circumstance, it is desirable to perform the anastomosis outside the irradiated field so that one end of the anastomosis has not been irradiated. The anastomosis should be buttressed with additional tissue, such as omentum or pedicled muscle, to aid healing and minimize leaks.

The choice of esophageal substitute may dictate the operative approach. Obese or very large patients may also influence the choice of approach. Prior operations may make certain approaches less desirable because of resultant scarring. Prior lobectomy may make transthoracic resection through the opposite chest impossible because of the inability to maintain adequate one-lung ventilation.

The two most important factors influencing choice of operation are (1) location of tumor and (2) the surgeon's preference. The surgeon's preference is governed by numerous factors, some of which have already been discussed.

The choice of incision is influenced by the ease of anastomosis and ability to mobilize the stomach and resect the esophagus. Tumors located in the middle third of the esophagus have traditionally been removed by a combined laparotomy and right thoracotomy—the *Ivor Lewis* approach; however, tumors in this location can also be approached by a transhiatal or a left thoracoabdominal technique.

HISTORICAL NOTE

The combined laparotomy and right thoracotomy, or Ivor Lewis esophagectomy, was proposed in 1946 at the Royal College of Surgeons' Hunterian Lecture by Ivor Lewis. This approach was quite a radical departure for an era fraught with many problems for surgery involving the thoracic cavity. The standard approach for middle third tumors at that time involved a blunt esophagectomy, cervical esophagostomy, gastrostomy, and subsequent skin tube reconstruction.

Lewis' original procedure involved a two-stage approach. The first stage involved a laparotomy and mobilization of the stomach based on the right gastric and right gastroepiploic arteries. The second stage, 1 to 2 weeks later, involved a right thoracotomy, resection of the esophagus, and esophagogastric anastomosis in the chest. The operation was successful in five of seven patients, a remarkable achievement for this era. The current technique has evolved to a single-stage procedure combining the basic elements of Lewis' two-stage procedure.

■ *HISTORICAL READING*

Lewis I: The surgical treatment of carcinoma of the oesophagus with special reference to a new operation for growths of the middle third. Br J Surg 34:18, 1946.

INDICATIONS

Any esophageal problem involving resection of the middle third of the esophagus is amenable to this approach. The primary indication is squamous or adenocarcinoma of the esophagus. Other indications include high-grade dysplasia in Barrett's esophagus, destruction of the distal esophagus by caustic ingestion, and failed myotomy for achalasia with sigmoid esophagus requiring near-total esophagectomy.

INVESTIGATIVE TECHNIQUES

Preoperative Evaluation

Because of the morbidity and mortality associated with this procedure, each patient must be carefully evaluated. Patients must be in reasonable medical condition and must have adequate pulmonary function. Despite great improvements in pain control, anesthesia, and postoperative care, patients with forced expiratory volume in 1 second under 1 L are probably not suitable candidates for this approach. Smoking should be stopped, and aggressive measures to treat underlying chronic obstructive lung disease should be instituted. Careful evaluation for underlying cardiac disease should be done in elderly or high-risk patients.

Radiologic Evaluation

Standard radiologic evaluation includes barium esophagography, computed tomography (CT) of the chest and upper abdomen, and, more recently, endoscopic ultrasound to assess depth of invasion and presence of enlarged lymph nodes (Rice et al, 1991).

Endoscopic Evaluation

Endoscopic evaluation is important in histologic diagnosis, assessment of the proximal and distal extent of tumor, and checking for the presence of Barrett's mucosa proximal to adenocarcinomas. The proximal extent of the tumor and abnormal mucosa is critical in determining surgical approach.

Endoscopy

Endoscopy is valuable in all patients with esophageal disease and should be performed by the surgeon. Endoscopy is most helpful in determining proximal extent of tumor. A 5-cm surgical margin is desirable for carcinoma of the esophagus. Distal tumors with proximal involvement above 30 cm may be technically difficult to resect from the left side. Tumor involvement of the esophagus between 30 and 35 cm represents the gray zone between application of the left-sided approach and the Ivor Lewis approach. Proximal margins should not be compromised, and therefore a left-sided supra-aortic anastomosis or the more traditional Ivor Lewis esophagectomy should be planned for tumors at this level.

In patients with adenocarcinoma arising in Barrett's mucosa, it is important to resect not only the tumor, including a 5-cm proximal margin, but also all of Barrett's mucosa. It is helpful to identify the proximal extent of Barrett's mucosa by endoscopically placing the nasogastric tube just above the squamocolumnar junction or to endoscope the patient intraoperatively to identify the location to ensure resection of all of Barrett's mucosa. Tumors extending above 30 cm may involve either the left mainstem bronchus or the trachea and should be evaluated with bronchoscopy. Surgeons should perform endoscopy to confirm these observations.

Mediastinoscopy has a limited role in the evaluation of suspected high mediastinal lymph nodes. A combined thoracoscopy-laparoscopy offers the potential for minimally invasive surgical staging of esophageal cancer, similar to that associated with mediastinoscopy for lung cancer (Krasna et al, 1996). Peritoneal or pleural seeding, lymph node involvement, and local extent of tumor can all be assessed. Pretreatment staging is necessary to better evaluate response to neoadjuvant therapy.

MANAGEMENT

Surgical Technique

With the patient supine, an upper midline abdominal incision is made, extending along the side of the xiphoid (Fig. 54–1). The abdomen is explored. If liver metastases or unresectable retroperitoneal nodes are found, resection should be abandoned and palliation of dysphagia should be achieved by other means. Palliation of dysphagia can be achieved by endoscopically placed salivary bypass tubes or by irradiation (Hancock and Glatstein, 1984; Richter et al, 1988).

If the tumor is resectable, an upper hand-type retractor elevates the superior aspect of the incision. The left triangular ligament of the liver is divided. The lesser sac is entered through the greater omentum, away from the right gastroepiploic artery. The omentum is then divided along the greater curvature, and the gastroepiploic artery is spared. An attempt is made to leave a piece of omentum on the greater curve for later use to wrap the anastomosis. By grasping the greater curve of the stomach (not the right gastroepiploic artery), the surgeon can elevate the stomach and can clamp and tie the short gastric vessels. Long clamps are useful for this sometimes difficult dissection. The use of hemoclips to control the short gastric arteries should be avoided because of their propensity to fall off. Care must be used so that the ties on the stomach do not include stomach wall, resulting in delayed necrosis and perforation.

The greater omentum can be dissected distally near the pylorus, but care must be taken not to injure the right gastroepiploic artery. Once dissection of the greater curvature is completed, the gastrohepatic ligament is divided. Care is taken to preserve the right gastric artery. The left gastric artery and vein are isolated and doubly ligated at their origin. Lymph nodes from this area are taken with the specimen.

Next, the hiatus and distal esophagus are dissected. It is wise to enlarge the hiatus at this time. It is very difficult to enlarge the hiatus from the right chest. Frequently, a large vein traverses the hiatus; it should be ligated to avoid postoperative hemorrhage. A Kocher maneuver is performed to ensure maximum mobility of the stomach. A pyloroplasty or pyloromyotomy is done and is covered with a lappet of nearby omentum. A feeding jejunostomy is inserted in high-risk or nutritionally depleted patients.

It is helpful to accomplish as much dissection of the lower esophagus as possible from the abdomen. This dissection facilitates the intrathoracic dissection of the lower esophagus, which can be difficult through a high right thoracotomy. An attempt should be made to advance the stomach and omentum into the posterior mediastinum before closing the abdomen to facilitate retrieval from the chest.

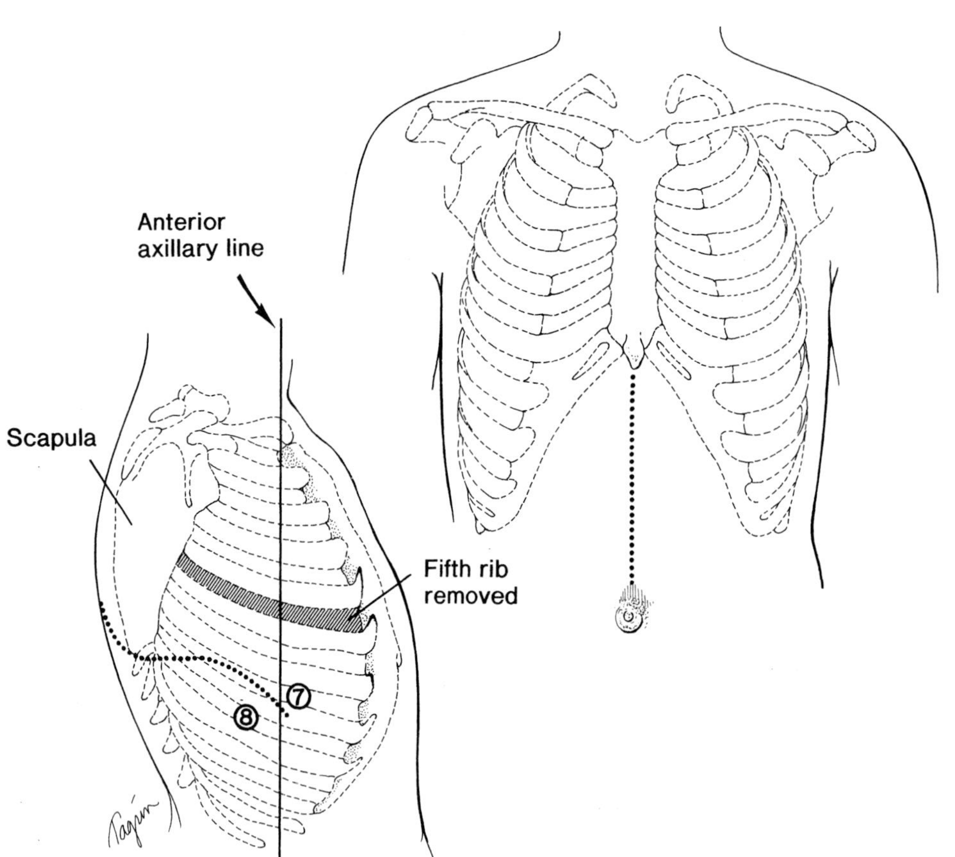

FIGURE 54–1 ■ Standard incisions for an Ivor Lewis esophagectomy. An upper midline abdominal incision is used to mobilize the stomach. A high right thoracotomy is used to resect the esophagus and do the esophagogastric anastomosis.

The patient is then placed in the left lateral decubitus position, and a standard posterolateral right thoracotomy is performed (see Fig. 54–1). The serratus muscle is spared, and the chest is entered through the fourth interspace. After the lung is examined for abnormalities, it is deflated and retracted anteriorly. The use of a double-lumen endotracheal tube allows the lung to be collapsed and affords excellent exposure for the esophageal dissection and subsequent anastomosis.

The azygos vein is divided. The esophagus is dissected from vertebral body to pericardium. All paraesophageal nodes, including subcarinal nodes, are included in the specimen. Structures should be ligated, rather than cauterized, to decrease the incidence of hemorrhage or chylothorax. Dissection is continued to the apex of the chest. The stomach is then pulled into the chest and divided. This step is usually done with a stapling device and reinforced with interrupted sutures. It is done only after all of the intrathoracic dissection has been completed to avoid any confusion about orientation of the stomach.

Great care must be taken to avoid pulling too much of the stomach into the chest. The excess stomach will fall into the costophrenic gutter and cause delayed emptying of the stomach. Pulling the stomach too taut may lead to severe kinking of the stomach at the level of the hiatus and to delayed emptying as well.

Anastomotic Technique

Churchill and Sweet (1942) described a triple-layer technique of esophagogastrostomy and conventional en bloc resection of the cancer and adjacent lymph nodes. Five years later, Sweet (1947) published his initial experience with surgical management of carcinoma of the esophagus in 141 patients. Operating in an era without sophisticated postoperative monitoring devices, mechanical ventilation, or broad-spectrum antibiotics, his results were remarkable: an operative mortality of 15%, anastomotic leaks in 1.4% of patients, and overall 5-year survival of 11%. These results served as a standard for many years. The low incidence of leaks and operative mortality was related to the reliability of the anastomosis.

Churchill and Sweet (1942) emphasized the details of technique and warned of factors predisposing to anastomotic leak. The lack of an esophageal serosal layer and the segmental blood supply of the esophagus make esophageal anastomosis more demanding than other intestinal anastomoses. Atraumatic handling of the tissues, preservation of the blood supply of both the esophagus and the stomach, avoidance of crushing clamps, interrupted sutures, cutting with a knife or other sharp instrument, and firm but gentle tying of sutures to avoid cutting tissues are all important details in the performance of an anastomosis. Churchill stated that

> . . . the mucous membrane sutures are placed with the exactitude and with the degree of tension that we would use in the fine plastic procedure on the lip. There must be no tension and there must be accuracy.

These words are still appropriate today.

The technique of esophageal anastomosis used at the

Massachusetts General Hospital today differs little from the technique Churchill and Sweet proposed nearly 60 years ago. A circle approximately 2 cm in diameter is scored on the surface of the stomach (Fig. 54–2*A*). The circular defect created should be 2 cm away from the stapled edge of the stomach to avoid compromise of the blood supply. Individual submucosal vessels are identified and ligated with fine silk sutures. This measure minimizes bleeding while the anastomosis is performed and allows for precise placement of sutures.

Interrupted horizontal mattress sutures of fine suture material (4–0 silk) are used to construct the back row of the anastomosis (Fig. 54–2*B*). Corner stitches are placed first, and the remaining sutures are evenly spaced between them. The sutures on the stomach include the seromuscular layers. The esophageal sutures should be deep enough to include both the longitudinal and circular muscles of the esophagus. The sutures should not be tied too tightly to avoid necrosis or cutting through the muscle.

The esophagus is opened sharply from one corner stitch to the other. The circular button of stomach is removed (Fig. 54–2*B*). The inner layer is completed with simple sutures, including just the mucosa of the esophagus and all layers of the stomach (Fig. 54–2*C*). The knots are on the inside, thereby allowing inversion or turning in of the mucosa of both the esophagus and stomach. This step is accomplished for the entire circumference of the anastomosis (Fig. 54–2*D*).

A nasogastric tube is passed into the stomach under direct vision before a single Connell stitch is placed for closure of the final opening. Healing of the inverted mucosa is an important feature in preventing leakage, and the location of the knots on the luminal side minimizes foreign body reaction with the actual tissues of the anastomosis. The outer row is completed using horizontal mattress sutures as described for the back row of the outer layer (Fig. 54–2*E*).

The omentum mobilized with the stomach is placed over the anastomosis anteriorly to provide an additional layer of coverage. A few sutures are placed between the stomach and the mediastinal pleura to avoid tension on the anastomosis when the patient is upright, particularly if the stomach is full. Sutures are also placed between the stomach and the diaphragmatic hiatus to prevent herniation of abdominal contents.

Viability of tissues on each edge of the anastomosis is best maintained if trauma is avoided. The edges are never crushed with clamps and, indeed, are handled with forceps as little as possible. Once the first stitch is placed and tied, traction on it permits placement of the next without the need for instrumental grasping of the mucosa. The surgeon ties the sutures by positioning the index finger cephalad to the anastomosis and lifting the stomach to the esophagus, avoiding pulling down on the fixed and more fragile esophagus. This step is especially important for the outer layer of the anastomosis because the esophagus lacks a serosal surface.

A nasogastric tube passed through the anastomosis for a short time avoids distraction at the suture line by a distended stomach. Gentle, periodic irrigation of the tube ensures its patency. Temporary gastric decompression more than compensates for any potentially deleterious effect of an intraluminal foreign body lying against the suture line for a short period.

Experience with this technique from the Massachusetts General Hospital in a consecutive series of 104 patients was reported (Mathisen et al, 1988). There were three postoperative deaths (2.9%), all attributable to pneumonia and respiratory failure.

Anastomotic Stricture

Dilatation was necessary in five patients for anastomotic stricture 3 to 6 weeks postoperatively. One to three dilatations were required for successful resolution of dysphagia. Delayed anastomotic stricture was not present in this group of patients.

Anastomotic Leaks

All patients underwent a postoperative barium swallow. There were no anastomotic leaks, even of the localized type. The reliability of this precise, two-layer anastomotic technique has been reported by others as well (Akiyama, 1973; Ellis et al, 1983).

Results

The greatest immediate concern is the fate of the intrathoracic anastomosis. It is undoubtedly this concern that has led to the popularity of the transhiatal esophagectomy, which places the anastomosis in the cervical area (Orringer and Orringer, 1983). We and others have shown that attention to the technical details of anastomosis leads to a very low incidence of leaks and subsequent mortality, stressing the importance of how the anastomosis is done rather than where it is done.

Transhiatal esophagectomy has become the popular alternative to Ivor Lewis esophagectomy. No direct randomized series have compared the two procedures. Muller and colleagues (1990) reviewed all published reports of surgical therapy of esophageal carcinoma from 1980 to 1988 (a summary of 59 published reports) and drew some conclusions about the two procedures. Others have compared the two procedures in a retrospective fashion within a single institution and provide some important insights into the relative merits of the two procedures (Lozac'h et al, 1997; Shahian et al, 1986).

In most reports, the risk of anastomotic leak from a *cervical* anastomosis is higher than that reported for an *intrathoracic* anastomosis (Muller et al, 1990). In patients experiencing leaks, however, morbidity and mortality related to the leak itself are lower if the anastomosis is located in the neck rather than in the chest. This finding is borne out in the Muller review. The anastomotic leak rate was 11% for intrathoracic anastomosis compared with 19% for cervical anastomosis. However, the mortality rate for an intrathoracic anastomotic leak was three times higher than that for a cervical anastomotic leak (69% versus 20%, respectively).

Cervical anastomotic leak rates for transhiatal esophagectomy without thoracotomy have been reported to be as low as 6% to 8% for operations performed for carcinoma of the intrathoracic esophagus (Orringer and Or-

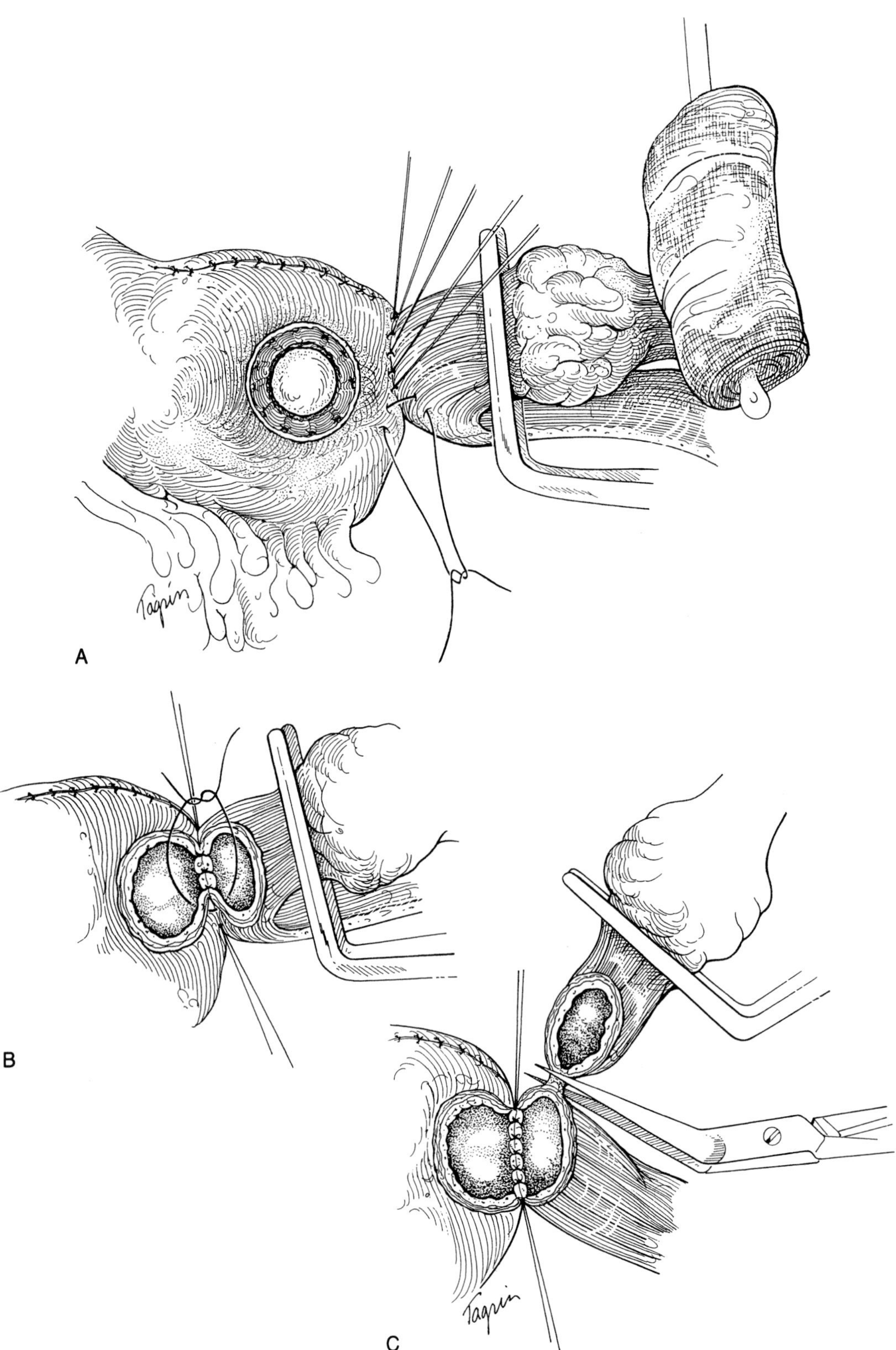

FIGURE 54–2 ■ Surgical technique. *A*, The serosa of the stomach has been scored, and the vessels have been ligated. The back row of sutures has been completed. *B*, The button of stomach has been removed, and the anterior wall of esophagus has been opened. *C*, The back row of the inner layer is completed, and the esophagus is transected.

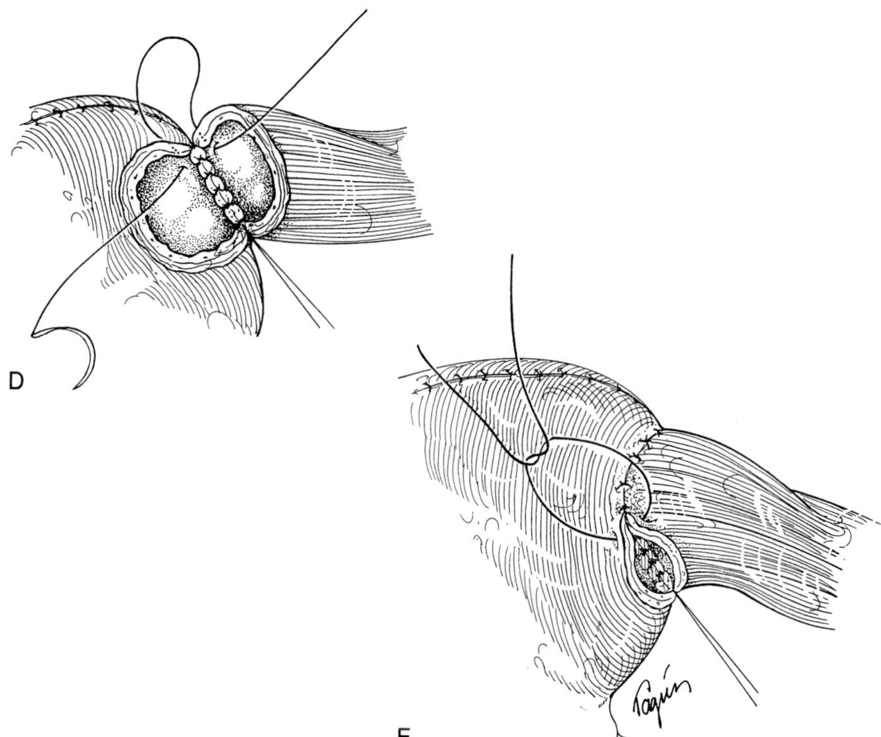

FIGURE 54–2 ■ *Continued. D,* The remainder of the inner layer is completed. A Connell stitch is used for closure of the final opening. A nasogastric tube is advanced across the anastomosis under direct vision before the inner layer is completed. *E,* The outer layer is nearly finished.

ringer, 1983), and leak rates from 0% to 2% have been reported for intrathoracic anastomosis (Akiyama, 1973; Ellis et al, 1983; Mathisen et al, 1988). Even within the same institution and with the same surgeons, cervical anastomosis is associated with a higher incidence of leaks. This finding is confirmed by the report from the Lahey Clinic, with a 15.4% leak rate for cervical anastomosis but 1.8% for intrathoracic anastomosis (Shahian et al, 1986).

Respiratory insufficiency and atelectasis occur more commonly after transthoracic esophagectomy, but the incidence of pneumonia is similar (Table 54–1). Transhiatal esophagectomy is associated with a high incidence of recurrent nerve paresis or palsy (6% to 24%) and is very uncommon after transthoracic esophagectomy. Chylothorax, posterior membranous tracheal tears, and increased blood loss are all more frequent after transhiatal esophagectomy. Most reports have not demonstrated the superiority of one procedure over another and view the procedures as alternative choices (Lozac'h et al, 1997; Shahian et al, 1986).

TABLE 54–1 ■ **Respiratory Complications After Right Transthoracic* Versus Transhiatal† Esophagectomy**

Complication	*Transthoracic (Mean % ± SD)*	*Transhiatal (Mean % ± SD)*
Pneumonia	21 ± 3	26 ± 22
Respiratory insufficiency	27 ± 19	13 ± 8
Atelectasis	23 ± 31	10 ± 7

* n = 2436.
† n = 1886.

Mortality

Muller and coworkers (1990) showed that overall postoperative mortality associated with surgical treatment of esophageal carcinoma was reduced by 50% during the 1980s compared with the rate in previous decades. This decrease can be attributed to advances in anesthesia, perioperative care, monitoring, and enteral and parenteral nutrition. For all types of surgical resections for carcinoma of the thoracic esophagus, there was no significant difference in the hospital mortality on the basis of location of the primary tumor in the esophagus or stage of disease at the time of resection. However, there was a significantly lower hospital mortality rate for resections performed with curative intent versus those with palliative intent (mean, 11% versus 19%, respectively) (Muller et al, 1990).

If the resective procedure involved a thoracotomy of any type, the hospital mortality rate was nearly identical whether or not the anastomosis was located in the neck (Table 54–2). However, the lowest mortality rate was found in patients who had undergone resection by transhiatal esophagectomy (mean 11%), even though, in some papers cited in the review, this procedure was restricted to those patients deemed at too high a risk for a transthoracic approach. Many institutions have reported operative mortality rates below 5% for either transthoracic or transhiatal resection (Akiyama, 1973; Ellis et al, 1983; Mathisen et al, 1988; Orringer and Orringer, 1983).

Survival

Despite the theoretical advantages of en bloc dissection and full lymphadenectomy, studies comparing these pro-

TABLE 54–2 ■ **Hospital Mortality Rate for Resection of Esophageal Carcinoma by Surgical Approach**

Procedure		*Mortality Rate (%)*
LTT/ITA	($n = 4161$)	17 ± 16
RTA/ITA	($n = 3410$)	16 ± 11
IT/CervA	($n = 5039$)	12 ± 10
THE	($n = 1402$)	11 ± 8

LTT/ITA, left transthoracic with intrathoracic anastomosis; RTA/ITA, right transthoracic with intrathoracic anastomosis; TT/CervA, transthoracic with cervical anastomosis; THE, transhiatal esophagectomy.

cedures with transhiatal esophagectomy show no difference in overall survival between these two approaches for esophageal carcinoma. Shahian and coworkers (1986) demonstrated no statistically significant difference in survival for all patients who underwent transthoracic versus extrathoracic esophagectomy for carcinoma (median, 14.1 versus 12.6 months; $P = .48$ NS), regardless of whether patients had stage I or stage III disease. In the review by Muller, only tumor stage at time of operation was a significant determinant of long-term survival; there was no significant difference in survival according to extent of surgery or type of resection (see Table 54–2). The same study showed no significant difference in survival for conventional resection without extensive lymph node dissection versus conventional resection with extensive lymph node dissection in 17,953 patients. Single-institution, nonrandomized series, however, have shown improved survival with transthoracic resection (Mathisen et al, 1988).

Complications

Anastomotic Leaks

Aggressive management of anastomotic leaks is required if fatalities are to be avoided. If the leak is small and contained or well drained by the chest tube, the patient should take nothing by mouth; antibiotic therapy and nutritional support should be continued, and barium swallow should be repeated 1 week later. CT is performed to identify any undrained collections. Small, undrained collections can be drained by percutaneous ultrasound-guided catheters. The catheters can be irrigated with sterile saline to clean the cavity. Early rib resection should be implemented to ensure complete drainage. This aggressive approach and the use of soft drainage catheters should reduce the risk of major hemorrhage from nearby great vessels.

The presence of a massive leak warrants urgent intervention. Considerable judgment is required to successfully manage this devastating complication. If the leak is related to necrosis of the stomach, the stomach should be resected to viable tissue and returned to the abdomen. A cervical esophagostomy should be done. Reconstruction of the gastrointestinal tract can be performed at a later date. Local repair in the presence of gross contamination of the pleural cavity can be expected to fail in most cases. If local repair is attempted, devitalized tissue should be débrided and the repair should be buttressed with healthy tissue such as omentum, chest wall muscles (serratus, pectoralis), or pedicled intercostal muscle. The lung should be decorticated, and wide drainage of the pleural cavity should be provided. Cervical esophagostomy may be appropriate if concern exists about the repair. This esophagostomy can be constructed in such a way that reanastomosis can be done between the divided ends of the esophagus in the neck, thus avoiding more complicated reconstructive methods (Heitmiller and Fraser, 1992).

Delayed Gastric Emptying

There are three main reasons for delayed gastric emptying after an Ivor Lewis esophagectomy:

1. Pyloric obstruction.
2. Obstruction at the level of the hiatus.
3. Redundant intrathoracic stomach lying in the posterior costophrenic gutter, resulting in a J-shaped configuration of the stomach before passage through the hiatus.

These problems are best avoided by an adequate drainage procedure at the time of operation, with the surgeon enlarging the hiatus, not pulling the stomach too tightly into the chest, and avoiding excess stomach in the chest.

When a drainage procedure has been done, pyloric obstruction usually resolves with time. Metoclopramide may be useful. Endoscopy and cautious balloon dilatation of the pylorus can be tried. Failure of conservative management requires reoperation and an adequate drainage procedure. Obstruction at the level of the hiatus usually demands re-exploration and enlargement of the hiatus. This procedure is often difficult, and great care must be taken to avoid injury to the blood supply of the stomach.

Late Functional Results

Although little information has been reported about late functional results after an Ivor Lewis esophagectomy, the Mayo Clinic did report early and late functional results in 100 patients (King et al, 1987). A pyloromyotomy (39 patients) or pyloroplasty (56 patients) was done in 95 patients. Early functional results were excellent, with development of dysphagia and gastroesophageal reflux in only 3% and 1% of patients, respectively. The mean follow-up of patients was 2.3 years. Late dysphagia occurred in 40 patients; in 5 patients it was related to anastomotic recurrence and in 35 to benign anastomotic narrowing, requiring dilatation. Dilatation (range, 1 to 22 dilatations; mean, 3.4 dilatations) relieved symptoms in all 35 patients with benign stenosis. Delayed presentation of reflux occurred in 14% of patients and dumping in 5%. All patients with reflux or dumping were treated successfully by standard medical therapy. Postoperative weight loss (median, 15.7 kg) occurred in 62% of patients. The authors believed that weight loss was multifactorial and not necessarily related to the procedure itself.

Ivor Lewis esophagectomy remains an excellent procedure for resection of the middle third of the esophagus with good long-term functional results. Proper patient selection, adequate preoperative preparation of the patient, attention to technical details of the operation, and diligent postoperative care allow this procedure to be performed safely with acceptable morbidity and mortality rates. A reliable anastomotic technique should be implemented to avoid intrathoracic anastomotic leaks, the source of greatest morbidity and mortality. Ivor Lewis esophagectomy offers potential advantages of wider, more complete resection for better staging information compared with transhiatal esophagectomy.

IVOR LEWIS–McKEOWN (THREE-STAGE) ESOPHAGECTOMY

Following the precedent of Ivor Lewis describing his two-stage technique of esophagectomy at the 1946 Hunterian Lecture, McKeown (1976) described the three-stage esophagectomy at a similar gathering in 1972. This variation allows for a slightly greater amount of esophagus to be excised and the prospect of the anastomosis to be placed in the neck but carries a greater risk of recurrent nerve injury and anastomotic leak.

The operation described by McKeown is carried out in three stages:

1. An abdominal stage to mobilize the stomach.
2. A right thoracotomy to excise the esophagus.
3. A right cervical incision through which to perform the esophagogastric anastomosis.

The first two stages are identical to those described for the Ivor Lewis approach, except for mobilizing the entire intrathoracic esophagus. At the apex of the chest, care must be taken to avoid injury to the right recurrent laryngeal nerve. Some dissection of the cervical esophagus can be done to facilitate the third stage of the operation. It is important to open the planes widely to allow ease of mobilization and delivery of the stomach into the neck.

Next, the stomach is delivered into the chest cavity. Care must be taken not to twist the stomach in its longitudinal axis. It is important to ascertain that the stomach will indeed reach the cervical incision. The true apex of the fundus should be identified with a suture for future reference. The stomach should be positioned as high in the chest as possible.

At this point, some prefer to close the thoracotomy and proceed to the cervical stage. Others divide the esophagogastric junction with a stapler and oversew the staple line. The true fundus is then carefully tacked to the esophagus to facilitate delivery of the stomach during the cervical stage of the operation. The choice of these two options depends on local factors and the preference of the surgeon.

The cervical phase of the operation can be approached through either the right (as described by McKeown) or the left side of the neck. The neck incision can be either the standard incision just anterior to the sternocleidomastoid muscle or a more cosmetic horizontal collar incision that favors the side chosen for the approach. The surgeon dissects the plane anterior to the sternocleidomastoid, ultimately retracting the carotid sheath and its contents laterally and the thyroid medially. Care must be taken not to place a retractor on the tracheoesophageal groove to avoid injury to the recurrent laryngeal nerve.

If sufficient dissection has taken place during the thoracotomy, it is easy to encircle the esophagus. If the esophagogastric junction has been divided, the esophagus is advanced and the stomach grasped. The tacking sutures are divided, and the remainder of the esophagus is delivered. If the gastroesophageal junction has not been divided, it must now be done, as described earlier. As the fundus of the stomach is delivered into the neck, it is important to keep the gastroesophageal junction to the patient's right and the dome of the fundus to the left to avoid the possibility of organoaxial rotation.

The cervical esophagogastric anastomosis is performed exactly as described earlier. I do try to place a few sutures between the stomach and the prevertebral fascia to anchor the stomach to reduce downward pull on the anastomosis. The fascial sutures should not be too deep to avoid contaminating this plane with bacteria.

Some subtle variations to the approach described by McKeown are worth mentioning. Preparing the right arm into the operative field allows access to the right neck. Exposure of the cervical esophagus can be achieved by extending the neck, bringing the arm to the side, and rotating the hips and shoulders to approximately 45 degrees to the table. The advantage of this approach is that it allows careful positioning of the stomach in the posterior mediastinum, facilitating delivery of the apex of the fundus of the stomach into the neck, avoiding excessive stretching of the stomach, and resulting in less manipulation of the tumor through the thoracic inlet. This is all achieved by having access to the stomach through the thoracotomy. Great care must be exercised to avoid injury to the recurrent laryngeal nerves as the cervical esophagus is encircled. This approach requires anticipation of a cervical anastomosis so that any lines can be avoided in the right arm and the patient can be positioned and prepared accordingly.

The other variation involves performing the right thoracotomy as the initial phase of the operation. This is especially effective if it is thought that the tumor might be unresectable because of invasion of local structures in the chest. The esophagus is mobilized thoroughly, as described earlier.

Once this step has been completed, the thoracostomy is closed in the standard fashion. The remainder of the operation is carried out as one would do for a transhiatal esophagectomy. The patient is returned to a supine position, and a thyroid bag or blankets are placed beneath the shoulders to extend the neck. The patient is prepared from chin to pubis. It is possible to have two teams work simultaneously in the neck and abdomen, although the situation may become crowded. The cervical esophagus is mobilized as described earlier through a left horizontal cervical incision. Care again must be exercised to avoid injury to the left recurrent laryngeal nerve.

As described earlier, the stomach is mobilized. With the hiatus enlarged, the stomach can be advanced through the posterior mediastinum to the neck. This can be accomplished in a variety of ways. I prefer to divide the esophagogastric junction with a stapling device and to oversew it with interrupted sutures. A large Penrose

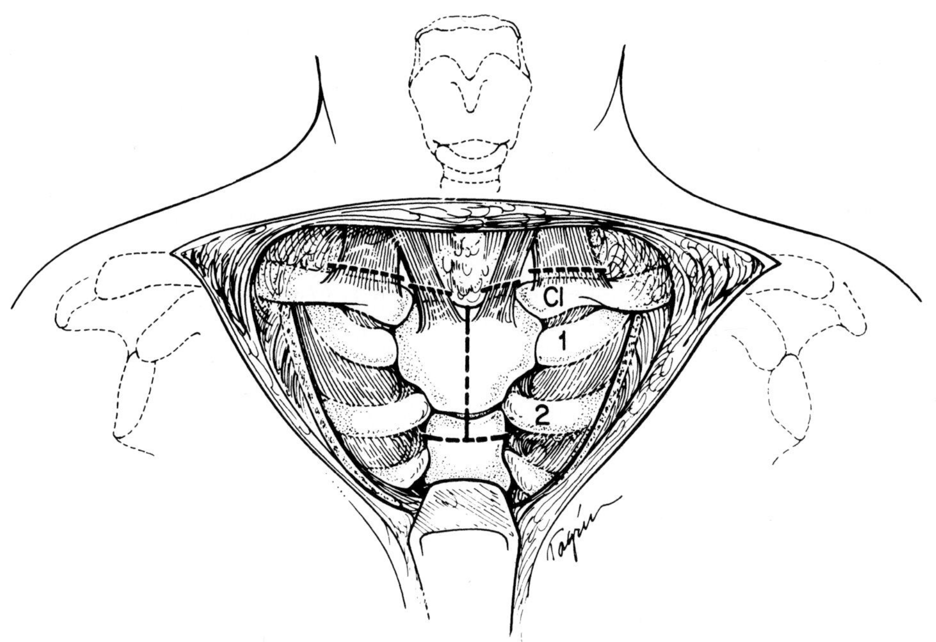

FIGURE 54–3 ■ *Dotted lines* represent the point of transection of the sternocleidomastoid muscle insertion in the clavicle and the division of the manubrium.

drain is sewn to the end of the esophagus. The esophagus is then delivered through the left cervical incision. The mobilized stomach is placed into a sterile plastic bag to facilitate passage through the posterior mediastinum. The true apex of the gastric fundus is determined, and this is positioned to be at the end of the bag. The distal end of the Penrose drain that has remained in the abdomen is sewn securely to the end of the bag that contains the fundus of the stomach.

The bag containing the stomach is manually delivered into the posterior mediastinum by a combination of advancing from below and pulling the Penrose drain from above. This technique has been very helpful in minimizing trauma and in ensuring proper alignment of the stomach.

Enlarging the Thoracic Inlet

In some patients, the thoracic inlet is too small to allow advancement of the stomach without excessive compression. This undoubtedly increases the risk of arterial insufficiency and venous congestion. The thoracic inlet can be

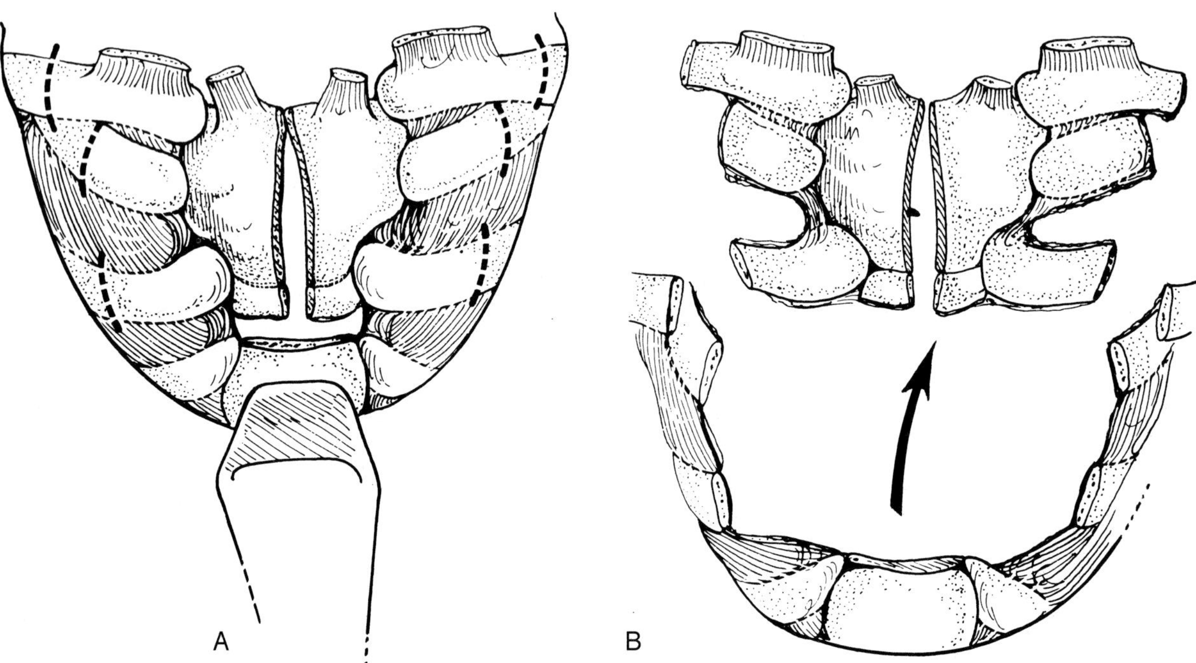

FIGURE 54–4 ■ *A* and *B*, Either one or both sides of the bony plate of chest wall can be removed to decompress the thoracic inlet.

enlarged to avoid this problem. The neck incision can be extended over the midline of the sternum to the second intercostal space. The muscular attachments to the medial head of the clavicle, sternum, and first and second costal cartilages are divided. The upper sternum is divided and then split vertically in the midline from notch to second interspace and across the second interspace transversely (Fig. 54–3). The clavicle is then divided 4 cm from the medial end by passing instruments carefully beneath the clavicle, avoiding injury to the underlying subclavian vein and dividing the bone with a Gigli saw or bone cutter. The first and second cartilages are divided after the intercostal muscle is freed from the junction of sternum and ribs.

Ideally, the pleura remains intact. If this does not provide enough room, the other half of the sternum, the clavicle, and the costal cartilages can be removed (Fig. 54–4).

COMMENTS AND CONTROVERSIES

Dr. Mathisen has described in admirable and meticulous fashion the technical details of the right thoracotomy approach for esophagectomy popularized by Ivor Lewis. The main advantage of this approach is the optimal surgical exposure of the midesophagus, which is essential for safe and complete resection of tumors that penetrate the esophageal wall or for achieving radical esophagectomy and lymph node resection if the surgeon believes that this approach increases the cure rate. In addition, as discussed by Dr. Mathisen, the intrathoracic anastomosis is far less prone to anastomotic leak than a cervical anastomosis, but the consequences of an intrathoracic leak are considerably more serious.

From a functional standpoint, an anastomosis high in the chest gives the same freedom from subsequent reflux symptoms as afforded by a cervical anastomosis. However, delayed gastric emptying from redundant intrathoracic stomach lying in the posterior costophrenic gutter or rotation of the stomach into the right chest is a significant potential disadvantage of the right thoracotomy approach.

Several years ago, at the University of Toronto, we did a retrospective comparison of outcome after the transhiatal approach compared with the right thoracotomy approach. Overall, morbidity and mortality were similar, but it was apparent that problems with delayed gastric emptying occurred much more frequently with the right thoracotomy approach than the transhiatal approach. This was reflected in the chest radiographs taken at subsequent patient follow-up. After transhiatal esophagectomy, the gastric silhouette was often not discernible on the chest radiograph, whereas an enlarged gastric silhouette, often with an air-fluid level, was not uncommon after the right thoracotomy approach.

I believe that the delayed gastric emptying seen is not related to pyloric obstruction but to the other two factors noted by Mathisen, namely, obstruction at the level of the hiatus or redundant stomach falling into the costophrenic gutter. In my own practice, I do not use either pyloromyotomy or pyloroplasty unless there is pyloric scarring from a previous peptic ulcer—an uncommon event with today's improved medical management of peptic ulcer disease.

When evaluating midesophageal tumors for possible involvement of the airway, I prefer the use of both rigid and flexible bronchoscopy. The rigid bronchoscope allows one to "feel" the laxity of the membranous wall of the airway when there is no tumor involvement and, conversely, to more easily identify rigidity and fixation of the membranous wall when there is adjacent tumor infiltration.

When resecting the esophagus in the presence of Barrett's epithelium, the surgeon should not only identify the upper level of columnar lining endoscopically but also should open the resected specimen in the operating room to visually confirm that the squamocolumnar junction is included in the resected specimen. The pathologist then further confirms this by quick section analysis of the proximal resection margin.

During the abdominal portion of the procedure, exposure of the upper abdomen is facilitated by using a fixed retractor with two blades, one on each costal arch for upper retraction. The harmonic scalpel is useful for dividing short gastric vessels, especially when exposure is difficult. I now use feeding jejunostomy in all cases, but this is not without potential complication. Careful attention to technical detail in fashioning the jejunostomy and attaching the jejunal loop to the anterior abdominal wall is important. Feeding with full-strength enteral feedings should be avoided in the first few days, as on rare occasions this is associated with impaction and gangrenous necrosis of the proximal jejunum.

During the thoracotomy portion of the procedure, Dr. Mathisen describes resection of the paraesophageal tissue "from vertebral body to pericardium." If dissection is indeed carried back to the vertebral bodies, injury to the thoracic duct commonly occurs. The possibility of this should be kept in mind, and if there is any doubt, ligation of the thoracic duct just above the diaphragm should be performed after the resection.

The three-stage procedure described by Dr. Mathisen gives the advantages of right thoracotomy exposure and location of the anastomosis in the cervical region. If this technique is to be used, I strongly recommend that the esophagogastric junction be divided through the thoracotomy approach because adequate resection and closure of the lesser curvature of the stomach can be difficult, if not impossible, through the cervical route.

Enlargement of the thoracic inlet is routinely recommended for bringing a gastric conduit to the neck through the retrosternal approach but is not commonly required for the posterior approach. When enlargement of the thoracic inlet is necessary, a somewhat lesser procedure than that depicted by Dr. Mathisen can be used, namely, resection of half of the manubrium and a segment of adjacent clavicle.

J. D. C.

KEY REFERENCES

Churchill ED, Sweet RH: Transthoracic resection of tumors of the stomach and esophagus. Ann Surg 115:897, 1942.

The lessons contained in Churchill and Sweet's description of the precise technical requirements of a safe anastomosis are as valid today as they were 60 years ago.

Mathisen DJ, Grillo HC, Wilkins EW, et al: Transthoracic esophagectomy: A safe approach to carcinoma of the esophagus. Ann Thorac Surg 45:137, 1988.

This paper describes the use of the single-stage Ivor Lewis procedure in 104 patients who underwent surgery with a 2.9% mortality and no leaks.

McKeown KC: Total three-stage oesophagectomy for cancer of the oesophagus. Br J Surg 63:259, 1976.

The technique of total three-stage esophagectomy is described fully. Points of detail in the procedure of the abdominal, thoracic, and cervical phases are emphasized. A brief note is made regarding the management of the respiratory situation at the end of the operation.

Sweet RH: Carcinoma of the esophagus and cardiac end of the stomach: Immediate and late results of treatment by resection of primary esophagogastric anastomosis. JAMA 135:485, 1947.

Operating without the modern support afforded by mechanical ventilation, monitoring devices, and antibiotics, Sweet achieved an operative mortality of 15%, a leak rate of 1.4%, and an overall 5-year survival of 11%. Sweet eschewed the right-sided approach to esophageal cancer.

■ *REFERENCES*

Akiyama H: Esophageal anastomosis. Arch Surg 107:512, 1973.

Carey RJ, Mathisen DJ: Long term follow-up of neoadjuvant therapy for squamous cancer of the esophagus. Cancer Invest 11:99, 1993.

Churchill ED, Sweet RH: Transthoracic resection of tumors of the stomach and esophagus. Ann Surg 115:897, 1942.

Ellis FH, Gibb SP, Watkins E Jr: Esophagogastrectomy: A safe, widely applicable, and expeditious form of palliation for patients with carcinoma of the esophagus and cardia. Ann Surg 198:531, 1983.

Forastiere AA, Heitmiller RF, Lee DJ, et al: Intensive chemoradiation followed by esophagectomy for squamous cell and adenocarcinoma of the esophagus. Cancer J Sci Am 3:144, 1997.

Hancock SL, Glatstein E: Radiation therapy of esophageal cancer. Semin Oncol 11:144, 1984.

Heitmiller R, Fraser C: Cervical esophago-esophageal anastomosis. Ann Thorac Surg 54:384, 1992.

King RM, Pairolero PC, Trastek VF, et al: Ivor Lewis esophagogastrectomy for carcinoma of the esophagus: Early and late functional results. Ann Thorac Surg 44:119, 1987.

Krasna MJ, Flowers JL, Attar S: Combined thoracoscopic and laparoscopic staging of esophageal cancer. J Thorac Cardiovasc Surg 111:300, 1996.

Lewis I: The surgical treatment of carcinoma of the oesophagus with special reference to a new operation for growths of the middle third. Br J Surg 34:18, 1946.

Lozac'h P, Topart P, Perramant M: Ivor Lewis procedure for epidermoid carcinoma of the esophagus: A series of 264 patients. Semin Surg Oncol 13:244, 1997.

Mathisen DJ, Grillo HC, Wilkins EW, et al: Transthoracic esophagectomy: A safe approach to carcinoma of the esophagus. Ann Thorac Surg 45:137, 1988.

McKeown KC: Total three-stage oesophagectomy for cancer of the oesophagus. Br J Surg 63:259, 1976.

Muller JM, Erasmi H, Stelzner M, et al: Surgical therapy of oesophageal carcinoma. Br J Surg 77:845, 1990.

Naunheim KS, Petruska PJ, Roy T, et al: Multimodality therapy for adenocarcinoma of the esophagus. Ann Thorac Surg 59:1085, 1995.

Orringer MS, Forastiere AA, Perez-Tamayo C, et al: Chemotherapy and radiation therapy before transhiatal esophagectomy for esophageal carcinoma. Ann Thorac Surg 49:348, 1990.

Orringer MB, Orringer JS: Esophagectomy without thoracotomy: A dangerous operation? J Thorac Cardiovasc Surg 85:72, 1983.

Rice TW, Boyce GA, Sivak MV: Esophageal ultrasound and the preoperative staging of carcinoma of the esophagus. J Thorac Cardiovasc Surg 101:536, 1991.

Richter JM, Hilgenberg AD, Mathisen DJ, et al: Endoscopic palliation of obstructive esophagogastric malignancy. Gastrointest Endosc 34:454, 1988.

Shahian DM, Neptune WB, Ellis FH, et al: Transthoracic versus extrathoracic esophagectomy: Mortality, morbidity, and long-term survival. Ann Thorac Surg 41:237, 1986.

Sweet RH: Carcinoma of the esophagus and cardiac end of the stomach: Immediate and late results of treatment by resection of primary esophagogastric anastomosis. JAMA 135:485, 1947.

Walsh TN, Noonan N, Hollywood D, et al: A comparison of multimodal therapy and surgery for esophageal adenocarcinoma. N Engl J Med 341:384, 1999.

Wright CD, Wain JC, Mathisen DJ, et al: Induction therapy for esophageal cancer with paclitaxel and hyperfractionated radiotherapy: A phase I and II study. J Thorac Cardiovasc Surg 114:811, 1997.

SYNCHRONOUS COMBINED ABDOMINOTHORACOCERVICAL ESOPHAGECTOMY

F. Griffith Pearson

DEFINITION

Synchronous combined abdominothoracocervical esophagectomy is a procedure in which the patient is placed supine with some elevation of the right side of the chest (Fig. 54–5). This position allows performance of an upper abdominal midline laparotomy, a right anterior thoracotomy in the third or fourth intercostal space, and a cervical incision on either the right or left side. In contrast to the Ivor Lewis (1946) and McKeown (1972) procedures, there is no need to reposition the patient during the abdominal, thoracic, or cervical stages of the operation. Furthermore, the abdominal, thoracic, and cervical components can be done synchronously with two surgical teams. With the patient in this position, the surgeon has the option of performing a transhiatal esophagectomy, a laparotomy, and a right anterior thoracotomy, with the anastomosis high in the right hemithorax, or a total thoracic esophagectomy using three incisions.

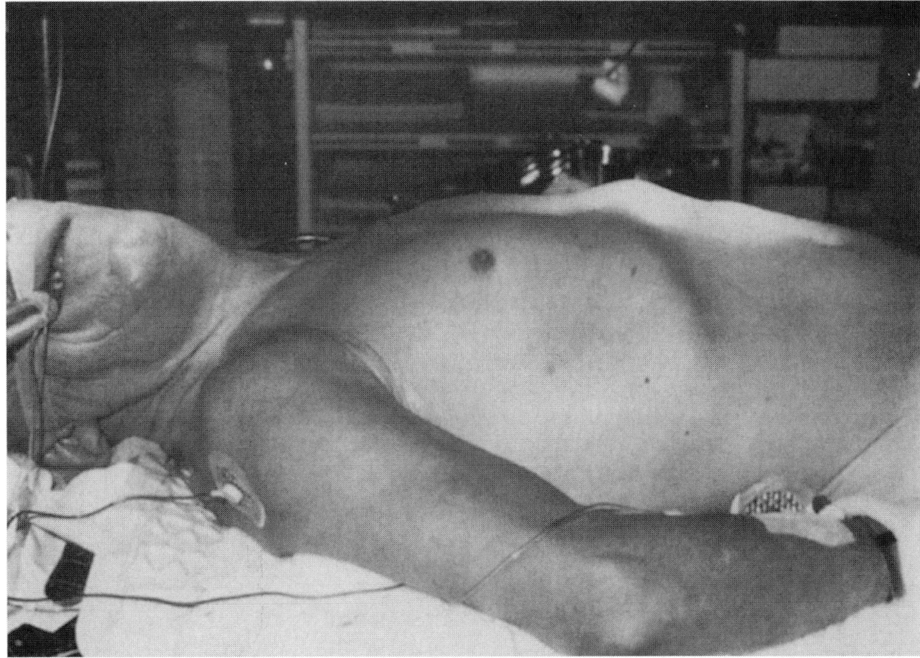

FIGURE 54–5 ■ Photograph illustrating the position and exposure of the patient. The right hemithorax is elevated slightly on a small bolster, and the right hand is placed under the small of the back with the elbow bent sufficiently to provide exposure of the right axilla. A double-lumen tube has been placed, and the patient's head has been turned to the right, which exposes the left neck for a left anterior stemomastoid incision. The surgical drapes extend from the abdomen below the level of the umbilicus along each side, with clear exposure of the right axilla as far back as the posterior axillary line, and along the line of the mandible and chin in the neck.

HISTORICAL NOTE

In 1946, Ivor Lewis described a technique of esophagectomy through a posterolateral right thoracotomy with the esophagogastric anastomosis in the right chest. McKeown (1972) described a modification of Lewis' technique, adding a third incision in the neck with a cervical anastomosis.

During the annual meeting of the Canadian Royal College of Physicians and Surgeons in 1965, Eric Nanson, in discussing a paper on esophageal cancer, described the "synchronous combined abdominothoracocervical technique" that he was using at that time. In the only reported publication describing this operation, Nanson (1975) stated that he had "routinely performed esophagectomy" by this synchronous combined approach since 1950. As I recall from personal discussion with Nanson at that meeting in 1965, he attributed its origin to Professor Robert Milnes-Walker of Bristol in the late 1940s. Nanson was Milnes-Walker's resident at that time. There is, however, no publication that verifies this origin.

Nanson recommended this operation for primary carcinoma of the distal two thirds of the esophagus and for benign strictures of peptic or corrosive origin that needed esophagectomy and replacement. In patients with adenocarcinoma of the cardia, Nanson recommended a left thoracoabdominal approach. At the time of Nanson's 1975 publication, adenocarcinoma in a columnar-lined distal esophagus was rarely reported.

In his original article, Nanson listed seven separate advantages of this synchronous combined approach: first and foremost among these, however, is the shortened operative time as a result of synchronous, two-team surgery, which avoids the need to reposition the patient during operation.

■ *HISTORICAL READINGS*

Lewis I: The surgical treatment of carcinoma of the oesophagus with special reference to a new operation for growths of the middle third. Br J Surg 34:18, 1946.

McKeown KC: Trends in oesophageal resection for carcinoma with special reference to total oesophagectomy. Ann R Coll Surg Engl 51:213–239, 1972.

Nanson EM: Synchronous combined abdomino-thoraco-cervical esophagectomy. Aust N Z J Surg 454:340, 1975.

INDICATIONS

The synchronous abdominothoracocervical approach provides exposure of the entire thoracic and cervical esophagus. From the abdominal side, the lower third of the thoracic esophagus can be mobilized through the dilated diaphragmatic hiatus. A right anterior thoracotomy through the third or fourth intercostal space provides access for dissection and mobilization of the upper and middle thirds of the thoracic esophagus. The addition of a cervical incision on either the left or the right side exposes the remainder of the organ.

With the patient supine and the thorax slightly elevated on the right side, the surgeon may choose to use only the upper abdominal and right anterior thoracic incisions, with creation of an esophagogastric anastomosis high in the right hemithorax. If the anastomosis is to be in the neck, this positioning allows either a transhiatal resection or the use of three incisions and two surgical teams for the synchronous combined abdominothoracocervical esophagectomy.

The operation is therefore suitable for resection of esophageal cancer at any level within the thoracic esophagus. This approach may also be used in patients requiring thoracic esophagectomy for benign disease, such as previously operated primary motor disorders complicated by unmanageable gastroesophageal reflux (e.g., achalasia with peptic stricture).

If the surgeon anticipates a difficult technical resection for cancer at and above the level of the carina, a full posterolateral thoracotomy can provide easier access.

TECHNIQUE

Anesthesia

Split-lung anesthesia is required so that the right lung may be collapsed at the time of right anterior thoracotomy.

Positioning the Patient

The patient is positioned as illustrated in Figure 54–5. The right elbow is slightly flexed, and the hand is placed beneath the small of the back. The right hemithorax is elevated with a small bolster, which provides access to the entire axilla. This positioning allows exposure for all three incisions illustrated in Figure 54–6 without the need to reposition and redrape the patient. A pillow is strapped firmly across the upper thighs to stabilize the patient so that the table may be rolled to the right or the left at any stage in the operation. The patient is usually maintained in 10 to 15 degrees of the reverse Trendelenburg position, which allows the viscera to drift inferiorly away from the diaphragm and operative area during the abdominal part of the operation.

Some form of bolster is placed between the shoulders to facilitate neck extension. My associates and I use an inflatable bag, which permits easy reversal of the neck extension at the end of the operation.

It is usually possible to turn the head to the patient's right, so that the left neck is exposed for performance of a left anterior sternomastoid incision. This left-sided exposure is less likely to result in injury to the ipsilateral recurrent laryngeal nerve from intraoperative traction.

Mattioli and colleagues (1997) reported experience with a modification of this position that is designed to further improve access and exposure for this operation. A custom-designed metal fitting, secured to the operating table, increases rotation of the thorax toward the left side and improves access for the right anterior thoracotomy.

The right axilla is exposed so that a submammary incision can be carried high in the axilla as far as the posterior axillary line. The field is isolated with use of four straight drapes. The exposed field extends from the chin and angle of the jaw above to the abdominal wall below the umbilicus inferiorly.

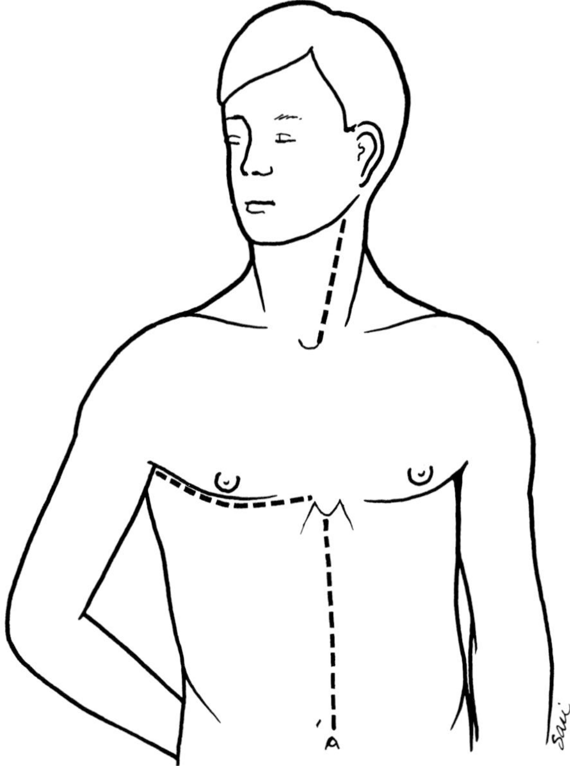

Figure 54–6 ■ Illustration of the three incisions that can be made without having to turn the patient with the need for repeated preparation and draping. The abdominal incision extends from the xiphoid to the umbilicus. The right anterior thoracotomy is usually made in the fourth interspace. It is carried medially to the sternal border and laterally to the posterior axillary line high in the axilla. The sternomastoid incision on the left side extends from the suprasternal notch below for about two thirds of the distance to the angle of the jaw above.

Laparotomy

A midline upper abdominal incision is made from the xiphoid above to the umbilicus below. A so-called upper-hand retractor is positioned (Fig. 54–7); this provides excellent exposure of the upper abdomen and the region of the diaphragmatic hiatus once the retaining retractors (Balfour and Harrington attachments) are secured in position (Fig. 54–8). The abdomen is explored, and at this point it is possible to confirm whether the malignancy is operable, at least from the abdominal side.

At this stage, the second surgical team may proceed with the right anterior thoracotomy. If, however, findings at laparotomy suggest that a transhiatal resection may be selected, the second team can then start the cervical exposure. The second team should have a separate instrument tray, including a second cautery, which can be positioned across the head of the patient. This second setup may be used for either the thoracotomy or the cervical components of the procedure. An additional scrub nurse is not necessary.

Stomach is usually used as a substitute and is prepared in the usual fashion with resection of at least two thirds of the lesser curvature side, including the lesser omentum and its contained lymph nodes. A pyloric drainage procedure may be performed, depending on the practice of the surgeon.

Right Anterolateral Thoracotomy

The skin incision is made in the submammary crease on the right side. The incision is carried medially to the right sternal border, with care taken to preserve the internal mammary vessels. The incision is carried laterally to the posterior axillary line in the skin, the underlying subcutaneous fat, and the chest wall muscles. The intercostal muscle, however, is freed from the upper border of the rib on the inferior side of the incision. Intercostal muscle can be freed from this rib posteriorly and medially almost to the level of the spine, which facilitates spreading of the ribs for subsequent exposure. The incision is

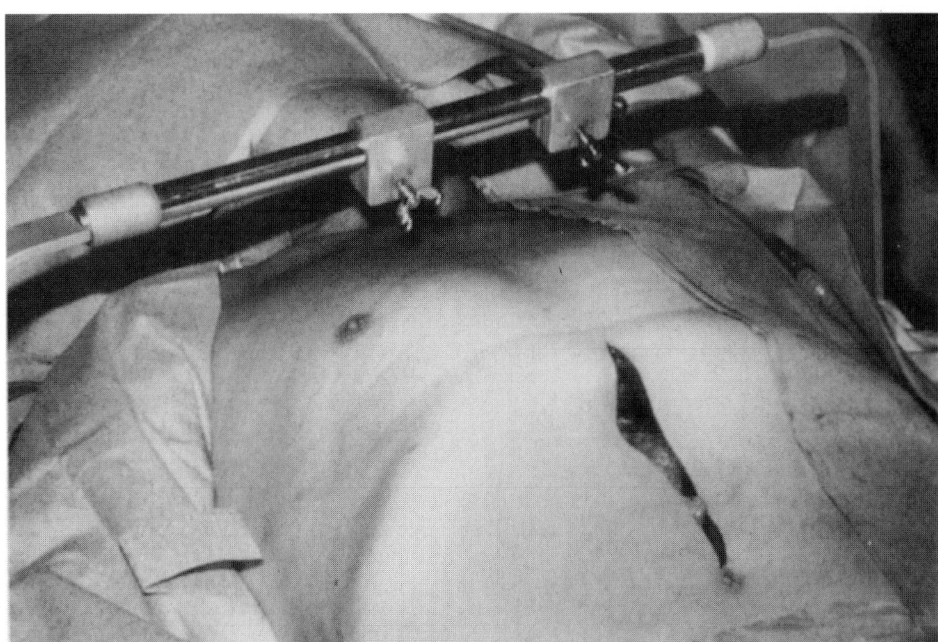

FIGURE 54–7 ■ The abdominal incision has been made and the upper-hand retractor has been positioned.

usually made in the fourth intercostal space, although the third space may be selected if a high and difficult dissection is anticipated. The margins of the thoracotomy incision are separated with a single retractor, which may be placed from either the anterior or posterior aspects of the incision.

The right lung is collapsed and can then be retracted anteriorly to expose the posterior mediastinum along the line of the mediastinal pleura overlying the esophagus. For the part of the dissection that lies at and above the level of the azygos vein, the right lung is retracted inferiorly. The inferior pulmonary ligament should be divided at the outset to facilitate anterior retraction of the lung. Strong anterior retraction may interfere with venous return and result in hypotension. This problem will obviously be identified by the anesthetist, and in some patients intermittent exposure is required for part of the esophagectomy.

Even though the incision is in the anterior half of the right hemithorax, surprisingly good exposure of the middle and upper thirds of the intrathoracic esophagus can be obtained in most patients. Access to this area is through the anterolateral part of the right chest, and the operating surgeon may achieve the best position by sitting on a stool. I find a headlight invaluable when operating in this "lateral" position.

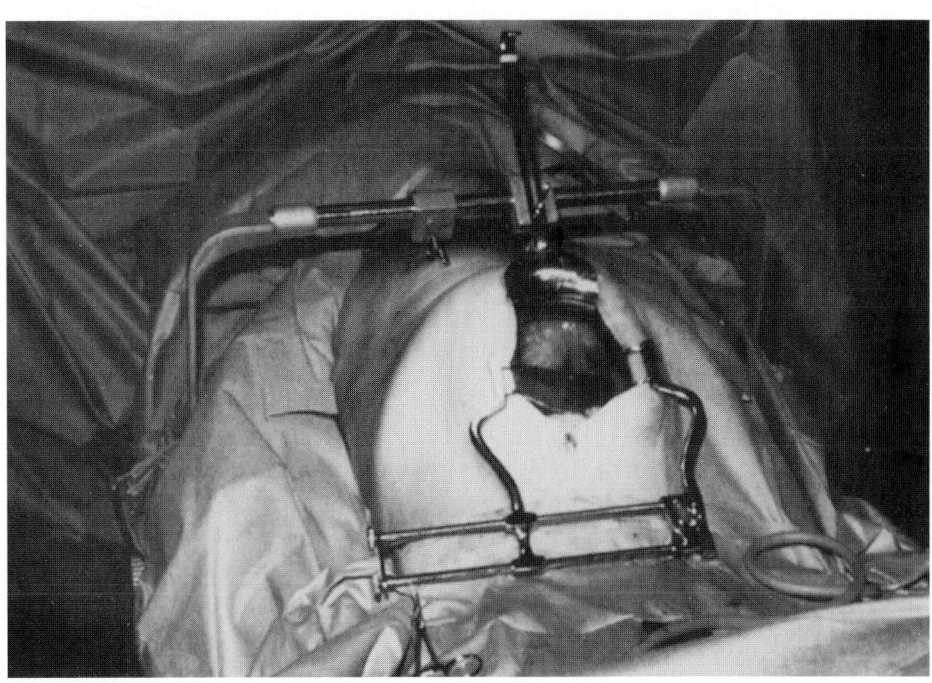

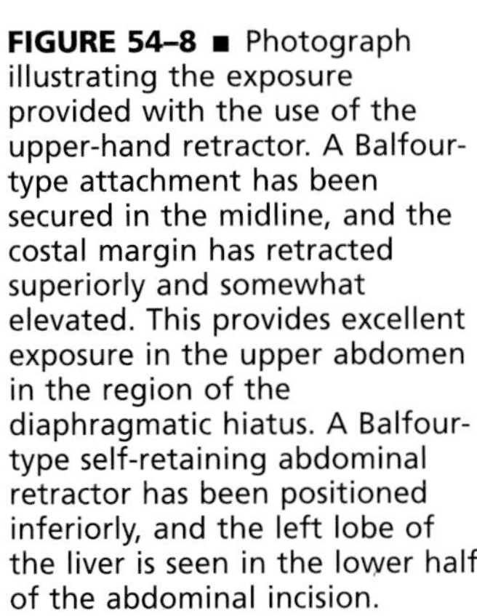

FIGURE 54–8 ■ Photograph illustrating the exposure provided with the use of the upper-hand retractor. A Balfour-type attachment has been secured in the midline, and the costal margin has retracted superiorly and somewhat elevated. This provides excellent exposure in the upper abdomen in the region of the diaphragmatic hiatus. A Balfour-type self-retaining abdominal retractor has been positioned inferiorly, and the left lobe of the liver is seen in the lower half of the abdominal incision.

Good visualization of the upper and middle thirds of the thoracic esophagus can be obtained, but the lower third lies hidden behind the right border of the heart and is relatively difficult to expose through this high anterior incision. In almost every case, however, the lower third of the esophagus can be accurately and well mobilized under direct vision from the abdominal side, through the dilated hiatus.

If the abdominal and thoracic components of the operation are done synchronously, it is desirable to have a team of four surgeons and one scrub nurse. There will be two operating surgeons, each with an assistant.

Cervical Incision

A left anterior sternomastoid incision is preferred. The omohyoid muscle and inferior thyroid arteries are divided to provide clear exposure, and the cervical esophagus is mobilized circumferentially, beginning just below the cricopharyngeal sphincter. The cervical esophagus is divided in the neck 3 or 4 cm distal to the cricopharyngeal sphincter, and the mobilized stomach is elevated into the neck through the bed of the resected esophagus in the posterior mediastinum. It is usually possible to judge that enough stomach has been mobilized by laying the gastric substitute across the front of the chest, with the top end of the gastric tube lying in the cervical incision (Fig. 54–9).

As soon as the mobilized stomach has been elevated into the right hemithorax, the abdominal incision can be closed; once the stomach has been elevated into the neck, the right thoracotomy can be closed. Once again, it is emphasized that this single exposure provides the opportunity for two surgical teams to operate synchronously in the abdominal, thoracic, or cervical areas.

Whenever possible, I prefer to secure the stomach in the posterior mediastinum by closing the mediastinal pleura on the right side. This obviates herniation of the stomach into the right hemithorax, which occasionally results in a redundant or retort-shaped stomach draped over the right hemidiaphragm, creating some angulation and obstruction at the pyloric end.

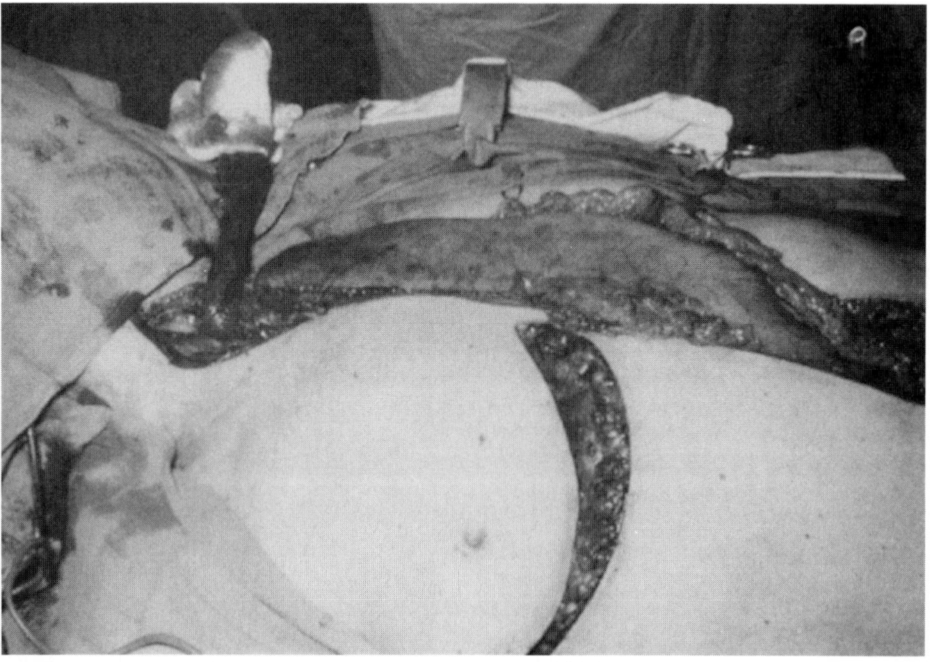

FIGURE 54–9 ■ Photograph taken before completion of the operation, with all three incisions demonstrated. The stomach has been mobilized on the right gastroepiploic arcade, and a long tube of stomach has been created by removal of the proximal two thirds of the lesser curvature side, including the lesser omentum and its contained lymph nodes. The stomach has been brought out through the abdominal incision and laid across the front of the midline of the chest. It easily reaches to the neck. The posterior mediastinal route will be used for the stomach, and this route is even shorter than the anterior cutaneous position seen in the photograph. The right anterior fourth interspace thoracotomy is visible. The skin incision was made in the submammary crease from the right sternal border to the posterior axillary line high in the axilla. The actual interspace opened, in this case, was the fourth. A tumor in the middle and lower thirds of the esophagus was resected; the middle-third component was mobilized through the anterior thoracotomy and the lower third through the dilated hiatus from the abdominal side. The cervical incision has been made; the esophagogastric junction has been divided below, and the entire thoracic esophagus, including the growth, has been elevated into the neck. The cervical esophagus and the segment containing the growth are seen in the upper right of the photograph. Most of the growth has been covered with a sponge.

Postoperative Care

Postoperative care is the same as that used for any thoracic esophagectomy. My own preference is to maintain continuous nasogastric suction for 3 to 5 days after operation. I use a single 28 French chest drain in the right hemithorax and remove the drain as soon as the effluent becomes relatively serous.

COMMENTS AND CONTROVERSIES

The operation described here for esophageal resection is a little known approach, with only two existing publications that describe the technique (Nanson, 1975). In concept, it does not differ greatly from the well-known and widely used procedures described by Lewis (1965) and McKeown (1972). The essential difference in this operation is the use of a high right anterior thoracotomy rather than the traditional posterolateral exposure.

There are several distinct advantages to positioning the thoracotomy anteriorly:

1. The patient can be positioned so that all three incisions may be made without any need for repositioning or repreparation.

2. Other than transhiatal esophagectomy (Orringer and Stirling, 1993), this is the only technique of thoracic esophagectomy in which two surgical teams may work synchronously with good effect. In experienced hands, this operation can be performed from "skin to skin" within about 3 hours.

3. During the operation, all three incisions are open and accessible at one time. This facility occurs with only one other technique, that of left thoracoabdominal and cervical resection (see Chapter 53, Part B).

4. With the patient positioned supine and prepared and draped from chin to lower abdomen, the exposure provides the options of synchronous combined abdominothoracocervical resection, transhiatal resection without thoracotomy, or resection using an abdominal incision and anterior thoracotomy with performance of the anastomosis in the upper part of the right hemithorax.

The disadvantages are due to the presumed impairment of access to the posterior mediastinum and esophageal bed at the level of the aortic arch and main carina. There is no doubt that a standard, full, right posterolateral thoracotomy may provide better technical exposure in some difficult cases, but this difference is not great in my experience and is of no consequence in a majority of resections in which the tumor lies in the middle third.

With experience, some of the apparent technical difficulties with access through an anterior thoracotomy are easily overcome.

F. G. P.

Dr. Pearson has given an excellent account of the procedure that we in the Toronto group locally used to refer to as the "three-hole" esophagectomy. For a number of years, it was my preferred approach for the reasons Dr. Pearson indicates, namely, the opportunity of exploring both the chest and the abdomen before making a final decision as to resection; the ability to use a two-team approach; and the time saved compared with the Ivor Lewis approach. For several reasons, however, I rarely employ this procedure at present.

First, with the increased incidence of early distal esophageal adenocarcinoma now seen, the transhiatal approach is commonly selected. This gives excellent exposure of the lower half of the esophagus, and the thoracotomy is generally not required. Second, the disadvantage of the "three-hole" approach is the difficult access to the upper portion of the esophagus both for dissection and for possible anastomosis. The thoracotomy portion of the procedure described by Dr. Pearson is an anterolateral approach. The right lung must be completely deflated and vigorously retracted anteriorly and inferiorly. This often leads to considerable manipulation of the lung, and if extensive adhesions are encountered in the chest, this can lead to significant difficulties. For this reason, I much prefer the right posterolateral thoracotomy, as employed in the Ivor Lewis procedure, for resecting tumors of the upper or middle esophagus. For relatively small tumors of the midesophagus, the approach described by Pearson may indeed be ideal.

Several years ago, we retrospectively compared results with the "three-hole" esophagectomy and the transhiatal approach. There was little difference in morbidity and mortality, but gastric functioning was much better in the transhiatal group because of the absence of gastric rotation into the right pleural space and draping of the stomach over the right hemidiaphragm with angulation at the hiatus, as described by Dr. Pearson. After transhiatal esophagectomy, it was rare to encounter the large fluid-filled poorly emptying stomach in the right chest, not uncommonly seen after a right thoracotomy approach.

J. D. C.

REFERENCES

Lewis I: The surgical treatment of carcinoma of the oesophagus with special reference to a new operation for growths of the middle third. Br J Surg 34:18, 1946.

Mattioli S, D'Ovidio F, Di Simone MP, et al: Patient position for a synchronous cervicothoracoabdominal two-team esophagectomy. Ann Thorac Surg 63:255–257, 1997.

McKeown KC: Trends in oesophageal resection for carcinoma with special reference to total oesophagectomy. Ann R Coll Surg Engl 51:213–239, 1972.

Nanson EM: Synchronous combined abdomino-thoraco-cervical esophagectomy. Aust NZ J Surg 45:340, 1975.

Orringer MB, Stirling MC: Transhiatal esophagectomy for benign and malignant disease. J Thorac Cardiovasc Surg 105:265, 1993.

CHAPTER **55**

Transhiatal Esophagectomy Without Thoracotomy

Mark B. Orringer

DEFINITION

After more than 50 years of experience with transthoracic esophagectomy, transhiatal esophagectomy without thoracotomy, more recently popularized by Orringer and Sloan (1978), Orringer and Orringer (1983), and Orringer (1984c), has emerged as an alternative operative approach that may be associated with substantially less risk and morbidity. Not only does transhiatal esophagectomy avoid the morbidity of a thoracotomy; the routine cervical esophageal anastomosis also virtually eliminates mediastinitis resulting from anastomotic disruption as a cause of postoperative death. Furthermore, the abdominal approach used for the esophagectomy provides access to all portions of the gastrointestinal tract used for esophageal substitution, giving the surgeon the option of using the stomach or any portion of the colon that might be needed for esophageal replacement.

The view that transhiatal esophagectomy is a safer alternative to traditional transthoracic resection was supported by Tryzelaar and colleagues (1982), Stewart and colleagues (1985), Baker and Schechter (1986), Hankins and colleagues (1987), Sabanathan and colleagues (1988), Finley and Inculet (1989), and Hankins and colleagues (1989). Others, such as Steiger and Wilson 1981), Caracci and colleagues (1983), Fok and colleagues (1984), and Shahian and colleagues (1986), challenged this view. Fok and coworkers (1984) in fact reported an 18% incidence of intraoperative bleeding severe enough to cause hypotension with transhiatal esophagectomy.

Katariya and colleagues (1994), in their collective review of the complications of transhiatal esophagectomy in 1353 reported patients, cited an overall 30-day mortality of 7.1%; a 1.3% incidence of massive intraoperative bleeding, necessitating conversion to a transthoracic procedure; an 11.3% incidence of recurrent laryngeal nerve injury; a 50% incidence of "thoracic or pulmonary complications"; and a 15.1% anastomotic leak rate. Seventy percent of the referenced papers, however, were series of 50 patients or less and therefore represented the initial phase of the authors' "learning curve" with this procedure. A more recent review of 1192 patients by Gandhi and Naunheim (1997) cites an average mortality rate of 6.7%, a 3% incidence of mediastinal hemorrhage, a 9% incidence of recurrent laryngeal nerve injury, a 12% incidence of respiratory complications, a 12% incidence of anastomotic leak, and a 15% incidence of cardiac complications. Fifty percent of the referenced papers were series of 100 or more patients. The University of Michigan report (1999) by Orringer and colleagues, on 1085 transhiatal esophagectomies for diseases of the intrathoracic esophagus, represents the largest published experience with this operation and provides a benchmark standard.

Critics of transhiatal esophagectomy have warned that the operation violates basic surgical principles of adequate hemostasis and exposure and falls short as a "cancer operation" because it precludes a complete en bloc mediastinal lymph node dissection, as advocated by Skinner (1983). However, growing experience has challenged these criticisms, and transhiatal esophagectomy has emerged, since the late 1970s, as an accepted method of esophageal resection. This chapter reviews the technique of transhiatal esophagectomy and cervical esophagogastrostomy, its indications and contraindications, and the results of this operation at the University of Michigan.

HISTORICAL NOTE

Using a vein stripper to avulse the esophagus from the posterior mediastinum, Denk (1913) first reported the performance of blunt transmediastinal esophagectomy without thoracotomy in cadavers and experimental animals. Turner (1933) carried out the first successful transhiatal esophagectomy for carcinoma and re-established continuity of the alimentary tract using an antethoracic skin tube at a second operation. As endotracheal anesthesia became established, thus permitting transthoracic esophagectomy under direct vision, transhiatal esophagectomy was essentially forgotten, being used only occasionally as a concomitant procedure with laryngopharyngectomy for pharyngeal or cervical esophageal carcinomas when the stomach was employed to restore continuity of the alimentary tract.

Ong and Lee (1960) and LeQuesne and Ranger (1966) reported the first successful primary pharyngogastric anastomoses after laryngopharyngectomy and thoracic esophagectomy. In these cases and in that reported by Akiyama and associates (1971), an essentially normal thoracic esophagus was being resected. Kirk (1974) used the transhiatal approach for palliation of incurable esophageal carcinoma in five patients. Thomas and Dedo (1977) treated four patients with severe chronic pharyngoesophageal caustic strictures by transhiatal esophagectomy, mobilizing the stomach through the posterior mediastinum and performing a pharyngogastric anastomosis. In general, however, throughout the world the most widely used technique of esophageal resection historically has consisted of a transthoracic approach with an intrathoracic esophagogastric anastomosis. The notion long prevailed that the mobilized stomach would not usually extend readily to the neck.

In an attempt to lessen the morbidity and mortality of esophageal resection and reconstruction, my colleagues and I adopted a policy of avoiding an intrathoracic esophagogastric anastomosis whenever possible. Regardless of the level of esophageal pathology, the entire thoracic esophagus was resected and a cervical esophageal anastomosis performed. Although this approach necessitated three incisions (cervical, thoracic, and abdominal), death from anastomotic disruption following esophagectomy virtually disappeared on our service.

In 1974, while mobilizing the stomach transabdominally in a patient with a sliding hernia and a small distal third esophageal adenocarcinoma in preparation for a standard transthoracic esophageal resection and esophageal reconstruction, I mobilized nearly 4 inches of esophagus out of the posterior mediastinum and into the abdomen through the diaphragmatic hiatus. My experience with mediastinoscopy for the evaluation of patients with carcinoma of the lung had taught me that the index finger could reach through a cervical incision into the mediastinum to the level of the carina. Therefore, in this particular obese patient, who was regarded as at high risk for thoracotomy, a cervical incision was made, and with one hand in the abdomen through the diaphragmatic hiatus and in the posterior mediastinum and the other hand in the superior mediastinum through the cervical incision, a "blunt" esophageal mobilization was performed and the esophagus extracted. The mobilized stomach was positioned in the posterior mediastinum in the original esophageal bed, and a cervical esophagogastric anastomosis was constructed.

The successful outcome of this initial experience with transhiatal esophagectomy without thoracotomy was the basis for the subsequent report by Orringer and Sloan (1978) of the procedure in 28 patients, of whom 4 had benign disease of the intrathoracic esophagus and 22 had carcinomas involving various levels of the esophagus. Since then, my group's experience with more than 1000 patients undergoing transhiatal esophagectomy without thoracotomy (Orringer, 1984a–c, 1985; Orringer and associates, 1993, 1999), as well as reports by Szentpetery and colleagues (1979), Bains and Spiro (1979), Cordiano et al, (1979), and others, has justified our current belief that there is seldom an indication for opening the thorax in patients requiring esophageal resection for either benign or malignant disease.

■ *HISTORICAL READINGS*

Akiyama H, Sato Y, Takahashi F: Immediate pharyngogastrostomy following total esophagectomy by blunt dissection. Jpn J Surg 1:225, 1971.

Bains MS, Spiro RH: Pharyngolaryngectomy, total extrathoracic esophagectomy and gastric transposition. Surg Gynecol Obstet 149:693, 1979.

Cordiano C, Fracastoro G, Mosciaro O, Mozzo W: Esophagectomy and esophageal replacement by gastric pull-through procedure. Int Surg 64:17, 1979.

Denk W: Zur Radikaloperation des Osophaguskarfzentralbl. Chirurg 40:1065, 1913.

Kirk RM: Palliative resection of esophageal carcinoma without formal thoracotomy. Br J Surg 61:689, 1974.

LeQuesne LP, Ranger D: Pharyngogastrectomy with immediate pharyngogastric anastomosis. Br J Surg 53:105, 1966.

Ong GB, Lee TC: Pharyngogastric anastomosis after oesophagopharyngectomy for carcinoma of the hypopharynx and cervical esophagus. Br J Surg 48:193, 1960.

Orringer MB: Transhiatal esophagectomy for benign and malignant disease. J Jpn Assoc Thorac Surg 36:656, 1988.

Orringer MB: Transhiatal esophagectomy for benign disease. J Thorac Cardiovasc Surg 90:649, 1985.

Orringer MB: Partial median sternotomy: Anterior approach to the upper thoracic esophagus. J Thorac Cardiovasc Surg 87:124, 1984a.

Orringer MB: Technical aids in performing transhiatal esophagectomy without thoracotomy. Ann Thorac Surg 38:128, 1984b.

Orringer MB: Transhiatal esophagectomy without thoracotomy for carcinoma of the thoracic esophagus. Ann Surg 200:282, 1984c.

Orringer MB, Marshall B, Stirling MC: Transhiatal esophagectomy for benign and malignant disease. J Thorac Cardiovasc Surg 105:265, 1993.

Orringer MB, Sloan H: Esophagectomy without thoracotomy. J Thorac Cardiovasc Surg 76:643, 1978.

Szentpetery S, Wolfgang T, Lower RR: Pull-through esophagectomy without thoracotomy for esophageal carcinoma. Ann Thorac Surg 27:399, 1979.

Thomas AN, Dedo HH: Pharyngogastrostomy for treatment of severe caustic stricture of the pharynx and esophagus. J Thorac Cardiovasc Surg 73:817, 1977.

Turner GG: Excision of thoracic esophagus for carcinoma with construction of extrathoracic gullet. Lancet 2:1315, 1933.

INDICATIONS AND CONTRAINDICATIONS

I regard virtually every patient in need of an esophagectomy for either benign or malignant disease as a potential candidate for transhiatal esophagectomy. Bronchoscopy is a routine part of the evaluation of every patient with an upper or middle third thoracic esophageal carcinoma, and endoscopic evidence of tracheobronchial invasion by the esophageal tumor is an absolute contraindication to transhiatal esophagectomy. As discussed in Chapter 60, for patients with cervicothoracic esophageal tumors in whom an anterior mediastinal tracheotomy is being contemplated, at least a 5-cm length of uninvolved trachea proximal to the carina after the resection is optimal and accurate bronchoscopic measurement of the distance between the tumor and the carina is a routine part of preoperative assessment of resectability.

Because of the extremely poor prognosis of patients with distant metastatic (stage IV) disease from esophageal carcinoma, I do not recommend an esophagectomy in patients with biopsy-proven metastases to either the liver, supraclavicular lymph nodes, or another site remote from regional lymph nodes. Although computed tomography (CT) is an important part of the assessment of the patient with esophageal carcinoma and is useful in suggesting pulmonary, hepatic, or distant intra-abdominal nodal metastases (which should nonetheless be confirmed with fine-needle aspiration), as reported by Quint and colleagues (1985), the CT scan is not a reliable indicator of the resectability of esophageal carcinoma. We have repeatedly been impressed by the fact that CT evidence of contiguity of the esophageal tumor and the adjacent aorta, prevertebral fascia, or tracheobronchial tree is not synonymous with *invasion*. Esophageal endoscopic ultrasonography (EUS) may provide additional information regarding likely invasion of adjacent vital structures.

However, our experience with more than 1000 transhiatal esophagectomies has indicated that the operation has been feasible in 98% of our patients in whom it has been attempted, based solely upon the findings of the barium esophagogram, esophagoscopy, and the CT scan.

Periesophageal fibrosis from prior esophageal operations, caustic injuries, or radiation therapy does not preclude a transhiatal esophagectomy. In patients with such a history, however, the surgeon must have a relatively low threshold for converting to a transthoracic esophageal resection if significant intrathoracic periesophageal adhesions are encountered upon assessment of the esophagus through the diaphragmatic hiatus. This is of particular importance in patients who have undergone a previous esophagomyotomy for either achalasia or esophageal spasm and in whom fusion between the exposed esophageal submucosa and the adjacent aorta may predispose to disastrous intraoperative bleeding at the time of esophagectomy. In every transhiatal esophagectomy, the surgeon's assessment of esophageal mobility on manual palpation of the esophagus through the diaphragmatic hiatus is the most important factor in determining whether it is appropriate to proceed or whether it is better to abandon the transhiatal route for a transthoracic resection under direct vision.

MANAGEMENT

Preoperative Preparation

An aggressive 2- to 3-week preoperative outpatient program of pulmonary physiotherapy, using an incentive inspirometer, and physical conditioning, by walking between 1 and 2 miles a day when possible, is initiated in patients with benign and malignant disease. Complete abstinence from cigarette smoking is mandatory. When the esophageal obstruction is high grade and precludes an adequate oral calorie intake of even liquid diet supplements, a nasogastric feeding tube is inserted through the tumor and into the stomach, and enteral feedings providing 2000 to 3000 calories/day are administered. In patients with a history of previous gastric disease or surgery that might preclude use of the stomach for esophageal replacement, a barium enema study is obtained to evaluate the suitability of the colon as an esophageal substitute, and the colon is prepared in the event that colonic interposition is required. This is not routine, however, since in patients with a normal stomach the gastric fundus readily reaches above the level of the clavicles for a cervical anastomosis.

Anesthesia

A radial artery catheter to monitor blood pressure during the esophagectomy and a thoracic epidural catheter for postoperative analgesia are inserted prior to induction of anesthesia. The arterial catheter is well secured and padded, since the patient's arms are kept at the sides during the operation to allow the surgeon access to the neck, chest, and abdomen. It is generally unnecessary to monitor central venous pressure; when required, however, it should be done through a right neck vein, away from the operative field on the left neck.

An *unshortened* standard endotracheal tube is generally used so that in the event of a posterior membranous tracheal tear during the transhiatal dissection, the end of the tube can be advanced until the balloon is beyond the tear and direct repair can then be performed. A double-lumen endotracheal tube is rarely used. Inhalation anesthetic agents are reduced and inspired oxygen concentration increased as the actual transhiatal dissection is performed to minimize the adverse affects of transient hypotension, which is not uncommon during the esophagectomy. The operation requires close cooperation between the anesthetist and the surgeon to minimize prolonged hypotension.

Operative Technique

The patient is positioned supine with a small folded sheet beneath the scapulae to extend the neck. The head is turned toward the right and stabilized with a head ring beneath the occiput. The arms are carefully padded to protect the intravenous and arterial catheters and are placed at the patient's sides. The skin is prepared and draped from the mandible to the pubis and anterior to both midaxillary lines. Even when there is concern that a transthoracic esophagectomy may be required (e.g., with upper or middle third esophageal tumors or with a history of a previous long esophagomyotomy), I prefer the patient to be supine. If a transthoracic approach is needed, the abdomen is closed and the patient is repositioned for a standard posterolateral thoracic incision. Use of a table-mounted, self-retaining (upper hand) retractor greatly facilitates exposure. Transhiatal esophagectomy has three separate phases: (1) abdominal, (2) mediastinal, and (3) cervical.

Abdominal Phase

The entire abdominal portion of the operation is performed through a supraumbilical incision (Fig. 55–1, *inset*). The triangular ligament of the liver is divided, and the left hepatic lobe is retracted to the right. It is quickly ascertained that the stomach is essentially normal, and the right gastroepiploic artery is identified early and protected. This is particularly important in patients with a history of previous abdominal surgery in whom the need to divide adhesions may jeopardize the gastric blood supply.

Mobilization of the greater omentum away from the stomach is begun at the midpoint of the greater curvature, and the lesser sac is entered through an avascular portion of omentum where the right gastroepiploic artery terminates as it enters the stomach or anastomoses with small branches of the left gastroepiploic artery. Separation of the omentum from the right gastroepiploic artery is carried out at least 1.5 to 2 cm inferior to the vessel to minimize the chance of injury to this artery.

The left gastroepiploic and short gastric vessels are divided and ligated along the high greater curvature of the stomach, which avoids injury to the spleen as well as gastric necrosis from ligation of these vessels too near the gastric wall. Distally, the greater omentum is separated from the stomach to the level of the pylorus, with

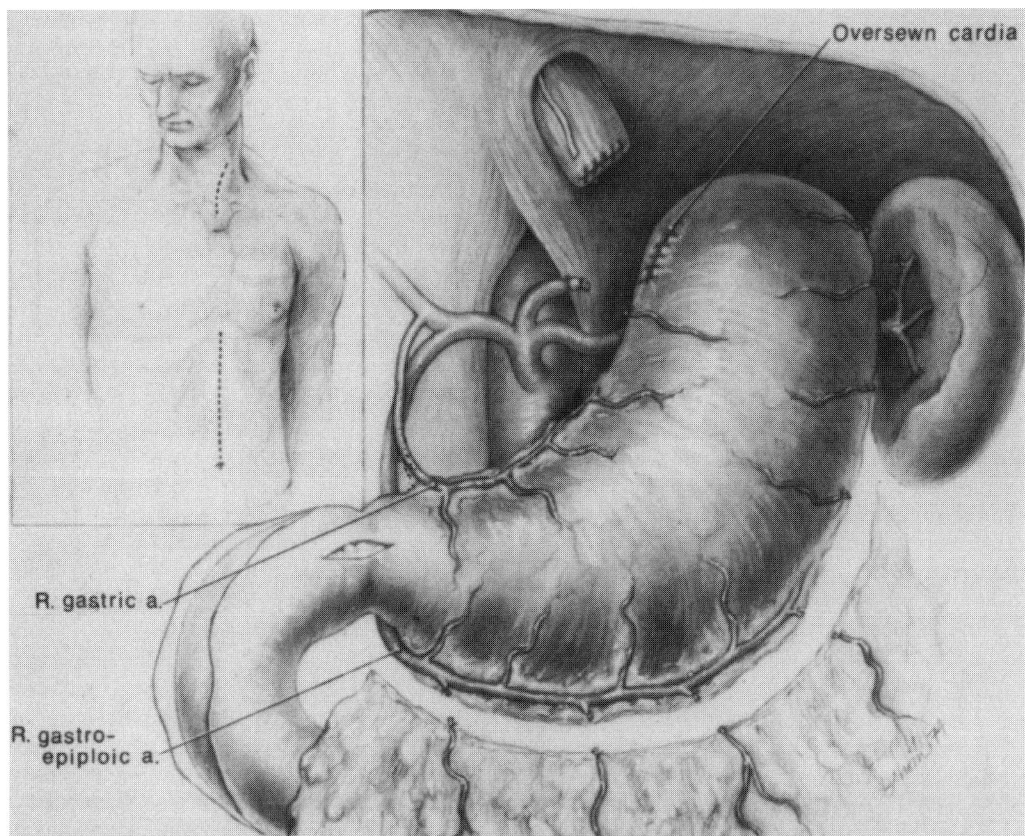

FIGURE 55–1 ■ Standard mobilization of the stomach for esophageal replacement, using either the substernal or posterior mediastinal route. The mobilized stomach is based upon the right gastric and right gastroepiploic vascular arcades after division of the left gastric artery and left gastroepiploic vessels. A pyloromyotomy and Kocher maneuver are performed routinely. The esophagus is separated from the lesser curvature of the stomach with the gastrointestinal anastomosis stapler, and the staple suture line is oversewn for reinforcement. *Inset*, standard left cervical incision paralleling the anterior border of the sternocleidomastoid muscle and the supraumbilical midline abdominal incision, used for substernal gastric interposition as well as transhiatal esophagectomy and esophageal replacement with the stomach in the posterior mediastinum. (From Orringer MB, Sloan H: Substernal gastric bypass of the excluded thoracic esophagus for palliation of esophageal carcinoma. J Thorac Cardiovasc Surg 70:836, 1975.)

care taken to avoid injury to the origin of the right gastroepiploic artery from the gastroduodenal artery. Once the greater curvature of the stomach is mobilized, the peritoneum overlying the esophageal hiatus is incised and the distal esophagus encircled with a 1-inch Penrose drain.

Proceeding downward now along the lesser curvature of the stomach, the surgeon incises the gastrohepatic omentum along the high lesser curvature, and the left gastric artery and vein are isolated, ligated, and divided. When the esophagectomy is being performed for carcinoma, the celiac axis lymph nodes are resected and submitted separately to the pathologist for staging purposes. When possible, the left gastric artery is divided near its origin from the celiac axis. If a large celiac axis lymph node mass is secondary to metastatic disease, however, cure is not possible: unless these lymph nodes are relatively easily resectable, they should be biopsied, but not totally excised, to lessen the risk of uncontrolled hemorrhage. The right gastric artery is protected as the remainder of the gastrohepatic omentum is divided inferiorly along the lesser curvature.

After the stomach has been mobilized, a generous Kocher maneuver is performed to provide sufficient duodenal mobility for the pylorus to be displaced from its usual position in the right upper quadrant of the abdomen to the level of the xiphoid process in the midline. A pyloromyotomy is then performed to avoid the possibility of delayed gastric emptying after the vagotomy that accompanies the esophagectomy. The pyloromyotomy begins with a 1.5-cm-long incision through gastric muscle and is carried through the pylorus and onto the duodenum for 0.5 to 1 cm (see Fig. 55–1). This is carried out with the cutting current of a needle-tipped electrocautery and a fine-tipped vascular mosquito clamp to dissect the gastric and duodenal muscle away from the underlying submucosa. Silver clip markers are placed at the level of the pyloromyotomy for future radiographic assessment of gastric emptying.

As in a transabdominal hiatal hernia repair or a standard Ivor-Lewis esophagogastrectomy, when possible the surgeon mobilizes the distal 5 to 10 cm of esophagus from the posterior mediastinum into the abdomen by retracting the esophagogastric junction downward with the encircling Penrose drain while dissecting upward along the esophageal wall into the mediastinum with the opposite hand (Fig. 55–2).

As experience is gained with transhiatal esophagectomy, less of the dissection of the distal half of the esophagus is done "bluntly." Rather, with narrow deep (Deaver) retractors inserted into the hiatus, the lateral periesophageal attachments are visually clamped with long 13-inch right-angle clamps, divided, and ligated. This direct esophageal mobilization is generally possible to at least the level of the carina.

When operating for carcinoma the surgeon assesses the mobility of the esophagus within the posterior mediastinum by grasping the tumor and "rocking" the esophagus from side to side to ascertain that it is not fixed to the prevertebral fascia, the aorta, or adjacent mediastinal structures. If there is no marked fixation of the esophagus, which would preclude a transhiatal resection, the mediastinal dissection is temporarily discontinued at this point. A 14-French rubber jejunostomy feeding tube is inserted 4 to 6 inches beyond the ligament of Treitz and is secured in place with a Weitzel maneuver. The jejunostomy tube is not brought out through the abdominal wall until the transhiatal esophagectomy is completed.

Cervical Phase

The cervical phase of the operation is performed through an oblique incision that parallels the anterior border of the left sternocleidomastoid muscle and extends from the suprasternal notch to the level of the cricoid cartilage (~ 5 to 6 cm). The platysma and omohyoid fascial layer are incised, the sternocleidomastoid muscle and carotid sheath and its contents are retracted laterally, and the larynx and trachea are retracted medially. No retractor should be placed against the recurrent laryngeal nerve in the tracheoesophageal groove during the entire cervical portions of this operation.

The middle thyroid vein and the inferior thyroid artery are usually ligated and divided. In patients with a "bull neck" habitus or those in whom cervical osteoarthritis prevents extension of the neck, an inadequate length of cervical esophagus may be available for the anastomosis. In such cases, addition of a partial upper sternal split provides the prerequisite access to the high retrosternal esophagus; however, this is not usually required.

The dissection proceeds directly posteriorly to the prevertebral fascia, which is followed by blunt finger dissection into the superior mediastinum. Dissection in the tracheoesophageal groove and injury to the left recurrent laryngeal nerve are avoided as the esophagus is retracted posteriorly away from the trachea; by gentle blunt dissection anteriorly and along the right lateral esophageal wall, the cervical esophagus is gradually encircled with a Penrose drain. This drain is retracted superiorly as blunt dissection of the upper thoracic esophagus from the superior mediastinum is carried out (see Fig.

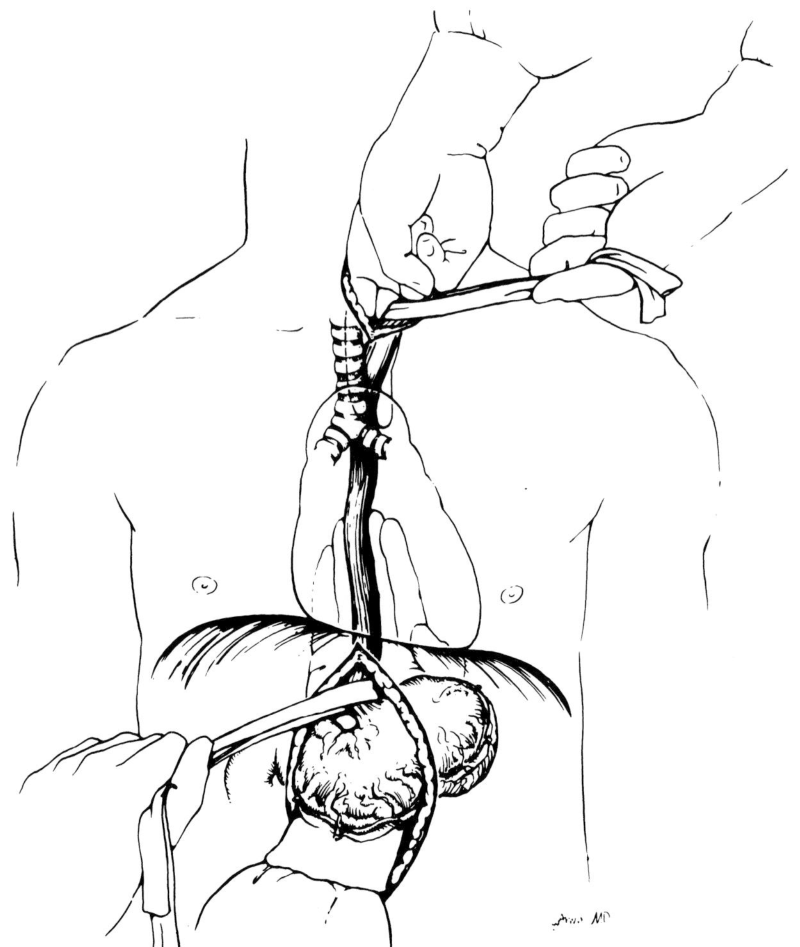

FIGURE 55–2 ■ The initial phase of transhiatal esophageal mobilization is carried out posterior to the esophagus along the prevertebral fascia, with the volar aspects of the fingers kept against the esophagus. (From Orringer MB: Surgical options for esophageal resection and reconstruction with stomach. In Baue AE, Geha AS, Hammond EL, et al [eds]: Glenn's Thoracic and Cardiovascular Surgery, 5th ed. East Norwalk, CT, Appleton & Lange, 1991, p 787.)

55–2). The volar aspects of the fingers are kept against the esophagus in the midline, and care is taken not to tear the posterior membranous trachea. With this technique, the upper thoracic esophagus is mobilized almost to the level of the carina through the neck incision.

Mediastinal (Transhiatal) Dissection

The transhiatal dissection of the esophagus is carried out in an orderly, sequential fashion. One hand in the abdomen is inserted through the diaphragmatic hiatus posterior to the esophagus as a "half sponge on a stick" is inserted into the superior mediastinum through the cervical incision along the prevertebral fascia (Fig. 55–3). The surgeon carries out the posterior esophageal dissection by sweeping the esophagus away from the prevertebral fascia from above until the sponge stick makes contact with the hand inserted through the diaphragmatic hiatus.

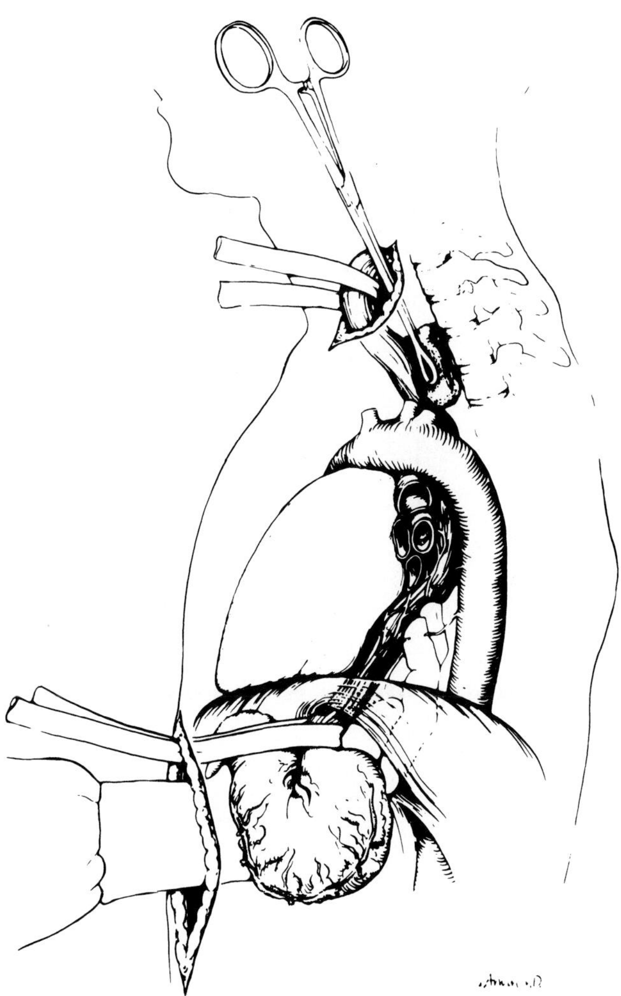

FIGURE 55–3 ■ The posterior transhiatal esophageal mobilization is facilitated by passing a "half sponge on a stick" through the cervical incision and along the prevertebral fascia until it makes contact with the hand inserted from below through the diaphragmatic hiatus. (From Orringer MB: Surgical options for esophageal resection and reconstruction with stomach. In Baue AE, Geha AS, Hammond EL, et al [eds]: Glenn's Thoracic and Cardiovascular Surgery, 5th ed. East Norwalk CT, Appleton & Lange, 1991, p 787.)

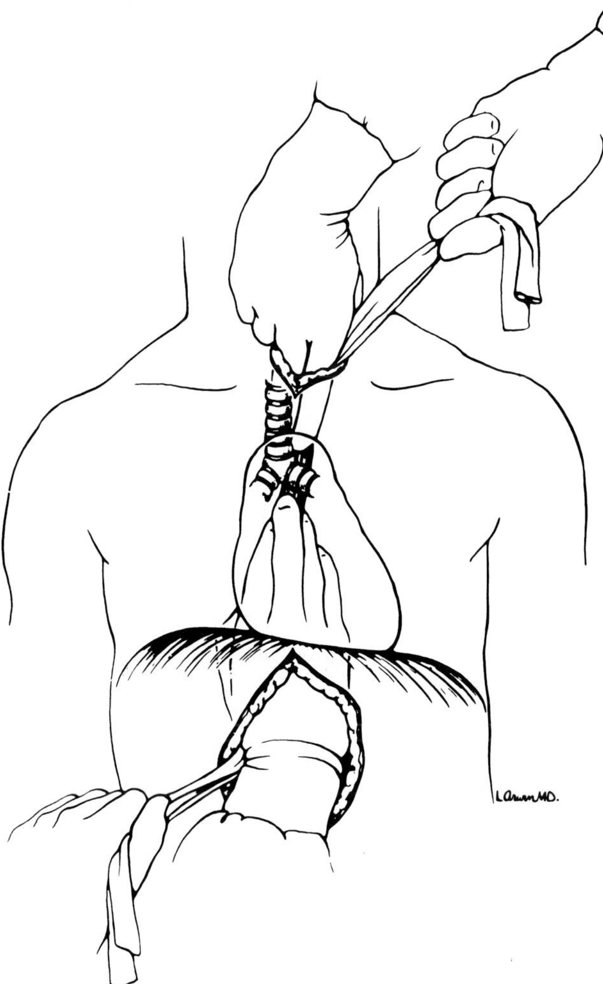

FIGURE 55–4 ■ As the anterior transhiatal esophageal mobilization is carried out, the surgeon minimizes the risk of injury to the posterior membranous trachea and left mainstem bronchus by keeping the volar aspects of the fingers against the esophagus. (From Orringer MB: Surgical options for esophageal resection and reconstruction with stomach. In Baue AE, Geha AS, Hammond EL, et al [eds]: Glenn's Thoracic and Cardiovascular Surgery, 5th ed. East Norwalk, CT, Appleton & Lange, 1991, p 787.)

Intra-arterial blood pressure is monitored continually during the esophageal dissection to avoid prolonged hypotension. Blood is evacuated from the posterior mediastinum by means of a 28-French Argyle Saratoga sump catheter inserted from the cervical incision downward into the mediastinum.

After the posterior esophageal dissection is completed, the anterior dissection is begun. The Penrose drain encircling the esophagogastric junction is retracted inferiorly as the surgeon's hand is inserted palm down against the anterior esophagus and is advanced into the mediastinum (Fig. 55–4). The esophagus is progressively mobilized away from the posterior aspect of the pericardium and the carina. The hand must be kept flattened and posterior to minimize cardiac displacement and hypotension. Simultaneous dissection through the abdominal and cervical incisions along the anterior surface of the esophagus

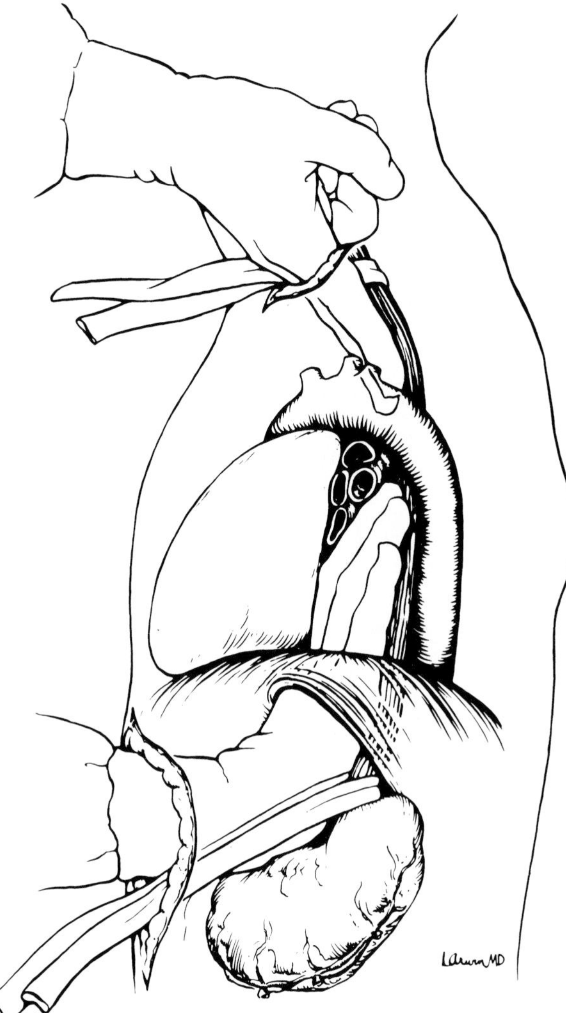

FIGURE 55–5 ■ In performing the anterior esophageal dissection, the surgeon should make a conscious effort to keep the hand as far posterior as possible to minimize hypotension due to cardiac displacement. (From Orringer MB: Surgical options for esophageal resection and reconstruction with stomach. In Baue AE, Geha AS, Hammond EL, et al [eds]: Glenn's Thoracic and Cardiovascular Surgery, 5th ed. East Norwalk, CT, Appleton & Lange, 1991, p 787.)

avulses the typically filmy attachments to the posterior trachea (Fig. 55–5).

With the anterior and posterior esophageal dissection complete, the remaining lateral esophageal attachments must now be divided. The surgeon gently tenses the cervical esophagus by placing upward traction on its encircling Penrose drain. The lateral upper esophageal attachments are gently dissected away from the esophagus as it is delivered progressively into the neck wound. In this fashion, approximately 5 to 8 cm of upper thoracic esophagus is circumferentially mobilized.

Next, with downward traction on the Penrose drain encircling the esophagogastric junction, one hand is inserted palm downward through the diaphragmatic hiatus anterior to the esophagus and is advanced into the superior mediastinum behind the trachea until the completely circumferentially mobilized upper esophagus and its intact lateral attachments are palpated (Fig. 55–6). The esophagus is "trapped" against the prevertebral fascia between the index and middle fingers, and a downward raking motion of the hand gently avulses the remaining periesophageal attachments and smaller vagal nerve branches (Fig. 55–7). Larger vagal branches are frequently palpated along the mid and distal esophagus, and their identification, division, and ligation under direct vision are facilitated by means of narrow, deep retractors again placed into the diaphragmatic hiatus.

At times, subcarinal or subaortic periesophageal adhesions or fibrosis prevents complete mobilization of a 1- to 2-cm segment of midesophagus. It may then be necessary to compress this tissue firmly between the index finger and thumb, thereby fracturing it. Alternatively, as originally described by Waddell and Scannell (1957) and later by Orringer (1984a), access to the upper thoracic esophagus to the level of the carina may be achieved by means of a partial upper sternal split, so that the re-

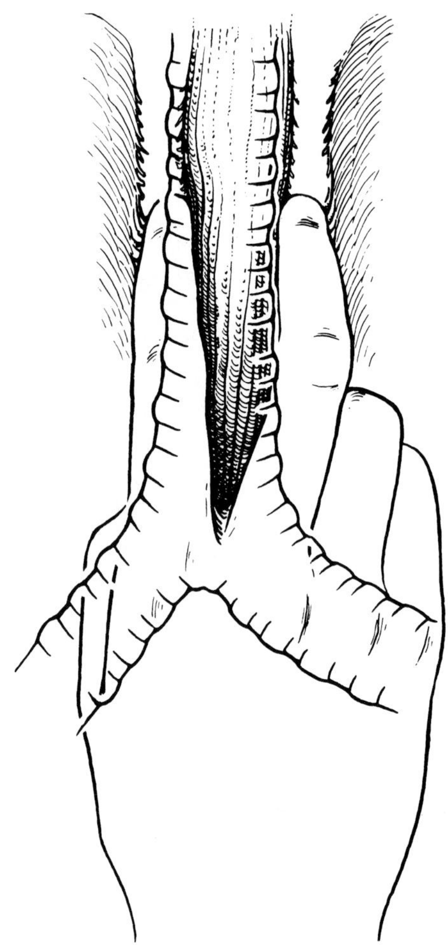

FIGURE 55–6 ■ Once the anterior and posterior esophageal attachments have been dissected, the hand inserted through the diaphragmatic hiatus is advanced superiorly into the mediastinum until the undivided lateral esophageal attachments at the thoracic inlet can be palpated. (From Orringer MB: Transhiatal blunt esophagectomy without thoracotomy. In Cohn LH [ed]: Cardiovascular Surgery. In Modern Techniques in Surgery, Vol 62. Mount Kisco, NY, Futura Publishing, 1983a, p 1.)

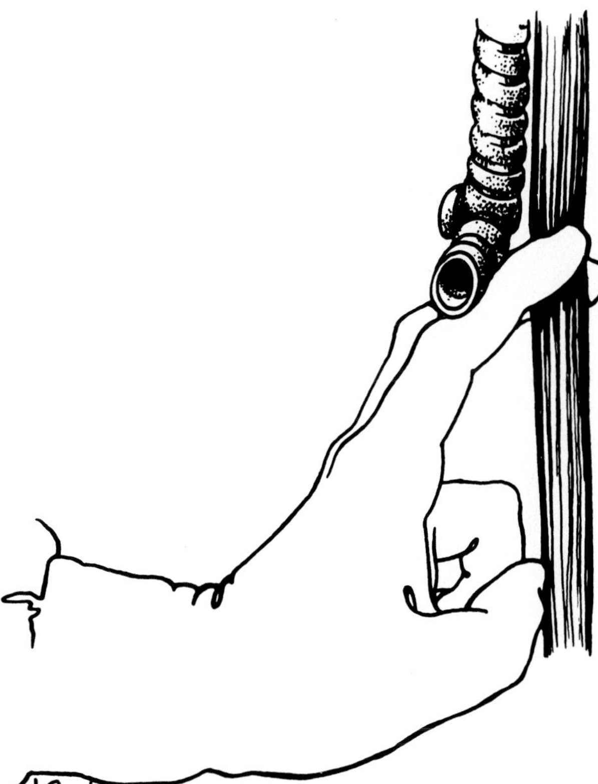

FIGURE 55–7 ■ The index and middle fingers are used to "trap" the esophagus against the prevertebral fascia, and, with a gentle but firm downward raking motion of the hand, the lateral esophageal attachments are gradually avulsed. (From Orringer MB: Transhiatal blunt esophagectomy without thoracotomy. In Cohn LH [ed]: Cardiovascular Surgery. In Modern Techniques in Surgery, Vol 62. Mount Kisco, NY, Futura Publishing, 1983, p. 1.)

maining periesophageal attachments can be divided under direct vision (Fig. 55–8).

When the entire intrathoracic esophagus has been mobilized, an 8- to 10-cm length is delivered into the cervical wound, and the esophagus is divided with the gastrointestinal anastomosis (GIA) surgical stapler. Whenever possible, the esophagus should be divided in the neck so as to leave a generous length of cervical and upper thoracic esophagus. If there is any difficulty with the stomach reaching to the neck, a partial upper sternal split can be made and the extra remaining length of upper esophagus can then easily reach to the gastric fundus. After the surgeon divides the esophagus with the GIA stapler, the stomach and lower thoracic esophagus are drawn out of the abdomen and placed upon the anterior thorax. Suturing a Penrose drain to the tip of the stomach to assist in drawing the stomach upward through the posterior mediastinum, as previously recommended, is no longer done in order to minimize trauma to the relatively ischemic gastric tip.

Once the esophagus has been removed from the mediastinum, and before attention is focused upon the specimen, narrow deep Harrington "sweetheart" retractors are placed in the diaphragmatic hiatus to allow direct inspection of the posterior mediastinum for bleeding and the mediastinal pleura for a tear. Blood is evacuated from the posterior mediastinum by means of the Argyle Saratoga sump catheter inserted from above through the cervical wound. Any bleeding aortic esophageal artery is identified, clamped, and ligated. If entry into either chest cavity has occurred during the esophageal dissection, as determined by direct inspection and palpation through the hiatus, a 32-French chest tube is inserted into the appropriate chest in the midaxillary line and connected to underwater chest tube suction. One or two large abdominal packs are pushed up through the hiatus into the posterior mediastinum and left there for hemostasis as preparation of the stomach continues.

The gastric fundus is retracted superiorly, and the lesser curvature of the stomach is cleaned of adjacent fat by dividing the vessels and fat at the level of the second vascular arcade ("crow's foot") from the cardia. The GIA stapler is used to divide the stomach beginning at this point (Fig. 55–9). When the partial proximal gastrectomy has been completed, the esophagus and attached upper stomach are removed from the field. The gastric staple suture line is oversewn with a running 4–0 polypropylene Lembert stitch.

The point along the greater curvature of the stomach that reaches most cephalad is identified (Fig. 55–10). As indicated, traction sutures in the tip of the stomach and suction devices to pull the stomach through the posterior mediastinum are avoided. Instead, after removing the posterior mediastinal packs and checking again for hemostasis, the mobilized stomach is gently pushed upward through the diaphragmatic hiatus and beneath the aortic arch into the superior mediastinum by one hand until the tip of the gastric fundus can be palpated by the finger of the other hand placed through the cervical incision. The gastric fundus is then gently grasped with a Babcock clamp and gently pulled upward while the other hand, inserted into the mediastinum from the abdomen, continually pushes the stomach upward (Fig. 55–11).

Care must be taken to avoid torsion of the stomach during its positioning in the posterior mediastinum. When the stomach is properly oriented, the oversewn gastric staple suture line is seen along the most medial aspect of the stomach in the neck wound and the greater curvature is toward the patient's left side (see Fig. 55–11, *inset*). The anterior surface of the stomach is also gently palpated through the hiatus and from the neck incision to ensure that no inadvertent twist of the stomach has occurred. In most patients, after the gastric fundus is mobilized so that its apex is several centimeters above the level of the clavicles, the pylorus comes to rest within 1 to 3 cm of the diaphragmatic hiatus in the abdomen.

Once the tip of the stomach has been mobilized into the neck wound, it generally remains there, although retraction back into the chest as the abdomen is being closed can be prevented by placing a moistened gauze posterior to the stomach along the prevertebral fascia at the thoracic inlet. Ideally, the gastric tip visible in the neck wound should be as pink and viable as it appeared in the abdomen before repositioning of the stomach.

Before the cervical anastomosis is performed, the abdominal phase of the operation is concluded. The diaphragmatic hiatus is narrowed with interrupted 0 silk

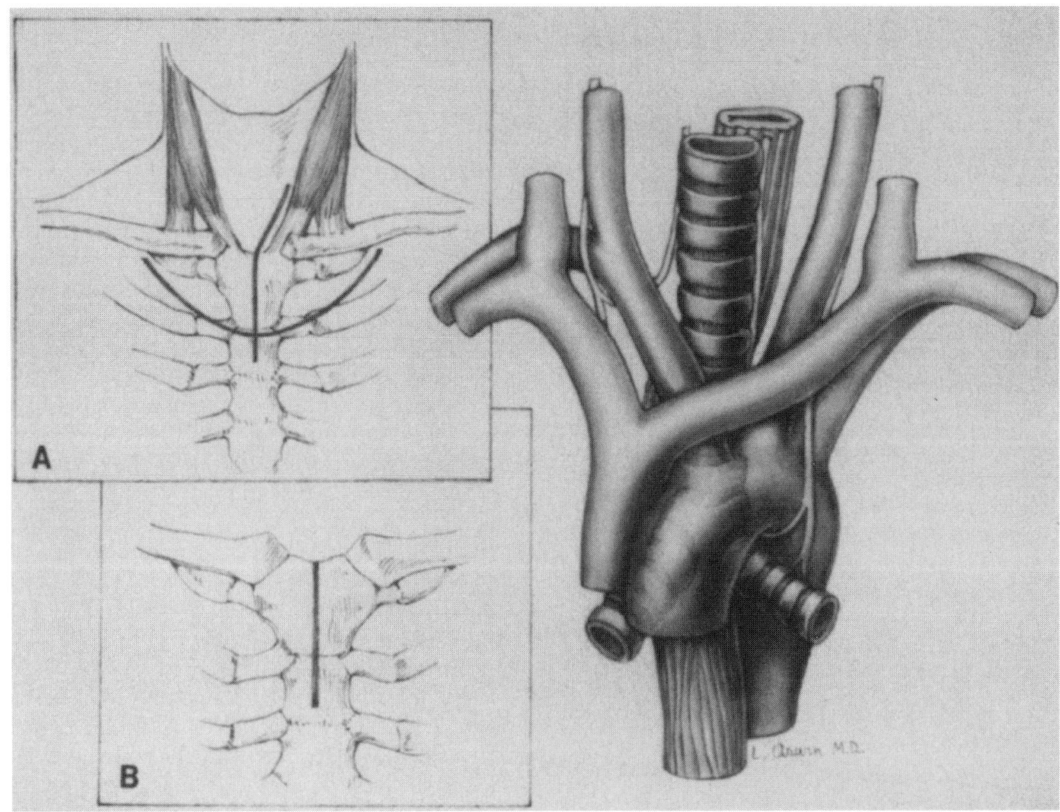

FIGURE 55–8 ■ In patients in whom exposure of the cervical esophagus is limited by cervical osteoarthritis that prevents extension of the neck or a "bull neck" habitus, an extension of the cervical incision onto the upper anterior thoracic esophagus or a more cosmetic curvilinear anterior thoracic skin incision *(inset A)* is used to carry out a partial upper sternal split across the sternomanubrial junction. A partial upper sternal split *(inset B)* provides exposure of the cervicothoracic esophagus almost to the level of the carina (main illustration). (From Orringer MB: Partial median sternotomy: Anterior approach to the upper thoracic esophagus. J Thorac Cardiovasc Surg 87:124, 1984.)

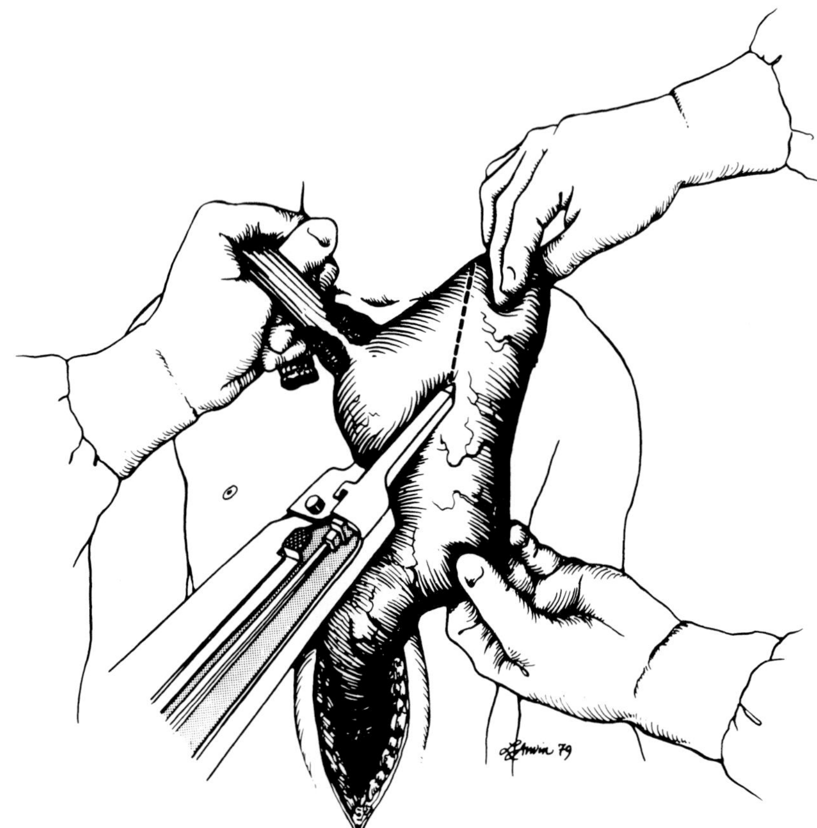

FIGURE 55–9 ■ Initially used only to obtain additional gastric margin in patients with carcinoma limited to the esophagogastric junction, this high gastric division beginning from the high lesser curvature and proceeding toward the high greater curvature is now performed routinely when the stomach is used to replace the esophagus after transhiatal esophagectomy. (From Orringer MB, Sloan H: Esophageal replacement after blunt esophagectomy. In Nyhus LM, Baker RJ [eds]: Mastery of Surgery. Boston, Little, Brown, 1984, p 426.)

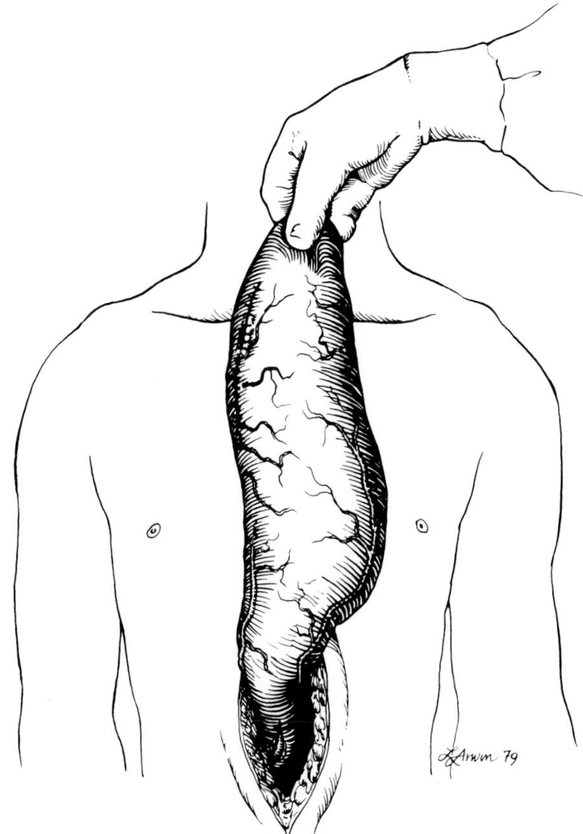

FIGURE 55–10 ■ The surgeon identifies the site along the high curvature of the stomach that will reach most cephalad to the neck by placing the mobilized stomach on the anterior chest. The stapled suture line of the lesser curvature has been oversewn. (From Orringer MB, Sloan H: Esophageal replacement after blunt esophagectomy. In Nyhus LM, Baker RJ [eds]: Mastery of Surgery. Boston, Little, Brown, 1984, p 426.)

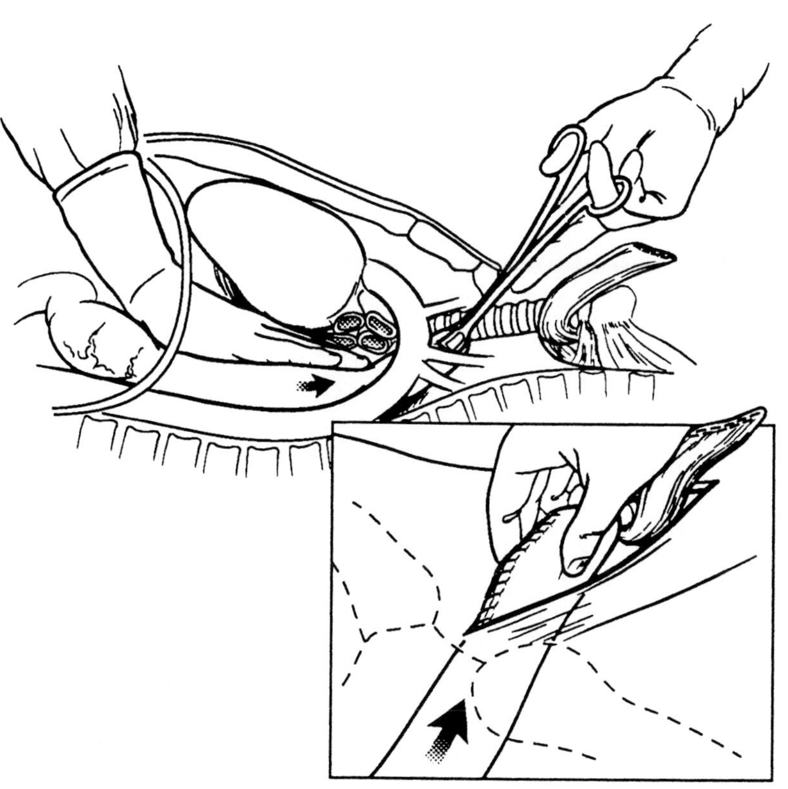

FIGURE 55–11 ■ The surgeon gently manipulates mobilized stomach through the posterior mediastinum in the original esophageal bed by placing one hand through the diaphragmatic hiatus. This hand gently pushes the stomach upward against the spine and underneath the aortic arch until the tip of the gastric fundus can be felt by the fingers of the other hand inserted through the cervical incision. The tip of the gastric fundus is then grasped with a Babcock clamp inserted through the cervical incision, and the stomach is gently delivered into the neck wound until it can be grasped by the fingertips *(inset)*. The upper stomach is delivered into the neck wound by pushing from below through the diaphragmatic hiatus rather than by traction on the stomach in the neck. (From Orringer MB, Marshall B, Iannettoni MD: Eliminating the cervical esophagogastric anastomotic leak with a side-to-side stapled anastomosis. J Thorac Cardiovasc Surg 119:277–288, 2000.)

sutures so that it easily admits three fingers alongside the stomach. The edges of the diaphragmatic hiatus are tacked to the anterior gastric wall with one or two 3–0 silk sutures to prevent subsequent herniation of intra-abdominal viscera into the chest. The left lobe of the liver is repositioned, and the previously divided triangular ligament is reattached to provide further closure of the hiatus. The pyloromyotomy is covered by adjacent omentum, which in turn is covered by the previously retracted left hepatic lobe.

The feeding jejunostomy tube is brought out through a separate left upper quadrant stab wound, and the jejunum is fixed to the anterior abdominal wall with several interrupted sutures. The surgeon closes and excludes abdominal incision from the field by covering it with a sterile towel and sheet. The last major portion of the operation, the cervical esophagogastric anastomosis, is now performed.

Cervical Esophagogastric Anastomosis

Attention now returns to the neck incision, where the end of the divided esophagus is grasped with an Allis clamp and retracted superiorly. Recently, as described by Orringer and associates (2000), use of a side-to-side stapled cervical esophagogastric anastomosis, rather than a manually sewn one, has dramatically reduced our anastomotic leak rate and is therefore now our technique of choice. When the stomach has been properly mobilized through the posterior mediastinum, a 4- to 5-cm length of gastric fundus is visible above the level of the clavicles (Fig. 55–12). A 3–0 silk traction suture is used to elevate the anterior gastric wall to the surface of the skin (see Fig. 55–12, *inset*). After carefully judging the point at which the esophagus will comfortably reach the stomach once the traction suture has been removed, the surgeon makes a 1.5-cm transverse gastrotomy on the anterior gastric wall (Fig. 55–13). The gastrotomy must be positioned far enough inferiorly from the tip of the stomach to allow the full insertion of the 3-cm-long staple cartridge. The cervical esophageal staple suture line is amputated obliquely, with the anterior tip of the divided esophagus being left slightly longer than the posterior corner (Fig. 55–14).

Two anastomotic stay sutures are placed (Fig. 55–15), and with downward traction of these stay sutures, a 3.0- to 3.5-staple cartridge loaded on a GIA II stapler is inserted into the stomach and the esophagus (Fig. 55–16*A*). The midpoint of the posterior wall of the cervical esophagus must be carefully aligned with the anterior wall of the stomach as the staple cartridge is advanced completely into the esophagus and stomach (Fig. 55–16*B*). After the jaws of the stapler are approximated, two "suspension sutures" between the stomach and esophagus are placed on either side (Fig. 55–17*A*). Firing the stapler results in a 3-cm-long side-to-side anastomosis (Fig. 55–17*B*). After placement of a 16-French nasogastric tube into the intrathoracic stomach by the anesthetist, the gastrotomy and remaining open esophagus are approximated in two layers (Fig. 55–18*A*, *B*). Silver clip markers are placed on either side of the anastomosis for future radiographic assessment, and the wound is closed loosely with interrupted sutures over a small Penrose drain. A portable chest radiograph is obtained in the operating

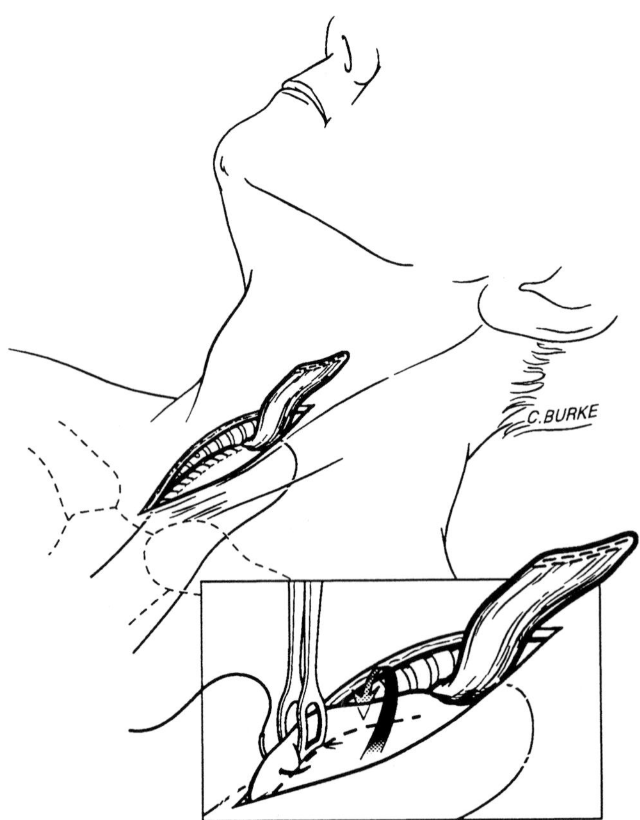

FIGURE 55–12 ■ The end of the divided cervical esophagus is retracted superiorly with an Allis clamp (not shown). The gastric staple suture line is toward the patient's right. *Inset*, A Babcock clamp is used to deliver the anterior surface of the stomach upward from the thoracic inlet and to rotate the gastric staple suture line even more medially *(inset)*. A 3–0 cardiovascular traction suture is placed distal to the clamp and is used to elevate the stomach to the surface of the wound for subsequent construction of the anastomosis. (From Orringer MB, Marshall B, Iannettoni MD: Eliminating the cervical esophagogastric anastomotic leak with a side-to-side stapled anastomosis. J Thorac Cardiovasc Surg 119:277–288, 2000.)

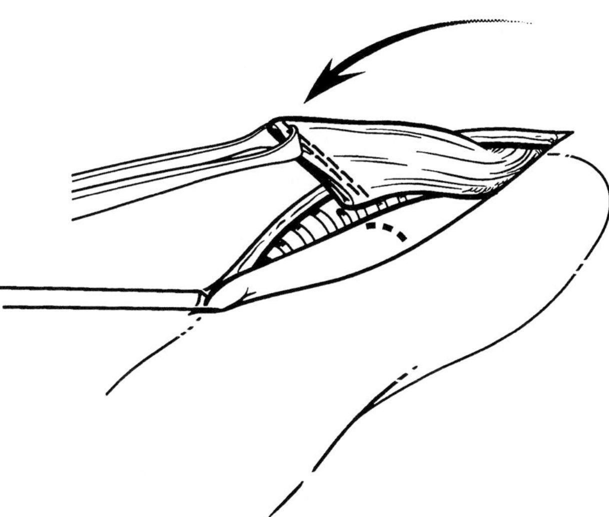

FIGURE 55–13 ■ The site of the subsequent anastomosis on the stomach is carefully selected, with some planned redundancy in the length of the remaining cervical esophagus. A 1.5-cm transverse gastrostomy *(dotted line)* is performed with a needle-tip electrocautery. (From Orringer MB, Marshall B, Iannettoni MD: Eliminating the cervical esophagogastric anastomotic leak with a side-to-side stapled anastomosis. J Thorac Cardiovasc Surg 119:277–288, 2000.)

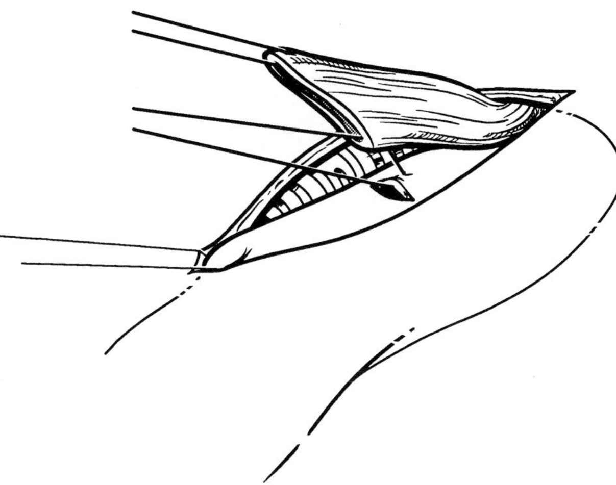

FIGURE 55–15 ■ Two full-thickness 4–0 anastomotic stay sutures are placed, one from the anterior tip of the cut cervical esophagus and one from the midpoint of the upper edge of the transverse gastrotomy and the posterior "corner" of the esophagus. The previously placed anterior gastric wall traction suture elevates the stomach from the depths of the cervical incision and helps to achieve apposition of the posterior wall of the cervical esophagus and the anterior wall of the stomach. (From Orringer MB, Marshall B, Iannettoni MD: Eliminating the cervical esophagogastric anastomotic leak with a side-to-side stapled anastomosis. J Thorac Cardiovasc Surg 119:277–281, 2000.)

room to ensure that no unrecognized hemograph or pneumothorax or large mediastinal hematoma is present and that the nasogastric, chest, and endotracheal tubes are in proper position.

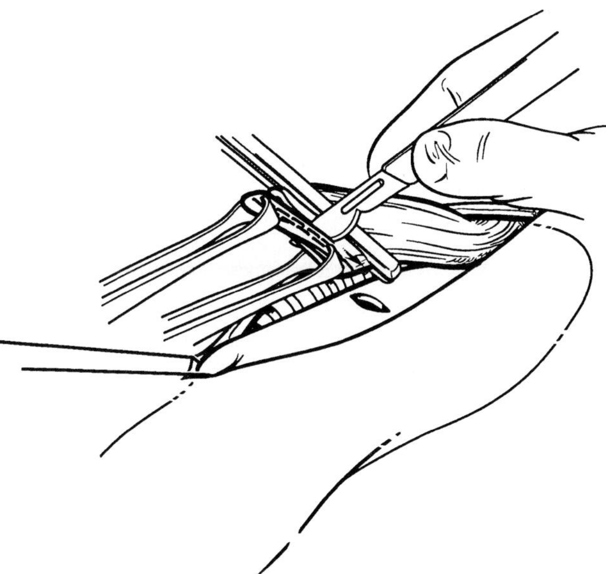

FIGURE 55–14 ■ The staple suture line is amputated with an atraumatic vascular forceps as a straight edge to ensure a clean cut. The anterior tip of the end of the divided esophagus is longer than the posterior tip. The amputated staple suture line is submitted to the pathology department as "the proximal esophageal margin." (From Orringer MB, Marshall B, Iannettoni MD: Eliminating the cervical esophagogastric anastomotic leak with a side-to-side stapled anastomosis. J Thorac Cardiovasc Surg 119:277–281, 2000.)

Transhiatal Esophagectomy for Carcinoma of the Esophagogastric Junction

The technique of transhiatal esophagectomy just described is applicable in most patients with carcinoma localized to the cardia and proximal stomach (Fig. 55–19). The traditional proximal hemigastrectomy performed for such tumors "wastes" valuable stomach that can be used for esophageal replacement, contributes little to the patient's longevity, and commits the surgeon to an intrathoracic esophageal anastomosis. In most cases it is possible to divide the stomach 4 to 6 cm distal to palpable tumor, thereby preserving the entire greater curvature of the gastric fundus. The narrowed remaining gastric "tube" functions well as an esophageal substitute. In this situation, with a narrower gastric tube, during construction of the cervical esophagogastric anastomosis, care must be taken to avoid placement of the stapler too close to the lesser curvature gastric staple line to avoid intervening ischemia of the anterior gastric wall.

The cervical esophagus should not be divided until the surgeon is satisfied that there will be adequate remaining stomach to reach to the neck. After the cervical esophagus is divided and the thoracic esophagus is removed, if the esophagogastric junction tumor is found to involve so much stomach that a proximal hemigastrectomy is required to remove it, there will be insufficient remaining gastric length to reach to the neck. Moreover, if the colon is not prepared, the patient will be left with a cervical esophagostomy and a feeding tube, a dismal outcome of an esophageal operation intended to relieve dysphagia.

POSTOPERATIVE CARE

The average operative time required for transhiatal esophagectomy is 3 to 5 hours, depending upon the patient's

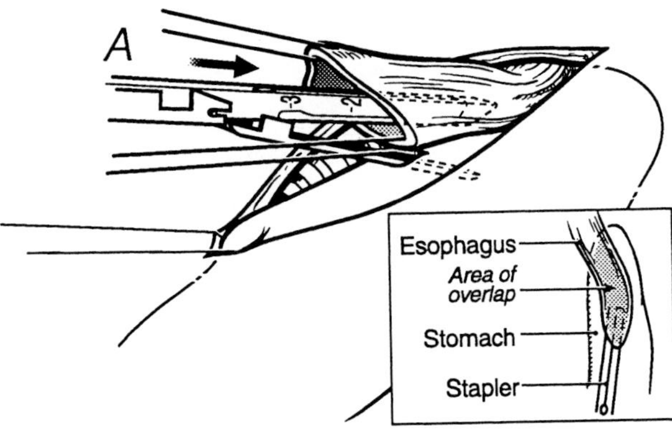

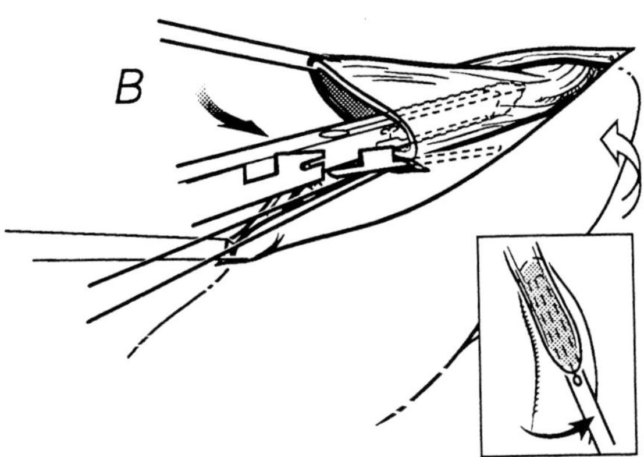

FIGURE 55–16 ■ *A*, As the two anastomotic stay sutures are retracted inferiorly, the endo-GIA 3.0–3.5 staple cartridge is inserted with the thinner "anvil" portion in the stomach and the thicker, staple-bearing portion in the esophagus. *B*, As the staple cartridge is advanced into the esophagus and stomach, the tip of the cartridge is gradually angulated toward the patient's right ear *(insets)*. The alignment of the esophagus and stomach must be parallel, and the gastric staple suture line should be well away from the anastomosis to avoid intervening ischemia between the gastric staple suture line and the anastomosis. (From Orringer MB, Marshall B, Iannettoni MD: Eliminating the cervical esophagogastric anastomotic leak with a side-to-side stapled anastomosis. J Thorac Cardiovasc Surg 119:277–281, 2000.)

size, the esophageal pathology, and the need for a partial upper sternal split. Although in the past mechanical ventilation was maintained overnight until the morning of the first postoperative day, for the past several years our patients have been extubated in the operating room and have been able to avoid an intensive care stay entirely. This is a function of preoperative preparation but, even more so, of the availability of epidural anesthesia to reduce postoperative pain and to facilitate optimal respiratory function.

Since the patient has been taught preoperatively the desirability and necessity of early postoperative ambulation and pulmonary hygiene, use of the incentive spirometer is resumed immediately after surgery and continued as it was preoperatively. Postoperative ileus seldom lasts longer than 24 to 48 hours. Therefore, feedings of 5% dextrose and water through the jejunostomy tube at a rate of 30 ml/hr are usually begun on the 2nd or 3rd postoperative day. If this is tolerated for 12 hours, half-strength jejunostomy tube feedings are begun, the volume is gradually increased, and full-strength feedings are initiated the next day. Usually by the 3rd postoperative day, the nasogastric tube drainage is less than 100 ml per 8-hr nursing shift, and the nasogastric tube is removed. Postoperative diarrhea may occur in response either to tube feedings or to the vagotomy that accompanies transhiatal esophagectomy. This is controlled with diphenoxylate (Lomotil) or tincture of opium (paregoric).

Within 3 to 5 days of operation, intravenous lines, the arterial catheter, the cervical wound drain, the Foley urethral catheter, and the nasogastric tube typically have been removed so that the patient can ambulate freely and practice unrestrained deep breathing. Within 24 hours of removal of the nasogastric tube, oral liquids are begun. Oral intake is progressively advanced, and, depending upon the patient's appetite and ability to take in adequate oral nutrition, the jejunostomy tube feedings are concomitantly decreased and then discontinued. On the 6th or 7th postoperative day, a barium swallow examination is performed to document that the anastomosis is intact and that gastric emptying through the pyloromyotomy is adequate (both areas having been marked intraoperatively with silver clips). If this study is satisfactory, the patient is discharged. The need for continuing jejunostomy tube feedings at home is individualized.

There is little justification for keeping the patient on nothing-by-mouth status until after a postoperative barium swallow on the 7th to 10th postoperative day. Since the patient is swallowing saliva from the moment of awaking from the operation, the fact that food is not being swallowed does not mean that oral contents are not crossing the anastomosis. Furthermore, at least one week is usually required for the patient to adjust to the initial retrosternal fullness, early satiety, or postvagotomy cramping and diarrhea ("dumping") that may occur; if one waits until after the barium swallow on the 7th to 10th postoperative day to feed the patient, another week of unnecessary hospitalization may be required.

The patient is now typically discharged after a satisfactory barium swallow on the 6th or 7th postoperative day. The jejunostomy feeding tube is removed at an outpatient visit 2 weeks later, approximately 4 weeks after operation. At times, if the patient is anorectic immediately after surgery, supplemental caloric intake with jejunostomy tube feedings at night may be continued for the first several weeks at home. Most patients, however, leave the hospital able to eat satisfactorily without the need for supplemental jejunostomy tube feedings.

COMPLICATIONS AND THEIR MANAGEMENT

The complications of transhiatal esophagectomy without thoracotomy occur in two broad categories:

1. Intraoperative, including pneumothorax, tracheal tear, and hemorrhage.
2. Postoperative, occurring in the first "critical" 10 days after operation and including hoarseness or impaired swallowing from recurrent laryngeal nerve injury,

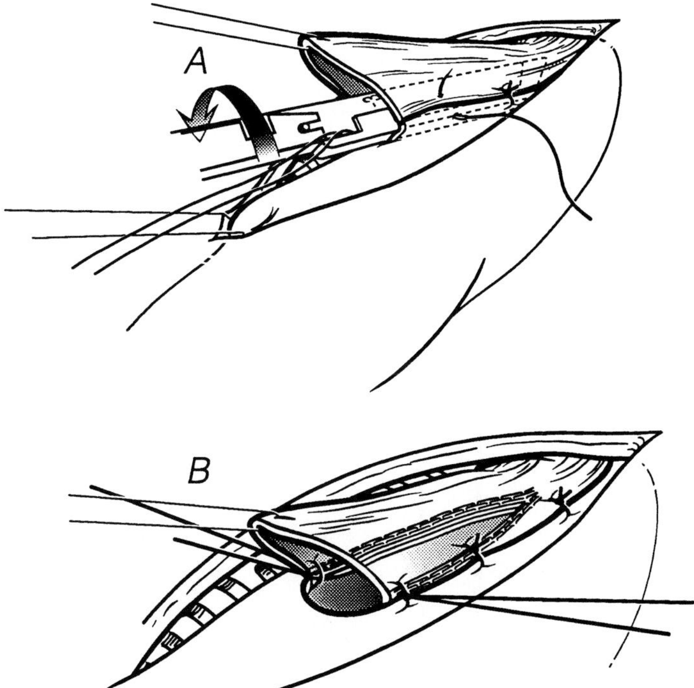

FIGURE 55–17 ■ *A*, The surgeon approximates the jaws of the staple cartridge by squeezing the handle of the stapler. Before it is fired, however, the stapler is rolled from side to side as two seromuscular sutures between the adjacent esophagus and stomach are placed on either side. These four sutures are now used instead of the initially advocated "suspension" sutures between the tip of the gastric fundus and the prevertebral fascia. *B*, Advancing the knife assembly of the stapler fires the cartridge and creates a 3-cm-long side-to-side anastomosis as the opposing wall of the esophagus and stomach is stapled and cut. The stapler is removed, the anastomosis inspected for bleeding, and a nasogastric tube inserted by the anesthetist and guided into the intrathoracic stomach. "Corner" sutures are placed in preparation for completion of the anastomosis. (From Orringer MB, Marshall B, Iannettoni MD: Eliminating the cervical esophagogastric anastomotic leak with a side-to-side stapled anastomosis. J Thorac Cardiovasc Surg 119:277–281, 2000.)

anastomotic disruption, chylothorax, supraventricular tachyarrhythmias, and sympathetic pleural effusion.

Entry into one or both pleural cavities during the mediastinal dissection occurs in nearly two thirds of patients undergoing transhiatal esophagectomy. Once the esophagectomy has been completed and before the stomach is positioned in the posterior mediastinum in the original esophageal bed, the pleura should be carefully inspected, both manually and by palpation through the diaphragmatic hiatus, to be certain that no tear has occurred. If the pleurae have been violated, immediate insertion of a 28 French chest tube or tubes generally provides effective therapy.

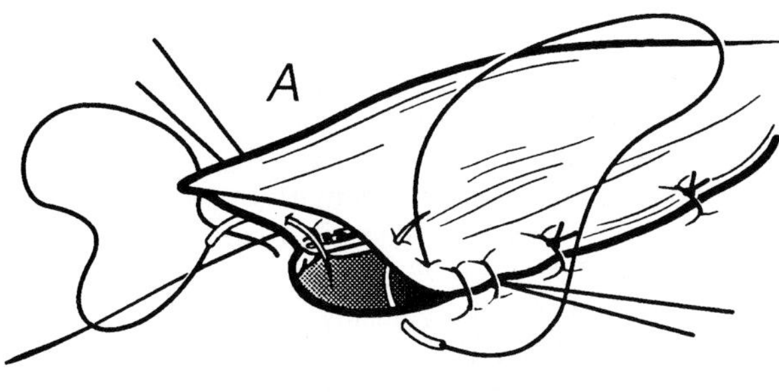

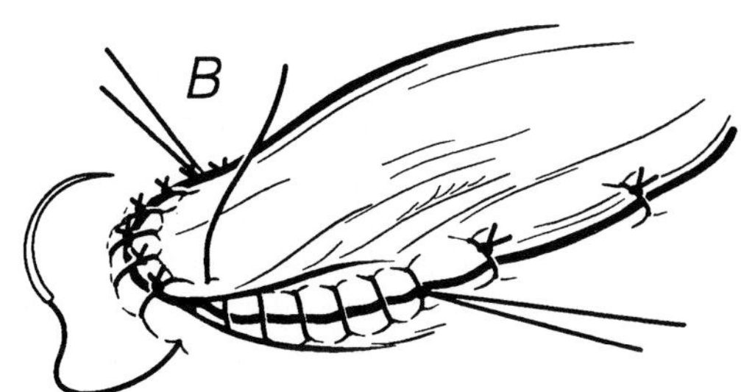

FIGURE 55–18 ■ The edges of the opened esophagus and stomach are approximated in two layers: a running inner layer of 4–0 monofilament absorbable suture *(A)* and an outer interrupted layer that incorporates the anterior wall of the upper esophagus *(B)*. (From Orringer MB, Marshall B, Iannettoni MD: Eliminating the cervical esophagogastric anastomotic leak with a side-to-side stapled anastomosis. J Thorac Cardiovasc Surg 119:277–281, 2000.)

Tracheal Tear

There are few more devastating experiences during transhiatal esophagectomy than the rush of air from the ventilator felt through a tear in the posterior membranous trachea. Tracheal tears occurring during this operation may vary from small, linear, and relatively easily sutured to ones that are irreparable injuries in some situations, as when the surgeon has wrongly attempted to resect a tumor that is densely adherent to or invading the trachea and major tracheobronchial disruption occurs.

If a tracheal tear occurs during esophagectomy, the endotracheal tube cuff should be deflated by the anesthetist, and the tube should then be advanced as the surgeon's hand, inserted through the hiatus and anterior to the esophagus to the level of the carina, guides it into the distal trachea or left mainstem bronchus so that the endotracheal tube cuff is distal to the tear. With control of the airway now re-established, the tear can be repaired in a more controlled fashion. A partial upper sternal split (see Fig. 55–8) provides ample exposure of the membranous trachea for most direct repairs. If possible, it is best to complete the transhiatal esophagectomy before attempting the tracheal repair, since exposure of the posterior trachea is better once the esophagus is removed.

If the tracheal tear is too extensive or involves the carina or mainstem bronchus, an anterior approach

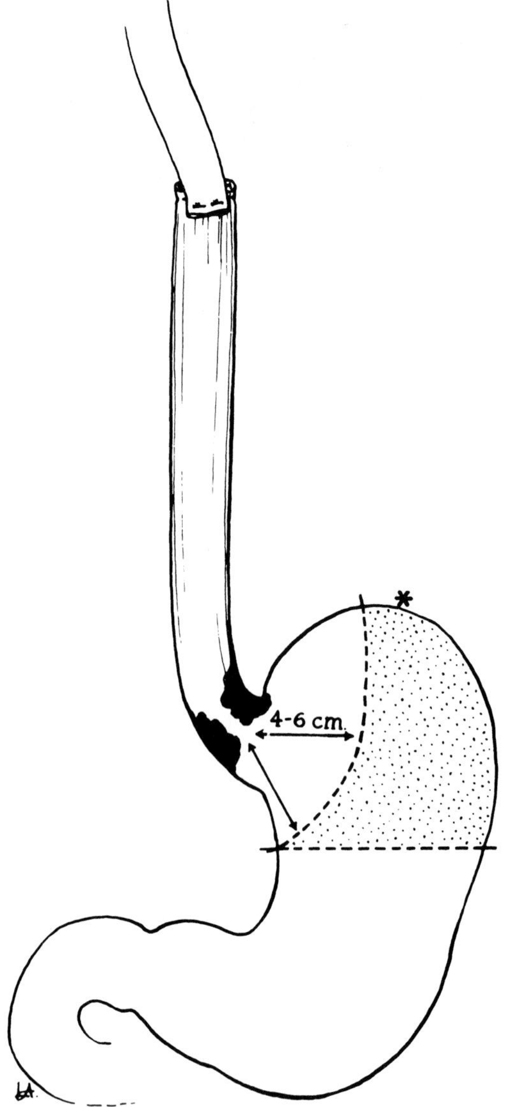

FIGURE 55–19 ■ Transhiatal esophagectomy, followed by cervical esophagogastric anastomosis, is applicable for localized tumors of the cardia and distal esophagus. The gastrointestinal anastomosis stapler is used to divide the high lesser curvature of the stomach 4 to 6 cm distal to palpable tumor. The *asterisk* indicates that point along the greater curvature that reaches most cephalad to the neck for the anastomosis. The *stippled area* represents the portion of stomach that traditionally has been resected when a standard hemigastrectomy is carried out for distal esophageal carcinoma, thereby precluding the possibility of a cervical esophagogastric anastomosis. (From Orringer MB, Sloan H: Esophagectomy without thoracotomy. J Thorac Cardiovasc Surg 76:643, 1978.)

through a partial upper sternal split will not be adequate. In such a situation, one-lung anesthesia, administered through the endotracheal tube inserted into the left mainstem bronchus, should be continued as a substernal gastric bypass is completed. Once alimentary continuity is established, the patient can be repositioned for a right thoracotomy, completion esophagectomy, and closure of the tracheal injury.

Bleeding

Average intraoperative blood loss for transhiatal esophagectomy is less than 700 ml, and major intraoperative bleeding is the exception rather than the rule. As shown in the elegant anatomic studies by Liebermann-Meffert and associates (1987), the aortic esophageal arteries branch into very small capillaries before they reach the wall of the esophagus, and when these smaller vessels are avulsed from the esophagus during transhiatal esophagectomy, natural hemostatic mechanisms of thrombosis and arterial contraction control bleeding. As one gains experience with the technique of transhiatal esophagectomy, progressively more of the dissection is performed under direct vision.

For example, with narrow retractors in either side of the diaphragmatic hiatus, the lateral esophageal attachments can be clamped, divided, and ligated, often to the level of the carina, by use of long, right-angled clamps. Major uncontrolled bleeding should occur rarely with this operation if the surgeon exercises judgment in selecting patients. When palpation of the esophagus through the diaphragmatic hiatus indicates dense fixation to the aorta or periesophageal tissues, the transhiatal approach should be abandoned.

Although I have not personally encountered uncontrolled intraoperative hemorrhage in the more than 1000 transhiatal esophagectomies that I have performed, I am aware of several anecdotal reports of aortal tears occurring during this procedure; none of these patients survived the operation. If major intraoperative bleeding occurs during the transhiatal dissection, the 28-French Argyle Saratoga sump catheter should be inserted through the cervical incision to help evacuate bleeding from above, and narrow deep retractors within the diaphragmatic hiatus should be used to inspect the mediastinum in an effort to identify and control the point of bleeding.

If hemostasis cannot be achieved, there is little alternative but to tamponade the mediastinum with large abdominal packs inserted through the diaphragmatic hiatus. The abdomen should be closed quickly with several large through-and-through heavy sutures, the wound covered with a plastic adhesive film, and the patient turned to the appropriate side for a thoracotomy. If bleeding has been encountered during dissection of the lower third of the esophagus, a left thoracotomy should be undertaken. Alternatively, if dissection of the mid or upper thoracic esophagus has resulted in bleeding, a right thoracotomy is more appropriate for control.

Recurrent Laryngeal Nerve Palsy

Recurrent laryngeal nerve injury during transhiatal esophagectomy and cervical esophagogastric anastomosis is a serious complication, which may have far greater consequences than simply a hoarse voice. Impaired cricopharyngeal motor function, with resulting cervical dysphagia and aspiration, may cause life-threatening aspiration pneumonia.

In my group's early experience with this operation, transient recurrent laryngeal nerve injury occurred frequently. The injury was initially attributed to "unavoidable" intraoperative stretching of the left recurrent laryngeal nerve beneath the aortic arch in the chest. However, it has subsequently become appreciated that such a mechanism of injury to the recurrent laryngeal nerve seldom occurs. Rather, almost inevitably, recurrent laryngeal nerve paresis or paralysis is the direct result of injury to the nerve during the cervical portions of the operation. It is therefore a preventable complication that can be avoided by not placing any metal retractor against the tracheoesophageal groove. This complication has occurred rarely in our hands since we adopted a policy of using only finger retraction against the tracheoesophageal groove during the cervical portions of the operation.

Cervical Anastomotic Leak

Cervical esophageal anastomotic leaks seldom occur after the 10th postoperative day, are typically associated with very little early postoperative morbidity, and are rarely fatal. If a fever of 101°F or more develops 48 hours after transhiatal esophagectomy, it is assumed that an anastomotic leak is present until proven otherwise, and an immediate contrast study of the esophagus is indicated. Water-soluble contrast material (Gastrografin) is used initially to identify a possible leak; if no leak is seen, dilute barium sulfate, which better defines the mucosal detail, is used. Alternatively, drainage of swallowed liquid or food from the cervical incision may be noted, and the diagnosis of a leak is then established on clinical grounds alone.

If such an anastomotic leak is diagnosed, the cervical wound is gently opened in its entirety at the bedside down to the prevertebral fascia, and the patient is asked to swallow water while a suction catheter is used to evacuate the fluid that issues from the neck wound, thereby flushing away associated debris. The neck wound is loosely packed with slightly moistened gauze several times a day, and nutrition is maintained with jejunostomy tube feedings. Leaks that occur between 7 and 10 days after operation are generally quite small.

Within 2 to 3 days of opening the neck wound, the patient is allowed to drink water after the wound has been unpacked, and observing the amount of water that exits through the wound gives an estimate of the size of the remaining fistula. As the fistula closes, the patient may swallow soft food while applying direct pressure over the packed cervical wound. A 46-French tapered Maloney esophageal dilator is passed through the anastomosis at the bedside at least once after the cervical wound is opened and before the patient is discharged to ensure that there is no element of distal obstruction (e.g., from local edema or fibrosis) associated with the fistula and to minimize the chance of anastomotic stricture development. As reported by Orringer and Lemmer (1986), passage of an esophageal dilator before the fistula has completely closed does not further damage the anastomosis and, in fact, is usually followed by total closure of the fistula in 2 to 5 days.

In fewer than 2% of patients with cervical esophagogastric anastomotic leaks, as reported by Iannettoni and colleagues (1995), catastrophic complications occur: gastric tip necrosis necessitating anastomotic takedown and cervical esophagostomy, vertebral body osteomyelitis, epidural abscess with neurologic impairment, internal jugular vein abscess, and tracheoesophagogastric anastomotic fistula. Patients who remain ill after bedside drainage of a cervical esophagogastric anastomotic leak should undergo cervical re-exploration in the operating room. Major gastric tip ischemia or necrosis, or both, may warrant takedown of the anastomosis, return of the intrathoracic stomach to the abdomen, resection of nonvisible stomach, and construction of a cervical esophagostomy. Esophageal reconstruction can be performed later if the patient survives this disastrous event.

Chylothorax

When chest tube drainage after transhiatal esophagectomy is excessive or prolonged, the diagnosis of chylothorax due to an injured thoracic duct should be considered. This diagnosis may not be apparent early after surgery before oral intake of fat has begun because the fluid draining from the chest tube is not "milky." However, if chest tube drainage exceeds 200 to 400 ml per 8-hr shift more than 48 hours after transhiatal esophagectomy, one should consider the possibility of a thoracic duct injury. The diagnosis is established by observing a change in the character of the chest tube drainage from a serous to a milky fluid after administration of 30 to 60 ml/hr of cream through the jejunostomy tube for 3 to 6 hours. In rare instances, it is necessary to determine cholesterol and triglyceride levels in the fluid to prove that a chylothorax has occurred.

There is little place for conservative management of chylothorax in the nutritionally compromised patient who has undergone esophagectomy for esophageal obstruction, as the loss of protein-rich chyle is poorly tolerated. As described by Orringer and colleagues (1988), unless the chylous drainage decreases dramatically within 3 to 5 days of instituting elemental jejunostomy tube feedings, thoracotomy and ligation of the injured thoracic duct most effectively manage the problem and minimize morbidity. After 60 to 90 ml/hr of cream has been administered through the jejunostomy tube for 6 hours and there is a sustained flow of milky fluid draining from the chest tube, a thoracotomy is performed. A double-lumen endotracheal tube permits one-lung anesthesia and exposure of the mediastinum through a more limited thoracotomy. The brisk flow of chyle from the injured thoracic duct makes identification of the tear and direct suture ligation a relatively simple undertaking. This direct approach often constitutes less of a physiologic insult to the patient than weeks of conservative management with intravenous hyperalimentation and chest tube suction.

Pleural Effusion

When the pleural cavity is not violated during transhiatal esophagectomy and no chest tube is therefore required, a sympathetic pleural effusion related to the mediastinal dissection may occur during the first postoperative week. If the effusion is asymptomatic and does not continue to enlarge, no treatment is necessary and spontaneous resolution follows. Alternatively, if significant dyspnea results from a large effusion, an occasional thoracentesis may be required. A recurrent pleural effusion, of course, must be differentiated from a chylothorax and treated accordingly.

RESULTS

In the largest reported series, Orringer and colleagues (1999) present data on 1085 patients in whom they have performed transhiatal esophagectomy without thoracotomy for diseases of the intrathoracic esophagus, 285 (26%) of whom had benign disease necessitating esophageal replacement and 800 (74%) had carcinoma (Table 55–1).

Transhiatal esophagectomy has been possible in 98.6% of patients in whom it has been attempted over a 22-year period. Fifteen patients required conversion to a transthoracic esophagectomy as a result of intrathoracic esophageal fixation or bleeding. Neither a history of prior radiation therapy nor chronic periesophageal fibrosis from prior esophageal operations has precluded transhiatal esophagectomy. Of the patients with carcinoma, 234 (29%) had a history of prior radiation therapy. Of the patients with benign disease, 146 (52%) had undergone one or more esophageal or periesophageal operations.

Stomach was used as the esophageal substitute in 96% of patients, a colon interposition being required in 39 patients who had either caustic gastric burns or a history of a prior gastric resection for peptic ulcer disease, precluding cephalad reach of the stomach to the neck for construction of a cervical anastomosis. The original esophageal bed in the posterior mediastinum was used for esophageal replacement in all but 20 patients with gross residual tumor or radiation fibrosis of the posterior mediastinum.

Morbidity

Three intraoperative deaths occurred as a result of mediastinal hemorrhage, which occurred during esophageal mobilization. Six other patients experienced inordinate intraoperative blood loss, ranging from 5850 to 18,440 ml. In three, the bleeding was from a torn azygos vein during mobilization of a mid-third carcinoma; in three others, the bleeding was intra-abdominal: two associated with portal hypertension from cirrhosis and one from splenic injury. If these latter six patients are excluded, the measured intraoperative blood loss averaged 689 ml (652 ml in the patients with carcinoma and 795 ml in those with benign disease).

TABLE 55–1 ■ **Indications for Transhiatal Esophagectomy (1085 Patients)**

		No. (%)
BENIGN CONDITIONS		**285 (26)**
Neuromotor dysfunction		93 (33)
Achalasia	70	
Spasm/dysmotility	22	
Scleroderma	1	
Stricture		75 (26)
Gastroesophageal reflux	42	
Caustic ingestion	19	
Radiation	4	
Other	10	
Barrett's mucosa with high-grade dysplasia		54 (19)
Recurrent gastroesophageal reflux		21 (7)
Recurrent hiatus hernia		14 (5)
Acute perforation		14 (5)
Acute caustic injury		6
Other		8
CARCINOMA OF INTRATHORACIC ESOPHAGUS		**800 (74)**
Upper third		36 (4.5)
Middle third		177 (28.0)
Lower third thoracic and/or cardia		587 (73.5)

From Orringer MB, Marshall B, Iannettoni MD: Transhiatal esophagectomy: Clinical experience and refinements. Ann Surg 230:392, 1999.

Intraoperative Complications

After removal of the esophagus from the mediastinum in 831 patients (77%), direct inspection through the diaphragmatic hiatus revealed entry into one or both pleural cavities, which was managed by placement of one or more chest tubes. Intraoperative membranous tracheal lacerations occurred in four patients; three of the lacerations involved the high membranous trachea and were exposed and successfully repaired through a partial upper sternal split. In the fourth patient, the tear involved the membranous carina. Management involved guiding the endotracheal tube into the left mainstem bronchus through the diaphragmatic hiatus, providing one-lung ventilation, and performing a substernal gastric bypass. The esophagectomy was then completed through a right thoracotomy, and the tracheal tear was successfully repaired.

A splenectomy was required in 34 patients (3%) because of intraoperative injury. The duodenal or gastric mucosa was entered during the pyloromyotomy in fewer than 2% of patients. Management consisted of suturing the hole with 5–0 polypropylene and buttressing the repair with adjacent omentum.

Postoperative Complications

Five patients (<1%), three with carcinoma and two with megaesophagus of achalasia, experienced *mediastinal hemorrhage*, requiring a thoracotomy for control of bleeding within 24 hours of transhiatal esophagectomy. *Recurrent laryngeal nerve injury* occurred in 74 patients (7%), which resolved spontaneously in 50 patients within 2 to 12 weeks. Hoarseness persisted in 24 patients (<1%), and 7 of these required vocal cord medialization procedures. During the past 10 years, since compulsively avoiding placement of metal retractors against the tracheoesophageal groove during the cervical portions of the operation, the incidence of postoperative hoarseness has been less than 3%. *Chylothorax* occurred in 18 patients (<1%), 12 with carcinoma and 6 with benign disease, and was managed successfully, as described previously by Orringer and associates (1988), with transthoracic ligation of the injured thoracic duct. Abdominal wound infection or dehiscence occurred in 29 patients (3%). Clinically significant *atelectasis* or *pneumonia* prolonging the hospitalization beyond 10 days occurred in 17 patients (2%).

Our overall *anastomotic leak* rate after a cervical esophagogastric anastomosis has been 13% (146 patients). All but nine of these anastomotic leaks were managed successfully by opening the cervical wound at the bedside, local wound packing, and early esophageal bougienage to prevent late stenosis, as described previously by Iannettoni and associates (1995). As indicated earlier, Orringer and associates (1999) reported that since initiation of the stapled side-to-side cervical esophagogastric anastomosis, the anastomotic leak rate has fallen to below 3%. *Necrosis of the upper stomach*, necessitating takedown of the intrathoracic stomach, resection of devitalized stomach, and a cervical esophagostomy, occurred in nine patients.

Mortality

The total hospital mortality among the 1085 patients was 4% (44 deaths). Among the 285 patients with benign disease, there were 8 deaths (2.8%); these were due to sepsis (5), myocardial infarction (1), respiratory insufficiency (1), and portal vein thrombosis (1). There were 36 deaths (4.5%) among the 800 patients with carcinoma; these resulted from hepatic failure (6), respiratory insufficiency (5), myocardial infarction (4), intraoperative hemorrhage (3), pneumonia (3), sepsis (3), intestinal ischemia (3), sudden death/cardiac arrest (3), pulmonary embolus (2), and posterior mediastinal abscess, peritoneal abscess, unrecognized brain metastasis, and delayed pyloromyotomy leak (1 each).

SUMMARY

In my group's experience, transhiatal esophagectomy has been applicable in virtually every situation requiring an esophagectomy for either benign or malignant disease. For example, this technique is being used increasingly in patients with failed esophagomyotomies for achalasia or those presenting with megaesophagus, as described by Orringer and Stirling (1989). Pinotti and colleagues (1981) advocated routine enlargement of the diaphragmatic hiatus by means of an incision from the anterior hiatus toward the xiphoid to facilitate transhiatal esophagectomy in their patients with megaesophagus or achalasia; however, we have rarely found this necessary. Gradual dilatation of the hiatus until it will accept the surgeon's hand (size 7 glove) generally provides ample exposure for the operation. The placement of narrow, deep retractors within the diaphragmatic hiatus permits dissection of the esophagus under direct vision, often to the level of the carina.

When the esophagus is found to be fixed to the aorta or to the tracheobronchial tree by invasive carcinoma or by fibrosis due to benign disease or multiple prior operations, the surgeon must be prepared to abandon the transhiatal route and convert to a transthoracic resection. Inflexible persistence with a transhiatal esophagectomy may have catastrophic consequences. In the end, it is the surgeon's judgment on palpation of the esophagus and assessment of its mobility that is the single most important factor in determining whether the transhiatal approach is appropriate for the esophagectomy.

This point having been made, however, increased experience leads to progressive gain in confidence. In our experience, we have been able to perform a transhiatal esophagectomy in 98.6% of all patients in whom it has been attempted in the past 20 years. Another important technical aid is the partial upper sternal split used to obtain access to the upper esophagus in patients with little or no length of cervical esophagus, for instance, in elderly patients with cervical osteoarthritis who cannot extend the neck, or the so-called bull neck ("no neck") individual in whom the cricoid cartilage (the level of the upper esophageal sphincter rests essentially at the level of the suprasternal notch).

From a functional standpoint, the stomach has emerged as the organ of choice for esophageal replacement for both benign and malignant disease. The almost inevitable occurrence of significant gastroesophageal reflux and esophagitis inherent in an intrathoracic esophagogastric anastomosis is rarely a clinically significant problem with a properly performed cervical anastomosis. The end-to-side cervical esophagogastric anastomotic construction appears at least in part to provide more of a "flap-valve" protection against regurgitation than does an end-to-end anastomosis between the tip of the gastric fundus and the cervical esophagus.

Long-term functional problems with colonic interposition (redundancy of the graft, delayed emptying, nocturnal regurgitation, aspiration) that have been well documented are far less frequent when the stomach is used as the esophageal substitute. As is the case after a partial gastric resection for peptic ulcer disease, gastric capacity after a cervical esophagogastric anastomosis is generally less and patients experience early satiety and frequently stabilize at a new lower weight after an initial period of weight loss.

It is important that patients be warned preoperatively about the possibility of postvagotomy dumping symptoms (postprandial cramping, diarrhea). In most cases, these symptoms can be controlled with (1) dietary modifications (avoidance of high-carbohydrate intake and dairy products and not stretching the stomach by drinking liquid with meals) or (2) medication (diphenoxylate for diarrhea, tincture of opium for spasm).

COMMENTS AND CONTROVERSIES

Over the past 15 years, I have gone from skeptic to convert regarding the use of the transhiatal approach for esophagectomy, as popularized and improved upon by Dr. Orringer and colleagues. Its increased application in my own practice is based on three factors: (1) getting over the learning curve, (2) the increasing incidence of esophagectomy for Barrett's esophagus with severe dysplasia and for the rapidly increasing incidence of adenocarcinomas at the esophagogastric junction, and (3) the development of instrumentation for minimally invasive surgery that is also applicable to this procedure, such as the harmonic scalpel and the endoscopic linear stapler.

An en bloc resection for a distal esophageal carcinoma is as easily accomplished through the hiatus as it is through the chest. However, radical resection of mediastinal lymph nodes is clearly not possible through the transhiatal approach; yet, many surgeons, including myself, remain skeptical of the value of a radical approach for most of the esophageal malignancies currently encountered. The harmonic scalpel not only facilitates division of the short gastric vessels but also is extremely useful for dissecting the esophagus through the hiatus, at least to the level of the carina. In some instances, the endoscopic stapler can also be used for this purpose.

With the use of long, thin retractors, as noted by Dr. Orringer, direct visualization to the level of the carina can be accomplished routinely. Somewhat surprisingly, a long, thin retractor, placed behind the pericardium, often provides much improved exposure without significant resulting hypotension.

As noted in commentaries to previous chapters on esophageal resection, I generally do not employ a pyloromyotomy or pyloroplasty. I share Dr. Orringer's concern regarding the suturing of a drain to the apex of the stomach to facilitate its traction into the neck. However, placing the stomach in a camera bag and tying the apex of the camera bag to an umbilical tape that is brought down from the neck by attachment to the distal severed end of the cervical esophagus allows the gentle, atraumatic retraction of the stomach through the mediastinum and into the neck along with concurrent pulsion from below, as described by Dr. Orringer.

The reduced operative time, potential for reduced morbidity by avoidance of thoracotomy, and superb long-term functional result achieved by the transhiatal esophagectomy must be balanced against the significantly higher incidence of anastomotic leakage following cervical anastomosis compared with intrathoracic anastomosis. Although such leakage is usually associated with minimum morbidity, this is not always true. The reason for the increased incidence of cervical anastomotic leakage remains uncertain. The general explanation is increased tension on the anastomosis due to its higher position and possible arterial or venous obstruction to the gastric circulation as it passes through the thoracic inlet. Another factor may be the fact that the cervical esophagus is generally transected at a fairly high level, with only a short distance of esophagus remaining between the larynx and the anastomosis. Thus, each time a patient swallows saliva or extends his or her head, direct traction is placed on the anastomosis without the "shock-absorbing" benefit provided by the longer length of esophagus remaining when an intrathoracic anastomosis is constructed. Dr. Orringer's recently described technique for a side-to-side staple anastomosis may be addressing this problem. As described, a longer than usual length of cervical esophagus must be preserved to utilize this technique. In addition, the three rows of staples on either side of this long anastomosis provide the ultimate in a tension-resistant anastomosis. The manually sewn portion, as depicted in the accompanying illustrations, cannot be subject to distraction because of the stapled portion of the anastomosis.

I would concur with the judgment that a postoperative chyle leak should be dealt with surgically unless it resolves within a few days. However, it is not necessary to ligate the thoracic duct at the site of injury; instead, use of a small right posterolateral thoracotomy to ligate the duct just above the hiatus inevitably solves the problem.

Dr. Orringer has made a major contribution to the field of esophageal surgery by his persistence in improving the technique, broadening the applicability, and reducing the morbidity associated with total esophagectomy for both benign and malignant conditions.

J. D. C.

■ *KEY REFERENCES*

Iannettoni MD, Whyte RI, Orringer MB: Catastrophic complications of the cervical esophagogastric anastomosis. J Thorac Cardiovasc Surg 110:1493, 1995.

Fewer than 2% of 856 patients undergoing transhiatal esophagectomy and cervical esophagogastric anastomosis experienced catastrophic cervical infectious complications. These 11 complications included vertebral body osteomyelitis (1), epidural abscess with neurologic impairment (2), pulmonary microabscesses from internal jugular vein abscess (1), tracheogastric anastomotic fistula (1), and major dehiscence necessitating anastomotic takedown (6). Although the generally low morbidity associated with a cervical esophagogastric anastomosis is emphasized, this sobering report of the prevention, presentation, and management of the serious complications that can occur merits review by those undertaking these operations.

Orringer MB, Marshall B, Iannettoni MD: Eliminating the cervical esophagogastric anastomotic leak with a side-to-side stapled anastomosis. J Thorac Cardiovasc Surg 119:277, 2000.

This report describes the authors' new technique of constructing the cervical esophagogastric anastomosis after transhiatal esophagectomy utilizing the Autosuture Endo GIA II stapler applied directly through the cervical wound. The anastomotic leak rate has been reduced to under 3% using this technique, and this has contributed to reduction in the average length of stay after an uncomplicated transhiatal esophagectomy to 7 days. Swallowing has been more comfortable, and ease of subsequent esophageal dilatation, if required, has been greater.

Orringer MB, Marshall B, Iannettoni MD: Transhiatal esophagectomy: Clinical experience and refinements. Ann Surg 230:392, 1999.

This report summarizes the authors' cumulative 22-year experience with 1085 transhiatal esophagectomies, the largest such reported series. Of these operations 800 were performed for carcinoma and 285 for benign disease. Stomach was used as the esophageal substitute in 96%. Overall hospital mortality rate was 4%. Blood loss averaged 689 ml. Major complications included anastomotic leak (13%), atelectasis/pneumonia (2%), intrathoracic hemorrhage, recurrent laryngeal nerve injury, chylothorax, and tracheal tear (<1% each). Late functional results have been excellent or good in 70%. Actuarial survival for patients with cancer equals or exceeds that reported after transthoracic esophagectomy.

Orringer MB, Sloan H: Esophagectomy without thoracotomy. J Thorac Cardiovasc Surg 76:643, 1978.

This preliminary report from the University of Michigan summarized the results of transhiatal esophagectomy in 26 patients (4 with benign disease and 22 with carcinomas involving various levels of the esophagus). It aroused renewed interest in a technique that had been virtually abandoned as the availability of endotracheal anesthesia permitted safe thoracotomy and esophagectomy under direct vision.

■ *REFERENCES*

Akiyama H, Sato Y, Takahashi F: Immediate pharyngogastrostomy following total esophagectomy by blunt dissection. Jpn J Surg 1:225, 1971.

Bains MS, Spiro RH: Pharyngolaryngectomy, total extrathoracic esophagectomy and gastric transposition. Surg Gynecol Obstet 149:693, 1979.

Baker JW, Schechter GL: Management of panesophageal cancer by blunt resection without thoracotomy and reconstruction with stomach. Ann Surg 203:491, 1986.

Caracci B, Garvin P, Kaminski DL: Surgical therapy of advanced esophageal cancer: A critical appraisal. Am J Surg 146:704, 1983.
Cordiano C, Fracastoro G, Mosciaro O, Mozzo W: Esophagectomy and esophageal replacement by gastric pull-through procedure. Int Surg 64:17, 1979.
Denk W: Zur Radikaloperation des Osophaguskarfzentralbl. Chirurg 40:1065, 1913.
Finley RJ, Inculet RI: The results of esophagogastrectomy without thoracotomy for adenocarcinoma of the esophagogastric junction. Ann Surg 21:535, 1989.
Fok M, Siu KF, Wong J: A comparison of transhiatal and transthoracic resection for carcinoma of the thoracic esophagus. Am J Surg 158:414, 1984.
Gandhi SK, Naunheim KS: Complications of transhiatal esophagectomy. Chest Surg Clin North Am 7:601, 1997.
Hankins JR, Attar S, Coughlin TR, et al: Carcinoma of the esophagus: A comparison of the results of transhiatal versus transthoracic resection. Ann Thorac Surg 47:700, 1989.
Hankins JR, Miller JE, Attar S, McLaughlin JS: Transhiatal esophagectomy for carcinoma of the esophagus: Experience with 26 patients. Ann Thorac Surg 44:123, 1987.
Iannettoni MD, Whyte RI, Orringer MB: Catastrophic complications of the cervical esophagogastric anastomosis. J Thorac Cardiovasc Surg 110:1493, 1995.
Katariya K, Harvey JC, Pina E, Beattie EJ: Complications of transhiatal esophagectomy. J Surg Oncol 57:157, 1994.
Kirk RM. Palliative resection of oesophageal carcinoma without formal thoracotomy. Br J Surg 61:689, 1974.
LeQuesne LP, Ranger D: Pharyngogastrectomy with immediate pharyngogastric anastomosis. Br J Surg 53:105, 1966.
Liebermann-Meffert DMI, Luescher U, Neff U, et al: Esophagectomy without thoracotomy: Is there a risk of intramediastinal bleeding? Ann Surg 206:184, 1987.
Ong GB, Lee TC: Pharyngogastric anastomosis after oesophagopharyngectomy for carcinoma of the hypopharynx and cervical oesophagus. Br J Surg 48:193, 1960.
Orringer MB: Anterior mediastinal tracheostomy with and without cervical exenteration. Ann Thorac Surg 54:628, 1992.
Orringer MB: Partial median sternotomy: Anterior approach to the upper thoracic esophagus. J Thorac Cardiovasc Surg 87:124, 1984a.
Orringer MB: Surgical options for esophageal resection and reconstruction with stomach. In Baue AE, Geha AS, Hammond EL, et al (eds): Glenn's Thoracic and Cardiovascular Surgery, 5th ed. East Norwalk, CT, Appleton & Lange, 1991, p 787.
Orringer MB: Technical aids in performing transhiatal esophagectomy without thoracotomy. Ann Thorac Surg 38:128, 1984b.
Orringer MB: Transhiatal blunt esophagectomy without thoracotomy. In Cohn LH (ed): Cardiovascular Surgery: Modern Techniques in Surgery, Vol 62. Mount Kisco, NY, Futura Publishing, 1983a, p 1.
Orringer MB: Transhiatal esophagectomy for benign and malignant disease. J Jpn Assoc Thorac Surg 36:656, 1988.
Orringer MB: Transhiatal esophagectomy for benign disease. J Thorac Cardiovasc Surg 90:649, 1985.
Orringer MB: Transhiatal esophagectomy without thoracotomy for carcinoma of the thoracic esophagus. Ann Surg 200:282, 1984c.
Orringer MB: Transmediastinal esophagectomy. In Dudley H, Pories WJ, Carter D (eds): Rob and Smith's Operative Surgery, 4th ed. London, Butterworth, 1983b, p 192.
Orringer MB, Bluett M, Deeb GM: Aggressive treatment of chylothorax complicating transhiatal esophagectomy without thoracotomy. Surgery 104:720, 1988.
Orringer MB, Lemmer JH: Early dilation in the treatment of esophageal disruption. Ann Thorac Surg 42:536, 1986.
Orringer MB, Marshall B, Iannettoni MD: Eliminating the cervical esophagogastric anastomotic leak with a side-to-side stapled anastomosis. J Thorac Cardiovasc Surg 119:277, 2000.
Orringer MB, Marshall BM, Iannettoni MD: Transhiatal esophagectomy: Clinical experience and refinements. Ann Surg 230:392, 1999.
Orringer MB, Marshall B, Stirling MC: Transhiatal esophagectomy for benign and malignant disease. J Thorac Cardiovasc Surg 105:265, 1993.
Orringer MB, Orringer JS: Transhiatal esophagectomy without thoracotomy—a dangerous operation? J Thorac Cardiovasc Surg 85:72, 1983.
Orringer MB, Sloan H: Esophageal replacement after blunt esophagectomy. In Nyhus LM, Baker RJ (eds): Mastery of Surgery. Boston, Little, Brown, 1984, p 426.
Orringer MB, Sloan H: Esophagectomy without thoracotomy. J Thorac Cardiovasc Surg 76:643, 1978.
Orringer MB, Sloan H: Substernal gastric bypass of the excluded thoracic esophagus for palliation of esophageal carcinoma. J Thorac Cardiovasc Surg 70:836, 1975.
Orringer MB, Stirling MC: Esophageal resection for achalasia—indications and results. Ann Thorac Surg 47:340, 1989.
Pinotti HW, Zilberstein B, Pollara W, Raia A: Esophagectomy without thoracotomy. Surg Gynecol Obstet 154:344, 1981.
Quint LE, Glazer GM, Orringer MB, Gross BH: Esophageal carcinoma: CT findings. Radiology 155:171, 1985.
Sabanathan S, Hashimi H, Pradhan GN: Transhiatal oesophagectomy in the management of carcinoma of the thoracic oesophagus. J R Coll Surg Edinb 33:192, 1988.
Shahian DM, Neptune WB, Ellis FH, Watkins E: Transthoracic versus extrathoracic esophagectomy: Mortality, morbidity, and long-term survival. Ann Thorac Surg 41:237, 1986.
Skinner DB: En bloc resection for neoplasms of the esophagus and cardia. J Thorac Cardiovasc Surg 85:59, 1983.
Steiger Z, Wilson RF: Comparison of the results of esophagectomy with and without a thoracotomy. Surg Gynecol Obstet 153:653, 1981.
Stewart JR, Sarr MG, Sharp KW, et al: Transhiatal (blunt) esophagectomy for malignant and benign esophageal disease: Clinical experience and technique. Ann Thorac Surg 40:343, 1985.
Szentpetery S, Wolfgang T, Lower RR: Pull-through esophagectomy without thoracotomy for esophageal carcinoma. Ann Thorac Surg 27:399, 1979.
Thomas AN, Dedo HH: Pharyngogastrostomy for treatment of severe caustic stricture of the pharynx and esophagus. J Thorac Cardiovasc Surg 73:817, 1977.
Tryzelaar JF, Neptune WB, Ellis FH Jr: Esophagectomy without thoracotomy for carcinoma of the esophagus. Am J Surg 143:486, 1982.
Turner GG: Excision of thoracic esophagus for carcinoma with construction of extrathoracic gullet. Lancet 2:1315, 1933.
Waddell WR, Cannon B: A technique for subtotal excision of the trachea and establishment of a sternal tracheostomy. Ann Surg 149:1, 1959.
Waddell WR, Scannell JG: Anterior approach to carcinoma of the superior mediastinal and cervical segments of the esophagus. J Thorac Surg 33:663, 1957.

CHAPTER **56**

Transabdominal Esophagogastrectomy

Manjit S. Bains

For patients with esophageal carcinoma, surgical resection provides the most dependable and durable palliation as well as a possibility of a cure. For curable patients, I prefer an Ivor Lewis approach, although in select cases a transhiatal esophagectomy with cervical anastomosis suffices. Both techniques impose a significant physiologic insult to the patient and a real potential for morbidity and mortality. These potential problems have stimulated interest in a technique for resection of the esophageal cancer and reconstruction of the esophagus to reduce morbidity and mortality, especially in those elderly patients requiring excellent palliation but who have little likelihood of cure.

Since 1981, for selected tumors involving the distal esophagus or gastroesophageal junction, I have performed an esophagogastrectomy through a transabdominal approach only, using the circular stapler to accomplish an end-to-end anastomosis. This technique is limited to physiologically compromised patients (e.g., very elderly, obese) with locally extensive but completely resectable tumors that can be mobilized from the abdomen through a dilated esophageal hiatus. Resection should provide histologically negative margins on frozen section, and the intent of this procedure is to provide immediate palliation.

A patient with good chance of cure undergoes a standard transthoracic resection to provide wider margins and a formal mediastinal node dissection. This limited technique reduces the operating time and spares the patient a thoracotomy or exploration of the neck with a corresponding reduction in morbidity. It has been employed in 31 patients with one death, early in our experience, as a result of an anastomotic leak and peritonitis. There have been no major complications since then.

OPERATIVE TECHNIQUE

A laparotomy is performed through a midline incision extending from the xiphoid process to the umbilicus, and the xiphoid process is excised for better exposure. The peritoneal cavity is carefully evaluated for any metastases, especially to the liver or the celiac nodes. The tumor is assessed for its extension into the adjacent viscera. The triangular ligament of the left lobe of the liver is divided, and the peritoneum is incised around the esophageal hiatus. The hiatus is dilated, and a plane is developed between the pericardium and the esophagus anteriorly. Dissection is continued superiorly into the mediastinum proximal to the tumor, as the surgeon determines the fixation of the tumor or extension into adjacent structures and availability of grossly tumor-free esophagus for an anastomosis. A decision is made at this point as to whether the tumor can be grossly resected with negative proximal and distal margins and whether an esophagogastrostomy anastomosis can be safely performed through this exposure.

The surgeon mobilizes the stomach along the greater curvature, preserving the right gastroepiploic vessels but ligating and dividing the left gastroepiploic and the short gastric vessels. Through the lesser sac, the peritoneum is incised along the superior border of the pancreas, and all the node-bearing tissue overlying the esophageal crurae and the abdominal aorta is swept up along with the mobilized stomach. The left gastric vessels are ligated and divided through the lesser sac. A pyloric drainage procedure is routinely performed. I prefer excising the anterior half of the pyloric muscular ring (pyloromyectomy), allowing the intact mucosa to bulge through the seromuscular defect (Bains and Spiro, 1979).

Esophageal mobilization is completed in the posterior mediastinum. Any tumor extension into the diaphragm is excised en bloc together with a rim of normal muscle. Tumor extension into the pericardium or the aorta is considered a contraindication for any resection. The distal esophagus is mobilized between the pericardium anteriorly, the aortic adventitia posteriorly, and the pleural reflections on either side (Fig. 56–1). Through the widened hiatus, this dissection can be easily performed under direct vision to above the level of the pulmonary vein with excellent exposure. A self-retaining Goligher retractor is very helpful in providing exposure (Figs. 56–2 and 56–3). Esophageal mobilization can be performed almost to the subcarinal region, but satisfactory peribronchial or subcarinal node dissection cannot be done. The esophagus is transected 5 to 7 cm above the tumor. Similarly, a margin of 7 to 10 cm is obtained along the lesser curvature of the stomach (Fig. 56–4). (The margins are confirmed to be free of tumor or frozen section.) The stomach is transected with the use of stapling devices, and the proximal half of the lesser curvature is excised. Esophagogastrostomy anastomosis is performed with a circular end-to-end anastomosis (CEEA) stapler (U.S. Surgical). This stapler is introduced into the stomach at a convenient point along the staple line for transection of stomach at the lesser curvature (Fig. 56–5). A purse-string suture is placed on the transected esophagus using 2–0 or 3–0 polypropylene or, if possible, a purse-string

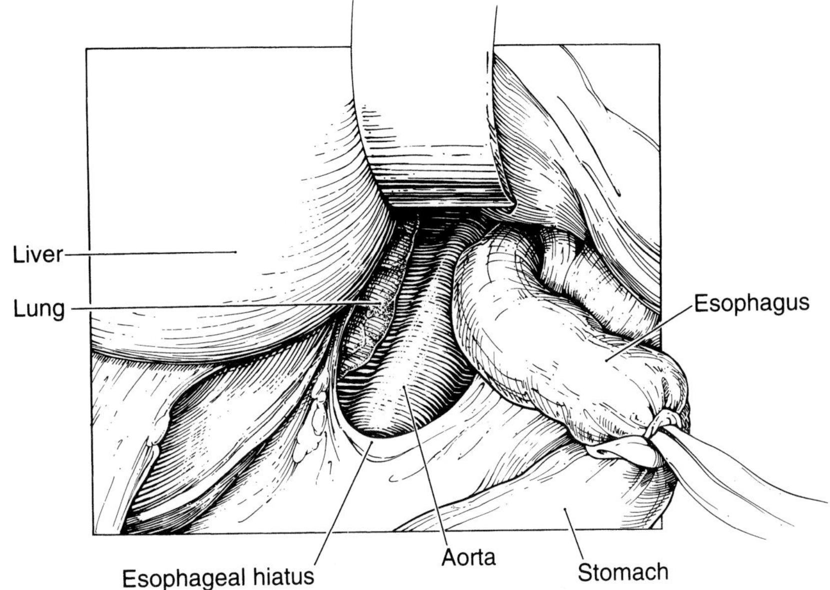

FIGURE 56–1 ■ Mobilization of the distal esophagus through a dilated esophageal hiatus. A retractor is used to retract the left lobe of the liver and the pericardium anteriorly and to keep the hiatus open. The esophagus has been mobilized off the aorta, the pleural reflexion, and the pericardium. A Penrose drain, tied at the gastroesophageal junction, provides traction on the esophagus.

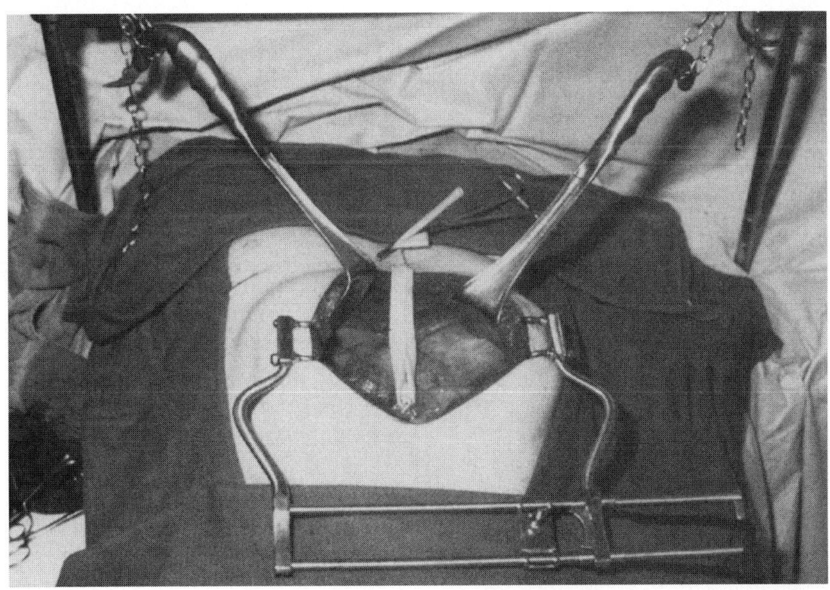

FIGURE 56–2 ■ A self-retaining Goligher retractor in place allows additional retractors to be anchored to it for a consistently reliable exposure.

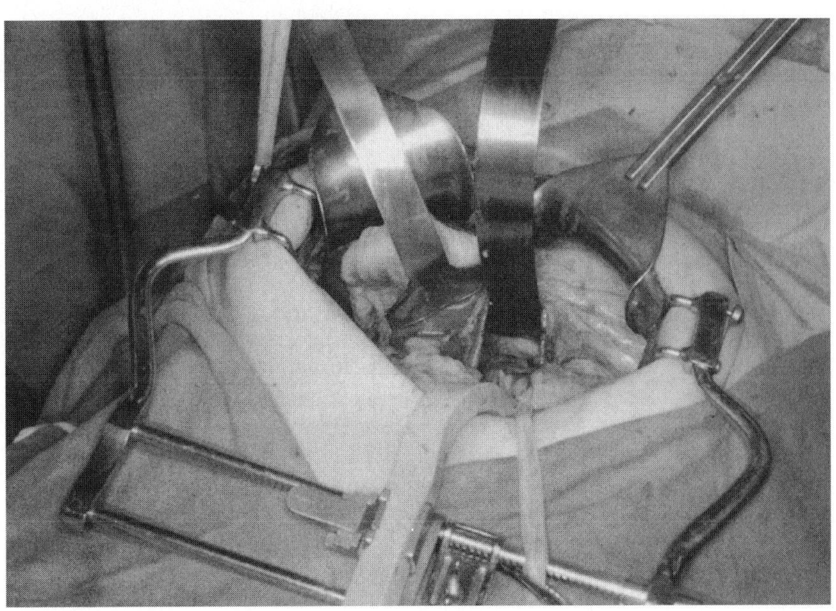

FIGURE 56–3 ■ Two Richardson retractors attached to a self-retaining Goligher retractor are pulling the costal arch, while a Harrington retractor, also supported by the Goligher retractor, keeps the esophageal hiatus open and retracts the pericardium anteriorly, providing excellent exposure to the distal esophagus.

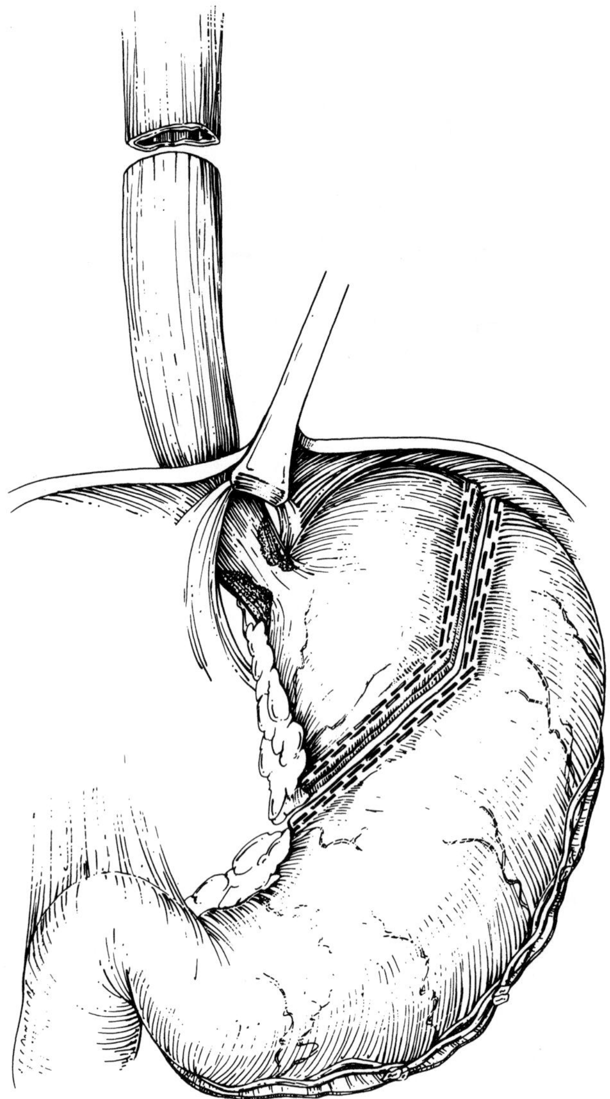

FIGURE 56–4 ■ The esophagus has been transected proximal to the tumor and the stomach and the fundus of the stomach and the lesser curvature have been distally resected, making a gastric tube along the greater curvature while ensuring an adequate margin from the tumor. A frozen section confirmation of tumor-free resection margins is essential.

instrument. Two traction sutures are placed at the 2 o'clock and 10 o'clock positions, and the lumen is triangulated, by use of an Allis clamp posteriorly. An end-to-end anastomosis stapler of appropriate size is introduced, and two satisfactory doughnuts of tissue must be obtained from the stapler. With a finger through the gastrotomy along lesser curvature and through the anastomosis as a guide, a Salem sump drain is advanced into the stomach for gastric decompression. The gastrotomy along the lesser curvature is closed, and the staple line along the lesser curvature is reinforced by a running 3–0 polydioxanone suture for seromuscular approximation. One of the pleural cavities is intentionally entered and drained. The stomach is loosely anchored to the diaphragm at the hiatus. The peritoneal cavity is not drained.

RESULTS

Since 1981, my associates and I have selected this procedure for 31 patients, or about 5% of all patients undergoing esophagectomy, usually with palliative intent. Almost all the patients had a stage T3 tumor, and the majority had adenopathy that was suspected for metastatic disease at the time of surgery. Four patients had complete obstruction and were found to have limited liver metastases not detected by computed tomography (CT). Another patient had a sigmoid lesion suggestive of a tumor. One patient died of peritonitis, secondary to anastomotic leak. Another patient died of a cerebral vascular accident while

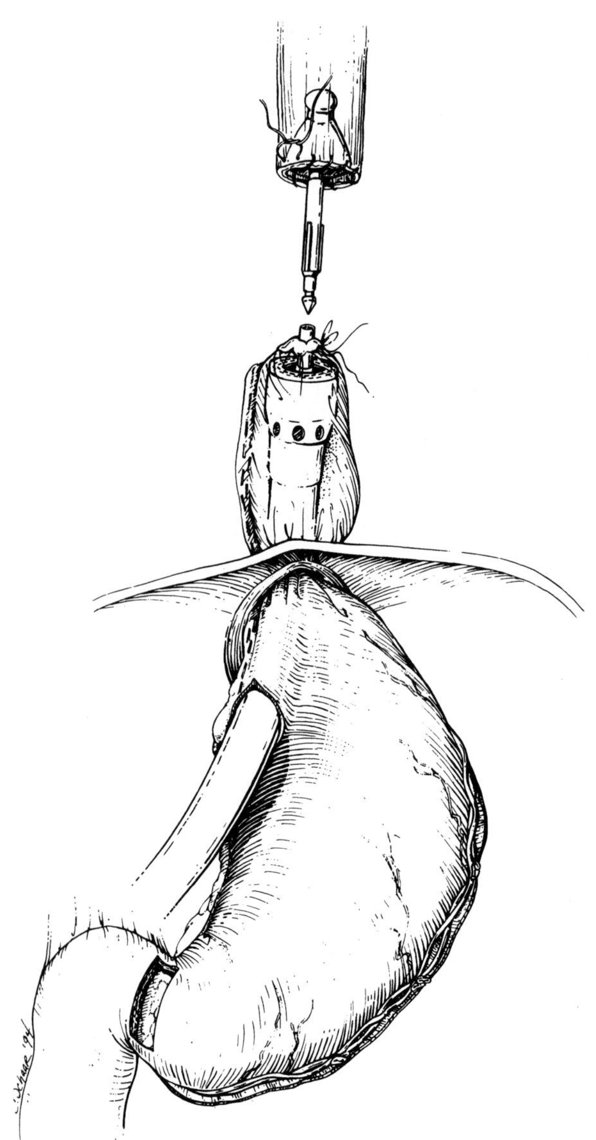

FIGURE 56–5 ■ A circular stapler is introduced through a gastrotomy along the lesser curvature staple line. An anterior hemipyloromyectomy has already been performed.

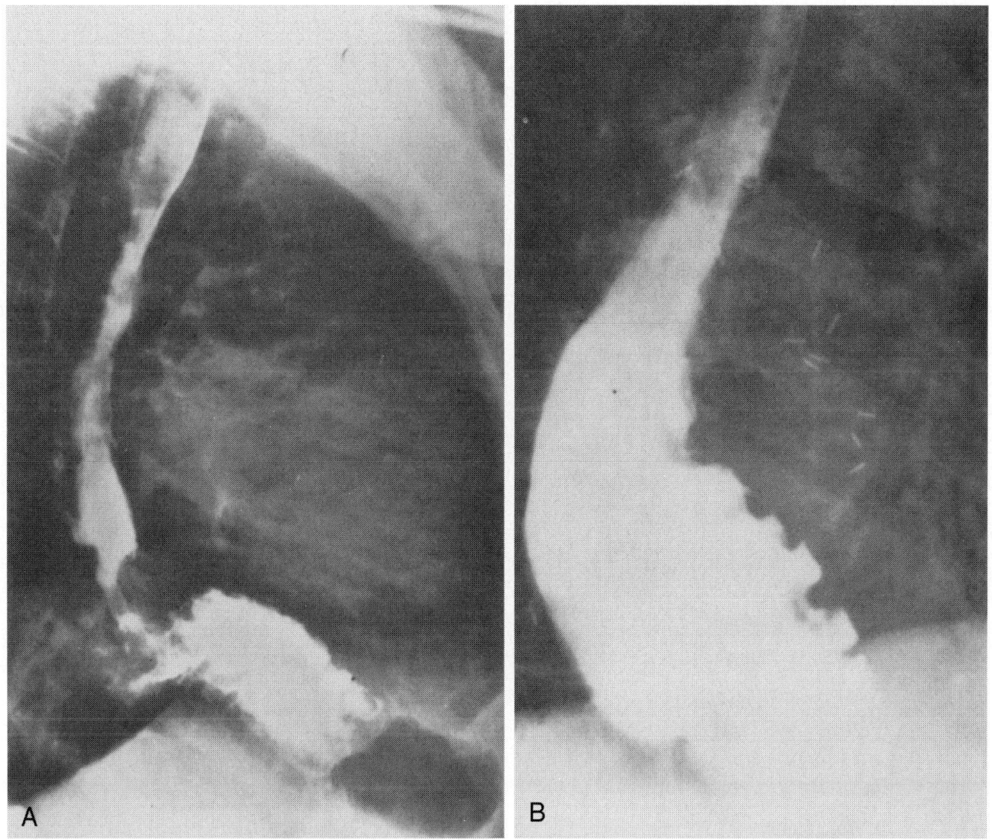

FIGURE 56–6 ■ Esophagram showing large tumor *(A)* at the gastroesophageal junction, with *(B)* the anastomosis almost at the level of the left main bronchus.

recovering from a postoperative pneumonia. One patient required a thoracotomy for closure of her disrupted staple line along the lesser curvature of the stomach, with subsequent uneventful postoperative course.

Relief of dysphagia has been very satisfactory. One patient has had significant complaints of reflux, requiring medical management. Two patients have survived for more than 10 years.

SPECIAL CONCERNS

Esophagectomy offers the most prompt and durable palliation, with chance of cure at least equal if not better than other modalities of therapy in treatment of cancer of the esophagus. Survival is dependent on the stage of disease as well as effectiveness of the treatment or completeness of resection in the case of surgery, and prospects remain dismal. Hence, it is important that any treatment proposed, while aiming for cure, should have the least morbidity or mortality, minimize hospital stay, and provide the ability to eat normally for effective palliation.

A number of approaches are used. The Ivor Lewis (Lewis, 1946) or laparotomy and right thoracotomy and the extrathoracic esophagectomy through a laparotomy and a cervical incision (Orringer, 1984) are the most popular ones. However, both of these approaches carry significant incidence of complications and mortality, which has stimulated an interest in exploring other techniques.

In a small number of patients with cancer in the distal thoracic esophagus or the gastroesophageal junction, with palliation as the primary goal, a grossly complete resection has been possible through a laparotomy and a transhiatal access to posterior mediastinum. A circular end-to-end stapler or the intraluminal stapler (ILS) (Ethicon) has enabled the anastomosis to be performed at or above the level of inferior pulmonary veins (Figs. 56–6 and 56–7). Manual anastomosis at this level would be quite difficult and unsatisfactory. It is important that all gross disease be excised and resection margins be assessed with a frozen section. The pleural cavity should be entered by dividing the mediastinal pleura to drain the posterior mediastinum rather than by allowing drainage to the peritoneal cavity. A decision to use this approach should be made at the time of surgery.

If there is any concern about the anastomosis allowing its completion, it should be addressed by proceeding with a thoracotomy. A similar approach has been reported by Misumi and colleagues (1989). This procedure is recommended for advanced but resectable disease involving the distal esophagus or the gastroesophageal junction in medically high-risk patients in whom palliation is the primary goal.

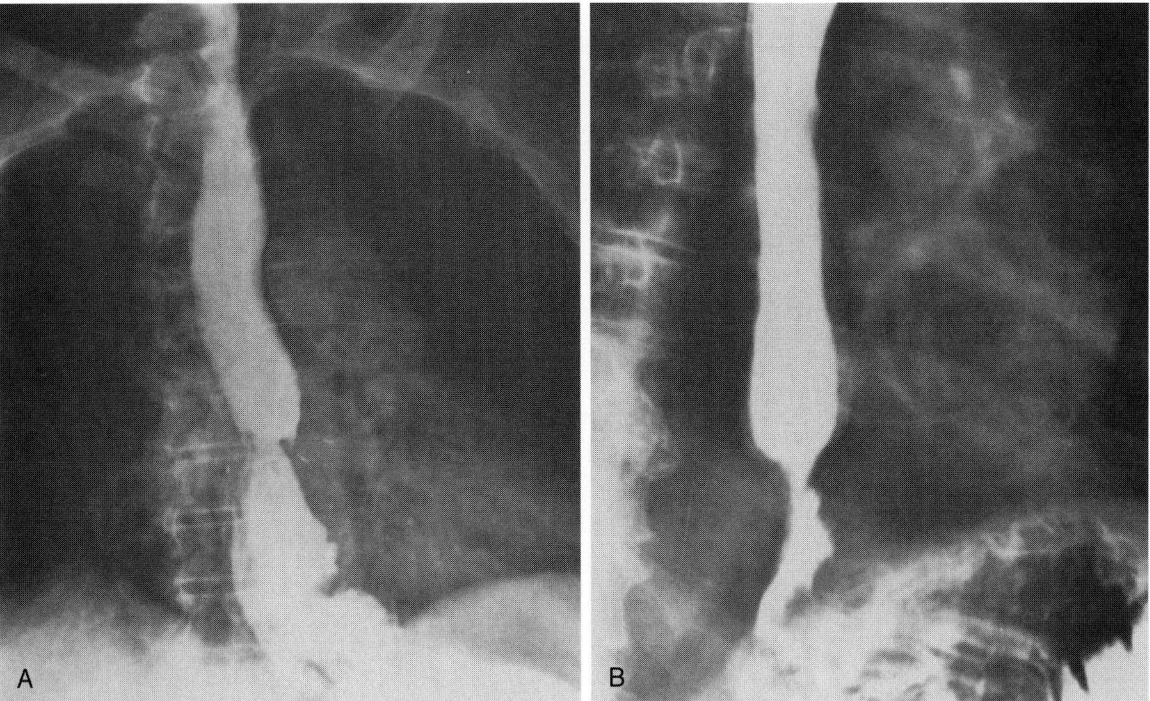

FIGURE 56–7 ■ *A*, Esophagram showing a large tumor at the gastroesophageal junction. *B*, Esophagram after resection, with the anastomosis above the level of the inferior pulmonary vein.

CONCLUSION

Resection of esophageal carcinoma with immediate reconstruction provides satisfactory palliation as well as a possibility of a cure. A technique is described for a select group of poor-risk patients with the tumor at the distal esophagus or the gastroesophageal junction, which spares the patients the added risks of a thoracotomy or neck exploration, to provide adequate palliation with acceptable morbidity and mortality.

■ *REFERENCES*

Bains MS, Spiro RH: Pharyngolaryngectomy, total extrathoracic esophagectomy, and gastric transposition. Surg Gynecol Obstet 149:693, 1979.

Lewis I: The surgical treatment of carcinoma of the oesophagus, with special reference to a new operation for growths of the middle third. Br J Surg 34:18, 1946.

Misumi A, Misumi K, Harada K, et al: Trans-abdominal operation for carcinoma of the gastric cardia: Application of pulling-up retractor and EEA stapler. Int Surg 75:223, 1989.

Orringer MD: Transhiatal esophagectomy without thoracotomy for carcinoma of the thoracic esophagus. Ann Surg 200:282, 1984.

CHAPTER **57**

En Bloc Resection for Esophageal Carcinoma

Nasser K. Altorki
David B. Skinner

In recent years, a variety of options have been advocated for treating esophageal carcinoma. These include several types of limited or more radical surgical resection, standard or high-dose radiation therapy, multidrug chemotherapy, and combinations of two or three modalities as well as local treatments that include laser, hot probe, stents, and mucosectomy. There is little agreement about the exact indications for any of these interventions. Treatment of esophageal cancer is evolving, imprecise, and more exciting than in past decades. This chapter presents our recommendation, based upon data, for the surgical treatment of patients with carcinoma of the esophagus.

HISTORICAL NOTE

In 1963, Logan reported the first surgical attempt to apply oncologic principles to the treatment of carcinoma of the cardia. He stressed obtaining adequate proximal and distal resection margins and a systematic removal of all tissues surrounding the cardia by an en bloc procedure. Although the operative mortality was high at that time, Logan reported the best 5-year survival yet achieved.

The first en bloc resection of the total intrathoracic esophagus was performed in 1965, but the patient did not survive to leave the hospital. Subsequently, from 1969 until 1981, 80 patients were treated by the principles of en bloc resection for lower, middle, and upper esophageal carcinoma. After sufficient experience had been obtained to demonstrate that the operation could be performed in a standardized fashion, safely, and with survival rates as good or better than previously achieved, the technique was published (Skinner, 1983) and underwent evaluation in other centers during the next decade (Akiyama, 1988; DeMeester et al, 1988; Siewert et al, 1988). With the advent of en bloc esophagectomy for attempted cure and the revival of esophagectomy without thoracotomy initially by Akiyama and associates (1971) and subsequently by Orringer and Sloan (1978), the stage was set for a debate of the different surgical strategies.

■ *HISTORICAL READINGS*

Akiyama H: Cardinals in the regional lymph node dissection in surgery of thoracic esophageal cancer. In Siewert JR, Holscher AH (eds): Disease of the Esophagus. Berlin, Springer-Verlag, 1988, p 416.

Akiyama H, Sato Y, Takahashi F: Immediate pharyngogastrostomy following total esophagectomy by blunt dissection. Jpn J Surg 1:225, 1971.

DeMeester TR, Zaninotto G, Johansson KE: Selective therapeutic approach to cancer of the lower esophagus and cardia. J Thorac Cardiovasc Surg 95:42, 1988.

Logan A: The surgical treatment of carcinoma of the esophagus and cardia. J Thorac Cardiovasc Surg 46:150, 1963.

Orringer MB, Sloan H: Esophagectomy without thoracotomy. J Thorac Cardiovasc Surg 76:643, 1978.

Siewert JR, Holscher AH, Roder JD, Bartels H: En bloc resektion der speiserohre beim Oesophaguscarcinom. Langenbecks Arch Chir 373:367, 1988.

Skinner DB: En bloc resection for neoplasm of the esophagus and cardia. J Thorac Cardiovasc Surg 85:59, 1983.

DIAGNOSIS

Staging

Pretreatment staging of esophageal cancer is essential to guide the selection of therapy and to permit a rational evaluation of the result of the various treatment options. Prior to 1987, the tumor factor (T) was determined by tumor size and degree of circumferential involvement and obstruction of the esophagus. All cases with full-thickness penetration into periesophageal tissue or with any positive lymph nodes were assigned to stage III disease, which contained a great majority of symptomatic patients. Applying this staging system to predict long-term survival demonstrated no significant differences between stage I and stage II classifications (Skinner et al, 1986).

A multifactorial analysis of proposed prognostic indicators in esophageal cancer led to the identification of the depth of esophageal wall penetration as the only independent predictor of prognosis for the primary tumor (T) (Skinner et al, 1982). Patients with 1 to 4 positive lymph nodes without full-thickness wall penetration had a significantly better prognosis after en bloc resection than did those with 4 or more positive lymph nodes, leading to a proposal to modify the N factor to N1 and N2 categories. This information was confirmed by studies of prognostic factors in Japan and elsewhere (Japanese Committee for Registration of Esophageal Carcinoma, 1985). It was proposed (Skinner et al, 1982, 1986) that the selection of operations for esophageal cancer be based upon this new staging system.

In 1987, the International Union Against Cancer changed the staging system to recognize depth of wall penetration for the T in addition to positive (N1) or negative lymph nodes (N0) and the presence (M1) or absence (M0) of systemic metastases. The (TNM) Tumor-Node-Metastasis system has also been adopted by the American Joint Committee on Cancer. The current international staging system for esophageal cancer designates *T0* as positive cytology without localization and *Tis* as intraepithelial or in situ carcinoma. *T1* disease is limited to the mucosa and submucosa. *T2* disease penetrates but does not extend through the muscular layers. *T3* is disease penetrating the full thickness of the esophageal wall to the periesophageal tissues, whereas *T4* tumors invade adjacent organs.

Using these TNM factors, the current staging system recognizes *stage I* as T1N0M0. *Stage II* is subdivided into two substages:

- *Stage IIA* includes T2N0 and T3N0
- *Stage IIB* includes T1–2N1

Stage III includes all patients with transmural disease and nodal metastases.

Stage IV is subdivided into two categories:

- *Stage IVA*, metastases present in the celiac or cervical nodes for carcinoma of the middle or lower thoracic esophagus
- *Stage IVB*, systemic visceral metastases present

A current proposal for modification of the staging system is to separate patients with one to four positive lymph nodes into an N1 category from those with more than four positive lymph nodes (N2). If this or similar modifications supported by the European and Japanese data are adopted, stage II esophageal cancer would be divided into stage IIA (T2–3N0M0) and stage IIB (T1–2N1M0). All N2 or T3N1 cases would be considered stage III esophageal carcinoma. This classification has a strong correlation with survival.

Earlier reports from our group emphasized the value of preoperative and intraoperative staging in the selection of the type of resection carried out in patients with esophageal cancer. That recommendation was based in part on the prolonged operating time and perceived high morbidity associated with en bloc resection. Accordingly, preoperative and intraoperative staging identified a subgroup of patients with favorable and potentially curable disease in whom en bloc resection was applied. Patients with obviously advanced disease were offered a more standard resection, since the limited expectation of cure in such instances did not appear to justify an extended resection. An interim analysis of our experience, however, suggested that not only were morbidity and mortality rates following en bloc and standard resection essentially identical but that there was a trend toward a survival advantage in patients with stage III disease following en bloc esophagectomy (Altorki et al, 1997). Our strategy has since evolved so en bloc resection is now considered the surgical procedure of choice in nearly all patients with no evidence of distant metastases and in whom no compelling medical contraindications exist for operation.

Preoperative Evaluation

A full staging workup is always carried out to determine the clinical TNM stage. A computed tomography (CT) scan of the chest and abdomen is performed primarily to exclude radiographic evidence of distant metastases. The value of CT scanning in determining malignant mural penetration is suboptimal. Blurring of the outer margin of the esophagus in the area of the tumor is suggestive of transmural disease; however, lesser degrees of penetration are less easily identified. Similarly, the CT scan is of limited value in predicting the presence of nodal disease, with an overall diagnostic accuracy of 50%. Endoscopic ultrasonography (EUS) is frequently used to define the T and N factors more accurately. The diagnostic accuracy of EUS in determining the T status is almost 80%, whereas nodal metastases are predicted with a 60% to 70% accuracy. Occasionally a transesophageal needle aspiration of suspected nodal areas can be done under EUS guidance. Although some have suggested that minimally invasive techniques, such as a laparoscopy or thoracoscopy, can be used for staging purposes, we have generally found such procedures time-consuming and of little added benefit and, possibly, harmful when the curative en bloc resection field is violated.

The principal causes of nontechnical morbidity and mortality are pulmonary and cardiovascular complications. Age alone is not a determining factor. Accordingly, detailed pulmonary function testing is carried out, as is a cardiologic evaluation, including stress testing. To evaluate choices for reconstruction, an upper gastrointestinal endoscopy or barium study determines the normality of the stomach or duodenum, and a colonoscopy or barium enema establishes the colon as an alternative organ for reconstruction.

Operative Technique

An en bloc resection entails excision of the tumor-bearing esophagus within a wide envelope of surrounding tissues, including the pericardium anteriorly, both pleural surfaces laterally, and the lymphatic tissues, including the thoracic duct, wedged dorsally between the esophagus and the spine. Additionally, an upper mediastinal and abdominal lymphadenectomy is performed.

For carcinoma of the cardia or of the lower esophagus, when 10-cm proximal margins can be obtained distal to the aortic arch as measured endoscopically, a left sixth interspace thoracotomy incision is performed. This incision provides the best exposure for thorough removal of all tissues surrounding the tumor-bearing cardia or distal esophagus. It enables the en bloc resection to be carried out through one incision. A thoracoabdominal incision is not necessary when the diaphragm is peripherally detached from the chest wall, extending from the pericardium medially to the spleen laterally, leaving a small cuff for later closure.

Retraction of the diaphragm through the phrenotomy gives excellent exposure to the entire left upper quadrant. It allows dissection of the splenic and hepatic artery lymph nodes in addition to division of the left gastric vessels at the celiac axis. All retroperitoneal tissues cephalad to the pancreas are dissected up into the hiatus, and a cuff of diaphragm muscle surrounding the tumor-bearing lower esophagus is removed (Fig. 57–1). The omentum is routinely resected, preserving the gastro-

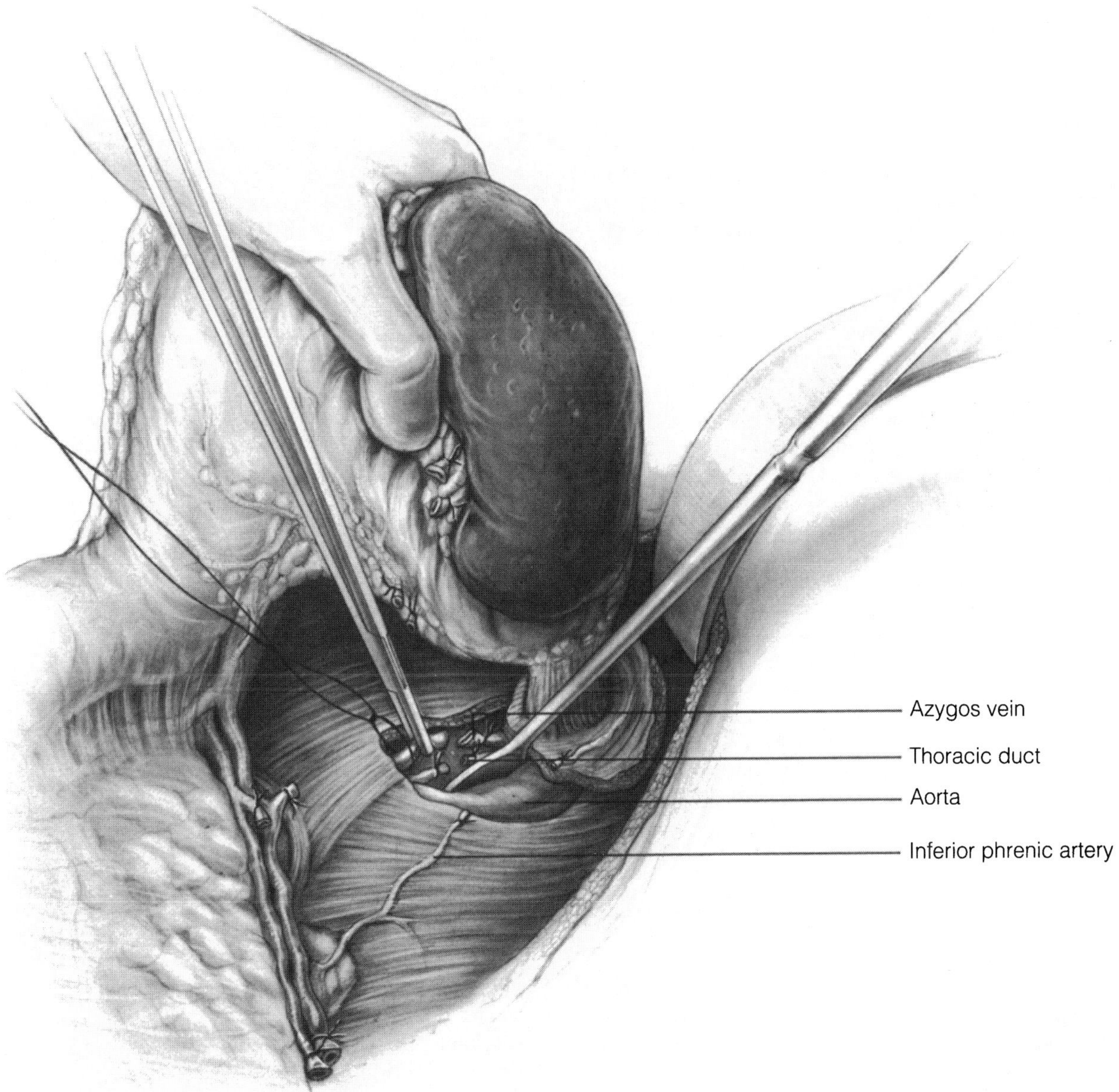

FIGURE 57–1 ■ Through a left thoracotomy with peripheral separation of the diaphragm, the celiac axis dissection is complete. Retroperitoneal tissues have been swept toward the cardia. A cuff of diaphragm around the distal esophageal tumor is incised, exposing the thoracic duct and azygos vein to start the mediastinal dissection. (From Skinner DB [ed]: In Atlas of Esophageal Surgery. New York, Churchill Livingstone, 1991, p 27.)

epiploic arcade for gastric blood supply. The mediastinal dissection is performed as described subsequently.

If the primary carcinoma in the lower esophagus is an adenocarcinoma, all glandular or Barrett's mucosa must be removed in addition to the 10-cm margin above the tumor. When an anastomosis is performed through this incision, it is preferable to employ an isoperistaltic segment of left colon for the interposition to avoid the complications of gastroesophageal reflux that occur in about one third of patients reconstructed with an esophagogastrostomy. When the dissection must be continued to the aortic arch or higher to achieve adequate margins or to remove columnar-lined esophagus, the final anastomosis is made in the neck. The organ for reconstruction, stomach or colon, is brought up through the left thoracotomy incision into the upper mediastinum and attached to the stump of the esophagus cephalad to the aortic arch. It is advanced further into the neck for subsequent anastomosis.

For carcinoma of the upper, middle, or lower esophagus within 10 cm of the aortic arch, the en bloc resection is performed through a right thoracotomy incision in the fifth interspace, removing a 1-cm segment of sixth rib posteriorly (Fig. 57–2). The mediastinal pleura is incised along the main trunk of the azygos vein throughout its course in the posterior mediastinum. Dissection is carried out anterior to the vein and medially toward the adventitia of the descending thoracic aorta. Although earlier en bloc resections have included resection of the azygos vein as well as the intercostal vessels, we have modified this portion of the procedure to preserve the intercostal vessels and the main trunk, but not the arch, of the azygos

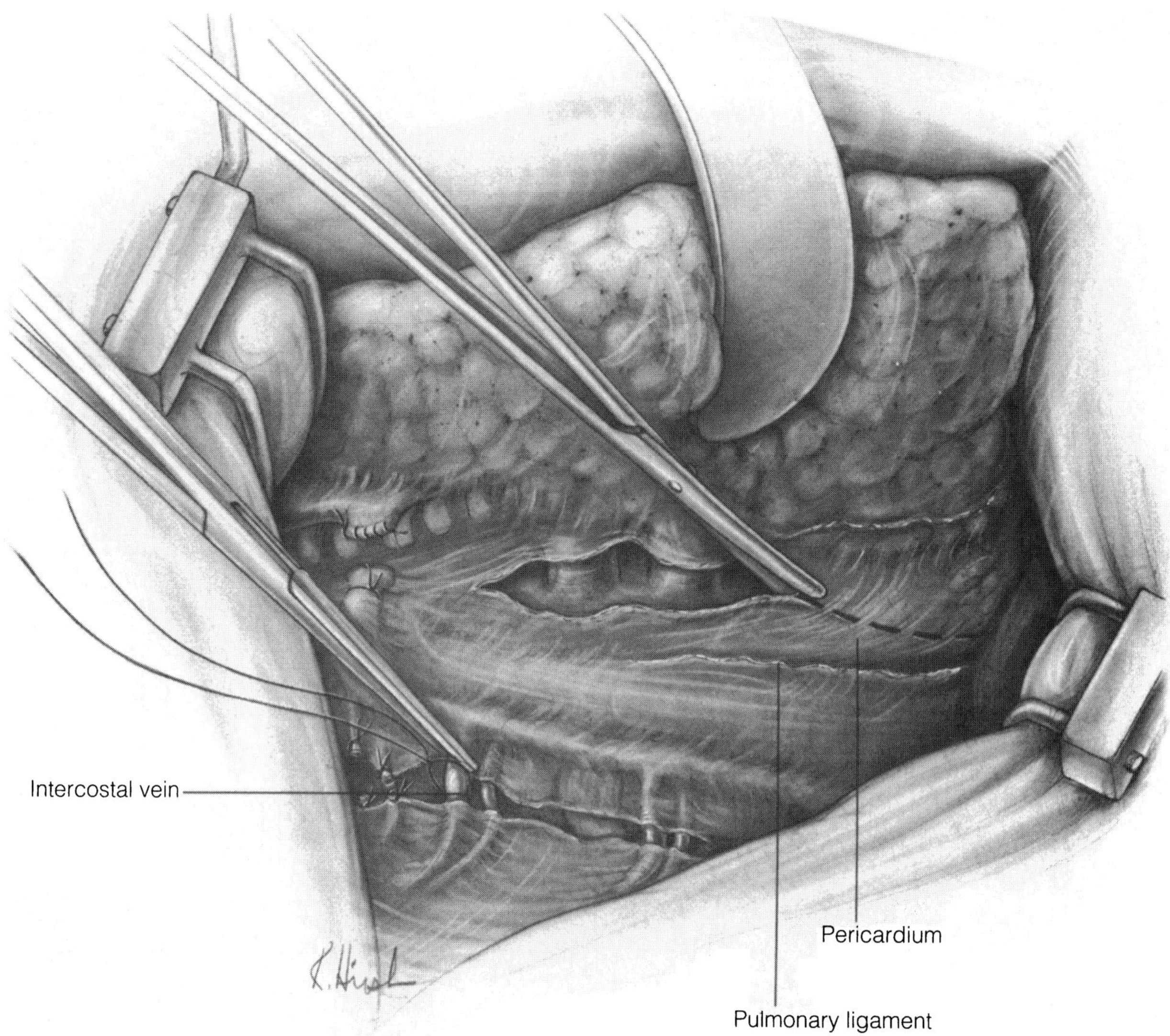

FIGURE 57–2 ■ For a middle third tumor, en bloc resection is done through a right thoracotomy. The tissues surrounding the esophagus are elevated from the vertebral body, and the pericardium is incised beginning on the superior pulmonary vein. (From Skinner DB [ed]: In Atlas of Esophageal Surgery. New York, Churchill Livingstone, 1991, p 33.)

vein. As the tissues are elevated anterior to the azygos vein, the dissection is carried across the mediastinum to the descending thoracic aorta. At the caudal end of this dissection, the thoracic duct is identified and ligated as it enters the mediastinum through the aortic hiatus of the diaphragm. Superiorly, both the azygos vein and the thoracic duct are divided at the level of the arch of the aorta.

In the superior mediastinum, the pleura is incised anteriorly at the tracheoesophageal groove. Particular care is taken to preserve the recurrent laryngeal nerves. The dissection continues down the tracheoesophageal groove, separating the esophagus from the membranous trachea, from the thoracic inlet to the carina. The arch of the azygos vein is divided flush with the superior vena cava and oversewn. The subcarinal lymph nodes are dissected toward the esophagus to expose the back of the pericardium. The pericardium is entered through its sleeve onto the superior pulmonary vein. The pericardium is incised caudally from the superior vein across the sleeve on the inferior vein and down to the level of the diaphragm (Fig. 57–3). The pericardium is then incised transversely at its cephalic extent to bring the incision to the sleeves extending onto the left pulmonary veins.

The surgeon completes the incision of an oval of pericardium by extending the pericardial incision on the left side distally and parallel to the incision onto the left pulmonary veins to the diaphragm. This step frees the entire specimen anteriorly. Several bronchoesophageal arteries are ligated flush with the aorta; the incision is carried anteriorly in front of the aorta onto the left pleural cavity, which is now entered.

At this point, the remaining attachment of the specimen is the left pulmonary ligament. This is the veil of tissue to the left lung between the incision into the left pleura, which is achieved through the pericardial resection, and the preaortic incision into the left pleural cavity. This tissue is divided, and now the entire intrathoracic esophagus, surrounded by an envelope of adjacent

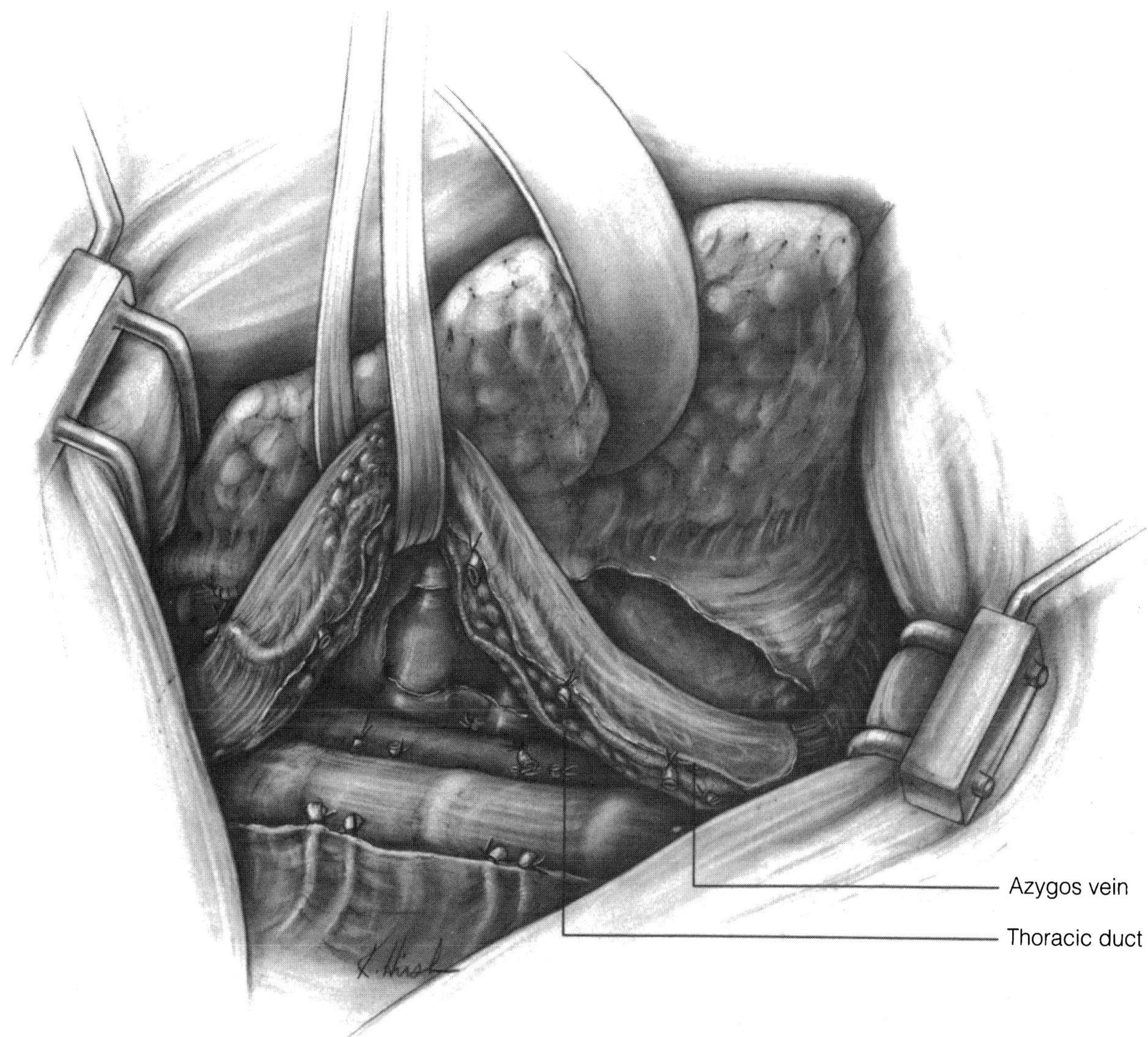

FIGURE 57–3 ■ En bloc resection of the entire midthoracic esophagus is complete. The esophagus is not seen except at the hiatus and at the base of the neck. All surrounding tissues, including azygos vein and thoracic duct with overlying pleura from both chests and pericardium, are part of the specimen. (From Skinner DB [ed]: In Atlas of Esophageal Surgery. New York, Churchill Livingstone, 1991, p 35.)

tissue, is ready for resection and removal. Except for the attachment of the esophagus to the membranous part of the trachea, the esophagus is not seen at any point throughout the dissection. The completely mobilized specimen is left in situ, and the thoracotomy is closed.

The patient is now repositioned for the next stage of the operation. The upper abdomen is opened, and a celiac, splenic, and hepatic lymph node dissection is done. The left gastric artery is divided at its origin from the celiac trunk. The neck is now opened through a low collar incision, and the previously mobilized esophagus is delivered into the wound and transected. The specimen is retrieved through the hiatus and transected distally. The distal transection line extends from the fundus of the stomach to the fourth branch of the left gastric artery. This step preserves the full length of the stomach for advancement into the neck if it is desired for reconstruction. Alternatively, and less frequently, a long segment of isoperistaltic left and transverse colon based on the ascending branches of the left colic artery can be prepared for advancement to the neck.

After the abdominal lymph node dissection is completed, the organ for reconstruction is advanced for anastomosis into the neck. This advancement can be achieved through either the substernal or the posterior mediastinal routes; the latter is the more direct and preferred approach. A single-layer, hand-sewn anastomosis is performed to the esophagus in the neck. The cervical and abdominal wounds are closed without drainage.

For carcinoma of the upper third of the esophagus, the curative approach begins with a right fifth interspace thoracotomy. After the surgeon has separated the tumor-bearing esophagus from the membranous trachea, the upper mediastinal nodes are dissected and an en bloc resection of the middle and lower mediastinum is carried out. Subsequently, a laparotomy is performed to prepare the esophageal substitute and advance it to the neck for the anastomosis.

Postoperative Care

Patients undergoing en bloc esophagectomy are routinely admitted to the intensive care unit for respiratory support for 24 to 48 hours. The removal of the thoracic duct and the mediastinal lymphatics leads to impressive sequestration of extracellular fluid and lymph and must be treated by aggressive fluid replacement during the first 48 hours after surgery. Pulmonary-lymphatic congestion is expected. Following congestion, a spontaneous diuresis heralds the mobilization of the extracellular fluid and intravenous fluid replacement must be cut back to maintenance levels to avoid the possibility of circulatory overload. After 3 to 5 days, the hemodynamic and fluid shifts are stabilized. The chest tubes should be left in place until the drainage is less than 200 ml/day.

Following en bloc resection and reconstruction with a colon or stomach, the patient is maintained without oral intake for 4 to 5 days. Clear liquids are started by mouth and, if tolerated for 24 hours, a barium swallow study is performed to confirm healing of the digestive tract anastomoses. The diet may then be advanced.

In addition to the possibility of an anastomotic leak, which occurs in approximately 10% of patients, other technical concerns exist, including ischemia or necrosis of the esophageal substitute. Lymphatic leak, or chylothorax, occurs in fewer than 1% of patients. Because the thoracic duct is ligated at the time of the initial procedure, there is almost never a need for reoperation, and most leaks cease with conservative management. If persistent, a chylothorax can be managed by a pleuroperitoneal shunt (Little et al, 1988).

Clinically evident cardiac arrhythmias occur in approximately 10% of patients following mediastinal dissection and are treated medically by means of close monitoring. Subcutaneous heparin is given preoperatively and during the recovery period to reduce the risks of venous thrombosis and pulmonary embolism. In an uncomplicated case, the patient spends 3 days in an intensive care unit and will be discharged from the hospital on a soft diet in 7 to 10 days. Complications that occur in approximately 50% of patients may prolong the intensive care or hospital stay, so that the average hospital duration in patients treated by en bloc esophagectomy is approximately 14 days.

Results

Over the past decade, 100 patients underwent en bloc resection for cancer of the thoracic esophagus at the Weill-Cornell Medical College. In-hospital mortality was 5%, whereas nonfatal complications occurred in 49% of patients. The principal morbidity was pulmonary and occurred in 27% of patients. Clinically detectable cardiac arrhythmias developed in 11% of patients, none of which were hemodynamically important. Anastomotic leaks developed in 12%, and all healed with simple drainage.

Overall survival, including operative mortality and non–cancer-related deaths, was 40% at 5 years. Survival by stage is shown in Table 57–1. Five-year survival for node-negative patients was 75% and was reduced to 25% in patients with nodal metastases. Tumor recurrence within the dissected fields (mediastinum or upper abdomen) or at the anastomosis was found in 8% of patients. This local recurrence rate compares favorably with the reported 25% to 40% local recurrence rate following less extensive resections (Kelsen et al, 1998).

TABLE 57–1 ■ En Bloc Resection: Survival by Stage

Stage	*n**	*Five-Year Survival*	*Median*
I	22	78%	n.r.
IIA	19	72%	n.r.
IIB	7	0%	30 mo
III	35	39%	53 mo
IVA	23	27%	20 mo

*Excluding operative mortality.
n.r., not reached.

Additional Therapy

At present, we do not recommend that patients receive preoperative therapy except in the context of a clinical trial. This view is supported by the results of several randomized trials that compared preoperative chemotherapy and preoperative chemoradiation with surgical resection alone. The bulk of the evidence from these studies shows that there is little added benefit beyond that achieved by surgical resection alone. Patients who are found to be node-negative following an R-O resection are not offered any postoperative therapy. Similarly, we do not recommend that postoperative chemotherapy be given to patients found to have nodal metastases if an R-O resection has been performed. Furthermore, because the local recurrence rate following en bloc resection is less than 10%, there appears to be little need for postoperative radiation therapy.

It is likely that the controversy about the surgical treatment of esophageal cancer will persist. Because staging depends on the amount of tissue removed for pathologic examination, it is not possible to have a precise comparison of competing therapies based on pathologic staging, and yet pathological staging is the principal determinant of long-term survival. Nonetheless, it appears unlikely that 5-year survival rates in the 40% range can be achieved using standard techniques of surgical resection. Further improvements in survival must probably await the advent of innovative and more effective adjuvant strategies.

COMMENTS AND CONTROVERSIES

This chapter describes, in clear detail, the en bloc resection for esophageal carcinoma currently employed by the authors. As they have indicated, the role of this type of radical resection remains controversial. Nonetheless, the results achieved to date are encouraging, and the application of this extensive procedure with an overall operative mortality of 5% is laudable.

As noted in previous commentaries, the use of positron emission tomography (PET) scanning for preoperative detection of metastatic esophageal carcinoma is rapidly gaining acceptance. In our own experience, the PET scan detects metastatic foci of esophageal cancer in 20% to 30% of patients in whom the CT scan was interpreted as showing no metastatic disease. As with any noninvasive technique, the PET scan is not infallible, and suspected metastatic foci should be confirmed pathologically before the patient is denied resection on the basis of PET scan findings alone. In this regard, we have used ultrasound-guided needle biopsy of nonpalpable, PET-positive supraclavicular nodes to confirm the presence of metastatic tumor detected by the PET scan.

Although the presumed advantages of the radical resection proposed by the authors remain unproven, the disadvantages of this approach are apparent for tumors in the distal esophagus or at the esophagogastric junction. The authors recommend more radical resection of stomach than is commonly employed and therefore require a colon interposition as the replacement conduit. Certainly, this adds risk, complexity, and a less satisfactory long-term functional outcome than the more commonly applied operation of total esophagectomy and a lesser degree of gastric resection, such that the remaining stomach can be brought safely to the neck for anastomosis.

The authors acknowledge the increased morbidity following this procedure, and this is reflected in a stay in the intensive care unit of 48 to 72 hours, an average mechanical respiratory support of 48 hours, and an average hospital stay of 14 days.

The authors do not recommend neoadjuvant therapy for most cases of esophageal carcinoma; indeed, convincing evidence for the benefit of such neoadjuvant therapy is currently lacking. Nonetheless, there is a definitely increasing, widespread trend to employ neoadjuvant chemotherapy and radiation therapy prior to esophageal resection for carcinoma. Ordinarily, such neoadjuvant therapy is well tolerated and does not appear to increase operative morbidity or mortality. However, such may not be the case should neoadjuvant therapy be employed prior to the resection described in this chapter, which, as noted carries increased inherent morbidity to begin with. In my own opinion, the authors have done a great service by pushing the limits of surgical resection in evaluating its potential benefit. This type of procedure should be done at a limited number of centers until we have a more clear appreciation of the risk-benefit ratio. It is not yet ready for prime time.

J. D. C.

■ REFERENCES

Akiyama H: Cardinals in the regional lymph node dissection in surgery of thoracic esophageal cancer. In Siewert JR, Holscher AH (eds): Disease of the Esophagus. Berlin, Springer-Verlag, 1988, p 416.

Akiyama H: Surgery for Cancer of the Esophagus. Baltimore, Williams and Wilkins, 1990.

Akiyama H, Sato Y, Takahashi F: Immediate pharyngogastrostomy following total esophagectomy by blunt dissection. Jpn J Surg 1:225, 1971.

Altorki NK, Girardi K, Skinner DB: En bloc eosphagectomy survival for stage III esophageal cancer. J Thorac Cardiovasc Surg 114:948, 1997.

Altorki NK, Skinner DB: The curative treatment of esophageal cancer. In Simmons RL, Udekwa AO (eds): Debates in Clinical Surgery. Chicago, Year Book Medical Publishers, 1990, p 167.

American Joint Committee on Cancer: Manual for Staging Cancer, 4th, ed. Philadelphia, JB Lippincott, 1992, p 57.

DeMeester TR, Zaninotto G, Johansson KE: Selective therapeutic approach to cancer of the lower esophagus and cardia. J Thorac Cardiovasc Surg 95:42, 1988.

Hagen JA, Peters JH, DeMeester TR: Superiority of extended en bloc esophagogastrectomy for carcinoma of the lower esophagus and cardia. J Thorac Cardiovasc Surg 106:850, 1993.

Hiebert C, Belsey RHR: Exclusive right approach to carcinoma of the mid-third of the esophagus. Ann Thorac Surg 18:1, 1974.

International Union Against Cancer: TNM Classification of Malignant Tumors, 4th, ed. Berlin, Springer-Verlag, 1987.

Japanese Committee for the Registration of Esophageal Carcinoma: A proposal for a new TNM classification of esophageal carcinoma. Jpn J Clin Oncol 19:625, 1985.

Kelsen DP, Ginsberg R, Pajak TF, et al: Chemotherapy followed by surgery compared with surgery alone for localized esophageal cancer. N Engl J Med 339:1979, 1998.

Lehr L, Rupp N, Siewert JR: Assessment of resectability of esophageal cancer by computed tomography and magnetic resonance imaging. Surgery 103:344, 1988.

Lerut T, Coosemans W, Van Raemdonck D, et al: Surgical treatment of Barrett carcinoma: Correlations between morphologic findings and prognosis. J Thorac Cardiovasc Surg 107:1059, 1994.

Lerut T, De Leyn P, Coosemans W, et al: Surgical strategies in esophageal carcinoma, with emphasis on radical lymphadenectomy. Ann Surg 216:583, 1992.

Little AG, Kadowaki MH, Ferguson MK, et al: Pleuroperitoneal shunting: Alternative therapy for pleural effusions. Ann Surg 208:443, 1988.

Logan A: The surgical treatment of carcinoma of the esophagus and cardia. J Thorac Cardiovasc Surg 46:150, 1963.

Orringer MB, Sloan H: Esophagectomy without thoracotomy. J Thorac Cardiovasc Surg 76:643, 1978.

Perachia A, Ruol A, Bardini R, et al: Lymph node dissection for cancer of the thoracic esophagus: How extended should it be? Dis Esoph 5:69, 1992.

Sannohe Y, Hiratsuka R, Doki K: Lymph node metastases in cancer of the thoracic esophagus. Am J Surg 141:216, 1981.

Siewert JR, Holscher AH, Roder JD, Bartels H: En bloc resektion der speiserohre beim Oesophaguscarcinom. Langenbecks Arch Chir 373:367, 1988.

Siewert JR, Roder JD: Lymphadenectomy in esophageal cancer surgery. Dis Esoph 5:91.

Skinner DB (ed): Atlas of Esophageal Surgery. New York, Churchill Livingstone, 1991.

Skinner DB: En bloc resection for neoplasm of the esophagus and cardia. J Thorac Cardiovasc Surg 85:59, 1983.

Skinner DB, Dowlatshahi KD, DeMeester TR: Potentially curable cancer of the esophagus. Cancer 50:2571, 1982.

Skinner DB, Little AG, Ferguson MK, et al: Selection of operation for esophageal cancer based on staging. Ann Surg 204:391, 1986.

Sugimachi K, Ohno S, Fujishiwa H, et al: Endoscopic ultrasonographic detection of carcinomatous invasion and of lymph nodes in the thoracic esophagus. Surgery 107:366, 1990.

Tanabe G, Baba M, Kuroshima K, et al: Clinical evaluation of esophageal lymph flow system based on the RI uptake of removed regional lymph nodes following lymphoscintigraphy. J Jpn Surg Soc 87:315, 1986.

CHAPTER **58**

Three-Field Lymph Node Dissection for Cancer of the Esophagus

Nasser K. Altorki

Toni Lerut

BACKGROUND

The concept of three-field lymph node dissection for carcinoma of the esophagus was introduced and practiced by Japanese surgeons since the early 1980s. This development was prompted by studies showing that the cervical lymph nodes were the site of tumor recurrence in 30% to 40% of patients in whom a curative resection had been performed (Isono et al, 1985). The extended procedure included dissection of the cervical, mediastinal and upper abdominal nodes in patients with carcinoma of the thoracic and abdominal esophagus. In 1991, Isono reported the results of a nationwide study on three-field dissection performed at 35 institutions throughout Japan. Nearly 1800 patients underwent esophagectomy with three-field lymph node dissection, whereas 2800 underwent two-field dissection. The following important observations were made:

1. Approximately, one third of patients had previously unsuspected metastasis to the cervical lymph nodes. The prevalence of cervical nodal metastases was highest for upper-third tumors (40%), but even patients with lower-third cancers had a 20% probability of metastatic carcinoma involving the cervical lymph nodes.
2. The frequency of nodal metastases increased with increasing depths of tumor penetration through the esophageal wall. Patients with intramucosal carcinoma had a 30% probability of nodal metastasis, whereas invasion into the submucosa, muscularis propria, and adventitia signaled a 50%, 60%, and 80% probability of nodal disease, respectively. Interestingly, a statistically higher prevalence of nodal metastases was observed after three-field lymph node dissection in patients with T1 and T2 tumors but not in patients with more advanced disease. This observation should cast some doubt on the logic of "limited disease = limited operation."
3. The cervical lymph nodes most frequently involved with metastatic carcinoma include the nodal chain along both recurrent nerves as well as the deep cervical nodes along the posterior aspect of the internal jugular vein. Supraclavicular nodal disease was infrequent and carried a distinctly poor outcome.

In light of these observations, it is clear that a large number of patients will be inaccurately staged after en bloc resection with isolated mediastinal and abdominal lymphadenectomy. Approximately a third of patients will have their tumor-node-metastasis (TNM) classification upstaged as a result of the extended procedure. Although most surgeons readily concede the impact of the extended lymphadenectomy on the tumor staging, its impact on survival is fervently disputed. Nonetheless, Japanese surgeons have provided a compelling argument for a positive impact on survival.

Akiyama and colleagues (1984) reported their experience with 717 patients in whom a complete (R-0) resection was performed using either a two-field (n = 393) or a three-field technique (n = 324). Five-year survival in node-negative patients was 84% after the three-field procedure compared to 55% after two-field lymphadenectomy (*P* = .004). Patients with node-positive disease also fared better after three-field dissection with a 5-year survival rate of 43% compared to a 28% 5-year survival rate after two-field dissection (*P* = .0008). The superior 5-year survival in node-positive patients clearly disposes of the argument that the improved survival rates are a function of simple stage migration. Similar results have been reported by a number of Japanese surgeons (Baba et al, 1994; Kato et al, 1991; Nishimaki et al, 1994). Significantly, most studies report a 5-year survival of 25% to 30% in patients with positive cervical lymph nodes. These impressive survival rates seem to argue that the recurrent laryngeal nodes should be considered a regional (N1) rather than distant site of disease for tumors of the intrathoracic and abdominal esophagus. Support for this notion is also suggested by data obtained from lymphoscintigraphy studies where a radiolabeled colloid is injected in the midthoracic esophagus (Aikou and Shimazu, 1989; Tanabe et al, 1986). Uptake was routinely detected by scintillation counting in the upper mediastinum and cervical nodes as well as in the left gastric nodes.

Despite these intriguing results reported by Japanese surgeons, most European and North American centers have greeted three-field dissection with skepticism. Several reasons might explain the lack of enthusiasm for the procedure:

1. A prevailing concept among Western surgeons is that patients with carcinoma of the esophagus have systemic disease at the time of presentation. Cure following

resection has often been considered a "chance phenomenon" that is dependent more on the biologic behavior of the tumor rather than the surgical strategy pursued.

2. Three-field lymph node dissection has been associated with a definite, albeit a statistically insignificant, increase in hospital morbidity. Foremost among the potential complications is injury to one or both recurrent nerves. Recurrent nerve injury has been reported in up to 50% of patients and in at least some patients has resulted in tracheostomy and prolonged mechanical ventilation. Furthermore, at least one study (Baba et al, 1998) examined the quality of life following esophagectomy with three-field lymph node dissection with particular emphasis on the effect of vocal cord paralysis. Twenty percent of patients reported severe hoarseness, restricted food intake, and reduced exercise tolerance up to 60 months postoperatively.

3. Notwithstanding the compelling data from Japan, nearly all were the result of retrospective studies that compared surgical therapy delivered over two different decades. Two randomized studies have been reported (Kato et al, 1991; Nishihira et al, 1998). The study by Nishihira showed no significant difference in survival between three-field and two-field lymph node dissection (65% versus 48%; $P = .1$). The study from the National Cancer Institute showed that 5-year survival was significantly better after three-field dissection (48% versus 33%; $P = .03$). Five-year survival in the group of patients with cervical nodal disease was an impressive 30%.

THE WESTERN EXPERIENCE

Esophagectomy with three-field lymph node dissection has been practiced at Cornell Medical College in New York since 1994 and at the University of Leuven since 1992. A prospective data base was established at both institutions to assess the feasibility of the procedure as well as to study the patterns of nodal metastasis and ultimate survival in a European and North American patient population. Particular emphasis was made to assess these criteria in adenocarcinoma of the esophagus, a disease rapidly increasing in incidence on both continents.

Patients were considered eligible for the procedure if the entire tumor was located within the tubular esophagus and there was no preoperative or intraoperative evidence of distant organ metastasis or confirmation of T4 disease. Additionally, the group at the University of Leuven evaluated the role of the procedure in patients with tumors of the gastroesophageal junction that extended aborally into the gastric cardia. Patients were carefully evaluated to assess their ability to undergo esophageal resection including a full pulmonary and cardiologic evaluation.

Advanced age by itself was not a contraindication to operation, although patients older than 75 years of age were often treated by en bloc two-field dissection. Computed tomography (CT) endoscopic ultrasonography, and more recently positron emission tomography (PET) were used to assess the extent of disease.

Surgical Procedure

The surgical approach is generally determined by the preference of the surgeon. A fifth interspace right thoracotomy is preferred by one of us (N.A.) for all tumors regardless of location. An alternative approach used at the University of Leuven is to perform an extended left thoracotomy for all tumors below the carina and tumors of the gastroesophageal junction. This sixth interspace thoractomy provides excellent access to the middle and lower mediastinum. A semilunar peripheral diaphragmatic incision provides excellent exposure of the upper abdomen. The peritoneum is incised, and the spleen, tail, and body of the pancreas are reflected medially. Dissection of the upper abdominal compartment commences at the level of the descending thoracic aorta and proceeds toward the celiac axis; to the superior mesenteric artery; and, in cases of gastroesophageal junction tumors, to the left renal vein and artery. This dissection clears all the lymphatics in the upper abdomen and extends medially to the nodal tissue along the common hepatic and splenic arteries.

In the chest, a posterior mediastinectomy is performed, including the thoracic duct and the nodes in the subcarinal region, the aortopulmonary window and along the main stem bronchi. Following resection of the specimen and advancement of the gastric tube to the neck, the thoracotomy is closed and the patient is repositioned. A U-shaped incision is made in the neck along with a manubrial split to access the lower neck and superior mediastinum. This third field of dissection includes the nodes lateral and posterior to the carotid sheath, the brachiocephalic nodes, and the supraclavicular nodes as well as dissection of the nodes along both recurrent nerves (Fig. 58–1).

When the operation is done through a right thoracotomy (routine at Cornell and for supracarinal lesions at Leuven), the previously described posterior mediastinectomy is initially performed up to the level of the arch of the azygos vein (Fig. 58–2). The prevertebral and retrotracheal attachments of the esophagus are divided and the organ mobilized to the neck. The left recurrent nerve is exposed near its origin at the level of the aortic arch and dissected to the thoracic inlet, thus allowing a left paratracheal node dissection. Finally, the right recurrent nerve is exposed as it loops around the right subclavian artery and the adjoining chain of nodes dissected well into the neck.

Although the recurrent laryngeal nodes are thought to have a cervical and superior mediastinal component, we believe that such distinction is arbitrary because the nodes form a contiguous group extending from the mediastinum to the neck. In fact, it is often possible to complete the dissection of these nodal groups well into the neck through the chest incision. The thoracotomy is closed, and a cervical and abdominal incision accomplish the abdominal and cervical nodal dissections previously described.

Postoperative Care

At the University of Leuven, patients are routinely admitted to the recovery room, where they are extubated in

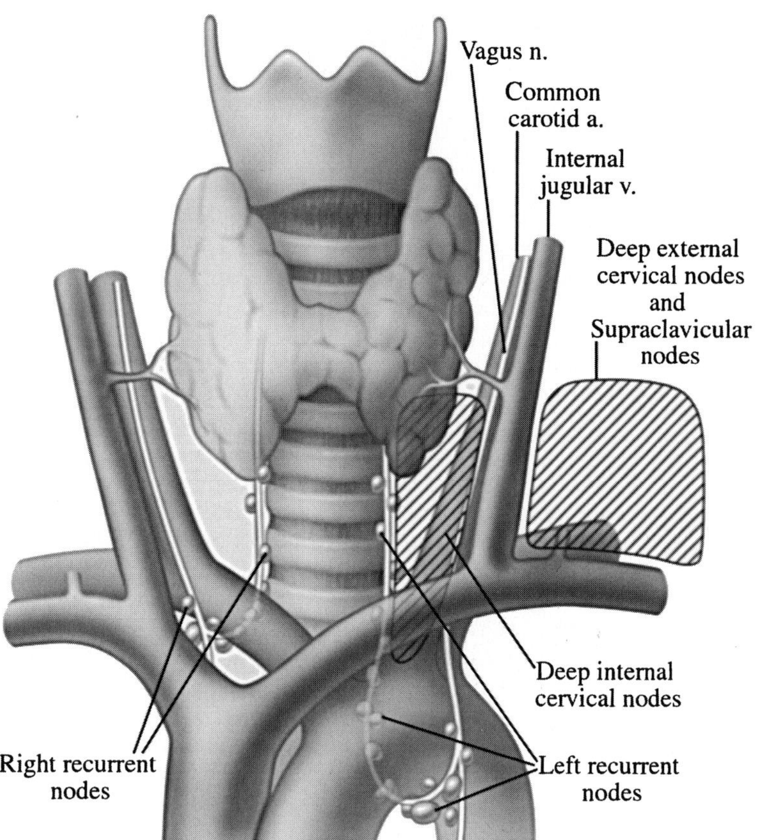

FIGURE 58–1 ■ Schematic representation of a view from a cervical incision combined with a partial sternal split for a three-field dissection.

the hours immediately after the operation. A mini-tracheostomy is routinely done at the end of the operation to facilitate extubation. Only at Cornell, patients are routinely admitted to the intensive care unit and receive mechanical ventilation for 24 to 48 hours. Following extubation, close attention is paid to bronchopulmonary hygiene, including bronchoscopy, if necessary, since bronchorrhea is commonly encountered. Patients are generally able to clear their own secretions by the 5th or 6th postoperative day in the absence of vocal cord palsy. Oral intake of liquids is usually begun on the 5th postoperative day and advanced to a general diet when the integrity of the anastomosis has been ascertained by a barium study. Hospital morbidity and mortality rates are shown in Table 58–1.

Patterns of Nodal Spread

A total of 69 patients with carcinoma of the esophagus were treated with esophagectomy and three-field dissection at Cornell Medical College (Altorki and Skinner 1997) and University of Leuven (Lerut et al, 1999). An average of 60 nodes were resected per case. Nodal metastasis was found in more than 70% of patients at both institutions. The most commonly affected nodal groups were, in order of frequency, the lesser curvature nodes, parahiatal nodes, and the recurrent nodes (Table 58–2). The prevalence of cervical nodal metastasis was essentially identical in both series and not dissimilar from the previously reported data from Japan. In the combined series, there were 32 patients with esophageal adenocarcinoma located mostly in the distal third. Ten patients (30%) had otherwise unsuspected metastases to the lymph nodes along the recurrent chain. The frequency of cervical nodal metastasis in patients with squamous cell

TABLE 58–1 ■ **Morbidity and Mortality of Three-Field Lymph Node Dissection**

	Cornell (n = 30)	*Leuven (n = 39)*
Operative mortality	1 (3.3%)	0
Pulmonary complications	11/30 (30%)	11/39 (28%)
Anastomotic leaks	6/30 (20%)	1/39 (2.5%)
Recurrent nerve injury	2/30 (6%)	2/39 (5%)
Infection complications	1/30 (3%)	5/39 (13%)

TABLE 58–2 ■ **Patterns of Nodal Spread**

	Cornell (n = 30)	*Leuven (n = 39)*
Resected nodes per patient	60	59
Patients with positive nodes (%)	70	78
Common sites of spread		
Left gastric nodes	57%	58%
Parahiatal nodes	42%	67%
Recurrent nodes	30%	28%
Squamous cell carcinoma with positive neck nodes	40% (6/15)	22% (5/22)
Adenocarcinoma with positive neck nodes	26% (4/15)	35% (6/17)

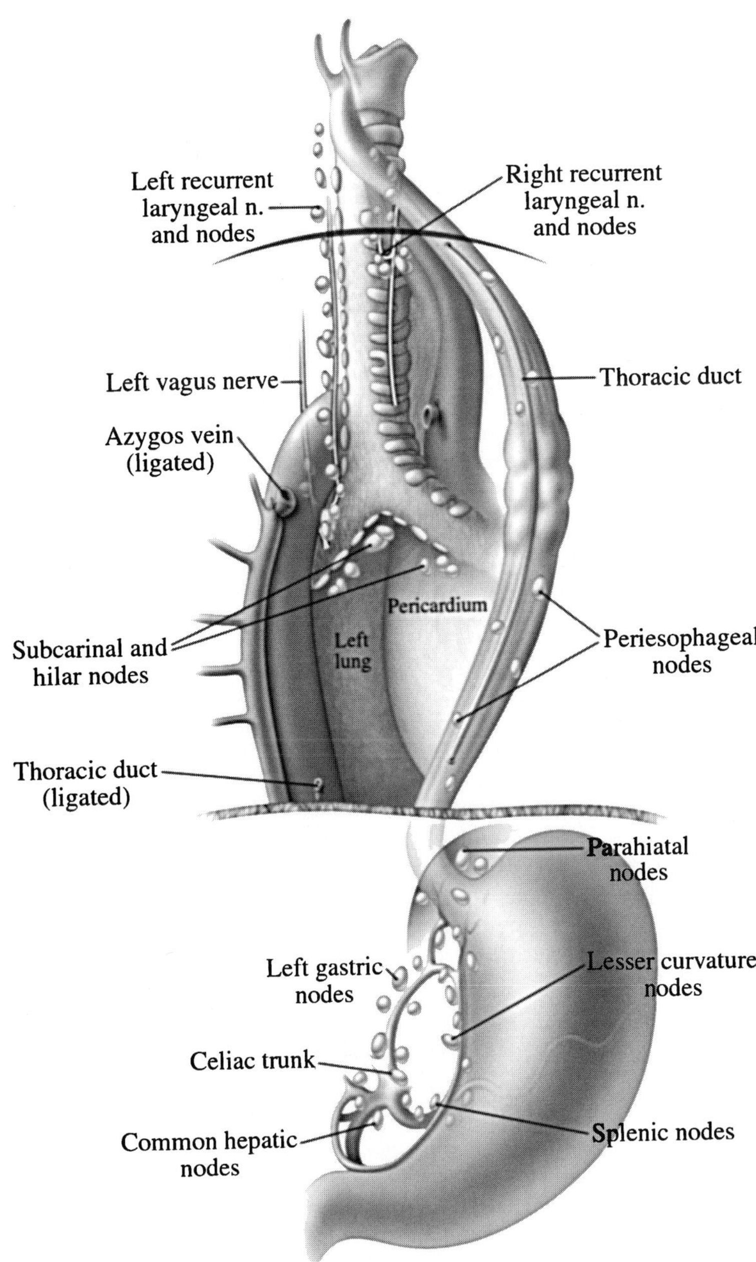

FIGURE 58–2 ■ The various nodal stations dissected through a right thoracotomy and laparotomy for a three-field node dissection. Further dissection is performed through a cervical incision.

carcinoma was nearly 30% (11/37). Overall, 16 of 69 patients (24%) were upstaged as a result of addition of the third field of dissection.

These data indicate that 30% of patients who undergo an en bloc two-field lymph node dissection would not be rendered disease-free at the conclusion of the operative procedure. Although the impact of three-field lymph node dissection on survival remains unproven, it seems difficult to construct a rational argument for an isolated two-field dissection that relegates 30% of the patients to an incomplete resection. There is overwhelming evidence that the ability to perform a complete (R-0) resection is an important determinant of survival. Furthermore, these findings shed some doubt on the significance of results obtained from various preoperative therapy trials. Indeed, the lack of a survival benefit in the combined therapy arm, reported by most of these studies, may be a function of an incomplete surgical resection rather than the result of an ineffective chemotherapy regimen.

Survival

Cornell Medical College

Thirty patients were treated with an esophagectomy and three-field lymph node dissection between August 1994 and July 1996. As of this writing, 14 patients (46%) are alive with minimum follow-up of 3 years; 13 are disease-free, and one is alive with stable metastasis to the thoracic vertebra. The survival for node-negative patients is 77% (7/9), whereas 7 of 21 (33%) node-positive patients are alive without evidence of disease recurrence. There appears to be no important difference in survival based on cell type. Nine out of 15 patients with adenocarcinoma and 5 of 15 with squamous cell cancer are alive. Interestingly, among 10 patients previously reported to have had metastasis to the cervical lymph node, 3 are alive without evidence of recurrent disease at 5 years, 5 years, and 3.5 years postoperatively. Twelve patients died of recurrent disease. Disease recurrence was at distant sites in 10 patients, local in 1 patient (mediastinal recurrence), and both local and distant in 1 patient (neck nodes and bones).

University of Leuven

Esophagectomy with three-field lymph node dissection was performed in 38 patients for whom a complete follow-up of 5 years is available. Overall, 3- and 5-year survival rates were 45% and 37%, respectively. Among eight patients without nodal metastases, six are alive (75%). Five-year survival for 30 patients with node-positive disease was 27%. Patients who had stage IV disease, based on distant nodal metastasis, had a 5-year survival of 20%.

CONCLUSION

Our combined experience suggests that three-field lymph node dissection for carcinoma of the esophagus can be performed with reasonably low mortality and morbidity. The procedure is technically demanding, and the surgeon must take great care in dissection of the recurrent nerves to avoid injury to these vulnerable structures. Our data regarding nodal metastasis are essentially identical to those reported by Japanese surgeons. The eventual impact on survival of this extended procedure remains to be determined, but preliminary results seem encouraging.

COMMENTS AND CONTROVERSIES

Drs. Altorki and Lerut have presented a balanced, thought-provoking review regarding the potential value of radical esophagectomy and lymph node dissection for carcinoma of the esophagus. The high percentage of unsuspected cervical lymph node metastasis even for lower esophageal tumors is important information, as is the upstaging, which occurs in a significant number of patients as a result of this procedure. The authors' own series are remarkable for the low operative mortality associated with the dissection.

As the authors suggest, there is no convincing evidence to date that radiacal resection improves outcome. No comment is made regarding the use of adjuvant therapies or whether the indication for such adjuvant therapies is altered by the postoperative staging resulting from the radical dissection. The indications for radical dissection also remain unclear and may logically be influenced by endoscopic ultrasound evaluation of tumor depth.

The Japanese experience cited by the authors suggests that a presence of positive cervical lymph nodes does not carry with it the ominous prognosis most of us assoicate with such a finding. It will be interesting to see how the increasing use of PET scanning, with its increased sensitivity to detect nodal metastases, influences the application of radical lymph node dissection. When previously unsuspected cervical lymph node metastases are identified on a preoperative PET scan, it is our practice to consider such patients inoperable. A randomized trial incorporating radical sugical resection in one arem and no surgery in the other arm would help determine the appropriate treatment for this group of patients.

J. D. C.

■ REFERENCES

Aikou T, Shimazu H: Difference in main lymphatic pathways from the lower esophagus and gastric cardia. Jpn J Surg 19:290–295, 1989.

Akiyama H, Tsurumaru M, Udagawa H, Kajiyama Y: Radical lymph node dissection for cancer of the thoracic esophagus. Ann Surg 220:364–373, 1994.

Altorki NK, Skinner DB: Occult cervical nodal metastasis in esophageal cancer: preliminary results of three-field lymphadenectomy. J Thorac Cardiovasc Surg 113:540–544, 1997.

Baba M, Aikou T, Yoshinaka H, et al: Long-term results of subtotal esophagectomy with three-field lymphadenectomy for carcinoma of the thoracic esophagus. Ann Surg 219:310–316, 1994.

Baba M, Aikou T, Natsugoe S, et al: H: Quality of life following esophagectomy with three-field lymphadenectomy for carcinoma, focusing on its relationship to vocal cord palsy. Dis Esoph 11:28–34, 1998.

Isono K, Onoda S, Okuyarna K, et al: Recurrence of intrathoracic esophageal cancer. Jpn J Clin Oncol 15:49–60, 1985.

Isono K, Sato H, Nakayama K: Results of a nationwide study on the three-field lymph node dissection of esophageal cancer. Oncology 48:411–420, 1991.

Kato H, Watanabe H, Tachimori Y, Iizuka T: Evaluation of the neck lymph node dissection for thoracic esophageal carcinoma. Ann Thorac Surg 51:931–935, 1991.

Lerut T, Coosemans W, De Leyn P, et al: Reflections on three field lymphadenectomy in carcinoma of the esophagus and gastro-esophageal junction. Hepatogastroenterology 46:717–25, 1999.

Nishihira T, Hirayama K, Mori S: A prospective randomized trial of extended cervical and superior mediastinal lymphadenectomy for carcinoma of the thoracic esophagus. Am J Surg 175:47–51, 1998.

Nishimaki T, Tanaka O, Suzuki T, et al: Patterns of lymphatic spread in thoracic esophageal cancer. Cancer 74:4–11, 1994.

Tanabe G, Baba M, Kuroshima K, et al: Clinical evaluation of esophageal lymph flow system based on the RI uptake of removal regional nodes following lymphoscintigraphy. J Jpn Surg Soc 87:315–323, 1986.

Van de Ven C, De Leyn P, et al: Three-field lymphadenectomy and pattern of lymph node spread in T3 adenocarcinoma of the distal esophagus and the gastroesophageal junction. Eur J Cardiothorac Surg 15:769–773, 1999.

CHAPTER **59**

Total Gastrectomy and Roux-en-Y Reconstruction

Hiroshi Akiyama
Harushi Udagawa

DEFINITION

Resection of the entire stomach is preferred by some surgeons for the management of selected patients with primary gastric malignancy. The operation frequently includes regional lymphadenectomy plus removal of the spleen and, if indicated, the distal half of the pancreas. The duodenal stump is closed, and gastrointestinal (GI) continuity is restored with Roux-en-Y esophagojejunostomy.

INDICATIONS

Gastrectomy (either proximal, distal, or total) is primarily indicated for patients with gastric cancer. The indications for total gastrectomy are complex. Factors that influence the choice of operation include:

- Location and extent of tumor involvement
- The need to resect other organs, such as the pancreas and spleen
- Extent of lymph node dissection

For early-stage cancer located in the cardia of the stomach, proximal gastrectomy with limited lymph node dissection in which distal pancreatectomy and even splenectomy are avoided is preferred. Regardless of the patient's status, total gastrectomy is recommended if the tumor is locally extensive or multiple (Maruyama et al, 1996).

Occasionally, the presence of concomitant lesions such as gastric ulcer may favor the selection of total gastrectomy. Even though the concomitant lesion is not malignant, it is hazardous to leave such disease in the gastric remnant. However, this situation has changed since histamine H_2-blockers and proton pump inhibitors became available, and small ulcer scars do not often influence the range of gastric resection in patients with good compliance.

Theoretically, advanced cancer that involves the proximal half of the stomach requires total gastrectomy, and at least splenectomy, when the surgeon intends to perform regional lymphadenectomy. This is particularly true for patients with cancer of the cardia. Tumor spread along the lesser curvature often influences the extent of gastric resection. Even when the tumor is well localized to the cardia, however, if it extends to the serosal layer, total gastrectomy with pancreaticosplenectomy is recommended to allow complete bursectomy. When the tumor extends to the esophagogastric junction, distal esophagectomy with inferior mediastinal lymph node dissection should be added.

Finally, when it is judged that recurrence is more likely to occur in the right epigastrium, Roux-en-Y reconstruction is preferable to jejunal interposition.

PREOPERATIVE EVALUATION AND PREPARATION

Preoperative evaluation includes both tumor staging and evaluation of the patient's general condition and operative risk. Tumor extent is evaluated with contrast esophagography, a GI series, endoscopy, conventional abdominal ultrasonography, endoscopic ultrasonography (if available), computed tomography (CT), and tumor markers. Barium enema is recommended when direct tumor invasion of the transverse colon is suspected. CT scanning of the lungs, bone scintigraphy, and cervical ultrasonography are also indicated when distant metastasis to the lungs, bone, or cervical lymph nodes is suspected. The patient's general condition and ability to withstand both laparotomy and thoracotomy should be evaluated.

OPERATIVE TECHNIQUE

Positioning the Patient

The patient is placed obliquely, between the right lateral decubitus and supine positions. Further adjustment can be made with rotation of the table as required. A rolled sponge is placed below the right subcostal area to elevate the left subcostal area for optimal exposure (Figs. 59–1 and 59–2).

Skin Incision

The skin incision is made obliquely from the epigastrium to the sixth or seventh intercostal space, depending on the location of the tumor and the patient's physical habitus. For advanced cancer, a small incision is initially made in the epigastrium to allow exploration (see Fig. 59–1, line A). As an alternative, the exploratory laparoscopy and laparoscopic ultrasonography can be performed but direct palpation is still required at times for the evaluation of resectability. Extensive metastasis that was not detected before surgery may contraindicate resection.

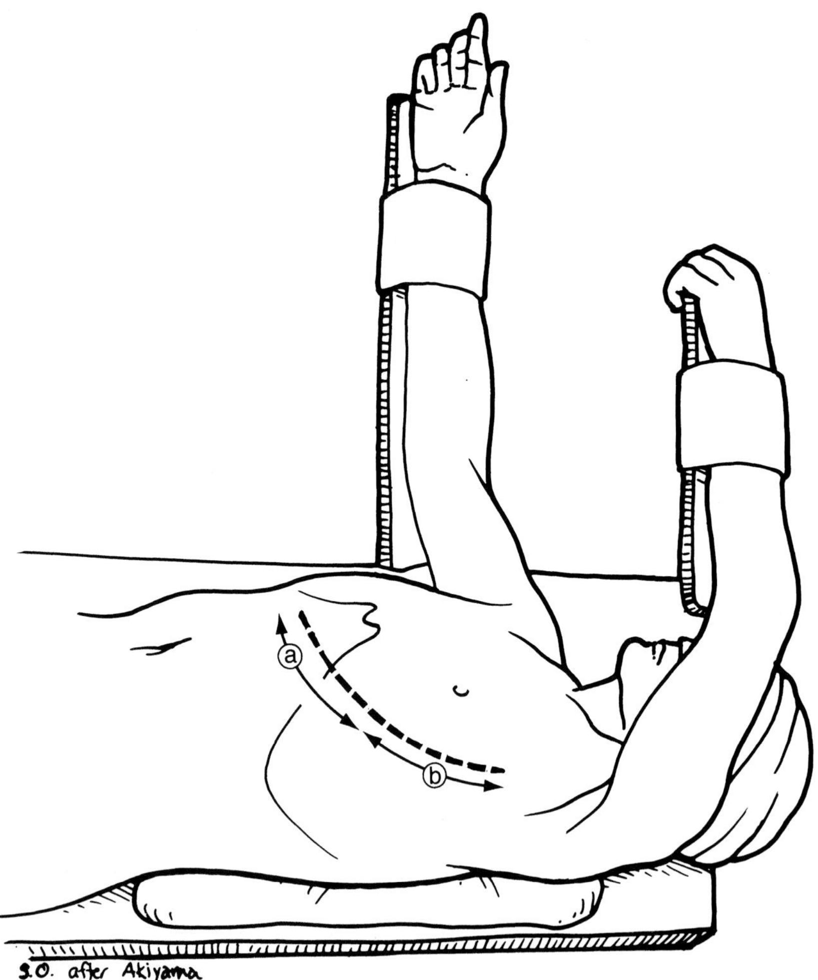

FIGURE 59–1 ■ Left thoracoabdominal approach for distal esophagectomy and total gastrectomy. Line "a" is for the initial abdominal exploration. When the tumor is resectable, the incision is extended (line "b").

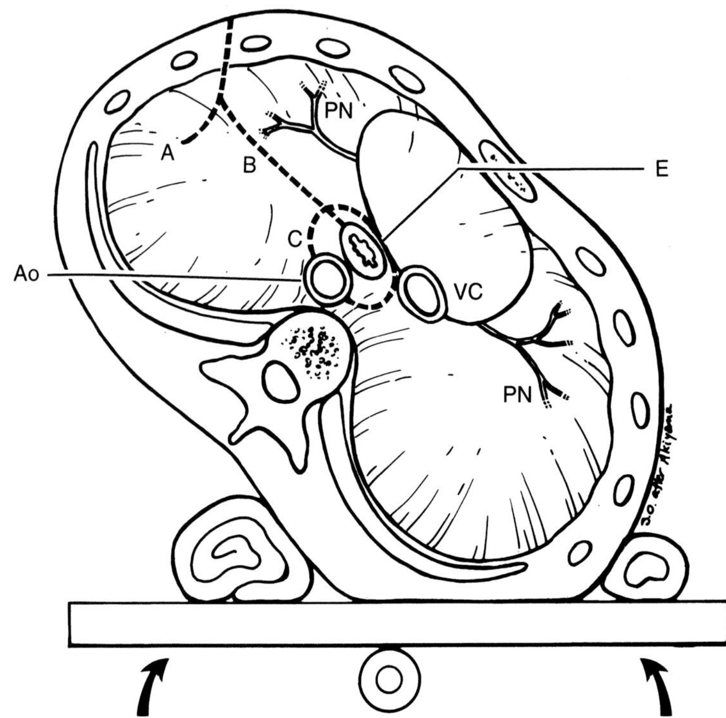

FIGURE 59–2 ■ Incision or partial resection of the diaphragm *(dotted lines)*. Position of the patient for the left and moderately advanced thoracoabdominal approach. *A,* Position for an early lesion. *B* and *C,* Position for a locally advanced lesion, which requires better exposure. *C,* Position for combined resection of the diaphragm. Rotation of the operating table is shown by two *black arrows*. (Ao, aorta; E, esophagus; PN, phrenic nerve.)

If the tumor is unresectable, the operation is terminated and the patient is spared a long thoracoabdominal incision. If the tumor is resectable, the abdominal incision is extended laterally and upward to the sixth or seventh intercostal space (see Fig. 59–1, line B). The external oblique muscle and portion of the serratus anterior muscle are exposed and divided. The underlying intercostal muscles are simultaneously exposed.

The costal cartilage between the sixth and seventh ribs is exposed at the costochondral junction and is not merely transected but resected (Fig. 59–3). Resection of this cartilage enhances surgical exposure and facilitates subsequent closure, which is made more secure and technically easier.

The surgeon opens the pleural cavity by incising the intercostal muscles along the upper border of the lower rib. Gentle retraction of the ribs is gradually performed with a self-retaining retractor while the diaphragm is being incised. A 10- to 15-cm diaphragmatic incision is sufficient for this approach. It is important that the position of the main trunk of the phrenic nerve be identified to avoid injury (Akiyama et al, 1979) (see Fig. 59–2).

To improve exposure, the cut edge of the diaphragm is temporarily sutured to the chest wall near the wound edge, thus effectively retaining the left lung inside the thoracic cavity and away from the operative field. If there is invasion of the diaphragm, the diaphragmatic incision is directed toward the esophageal hiatus and the appropriate segment of diaphragm is resected (see Fig. 59–2). The surgeon incises the full length of the diaphragm to enhance exposure by converting the pleural and abdominal cavities into one surgical field.

Resection

Extent of Serosal Invasion and Indications for Resection of the "Omental Bursa"

The serosal surface of the gastric cardia is examined for tumor invasion. If serosal invasion is apparent or suspected, the mass is wrapped with a thick, dry towel to prevent contamination of the surgical field by tumor cells during subsequent manipulation. A window is created in the greater omentum to evaluate the lesser sac. If the tumor also invades the bursa (lesser sac), the space is packed with a dry towel to prevent tumor cell contamination, and the omental window is closed. Further unnecessary manipulation of the tumor is avoided during subsequent gastrectomy and omental "bursectomy."

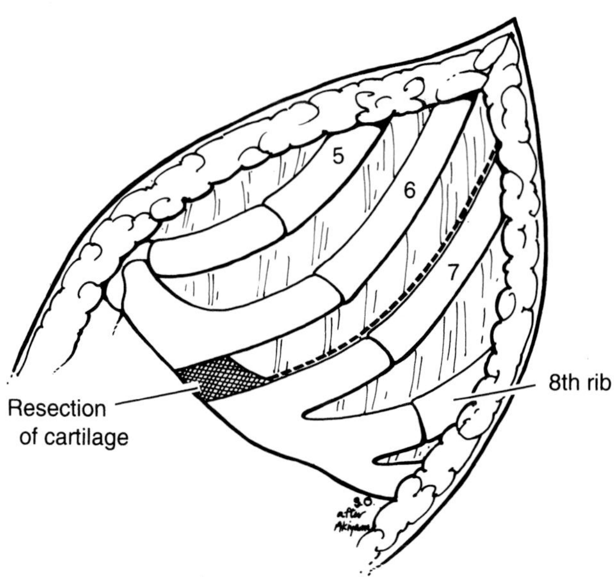

FIGURE 59–3 ■ Resection of the costal cartilage for an optimal operative field.

Freeing of the Greater Curvature and Transection of the Duodenum

The gastrocolic ligament is divided along the avascular border of the transverse colon. Dissection is continued toward the left side, and the peritoneum along the splenic flexure of the colon is incised. On the right side, the hepatic flexure of the colon is freed from the head of the pancreas. The right gastroepiploic vessels are isolated and divided at their origin. Infrapyloric lymph nodes are freed from the surface of the pancreas. The gastroduodenal artery is identified and traced to its origin from the common hepatic artery, and the regional lymph nodes at this site are identified. The right gastric artery is transected at the level of the first portion of the duodenum.

Lymph nodes from the gastric side of the divided vessels are removed together with the stomach. The distal portion of the transected right gastric artery and the lymph nodes along it are extirpated during subsequent dissection of the hepatoduodenal ligament when necessary. The duodenum is then transected. For Roux-en-Y reconstruction, the duodenal stump is stapled and closed.

When bursectomy is planned, division of the gastrocolic ligament is started near the right end of the greater omentum. The layer between the most superior leaf of the transverse mesocolon and the middle colic vessels is entered without opening the omental bursa, and with continuous dissection, the peritoneum on the pancreatic head is peeled off, starting from the gastroduodenal artery side toward the left.

Lymph Node Dissection

The lesser omentum is divided along the inferior edge of the liver up to the cardioesophageal junction. As the dissection is continued medially, lymph nodes along the common hepatic, splenic, left gastric, and celiac arteries are freed and dissected. The left gastric artery is doubly ligated and cut at its origin. The extent of lymph node dissection is indicated in Figure 59–4 (dotted line), and the frequency of metastasis in each lymph node station is shown in Table 59–1.

Pancreaticosplenectomy and Its Alternative

Resection of the distal half of the pancreas and the spleen together with the splenic vessels is the most certain way to dissect the lymph nodes along the splenic, short gastric, left gastroepiploic, and posterior gastric arteries. Bursectomy is difficult, if not impossible, without distal pancreatectomy. The drawbacks to this procedure are the risk of pancreatic fistula and decreased endocrine function of the pancreas. This procedure is definitely indi-

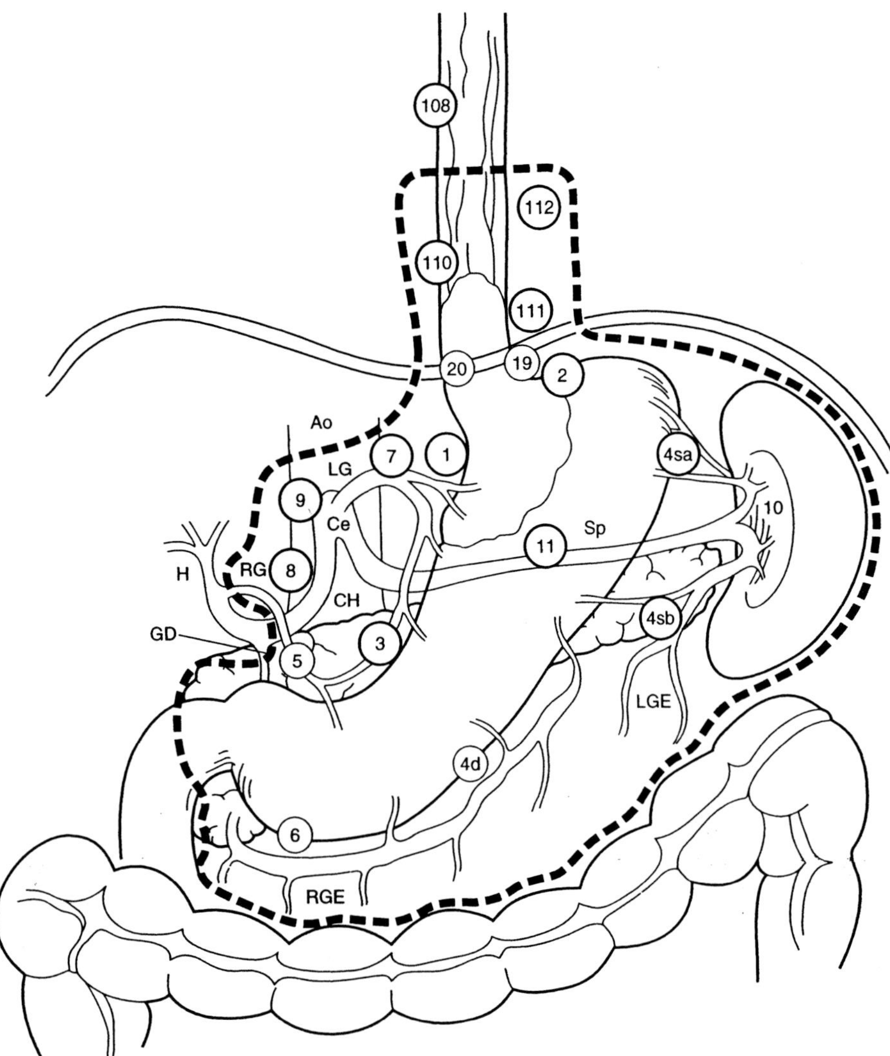

FIGURE 59–4 ■ Extent of resection and lymph node dissection. The *dotted line* represents the resection line. Numbers are explained in Table 59–1. (Ao, aorta; Ce, celiac trunk artery; CH, common hepatic artery; GD, gastroduodenal artery; H, hepatic artery; LG, left gastric artery; LGE, left gastroepiploic artery; RG, right gastric artery; RGE, right gastroepiploic artery; Sp, splenic artery.)

cated when the tumor or metastatic lymph nodes show direct invasion of the distal pancreas or the splenic artery or when a gastric tumor with a higher location shows serosal exposure on the posterior gastric wall. It is mandatory that all of the tumor (primary or metastatic) be eradicated, at least macroscopically.

When pancreaticosplenectomy is performed, the surgeon first mobilizes the spleen and the distal half of the pancreas from the retroperitoneum. The peritoneal reflection behind the spleen is cut longitudinally, and the avascular plane behind the pancreas and spleen and anterior to the adrenal gland is dissected until the posterior surface of the abdominal esophagus and the root of the splenic artery are exposed. The left thoracoabdominal approach is the most suitable for this procedure because mobilization can be achieved under direct vision from the left lateral aspect of the spleen.

The splenic artery is doubly ligated and transected at its origin. The accompanying splenic vein is also doubly ligated and is cut at the level of the root of the splenic artery. The vein is easily identified on the posterior surface of the body of the pancreas. The junction of the splenic and inferior mesenteric veins is usually on the right side of the resection line. The pancreas is cut with a linear stapling device at the line of resection. When bursectomy is planned, the peritoneum overlying the pancreas should be peeled off from right to left, as mentioned, beyond the resection line of the pancreas. When bleeding points are identified on the cut surface of the proximal pancreas, they are controlled by suturing with an atraumatic needle.

The alternative to pancreaticosplenectomy is splenectomy and lymph node dissection along the splenic artery without pancreatectomy. The first step also is dissection of the same avascular plane behind the pancreas. The surgeon performs the splenectomy by dividing the vessels that enter the splenic hilum while taking care to not injure the pancreatic tail. Lymph node dissection along the splenic artery is performed with meticulous hemostasis of all of the small posterior gastric vessels encountered during removal of the lymph nodes that lie on the splenic artery. It is possible and sometimes easier to remove the splenic artery with attached lymph nodes while leaving the pancreas.

TABLE 59–1 ■ Frequency of Lymph Node Metastases in Adenocarcinoma of the Stomach with Esophageal Invasion Resected by the Left Thoracoabdominal Approach

No. and Name of Lymph Node*	*Percent per No. Cases of Adenocarcinoma with Esophageal Invasion (n = 256)*
1 Right cardial nodes	39.8
2 Left cardial nodes	39.5
3 Nodes along the lesser curvature	44.9
4sa Nodes along the short gastric artery	15.6
4sb Nodes along the left gastroepiploic artery	5.9
4d Nodes along the right gastroepiploic artery	18.8
5 Suprapyloric nodes	8.6
6 Infrapyloric nodes	10.6
7 Nodes along the left gastric artery	32.4
8 Nodes along the common hepatic artery	14.5
9 Nodes around the celiac artery	23.8
10 Nodes at the splenic hilum	18.4
11 Nodes along the splenic artery	29.7
19 Infradiaphragmatic nodes	†
20 Nodes in the esophageal hiatus	†
108 Paraesophageal nodes in the middle thorax	1.2
110 Paraesophageal nodes in the lower thorax	5.9
111 Supradiaphragmatic nodes	5.9
112 Posterior mediastinal nodes	8.6

*See Figure 59–4 and Japanese Research Society for Gastric Carcinoma: Japanese Classification of Gastric Carcinoma. Tokyo, Kanehara & Co, Ltd, 1995.

†Data not available (recently subclassified).

Dissection of the Lower Mediastinum

After the abdominal portion of the procedure is completed, dissection is extended into the mediastinum. First, the anchoring stitch is removed from the diaphragm and a tape is passed through the hiatus. The tape then is pulled down to achieve good exposure of the left thoracic cavity. After gentle division of the pulmonary ligament, with care taken to not injure the pulmonary vein, the left lung is gently retracted superiorly for increased exposure. The pleura that covers the lower thoracic esophagus is incised. Loose connective tissue in the lower mediastinum, including mediastinal, paraesophageal, para-aortic, and diaphragmatic lymph nodes, is dissected free of the pericardium, aortic adventitia, and left mediastinal pleura (Fig. 59–5; see Fig. 59–4). Injury to the azygos vein and the thoracic duct should be avoided.

Determination of the Level of Esophageal Transection

Although the extent of intramural esophageal tumor spread is usually detected with preoperative endoscopic examination, the level of esophageal resection must be decided during intraoperative examination. This is particularly true for invasive tumors. As Shefton and coworkers (1977) have stated:

> Although the lesion was demonstrated roentgenologically in all patients, no reliable indication of its limits could be obtained, and spread was seriously underestimated by both preoperative barium studies and direct examination at operation.

Even if the surgeon obtains precise information from the endoscopist about the endoscopic tumor margins, the surgeon may encounter difficulty in determining the level of transection to obtain a clear resection margin. When the proximal margin is uncertain, intraoperative esophagotomy is performed before esophageal transection to determine the level for a clear surgical margin (Akiyama et al, 1974) (Fig. 59–6). Frozen section studies may be useful when needed.

En Bloc Tumor Resection

The distal cut end of the esophagus is wrapped in a sterile towel and pushed down into the abdomen through the hiatus. The lower esophagus, the stomach, the spleen, and the distal half of the pancreas are then removed en bloc from the abdomen. When omental bursectomy is performed, the undissected peritoneum of the omental bursa on the left half of the transverse mesocolon is peeled off in a peripheral direction from the central to the middle colic vessels. This completes resection of the tumor.

Gonzalez and associates (1981) recommend more radical surgical intervention, encompassing total esophagogastrectomy and resection of the distal pancreas, spleen, and regional lymph nodes. In their operation, total esophagectomy was performed transhiatally, without thoracotomy.

Roux-en-Y Reconstruction

Roux-en-Y jejunal reconstruction is one of the favored methods after total gastrectomy. Although there are many alternatives, including jejunal interposition (with and without a jejunal pouch) and ileocolic interposition, Roux-en-Y reconstruction has the advantage of simplicity. The transected duodenal stump is closed, and the elevated jejunal limb is constructed in Roux-en-Y fashion from a jejunal loop and anastomosed to the esophagus via the retrocolic route. To prevent reflux, the recommended interval between the esophageal hiatus and the jejunojejunostomy is approximately 30 cm.

Techniques for Esophagojejunostomy

The crucial anastomosis is the esophagojejunostomy. After its completion, subsequent jejunojejunostomy is usually performed without difficulty. Initially, the esophagojejunal anastomosis was fashioned by manual suturing; however, after the development of mechanical stapling devices, the stapled GI anastomosis (Ravitch and Steichen, 1979; Steichen and Ravitch, 1980) gained widespread acceptance. The significant advantages of mechanical staplers, such as procedural uniformity and a shorter operating time, are well recognized.

Among the different methods of constructing the esophagojejunostomy, whether with a stapler or manually, the end-to-side technique is preferred to the end-to-end anastomosis (EEA). In a stapled GI anastomosis, the

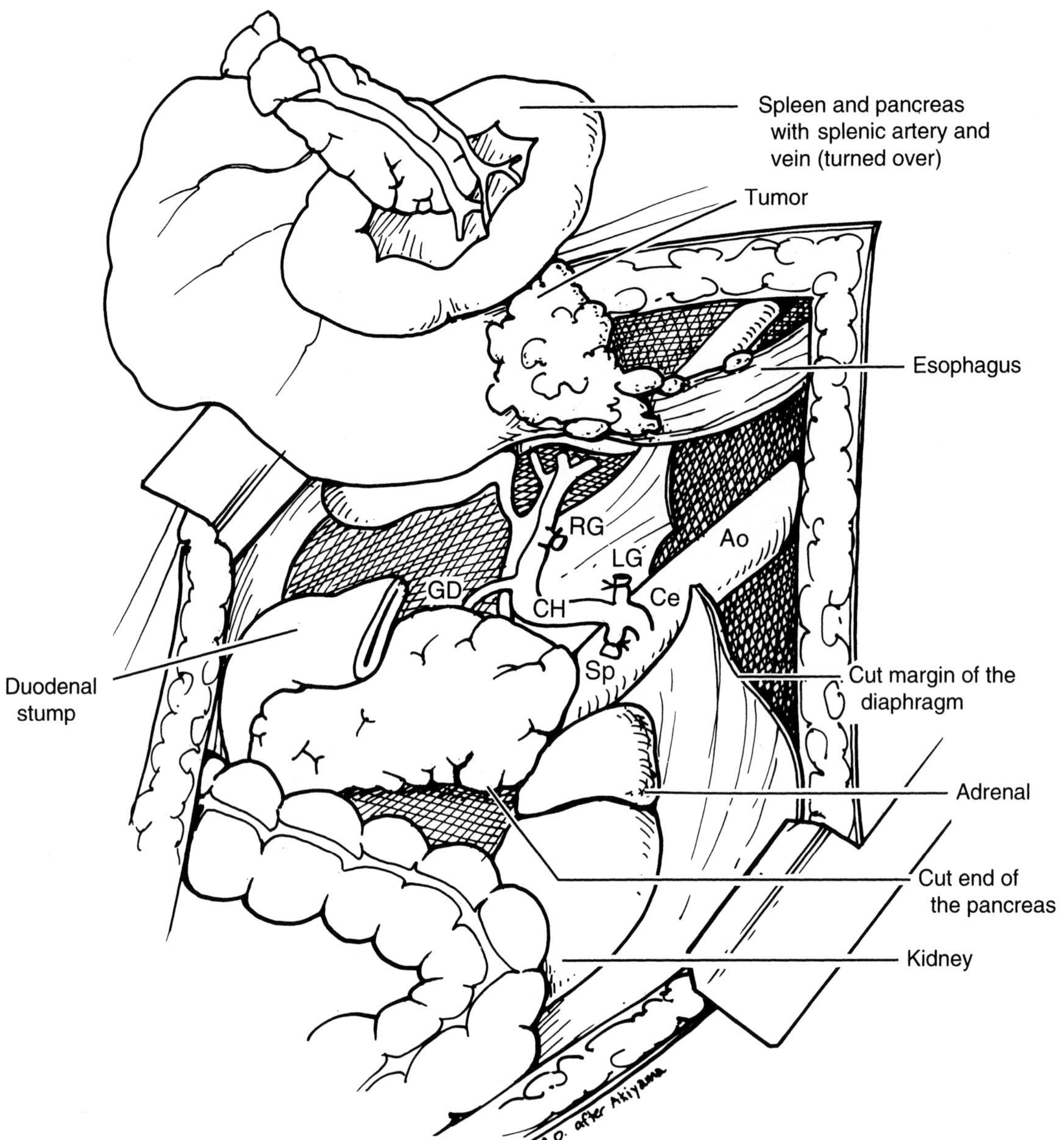

FIGURE 59–5 ■ Completion of lymph node dissection. The esophagus is ready to be transected. (Ao, aorta; Ce, celiac trunk artery; CH, common hepatic artery; GD, gastroduodenal artery; LG, left gastric artery; RG, right gastric artery; Sp, splenic artery.) (Adapted from Akiyama H, Kogure T, Itai Y: Role of esophagotomy in the surgical treatment of esophageal cancer. Intern Surg 58:478, 1974.)

surgeon accomplishes end-to-side esophagojejunostomy by inserting the EEA instrument through the transected end of the jejunum. The same anastomosis performed manually has the advantage of creating a lumen in the jejunal wall that corresponds to the size of the esophageal lumen. Because the site of anastomosis is on the antimesenteric border of the jejunum, the blood supply is not compromised.

Preparation of the Jejunal Loop

A tension-free intestinal loop with sufficient blood supply should be chosen. The intestinal loop is usually elevated to the level of the inferior pulmonary vein via the retrocolic route. The adequacy of the esophageal hiatus for passage of the jejunum should be ensured. If the hiatal opening is judged to be too tight, an additional incision can be made to widen it. The mesenteric axis of the elevated intestinal loop should not be twisted because this compromises the blood supply.

Purse-String Suturing of the Transected Esophagus

In preparation for EEA, a purse-string suture is placed at the cut end of the esophagus. Manual suturing is preferred. Akiyama's esophageal clamp (Fig. 59–7) is applied approximately 1.5 cm proximal to the cut end of the esophagus, and the purse-string suture is placed around the cut end, beginning with the needle inside the lumen and directed outward, as shown in Figure 59–7. With this method, the mucosal layer is certain to be caught with each stitch.

The ideal material for the purse-string suture should be easy to handle, strong, adequately slippery, and secure when knotted. A 1–0 silk suture impregnated with sterile glycerin and an atraumatic needle are usually used. A meticulous technique is needed because each stitch must be placed on a line approximately 3 mm from the cut end at intervals of 4 to 5 mm with the margins on stretch. Technical faults, such as too few stitches, result in failure of the purse-string to secure the full circumference of the mucosa, whereas too many stitches lead to difficulty in securing the purse-string knot.

The distance between the cut end and the "seam line" should vary according to the size of the stapler used and should be directly proportional to the unit size. Otherwise, excessive tissue will protrude beyond the suture after the purse-string suture is pulled tight around the center rod.

Insertion of the Instrument into the Jejunum

A small intestinal clamp is applied distally across the jejunum, and the cut end of the intestine is stabilized at four corners with hemostats. The diameter of the lumen is checked to select the appropriate cartridge size. Several factors, such as diameter, spasticity, stretchability, and

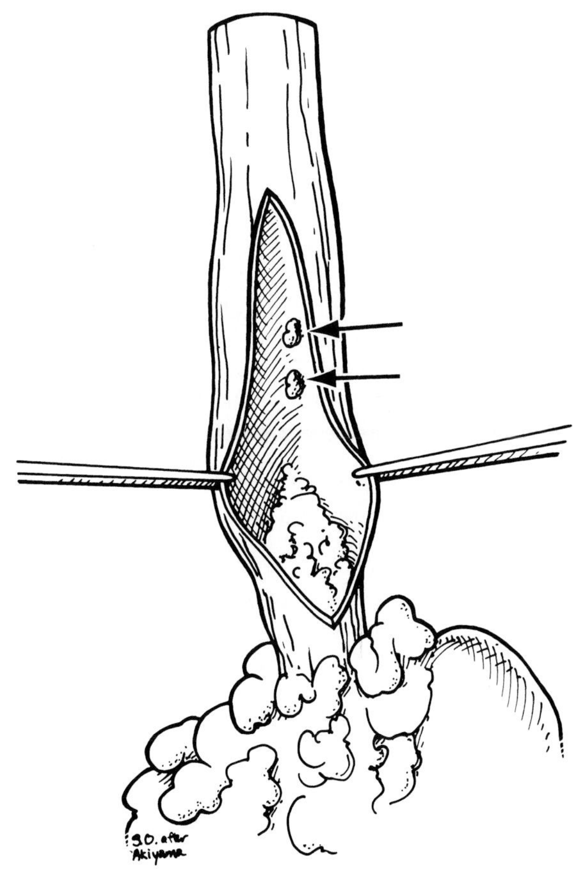

FIGURE 59–6 ■ Exploratory esophagotomy for observing intramural tumor extension. Total esophagectomy by blunt dissection may be carried out for high or multiple skip lesions if present *(arrows)*.

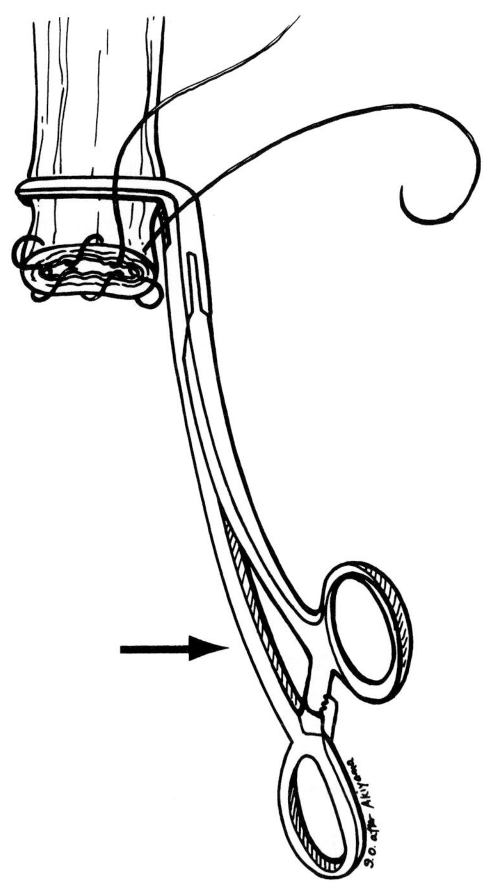

FIGURE 59–7 ■ Manual purse-string suture (interval, approximately 6 mm) using Akiyama's esophageal clamp *(arrow)*.

mucosal strength of both the jejunal and esophageal walls, should be evaluated for selection of cartridge size. The most common size used is 28 mm in diameter.

The center rod of the EEA instrument is inserted into the jejunal lumen with its tip toward the antimesenteric surface of the bowel wall.

Management of the Esophagus and Esophagojejunostomy

Stretching the esophageal lumen to its fullest extent with traction exerted by "soft" grasping devices (we usually use four pulmonary clamps) is essential to obtain the widest lumen for easy instrument insertion. This is done after the removal of Akiyama's esophageal clamp.

With a large esophageal lumen, no difficulty is encountered during insertion of the instrument; however, when the esophagus is narrow and fragile, various maneuvers are required to achieve atraumatic insertion. One should remember that the lateral cross-sectional area of the anvil is smaller than the transverse or horizontal cross-sectional area. Actually, the center rod can be directed only obliquely along the axis of the esophagus because of the limited operating field. After a portion of the rim of the anvil has been inserted into the lumen, the central portion of the anvil is advanced into the lumen while the anterior esophageal wall is distended by the inserted rim (Fig. 59–8*A*). The remaining portion of the rim is then eased into the lumen by a downward tilt of the center rod (Fig. 59–8*B*). Gentle traction on the atraumatic hemostats stretching the esophageal wall facilitates insertion of the instrument (Fig. 59–8*C*).

After the instrument has been successfully inserted, the purse-string suture is tightened around the center rod and tied. When the anvil is screwed down, care should be taken to not bite the jejunal mucosa of the mesenteric side (Fig. 59–9). After the usual precautions are taken, the trigger is fired and the stapling mechanism is activated. During withdrawal of the instrument, the same principles are followed as during insertion. The anvil is loosened from the cartridge with only 360 to 540 degrees of rotation of the screw, and the instrument is pushed slightly to either the right or the left to free the rim of the anvil on the opposite side. The instrument is then withdrawn with rotatory motion, with unnecessary trauma to the anastomosis avoided.

Immediately after completion of a stapled anastomosis, the intact rings of tissue from the jejunal and esophageal walls are examined and satisfactory status is verified. When continuous bleeding from the nasogastric tube begins or expansion of the jejunum below the EEA anastomosis occurs, arterial bleeding at the anastomosis line is suspected. The jejunal end through which the EEA instrument was inserted should be opened and the bleeding point in such a case identified. Bleeding then can be controlled with a suture ligature from the inside.

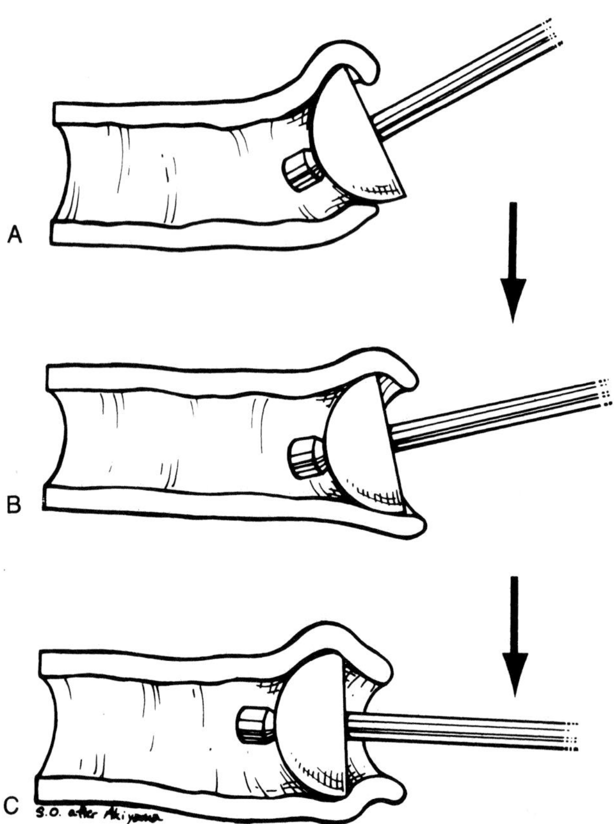

FIGURE 59–8 ■ *A–C*, Insertion of the anvil in instrumental anastomosis (see text).

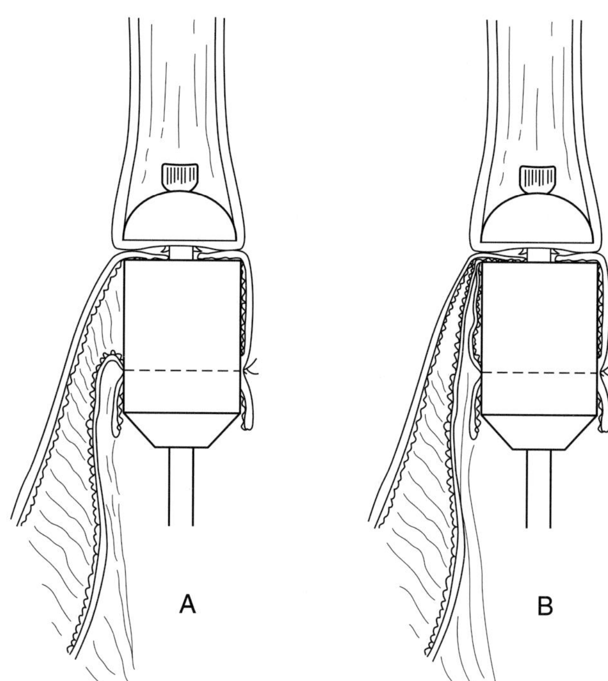

FIGURE 59–9 ■ Caution is necessary in approximating the anvil and the cartridge. Biting the jejunal mucosa of the mesenteric side *(B)* results in intractable stricture.

During end-to-side esophagojejunostomy, closure of the jejunal limb creates a pouch, which should be neither too long nor too short. Jejunojejunostomy is performed 30 cm distal to the esophageal hiatus (Fig. 59–10).

Closure

A small chest tube is inserted via the eighth intercostal space in the posterior axillary line before closure of the thoracotomy wound. The incised diaphragm is repaired with a heavy running suture of the surgeon's choice, and the final 4 to 5 cm is closed with interrupted sutures from the abdominal side. These sutures should be left unknotted until the incised intercostal space has been approximated with one or two heavy 1–0 sutures through the lower rib and the superior border of the upper rib. The chest wall is then closed in layers.

When distal pancreatectomy has been performed, two soft drains are placed near the cut end of the pancreas—one running from the left flank toward the left subphrenic space and the other running from the epigastrium and under the lateral segment of the liver toward the gap between the jejunal Roux limb and the descending aorta. A small enteral tube is inserted into the jejunal loop for postoperative decompression and subsequent tube feeding.

POSTOPERATIVE MANAGEMENT

Postoperatively, intestinal decompression is accomplished with the placement of a nasal tube in the jejunal loop for 3 or 4 days until bowel function returns. Thereafter, the tube is used for enteral feeding. Total parenteral nutrition

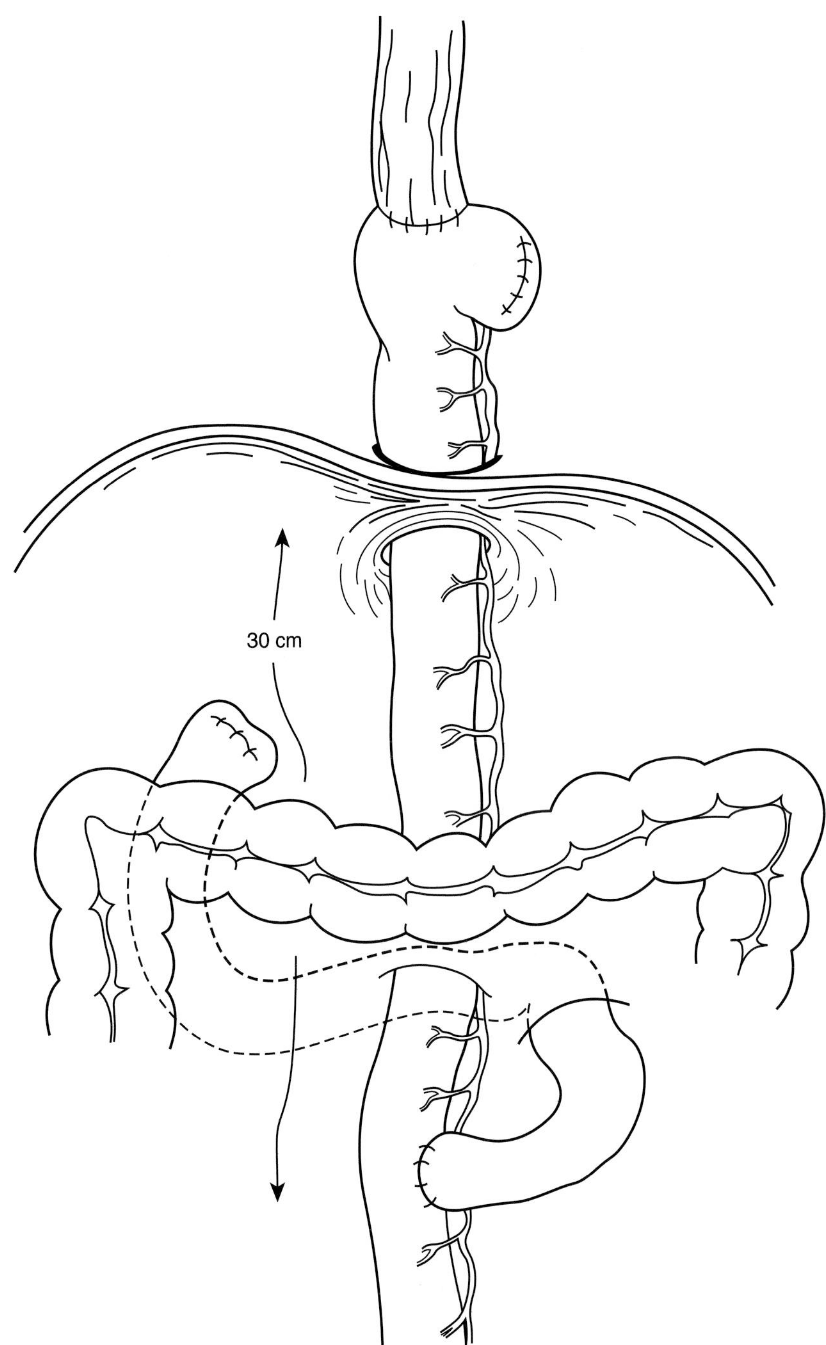

FIGURE 59–10 ■ Completion of total gastrectomy and Roux-en-Y diversion. The "handle of a stick" in the Roux-en-Y loop should not be too short or too long.

is preferred to provide a high-calorie food source in addition to tube feeding. Parenteral feeding is combined with tube feeding, and oral intake usually begins on the 10th postoperative day after contrast radiographic examination of the anastomosis. Broad-spectrum antibiotics are administered for prophylaxis for a total of 4 days, including the day of the operation. Long-term antibiotic therapy is avoided.

For patients with a malignancy, follow-up examination is usually carried out at intervals of 6 months. Examinations include ultrasonography, chest radiography, and blood tests for tumor markers. CT scanning and bone scintigraphy are also performed when recurrence is strongly suspected. Follow-up is usually continued for 5 years after surgery.

■ *REFERENCES*

Akiyama H, Kogure T, Itai Y: Role of esophagotomy in the surgical treatment of esophageal cancer. Int Surg 59:478, 1974.

Akiyama H, Miyazono H, Tsurumaru M, Hashimoto C: Thoracoabdominal approach for carcinoma of the cardia of the stomach. Am J Surg 137:345, 1979.

Gonzalez EM, Garcia JI, Selas PR, et al: Extended esophagogastrectomy as surgical treatment for carcinoma of the cardia. Jpn J Surg 11:311, 1981.

Maruyama K, Sasasko M, Kinoshita T, et al: Surgical treatment for gastric cancer: The Japanese approach. Semin Oncol 23:360, 1996.

Ravitch MM, Steichen FM: A stapling instrument for end-to-end inverting anastomoses in the gastrointestinal tract. Ann Surg 189:791, 1979.

Shelton GK, Grech P, Giddings AEB: Assessment and resection of carcinoma at the gastroesophageal junction. Surg Gynecol Obstet 144:563, 1977.

Steichen FM, Ravitch MM: Mechanical sutures in esophageal surgery. Ann Surg 191:373, 1980.

CHAPTER **60**

Resection of Carcinoma Involving the Cervicothoracic Esophagus: Cervical Exenteration

Mark B. Orringer

DEFINITION

Involvement of the cervicothoracic esophagus at the thoracic inlet by tumors of laryngotracheal, esophageal, or thyroid origin results in compromise not only of the ability to swallow but also, in many instances, of the airway. Techniques derived from a variety of surgical specialties (i.e., thoracic surgery, otolaryngology, plastic surgery, and general surgery) have been applied in the management of these tumors. Removal of the esophagus is often the least difficult part of the entire procedure. Laryngectomy and resection of the proximal trachea may be required, often with the adjacent anterior cervical skin that is involved by local tumor recurrence (e.g., a tracheal stomal recurrence after laryngectomy). The reconstructive phase of this "cervical exenteration" procedure is technically challenging because it involves restoration of alimentary continuity, coverage of the great vessels of the neck and superior mediastinum, and establishment of a satisfactory airway.

The magnitude of the operative undertaking required to resect a cervicothoracic esophageal malignancy, to reestablish alimentary continuity, and to provide a satisfactory airway should not be underestimated, and considerable expertise is required. The results of surgical therapy in these patients, many of whom have not responded to radiation therapy for control of the primary tumor, are not nearly as good as those achieved when only an esophagectomy and visceral esophageal substitution are required. Despite the magnitude of the operative undertaking required to treat these tumors successfully, gratifying palliation and, at times, cure can be achieved with a systematic and organized approach.

HISTORICAL NOTE

The first reconstruction of a cervical pharyngoesophageal defect was reported in 1908 by von Hacker (1908); a long cervical skin flap was used. This technique was popularized by Wookey (1949), who developed a two-stage reconstruction that mobilized local skin flaps. Bakamjian (1965) described the use of a medially based deltopectoral flap for esophageal reconstruction in 1965, which also required a two-stage procedure. However, it was subsequently demonstrated that total cervicothoracic esophageal reconstruction by this approach could be performed effectively in a single stage in 90% of patients.

Jianu (1912) first suggested the use of a tubed gastric pedicle for esophageal bypass. In 1951, Gavriliu and Georgescu (1955) used a reversed gastric tube for similar indications. The first report of transposition of the entire stomach with its intact blood supply through the posterior mediastinum into the neck with a pharyngogastric anastomosis was by Ong and Lee (1960). Many modifications and alterations in technique have been described since that time.

Various free abdominal visceral pedicles have been transposed to the neck, including gastric antrum and different segments of colon, but the most popular one that has stood the test of time is the free jejunal graft, use of which was first reported in 1961 by Roberts and Douglass (1961) and popularized by Jurkiewicz (1965) in North America.

There are proponents of both free jejunal transplantation and gastric transposition with orthotopic placement after total esophagectomy.

■ HISTORICAL READINGS

Bakamjian VY: A two-stage method for pharyngoesophageal reconstruction with a primary pectoral skin flap. Plast Reconstr Surg 36:173, 1965.

Gavriliu D, Georgescu L: Esophagoplastic direction a material gastric. Rev Stiintelor Med (Bucharest) 3:33, 1955.

Jianu A: Gastronstine u Oesophagosplastik. Dtsch Z Chir 118:383, 1912.

Jurkiewicz MJ: Vascularized intestinal graft for reconstruction of the cervical esophagus and pharynx. Plast Reconstr Surg 36:509, 1965.

Roberts RE, Douglass FM: Replacement of the cervical esophagus and hypopharynx by a revascularized free jejunal segment. N Engl J Med 264:342, 1961.

von Hacker V: Über Resection und Plastik am Halsabschnitt der Speiserone insbesondere beim Carcinom. Arch Klin Chir 82:257, 1908.

Wookey H: The surgical treatment of carcinoma of the pharynx and upper esophagus. Surg Gynecol Obstet 75:499, 1949.

TECHNICAL CONSIDERATIONS

The best method of restoring alimentary continuity after laryngopharyngectomy has been debated by Frederickson et al (1981), Withers et al (1981), Moores et al (1983), Spiro et al (1983), Harrison and Thompson (1986), Gomes et al (1987), Goldberg et al (1989), Spiro et al (1991), Cahow and Sasaki (1994), Sasaki et al (1995), Azurin et al (1997), and others who prefer gastric transposition.

Reported mortality rates have ranged from 5% to 31% and anastomotic leakage rates from 7% to 37%. Lam and associates (1981) reported a 14-year experience with 157 pharyngogastric anastomoses after pharyngolaryngo-esophagectomy. Overall hospital mortality was 31% (18% in the last 2 years of the study) and the anastomotic leak rate was 23%. The authors did not mention postoperative regurgitation as a significant functional problem. More recently, Sullivan and associates (1999) reported a series of 32 pharyngogastric reconstructions with an operative mortality of 12% and an anastomotic leak rate of 31%. Postoperative functional results are not discussed.

As microsurgical technique has improved, however, the free jejunal transfer has become the most popular method of pharyngeal reconstruction after resection of proximal lesions of the hypopharynx, pharynx, larynx, and esophagus above the thoracic inlet. A number of authors (Carlson et al, 1992; Coleman et al, 1984; Flynn et al, 1989; Jurkiewicz, 1984; Paletta and Jurkiewicz, 1991; Salamoun et al, 1987; Sasaki et al, 1980) reported successful re-establishment of alimentary continuity in approximately 95% of patients with morbidity similar to that reported after gastric transposition.

Several studies (de Vries et al, 1989; Schusterman et al, 1990) have compared jejunal transfer and pharyngo-gastric anastomosis and have demonstrated relatively similar morbidity and results. Fujita and coworkers (1999) compared total esophagectomy with pharyngogastric anastomosis and proximal esophagectomy with jejunal transfer for esophageal cancer at the cervicothoracic junction. They reported no significant difference in the incidence of local recurrence and lower hospital mortality (13% versus 50%) in those patients undergoing proximal versus total esophagectomy, respectively. What has emerged is a general consensus that for relatively short-length reconstruction above the thoracic inlet, a free jejunal transfer is the operation of choice. Tumors extending to or below the thoracic inlet or requiring a total esophagectomy are best treated with either a gastric or colonic interposition.

Mediastinal Tracheostomy

When a tumor invades the esophagus at the thoracic inlet (Fig. 60–1), the high retrosternal trachea at the same level may also be involved. Therefore, if a concomitant laryngopharyngectomy is required, construction of a standard tracheostomy may not be possible because the remaining tracheal stump distal to the tumor will not reach to the level of the suprasternal notch. This creates the need to establish an airway in the intrathoracic trachea.

Watson (1942), Sloan and Cowley (1951), Kleitsch (1952), Minor (1952), and Waddell and Cannon (1959) described the earliest attempts to achieve an intrathoracic tracheal airway. Sission and coworkers (1962) removed the clavicles and manubrium to gain access to the thoracic trachea in six patients with stomal recurrences and rotated skin and pectoral muscle flaps to construct an anterior mediastinal tracheostomy. Sisson (1967), Sisson and coworkers (1975, 1977), and Krespi and coauthors (1985) subsequently reported one of the most extensive experiences with anterior mediastinal tracheostomy for laryngotracheal and cervical esophageal carcinoma. Grillo (1966) popularized the bipedicled upper thoracic apron flap with resection of the anterior breastplate for construction of an anterior mediastinal tracheostomy. Stell and associates (1970) modified this approach and used a wider bipedicled upper thoracic apron flap and resection of only one half of the manubrium and the clavicle and the first rib on only one side.

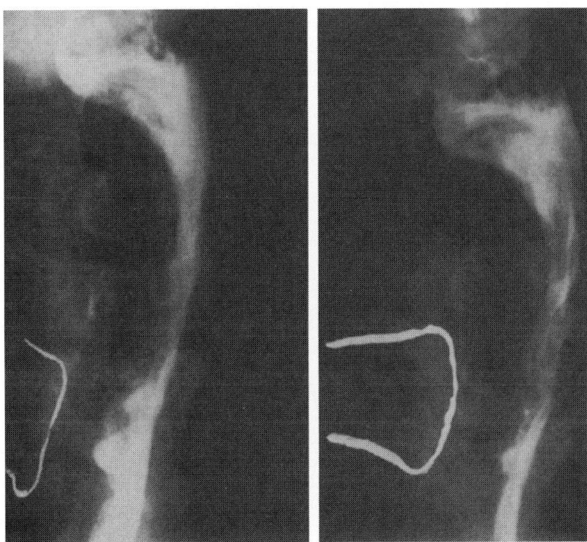

FIGURE 60–1 ■ Cervicothoracic esophageal squamous cell carcinoma straddling the thoracic inlet and extending behind the level of the head of the clavicle, which has been highlighted. (From Orringer MB: Transhiatal esophagectomy without thoracotomy. In Zuidema GD, Orringer MB [eds]: Shackelford's Surgery of the Alimentary Tract, 3rd ed. Philadelphia, WB Saunders, 1991, p 408.)

Orringer and Sloan (1979) used the Grillo approach, removing the anterior "breastplate," that is, the medial clavicles, upper manubrium, and adjacent medial first (and occasionally second) ribs, for construction of an anterior mediastinal tracheostomy. This technique was also found to facilitate the resection of cervicothoracic esophageal malignancies by providing a wide exposure of the superior mediastinum and its contents (Figs. 60–2 and 60–3). With this approach, the retrosternal trachea can be divided for the construction of an anterior mediastinal tracheostomy and a laryngopharyngectomy, and transhiatal esophagectomy can be carried out.

I previously reported my preference for use of the stomach whenever possible (Orringer, 1992) to re-establish alimentary continuity (Figs. 60–4 and 60–5). However, construction of a pharyngogastric anastomosis requires that the mobilized stomach reach cephalad to its limit, and tension on the anastomosis may be responsible for the relatively high incidence of anastomotic leaks (up to one third) with this approach.

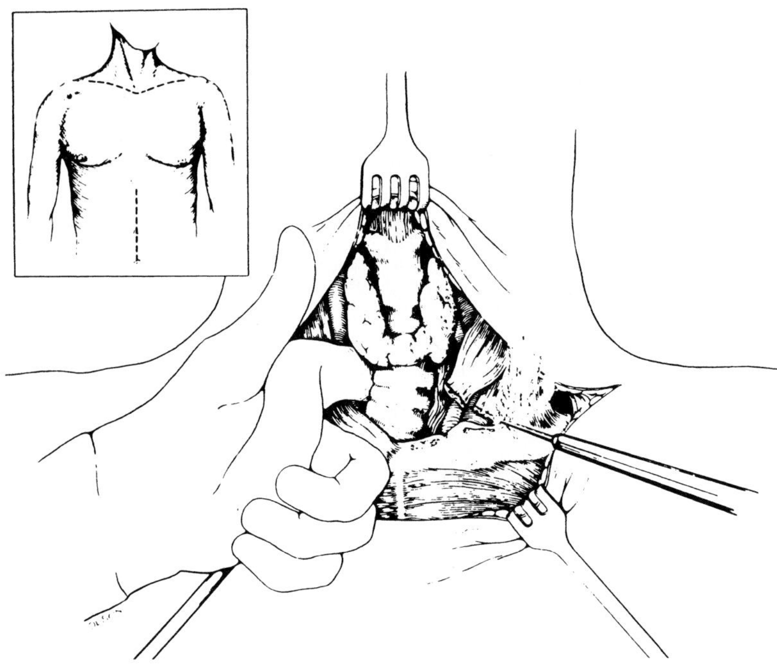

FIGURE 60–2 ■ Anterior mediastinal tracheostomy: initial approach. Extended supraclavicular collar incision *(inset)*. After the cervicothoracic esophageal tumor was determined to be free from the carotid sheaths and prevertebral fascia, the anterior cervical skin and platysma are elevated and the sternocleidomastoid muscles detached from the clavicles and sternum. Grillo's bipedicled upper thoracic visor flap is no longer used. (From Orringer MB: Anterior mediastinal tracheostomy with and without cervical exenteration. Ann Thorac Surg 54:628, 1992.)

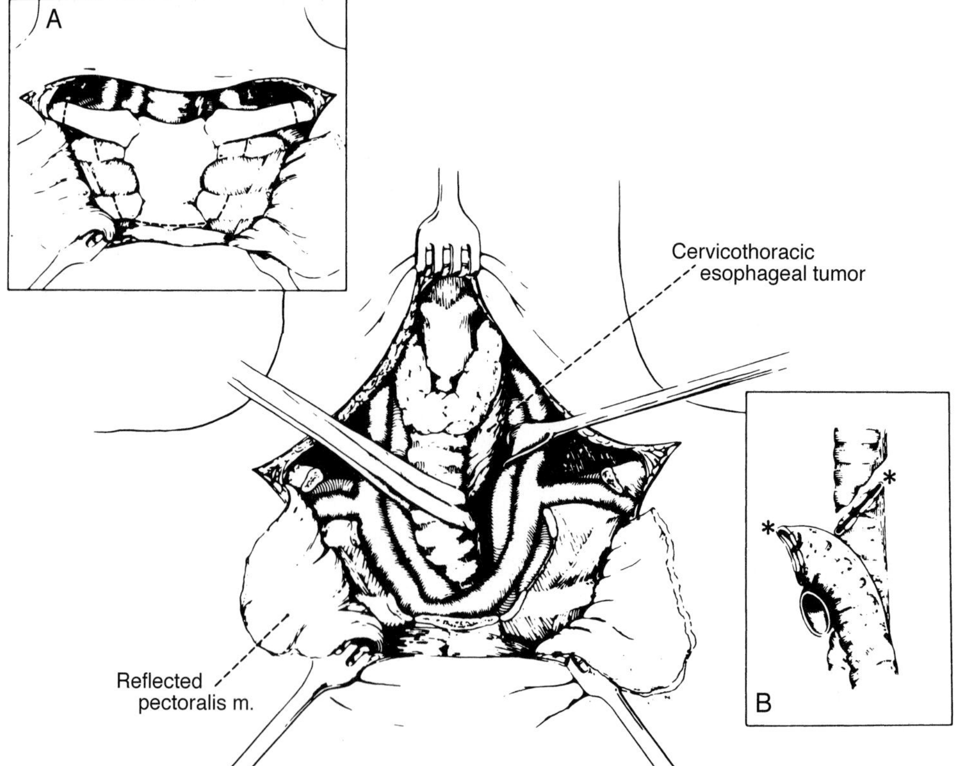

FIGURE 60–3 ■ The anterior thoracic "breastplate" resected for construction of an anterior mediastinal tracheostomy includes the medial clavicles, short segments of the first rib cartilages, manubrium, and occasionally also the medial second ribs. Removal of the anterior breastplate provides unequaled exposure of the superior mediastinum, the trachea, cervicothoracic esophagus, and associated great vessels *(inset A)*. The trachea must be divided obliquely to preserve the posterior membranous tracheal length *(asterisk, Inset B)*, which must reach most anteriorly when the end of the divided trachea is sutured to the skin. (From Orringer MB, Sloan H: Anterior mediastinal tracheostomy. J Thorac Cardiovasc Surg 78:850, 1979.)

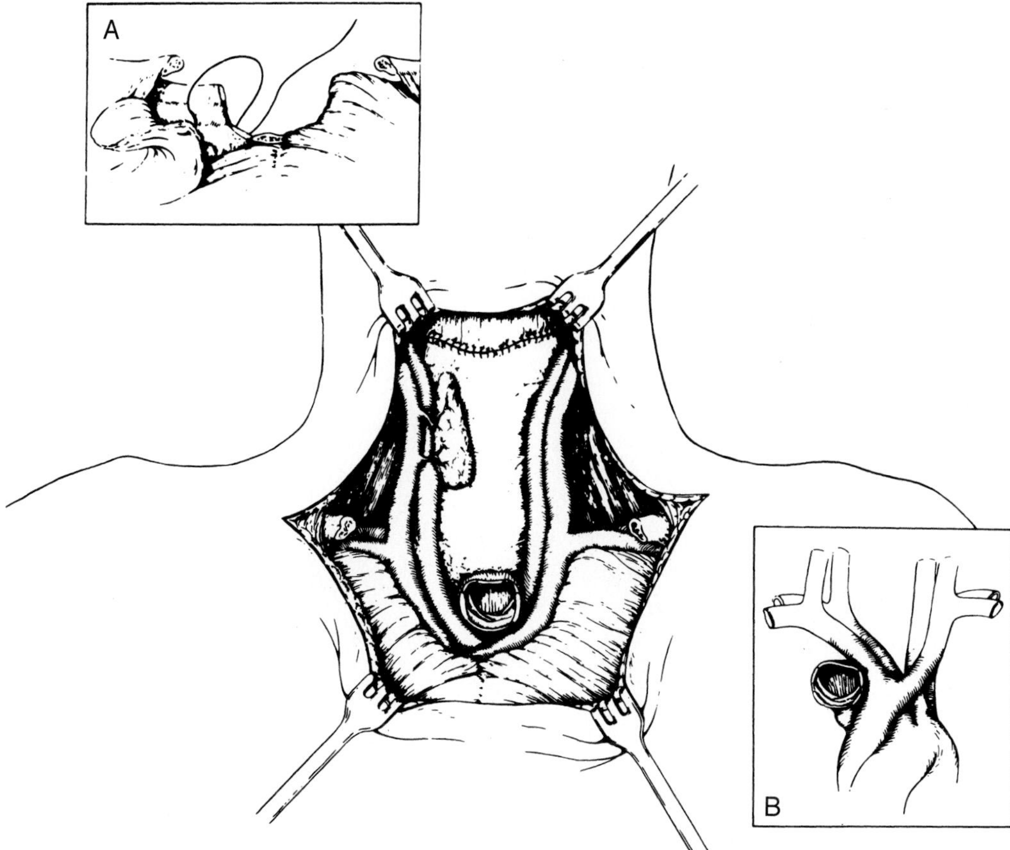

FIGURE 60–4 ■ The pharyngogastric anastomosis has been completed, one lobe of the thyroid gland and associated parathyroid glands preserved, and the trachea positioned for construction of the anterior mediastinal tracheostomy. The previously elevated pectoralis major may be sutured over the edges of the divided bony chest wall, although this is not essential *(inset A)*. Tracheal stump transposition inferior and to the right of the innominate artery and vein is used liberally to minimize tension between the divided trachea and innominate artery and resultant innominate artery erosion *(inset B)*. (From Orringer MB, Sloan H: Anterior mediastinal tracheostomy. J Thorac Cardiovasc Surg 78:850, 1979, with permission.)

Although a relatively small pharyngogastric anastomotic leak generally heals with the use of continuous subcutaneous drainage catheters, a major anastomotic dehiscence at times necessitates construction of a pharyngostome and a later attempt at restoring alimentary continuity. Of equal, if not greater, concern is the functional result of a pharyngogastric anastomosis. This is in sharp contrast to the results with a standard cervical esophagogastric anastomosis after transhiatal esophagectomy in which my colleagues and I (1999) reported an incidence of clinically troublesome gastroesophageal reflux in fewer than 10%. Loss of the upper esophageal (cricopharyngeal) sphincter, which occurs in patients undergoing construction of a pharyngogastric anastomosis, results in nearly uniform postoperative regurgitation of gastric contents during coughing, bending, and reclining, and this becomes a major complaint of the survivors of these operations. Primarily for this latter reason, although it is possible to mobilize sufficient gastric length for performance of a pharyngeal anastomosis in virtually every patient, I now believe that a colon interposition is the preferred method for restoring alimentary continuity after a laryngopharyngectomy (Orringer, 1999). This view is consistent with that of Grillo and Mathisen (1990), who favor colonic esophageal replacement in patients who undergo cervical exenteration. Although the operation is technically more complex, the anastomotic leak rate is lower and the functional results are better.

As we have gained facility with the technique of anterior mediastinal tracheostomy, we have found it unnecessary to construct the “visor” or bipedicled apron flap described by Grillo (1966, 1970). Rather, as I had reported (Orringer, 1992), resection of the anterior chest wall, which is required for construction of the mediastinal tracheostomy, is achieved through an extended low collar incision performed with the patient's neck flexed and the skin of the upper anterior chest retracted downward (see Fig. 60–2). This results in better vascularized anterior thoracic skin rather than the bipedicled apron flap for construction of the tracheostomy. When there is a local tracheal stomal recurrence after a laryngectomy for carcinoma (Figs. 60–6 and 60–7), resection of a 3- to 5-cm margin of skin around the stoma and recurrence is required. In such cases, after the tracheostoma and involved adjacent skin are resected, a thoracoacromial “nipple” flap, as originally described by Conley (1960) and Sisson (1967), is used to resurface the anterior neck and superior mediastinum (Figs. 60–8 and 60–9).

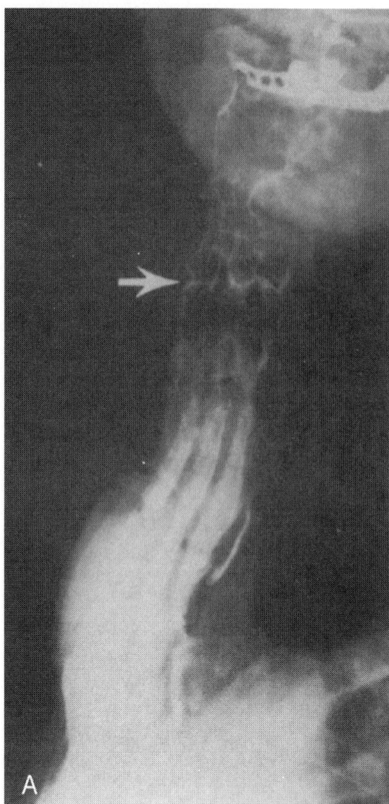

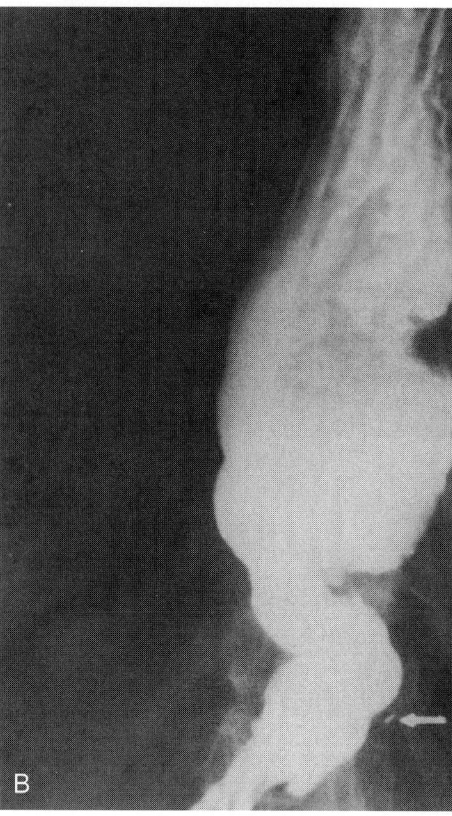

FIGURE 60–5 ■ Completed pharyngogastric anastomosis *(A)* *(arrow)* and level of pyloromyotomy *(B)* *(arrow)* after laryngopharyngo-esophagectomy and anterior mediastinal tracheostomy in patient shown in Figure 60–1. (From Orringer MB: Transhiatal esophagectomy without thoracotomy. In Zuidema GD, Orringer MB [eds]: Shackelford's Surgery of the Alimentary Tract, 3rd ed. Philadelphia, WB Saunders, 1991, p 408.)

From a technical standpoint, a minimum 5-cm length of residual distal trachea above the carina is ideal to reach to the skin for the construction of an anterior mediastinal tracheostomy. Precise preoperative bronchoscopic measurements are therefore used to determine the distance between the carina and the tumor and to establish operability.

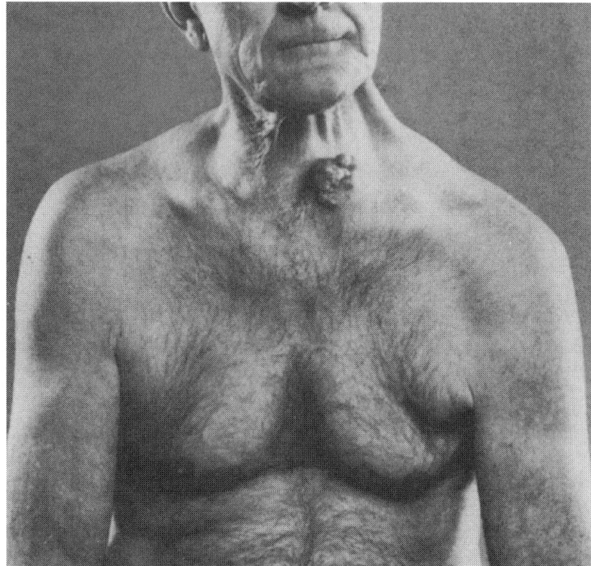

FIGURE 60–6 ■ Stomal recurrence of laryngeal squamous carcinoma in a 60-year-old man who had undergone a laryngectomy 2 years earlier. (From Orringer MB: Transhiatal esophagectomy without thoracotomy. In Zuidema GD, Orringer MB [eds]: Shackelford's Surgery of the Alimentary Tract, 3rd ed. Philadelphia, WB Saunders, 1991.)

Since his earliest description of anterior mediastinal tracheostomy, Grillo (1966, 1970) has expressed concern about innominate artery erosion as a possible major postoperative complication in these patients. He and Mathisen (1990) even advocated (1) prophylactic division of the innominate artery after preoperative aortic arch angiography and (2) intraoperative electroencephalographic monitoring after clamping the vessel before it is divided.

Mathisen and coauthors (1988) also advocated the use of an omental pedicle to cover the mediastinal great vessels and prevent subsequent erosion. The complication of tracheoinnominate artery erosion after mediastinal tracheostomy, however, results because of tension between the innominate artery and the divided trachea, which has been pulled forward over the top of the artery and has been sutured to the skin. This can be avoided. If there is the least concern about pressure on the innominate artery by the overlying trachea, the remaining tracheal stump should be transposed beneath and to the right of the innominate artery (see Fig. 60–4*B*), as originally described by Waddell and Cannon (1959). There cannot be pressure necrosis of the trachea against the innominate artery if the trachea is angled forward to reach the skin beneath the artery. Thus, in my experience (Orringer, 1992), in a report of 47 malignancies that involved the cervicothoracic esophagus, an anterior mediastinal tracheostomy was required in 33 patients (70%), and there was one postoperative innominate artery erosion early before "tracheal transposition" was used more liberally.

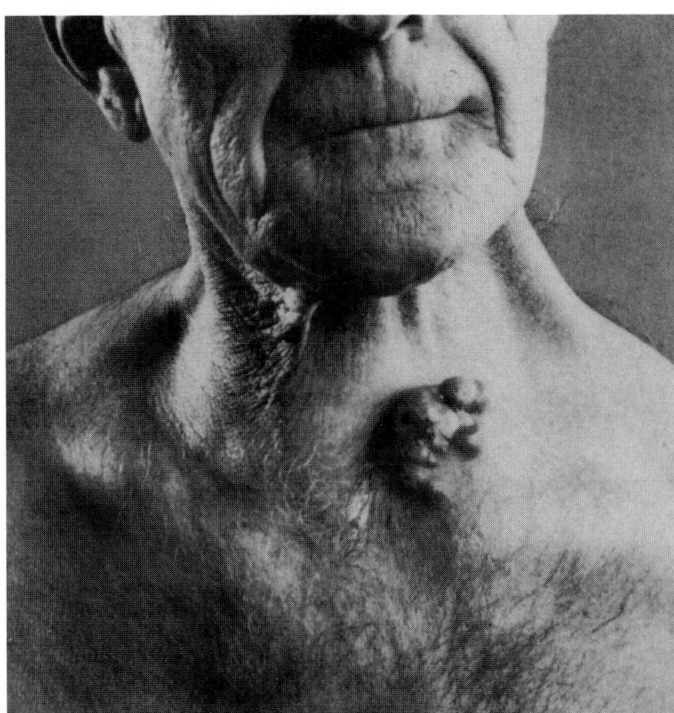

FIGURE 60–7 ■ Detail of tracheal stomal recurrence in same patient as shown in Figure 60–6. The tumor involved the adjacent esophagus, which was also resected with the tracheostome and surrounding skin. (From Orringer MB: Transhiatal esophagectomy without thoracotomy. In Zuidema GD, Orringer MB [eds]: Shackelford's Surgery of the Alimentary Tract, 3rd ed. Philadelphia, WB Saunders, 1991, p 408.)

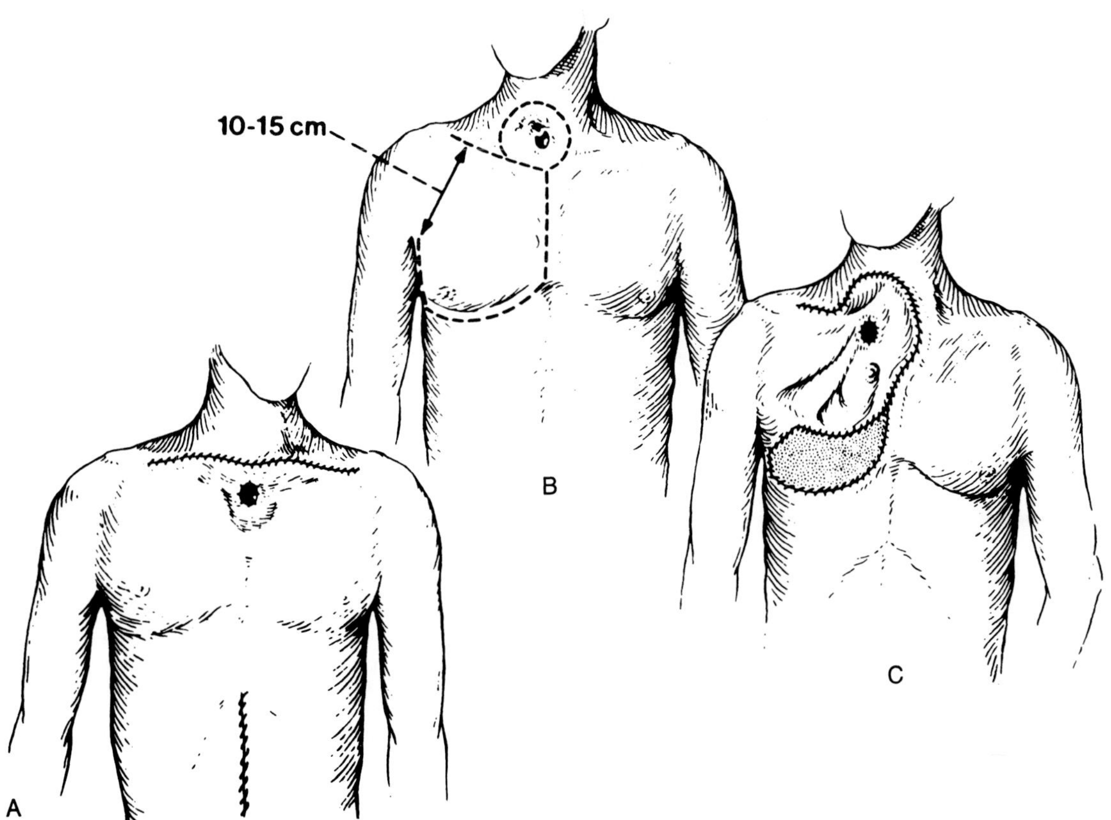

FIGURE 60–8 ■ Skin flaps used for construction of anterior mediastinal tracheostomy. *A*, Extended collar incision with completed anterior mediastinal tracheostomy and upper midline abdominal incision after cervical exenteration, transhiatal esophagectomy, and pharyngogastric anastomosis. The tracheostome may either be constructed as shown through a separate opening in the upper thoracic skin flap or incorporated into the cervical incision closure. *B*, When there is recurrent tracheal stomal carcinoma, a 3- to 5-cm margin of anterior skin around the tumor must be resected. In such cases, a thoracoacromial nipple flap is used to resurface the anterior neck and superior mediastinum. *C*, The anterior mediastinal tracheostomy is constructed, and a split-thickness skin graft is used to resurface the anterior thorax if necessary. (From Orringer MB: Anterior mediastinal tracheostomy with and without cervical exenteration. Ann Thorac Surg 54:628, 1992.)

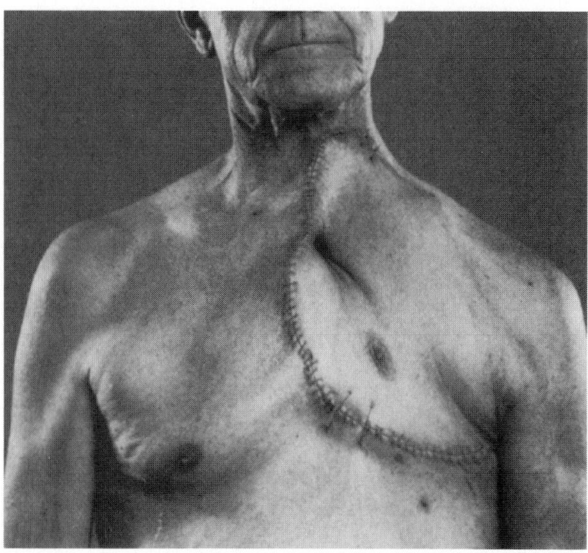

FIGURE 60–9 ■ Completed anterior mediastinal tracheostomy and left thoracoacromial nipple flap after pharyngo-esophagectomy, resection of the tracheostome and adjacent skin, and pharyngogastrostomy in the patient shown in Figures 60–6 and 60–7. (From Orringer MB: Transhiatal esophagectomy without thoracotomy. In Zuidema GD, Orringer MB [eds]: Shackelford's Surgery of the Alimentary Tract. 3rd ed. Philadelphia, WB Saunders, 1991, p 408.)

Cervical exenteration combined with anterior mediastinal tracheostomy and pharyngogastrostomy is a formidable technical undertaking. Although long-term survival for patients with most cervicothoracic esophageal and tracheal malignancies is seldom achieved, this approach provides effective palliation and occasional cure. With judicious patient selection, meticulous attention to operative detail, and intensive postoperative care, meaningful palliation is possible in these unfortunate patients who have compromise of both their ability to swallow and their airway. In recent years, as chemo-radiotherapy has emerged as the preferred approach in patients with squamous cell carcinoma of the cervicothoracic esophagus, the need for radical surgery has diminished substantially.

Preservation of Thyroid and Parathyroid Gland Function

Every attempt is made to preserve some degree of thyroid and parathyroid gland function, if necessary, by a dissection of some of the parathyroid glands from the specimen and their reimplantation into either adjacent pectoral muscle or the subcutaneous tissue of the forearm. Unfortunately, given the extent of the tumor or the degree of prior radiation therapy that many of these patients have had, it is often impossible to identify the parathyroid glands within the indurated cervical tissues. If iatrogenic hypoparathyroidism results from the cervical exenteration, lifelong calcium and vitamin D replacement is required.

COMMENTS AND CONTROVERSIES

The combined resection of the cervicoesophagus along with the larynx and upper trachea is a daunting undertaking associated with a high mortality and fraught with difficult-to-manage complications. This is especially so, as most of these procedures are carried out for residual or recurring tumor after previous high-dose radiotherapy. Frequent and persistent anastomotic leakage and airway necrosis are among the most dread complications.

Dr. Orringer in this chapter has emphasized the importance of a multidisciplinary approach involving thoracic surgery, otolaryngology, and plastic surgery. As he notes, combined chemotherapy with radiation therapy is generally considered the preferred approach for treatment of squamous cell carcinoma of the cervical esophagus. Improved results with this modality, fortunately, have reduced the need for employing the exenteration techniques that he so well describes. Of particular importance is his observation that jejunal or colonic interposition results in a better functional result than use of the whole stomach for reconstruction. We have also found the forearm flap, based on the radial artery, to be excellent for replacement of a short segment of the cervical esophagus. In the face of previous radiation to the cervical region, subsequent excision of the cervical esophagus often renders the adjacent membranous wall of the trachea severely ischemic. For this reason also, a short-segment jejunal interposition or forearm flap may be preferable to transhiatal esophagectomy and gastric transposition to the pharynx.

J. D. C.

■ KEY REFERENCES

Grillo HC, Mathisen DJ: Cervical exenteration. Ann Thorac Surg 49:401, 1990.

This is an outstanding, well-illustrated review of the operative technique and the authors' clinical experience with 18 patients undergoing cervical exenteration. The use of the bipedicled upper thoracic "apron" flap for performance of an anterior mediastinal tracheostomy in 14 patients is described. The innominate artery was divided in seven patients. Colon was used to replace the esophagus. There was one operative death and two anastomotic leaks.

Orringer MB: Anterior mediastinal tracheostomy with and without cervical exenteration. Ann Thorac Surg 54:628, 1992.

This is a comprehensive, well-illustrated review of the author's experience with 44 anterior mediastinal tracheostomies, 34 performed consistently with cervical exenteration (laryngopharyngoesophagectomy) for laryngeal, tracheal, or cervicothoracic esophageal malignancies. Avoidance of the complication of tracheoinnominate artery erosion by transposing the divided tracheal stump beneath and to the right of the innominate artery is described in 14 patients. The hospital death rate was 14% (6 deaths), and of 31 pharyngogastric anastomoses there were 9 (29%) anastomotic leaks. The desirability of performing the anterior mediastinal tracheotomy using a low collar incision rather than the Grillo bipedicled apron flap is emphasized.

■ REFERENCES

Azurin DJ, Go LS, Kirkland ML: Palliative gastric transposition following pharyngolaryngoesophagectomy. Am Surg 63:410, 1997.

Bakamjian VY: A two-stage method for pharyngoesophageal reconstruction with a primary pectoral skin flap. Plast Reconstr Surg 36:173, 1965.

Cahow CE, Sasaki CT: Gastric pull-up reconstruction for pharyngo-laryngo-esophagectomy. Arch Surg 129:425, 1994.

Carlson GW, Schusterman MA, Guillamondegui OM: Total reconstruction of the hypopharynx and cervical esophagus: A 20-year experience. Ann Plast Surg 29:408, 1992.

Coleman JJ, Searles JM Jr, Hester TR, et al. Ten years experience with free jejunal autograft. Am J Surg 154:394, 1987.

Conley JJ: The use of regional flaps in head and neck surgery. Ann Otol Rhinol Laryngol 69:1223, 1960.

deVries EJ, Stein DW, Johnson JT, et al: Hypopharyngeal reconstruction: A comparison of two alternatives. Laryngoscope 99:614, 1989.

Flynn MB, Banis J, Acland R: Reconstruction with free bowel autografts after pharyngoesophageal or laryngopharyngoesophageal resection. Am J Surg 158:333, 1989.

Frederickson JM, Wagenfeld DJH, Pearson G: Gastric pull-up vs. deltopectoral flap for reconstruction of the cervical esophagus. Arch Otolaryngol 107:613, 1981.

Fujita H, Kakegawa T, Yamama H, et al: Total esophagectomy versus proximal esophagectomy for esophageal cancer at the cervicothoracic junction. World J Surg 23:486, 1999.

Gavriliu D, Georgescu L: Esophagoplastic direction a material gastric. Rev Stiintelor Med (Bucharest) 3:33, 1955.

Goldberg M, Freeman J, Gullane PJ, et al: Transhiatal esophagectomy with gastric transposition for pharyngolaryngeal malignant disease. J Thorac Cardiovasc Surg 97:327, 1989.

Gomes MN, Krole S, Spear SL: Mediastinal tracheostomy. Ann Thorac Surg 43:539, 1987.

Grillo HC: Surgery of the trachea. In Ravitch M (ed): Current Problems in Surgery. Chicago, Year Book Medical Publishers, 1970.

Grillo HC: Terminal or mural tracheostomy in the anterior mediastinum. J Thorac Cardiovasc Surg 51:422, 1966.

Harrison DF, Thompson AE: Pharyngolaryngoesophagectomy with pharyngogastric anastomosis for cancer of the hypopharynx: Review of 101 operations. Head Neck Surg 8:418, 1986.

Jianu A: Gastronstine u Oesophagosplastik. Dtsch Z Chir 118:383, 1912.

Jurkiewicz MJ: Reconstructive surgery of the cervical esophagus. J Thorac Cardiovasc Surg 88:893, 1984.

Jurkiewicz MJ: Vascularized intestinal graft for reconstruction of the cervical esophagus and pharynx. Plast Reconstr Surg 36:509, 1965.

Kleitsch WP: Anterior mediastinal tracheostomy. J Thorac Cardiovasc Surg 24:38, 1952.

Krespi YP, Wurster CF, Sisson GA: Immediate reconstruction after total laryngopharyngectomy and mediastinal dissection. Laryngoscope 95:156, 1985.

Lam KH, Wong J, Lim ST, Ong GB: Pharyngogastric anastomosis following pharyngolaryngoesophagectomy: Analysis of 157 cases. World J Surg 5:509, 1981.

Mathisen DJ, Grillo HC, Vlahakes GJ, Daggett WM: The omentum in the management of complicated cardiothoracic problems. J Thorac Cardiovasc Surg 95:677, 1988.

Minor GR: Trans-sternal tracheal excision for carcinoma. J Thorac Cardiovasc Surg 24:88, 1952.

Moores DWO, Ilves R, Cooper JD, et al: One-stage reconstruction for pharyngolaryngectomy: Esophagectomy and pharyngogastrostomy without thoracotomy. J Thorac Cardiovasc Surg 85:330, 1983.

Ong GB, Lee TC: Pharyngogastric anastomosis after oesophagopharyngectomy for carcinoma of the hypopharynx and cervical esophagus. Br J Surg 48:193, 1960.

Orringer MB: Anterior mediastinal tracheostomy with and without cervical exenteration. Ann Thorac Surg 54:628, 1992.

Orringer MB: Anterior mediastinal tracheostomy with and without cervical exenteration: Update in 1998. Ann Thorac Surg 68:591, 1999.

Orringer MB: Transhiatal esophagectomy without thoracotomy. In Zuidema GD, Orringer MB (eds): Shackelford's Surgery of the Alimentary Tract, 3rd ed. Philadelphia, WB Saunders, 1991, p 408.

Orringer MB, Marshall B, Iannettoni MD: Transhiatal esophagectomy: Clinical experience and refinements. Ann Surg 230:392, 1999.

Orringer MB, Sloan H: Anterior mediastinal tracheostomy: Indications, techniques, and clinical experience. J Thorac Cardiovasc Surg 78:850, 1979.

Paletta CE, Jurkiewicz MJ: Esophageal replacement: Microvascular jejunal transplantation. In Baue AE, Geha AS, Hammond GL, et al (eds): Glenn's Thoracic and Cardiovascular Surgery, 5th ed. Norwalk, CT, Appleton & Lange, 1991, p 819.

Roberts RE, Douglass FM: Replacement of the cervical esophagus and hypopharynx by a revascularized free jejunal segment. N Engl J Med 264:342, 1961.

Salamoun W, Swartz WM, Johnson JT, et al: Free jejunal transfer for reconstruction of the laryngopharynx. Head Neck Surg 96:149, 1987.

Sasaki CT, Salzer SJ, Cahow E, et al: Laryngopharyngoesophagectomy for advanced hypopharyngeal and esophageal squamous cell carcinoma: The Yale experience. Laryngoscope 105:160, 1995.

Sasaki TM, Baker HW, McConnell DB, Vetto RM: Free jejunal graft reconstruction after extensive head and neck surgery. Am J Surg 139:650, 1980.

Schusterman MA, Shestak K, deVries EJ, et al: Reconstruction of the cervical esophagus: Free jejunal transfer versus gastric pull-up. Plast Reconstr Surg 85:16, 1990.

Sisson GA: Flaps and grafts in head and neck surgery. Minn Med 50:952, 1967.

Sisson GA, Bytell DE, Becker SP: Mediastinal dissection 1976: Indications and newer techniques. Laryngoscope 87:751, 1977.

Sisson GA, Edison BD, Bytell DE: Trans-sternal radical neck dissection, postoperative complications and management. Arch Otolaryngol 101:46, 1975.

Sisson GA, Straehley CJ Jr, Johnson NE: Mediastinal dissection for recurrent cancer after laryngectomy. Laryngoscope 72:1064, 1962.

Sloan H, Cowley RA: Posterior mediastinal tracheostomy. J Thorac Surg 21:602, 1951.

Spiro RH, Bains MS, Shah JP, Strong EW: Gastric transposition for head and neck cancer: A critical update. Am J Surg 162:348, 1991.

Spiro RH, Shah JP, Strong BW, et al: Gastric transposition in head and neck surgery: Indications, complications, and expectations. Am J Surg 146:483, 1983.

Stell PM, Bickford BJ, Brown GA: Thoracotracheostomy after resection of the larynx and cervical trachea for cancer. J Laryngol Otol 84:1097, 1970.

Sullivan MW, Talamonti MS, Sithanandam K, et al: Results of gastric interposition for reconstruction of the pharyngoesophagus. Surgery 126:666, 1999.

von Hacker V: Über Resection und Plastik am Halsabschnitt der speiserone insbesondere beim carcinom. Arch Klin Chir 82:257, 1908.

Waddell WR, Cannon B: A technique for subtotal excision of the trachea and establishment of a sternal tracheostomy. Ann Surg 149:1, 1959.

Watson WL: Cancer of trachea fifteen years after treatment for cancer of larynx. J Thorac Cardiovasc Surg 12:142, 1942.

Withers EH, Davis JL, Lynch JB: Anterior mediastinal tracheostomy with a pectoralis major musculocutaneous flap. Plast Reconstr Surg 67:381, 1981.

Wookey H: The surgical treatment of carcinoma of the pharynx and upper esophagus. Surg Gynecol Obstet 75:499, 1949.

CHAPTER **61**

Video-Assisted Approaches for Resection of Carcinoma of the Esophagus

James D. Luketich
Neil Christie
Ninh T. Nguyen

Conventional esophagectomy requires either a laparotomy with a transhiatal dissection or a laparotomy combined with thoracotomy, and it is associated with significant morbidity and mortality (Millikan et al, 1995). Reductions in complication rates have been reported in centers with a high volume of esophageal surgery, but morbidity remains considerable (Patti et al, 1998). As advances in minimally invasive surgical instrumentation and technique continue, some surgeons have reported the application of minimally invasive techniques to resection of the esophagus in an attempt to decrease further the associated morbidity of esophagectomy. Most of these case studies or small series have used video-assisted thoracoscopy to mobilize the thoracic esophagus in combination with a standard open laparotomy to complete the esophagectomy (Akaishi et al, 1996; Dexter et al, 1996; Luketich et al, 1998d). Clear advantages of thoracoscopic esophageal mobilization over thoracotomy or laparotomy alone with transhiatal dissection were not demonstrated in these studies. In one study, thoracoscopic esophagectomy was associated with less postoperative pain and more complete recovery of vital capacity compared with open surgery (Akaishi et al, 1996).

DePaula was the first surgeon to report a large series of 48 patients undergoing a total laparoscopic transhiatal esophagectomy (DePaula et al, 1996). In two patients, conversion to open surgery was required and two others required thoracoscopic assistance. Swanstrom and Hansen (1997) reported nine cases of laparoscopic total esophagectomy. There were no conversions to laparotomy, but one patient required a right thoracoscopy with intrathoracic anastomosis due to poor viability of the gastric tube. We have also reported this total laparoscopic approach; however, we found that the completion of the thoracic esophageal mobilization and lymph node dissection was unsatisfactory and that the addition of thoracoscopy was very helpful (Luketich et al, 1998a). We have now reported the results of this operation in 77 patients with a zero operative mortality (Luketich et al, 1998b, 1998c, 2000; Nguyen et al, 1999). To our knowledge, prior to our work, there have been no published series of combined thoracoscopic and laparoscopic esophagectomy performed without the addition of either standard thoracotomy or laparotomy.

PATIENT SELECTION

Patients are selected for minimally invasive esophagectomy after laparoscopic and thoracoscopic staging and endoscopic ultrasound have excluded metastases and confirmed the presence of a resectable esophageal carcinoma. Our initial experience was primarily in patients with Barrett's high-grade dysplasia but has evolved to include most patients with resectable lesions, including those with limited nodal involvement. In some cases, patients with bulky tumors or extensive nodal involvement or those who had undergone prior surgery are approached via standard laparotomy and thoracotomy or with palliative measures.

TECHNIQUE OF COMBINED LAPAROSCOPIC AND THORACOSCOPIC APPROACH TO ESOPHAGECTOMY

The patient is intubated with a double-lumen tube for single-lung ventilation and is positioned in the left lateral decubitus position. Four thoracoscopic ports are introduced (Fig. 61–1). The camera port (10 mm) is placed at the seventh intercostal space, midaxillary line. A 5-mm port is placed at the eighth or ninth intercostal space 2 cm posterior to the posterior axillary line for the ultrasonic coagulating shears (U.S. Surgical, Norwalk, CT). Two additional 5-mm ports are placed, one posterior to the tip of the scapula and one at the fourth intercostal space at the anterior axillary line for retraction and countertraction during the esophageal dissection. Next, a single retracting suture, O-Surgitek (U.S. Surgical), is placed in the central tendon of the diaphragm and brought out of the inferior anterior chest wall through a 1-mm skin nick using the endovascular closing device (Endoclose, U.S. Surgical). This traction suture allows downward retraction on the diaphragm without the need for a retractor and produces good exposure of the distal esophagus.

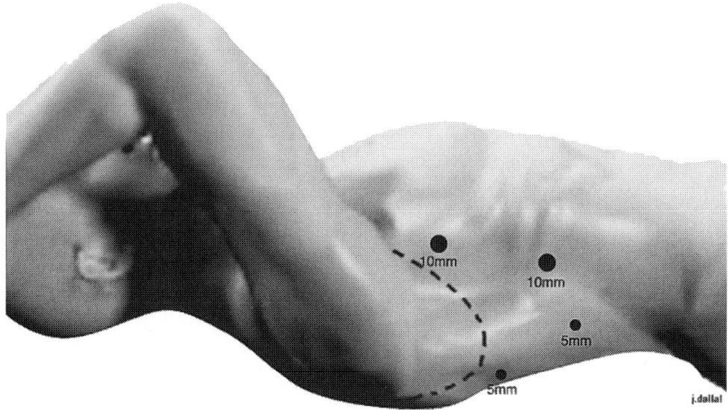

FIGURE 61–1 ■ Thoracic trocar position on the right chest for thoracoscopic exposure.

The mediastinal pleura overlying the esophagus is divided, and the entire thoracic esophagus is exposed. A Penrose drain is placed around the esophagus to facilitate traction and exposure (Fig. 61–2). The surgeon divides the azygos vein using an endoscopic vascular stapler (Endo-GIA, U.S. Surgical). Circumferential mobilization of the esophagus with all surrounding lymph nodes and periesophageal tissue and fat is performed from the diaphragmatic reflection to the thoracic inlet. A single 28 French chest tube is inserted through the camera port, the other port sites are closed, and the patient is turned to the supine position.

In the supine position, five abdominal ports are placed on the anterior abdominal wall in an approach similar to that of a laparoscopic Nissen fundoplication (Fig. 61–3). The surgeon retracts the left lobe of the liver upward to expose the esophageal hiatus using a Diamond-Flex retractor (Snowden Pencer, Tucker, GA) and holds it in

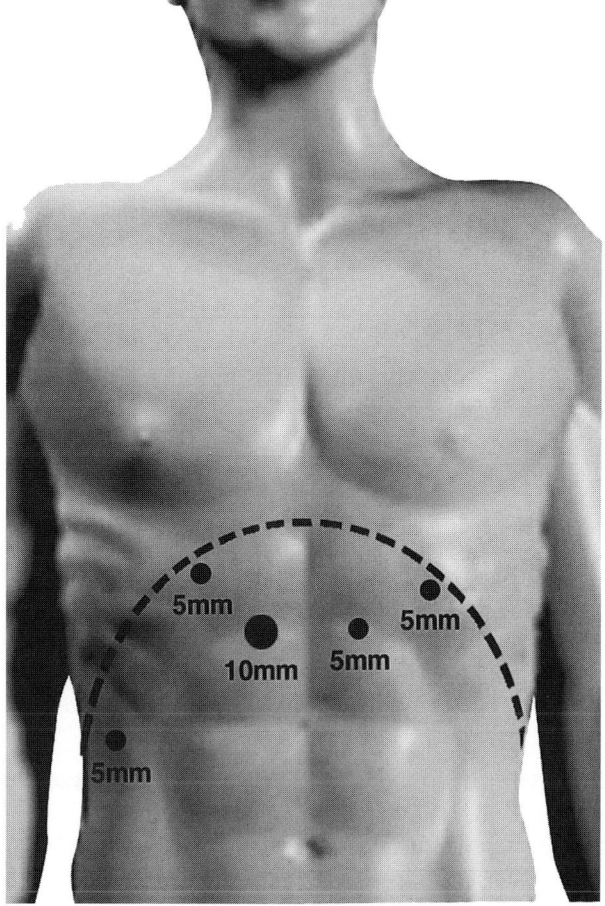

FIGURE 61–3 ■ Abdominal trocar position for laparoscopic transhiatal dissection.

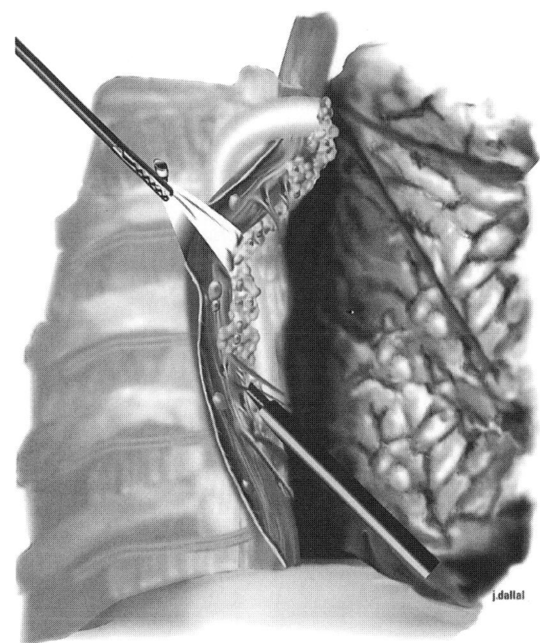

FIGURE 61–2 ■ Thoracoscopic mobilization of the thoracic esophagus and mediastinal lymph nodes.

place with a self-retaining system (Mediflex, Velmed, Inc., Wexford, PA). The surgeon begins by dissecting the gastrohepatic ligament and exposing the right crus of the diaphragm. Ultrasonic coagulating shears (U.S. Surgical) are used to divide the short gastric vessels. The dissection continues along the greater curvature of the stomach, and the right gastroepiploic arcade is preserved. The stomach is retracted superiorly, allowing lymph node dissection of the celiac and gastric vessels. Once the gastric artery and vein are exposed, the endoscopic vascular stapler is used to divide them.

The surgeon then performs the pyloroplasty using ultrasonic shears (Fig. 61–4*A* and *B*), and uses transverse sutures (Endostitch, U.S. Surgical) to close the incision. The lesser curve fat and nodes are dissected en bloc with the stomach. The surgeon then constructs the gastric tube by dividing the stomach, starting at the distal lesser curve and preserves the right gastric vessels using the 4.8-mm endoscopic stapler (Endo-GIA II, U.S. Surgical) (Fig. 61–5). The gastric tube is attached to the esophageal and esophagogastric specimen using two sutures (Endostitch) (Fig. 61–6). An additional suture is placed on the anterior proximal gastric tube to prevent twisting as the tube is brought up to the neck.

The surgeon places a laparoscopic jejunostomy tube by first attaching a limb of proximal jejunum to the

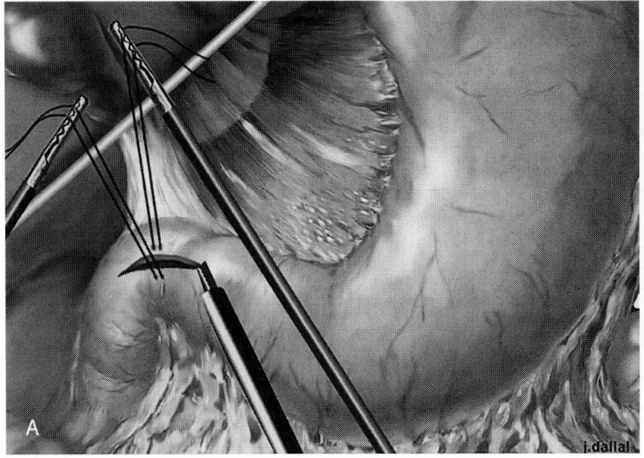

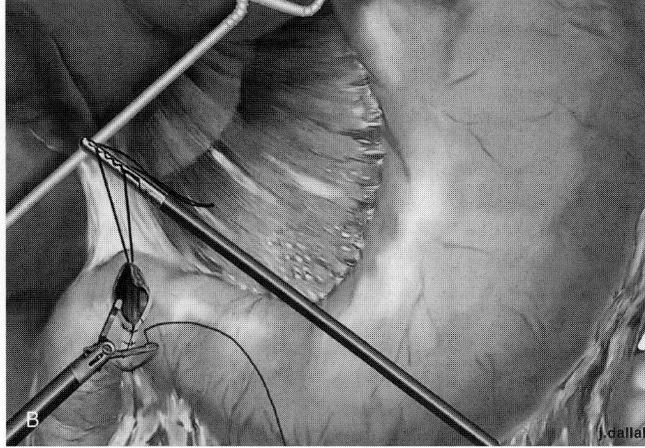

FIGURE 61–4 ■ Pyloroplasty. *A,* Ultrasonic shears are used. *B,* Closure is achieved with sutures (Endostitch).

anterior abdominal wall using the Endostitch. A needle catheter kit (Compat Biosystems, Minneapolis) is placed percutaneously into the peritoneal cavity under direct laparoscopic vision and is directed into the loop of jejunum. The guidewire and catheter are threaded into the jejunum. The jejunal puncture area is tacked completely to the anterior abdominal wall for a distance of several centimeters. The last step in the abdominal operation is the final dissection of the right and left crural areas to open the plane into the thoracic cavity. This step is completed last to minimize loss of pneumoperitoneum into the mediastinum. We also divide the right and left crurae to widen the hiatus to prevent gastric outlet obstruction.

A 4- to 6-cm horizontal neck incision is made just above the suprasternal notch, and the cervical esophagus is mobilized and exposed. Finger dissection is continued distally until the thoracic dissection plane is encountered. The surgeon divides the esophagus using the automatic purse string device (U.S. Surgical), and the esophagus is pulled up out of the wound, and as traction is applied to the specimen from the neck, another surgeon guides the specimen in its proper alignment into the mediastinum. The specimen is removed from the field. An anastomosis is performed between the esophagus and the gastric tube with the use of a 25-mm end-to-end anastomosis stapler (U.S. Surgical) placed through a small anterior gastrotomy. The remaining gastrotomy is closed with a stapler. The completed reconstruction is shown in Figure 61–7.

RESULTS

We have performed minimally invasive esophagectomy in more than 150 patients. We next review the results of our first 77 patients operated on from August 1996 to June 1999, which have been recently reported. Indications for esophagectomy included esophageal carcinoma (n = 52), Barrett's esophagus with high-grade dysplasia (n = 19), and benign esophageal disorders (n = 6). The mean age was 65.1 years, with an age range of 30 to 89 years. Fifty patients (65%) had undergone prior surgery involving the abdominal or thoracic cavity. Twenty of these patients had had esophageal surgery: hiatal hernia repair in 4, laparoscopic staging for esophagus cancer in 16, and laparoscopic Heller myotomy in 2.

Minimally invasive approach to esophagectomy included total laparoscopic transhiatal esophagectomy (n = 9), thoracoscopic combined with laparoscopic esophagectomy (n = 60), and laparoscopic gastric mobilization with right muscle-sparing minithoracotomy (n = 8). Conversion to laparotomy was necessary in 4 patients as a result of dense adhesions. Pyloromyotomy was performed in 27 patients, and pyloroplasty was performed in 46 patients. A laparoscopic jejunostomy tube was placed in 56 patients.

The mean operative time was 7.5 hours (range, 4.0 to 13.6 hours). The mean intensive care unit stay was 1 day (range, 0 to 60 days). The mean hospital stay was 7 days (range, 4 to 73 days). The 30-day operative mortality was zero. There were no intraoperative emergencies requiring urgent conversion. Major complications occurred in 21 (27%) of patients (Table 61–1).

Six of the seven anastomotic leaks in the neck were

TABLE 61–1 ■ **Complications Following Resection of Esophageal Carcinoma**

Minor Complications	*No. of Cases*	*Major Complications*	*No. of Cases*
Transfusion	5	Hypopharynx laceration	1
Urinary retention	1	Small-bowel perforation	1
Air leak	3	Tracheal tear	1
Atelectasis	5	Recurrent laryngeal nerve injury	2
Aspiration requiring NG tube	1	Chylothorax	3
Pleural effusion	18	Anastomotic leak	7
Atrial fibrillation	8	Abscess (1 mediastinal, 1 abdominal)	2
Dislodged J-tube	1	Pyloric leak	1
J-tube infection	2	Delayed gastric emptying†	3
Delayed gastric emptying*	1	Deep vein thrombosis	1
Stricture requiring dilation	1	Pulmonary embolus	1
Clostridium difficile colitis	1	Myocardial infarction	2
Wound infection	1	Adult respiratory distress syndrome	1
		Pneumonia	4
		Acute respiratory failure	2

*Resolved after pyloric dilation.
†Laparoscopic pyloroplasty required.

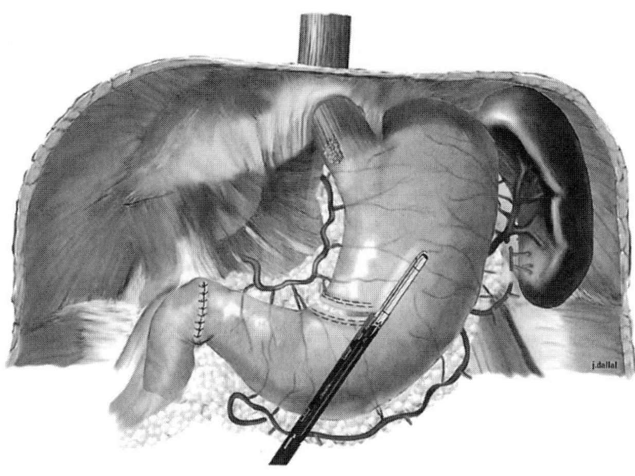

FIGURE 61–5 ■ A gastric conduit is created by an endoscopic stapler.

managed by conservative measures. A descending perigastric tube abscess in one patient developed and resolved with open neck drainage and drain placement. The single hypopharyngeal perforation was secondary to a malpositioned esophageal temperature probe and was repaired primarily at the time of esophagectomy with no further sequelae.

One patient suffered a tracheal tear on postoperative day 6 during reintubation for respiratory distress. The reintubation injury was due to malposition of the stylet of the endotracheal tube. This was repaired by right thoracotomy and was followed by a prolonged hospital stay of 50 days; ultimately, the patient recovered. Two patients experienced permanent recurrent laryngeal injury requiring vocal cord injections with polytetrafluoroethylene (Teflon). Minor complications in the perioperative period occurred in 55% (see Table 61–1).

Delayed complications (>30 days after surgery) occurred in four patients. Two patients who had had an initial pyloromyotomy suffered persistent delayed gastric emptying that necessitated laparoscopic pyloroplasty with good results. One patient experienced delayed gastric emptying with holdup of contrast material at the crural level; laparoscopic crural division was performed with good results. One patient, presenting with a moderately symptomatic diaphragmatic herniation of bowel into the right chest, underwent elective laparoscopic reduction and repair with good results.

The final pathologic stage of the cancer patients included stages 0 (4), I (10), IIA (16), IIB (10), III (30),

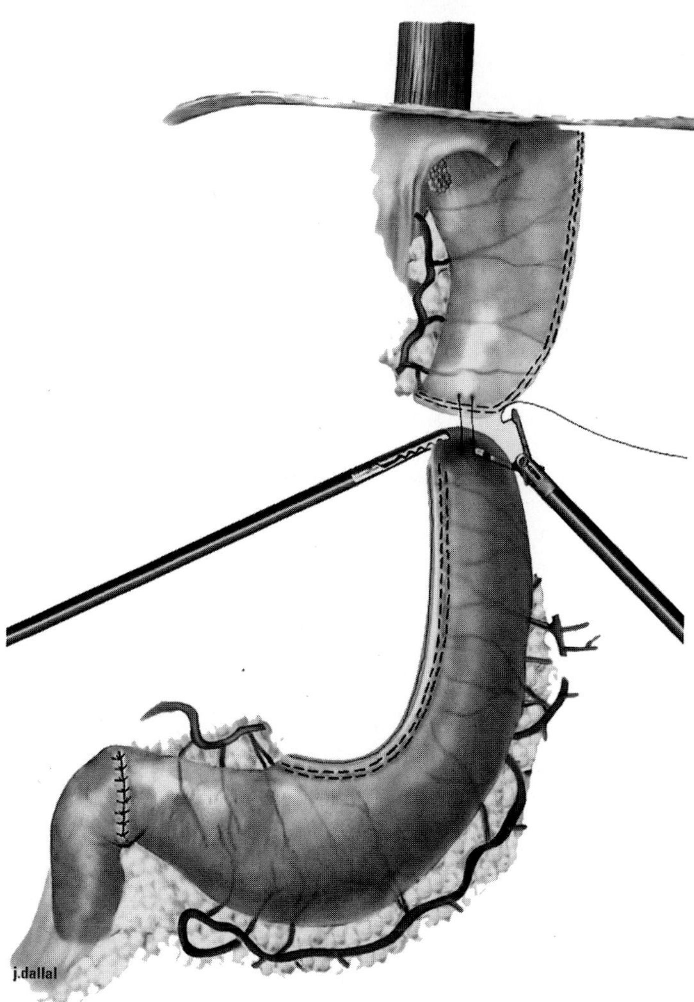

FIGURE 61–6 ■ Removal of an esophageal specimen en bloc with transhiatal pull-through of the gastric conduit through the cervical incision.

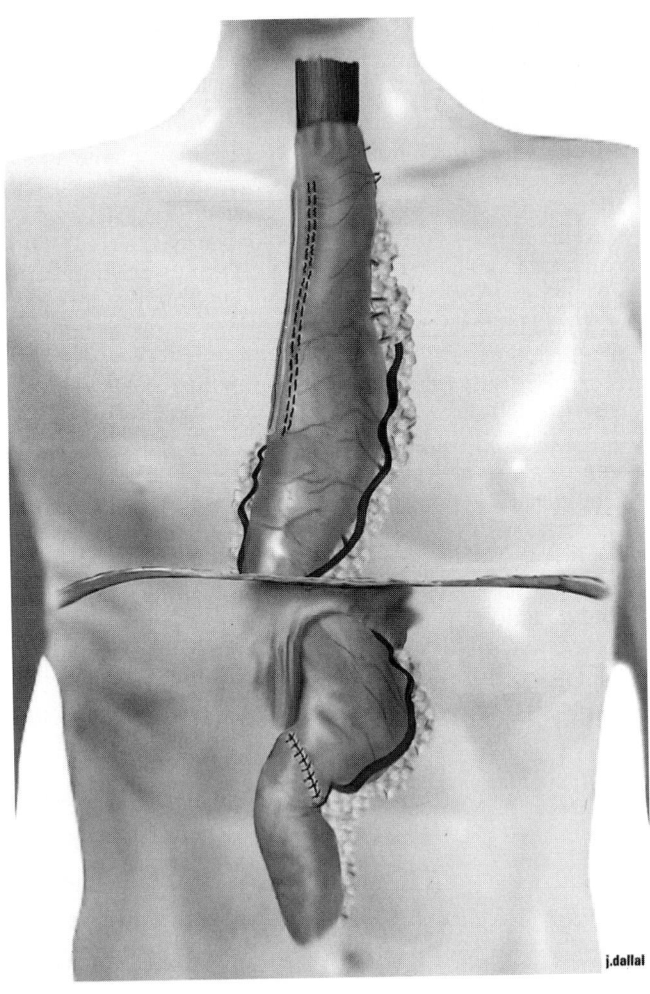

FIGURE 61–7 ■ Completed reconstruction. *Note:* The closed gastrotomy site for the stapled cervical anastomosis is not shown.

and IV (1). Histologic subtypes included adenocarcinoma of the gastroesophageal junction, present in 90% of cases; 10% had midesophageal squamous cell carcinoma. No cases of cervical esophageal cancer were included. In all cases, surgical margins were negative on frozen section. The final pathologic examination revealed microscopic disease at the adventitial margin in three patients. The average number of lymph nodes removed with the specimen was 16 (range, 10 to 51). Approximately 60% of the lymph nodes were from the laparoscopic dissection and 40% were from the chest. The six patients with benign indications were all alive at 20-month follow-up.

The cancer group (71 patients) had an overall survival rate of 81% at a median follow-up of 20 months. There have been 18 patients with cancer recurrence. In eight, only distant disease was present, and in eight there was local and distant recurrence. In the two patients with local recurrence only, one had extensive Barrett's esophagus preoperatively and ultimately underwent resection for an apparent new primary tumor within residual Barrett's extending into the cervical esophagus. The other patient had extensive recurrence of invasive carcinoma along the gastric tube and has been receiving palliative photodynamic therapy. Survival by stage is illustrated in Figure 61–8.

DISCUSSION

Our initial results in 77 patients confirmed the feasibility and safety of performing esophagectomy using minimally invasive technique (Luketich et al, 2000). Our technique continues to evolve, and currently our preferred approach is the combined laparoscopic and thoracoscopic technique. The thoracoscopic approach improves our ability to perform a more extensive lymph node dissection and to easily mobilize the middle and proximal third of the

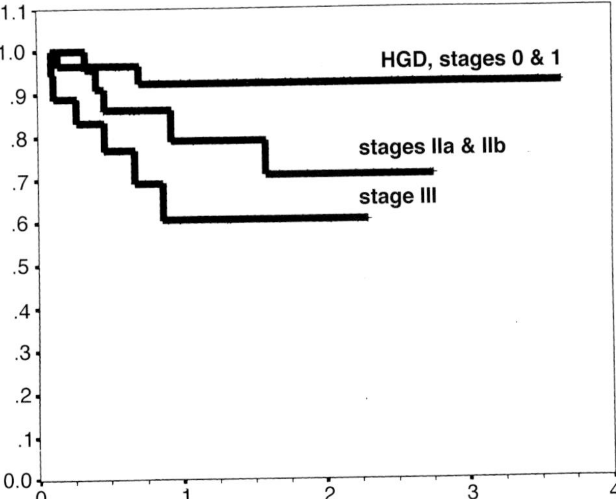

FIGURE 61–8 ■ Kaplan-Meier survival curves for 71 patients with cancer resections. Stage I (n = 14); stage IIA and IIB (n = 26); stage III (n = 30). (HGD, carcinoma in situ.)

esophagus. Our average lymph node count is now between 20 and 30; this is in excess of what we routinely obtain with a transhiatal esophagectomy. The azygos vein is divided to facilitate dissection of the upper third of the esophagus. Laparoscopy is performed following thoracoscopy. The laparoscopic transhiatal technique was our initial approach, but limitations of a small working space through the esophageal hiatus and difficulty in dissection of the middle and upper third esophagus led to our routine addition of thoracoscopy.

Minimally invasive esophagectomy is a technically demanding operation requiring advanced laparoscopic and thoracoscopic surgical skills. The routine performance of advanced laparoscopic and thoracoscopic procedures allowed us to perform this operation safely (Luketich et al, 1997a, 1997b, 2000; Nguyen et al, 1998). For example, we have performed more than 1000 laparoscopic antireflux procedures, 150 staging procedures for esophageal carcinoma, 75 esophageal myotomies, and many other procedures that allowed us to gain experience in esophageal mobilization. We recommend that any minimally invasive procedure on the esophagus be performed only by surgeons with extensive experience in open esophageal surgery and having significant laparoscopic and thoracoscopic skills.

There is a significant learning curve to this procedure, as demonstrated by our initial operative times, which were frequently in excess of 7 to 8 hours; however, we have now demonstrated that surgeons in our group who have performed more than 20 of these procedures can accomplish the operation in under 5 hours. Appropriate instrumentation, including the ultrasonic shears, the endoscopic stapler, and the liver retractor, is necessary to perform this procedure.

Our series, similar to those of DePaula and Swanstrom, confirms that esophagectomy can be safely performed by the total laparoscopic or thoracoscopic approach in selected cases in centers specializing in minimally invasive esophageal surgery (DePaula et al, 1996; Swanstrom and Hansen, 1997). Prospective trials with longer follow-up will be required to confirm any advantages of minimally invasive esophagectomy over conventional approaches, and open surgical approaches should remain the standard operation for esophagectomy in most institutions. However, in comparing our patients undergoing minimally invasive esophagectomy to open, we believe that there is less pain, a shorter hospital stay, and a more rapid recovery to full activity following minimally invasive esophagectomy.

COMMENTS AND CONTROVERSIES

The preceding chapter by Drs. Luketich and coauthors is a dramatic illustration of how far minimally invasive instrumentation and techniques have advanced in such a short time. The issues raised by this chapter, in my mind, have more to do with how we approach and assess new technology and procedures and less with issues regarding the best surgical approach for patients with carcinoma of the esophagus. Dr. Luketich and colleagues have demonstrated what can be done with minimally invasive techniques, but there is much room to debate what evidence is required to determine whether this approach in fact should be done.

The short-term results reported, in terms of hospital stay, morbidity, and mortality, are not dissimilar from those reported with open surgical techniques. There are some apparent disadvantages to the procedure described for those patients in the series operated on for benign disease, high-grade dysplasia, or very early carcinoma in whom a transhiatal approach would ordinarily be employed. These disadvantages include the thoracoscopic component with its need for a double-lumen tube, entrance into the right pleural space, and use of intercostal instrumentation with its potential for long-term post-thoracotomy pain from intercostal neuralgia. In addition, the long operative times and the extensive use of thoracoscopic and laparoscopic instrumentation adds a very significant cost to the procedure. Finally, the ultimate assessment of this type of newer technique must be made on the basis of comparative long-term results in terms of functional and oncologic outcome.

The question is: How should this type of procedure be responsibly introduced and evaluated? Since there are existing techniques to accomplish the same goal, how should such a technique with its uncertain benefit and risk be introduced without inhibiting the ability of the surgeon to innovate on the one hand while avoiding unnecessary risks and unjustified claims of benefit on the other? In my opinion, this should be done at a limited number of centers, where appropriately selected patients are randomized from the outset to either the new procedure or the more traditional approach, with careful analysis of morbidity, mortality, cost, and long-term outcome. This is, in fact, consistent with the author's conclusion that "prospective trials with longer follow-up will be required to confirm any advantages of minimally invasive esophagectomy over conventional approaches, and open surgical approaches should remain the standard operation for esophagectomy in most institutions."

J. D. C.

REFERENCES

Akaishi T, Kaneda I, Higuchi N, et al: Thoracoscopic en bloc total esophagectomy with vertical mediastinal lymphadenectomy. J Thorac Cardiovasc Surg 112:1533–1541, 1996.

DePaula AL, Hashiba K, Ferreira EAB, et al: Trans-hiatal approach for esophagectomy. In Toouli J, Gossot D, Hunter JG (eds): Endosurgery. New York, Churchill Livingstone, 1996, pp 293–299.

Dexter SPL, Martin IG, McMahon MJ: Radical thoracoscopic esophagectomy for cancer. Surg Endosc 10:147–151, 1996.

Luketich JD, Kassis ES, Landreneau R, et al: A comparison of total video thoracoscopic lobectomy and standard thoracotomy for early stage non–small cell lung cancer (NSCLC) [Abstract]. Lung Cancer 18:98, 1997a.

Luketich JD, Schauer P, Landreneau R, et al: Minimally invasive surgical staging is superior to endoscopic ultrasound in detecting lymph node metastases in esophageal cancer. J Thorac Cardiovasc Surg 114:817–823, 1997b.

Luketich JD, Nguyen NT, Schauer P: Laparoscopic transhiatal esophagectomy for Barrett's esophagus with high-grade dysplasia. J Soc Laparoendosc Surg 2:75–77, 1998a.

Luketich JD, Nguyen NT, Weigel TL, et al: Minimally invasive approach to esophagectomy. J Soc Laparoendosc Surg 2:243–247, 1998b.

Luketich JD, Nguyen NT, Weigel TL, et al: The role of laparoscopy and video-assisted thoracoscopy in esophagectomy [Abstract]. Surg Endosc 12:554, 1998c.

Luketich JD, Schauer PR, Urso K, et al: Future directions in esophageal cancer. Chest 113 (1 suppl):1205–1225, 1998d.

Luketich JD, Schauer PR, Christie NA, et al: Minimally invasive esophagectomy. Ann Thorac Surg 70:906–912, 2000.

Millikan KW, Silverstein J, Hart V, et al: A 15-year review of esophagectomy for carcinoma of the esophagus and cardia. Arch Surg 130:617–624, 1995.

Nguyen NT, Schauer PR, Hutson W, et al: Preliminary results of thoracoscopic Belsey-Mark IV anti-reflux procedure. Surg Laparosc Endosc 8:185–188, 1998.

Nguyen NT, Schauer PR, Luketich JD: Combined laparoscopic and thoracoscopic approach to esophagectomy. J Am Coll Surg 188:328–332, 1999.

Patti MG, Corvera C, Glasgow RE, et al: A hospital's annual rate of esophagectomy influences the operative mortality rate. J Gastrointest Surg 2:186–192, 1998.

Swanstrom LL, Hansen P: Laparoscopic total esophagectomy. Arch Surg 132:943–949, 1997.

CHAPTER **62**

Esophageal Bypass

Alex G. Little

Esophageal carcinoma presents a dichotomous therapeutic challenge to the surgeon that requires the consideration of both curative and palliative treatment strategies. Potentially curative therapeutic alternatives are presented in other chapters, and all include surgical resection. Unfortunately, 40% to 60% of patients are not realistic candidates for a curative operation because they present with advanced local or metastatic disease, specifically stage III or stage IV cancer. Despite their limited life expectancy, these patients deserve and require palliation for the devastating sequelae of esophageal obstruction. Options include, alone or in combination, palliative resection, endoscopic laser ablation, brachytherapy, external beam radiation therapy, chemotherapy, intubation or stenting of the esophagus with prostheses, and surgical bypass of the esophagus.

It is my belief that surgical resection is not only important as part of a curative therapeutic strategy but also for palliation alone when the primary tumor is technically resectable but cure is unlikely. This conclusion is supported by the reports of Abe and associates (1989), Belsey (1980), Lorentz and colleagues (1989), Skinner (1980), and Wong (1987). With one intervention, the obstructive tumor is removed and unimpeded swallowing is restored with reasonable surgical morbidity and mortality risks. This approach applies to patients with T4 tumors that invade resectable strictures, such as the diaphragm, and to patients with N1 disease with involvement of regional lymph nodes. Cure is not a realistic surgical goal in these patients, but the resection of gross local disease is possible and constitutes the ideal palliative option. Only when esophagectomy is impossible—that is, when truly unresectable disease is present, such as when the celiac axis is encased by malignant lymph nodes or the primary tumor involves the aorta are the alternative palliative approaches preferable.

External beam radiation therapy frequently causes tumor shrinkage but provides only modest palliation as the tumor is replaced by fibrous tissue and stricture formation and dysphagia persists. Chemotherapeutic regimens that include cisplatin produce a complete or partial response in 50% to 70% of patients with localized tumors. Efficacy is less than that for metastatic disease or for extensive local disease, and the side effects limit the palliative role, although Herskovic and colleagues (1992) document impressive results with chemoradiation, and this combination may yet prove its efficacy and sufficiency. Endoscopic laser treatment effectively restores a swallowing tube, but rapid tumor regrowth is typical. As shown by Low and co-workers (1998), the recent introduction of both covered and uncovered metal stents has made stenting a more attractive option than when rigid plastic stents were used. The role of brachytherapy is essentially experimental and not yet defined.

This chapter covers the palliative option of bypass for patients whose cancer is (1) technically unresectable because of tumor invasion of structures such as the trachea or aorta or because their physiologic status is insufficient to withstand an esophagectomy or (2) who have metastatic esophageal cancer or another disease process that foretells such a short remaining life span that exposure to the risks and hospitalization stay associated with an esophagectomy is not reasonable.

HISTORICAL NOTE

As described by Kirschner (1920) and Yudin (1944), before the feasibility and safety of extraction of the esophagus were established, surgical methods of reestablishing gastrointestinal tract continuity when the esophagus was obstructed by cancer or nondilatable stricture were routinely based on esophageal bypass techniques. As reviewed by Segalin and colleagues (1989), complicated plastic operations with the formation of chest wall skin tubes or long segments of jejunum passed subcutaneously were the most widely used methods to link the cervical esophagus with the stomach. Complications were excessive, results were poor, and enthusiasm was contained.

With the maturation and evolution of thoracic oncologic surgery, the development of successful techniques for esophagectomy alleviated the need for bypass in most patients because of the benefits of tumor removal compared with bypass alone. As this chapter discusses, however, the need for palliation remains for patients in whom esophagectomy is not possible.

HISTORICAL READINGS

Kirschner M: Ein neues verfahren der oesophagoplastik. Arch Klin Chir 114:606, 1920.

Yudin SS: The surgical construction of 80 cases of artificial esophagus. Surg Gynecol Obstet 78:361, 1944.

MANAGEMENT

Patient Selection

The identification of esophageal cancer that is technically unresectable because of invasion of structures such as the trachea or aorta can occur preoperatively or, as pointed out by Lam and associates (1982) and Wong and colleagues (1982), intraoperatively. These patients are candidates for surgical bypass. Patients with involvement of regional nodes or even with minimal metastatic disease, such as a single liver nodule, are best served by resection and reconstruction rather than bypass alone. Perhaps the ideal candidate for esophageal bypass is a patient with a malignant esophagorespiratory fistula. As reviewed by Duranceau and Jamieson (1984), these fistulas are a relatively common event in the natural history of esophageal cancer and are diagnosed in 5% to 10% of patients. They usually involve the distal trachea or left mainstem bronchus and obviously preclude resection. Patients are rendered particularly miserable as they continually aspirate ingested foods, their own saliva, and refluxed gastric contents. This aspiration provokes continuous coughing, which is unpleasant in itself and makes sleep impossible, and eventually causes aspiration pneumonia. On the other hand, in the absence of metastatic disease, life expectancy is 3 to 18 months if the fistula is controlled. Consequently, an aggressive approach that includes bypass is appropriate for patients without metastases. Staging examinations must be sufficient to reasonably exclude metastatic or extensive nodal spread.

When either a complete or an impending fistula has been identified by barium swallow radiography (Fig. 62–1) or bronchoscopic documentation of invasion of the airway, surgical intervention should take place as soon as possible after completion of the staging process, because the patient's condition will deteriorate with the passage of time as a result of continued soilage of the lungs.

Once a commitment to esophageal bypass is established, three separate and independent surgical considerations must be taken into account: (1) the route of bypass, (2) the conduit used for bypass, and (3) the handling of the bypassed, isolated esophageal segment. In addition, these are typically fragile patients who are nutritionally depleted, with exhausted energy stores and compromised immunologic capability, and who have insulted lungs. A feeding jejunostomy should be placed in all patients during surgery for early postoperative institution of enteral nutrition and for continued support if oral alimentation is delayed by a need for prolonged mechanical ventilation or an anastomotic leak.

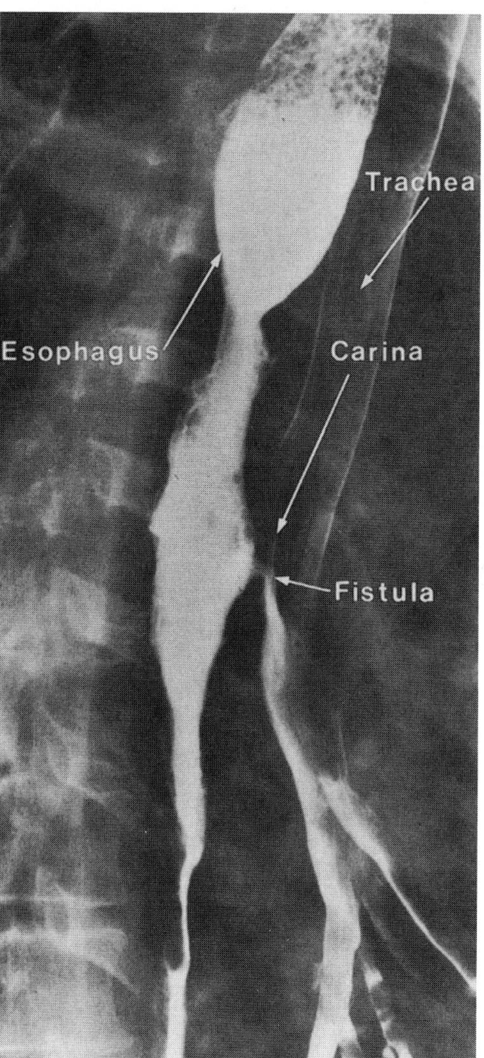

FIGURE 62–1 ■ Barium swallow radiograph demonstrating a malignant tracheoesophageal fistula. Not only is the fistula tract identifiable, but the absence of barium in the upper trachea eliminates the possibility of aspiration as the cause of contrast material in the bronchial tree.

Bypass Routes

The three possible anatomic bypass routes are (1) the posterior mediastinum, (2) the anterior mediastinum or retrosternal space, and (3) subcutaneously (antesternally) over the sternum.

Posterior Mediastinum Route

Although the posterior mediastinum represents the shortest distance between the neck and the abdomen and is the location most often used after esophagectomy, this route is obviously not available because it is occupied by the primary tumor and the esophagus. A pleural location for the interposed organ is possible but is not ideal because a thoracotomy is required and gastric or colonic distention is common, presumably because of the negative thoracic pressure. This complication further compromises the already tenuous respiratory status of the typical patient, decreasing the attractiveness of this location for the interposed segment.

Anterior Mediastinum (Retrosternal) Route

The anterior mediastinal or retrosternal location is, by default, the route of choice for placement of the esophageal substitute in most bypass operations. The neck-to-abdomen distance is slightly longer than the posterior mediastinal route, but both the stomach and colon segments are reliably able to bridge this gap. A benefit of this location is that it is anatomically separated from the tumor, which affords protection against obstruction by the tumor of the bypass segment.

The operation is performed through a neck and an upper abdominal midline incision, which spares the patient a thoracotomy and is generally tolerated even by

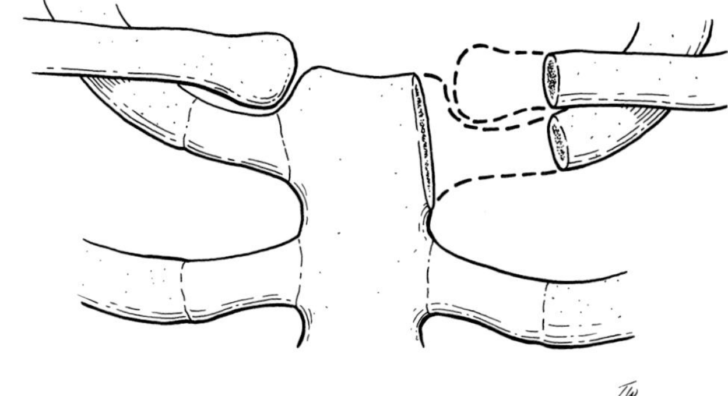

FIGURE 62–2 ■ Anatomy of the thoracic outlet following resection of the head of the left clavicle and the indicated portion of the manubrium and first rib. This important maneuver opens the space considerably for any substernal visceral esophageal substitute, especially the anterior-posterior dimension.

patients with marginal pulmonary function. The cervical esophagus and stomach are mobilized. The anterior fibers of the diaphragm are detached from the xiphisternum with electrocautery, and a substernal tunnel is bluntly developed by hand. The stomach or colon is brought over the liver and through the tunnel into the neck, where a cervical anastomosis is constructed. The interposed organ (stomach or colon) should be passed up the substernal tunnel by hand rather than being pulled up from above.

I do suture the stomach or colon to a malleable retractor with two holes in its end and use this to ensure its correct orientation. Traction from above, however, may tear and should be avoided. As shown in Figure 62–2, resection of the head of the left clavicle and first rib with an oscillating saw, including a portion of the manubrium, is an important feature of this undertaking, because it decompresses the thoracic inlet. This minimizes pressure on the interposed organ and its blood supply.

Subcutaneous (Antesternal) Route

The subcutaneous or antesternal approach for esophageal bypass can be used when necessary, such as when the anterior mediastinal compartment is not available because of previous cardiac surgery. The operation is similar to the retrosternal procedure, except that the tunnel that connects the abdomen to the neck is developed by elevating the skin from the muscular fascia over the sternum. The distance from the abdomen to the neck is a few centimeters longer than that for the substernal route, but the stomach is usually of sufficient length to bridge this gap and functions adequately. The final cosmetic result is acceptable, although a bulge is evident over the anterior chest.

Choice of the Esophagus Substitute

Stomach

The stomach is the first choice as substitute, primarily because of the reliability of its blood supply. Mobilization and preparation of the stomach are described in other chapters. Two important specific steps are emphasized:

1. A gastric emptying procedure, either a pyloromyotomy or a short pyloroplasty, is routine because these patients poorly tolerate a reoperation if delayed gastric emptying secondary to pylorospasm develops postoperatively.

2. The entire stomach, rather than a tubularized version, should be used to ensure that sufficient length is available. To accomplish this step, the surgeon separates the stomach from the esophagus by transection exactly at, or slightly on the gastric side of, the gastroesophageal junction. Release of the lesser curve by division of the lesser curve mesentery, which contains the vagal nerve and left gastric artery branches, helps to provide maximum gastric length. Figure 62–3 illustrates these steps, and Figure 62–4 shows the stomach attached to the malleable retractor, which keeps the stomach oriented as

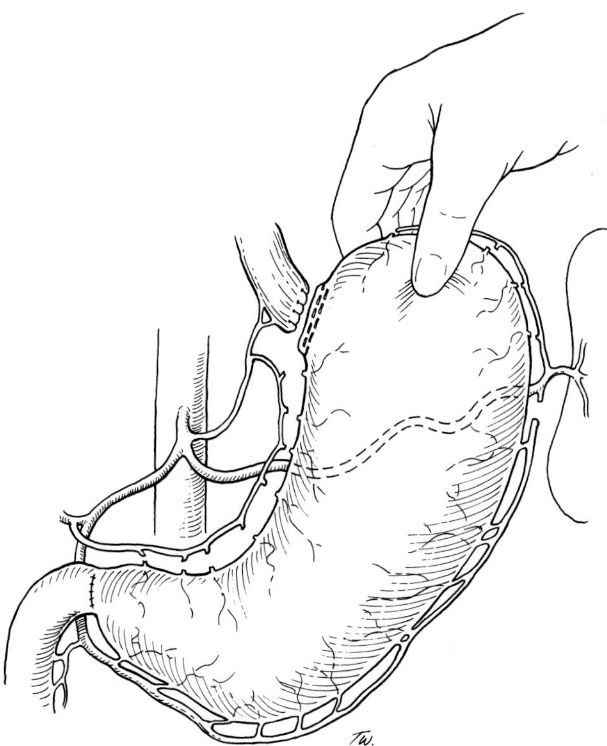

FIGURE 62–3 ■ Appearance of the stomach being prepared for substernal positioning. A short pyloroplasty has been performed, and detachment from the esophagus is taking place at the gastroesophageal junction. The division of the lesser curve mesentery, which allows greater stretch, is indicated. The hand is holding the apex of the fundus, which is used for the final esophageal anastomosis.

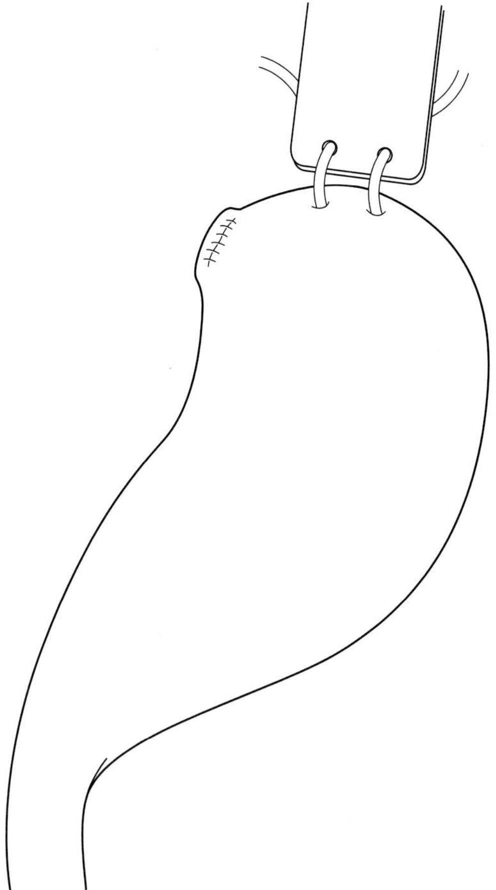

FIGURE 62–4 ■ A method of passing the stomach to the neck is depicted. After the substernal space is opened by manual dissection, a malleable retractor is passed through it. The stomach is sutured to the distal end through two holes in the retractor. The stomach is grasped and manually delivered into the neck from below as gentle traction is applied to the retractor to preserve the correct orientation of the stomach so that it does not twist on itself.

it is passed by hand up the substernal tunnel from below. Figure 62–5 shows the final appearance after completion of the esophagogastrostomy in the neck.

Results of gastric bypass have steadily improved. In the past, excessively high complication rates were associated with this procedure, with hospital mortality rates as high as 30% to 40% and morbidity rates in excess of 60% (Orringer, 1984; Robinson et al, 1981). Improvements in technique and perioperative care have decreased the morbidity and mortality rates as shown by many: Akyama and Hiyama (1974), Conlan and colleagues (1983 and 1984), Ong and associates (1982), Roeher and Horeyseck (1981), Sugimachi and colleagues (1982), and Meunier and co-workers (1996).

A large series by Mannell and associates (1988) reported an 11% hospital mortality rate. Eighty-nine percent of survivors were able to eat a normal, unrestricted diet, and the 6-month survival rate was 60%. Survival however, is limited in these patients with advanced malignant disease, and they present a higher risk for surgery because of the detrimental effects of pulmonary contamination. A judgment must be made regarding the risk—in terms of treatment morbidity and mortality—versus the palliative efficacy of bypass operations. Illustrative of this consideration is the report by Burt and colleagues (1991). Their operative mortality rate for bypass procedures, using stomach and colon, was no less than 25%, but the patients had a longer median survival than did any other treatment group. Palliation was judged to have been better as well.

Colon

If the stomach is not available for use because of intrinsic disease or previous gastric surgery, the colon is an acceptable second choice. Careful preparation of a colon segment based on the left colic artery usually results in a sufficient length to reach the neck and allows an isoperistaltic orientation. As shown in Figure 62–6, it is necessary to divide the middle colic vessels below their bifurcation to achieve reliable vascularization to the hepatic side of the transverse colon.

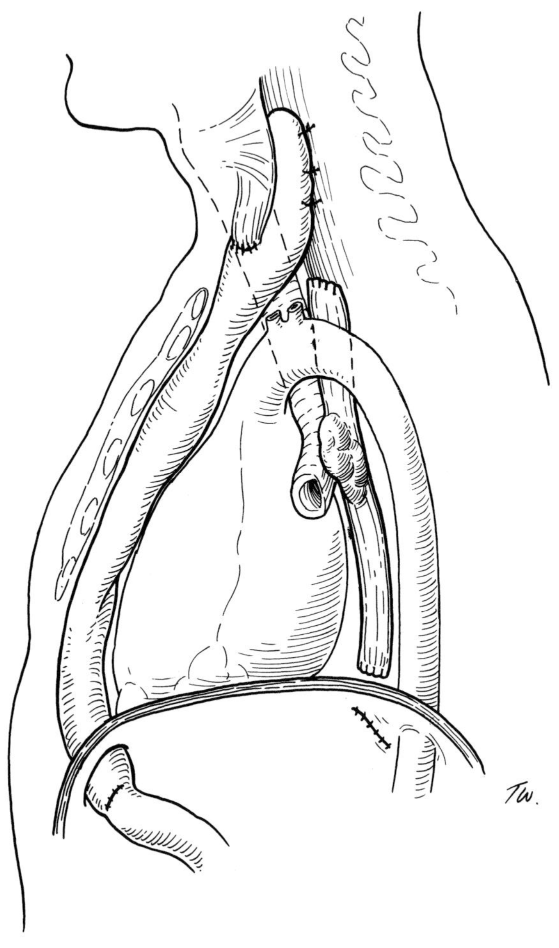

FIGURE 62–5 ■ Lateral schematic view showing the final appearance of a substernal gastric bypass. As discussed in the text, it is frequently necessary to drain the isolated esophageal segment with a catheter unless the esophagorespiratory fistula is large enough to accommodate free drainage from the esophagus.

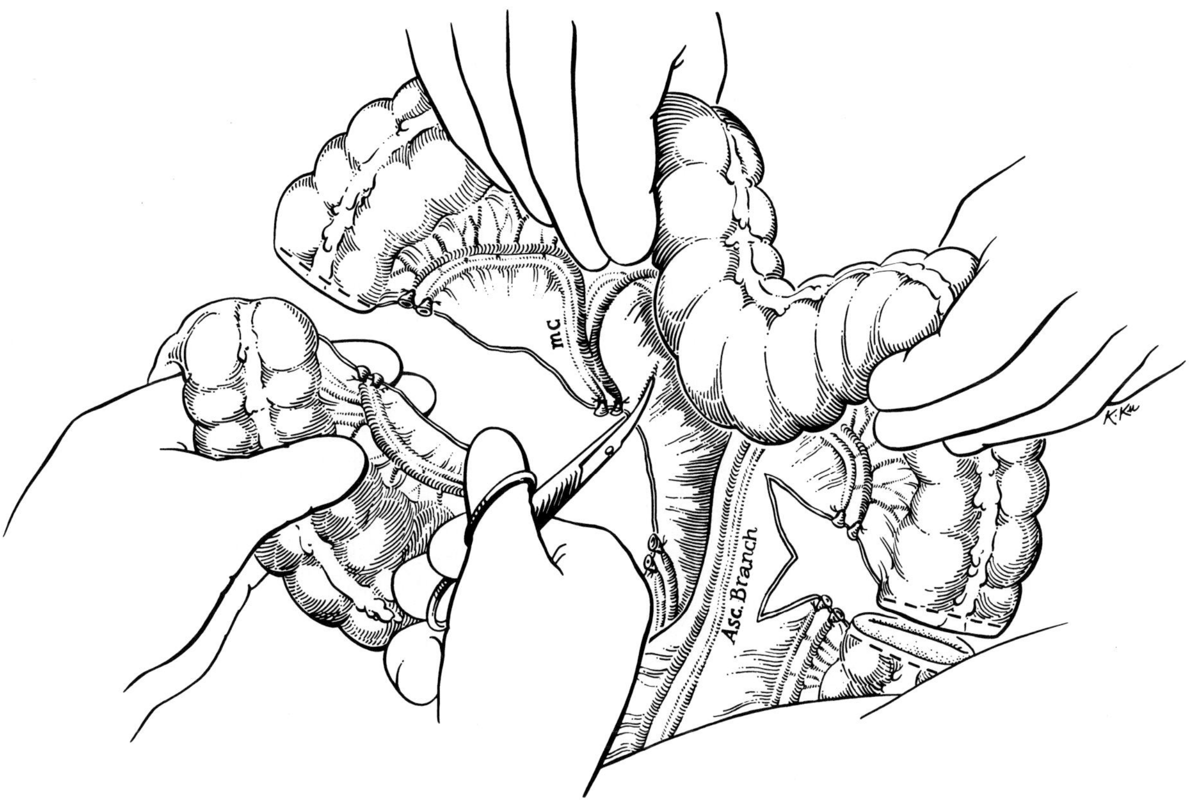

FIGURE 62–6 ■ As shown here, in preparing a colon segment long enough to reach the neck, the middle colic vessels must be divided below their bifurcation so that flow is preserved to the right side of the colon segment.

If colon is used, it should be oriented in an isoperistaltic manner whenever possible. Antiperistaltic placement, such as when a right colon segment is based on the right colic blood supply, can result in dilatation and nonfunction, causing dysphagia. Disadvantages of using the colon instead of the stomach include the need for three anastomoses: anastomosis of the colon segment to the esophagus and the stomach as well as colocolostomy; however, the only contraindication to the use of colon is intrinsic colon pathology, such as cancer, polyps, and diverticulosis.

Results of colon use can be equivalent to those achieved with the use of the stomach (Little et al, 1984). However, complications and related morbidity are more likely for colon interposition than for gastric interposition (Curet-Scott et al, 1987; Santos, 1991). Accordingly, there has been a definite trend toward preferential use of the stomach rather than the colon for esophageal replacement or bypass.

Jejunum is not usually a realistic option because of the inability to obtain sufficient length to reach the upper esophagus because of the inconsistent, segmental distribution of its vascular supply. Only if the stomach and colon are unavailable, if the patient is fit enough to tolerate a thoracotomy, and if the tumor is very low in the mediastinum can the jejunum be a consideration. When jejunal interposition is successful, the results are similar to those of other bypass procedures. It is noteworthy that in one report by Lorentz and associates (1989), the anastomotic leakage late for jejunum was less than that for either stomach or colon.

The Excluded Esophagus

When the esophagus is excluded and left in situ, several surgical options are available. If there is an open fistula to the trachea or bronchus, it is safe to simply close both esophageal ends and leave the esophageal remnant as a pseudodiverticulum of the respiratory tract. The remnant does not become an abscess or a mucocele because of free communication and drainage of esophageal secretions through the fistula. The addition of this small amount of lung dead space does not affect pulmonary function.

If there is no fistula or if one is present but small, esophageal drainage is prudent to avoid abscess or mucocele development within the blind esophageal segment or a blowout of the distal end. Kirschner (1920) described esophagojejunostomy as a solution, but this maneuver requires an investment of the time and effort necessary to construct an anastomosis and exposes the patient to the risk of anastomotic leak. Alternatively, Little and associates (1984) describe the placement of a red rubber catheter through the divided esophagus in the superior mediastinum, through the neck, and closure of the esophagus around the tube. This tube then is brought out through a separate incision as a cervical esophagostomy (Fig. 62–7). The catheter is simply attached to a Foley drainage bag after surgery and is gradually advanced and

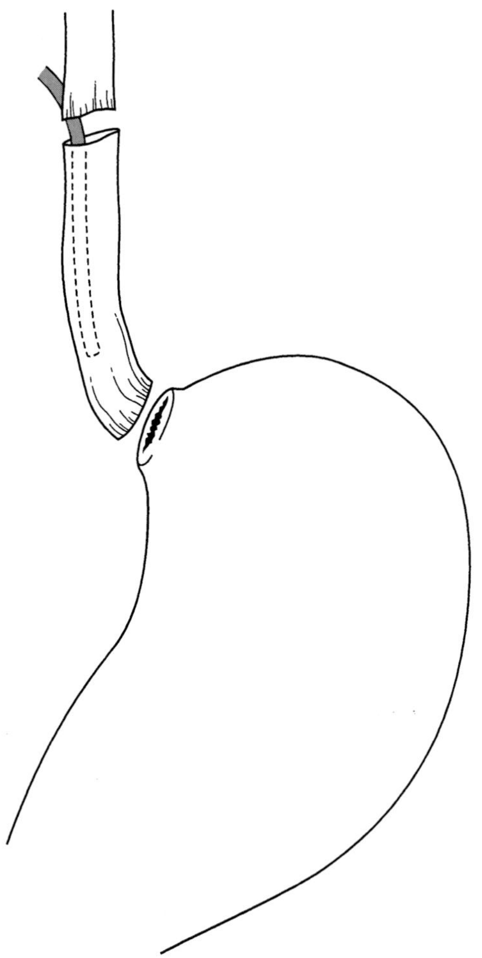

FIGURE 62–7 ■ Placement of a red rubber catheter in the excluded esophagus is illustrated. The stomach is subsequently brought into the neck via the substernal route for an anastomosis to the esophagus.

removed during the second or third postoperative week. Rarely does drainage persist after final removal of the tube.

COMMENTS AND CONTROVERSIES

Dr. Alex Little addresses a difficult surgical and philosophical problem—namely, the optimal palliation for unfortunate individuals with unresectable carcinoma of the esophagus. I am reminded of the comments of one of my mentors in the field of esophageal surgery who felt that it was his obligation to either palliate such patients or "put them out of their misery in the attempt." As I recall, his success rate approached 100%. In his introduction, Dr. Little espouses the view that palliative resection should be considered even when it is apparent from the outset that cure is not possible. Given the high mortality, and especially the prolonged morbidity so often associated with that type of resection, it is my opinion that a combination of chemotherapy and radiotherapy, along with palliative esophageal intubation as necessary, is a preferred approach.

The main subject of the chapter is esophageal bypass, a procedure that is seldom used, however, I strongly agree with Dr. Little's advocacy of this approach for selected patients with malignant tracheoesophageal fistula in the absence of extensive metastatic disease. I also concur that the use of the whole stomach for the bypass is ideal. However, if after preparation of the stomach it proves too short to bridge the gap, extra length can be achieved through excision of the lesser curvature of the stomach, which untethers the greater curvature and allows it to be brought up to a higher level.

Regarding the excluded esophagus in the presence of a malignant tracheoesophageal fistula, I do not believe that closing both ends is a good option because this often leads to breakdown of the distal closure. Furthermore, a fair amount of mucus can accumulate in the excluded esophagus and sudden dumping of this into the respiratory tract may cause repeated respiratory embarrassment and infection. Therefore, it is preferred that the distal end of the esophagus be drained into the gastrointestinal tract. This can be accomplished with either a Roux-en-Y anastomosis to the distal esophagus or a nonreversed gastric tube bypass, which leaves the esophagogastric junction intact for drainage while diverting the ingested food stream to the antral region of the stomach, since this is the junction between the gastric bypass tube and the residual stomach.

J. D. C.

■ REFERENCES

Abe S, Tachibana M, Skimokuwa T, et al: Surgical treatment of advanced carcinoma of the esophagus. Surg Gynecol Obstet 168:115, 1989.

Akyama H, Hiyama M: A simple esophageal bypass operation by high gastric division. Surgery 25:674, 1974.

Belsey RH: Palliative management of esophageal carcinoma. Am J Surg 139:789, 1980.

Burt M, Diehl W, Martini N, et al: Malignant esophagorespiratory fistula: Management options and survival. Ann Thorac Surg 52:222, 1991.

Conlan AA, Nicolaou N, Deliharias PG, Pool R: Pessimism concerning palliative bypass procedures for established malignant esophagorespiratory fistulas: A report of 18 patients. Ann Thorac Surg 37:108, 1984.

Conlan AA, Nicolaou N, Hammond CA, et al: Retrosternal gastric bypass for inoperable esophageal cancer: A report of 71 patients. Ann Thorac Surg 36:396, 1983.

Curet-Scott MJ, Ferguson MK, Little AG, Skinner DB: Colon interposition for benign esophageal disease. Surgery 102:568, 1987.

Duranceau A, Jamieson GG: Malignant tracheoesophageal fistula. Ann Thorac Surg 37:346–354, 1984.

Herskovic A, Marty K, Al-Sarraf M, et al: Combined chemotherapy and radiotherapy compared with radiotherapy alone in patients with cancer of the esophagus. N Engl J Med 326:1593, 1992.

Kirschner M: Ein neues verfahren der oesophagoplastik. Arch Klin Chir 114:606, 1920.

Lam KH, Wong J, Lim STK, Ong GB: Intrathoracic gastric bypass for carcinoma of oesophagus found unresectable at exploration. Br J Surg 69:71, 1982.

Little A, Ferguson M, DeMeester T, et al: Esophageal carcinoma with respiratory tract fistula. Cancer 53:1322, 1984.

Lorentz T, Fok M, Wong J: Anastomotic leakage after resection and bypass for esophageal cancer: Lessons learned from the past. World J Surg 13:472, 1989.

Low DE, Kozarek RA: Comparison of conventional and wire mesh expandable prostheses and surgical bypass in patients with malignant esophagorespiratory fistulas. Ann Thorac Surg 65:919, 1998.

Mannell A, Becker P, Nissenbaum M: Bypass surgery for unresectable oesophageal cancer: Early and late results in 124 cases. Br J Surg 25:283, 1988.

Meunier B, Spilopoulos Y, Stosik C, et al: Retrosternal bypass operation for unresectable squamous cell cancer of the esophagus. Ann Thorac Surg 62:373, 1996.

Ong GB, Lam KH, Lim STK, Wong J: Jejunal loop bypass and fundoplication for malignant esophagobronchial fistula. Surg Gynecol Obstet 154:165, 1982.

Orringer M: Substernal gastric bypass of the excluded esophagus: Results of an ill-advised operation. Surgery 96:467, 1984.

Robinson J, Isu S, Everett M, et al: Substernal gastric bypass for palliation of esophageal carcinoma: Rationale and technique. Surgery 97:305, 1981.

Roeher HD, Horeyseck G: The Kirschner bypass operation: A palliation for complicated esophageal carcinoma. World J Surg 5:543, 1981.

Santos G: Late volume changes in retrosternal colon bypass. Ann Thorac Surg 51:296, 1991.

Segalin A, Little A, Ruol A, et al: Surgical and endoscopic palliation of esophageal carcinoma. Ann Thorac Surg 48:267, 1989.

Skinner D: Esophageal reconstruction. Am J Surg 139:810, 1980.

Sugimachi K, Ueo H, Kac H, et al: Problems in esophageal bypass for unresectable carcinoma of the thoracic esophagus. J Thorac Cardiovasc Surg 84:62, 1982.

Wong J: Esophageal resection for cancer: The rationale of current practice. Am J Surg 153:18, 1987.

Wong J, Lim T, Ong G: Intrathoracic gastric bypass for carcinoma of the esophagus found unresectable at exploration. Br J Surg 69:71, 1982.

Yudin SS: The surgical construction of 80 cases of artificial esophagus. Surg Gynecol Obstet 78:361, 1944.

CHAPTER **63**

Esophageal Intubation

Juan A. Cordero, Jr.
Darroch W. O. Moores

Esophageal obstruction from any cause remains a challenging clinical problem. Malignant esophageal obstruction is most commonly caused by primary esophageal carcinoma and rarely by a metastatic tumor within the mediastinum that invades or compresses the esophagus. Palliation to relieve dysphagia and odynophagia is the primary goal for patients with unresectable or inoperable tumors. Tumors may be unresectable and incurable because of local invasion, regional lymph node metastases, distant metastases, or irreversible cardiopulmonary conditions that preclude surgical resection. Palliation can be achieved with repeated dilatations, surgery, radiation therapy alone, laser therapy, photodynamic therapy, chemotherapy, combination chemotherapy and radiation therapy, or endoesophageal prostheses.

The use of bypass procedures, as documented by Orringer (1984) and Ginoux and Segal (1984), is associated with high morbidity and mortality rates and poor results. It is difficult to justify major surgical intervention in this group of patients with short life expectancies and significant comorbidities. Hahl and associates (1991), Buset and colleagues (1987), and Sankar and associates (1991) reported on the use of lasers in patients with malignant esophageal obstruction. Lasers are successful in relieving dysphagia and in providing good palliation, but patients usually require multiple tedious, time-consuming sessions. Radiation therapy can relieve esophageal obstruction with a response rate of approximately 80%; however, as reported by Earlam and Cunha-Melo (1980), an adequate response may take several weeks and relief is often short-lived. Multiagent chemotherapy can achieve good results and can relieve dysphagia, usually at the expense of significant toxicity. As reported by Herskovic and associates (1992), combination chemotherapy was associated with life-threatening side effects in 20% of patients, and only 58% of patients experienced improvement in the ability to swallow.

The method of palliation chosen for this group of very ill patients is usually dictated by (1) the location and extent of the tumor, (2) the patient's age and performance status, and (3) the experience of the treating physician. In our opinion, esophageal intubation by the use of an endoprosthesis is the least expensive, simplest, and most effective treatment of immediate and durable palliation for obstructing esophageal carcinoma.

HISTORICAL NOTE

The use of esophageal intubation for malignant obstruction dates back to the mid 19th century. In the late 1880s, Symonds (1887) described his experience with the intubation of malignant strictures using ivory and silver prostheses. In 1924, Soutter described esophageal intubation with metallic tubes after dilatations with bougies. These tubes were small in diameter and difficult to insert. These early attempts were associated with a high rate of esophageal perforation and failed to gain wide acceptance.

In the 1950s, Mousseau and Celestin popularized traction (pull-through) tubes in the treatment of esophageal obstruction. Mousseau and associates (1956) developed an elongated prosthesis with a long tapered end that required a laparotomy and gastrostomy for its placement and anchoring. Celestin (1959) modified the Mousseau tube by creating a longer tube with a detachable polyethylene bougie. The Celestin tube was in widespread use during the 1960s and 1970s, but the advent of modern push-through tubes relegated this type of tube to the archives of history.

Atkinson and Ferguson (1977) introduced a pulsion tube, similar to the Celestin tube, which was placed during fiberoptic endoscopy. The major advantage of the Atkinson tube was that it could be placed safely without the need for laparotomy. The Atkinson tube and the Wilson-Cook tube (Fig. 63–1) gained widespread acceptance and have been in use throughout the world.

Girardet and colleagues (1974) published a collective review of 2459 patients who were treated with esophageal tubes. The mortality rate for the entire group of patients was 13.9%. Traction tubes were associated with a mortality rate of 23.5%, whereas pulsion tubes were associated with a mortality rate of 11%. The most common complications were tube obstruction and tube dislodgment; the overall complication rate was 25.4%. Average survival for the entire group after the placement of an esophageal stent was 4.2 months. More than half of the patients had satisfactory improvement in their ability to swallow.

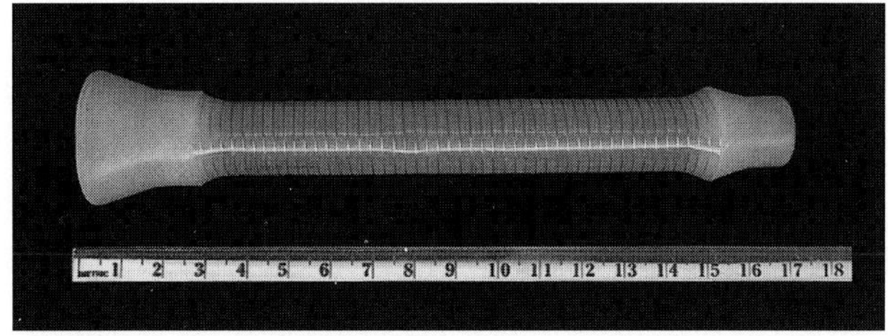

FIGURE 63–1 ■ Wilson-Cook tube.

■ HISTORICAL READINGS

Atkinson M, Ferguson R: Fiberoptic endoscopic palliative intubation of inoperable oesophagogastric neoplasms. Br Med J 1:266, 1977.

Mousseau M, Le Forestier J, Barbin J, et al: Place de l'intubation à demeure dans le traitement palliatif du cancer de l'oesophage. Arch Fr Mal Appl Dig 45:208, 1956.

Symonds CJ: The treatment of malignant stricture of the oesophagus by tubage or permanent catheterism. Br Med J 1:870, 1887.

SELF-EXPANDING METALLIC STENTS

The recent development of self-expanding metallic stents, which were previously used for vascular and biliary strictures, has provided an attractive alternative to the conventional plastic endoprostheses (Atkinson and Wilson-Cook tubes) in the management of malignant esophageal obstruction. The placement of conventional plastic esophageal stents requires dilatation to 52 French. Placement of the Microinvasive second-generation Wallstents and the Ultraflex stents calls for only minimal dilatation (27 French), which makes these stents easier and safer to deploy. The internal diameter of conventional plastic endoprostheses is only 12 mm, whereas the new self-expanding stents have internal diameters of 20 mm, which affords the patient better palliation.

Five metallic stents are available commercially (Table 63–1):

- Gianturco Z Stent (Wilson-Cook, Winston-Salem, N.C.)
- EsophaCoil Stent (InStent, Eden Prairie, Minn.)
- Ultraflex Stent (Microinvasive, Watertown, Mass.)
- Wallstent, first and second generations (Microinvasive)

These self-expanding metal prostheses are easily placed endoscopically, with the patient under either local or general anesthesia. The original self-expanding metallic stents for esophageal obstruction were not covered and allowed tumor ingrowth through the metal interstices, which led to a significant incidence of repeated obstruction. The development of covered stents essentially eliminated tumor ingrowth, allowing longer periods of palliation. Available covered stents have silicone incorporated between two layers of wire mesh. Early reports of fragmentation of the silicone have been eliminated with improvements in design.

TECHNIQUES AND RESULTS

In our series, 59 patients underwent placement of self-expanding covered esophageal stents (50 first-generation Wallstents, 5 second-generation Wallstents, and 4 nitinol Ultraflex stents) between December 1994 and December 1998 (Figs. 63–2 to 63–4). There were 36 men and 23 women in the series (age range, 41 to 94 years). Fifty-one patients had obstruction from primary esophageal carcinoma (unresectable disease in 45, recurrent anastomotic disease in 4, and bronchoesophageal fistula in 2), 3 patients had other obstructive carcinomas (gastric, lung, and mesothelioma), and 5 patients had benign disease (peptic stricture in 3 and anastomotic stricture in 2). All patients underwent esophageal dilatation by means of a flexible gastroscope and Savary bougies. After dilatation, the length of the obstruction was marked fluoroscopically with paper clips taped to the skin and placement of the esophageal Wallstent was performed under fluoroscopic control (Fig. 63–5). These stents self-expand and do not require additional dilatation after placement. All patients underwent barium esophagography after placement of the stent to ensure adequate placement and luminal patency (Fig. 63–6).

Follow-up was complete in all patients, ranging from 4 weeks to 12 months. Successful stent placement was achieved in all patients. There was one postoperative death secondary to cardiac arrest in a patient with a bronchopleural fistula. Stent migration occurred in one patient with hiatal hernia, peptic stricture, and severe inoperable coronary artery disease. A 4-cm, first-generation Wallstent migrated into the stomach as a result of

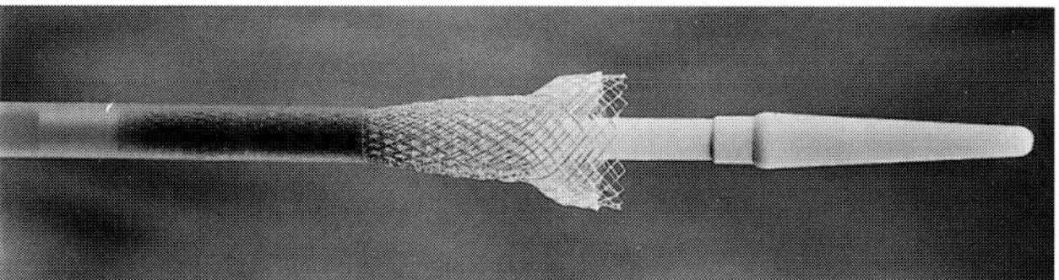

FIGURE 63–3 ■ Partially deployed Wallstent. (From Moores DWO, Ilves R: Treatment of esophageal obstruction with covered, self-expanding esophageal Wallstents. Ann Thorac Surg 62:963, 1996. Reproduced by permission of the Society of Thoracic Surgeons.)

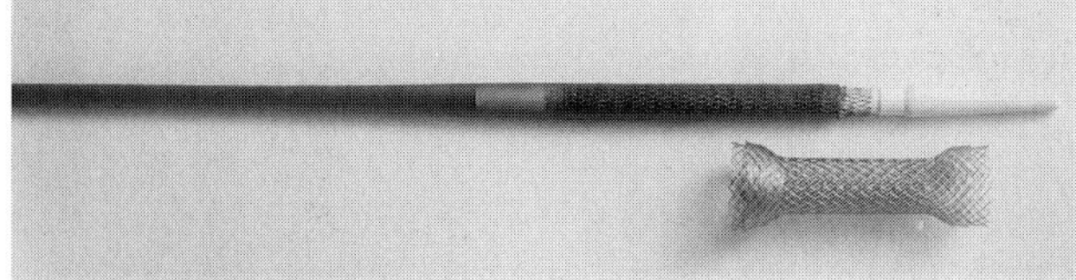

FIGURE 63–2 ■ Wallstent within an introducer. (From Moores DWO, Ilves R: Treatment of esophageal obstruction with covered, self-expanding esophageal Wallstents. Ann Thorac Surg 62:963, 1996. Reproduced by permission of the Society of Thoracic Surgeons.)

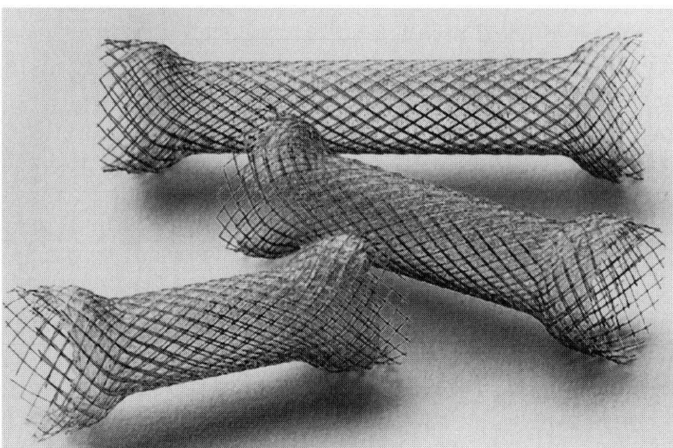

FIGURE 63–4 ■ Wallstents measuring 4, 6, and 9 cm long. (From Moores DWO, Ilves R: Treatment of esophageal obstruction with covered, self-expanding esophageal Wallstents. Ann Thorac Surg 62:963, 1996. Reproduced by permission of the Society of Thoracic Surgeons.)

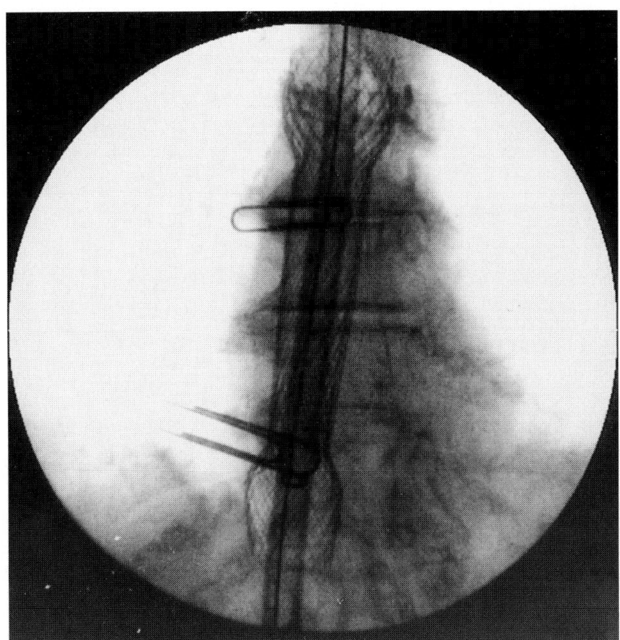

FIGURE 63–5 ■ Fluoroscopic picture of a Wallstent between radiopaque markers. (From Moores DWO, Ilves R: Treatment of esophageal obstruction with covered, self-expanding esophageal Wallstents. Ann Thorac Surg 62:963, 1996. Reproduced by permission of the Society of Thoracic Surgeons.)

low placement. The stent was removed via a limited laparotomy with the subsequent placement of a 6-cm stent. The patient experienced no further problems. The remainder of the stents were well tolerated, and patients in the series were able to eat normally, including solid foods.

Similar results with covered metallic stents have been published. Song and associates (1994) reported on 132 Gianturco metallic stents placed in 116 patients with malignant esophageal obstruction. Placement of the stent was successful in 100% of cases. Most of the patients (78%) could ingest solid food, and the remainder (20%) tolerated soft food. Complications included tube blockage (13 patients) and tube migration (12 patients).

Ell and colleagues (1994) had similar results in a series of 31 stents placed in 23 patients. Technical success was achieved in all patients, and the relief of dysphagia occurred in most patients. Stent migration was the primary complication and occurred in one patient.

Data from a controlled trial of expansile metallic stents were reported by Knyrim and associates (1993). In this series, 42 patients with malignant esophageal obstruction were randomly assigned to treatment with either a Wilson-Cook plastic prosthesis or an expansile metal mesh stent. Complications were found to be much less frequent in the expansile metal stent group than in the plastic prosthesis group (no complications versus nine reports of complications). Relief of dysphagia was similar in the two groups of patients. Hospital stays were significantly longer in patients receiving a plastic prosthesis. The authors concluded that despite the higher initial cost ($1500 versus $200), the metallic stents were cost-effective because of the lack of fatal complications and the decreased length of hospital stay.

DISCUSSION

Patients with inoperable carcinoma of the esophagus require palliation to provide comfort and to restore gastrointestinal continuity. Surgery, radiation therapy, laser therapy, combination chemotherapy, and endoesophageal prostheses are the primary modalities of treatment for this group of patients. Endoluminal esophageal prostheses for malignant esophageal obstruction have been in use for more than a hundred years. Plastic endoprostheses of the pulsion and traction variety are used worldwide. However, these tubes continue to be associated with significant morbidity and mortality, as reported by Gasparri and colleagues (1987) and Fell and associates (1966). The self-expanding metal endoprostheses for esophageal stenting offer an attractive alternative in the treatment of malignant esophageal obstruction.

In our reported series (Moores and Ilves, 1996), patients with malignant obstruction had unresectable and inoperable primary esophageal tumors, recurrent malignant anastomotic stricture, or metastatic disease in the mediastinum that caused invasion or obstruction of the esophagus. We placed stents at all levels of the esophagus, including the cervical esophagus and the gastroesophageal junction, with excellent palliation.

Caution must be exercised when stents are placed through the gastroesophageal junction because stents in this location cause free gastroesophageal reflux and are associated with a higher incidence of migration. After stent placement through the gastroesophageal junction, patients should be managed with elevation of the head of the bed and long-term antacid therapy. Using this regimen in patients with stents through the gastroesophageal junction, we have noted no episodes of significant aspiration or further esophageal stricture formation proximal to the stents.

TABLE 63–1 ■ **Self-Expanding Metallic Stents**

Characteristic	*Gianturco Z Stent*	*EsophaCoil Stent*	*Wallstent*	*Ultraflex Stent*
Material	Stainless steel	Nitinol	Elgiloy	Nitinol
Deployment diameter (mm)	31	31	38	24
Expanded internal stent diameter (mm)	18	18	18	18
Total stent lengths (mm)	60, 80, 100, 120, 140	100, 150	80, 100, 130, 150	100, 150
Covered stent lengths (mm)	60, 80, 100, 120, 140	Uncovered	60, 80, 110, 130	70, 120

Adapted from Franco KL, Putnam JB (eds): Advanced Therapy in Thoracic Surgery. Philadelphia, BC Decker, 1998, p 443.

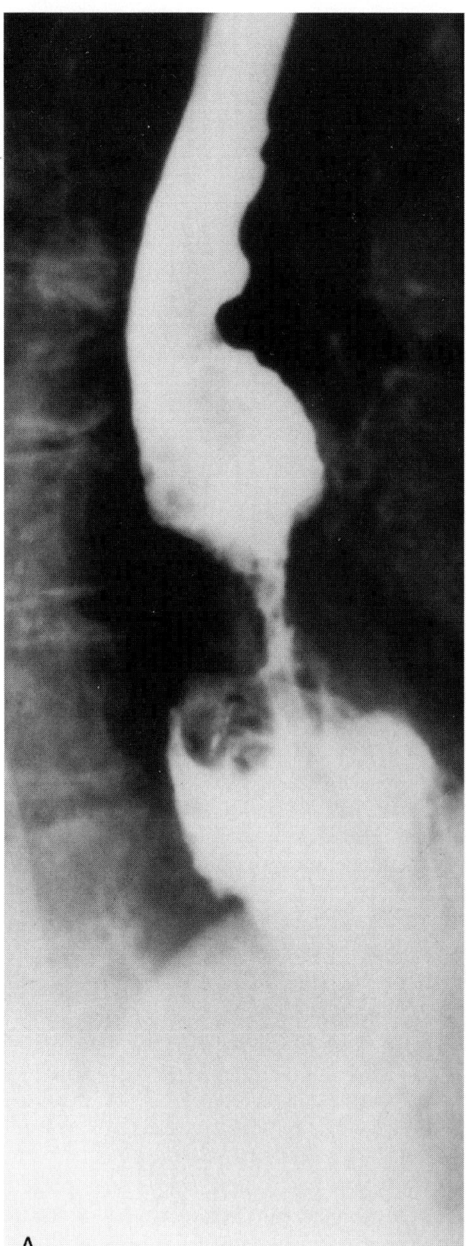

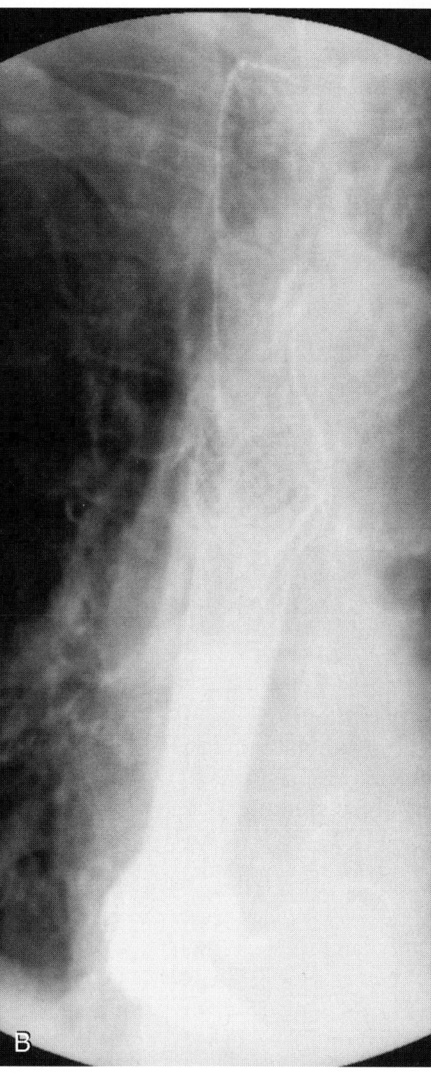

FIGURE 63–6 ■ *A,* Primary esophageal carcinoma treated with a Wallstent in a 94-year-old woman. *B,* After Wallstent placement, she survived for 4 months without further dysphagia. (From Moores DWO, Ilves R: Treatment of esophageal obstruction with covered, self-expanding esophageal Wallstents. Ann Thorac Surg 62:963, 1996. Reproduced by permission of the Society of Thoracic Surgeons.)

Obstruction in the cervical esophagus is believed to be a contraindication to the placement of conventional plastic esophageal stents (Mehran and Duranceau, 1994). Patients in our series who underwent the placement of covered self-expanding stents in the cervical esophagus tolerated the prosthesis well, without evidence of erosion into the trachea or migration of the stent proximally across the cricopharyngeus. If a stent is required high in the cervical esophagus, care must be taken to ensure that the stent be placed below the cricopharyngeus (Fig. 63–7). The Wallstent cannot be moved once it is fully deployed. The Ultraflex stent can be manipulated and removed after deployment and is thus our stent of first choice (Fig. 63–8).

Placement of a self-expanding metal esophageal prosthesis does not prevent or preclude the patient from undergoing subsequent chemotherapy or radiotherapy. Tube dislodgment secondary to postinsertion radiotherapy has been reported in patients with conventional stents. An advantage of the covered esophageal self-expanding stent is its ability to expand in response to tumor shrinkage after radiotherapy. Two of the patients in our series underwent extensive chemotherapy after successful stent placement. Despite a reduction in tumor size, the Wallstent remained in place and did not migrate.

Conventional plastic prostheses have an outer diameter of 16 mm and an inner diameter of only 12 mm. The surgeon must dilate the esophageal obstruction to 52 French to place one of these rigid tubes. The second-generation Wallstent stent (Fig. 63–9) and the Ultraflex stent require dilatation to only 27 French for safe deployment. Once deployed, the self-expanding stents can expand up to a maximum internal diameter of 20 mm. This large internal diameter allows much better swallowing

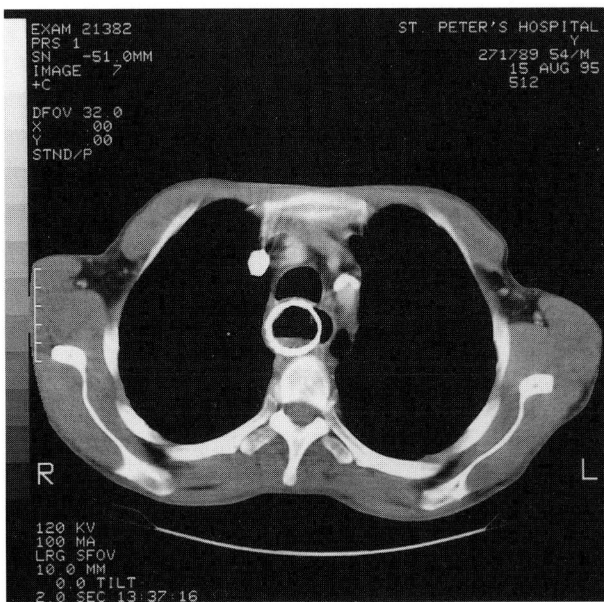

FIGURE 63–7 ■ Computed tomographic scan showing cross-section of a Wallstent in the upper esophagus. The esophageal lumen is widely patent with no tracheal compression. (From Moores DWO, Ilves R: Treatment of esophageal obstruction with covered, self-expanding esophageal Wallstents. Ann Thorac Surg 62:963, 1996. Reproduced by permission of the Society of Thoracic Surgeons.)

than the rigid conventional tubes. Self-expanding stents may be stacked on end to treat very long lesions.

CONCLUSION

Self-expanding metallic covered stents offer an attractive alternative in the palliation of malignant esophageal obstruction. The expandable stents are safe and easy to place. In our experience, they provide excellent and durable palliation of malignant esophageal obstruction at all levels. These stents are compatible with antineoplastic therapy and may be stacked during the treatment of long lesions. Self-expanding metallic stents are our treatment

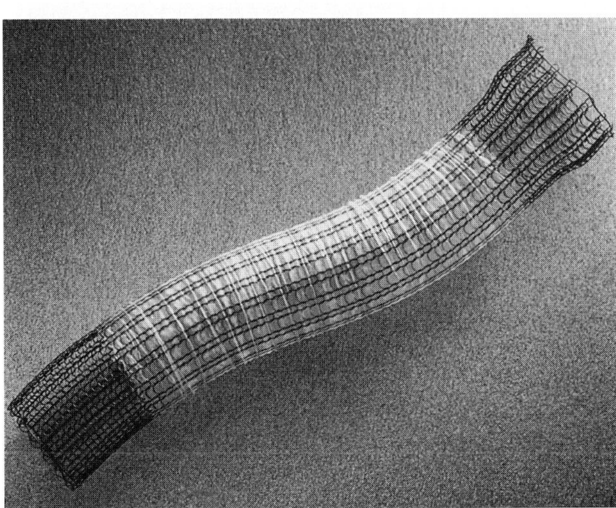

FIGURE 63–8 ■ Ultraflex stent.

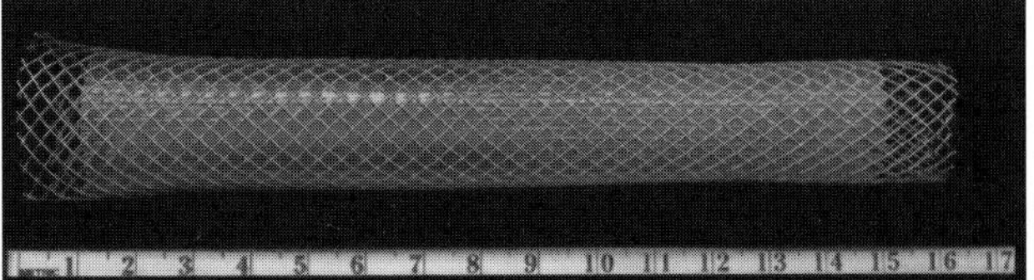

FIGURE 63–9 ■ Second-generation Wallstent.

of choice for endoscopic palliation of malignant esophageal obstruction at all levels of the esophagus.

COMMENTS AND CONTROVERSIES

Drs. Cordero and Moores succinctly review the endoesophageal prostheses available for palliation of malignant obstruction and appropriately conclude that the expandable, coated nitinol (Ultraflex) stent is the prosthesis of choice. This device is easy to place and consists of a single strand of woven material, which facilitates its subsequent removal if necessary. The previously popular Wallstent was composed of numerous interwoven wires with sharp, bare ends that made them difficult to reposition and almost impossible to remove.

The most dangerous aspect of endoesophageal prosthetic insertion is the dilatation required for their insertion. Rupture of the esophagus was more common when earlier plastic tubes required dilatation to a large diameter.

Special care must be taken in the presence of tumor penetration into the back wall of the trachea with or without the presence of an established malignant fistula between the esophagus and the airway. Excessive dilatation of the esophagus may create a fistula where none previously existed or may markedly enlarge an existing fistula.

The presence of an uncoated flared skirt at the top end of the expandable stents makes them difficult to place for very high esophageal lesions. A device with no more than 1 cm of uncoated skirt at the top end of the prosthesis would be advantageous in this situation.

J. D. C.

REFERENCES

Atkinson M, Ferguson R: Fiberoptic endoscopic palliative intubation of inoperable oesophagogastric neoplasms. Br Med J 1:266, 1977.

Buset M, des Marez B, Baize M, et al: Palliative endoscopic management of obstructive esophagogastric cancer: Laser or prosthesis? Gastrointest Endosc 33:357, 1987.

Celestin LR: Permanent intubation in inoperable cancer of the esophagus and cardia: A new tube. Ann R Coll Surg 25:165, 1959.

Earlam R, Cunha-Melo JR: Oesophageal squamous cell carcinoma: II. A critical review of radiotherapy. Br J Surg 67:457, 1980.

Ell C, Hochberger J, May A, et al: Coated and uncoated self-expanding metal stents for malignant stenosis in the upper GI tract: Preliminary clinical experiences with Wallstents. Am J Gastroenterol 89:1496, 1994.

Fell SC, Grunwald RP, Hurwitt ES: Palliation of esophageal carcinoma by prosthetic intubation. J Thorac Cardiovasc Surg 51:272, 1966.

Gasparri G, Casalegno PA, Camandona M, et al: Endoscopic insertion of 248 prostheses in inoperable carcinoma of the esophagus and cardia: Short-term and long-term results. Gastrointest Endosc 33:354, 1987.

Ginoux M, Segal P: Palliative surgical treatment for carcinoma of the esophagus. Int Surg 69:257, 1984.

Girardet RE, Ransdell HT Jr, Wheat MW Jr: Palliative intubation in the management of esophageal carcinoma. Ann Thorac Surg 18:417, 1974.

Hahl J, Salo J, Ovaska J, et al: Comparison of endoscopic Nd:YAG laser therapy and oesophageal tube in palliation of oesophagogastric malignancy. Scand J Gastroenterol 26:103, 1991.

Herskovic A, Martz K, al-Sarraf M, et al: Combined chemotherapy and radiotherapy compared with radiotherapy alone in patients with cancer of the esophagus. N Engl J Med 326:1593, 1992.

Knyrim K, Wagner HJ, Bethge N, et al: A controlled trial of an expansive metal stent for palliation of esophageal obstruction due to inoperable cancer. N Engl J Med 329:1302, 1993.

Mehran RJ, Duranceau A: The use of endoprosthesis in the palliation of esophageal carcinoma. Chest Surg Clin North Am 4:331, 1994.

Moores DWO, Ilves R: Treatment of esophageal obstruction with covered, self-expanding esophageal Wallstents. Ann Thorac Surg 62:963, 1996.

Mousseau M, Le Forestier J, Barbin J, et al: Place de l'intubation à demeure dans le traitement palliatif du cancer de l'oesophage. Arch Fr Mal Appl Dig 45:208, 1956.

Orringer MB: Substernal gastric bypass of the excluded esophagus: Results of an ill-advised operation. Surgery 96:467, 1984.

Sankar MY, Joffe SN: Endoscopic contact Nd:YAG laser resectional vaporization (ECLRV) and esophageal dilatation (ED) in advanced malignant obstruction of the esophagus. Am Surg 57: 259, 1991.

Song HY, Do YS, Han YM, et al: Covered, expandable esophageal metallic stent tubes: Experiences in 119 patients. Radiology 193:689, 1994.

Soutter HS: A method of intubating the oesophagus for malignant stricture. Br Med J 1:782, 1924.

Symonds CJ: The treatment of malignant stricture of the oesophagus by tubage or permanent catheterism. Br Med J 1:870, 1887.

CHAPTER **64**

Laser Therapy for Carcinoma of the Esophagus

Gilles Beauchamp
Denise Ouellette

Since the 1980s, laser technology has found a place in the treatment of esophageal carcinoma and cancer of the esophagogastric junction.

The word *laser* is an acronym for *l*ight *a*mplification by *s*timulated *e*mission of *r*adiation. A laser is a device that produces light with special properties that differ from those of incandescent or fluorescent light; these properties are (1) monochromaticity, (2) coherence, (3) brightness, and (4) directional power.

Carcinomas of the esophagus and gastric cardia are increasingly common and are usually advanced at presentation. For many patients, curative surgical resection or curative radiotherapy is not possible. Dysphagia is usually prominent and calls for palliation with minimal morbidity (Reed, 1995).

Historically, surgery was considered to be a primary modality for the palliative treatment of advanced esophageal cancer. Unfortunately, most patients with advanced disease are unsuitable for surgery because of extensive disease, advanced age, or poor surgical risk. The success rate of palliation for both bypass and esophagectomy is high, but mean survival often is less than 1 year. The main problems with surgery are related to the need for hospitalization and high morbidity and mortality rates.

Dilatation has very limited and short-lived effects and should be considered only as complementary to another endoscopic modality, such as esophageal stenting or tumor-ablation procedures.

Radiotherapy is an alternative to palliation; however, it is associated with several disadvantages:

1. Results are not obtained rapidly.
2. Response rates are often incomplete.
3. Recurrence rates are high.
4. Duration of the treatment varies between 3 and 5 weeks.
5. The patient must be in the radiotherapy suite each day.
6. Esophagitis, a common development, may be severe, causing esophageal stenosis, which must be treated by endoscopic dilatation, and sometimes causing tracheoesophageal fistula.

Bicap tumor probe delivers bioplar electrocoagulation energy to the tumor and is helpful to relieve dysphagia. It carries a very low range of complications. The Bicap tumor probe apparatus is much less cumbersome than the neodymium:yttrium-aluminum-garnet (Nd:YAG) laser, the cost is low, and it is useful in treating circumferential esophageal tumors.

Intratumoral injection of ethanol allows improved swallowing in most patients treated, with a low complication rate. The procedure is easy to perform, does not require special equipment or special skills, and is inexpensive. The main drawback is the difficulty in judging the extent of damage after injection and the total volume of injected ethanol required. Excessive injection can produce perforation or fistula. Fibrotic tumors are usually difficult to treat.

Endoscopic intubation with metal stents is widely used and is associated with relatively low mortality and morbidity (see Chapter 65). Prosthetic insertion can be performed successfully in almost all patients, with improvement of dysphagia noted in 90% to 95% of cases. The use of self-expanding metal stents presents several advantages over older types of prostheses.

1. They create a larger lumen for better relief of dysphagia.
2. They are easier and less traumatic to introduce.
3. A lower complication rate is well recognized.

The main problems with metal stents are their high costs and the possible repeated obstruction of the lumen due to neoplastic regrowth or displacement of the prosthesis after adjuvant treatment (Dittler, 1996).

For many surgeons, metal stents are the first choice for palliation of esophageal carcinoma, but endoscopic laser ablation offers an alternative in certain situations. It may help when it is impossible to use a prosthesis, or it may be useful in combination with a prosthesis or radiotherapy. It may also be used for immediate control of dysphagia before any treatment.

Endoscopic laser therapy is based on the use of high-energy output directed to tumor tissue under direct vision to produce a photothermal destruction and reopening of the esophageal lumen. Laser radiation induces heat production in the target tissue and causes direct coagulation and vaporization.

HISTORICAL NOTE

Although the application of laser therapy in medicine is relatively new, the original theory of laser was first suggested by Neils Bohr, who postulated that as an atom falls from a high- to a low-energy level, it emits a quantum of energy in the form of light or electromagnetic radiation.

Einstein, working on Bohr's theory, speculated that an excited atom could be stimulated to emit a photon if struck by an identical photon. The identical photon would propagate onward in a parallel path in synchrony with the emitted photon. This is the *stimulated emission* that is found in the definition of the word *laser.*

In 1960, Maiman constructed the first laser in the United States by using a rod of ruby. The Nd:YAG laser was first described by Snitzer (1966). It was introduced in Europe in the late 1970s to deliver radiation with a wavelength of 1064 μm, suitable for conduction by quartz fiber and thus for transmission through the flexible gastroscope. Fleischer and Kessler (1983) were two of the first to introduce the Nd:YAG laser for the palliation of esophageal cancer in North America.

■ *HISTORICAL READINGS*

Fleischer D, Kessler F: Endoscopic Nd:YAG laser therapy for carcinoma of the esophagus: A new form of palliative treatment. Gastroenterology 85:600–606, 1983.

Maiman TH: Optical and microwave-optical experiments in ruby. Phys Rev Lett 4:564, 1960.

Snitzer E: Glass lasers. Appl Optics 5:1847, 1966.

LASER PRINCIPLES

Physics Terminology

To help the reader understand the principles of laser therapy, we now review a few terms and concepts from modern physics.

Molecular systems contain only certain discrete amounts of energy. A molecule with the lowest possible amount of energy is said to be in the *ground state*; molecules with more than this amount of energy are said to be in an *excited state*. Any molecule in an excited state tends to lose energy. One way in which an excited molecule can lose energy is through the emission of a light wave or photon (Doiron and Profio, 1985; Polanyi, 1985).

The wavelength of a given photon is characteristic of the energy difference between the particular excited state from which it was emitted and the lower-energy state in which it leaves the molecule.

Each lasting medium emits a specific wavelength, which interacts with biologic tissues in different ways. Coherent monochromatic light can be focused onto an extremely small spot, much smaller than can be achieved with the incoherent and polychromatic light from familiar sources. This makes it possible to achieve very high-power densities in the focal spot of the laser beam that are capable of vaporizing any material.

To obtain a special light (laser) that has the characteristic of being monochromatic, coherent, and bright with directional power, three conditions are required:

1. An active medium (gas, solid, or liquid) with special properties must be present.
2. The medium used must be pumped, or energized, and must produce an inverted population of atoms.
3. The medium must be included within a resonator.

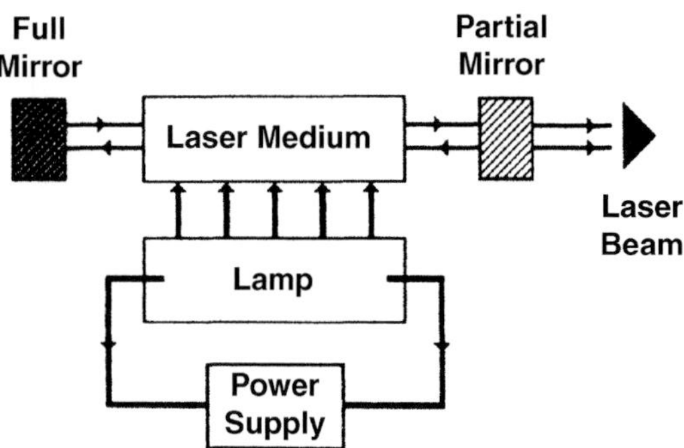

FIGURE 64–1 ■ Schematic showing principle of laser light. The power source activates the lamp, which stimulates the laser substance.

These three elements are the basis of a laser device (Reilly and Fleischer, 1991) and are represented in Figure 64–1. Each component is examined next.

Laser Components

Active Medium

The active medium of the laser refers to the collection of atoms, molecules, or ions that are stimulated to emit a beam of monochromatic and coherent light.

Carbon dioxide and Nd:YAG represent two of the most important active media used in laser instruments for the treatment of esophageal cancer. The name attached to the type of laser refers to the material that is used as the *lasing* medium, the solid or gas component that determines the wavelength of the laser emission.

Pump

To obtain lasing, the active medium must be able to have more atoms in an excited state. This requires the pumping of molecules or electrons in the excited state. The pumping is simply a form of electromagnetic energy that is capable of being absorbed by atoms in the active medium.

After the atoms of the active medium have absorbed the energy from the pump source, they spontaneously emit light in all directions. If a sufficient number of atoms are excited, the photons that travel along the axis of the cavity collide with other excited atoms, resulting in two photons of light that travel in phase with each other in the same direction. These two photons collide with other atoms, increasing the number of photons that travel in phase with one another and multiplying the number of coherent photons. The presence of more molecules in an excited state than in another state of lower energy is called an *inverted population.*

Resonator

Amplification takes place inside an optical resonator, a cavity in which light may travel back and forth. The randomly emitted light from the active medium is reflected by the mirrors placed at both ends of the resonator. The photons of light become excited in the active medium and stimulate the molecules to become excited and emit photons that maintain a fixed relationship to the stimulating photons and create amplification. With the arrangements of the mirrors, only a small portion of photons can be released from the resonator in a narrow fixed direction localized to a small cross-sectional area.

The laser device, which is the combination of an active medium stimulated by a pump source inside a resonator, creates a light that has coherence, brightness, and monochromaticity and that is highly concentrated in a specific direction.

Laser Type

The emitted wavelength is governed by the active medium within the resonator. The Nd:YAG laser uses a crystal of yttrium-aluminum-garnet which contains a small proportion of ions of the rare earth metal neodymium. It produces a near-infrared wavelength, which is invisible to the human eye.

For example, consider a tube that contains a solid medium such as Nd:YAG on which an electrical discharge can be made to excite the molecule of Nd:YAG. In this discharge, there is a population inversion between two of the excited states of the Nd:YAG molecule. If carefully aligned mirrors are placed at each end of the tube, a photon that happens to be emitted exactly along the axis of the tube via spontaneous emission from one of the molecules in the inverted state can bounce back and forth between the mirrors, each time stimulating the emission of additional photons by other molecules in the inverted state. The intensity of the beam can grow very large.

The carbon dioxide laser uses a mixture of carbon dioxide and nitrogen gas to produce far-infrared radiation. Both the carbon dioxide laser and the Nd:YAG laser have been widely used in medicine as tools that cut and coagulate.

There are two fundamental varieties of laser energy output:

- Continuous-wave, in which a constant laser beam is produced
- Pulse output, in which energy is emitted in short high-energy bursts

Delivery Devices

The laser delivery system should enable the delivery of light, energy, or both in close proximity to the tissue. The development of flexible quartz fibers allows the laser light beam to be easily carried from the laser source to the treatment site via any endoscope. Fibers contain a central core of high-quality glass coated with a thin layer at a slightly lower refractive index. The light is transmitted along the fiber via total internal reflection. The fibers have diameters that range from 0 to 1 mm. The fibers are inserted into a plastic catheter that is designed to allow gas flow through a small space between the actual fiber and the catheter. This coaxial system permits insufflation of gas to cool down the fiber and to prevent deposit of debris on its tip. Debris on the fiber tip heats up rapidly and melts as the laser is fired, thus occasionally destroying the fibers.

Laser-Tissue Interactions

The individual properties of the available lasers result from the individual wavelengths. The level of tissue absorption and depth of tissue penetration depend on the laser wavelength. The tissue effect produced by the laser involves an interaction with water and hemoglobin, which in turn depends on individual laser wavelengths. When the laser light interacts with tissue, it converts the light to thermal energy (Sliney, 1985).

In fact, laser light creates a molecular agitation in biologic tissue that eventually produces heat. The level of molecular agitation induced by light is directly related to the light absorbed into the tissue. The depth of tissue penetration depends on the amount of light absorbed.

Laser radiation has several effects on tissue. It can produce hemostasis, tissue destruction, or both. These effects are secondary to the temperature level achieved in the tissues.

When the critical temperature of 80°C is reached in a particular layer of tissue, it results in the denaturation of collagen and the constriction of blood vessels. When the temperature reaches 100°C, the water in the tissue boils and results in vaporization of tissue. When the temperature reaches 210°C, dehydration of tissue and burning occur.

When the energy generated by the laser is absorbed by a unit of volume of tissue, its characteristics change. With high intensity, tissue devitalization or vaporization takes place. These effects on tissue are controlled by changing parameters of the laser beam, such as power, spot size, exposure time, and wavelength.

Tissue injury and necrotization through heating are the primary effects of Nd:YAG laser irradiation. With the Nd:YAG laser, the constitutions of tissues change as they are coagulated; cellular water is brought to boil, and desiccation and carbonization take place. The redistribution of the radiation through scattering can lead to a maximum concentration of thermal energy in a volume just below the tissue surface. Rapid expansion of the cellular water in this volume leads to a breaking or popping of the superficial layer; this was called the *popcorn effect*. The heating of tissues is slow and focused to spot sizes of a few millimeters in diameter. Tissue damage also extends laterally. Vaporization of a fraction of the tissue volume affected by the radiation follows tissue desiccation and carbonization.

PATIENT EVALUATION

When endoscopic laser therapy is considered for a new patient with esophageal or esophagogastric cancer, the patient must undergo an evaluation to determine whether endoscopic therapy is appropriate and whether laser therapy is the best choice. A contrast radiograph provides information about the location, length, shape, and nature of the esophageal cancer and often is the best method of identifying angulations and distortions.

Endoscopic evaluation with biopsy allows a precise tissue diagnosis and allows the surgeon to determine the exact geometry of the tumor. How exophytic is the tumor? Is there any polypoid component?

The standard of evaluation has been computed tomography (CT) with oral contrast medium as well as ultrasonography of the liver to evaluate for the presence of metastasis. Magnetic resonance imaging (MRI) does not provide additional information. Endoscopic ultrasonography may be used to determine the stage of the disease before treatment. The use of positron emission tomography (PET) scanning has been shown to be more sensitive than CT scanning for the detection of metastases.

Finally, a global evaluation of the patient, including cardiopulmonary and hemostatic functioning, must be carried out before the patient undergoes any treatments.

DELIVERY OF LASER

The gastroscope is advanced to the proximal margin of the tumor. The quartz fiber is then passed through the biopsy channel of the endoscope. The Nd:YAG laser is set at 80 to 100 W for a 1.5- to 2-second pulse. The tip of the fiber is positioned 1 cm from the tissue surface as treatment is applied. The beam usually exits the fiber tip at a fixed divergence angle, about 10 degrees. The laser beam that strikes the tissue, therefore, has the configuration of a cone with its apex at the end of the fiber. The diameter of the circular base of the cone *(spot size)* decreases as the fiber moves closer to the tissue; the reverse occurs as the fiber moves away. As the spot size decreases, the laser energy is confined to a smaller area.

If the output of the laser remains constant, the degree of tissue heating is greater per unit of time. This means that the range of tissue damage that occurs in response to laser energy can be controlled to a certain degree by varying the distance between the end of the laser fiber and the tissue surface. Most medical lasers have a *pilot light*, which is a second laser that provides a circle of visible light on the tissue surface corresponding to the spot size of the laser light.

A foot pedal is used to fire the laser. We usually set the maximum duration of the laser pulse at 2 seconds. In actual practice, most pulses are of shorter duration. Depending on spot size, a pulse of 2 seconds produces tissue vaporization as well as smoke, which may obscure the endoscopic field. As noted, the resulting tissue effect also is a function of the spot size, which can be changed by varying the distance between the fiber tip and the tissue surface. A small spot size tends to vaporize tissue rapidly but with a great amount of smoke. A larger spot size tends to cause coagulation.

During treatment, the endoscope should be periodically advanced into the stomach to evacuate smoke and gas. Some endoscopists advocate placing a small nasogastric tube along the tip of the endoscope to draw out the gas and smoke; however, this may be dangerous and we have not found this measure to be necessary.

It is useful to keep the tip of the fiber close to the end of the endoscope. As long as the fiber tip can be seen during firing, the endoscope does not become damaged.

The distal end of commonly used noncontact fibers disintegrates if the laser is fired while the tip is in contact with tissue or fluid or if the end of the fiber is covered with charred tissue. The distal end should be inspected frequently during the procedure and cleaned with a small brush as necessary.

During a laser ablation procedure, a cloud of smoke may exit via the instrument channel of the endoscope or around the endoscope. A mechanism must be available to remove the considerable amount of smoke that may develop. A commercially available smoke evacuator connected to a large plastic suction is placed near the patient's mouth or on the endoscope itself to reduce smoke in the procedure room. Other equipment often needed during the procedure includes guidewires, dilators, foreign body extractors, and cleaning brushes.

For security considerations, optical filters that fit over the ocular portion of a fiberoptic endoscope or special goggles must always be used during calibration of the laser to avoid inadvertent injuries to the eye.

The prograde approach was originally described by Fleischer and colleagues (1982). The endoscope is advanced into the proximal end of the tumor, and photocoagulation is then carried out, starting at the top of the tumor. Usually 1 to 2 cm of tumor can be coagulated and destroyed. Forty-eight hours later, a second treatment is performed, with gradual progression down the length of the obstructing esophageal neoplasm. Two or three laser sessions are usually required to remove the majority of the tumor (Ell and Demling, 1987).

With the retrograde approach, a guidewire is first passed down under direct vision through the biopsy channel of the endoscope. It is sometimes passed through the tumor and into the stomach under fluoroscopic control. Dilatation of esophageal tumor is carried out with Savary-type dilators, with progression from a 3-mm dilator to 15-mm dilators.

The endoscope is then reintroduced over the guidewire, is left in place, and is passed down the esophagus into the stomach. After this step, the endoscope is gradually withdrawn until the distal tumor comes into view.

The endoscopist treats the tumor beginning with the distal portion and working proximally. Vigorous débridement and irrigation are also performed and continued along the entire aspect of the tumor as the endoscopist slowly withdraws the endoscope in an attempt to treat the entire lesion in a single session. The goal is to produce a luminal diameter of approximately 1.5 cm, coagulating the tumor to a depth of 5 to 7 mm (Ell and Demling, 1987).

The main advantage of the retrograde approach is that the entire procedure can be performed in a single session, which allows greater control of luminal diameter and provides a decreased risk of esophageal perforation.

Mitty and associates (1996) showed that effective palliation of obstructing esophageal carcinoma can be achieved in one session with a one-stage retrograde approach using the Nd:YAG laser with the patient under general anesthesia. They used the procedure in 62 consecutive patients; 93% of the patients showed symptomatic improvement, and 50% of the patients experienced effective palliation with only one procedure during the course of their illness.

Lightdale and associates (1987) and Ferraro and colleagues (1990, 1995) showed that endoscopic Nd:YAG laser therapy, coupled with initial dilatation, is feasible in an outpatient setting, with no increase in morbidity or complications. In view of the limited survival time of these patients, outpatient management is highly desirable.

We perform laser therapy using general anesthesia. With local anesthesia, there is a potential for patient discomfort because laser therapy may take 20 to 60 minutes and dilatation may be required initially. A large-diameter endoscope is commonly used, and insufflation of gas from the laser fibers causes abdominal distention. The heat generated by the treatment may be absorbed by the normal esophagus and may cause pain. Thus, patients require greater sedation during laser procedures, although some patients tolerate the procedure without any sedation.

Keon (1992) reviewed the anesthetic management during laser therapy and indicated the type of ventilation needed and the complications related to laser surgery, which can be kept to a minimum with proper expertise.

LIMITS OF TREATMENT

Photoablation is terminated when most of the narrowing has been treated or when the patient becomes intolerant to the procedure. There is no absolute upper limit of the amount of energy that can be delivered in a single session, although rarely has more than 15,000 joules been applied in one session, and 3000 to 8000 joules is most often used. In published reports, the mean energy delivered per treatment session ranges from 2500 to 8500 joules. When a patient has undergone laser treatment in the preceding few days, it often is necessary to débride necrotic tumor before further treatment.

The general strategy of laser treatment is to establish an adequate lumen as quickly as possible; usually, two or three treatment sessions are needed to establish a lumen through a tumor. The evaluation of the results often is subjective, consisting of the relief of dysphagia. If the patient experiences minimal or no improvement in the ability to swallow despite adequate lumen diameter, further laser therapy may not be useful and other treatments should be chosen. If the patient improves with some relief of dysphagia, it is necessary to periodically reassess the patient and to treat him or her again to maintain luminal patency. The interval between reassessment usually is about 1 month but varies among patients.

Generally, a period of 48 hours is recommended between treatments, which allows for maximal tissue necrosis. When the treatment area is examined 48 hours later, it looks like a whitish yellow, soft, necrotic mass. This portion of destroyed tumor tissue can be removed with the use of various forceps. After the necrotic tissue is removed, treatment is begun on the underlying, previously untreated area. This approach is continued until the lumen is opened sufficiently to allow for passage of the endoscope freely into the stomach.

In some patients, laser therapy becomes progressively less effective with time; this usually occurs at about 4 months. The interval between treatment sessions shortens, and the dysphagia-free interval between treatments becomes brief; at this time, laser therapy is rarely useful for relieving dysphagia.

The success rate of palliation with laser therapy to restore luminal patency is greater than 90%, but the functional success rate varies between 70% and 85%. The extent of disease, the anatomic location of the tumor, and the patient's general performance status contribute to the success of palliation.

COMPLICATIONS

Laser therapy is a relatively safe method of palliation. Minor complications include transient fever, mild chest pain during the procedure, and sometimes a transient initial worsening of dysphagia due to tissue edema.

The complication rate after laser therapy varies from 1.5% to 18%, and the mortality rate ranges from 0% to 2% (Brennan et al, 1990; Maunoury et al, 1992; Rutgeerts et al, 1988). An international inquiry regarding 1359 patients from 47 centers reported a complication rate of 4.1% (Ell and Demling, 1987). Half of the complications were perforations, but fistula, hemorrhage, and sepsis were also reported. The mortality rate was 1% (Sander and Poest, 1993), and these authors reported a complication rate of less than 10% in 130 patients.

One of the major complications of laser therapy is perforation (Tyrrell et al, 1995). Perforation occurs in 1% to 9% of patients who undergo endoscopic laser therapy (Carter et al, 1993). Most patients undergo esophageal dilatation before endoscopic laser therapy, and perforation may result from dilatation rather than from the laser therapy.

Although hemorrhage is usually minor and self-limiting, it can be delayed up to several days after laser therapy because tumor sloughing occurs. Occasionally, an iatrogenic Mallory-Weiss tear develops and causes some bleeding. Tracheoesophageal fistulas may occur up to 6 weeks after laser therapy. Laser therapy may contribute to fistula formation by destroying the tumor present between the esophagus and the trachea, and laser therapy of lesions in areas previously treated with radiation therapy may increase the risk of fistula. However, fistula formation can occur in 5% to 10% of patients as part of the natural progression of the disease.

After treatment, strictures may develop in patients with circumferential submucosal lesions requiring repeated laser sessions. These strictures may contribute to recurrent dysphagia.

RESULTS

Factors Affecting Outcome

Fleischer and Sivak (1985) assessed patients with esophageal and esophagogastric cancer, seeking parameters that would affect the initial outcome of palliative treatment with Nd:YAG laser therapy. There were no differences in the treatment response between patients with squamous cell carcinoma and those with adenocarcinoma of the esophagus. The best response was found in tumors of the mid and distal esophagus, especially in tumors less than 5 cm in length.

Rutgeerts and associates (1988) obtained very good short- and long-term results in patients with recurrent cancer at the esophagogastric or esophagojejunal anastomosis.

In 1990, Mathus-Vliegen and Tytgat noted that circumferential growth and location of the carcinoma at the cardiac junction represent unfavorable factors in palliation of dysphagia. Good outcomes, in the experience of Brennan and colleagues (1990), were more likely when the length of the tumor was less than 5 cm, when the lumen was straight, and when the lesion was predominantly exophytic.

In 1995, Spinelli and associates also reported good results obtained in patients with tumors in the distal esophagus and gastric cardia and for stenoses of less than 5 cm.

Clinical versus Functional Success

Several factors relating to a better functional outcome have been identified. Mellow and Pinkas (1985) reported that luminal patency was achieved in 97% of cases, but functional success, which allowed patients to eat comfortably and to leave the hospital, was achieved in 70% of patients.

The patient's condition before treatment played an important role in outcome when a proximal esophageal tumor was present (Alexander et al, 1994). Patients who were in good condition before treatment showed a 70% chance of complete relief of dysphagia.

Quality of life was examined prospectively by Loizou and colleagues (1992) and Barr and associates (1990). The Loizou team concluded that although laser therapy resulted in a significant initial improvement in quality of life, the improvement was transient and quality of life worsened significantly as a patient's general condition deteriorated during the final stage of the illness.

Barr and Krasner (1991), after evaluating 40 patients, concluded that the patient's swallowing ability and quality of life were improved significantly at some point in time after laser therapy. The mean survival time was 16 weeks, with 58% of patients dying at home, 28% dying in the hospital, and 18% dying in a hospice.

Spinelli and associates (1995) reported good relief of dysphagia in 74% of patients. The worst results were observed when the tumor was located in the upper third of the esophagus or was longer than 10 cm. In 1987, Lightdale and colleagues reported that palliation was less effective when tumors involved the cervical esophagus, were longer than 8 cm, and were primarily infiltrating or extraluminal.

Duration of Palliation

It appears that laser photoablation improves the overall quality of life in patients with malignant dysphagia for only a short time. Spinelli and associates (1995) reported that duration of palliation depended on tumor length. The average dysphagia-free interval was 8 weeks in lesions less than 5 cm and 6 weeks in lesions more than 5 cm.

The main drawback of the laser treatment is the need for repeated treatments to obtain a good functional result. The mean interval between treatments is usually 3 to 8 weeks (Lightdale et al, 1987; Spinelli et al, 1995).

Survival

To investigate whether laser treatment prolonged survival times, Karlin and associates (1987), comparing 10 laser-treated patients with 20 historical control subjects in a retrospective study, suggested that endoscopic laser therapy significantly prolonged survival time in patients with squamous cell carcinoma of the esophagus. Stange and colleagues (1989), analyzing survival time in 59 patients, found that survival was statistically independent of tumor histology, location, length, and previous treatment. Survival was related to the degree of tumor stenosis and dysphagia before and after laser treatment. There was no causal relationship between improvement in dysphagia and survival.

In the literature, long-term survival has been reported to be mostly related to tumor length (<6 cm) (Alderson and Wright, 1990; Naveau et al, 1990).

Endoscopic Laser Therapy and Combined Treatment

To prolong the treatment interval in patients who underwent laser therapy, Sargeant and colleagues (1992) combined laser photocoagulation with external beam radiotherapy. The median dysphagia grade improved after laser treatment, and this improvement was maintained with radiotherapy. The median dysphagia-free interval was 9 weeks. The combined modality significantly prolonged survival compared with historical controls.

Bader and associates (1986) investigated the combination of laser and afterload therapy with iridium 192. They reported that up to 80% of patients remained free of restenosis and that radiation-induced side effects were not observed. A prospective, randomized, controlled study on the use of laser alone versus laser with afterloading radiation with iridium 192 did not confirm the previously published results; survival was not prolonged after endoluminal irradiation (Sander et al, 1991). Renwick and colleagues (1992) treated 21 patients using laser combined with brachytherapy with cesium 137 and achieved good relief of dysphagia. Harper and associates (1992) treated 59 patients with advanced metastatic gastroesophageal adenocarcinoma with laser alone or laser therapy in combination with chemotherapy; the latter group showed some improvement.

Laser therapy was compared with other types of palliative treatments. A prospective, randomized clinical trial conducted by Low and Pagliero (1992) compared brachytherapy with treatment with iridium 192 and laser. Both modalities were well tolerated. Initial improvement of dysphagia was observed in 83% of patients after brachytherapy and 91% of patients after iridium 192 and laser treatment. Repeated treatments were three times as common with laser therapy, but overall treatment failure rates were equal in the two groups. No differences were observed in regard to duration of the palliative effect and in the improvement of the performance score.

Laser therapy has been compared with other endoscopic tumor-debulking procedures. Jensen and colleagues (1988) compared the use of Nd:YAG laser and Bicap tumor probe. Relief of dysphagia was obtained in 85% of patients, with no differences between the two groups. Angelini and associates (1991) conducted a prospective, randomized study to compare the results of laser therapy with those of local injection of polidocanol. After the first session of treatment, 88.8% of patients underwent laser therapy and 81.5% of patients treated by injection reported relief of dysphagia. A significant decrease in the need for further treatments was observed in the polidocanol-treated group.

Banerjee and colleagues (1993) compared the results of the use of laser alone with those of laser therapy combined with ethanol injection. Symptomatic improvement was observed in all patients, but the amount of laser energy required to obtain luminal patency was 40% lower in patients who also were treated with ethanol injection.

In a multicenter phase III trial (Lightdale, 1993), photodynamic therapy and Nd:YAG laser therapy were compared. Improvements in dysphagia at 1 week and at 1 month were similar, but better results in the photodynamic therapy group were observed when the lesion was longer than 10 cm and when the tumor was located in the cervical esophagus. Complication rates and median survival times were similar.

In a study comparing photodynamic therapy and laser, Heier and associates (1995) showed that both modalities provided the restoration of luminal patency with a low complication rate. Photodynamic therapy allowed for better dietary performance with better status performance. Duration of the palliative effects was longer with photodynamic therapy. There were no differences in survival.

Nd:YAG laser therapy was compared with the placement of endoesophageal plastic prosthesis (Ritcher et al, 1988). Post-treatment swallowing was better in patients treated with laser.

In a prospective, nonrandomized study that compared laser therapy with endoscopic placement of an Atkinson tube, Loizou and colleagues (1991) found no significant differences in the improvement of dysphagia when the tumor was located in the thoracic esophagus. Intubation was more successful for lesions of the cardia. In patients who received palliative treatment over a long period, however, the mean dysphagia grade was significantly better in the laser group, although these patients required more procedures.

Hahl and associates (1991) reported a comparison between endoprosthesis treatment and laser therapy. Complications occurred in 48% of intubated patients, with a mortality rate of 11% compared with 8.7% of the laser-treated patients. Carter and associates (1992) reported that the best swallowing grade was achieved with laser recanalization in comparison with a prosthesis. There were no statistical differences regarding median survival. Fuchs and colleagues (1991) studied 40 patients to evaluate the quality of life for patients treated with laser versus endoprosthesis. They found no significant differences between laser and endoprosthesis treatment with regard to survival, food passage, or quality of life.

Barr and associates (1990) reported a prospective, randomized trial that compared laser and Atkinson tube therapies. No differences in quality of life were observed between the two groups. The recurrent dysphagia rate was higher in the prosthesis group of patients, who required fewer endoscopic procedures. The complication rate was significantly lower in patients treated with laser alone.

CONCLUSION

The use of endoscopic laser photocoagulation for the relief of dysphagia in patients with esophageal and gastric cardiac tumors remains an option. The feasibility of using an Nd:YAG laser has been demonstrated to achieve relief of obstruction in a relatively safe manner. Recanalization of the lumen can usually be obtained.

Today, one must admit that self-expanding metal stents appear to be superior, although not all data are available to make an accurate comparison of the various palliative modalities. Laser therapy remains another option for the surgeon to use in appropriately selected patients.

■ *REFERENCES*

Alderson D, Wright PD: Laser recanalization versus endoscopic intubation in the palliation of malignant dysphagia. Br J Surg 77:1151–1153, 1990.

Alexander GL, Wang KK, Ahlquist DA, et al: Does performance status influence the outcome of Nd:YAG laser therapy of proximal esophageal tumors? Gastrointest Endosc 40:451–454, 1994.

Angelini G, Fratta Pasini A, Ederle A, et al: Nd:YAG laser versus polidocanol injection for palliation of esophageal malignancy: A prospective, randomized study. Gastrointest Endosc 37:607–610, 1991.

Bader M, Dittler HJ, Ultsch B, et al: Palliative treatment of malignant stenoses of the upper gastrointestinal tract using a combination of laser and afterloading therapy. Endoscopy 18(Suppl 1):27–31, 1986.

Banerjee B, Tokunaga K, Tahira A, et al: Combined treatment with Nd:YAG laser and absolute ethanol injection compared to Nd:YAG laser therapy alone in malignant esophageal and rectal obstruction. Gastrointest Endosc 39:248, 1993.

Barr H, Krasner N: Prospective quality-of-life analysis after palliative photoablation for the treatment of malignant dysphagia. Cancer 68:1660–1664, 1991.

Barr H, Krasner N, Raouf A, Walker RJ: Prospective randomised trial of laser therapy only and laser therapy followed by endoscopic intubation for the palliation of malignant dysphagia. Gut 31:252–258, 1990.

Brennan FN, McCarthy JH, Laurence B: Endoscopic Nd:YAG laser therapy for palliation of upper gastrointestinal malignancy. Med J Aust 153:27–31, 1990.

Carter R, Smith JS, Anderson JR: Laser recanalization versus endoscopic intubation in the palliation of malignant dysphagia: A randomized prospective study. Br J Surg 79:1167–1170, 1992.

Carter R, Smith JS, Anderson JR: Palliation of malignant dysphagia using the Nd:YAG laser. World J Surg 17:608–614, 1993.

Dittler HJ: Palliation of esophageal cancer: Stents and tubes. Dis Esophagus 9:105–116, 1996.

Doiron DR, Profio AE: Laser instrumentation and safety. Clin Chest Med 6:209, 1985.

Ell Ch, Demling L: Laser therapy of tumor stenoses the upper gastrointestinal tract: An international inquiry. Lasers Surg Med 7:491–494, 1987.

Ferraro P, Beauchamp G, Aumais G: Endoscopic Nd:YAG laser therapy of malignant esophageal obstruction on an outpatient basis. Can J Surg 33:479–482, 1990.

Ferraro P, Beauchamp G, Ouellette D, et al: Le laser YAG endoscopique et la thérapie palliative du cancer de l'oesophage. Ann Chir 49:1, 1995.

Fleischer D, Kessler F: Endoscopic Nd:YAG laser therapy for carcinoma of the esophagus: A new form of palliative treatment. Gastroenterology 85:600–606, 1983.

Fleischer D, Kessler F, Haye O: Endoscopic Nd:YAG laser therapy for carcinoma of the esophagus: A new palliative approach. Am J Surg 143:280–283, 1982.

Fleischer D, Sivak MV: Endoscopic Nd:YAG laser therapy as palliation for esophagogastric cancer. Gastroenterology 89:827–831, 1985.

Fuchs KH, Freys SM, Schaube H, et al: Randomized comparison of endoscopic palliation of malignant esophageal stenoses. Surg Endosc 5:63–67, 1991.

Hahl J, Salo J, Ovaska J, et al: Comparison of endoscopic Nd:YAG laser therapy and oesophageal tube in palliation of oesophagogastric malignancy. Scand J Gastroenterol 26:103–108, 1991.

Harper PG, Highley M, Houston S: Significant palliation of advanced gastric/oesophageal adenocarcinoma with laser endoscopy and combination chemotherapy. Proc Ann Meet Am Soc Clin Oncol 11:A472, 1992.

Heier SK, Rothman KA, Heier LM, Rosenthal WS: Photodynamic therapy for obstructing esophageal cancer: Light dosimetry and randomized comparison with Nd:YAG laser therapy. Gastroenterology 109:63–72, 1995.

Jensen DM, Machicado G, Randall G, et al: Comparison of low-power YAG laser and Bicap tumor probe for palliation of esophageal cancer strictures. Gastroenterology 94:1263–1270, 1988.

Karlin DA, Fisher RS, Krevsky B: Prolonged survival and effective palliation in patients with squamous cell carcinoma of the esophagus following endoscopic laser therapy. Cancer 59:1969–1972, 1987.

Keon TP: Anesthetic management during laser surgery. Intern Anesthesiol Clin 30:99–107, 1992.

Lightdale C, Heier S, Marcon N, et al: A multicenter phase III trial of photodynamic therapy vs Nd:YAG laser in the treatment of malignant dysphagia. Gastrointest Endosc 39:283, 1993.

Lightdale CJ, Zimbalist E, Winawer SJ: Outpatient management of esophageal cancer with Nd:YAG laser. Am J Gastroenterol 82:46–50, 1987.

Loizou LA, Grigg D, Atkinson M, et al: A prospective comparison of laser therapy and intubation in endoscopic palliation for malignant dysphagia. Gastroenterology 100:1303–1310, 1991.

Loizou LA, Rampton D, Atkinson M, et al: A prospective assessment of quality of life after endoscopic intubation and laser therapy for malignant dysphagia. Cancer 70:386–391, 1992.

Low DE, Pagliero KM: Prospective randomized clinical trial comparing brachytherapy and laser photoablation for palliation of esophageal cancer. J Thorac Cardiovasc Surg 104:173–179, 1992.

Maiman TH: Optical and microwave-optical experiments in ruby. Phys Rev Lett 4:564, 1960.

Mathus-Vliegen EMH, Tytgat GNJ: Analysis of failures and complications of neodymium:YAG laser photocoagulation in gastrointestinal tract tumors. Endoscopy 22:17–23, 1990.

Maunoury V, Brunetaud JM, Cochelard D, et al: Endoscopic palliation for inoperable malignant dysphagia: Long term follow up. Gut 33:1602–1607, 1992.

Mellow MH, Pinkas H: Endoscopic laser therapy for malignancies affecting the esophagus and gastroesophageal junction. Arch Intern Med 145:1443–1446, 1985.

Mitty RD, Cave Dr, Birkett DH: One-stage retrograde approach to Nd:YAG laser palliation of esophageal carcinoma. Endoscopy 28:350–355, 1996.

Naveau S, Chiea A, Poynart T, Chaput JC: Endoscopic Nd:YAG laser therapy as palliative treatment for esophageal and cardial cancer: Parameters affecting long term outcome. Dig Dis Sci 35:294–301, 1990.

Polanyi TG: Physics of surgery with lasers. Clin Chest Med 6:179, 1985.

Reed CE: Comparison of different treatments for unresectable esophageal cancer. World J Surg 19:828–835, 1995.

Reilly HF, Fleischer DE: Palliative treatment of esophageal carcinoma using laser and tumor probe therapy. Gastroenterol Clin North Am 20:731–742, 1991.

Renwick P, Whitton V, Moghssi K: Combined endoscopic laser therapy and brachytherapy for palliation of esophageal carcinoma: A pilot study. Gut 33:435–438, 1992.

Ritcher JM, Hilgenberg AD, Christensen MR, et al: Endoscopic palliation of obstructive esophagogastric malignancy. Gastrointest Endosc 34:454–458, 1988.

Rutgeerts P, Vantrappen G, Broeckaert L, et al: Palliative gastroesophageal junction: Impact on the quality of remaining life. Gastrointest Endosc 34:87–90, 1988.

Sander R, Hagenmueller F, Sander C, et al: Laser versus laser plus afterloading with iridium-192 in the palliative treatment of malignant stenosis of the esophagus: A prospective randomized and controlled study. Gastrointest Endosc 37:433–440, 1991.

Sander RR, Poest H: Cancer of the oesophagus-palliation-laser treatment and combined procedures. Endoscopy 25(Suppl):679–682, 1993.

Sargeant IR, Loizou LA, Tobias JS, et al: Radiation enhancement of laser palliation for malignant dysphagia: A pilot study. Gut 33:1597–1601, 1992.

Sliney DH: Laser-tissue interactions. Clin Chest Med 6:203, 1985.

Snitzer E: Glass lasers. Appl Optics 5:1847, 1966.

Spinelli P, Mancini A, Dal Fante M: Endoscopic treatment of gastrointestinal tumors: Indications and results of laser photocoagulation and photodynamic therapy. Semin Surg Oncol 11:307–318, 1995.

Stange EF, Dylla J, Fleig WE: Laser treatment of upper gastrointestinal tract carcinoma: Determinants of survival. Endoscopy 21:254–257, 1989.

Tyrrell MR, Trotter A, Adam A, Mason RC: Incidence and management of laser-associated oesophageal perforation. Br J Surg 82:1257–1258, 1995.

CHAPTER **65**

Colon Replacement

Thomas W. Rice

The principal function of the esophagus is the rapid unidirectional transit of food from the hypopharynx to the stomach. Unlike other segments of the gastrointestinal (GI) tract, the esophagus has no digestive, absorptive, or endocrine activities. Despite this seemingly rudimentary task and the deceptively simple arrangement of a muscle pump between two sphincters, it is difficult to replicate esophageal function with other portions of the GI tract.

A segment of colon is one of the options for the replacement or bypass of the esophagus. The advantages of colon replacement are few. An adequate length of colon is usually available. The blood supply, although less reliable than that of the stomach, is easily assessed and generally adequate.

The disadvantages of colon replacement are multiple. The preoperative evaluation and preparation of the colon are more demanding than the evaluation or preparation of either the stomach or jejunum because of the frequent occurrence of intrinsic colonic disease and the abundant bacterial colonization of the colon.

Colon replacement is a more complex operation than either gastric or simple jejunal replacement. Three anastomoses are mandatory to reestablish GI continuity in colon and jejunal replacements; only one anastomosis is required in gastric substitution. The early complication of colonic graft necrosis is uniformly lethal if it is not recognized early and treated by excision of the colon replacement. There is a propensity to late complications as a result of the limited acid resistance of the colonic mucosa and the tendency of the colon replacement to dilate and form redundant loops.

The colon should be considered for esophageal replacement only in patients with a potential for long-term survival and an otherwise functional GI tract. The segment of colon used (e.g., right, transverse, or left) and the direction of replacement (e.g., isoperistaltic or antiperistaltic) are determined by the state of the colon and the surgeon's preference and experience. The route of reconstruction, which may be in the posterior mediastinum through the bed of the esophagus, in the pleural space along the pulmonary hilum, in the retrosternal space, or subcutaneous, is determined on the basis of the primary esophageal condition and the length of colon available. When indicated and if correctly constructed, a colon replacement functions as an adequate esophageal substitute despite the vastly different physiologic properties of these two markedly dissimilar GI organs.

HISTORICAL NOTE

Early attempts at esophageal resection and reconstruction were limited to the cervical esophagus. Czerny (1877) reported the first successful resection of a cervical esophageal carcinoma. Mikulicz (1886) was the first to reconstruct the cervical esophagus. In early esophageal reconstructions, pedicled skin flaps were used. These operations were soon followed by resections of the esophagogastric junction and intra-abdominal reconstructions using the stomach or jejunum. During this period, attempts to resect the intrathoracic esophagus were uniformly fatal because of the inability to control the pleural space during and after the thoracic procedure. Most of the patients died perioperatively from the complications of pneumothorax. Thus, resection of the thoracic esophagus was abandoned, and subcutaneous or retrosternal esophageal bypass became the favored procedure for both benign and malignant esophageal strictures.

In 1911, Kelling performed the first stage of an unplanned operation using isoperistaltic transverse colon brought subcutaneously to the nipple level and a skin tube to bypass an esophageal carcinoma. One month later, before GI continuity could be successfully re-established between the cervical esophagus and the skin tube, the patient died. In the same year, Vulliet, based on his work with cadaver dissections, proposed the use of antiperistaltic right colon for esophageal bypass.

von Hacker (1914) constructed the first clinically successful colon bypass of the esophagus. Ochsner and Owens (1934) reviewed the published experience with antethoracic esophageal bypass. There were only 20 reported colon replacements at that time, which represented just 8% of all esophageal bypasses. Although the records are incomplete, there was a 22% mortality rate, the operation was completed in only 61% of patients, and 54% of patients had fair to excellent results. Although these were the best results of any substitute in this report, Ochsner and Owens (1934) concluded that

> a distinct disadvantage in the use of the colon is the extremely slow emptying time, the ingested food remaining in it for long periods of time before entering the stomach. von Hacker in one of his cases found that after a contrast meal more barium remained in the colonic oesophagus than had passed into the stomach.

The development of positive-pressure ventilation and endotracheal intubation and the appreciation of the importance of chest tube drainage of the pleural space allowed thoracic surgery to be conducted safely. However, intrathoracic esophageal surgery did not advance until improvement of infection control because it was believed that the esophagus could not be opened in the thoracic cavity without lethal contamination (May and Samson, 1969). The integration of these advancements allowed the reintroduction of esophageal resection and the resurgence of the colon as an esophageal replacement. May and Samson reported that "the colon has been the most commonly used visceral esophageal substitute since 1950. Its use increased rapidly with the advent of antibiotics and improved bowel preparation."

The complexity of colon replacement and the increased experience with gastric replacement have caused a progressive decrease in the use of the colon as an esophageal substitute. Postlethwait (1983) reported that the

> results of a survey of current reports, as well as my own personal experience, indicate that, at present, the stomach is the organ used most frequently for substitution or bypass of the esophagus. Replacement of the esophagus with colon, an operation which is now performed less frequently than in the past, should have a role in this area of surgery.

Today colon replacement has been relegated to an important but secondary role in esophageal replacement (Thomas et al, 1997).

■ *HISTORICAL READINGS*

Czerny V: Neue Operationen. Zentralbl Chir 4:443, 1877.

Kelling G: Àsophagoplastik mit Hilfe des Querkolon. Zentralbl Chir 38:1209, 1911.

May IA, Samson PC: Esophageal reconstruction and replacements. Ann Thorac Surg 7:249, 1969.

Mikulicz J: Ein Fall yon Resections des carcinomatosen Oesophagus mit plastichem Ersatz des excirdirten Stückes. Prager Med Wochenschr 11:93, 1886.

Ochsner A, Owens N: Anterothoracic esophagoplasty for impermeable stricture of the esophagus. Ann Surg 100:1055, 1934.

Postlethwait RW: Colonic interposition for esophageal substitution. Surg Gynecol Obstet 156:377, 1983.

von Hacker V: Ueber Oesophagoplastik im allgemeinen und über den Ersatz der Speiseröhre durch antithorakale Haut-dick-darmschlauchbildung im besonderen. Arch Klin Chir 105:973, 1914.

Vulliet H: De l'oesophagoplastie et de ses diverses modifications. Semain Med 45:529, 1911.

BASIC SCIENCE

The colon receives the entire small bowel effluent. From this, it absorbs water and electrolytes and stores the resultant fecal matter until an opportunity for defecation is available. The motility patterns that allow these functions can be divided into three activities that are located in three distinct areas (Christensen, 1987):

1. *Retrograde annular contractions* result in a rhythmic antiperistaltic mixing activity, which aids in the absorption of fluids and electrolytes in the cecum and ascending colon.
2. In the transverse and descending colon, *annular contractions* segment the feces and slowly propel them toward the rectum.
3. In the distal colon, *strong contractions* move the feces into the rectum.

If these motility patterns have been maintained in colon replacements, the use of antiperistaltic right colon and isoperistaltic left colon would be indicated. In most patients, however, the colon functions as a passive conduit and empties much more slowly than the normal esophagus (Table 65–1). Transit through colon replacements is mainly under the influence of gravity. Segmental contractions give the appearance of peristalsis; occasionally, colonic contractions are propulsive, especially when stimulated by the introduction of acid into the colonic lumen (Benages et al, 1981; Clark et al, 1976; Corazziari et al, 1977). Propulsive contractions were recorded early postoperatively after right colon replacement; because of this finding, Myers and colleagues (1998) suggest an isoperistaltic replacement whenever possible. However, antiperistaltic and isoperistaltic grafts have similar transit times (Isolauri et al, 1987).

Passive function of colon replacements has been reported when colon is used as an esophageal replacement in children (Sieber and Sieber, 1968; Sutton et al, 1989). Although motility is maintained in the ileal portion of right colon replacements and is preferred by some pediatric surgeons (Calleja et al, 1988; Raffensperger et al, 1996; Yararbai et al, 1998), the use of segments of terminal ileum longer than 10 cm is responsible for vitamin B_{12} deficiencies in children (Rodgers et al, 1978). Children are also susceptible to anemia as a result of suppressed serum iron concentrations, which is unrelated to the use of terminal ileum.

Peculiar to the colon is the abundance of bacterial colonization, consisting predominantly of gram-negative anaerobic organisms. Native colon bacterial flora necessitates a rigorous bowel preparation not required for the stomach or jejunum, and this may be responsible for or may be an aggravating factor in the early and late complications of colon replacement. The goblet cells of the colonic mucosa secrete a mucus that is protective in the normal colonic environment; however, this mucus is inadequate to prevent acid injury.

The predictable and adequate arterial supply and venous drainage of the colon allow it to be used as an

TABLE 65–1 ■ **Colon Graft and Esophageal Emptying Measured as 50% and 25% Activity Levels in Colon Graft and Esophageal Thirds**

	50% Upper Third	*Middle Third*	*Lower Third*	*25% Upper Third*	*Middle Third*	*Lower Third*
Colon replacement (n = 25)	5.4 ± 7.9	30.6 ± 57.9	400 ± 527*	40 ± 155	190 ± 420	456 ± 518†
Normal esophagus (n = 10)	2.8 ± 1.3	4.7 ± 1.5	5.2 ± 1.4	3.3 ± 1.4	5.6 ± 1.3	6.4 ± 1.3

*The lowermost third of the colon graft did not reach the 50% activity level in 2 patients.
†The lowermost third of the colon graft did not reach the 25% activity level in 10 patients.
Adapted from Isolauri J, Koskinen MO, Markkula H: Radionuclide transit in patients with colon interposition. J Thorac Cardiovasc Surg 94:521, 1987.

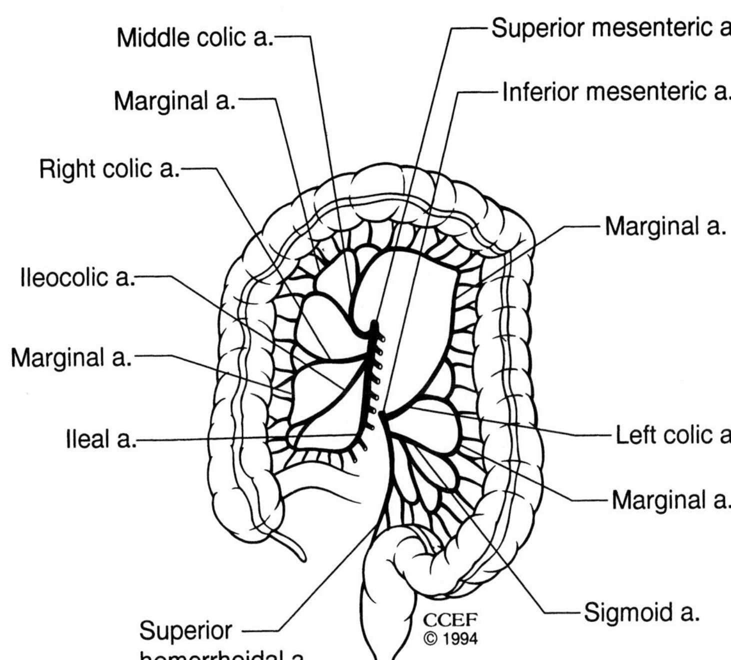

FIGURE 65–1 ■ Arterial blood supply of the colon. (Copyright, Cleveland Clinic Foundation, 1994.)

esophageal replacement (Fig. 65–1). The right colon and the transverse colon are supplied by the superior mesenteric artery through its branches: the ileocolic, right colic, and middle colic arteries. The transverse, descending, and sigmoid colon segments are supplied by the inferior mesenteric artery through its branches, the left colic, sigmoid, and superior hemorrhoidal arteries. As these main arteries reach the colon, they bifurcate 1 to 3 cm from the mesenteric border of the colon to form anastomosing arcades with adjacent branches. A continuous chain of communicating vessels ring the colon, and it is this marginal artery that allows long segments of the colon to be used for replacement.

Although three colonic branches of the superior mesenteric artery are seen in 68% of patients, anomalies in this arterial supply are common. In order of frequency, these anomalies are (1) absence of the right colic artery (12.4%), (2) multiple right colic arteries (8.9%), (3) multiple middle colic arteries (6.2%), (4) absence of the middle colic artery (3.6%), and (5) multiple middle and right colic arteries (0.5%) (Sonneland et al, 1958). A discontinuous marginal artery of the right colon has been reported in 5% to 70% of patients (Steward and Rankin, 1933; Ventemiglia et al, 1977). Absence of the marginal artery, which connects the superior and inferior mesenteric arteries at the splenic flexure, is infrequent. In one report, this anomaly was seen in 2% of patients (Robillard and Shapiro, 1947). Other large series have not reported this anomaly (Beck and Barnofsky, 1960; Steward and Rankin, 1933).

Even though this portion of the marginal artery is constant, the inferior mesenteric artery and its branches are susceptible to atherosclerosis. In patients with significant peripheral vascular disease, the interior mesenteric artery and its branches may be occluded. In this situation, although the left colon usually is adequately supplied through the marginal artery, it is unacceptable for esophageal replacement.

The venous drainage follows the arterial supply in the colonic mesentery. The superior mesenteric vein drains directly into the portal vein. A lack of sufficient marginal venous drainage in the right colon has been implicated in the complications of colon infarction and anastomotic leakage in as many as 25% of patients who undergo right colonic esophageal replacement (Nicks, 1967). The left colic vein drains into the splenic vein. Excellent marginal venous drainage of the left colon was reported in 100% of patients studied. If there has been previous splenic or pancreatic surgery, possible compromise of the inferior mesenteric venous drainage should be considered.

The more constant and reliable arterial supply and venous drainage of the left colon led to its preferential use for esophageal replacement. The smaller diameter of the left colon more closely approximates the esophageal diameter, and this may be a beneficial attribute in colon replacement (Belsey, 1965). However, the claim that the left colon is better able to propel a solid bolus is of little clinical significance because colon replacements have minimal motility and in general function as passive conduits. When a colon replacement is indicated, the right or transverse colon should be reserved and used when the left colon is not available or is inadequate for esophageal substitution.

MANAGEMENT

Indications for Colon Replacement

Colon replacement of the esophagus is indicated for GI reconstruction after resections of primary esophageal malignancies only if the stomach is unacceptable for this substitution. Traditionally, bypass of unresectable esophageal carcinomas with colon was the most frequent use of this conduit. However, the magnitude of this operation frequently overshadows any palliation gained. With the improved means of palliation for unresectable periesophageal and esophageal malignancies, colon bypass of the esophagus is rarely, if ever, indicated.

Colon replacement for benign esophageal disease is one of the options of esophageal substitution. The increasing use of gastric replacement for benign esophageal disease has demonstrated its equivalence or superiority to colon replacement. A colon replacement is an alternative and may be indicated for esophageal replacement in the therapy of long-gap esophageal atresia that is not amenable to standard reconstructive techniques, undilatable benign strictures (e.g., caustic, peptic, and others), end-stage functional disorders, and multiple failed esophageal surgeries in which esophageal function cannot be salvaged. The colon is contraindicated for esophageal replacement if there is underlying primary colonic disease or if there is inadequate arterial supply or venous drainage of the colon.

Preoperative Preparations

After the primary esophageal pathologic condition is determined to be potentially resectable, the colon and route of reconstruction must be evaluated. This process begins with a careful history and physical examination. A history of significant colonic symptoms, treatment of primary colon disorders, or previous abdominal operations suggests that the colon may be unsatisfactory for esophageal replacement. Severe constipation, especially in elderly patients, should signal that the colon may not be an appropriate esophageal substitute (Belsey, 1965). Previous surgery or inflammatory conditions in the esophageal bed, left pleural space, anterior mediastinum, or chest or abdominal wall may render these routes unavailable for esophageal reconstruction.

It is essential that the colonic mucosa be inspected before it is used. An air-contrast barium enema is the minimum examination permissible. Colonoscopy provides a superior examination of the mucosa and allows a biopsy of the mucosal abnormalities to be performed and any colonic polyps to be removed. Colonoscopy has replaced barium enema in most practices. Because the arterial blood supply and venous drainage of the colon play such a vital role in a successful operation, most consider preoperative angiography to be a prerequisite examination.

The routine use of angiography has reduced the operating time and perhaps the incidence of anastomotic complications (Ventemiglia et al, 1977). If angiography is not used routinely, it is required in any patient in whom the colonic vasculature may have been compromised by previous abdominal surgery or in any patient with a history of significant cerebral, coronary, or peripheral vascular disease.

The route of reconstruction should be considered and investigated. Underlying esophageal disease and adjacent mediastinal pathologic findings may preclude the use of the posterior mediastinum. Previous thoracotomy or inflammatory or infectious diseases of the lung or pleura may exclude the use of the pleural space. Previous surgery or anterior mediastinal pathologic conditions may limit the use of the retrosternal space. The subcutaneous route is the least acceptable of these routes of reconstruction, but it is almost always available. These areas should be studied in the preoperative computed tomography (CT) scan.

The length of colon required for esophageal substitution is determined by the extent of esophageal resection and the route of reconstruction. As the route of reconstruction moves from the posterior mediastinum to the subcutaneous space, the length of colon that is required increases. However, the difference in length between the subcutaneous and posterior mediastinal routes differs by only 4 cm (Ngan and Wong, 1986). Meticulous colon preparation is required and should consist of both a mechanical and an antibiotic component. A short and quick preparation is desirable to avoid excessive colonic secretions and mucus production. Otherwise, the investigations and preparations are similar to those for any patient who is undergoing major abdominal or thoracic surgery.

Operative Technique

An upper midline abdominal incision and a neck incision allow the transhiatal resection of the esophagus and the preparation and use of any colonic segment for esophageal substitution. This also is the preferred approach for the second stage of a staged colon replacement after esophageal resection. A left thoracoabdominal incision is an excellent option for esophageal excision and left colon replacement. A left neck incision may be added if required because of the underlying esophageal condition or the need for an esophagocolic anastomosis in the neck. For esophageal excision and right colon replacement, three incisions are usually required. A right thoracotomy followed by an upper midline abdominal and a neck incision or a simultaneous laparotomy, right anterior thoracotomy, and neck incision may be used.

If resection and reconstruction of the esophagus are planned, resectability of the esophagus should be assessed first; then the suitability of the colon for interposition should be evaluated. Palpation of the colon ensures that it is free of any significant pathologic findings and allows an assessment of the mechanical bowel preparation. The entire colon then is mobilized by division of the developmental attachments so that the proposed segment and adjacent areas can be evaluated. The mesentery should be inspected to ensure that there is adequate length with no mesenteric shortening or fibrosis. The arterial supply of the segment of colon to be used is inspected and transilluminated to guarantee an adequate and complete marginal artery (Fig. 65–2). When it is confirmed that the colon is acceptable for esophageal substitution, the esophageal resection is completed.

Left Colon

The greater omentum is removed from the splenic flexure and the distal two thirds of the transverse colon. The arterial supply of the omentum from the stomach and hepatic flexure is maintained so that the omentum is available for later use if required.

The length of colon necessary for esophageal replacement is estimated by the placement of an umbilical tape

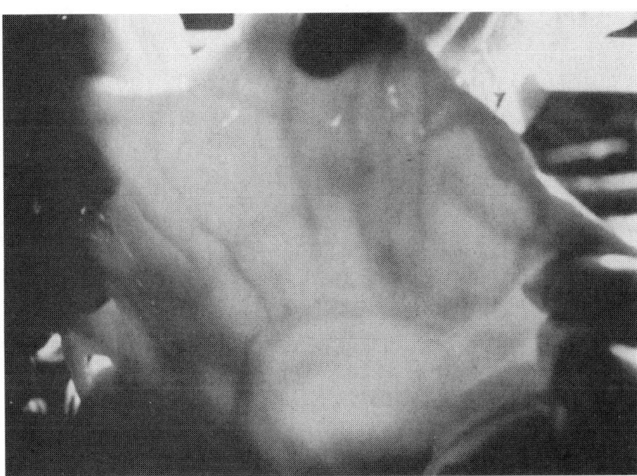

FIGURE 65–2 ■ The mesentery of the colon is transilluminated to allow inspection of the marginal artery.

along the prepared surface of the skin over the proposed route of reconstruction from the midportion of the gastric remnant or the jejunal loop (if the stomach has been removed) to the distal end of the esophagus or pharynx. Because the subcutaneous route requires the longest segment of colon, this estimate should be adequate for other routes. This marked length of umbilical tape is then placed along the antimesenteric border of the colon to provide an approximate estimate of the length of colon needed. The marginal artery proximal and distal to these marked areas is exposed. If the proximal line of transection is to the right of the middle colonic artery, the base of this artery must be exposed proximal to the marginal artery. Atraumatic vascular clamps are then placed on the proximal and distal segments of the marginal artery and, if necessary, the middle colic artery.

Next, the viability of this segment of colon, now supplied solely by the left colic artery, is assessed. Fluorescein angiography with Wood's light examination may be used for intraoperative arterial assessment. If the segment of colon does not have an adequate blood supply, an alternate segment of colon or a different organ of substitution must be sought.

Once adequate vascularity of the left colon segment has been determined, the middle colic artery is ligated and divided (if required) proximal to its branching into the marginal artery, and the proximal and distal portions of the marginal artery are ligated and divided (Fig. 65–3). The peritoneum and the fatty mesentery are divided from the colonic wall to the base of the mesentery at the proposed proximal and distal areas of transection. The colon segment is then isolated by transection of the colon at the proximal and distal margins with a linear cutting stapler.

Right Colon

The greater omentum is removed from the hepatic flexure and the proximal two thirds of the transverse colon. The arterial supply of the omentum from the stomach and splenic flexure is maintained so that the omentum is available for later use if required. The length of colon necessary for esophageal replacement is estimated as previously described. The marginal artery proximal and distal to these marked areas is exposed. The base of the ileocolic, right colic, and ileal (if required) arteries are exposed proximal to the marginal artery. Atraumatic vascular clamps are then placed on these arteries, and the viability of this segment of colon, now supplied solely by the middle colic artery, is assessed.

Once adequate vascularity of the right colon segment has been ensured, the ileocolic and right colic arteries are ligated and divided proximal to their branching to form the marginal artery, and the proximal and distal portions of the marginal artery are ligated and divided (Fig. 65–4). The peritoneum and the fatty mesentery are divided from the colonic wall to the base of the mesentery at the proposed proximal and distal areas of transection. The colon segment is then isolated by transection of the colon at the proximal and distal margins with a linear cutting stapler.

Transverse Colon

The transverse colon is used much less frequently than the left or right colon segments for esophageal substitution. The greater omentum is removed from the transverse colon and the hepatic and splenic flexures. The arterial supply of the omentum from the stomach is maintained so that the omentum is available for later use if required.

The length of colon necessary for esophageal replacement is estimated as previously described. If the segment is based on the left colic artery, mobilization is similar to that described for a left colon replacement. If it is based on the middle colic artery, mobilization is similar to that described for a right colon replacement (Fig. 65–5).

Replacement

The colonic segment is then placed along the same cutaneous path, previously marked with the umbilical tape, to ensure that it is of adequate length (Fig. 65–6). The route of reconstruction is prepared. If the posterior mediastinum has been selected, the preceding esophageal resection has usually adequately prepared this route.

The *transpleural* route is the only route that passes through a true space. The lower entry into the pleural space is through the esophageal hiatus or through an anterior phrenotomy. The colon replacement may pass anterior to the pulmonary hilum to leave the pleural space through the superior entry site at the thoracic inlet behind the junction of the clavicle and manubrium. In this position, it may be necessary to excise the head of the clavicle, the cartilaginous portion of the first rib, and the lateral portion of the manubrium to eliminate compression of the colon segment and its mesentery and to prevent arterial or venous insufficiency of the colon replacement. The transpleural route also allows the colon replacement to pass behind the pulmonary hilum outside the aortic arch. The esophagocolic anastomosis may be constructed in the pleural space, or the colon segment may leave the pleural space through the bed of the resected esophagus.

The *retrosternal* route is entered by a detachment of

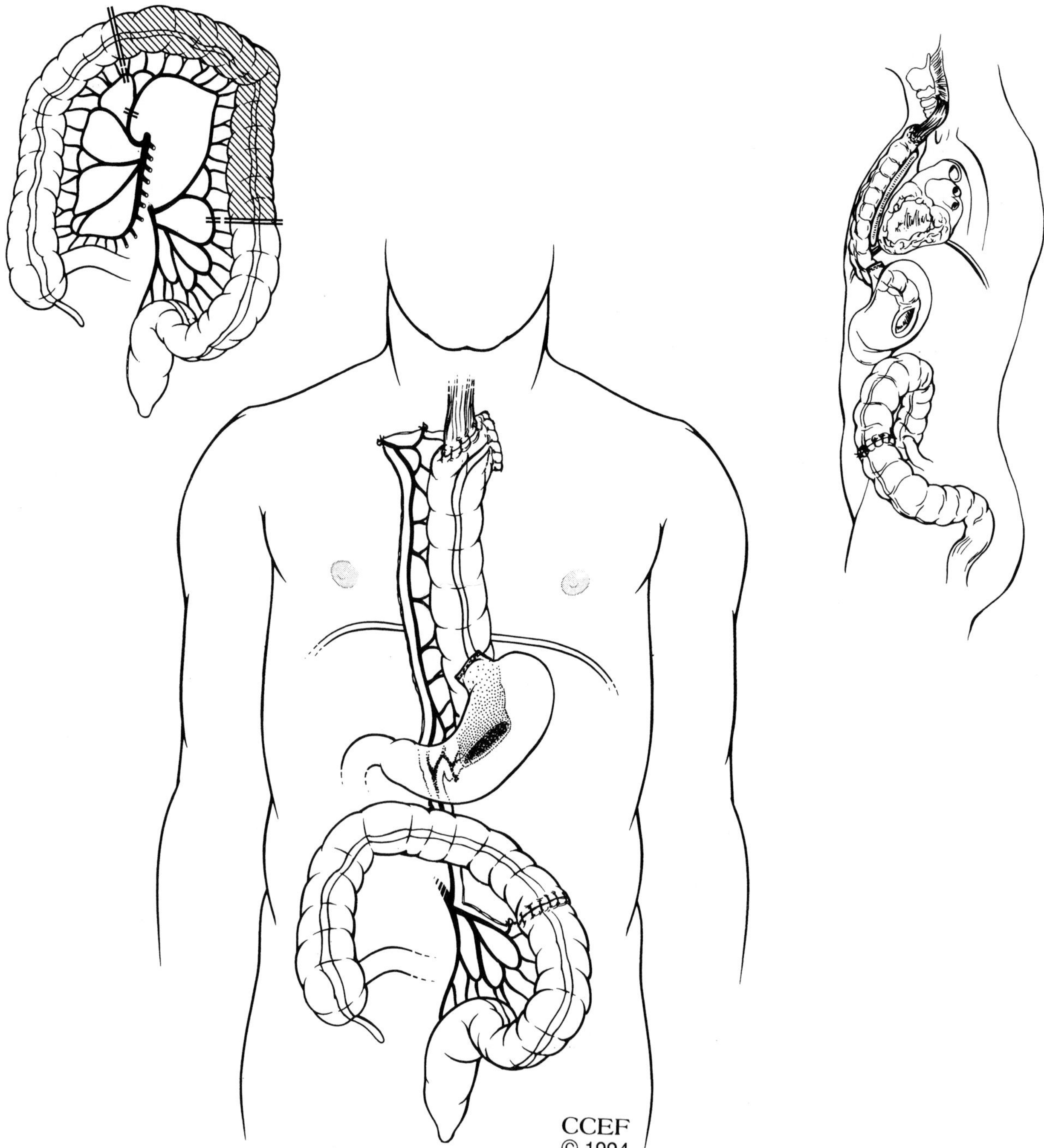

FIGURE 65–3 ■ An isoperistaltic, subcutaneous left colon replacement of the esophagus. The preparation of the arterial supply based on the left colic artery *(left inset)*; the subcutaneous route of the completed left colon replacement is depicted in the lateral view *(right inset)*. Anteroposterior view of this isoperistaltic left colon replacement *(main figure)*. (Copyright, Cleveland Clinic Foundation, 1994.)

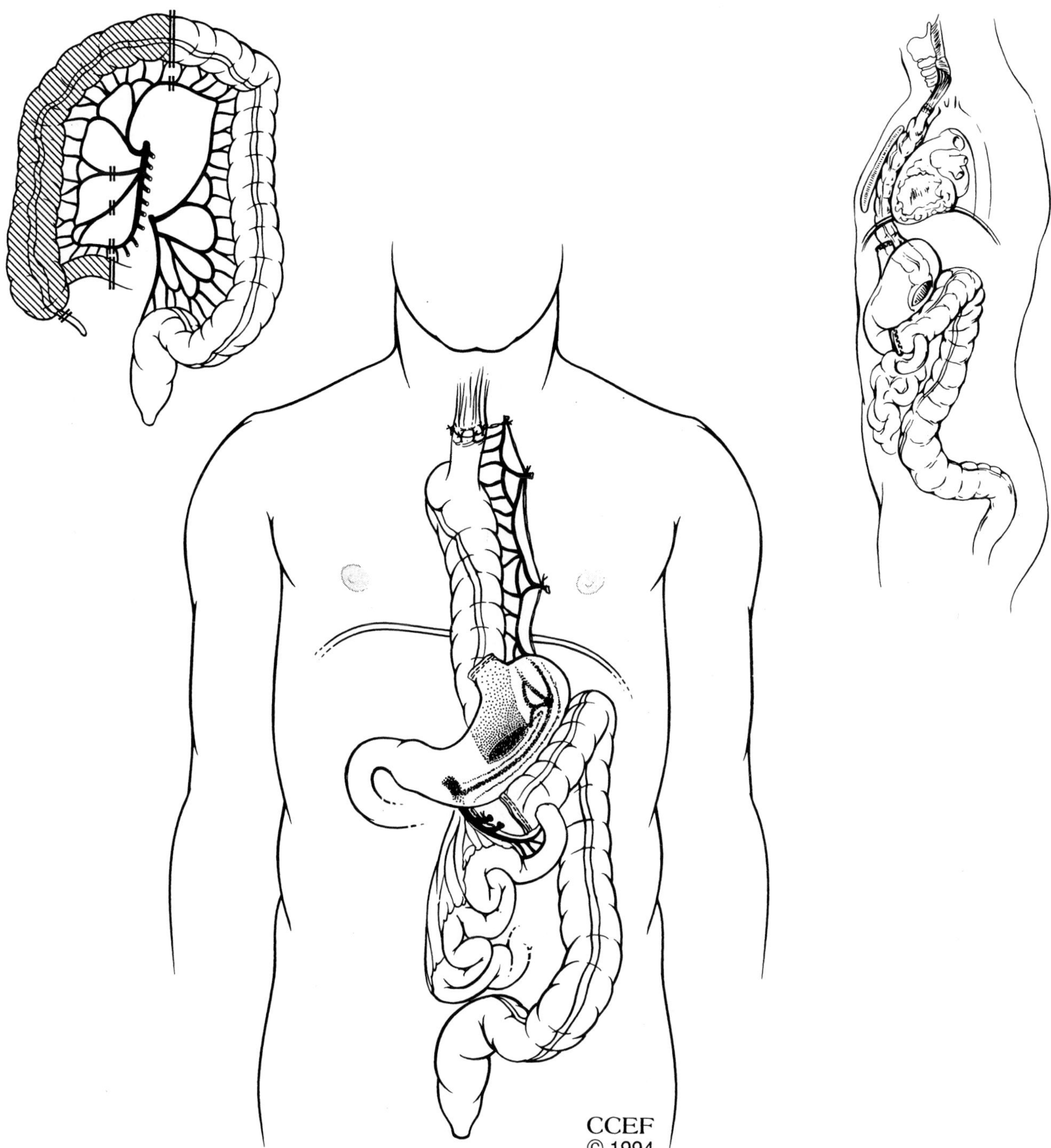

FIGURE 65–4 ■ Isoperistaltic, retrosternal right colon replacement of the esophagus. Preparation of the arterial blood supply is based on the middle colic artery *(left inset)*. The retrosternal route of the completed right colon replacement is depicted in the lateral view *(right inset)*. Anteroposterior view of this isoperistaltic right colon replacement *(main figure)*. (Copyright, Cleveland Clinic Foundation, 1994.)

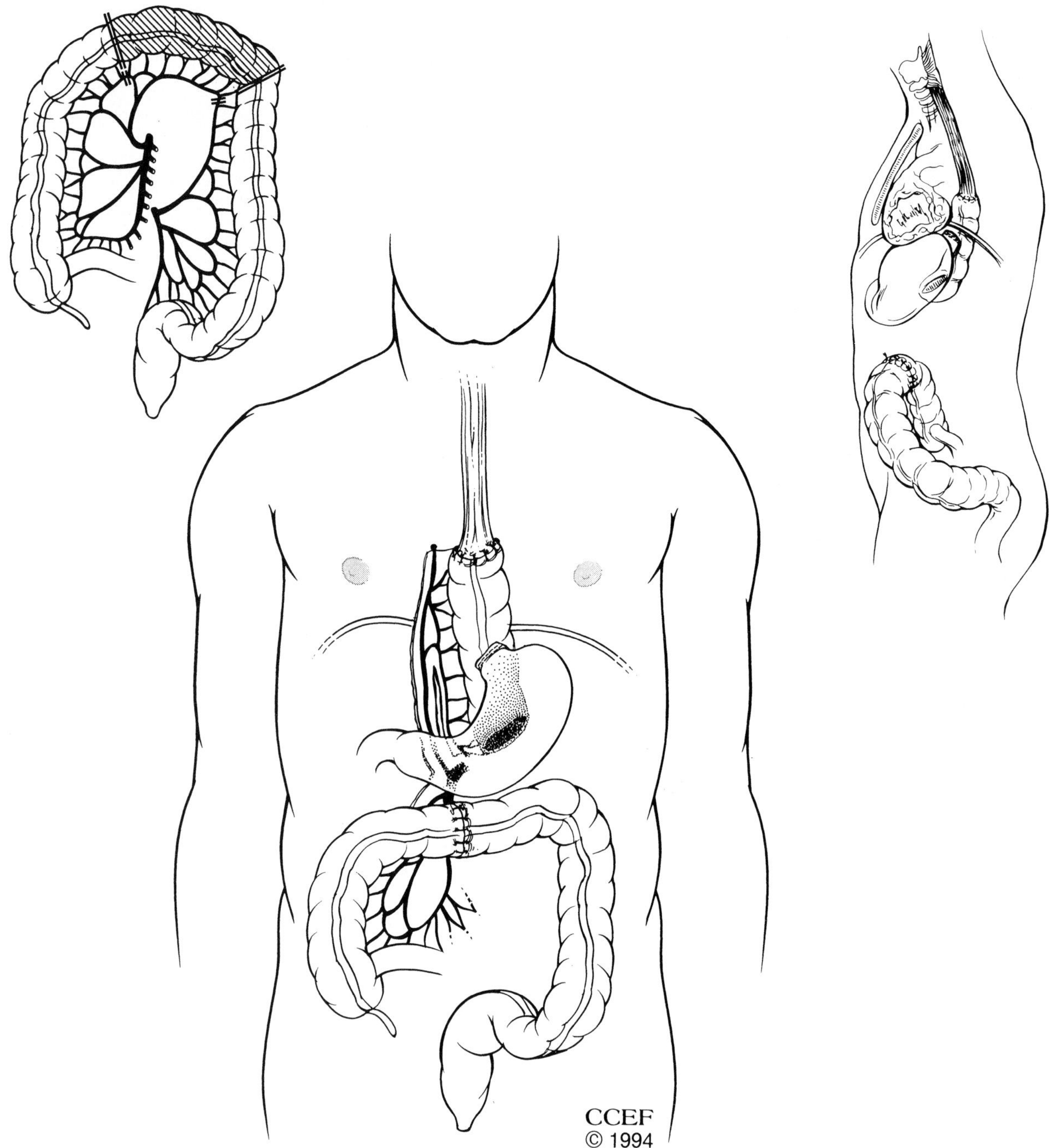

FIGURE 65–5 ■ Isoperistaltic, short-segment, transverse colon replacement of the esophagus. Preparation of the arterial blood supply is based on the middle colic artery *(left inset)*. The posterior mediastinal route in the bed of the esophagus of this short-segment, transverse colon replacement is depicted in this lateral view *(right inset)*. Anteroposterior view of this isoperistaltic transverse colon replacement *(main figure)*. (Copyright, Cleveland Clinic Foundation, 1994.)

the diaphragm from the sternum below the xiphoid process. The superior entry site is prepared by a division of the deep layer of the cervical fascia and entry into the retrosternal space in the midline behind the manubrium. The retrosternal tunnel is then prepared by blunt digital dissection from the superior and inferior entry sites. If the upper entry site of the retrosternal tunnel is constricting, the head of the clavicle, anterior portion of the first rib, and the lateral portion of the manubrium may be excised to widen the thoracic inlet.

The *subcutaneous* route requires an obligatory ventral hernia to allow passage of the colon replacement from the subcutaneous space into the abdominal cavity. The surgeon constructs the subcutaneous tunnel by dividing the attachment between the subcutaneous tissue and the sternum and chest wall musculature. The superior and inferior entry sites of the subcutaneous tunnel are connected by the passage of a blunt dissector. This tunnel is further widened by the passage of a long laparotomy sponge through the tunnel. The sponge is left in the

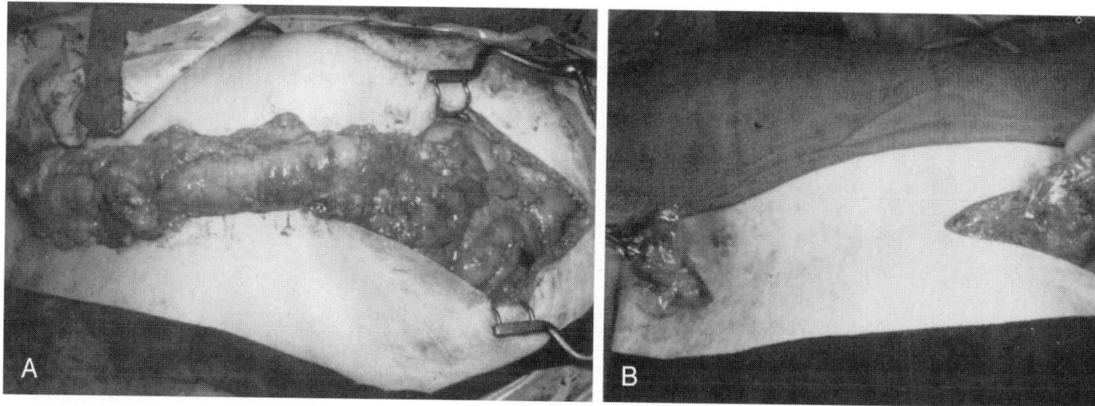

FIGURE 65–6 ■ *A,* The colon segment is placed along the cutaneous route previously marked with the umbilical tape to ensure adequate length of the harvested replacement. *B,* The colon replacement is delivered to the neck through the retrosternal route with the help of a large sterile plastic bag.

tunnel for 5 to 10 minutes to aid in hemostasis. The tunnel should be widened until it allows passage of the colon segment and its mesentery without compression (Fig. 65–7).

The colon segment is inspected and prepared for passage through the tunnel. This is facilitated by the placement of the colon segment into a large sterile plastic bag, and the bag is drawn through the prepared replacement route (Celerier et al, 1986; Inculet et al, 1988) (see Fig. 65–6). The proximal esophagocolic anastomosis is constructed usually in an end-to-side fashion along the antimesenteric tenia of the colon (Fig. 65–8). Because a stapled anastomosis is difficult to perform high in the neck, an interrupted sutured anastomosis of single-layer monofilament absorbable suture is the preferred technique. The correct length of the colon segment is then reconfirmed, and any redundant colon is pulled back into the abdomen.

The colon is tacked to the edges of the tunnel (diaphragm) with three stitches, each applied to one of the teniae. Any excess colon is excised along the mesenteric border to protect the vascularity of the colon replacement (see Fig. 65–8). The cologastric or colojejunal anastomosis is then constructed. To minimize reflux into the colon replacement, the anastomosis can be constructed on the posterior gastric wall at the junction of the upper and middle thirds of the gastric remnant (see Fig. 65–8). The weight of the full stomach rests on this anastomosis and provides some reflux protection. The construction of a partial fundoplication about this anastomosis provides further reflux control (Butterfield and Massi, 1972). The anterior wall of the stomach is an alternative site for the cologastric anastomosis. The cologastric anastomosis is more amenable to stapling than is the esophagocolic anastomosis.

The last of the three anastomoses re-establishes GI

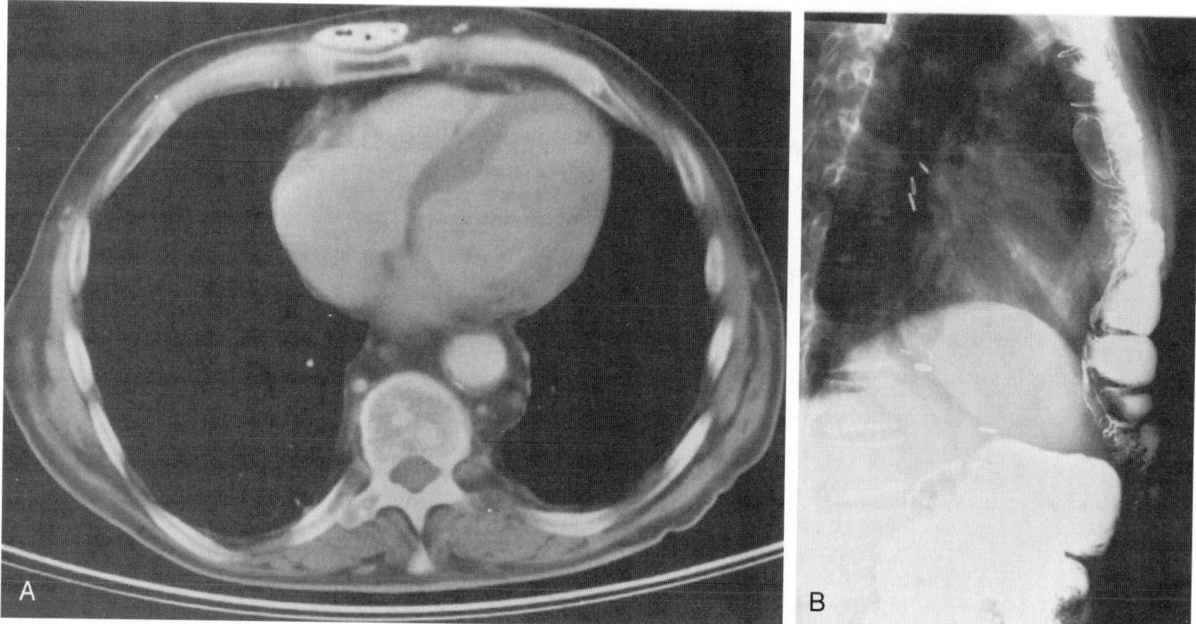

FIGURE 65–7 ■ *A,* A subcutaneous colon replacement is seen anterior to the sternum in this CT scan of the chest. *B,* Barium "esophogram" of a subcutaneous colon replacement.

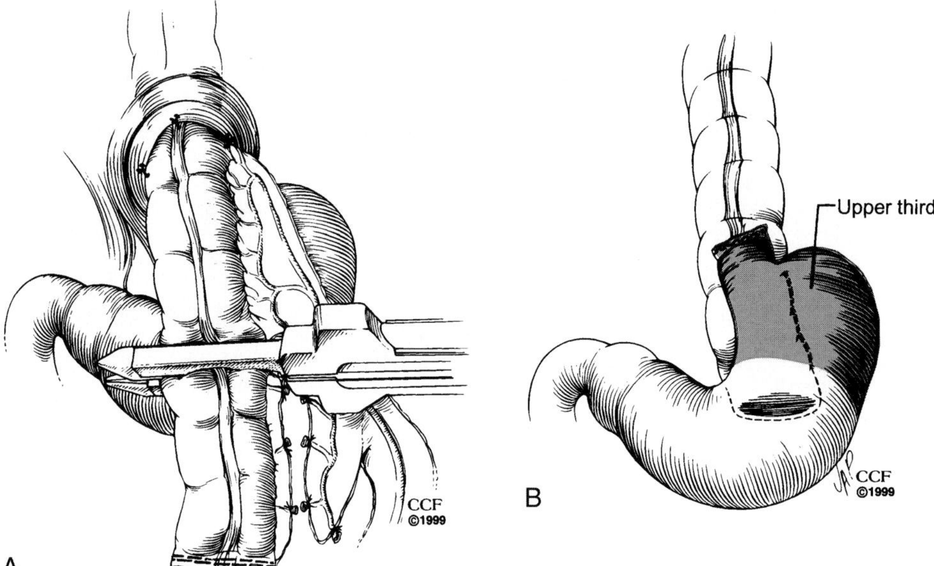

FIGURE 65–8 ■ *A,* Excess colon is excised along the mesenteric border, protecting the vascularity of the interposition. *B,* The cologastric anastamosis is constructed to minimize reflux of gastric contents into the colon interposition. The anastamosis is made on the posterior wall of the stomach at the junction of the upper and middle thirds of the gastric remnant. The weight of the full stomach rests on the anastamosis and distal colon and provides some reflux protection. Construction of a partial fundoplication around this anastomosis may provide further reflux control. (Copyright, Cleveland Clinic Foundation, 1999.)

continuity and is either *ileocolic* or *colocolic*. The colonic mesenteric defect is then closed with absorbable interrupted suture. A feeding jejunostomy should be constructed at this time.

The incisions are closed. If the operation is the second stage of a two-stage operation, the wound at the site of the end-esophagostomy, the location of the upper anastomosis (esophagocolic), is best managed with loose closure of the wound or, more appropriately, packing of the wound with delayed secondary closure. This minimizes wound infections and the possibility of anastomotic complications.

Results

As many as 65% of patients experience postoperative complications after colon replacement (Thomas et al, 1997). In addition to the complications that may occur after any thoracic operation, the specific early complications of colon replacement of the esophagus are anastomotic leak and necrosis of the colon graft. Anastomotic leakage is variable and complicates 2% to 40% of operations (Khan et al, 1998; Lortat-Jacob and Giuli, 1973).

As with other GI anastomoses, the reasons for the failure of an anastomosis in a colon replacement are multifactorial. Commonly implicated factors include ischemia, technical error, anastomotic tension, infection, and distraction of the anastomosis as a result of swallowing and excessive head and neck motion. Anastomotic leakage usually occurs at the esophagocolic anastomosis. It is uncommon to have failure of the cologastric, colojejunal, ileocolic, or colocolic anastomosis. Therapy requires the placement of the anastomosis at rest, adequate drainage, administration of antibiotics, and nutritional support. In the absence of complete disruption of the anastomosis, proximal colonic necrosis, or mediastinitis, surgical intervention is seldom required. Most fistulas heal spontaneously, but as many as 50% are complicated by anastomotic strictures that require dilatation (Wain et al, 1999). Repeated surgery with anastomotic revision is uncommon (Loinaz and Altorki, 1997).

Vascular compromise is usually precipitated by venous insufficiency and thrombosis and, less commonly, by arterial insufficiency. This problem is magnified by the bacterial contamination of the colon and results in necrosis of the colon graft in up to 16% of patients, a significantly greater incidence than that seen with gastric replacement (1%) (Yoshino et al, 1996). This complication is uniformly fatal if not recognized and treated with immediate graft excision. Colon necrosis is a major cause of death after this procedure. The conditions that mandate a presternal right colon replacement may place the patient at an increased risk of graft necrosis (Yoshino et al., 1996). Ischemic complications of the esophagocolonic anastomosis may be reduced by supercharging (augmenting) the colonic arterial supply and venous drainage with microvascular anastomosis of cervical vessels to the colonic mesenteric vessels (Golshani et al, 1999; Kiyokawa, et al, 1997).

Hospital mortality rates for colon replacement vary from 0% to 23% (Griffiths and Shaw, 1973; Hankins et al, 1984). The incidence of operative death has decreased with time, in part because of improved preoperative preparation, operative technique, and postoperative care, but also as a result of better patient selection. The operation has been reserved for patients with benign esophageal diseases, and the practice of colon bypass of unresectable malignancies has been abandoned. Patient-related factors cause operative mortality rates for esophageal resection and colon replacement of malignant esophageal disease to be two to four times those for benign disease.

The major late complications of colon replacement of the esophagus are stricture (Fig. 65–9), graft redundancy, and poor function of the colon replacement (Figs. 65–10 and 65–11). The same factors that foster anastomotic leakage may cause anastomotic stricture. In addition, reflux of gastric contents may cause ulceration and stricture of the lower portion of the replacement. Peptic

Dysfunction of the colon replacement results in persistent dysphagia or development of upper GI and respiratory symptoms. Evaluation of the long-term relief of dysphagia through colon replacement should not be based on experience in the therapy of malignant disease because of the poor survival rates in most patients with cancer and the practice of the use of colon bypass for palliation of patients with esophageal malignancies (Higton and Lord, 1970). Good to excellent results with colon replacement are achieved in 75% to 85% of patients with benign esophageal disease. In a review of 45 patients treated for benign disease with colon replacement, 24% had no GI symptoms during follow-up. Regurgitation, vomiting, and dumping occurred in 22%, 31%, and 18% of patients, respectively (Isolauri et al, 1986).

Perhaps the best determination of a successful colon replacement is the ability of a patient to gain and maintain weight. In children, this capacity can be monitored by growth. Stone and colleagues (1986) reported that 89% of 36 children who underwent colon replacement increased their weight percentile. Colon replacement has been reported to increase the weight percentile in children with esophageal atresia, on average from the 12th to the 33rd percentile, while maintaining the 50th percentile in children with lye strictures (Kelly et al, 1983). In five of six children who underwent colon replacement, however, poor absorption of fat was implicated as a cause of poor weight gain (Louhimo et al, 1969).

Quality of life has been assessed in patients treated for esophageal atresia with both primary repair and colon interposition (Ure et al, 1998). Patients undergoing primary repair had quality-of-life scores similar to those of healthy control subjects, whereas scores in patients with colon interposition were significantly lower because of increased GI and respiratory symptoms. Despite increased symptoms compared with the primary repair group, however, the colon replacement group had similar physical, social, and emotional functions and no differences in inconvenience or need for medical therapy.

COMMENTS AND CONTROVERSIES

An esophageal substitute must provide swift, predominantly unidirectional transit of liquids and solids from the hypopharynx to the stomach. The colon serves as a true esophageal substitute when it is used to replace or bypass the esophagus. However, technical difficulties and the vastly different physiologic properties of the colon and esophagus can result in poor transit in a colon replacement. In contradistinction, when the stomach is used to replace or bypass the esophagus, it does not function as a true esophageal substitute. In a gastric replacement of the esophagus, the esophagus is shortened and the esophagogastric junction is translocated from the abdomen into the thorax or neck. If the esophagogastric junction is adequately reconstructed, there is minimal delay in the transit of liquids and solids from the hypopharynx to the stomach. The intrathoracic position of the stomach and the difficulties in the emptying of this denervated organ cause many of the complications of gastric replacement of the esophagus. For most physicians and surgeons, the long-term management of gastric-emptying abnormalities in a gastric replacement is better accomplished than the management of delayed transit in a redundant colon replacement.

In addition, the increased complexity of a colon replacement compared with that of a gastric replacement, in every phase of its use (initial evaluation, preoperative preparation, operative management, and the postoperative care), has led most surgeons to choose the stomach as the primary esophageal substitute in malignant esophageal disease and has caused many to abandon the colon in favor of the stomach as the primary esophageal replacement in benign disease (Anderson, 1986; Ein et al, 1978; Goon et al, 1985; Orringer, 1985; Pineschi et al, 1985a, 1985b; Wolfstein et al, 1979). For most esophageal surgeons, the colon is a "second-line" esophageal substitute that is used only if the stomach is not acceptable for esophageal reconstruction.

T. W. R.

Dr. Rice has clearly summarized and illustrated the use of colon replacement as an esophageal substitute. He has also correctly concluded that the use of this procedure is rarely indicated today, being reserved for circumstances in which the stomach or the combination of stomach and jejunal graft is not available. From a functional standpoint, use of the stomach for reconstruction provides excellent long-term results. By contrast, the use of the colon is associated with increasing long-term functional problems secondary to lengthening, dilatation, redundancy, and poor propulsion.

In the previous edition of this textbook, Dr. Pearson, commenting on use of the colon, cautioned that the use of an antiperistaltic segment of colon may be associated with painful spasm and functional obstruction because of muscle spasm in the segment during deglutition. On the basis of personal observation, I echo his cautionary statement regarding the use of an antiperistaltic segment of right colon.

Notwithstanding these comments, the use of a long segment of colon remains an important option for reconstruction when the stomach is not available. This important chapter by Dr. Rice clarifies the role of the colon and well illustrates its use when necessary.

J. D. C.

KEY REFERENCES

Belsey RHR: Reconstruction of the esophagus with left colon. J Thorac Cardiovasc Surg 49:33, 1965.

This is the largest report of the technique and results of isoperistaltic left colon replacement of the esophagus.

Jeyasingham K, Lerut T, Belsey RHR: Functional and mechanical sequelae of colon interposition for benign oesophageal disease. Eur J Cardiothorac Surg 15:327, 1999a.

The long-term results of the Bristol experience with colon interposition for benign esophageal diseases are reported. Obstructive complications and graft redundancy are significant complications in patients with long-segment colon replacement.

May IA, Samson PC: Esophageal reconstruction and replacements. Ann Thorac Surg 7:249, 1969.

This is an excellent historical review of esophageal replacement.

Postlethwait RW: Colonic interposition for esophageal substitution. Surg Gynecol Obstet 156:377, 1983.

This is a current review of the results of colon replacement of the esophagus.

■ REFERENCES

Anderson KD: Gastric tube esophagoplasty. Prog Pediatr Surg 19:55, 1986.

Beck AR, Baronofsky ID: A study of the left colon as a replacement for the resected esophagus. Surgery 48:499, 1960.

Benages A, Moreno-Ossett E, Paris F, et al: Motor activity after colon replacement of esophagus: Manometric evaluation. J Thorac Cardiovasc Surg 82:335, 1981.

Butterfield WC, Massi J: Gastric reflux in colon interpositions: A method of treatment. J Thorac Cardiovasc Surg 64:229, 1972.

Calleja IJ, Moreno E, Santoyo J, et al: Long esophagoplasty: Functional study. Hepatogastroenterology 35:279, 1988.

Celerier M, Sarfati E, Gossot D: A new sleeve to lead the stomach or the colon through the chest (Letter). J Thorac Cardiovasc Surg 91:939, 1986.

Christensen J: Motility of the colon. In Johnson LR (ed): Physiology of the GI Tract, 2nd ed. New York, Raven Press, 1987, p 665.

Clark J, Moraldi A, Moossa AR, et al: Functional evaluation of the interposed colon as an esophageal substitute. Ann Surg 183:93, 1976.

Corazziari E, Mineo TC, Anzini F, et al: Functional evaluation of colon transplants used in esophageal reconstruction. Am J Dig Dis 22:7, 1977.

Curet-Scott MJ, Ferguson MK, Little AG: Colon interposition for benign esophageal disease. Surgery 102:568, 1987.

Czerny V: Neue Operationen. Zentralbl Chir 4:443, 1877.

Ein SH, Shandling B, Simpson JS, et al: Fourteen years of gastric tubes. J Pediatr Surg 13:638, 1978.

Golding-Wood DG, Randall CJ: Pouch formation in the interposed colon. J Laryngol Otol 99: 1043, 1985.

Golshani SD, Lee C, Cass D, et al: Microvascular "supercharged" cervical colon: Minimizing ischemia in esophageal reconstruction. Ann Plastic Surg 43:533, 1999.

Goon HK, Cohen DH, Middelton AW: Gastric tube oesophagoplasty—a long-term assessment. Z Kinderchir 40:21, 1985.

Griffiths JD, Shaw HJ: Cancer of the laryngopharynx and cervical esophagus: Radical resection with repair by colon transplant. Arch Otolaryngol Head Neck Surg 97:340, 1973.

Hankins JR, Cole FN, McLaughlin JS: Colon interposition for benign esophageal disease: Experience with 23 patients. Ann Throac Surg 37:192, 1984.

Higton DIR, Lord IJ: Dysphagia following colon pedicle grafts. Br J Surg 57:825, 1970.

Inculet RI, Finley RJ, Cooper JD: A new technique for delivering the stomach or colon to the neck following total esophagectomy. Ann Thorac Surg 45:451, 1988.

Isolauri J, Harju E, Markkula H: Gastrointestinal symptoms after colon interposition. Am J Gastroenterol 81:1055, 1986.

Isolauri J, Koskinen MO, Markkula H: Radionuclide transit in patients with colon interposition. J Thorac Cardiovasc Surg 94:521, 1987.

Jeyasingham K, Lerut T, Belsey RHR: Revisional surgery after colon interposition for benign oesophageal disease. Dis Esophagus 12:7–9, 1999b.

Kelling G: Àsophagoplastik mit Hilfe des Querkolon. Zentralbl Chir 38:1209, 1911.

Kelly JP, Shackelford GD, Roper CL: Esophageal replacement with colon in children: Functional results and long-term growth. Ann Thorac Surg 36: 634, 1983.

Khan AR, Stiff G, Mohammed AR, et al: Esophageal replacement with colon in children. Pediatr Surg Int 13:79, 1998.

Kiyokawa K, Tanabe HY, Tai Y, et al: Impact on outcome of additional microvascular anastomosis–supercharge–on colon interposition for esophageal replacement: Comparative and multivariate analysis. World J Surg 21:998, 1997.

Loinaz C, Altorki NK: Pitfalls and complications of colon interposition. Chest Surg Clin North Am 7:533, 1997.

Lortat-Jacob JL, Giuli R: Esophageal replacement. Prog Surg 12:77, 1973.

Louhimo I, Pasila M, Visakorpi JK: Late gastrointestinal complications in patients with colonic replacement of the esophagus. J Pediatr Surg 4:663, 1969.

Malcolm JA: Occurrence of peptic ulcer of the esophagus in colon used for esophageal replacement. J Thorac Cardiovasc Surg 55:763, 1968.

May IA, Samson PC: Esophageal reconstruction and replacements. Ann Thorac Surg 7:249, 1969.

Mikulicz J: Ein Fall von Resections des carcinomatosen Oesophagus mit plastichem Ersatz des excirdirten Stückes. Prager Med Wochenschr 11:93, 1886.

Myers JC, Matthew G, Watson JI, et al: Peristalsis in an interposed colonic segment immediately following total oesophagogastrectomy. Aust N Z J Surg 68:278, 1998.

Ngan SY, Wong J: Lengths of different routes for esophageal replacement. J Thorac Cardiovasc Surg 91:790, 1986.

Nicks R: Colonic replacement of the oesophagus: Some observations on infarction and wound leakage. Br J Surg 54:124, 1967.

Ochsner A, Owens A: Anterothoracic esophagoplasty for impermeable strictures of the esophagus. Ann Surg 100:1055, 1934.

Orringer MB: Transhiatal esophagectomy for benign and malignant disease. J Thorac Cardiovasc Surg 90:649, 1985.

Pineschi A, Pini M, Torre G, et al: Gastric tube oesophagoplasty for oesophageal atresia: A follow-up study: Part II. Radiologic, endoscopic and histologic controls. Kinderchir 40:16, 1985a.

Pineschi A, Torre G, Levi N: Gastric tube oesophagoplasty for oesophageal atresia: A follow-up study: Part I. Clinical controls. Z Kinderchir 40:13, 1985b.

Postlethwait RW: Colonic interposition for esophageal substitution. Surg Gynecol Obstet 156:377, 1983.

Raffensperger JG, Luck SR, Reynolds M, et al: Intestinal bypass of the esophagus. J Pediatr Surg 31:38, 1996.

Robillard GL, Shapiro AL: Variational anatomy of the middle colic artery: Its significance in gastric and colonic surgery. J Int Coll Surg 10:157, 1947.

Rodgers BM, Talbert JL, Moazam F, et al: Functional and metabolic evaluation of colon replacement of the esophagus in children. J Pediatr Surg 13:35, 1978.

Sieber AM, Seiber WK: Colon transplants as esophageal replacement: Cineradiographic and manometric evaluation in children. Ann Surg 168:116, 1968.

Sonneland J, Anson BJ, Beaton LE: Surgical anatomy of the arterial supply to the colon from the superior mesenteric artery based upon a study of 600 specimens. Surg Gynecol Obstet 106:385, 1958.

Steward JA, Rankin FW: Blood supply of the large intestine. Arch Surg 26:843, 1933.

Stone MM, Mahour GH, Weitzman JJ, et al: Esophageal replacement with colon interposition in children. Ann Surg 203:346, 1986.

Sutton R, Sutton H, Ackery DM, et al: Functional assessment of colonic interposition with ^{99m}Tc-labeled milk. J Pediatr Surg 29:874, 1989.

Thomas P, Fuentes P, Giudicelli R, et al: Colon interposition for esophageal replacement: Current indications and long-term function. Ann Thorac Surg 64:757, 1997.

Ure BM, Slaney E, Eypasch EP, et al: Quality of life more than 20 years after repair of esophageal atresia. J Pediatr Surg 33:511, 1998.

Ventemiglia R, Khalil KG, Frazier OH, et al: The role of preoperative mesenteric arteriography in colon interposition. J Thorac Cardiovasc Surg 74:98, 1977.

von Hacker V: Ueber Oesophagoplastik im allgemeinen und über den Ersatz der Speiseröhre durch antithorakale Haut-dickdarmschlauchbildung im besonderen. Arch Klin Chir 105:973, 1914.

Vulliet H: De l'oesophagoplastic et de ses diverses modifications. Semain Med 45:529, 1911.

Wain JC, Wright CD, Kuo EY, et al: Long-segment colon interposition for acquired disease. Ann Thorac Surg 67:313, 1999.

Wolfstein I, Rabau MY, Avigad I, et al: Esophageal replacement in children: 10 years' experience. Isr J Med Sci 15:742, 1979.

Yararbai O, Osmanodlu H, Kaplan H, et al: Esophagocoloplasty in the management of postcorrosive strictures of the esophagus. Hepatogastroenterology 45:59, 1998.

Yoshino K, Kawano T, Nagai K, et al: Diagnosis and treatment of complications after oesophagoplasty. Eur J Surg 162:791, 1996.

CHAPTER **66**

Long-Term Results of Colon Replacement

K. Jeyasingham

HISTORICAL NOTE

When the occasion arises for the esophagus to be replaced in part or in whole by a suitable hollow viscus, the colon is one of several options available to the surgeon. Since Kelling (1911) and Vuillet (1911) described the technique, numerous authors have presented the short-term results of the procedure (Belsey, 1965; Neville and Clowes, 1958; Waterston, 1965). With increasing long-term survival of patients after the procedure, others have described the long-term results of colon interposition in children (German and Waterston, 1976).

The colon is a thin-walled organ that contracts sluggishly and is normally located in a positive-pressure environment in the abdomen, so it behaves differently than the esophagus. The esophagus is a relatively thick-walled organ that is located in a negative-pressure environment and has a lumen that is normally collapsed and that empties its contents not only by bolus-induced contraction but also by gravity. The functional efficacy of the colon as an esophageal substitute has attracted the attention of gastroenterologists, physiologists, and radiologists, not to mention the surgeons themselves.

Despite these attentions, colon replacement of the esophagus is widely practiced for varying indications (Tables 66–1 and 66–2).

■ *HISTORICAL READINGS*

Belsey RHR: Reconstruction of the esophagus with left colon. J Thorac Cardiovasc Surg 49:33, 1965.

German JC, Waterston DJ: Colon interposition for the replacement of the esophagus in children. J Pediatr Surg 11:227–234, 1976.

Kelling GE: Oesophagoplastik mit Hilfeder Querkolon Zentralbl Chirurgie 38:1209, 1911.

Neville WE, Clowes GHA: Reconstruction of the esophagus with segments of colon. J Thorac Surg 35:2, 1958.

Vuillet H: De l'oesophagoplastic et des diverses modifications. Semin Med 31:529, 1911.

Waterston D: Colonic replacement of the esophagus (interthoracic). Surg Clin North Am 44:1441–1447, 1965.

TABLE 66–1 ■ **Indications for Colon Replacement of the Esophagus**

Congenital atresia
Corrosive strictures
Recurrent hiatal herniation
Short esophagus with gastroesophageal reflux
Columnar-lined esophagus with marked dysplasia
Carcinoma of the esophagus

TABLE 66–2 ■ **Age Distribution in Relation to Etiology and Extent of Colon Interposition in 365 Patients with Benign Esophageal Disease**

	Age	*Extent*	*n*
CHILDREN			
Atresia	2–5 yr	Long-segment colon	44
Stricture	5–13 yr	Short-segment colon	84
Recurrent hiatal hernia	5–13 yr	Short-segment colon	6
ADULTS			
Corrosive strictures	13–70 + yr	Long-segment colon	25
Recurrent hiatal hernia and peptic stricture	13–70 + yr	Short-segment colon	206

DEFINITION

Depending on whether a portion or all of the esophagus is to be replaced, a *short* or *long* segment of the organ may have to be transposed to bridge the gap between the cut ends of the esophagus and stomach. The anatomy and vascular supply of the colon lend themselves to such tailoring of the segment of colon that must be mobilized (Fig. 66–1*A–D*). The right hemicolon may be mobilized based on the right colic vasculature; the transverse colon, based on the middle colic vasculature, and the left hemicolon based on the left colic vessels. When it is adequate to mobilize the splenic flexure alone, the upper left colic vessels provide a suitable pedicle of blood supply.

When a short length of colon is used, the procedure is called a *short-segment colon interposition*; when the esophagus is being replaced totally or subtotally, a *long-segment colon interposition* is required. This distinction is extremely important in evaluation of the long-term results of colon interposition for the various indications. The short-segment colon interposition is usually required to bridge the gap after resection of a benign esophageal stricture or esophagogastric junctional carcinoma (Fig. 66–2). The long segment is used more often to replace a congenitally atretic esophagus or a corrosive stricture or when the seat of malignancy is in the middle or upper third of the esophagus (Fig. 66–3).

In a retrospective study (Jeyasingham et al, 1999a, 1999b) of 365 patients who survived colon interposition

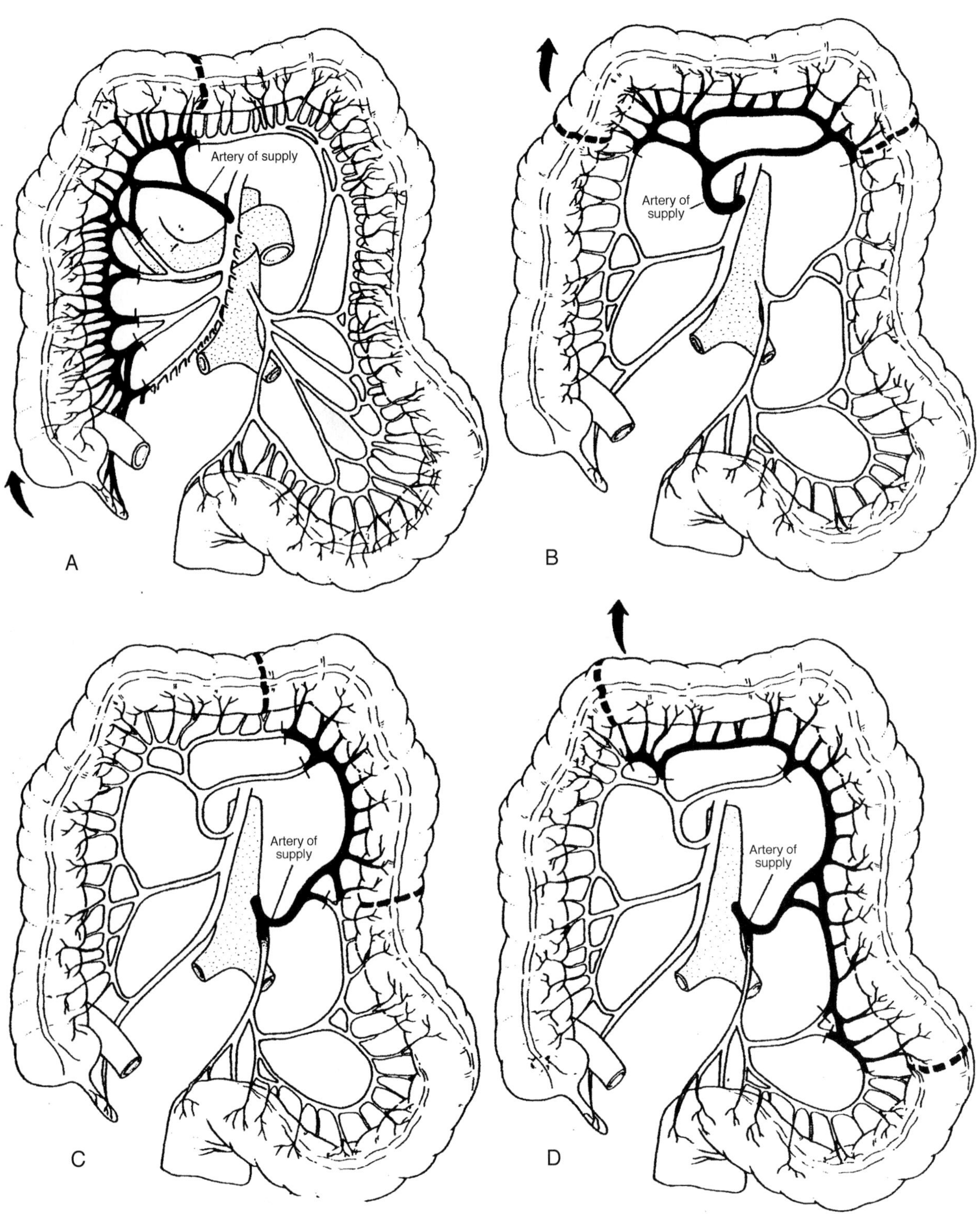

FIGURE 66–1 ■ *A–D,* The anatomy of the colon in relation to its blood supply to demonstrate the appropriate vascular pedicles required for various lengths of colon used in interposition surgery.

of the esophagus performed by members of one thoracic surgery department over 30 years, we evaluated the long-term results and assessed the need for revisional surgery for problems that could not be managed conservatively. Follow-up incorporated a 7- to 38-year period. Sixty-nine of the patients had undergone a long-segment colon interposition, and 296 had undergone a short-segment interposition. In all cases, the colon was interposed in an isoperistaltic manner and positioned in the posterior mediastinum. All 365 patients were reviewed regularly. Those who presented with upper gastrointestinal symptoms were investigated radiologically and endoscopically and, in selected instances, with ambulatory manometry and pH monitoring. It was thus possible to study the mechanical and functional sequelae that required pharmacologic or surgical intervention.

ESOPHAGEAL LABORATORY STUDIES

In an earlier study that contributed to an understanding of the normal physiology of the transposed colon, 10 asymptomatic adults who had undergone short-segment colon interposition up to 20 years previously underwent ambulatory monitoring manometry in the esophageal laboratory over 23 hours (Fig. 66–4). Low-amplitude contractions of a repetitive and sporadic nature occurred at different levels of the colon. These contractions did not appear to propagate along the length of the bowel. Apart from these contractions, the colon showed narrow-based high-peaked contractions that occurred simultaneously at different levels and a broad-based, bell-shaped, medium-amplitude contraction. Another significant waveform that was noted was the high-amplitude contractions observed with an amplitude of approximately 100 to 200 mm Hg at a frequency of about 4.4 waves per 24 hours. These contractions occurred in the early morning hours and were accompanied by the urge to defecate (Peppas et al,

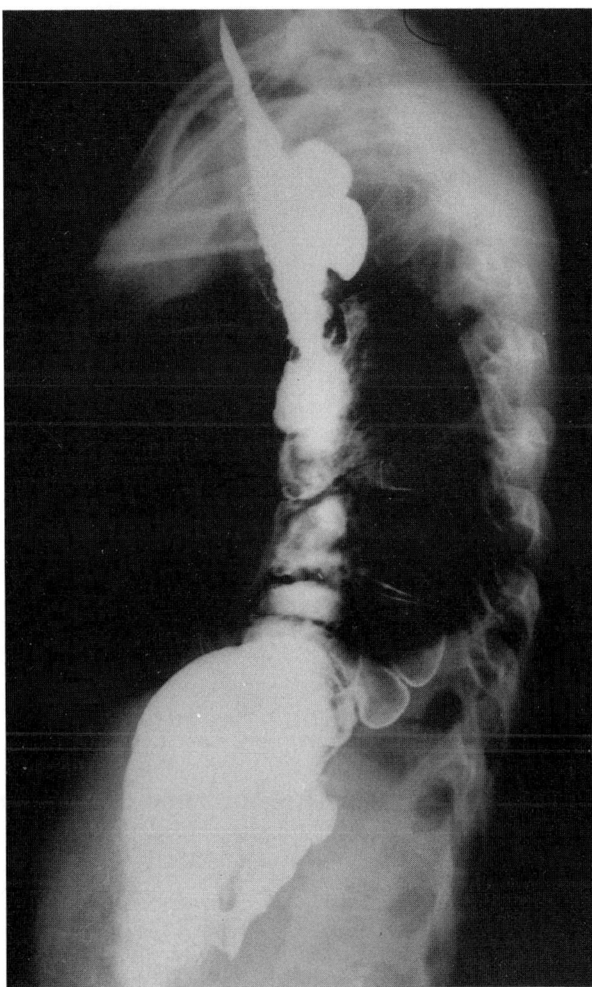

FIGURE 66–3 ■ Barium study in a patient who had undergone long-segment colon interposition showing an equally satisfactory early result.

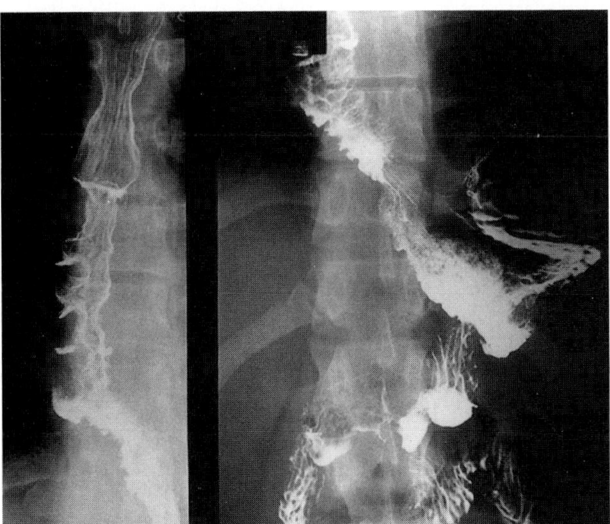

FIGURE 66–2 ■ Barium study of short-segment colon interposition for a lower third stricture associated with a columnar lining with marked dysplasia. Note the vertical disposition of the colon without any tortuosity in the chest and the low level of cologastric anastomosis in the abdomen.

1993). Ambulatory pH manometry in the asymptomatic patient did not reveal any acid reflux into the intrathoracic colonic segment. No measurements, however, were obtained from the intra-abdominal segment of colon in any of these 10 patients. Endoscopic examination of the upper gastrointestinal tract by esophagocologastroscopy in the same patients did not reveal any evidence of peptic ulceration in the residual esophagus, colon, or anastomotic cologastric stoma.

SYMPTOMATIC SEQUELAE

Of the 296 short-segment colon interpositions, five iatrogenic long-term sequelae were manifest in the form of *transhiatal herniation* of abdominal viscera at 3 and 10 years after surgery. One patient developed a delayed *incisional herniation* of the abdominal viscera through a peripheral incision in the diaphragm 2 years after the original operation. All three patients had undergone surgery in the early years of the series and had experienced vague abdominal symptoms for some months before presentation. *Septic complications* were manifested not only in the early postoperative period but also as delayed sequelae

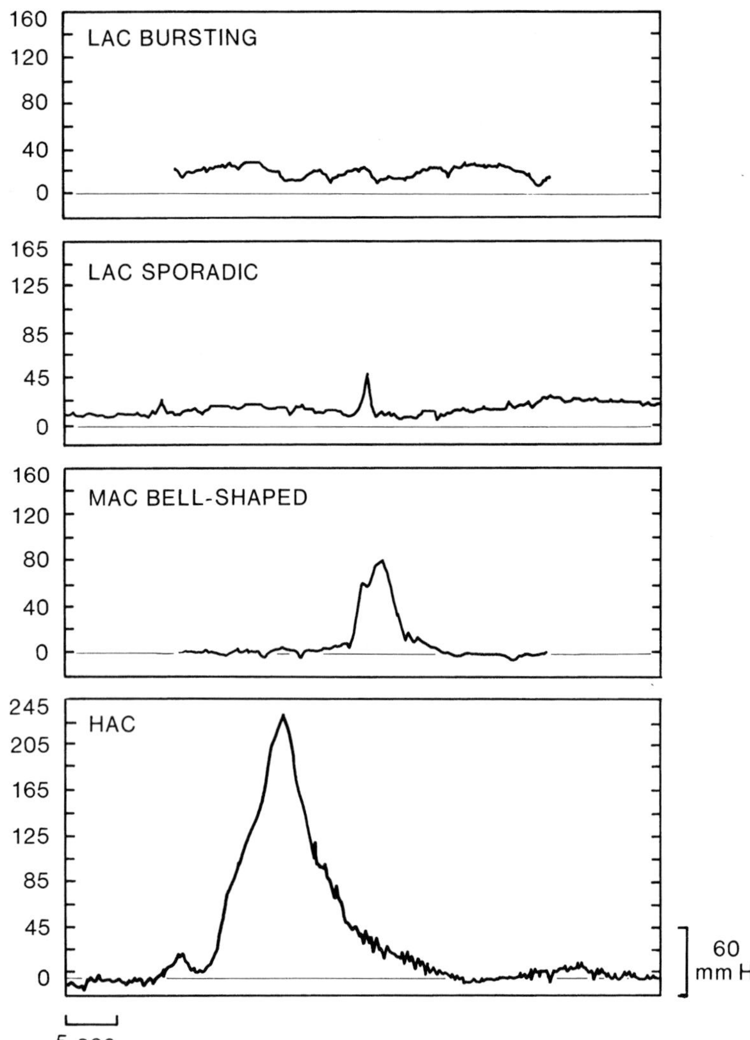

FIGURE 66–4 ■ Waveforms noted in ambulatory manometry in the long-term follow-up of asymptomatic short-segment colon interposition. HAC, high-amplitude contraction; LAC, low-amplitude contraction; MAC, medium-amplitude contraction.

several years after surgery, as demonstrated in two of our patients with *colocutaneous fistulas* that required surgical intervention. *Colobronchial fistulas* manifested in two patients at 2 and 14 years after the original operation and required excision of the tract. *Neoplastic transformation* can manifest in the cologastric junction, as occurred in two patients with short-segment colon interpositions (Table 66–3).

Although long-term sequelae in the 296 patients with short-segment colon interposition were few, the 69 patients who underwent long-segment colonic interposition had far more problems. *Esophagocolic strictures* occurred in four patients, of whom two had recurrence after surgery and required further revision. *Cologastric strictures* occurred in seven patients, requiring either revision of the anastomosis or bypass between the colon in the intra-abdominal portion and posterior surface of the stomach.

Mechanical delays in long-segment colonic interposition often occur in conjunction with functional delays and can occur at various levels—at the thoracic inlet, at the aortic arch crossing, and at the hiatal orifice. Likewise, *redundancy* tends to occur above the aortic arch level, at the supradiaphragmatic area, and in the infradiaphragmatic segment. Redundancy of the colon tends to recur despite revision or diversionary surgery (Fig. 66–5; see Table 66–3).

Iatrogenic sequelae are predominantly avoidable by paying meticulous attention to detail during the initial operation. Neoplastic changes in the colonic segment or in the cologastric junction are, however, unavoidable and merely manifest the characteristic tendency of glandular epithelium anywhere in the gastrointestinal tract.

The long-term sequelae of short-segment colon interpositions are rare and are iatrogenic, septic, or neoplastic,

TABLE 66–3 ■ **Long-Term Sequelae in 296 Short-Segment Colon Interpositions for Benign Disease**

Sequela	*n*
Diaphragmatic herniation	
Transhiatal	2
Incisional	1
Cologastric adenocarcinoma	2
Septic colocutaneous fistula	2
Colobronchial fistula	2

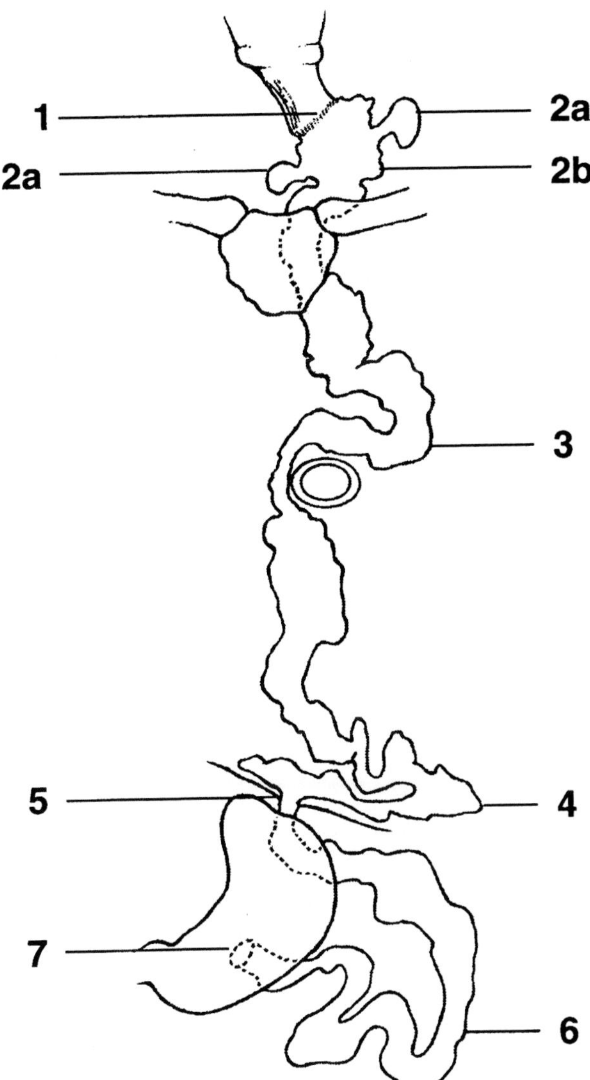

FIGURE 66–5 ■ Diagram showing the various levels at which mechanical and functional sequelae occur in long-segment colon interpositions. 1, esophagocolic stricture; 2a, cervical colonic pouch; 2b, dilatation proximal to thoracic inlet; 3, supra-aortic redundancy; 4, supradiaphragmatic redundancy; 5, hiatal obstruction; 6, subdiaphragmatic redundancy; 7, cologastric stricture.

but the long-term sequelae of long-segment colonic interposition are different. Ischemic stenosis frequently occurs at the cervical esophagogastric anastomosis and the intra-abdominal cologastric anastomosis. When the intra-abdominal segment of colon is positioned posterior to the stomach and the anastomosis is performed low on the body of the stomach, combined with pyloroplasty, gastrocolic acid reflux is minimal and acid ulceration in the colon is unlikely. A few reports, however, have suggested that should reflux occur into the colon, the colonic mucosa shows little resistance to acid ulceration. This situation is likely to prevail if the cologastric anastomosis is performed high on the body of the stomach or at the transected cardia.

When the left hemicolon is mobilized on the left colic vasculature for an isoperistaltic transposition, the colonic visceral length far outstretches the length of the vascular pedicle. The vascular mesocolon remains in the posterior mediastinum as a taut sheet, but the colon assumes a tortuous convoluted shape in the thorax and neck. The cervical anastomosis is far removed from the source of the vessel in the abdomen and is therefore susceptible to stricture formation even if immediate postoperative anastomotic subclinical leaks are overcome by drainage of the cervical tissues. Four of the 69 patients who underwent long-segment colon interposition presented with delayed cervical esophagocolic anastomotic strictures, and 2 of them required revision of the stenosis twice and still required endoscopic dilatations.

The causes of redundancy and hold-up are multiple. The colon is a thin-walled, hollow viscus that responds to the negative intrathoracic pressure by passively dilating above any potential obstruction, anatomic or otherwise. Such landmarks occur at the cervical inlet at the aortic arch level, the crossing of the descending aorta and left diaphragmatic hiatus. With increasing age, the colon appears to elongate as well as to dilate in this new environment. The disproportion of the colonic length to the vascular pedicle renders the dilatation and tortuosity more likely, as is demonstrated in 15 patients who required 17 procedures to correct increasing symptomatic redundancy several years after the original procedure (Fig. 66–6 and Table 66–4).

In a series of 112 children studied over 30 years, Ahmed and Spitz (1986) observed stricture formation in 34 (30.3%) of their patients and the need for revision of the esophagocolic anastomosis in the neck in 20 of these 34 patients (Table 66–5). Although excellent results were reported by German and Waterston (1976) and by Pampeo and associates (1997), in a multivariate analysis of 50 patients who underwent colon interposition for a variety of indications, Thomas and colleagues (1997) concluded that the single independent predictor of a good functional result was the placement of the colon in the posterior mediastinum (Table 66–6).

Objective functional evaluation of the results of colon interposition were carried out with manometry using a fluid-filled system (Benages et al, 1981). The presence of segmental contractions prompted the authors to conclude that these contractions could propel the contents of the

TABLE 66–4 ■ **Long-Term Sequelae After 69 Long-Segment Colon Interpositions for Benign Disease**

Sequela	*n*
Esophagic colic anastomotic stricture	4
Thoracic inlet obstruction	2
Colonic adenocarcinoma (intrathoracic)	1
Supra-aortic redundancy	4
Supradiaphragmatic redundancy	11
Hiatal obstruction	2
Subdiaphragmatic redundancy	2
Cologastric anastomotic stricture	7
Hemorrhagic peptic ulceration in the redundant segment	1
Anastomotic hemorrhage (after revision)	1

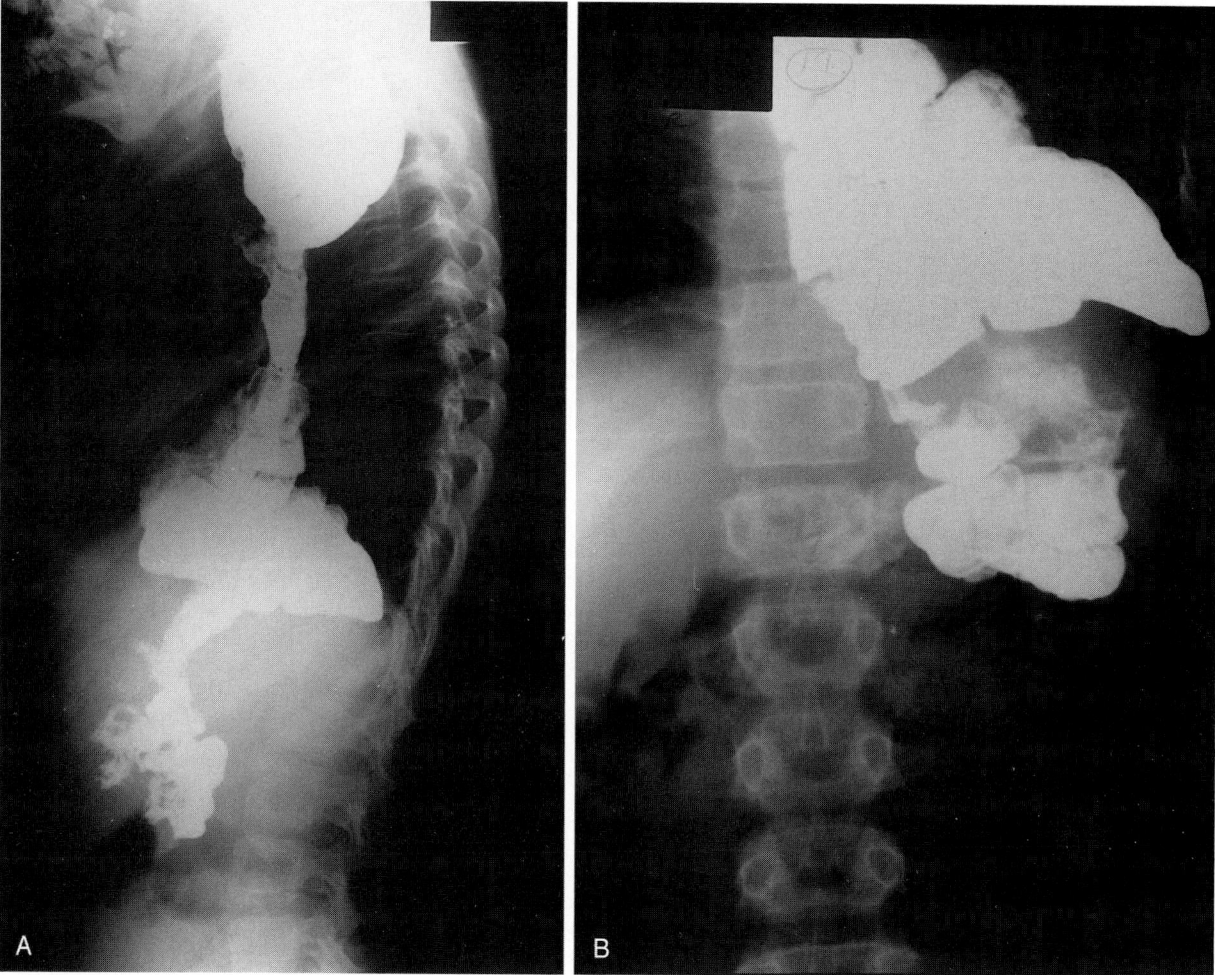

FIGURE 66–6 ■ *A* and *B*, Barium study of long-segment colon interposition several years after surgery shows a tendency for delay above the aortic arch and, again in the same patient, above the diaphragmatic hiatus.

colon into the stomach. The same group (Moreno-Osset et al, 1986) compared an isoperistaltic tube of stomach, jejunum, and colon as esophagus substitutes and concluded that the steady, homogeneous colonic responses played an active role in the transit of the food bolus.

Using a similar fluid-filled system combined with pH monitoring, Isolauri and associates (1987) considered the rarity of reflux of acid from the stomach into the colon as being the result of the vagotomy associated with the surgery and the availability of the alkaline colonic mucus. Peppas and colleagues (1993) used ambulatory manometry and pH monitoring in patients who had undergone short-segment colon interposition and confirmed the earlier observations of Narducci and associates (1987) in the normally situated abdominal colon. However, in addition to three main types of contractions—synchronous, sequential, and segmental—five subtypes were observed based on the amplitude of contractions. Ten years after his original interposition operation, one patient manifested a high-amplitude, long-duration contraction that

TABLE 66–5 ■ **Revision Surgery for Iatrogenic and Neoplastic Long-Term Complications**

Operation	*n*
Reduction and repair of transhiatal hernia	2
Reduction and repair of incisional hernia	1
Release of hiatal obstruction	2
Exploration for cologastric neoplastic change	2
Resection and repair of colobronchial fistula	2

TABLE 66–6 ■ **Revision Surgery for Functional Sequelae After Long-Segment Colon Interposition**

Operation	*n*
Revision of cervical esophagocolic anastomosis	4
Release of thoracic inlet delay	2
Resection and reconstruction of supra-aortic redundancy	4
Resection and reconstruction of supradiaphragmatic redundancy	11
Resection and reconstruction of subdiaphragmatic redundancy	3
Cologastric diversion of subdiaphragmatic redundancy	4
Resection and reconstruction of subdiaphragmatic redundancy	3

was probably associated with an obstructive effect of the diaphragmatic hiatus, but the only symptom in this patient was an urge to defecate simultaneously with the appearance of the high-amplitude contraction.

Although patients who underwent short- and long-segment colonic interpositions for benign disease were available for the study of long-term sequelae, this does not seem to hold true for patients who undergo colonic interposition for malignant disease. Most long-term studies therefore have been conducted in patients who underwent surgery for benign disease, and it is therefore not clear whether patients who survive long-term sequelae would be similar in surgery for malignancy.

COMMENTS AND CONTROVERSIES

This chapter by Jeyasingham nicely complements the previous chapter by Dr. Rice, because it illustrates indications for short-segment and long-segment colon interpositions and documents the problems associated with the use of colon as an esophageal substitute. The extensive experience with the use of short-segment colon for distal esophageal replacement was acquired during an era when it was recognized that an esophagogastric anastomosis low in the chest was associated with a very poor functional outcome and before it was recognized that an esophagogastric anastomosis high in the chest, or in the neck, is associated with an excellent functional outcome.

The long-term follow-up of the patients in this remarkable series of colon interpositions provides a unique and invaluable perspective on its application.

J. D. C.

REFERENCES

Ahmed A, Spitz L: Outcome of colonic replacement of the esophagus in children. Prog Pediatr Surg 19:37–54, 1986.

Belsey RHR: Reconstruction of the oesophagus with left colon. J Thorac Cardiovasc Surg 49:33, 1965.

Benages A, Moreno-Osset E, Paris F, et al: Motor activity after colon replacement of esophagus: Manometric evaluation. J Thorac Cardiovasc Surg 82:335–340, 1981.

German JC, Waterston DJ: Colon interposition for the replacement of the esophagus in children. J Pediatr Surg 11:227–234, 1976.

Isolauri J, Reimkarnem P, Markkula H: Functional evaluation of interposed colon in oesophagus: Manometric and 24-hour pH observations. Acta Chir Scand 153:21–24, 1987.

Jeyasingham K, Lerut T, Belsey RH: Mechanical and functional sequelae of colon interposition for benign oesophageal disease. Eur J Cardiothorac Surg 15:327–332, 1999a.

Jeyasingham K, Lerut T, Belsey RH: Revisional surgery after colon interposition for benign oesophageal disease. Dis Esophagus 12:7–9, 1999b.

Kelling GE: Oesophagoplastik mit Hilfeder Querkolon Zentralbl Chirurgie 38:1209, 1911.

Moreno-Osset E, Tomas-Ridocci MT, Paris F, et al: Motor activity of esophageal substitute (stomach, jejunal, and colon segments). Ann Thorac Surg 41:515–519, 1986.

Narducci F, Bassotti G, Gaburri M, Morelli A: Twenty-four hour manometric recording of colonic motor activity in healthy men. Gut 28:17–25, 1987.

Neville WE, Clowes GHA: Reconstruction of the esophagus with segments of colon. J Thorac Surg 35:2, 1958.

Pampeo E, Coosemans W, De Leyn P, et al: Esophageal replacement with colon in children using either the intrathoracic or retrosternal route: An analysis of both surgical and long-term results. Surg Today 27:729–734, 1997.

Peppas G, Payne HR, Jeyasingham K: Ambulatory motility patterns of the transposed short segment colon. Gut 34:1572–1575, 1993.

Thomas P, Fuentes P, Guidicelli R, Reboud E: Colon interposition for esophageal replacement: Current indications and long-term function. Ann Thorac Surg 64:757–764, 1997.

Vuillet H: De l'oesophagoplastic et des diverses modifications. Semin Med 31:529, 1911.

Waterston D: Colonic replacement of the esophagus (intrathoracic). Surg Clin North Am 44:1441–1447, 1965.

CHAPTER 67

Free Vascularized Grafts in Esophageal Reconstruction

Bruce H. Haughey

Timothy S. Lian

Reconstruction of the circumferential pharyngoesophageal and cervical esophageal defects has as its primary goal the reconnection of the pharynx to the esophagus with an epithelium-lined conduit. With a healed, well-vascularized, and pliable tissue tube in place, patients will predictably swallow by mouth after a single reconstructive procedure.

The various techniques of pharyngoesophageal and cervical esophageal reconstruction have used a hierarchy of tissues from all levels of the "reconstructive ladder," with skin grafts and local, regional, and distant tissues employed to form a tubular connection between the pharynx and the esophagus. This chapter focuses on microvascular free tissue transfer reconstruction of the pharyngoesophageal and cervical esophageal circumferential defect. Total esophagectomy and thoracic esophageal defects are best reconstructed with gastric pull-up or colonic interposition procedures, discussed elsewhere in this text.

Construction of the neopharynx and cervical esophagus improves a patient's quality of life. Immediate reconstruction of a circumferential defect facilitates early oral alimentation and allows oral speech after a tracheoesophageal puncture (Haughey, 1995). Connection of the pharynx with the esophagus prevents soiling of the neck and chest with saliva and food and eliminates maceration of the skin. Aspiration of saliva into the tracheostoma with pneumonia is also avoided. Elimination of a pharyngostoma avoids the requisite packing and dressing, with their attendant costs and social stigmatism.

PREOPERATIVE EVALUATION

Generally, patients who require a total or partial laryngopharyngectomy and cervical esophagectomy have one or more major systemic illnesses. Derangement of the pulmonary, cardiac, renal, airborne, vascular, hepatic, or hematopoietic systems carries inherent perioperative risk. Tobacco and ethanol abuse, the usual etiologic factors for head and neck cancer, are commonly coupled with long-standing malnutrition. Timely general medical clearance is mandatory before surgery for risk assessment, intervention, and anesthetic treatment planning. A percutaneous gastrostomy (PEG) tube may be placed several weeks ahead of the anticipated procedure to fortify a patient's nutritional status. Dental evaluation is also a requisite, especially if the dentate oral cavity is within the intended radiation portal. Social service input is helpful for postoperative home care.

Site-specific problems of the neck are usually related to prior surgery or radiation therapy, but these problems may have systemic implications. Up to 15% of head and neck cancer patients have occult hypothyroidism, which if untreated could precipitate a perioperative cardiopulmonary event or result in delayed or failed wound healing. Radiation-induced atherosclerosis may cause subtotal occlusion of the carotid vasculature, with possible cerebral ischemia after manipulation. External carotid donor vessels may be similarly diseased and require an alternate donor vessel for flap viability. A neck previously dissected on both sides should be considered for a carotid and/or aortic angiogram to aid in the search for appropriate donor vessels.

DONOR SITES

A donor site is selected based on defect size, patient age, gender, body habitus, hair pattern, occupation, and preference of both patient and surgeon (Fig. 67–1). The preferred donor site is the radial forearm; a reasonable alternative is the lateral thigh.

The radial forearm free flap (RFFF) allows a two-team approach, leaves few donor site problems, and imports new skin for the neopharynx and/or neck closure; however, this flap requires a skin graft for donor site closure. Some reports recommend harvest within the subcutaneous plane to maximize preservation of tendon and sensory nerve function (Chang et al, 1996).

The lateral thigh free flap (LTFF) is usually closed primarily, even for a large skin donor paddle, and does not have the same concern with adequacy of vascular perfusion of the extremity as does the RFFF (Hayden, 1993). The LTFF may be relatively contraindicated in an obese patient because this donor site is a usual location for the accumulation of fatty "saddlebags," especially in women. If such is the case, free jejunal transfer is a reasonable option at the expense of a laparotomy.

Vascular compromise of the extremity should be a minimal issue with the RFFF, provided that a favorable preoperative Allen test is obtained and an intraoperative evaluation of vascular perfusion of the hand is performed after division of the radial artery (Brown et al, 1996). A

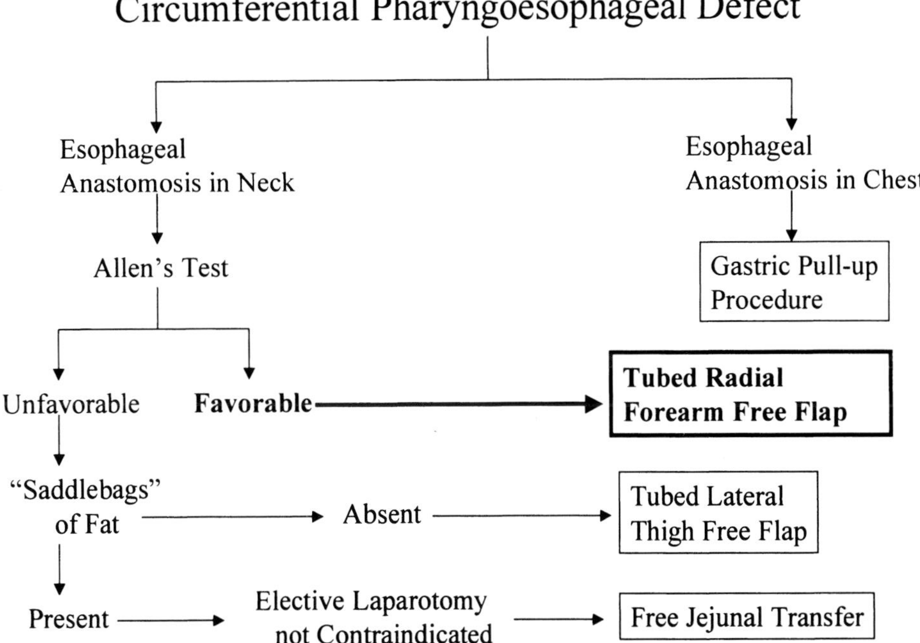

FIGURE 67–1 ■ Reconstructive options for the circumferential pharyngoesophageal defect are shown on the algorithm. The preferred reconstruction, shown in bold type, is the tubed radial forearm free flap.

compartment syndrome caused by an expanding hematoma, tight dressing, or splint is also possible. In contrast, without a laparotomy, there is no issue of a donor site–related ileus, abdominal abscess, enteric anastomotic leak, abdominal bleeding, or peritonitis.

RADIAL FOREARM FREE FLAP

The radial fasciocutaneous flap was first introduced by Yang and associates in 1981. For pharyngoesophageal reconstruction, the RFFF skin paddle typically measures 8 × 12 cm centered longitudinally over the radial artery (Colin and Haughey, 1998). The distal edge stops 3 to 4 cm from the proximal wrist skin crease to allow for coverage with a shirt sleeve, and for a watch or jewelry to be worn over native wrist skin. Under tourniquet control for no more than 1.5 hours, the flap is elevated medially and laterally; the surgeon takes care to preserve the paratenon and epimysium for subsequent skin grafting. The superficial radial (sensory) nerve is preserved, and the cephalic vein is incorporated into the skin paddle.

The radial artery is temporarily occluded on the distal end of the skin paddle with two microvascular clamps, and then the artery is divided. After release of the tourniquet, the hand and thumb are examined to confirm adequate vascular perfusion, and the distal radial artery backflow is assessed. Only then is the distal radial arterial stump suture-ligated. If perfusion is inadequate, the radial artery can be reanastomosed, the hand is reperfused, and an alternate donor site is chosen.

The pedicle is elevated from between the tendons and muscle bellies of the brachioradialis and flexor carpi radialis, with careful preservation of its attachment to the flap. The flap then remains attached only by the radial artery and veins while the initial flap contouring is being done and perfusion continues in situ. The skin paddle is folded lengthwise upon itself, skin inside, thus forming an epithelium-lined tube on the forearm (Fig. 67–2); 3–0 polyglactin 910 interrupted vertical mattress sutures are used in this closure every 0.5 cm.

Recipient vessels are chosen and prepared in the neck in anticipation of the microvascular fee tissue transfer. Branches of the external carotid artery are evaluated for diameter, length, patency, pulsatile flow, and lie of the vessel, including its relationship to any potential recipient vein. Typically, the linguofacial trunk or superior thyroid artery is chosen. The former vessel is turned beneath and then superficial to the hypoglossal nerve to help set up an unencumbered arterial anastomosis. A suitable recipient vein such as the external jugular or tributary into the internal jugular is selected and left in situ.

After flap harvest, the yet-to-be revascularized skin tube is oriented with the lengthwise suture line against the prevertebral fascia. Usually, the proximal part of the skin paddle can be made 2 to 3 cm wider than the distal paddle, which allows a wide open inlet to the prefabricated skin tube at the tongue base. The whole skin tube is then tacked to local tissue, and the vascular pedicle is properly draped. Attention is then directed to the microvascular anastomoses.

An interrupted or running continuous 9–0 nylon suture is used to perform an end-to-end anastomosis of the artery, and a mechanical coupling device (e.g., the 3M Precise system) is used to perform the venous anastomoses. Ischemia time is routinely under 1.5 hours. The proximal and distal flap anastomoses to the pharynx and esophagus are performed usually over a nasogastric tube salivary stent. The longitudinal suture line uniting the side of the flap into a tube is carefully positioned against the prevertebral fascia to ensure an immobile base (Fig. 67–3). The repair is then insufflated via the nostril with water or hydrogen peroxide, and the suture lines are assessed for leakage. Additional sutures are placed as necessary.

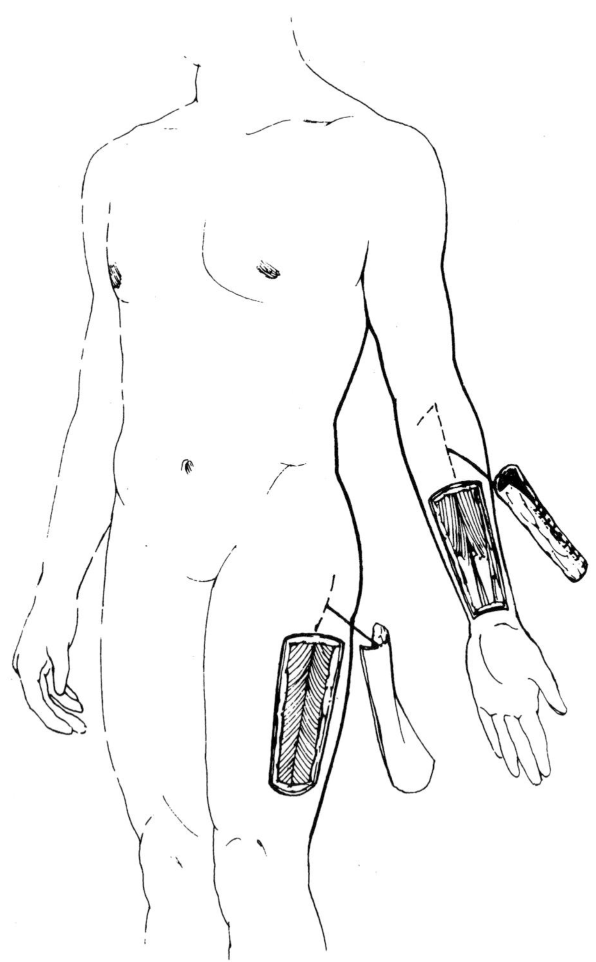

FIGURE 67–2 ■ The preferred donor sites for pharyngoesophageal reconstruction are depicted. The radial forearm free flap has been tubed while perfusion continues by the native radial vessels before transfers to the neck.

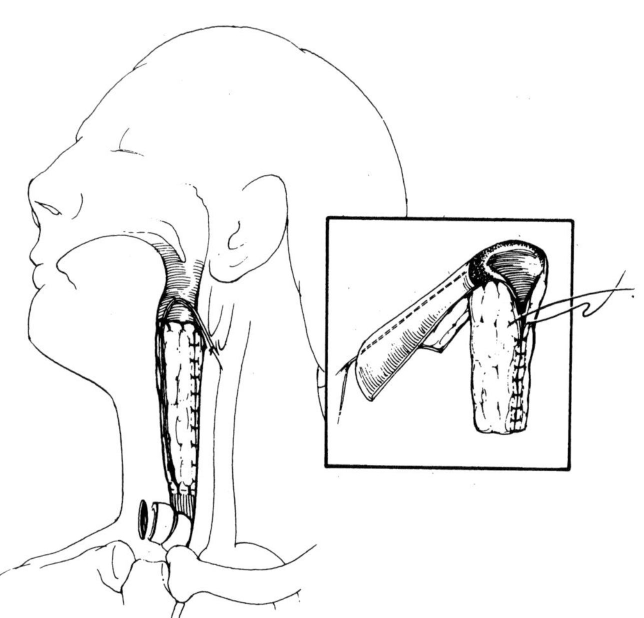

FIGURE 67–3 ■ The prefabricated fasciocutaneous tube has been inset to reconnect the pharynx and esophagus. Note that the vertical suture line is overlying the prevertebral fascia. *Inset,* A tubed flap, a de-epithelialized skin segment, and an attached skin paddle are shown. This technique allows pharyngoesophageal reconstruction along with resurfacing of deficient neck skin by a single free tissue transfer.

The neck flaps are reapposed over drains, and a marking suture is placed in the skin overlying a distal portion of the reconstruction where the Doppler signal is easily heard for postoperative monitoring.

LATERAL THIGH FREE FLAP

The lateral thigh flap was introduced by Baek in 1983, and its use for reconstruction of pharyngoesophageal defects was first described by Hayden in 1984. The skin of the lateral thigh receives its arterial blood supply from cutaneous branches of the perforators from the profunda femoris artery. The principal arterial supply to the lateral thigh is the third perforator, although in a very small minority of patients the fourth cutaneus perforator is the dominant pedicle. Venous drainage from the lateral thigh is through venae comitantes that accompany each of the arterial perforators. There are almost always two venae comitantes traveling with the arterial perforator, but more proximally, they join to become one large vein that ultimately accompanies the profunda femoris artery.

The third cutaneous perforator of the profunda femoris artery arborizes deep to the superficial fascia and the fat of the lateral thigh. It supplies an elliptical distribution in the lateral thigh, allowing for flaps of at least 27 × 14 cm to be harvested without any peripheral necrosis.

Flap design is similar to the RFFF as just described. The microvascular technique and insetting of the cutaneous portion of the LTFF follow the same principles described for the RFFF.

Once the flap has been harvested and transferred to the head and neck, closure of the leg defect is carried out by wide undermining and primary closure, resulting in a linear scar of the lateral thigh. The skin is usually thin and pliable and is frequently hairless, especially in women. With thin, pliable skin, the flap can be easily tubed to provide an epithelium-lined conduit for pharyngoesophageal and cervical esophageal repair. Because the donor site is usually closed primarily, scarring is minimal.

The distant location of this flap from the head and neck allows for synchronous double-team surgery. In obese patients in whom a very thin and pliable flap is required and large thigh fat deposits are encountered, this flap may not be appropriated.

JEJUNAL FREE FLAP

Autotransplantation of a segment of the jejunum was first described by Seidenberg and colleagues in 1959. This procedure was first done in dogs and thereafter successfully performed in humans. It involves harvest of a segment of the second loop of jejunum with its mesenteric arcade of vessels, transplantation to the neck region, and microsurgical revascularization. It is an appropriate choice for pharyngoesophageal replacement, because the jejunum is yet another mucosa-lined conduit from the alimentary tract, the caliber of which closely approximates that of the pharyngoesophagus. Digestion is not disturbed by sacrifice of the small segment of jejunum; primary reanastomosis in the abdomen is fairly straightforward. It is a reliable flap that, once revascularized, has an excellent blood supply.

Much has been written about placement of the jejunum in the neck in an isoperistaltic direction; some authors believe that an isoperistaltic direction causes problems with swallowing. It has been difficult to validate this premise because peristalsis of the jejunal segment, once it has been transplanted, is in no way coordinated with the oral or esophageal phase of swallowing. Nonetheless, it is easy enough to mark the jejunal segment before harvest and to place it in the neck in the proper orientation.

In all large head and neck operations in which the pharynx is entered, perioperative systemic antibiotics should be administered. Preparation of the bowel for its sterilization, however, is more controversial. In 1959, Lillehei and colleagues demonstrated that bowel sterilization did not increase survival in dogs that had their superior mesenteric arteries clamped for 5 hours. McGill and co-workers (1979) also showed that intraluminal antisepsis of isolated dog jejunum clamped for 90 minutes did not decrease the extent of the resulting mucosal injury. Despite this, Wang and associates, as recently as 1986, recommended irrigation of the isolated jejunal lumen with germanium bromide and neomycin. Although a few authors have advocated preoperative bowel preparation, the majority do not consider it necessary for small intestinal transfers (Coleman et al, 1989). A two-team approach generally is used in autografting, with one group harvesting the segment of jejunum while the other performs the cancer ablation procedure. As always, it is imperative that the ablative team be sensitive to the needs of the microvascular surgeon in preserving a suitable recipient artery and vein.

The segment of jejunum to be harvested should be supplied by a single vascular arcade of adequate dimensions. Some authors identify the appropriate arcade by transilluminating the mesentery (Deane et al, 1987). Considerable controversy exists regarding the best segment of jejunum to be harvested. Jejunal segments have been isolated from just distal to the ligament of Treitz, from the fourth jejunal arcade, and from 20 cm, 28 cm, 45 to 60 cm, and even 100 to 150 cm distal to the ligament of Treitz (Hester et al, 1984).

After the jejunal segment is isolated, the vascular pedicle is dissected proximally to a point close to the origin from the superior mesenteric vessels. This yields the largest vessel diameter and length to provide flexibility and ease of vascular anastomoses. The jejunal segment is divided and left vascularized by its arcade until the recipient site has been prepared.

After the donor and recipient vessels have been placed in approximating clamps, the head should be manipulated to assess the effect that any changes in position may have on the vessels. This should be performed again after the anastomoses have been completed. If the vessels approximate with tension, an interpositional vein graft may be needed.

The proximal enteric anastomosis usually is hand sewn in an end-to-end fashion with interrupted sutures. If the circumference of the hypopharynx is greater than that of the jejunal graft, the cephalad jejunum can be opened along its antimesenteric border to improve the size match. Although enteric stapling of the pharyngojejunal anastomosis has been reported, in most cases this is a difficult undertaking because of problems in inserting the stapling device through the oral cavity and in obtaining a watertight seal because of discrepancies in the size of the apposing pharyngeal and enteric lumina. The distal suture line can be stapled or hand-sewn with interrupted sutures. After the vascular and enteric anastomoses are performed, any redundant mesentery should be wrapped around the enteric anastomoses. This has been shown to decrease the incidence of postoperative fistulas (Nahai et al, 1984). After the reconstruction is completed the wounds are closed and drained in standard fashion.

POSTOPERATIVE CARE

After microvascular free tissue transfer reconstruction, the patient is sent to an intensive care unit for 1 to 2 days. Low doses of intravenous heparin (50 units/hr), aspirin per rectum (600 mg/day), hetastarch (500 ml/day), and dexamethasone (6 mg every 6 hours) are given for 3 days. The flap is checked hourly for clinical evidence of arteriovenous insufficiency by assessing the adequacy of the Doppler signal and by inspection, capillary refill, and needle prick testing of any visible paddle on the neck. The neopharyngoesophageal reconstruction is also evaluated by daily inspection of the pharyngoesophageal lumen using fiberoptic nasopharyngoscopy. The donor site is also evaluated to ensure adequacy of distal limb perfusion in the case of RFFF reconstruction and to monitor for wound infection.

Patients are begun on oral feeding with clear liquids at 10 days after their reconstruction or 14 days if there is a history of prior irradiation. If no fever or neck tenderness develops, then the diet is advanced daily as tolerated. A speech pathology consultation may be necessary for swallowing instructions.

COMPLICATIONS

The most common major complication of any type of pharyngoesophageal and cervical esophageal reconstruction is the pharyngocutaneous fistula. A low cervical fistula carries risks of aspiration, mediastinitis, and erosion of the vessels of the neck and chest. Fistulas develop because of previous irradiation, residual tumor, nonhealing recipient tissue, flap tissue loss, or poor surgical technique. Tissue trauma, wound tension, mucosal inversion, hematoma formation, or infection contribute to development of a fistula.

Once recognized, most fistulas respond to conservative treatment. This requires protecting the airway with a cuffed tracheotomy tube, administration of culture-directed intravenous antibiotics, and possible biopsy to rule out recurrent disease. The fistula should be diverted away from the great vessels and tracheostomy by packing, wound revision, and pressure dressings. A suction drain, salivary bypass tube, or T tube may be helpful to reduce the amount of soilage of the neck tissues.

If the fistula is persistent, relatively small, and not exposed previously to radiation, local turn-in flaps may have value. For larger lesions, the time-honored technique is to create a controlled pharyngostomy or esophagostomy, which when matured can be closed with regional myofascial tissue such as the pectoralis major flap and covered with a skin graft.

COMMENTS AND CONTROVERSIES

This chapter documents the recent evolution in reconstruction of the pharyngoesophageal region after pharyngolaryngectomy. Until about 10 years ago, the use of the stomach for pharyngogastric anastomosis was considered the standard method of reconstruction. With proper mobilization of the stomach, and resection of a portion of the lesser curvature, adequate length can usually be obtained for anastomosis, even high in the pharynx. On occasion, however, the use of stomach may cause the anastomosis to be under tension. In addition, gastric ischemia or venous congestion may present a problem for a high pharyngogastric anastomosis. The use of the vascularized forearm, the thigh skin flap, or an isolated jejunal or gastric segment obviates these problems.

From my own experience, working with one of the authors (Dr. Haughey), I can attest that the radial forearm free flap gives excellent results when used as either a lateral patch or a tubed conduit. The use of this flap, compared with the use of stomach, has the further great advantage of simplifying the operation and reducing morbidity by eliminating the need for esophagectomy, laparotomy, and gastric mobilization. For the thoracic surgeon, the importance of incorporating the otolaryngologist and plastic surgeon as part of a multidisciplinary approach to reconstruction of the cervical esophagus is obvious.

REFERENCE

Hiebert CA, Cummings GO Jr: Successful replacement of the cervical esophagus by transplantation and revascularization of a free graft of gastric antrum. Ann Surg 154:103, 1961.

J. D. C.

■ REFERENCES

Baek SM: Two new cutaneous free flaps: The medial and lateral thigh flaps. Plast Reconstr Surg 71:354, 1983.

Brown MT, Cheney ML, Gliklich RL, et al: Assessment of functional morbidity in the radial forearm free flap donor site. Arch Otolaryngol Head Neck Surg 122:991, 1996.

Chang SC, Miller G, Halber CF, et al: Limiting donor site morbidity by suprafascial dissection of the radial forearm flap. Microsurgery 17:136, 1996.

Coleman JJ, Tan K, Searles JM, et al: Jejunal free autograft: Analysis of complications and their resolution. Plast Reconstr Surg 84:589, 1989.

Colin WB, Haughey BH: Pharyngoesophageal Reconstruction, The Method of Bruce H. Haughey. In Gates G (ed): Current Therapy in Otolaryngology Head and Neck Surgery, 6th ed. St. Louis, Mosby–Year Book, 1998, pp 285–288.

Deane LM, Gilbert DA, Schecter GL, et al: Free jejunal transfer for the reconstruction of pharyngeal and cervical esophageal defects. Ann Plast Surg 19:499, 1987.

Haughey BH: Vibratory segment function after free flap reconstruction of the pharyngoesophagus. Laryngoscope 105:487, 1995.

Hayden RE: The lateral thigh flap to total pharyngeal reconstruction. Paper presented at the International Microsurgical Congress, Pittsburgh, PA, 1984.

Hayden RE: Reconstruction of the hypopharynx. In Cummings C, Fredrickson JM, Harker LA, et al (eds): Otolaryngology–Head and Neck Surgery, 2nd ed. St. Louis, Mosby–Year Book, 1993, p 2178.

Hester TR, McConnel F, Nahai F, et al: Pharyngoesophageal stricture and fistula. Ann Surg 199:762, 1984.

Lillehei RC, Goott B, Miller FA: The physiological response of the small bowel of the dog to ischemia including prolonged in-vitro preservation of the bowel with successful replacement and survival. Ann Surg 150:543, 1959.

McGill CW, Taylor BH, Flynn MB, et al: Effects of cooling and intraluminally administered antiseptics on surgically induced ischemia of the intestine in dogs. Surg Gynecol Obstet 149;377, 1979.

Nahai F, Stahl RS, Hester TR, et al: Advanced applications of revascularized free jejunal flaps for difficult wounds of the head and neck. Plast Reconstr Surg 74:778, 1984.

Seidenberg B, Hurwitt ES, Som ML: Immediate reconstruction of the cervical esophagus by a revascularized isolated jejunal segment. Ann Surg 149:162, 1959.

Wang ID, Sun YE, Chen Y: Free jejunal grafts for reconstruction of the pharynx and cervical esophagus. Ann Otol Rhinol Laryngol 95:348, 1986.

Yang G, Chen B, Gao U, et al: Forearm free skin flap transplantation. Natl Med J China 61:139, 1981.

CHAPTER **68**

Gastric Tubes: Reversed and Nonreversed

Stanley C. Fell

Manoel Ximenes-Netto

For anatomic and physiologic reasons, the ideal esophageal replacement may be a tube constructed from the greater curvature of the stomach and vascularized by the gastroepiploic arcade.

In adults, either pre-existing colonic disease or prior colon resection prohibits the use of a colon conduit. Infants with esophageal atresia may have an associated high imperforate anus and require reconstructive colon surgery. Anomalous arterial patterns or a poor marginal artery make colon interposition hazardous. In contrast, the stomach has an excellent arterial supply in a predictable pattern (Fig. 68–1). The gastroepiploic arcade, which is situated peripheral to the greater curvature of the stomach and thus has a greater arc, lengthens when the gastric tube is created and straightened and does not limit the length of the conduit. The colon and jejunum, with their fan-shaped mesenteries, are longer than their vascular arcades and therefore tend to be redundant when interposed between the esophagus and stomach. In contrast to the gastroepiploic vessels, which are closely applied to the stomach, these mesenteries are subject to tension and torsion.

Colon interposition, even if not redundant when first performed, dilates and becomes redundant years later, with attendant problems of stasis and poor emptying. This phenomenon has not been noted with the gastric tube.

An earlier gastrostomy is not a contraindication to the construction of a gastric tube. In fact, it is a great advantage, because the stomach may be dilated when a large amount (1000 to 1500 mL) of a liquid diet is offered

Supported by the Feldesman Fund for Thoracic Surgery at the Albert Einstein College of Medicine.

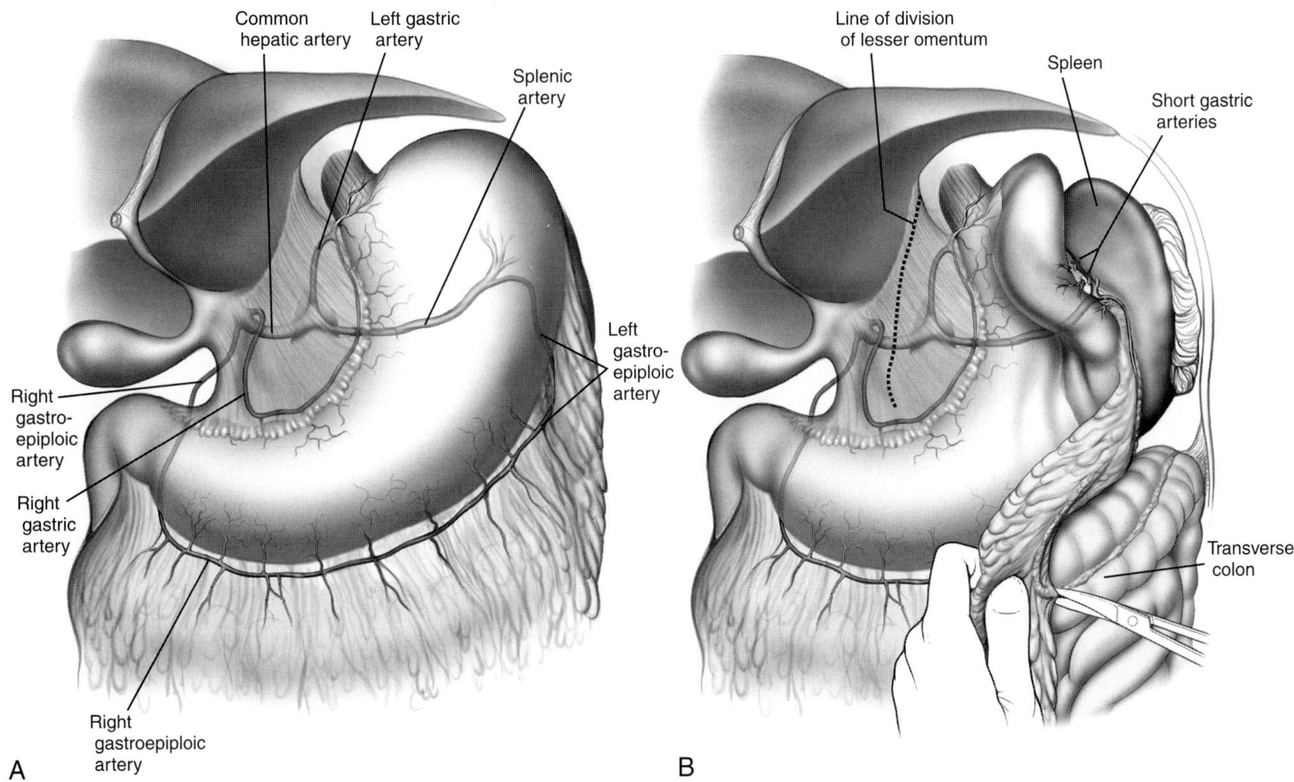

FIGURE 68–1 ■ *A,* Arterial supply of the stomach. *B,* The greater omentum is mobilized.

every 3 or 4 hours during waking hours. In 2 to 3 months, the stomach is so enlarged that there is abundant stomach available for esophageal replacement. If this form of reconstruction is anticipated and prior gastrostomy is required, preferably it should be performed toward the lesser curvature of the stomach. The location of the gastrostomy is of little consequence, provided that the stomach is dilated as described. Prior gastric resection or outlet obstruction usually is a contraindication to the application of the gastric tube for esophageal reconstruction.

HISTORICAL NOTE

In experiments on cadaver dogs, Beck and Carrel (1905) demonstrated that a tube constructed from the greater curvature of the stomach based on the left gastroepiploic artery could reach the cervical esophagus. Jianu (1912) successfully performed *reversed gastric tube* (RGT) esophagoplasty in living dogs, but his two attempts in humans in 1914 failed. In 1951, Gavriliu performed the first successful RGT in a human; since then, he has performed 718 of these procedures (Gavriliu, 1988).

Independently, Heimlich and Winfield (1955) in the United States, repeated the experimental work of Jianu and subsequently reported their experience in humans (Heimlich, 1961). Sanders (1962) was the first to use the RGT for esophageal replacement in a child. Anderson and Randolph (1978) reported excellent results in pediatric cases. Postlethwait (1979) developed and popularized the use of the *nonreversed gastric tube* (NRGT) based on the work of Mes (1948). A comprehensive review of the history of the RGT was published by O'Connor (1983).

■ *HISTORICAL READINGS*

Anderson KD, Randolph JG: Gastric tube interposition: A satisfactory alternative to the colon for esophageal replacement in children. Ann Thorac Surg 25:521, 1978.

Beck C, Carrel A: Demonstration of specimens illustrating a method of formation of a prethoracic esophagus. Ill Med J 7:463, 1905.

Gavriliu D: The replacement of the esophagus by a gastric tube. In Jamieson G (ed): Surgery of the Oesophagus. New York, Churchill Livingstone, 1988, p 765.

Heimlich HJ: Replacement of the entire esophagus for malignant or benign stenosis. Am J Gastroenterol 35:311, 1961.

Jianu A: Gastrostomie and Oesophagoplastik. Dtsch Z Chir 118:383, 1912.

Mes G: New method of esophagoplasty. J Int Coll Surg 11:270, 1948.

O'Connor TW: A historical review of reversed gastric tube esophagoplasty. Surg Gynecol Obstet 156:371 1983.

Postlethwait RW: Technique for isoperistaltic gastric tube for esophageal bypass. Ann Surg 189:673, 1979.

Sanders GB: Esophageal replacement with reversed gastric tube, utilization for bleeding esophageal varices in a 4 year old child. JAMA 181:944, 1962.

MANAGEMENT: OPERATIVE TECHNIQUE

The patient is positioned supine with a foot board on the table. During the course of mobilization of the stomach, it is helpful to tilt the patient 30 degrees, feet down, to facilitate access to the proximal portion of the stomach.

Laparotomy is performed through a midline incision that extends from the xiphoid to below the umbilicus. A self-retaining retractor is inserted, and the stomach and omentum are drawn into the operative field. The vascular arcade and the greater curvature are inspected and palpated. A decision is made in regard to which gastroepiploic artery will vascularize the tube.

The RGT is based on the left gastroepiploic artery, and the NRGT is based on the right gastroepiploic artery. The gastrohepatic ligament is opened, and a hand is placed in the lesser sac, passing superficial to the pancreas, with the fingers exiting the omentum on the greater curvature inferior to the vascular arcade.

The greater omentum is dissected from the transverse colon and both hepatic and splenic flexures, with care taken to avoid injury to the middle colic artery. The resultant omental flap is left attached to the gastric tube (GT), to be elevated into the neck and wrapped about the cervical anastomosis to protect against anastomotic leak (Figs. 68–2 and 68–3). The spleen is retracted medially, and a large, moist pad is placed between it and the posterior abdominal wall, thus relieving tension on the vasa brevia.

At the level of the spleen, the gastroepiploic artery is no longer present on the greater curvature and only the short gastric arteries must be isolated individually and divided. This may not be necessary in children.

The vessels are divided close to the spleen with clips for the splenic end and silk ties for the gastric end of the vessels. Although splenectomy was an integral part of the surgical procedure, as originally described (see later), it is not required unless there is an irreparable splenic laceration. Once the stomach is dilated by means of a previous gastrostomy, the greater curvature does not come near the hilum of the spleen, thus making splenectomy unnecessary.

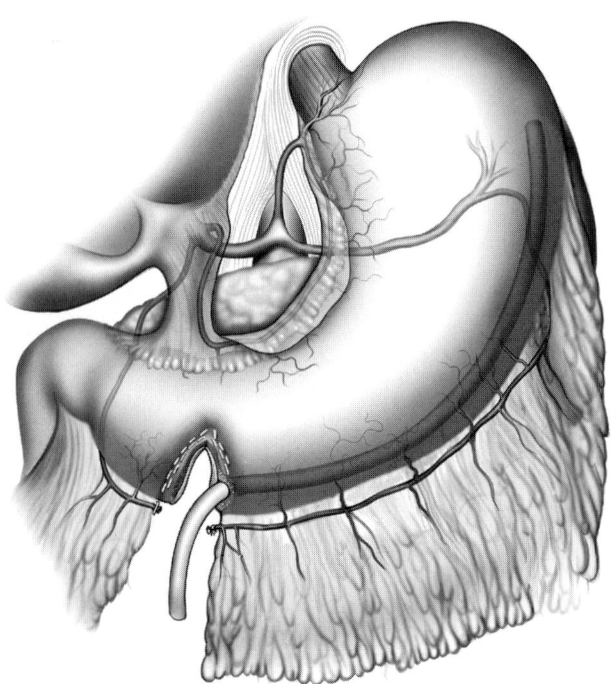

FIGURE 68–2 ■ The reversed gastric tube is constructed over the catheter commencing 4 cm proximal to the pylorus.

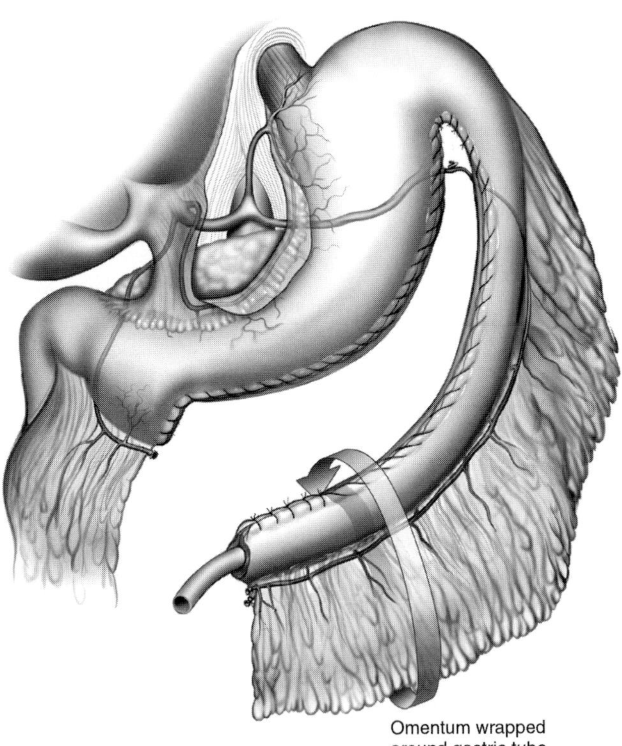

FIGURE 68–3 ■ The omentum, preserved to buttress the cervical anastomosis, is wrapped about the tube to facilitate its transposition to the neck.

If possible, the abdominal esophagus is mobilized and encircled with a Penrose drain. When the drain is retracted to the right, the ligation and division of the vasa brevia is facilitated. The gastrophrenic attachments are divided, and the stomach is freed from its avascular adhesions to the pancreas. This mobilizes the entire greater curvature and fundus.

To prepare the RGT, the right gastroepiploic artery is ligated and divided approximately 4 cm from the pylorus (see Fig. 68–2). This area of the antrum must be sufficiently wide to allow emptying of the gastric remnant. A linear stapling instrument is placed at that point at a right angle to the greater curvature. In adults, a 2.5-cm double row of staples is inserted. The distal staple line is oversewn with a continuous 3–0 polypropylene suture. Several of the staples are removed from the proximal staple line to allow for the insertion of a 40 French rubber catheter, which is advanced proximally to the fundus. In children, a 20 to 26 French catheter is used, depending on the child's age.

The RGT is constructed with multiple applications by a linear stapling instrument in loose proximity to the catheter to avoid tension on the staple line. A 2.5-cm-diameter tube long enough to reach the cervical esophagus is thus created. Usually, four applications of the stapling device are required to construct the tube.

The staple line of the newly formed greater curvature of the stomach is oversewn with a continuous 3–0 polypropylene suture. The staple line of the RGT is similarly oversewn (see Fig. 68–3). Interrupted sutures are used at the angle where the tube joins the stomach. Keeping the tube stretched to its full length on the catheter ensures that it is not shortened by the application of the suture. The continuous suture is completed 5 cm from the end of the tube. At this point, interrupted sutures are used again; this allows the excision of redundant tube if necessary. The tube may be placed on the anterior chest wall to verify that its length is sufficient for the cervical anastomosis.

If an additional 5-cm length is required, two techniques are available. The pylorus and first portion of the duodenum may be included in the RGT (Gavriliu, 1975). A Kocher maneuver is performed, and the right gastric artery is divided. A terminal branch of the right gastroepiploic artery in the pyloric area also requires division before transection of the duodenum 2 cm distal to the pylorus. The 40 French catheter is then inserted through the duodenum, and the RGT is constructed, as previously described. A Bilroth I gastroduodenostomy is then performed to the gastric remnant.

In cases of caustic stricture, Ximenes-Netto and associates (1998) transected the esophagogastric junction, closing both defects with staple lines and oversewing. This maneuver allows the fundus to be positioned anteriorly, thus effecting a 40% increase in tube length for anastomosis to the pharynx. In their experience, decompression of the distal esophagus via external tube drainage or anastamosis to the jejunum has not been necessary because the esophageal mucosa has been effectively destroyed by the initial injury.

The omentum is inspected. Any devascularization should be excised. The remaining omentum is wrapped about the tube to facilitate its transposition to the neck. This is accomplished by shielding the tube and catheter in a plastic sleeve. The tube may be transposed via the substernal, transthoracic, or transhiatal route as circumstances dictate.

Three possibilities exist regarding the cervical anastomosis of the RGT, depending on the extent of fibrosis that results from the caustic injury. The anastomosis may be performed above the hyoid bone, through it after its removal, or below it (Fig. 68–4). When the anastomosis is made to the pharynx, Ximenes-Netto and associates (1998) use the Montgomery T tube to stent the anastomosis; the tube is left in place for at least 3 months. The higher the anastomosis, the more difficulties are encountered and, therefore, the more frequent findings of leaks and strictures.

The cervical anastomosis is wrapped with omentum. Closed suction drainage of the cervical incision is advisable, and the wound is loosely closed.

A feeding jejunostomy is constructed, and feedings are begun on the 3rd postoperative day. An oral contrast study is performed on the 7th postoperative day. If the results of the study are satisfactory, a soft diet is begun.

To prepare the NRGT, an extensive Kocher maneuver is performed to free the duodenum and the head of the pancreas so that the pylorus approaches the midline. The greater omentum and vasa brevia are managed, as previously described, and the gastric fundus is freed from its diaphragmatic attachments and the pancreas. The prepyloric region is examined for an area that is sufficiently wide to allow the construction of a tube 2.5 cm in

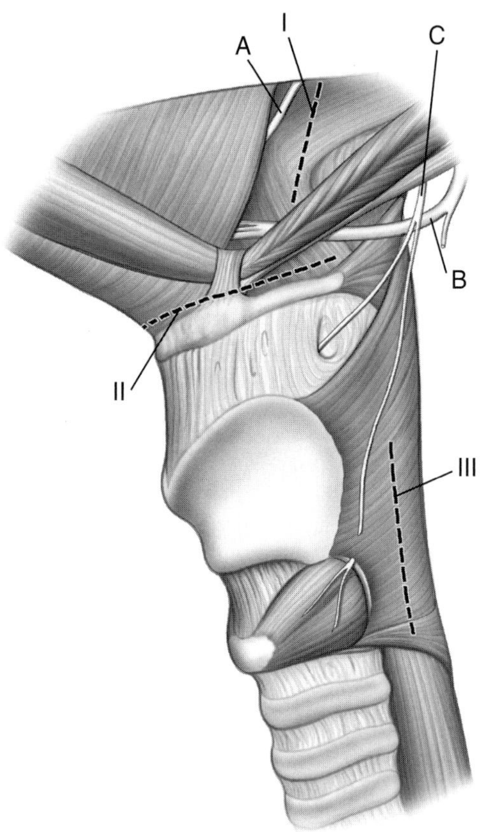

FIGURE 68–4 ■ The cervical anastomosis may be performed either above the hyoid bone (I), through it after its removal (II), or laterally (III). Also demonstrated are the lingual nerve (*A*), the hypoglossal (*B*) and superior laryngeal (*C*) nerves. (Redrawn from Popovici Z: Aspects particulleres de la colo-oesophagoplastie dans les stenoses oesophagennes post caustiques. J Chir (Paris) 113:269, 1977.)

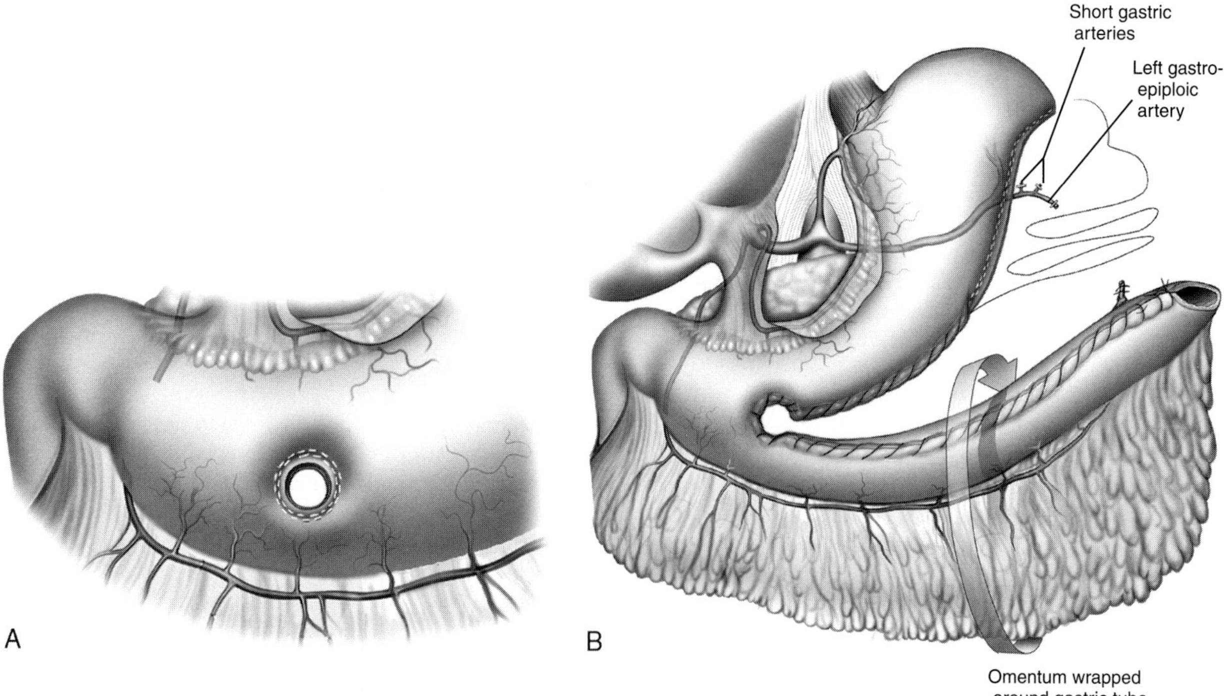

FIGURE 68–5 ■ *A,* Preparation of the nonreversed gastric tube. The circular stapler creates the defect required for insertion of the linear stapler. *B,* Omental wrap of the nonreversed gastric tube prior to cervical transposition.

diameter, with at least an equal amount for the remaining antrum. At that point, the anterior and posterior walls of the stomach are opened with cautery to allow the insertion of a linear stapling instrument. Alternatively, a 25-mm circular stapling instrument is inserted with the anvil applied to the posterior wall of the stomach (Fig. 68–5*A*).

The linear stapler is inserted through the defect created by the circular stapler. The tube is not constructed over a catheter; therefore, its width must be carefully appraised before each application of the stapling device. It is helpful to mark the line of staple application on the anterior wall of the stomach with needle tip cautery at the low power setting.

The final application of the stapling instrument is oblique in the fundic area. The staple closure of the stomach and the tube are reinforced with a continuous polypropylene suture, as previously described (Fig. 68–5*B*). Interrupted sutures are used at the fundic end so that any excess tube may be excised if necessary.

RESULTS

Anastomotic leak and stricture have been common occurrences in cases of gastric tube esophagoplasty, just as they are after transhiatal interposition of the entire stomach to the neck. Orringer and Iannettoni (2000) reported a 10% to 15% leak rate in more than 1000 patients undergoing transhiatal esophagectomy. Leaks do not necessarily result in stricture, and the reverse is also true.

Gavriliu (1975) reported a 20% incidence of cervical fistulas in his early cases. This rate decreased to 6% in his last 300 cases, but he stated that "the leaks are not included in these statistics." Heimlich (1972) reported eight leaks in 53 cases of RGT and nine strictures, of which four occurred after leaks.

Ximenes-Netto and associates (1998) reported a 10% (eight cases) fistula rate in 80 cases of RGT, but only three required reoperation. The esophageal transit time, when measured with technetium 99m pertechnetate in 16 patients, averaged 15.6 seconds (normal, 8.8 ± 6 seconds) with partial retention in the distal third. No reflux was seen in this group of individuals on whom these studies were performed (Fig. 68–6). Posthlethwait (1979) reported 13 leaks in 30 cases of NRGT interposition; the leaks closed in 1 to 4 weeks.

Anastomotic leaks are also common in pediatric cases. Ein and colleagues (1987) noted 24 leaks (66%) and 15 strictures (41%) in 36 cases. All but one leak closed within 3 months; however, nine children required surgery. Nine cases of stricture required surgical revision. In 29 of the 36 cases, gastric tube interposition was performed in two stages. The gastric tube was constructed in the first stage, and the cervical anastomosis was performed 2 weeks to 2 months later (Cohen et al, 1974). This protocol allows the mediastinum to seal and obviates the risk of cervical leak, which results in mediastinal sepsis. In the interval between stages, the child is fed through a gastrostomy.

Regardless of how the gastric tube is constructed, it is a vagotomized structure. Peristalsis has not been noted in the gastric tube. It is erroneous to term the RGT "antiperistaltic" and the NRGT as "peristaltic"; both tubes serve only as conduits. The RGT has a theoretic advantage. It has mucus-secreting antral mucosa anastomosed to the esophagus and acid-secreting fundic tissue at the suture line. Nevertheless, no long-term clinical differences between the two procedures have been found.

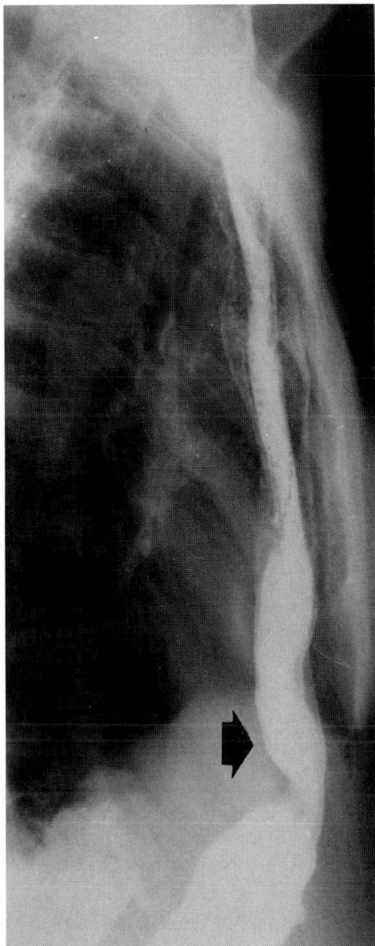

FIGURE 68–6 ■ Lateral view of the reversed gastric tube, demonstrating its intra-abdominal portion (*arrow*).

Reflux is common, especially in children, who may require elevation of the head of the bed during sleep. Lindahl and colleagues (1990) performed upper gastrointestinal endoscopy on 14 children who had undergone gastric tube esophagoplasty for esophageal atresia performed more than 2 years earlier. Ten patients were noted in biopsy specimens to have Barrett's metaplasia. In no case was there severe dysplasia or intestinal metaplasia. It was concluded that the vagotomized tube secretes acid in response to the influence of the residual stomach, which has normal vagal innervation and secretes gastrin, thus stimulating acid production by the parietal cells of the tube. Therefore, cervical esophagitis and gastric metaplasia may occur in the absence of gastrotubal reflux. The long-term risk of this finding has not yet been determined. Barrett's epithelium has also been noted in 8% of patients with esophageal atresia treated by conventional repair.

COMMENTS AND CONTROVERSIES

Given that no substitute performs as well as a healthy native esophagus, the gastric tube has advantages over other conduits in addition to the anatomic reasons previously mentioned. The diameter of the tube is similar to that of the esophagus and occupies less space in the thorax and neck than does the colon or whole stomach. Reflux may occur in all conduits, but it is better tolerated in the gastric tube than in the colon, which may develop ulceration. Colon interposition requires three enteric suture lines; the gastric tube has only one. Gastric tube interposition is technically easier to perform, takes less operating time, and does not require bowel preparation.

The major deficiency of the gastric tube esophagoplasty is the frequent occurrence of anastomotic leak or stricture. These complications, reported by all who use this method of reconstruction, imply that the impaired vascularity of the gastric tube is the cause, whether or not the tube is reversed or nonreversed. Gavriliu (1975) and Heimlich (1972) suggested that splenectomy augments flow to the left gastroepiploic artery. There is no physiologic evidence that this occurs, nor has splenectomy reduced the incidence of anastomotis failure.

Splenectomy has its own risks, not the least of which is impaired resistance to infection by encapsulated organisms, such as pneumococci. Accordingly, it is rarely performed in pediatric cases. It is not indicated in the preparation of the NRGT and is not a requirement for a successful RGT.

The anatomic studies of Liebermann-Meffert and associates (1992) are a notable contribution to the understanding of the vascular deficiencies of the gastric tube. By means of corrosion casts, the authors demonstrated that the right gastroepiploic artery is the exclusive conduit of blood to the tube and that the right gastric artery makes an inconsequential contribution. The branches of the left gastroepiploic artery vascularize the midportion of the tube, and there is only a weak connection between the right and left gastroepiploic arteries. The arterial supply of the upper 20% of the gastric tube (fundus) is through arterioles and capillaries. Arterial communication between the right and left gastroepiploic arteries thus occurs via retrograde flow if either of these vessels is divided. The arterial supply of the fundus is also retrograde after division of the vasa brevia. Liebermann-Meffert and associates (1992) further demonstrated that the right gastroepiploic artery, besides receiving flow from the gastroduodenal artery, receives equal inflow from the pancreatic branches of the superior mesentery artery.

This anatomic study suggests that the right gastroepiploic artery, the vascular pedicle of the NRGT, provides better arterial inflow and more efficient retrograde perfusion of the left gastroepiploic artery than would occur in the reverse situation. Furthermore, division of the right gastric artery allows for a more extensive Kocher maneuver and brings the pylorus to the midline, making elevation of the tube easier and tension-free. After this step, the fundic area of the tube (the upper 20%), which has the poorest blood supply, can be shortened.

If the gastric tube is to be placed substernally, the thoracic inlet should be widened by a resection of the sternal attachments of the strap muscles and the sternomastoid muscle if necessary. This maneuver prevents compression of the arterial supply and venous drainage of the tube.

It is hoped that the techniques described might improve the vascularity of the gastric tube and decrease the incidence of anastomotic leak or stricture.

S. C. F.
M. X. N.

The preceding chapter and its beautiful illustrations demonstrate a little-used, but nonetheless very important, option for esophageal bypass. This option has the major advantage of retaining the esophagogastric junction for drainage of the excluded or bypassed esophagus. The authors describe its use mainly for benign conditions such as lye stricture or esophageal atresia, but one of its appropriate applications is for bypass of malignant tracheoesophageal fistula.

The authors note the anatomic studies of gastric vasculature by Liebermann-Meffert and colleagues (1992), indicating that based on an intact right gastroepiploic artery, the NRGT is more likely to result in a well-vascularized gastric tube. In fact, this is borne out by experience, and it is generally accepted that the NRGT is by far a better option than the RGT. As noted by the authors, mobilization of the duodenum, which allows the antrum to be reflected proximally, allows the gastric tube to more easily reach the neck. Another advantage of the RGT is that the ingested material empties into the antrum well away from the esophagogastric junction, and this may be of special importance in reducing reflux of gastric contents up into the esophagus.

The authors note the uniformly high rate of anastomotic leakage at the esophagogastric junction after use of either the RGT or the NRGT. For this reason, a two-stage operation in which the gastric tube is brought to the neck in the first stage and the esophagogastric anastomosis is performed 7 to 10 days later should be strongly considered. This is particularly appropriate if there is a preexisting cervical esophagostomy.

J. D. C.

KEY REFERENCES

Ein SH, Shandling B, Stephens CA: Twenty-one year experience with the pediatric gastric tube. J Pediatr Surg 22:77, 1987.

This report presents the technique, complications, and results of gastric tube esophagoplasty in pediatric cases.

Gavriliu D: Aspects of esophageal surgery. Curr Probl Surg 12:36, 1975.

This article is of historical interest yet furnishes important details of the operative technique for the creation of the RGT. Some aspects of the technique are controversial, and the complications are not well described.

Liebermann-Meffert D, Meier R, Siewert J: Vascular anatomy of the gastric tube used for esophageal reconstruction. Ann Thorac Surg 54:1110, 1992.

An elegant laboratory study of the blood supply of the stomach when it is used as an esophageal substitute.

Postlethwait RW: Technique for isoperistaltic gastric tube for esophageal bypass. Ann Surg 189:673, 1979.

This is the first article to describe the technique of the NRGT gastric tube in adults.

Ximenes-Netto M, Silva RO, Vieira LF, Gregorcic A: The reversed gastric tube revisited: A useful replacement for benign disease. South Am J Thorac Surg 5:22, 1998.

This article describes the results in 80 cases of RGT for replacement of the esophagus and pharynx for benign diseases. The hospital mortality rate was 3.7% (three cases), and excellent to good results were obtained in 85.2% of the surviving patients.

■ REFERENCES

Anderson KD, Randolph JG: Gastric tube interposition: A satisfactory alternative to the colon for esophageal replacement in children. Ann Thorac Surg 25:521, 1978.

Beck C, Carrel A: Demonstration of specimens illustrating a method of formation of a prethoracic esophagus. Ill Med J 7:463, 1905.

Cohen DH, Middleton AW, Fletcher J: Gastric tube esophagoplasty. J Pediatr Surg 9:451, 1974.

Gavriliu D: The replacement of the esophagus by a gastric tube. In Jamieson G (ed): Surgery of the Oesophagus. New York, Churchill Livingstone, 1988, p 765.

Heimlich HJ: Replacement of the entire esophagus for malignant or benign stenosis. Am J Gastroenterol 35:311, 1961.

Heimlich HJ: Esophagoplasty with reversed gastric tube. Am J Surg 123:80, 1972.

Heimlich HJ, Winfield JM: The use of gastric tube to replace or bypass the esophagus. Surgery 37:549, 1955.

Jianu A: Gastrostomie and Oesophagoplastik. Dtsch Z Chir 118:383, 1912.

Lindahl H, Rintala R, Sariola H, Louhimo L: Cervical Barrett's esophagus: A common complication of gastric tube reconstruction. J Pediatr Surg 25:446, 1990.

Mes G: New method of esophagoplasty. J Int Coll Surg 11:270, 1948.

O'Connor TW: A historical review of reversed gastric tube esophagoplasty. Surg Gynecol Obstet 156:371, 1983.

Orringer MB, Iannettoni MD: Eliminating the cervical esophagogastric leak with a side-to-side stapled anastamosis. J Thorac Cardiovasc Surg 119:277, 2000.

Postlethwait RW: Technique for isoperistaltic gastric tube for esophageal bypass. Ann Surg 189:673, 1979.

Sanders GB: Esophageal replacement with reversed gastric tube: Utilization for bleeding esophageal varices in a 4-year-old child. JAMA 181:944, 1962.

INDEX

Note: Page numbers followed by the letter f refer to figures and those followed by t refer to tables.

A

B

E

G

M

O

P

Q

R

S

U